TEXTBOOK OF MEDICAL PHYSIOLOGY

Fourth Edition

TEXTBOOK OF MEDICAL PHYSIOLOGY

Indu Khurana, MD
Professor Emeritus
SGT University, Budhera, Gurugram, Haryana, India
Formerly Dean-cum-Principal and Professor, Physiology
World College of Medical Sciences and Research
Jhajjar, Haryana, India
Formerly Professor and Head, Department of Physiology
Pt BD Sharma Postgraduate Institute of Medical Sciences
Rohtak, Haryana, India

Arushi Khurana, MD
Advanced Fellowship in Haematology and Lymphoma
Faculty, Medical Oncology Services, Department of Medicine
Mayo Clinic, College of Medicine and Science
Rochester, Minnesota, USA

Narayan Gurukripa Kowlgi, MD
Cardiac Electrophysiology Fellowship
Faculty, Heart Rhythm Services, Department of Cardiovascular Medicine
Mayo Clinic, College of Medicine and Science
Rochester, Minnesota, USA

ELSEVIER

ELSEVIER

RELX India Private Limited
Registered Office: 818, 8th Floor, Indraprakash Building, 21, Barakhamba Road, New Delhi 110001
Corporate Office: 14th Floor, Building No. 10B, DLF Cyber City, Phase II, Gurgaon-122002, Haryana, India

Textbook of Medical Physiology, 4e, Indu Khurana, Arushi Khurana and Narayan Gurukripa Kowlgi

Publisher's note: Elsevier takes a neutral position with respect to territorial disputes or jurisdictional claims in its published content, including in maps and institutional affiliations.

Previous editions copyrighted 2020, 2015, 2011 by Elsevier, A division of Reed Elsevier India Private Limited.

ISBN: 978-81-312-6865-0
e-book ISBN: 978-81-312-6866-7

Content Strategist: Chandan Kumar
Content Project Manager: Goldy Bhatnagar
Sr Production Executive: Dhan Singh
Sr Graphic Designer: Gopalakrishnan Venkatraman

Typeset by GW India

Printed and bound at Rajkamal Electric Press, Kundli, Haryana-131 028

To

The Teachers and Residents in Physiology for Their Endeavour to Dissipate and Acquire Knowledge

My Parents and Teachers for Their Blessings

Preface to the Fourth Edition

Fourth edition of *Textbook of Medical Physiology* has been thoroughly revised and updated. The recent advances and molecular aspects have been added in each chapter, without changing its general organization and format. To cater the needs of postgraduate students, applied physiology has been updated with recent concepts on path-physiology, and the recent advances in investigative and therapeutic principles. In the Section on Specialized Integrated Physiology a new chapter on "Physiology of Yoga" has been added. For better understanding of applied physiology, relevant clinical cases have been added. For self-assessment of understanding the basic and applied physiology long and short questions have been added at the end of each chapter. Though the book is meant for postgraduate students of Physiology, undergraduate students will also find this an authentic resource for in depth understanding of the subject as well as for preparation of postgraduate entrance tests.

Salient features of fourth edition:

- This book is thoroughly revised and updated, retaining its well-accepted style of organization of the text in 12 Sections.
- A brief overview is given in the beginning of each section, highlighting the topics covered.
- Chapter outline given in the beginning of each chapter provides clear layout of the text included.
- Relevant functional anatomy given in the beginning of each chapter is quite useful in conceptualizing the subject.
- Presentation of the text with various levels of headings, sub-headings, boldface and italics given in the text will be helpful for the students to understand, retain and reproduce.
- To emphasize the clinical significance of physiology, relevant applied aspects have been adequately covered in each chapter and highlighted separately in boxes.
- Additional important information has been highlighted in the form of important notes.
- The text is illustrated with plenty of clear line diagrams that provide vivid and lucid details.
- To further upgrade the book, many new figures, tables and flowcharts have been added.

This edition of the book has been possible because of feedback, active criticism, suggestions and generous help of many faculty members specially Dr Sushma Sood, Prof Emeritus, NC Medical College, Israna (Haryana), Prof Latika Mohan, HOD, AIIMS, Rishikesh, Prof Neeta Mehta, HOD, Government Medical College, Ahemdabad, Prof Mridu, HOD, Government Medical College, Amritsar, Prof Anuradha Iyer, HOD, Government Medical College, Nalhar, Mewat, Prof Jyoti Sethi, HOD, Government Medical College, Karnal, and students. I sincerely thank them all. Having Dr Arushi Khurana, and Dr Narayan Gurukripa Kowlgi, Assistant Professors Department of Internal Medicine Mayo Clinic, College of Medicine and Science, Rochester, Minnesota, USA, as coauthors have been very helpful in updating the text and providing photographs of echocardiography, colour Doppler echocardiography and angiography especially for the applied aspects.

I bow with reverence to my teachers for grooming me for this task. I express indebtedness to my greatest source of inspiration, my husband Dr AK Khurana, Director, Khurana Eye Centre, Rohtak, former Senior Professor and Head, Regional Institute of Ophthalmology, PGIMS, Rohtak, for his invaluable guidance and unconditional help at every step and contributing chapter on 'Physiology of Vision' in this book. My son Aruj K Khurana, Vitreoretinal Surgeon, Khurana Eye Centre, Rohtak and Assistant Prof faculty of Medical Sciences SGT University, Gurugram and daughter-in-law Dr Bhawna Piplani Khurana, Squint and Oculoplasty Surgeon, Khurana Eye Centre, Rohtak and Associate Prof faculty of Medical Sciences, SGT University, Gurugram, and my awesome little grandchildren Agastya, Abhinaman and Amayra need to be complimented for keeping me energized by their never-ending love and affection.

I also thank Shri Manmohan Singh Chawla, Managing Trustee; Ms Madhupreet Chawla, Chairperson; Shri Ram Bahadur Rai, Chancellor; Professor Sham Singla, Advisor; Professor Gen. Dheeraj Behl, Dean FHMS; Shri GL Khanna, Head, HR Department, SGT University, for their encouragement and providing atmosphere conducive to such academic activities.

It is my special pleasure to acknowledge with gratitude the most assured co-operation and skill from the staff of RELX India Pvt Ltd, especially, Chandan Kumar (Content Strategist) and Goldy Bhatnagar (Content Project Manager), to complete the project in assigned time.

Sincere efforts have been made to verify correctness of the text. However, in spite of best efforts some inaccuracies, ambiguities and typographical mistakes are likely to be noticed by the readers. Therefore, feedback and suggestions from the teachers and students are invited for improving the future edition. Feedback received will be highly appreciated and duly acknowledged.

Indu Khurana

Preface to the Third Edition

The third edition of *Textbook of Medical Physiology* has been thoroughly revised and updated. The recent advances and molecular aspects have been added in each chapter, without changing its general organization and format. To cater to the needs of postgraduate students, applied physiology has been updated with recent concepts on pathophysiology, and so also the recent advances in investigations and therapeutic principles. Undergraduate students will find this an authentic resource for indepth understanding of the subject as well as for preparation of postgraduate entrance tests.

Salient features of the third edition:

- This book is thoroughly revised and updated, retaining its well-accepted style of organization of the text in 12 sections.
- A brief overview is given in the beginning of each section, highlighting the topics covered.
- Chapter outline given in the beginning of each chapter provides clear layout of the text included.
- Relevant functional anatomy given in the beginning of each chapter is quite useful in conceptualizing the subject.
- Presentation of the text with various levels of headings, subheadings, boldface and italics given in the text will be helpful for the students to understand, retain and reproduce.
- To emphasize the clinical significance of physiology, relevant applied aspects have been adequately covered in each chapter and highlighted separately in boxes.
- Additional important information has been highlighted in the form of 'important notes'.
- The text is illustrated with plenty of clear line diagrams that provide vivid and lucid details.
- To further upgrade the book, many new figures, tables and flowcharts have been added.

The third edition of this book has been possible because of feedback, active criticism, suggestions and generous help of many faculty members and students. I sincerely thank them all. Having Dr Arushi Khurana, MD, an Advance Hematology Fellow in Lymphoma at Mayo Clinic, Rochester, MN, USA, former Chief Resident, Department of Internal Medicine, University of Connecticut, USA, and Fellow, Hematology–Oncology, Massey Cancer Center, Virginia Commonwealth University, Richmond, VA, and Dr Narayan Gurukripa Kowlgi, Cardiac Electrophysiology Fellow at Mayo Clinic, Rochester, MN, USA, former Chief Resident, Department of Internal Medicine, University of Connecticut, USA, and Fellow in Cardiovascular Diseases at Pauley Heart Center, Virginia Commonwealth University, Richmond, VA, as coauthors have been very useful in updating the text, especially the applied aspects.

I bow with reverence to my teachers for grooming me for this task. I express indebtedness to my greatest source of inspiration, my husband Dr A.K. Khurana, former Senior Professor, Regional Institute of Ophthalmology, PGIMS, Rohtak, for his invaluable guidance and unconditional help at every step and contributing chapter on 'Physiology of Vision' in this book. My son Aruj K. Khurana, Vitreoretinal Surgeon, NEI, Rishikesh, presently working as Assistant Professor at World College of Medical and Research, Jhajjar, daughter-in-law Dr Bhawna Piplani Khurana, Oculoplastic Surgeon, worked at AIIMS Rishikesh and NEI Rishikesh, and as Assistant Professor, Ophthalmology at SGRRIMHS, Dehradun, and my awesome little grandson Agastya need to be complimented for keeping me energized by their never-ending love and affection.

I am highly thankful to Dr (Mrs) Ritu Singh, Trustee, and Dr Narender Singh, Chairman, World College of Medical Sciences and Research, Jhajjar, for their encouragement and for infusing an academic atmosphere.

It is my special pleasure to acknowledge with gratitude the most assured co-operation and skill from the staff of RELX India Pvt Ltd, especially Arvind Koul (Content Strategist), Shabina Nasim (Head of Content Project Management) and Goldy Bhatnagar (Content Project Manager), to complete the project in time.

Sincere efforts have been made to verify correctness of the text. However, in spite of best efforts some inaccuracies, ambiguities and typographical mistakes are likely to be noticed by the readers. Therefore, feedback and suggestions from the teachers and students are invited for improving the future edition. Feedback received will be highly appreciated and duly acknowledged.

Indu Khurana

Contents

PART I

GENERAL PHYSIOLOGY

PART OUTLINE

GENERAL PHYSIOLOGY

SECTION 1

SECTION OUTLINE

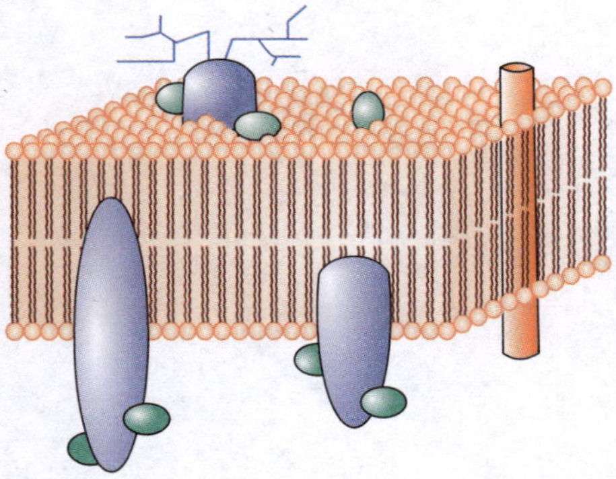

INTRODUCTION

Physiology, in simple terms, refers to the study of normal functioning of the living structures. The *human physiology* is concerned with the way the various systems of the human body function, and the way each contributes to the functions of the body as a whole. In other words, the human physiology is concerned with specific characteristics and mechanisms of the human body that make it a living being, and the mechanisms which help in adaptation and homeostasis, which are the two fundamental features of life.

The *general physiology* envisages the general concepts and principles that are basic to the functions of all the systems. As we know, the fundamental unit of human body is a cell; therefore, this section includes a short review of fundamental aspects of the cell physiology. Before studying the general biophysiological processes and the cell physiology, it will be worthwhile to have a brief knowledge about the functional organization, composition and internal environment of the human body.

1.1 Functional Organization, Composition and Internal Environment of Human Body

CHAPTER OUTLINE

FUNCTIONAL ORGANIZATION OF THE HUMAN BODY

The human body is actually a social order of about 100 trillion cells organized into different functional structures, some of which are called organs; some organs collectively form a system. For convenience of description, the human body can be considered to be functionally organized into various systems.

1. Skin and its appendages Skin is the outermost covering of the human body. Its appendages include hairs, nails, sebaceous glands and sweat glands. In addition to providing mechanical protection to the underlying tissues, the skin performs following important functions:

- It acts as a physical barrier against entry of microorganisms and other substances.
- It prevents loss of water from the body.
- It is a very important sensory organ, containing receptors for touch and related sensations.
- It plays an important role in regulating body temperature.

2. Skeletal system The basic framework of the body is provided by a large number of bones that collectively form the *skeleton*. At joints, the bones are united to each other by fibrous bands called *ligaments*. In addition to the bones and joints, the skeletal system also includes the *cartilages* present in the body.

3. Muscle system Overlying and usually attached to the bones are various muscles. Muscles are composed of many elongated cells called *muscle fibres,* which are able to contract and relax. Three distinct types of muscles can be identified: skeletal muscles, smooth muscles and cardiac muscles.

4. Nervous system The nervous system is, predominantly, made up of tissues that have the special property of being able to conduct impulses rapidly from one part of the body to another. The specialized cells that constitute the functional units of the nervous system are called *neurons.* The nervous system may be divided into: (i) the *central nervous system,* made up of brain and spinal cord, and (ii) the *peripheral nervous system,* consisting of the peripheral nerves and the ganglia associated with them. The nerves supplying the body wall and limbs are often called *cerebrospinal nerves.* The nerves supplying the viscera, along with the parts of the brain and spinal cord related to them, constitute the *autonomic nervous system.* The autonomic nervous system is subdivided into two major parts: the *sympathetic* and the *parasympathetic* nervous system.

5. Cardiovascular system The cardiovascular system consists of the *heart* and the *blood vessels.* The blood vessels that take blood from the heart to various tissues are called *arteries.* The smallest arteries are called *arterioles.* Arterioles open into a network of *capillaries* that perfuse the tissues. Exchange of various substances between the blood and the tissues take place through the walls of capillaries. In some situations, capillaries are replaced by slightly different vessels called *sinusoids.* Blood from capillaries (or from sinusoids) is collected by small *venules* which join to form *veins.* The veins return blood to the heart.

6. Respiratory system The respiratory system consists of the lungs and the passages through which air reaches them. The passages are nasal cavities, the pharynx, the trachea, the bronchi and their intrapulmonary continuations.

7. Digestive system The digestive or the so-called alimentary system includes all those structures that are concerned with eating, and with the digestion and absorption of food. The system consists of an alimentary canal which starts at the mouth and ends at the anus. The alimentary canal includes the oral cavity, pharynx, oesophagus, stomach, small intestine and large intestine. Other structures included in the digestive system are the liver, the gall bladder and the pancreas.

8. Excretory system *Excretion* is the removal of waste products of metabolism from the body. *Egestion* (or defaecation) is the removal of undigested food from the gut and is not regarded as excretion because the material taken into the gut through the mouth is not made by the body itself. The organs forming the excretory system are the kidney, the ureters, the bladder and the urethra.

9. Reproductive system Reproduction is the production of a new generation of individuals of the same species. It involves the transmission of genetic material from one generation to the next. The *male reproductive organs* are the testes, the epididymis, the ductus deferens, the seminal vesicles (which are paired), the prostate, the male urethra and the penis (which are unpaired). *The female reproductive organs* are the right and left ovaries and uterine tubes, the uterus, the vagina, the external genitalia and the mammary glands.

10. Endocrine system Endocrine tissue is essentially made up of cells that produce secretions which are poured directly into blood. The secretions of the endocrine cells are called *hormones*. Some organs are entirely endocrine in function. They are referred to as *endocrine glands* (or *ductless glands*). Those traditionally included under this heading are the hypophysis cerebri (pituitary gland), the pineal gland, the thyroid gland, the parathyroid glands and the suprarenal (adrenal) glands. Groups of endocrine cells may be present in the organs that have other functions. These include the *islets of Langerhans* of pancreas, the interstitial cells of the testis, the follicles and corpora lutea of the ovaries. Hormones are also produced by some cells in the kidney, the thymus and the placenta. Some workers describe the liver as being partly an endocrine gland.

11. Blood and immune system *Blood* is regarded as a modified connective tissue because the cellular elements in it are separated by a considerable amount of 'intercellular substance' and because some of the cells in it have close affinities to cells in general connective tissue.

Circulating blood normally contains three main types of cells which perform their respective physiologic functions: (i) the red cells (*erythrocytes*) are largely concerned with oxygen transport, (ii) the white cells (*leucocytes*) play various roles in the body defence against infection and tissue injury and (iii) platelets (*thrombocytes*) which are primarily involved in maintaining integrity of blood vessels and in preventing blood loss. Detailed physiology of each organ system is considered in the relevant chapters.

BODY COMPOSITION

The normal body in an average adult male is composed of *water* (60%), *minerals* (7%), *protein* and related substances (18%) and *fat* (15%). The water, denoted by the term total body water (TBW), and the electrolytes need special emphasis.

TOTAL BODY WATER

Water is the principal and essential constituent of the human body. The TBW is about 10% less in a normal young adult female (average 50%) than that in average adult male (60%) due to relatively greater amount of adipose tissue in the females. In both sexes, the value tends to decrease with age (Table 1.1.1).

Table 1.1.1 Total body water (% of body weight in relation to age and sex)

Age (years)	TBW (%) Male	TBW (%) Female
10–18	59	57
18–40	61	51
40–60	55	47
Above 60	52	46

The Body Fluid Compartments

TBW is distributed into two main compartments of the body fluids separated from each other by membranes freely permeable to water (Fig. 1.1.1; Table 1.1.2):

1. Intracellular fluid compartment The intracellular fluid (ICF) compartment comprises about 40% of the body weight, the bulk of which is contained in the muscles.

2. Extracellular fluid compartment The extracellular fluid (ECF) compartment constitutes about 20% of the body weight. The ECF compartment comprises the following:

i. Plasma. It is the fluid portion of the blood (*intravascular fluid)* and comprises about 5% of the body weight (i.e. 25% of the ECF). On an average out of 5 L of total blood volume, 3.5 L is plasma.

ii. Interstitial fluid including lymph. It constitutes the major portion (about three-fourth) of the ECF. The composition of interstitial fluid is the same as that of plasma except it has little protein. Thus, interstitial fluid is an ultrafiltrate of plasma.

iii. Transcellular fluid. It is the fluid contained in the secretions of the secretary cells and cavities of the body, e.g. saliva, sweat, cerebrospinal fluid (CSF), intraocular fluids (aqueous humour and vitreous humour), pericardial fluid, bile, present between the layers (pleura, peritoneum and synovial membrane), lacrimal fluid and luminal fluids of the gut, thyroid and cochlea.

Transcellular fluid volume is relatively small, about 1.5% of the body weight, i.e. 15 mL/kg body weight (about 1 L in a person weighing 70 kg).

iv. Mesenchymal tissue fluid. The mesenchymal tissues such as dense connective tissue, cartilage and bones contain about 6% of the body water.

The interstitial fluid, transcellular fluid and mesenchymal tissue fluid combine to form 75% of ECF.

The normal distribution of TBW in the fluid compartments is kept constant by two opposing sets of forces: osmotic and hydrostatic pressure.

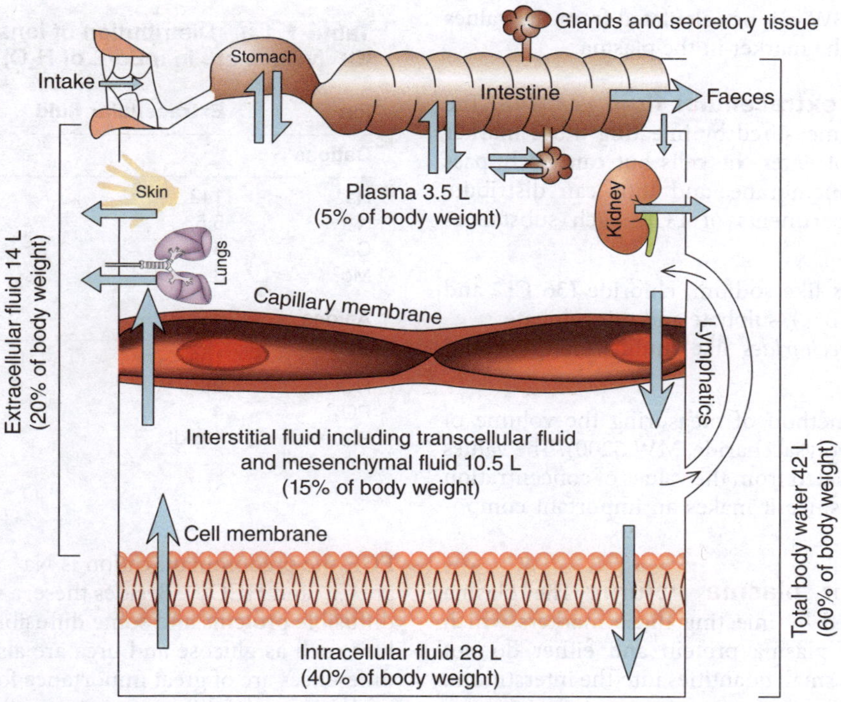

Fig. 1.1.1 Distribution of total body water in different compartments. Arrows indicate fluid movement.

Table 1.1.2 Distribution of total body water in a normal 70-kg person

	Volume (L)	Body weight (%)	Body water (%)
Total body water (TBW)	42	60	100
• Intracellular fluid (ICF)	28	40	67
• Extracellular fluid (ECF)	14	20	33
• Plasma (25% of ECF)	3.5	5	08
• Interstitial fluid, transcellular fluid and mesenchymal tissue fluid (75% of ECF)	10.5	15	25

Measurement of Body Fluid Volumes

Theoretically, it is possible to measure the volume of each fluid component by injecting a substance (indicator) that will stay in only one compartment (provided the concentration of the substance in the body fluid and the amount removed by excretion and metabolism can be accurately measured) as:

$$V = \frac{A_1 - A_2}{C}, \text{ where:}$$

V = Volume of fluid compartment
A_1 = Amount of indicator injected in the fluid
A_2 = Amount of indicator removed by excretion and metabolism
C = Concentration of the indicator in the fluid

For example, if 150 mg of sucrose (A_1) is injected into a 70-kg man, 10 mg sucrose (A_2) has been excreted or metabolized and the concentration of plasma sucrose (C) measured is 0.01 mg/mL; then the volume distribution of sucrose is

$$\frac{150 \text{ mg} - 10 \text{ mg}}{0.01 \text{ mg/mL}} = 14{,}000 \text{ mL}$$

Prerequisites for Accurate Body Fluid Measurement

Although the formula described above for measuring the body fluid volume appears simple, the material injected (indicator) should have the following characteristics:

- It should be nontoxic.
- It must mix evenly throughout the compartment being measured.
- It should be relatively easy to measure its concentration.
- It must have no effect of its own on the distribution of water or other substances in the body.
- Either it must be unchanged by the body during the mixing period or the amount changed (excreted and/or metabolized) must be known.

This method of measuring body fluids is called *'indicator dilution method'* and can be used to measure the volume of different compartments of the body fluid by using suitable indicators/markers which will get distributed in that particular compartment as follows:

1. Measurement of total body water volume The volume of TBW can be estimated by measuring the distribution of isotopes of water. The injected marker should be evenly distributed in all the compartments of body fluid. Such markers include:

- Deuterium oxide (D_2O)
- Tritium oxide (T_2O)
- Aminopyrine

The volume of the TBW can be calculated from the values of the concentration of the marker in the plasma.

2. Measurement of extracellular fluid volume The volume of ECF can be measured by injecting those marker substances which cannot enter the cells but can freely pass through the capillary membrane, and thus can distribute evenly in all the compartments of ECF. Such substances include:

- *Radioactive substances* like sodium, chloride (36 Cl^- and 38 Cl^-), bromide (82 Br^-), sulphate and thiosulphate
- *Non-metabolizable saccharides* like inulin, mannitol and sucrose

The most accurate method of measuring the volume of ECF is by using *inulin* (polysaccharide, MW 5200). The values of ECF volume are calculated from the values of concentration of *inulin* in the plasma since it makes an important component of the ECF.

3. Measurement of plasma volume The plasma volume can be measured by injecting those markers which bind strongly with the plasma protein and either do not diffuse or diffuse only in small quantities into the interstitium. These substances are

- Radioactive iodine: ^{131}I
- The dye Evan's blue: T-1824

The plasma volume can also be calculated from the values of the RBCs which can be measured using radioactive isotopes of chromium (^{51}Cr).

4. Measurement of intracellular fluid volume The volume of ICF cannot be measured directly, since there is no substance which can be confined exclusively to this compartment after intravenous injection. Therefore, values of ICF volume are calculated from the values of TBW and ECF as:

$$\text{ICF volume} = \text{TBW volume} - \text{ECF volume}$$

5. Measurement of interstitial fluid volume Like ICF volume, the volume of interstitial fluid also cannot be measured directly for the same reasons. Its values can be roughly calculated from the values of ECF volume and plasma volume as:

$$\text{Interstitial fluid volume} = \text{ECF volume} - \text{plasma volume}$$

Important Note

The ECF volume/ICF volume ratio is larger in infants and children compared to adults, but absolute volume of ECF in children is smaller than in adults. Therefore, dehydration develops rapidly, more frequently and severely in children than in adults.

BODY ELECTROLYTES

The electrolytes constitute about 7% of the total body weight and they perform many major functions in the body. The distribution of electrolytes in various compartments differs markedly. Table 1.1.3 shows the distribution of electrolytes in two major compartments of body fluid: the ECF and the ICF.

From Table 1.1.3, it may be noted that in the ICF the main cations are K^+ and Mg^{2+} and the main anions are PO_4^{3-} and proteins. It has low concentration of Na^+ and Cl^-. While in ECF, the predominant cation is Na^+ and the principal anions are Cl^- and HCO_3^-. Besides these, a small proportion of nondiffusible proteins and some diffusible nutrients and metabolites such as glucose and urea are also present in ECF. These differences are of great importance for the survival of tissues.

Table 1.1.3 Distribution of ions in the ECF and ICF (values are in mEq/L of H_2O)

Ion	Extracellular fluid	Intracellular fluid
Cations		
Na^+	142	14
K^+	5.5	150
Ca^{2+}	5	<1
Mg^{2+}	3	58
Anions		
Cl^-	103	4
HCO_3^-	28	10
PO_4^{3-}	4	75
Proteins	1 g/dL	5 g/dL

The essential difference between the two main subdivisions of ECF is the higher protein content in plasma than in the interstitial fluid which plays important role in maintaining fluid balance.

Important Notes

It is important to note that

- Essentially all of the body K^+ is in the exchangeable pool.
- Only 65%–70% of the body Na^+ is exchangeable.
- Almost all of the body Ca^{2+} and Mg^{2+} are nonexchangeable.
- Only the exchangeable solutes are osmotically active.
- Although there is difference in the ionic composition of different fluid compartments, the osmolality remains same, i.e. 290 mOsm/kg H_2O.
- Electrolyte balance is very important to maintain homeostasis. For detail see page 527.

Functions of Electrolytes

1. Electrolytes are the main solutes in the body fluids for maintenance of acid–base balance.
2. Electrolytes maintain the proper osmolality and volume of body fluids.
3. The concentration of certain electrolytes determines their specific physiologic functions, e.g. the effect of calcium ions on neuromuscular excitability.

INTERNAL ENVIRONMENT AND HOMEOSTASIS

INTERNAL ENVIRONMENT

Claude Bernarde (1949), the great French physiologist, introduced the term *internal environment* of the body or the *milieu interieur* for the ECF of the body. He said so since all the body cells essentially depend on the ECF for maintenance of cellular life. Cells are capable of living, growing and performing their special functions as long as the proper concentration of oxygen, glucose, different ions, amino acids, fatty substances and other constituents are available in the internal environment.

The composition of ECF vis-à-vis ICF has been discussed in page 6.

HOMEOSTASIS

Homeostasis, a term introduced by W.B. Cannon in 1926, refers to the mechanism by which the constancy of the internal environment is maintained and ensured. For this purpose, living membranes with varying permeabilities such as vascular endothelium and cell membrane play important roles in the exchange of fluids, electrolytes, nutrients and metabolites across the compartments of body fluids.

The factors involved in the maintenance of internal environment can be summarized as:

- Maintenance of pH of ECF (acid–base balance)
- Regulation of temperature
- Maintenance of water and electrolyte balance
- Supply of nutrients, oxygen, enzymes and hormones
- Removal of metabolic and other waste products

Role of Different Systems of the Body in Homeostasis

Almost all the systems of the human body play vital roles in the maintenance of the internal environment. The details of the role played by each system are described in the relevant chapters. The outlines of the contributions to different mechanisms of homeostasis made by different functional systems of the body are summarized as follows:

1. ***Transport of ECF:*** The circulatory system plays the most vital role in the transport of ECF in the body. In this way, the ECF, everywhere in the body – both the plasma and the interstitial fluid, is continually being mixed, thereby maintaining almost complete homogeneity throughout the body.
2. ***Supply of oxygen and nutrients to ECF:*** The nutrients and oxygen are must to provide energy for various cell activities for the growth of the tissue. The respiratory system, digestive system, circulatory system and the musculoskeletal system play major roles in the supply of adequate amount of oxygen and nutrients. Hormones play an essential role in the metabolism of nutrients and other substances necessary for the cells.
3. ***Removal of metabolic end products and waste:*** Kidneys and other excretory organs are involved in the excretion of end products of metabolism and other waste products. Respiratory system plays a role in the removal of carbon dioxide from the body.
4. ***Water and electrolyte balance:*** It is maintained in the body by a combined effort of kidneys, skin, lungs, salivary secretion and digestive system.
5. ***The pH of blood and acid–base balance:*** These are maintained by the respiratory system, kidneys, blood and the various buffer systems in the body.
6. ***The temperature of the body:*** It is maintained affirmably by a combined effort of the skin, cardiovascular system, respiratory system, digestive system, excretory system, skeletal muscle system and the nervous system.
7. ***Regulation of body functions:*** It is very important for homeostasis. The nervous system and the hormonal system of regulation play key roles. The autonomic nervous system regulates all the vegetative functions of the body essential for homeostasis.
8. ***Reproduction:*** Reproduction is not considered a homeostatic function. However, it does help to maintain static conditions by generating new beings to take the place of those that are dying. This perhaps sounds like a permissive usage of the term homeostasis, but it does illustrate that essentially all body structures are so organized that they help to maintain the automaticity and continuity of life.

Mode of Action of Homeostatic Control System

Homeostasis is a complex phenomenon. The above-mentioned examples of homeostatic control mechanisms are only a few of the many hundreds to thousands in the body, all of which have certain characteristics in common. The mode of operation of all the systems, which are involved in the homeostasis, is through 'feedback' mechanism and the adaptive control system. Feedback mechanism is of two types: the negative feedback mechanism and the positive feedback mechanism.

Negative Feedback Mechanism

Most control systems of the body act by negative feedback, i.e. in general if the activity of a particular system is increased or decreased, a control system initiates a negative feedback, which consists of a series of changes that return the activity towards normal.

The degree of effectiveness with which a control system maintains constant conditions is determined by the gain of the negative feedback.

Examples of feedback mechanism are:

1. When the blood pressure suddenly rises or lowers, it initiates a series of reactions that try to bring the blood pressure to normal levels.
2. When thyroxine secretion is in excess, it inhibits the secretion of thyroid-stimulating hormone (TSH) from pituitary so that thyroxine is not secreted from the thyroid gland. (For details see page 689.)

Effectiveness of control system is the degree or gain by which control system maintains homeostasis. The simple formula for assessing the gain is

$$\text{Gain of control system} = \text{Correction/Error}$$

Interpretation: If the gain of control system is more, then the error is less, meaning thereby the effectiveness of the control system is more.

Positive Feedback Mechanism

Positive feedback is better known as a vicious circle. Usually, it is harmful and in some instances even death can occur due to positive feedback. For example, as shown in Fig. 1.1.2, when a person has suddenly bled 2 L of blood, a vicious circle of progressively weakening of the heart is set in motion, which ultimately causes death.

A mild degree of feedback can be overcome by the negative feedback control mechanisms of the body, and a vicious cycle fails to develop. For example, when a patient bleeds 1 L of blood instead of 2 L, the negative feedback mechanisms of controlling the blood pressure may overcome the positive

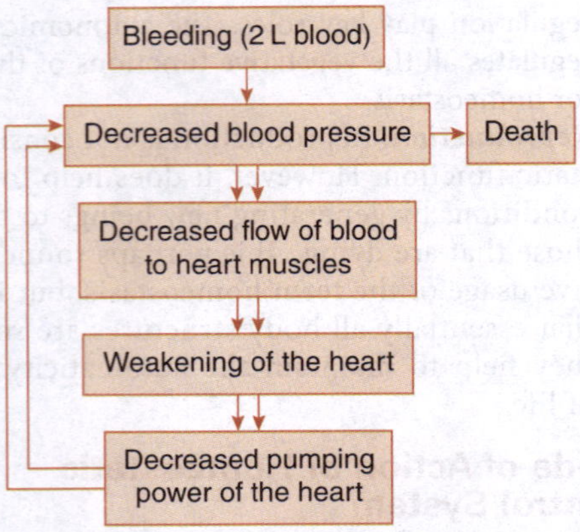

Fig. 1.1.2 Shows how a positive feedback mechanism can cause death.

feedback, and the blood pressure will return to normal, as shown in Fig. 1.1.2.

Furthermore, sometimes positive feedback can serve useful purposes, e.g. under following circumstances:

- *Clot formation* following rupture of vessels is accelerated by a vicious cycle of thrombin formation (for details see page 203). This stops the bleeding.
- *Child birth* during labour is facilitated by progressively increasing uterine contractions due to positive feedback from stretching of cervix by head of the baby (for details see page 856).
- *Generation of nerve signals* by the vicious cycle of progressive leakage of Na^+ ions from the channels set up following stimulation of membrane of nerve fibre is due to the positive feedback.

Adaptive Control System

Adaptive control system refers to a delayed type of negative feedback mechanism. This is seen in nervous system (for details see page 910). For example, when some movements of the body occur very rapidly, there is not enough time for nerve signals to travel from the peripheral parts of the body all the way to the brain and then back to the periphery again in time to control the movements. Under such circumstances, the brain uses a principle called *feed-forward control* to cause the required muscle contraction, which retrospectively is conveyed to the brain by the sensory nerve signals from the moving part. If the movement performed is found incorrect, then the brain corrects the *feed-forward signals* that it sends to the muscle the next time the movement is required. Such a correction made by successive retrospective feedback mechanism is called *adaptive control.*

Self-Assessment

1. Discuss the total body water, its distribution and measurement.
2. Discuss the homeostasis and its regulation.
3. Describe body electrolytes and its significance.

Clinical Cases

Case 1

A 1-year-old child suffering with diarrhoea is brought to emergency. On examination, it was found that the child is severely dehydrated.

Q1. What is the reason for severe dehydration?

Q2. Why does dehydration develop rapidly in infants compared to adults?

Case 2

A young 22-year-old boy met with an accident and was brought to hospital emergency. On examination, it was found that his pulse was very feeble and low volume; BP systolic 40 mm Hg, diastolic not recordable; respiration gasping (air hunger). Before starting the treatment, he was declared dead.

Q1. In this case, due to which feedback mechanism did death of the patient occur?

1.2 The Cell Physiology

CHAPTER OUTLINE

CELL STRUCTURE

The cell is the smallest structural and functional unit of the body. The human body contains about 100 trillion cells. Different types of cells of the body possess features which distinguish one type from the other, and are specially adapted to perform one or a few particular functions, e.g. the red blood cells transport oxygen from lungs to the tissues, the muscle cell is specialized for the function of contraction and the intestinal mucosal cells are specialized for absorption of foodstuff. However, most mammalian cells have an overall common structure and certain basic characteristics are described.

Under normal conditions, cells are dynamic structures existing in fluid environment. A typical cell, as seen by the light microscope, consists of three basic components:

- Cell membrane
- Cytoplasm
- Nucleus

CELL MEMBRANE

Cell membrane or the plasma membrane is the protective sheath enveloping the cell body. It separates the contents of the cell from the external environment and controls exchange of materials between the fluid outside the cell (extracellular fluid) and the fluid inside the cell (intracellular fluid). A detailed knowledge of its structure (Fig. 1.2.1) is essential for the understanding of cell functions. Therefore, it will be discussed separately (see page 15).

CYTOPLASM

Cytoplasm is an aqueous substance (cytosol) containing a variety of cell organelles and other structures. In eukaryotic cells, the nucleus and cytoplasm together form the protoplasm. The structures dispersed in the cytoplasm can be broadly divided into three groups – organelles, inclusion bodies and cytoskeleton.

Organelles

The organelles are the permanent components of the cells that are bounded by limiting membrane and contain enzymes, hence participating in the cellular metabolic activity. These include the mitochondria, the endoplasmic reticulum (ER), ribosomes, the Golgi apparatus, peroxisomes, centrosomes and centrioles.

1. Mitochondria Mitochondria are the major sites for aerobic respiration. These are oval structures about 5–12 μm in length and 0.5–1 μm in diameter, and more numerous in metabolically active cells.

Structure. The mitochondria consist of:

Membranes. There are two layers of the membrane: the outer smooth and inner folded into incomplete septa called cristae (Fig. 1.2.1A). Chemically and structurally, the membranes of mitochondria are similar to the cell membrane. The inner membrane, in addition, contains lollipop-shaped globular structures present between the layers of the membrane.

Matrix of the mitochondria contains enzymes required in Krebs cycle or tricarboxylic acid cycle (TCAC), by which products of carbohydrate, fat and protein metabolism are oxidized to produce energy, which is stored in the form of ATP in the lollipop-like globular structures.

Functions. In addition to their role as power-generating units, the mitochondria may have a role in synthesizing membrane-bound proteins since they also possess deoxyribonucleic acid (DNA) and ribosomes. The mitochondria have their own genome; however, the DNA of mitochondrial genome is much less than the nuclear genome. Mitochondrial DNA encodes 13

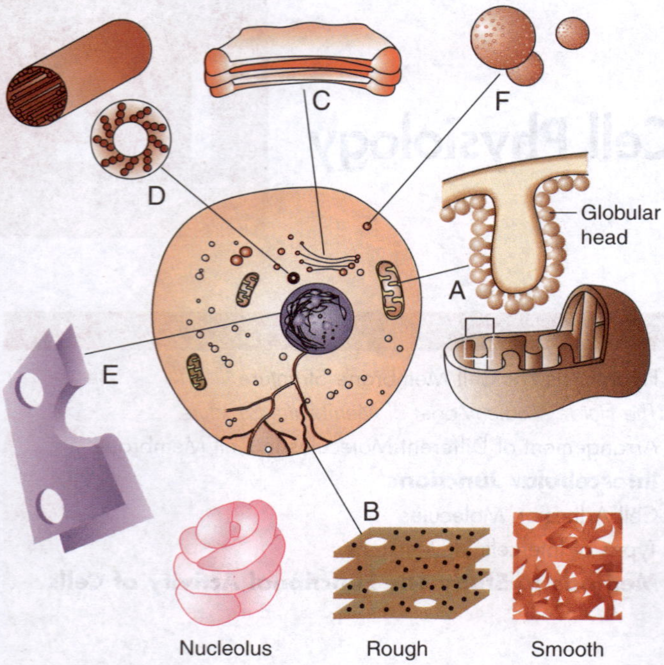

Fig. 1.2.1 Structure of a typical cell (in the centre) showing various organelles: **A,** mitochondrion; **B,** endoplasmic reticulum (rough and smooth); **C,** Golgi apparatus; **D,** centrosome; **E,** nucleus; and **F,** secretory granules.

protein subunits which are associated with proteins and are coded by nuclear genes to form enzyme complexes and ribosomal transfer ribonucleic acid (RNA) (needed by intramitochondrial ribosomes for protein synthesis). The enzyme complexes responsible for oxidative phosphorylation include:

- Complex I: Reduced nicotinamide adenine dinucleotide dehydrogenase (NADH)
- Complex II: Succinate dehydrogenase ubiquinone oxidoreductase
- Complex III: Ubiquinone-cytochrome C reductase
- Complex IV: Cytochrome C oxidase
- Complex V: ATP synthetase

The complexes I, III and IV pump protons (H^+) into intermembranous spaces during electron transfer, and complex II along with complexes III and IV acts with complex I, coenzyme Q and cytochrome C and convert metabolites to carbon dioxide and water. Complex V converts ADP and inorganic phosphate to ATP.

Mechanism of oxidative phosphorylation. According to chemiosmotic theory proposed by Peter Mitchell in 1961, for ATP formation H^+ moves across the inner mitochondrial membrane through selectively permeable membrane down the electrochemical gradient.

Mitochondria also have a role in apoptosis (programmed cell death).

Important Note

Mitochondrial DNA repair system is ineffective and mutation rate is higher as compared with nuclear DNA (10 times). Therefore, a large number of rare diseases due to mitochondrial DNA mutation have been traced, particularly in disorders of tissue associated with high metabolic rate.

Applied Aspects

Mitochondrial disease is a genetic disorder that occurs when mitochondria fail to produce enough energy for the body to function properly. It is caused by mutation in mitochondrial DNA. ***Symptoms*** include poor growth, developmental delay, muscle weakness, muscle pain, decreased muscle tone, vision and hearing problem and mental retardation.

The examples of mitochondrial disease include:

- Infantile mitochondrial myopathy occurs due to deficiency of NADH Coenzyme Q (CoQ) oxidoreductase and cytochrome oxidase
- Mitochondrial myopathy
- Diabetes mellitus and deafness
- Leber hereditary optic neuropathy (LHON)
- Neuropathy, ataxia, retinitis pigmentosa and ptosis (NARP)
- Myoneurogenic gastrointestinal encephalopathy (MMGIE)

Treatment: There is no specific cure for mitochondrial disease; however, physiotherapy and medication can manage the symptoms. The use of supplements and coenzyme Q10, also known as ubiquinone, which is an electron, can help.

2. Endoplasmic reticulum (ER) is a system of flattened, membrane-bound vesicles and tubules called *cisternae* (Fig. 1.2.1B). It is continuous with the outer membrane of the nuclear envelop, with Golgi apparatus and possibly with the cell membrane. Morphologically, two types of ER can be identified: rough or granular and smooth or agranular.

(I) Rough endoplasmic reticulum. The rough ER is characterized by presence of a number of ribosomes on its surface and transports proteins made by the ribosomes through the cisternae. Thus, the rough ER is especially well developed in cells active in protein synthesis, e.g. Russell bodies of plasma cells, Nissl granules of nerve cells and acinar cells of pancreas.

(II) Smooth endoplasmic reticulum. Smooth ER is devoid of ribosomes on its surface. It is a site of lipid and steroid synthesis. Therefore, it is found in abundance with Leydig cells and cells of the adrenal cortex. In the skeletal and cardiac muscles, smooth ER is modified to form sarcoplasmic reticulum, which is involved in the release and sequestration of calcium ions during muscular contraction.

3. Golgi apparatus The Golgi apparatus or complex is a collection of membranous vesicles, sacs or tubules. This was first reported by Camillo Golgi in 1898, which is generally located close to the nucleus. It is continuous with the ER. Golgi apparatus is particularly well developed in exocrine glandular cells (Fig. 1.2.1C).

Functions. Its main functions are as follows:

- Synthesis of carbohydrates and complex proteins.
- Packaging of proteins synthesized in the rough ER into vesicles.
- Site of formation of lysosomal enzymes.
- Transport of the material to the other parts of cell or to cell surface membrane and secretion.
- Glycosylation of proteins to form glycoproteins.

Table 1.2.1 Lysosomal enzymes and cell components as their substrates

Enzyme	Substrates
Deoxyribonuclease	DNA
Ribonuclease	RNA
Glycosidases	Glycosides and polysaccharides
Collagenases	Collagen
Arylsulphatases	Sulphate esters
Cathepsins	Proteins

Important Note

Camillo Golgi's Black Reaction: In 1873, in Italy, Camillo Golgi first discovered that nerve cells could be stained with silver nitrate turning into black against yellow background. The black stained neurons led him to name this technique as Camillo black reaction.

4. Ribosomes Ribosomes are spherical particles, 15 nm in diameter, which contain 80%–85% of the cell's RNA. They may be present in the cytosol in free (unattached) or in bound form (attached to the membrane of ER). Slightly smaller forms of ribosomes are also found in mitochondria.

Functions. They are the site of protein synthesis. They synthesize all transmembrane proteins, secreted proteins and most proteins that are stored in Golgi apparatus, lysosomes and endosomes.

5. Lysosomes Lysosomes are rounded to oval membrane-bound organelles 250–750 nm in diameter, containing powerful lysosomal digestive (hydrolytic) enzymes. They are formed by the Golgi apparatus. As many as 40 different lysosomal enzymes have been synthesized. Some are listed in Table 1.2.1. These enzymes are acidic hydrolases and act best at acidic pH. The interior of lysosome is acidic (pH 5) as compared to rest of the cytosol (pH 7.2). The lysosomal acidic nature is maintained by proton pump or H^+-ATPase.

Lysosomes are particularly abundant in the cells involved in phagocytic activity, e.g. neutrophils and macrophages. There are three forms of lysosomes:

Primary lysosomes or storage vacuoles are formed from the various hydrolytic enzymes synthesized by rough ER and packaged in the Golgi apparatus.
Secondary lysosomes or autophagic vacuoles are formed by fusion of primary lysosomes with parts of damaged or worn-out cell components.
Residual bodies are undigestible materials in the lysosomes.

Applied Aspects

Lysosomal storage disorders (LSD) are genetic disorders which occur due to defective/absent activity of lysosomal enzymes. Lysosomal enzymes are signal/controllers/regulators of autophagy (i.e. clearance of damaged cellular organelle or unmetabolized cellular substances).

Pathophysiology: The latest concept of pathobiology of LSD is that reactive oxygen species (ROS) damage the cell components and it is necessary to be cleared through autophagy. Transcription factor EB (TFEB), the signalling factor, is responsible for clearance. The mutation of TFEB leads to defective synthesis of lysosomal enzymes resulting in accumulation of damaged cellular components.

Examples:

- *Gaucher disease* occurs due to deficiency of β-galactosidase.
- *Tay–Sachs disease* occurs due to hexosaminidase deficiency, which causes mental retardation and blindness.

Important Note

Acidic pH of lysosome is a safety feature for the cell, because if there is leakage of lysosomal contents into the cytosol, lysosomal enzymes are not effective at pH 7.2, and thus would not be able to digest cytosolic enzymes.

6. Peroxisome Peroxisomes, also known as microbodies, are spherical structures enclosed by a single layer of unit membrane. These are predominantly present in hepatocytes and tubular epithelial cells.

Functions. They essentially contain two types of enzymes:

- *Oxidases* which are active in oxidation of lipid, such as amino acid oxidase and urate oxidase.
- *Catalases* which act on hydrogen peroxide to liberate oxygen. They destroy oxygen free radicals.

Applied Aspects

Deficiency of urate oxidase causes rise in uric acid level leading to gout.
Gout is an inflammatory arthritis characterized by deposition of urate crystals in the joints (especially small joints of toes) due to defective metabolism of uric acid leading to hyperuricaemia. Gout is of two types:
Primary gout occurs due to deficiency of urate oxidase.
Secondary gout occurs due to kidney disease due to decreased excretion of uric acid in the urine.

7. Centrosome The centrosome consists of two short cylindrical structures called centrioles (Fig. 1.2.1D). It is situated near the centre of the cell, close to the nucleus. The two centrioles are arranged at right angle to each other. During cell division, centrosomes duplicate themselves and move apart towards poles as mitotic spindles.

The centrioles are responsible for movement of chromosomes during cell division.

Cytoplasmic Inclusions

The cytoplasmic inclusions are the temporary components of certain cells. These may or may not be enclosed in the membrane. A few examples of cytoplasmic inclusions:

- *Lipid droplets.* These are seen in the cells of adipose tissue, liver and adrenal cortex.
- *Glycogen.* It is seen in the cells of liver and skeletal muscles.

- *Proteins as secretory granules* are seen in the secretory glandular cells (Fig. 1.2.1F).
- *Melanin pigment* is seen in the cells of epidermis, retina and basal ganglia.
- *Lipofuscin.* It is a yellow-brown pigment believed to be derived from secondary lysosomes and is seen in the cardiac muscle and brain cells of elderly people.

Cytoskeleton

The cytoskeleton is a complex network of fibres that maintains the structure of the cell and allows it to change shape and move. It primarily consists of microtubules, intermediate filaments and microfilaments, along with proteins, which anchor and tie them together (Fig. 1.2.2).

1. Microtubules Microtubules are long hollow tubular structures without limiting membrane, about 15–25 nm in diameter. These are made up of two globular protein subunits, α- and β-tubulin. The bundles of tubulin give structural strength to the cells. Microtubules form the transport system of the cells. Microtubules possess two ends; polar end where subunits of microtubules aggregate is known as positive (+) end or assembling end and where subunits disassemble/segregate is called negative (–) end.

Some of the other organelles and protein molecules move to different parts of the cell through the microtubules. *Kinesin* and *dynein,* known as molecular motors, help in the movement of molecules through the microtubules.

> **Important Note**
>
> ***Colchicine,*** an antimitotic drug, prevents assembly of microtubules, thus blocking mitotic activity of cells at metaphase phase.
>
> ***Paclitaxel,*** an anticancer drug, binds to microtubules and stabilize them by polymerization producing defect in mitotic spindles, thus stopping cancer cells from separating into two new cells.

The *cilia and flagella,* which project from the surface of certain cells (spermatozoa, respiratory mucosa and fallopian tubes), are also composed of microtubules enclosed in plasma membrane. Structurally, a cilium consists of axoneme having nine outer microtubules duplets and two inner microtubules. The basal body of axoneme is at the base. The ciliary activity helps in cell movement.

> **Applied Aspects**
>
> **Primary ciliary dyskinesia (immobile cilia syndrome)** is an autosomal recessive disease. In this condition, axonemal activity is affected due to defective structure of cilia.
>
> ***Characteristic features:***
> - Lung infection due to reduction/absence of ciliary mucosal clearance from lungs
> - Infertility in males
> - Altered sense of smell
> - Hearing loss
>
> **Kartagener's syndrome** is a rare autosomal recessive genetic disorder comprising of triad due to defective action of cilia.
> - Chronic sinusitis
> - Situs inversus (body organs are placed on opposite side)
> - Bronchiectasis

2. Intermediate filaments Intermediate filaments are filamentous structures about 10 nm in diameter. Some of these filaments connect the nuclear membrane to the cell membrane. Their main function is to mechanically integrate the cell organelles within the cytoplasm. In their absence, cells rupture more easily, and when they are abnormal in humans, blistering of the skin is common.

3. Microfilaments Microfilaments are long solid filamentous structures having a diameter of 6–8 nm. These are made up of contractile proteins, actin and myosin. Actin is the most abundant protein in the mammalian cell. It attaches to various parts of the cytoskeleton by other proteins (anchor proteins). These are identified by numbers such as 4.1, 4.2, 4.9 (Fig. 1.2.2). The actin filaments interact with integrin receptors to form focal adhesion complexes. The microfilaments are scattered in an unorganized network. Extension of microfilaments along with the plasma membrane on the surface of the cells forms *microvilli,* which increase the absorptive surface of the cells (e.g. intestinal epithelium). In the skeletal muscle, the presence of actin and myosin filaments is responsible for their contractile property.

Molecular Motors

Molecular motors are proteins, 100–500 KDa ATPases. They bind to microtubules and move along them by hydrolysing ATP. The molecular motors help in the transport of different

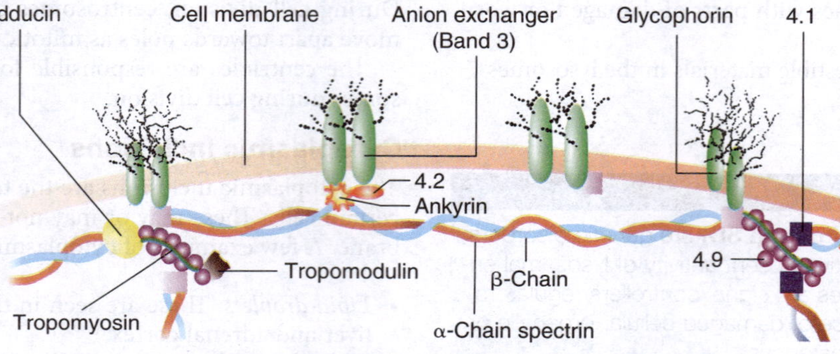

Fig. 1.2.2 Cytoskeleton showing various proteins.

proteins, organelles and their cargo (including membranous vesicles and protein complexes) to other parts of the cell. Broadly, the molecular motors can be divided into two types:

1. Microtubule-based molecular motors This is a superfamily of many forms of molecular motors that produce motion along the microtubules. Following are the two important molecular motors of this family:

i. Conventional kinesin It is a double-headed molecule that moves its cargo towards the positive ends of microtubules.

ii. Dyneins These have two heads with their neck pieces embedded in a complex of proteins. These include:

- ***Cytoplasmic dynein:*** It moves particles and membranes towards the negative end of the microtubule.
- ***Axonemal dynein:*** It can oscillate, and is thus responsible for beating of flagella and cilia which project from the surface of certain cells.

2. Actin-based molecular motors This is a superfamily of many molecular motors that produce motion along the actin. The important example of this group is *myosin*.

Myosin The superfamily is further divided into 15 classes. The two important members of this family are myosin-I and myosin-II, which are described briefly:

Myosin-I: Its molecules have a single head. Myosin-I is associated with actin in many cells.

Myosin-II: Its molecules have two heads, but only one head is active in a molecule. Myosin-II is associated with skeletal muscle.

Mechanism of action The myosins form cross-bridges to the actin molecules, and the myosin heads move generating force which is responsible for movement of various cells such as:

- Contraction of intestinal villi
- Contraction of skeletal, cardiac and smooth muscles

NUCLEUS

Nucleus is present in all eukaryotic cells. It controls all the cellular activities, including reproduction of the cell. Most of the cells are uninucleated, except a few types of cells like skeletal muscle cells, which are multinucleated. Mostly, nucleus is spherical and situated in the centre of the cell; however, its shape and location may vary in different types of cells. The nucleus consists of an outer nuclear membrane enclosing nucleoplasm and nucleoli (Fig. 1.2.1E).

1. Nuclear membrane The nuclear membrane is a double-layered porous structure having a 40–70 nm wide space called *perinuclear cistern* which is continuous with the lumen of ER. The outer layer of the nuclear membrane is continuous with ER. The nuclear membrane contains nuclear membrane complexes. Each complex is made up of proteins organized in the form of tunnel. The exchange of materials between nucleoplasm and cytoplasm occurs through these tunnels.

2. Nucleoplasm The nucleoplasm or the nuclear matrix is a gel-like ground substance containing large quantity of genetic material in the form of DNA. When a cell is not dividing, the nucleoplasm appears as a dark staining thread-like material called nuclear *chromatin*. During cell division, the chromatin material is converted into rod-shaped structures, the chromosomes. There are 46 chromosomes (23 pairs) in all the dividing cells of the body, except the gamete (sex cells) which contains only 23 chromosomes (haploid number). Each chromosome is composed of two chromatids connected at the centromere to form 'X' configuration having variation of the location of centromere. The chromosomes are composed of three components – DNA, RNA and other nuclear proteins. The nuclear DNA carries the genetic information which is passed via RNA into the cytoplasm for synthesis of proteins of similar composition.

3. Nucleolus The nucleus may contain one or more rounded bodies called nucleoli. The nucleoli are the site of synthesis of ribosomal RNA. The nucleoli are more common in growing cells or in cells actively synthesizing proteins.

THE CELL MEMBRANE

An understanding of the structure and properties of the cell membrane is most essential to understand the various physiological activities of the cell, including transport across cell membrane. Electron microscopy has shown that cell membrane/plasma membrane has a *trilayer* structure having total thickness of 7–10 nm (70–100 Å) and is known as *unit membrane*. The three layers consist of *two electron dense layers* separated by an *electron-lucent layer* (clear zone). Biochemically, the cell membrane is composed of complex mixture of lipids (40%), proteins (55%) and carbohydrates (5%).

HYPOTHESIS FOR CELL MEMBRANE STRUCTURE

A few hypotheses have been proposed to explain the distribution of various biochemical components in the cell membrane. The most important hypothesis is the fluid mosaic model of Singer and Nicolson.

The Fluid Mosaic Model of Membrane Structure

In 1972, Singer and Nicolson put forward the fluid mosaic model of membrane structure (Fig. 1.2.3), which is presently the most accepted one. According to this model:

Phospholipid bilayer is the basic continuous structure forming the cell membrane. The phospholipids are present in fluid form. This fluidity makes the membrane quite flexible and thus allows the cells to undergo considerable changes in the shape without disruption of structural integrity.

The protein molecules are present as a discontinuous mosaic of globular proteins which float about in the fluid phospholipid bilayer forming a *fluid mosaic pattern*.

ARRANGEMENT OF DIFFERENT MOLECULES IN CELL MEMBRANE

The arrangement of molecules of phospholipids, proteins and carbohydrates forming the cell membrane is as follows:

Arrangement of Lipid Bilayer of the Cell Membrane

Each lipid molecule in the lipid bilayer of the cell membrane primarily consists of phospholipid, cholesterol and glycolipids.

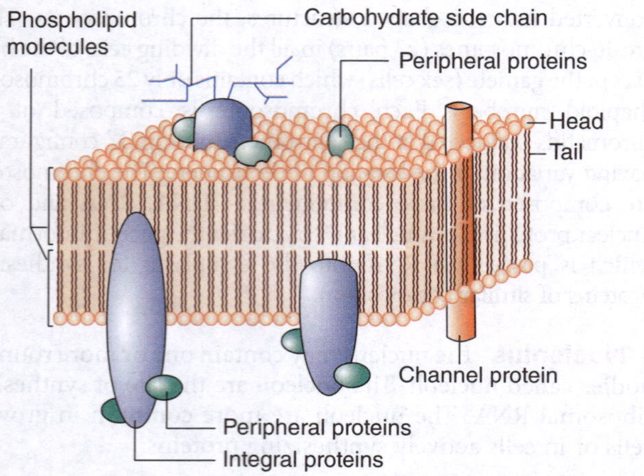

Fig. 1.2.3 Fluid mosaic model of the cell membrane structure.

The presence of cholesterol is responsible for the characteristic which has the consistency of olive oil. The lipid molecule is clothes-pin shape and consists of a *head end* and a *tail end*.

The head end or the globular end of the molecule contains phosphate moiety of phospholipid or hydroxyl radicle of cholesterol. It is positively charged and quite soluble in water (i.e. *polar* or *hydrophilic)*. The tail end consists of two chains of fatty acids or steroid radicle of cholesterol. It is quite insoluble in water (nonpolar or hydrophobic). These lipid molecules are arranged as bilayers in such a way that their nonpolar hydrophobic tail ends are directed towards the centre of the membrane, whereas their polar hydrophilic head ends are directed outwards on either side of the membrane (Fig. 1.2.3). In this way, head ends of molecules face the aqueous phase, i.e. extracellular fluid on the outside and the intracellular fluid (cytoplasm) on the inner side. The major types of phospholipids are *phosphatidyl choline, phosphatidyl ethanolamine, glycosphingolipids, sphingomyelin* and *cholesterol*.

Functional significance of the lipid bilayer The lipid bilayer of the cell membrane makes it a semipermeable membrane which constitutes the major barrier for the water-soluble molecules like electrolytes, urea and glucose. On the other hand, fat-soluble substances like oxygen, fatty acids and alcohol can pass through the membrane with ease.

Arrangement of Proteins in the Cell Membrane

Most protein molecules float about in the phospholipid bilayer forming a fluid mosaic pattern. The proteins are attached on the surface the cell membrane by anchors such as glycosylphosphatidylinositol (GPI). The two types of proteins recognized in the cell membrane are as follows:

Lipoproteins, i.e. the proteins containing lipids, are lipidated proteins having specific lipids attached to them; therefore, these proteins may be myristoylated, palmitoylated or prenylated, which function as enzymes and ion channels.
Glycoproteins, i.e. the proteins containing carbohydrates, which function as receptors for hormones and neurotransmitters.

The proteins in the cell membrane are described as:

1. Peripheral proteins These are present peripheral to the lipid bilayer, both inside and outside to it.

(i) ***Intrinsic proteins:*** These are located in the inner surface of the lipid bilayer and serve mainly as enzymes. Some of these are anchored to the cytoskeleton of the cell (Fig. 1.2.2).

(ii) ***Extrinsic or surface proteins:*** These are the proteins located on the outer surface of the lipid bilayer. These protein molecules are not associated tightly with the cell membrane, and thus can dissociate readily from the cell membrane. Some of these proteins serve as *cell adhesion molecules* (CAMs), i.e. GPI that anchor cells to neighbouring cells and to the basal lamina.

2. Integral proteins or transmembrane proteins

These are the proteins that extend into the lipid bilayer. The proteins stay in the membrane because they have regions of hydrophobic amino acids which interact with fatty acid tails to exclude water. The rest of the proteins are hydrophilic and face into the cell or out into the external environment, both of which are aqueous (Fig. 1.2.3). Some proteins penetrate only part of the way into the membrane, while others penetrate all the way through. The integral proteins, on the basis of functions they serve, have been described as follows:

Channel proteins: Some of the integral protein molecules serve as channels for water-soluble substances like glucose and electrolytes. These are also called the channel proteins.
Carrier proteins: The protein molecules that help in transport of substances across the cell membrane by means of active and passive (facilitated diffusion) transport are called carrier proteins.
Receptor proteins: Some of the proteins function as receptors that bind neurotransmitters and hormones, initiating physiologic changes inside the cell. The number of receptors of a cell are not constant, but keep on increasing (upregulation) or decreasing (downregulation) in response to various stimuli. Some of receptor proteins span (up and down movement) the entire thickness of the membrane several times like a sound wave and help in transport of substances.
Antigens. Some proteins in the cell membrane also act as antigens. These are glycoproteins with branching carbohydrate side chains like antennae. There are an enormous number of possible shapes to these side chains, so each type of cell can have its own specific marker. This enables cells to recognize other cells and behave in an organized way, e.g. during development of tissue and organ in multicellular organisms. It also means that foreign antigen can be recognized. Thus, these proteins help in processing the antibodies and distinguish self from nonself.
Pumps. There are certain proteins in the cell membrane which act as pumps, and form the active transport system of the cell, e.g. Na^+–K^+-ATPase pump, K^+–H^+-ATPase pump and Ca^{2+} pump.

Arrangement of Carbohydrates in the Cell Membrane

The carbohydrates are attached either to the proteins (glycoproteins) or the lipids (glycolipids). Throughout the surface of cell membrane, carbohydrate molecules form a thin loose covering called *glycocalyx*.

Functions of cell membrane carbohydrates are:

- Being negatively charged, the carbohydrate molecules of the cell membrane do not allow the negatively charged particles to move out of the cell.

- The glycocalyx helps in tight fixation of the cells with one another.
- Some of the carbohydrate molecules also serve as *receptors.*

INTERCELLULAR JUNCTIONS

The cell membranes of the neighbouring cells are connected with one another through the *intercellular junctions* or the junctional complexes, which are of three types.

Before describing the types of intercellular junctions, it will be worthwhile to have some information about CAMs.

CELL ADHESION MOLECULES

CAMs are the prominent parts of the intercellular connections by which the cells are attached to basal lamina and to each other.

Types of CAMs. The CAMs have been variously classified. Most simply, they can be divided into four broad families:

1. ***Integrins:*** These are heterodimers that bind to various receptors.
2. ***Adhesion molecules of IgG subfamily:*** Through these molecules, the IgG immunoglobulins bind to various antigens.
3. ***Cadherins:*** These are Ca^{2+}-dependent molecules that mediate cell-to-cell adhesions by haemophilic reactions.
4. ***Selectins:*** These are lectin-like domains that bind carbohydrates.

Mechanism of adhesions. The CAMs act as adhesion proteins by following mechanisms:

- *Anchorage with cytoskeleton:* Many CAMs pass through the cell membrane and are anchored to the cytoskeleton inside the cell.
- *Homophilic binding,* i.e. some CAMs bind to like molecules on the other cells.
- *Heterophilic binding,* i.e. some CAMs bind to different molecules on the other cells.
- *Binding to laminins:* Many CAMs bind to laminins, a family of large cross-shaped molecules with multiple receptor domains in the extracellular matrix.

Functions of CAMs. In addition to *binding the neighbouring cells* to each other, the CAMs perform following other functions:

- They transmit signals into and out of the cells.
- They play a role in embryonic development and formation of the nervous system and other tissue.
- They hold tissue together in adults.
- They play an important role in inflammation and wound healing.
- They also play a role in metastasis of tumours.

TYPES OF INTERCELLULAR JUNCTIONS

1. Tight junction. This is also called *zona occludens* or the *occluding zone* (Fig. 1.2.4A). In this type of intercellular junction, the outer layer of the cell membrane of the neighbouring cells fuse with each other, thus obliterating the space between the cells. A tight junction is composed of parallel strands of tightly packed transmembrane proteins (mainly occludin, junctional adhesion molecules and claudins). Such junctions form a barrier to the movement of ions and other solutes from one cell to another. Following are a few examples of the cells where tight junctions are present:

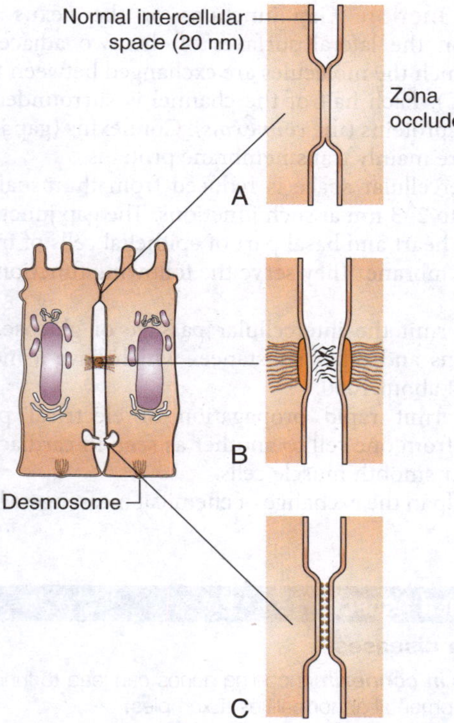

Fig. 1.2.4 Schematic diagram of a cell showing various intercellular junctions: **A,** tight junction; **B,** adherens junction; and **C,** gap junction.

- Apical margins of epithelial cells, such as the intestinal mucosa.
- The renal tubular epithelial cells.
- Capillary endothelium in the brain forming the blood–brain barrier.
- Blood–aqueous barrier formed by the tight junctions between the cells of the inner nonpigmented epithelium of the ciliary body.
- Outer blood–retinal barrier formed by the tight junctions between adjacent cells of the retinal pigment epithelium.

2. Adherens junction. This is also called *zonula adherens.* In this type of junction, cell membrane of the adjacent cells are separated by a 15- to 20-nm wide space which is at focal places obliterated by the dense accumulation of the proteins (cadherin and extracellular part of several transmembrane proteins) at the cell surface. Bundles of intermediate filaments project from the intercellular functional areas and radiate into the cytoplasm. This holds the adjacent cells at these focal places. These are of two types:

Desmosomes are the adherens junctions where thickened focal areas are formed on both the opposing cell membranes (Fig. 1.2.4B).

Hemidesmosomes are the adherens junctions where focal thickening is seen only on the membrane of one of the two adjacent cells. So, this is also known as half-desmosome. Adherens junctions are seen in the cells of epidermis. Focal adhesions attach the cell to the basal lamina and also to actin filaments present inside the cell, and thus help in cell movement.

3. Gap junction. Gap junctions or the nexus are the channels on the lateral surfaces of the two adjacent cells through which the molecules are exchanged between the cells (Fig. 1.2.4C). Each half of the channel is surrounded by six subunits of proteins (the *connexins).* Connexins (gap junction proteins) are mainly transmembrane proteins.

The intercellular space is reduced from the usual size of 15–20 nm to 2–3 nm at such junctions. The gap junctions are seen in the heart and basal part of epithelial cells of intestinal mucous membrane. They serve the following functions:

- These permit the intercellular passage of glucose, amino acids, ions and other substances which have a molecular weight of about 1000.
- These permit rapid propagation of electrical potential changes from one cell to another as seen in cardiac muscle and other smooth muscle cells.
- These help in the exchange of chemical messengers between the cells.

Applied Aspects

Connexin diseases

Mutations in connexin encoding genes can lead to functional and developmental abnormalities. Examples:

- Connexin Cx43 is the main cardiac connexin found in ventricular myocardium, mutation in Cx43 is linked with oculodental digital dysplasia.
- Connexin Cx40 mutation is linked to atrial fibrillation.

Connexin deletions results in defects in electrophysiological changes in the heart causing sudden cardiac death, female sterility, cataract, hearing loss, abnormal bone, development, etc.

METHODS TO STUDY THE FUNCTIONAL ACTIVITY OF CELLS

Various methods have been prescribed to study/demonstrate the cellular functional activity:

1. Microscopic studies include:

- Light microscopy
- Electron microscopy
- Bright field microscopy
- Phase contrast microscopy
- Fluorescence microscopy
- Confocal microscopy

2. Biopsy with microscopy: The biopsy sample is either chemically treated or frozen and sliced into very thin sections. The sections are placed on the slides, stained to enhance the contrast and studied under the microscope.

3. Assessment of bioelectrical activity: Bioelectricity is the electrical currents or electrical potentials generated by or occurring within living cells, tissues and organisms. The bioelectric activity can be studied by:

- Patch clamp technique
- Voltage clamp technique

For details see page 21.

4. Genetic functions of the cells are assessed by:

- Karyotyping
- Polymerase chain reaction (PCR)
- Blot technique

5. Cell growth studies in culture media: The cells are grown and maintained in controlled conditions. The culture medium provides adequate environment for cell growth. By this the microorganisms such as bacteria, yeast, human/plant or animal cells in laboratory. Cell cultures may be used to diagnose infections to test new drugs and in research.

6. Assessment of cellular secretory activity: The secretary activity can be assessed by:

- Blood/plasma levels
- Bioassay
- Immunoassay

7. Biomarkers: The biomarkers are the measurable genes or molecules used to determine the abnormal cells to assess risk of the disease. For example:

- BRCA-1 and BRCA-2 genes indicate risk of breast and ovarian cancer.
- Mutation of amyloid precursor gene indicates Alzheimer disease.

Self-Assessment

1. Discuss the structure, composition and functional significance of the components of cell membrane.
2. Discuss the structure, types and functions of intercellular junctions.
3. Describe:
   (a) Molecular motor
   (b) Method to study cellular activity

Clinical Cases

Case 1

A 36-year-old male married, for the last 8 years, complains of alteration in the sense of smell, hearing loss, frequent lung infection and unable to pregnant his wife.

Q1. What is the probable diagnosis?

Q2. What type of disease is it and what is its cause?

Case 2

A patient was diagnosed a case of Gaucher disease.

Q1. What is the cause of this disease?

Q2. It occurs mainly in the defect of which organelle?

Case 3

A female patient presents with pain, redness and swelling of joints of her fingers and toes. The patient is thoroughly examined, investigated and diagnosed a case of gout.

Q1. What is the reason for redness and swelling of joints?

Q2. Basically, gout is related to defect of which organelle?

1.3 Transport Through Cell Membrane

CHAPTER OUTLINE

The physiological activities of a cell depend on substances like nutrients, oxygen and water, which must be transported into the cell, and at the same time, metabolic waste must be transported out of the cell. Various processes involved in the transport of substances across the cell membrane may be grouped as follows:

- Passive transport
- Active transport
- Vesicular transport

PASSIVE TRANSPORT

Passive transport refers to the mechanism of transport of substances along the gradient without expenditure of any energy. It depends on the physical factors like concentration gradient, electrical gradient and pressure gradient. Since the transport of substances occurs along the gradient, this process is also called *downhill movement*. The passive transport mechanisms operating at the cell membrane level are diffusion and osmosis.

DIFFUSION

Diffusion refers to passive transport of molecules from areas of higher concentration to areas of lower concentration. Diffusion through cell membrane is divided into two subtypes – simple diffusion and facilitated diffusion.

Simple Diffusion

In simple diffusion, transport of atoms or molecules occurs from one place to another due to their random movement. All the molecules, whether dissolved or undissolved, are at constant random movement except at absolute zero temperature. Due to constant random movement, the molecules collide with each other and also strike with the cell membrane. The frequency of collision and the probability of striking to the cell membrane will be higher on the side of the membrane having higher concentrations of that particular molecule. In this process, there occurs a net flux of the molecules from the areas of high concentration to areas of low concentration. The net movement of the molecules ceases when the concentration of molecules are equal, and there occurs a condition of *diffusional equilibrium*. Quantitatively, the net movement of the molecules across a permeable membrane where only simple diffusion is occurring is expressed by *Fick's law of diffusion*, which states that rate of diffusion (J) is directly proportional to the difference in the concentration of the substance in two regions (concentration gradient, i.e. $C_1 - C_2$) and cross-sectional area (A) and inversely proportional to the distance to be travelled (thickness of the membrane, T).

Thus, $J = D\dfrac{A(C_1 - C_2)}{T}$, where D is the diffusion coefficient.

The diffusion of molecules across the biological membranes differs depending on the lipid solubility, water solubility, type of electrical charge and size of the molecules. Furthermore, selective permeability of the semipermeable cell membrane also affects the diffusion of different molecules. How the different molecules diffuse across a cell membrane is discussed as follows.

Simple Diffusion of Lipid-Soluble Substances Through the Cell Membrane

The rate of diffusion through the lipid bilayer of the cell membrane is directly proportional to the solubility of a substance in lipids. Therefore, molecules of substances like oxygen, nitrogen, carbon dioxide, alcohol, steroid hormones and weak organic acids and bases, being lipid soluble, diffuse very rapidly through the lipid bilayer of the cell membrane.

Simple Diffusion of Water and other Lipid-Insoluble Molecules through the Cell Membrane

Astonishingly, water and other lipid-insoluble substances can also pass easily through the cell membrane. It has been shown that it is possible due to the presence of the so-called *protein channels* (made from transmembrane proteins) in the cell membrane.

Diffusion through protein channels The protein channels are tube-shaped channels that extend in the cell membrane from the extracellular to the intracellular ends (Fig. 1.3.1). Therefore, even the highly lipid-insoluble substances can diffuse by simple diffusion directly through these channels of the cell membrane. However, permeability of such substances depends on their molecular size, shape and charge.

The protein channels are equipped with following characteristics:

- Selective permeability
- Gating mechanism

Selective permeability of protein channels. The protein channels are highly selective, i.e. each channel can permit only one type of ion to pass through it. This results from the characteristics of the channel itself, such as, its diameter, its shape and nature of electrical charges along its inside surfaces. Examples of some selective channels are sodium and potassium channels:

Sodium channels are specifically selective for the passage of sodium ions. These are 0.3 × 0.5 nm in size and their inner surfaces are *strongly negatively charged* (Fig. 1.3.2). As voltage-gated sodium channels are made up of a single polypeptide with four homogenous domains. Each domain contains six membrane spanning alpha helices; one of these helices is S_4 voltage-sensitive helix.

> *Note:*
> - Terodotoxin (TTX) is a potent toxin, which specifically binds to voltage-gated sodium channels and physically blocks the flow of sodium ions, thereby preventing generation and conduction of action potential (AP).
> - Inactivation of Na^+ channels by local anaesthetics are use dependent (i.e. degree of block is proportional to the rate of stimulation). This indicates that more number of drug molecules (ion form) enter through sodium channel when the channel is open and cause more inactivation.

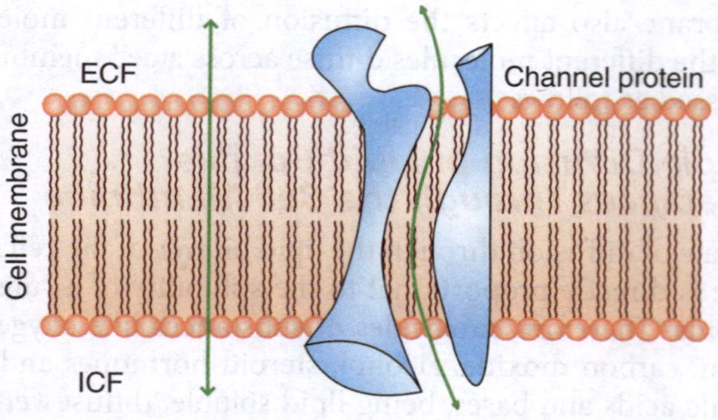

Fig. 1.3.1 Simple diffusion.

Potassium channels are specifically selective for the passage of potassium ions. These are 0.3 × 0.3 nm in size and *not negatively charged* (Fig. 1.3.3). Structurally, voltage-gated potassium channels are tetrameric structure having four protein subunits associate to form a symmetrical (C_4) complex arranged around a central conducing pore. Each subunit is composed of six membranes spanning hydrophobic α-helical sequence and voltage sensors in S_1–S_4.

Gating mechanism in protein channels. Some protein channels are continuously open, whereas most others are 'gated', i.e. they are equipped with actual gate-like extensions of the transport protein molecule that can open and close as per requirement. This gating mechanism is a means of controlling the permeability of the channels. The opening and closing of gates are controlled in three principal ways:

1. Voltage-gated channels: These respond to the electrical potential across the cell membrane. As shown in Fig. 1.3.2, in the case of sodium channels, the gates are located at the outer end of the channels and these remain tightly closed, when there is a strong negative charge on the inside of cell membrane. When the inside of cell membrane loses its negative charge, these gates open and there occurs a tremendous inflow

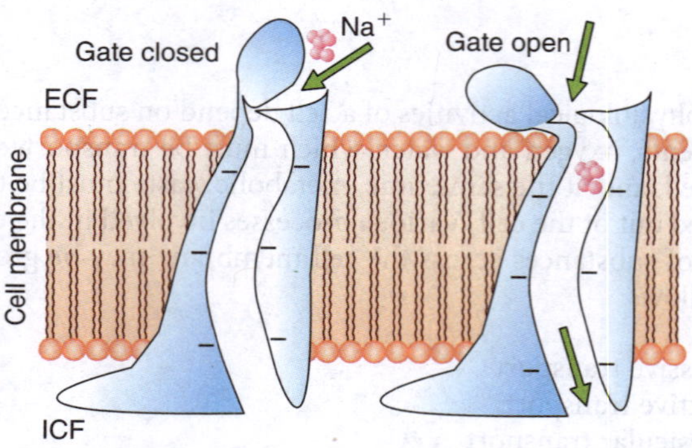

Fig. 1.3.2 Voltage-gated sodium channels.

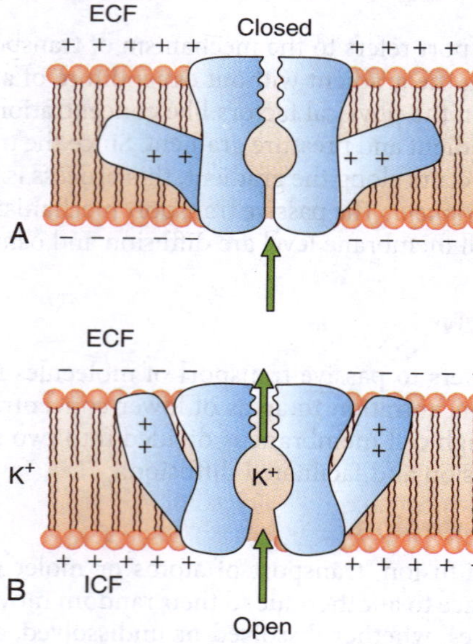

Fig. 1.3.3 Voltage-gated potassium channels: **A**, closed; **B**, open.

of sodium ions. This is the basis of occurrence of AP in nerves that are responsible for nerve signals.

In the case of potassium channels, the gates are located at the inner end of the channel (Fig. 1.3.3) and they too open when the inside of the cell membrane loses its negative charge, but this response is much slower than that for the sodium channel. The opening of potassium channel gates is partly responsible for terminating the AP.

The ion current flow through a single voltage-gated channel protein can be recorded by the patch clamp technique.

Patch clamp method is a simple method in which a micropipette of tip diameter 1–2 μm is abutted against the outer surface of the membrane and suction is applied to suck small membrane inside the pipette, the edges of the pipette tip touching the membrane, creating a tight sealing. The patch of membrane inside the tip of the pipette contains 1–2 channel proteins. Following are three different types of patches:

- *Cell-attached patch:* In this type, the patch remains intact with the cell (Fig. 1.3.4A).
- *Inside-out patch:* In this type, the patch is pulled loosely from the cell forming inside-out patch (Fig. 1.3.4B).
- *Whole-cell patch:* In this type, the patch sucked out in the pipette is still attached on to the rest of the cell membrane, thus providing direct access to the interior of the whole cell and is also known as whole cell recording (Fig. 1.3.4C).

These patches are so small that they contain only single channel proteins and that can be studied by varying the concentration of ions, as well as voltage, across the membrane. The transport characteristics and also the opening and closing of gates can be studied (Fig. 1.3.4D).

2. Ligand-gated channels: Gates of these channels open when some other chemical molecule binds with the gate proteins, which is why this is also called *chemical gating*. The ligand (binding molecules) may be internal or *external*.

- The external or extracellular ligands are also called *first messengers*. One of the most important examples of external ligand channel gating is the effect of acetylcholine on the so-called *acetylcholine channels*. This gate plays an important role in transmission of nerve signals from one nerve cell to another and from nerve cells to muscle cells.
- The internal or the intracellular ligands are also called *second messengers*. The examples include intracellular Ca^{2+}, cAMP or G protein produced in the cells. The second messenger generally activates protein kinases.

3. Mechanically gated channels: Some protein channels are opened by mechanical stretch. These mechanosensitive channels play an important role in cell movements.

Applied Aspects

Channelopathies: Mutations in single-ion channel results in wide varieties of channelopathies.

Examples:

- Periodic paralysis occurs due to defect in one subunit of K^+ channel.
- Myasthenia occurs due to defective nicotinic acetylcholine receptors.
- Malignant hyperthermia occurs due to defect in ryanodine (Ca^{2+} channels).
- Long QT syndrome occurs due to defect in both Na^+ and K^+ channels.
- Bartter syndrome occurs due to defect in K^+ channel subunits.

Facilitated Diffusion

The water-soluble substances having larger molecules, such as glucose, cannot diffuse through the protein channels by simple diffusion. Such substances diffuse through the cell membrane with the help of some carrier proteins. Therefore, this type of diffusion is called facilitated or carrier-mediated diffusion. There are many types of carrier proteins in the cell membrane, each type having binding sites that are specific for a particular substance. Among the most important substances that cross cell membranes by facilitated diffusion are *glucose* and most of the *amino acids*.

Mechanism of facilitated diffusion Postulated mechanism for facilitated diffusion is shown in Fig. 1.3.5. As shown in the figure, a conformational change occurs in the carrier protein after the molecule to be transported is bound at the receptor site. The repetitive spontaneous configurational changes allow the diffusion of the molecule. Earlier, belief was that the carrier protein acts like a shuttle between the outer and inner surfaces of the cell membrane, which has been discarded now.

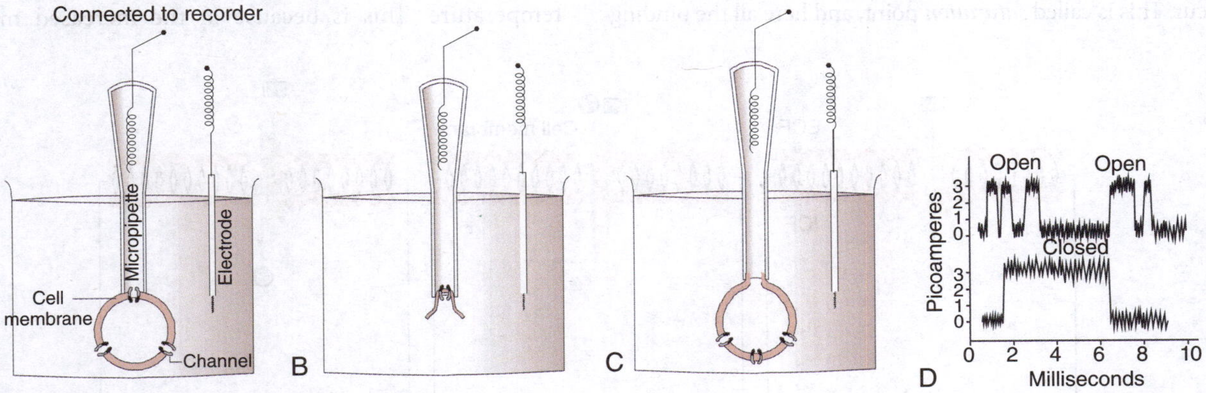

Fig. 1.3.4 Various types of patch clamps used to study the activity of ion channels across the membrane: **A,** cell-attached patch; **B,** inside-out patch; **C,** whole-cell patch. **D,** Note the changes in the membrane current with time and its flow through sodium channels.

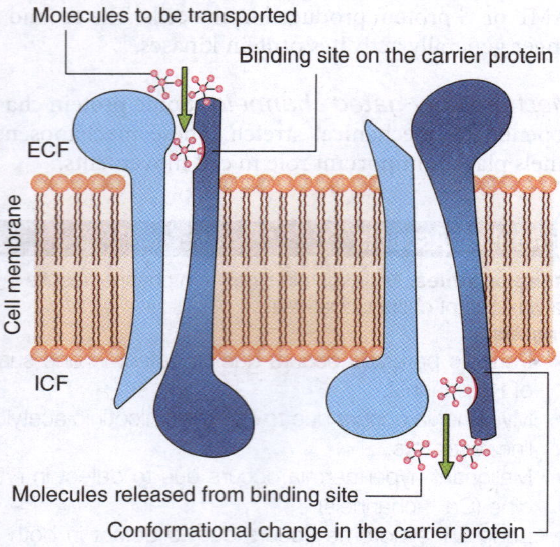

Fig. 1.3.5 Postulated mechanism of facilitated diffusion.

Types of carrier protein systems. Three types of carrier protein systems are known – uniport, symport and antiport (Fig. 1.3.6). The symports and antiport are together known as cotransport.

1. ***Uniport:*** In this system, the carrier proteins transport only one type of molecules.
2. ***Symport:*** In this system, transport of one substance is linked with transfer of another substance. For example, facilitated diffusion of glucose in the renal tubular cells is linked with the transport of sodium.
3. ***Antiport:*** In this system, the carrier proteins exchange one substance for another. For example, Na^+–K^+ exchange or Na^+–H^+ exchange in the renal tubules.

Differences between Simple and Facilitated Diffusions

1. ***Specificity:*** The carrier proteins are highly specific for different molecules.
2. ***Saturation:*** As shown in Fig. 1.3.7, in simple diffusion, the rate of diffusion increases proportionately with the increase in the concentration of the substance and there is no limit to it. However, in facilitated diffusion, the rate of diffusion increases with increase in concentration gradient to reach a limit beyond which a further increase in the diffusion cannot occur. This is called *saturation* point, and here all the binding sites on the carrier proteins are occupied and the system operates at its maximum capacity.
3. ***Competition:*** When two molecules, say A and B, are carried by the same protein, there occurs a competition between the two molecules for the transport. Thus, an increase in the concentration of 'A' molecule will decrease the transport of molecule 'B', and vice versa. No such competition is known to occur in simple diffusion.

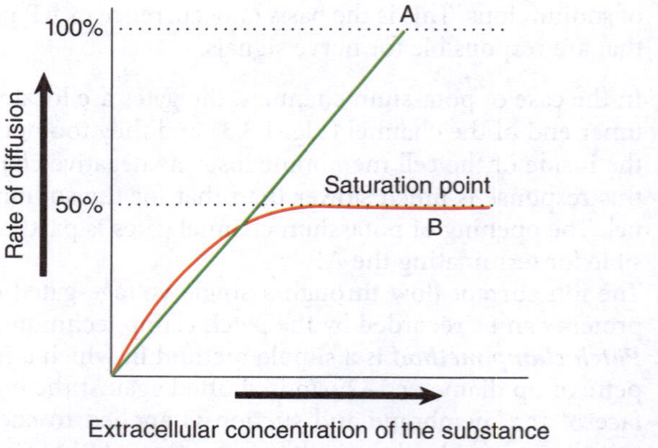

Fig. 1.3.7 Effect of concentration of substance on rate of diffusion in simple diffusion **(A)** and facilitated diffusion **(B)**.

Factors Affecting Net Rate of Diffusion

The mechanisms described above deal with the diffusion of substances through the cell membrane. The diffusion of the substance can occur either way, i.e. extracellular fluid (ECF) to intracellular fluid (ICF) or vice versa, depending on the prevailing environment. The factors that affect the net rate of diffusion in the desired direction are summarized as follows:

1. Cell membrane permeability: Permeability of the cell membrane (*P*) is the major determining factor for the net diffusion, which in turn depends on the following factors:

Thickness of the membrane: The diffusion is inversely proportional to the thickness of the cell membrane, i.e. the greater the thickness, lesser is the rate of diffusion.

Lipid solubility: Diffusion is directly proportional to the lipid solubility of the substance.

Distribution of protein channels in the cell membrane: The rate of diffusion of lipid-insoluble substance is directly proportional to the number of channels per unit area of the cell membrane.

Temperature: Rate of diffusion increases with increase in the temperature. This is because of the increased motion of

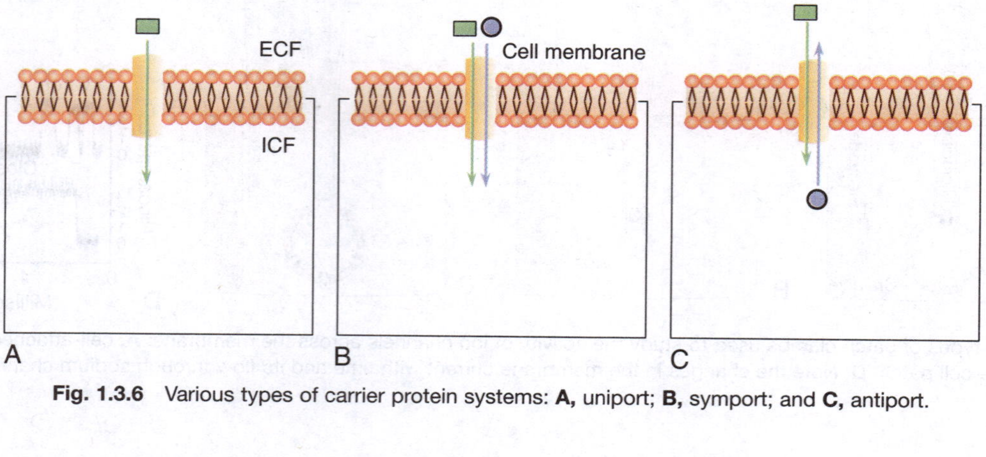

Fig. 1.3.6 Various types of carrier protein systems: **A,** uniport; **B,** symport; and **C,** antiport.

the molecules and ions of the solution with increase in temperature.

Size of the molecules: Rate of simple diffusion is inversely proportional to the size of molecules.

Area of the membrane: The net diffusion of the substance is directly proportional to the total area of the membrane.

The total permeability is often expressed as the *diffusion coefficient (D)* of the entire membrane. It is calculated by multiplying the permeability through a unit membrane area with total area of the cell membrane (*A*). Thus:

$$D = P \times A$$

2. Concentration gradient: The simple diffusion is directly proportional to the concentration gradient (Fig. 1.3.8A) and is denoted by:

Net diffusion α D $(C_o - C_i)$, where C_o is concentration of the substance outside, C_i is concentration of the substance inside and D is the diffusion coefficient of the cell membrane for the substance.

The facilitated diffusion, however, has certain limitations beyond a certain level of concentration gradient (Fig. 1.3.7B).

3. Electrical potential gradient: Electrical potential across the cell membrane is another important factor which affects the diffusion of ions across the cell membrane.

As shown in Fig. 1.3.8B, the concentrations of negative ions are the same on both sides of the membrane, but there is an

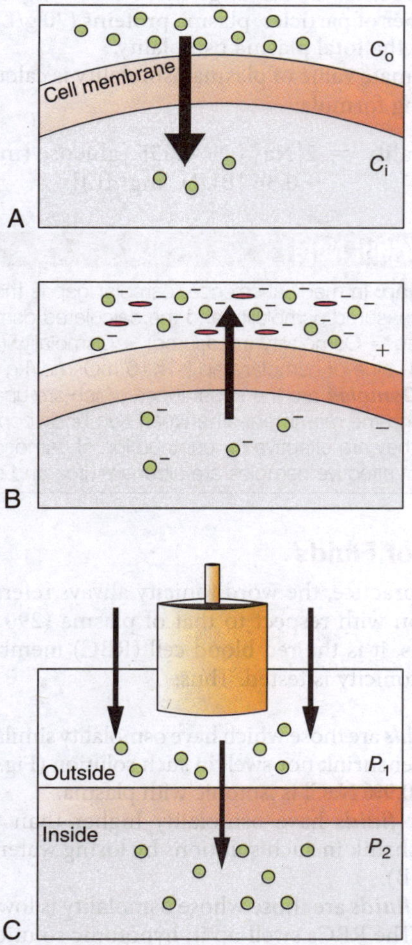

Fig. 1.3.8 Factors affecting net rate of diffusion: **A,** concentration gradient; **B,** electrical gradient; and **C,** pressure gradient.

electrical gradient across the cell membrane because of positive charge outside and negative charge inside the membrane. The positive charge attracts the negative ions, whereas the negative charge repels them. Therefore, net diffusion occurs from inside to outside till the concentration gradient created balances the electrical gradient. In other words, net diffusion of any ion across the cell membrane (*J*) will be the resultant of the combined effect of concentration gradient and electrical potential gradient, and is denoted by the following equation:

$$J = -DA\left[dc/dx + \left(\frac{CF}{RT}\right)dv/dx\right], \text{ where}$$

J is rate of ion diffusion
D is diffusion coefficient
A is area of plane through which ion movement is taking place
dc/dx is concentration gradient
Z is valency of the ion
C is ion concentration
F is Faraday constant (96,500 coulomb per mol of ion)
R is gas constant (8.316 joules per degree)
T is absolute temperature
dv/dx is electrical potential gradient

At normal body temperature (37°C), the electrical gradient that will balance the concentration gradient of a univalent ion can be determined by *Nernst equation:*

$$\text{EMF (in millivolts)} = \pm 61 \log \frac{C_o}{C_i}, \text{ where}$$

EMF is the electromotive force between outside and inside of the membrane
C_0 is the concentration of ion outside the membrane
C_1 is the concentration of ion inside the membrane

This equation is extremely important in understanding the membrane potential, hence discussed in detail in the relevant section (page 31).

4. Pressure gradient: It has been observed that the increased amounts of energy are available to cause net movements of molecules from the high pressure side towards the low pressure side. The pressure-gradient effect is demonstrated in Fig. 1.3.8C, which shows that high pressure developed by the piston on one side of the cell membrane causes greater number of molecules to strike the membrane resulting in net diffusion to the other side.

OSMOSIS

Osmosis refers to diffusion of water or any other solvent molecules through a semipermeable membrane (i.e. membrane permeable to solvent but not to the solute) from a solution containing lower concentration of solutes towards the solution containing higher concentration of solutes, Fig. 1.3.9 shows osmosis across a selective permeable membrane. When a sodium chloride solution is placed on one side of the membrane and water on the other side (Fig. 1.3.9A), net movement of water occurs from the pure water into the sodium chloride solution (Fig. 1.3.9B).

Osmotic Pressure

Osmotic pressure refers to the minimum pressure which when applied on the side of higher solute concentration prevents the osmosis. Fig. 1.3.9C shows that when appropriate

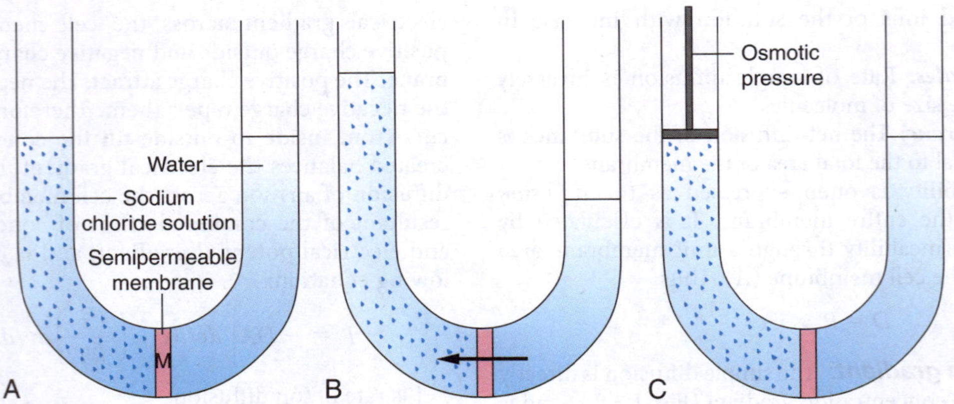

Fig. 1.3.9 Diagrammatic representation of phenomenon of osmosis: **A,** semipermeable membrane 'M' separates sodium chloride solution from pure water; **B,** net movement of water occurs through M from pure water side into the sodium chloride solution side; and **C,** demonstration of osmotic pressure (net movement of water from pure water side to sodium chloride solution is prevented by applying appropriate pressure on the solution side).

pressure is applied, the net diffusion of water into the sodium chloride solution is prevented.

The osmotic pressure in the body fluids refers to the pressure exerted by the solutes dissolved in water or other solvents. The osmotic pressure exerted by the colloidal substances in the body is called *colloidal osmotic pressure.* The colloidal osmotic pressure due to plasma colloids (proteins) is called *oncotic pressure.*

The osmotic pressure depends on the number of molecules or ions dissolved in a solution rather than their size, type or chemical composition. In case of nondissociated solutes, 1 g molecular weight of any substance will contain similar number of molecules, and hence exert similar degree of osmotic pressure, i.e. equal to 22.4 atmospheres, whereas in case of dissociated solutes, the osmotic pressure depends on the number of ions resulting from its dissociation.

Osmole, Osmolality and Osmolarity

Osmole: It is the unit used in place of grams to express the concentration in terms of number of osmotically active particles in a given solution. One osmole is equal to the molecular weight of a substance in grams divided by the number of freely moving particles liberated in solution by each molecule. Thus:

- A molar solution of glucose contains 1 mole and exerts osmotic pressure of 1 atmosphere.
- A molar solution of NaCl contains 2 osmoles (1 mole of Na^+ and 1 mole of Cl^-) and exerts osmotic pressure of 2 atmospheres.
- A molar solution of $CaCl_2$ contains 3 osmoles (1 mole of Ca^{2+} and 2 moles of Cl^-) and thus exerts osmotic pressure of 3 atmospheres.
- One milliosmole (mOsm) is 1/1000 of an osmole.

Osmolality of a solution refers to the number of osmotically active particles (osmoles) per kilogram (kg) of a solution, while ***osmolarity*** refers to the number of osmoles per litre (L) of a solution. Therefore, osmolarity is affected by the volume of the various solutes in the solution and the temperature, while osmolality is not. The osmotic pressure is determined by the osmolality and not osmolarity. However, the quantitative differences between the osmolarity and osmolality are less than 1%. In practice, *osmolarity* is more frequently used in physiological studies, since it is far easier to measure osmolarity vis-à-vis osmolality.

Normal plasma osmolality: The normal osmolality of the ECF and ICF is 290 mOsm/kg. In the plasma of the total osmolality, 270 mOsm are contributed by Na^+, Cl^- and HCO_3^-. The remaining 20 mOsm are contributed by glucose and urea. Because of the large molecular weight and hence lesser number of particles, plasma proteins (70 g/L) contribute 2 mOsm to the total plasma osmolality.

Approximate value of plasma osmolality is calculated using the following formula:

$$\text{Osmolality} = 2[Na^+] + 0.055\ [\text{glucose (mg/mL)}] + 0.36\ [\text{BUN (mg/dL)}]$$

Important Note

Osmolar gap: In medical science, osmolar gap is the difference between measured osmolality and the calculated osmolality, i.e.:
Osmolar gap = Osmolality (measured) − Osmolality (calculated)
The normal value of osmolar gap is <10 mOsmol/kg H_2O
Effective Osmoles are the substances which are unable to cross through the membranes between two body compartments. Therefore, they are effective for contribution of osmotic gradient. Examples of effective osmoles are albumin, urea and ethanol.

Tonicity of Fluids

In clinical practice, the word tonicity always refers to tonicity of a solution with respect to that of plasma (290 mOsm). In other words, it is the red blood cell (RBC) membrane across which the tonicity is tested. Thus:

Isotonic fluids are those which have osmolality similar to plasma. RBCs neither shrink nor swell in such solution (Fig. 1.3.10A). A solution of 0.9% NaCl is isotonic with plasma.

Hypertonic fluids have osmolality higher than the plasma. The RBCs shrink in such solutions by losing water by osmosis (Fig. 1.3.10B).

Hypotonic fluids are those whose osmolality is lower than that of plasma. The RBCs swell up in hypotonic solutions by gaining water by osmosis (Fig. 1.3.10C).

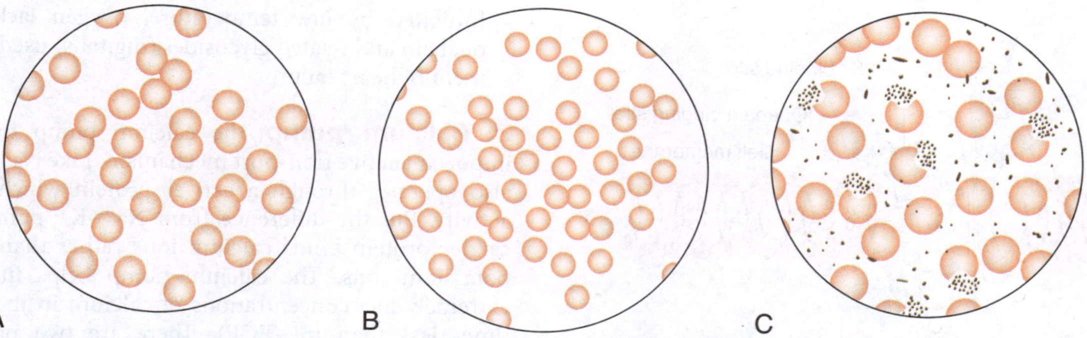

Fig. 1.3.10 Tonicity of fluids: **A,** isotonic fluid (0.9% NaCl) has osmolarity similar to plasma, RBCs neither shrink nor swell in it; **B,** hypertonic fluid (2% NaCl) has osmolarity higher than plasma, RBCs shrink in it; and **C,** hypotonic fluid (0.3% NaCl) has osmolarity lower than plasma, RBCs swell in it and burst open.

Applied Aspects

- The total plasma osmolality may increase in patients with severe dehydration.
- Increased blood glucose level in patients with severe diabetes also increases the plasma osmolality.
- Excessive intravenous administration of 5% glucose decreases plasma osmolality leading to swelling of the body tissues.
- Hyperosmolality can cause coma by causing water to flow out of the brain cells (hyperosmolar coma).
- Raised plasma levels of urea in patients with renal diseases also cause hyperosmolality.

ACTIVE TRANSPORT

Active transport refers to the mechanism of transport of substances against the chemical and/or electrical gradient. Active transport involves expenditure of energy which is liberated by breakdown of high energy compounds like adenosine triphosphate (ATP). Since the transport of substances occurs against the electrochemical gradient, this process is also called *uphill movement.*

MECHANISM OF ACTIVE TRANSPORT

Active transport is also carrier mediated, but its mechanism is different from that of facilitated diffusion. However, since the carrier proteins are involved in the transport mechanism, so like facilitated diffusion, the active transport also shows specificity, saturation and competition.

Since the active transport mechanism involves the expenditure of energy, the transporting carrier protein system is also called the '*active pump mechanism*'. The substance to be transported combines with the specific carrier protein on the cell membrane. The complex so formed undergoes conformational changes and is actively pumped towards the inner surface of cell membrane, where the substance is released and the carrier protein moves back to the outer surface to transport another molecule.

Substances transported actively across the cell membrane include:

Ionic substances such as Na^+, K^+, Ca^{2+}, Cl^- and I^-
Nonionic substances such as glucose, amino acids and urea

TYPES OF ACTIVE TRANSPORT

The active transport is of two types:

- Primary active transport
- Secondary active transport

A. Primary Active Transport Processes

In primary active transport process, the energy is derived directly from the breakdown of ATP or some other high-energy phosphate compound. Following are some of the important pumps involved in the primary active transport processes:

- Sodium–potassium pump
- Calcium pump
- Potassium–hydrogen pump

1. Sodium–potassium pump Sodium–potassium (Na^+–K^+) pump is present in all the cells of the body. It is involved with the active transport of sodium ions outwards through the cell membrane and potassium ions inwards, simultaneously. Thus, this pump is responsible for maintaining the Na^+ and K^+ concentration differences across the cell membrane and for establishing a negative electrical potential inside the cells.

Structure of Na^+–K^+ pump (Fig. 1.3.11). The carrier protein involved in Na^+–K^+ pump is a complex, consisting of two separate protein units, a larger the α-subunit (molecular weight approximately 100,000) and a smaller β-subunit (molecular weight approximately 55,000). The α-subunit is mainly concerned with Na^+–K^+ transport. It has the following binding sites:

- Three intracellular sites, one each for binding sodium ions ($3Na^+$) and ATP, and one phosphorylation site.
- Two extracellular sites, one each for binding potassium ions ($2K^+$) and ouabain.

Mechanism of operation of Na^+–K^+ pump (Fig. 1.3.12). The functioning of Na^+–K^+ pump involves the use of enzyme ATPase. The enzyme ATPase is activated when three sodium ions and one ATP molecule bind to their respective binding sites. The activated ATPase catalyses the hydrolysis of ATP to ADP and liberates a high-energy phosphate bond of energy (phosphorylation). The energy so liberated is believed to cause a conformational change in the carrier protein molecule extruding sodium into the ECF. This is followed by binding

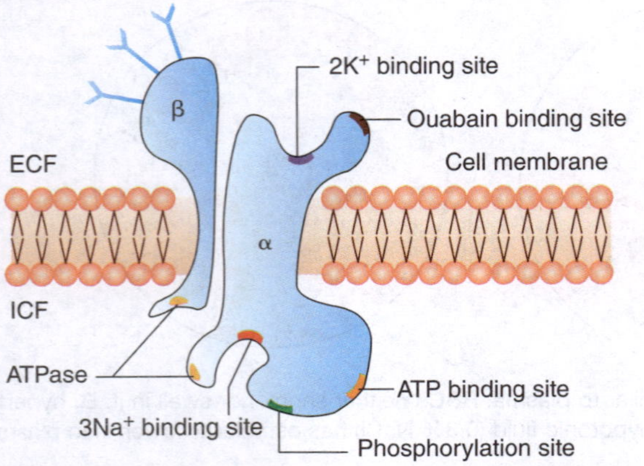

Fig. 1.3.11 Structure of sodium–potassium-ATPase pump.

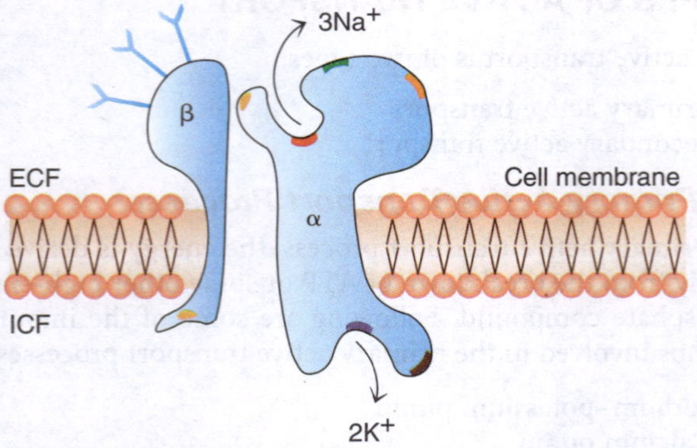

Fig. 1.3.12 Mechanism of operation of sodium–potassium-ATPase pump.

of two potassium ions to the receptor site on extracellular surface of the carrier protein and dephosphorylation of α-subunit which returns to its previous conformation, releasing potassium into the cytoplasm.

Functions of Na^+–K^+ pump. The Na^+–K^+ pump subserves two main functions:

1. ***Controlling the cell volume:*** It is the most important function of the Na^+–K^+ pump, without which most cells of the body will swell up until they burst. Inside the cells are large number of proteins and other organic compounds that cannot escape from the cell. Being negatively charged these also collect large number of positive ions. All these substances cause osmosis of water to the interior of the cell, which is prevented by the Na^+–K^+ pump. When the Na^+–K^+ pump fails, the cells swell up and burst.
2. ***Electrogenic activity.*** Na^+–K^+ pump acts as electrogenic pump since it produces a net movement of positive charge out of the cell ($3Na^+$ out and $2K^+$ in), thus creating electrical potential across the cell membrane. This is a basic requirement in nerves and muscles to transmit the signals.

Regulation of Na^+–K^+ pump. The activity of Na^+–K^+ pump is affected as:

- Increased by cAMP, diacylglycerol (DAG), thyroid hormone, aldosterone, insulin and G actin
- Inhibited by low temperature, oxygen lack, dopamine, ouabain and related glycosides (digitalis) used for the treatment of heart failure

2. Calcium pump The calcium pump forms another important active transport mechanism. Like Na^+–K^+ pump, it also operates through a carrier protein which has ATPase activity. But the difference from Na^+–K^+ pump is that the carrier protein binds calcium ions rather than sodium and potassium ions. The calcium pump helps in maintaining extremely low concentrations of calcium in the ICF (10,000 times less than the ECF). There are two primary active transport calcium pumps:

- One is in the cell membrane which extrudes Ca^{2+} out of the cell.
- The other is calcium pump which actively transports cytoplasmic calcium into the one or more of the cellular organelles like sarcoplasmic reticulum of the muscle cells and mitochondria of all the cells.

3. Potassium–hydrogen pump The primary active transport system of hydrogen ion also operates through ATPase (K^+–H^+-ATPase) activity. These are present at following two places in the human body:

Parietal cells of gastric glands: The K^+–H^+ pump located in these cells actively transports H^+ out of the cells into the lumen of gastric glands and K^+ into the cell from the lumen. The H^+ combines with Cl^- to form HCl in the lumen of gastric glands (for details see page 579).
Renal tubules: The K^+–H^+ pump is located in the intercalated cells of late distal tubules and cortical collecting ducts. Here, large amounts of H^+ are secreted into the tubules to eliminate them from the body for the purpose of controlling blood H^+ concentration (for details see page 492).

B. Secondary Active Transport

In secondary active transport processes, the energy is derived secondarily from the energy which has been stored in the form of ionic concentration differences between the two sides of a membrane, created in the first place by primary active transport. At many areas in the body, transport of some other substance is coupled with the active transport of Na^+, i.e. the same carrier protein which is involved in the active transport of Na^+ also secondarily transports some other substance. The secondary active transport of substance may occur in the form of sodium cotransport or sodium counter-transport.

Sodium cotransport The carrier protein here acts as symport, i.e. transports some other substance along with the sodium. Substances carried by sodium cotransport include glucose, amino acids, chloride and iodine.

Sodium cotransport of glucose. The glucose is transported into most cells against large concentration gradient. As shown in Fig. 1.3.13A, the carrier protein has two receptor sites on the outer surface, one for sodium and other for glucose. The special feature of the carrier protein is that the conformational change in it occurs only when both the sodium and glucose molecules are attached to it. Due to conformational change in the carrier protein, both the sodium and the glucose are transported simultaneously inside the cell (Fig. 1.3.13B). The cotransport of glucose occurs during

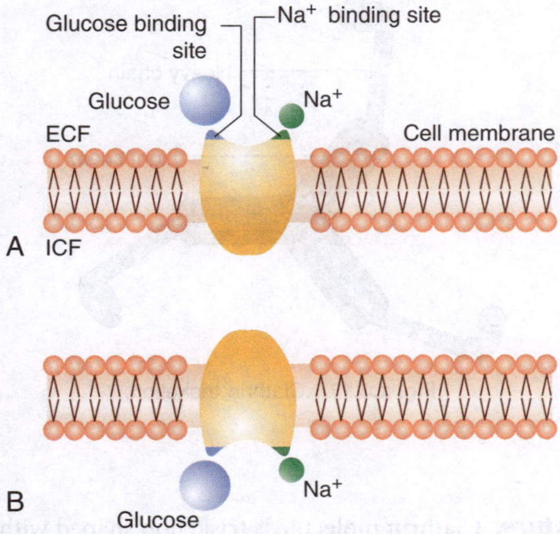

Fig. 1.3.13 Postulated mechanism of sodium cotransport of glucose (secondary active transport): **A,** carrier protein has two receptor sites, one for sodium and one for glucose; and **B,** conformational change in carrier protein causes transport of both glucose and sodium inside the cell simultaneously.

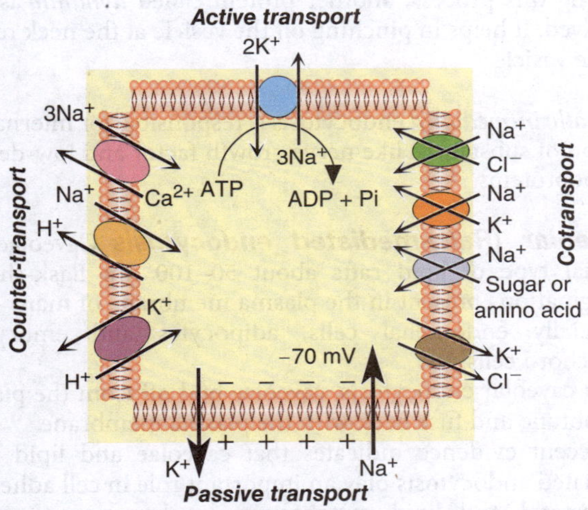

Fig. 1.3.14 Composite diagram of the cell showing the various cotransport and counter-transport mechanisms and maintenance of membrane potential as an effect of primary active transport of Na^+ and K^+.

its absorption from the intestine into the blood and during the reabsorption of glucose from renal tubule in the blood (Fig. 1.3.14). (For details, see page 642.)

Sodium cotransport of amino acids. It occurs especially in the epithelial cells of intestinal tract and renal tubules during absorption of the amino acids into the blood. The mechanism of sodium cotransport of amino acids is similar to that of glucose, except that the carrier proteins involved are different. There are five sets of carrier proteins in the cell membrane, each transporting different amino acids depending on their molecular weights.

Sodium counter-transport The carrier protein involved here acts as *antiport,* i.e. sodium ion is exchanged for some other substance. Some of the sodium counter-transport mechanisms occurring in the body are as follows:

1. ***Sodium–calcium counter-transport*** is known to occur in almost all cell membranes with sodium ions moving inside and calcium outside the cell (Fig. 1.3.14). The transport of these ions in the opposite direction is carried by the same carrier protein.
2. ***Sodium–hydrogen counter-transport*** is especially known in the proximal tubules of kidney. Here, the Na^+ ions move inside the cell and the H^+ ions move out of the cell by the same carrier protein.
3. ***Other counter-transport systems*** which exist somewhere in the body are sodium–potassium counter-transport system, sodium–magnesium counter-transport, calcium–magnesium counter-transport system and chloride–bicarbonate counter-transport system.

VESICULAR TRANSPORT

Vesicular transport mechanisms are involved in the transport of macromolecules such as large protein molecules which can pass through the cell membrane neither by diffusion nor by active transport mechanisms. The vesicular transport mechanisms include endocytosis, exocytosis and transcytosis.

ENDOCYTOSIS

Endocytosis is the process in which the substance is transported into the cell by infolding of the cell membrane around the substance and internalizing it (Fig. 1.3.15). It is further of three types:

1. ***Pinocytosis,*** i.e. cell drinking, refers to the process of engulfing liquid substances by the enfolding of cell membrane, e.g. reabsorption by renal tubular epithelial cells.
2. ***Phagocytosis,*** i.e. cell eating, is the process of engulfing of solid particles such as bacteria, dead tissue and foreign particles by the cells. The process of phagocytosis involves three steps – (i) the attachment stage, (ii) the engulfment stage and (iii) killing or degradation stage (see page 162).
3. ***Receptor-mediated endocytosis:*** In this process, the substance to be transported binds with the special receptor proteins present on the cell surface. The receptor protein–substance complex is then engulfed by the cell membrane by the process of endocytosis. Transport of iron and cholesterol into the cells occurs by receptor-mediated endocytosis.

Mechanism of Endocytosis

There are two pathways by which endocytosis takes place:

1. Constitutive pathway (constitutive endocytosis): In this process, the molecule (substance) first makes contact with the cell membrane, then the cell membrane invaginates to form *endocytic vesicle* followed by fusion of noncytoplasmic sides of the cell membrane, and invagination is pinched off (Fig. 1.3.15).

2. Clathrin-mediated pathway (clathrin-mediated endocytosis): Clathrin-mediated endocytosis occurs at the specific sites (indentation) on the cell membrane where clathrin (a protein) accumulates (Fig. 1.3.16A–D).

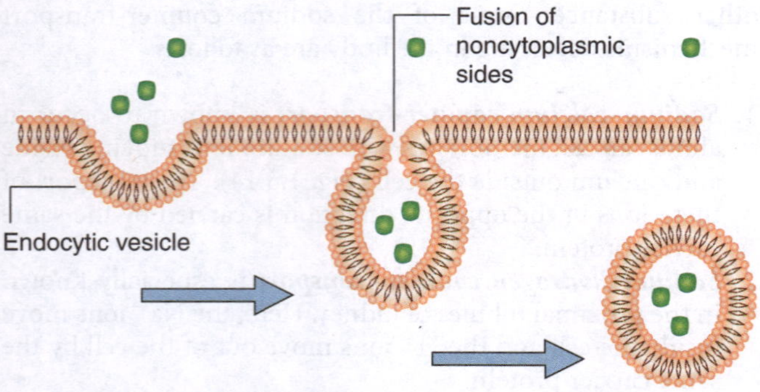

Fig. 1.3.15 Constitutive pathway of endocytosis.

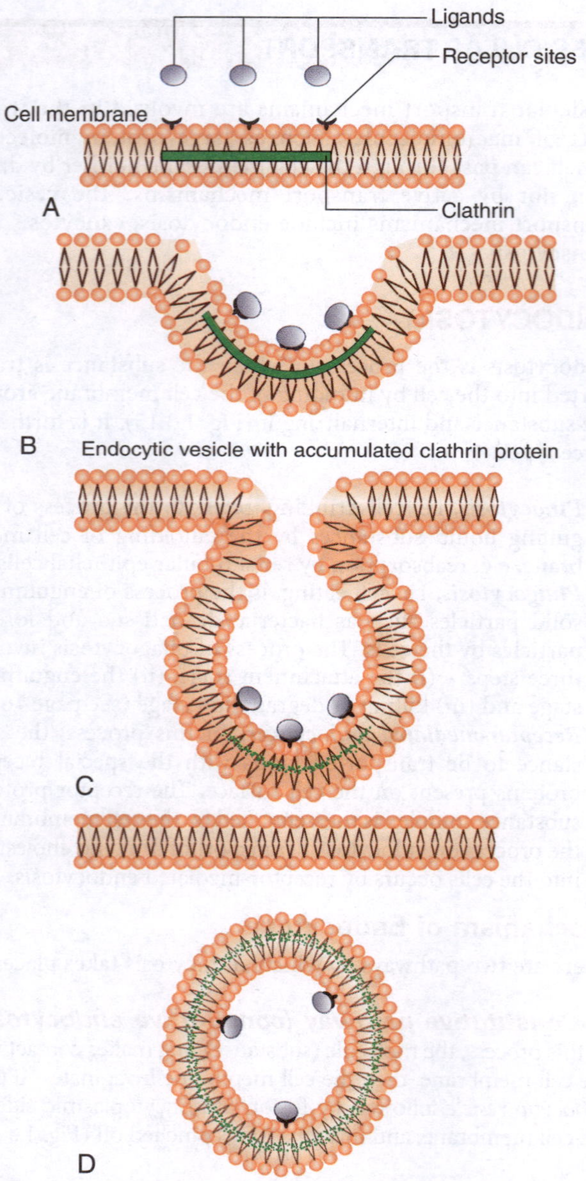

Fig. 1.3.16 Clathrin-mediated endocytosis: **A,** the cell membrane showing receptors (to which the substance binds) and accumulation of clathrin; **B** and **C,** formation of endocytic vesicle; and **D,** complete internalization.

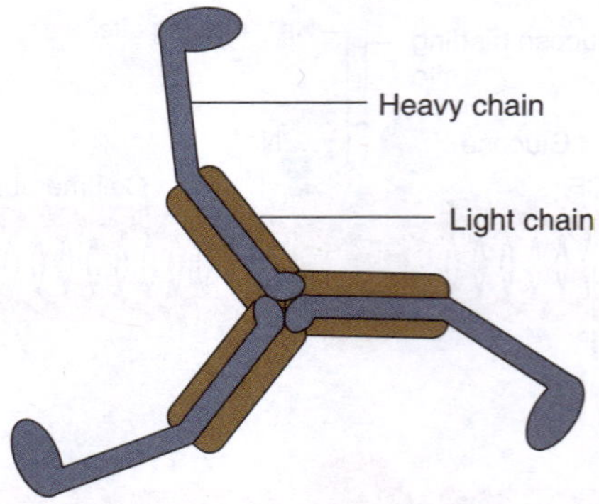

Fig. 1.3.17 Clathrin triskelion.

Structure: Clathrin molecule is triskelion shaped with three legs radiating from the central hub (Fig. 1.3.17).

Role of clathrin: As the endocytosis progresses, clathrin molecule forms a geometrical array and surrounds the endocytic vesicle. After complete formation of the vesicle, the clathrin molecule falls off recycle to form another vesicle. During this process, another protein called *dynamin* is also involved. It helps in pinching off the vesicle at the neck region of the vesicle.

- *Clathrin-mediated* endocytosis is responsible for internalization of substances like nerve growth factor and low-density lipoproteins.

Caveolar (Raft)-mediated endocytosis Caveolae are special type of lipid rafts about 50–100 nm flask-shaped invaginations present in the plasma membrane of many cells, especially endothelial cells, adipocytes and embryonic notochord cells.

In caveolar endocytosis, caveolae bud off from the plasma membrane and fuse back with the plasma membrane.

Recent evidence indicates that caveolae and lipid raft–mediated endocytosis play an important role in cell adhesion, cholesterol and lipid metabolism, mechanosensation and cellular signalling.

The cell membrane also contains small caveolae, indentations coated with protein caveolin involved in ingestion of various amino acids and peptides. Receptor-mediated endocytosis also occurs by this mechanism.

EXOCYTOSIS

Exocytosis (Fig. 1.3.18) is reverse of endocytosis, i.e. by this process the substances are expelled from the cell without passing through the cell membrane. In this process, the substances which are to be extruded are collected in the form of granules or vesicles which move towards the cell membrane. Their membrane then fuses with the cell membrane. The area of fusion breaks down releasing the contents to the exterior and leaving the cell membrane intact. Release of hormones and enzymes by secretory cells of the body occurs by exocytosis. The process of exocytosis requires Ca^{2+} and energy along with docking proteins. Excretion of specific hormones and granules by the cells is termed *emiocytosis*.

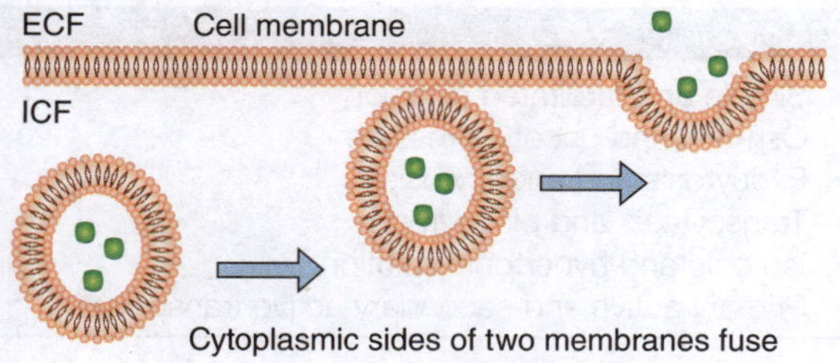

Fig. 1.3.18 Exocytosis.

There are two pathways by which secretion from the cell occurs.

1. Nonconstitutive pathway: In this process, the proteins from the Golgi apparatus initially enter in the secretory granules, where processing of prohormones to mature hormones occurs before exocytosis.

2. Constitutive pathway: It involves the prompt transport of proteins to the cell membrane in vesicles, with little or no processing or storage.

TRANSCYTOSIS

Vesicular transport within the cell is called transcytosis or cytopempsis. It is quite similar to exocytosis and endocytosis. Three basic steps involved in this process are (i) vesicle formation, (ii) vesicle transportation and (iii) docking in the cell.

Role of various proteins in vesicular transport The vesicles involved in the transport are coated with proteins. The different types of coating proteins which have been identified are as follows:

- *AP-1 clathrin:* It is present in vesicles involved in transportation from Golgi apparatus to lysosomes.
- *AP-2 clathrin:* It exists in endocytic vesicles involved in transportation to endosomes.
- *CO-PI and CO-PII:* These are coating proteins present in vesicles involved for transportation between endoplasmic reticulum and Golgi apparatus.
- *Dynamin:* It appears to be involved in vesicle formation from Golgi apparatus and also from cell membrane.
- *Docking protein:* Each target cell has a set of docking proteins (v SNARE protein) and latch proteins (t SNARE protein). When the vesicle reaches its target cell, these proteins ensure that the vesicle will dock with the corresponding set of docking proteins.

OTHER TRANSPORT PROCESSES

So far we have considered transport across the cell membrane, i.e. movement of substances between the ICF and ECF through the cell membrane. In addition to it, there are many situations in the body where transport of substances occurs through the epithelia and the capillary endothelial cell membrane. Some of these processes are discussed briefly:

- Transport across epithelia
- Ultrafiltration

TRANSPORT ACROSS EPITHELIA

Transport across epithelia involves movement of the substances from one side of the epithelium to the other. The transepithelial transport occurs in body cavities lined by continuous sheet of cells such as in gastrointestinal tract, renal tubules, pulmonary airways and other structures. For transepithelial transport to occur, the cells need to be bound by tight junctions, and have different ion channels and transport protein in different parts of their membrane. Transport across epithelia may occur in two ways:

1. Transport through the cells proper (transcellular): In gastrointestinal tract and in urinary tubules, substances are transferred from the lumen into the epithelial cells at their apical borders and then from the basal borders of the cells into interstitial fluid. From the interstitial fluid, the substances are finally transported into the blood through the capillaries.

2. Transport across the tight junctions: It has been identified that in the epithelia of small intestine, proximal renal tubules and gall bladder, most of the sodium chloride passes through the tight junctions (areas of tight adherence between the two adjacent cells) rather than traversing the whole length of the epithelial cells. This type of transport is also known as paracellular transport.

ULTRAFILTRATION

When a solution of protein and salt is separated from plain water or a less concentrated salt solution by a membrane permeable to salt and water and not to the protein, there will be a net movement of water on the protein side by diffusion and a movement of salt away from the protein side. This process is called dialysis (Fig. 6.5.7).

Ultrafiltration refers to the occurrence of dialysis under hydrostatic pressure (Fig. 4.4.26). Ultrafiltration occurs at the capillary level in the body. The capillary blood is under hydrostatic pressure. The pressure is 35 mm Hg near the arteriolar end and gradually declines to 12 mm Hg near the venous end of the capillary. Through the capillaries, ultrafiltration of all the constituents of the plasma occurs except the proteins into the interstitial spaces. Ultrafiltration plays an important role in the formation of body fluids. Plasma proteins, to which the capillary wall is not permeable, exert an osmotic pressure of about 25 mm Hg. This osmotic pressure opposes the hydrostatic pressure, resulting in limitation of outflow of fluid from the capillaries near the arteriolar end and backflow of interstitial fluid into capillaries (by osmosis) near their venous end where osmotic pressure (25 mm Hg) is greater than the hydrostatic pressure of blood (12 mm Hg) (Fig. 4.4.26).

Self-Assessment

1. Describe the mode of transport of water-soluble substances across the cell membrane.
2. Describe the gating mechanism of protein channels.
3. Describe the mechanism of action of Na^+–K^+-ATPase.
4. Differentiate between:
   - Active and passive transport
   - Simple and facilitated diffusion
   - Osmotic and oncotic pressure
   - Exocytosis and endocytosis
   - Transcytosis and pinocytosis
   - Isotonic and hypertonic solution
   - Primary active and secondary active transport

Clinical Cases

Case 1

A 70-year-old diabetic woman is brought in the emergency with the following signs and symptoms:

- Comatose
- Pulse weak and feeble
- Breathing rapid and sallow
- Dry skin

Investigations reveal blood glucose 420 mg/dL, marked glycosuria and low plasma proteins.

Q1. What is the diagnosis?

Q2. What is plasma osmolality in this condition?

Q3. Is there any other condition in which plasma osmolality increases or decreases?

Case 2

In medicine OPD a 60-year-old male patient presented with breathlessness, fatigue and muscle weakness. On examination, the patient presents hepatomegaly, cardiomegaly and low BP. The sign and symptoms and investigation are suggestive of chronic heart failure. To relieve symptoms cardiac glycosides (digitalis) were prescribed.

Q1 What is the mechanism of action of the drug for improvement in the symptoms?

Case 3

A 65-year-old patient on drug digitalis for atrial arrhythmia is instructed by his cardiologist to get blood analysis for K^+ on regular basis because hypokalaemia increases the risk of digitalis toxicity.

Q1 How does hypokalaemia increase the risk of digitalis toxicity?

Membrane Potential

1.4

CHAPTER OUTLINE

INTRODUCTION

There exists a potential difference across the membrane of all living cells with the inside being negative in relation to the outside. This potential difference is named *membrane potential,* because the cations and anions arrange themselves along the outer and inner surfaces of the cell membrane. The magnitude of membrane potential varies from cell to cell and in a particular cell varies according to its functional status. For example, a nerve cell has a membrane potential of −70 mV (inside negative) at rest, but when it gets excited, the membrane potential becomes about +30 mV (inside positive). The membrane potential at rest is called *resting membrane potential* (RMP) or resting transmembrane potential or simply resting potential. The term rest does not imply that the cell is metabolically quiescent but that it is not undergoing any electrical change. The membrane potential measured during the excited state of the cell is called *action potential.* For details of action potential, see page 59.

GENESIS OF MEMBRANE POTENTIAL

Membrane potential is basically due to unequal distribution of ions across the cell membrane, which in turn results due to the combined effect of various forces acting on the ions. Following are the factors involved in the genesis of membrane potential which need elaboration:

- Selective permeability of the cell membrane
- Gibbs–Donnan equilibrium
- Nernst equation
- Constant field Goldman equation
- Sodium–potassium-ATPase pump

SELECTIVE PERMEABILITY OF THE CELL MEMBRANE

The cell membrane is selectively permeable, i.e. to some ions it is freely permeable, to others impermeable and to some others it has variable permeability as:

- Ions like Na^+, K^+, Cl^- and HCO_3^- are diffusible ions. The cell membrane is freely permeable to K^+ and Cl^- and moderately permeable to Na^+.
- Though the particle size of K^+ is larger (atomic weight 39) as compared to Na^+ (atomic weight 23), the permeability for K^+ is approximately 50–100 times greater than that for Na^+. This is because hydrated K^+ is smaller than hydrated Na^+. In other words, the energy required to separate water from Na^+ is greater as compared to K^+, so the K^+ permeability is higher than Na^+.
- The cell membrane is practically impermeable to intracellular proteins and organic phosphate, which are negatively charged ions.
- The presence of gated channels in the cell membrane is responsible for the variable permeability of certain ions in different circumstances.

GIBBS–DONNAN MEMBRANE EQUILIBRIUM

According to Gibbs–Donnan membrane equilibrium, when two ionized solutions are separated by a semipermeable membrane, at equilibrium:

- Each solution shall be electrically neutral, i.e. total charges on cations will be equal to total charges on anions.

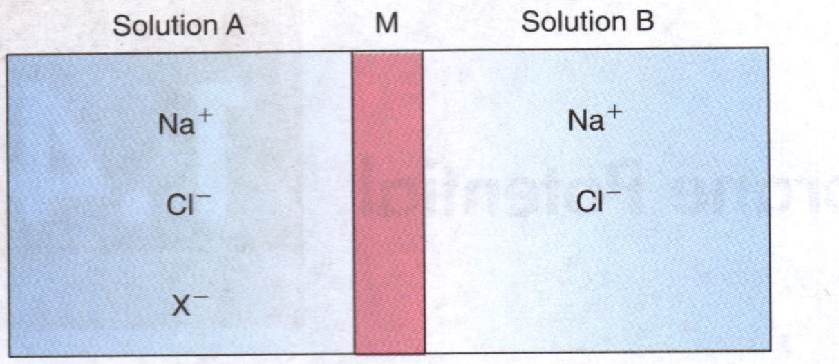

Fig. 1.4.1 Semipermeable membrane 'M' separates ionic solutions of sodium chloride **A** and **B**.

- The product of diffusible ions on one side of the membrane will be equal to the product of diffusible ions on the other side of the membrane.

To understand, let us consider 'M' as a semipermeable membrane separating two ionized solutions of sodium chloride A and B (Fig. 1.4.1). Then, according to Gibbs–Donnan equilibrium:

1. Each solution is electrically neutral, i.e.

$$(\text{cations})_A = (\text{anions})_A, \text{ and } (\text{cations})_B = (\text{anions})_B$$
OR
$$(Na^+)_A = (Cl^-)_A \text{ and, } (Na^+)_B = (Cl^-)_B$$

2. The product of diffusible ions on both sides will be equal, i.e.

$$(\text{diffusible cations})_A \times (\text{diffusible anions})_A = (\text{diffusible cations})_B \times (\text{diffusible anions})_B$$
OR
$$[(Na^+)_A \times (Cl^-)_A] = [(Na^+)_B \times (Cl^-)_B]$$

From the above, the ratio of diffusible ions will be as follows:

$$\frac{(\text{diffusible cations})_A}{(\text{diffusible cations})_B} = \frac{(\text{diffusible anions})_B}{(\text{diffusible anions})_A}$$
OR
$$\frac{[Na^+]_A}{[Na^+]_B} = \frac{[Cl^-]_B}{[Cl^-]_A}$$

Thus, there will be symmetrical distribution of ions at equilibrium. But if one or more nondiffusible ions 'X' are present on one side (A side) of the membrane, according to Gibbs-Donnan, at equilibrium the distribution of diffusible ions will be as follows:

1. Both solutions will be electrically neutral, i.e.

$$(Na^+)_A = (Cl^-)_A + (X^-)_A \text{ and } (Na^+)_B = (Cl^-)_B$$
$$\text{So, } (Na^+)_A + (Cl^-)_A + (X^-) > (Na^+)_B + (Cl^-)_B \text{..........(1)}$$

2. The product of diffusible ions on two sides will be equal, i.e.

$$(Na^+)_A \times (Cl^-)_A = (Na^+)_B \times (Cl^-)_B \text{..........(2)}$$

From the relationship of (1) and (2), it is found that:
- $(Na^+)_A > (Na^+)_B$
- $(Cl^-)_A < (Cl^-)_B$

Hence, there is unequal distribution of diffusible ions (asymmetrical). At equilibrium, Na^+ is greater on the side which contains nondiffusible anions 'X^-' (side A) and anion Cl^- is greater on the other side (side B). However, their concentration ratios are equal.

Since the intracellular fluid (ICF) contains nondiffusible anions like proteins and organic phosphate, according to Gibbs–Donnan equilibrium, there should be an asymmetrical distribution of diffusible ions across the cell membrane with cations being more inside than the outside. However, in reality, the interior of the cell is negatively charged which will be explained in the ensuing discussion.

NERNST EQUATION

The asymmetrical distribution of diffusible ions across the cell membrane in the form of excess diffusible cation inside due to Gibbs–Donnan equilibrium (as explained above) results in a concentration gradient. As a result of this, diffusible cations (K^+) will try to diffuse back into the extracellular fluid (ECF) from ICF, but are counteracted by the electrical gradient, which will be created due to the presence of nondiffusible anions inside the cell. Thus, equilibrium will be reached between the concentration gradient and the electrical gradient resulting in diffusion potential (equilibrium potential) across the cell membrane. The magnitude of this equilibrium potential can be determined by Nernst equation as:

$$E_{(m)} = -\frac{RT}{ZF} \ln \frac{(\text{Conc})_i}{(\text{Conc})_o}$$

where:

$E_{(m)}$	Equilibrium potential (in millivolts) of the ions at which efflux and influx of the ions are equal
R	The natural gas constant and its value is 8.316 J/degree
T	The absolute temperature
F	The Faraday constant and its value is represented as number of C/mole of charge (96,500 C/mole)
Z	The valency of the ion
ln	Symbol for natural logarithm
$(\text{Conc})_i$	The concentration of the ions in the intracellular fluid (inside)
$(\text{Conc})_o$	The concentration of the ions in the extracellular fluid (outside)

At normal body temperature (37°C), converting from the natural log to the base 10 log and replacing some of the constants with numerical values, the equation can be simplified to:

$$E_{(m)} = \pm 61 \ln \frac{(\text{Conc})_i}{(\text{Conc})_o}$$

The equilibrium potential ($E_{(m)}$) for some of the important ions in the mammalian spinal motor neuron calculated from the simplified Nernst equation is shown in Table 1.4.1.

Important Note

- Regarding Nernst equation, an ion always diffuses in the direction to bring RMP towards its equilibrium.
- RMP is usually approaches the $E_{(m)}$ of most permeable ion.

Table 1.4.1 Equilibrium potential [$E_{(m)}$] for important ions in a mammalian spinal motor neuron

	Concentration (in mmol/L of H_2O)		
Ion	Outside the cell	Inside the cell	Equilibrium potential (in mV)
Na^+	150	15	+60
K^+	05.5	150	−90
Cl^-	125	09	−70
Ca^{2+}	5	<1	+130

GOLDMAN–HODGKIN–KATZ EQUATION

The Nernst equation helps in calculating the equilibrium potential for each ion individually. However, the magnitude of the membrane potential at any given time depends on the distribution of Na^+, K^+ and Cl^- and the permeability of each of these ions. The integrated role of different ions in the generation of membrane potential can be described accurately by the *Goldman constant field equation* or the so-called Goldman–Hodgkin–Katz (GHK) equation:

$$V = \frac{RT}{F} \ln \frac{P_k[K^+]_i + P_{Na^+}[Na^+]_i + P_{Cl^-}[Cl^-]_o}{P_k[K^+]_o + P_{Na^+}[Na^+]_o + P_{Cl^-}[Cl^-]_i}$$

where:

V is the membrane potential
R is the gas constant
T is the absolute temperature
F is Faraday constant
P_{K^+}, P_{Na^+} and P_{Cl^-} are the permeabilities of the membrane to K^+, Na^+ and Cl^-, and brackets signify concentration and i and o refer to inside and outside of the cell, respectively

Inferences of Goldman constant field equation

Following important inferences can be drawn from the Goldman constant field equation:

1. ***Most important ions for development*** of membrane potentials in nerve and muscle fibres are sodium, potassium and chloride. The voltage of membrane potential is determined by the concentration gradient of each of these ions.
2. ***Degree of importance*** of each of the ions in determining the voltage depends on the membrane permeability of the individual ion. For example, if the membrane is impermeable to K^+ and Cl^-, then the membrane potential will be determined by the Na^+ gradient alone and the resulting potential will be equal to the Nernst potential for sodium.
3. ***Positive ion concentration from inside the membrane to outside*** is responsible for electronegativity inside the membrane. This is because of the fact that due to concentration gradient, the positive ions diffuse outside leaving the non-diffusible negative ions inside the cell.
4. ***Signal transmission*** in the nerves is primarily due to change in the sodium and potassium permeability because their channels undergo rapid change during conduction of the nerve impulse and not much change is seen in the chloride channels.

ROLE OF NA^+–K^+-ATPASE PUMP

The role of Na^+–K^+-ATPase lies in building the concentration gradient. It serves to pump back the Na^+ that diffuses into the cell and K^+ that diffuses out of the cell. In the resting membrane, these diffusions are negligible, so the Na^+–K^+ pump works very feebly in this stage. Furthermore, although the Na^+–K^+ pump is potentially electrogenic (since it pumps out three Na^+ ions for two K^+ ions), at no stage is the pump able to build up a significant membrane potential. This is because of the fact that as soon as the pump creates a negative potential inside the cell, chloride ions rush out of the cell and restore electroneutrality. Thus, in other words, this pump, pumps out three Na^+ ions and one Cl^- ion for every two K^+ ions it pumps in.

RECORDING OF MEMBRANE POTENTIAL

INSTRUMENTS USED FOR RECORDING

The essential instruments used in recording the activity of an excitable tissue:

- Microelectrodes
- Electronic amplifiers
- Cathode ray oscilloscope (CRO)

Basic principles of the functioning of these instruments are described on page 67.

TECHNIQUE OF RECORDING

Technique of recording of membrane potential is described on page 68.

Self-Assessment

1. Discuss the genesis of resting membrane potential.
2. Describe the significance of Gibbs–Donnan membrane equilibrium, Nernst equation and Goldman–Hodgkin–Katz equation?

Clinical Case

Case 1

An 82-year-old woman is brought to the emergency room with complaints of extreme thirst and generalized weakness she has consumed large quantity of orange juice to quench the thirst. Laboratory investigations reveal hyperkalaemia.

Q1. What will happen to the membrane potential of nerve?

1.5 Genetics: An Overview

CHAPTER OUTLINE

INTRODUCTION

Genetics may rightly be claimed to be one of the most important branches of biology. Foundation for the present day genetics was laid by the Mendel's work published in 1866. He demonstrated that characteristics do not blend but pass from parents to offspring as discrete (separate) units. These units, which appear in the offspring in pairs, remain discrete and are passed on to subsequent generations by the male and female gametes each of which contain a single unit. The Danish botanist Wilhelm Ludvig Johannsen called these units genes in 1909 and the American geneticist Thomas Hunt Morgan, in 1912, demonstrated that they are carried on chromosomes. Since the early 1900, the study of genetics has made great advances. An overview of this is given here in brief.

STRUCTURAL AND FUNCTIONAL CHARACTERISTICS OF SUBSTRATE FOR GENETICS

CHROMOSOMES

Waldeyer in 1888 coined the term chromosomes to denote the thread-like structures present in the nucleus of eukaryotic cells during division. It is now established that the chromosomes are responsible for the transmission of the hereditary information from one generation to next. There are 46 chromosomes (23 pairs) in all the dividing cells of the body except the gametes (sex cells which contain only 23 chromosomes) haploid number.

Morphology of chromosomes Each chromosome is composed of two chromatids connected at the *centromere.* Each chromatid consists of two *chromonemes. Telomeres* are the terminal ends of chromosome DNA molecules.

Morphological types of chromosomes. Depending on the location of the centromere, four morphological types of chromosomes are recognized (Fig. 1.5.1):

- *Metacentric chromosomes:* The centromere divides the chromosomes into two equal arms (Fig. 1.5.1A).
- *Submetacentric chromosomes:* The centromere divides the chromosomes into two unequal arms (Fig. 1.5.1B).
- *Acrocentric chromosomes:* The centromere is located in such a way that a very short arm of chromosomes is visible (Fig. 1.5.1C).
- *Telocentric chromosomes:* The centromere is located at one end (Fig. 1.5.1D).

Functional types of chromosomes. There are three types of eukaryotic chromosomes:

- *Autosomes* are the chromosomes present in somatic cells. The number of autosomes in a cell is fixed and is expressed as 2*n* or *diploid number.*
- *Sex chromosomes* are present in the sex cells and are responsible for determining the sex of an individual.
- *Supernumerary or redundant chromosomes* are also found in eukaryotic cells but their occurrence is quite uncommon.

Chemical structure of chromosomes The chromosomes are mainly composed of DNA. The chromosome also contains RNA, basic proteins called histones, complex proteins including enzymes, some organic phosphorus compounds and inorganic salts. The amount of DNA in a haploid cell is half the amount present in a diploid cell of the same species. Furthermore, the concentration of DNA in any cell remains constant in every circumstance. An important feature of DNA is that it is metabolically stable.

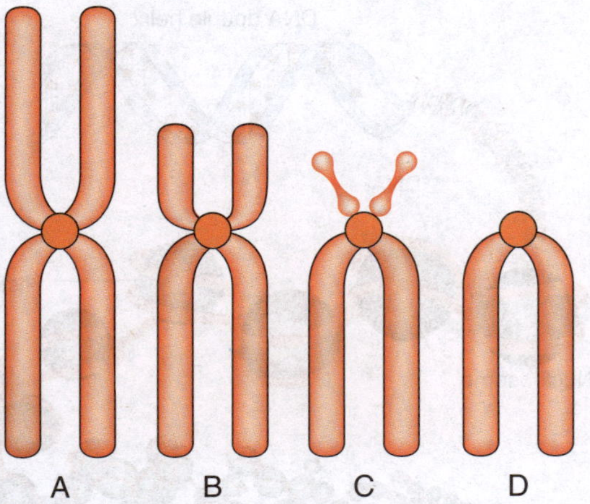

Fig. 1.5.1 Morphological types of chromosomes: **A,** metacentric; **B,** submetacentric; **C,** acrocentric; **D,** telocentric.

STRUCTURE AND FUNCTION OF DNA AND RNA

DNA

DNA, i.e. deoxyribonucleic acid, is a molecule of inheritance and thus may be regarded as the 'Reserve Bank' of genetic information. It is exclusively responsible for maintaining the identity of different species of organisms for millions of years.

Structure of DNA DNA is a polymer of four monomeric deoxyribonucleotides, namely, deoxyadenylate (dAMP), deoxyguanylate (dGMP), deoxycytidylate (dCMP) and deoxythymidylate (dTMP). Each deoxyribonucleotide in turn is composed of a nitrogenous base purine or pyrimidine (A, G, C or T), a pentose sugar, i.e. deoxyribose, and a phosphate. Each molecule of DNA has equal number of adenine and thymine residues (A = T) and equal number of guanine and cytosine residues (G = C). This is known as *Chargaff's rule.*

Watson–Crick model of DNA structure. The salient features of Watson–Crick model of DNA (now known as B-DNA) are as follows (Fig. 1.5.2):

Double helix structure: Each DNA molecule is a right-handed double helix composed of two polydeoxyribonucleotide chains (strands) twisted around each other on a common axis.

Antiparallel chains: The two chains of each DNA molecule are antiparallel, i.e. one chain runs in the 5′ to 3′ direction while the other in 3′ to 5′ direction.

Dimensions: The width of a double helix is 20 Å (2 nm). Each turn (pitch) of the helix contains 10 pairs of nucleotides, each placed at distance of about 3.4 Å (0.34 nm); thus, each turn is 34 Å (3.4 nm) in dimension.

Arrangement of base, sugar and phosphate molecule: Each chain has a sugar–phosphate backbone with bases that project at right angles and hydrogen bond with the bases of the opposite chain across the double helix (Fig. 1.5.3).

Complementary chains: The two polynucleotide chains are not identical but complementary due to base pairing.

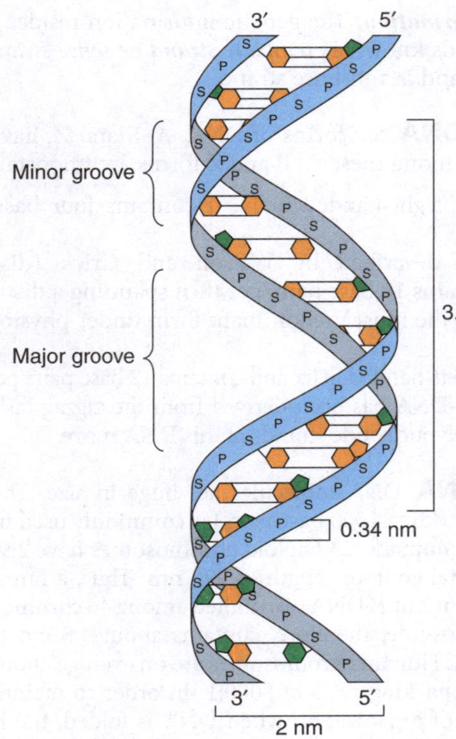

Fig. 1.5.2 Watson–Crick model of DNA structure.

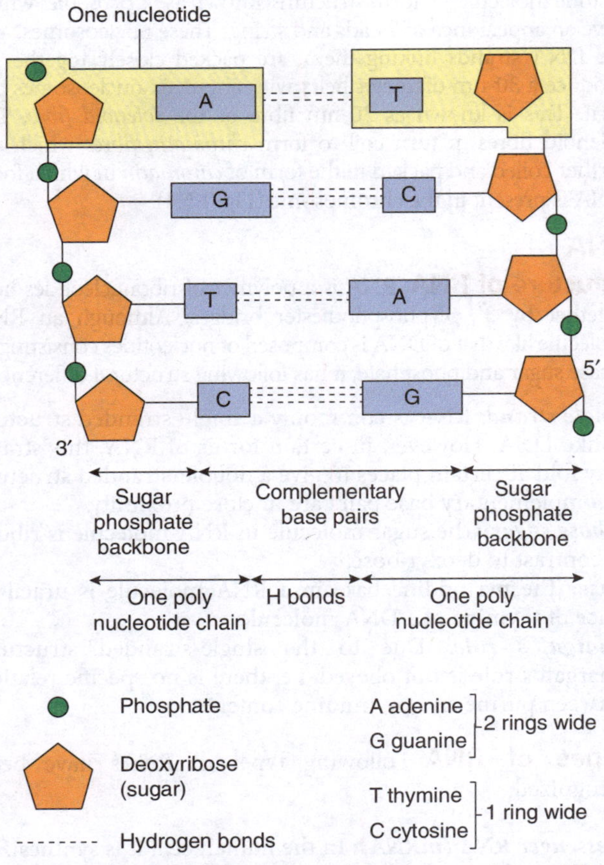

Fig. 1.5.3 Diagrammatic structure of straightened chains of DNA.

Genetic information: The genetic information resides in one of two strands known as *template strand* or *sense strand.* The opposite strand is antisense strand.

Types of DNA Six forms of DNA, A–E and Z, have been identified. Among these A, B and Z forms are important.

A-DNA is a right-handed helix. It contains four base pairs per turn.

B-DNA, as described by Watson and Crick (discussed above), contains 10 base pairs per turn spanning a distance of 3.4 nm. It is the most predominant form under physiological conditions.

Z-DNA is a left-handed helix and contains 12 base pairs per turn. The name Z-DNA has been derived from the zigzag fashion in which the polynucleotide strands of this DNA move.

Size of DNA DNA molecules are huge in size. The term kilobase pair (kb = 1000 base pairs) is commonly used in DNA structure. In humans, 23 haploid chromosomes have 2,900,000 kb with a total contour length of 990 nm. Thus, a human cell contains about 2 m of DNA distributed among 46 chromosomes. Each chromosome, therefore, contains about 4.8 cm (48,000 μm) of DNA. Human chromosomes are on average about 6 μm long, with a packing ratio of 8000:1. In order to maintain the high degree of organization when DNA is folded, the histone proteins form a precise architectural scaffolding for the DNA.

Organization of DNA in the cell In human cells, the DNA is found in association with positively charged protein molecules called *histones.* Each DNA helix combines with a group of eight histone molecules to form structures known as *nucleosomes* which have an appearance of 'beads and string'. These nucleosomes, and the DNA strands linking them, are packed closely together to produce a 30-nm diameter helix with about six nucleosomes per turn. This is known as 30-nm fibre or the *solenoid fibre.* The solenoid fibres in turn coil to form *chromatin fibres* which are further coiled and packed in the form of *chromatin* in which form DNA is present in the chromosome (Fig. 1.5.4).

RNA

Structure of RNA RNA is a polymer of ribonucleotides held together by 3′, 5′-phosphodiester bridges. Although an RNA molecule like that of DNA is composed of nucleotides consisting of a base sugar and phosphate, it has following structural differences:

Single strand: RNA is commonly a single-stranded structure unlike DNA. However, in certain forms of RNA, this strand may fold at certain places to give a double-stranded structure if complementary base pairs are in close proximity.

Ribose sugar: The sugar molecule in RNA molecule is ribose in contrast to deoxyribose.

Base: The pyrimidine base in a RNA molecule is uracil in place of thymine of a DNA molecule.

Chargaff's rule: Due to the single-stranded structure, Chargaff's rule is not obeyed, i.e. there is no specific relation between purine and pyrimidine contents.

Types of RNA Following types of RNAs have been recognized:

Messenger RNA (mRNA): In the human cell, it is synthesized in the nucleus and enters the cytoplasm to participate in protein synthesis.

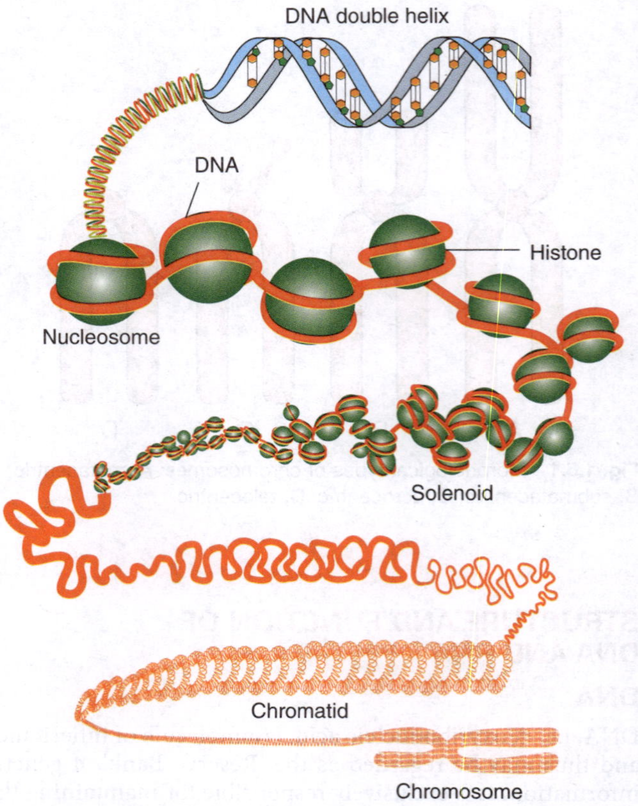

Fig. 1.5.4 Diagrammatic organization of DNA in a chromosome of the human cell.

Transfer RNA (tRNA): There are about 20 species of tRNA corresponding to 20 amino acids present in protein structure. The structure of tRNA resembles that of clover leaf with four arms. tRNA delivers amino acids for protein synthesis.

Ribosomal RNA (rRNA): rRNAs are present in ribosomes (factories of protein synthesis). It is believed that rRNAs play a significant role in binding of mRNA to ribosomes in protein synthesis.

MicroRNA (μRNA) has 20–25 nucleotides. Its main role is regulation of gene expression at post-transcriptional stage.

DNA REPLICATION

DNA replication is a process by which each original DNA molecule gives rise to two copies with identical structure. The method by which the DNA replicates is called *semiconservation replication* since each new double helix retains (conserves) one of the two strands of the original DNA double helices. Steps involved in the DNA replication are as follows (Fig. 1.5.5):

1. Initiation of replication. The site from where the replication of DNA is initiated is called *origin of replication.* In prokaryotes, DNA replication initiates from only one site, hence called monorepliconic replication, and in eukaryotes it starts from multiple sites (*multirepliconic replication*). The origin of replication mostly consists of A–T base pairs. When a specific binding protein (dna protein) binds to the site of replication then there occurs separation of double-stranded DNA, and separated strands of DNA form a bubble at the site of origin.

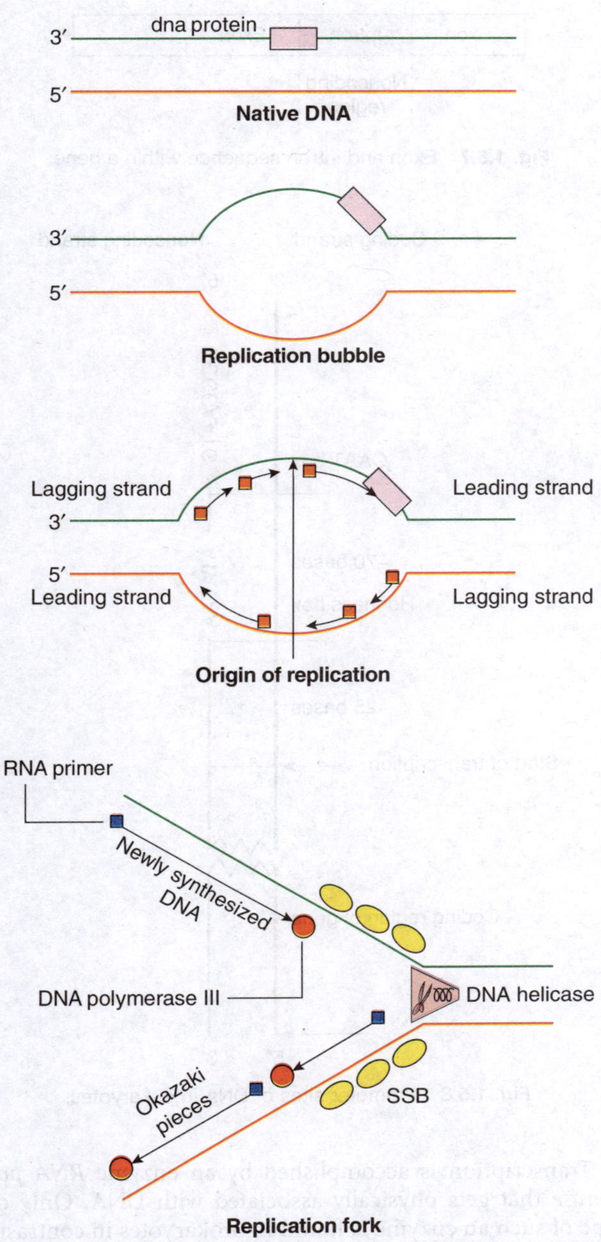

Fig. 1.5.5 Simplified diagram showing main steps of DNA replication.

2. Formation of replication fork and replication eye. The next step in the DNA replication is unwinding of double helix leading to formation of either Y-shaped *replication fork* (when DNA replication initiates from the terminal end of the double helix), or θ-shaped replication eye (when DNA replication starts from the intercalary position). This step is controlled by an enzyme called *helicase* and a protein called *single-strand binding* (SSB) protein.

Role of DNA helicases: These enzymes bind to both the strands of DNA at replication fork and move along the DNA helix and separate the strands of the DNA double helix. The function of helicases can be compared to a zip opener.

Role of single-strand DNA binding (SSB) proteins: As the name indicates, SSB protein binds only to single-stranded DNA (separated by helicase). Main function of this protein is to keep the two DNA strands separate, hence, also called helix destabilizing protein. SSB protein also provides template for new DNA synthesis and prevent degradation of single-stranded DNA.

3. Formation of RNA primer. RNA primer consists of a short fragment of RNA (about 5–50 nucleotides). It is required for synthesis of new DNA. The RNA primer is synthesized on DNA template by specific *RNA polymerase* (primase).

4. DNA synthesis along the replication fork. DNA replication occurs simultaneously in both the leading as well as lagging strands of Y-shaped replication fork and is of two types:

Continuous DNA replication: In the leading strand, DNA polymerase III binds to the single-stranded DNA and starts to move along the strand. Each time it meets the next base on DNA, free nucleotides approach the DNA strand, and one with the correct complementary base hydrogen bonds to the base in the DNA. The free nucleotide is then kept in place by the enzyme until it binds to the preceding nucleotide thus extending the new strand of DNA. The enzyme continues to move along one base at time with new DNA strand growing as it does so.

Discontinuous DNA replication: Occurs in the lagging strand, the fragments or pieces of DNA are called Okazaki fragments.

GENES

General Considerations

Gene is the functional unit of DNA. A gene could therefore be defined as a piece of DNA which codes for a protein. In strictest sense, the gene can be defined as the DNA code for a single polypeptide chain. Since some proteins are made up of more than one polypeptide chain, they are therefore coded for by more than one gene.

Genome

The term genome refers to total genetic information contained in a cell.

Human genome For humans, the genome is essentially equivalent to all of the genetic information which is present in a single set of 23 chromosomes.

Human genome project (1990–2003). The human genome project (HGP) was an international 13 years' effort to discuss complete set of human genes and make them accessible for further biological study and to determine the complete sequence of DNA basis in the human genome. The human genome project (HGP), which completed on 14 April 2003, has accomplished the following goals:

- Identified all the *approximate 30,000 genes in human DNA*.
- Determined the sequences of 3 billion chemical base pairs that make the human DNA.

Functional genomics. Understanding the functions of genes and other parts of genome is known as functional genomics.

Comparative genomics. Comparative genomics is the analysis and comparison of genome from different species.

Constitutive and inducible genes. The genes are generally considered under two categories:

Constitutive. The products (proteins) of these genes are required all the time in a cell. Therefore, the constitutive genes (or housekeeping genes) are expressed more or less at a constant rate in almost all the cell and, furthermore, they may not be subjected to regulation, e.g. enzymes of citric acid cycle.

Inducible genes. The concentration of the proteins synthesized by inducible genes is regulated by various molecular signals. An inducer increases the expression of these genes while a repressor decreases, e.g. tryptophan pyrrolase of liver is induced by tryptophan.

Gene Expression: Central Dogma

As mentioned above, each cell of human body contains the entire genome, yet the genetic expression is very selective and different patterns of protein synthesis occur in different tissues. Not only this, even in the same tissue there is wide variation in the proteins produced during the course of development.

The expression of genetic material occurs through the production of proteins. This involves two consecutive steps transcription and translation. In transcription, the genetic information, stored in DNA, is transferred to an RNA intermediate, which in turn uses this information to direct the synthesis of proteins during translation. This unidirectional flow of information was described by F.H.C. Crick in 1958 as the central dogma of molecular biology (Fig. 1.5.6). However, an important modification of this information flow was given by David Baltimore and H. Temin, who described reversible sequence through reverse transcription or feminism in the presence of transcripts (revised central dogma).

Transcription

Transcription is a process in which RNA is synthesized from DNA. All the three types of RNAs (mRNA, tRNA and rRNA) are produced through transcription. The transcription process is selective, i.e. the entire molecule of DNA is not expressed in transcription, but the RNAs are synthesized only for selected regions of DNA. The strand of DNA that directs the synthesis of mRNA via complementary base pairing is called the *template strand* or *coding* or sense strand, and the other strand is known as *noncoding strand* or *antisense strand.* In eukaryotes, the genes that direct the formation of proteins fragmented into several segments known as exons. The exons are separated by introns which are not translated (Fig. 1.5.7).

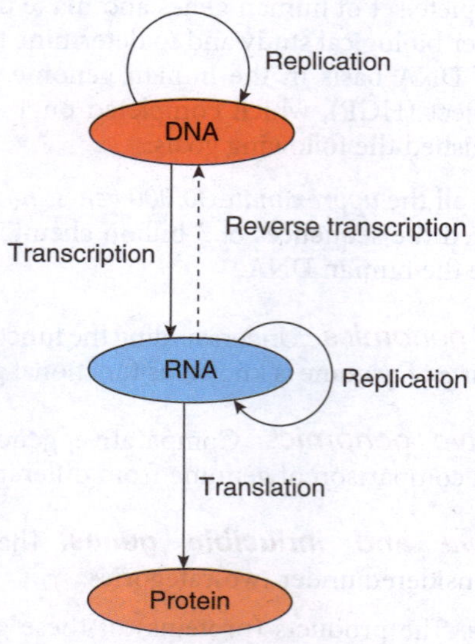

Fig. 1.5.6 Central dogma: the flow of genetic information.

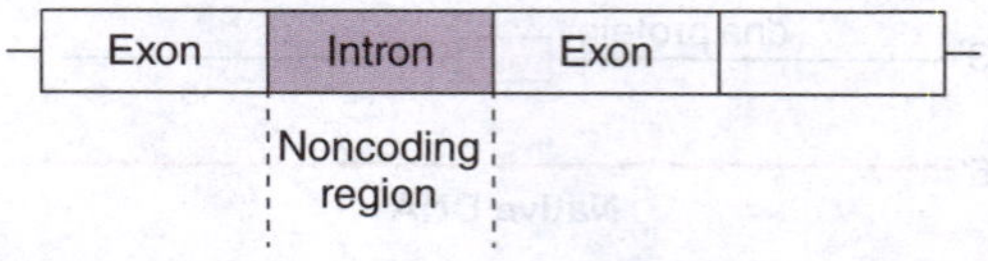

Fig. 1.5.7 Exon and intron sequence within a gene.

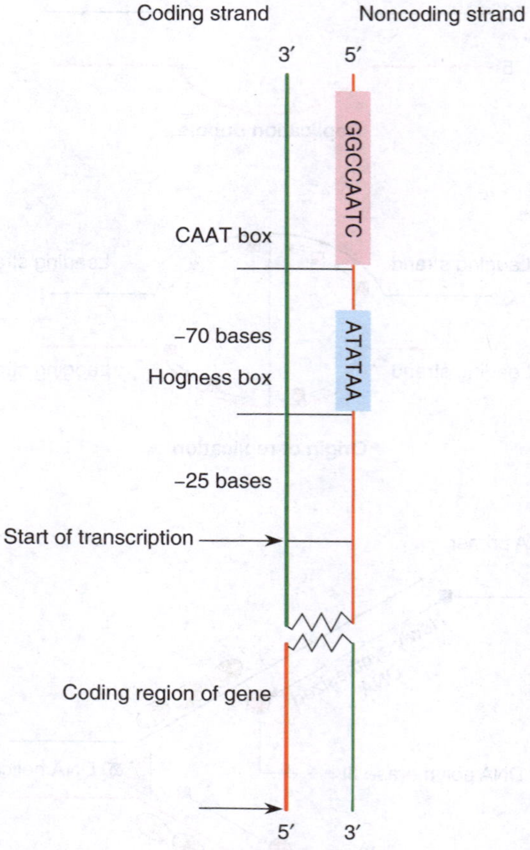

Fig. 1.5.8 Promoter sites of DNA in eukaryotes.

Transcription is accomplished by an enzyme *RNA polymerase* that gets physically associated with DNA. Only one type of such an enzyme is found in prokaryotes in contrast to eukaryotes (where three different forms of RNA polymerase are found). RNA I, II and III catalyse the synthesis of rRNA, mRNA and tRNA, respectively.

Promoter sites. RNA polymerase binds to a region of DNA called promoter site. In eukaryotes, a sequence of DNA bases has been identified. This sequence, known as Hogness box or TATA box (Fig. 1.5.8), is located on left about 25 nucleotides away (upstream) from the starting site of mRNA synthesis. There also exists another site of recognition between 70 and 80 nucleotides upstream from the start of transcription. This second site is referred to as CAAT box. One of these two sites (or sometimes both) helps RNA polymerase II to recognize requisite sequence of DNA for transcription.

Salient features of transcription in eukaryotes

- Premotor site is the site at which RNA polymerase is attached and catalyses the process of transcription.
- TATA sequence ensures the proper point where transcription starts.

- mRNA consists of pre-RNA cap at 5′ end followed by RNA sequence and poly(A) tail at 3′ (that stabilize the RNA).
- Immediately after formation of mRNA from DNA, post-transcriptional modification occurs.
- Transcription in eukaryotes unlike prokaryotes occurs within the nucleus and mRNA moves out of the nucleus into the cytoplasm for translation.
- The initiation and regulation of transcription in eukaryotes is more extensive than prokaryotes.

Post-transcriptional modifications. The post-transcriptional modification of primary (pre-mRNA) is a regulated process in which splicing occurs to form many mRNA from a single pre-mRNA.

- The mRNA in eukaryotes is processed from the primary RNA transcript, a process called maturation which includes:
- Releases of the introns and joining with two adjacent exons to produce mature mRNA.
- The introns are eliminated by spliceosomes (complex units made up of mRNA and protein) or by self-splicing by RNA.
- Then mature mRNA move out of the nucleus into the cytoplasm.

RNA editing: Besides, these two post-transcriptional modifications, RNA editing may also take place before translation begins.

Reverse transcription. It refers to the formation of DNA from RNA. Reverse transcription is known to occur in retroviruses which include human immunodeficiency virus (HIV) that causes acquired immunodeficiency disease (AIDS). The enzyme *reverse transcriptase* is responsible for this process. The DNA so formed is complementary (cDNA) to viral RNA and can be transmitted to host DNA.

Translation: Biosynthesis of Proteins

Translation is the process by which genetic message carried by mRNA from the DNA is converted in the form of a polypeptide chain having specific sequence of amino acids. Before discussing the process of translation, it will be worthwhile to know something about the genetic code.

Genetic code. Process by which the information coded in the mRNA is decoded into polypeptide is referred to as *deciphering the genetic code.* Dr Hargobind Khorana shared 'Nobel Prize' in 1968 with Marshall W Nirenberg and Robert W Holly for the discovery of genetic code. The genetic code (codon) is formed by three nucleotides (triplet) base sequences in mRNA. The codons are formed of four nucleotide base (A, G, C and U). These four bases produce 64 different combinations of three base codons. Of the 64 codons, 61 codons code for 20 amino acids found in proteins and 3 codons (UAA, UAG and UGA) are *termination codons* which act as stop signals in protein synthesis. The codons AUG and sometimes GUG act as *initiating codons.*

Characteristics of genetic code:

Universality, i.e. same codons are used to code for the same amino acids in all the living organisms with a few exceptions.

Specificity, i.e. a particular codon always codes for the same amino acid, e.g. AUG is the codon for methionine.

Nonoverlapping, i.e. the genetic code is read from a fixed point as a continuous base sequence.

Degenerate, i.e. one amino acid is coded by more than one codon. The codons that designate the same amino acid are called synonyms.

Process of protein biosynthesis. The process of protein synthesis in addition to mRNA requires amino acids tRNA, energy sources (ATP and GTP) and protein factors. Protein synthesis occurs over ribosomes which are also called *protein factories.* The protein biosynthesis involves three processes:

I. Activation of amino acids: Amino acids are activated and attached to tRNA in a two-step reaction. A group of enzymes, namely aminoacyl tRNA synthetases, is required for this process. In the first step, an amino acid reacts with ATP in the presence of specific amino acid tRNA to form *enzyme–AMP–amino acid complex.* This complex then reacts with a specific tRNA and the amino acid is transferred to 3′ end of the tRNA to form aminoacyl tRNA.

II. Translation proper involves three steps – initiation, elongation and termination (Fig. 1.5.9).

1. ***Initiation:*** The translation of mRNA begins with the formation of initiation complex.
2. ***Elongation:*** Ribosomes elongate the polypeptide chain by a sequential addition of amino acids to the growing carboxyl end. The elongation process is repeated again and again with addition of one amino acid each time till signal for termination is reached.
3. ***Termination*** of polypeptide synthesis is evoked by a nonsense or termination codon (UAA, UAG or UGA).

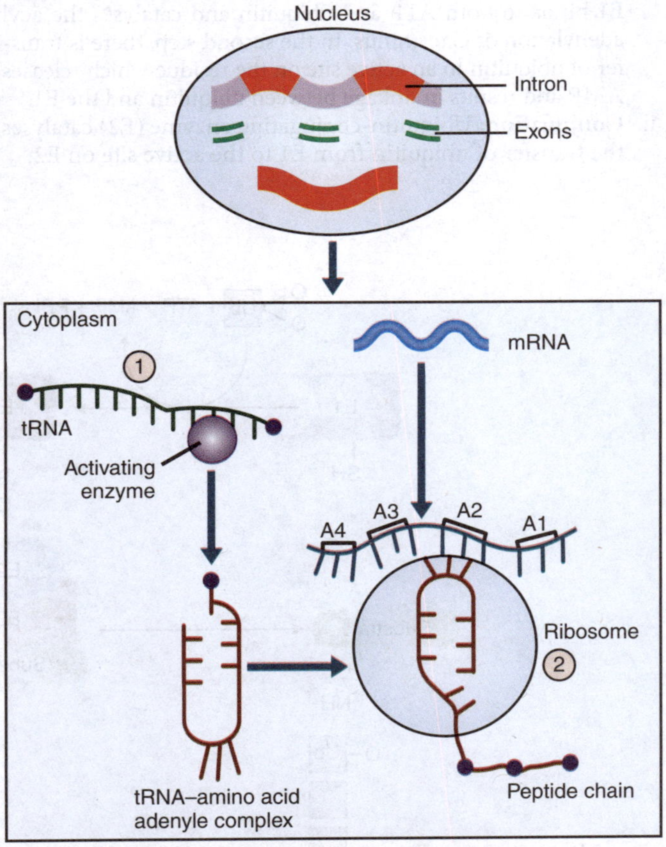

Fig. 1.5.9 Stages of translation process: 1, formation of initiation complex; 2, elongation of polypeptide chain.

III. Post-translational modifications: The proteins synthesized in translation are as such not functional. Many changes take place in the polypeptides after the initiation of their synthesis or, most frequently, after the protein synthesis is completed. Post-translational modification includes:

- Proteolytic degradation
- Covalent modifications (phosphorylation, hydroxylation and glycosylation)
- Packaging and folding

Ubiquitination and Protein Degradation

Protein degradation like protein synthesis is important and very well regulated. Ubiquitin is a small protein that is found in almost all cellular tissues in human and other eukaryotic organisms. Ubiquitin is discovered by Gideon Goldstein in 1975 in New York. Four genes in human genome code for ubiquitin: UBB, UBC, BA^{52} and RP^{527A}. Ubiquitin plays an important role in destruction of defective proteins and or aged proteins. Ubiquitination or ubiquitylation is an enzymatic post-translation modification in which ubiquitin is attached to a substrate protein. Ubiquitination requires three types of enzymes:

Ubiquitin-activating enzyme (E1s)
Ubiquitin-conjugating enzyme (E2s)
Ubiquitin ligases (E3s)

Process of ubiquitination mainly consists of following three steps (Fig. 1.5.10)

i. **Activation of ubiquitin by ubiquitin-activating enzyme (E1),** which is a two-step reaction dependent on ATP. In the initial step, there is production of adenylate intermediate. The E1 binds to both ATP and ubiquitin and catalyses the acyl adenylation of C terminus. In the second step, there is transfer of ubiquitin to an active site on the residue which releases AMP and results in linkage between ubiquitin and the E1.
ii. **Conjugation:** Ubiquitin-conjugating enzyme (E2) catalyses the transfer of ubiquitin from E1 to the active site on E2.
iii. **Ligation:** Ubiquitin ligases (E3s) catalyse the final step of ubiquitination cascade.

Ubiquitination affects proteins in many ways: it can mark them for degradation via proteasomes, alter their cellular location, affect their activity and promote or prevent protein interaction.

Regulation of Gene Expression

As discussed earlier, each nucleated somatic cell in the body contains full genetic message, yet there is great differentiation and specialization in the functions of various types of adult cells. It is because of the fact that there exists a foolproof system for regulation of gene expression that maintains orderly growth in cells and prevents uncontrolled growth. The genes are controlled both spatially and temporally. The regulation of gene expression is thus absolutely essential for growth, development and differentiation of an organism. The positive regulator increases the gene expression whereas the negative regulator decreases it.

Regulation of gene expression in prokaryotes In prokaryotes, gene expression is regulated by operon system. Operons are segments of genetic material which function as regulated units that can be switched on and switched off. The operon systems are of two types:

1. ***Inducible operon system*** (lac operon system): An inducible operon system is that regulated genetic material which remains switched off normally but becomes operational in the presence of an inducer. It occurs in catabolic pathway.
2. ***Repressible operon system*** (tryptophan operon system): A repressible operon system is that regulated genetic material which normally remains active/operational. It usually occurs in anabolic pathways.

Regulation of gene expression in eukaryotes The regulation of gene expression in eukaryotes is very complex

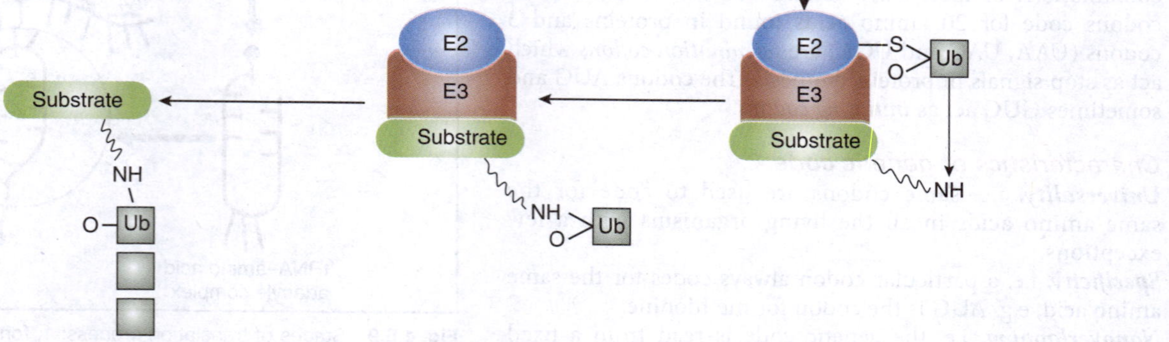

Fig. 1.5.10 The ubiquitination process.

and involves various mechanisms. Some of the mechanisms are as follows:

1. ***Gene amplification:*** In this mechanism, the expression of gene is increased several folds. An example of gene amplification in humans includes development of drug resistance by the malignant cells to long-term administration of methotrexate. This occurs by amplifying the gene coding for dihydrofolate reductase.
2. ***Gene rearrangement:*** The process of gene rearrangement is responsible for the generation of 10 billion antigen-specific immunoglobulins.
3. ***Regulation of gene expression through transcription factors:*** Transcription factors are products of other genes and hence mediate transregulation by binding to specific DNA segments. This specific interaction of protein to DNA in over 80% of the nontranscription factors is brought about by one of the four DNA-binding motifs: zinc finger motif, lucine zipper motif, helix–turn–helix motif and helix–loop–helix motif.
4. ***Regulation of gene through mRNA:*** Gene expression is also regulated by regulation of synthesis transport, processing and stability of mRNA.

Applied Aspects

Applied Genetics

Applications of genetics are many more and beyond the scope of a book on physiology; only a few of interest described here include some aspects of:

- *Molecular genetics and biotechnology*
- *Molecular genetics and medicine*

Molecular Genetics and Biotechnology

Biotechnology involves use of living organisms or products of living organisms for the welfare of human. Presently, molecular biology has combined with genetics to give us more powerful biotechnology. The tools of molecular genetics have provided improved way to make use of living organisms for the benefit of humans. The subject of molecular genetics and biotechnology is expanding fast and has already become very vast. The present discussion includes only a few important aspects, i.e.:

- Genetic engineering/recombinant DNA technology (RDT)
- Polymerase chain reaction (PCR)
- Blotting techniques
- Cloning
- Apoptosis

Genetic Engineering/Recombinant DNA Technology

The terms genetic engineering, RDT, DNA cloning, molecular cloning, gene cloning all refer to the process of transfer of a DNA fragment of interest from one organism to a self-replicating genetic element such as a bacterial plasmid. In other words, this technology involves cutting, modifying and joining DNA molecules using enzymes such as restriction enzymes and DNA ligase.

Stages of recombinant technology

Stage 1: Generation of a copy of gene required. This is the most difficult part of the process. Three methods are used to get a copy of a gene:

- Making a copy of the gene from its mRNA, using reverse transcriptase
- Synthesizing the gene artificially
- Using a *shotgun approach* which involves chopping up the DNA with *restriction enzymes* and searching for the piece with the required gene (Fig. 1.5.11)

Stage 2: Joining the gene to a vector or carrier molecule. A vector is a carrier of a DNA molecule to which the generated gene is attached for cloning. Following are three commonly used vectors in RDT (Fig. 1.5.11)

- Plasmids
- Bacteriophages
- Cosmids

Stage 3: Introduction of vector DNA into the host cell to produce chimeric DNA. The main aim of genetic engineering is to insert a DNA of interest (generated gene) into a vector DNA so that the DNA fragment replicates along with the vector after annealing. This hybrid combination of two fragments of DNA is referred to as *chimeric DNA* or *hybrid DNA* or *recombinant DNA.*

Stage 4: Cloning of chimeric DNA (Fig. 1.5.12). A clone is a large population of identical molecules, bacteria or cells that arise from

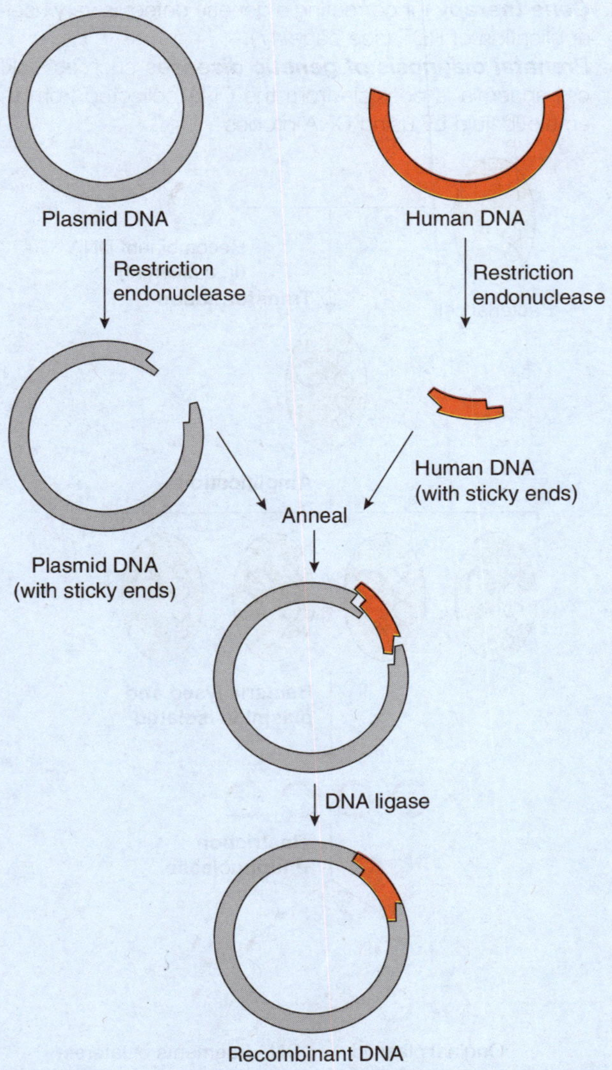

Fig. 1.5.11 Stages of recombinant DNA technology.

a common ancestor. The chimeric DNA contained in a plasma (vector) can be introduced into bacterial cells by a process called *transfection*. The replicating bacterial cell (host cell) permits the amplification of the chimeric DNA of the vector. In this way, cloning results in the production of large number of identical target DNA molecules. The cloned target DNA is released from the vector by cleavage (using appropriate restriction endonucleases), isolated, characterized and used for various purposes.

Applications of genetic engineering Genetic engineering has revolutionized the application of molecular biology to medical/agricultural sciences that has immensely benefitted the mankind. A few important applications are as follows:

1. ***Production of proteins/hormones:*** It is possible to produce proteins/hormones in large amount for therapeutic purposes. These include insulin, growth hormone, erythropoietin, interferons, vaccines and blood clotting factors.
2. ***Molecular analysis of diseases*** such as sickle cell anaemia, thalassaemia, cystic fibrosis using RDT has led to better understanding of these diseases.
3. ***Laboratory diagnostic applications:*** Using this technique, the diagnosis of diseases like AIDS has become simple and rapid.
4. ***Gene therapy*** for correcting a genetic defect is very useful application of RDT (see page 47).
5. ***Prenatal diagnosis of genetic diseases*** such as sickle cell anaemia is possible from the DNA collected from the amniotic fluid by using DNA probes.

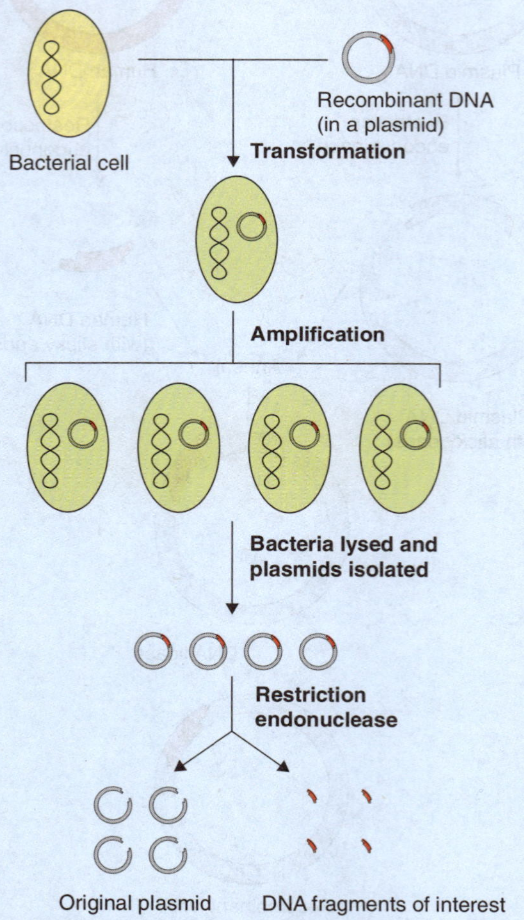

Fig. 1.5.12 Cloning of a recombinant DNA.

6. ***Transgenesis*** refers to transfer of genes into the fertilized ovum which will be found in somatic as well as germ cells and passed on to successive generation.
7. ***Application in forensic medicine:*** *DNA fingerprinting* applying Southern blot technique is useful in identifying criminals and settling the disputes of parenthood of children.
8. ***Industrial applications:*** Enzymes synthesized by this technology are used to produce sugar, cheese and detergents.
9. ***Agricultural applications*** include development of genetically engineered plants to increase the yield of crops, to resist draught and to resist diseases.
10. ***Evolution:*** This technique helps in bridging several missing links in the evolution by amplifying the DNA by PCRs from the archaeological sample of extinct animals.

Polymerase Chain Reaction

PCR is a sensitive, selective and extremely rapid method of amplifying a target sequence of DNA.

Technique of PCR involves the following steps:

- *Denaturation of DNA* refers to separation of double-stranded target DNA into single strand by heating.
- *Annealing with two primers* (one for each strand) is allowed to occur after cooling the single DNA strand.
- *DNA amplification* occurs by synthesis of new DNA strand in the presence of enzyme DNA polymerase and the substrates deoxyribonucleotide triphosphates. These strands are compliments to the target DNA. The cycle of DNA amplification is repeated again and again. The Taq DNA polymerase is *heat resistant;* this special feature makes it suitable for automation of PCR. PCR results in the amplification of target DNA by about a million (10^6) fold with high specificity.

Application of PCR. PCR is highly sensitive; it can detect even the presence of a single molecule of DNA. PCR amplification of sequences of human genomic DNA produces an amount of target DNA (up to 1 mg) which is sufficient for direct application in any one of a wide range of molecular biological procedures, including direct DNA sequencing. PCR has several applications:

- Rapid diagnosis of AIDS
- DNA fingerprinting is useful in kinship analysis and in the identification of crime suspects
- Prenatal diagnosis of genetic diseases
- Study of evolution from DNA of archaeological samples
- Sex identification

Blotting Techniques

Blotting techniques refer to the analytical techniques used for the identification of a special DNA, or RNA or a protein. These include:

- Southern blotting (for DNA)
- Northern blotting (for RNA)
- Western blotting (for protein)

Southern blotting Southern blotting technique is named after the scientist who identified it, while the northern and western blot techniques are the laboratory jargons which are now accepted.

Steps of Southern blotting includes:
- *Extraction of DNA* from the cells (say leucocytes).
- *Cleavage of DNA* into fragments by restriction endonucleases.
- *Separation of the fragments* of DNA is done by gold electrophoresis.
- *Denaturation of DNA* is done either prior to or during transfer by placing the gel in an alkaline solution (NaOH).
- *Transfer of DNA fragments to a sheet of nitrocellulose paper* from the agarose gel is done by blotting (hence the name blot).
- *Fixation of DNA fragments to the membrane* is then done by any of the following methods:
  - Oven baking 80°C
  - Ultraviolet cross-linking
- *Formation of labelled DNA hybrid complexes:* After fixing the DNA fragments, the membrane is placed in a solution of labelled DNA probe. This leads to hybridization reaction forming labelled DNA hybrid complexes.
- *Identification of labelled DNA hybrid complex:* After the hybridization reaction has been carried out, the membrane is washed to remove unbounded radioactivity and regions of hybridization are identified *by autoradiography* by placing the membrane in contact with X-ray film.

Applications. Important applications of Southern blotting:
- DNA fingerprinting
- Detection of mutant gene causing cystic fibrosis

Northern blotting Northern blotting is similar to Southern blotting except that it is for RNA instead of DNA.

Applications. Important applications of northern blotting are analysis of the expression of a gene in a particular tissue.

Western blotting Western blotting is the technique for identification of a specific protein. It involves the transfer of electrophoresed protein bands from SDS polyacrylamide gel onto a nitrocellulose membrane followed by probing using a labelled antibody probe.

Applications. Western blot test is widely used as confirmatory test of HIV. In combination with a positive enzyme-linked immunosorbent assay (ELISA), a positive western blot is 99.9% accurate in detecting HIV infection.

Cloning

Cloning refers to making many identical copies of a molecule.

Certain terms which need to be defined before discussing the different types of cloning include:
- *Transformation* refers to introduction of any DNA molecule into any living cell.
- *Transfection* refers to introduction of purified DNA molecules into cultured cells.
- *Transduction* is the transfer of genetic material or DNA from one cell to another with the help of a virus.
- *Microinjection* is a method of introducing new DNA into a cell by injecting it directly into the nucleus.
- *Biolistics* refers to the means of introducing DNA into cells that involves bombardment with high-velocity microprojectiles located with DNA.

Types of cloning. Some important types of cloning:
- Gene cloning/DNA cloning
- Reproductive cloning
- Therapeutic cloning
- Tissue culture

Gene cloning Gene cloning refers to the process of transfer of a DNA fragment of interest from one organism to a self-replicating genetic element (cloning vector) such as bacterial plasmid and subsequent propagation of the recombinant DNA molecule in the host organism (Fig. 1.5.12). Other terms used to denote gene cloning are DNA cloning and RDT.

Details of this process have already been described on page 41.

Applications of gene cloning, i.e. RDT have already been highlighted. Important genetic applications include:
- Gene therapy
- Gene engineering of organisms
- Sequencing genomes

Reproductive cloning Reproductive cloning is a technology used to generate an animal that has same nuclear DNA as another currently or previously existing animal.

Technique. Reproductive cloning uses the technique of somatic cell nuclear transfer (SCNT). In this technique, genetic material is transferred from the nucleus of a donor adult cell to an egg whose nucleus, and thus its genetic material, has been removed. The reconstructed egg containing the DNA from a donor cell is then treated with chemicals or electric current to stimulate cell division. Once the cloned embryo reaches a suitable stage, it is transferred to the uterus of a female host where it continues to develop until birth. A sheep (Dolly) was created by SCNT process from a cell taken from the parent's udder by the research team at the Roslin Institute in Edinburgh (Scotland) in February 1997.

Applications. Reproductive cloning can be used to repopulate endangered animals or animals that are difficult to breed. Examples are as follows:
- In 2001, the first clone of an endangered animal, a wild ox called a *gaur* was born. The young gaur died from an infection about 48 hours after its birth.
- In Italy (2001), a successful cloning of a healthy baby *mouflon,* an endangered wild sheep was reported. The cloned mouflon is living at a wild centre in Sardinia.

Embryo cloning (therapeutic cloning) Therapeutic cloning refers to the production of human embryos for use in research.
- This process is aimed at harvesting stem cells that can be used to study human development and to treat diseases rather than to create a cloned human being.
- Stem cells are extracted from the egg at the blastocysts stage of development and can be used to generate virtually any type of specialized cells in the human body.
- First human embryo for the purpose of therapeutic research was cloned in November 2001 by the scientists from Advanced Cell Technology (ACT), a biotechnology company in Massachusetts.

Applications. Stem cells can be used to serve as replacement cells to treat heart disease, Alzheimer disease, cancer and other diseases.

Tissue culture Cells may also be cloned for special purposes. This technique is called *tissue culture.* Certain cells when placed in a suitable medium can be cultured indefinitely.

Applications. The use of cloned cells allows the study of the action of such chemicals as hormones, drugs, antibiotics, cosmetics and pharmaceutical products to be made on cells. Such a technique is a useful substitute for laboratory animals such as rats, cats and dogs.

Apoptosis

Apoptosis, also called as programmed cell death (PCD), occurs under genetic control. Since the cell's own genes play an active role in its demise, so apoptosis can also be called *cell suicide.* It should be distinguished from necrosis in which the healthy cells are destroyed by some injury inflicted on the cells, e.g. inflammation. Since necrosis is caused by some external process, it can be also called *cell murder*. Thus, apoptosis is a natural process while necrosis is an unnatural process. Consequently, apoptosis does not induce a local inflammatory response while cell necrosis does.

Need and examples of apoptosis: Apoptosis is a very common process during development as well as adulthood, the need of which is highlighted with some examples:

1. Apoptosis for proper development of tissues

- *In the central nervous system,* large number of neurons are produced and then die during the remodelling that occurs during development and synapse formation.
- *During formation of the fingers and toes* of the fetus, the apoptosis plays an important role of removing the web tissue between the finger and toes.
- *During sexual development* in fetal life, apoptosis is responsible for regression of duct systems.

2. Apoptosis for normal functioning of adult tissues. For example:

Cyclic breakdown of endometrium that leads to start of menstruation is caused by apoptosis.

Epithelial cells that lose their connection to the basal lamina and surrounding cells undergo apoptosis.

Enterocytes sloughed off the tips of intestinal villi undergo apoptosis.

3. Apoptosis to destroy the cells that represent a threat to the integrity of the organism. For examples:

- Apoptosis of the cells infected with virus
- Apoptosis of the cells of the immune system to prevent them from attacking body constituents
- Apoptosis of the cells with DNA damage
- Apoptosis of the cancer cells

Mechanism of apoptosis The final common pathway leading to apoptosis is the activation of a group of cysteine proteases called *caspases* which exist in cells as inactive proenzymes (Fig. 1.5.13).

Triggering stimuli: Apoptosis can be triggered by external and internal stimuli (Fig. 1.5.13).

Internal stimuli: One of the important pathways goes through the mitochondria, which release *cytochrome* and a protein called smac/DIABLO, causing activation of the *caspase 9.*

Apoptosis-inducing factor (AIF) located in the intermembrane space of mitochondria migrates to nucleus and destroys DNA after binding leading to cell death.

External stimuli: One ligand that activates receptors triggering apoptosis is FAS (a transmembrane protein that projects from natural killer cells and T lymphocytes but also exists in circulating form). Another ligand is tumour necrosis factor (TNF). These activate the enzyme caspase 8 followed by cascade of caspase activation.

Net result of caspase activation is DNA fragmentation, cytoplasmic and chromatin condensation and eventually membrane bleb formation with cell breakup and removal of the debris by phagocytosis (Fig. 1.5.13).

Molecular Genetics and Medicine

Clinical applications of molecular genetics in medicine are rapidly increasing owing to research and advances in the molecular aspect of genetics, regulation of gene expression and protein synthesis. Some of the aspects in relation to molecular genetics and medicine described here:

- Mutations and genetic human diseases
- Detecting human genetic variations (genetic screening)
- Genetics and cancer
- Gene therapy

Mutations and genetic human diseases

Mutations Mutation refers to a change in the DNA structure of a gene. The substances or factors that are responsible for the mutations are called *mutagens,* e.g. X-rays, ultraviolet light and certain chemicals. There are two major types of mutations:

1. Point mutations: In this type, one base pair of DNA is replaced by another. Point mutations are further of two subtypes: transitions and transversions.

- *Transitions.* In this type of mutation, purine or pyrimidine is replaced by another purine or pyrimidine, respectively.
- *Transversions:* In this type of mutation, a purine is replaced by pyrimidine or pyrimidine is replaced by purine.

Effects of point mutations: Point mutations can lead to one of the following effects:

a. *Silent mutation:* No detectable effect is produced when the codon (of mRNA) containing change base codes for same amino acid. For example, UCA codes for serine but when there is change in third base (UCU), still it codes for serine. Therefore, when no effect is detected it is called *silent mutation.*

b. *Missense mutation:* This occurs when altered base codes for different amino acid and that amino acid in a protein molecule may be acceptable or partially acceptable or not acceptable as far as the action of protein molecule is concerned. The amino acid so formed is called *mistaken* or *missense amino acid*. The classical example of effect of missense mutation is sickle cell anaemia.

c. *Nonsense mutation:* When the codon with changed base may become the *termination codon* and acts as stop signal and thus causes termination of protein synthesis at that point, the effect produced is called nonsense mutation.

2. Frame shift mutations: This occurs when one or more than one base pairs are either deleted or inserted into the DNA

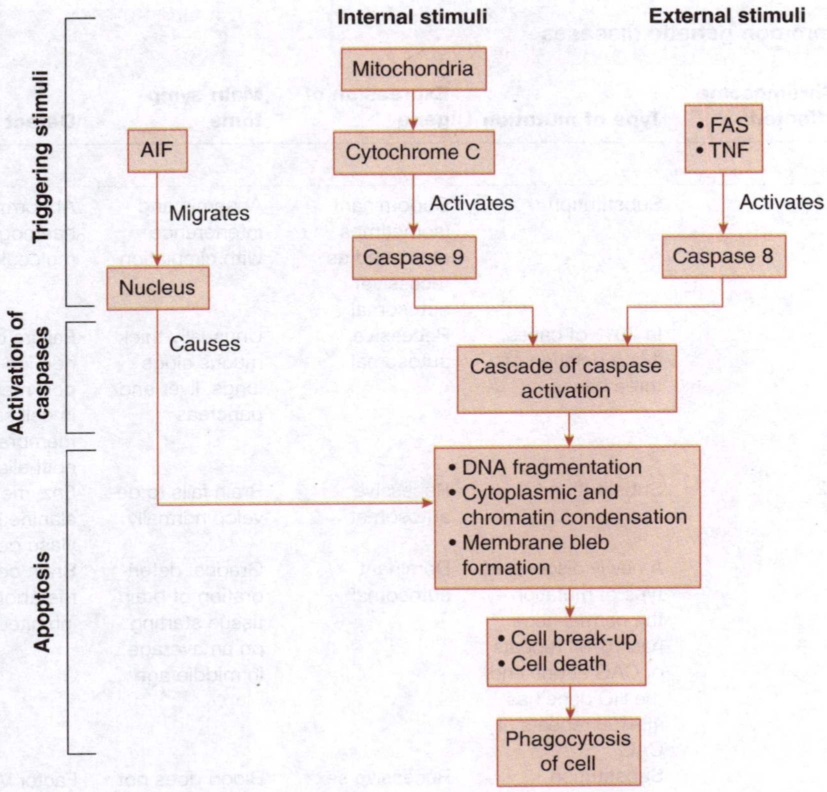

Fig. 1.5.13 Steps involved in apoptosis.

of gene. Therefore, frame shift mutations are also called deletion or insertional mutations.

Effects of frame shift mutations: The consequences as a result of insertion or deletion of a base in a gene cause altered reading frame of the mRNA. Thus, the machinery of mRNA (containing codon) is unable to recognize that a new base is added or missing. Since there is no punctuation in reading of codons, translation continues and as a result of that the proteins synthesized will have many altered amino acids and/or premature terminated proteins.

Genetic human diseases Salient aspects of some common genetic human diseases associated with mutations are summarized in Table 1.5.1.

Genetic Screening Genetic screening refers to detection of mutant genes in an individual (detecting human genetic variations). Modern genetics is making this much earlier than it was in the past.

Field of genetic screening There are three situations where genetic screening is of particular relevance:

1. *Prenatal diagnosis.* Prenatal diagnosis aims at identifying the health problems of unborn babies. Parents can be provided counselling and option for abortion as per situation. Techniques of prenatal diagnosis include:

- Chorionic villus sampling (CVS)
- Amniocentesis
- Preimplantation diagnosis

2. *Carrier diagnosis.* This is the identification of people who carry a particular genetic disease, usually with no visible symptom or harm to themselves. Examples include sickle cell anaemia, cystic fibrosis and phenylketonuria (PKU).

3. *Predictive diagnosis.* This is the prediction of a future disease from which one is likely to suffer. The classic example of this 'genetic time bomb' is Huntington chorea where the onset of disease occurs in middle age.

Genetics and Cancer

Cancer is a disease characterized by uncontrolled cell growth.

Points favouring genetic basis for cancer include:

- *Hereditary predisposition* is noted in some cancers like colon cancer and retinoblastoma.
- *Chromosomal abnormalities* are noted in many forms of cancers like Burkitt lymphoma and acute myeloid leukaemia.
- *Defective DNA repair mechanisms* have been associated with occurrence of cancers.
- *Genetic damages* (mutagenesis) by the action of various agents like ionizing radiations and UV rays are associated with occurrence of cancer.

Genes and molecular factors involved in pathogenesis of cancer include:

1. *Oncogenes.* Over 100 oncogenes (cancer-causing genes) have been described. These genes are derived by somatic

Table 1.5.1 Some common genetic diseases

Genetic disease/ disorder	Chromosome affected	Type of mutation	Expression of gene	Main symptoms	Defect	Frequency at birth
Gene mutations						
Sickle cell anaemia	11	Substitution	Codominant (sometimes described as recessive) autosomal	Anaemia and interference with circulation	Abnormal haemoglobin molecule	1 in 1600 among black people
Cystic fibrosis	7	In 70% of cases, it is a deletion of three bases	Recessive autosomal	Unusually thick mucus clogs lungs, liver and pancreas	Failure of chloride ion transport mechanism in cell surface membranes of epithelial cells	1 in 1800 among white people
PKU (phenylketonuria)	12	Substitution	Recessive autosomal	Brain fails to develop normally	Enzyme phenylalanine hydroxylase defective	1 in 18,000
Huntington chorea (disease)	4	A newly discovered type of mutation – the normal gene has 10–34 repeats of CAG at one end, the HC gene has 42–100 repeats of CAG	Dominant autosomal	Gradual deterioration of brain tissue starting on an average in middle age	Brain cell metabolism is inhibited	1 in 10,000 to 1 in 20,000 worldwide
Haemophilia	X	Substitution	Recessive sex linked	Blood does not clot	Factor VIII or IX protein defective	1 in 7000
Chromosome mutations						
Down syndrome	21	Extra chromosome (trisomy 21)		Reduced intelligence, characteristic facial features		1 in 750
Klinefelter syndrome (XXY)	Sex	Extra X chromosome in male (trisomy)		Feminized male		1 in 500
Turner syndrome (XO)	Sex	Missing X chromosome in female (monosomy)		Sterile female		1 in 2500

Notes: **Autosomal –** affecting non-sex chromosome (autosome); **monosomy –** one chromosome missing ($2n - 1$); **trisomy –** one extra chromosome ($2n + 1$). Monosomy and trisomy are examples of **aneuploidy,** where the total number of chromosomes is not an exact multiple of the haploid number.

mutations from the closely related *proto-oncogenes* (normal genes that encode proteins having a role in cell's normal activities). The genetic changes converting proto-oncogenes into oncogenes:

Missense mutation, i.e. change in the amino acid sequence of proto-oncogene protein converts it into oncogene.

Gene amplification, e.g. Myc genes have been amplified in human leukaemia, breast, stomach, lung and colon cancer.

Chromosomal translocations, e.g. in Burkitt lymphoma, a region of chromosome 8 is translocated to either chromosome 2, 14 or 22. The breakpoint in chromosome 8 causes the overexpression of c-myc gene.

Retroviral integration, e.g. in avian lymphomas, the integration of the avian leucosis virus can enhance the transcription of the c-myc gene.

2. Tumour suppressor gene (antioncogenes). Over 10 tumour suppressor genes have been described which produce proteins that suppress a tumour. When a tumour suppressor gene becomes inactivated by mutation, it becomes more likely that cancer will occur. It is important to note that for causing cancer, both alleles of tumour suppressor genes should be mutated. The most studied of these genes are RB gene (retinoblastoma gene) and P^{53} gene.

RB gene: Retinoblastoma (RB) gene functions as cancer suppressor. After two mutations (Knudson's two-hit hypothesis) when both copies of the gene at the retinoblastoma locus (14.1 band on the long arm of chromosome 13, i.e. 13q 14.1) are lost, deleted or inactivated, retinoblastoma (tumour of retina occurring in early childhood) develops.

P^{53} gene: About 50% of all human cancers are associated with defects in P^{53} gene. Induction of the P^{53} gene leads to the synthesis of P^{53} protein that functions as a transcription factor and can:

- Activate genes that promote DNA repair.
- Activate genes that arrest cell division and may generally repress other genes that are required for cell division.
- Activate genes that promote apoptosis.

Mutation in P^{53} gene leads to production of P^{53} protein that fails to perform the aforementioned functions and permit other mutations in DNA to persist. The accumulated mutations eventually cause cancer.

3. Mutator genes. Normal cells have caretaker genes that regulate DNA repair, i.e. they prevent faulty DNA transcription and regulation. The mutated version or mutator gene is characterized by loss of normal surveillance function that renders DNA susceptible to accumulation of mutation, and therefore progression of cancer.

4. Telomeres in cancer. Telomeres take care of the terminal tips of the chromosomes, which progressively shorten due to repetitive cell division. Telomerase is the enzyme required for continued recognition of telomere in successive cell divisions. Cancer cell expresses telomerase with consequent telomerase lengthening and this helps the transformed cells to maintain their cancerous state.

Conclusion To conclude, cancer is a multistep phenomenon where series of genetic changes with or without virus infection cause the development of final cancerous state (Fig. 1.5.14). These genetic changes can be produced by:

- Ionizing radiations
- Chemic carcinogens
- Radioactive material
- Spontaneous mutations
- Inherited mutations

Gene Therapy

Gene therapy is the name given to methods that aim to cure an inherited disease by providing the patient with a correct copy of the defective gene. Gene therapy has now been extended to include the attempts to cure any disease by introduction of a cloned gene into the patient.

Basic principles Basic principles involved in correcting a genetic defect:

Gene replacement, i.e. replacement of a mutant gene with a normal gene

Gene correction, i.e. correction of the mutated area (specific bases) of DNA leaving the rest of DNA unchanged

Gene augmentation, i.e. insertion of a foreign DNA into the genome of a cell to rectify the genetic defect

Basic approaches to gene therapy:

Germ line therapy can be carried out by microinjection of DNA into the isolated egg cell that is reimplanted into the mother. If successful, the gene is present and expressed in all cells of the resulting individual. Thus, theoretically the germ line therapy can be used to treat any inherited disease. At the moment, such treatment is regarded as unethical in humans because the gene would be passed on to future generations.

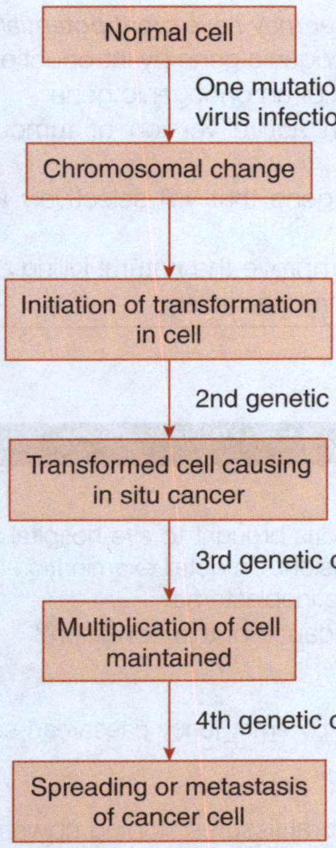

Fig. 1.5.14 Multistep phenomena of series of genetic changes leading to development of cancer.

Somatic cell therapy: In humans, at the moment the focus is on somatic cell therapy. This involves changing some, though not all, of the somatic cells which are non-sex cells of the body. Changes in these cells cannot be inherited. The patients treated will therefore be cured but they will still be able to pass the faulty gene on to their offspring. Steps involved in this therapy are as follows:

- Isolation of the cells with the gene defect from a patient
- Growing the isolated cells in culture
- Transfecting the isolated cell with a remedial gene construct
- Selecting, growing and testing the transfecting cells
- Either transplanting or transfusing the transfecting cells back into the patients

Examples of successful trials of gene therapy ***Somatic cell therapy in cystic fibrosis of the lung:*** The gene (cDNA) cloned in adenovirus vectors or contained in liposomes, when introduced into the respiratory tract via an inhaler, is taken up by the epithelial cells. These epithelial cells then synthesize normal protein called cystic fibrosis transmembrane conductance regulator (CFTR). Probably, 10% of the cells need to be corrected to eliminate the problem.

Somatic cell therapy in severe combined immunodeficiency disease (SCID): In this disease, the mutated gene is unable to synthesize the enzyme ADA (adenosine deaminase). ADA is needed by the white blood cells (lymphocytes) responsible for immunity against infection. Without ADA, the child develops SCID and dies of infection in the early childhood.

Two children, aged 4 and 9 years, suffering from SCID, were selected for gene therapy in the USA in 1990. Lymphocytes were isolated from the children, then a normal gene was introduced by means of a retrovirus vector and the cells were replaced. These children had shown significant improvement after 1 year of therapy, repeated every 1–2 month.

Gene therapy in cancer may have great potentiality:
- Inactivation of oncogenic gene by introduction of a gene or an antisense RNA of an oncogenic gene
- Introduction of an active version of tumour suppressor gene
- Introduction of a gene that will selectively kill the cancer cells
- Gene therapy to improve the natural killing of cancer cells by the patient's immune system

Self-Assessment

Q1. Discuss the process of biosynthesis of proteins.
Q2. Discuss the role of genes and molecular factors in pathogenesis of cancer.
Q3. Discuss the significance of gene therapy in treatment of diseases.
Q4. Write notes on:
1. Polymerase chain reaction
2. Genetic engineering and its application
3. Apoptosis

Clinical Cases

Case 1

A 2-year-old male child is brought to eye hospital with bulging of right eye and loss of vision. On detail examination and testing it is diagnosed a case of retinoblastoma.

Q1 What is genetic cause of this condition?

Case 2

A male baby is borne by emergency caesarean section with the following features:
- Flattened face
- Small eyes, palpebral fissures sloping upwards
- Small ears
- Single palmer crease across the palm of the hand

The newborn baby is diagnosed a case of Down syndrome.

Q1. Down syndrome, a genetic disorder, occurs due to which abnormality?

Case 3

A male baby developed the following features in his first year of life:
- Chronic diarrhoea
- Oral thrush
- History of frequent respiratory tract infection not relieving even with 2 months of antibiotic treatment

The provisional diagnosis made is severe combined immunodeficiency disease (SCID); for conformation gene sequencing is advised.

Q1. What type of disease is SCID?
Q2. For confirmation of diagnosis what further tests are to be advised?
Q3. How can this disease be treated?

PART II

SYSTEMIC PHYSIOLOGY

PART OUTLINE

NERVE MUSCLE PHYSIOLOGY

SECTION 2

SECTION OUTLINE

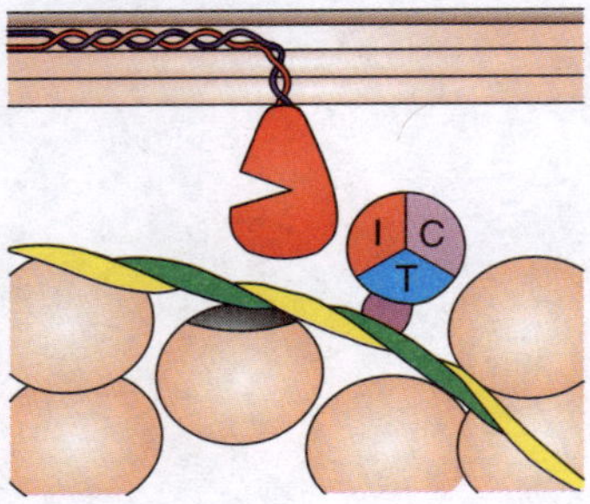

INTRODUCTION

The nerve and muscle cells are *excitable*, that is, capable of generation of electrical impulses at their membranes. For this very reason, the physiological aspects of these excitable tissues are discussed together in this section.

The electrical impulses generated in the excitable tissues, in most instances, can be used to transmit signals along the membranes. A neuron is the basic unit of nervous tissue. It is specialized for the function of reception, integration and transmission of information in the body. Muscles, like neurons, are excitable tissues but are characterized by the fact that a mechanical contraction follows an action potential.

To understand the physiological aspects, it is imperative to have knowledge about the *functional anatomy* and physiological properties of the nerve, the muscle and the neuromuscular junction. Furthermore, to understand the fundamental aspects of generation of the electrical impulses by the excitable tissues, it will be worthwhile to revise the basics of membrane potential which have been described in Chapter 1.4 (page 34).

The Nerve 2.1

CHAPTER OUTLINE

FUNCTIONAL ANATOMY

NEURON

Neuron or the nerve cell is the structural and functional unit of the nervous system. An aggregation of the neuronal cell bodies located inside the central nervous system (CNS) is called a *nucleus* and that located outside the CNS is called a *ganglion*. The nervous system of humans is made up of innumerable neurons. The total number of estimated neurons in the human brain is more than 10^{12}. The neurons are linked together in a highly intricate manner. It is through these connections that the body is made aware of changes in the environment or of those inside the body itself, and appropriate responses to such changes are produced.

Structure

Neurons vary considerably in size, shape and other features. However, most of them have some major features in common. The neuron is like any other cell in the body, except that it has processes. The basic structure of a neuron is best studied in a spinal motor neuron. A neuron primarily consists of the cell body and processes called *neurites*, which are of two kinds, the dendrites and the axon (Fig. 2.1.1).

Cell body The cell body of a neuron is also called the *soma* or *perikaryon* and may be round, stellate, pyramidal or fusiform in shape. Like any other cell, it consists of a mass of cytoplasm with all its principal constituents surrounded by a cell membrane. The cell body contains a large nucleus with one or two nucleoli but there is no centrosome. The absence of centrosome indicates that the neuron has lost ability for division. Thus, neurons once destroyed are replaced by neuroglia only. In addition to the general features of a typical cell (page 11), the cytoplasm of a neuron has the following distinctive characteristics (Fig. 2.1.1).

Nissl granules/bodies. These are basophilic granules, and when seen under electron microscope, these bodies seem to be composed of rough-surfaced endoplasmic reticulum. The presence of abundant granular endoplasmic reticulum is an indication of the high level of protein synthesis in neurons. The proteins are needed for the maintenance and repair and for the production of neurotransmitters and enzymes. The Nissl bodies are present in the dendrites as well, but are usually absent from axon hillock and the axon. These bodies disintegrate into fine dust and finally disappear (*chromatolysis*) on fatigue, due to the effect of certain poisons and on sectioning of the axon.

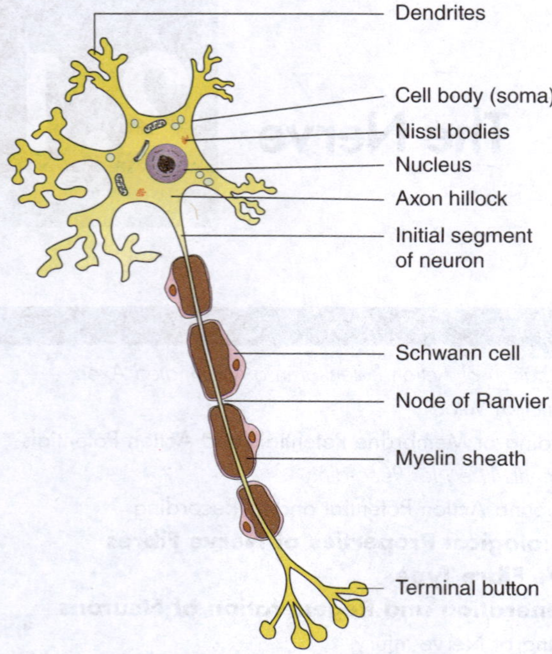

Fig. 2.1.1 Structure of a typical neuron.

Neurofibrillae. The presence of a network of neurofibrillae in the cytoplasm of the neuron is another distinctive feature. These consist of microfilaments and microtubules. In certain degenerative diseases like Alzheimer disease, the neurofilament protein gets altered, resulting in the formation of characteristic lesions called *neurofibrillary tangles*.

Pigment granules. These are seen in some neurons. For example, *neuromelanin* is present in the neurons of substantia nigra. Ageing neurons contain the pigment *lipofuscin*.

Dendrites The dendrites are multiple, small, branched processes. Dendrites contain Nissl bodies and neurofibres. These often look thorny due to numerous minute projections called *spines* present on their surface. The spines are the site of synaptic contact.

Dendrites are the *receptive processes* of the neuron receiving signals from other neurons via their synapses with axon terminals. The synaptic inputs produce *graded local potentials* which get algebraically summated on the surface of dendrites. Dendrites usually do not produce action potentials. They mostly conduct graded potentials. Some very long dendrites like axons may conduct action potentials.

Axon The axon is the single longer process of the nerve cell. It varies in length from a few micrometres to 1 m. It arises from the conical extension of the cell body called *axon hillock*, which is devoid of Nissl bodies. The part of the axon between the axon hillock and the beginning of the myelin sheath is called the *initial segment*. In the axon, the cell membrane continues as *axolemma* and the cytoplasm as *axoplasm*. The axon terminates by dividing into a number of branches, each ending in a number of *synaptic knobs* also known as *terminal buttons* or axon telodendria. Synaptic knobs contain microvesicles in which chemical neurotransmitters are stored.

Axons perform the specialized function of conducting impulses away from the cell body. They transmit propagated impulses (all-or-none transmission).

Myelogenesis Myelogenesis is the formation and development of myelin sheath in the nervous system. The myelin sheath of axons are produced by specialized glial cells – in the CNS by oligodendrocytes and Schwann cells in the peripheral nervous system. Myelogenesis begins during fifth fetal month and continues throughout life.

Process of myelogenesis Myelin sheath is present around the axons in the so-called myelinated nerve fibres (Fig. 2.1.2A).

Myelin sheath consists of protein–lipid complex, which is produced by glial cells called *Schwann cells* which encircle the axon and forms a thin sleeve around it (Fig. 2.1.2B). The Schwann cell wraps its membranes about 100 times around an axon and then the myelin is compacted by an extracellular membrane protein called protein zero (Po). Each Schwann cell provides the myelin sheath for a short segment of the axon. At the junction of any two such segments, there is a short gap (i.e. periodic 1 μm constrictions at about 1 mm distance). These gaps are the *nodes of Ranvier*. In the CNS of mammals, myelin sheath is formed by oligodendrocytes rather than Schwann cells. There are some axons which are devoid of myelin sheath. These *unmyelinated* axons invaginate into the cytoplasm of Schwann cells (Fig. 2.1.2C).

Functions The myelin sheath serves the following functions:

- Its fatty protein coating provides protective insulation for nerve cells.
- It decreases axonal electrical capacitance, altering conduction properties and reducing the energy requirement for action potential propagation.

Myelination of axons increases the speed of conduction and greatly increases their diameter. In motor nerves, speed is important. Hence, motor neurons to muscles and sensory (proprioceptive) fibres from muscles are heavily myelinated.

Applied Aspects

Multiple sclerosis (MS) is a demyelinating autoimmune disease in which antibodies and white blood cells attack the myelin sheath leading to inflammation and injury to myelin sheath. Due to loss of myelin sheath, there is leakage of K^+ through voltage-gated channels resulting in hyperpolarization and thus failure of action potential conduction.

Sign and symptoms: In patients with MS, the physiological deficit consists of muscle weakness, fatigue, diminished motor function and sensory disturbances. The diagnosis of these patients is based on the following tests:

i. *Blood tests* help to rule out other diseases with symptoms similar to MS.
ii. *Nerve conduction tests* detect slow conduction in motor and sensory pathways.
iii. *Cerebrospinal fluid analysis* detects oligoclonal bands indicative of an abnormal autoimmune response against myelin sheath.
iv. *Magnetic resonance imaging (MRI) assessment* visualizes multiple sclerotic area in the brain.

Treatment: Although there is no specific treatment of MS, drugs like *interferon* can suppress autoimmune response.

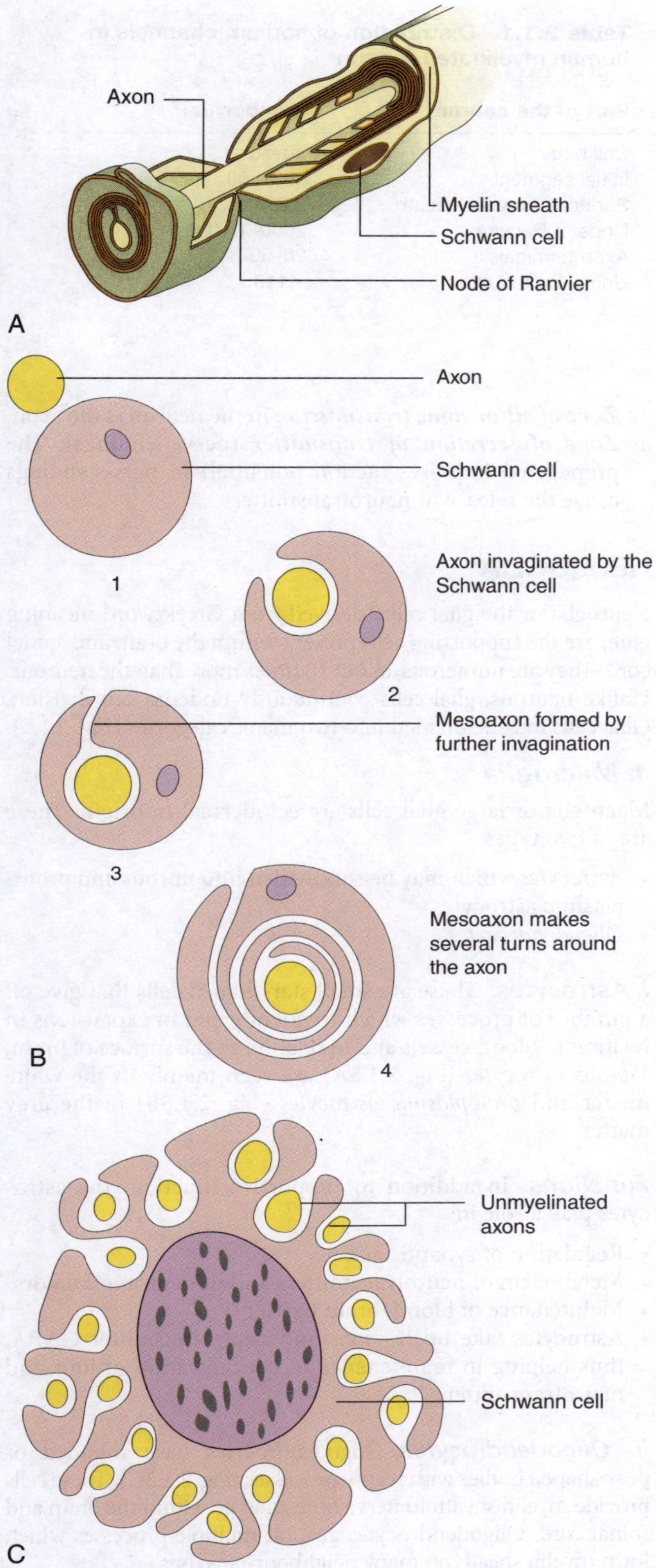

Fig. 2.1.2 Structure of a myelinated neuron: **A**, Schwann cell encircles the axon to form myelin sheath; **B**, stages of myelination; and **C**, structure of an unmyelinated neuron. **Note:** Unmyelinated axons invaginate cytoplasm of Schwann cell.

Types of Neurons

Neurons have been variously classified as follows.

I. Depending on the number of poles Depending on the number of poles from which processes arise, neurons are divided into unipolar, bipolar and multipolar (Fig. 2.1.3):

1. ***Unipolar neurons*** have a single pole, from which both the processes – axons and dendrites – arise (Fig. 2.1.3A). True unipolar cells are present only in embryonic stage in human beings. However, the primary sensory neurons (neurons conveying impulses from a sensory receptor to spinal cord) are *pseudounipolar* (Fig. 2.1.3B).
2. ***Bipolar neurons*** have two poles, one for axons and the other for dendrites (Fig. 2.1.3C). Bipolar neurons are found in the vestibular and cochlear ganglia and in the nasal olfactory epithelium and as bipolar cells in the retina.
3. ***Multipolar neurons*** have many poles. One of the poles gives rise to axons and all others to dendrites (Fig. 2.1.3D). Most vertebrate neurons, especially in the CNS, are multipolar. The dendrites branch profusely to form the dendritic tree.

II. Depending on the function Depending on the functions, the neurons are of two types – motor and sensory.

1. ***Motor neurons***, also known as efferent nerve cells, carry the motor impulses from CNS to the peripheral effector organs like muscles, glands and blood vessels. These neurons have very long axons and short dendrites.
2. ***Sensory neurons***, also known as afferent nerve cells, carry sensory impulses from periphery to the CNS. These neurons have short axons and long dendrites.

III. Depending on the length of axons Depending on the length of axons, the neurons are divided into Golgi type I and Golgi type II.

1. ***Golgi type I neurons***, also known as projection neurons, have long axons. Their cell body lies in the CNS and axons reach the remote peripheral organs. They include the neuron forming peripheral nerves and long tracts of brain and spinal cord.
2. ***Golgi type II neurons***, also known as *short circuit neurons* have short axons. They are usually small and especially numerous in the cerebral cortex, cerebellar cortex and retina.

Zones of The Neuron

From the functional point, each neuron is divided into four zones (Fig. 2.1.4):

1. ***Receptor zone*** (dendritic zone) is the region where local potential changes are generated by integration of the synaptic connections.
2. ***Site of origin of conducted impulse*** is the site where propagated action potentials are generated. In case of spinal motor neurons, *initial segment* and in cutaneous sensory neurons, the *first node* of Ranvier is the site of origin of conducted impulses. The distribution of ion channels along the axon plays an important role in initiation of propagated action potential. The concentration of voltage-gated Na^+ channels is very high in the initial segment and the first node of Ranvier. The estimated distribution of Na^+ channels in different parts of a mammalian myelinated neuron is shown in Table 2.1.1.

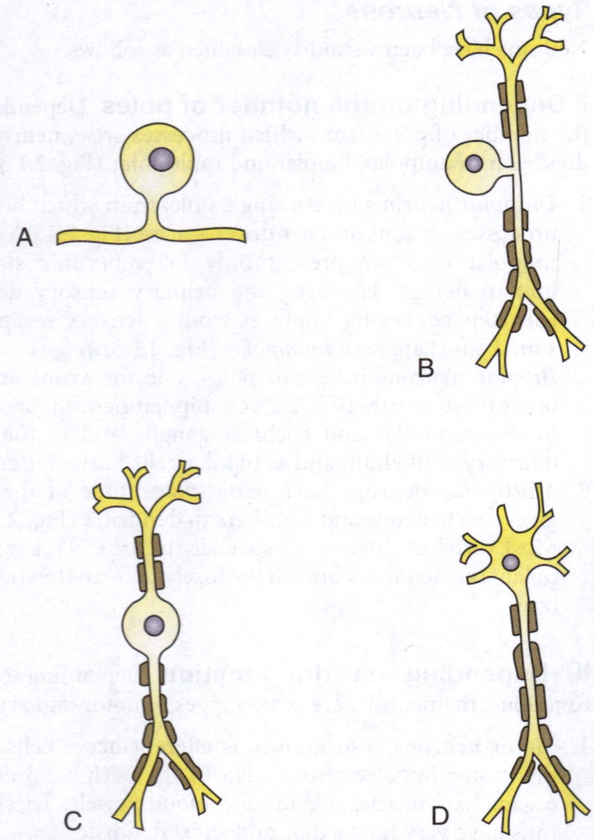

Fig. 2.1.3 Different types of neurons: **A**, unipolar; **B**, pseudounipolar; **C**, bipolar; and **D**, multipolar.

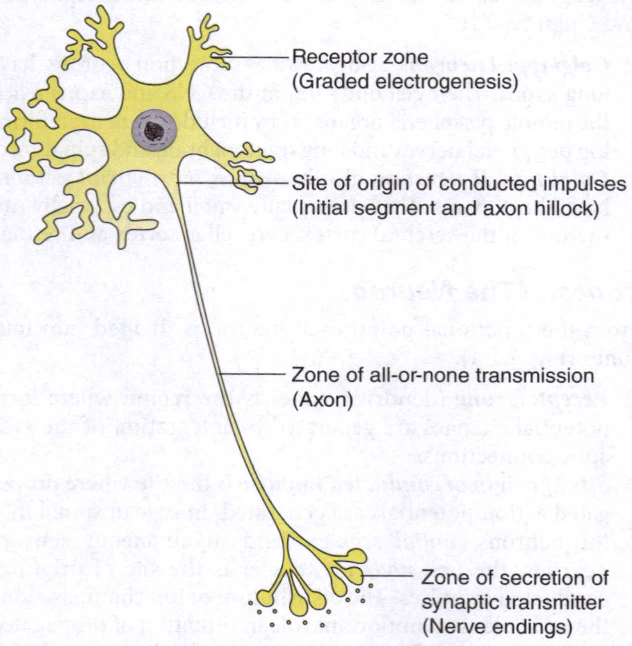

Fig. 2.1.4 Functional zones of the neuron.

Table 2.1.1 Distribution of sodium channels in human myelinated neuron

Part of the neuron	Number/μm²
Cell body	50–75
Initial segment	350–500
Surface of myelin sheath	<25
Node of Ranvier	2000–12,000
Axon terminals	20–50
Unmyelinated axon	~110

3. ***Zone of all-or-none transmission*** in the neuron is the axon.
4. ***Zone of secretion of transmitter*** (nerve endings). The propagated impulses (action potential) to nerve endings cause the release of neurotransmitter.

NEUROGLIA

Neuroglia or the glial cells (derived from Greek word meaning glue) are the supporting cells present within the brain and spinal cord. They are numerous, about 10 times more than the neurons. Unlike neurons, glial cells continuously undergo cell division. Glial cells may be divided into two major categories (Fig. 2.1.5).

1. Macroglia

Macroglia or large glial cells are ectodermal in origin. These are of two types:

- *Astrocytes* which may be subdivided into fibrous and protoplasmic astrocytes
- *Oligodendrocytes*

i. Astrocytes. These are small star-shaped cells that give off a number of processes which frequently end in expansions in relation to blood vessels and in relation to the surface of brain. *Fibrous astrocytes* (Fig. 2.1.5A) are seen mainly in the white matter and *protoplasmic astrocytes* (Fig. 2.1.5B) in the grey matter.

Functions. In addition to supportive function, the astrocytes play a role in:

- Regulation of synaptic activity
- Metabolism of neurotransmitters and of neuromodulators
- Maintenance of blood–brain barrier
- Astrocytes take up K^+ ions and neurotransmitter GABA, thus helping in maintenance of concentration of ions and neurotransmitter

ii. Oligodendrocytes. Oligodendrocytes have rounded or pear-shaped bodies with scanty processes (Fig. 2.1.5C). These cells provide myelin sheath to nerve fibres that lie within the brain and spinal cord. Oligodendrocytes give off multiple processes which form myelin sheath on many neighbouring axons.

2. Microglia

Microglia or the small glial cells are mesodermal in origin. Microglial cells are formed from the monocytes which get settled into the brain. These are the smallest neuroglial cells having flattened cell bodies and short processes (Fig. 2.1.5D). They are more numerous in grey matter than in white matter.

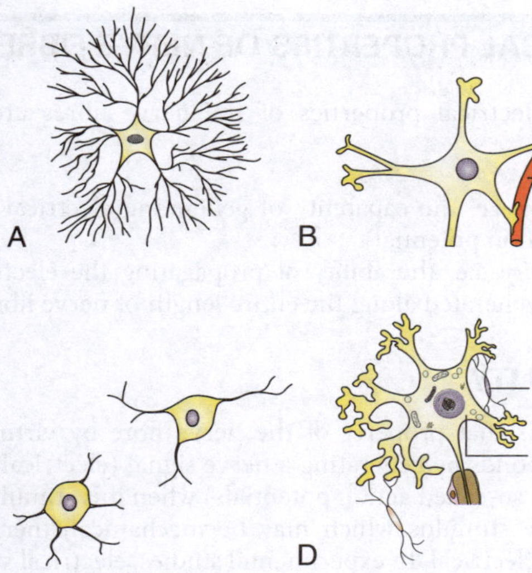

Fig. 2.1.5 Different types of glial cells: **A**, fibrous astrocyte; **B**, protoplasmic astrocyte; **C**, oligodendrocyte; and **D**, microglial cells.

Functions The following are the functions subserved by microglia:

- Scavenging and phagocytosis
- Microglial cells release cytokines (IL-1), which destroy the bacteria and viruses and damaged neurons by releasing substances like H_2O_2 and NO
- Microglia help in repair and growth of neurons
- Microglial cells act as effective antigen-presenting cells when activated

PERIPHERAL NERVE

A compact bundle of axons located outside the CNS is called a nerve. In a nerve, the axons are arranged in different bundles called fasciculi (Fig. 2.1.6).

- Each axon or nerve fibre is covered by *endoneurium* which is bound internally by basal lamina around the Schwann cells and externally by the relatively impermeable inner basal lamina of the perineurium.
- Each fasciculus is covered by *perineurium*. The cells of perineurium are tightly adherent and act as a barrier to passage of particulate traces, dye molecules or toxins into the endoneurium.
- The whole nerve is covered by *epineurium* which is a tubular sheath formed by areolar membrane. It limits the extent to which the nerve can be stretched by body movements or external pressure, thereby protecting the fragile axons inside the nerve.

BIOLOGICAL ACTIVITIES

PROTEIN SYNTHESIS

The cell bodies (soma) of all the neurons contain cellular apparatus required for protein synthesis, i.e. the ribosomes and the Golgi apparatus. Since the axons do not have these organelles, all the proteins including the neurotransmitters are synthesized in the cell body and then transported along the axon to the synaptic knobs by the process of *axoplasmic flow*, as discussed in the subsequent text. Thus, the cell body maintains the functional and anatomic integrity of the axon.

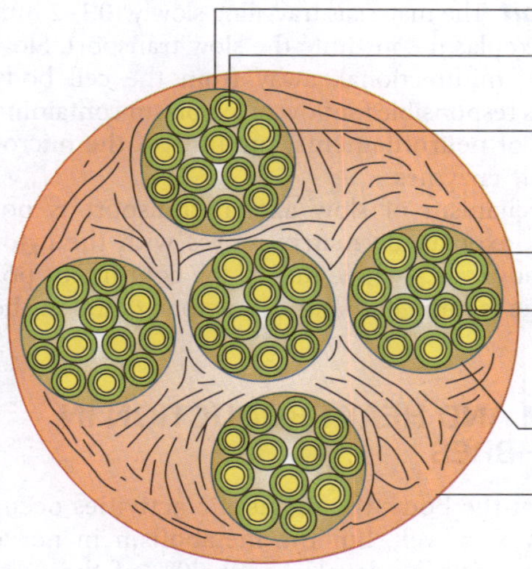

Fig. 2.1.6 Cross-section of a peripheral nerve.

Therefore, if the axon is cut, the part distal to cut degenerates (Wallerian degeneration).

Axoplasmic Transport

Axoplasm, the cytoplasm of the neurons, is in constant motion. The axoplasmic transport is vital to nerve cell functions, since movement of various materials occur through it. The axoplasmic transport is of two types: rapid and slow.

1. Rapid transport Some materials travel 100–400 mm/day along the axoplasm and constitute the rapid transport. Microtubules play an important role in this form of transport. Rapid transport is bidirectional, i.e. both away from and towards the cell body.

i. ***Anterograde or orthograde rapid transport*** occurs from the neuron cell body to the axon terminal. It is driven by the molecular motors *kinesin* and *dynein*. The materials transported by anterograde rapid transport include membrane-bound organelles like short tubules of reticulum, mitochondria, small vesicles, actin, myosin and the clathrin used in recycling of synaptic vesicle membrane.

ii. ***Retrograde rapid transport*** occurs from the nerve terminals towards the cell body of the neuron, returning materials for degradation or reuse. Retrograde rapid transport is driven by the molecular motor *dynein*, and has a velocity 200 mm/day. The materials transported by this mode include proteins and small molecules picked up by the axon terminals.

Important Notes

- Retrograde axoplasmic flow may also carry tetanus toxin and neurotropic viruses (e.g. polio, herpes simplex and rabies) along the axon into the neuronal cell bodies in the CNS.
- It has also been employed by neuroanatomists for charting out neural pathways.
- Nerve growth factor taken up by endocytosis at the ending is transported back to the soma, where it helps in neuronal growth, its survival and prevents apoptosis.

2. Slow transport The materials travelling slowly (0.1–2 mm in a day) in the axoplasm constitute the slow transport. Slow transport is only unidirectional, away from the cell body (anterograde). It is responsible for flow of axoplasm containing protein subunits of neurofilaments, tubulins of the microtubules and soluble enzymes.

The exact mechanism of slow axonal transport is not known. Probably, axoplasmic matrix moves with the cytoskeleton which moves as a whole due to the continuous polymerization at the leading end and depolymerization at the trailing end.

METABOLISM AND HEAT PRODUCTION IN THE NERVE FIBRES

Like other cells of the body, the metabolic activities occur in the nerve fibres as well, but the metabolism in nerve fibres occurs at a very low level. About 70% of the total energy required is used to maintain polarization of the membrane by the action of Na^+–K^+-ATPase pump. The energy required to maintain polarization of the resting membrane is supplied mainly by combustion of sugars and phospholipids.

During nerve activity, the ATP and creatine phosphate break down, i.e. undergo hydrolysis, and supply energy for the propagation of the nerve impulse. At maximum activity, the metabolic rate of nerve fibres just doubles the metabolic rate at resting stage, whereas in skeletal muscles, the metabolic rate may increase by 100 times as compared to the metabolic rate at rest. However, the chemical changes during metabolic activity are almost the same in a nerve and a muscle, i.e. if oxygen supply is deficient, pyruvic acid and lactic acids are formed and accumulate. The nerve fibres are rich in vitamin B_1, which is essential for complete oxidation of pyruvic acid and lactic acids. Furthermore, unlike muscles, even in the absence of oxygen, processes like excitability, conductivity and recovery can go on in a nerve for a considerable period.

Heat production in the nerve fibres As discussed earlier, the metabolism in the nerve fibre is very slow; therefore, during resting phase, only a small amount of heat is produced, which increases to some extent during phase of activity. In a nerve fibre, heat is produced in three phases:

1. ***Resting heat*** is the amount of heat produced during the inactive stage.
2. ***Initial heat*** is the amount of heat produced during action potential (stage of activity). It is about 10% of the total heat produced. It results from anaerobic metabolic activity due to breakdown of ATP and creatine phosphate.
3. ***Delayed or recovery heat*** is produced during the recovery phase which follows the phase of activity. The energy is produced by aerobic metabolic activities and is about 30 times the initial heat. The delayed heat is produced in two stages: the first stage lasts for a few seconds and produces only a small amount of heat, and the second stage lasts for 10–30 minutes and contributes the major amount of the total heat produced. The energy produced during recovery stage is used for resynthesis of ATP and creatine phosphate and as such for restoring the normal excitability of the nerve fibre.

ELECTRICAL PROPERTIES OF NERVE FIBRE

The main electrical properties of the nerve fibres are as follows:

- *Excitability*, i.e. the capability of generating electrical impulses (action potential)
- *Conductivity*, i.e. the ability of propagating the electrical impulses generated along the entire length of nerve fibres

EXCITABILITY

Excitability is that property of the nerve fibre by virtue of which it responds by generating a nerve signal (electrical impulses or the so-called action potentials) when it is stimulated by a suitable stimulus which may be mechanical, thermal, chemical or electrical. In experimental studies, electrical stimulus is more frequently employed since its strength and frequency can be accurately controlled.

Before discussing the excitability (production of action potential), it will be useful to know about the electrical potential in the nerve fibre at rest, i.e. before it is stimulated (resting membrane potential [RMP]). Furthermore, when the stimulus is subthreshold, it does not produce action potential but it causes some change in the RMP termed electrotonic potential. After discussing the production of action potential, various characteristics of the stimulus which can affect the production of action potential will be discussed.

Resting Membrane Potential

There exists a membrane potential of −70 mV (inside negative) across the membrane of nerve fibre at rest. This is called *RMP*. The study of electrical activity of a tissue has been made possible due to advances in the method of the recording electrical potentials, especially the development of microelectrodes and 'cathode ray oscilloscope (CRO)'. For details, see page 67.

As shown in Fig. 2.1.7A, when two electrodes are placed on the surface of a nerve fibre and connected to a CRO, no potential difference is observed. However, if one of the microelectrodes is inserted inside the nerve fibre (Fig. 2.1.7B), a steady potential difference of −70 mV (inside negative) is observed on the CRO. This is RMP and indicates the resting state of cell also called *state of polarization*.

Ionic Basis of Resting Membrane Potential

The details of the processes concerned with the ionic basis of RMP, i.e. selective permeability of cell membrane, Gibbs–Donnan equilibrium, Nernst equation, Goldman's constant field equation and role of Na^+–K^+ pump, have been discussed in Chapter 1.4 on membrane potentials (page 34). However, the ionic basis of RMP is summarized here.

In a nutshell, the distribution of ions across the cell membrane and the nature of cell membrane are responsible for the RMP. Basically, RMP is diffusion potential modified to some extent by the activity of Na^+–K^+ pump as follows:

- Because of large concentration gradient, the K^+ ions diffuse out of the membrane via K^+ channels, but the electrical gradient created opposes it.

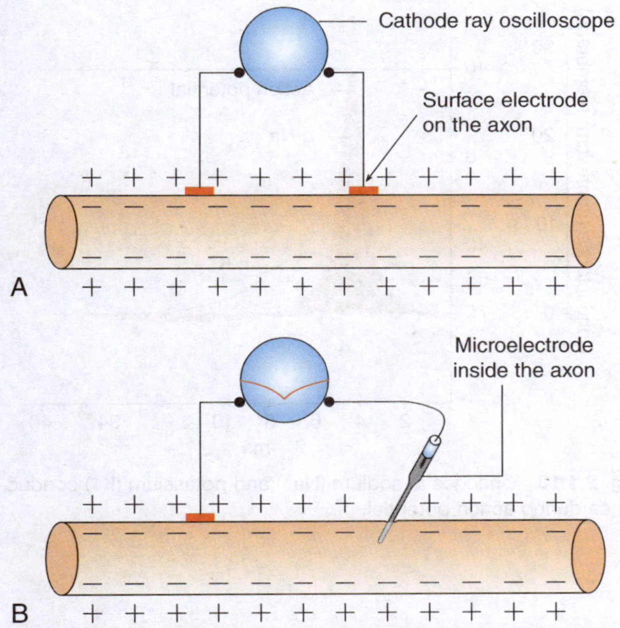

Fig. 2.1.7 Recording of resting membrane potential: **A**, both electrodes are on the surface of axon, no potential difference is recorded; and **B**, one electrode on the surface and other inserted inside the axon, potential difference (−70 mV) is recorded.

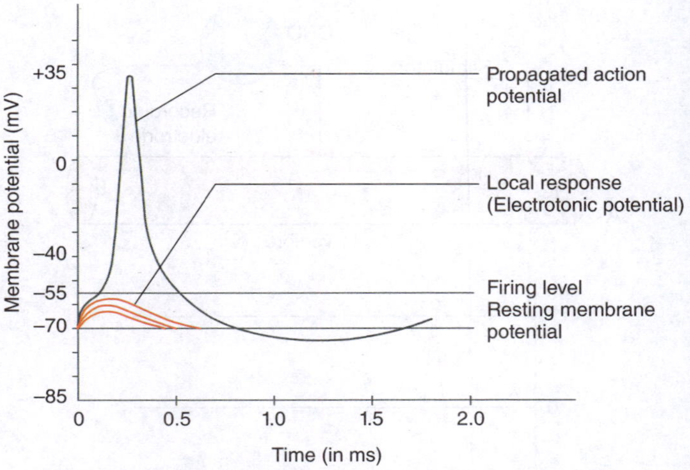

Fig. 2.1.8 Electrotonic potentials (local response).

- Consequently, equilibrium is reached where the potential difference is such that it effectively balances the outward diffusion of K^+ due to concentration gradient.
- At the equilibrium, there is slight excess of cations on the outside and anions on the inside. This condition is maintained by Na^+–K^+ pump, which pumps Na^+ back and keeps the intracellular concentration of Na^+ low.
- Na^+–K^+ pump being electrogenic (because it pumps three Na^+ ions out of the cell for every two K^+ ions it pumps in), it also contributes a small amount to the membrane potential by itself.

At rest, membrane permeability to K^+ is greater due to more opened K^+ channels than the Na^+ channels. Therefore, the intracellular and extracellular K^+ concentration is the main determinant of RMP and that is why RMP is closed to equilibrium potential for K^+.

Action Potential

When the stimulus is subminimal or subthreshold, it does not produce action potential, but does produce some changes in the RMP. There is slight depolarization for about 7 mV which cannot be propagated, since propagation occurs only if the depolarization reaches a firing level of 15 mV (-55 mV). Therefore, this is a local response or phenomenon termed the *electrotonic potential.* As depicted in Fig. 2.1.8, the electrotonic potential does not obey all-or-none law. As is clear from Fig. 2.1.8, when the intensity of stimulus is increased gradually, every time there is an increase in the amplitude of the local response till firing level of 15 mV is reached. Once the firing level is reached, there occurs action potential, i.e. there occurs abrupt depolarization with propagation (action potential) of the cell membrane which was in a polarized state. The adequate strength of stimulus necessary for producing the action potential in a nerve fibre is known as *threshold* or *minimal stimulus.* In other words, the *action potential* may be defined as the brief sequence of changes which occur in the RMP when stimulated by a threshold stimulus.

Phases of Action Potential

The action potential basically occurs in two phases: depolarization and repolarization. When the nerve is stimulated, the polarized state (−70 mV) is altered, i.e. RMP is abolished and the interior of the nerve becomes positive (+35 mV) as compared to the exterior. This is called *depolarization phase.* Within no time, a reverse to the nearly original potential occurs and this second phase of action potential is called *repolarization phase.*

Action potential curve obtained when RMP is being recorded on a CRO and the nerve fibre is stimulated at a short distance away from the recording electrode (Fig. 2.1.9A) has the following components (Fig. 2.1.9B):

1. ***RMP.*** It is recorded as a straight baseline at −70 mV.
2. ***Stimulus artefact.*** It is recorded as mild deflection of the baseline as soon as the stimulus is applied. The stimulus artefact occurs due to leakage of current from the stimulating electrode to the recording electrode.
3. ***Latent period.*** It is recorded as short isoelectric period (0.5–1 milliseconds) following the stimulus artefact. It represents the interval between the application of stimulus and the onset of action potential. It depends on the distance between the site of stimulation and the point of recording and the velocity of action potential along the particular axon.
4. ***Firing level.*** After the latent period, phase of depolarization starts. To begin with, depolarization proceeds relatively slow up to a level called the *firing level* (−55 mV), at which depolarization occurs very rapidly.
5. ***Overshoot.*** From the firing level, the curve reaches the zero potential rapidly and then *overshoots* the zero line up to +35 mV.
6. ***Spike potential.*** After reaching the peak (+35 mV), the phase of depolarization is completed and the phase of

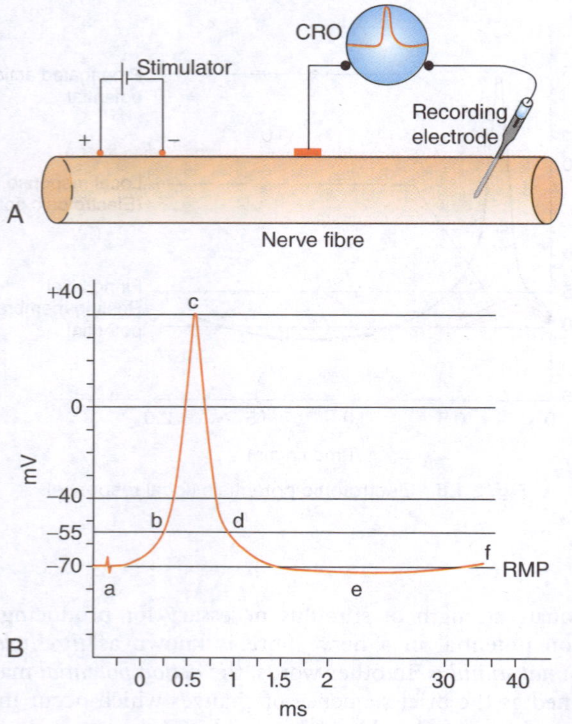

Fig. 2.1.9 Recording of action potential of a large mammalian myelinated nerve fibre: **A**, arrangement for recording action potential; and **B**, various phases (components) of action potential (a, stimulus artefact; b, firing level; b to c, depolarization; c to d, repolarization; d to e, after-depolarization; and e to f, after-hyperpolarization).

repolarization starts and the potential descends quickly near firing level. The phase of rapid rise of potential in depolarization and a rapid fall in repolarization phase combinedly constitute the so-called *spike potential.* Its duration is approximately 1 millisecond in an axon.

7. ***After-depolarization.*** It is the slow repolarization phase which follows a rapid fall in spike potential and extends up to attainment of RMP level. It is called phase of *negative afterpotential* and lasts for about 4 milliseconds.
8. ***After-hyperpolarization.*** After reaching the resting level (−70 mV), the potential further falls and becomes more negative (−72 mV). This phase is called *after-hyperpolarization* or phase of *positive* afterpotential. It lasts for a prolonged period (35–40 milliseconds). Finally, the RMP is restored.

Ionic Basis of Action Potential

Role of voltage-gated Na^+ and K^+ channels. The development of action potential was studied by Hodgkin and Huxley using the *voltage clamp technique.* According to *Hodgkin–Huxley theory*, the sequence of events is as follows.

Polarization phase. RMP (−70 mV) is due to distribution of more cations outside the cell membrane and more anions inside the cell membrane. At this point, though Na^+ is more in extracellular fluid (ECF), it cannot enter the cell due to the impermeability of the membrane.

Depolarization phase. When threshold stimulus is applied to the cell membrane, at the point of stimulation (Fig. 2.1.10), the permeability of the membrane for Na^+ ions

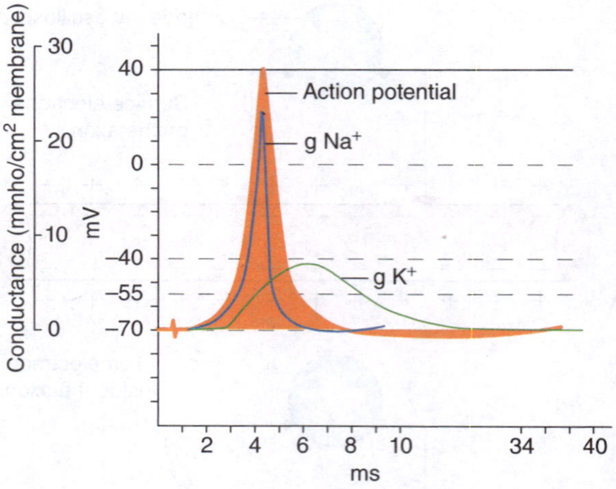

Fig. 2.1.10 Changes in sodium (Na^+) and potassium (K^+) conductance during action potential.

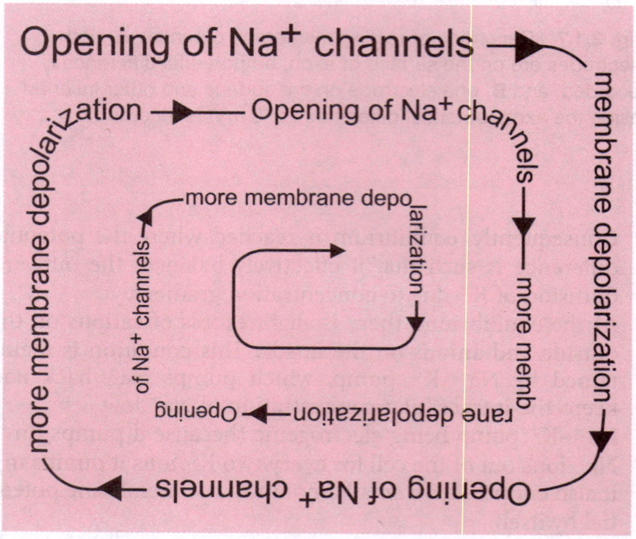

Fig. 2.1.11 Positive feedback spiral (Hodgkin cycle).

increases. At first, the rise of permeability for Na^+ is slow till it reaches *firing level.* When the membrane potential depolarizes, the Na^+ channels start opening up. The opening of the Na^+ channels depolarizes the membrane further, leading to the opening of greater numbers of Na^+ channels. Thus, there is *positive feedback spiral*, the so-called Hodgkin cycle (Fig. 2.1.11), resulting in rapid change in membrane potential. Once firing level is reached, the voltage-gated Na^+ channels open massively and as the concentration gradient and electrical gradient of this ion are directed inward, there occurs a rapid influx of Na^+ ions into the cell (Fig. 2.1.12A). This rapid entry of Na^+ is sufficient to overwhelm the repolarizing forces and the membrane potential seems to be carried towards the equilibrium potential of Na^+ (+60 mV). However, the depolarization does not reach a value greater than +35 mV because of the following reasons:

- Na^+ channels are inactivated in a fraction of millisecond and the gates close again.

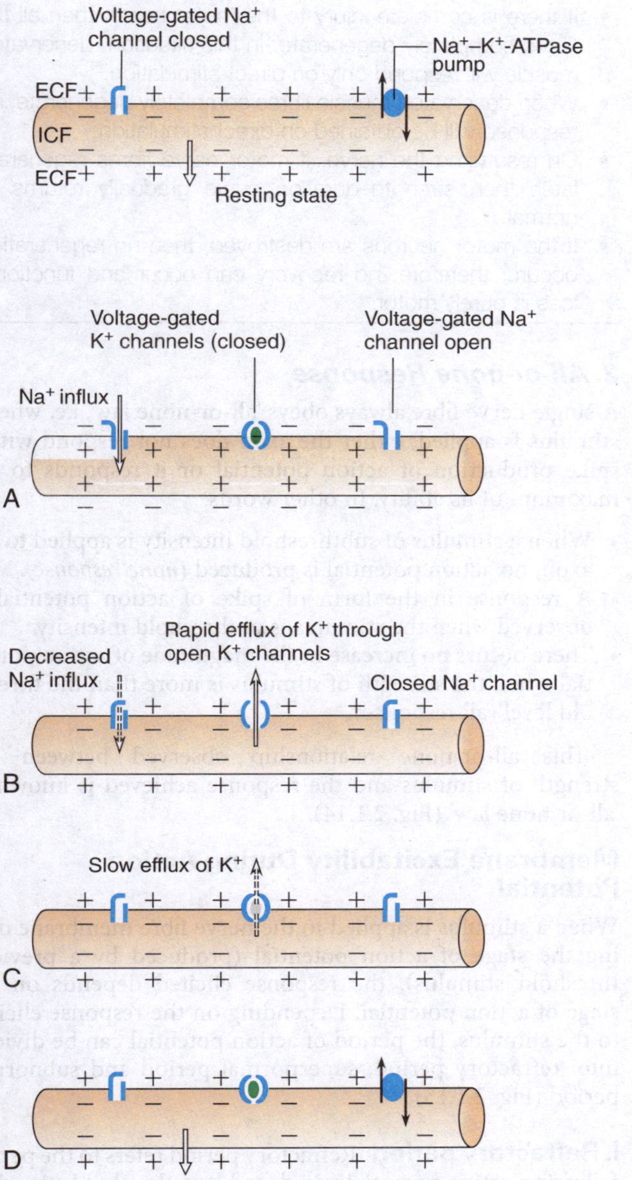

Fig. 2.1.12 Schematic diagram to show the role of voltage-gated ion channels in resting state (Na^+–K^+-ATPase pump active); **A**, during depolarization phase (Na^+ channels open up and K^+ channels remain closed); **B**, during rapid repolarization phase (K^+ channels open up resulting in rapid efflux of K^+ and Na^+ influx decreases); **C**, during after-depolarization and hyperpolarization phases (Na^+ channels get closed, K^+ efflux slows down); and **D**, restoration of resting membrane potential by activation of Na^+–K^+-ATPase pump (resulting in efflux of **three** Na^+ and influx of **two** K^+).

- Due to rapid influx of Na^+, the concentration gradient diminishes and during overshoot phase the electrical gradient for Na^+ also reverses.
- Change in the membrane potential during depolarization results in opening of voltage-gated K^+ channels (Fig. 2.1.12B). Therefore, within a fraction of millisecond of the threshold excitation, K^+ leaves the cell along its concentration gradient.

Repolarization phase. Repolarization occurs due to decrease in further Na^+ influx and K^+ efflux through the voltage-gated K^+ channels which open later than Na^+ channels but remain activated for a prolonged period (Figs 2.1.10 and 2.1.12B).

Decrease in Na^+ influx and efflux of K^+ cause net transfer of positive charge out of the cell that serves to complete the repolarization.

After-depolarization. After the rapid initial repolarization (spike potential), further repolarization occurs slowly. This is due to the fact that rate of K^+ efflux slows down as the electrical gradient responsible for initial rapid diffusion declines. This last phase of slow repolarization due to slow efflux of K^+ is called *after-depolarization* (Fig. 2.1.12C).

After-hyperpolarization. The slow efflux of K^+ continues even after the RMP is reached, resulting in a prolonged phase of *hyperpolarization* during which the membrane potential falls up to −72 mV. However, little after, the voltage-gated K^+ channels also shut down. The final ionic distribution is brought to the resting state by the action of Na^+–K^+ pump and the leak channels (K^+ and Cl^-) (Fig. 2.1.12D).

Role of calcium ions. In addition to Na^+ and K^+ ions, the Ca^{2+} ions also play some role in the development of action potential. The concentration of Ca^{2+} in ICF is very low as compared to that in ECF. Therefore, when Na^+ channels are open, some Ca^{2+} ions also move inside the cell through these opened-up Na^+ channels. Furthermore, a separate class of channels known as *slow calcium channels* also exists in the cell membrane. These calcium channels also open up admitting Ca^{2+} during development of action potential.

Important Notes

- Low extracellular Na^+ concentration decreases the amplitude (size of action potential); however, there is little/no effect on resting membrane potential.
- Low extracellular Ca^{2+} concentration increases the excitability of nerve and muscle by decreasing the amount of depolarization necessary for initiating changes in Na^+ and K^+ conductance required for action potential.
- Increase in Ca^{2+} concentration stabilizes the membrane by decreasing excitability.

The *calcium channels* are especially important in cardiac and smooth muscles where these are in abundance. In fact, in some types of smooth muscles, the fast sodium channels are hardly present, so the action potentials then are caused almost entirely by activation of the slow calcium channels.

Characteristics of Nerve Excitability vis-à-vis Characteristics of the Stimulus

The excitable nerve fibre exhibits some peculiar characteristics of the excitability depending on the strength and duration of the stimulus used and the electrogenic state of the nerve fibre when stimulus is applied. Some of the important excitability characteristics are described.

1. Strength–Duration Curve

It has been observed experimentally that an action potential is produced if the nerve fibre is stimulated by a stimulus of adequate strength (intensity) and duration. The minimal intensity of stimulating current acting for a given duration producing an action potential is called *threshold intensity*. The

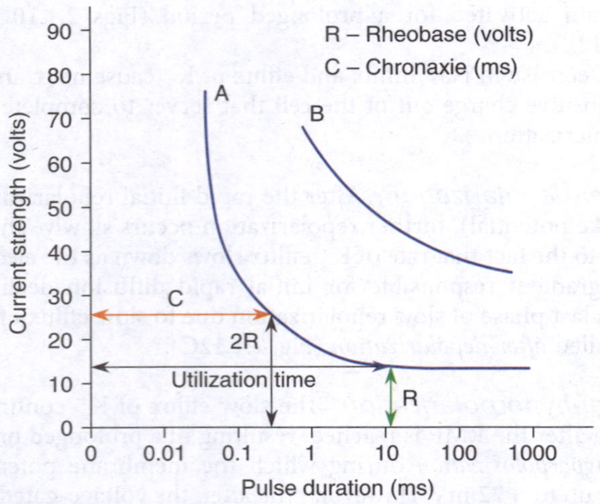

Fig. 2.1.13 Strength–duration curves: (A) for nerve; and (B) for muscle.

relationship between the strength and duration of a stimulus has been studied by varying the duration of a stimulus and finding out the threshold strength for each duration. The record of results plotted on a semilog graph paper gives the *strength–duration curve* (Fig. 2.1.13). The following inferences can be drawn from the strength–duration curve:

Rheobase (R) refers to the minimum intensity of stimulus which if applied for adequate time (utilization time) produces a response.

Chronaxie (C) refers to the minimum duration for which the stimulus of double the rheobase intensity must be applied to produce a response. Within limits, chronaxie of a given excitable tissue is constant. In other words, the chronaxie is an index of the excitability of a tissue and can be used to compare the excitability of various tissues. For example, a nerve fibre has far shorter chronaxie value than a muscle fibre indicating greater excitability of the former.

- When a stimulus of weaker intensity than the rheobase is applied, it will not produce a response, no matter how long the stimulus is applied.
- Stimulus of extremely short duration will not produce any response, no matter how intense that may be.

Important Notes

Chronaxie is dependent on the density of voltage-gated Na^+ channels that is why:

- Chronaxie value of white muscle fibres is shorter than red muscle fibres.
- Chronaxie value of infant's muscle fibres is 10 times more than in adults.

Applied Aspects

Plotting of strength–duration curve has significance in the following situations:

- Nerve injury: Following an injury, the affected nerve fibres become inexcitable after a few days. If only most excitable fibres get injured, then the strength–duration curve will represent the response of intact less excitable fibres.
- If there is complete injury to the motor nerve, then all the fibres completely degenerate. In this situation, denervated muscle will respond only on direct stimulation.
- When denervated muscle fibres completely degenerate, no response will be obtained on direct stimulation.
- On resuturing the nerve, if motor nerve fibres regenerate later, then strength–duration curve gradually returns to normal.
- If the motor neurons are destroyed, then no regeneration occurs; therefore, no recovery can occur and functional loss is purely motor.

2. All-or-none Response

A single nerve fibre always obeys 'all-or-none law', i.e. when a stimulus is applied, either the axon does not respond with a spike production of action potential or it responds to the maximum of its ability. In other words:

- When a stimulus of subthreshold intensity is applied to the axon, no action potential is produced *(none response)*.
- A response in the form of spike of action potential is observed when the stimulus is of threshold intensity.
- There occurs no increase in the magnitude of action potential when the strength of stimulus is more than the threshold level (all response).

This all-or-none relationship observed between the strength of stimulus and the response achieved is known as 'all-or none law' (Fig. 2.1.14).

Membrane Excitability During Action Potential

When a stimulus is applied to the nerve fibre membrane during the stage of action potential (produced by a previous threshold stimulus), the response elicited depends on the stage of action potential. Depending on the response elicited to the stimulus, the period of action potential can be divided into: refractory period, supernormal period and subnormal period (Fig. 2.1.15).

I. Refractory period Refractory period refers to the period following action potential (produced by a threshold stimulus) during which a nerve fibre either does not respond or responds subnormally to a stimulus of threshold intensity or greater than threshold intensity. It is of two types.

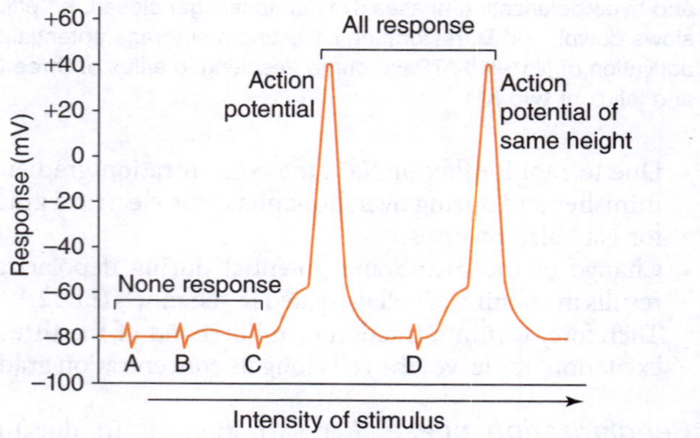

Fig. 2.1.14 All-or-none response in a single nerve fibre: (A and B) subthreshold; (C), threshold; and (D) suprathreshold stimuli.

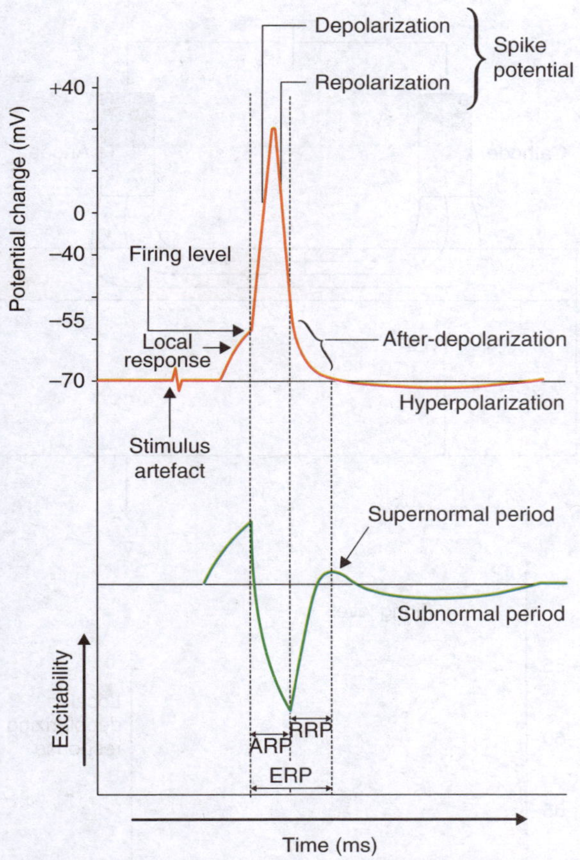

Fig. 2.1.15 Membrane excitability during different phases of action potential: absolute refractory period (ARP), relative refractory period (RRP) and effective refractory period (ERP).

Absolute refractory period. It is a short period following action potential during which second stimulus, no matter how strong it may be, cannot evoke any response (another action potential). In other words, during absolute refractory period (ARP), the nerve fibre completely loses its excitability. The ARP corresponds to the period of action potential from firing level until repolarization is almost one-third complete (spike potential). During this period, neither a fresh impulse can be generated nor an impulse generated elsewhere can pass through this area.

Ionic basis of absolute refractory period. During upstroke of action potential (depolarization), the *m gates* of sodium channels in the membrane of nerves are opened rapidly. During downstroke (early repolarization), the channels are closed by closure of inactivation *(h) gates* of the sodium channel and slow potassium channels are not yet opened. These sodium channel gates do not open unless potential comes back to resting level. Therefore, during this period (ARP), the nerve fibre is not stimulated at all.

Relative refractory period. Relative refractory period (RRP) is a short period during which the nerve fibre shows response if the strength of stimulus is more than normal. It extends from the end of ARP to the start of *after-depolarization* of the action potential.

Ionic basis of relative refractory period. During this stage, the Na^+ channels are coming out of inactivated stage and voltage-gated potassium channels are still open. The stronger stimulus (suprathreshold) at this stage is able to open more Na^+ channels through 'm' gates and thus excites a response. The action potential elicited during this period, however, has a lower upstroke velocity and lower overshoot potential than the normal action potential.

Effective refractory period. The effective refractory period (ERP) includes the ARP and the early part of RRP. At the end of an ERP, the nerve membrane is able to produce and conduct the action potential.

II. Supernormal period During supernormal period, the membrane is hyperexcitable, i.e. the threshold of stimulus is decreased. This period corresponds with the *after-depolarization* phase of the action potential.

Ionic basis of supernormal period. During 'after-depolarization' phase, the Na^+ channels have come out of inactivated state but the K^+ channels (voltage gated) are mostly closed and the membrane potential is nearer to the firing level, so a stimulus of low intensity will be able to excite action potential. In other words, the threshold level of stimulus is decreased during this stage.

III. Subnormal period During this period, the membrane excitability is low, i.e. the threshold of stimulus is increased. This period corresponds with the *after-hyperpolarization* stage of the action potential.

Basis of subnormal period. During *after-hyperpolarization* phase, the intracellular negativity further increases (approximately −72 mV). Thus, the membrane potential goes farther away from the firing level and so the threshold of stimulus increases. This phase of subnormal period lasts for about 40 milliseconds.

3. Accommodation

We have studied that when a stimulus of sufficient strength (threshold level) is applied quickly, the action potential is produced. However, when the stimulus strength is increased slowly to the firing level (during constant application), no *action potential is produced*. This is because of the fact that firing level of depolarization of the nerve fibre is not reached as the membrane adapts to the applied stimulus. This phenomenon of adaptation to the stimuli is called *accommodation*. Therefore, a *square pulse stimulus* (Fig. 2.1.16A) which rises sharply to its peak level effectively triggers an action potential, whereas a *sawtooth pulse* stimulus (Fig. 2.1.16B), which rises to its peak slowly, often fails to trigger an action potential.

Ionic basis of accommodation. When the membrane depolarizes, both Na^+ and K^+ channels open up. If depolarization occurs rapidly, the opening of the Na^+ channels overwhelm the repolarizing forces and the typical action potential is produced. However, when the induced depolarization is produced slowly, more and more Na^+ channels open up, only to get inactivated after 1 millisecond, whereas the K^+ channels remain open which tend to restore the membrane potential. Thus, the repolarizing forces overwhelm the depolarizing forces and so the action potential is not produced.

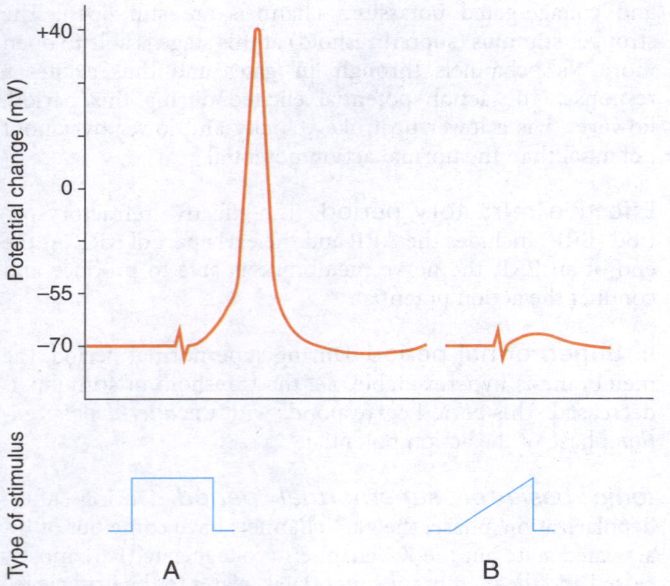

Fig. 2.1.16 Single nerve fibre response to **A**, square pulse stimulus; and **B**, sawtooth pulse stimulus.

4. Infatiguability

A nerve fibre cannot be fatigued, even if it is stimulated for a long time. This property of infatiguability is due to the fact that during action potential, neither a fresh impulse (action potential) can be generated nor the action potential can be conducted through the nerve fibre. In other words, once stimulated, the nerve cannot be stimulated immediately again due to ARP (see page 63) and thus cannot be fatigued.

Electrotonic Potential and Local Response

When a nerve fibre is stimulated by subminimal or subthreshold stimuli, the action potential is not produced, but there do occur some changes in the RMP. These local nonpropagated changes are called *electrotonic potentials or acute subthreshold potentials*.

Types of electrotonic potentials. Depending on the nature (negative or positive) of subthreshold level current used to stimulate (Fig. 2.1.17), the electrotonic potentials are of two types:

Catelectrotonic potential. Catelectrotonic potentials are localized depolarizing potential changes in the membrane potential produced when the stimulus of subthreshold strength is applied with cathode. This potential change rises sharply and then decays exponentially with time.

Anelectrotonic potential. Anelectrotonic potentials are the localized hyperpolarizing potential changes in the membrane potential when anodal subthreshold current is applied.

Production of Electrotonic Potentials

The electrotonic potentials are produced due to passive changes in the membrane polarization caused by addition or subtraction of the charge by the particular electrode.

Graded potentials As shown in Fig. 2.1.17, the electrotonic potentials produced by varying intensities of stimuli are proportionate to the magnitude of stimulation. Therefore, these are also known as *graded potentials*. The graded response is achieved at both cathode and anode up to

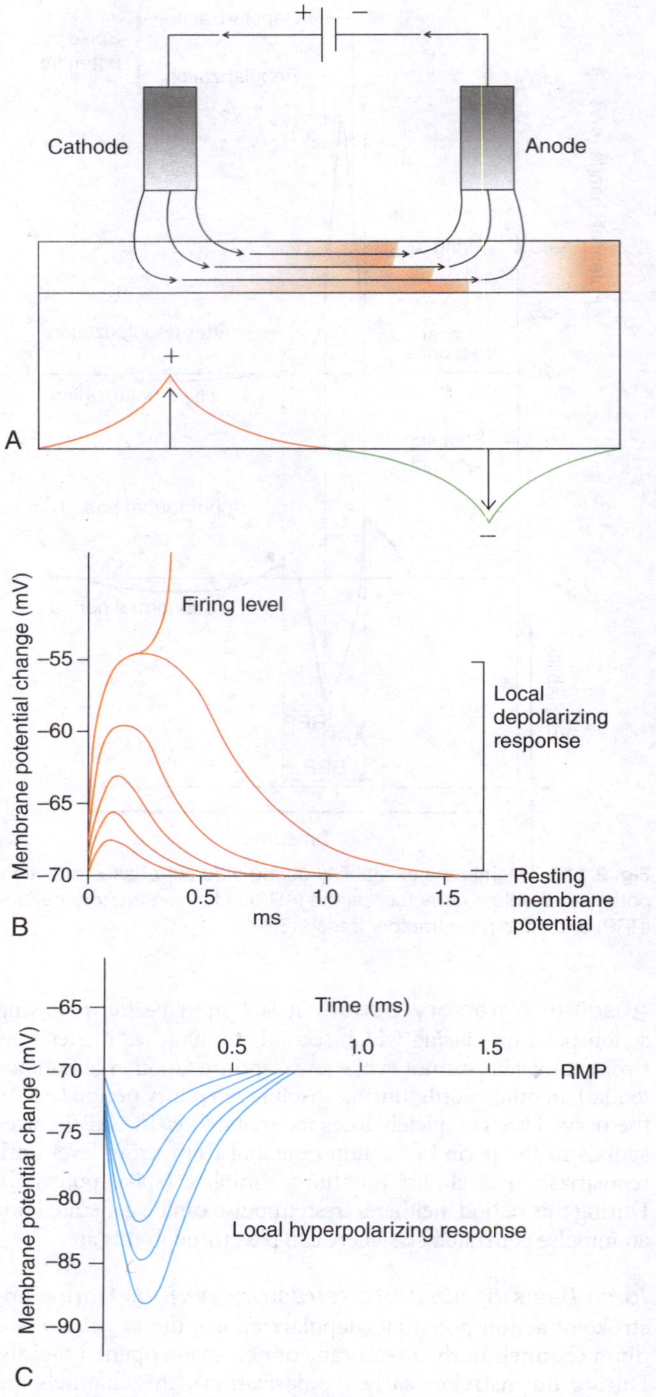

Fig. 2.1.17 Electrotonic potential: **A**, arrangement of recording electrotonic potentials; **B**, catelectrotonic potential recorded by application of subthreshold stimuli (varying intensities) at cathode; and **C**, anelectrotonic potential recorded by application of stimuli (varying intensities) at anode.

7 mV of depolarization or hyperpolarization. At anode, the graded response is achieved even with stronger stimuli. However, the cathodal responses become greater than the proportionate increase in the stimulus intensities to produce depolarization of 7–15 mV. This disproportionate response at cathode occurs due to opening of more voltage-gated Na^+ channels, and is called *local response*. A further increase in the intensity of cathodal stimulus may produce *firing level* (15 mV) initiating the action potential (Fig. 2.1.17B).

Table 2.1.2 Differences between graded potential and action potential

Graded potential	Action potential
1. The amplitude of graded potential is proportionate to the intensity of the stimulus and can get summated	The amplitude of action potential remains constant with increasing intensity of stimulus; therefore, it cannot be summated
2. Graded potentials can be either depolarizing or hyperpolarizing	Action potential is always depolarizing
3. Graded potential can be generated either spontaneously or in response to either physical or chemical stimuli	Action potential is generated only in response to membrane depolarization
4. Graded potentials cannot conduct impulse	Action potential can conduct impulses
5. Examples • Receptor potential at sensory nerve endings • Motor end-plate potential	Examples • Action potential of a nerve fibre, skeletal muscle and cardiac muscle

Differences between graded potentials and action potential are summarized in Table 2.1.2.

Changes in Excitability During Electrotonic Potential

1. ***During catelectrotonic potential***, the threshold of neuron to stimulation decreases, i.e. the excitability increases. The cathodal currents move the membrane potential towards firing level. Therefore, when cathodal stimuli of subthreshold strength are applied in quick succession, the passive depolarizing potential is added up (summated) and firing level may be reached. At this potential, depolarizing forces are stronger than repolarizing forces. This property is called *summation of subminimal stimuli* (Fig. 2.1.17B).
2. ***During anelectrotonic potential***, threshold of neuron stimulation is elevated, i.e. the membrane excitability is decreased. It is because the anodal currents take the membrane potential farther away from the firing level (i.e. the membrane potential becomes about −85 mV) and thus inhibit impulse formation (Fig. 2.1.17C). The size of anelectrotonic potential is proportionate to the magnitude of anodal current strength. When stimulation with anodal current is stopped, it may lead to overshoot of membrane potential towards depolarization direction. This *rebound depolarization* response is sometimes so large that the firing level may be reached producing the action potential.

Important Notes

There are certain factors which effect the excitability of the nerve fibres:

1. ***High extracellular calcium concentration.*** A high extracellular Ca^{2+} concentration decreases membrane permeability to Na^+ ions, thereby decreasing the membrane excitability.
2. ***Hypocalcaemia (low concentration of extracellular Ca^+)*** increasing excitability of nerve fibres by decreasing amount of depolarization required for opening of voltage-gated Na^+ channels.
3. ***Local anaesthetics.*** Local anaesthetic agents like *procaine, tetracaine* and *lidocaine* act directly by binding to the activation gates of the Na^+ channels. These agents block the Na^+ channels, thus reducing the membrane excitability. Therefore, effect of local anaesthetics on membrane excitability depends on the distribution or density of Na^+ channels. For example, in myelinated nerves, the density of Na^+ channels is high at *node* of Ranvier. The local anaesthetics are unable to block all the Na^+ channels; hence, myelinated nerve fibres are less sensitive to local anaesthetics, whereas unmyelinated nerve fibres are highly susceptible to local anaesthesia.

CONDUCTIVITY

Conductivity refers to propagation of nerve impulse (action potential) in the form of a wave of depolarization through the nerve fibre. Normally in the body, the action potential is transmitted through nerve fibre in one direction, but in experimental conditions when nerve fibre is stimulated in the middle, the action potential initiated is conducted equally in either direction (Fig. 2.1.18B). Mechanism of conduction of action potential along an unmyelinated nerve fibre and a myelinated nerve fibre is described as follows.

Propagation of Action Potential in an Unmyelinated Axon

The steps of propagation of action potential along an unmyelinated axon are summarized as follows:

- In the resting phase (polarized state), the axonal membrane is outside positive and inside negative (Fig. 2.1.18A).
- When an unmyelinated axon is stimulated at one site by a threshold stimulus, action potential occurs at that site, which means that the site is depolarized. In other words, the outside of that site becomes negative and the inside positive (reversal of polarity) but the neighbouring areas up to now remain in polarized state (Fig. 2.1.18C).
- As both ECF and ICF are conductive to electricity, a current will flow from positive polarized area to negative activated area through ECF and in the reverse direction in ICF (Fig. 2.1.18C). Thus, a *local circuit current* flows between the resting polarized site to the depolarized site of the membrane (current sink).
- This circular current flow depolarizes the neighbouring area of the membrane up to firing level and a new action potential is produced which in turn depolarizes the neighbouring area ahead. Thus, due to successive depolarization of the neighbouring area, the action potential is propagated along the entire length of the axon (Fig. 2.1.18D). This type of conduction is known as *electrotonic conduction*. Once initiated, the moving impulse cannot spread to reverse direction because the proximal site is in *refractory state* and thus the distal sites being in polarized state keep on getting depolarized. Thus, the direction of propagation of impulse is that of current flow inside the nerve fibre (Fig. 2.1.18E).
- The depolarization remains at any site for some length of time; therefore, portion which depolarizes first also repolarizes first. Thus, the repolarization is also propagated following the depolarization (Fig. 2.1.18F).

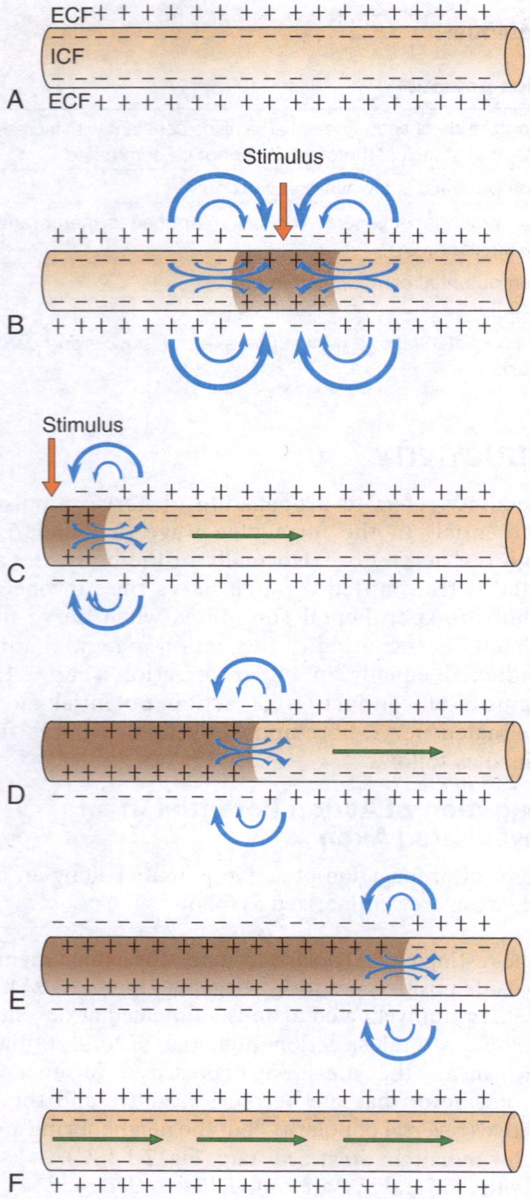

Fig. 2.1.18 Electrotonic conduction of impulse in an unmyelinated nerve fibre: **A**, resting phase (polarized state); **B**, conduction of impulse in both directions when stimulus applied at the middle of nerve fibre; **C**, when stimulus applied at one end of the nerve fibre; **D** and **E**, propagation of impulse in one direction along the nerve fibre; and **F**, repolarization (occurs in same direction).

- The magnitude of action potential does not change as it is conducted along the membrane, because the new action potentials are being generated constantly. However, the speed of propagation of action potential varies in different tissues.

Propagation of Action Potential in a Myelinated Axon

As discussed in the section 'Functional Anatomy', the myelinated nerve fibres have a wrapping of myelin sheath with gaps at regular intervals which are devoid of myelin sheath (nodes of Ranvier). The axonal membrane in the naked area (nodes of Ranvier) bears densely packed ion channels. The myelin

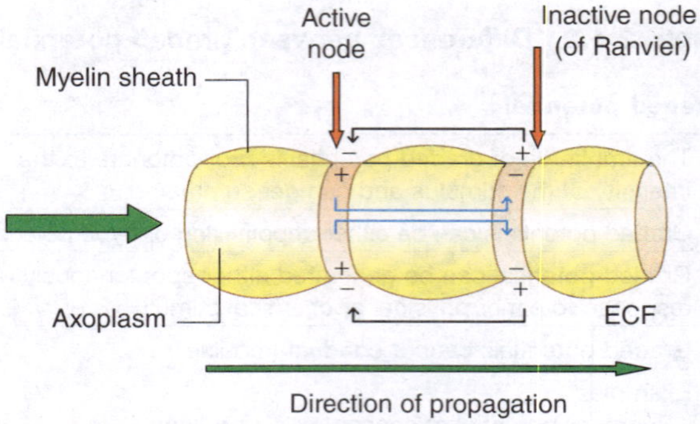

Fig. 2.1.19 Saltatory conduction along a myelinated nerve fibre.

sheath acts as an insulator and does not allow the current flow. Therefore, in myelinated nerve fibres, the *local circuit of current flow* occurs only from one node of Ranvier to the adjacent node (Fig. 2.1.19). That is, the impulse (action potential) jumps from one node of Ranvier to next. This is known as *saltatory conduction*. Since the impulse jumps from one node to other, the speed of conduction in myelinated fibres is rapid (50–100 times faster) than that in the unmyelinated fibre.

Orthodromic Versus Antidromic Conduction

Normally, the action potential is propagated in one direction. That is, usually the nerve impulse from the receptors or synaptic junctions travels along the entire length of the axon to their termination. This type of conduction is called *orthodromic conduction*. The conduction of nerve impulse in the opposite direction, as seen in the sensory nerve supplying the blood vessels, is called *antidromic conduction*.

Conduction Velocity

Factors Affecting Conduction Velocity

The velocity of conduction in nerve fibres varies from as little as 0.25 m/s in very small unmyelinated fibres to as high as 100 m/s in very large myelinated fibres. In general, the factors affecting conduction velocity are as follows.

A. Factors attributable to action potential generation are:

1. ***Temperature:*** It affects conduction velocity by its effect on the duration of the action potential. A decrease in temperature causes a marked increase in the duration of action potential (specially the spike) and thus delays conduction, i.e. slows down the conduction velocity.
2. ***Level of RMP:*** It affects the conduction velocity variably. Where the RMP is less negative, it slows down both generation of action potential and electrotonic conduction. When RMP is more negative, it slows down the generation of action potential but speeds up electrotonic conduction. The resultant effect on conduction velocity is variable but usually a decrease.
3. ***Level of threshold potential (firing level):*** If it is low, the conduction velocity is increased. It is due to the fact that at low firing level, one action potential can trigger a second action potential a distance away where the local currents are feeble. A decrease in the firing level occurs when the concentration of divalent ion in the ECF decreases.

B. Factors attributable to electrotonic conduction are:

1. ***Axon diameter*** affects the conduction velocity through the *resistance offered by the axoplasm* (Ri) to the flow of

axoplasmic current. Greater this resistance, weaker is the electrotonic conduction. If the diameter of the axon is greater, the axoplasmic resistance (Ri) is lesser and hence the velocity of conduction is higher.

- In an unmyelinated nerve fibre, the conduction velocity is directly proportional to the square root of the fibre diameter (*D*), i.e.

$$\text{Conduction velocity} \propto \sqrt{D}$$

2. ***Myelination*** increases conduction velocity by its following effects:
   - By increasing the axon diameter.
   - By the saltatory conduction produced due to its insulating effect (as discussed above).
   - *Resistance offered by the membrane* (Rm) is high in thick myelinated nerve fibres. When Rm is high, the membrane current falls, resulting in higher axoplasmic current and stronger electrotonic conduction.
   - Electrical capacitance (Cm) is low in thick myelinated nerve fibres. The lesser the membrane capacitance, the stronger the electrotonic conduction.

   In a myelinated nerve fibre, the conduction velocity is directly proportional to the fibre diameter as follows:

$$\text{Conduction velocity (in m/s)} = 6 \times \text{axonal diameter (in } \mu\text{m)}$$

3. ***Resistance offered by ECF (Ro)*** to the outer longitudinal current also affects the conduction velocity. Greater this resistance (Ro), weaker is the electrotonic conduction. However, Ro usually remains constant.

RECORDING OF MEMBRANE POTENTIALS AND ACTION POTENTIALS

The recording of membrane excitation and action potential is made possible by the use of highly sophisticated equipment. The mammalian axons are about 20 μm or less in diameter, so being relatively small, it is very difficult to separate them out from other axons. Certain invertebrate species like crab (*Carcinus*), cuttlefish (*Sepia*) and squid (*Loligo*) have giant cells. The largest axon found in the neck region of *Loligo* is about 1 mm in diameter. The fundamental properties are quite similar to those of human axons. Therefore, these animals can be used for recording various events.

Instruments Used for Recording

The membrane potential changes during activities of nerve fibre are very rapid (occurring in less than a second); therefore, the recording instrument should be capable of responding extremely rapidly, i.e. it must be inertialess. Furthermore, the potential changes occurring are in millivolts and hence need to be amplified before being recorded. The essential instruments used in recording the activity of excitable tissue are as follows:

- Microelectrodes
- Electronic amplifiers
- CRO

Basic principles of the functioning of these instruments are discussed briefly.

1. Microelectrodes. Microelectrodes are usually very small pipettes (micropipette) of tip size less than 1 mm diameter, filled with strong electrolyte solution (KCl) and having very high resistance (1 billion Ω) to electrical flow. The tip of micropipette electrode is impaled through the cell membrane of the nerve fibre. Another electrode called *indifferent electrode* is placed in the ECF (Fig. 2.1.20).

The microelectrode can be connected to CRO through a suitable amplifier for recording rapid changes in membrane potential during nerve impulse transmission.

2. Electronic amplifier. This device can magnify the potential changes of the tissue to more than thousand times so that these can be recorded on the oscilloscope screen.

3. Cathode ray oscilloscope. CRO is almost an inertialess instrument which can record and measure the electrical events of living tissues instantaneously. It primarily consists of a glass tube with a cathode, fluorescent surface (screen) and two sets of electrically charged plates (Fig. 2.1.20).

Cathode is in the form of an electronic gun. When connected to a suitable anode and electric current is passed, the electronic gun emits electrons.

Fluorescent surface (the face of glass tube coated with fluorescent material) acts as a screen. The electrons emitted from the cathode are directed into a beam which hits this screen.

Electrically charged plates are arranged in two sets: vertical and horizontal.

- *Horizontal deflection plates* are placed on either side of the electron beam. These are connected to sweep generator (*electronic sweep circuit*). When a voltage is applied across these plates, the beam of electrons (being negatively charged) is attracted towards the positively charged plate and repelled away by the negatively charged plate. If 'sawtooth voltage' (i.e. voltage increased slowly, then suddenly reduced, and again slowly increased) is applied, the electron beam will steadily move towards the positively charged plate (with slowly increasing voltage), then back to its original position (with sudden reduction in the voltage), and again move towards the positively charged plate. In this way, the electron beam is

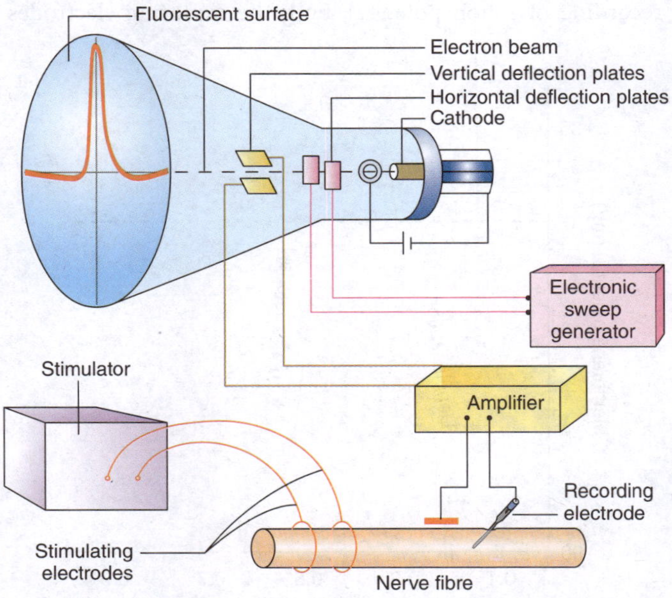

Fig. 2.1.20 Cathode ray oscilloscope and simplified diagram to record action potential from a nerve fibre.

made to sweep across the fluorescent screen horizontally, which will give a continuous marking of line of glowing light.

- *Vertical deflection plates* are placed above and below the electron beam. These are connected to recording electrodes placed on the nerve through an electronic amplifier. The potential change occurring in the nerve will charge these plates which will cause vertical (upward and downward) deflection of the electron beam. The magnitude of deflection will be proportional to the potential difference between the two plates. Thus, action potential is recorded as vertical deflection of the beam as it moves across the fluorescent screen of the CRO.

Recording of Resting Membrane Potential

The arrangement of electrodes for recording membrane potential is shown in Fig. 2.1.7. The electrical potential is recorded at the surface of the membrane (exterior) and inside the membrane at each point in a nerve fibre. Starting from one end of the nerve fibre (left side of the figure) and passing to the other end (right side) and when both the electrodes (indifferent and microelectrodes) are on the surface (outside) of the nerve fibre membrane, no potential difference was recorded (zero potential), which is potential of ECF. However, when microelectrode is made to penetrate into the interior of cell, a constant potential difference (−70 mV) is observed. This is known as RMP (Fig. 2.1.7).

Recording of Action Potential

Monophasic recording of action potential. For monophasic recording of action potential, one microelectrode is placed inside the nerve fibre and the other electrode on the outside surface. These electrodes are then connected to the CRO (Fig. 2.1.20). When the nerve is stimulated, as shown in Fig. 2.1.21, a typical monophasic record of action potential obtained has the following components:

- Depolarization
- Repolarization

It has been described in detail on page 59.

Biphasic recording of action potential. For biphasic recording of action potential, both the exploring electrodes

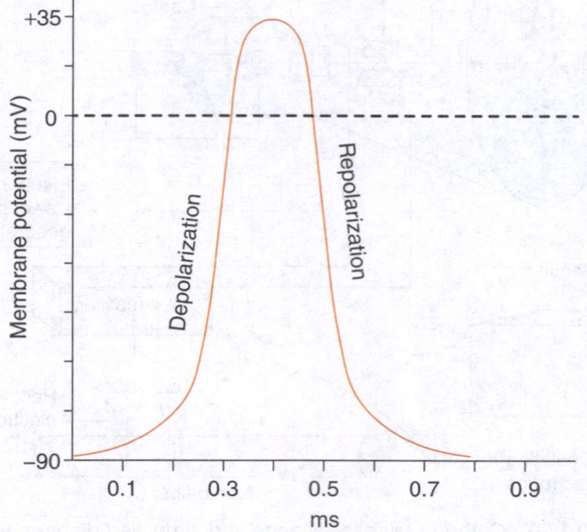

Fig. 2.1.21 A typical monophasic record of action potential.

(x and y) are placed on the outside surface of nerve fibre, and they are connected to a CRO (Fig. 2.1.22). When the nerve is stimulated, the excitation of one electrode will cause deflection opposite to that of another during the passage of impulse. Record of this alternate deflection (one negative below the baseline and one positive above the baseline, called *biphasic action potential*) is depicted as follows:

- During *resting state*, only baseline is recorded as both electrodes are equipotential (Fig. 2.1.22A).
- When a threshold stimulus is applied, an action potential is initiated and first the membrane under electrode x gets depolarized (outside −ve) but the membrane under electrode y is still polarized (outside +ve). Because of the potential difference between the two electrodes, a downstroke is recorded by CRO (Fig. 2.1.22B).
- When impulse passes beyond 'x' but has not reached 'y', and membrane under electrode x is repolarized (outside +ve), the record comes back to a baseline as again the membrane under the two electrodes becomes equipotential (Fig. 2.1.22C).
- As shown in Fig. 2.1.22D, when the impulse reaches y electrode, the membrane under it gets depolarized (outside −ve). Since at x the membrane is repolarized (outside +ve), the potential difference between the two electrodes is recorded as upstroke by CRO.
- When impulse passes beyond 'y', and membrane under it is repolarized (outside +ve), once again the record comes to baseline as both electrodes are again equipotential (Fig. 2.1.22A).
- A typical complete record of biphasic action potential is shown in Fig. 2.1.23.

Advantages of biphasic recording are:

- Comparatively easy process, since both the electrodes are placed on the outside surface of the nerve.
- Propagation of action potential can also be recorded.

Disadvantages of biphasic recording are:

- Graph obtained is variable depending on the distance between the electrodes and the rate of conduction of impulse in the nerve fibre.
- Proper analysis of action potential cannot be done as can be done in monophasic recording.
- Potential difference recorded is somewhat smaller than actual, as nerve fibre has to be kept in a solution to prevent drying.

COMPOUND ACTION POTENTIAL AND ITS RECORDING

Compound action potential is the monophasic recording of action potential from a *mixed* nerve which contains different types of nerve fibres with varying diameter. Therefore, the compound action potential represents an algebraic summation of the all-or-none action potentials of many axons.

Response of a mixed nerve to stimulus Response of a mixed nerve to a stimulus will depend on the thresholds of the individual axon in the nerve and their distance from the stimulating electrode as follows (Fig. 2.1.24):

Subthreshold stimulus stimulates none of the axons and thus no response is observed.

Threshold intensity stimulus makes the axons with low threshold to fire and thus a small potential change is observed.

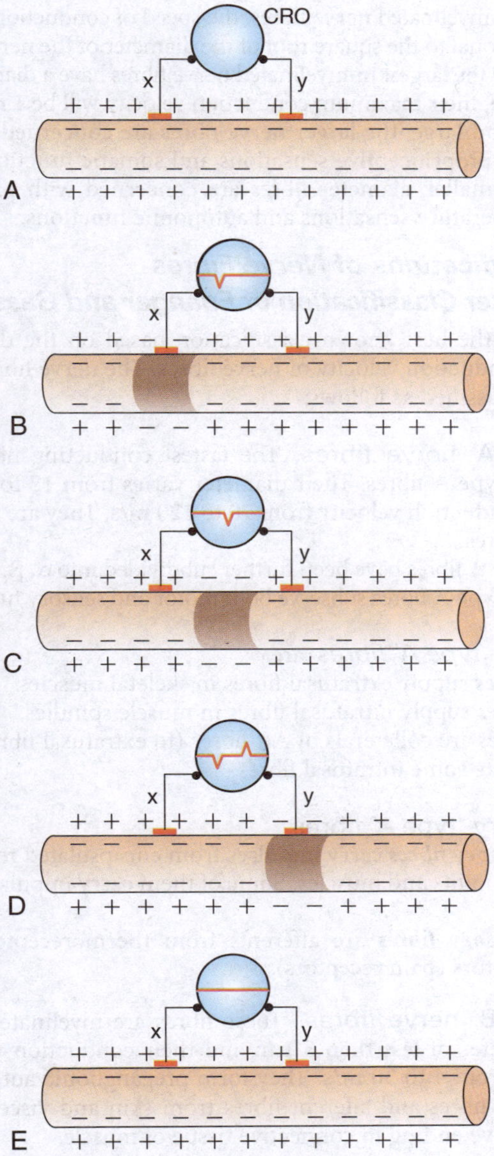

Fig. 2.1.22 Arrangement for recording biphasic action potential (recording electrodes x and y are on the surface of nerve fibre connected to cathode ray oscilloscope): **A**, resting state; **B**, on stimulation when wave of excitation reaches electrode 'x'; **C**, when impulse passes beyond electrode 'x'; **D**, when impulse reaches electrode 'y'; and **E**, when impulse passes away from electrode 'y'.

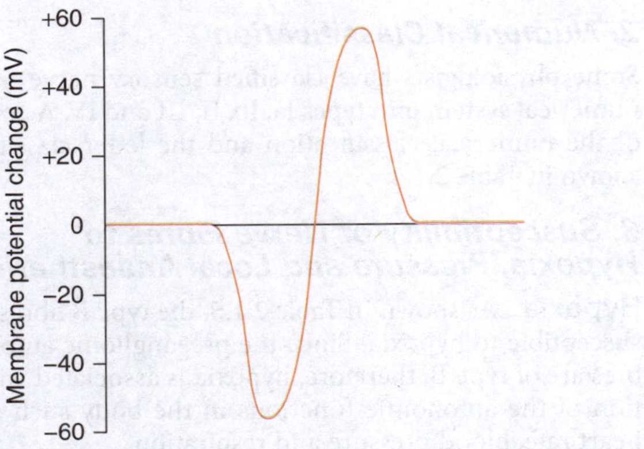

Fig. 2.1.23 A typical complete record of biphasic action potential.

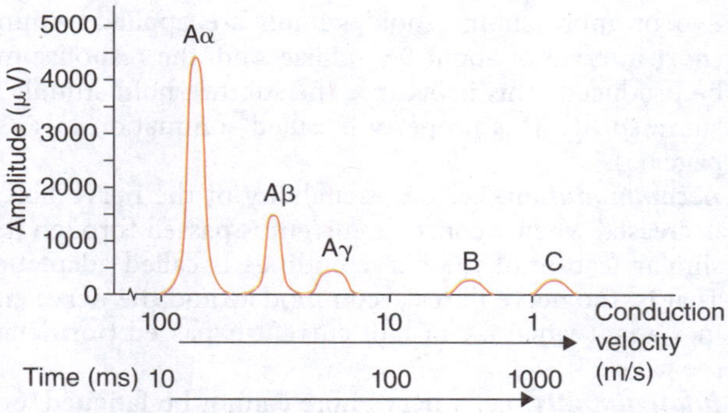

Fig. 2.1.24 Typical record of compound action potential (recorded from a mixed nerve) showing multiple peaks.

With further increase in the intensity of stimulus, the axons with higher thresholds also fire. The electrical response increases proportionately until the stimulus is strong enough to excite all of the axons in the nerve. The stimulus which excites all the axons is called *maximal stimulus*.

Supramaximal stimulus does not produce any further increase in the potential.

Features of a compound action potential

- It has a unique shape (multiple peaks), because a mixed nerve is made up of different fibres with various speeds of conduction.
- The number and size of the peaks vary with the types of fibres in the particular nerve being studied.
- When less than maximal stimuli are used, the shape of compound action will depend on the number and type of fibres stimulated.
- Thus, a typical record of compound action potential will contain three different curves labelled as α, β and γ (Fig. 2.1.24).

PHYSIOLOGICAL PROPERTIES OF NERVE FIBRES

The properties of the nerve fibres are mainly because of the nerve cells being excitable tissue, i.e. having a low threshold for excitation. Therefore, the main properties of the nervous tissue are excitability and conductivity and all other properties are secondary to these. After studying the electrical activities of the nerve fibres in detail, their important physiological properties can be summarized as follows:

1. ***Excitability***, i.e. the nerve fibres when stimulated produce waves of depolarization, called *excitation impulse* (for details, see page 58).
2. ***All-and-none response***, i.e. when stimulated, the nerve fibre either shows no excitation or responds to the maximum of its ability (for details, see page 62).
3. ***Refractory period***, i.e. when the nerve fibre is stimulated by two successive stimuli of more than threshold intensity:
   - It responds to the first stimulus.
   - It is unable to respond to the second stimulus for quite some time, called the refractory period (for details, see page 62).
4. ***Summation***, i.e. response to the successive subthreshold stimuli can be summated. When one subthreshold stimulus is applied, the nerve fibre does not respond. However, if

two or more subthreshold stimuli are applied within a short interval of about 0.5 millisecond, the response may be produced. This is because the subthreshold stimuli are summed up. This property is called summation (also see page 65).

5. ***Accommodation***, i.e. the excitability of the nerve fibre is decreased when a constant current is passed through it. A similar feature of the nerve endings is called adaptation. That is, the nerve fibres accommodate and the nerve endings adapt when a constant current is passed (for details, see page 63).
6. ***Infatiguability***, i.e. a nerve fibre cannot be fatigued, even if it is stimulated continuously for a long time (also see page 64).
7. ***Conductivity***, i.e. the nerve fibres possess the ability to transmit the excitation impulse along their entire length (for details, see page 65).

NERVE FIBRE TYPES

Various schemes for classification of nerve fibres on the basis of their diameter and their conduction velocity have been proposed. The best known classification is of Erlanger and Gasser. Before discussing this important classification, it will be useful to be familiar with the various terminologies used in relation to nerve fibres and certain facts about the conduction velocity in nerve fibres.

Terminology Used in Relation to Nerve Fibres

Myelinated versus nonmyelinated fibres. The myelinated nerve fibres are covered by a myelin sheath while the nonmyelinated nerve fibres have no such sheath.

Somatic versus visceral nerve fibres. Somatic nerve fibres supply the skeletal muscles of the body while visceral nerve fibres supply the various internal organs (viscera).

Cranial versus spinal nerves. Nerve fibres arising from the brain form the cranial nerves while those arising from the spinal cord form the spinal nerves.

Motor versus sensory nerve fibres. Motor nerve fibres, also known as *efferent fibres*, carry motor impulses from CNS to different parts of the body. The sensory nerve fibres, also known as *afferent fibres*, carry sensory impulses from different parts of the body to CNS.

Adrenergic versus cholinergic nerve fibres. Adrenergic nerve fibres secrete noradrenaline while cholinergic fibres secrete acetylcholine as neurotransmitter.

Certain Facts About the Conduction Velocity in Nerve Fibres

- Fibres of larger diameter conduct impulses more rapidly than those of smaller diameter.
- The impulse conducted through larger diameter nerve fibres will have greater magnitude and lesser duration of spike, lesser threshold of excitation and lesser refractory period, as compared to the impulses conducted through nerve fibres of smaller diameter.
- The speed of conduction is about six times the diameter of a myelinated nerve fibres. Since the diameter of myelinated nerve fibres varies from 1 to 20 μm, the conduction velocity will vary from 6 to 120 m/s.
- In unmyelinated nerve fibres, the speed of conduction is proportional to the square root of the diameter of the nerve fibre. Since the largest unmyelinated nerve fibres have a diameter of 1 μm, their maximum conduction velocity will be 1 m/s.
- By and large, the larger nerve fibres are concerned mainly with proprioceptive sensations and somatic functions, and the smaller diameter fibres are concerned with pain and temperature sensations and autonomic functions.

Classifications of Nerve Fibres

1. Letter Classification of Erlanger and Gasser

This is the best known classification based on the diameter and conduction velocity of nerve fibres. The nerve fibres have been classified as follows:

'Type A' nerve fibres. The fastest conducting fibres are called type A fibres. Their diameter varies from 12 to 20 μm and conduction velocity from 70 to 120 m/s. They are myelinated fibres.

Type A fibres have been further subdivided into α, β, γ and δ fibres. Type A fibres subserve both motor and sensory functions.

Motor 'type A' fibres are:

Aα fibres supply extrafusal fibres in skeletal muscles.

Aγ fibres supply intrafusal fibres in muscle spindles.

Aδ fibres are collaterals of Aα fibres (to extrafusal fibres) that innervate some intrafusal fibres.

Sensory 'type A' fibres

Aα sensory fibres carry impulses from encapsulated receptors in skin, joints and muscles. Some of them carry impulses from the gut.

Aδ sensory fibres are afferents from thermoreceptors and nociceptors (pain receptors).

'Type B' nerve fibres. These fibres are myelinated, have a diameter of less than 3 μm and their conduction velocity varies from 4 to 30 m/s. They form preganglionic autonomic efferent fibres and afferent fibres from skin and viscera, and free nerve ending in connective tissue of muscle.

'Type C' nerve fibres. These are unmyelinated, have a diameter of 0.4–1.2 μm and their conduction velocity varies from 0.5 to 4 m/s. These form the postganglionic autonomic fibres, some sensory fibres carrying pain sensations, some fibres from thermoreceptors and some from viscera.

The salient features of type A, B and C nerve fibres are summarized in Table 2.1.3.

2. Numerical Classification

Some physiologists have classified sensory nerve fibres by a numerical system into types Ia, Ib, II, III and IV. A comparison of the numerical classification and the letter classification is shown in Table 2.1.4.

3. Susceptibility of Nerve Fibres to Hypoxia, Pressure and Local Anaesthetics

Hypoxia. As shown in Table 2.1.5, the type B fibres are most susceptible to hypoxia. Since the preganglionic autonomic fibres are of type B, therefore, hypoxia is associated with alteration of the autonomic functions in the body such as rise in heart rate, blood pressure and respiration.

Table 2.1.3 Salient features of type A, B and C nerve fibres

Fibre	Type	Myelinated/ nonmyelinated	Fibre diameter (μm)	Conduction velocity (m/s)	Spike duration (ms)	Absolute refractory period (ms)	Functions: Efferent	Functions: Afferent
A	α	Myelinated	12–20	70–120	0.4–0.5	0.4–1	Somatic motor	Proprioception
	β	Myelinated	5–12	30–70	0.4–0.5	0.4–1	–	Touch and pressure
	γ	Myelinated	3–6	15–30	0.4–0.5	0.4–1	Motor to muscle spindles	–
	δ	Myelinated	2–5	12–30	0.4–0.5	0.4–1	–	Pain, cold and touch
B	–	Myelinated	<3	3–15	1.2	1.2	Preganglionic autonomic	–
C	–	Nonmyelinated	0.4–1.2	0.5–2	2	2	Postganglionic autonomic (sympathetic)	Pain, temperature, some mechanoreceptors and reflex responses

Table 2.1.4 Numerical vis-à-vis letter classification of sensory nerve fibres

Types of nerve fibre: Numerical classification	Letter classification	Origin
Ia	Aα	Muscle spindle (annulospiral endings)
Ib	Aα	Golgi tendon organ
II	Aβ	Muscle spindle (flower spray endings), touch and pressure
III	Aδ	Pain and cold receptors, some touch receptors
IV	C	Pain, temperature and other receptors

Pressure. Type A fibres are most susceptible to pressure and the type C least. Therefore, pressure on a nerve can produce temporary paralysis due to loss of conduction in motor, touch and pressure fibres (type A), while pain sensation (carried by type C fibres) remains relatively intact. This is a common observation after sitting cross-legged for long periods and after sleeping with arms under the head.

Local anaesthetics. Type C fibres (conducting pain, touch and temperature sensations generated by cutaneous receptors) are most susceptible to local anaesthetics. This fact is useful for surgical interventions under local anaesthesia.

DEGENERATION AND REGENERATION OF NEURONS

When the axon of neuron is injured, a series of degenerative changes are seen at three levels:

- In the axon distal to injury
- In the axon proximal to injury
- In the cell body

Table 2.1.5 Susceptibility of nerve fibres to hypoxia, pressure and local anaesthetics

Sensitivity to	Type of nerve fibre: Most susceptible	Intermediate susceptible	Least susceptible
Hypoxia	B	A	C
Pressure	A	B	C
Local anaesthetics	C	B	A

Along with the degenerative changes, the reparative process (regeneration) also starts soon if the circumstances are favourable. The effects of injury to a nerve and the occurrence of regenerative changes thereafter will depend on the degree and type of damage.

GRADING OF NERVE INJURY

Common causes of nerve injury are transection (through and through cut), crushing of nerve fibres, local injection of toxic substances, ischaemia due to obstruction of blood flow and effects of hyperpyrexia on the neurons. For grading/classification of nerve injury, two systems exist: Seddon classification system (1942) and Sunderland classification system (1951).

Seddon Classification

According to Seddon system, the nerve injury is presented in three forms:

I. Neurapraxia
II. Axonotmesis
III. Neurotmesis

Neurapraxia (transient block)

- This is the mildest form of nerve injury, in which some type of sensory and motor loss occurs. There is reversible physiological conduction block.
- It occurs due to mechanical pressure causing regional demyelination.

- Spontaneous recovery occurs after few days/weeks.
- Typically seen in crush palsy/pressure palsy (in state of drunkenness, Saturday night palsy and in mild type of tourniquet palsy).

Axonotmesis (lesion in continuity)

- This is more severe injury than neurapraxia. Axonotmesis usually occurs due to crush injury.
- There is complete interruption of axon, so there is loss of conduction in the nerve fibre.
- The neural connective tissues (myelin sheath, endoneurium and perineurium) are intact and functional.
- Wallerian degeneration occurs because of loss of axonal flow.
- Regeneration occurs at the rate of 1.5–3 mm/day.
- Recovery occurs within weeks/months.

Neurotmesis (division of a nerve)

- This is most severe form of nerve injury.
- If nerve is completely transected, then no recovery is possible unless surgically resutured.
- Histologically all supportive neural connective tissues are destroyed.
- Recovery is unpredictable.

Sunderland Classification

Sunderland had graded the injury to nerve fibres in order of severity into the following degrees:

First-degree injury involves only transient loss of function resulting from a mild pressure on the nerve. The temporary loss of function is caused by local anoxia produced by ischaemia following obstruction to the blood flow. The lost function of the nerve fibres returns within few hours to few weeks of the removal of the causative pressure, since the axon is not destroyed.

Second-degree injury includes severe nerve damage with intact endoneural tube. It results from a severe and prolonged pressure on the nerve. The nerve fibre is severely damaged at the pressure point and is followed by degenerative changes. However, the regeneration and restoration of the function of the nerve are facilitated as the endoneural tube remains intact.

Third-degree injury includes severe damage to the nerve fibre with interruption of the endoneural tube.

Fourth-degree injury refers to a severe damage to the nerve fibres associated with disorganization of nerve fasciculi.

Fifth-degree injury is labelled when there occurs complete transection, i.e. the nerve fibres are cut through and through. Degenerative changes are initiated very early following fifth-degree injury to the nerve fibres.

It is however important to note that any nerve injury is usually mixed. Both Seddon and Sunderland classifications are depicted in Table 2.1.6.

STAGE OF DEGENERATION

The degenerative changes which occur in the part of axon distal to the site of injury are referred to as *anterograde degeneration* or Wallerian degeneration (after the discoverer A. Waller, 1862). The degenerative changes occurring in the neuron proximal to the injury are referred to as *retrograde degeneration*. These changes take place in the cell body and in the axon proximal to injury.

Changes in The Part of Axon Distal to Injury

Degenerative changes in the part of axon distal to injury, also known as anterograde degeneration or Wallerian degeneration, occur within few hours of injury. The changes take place in the entire length of this part of the axon simultaneously. The degeneration changes start within few hours of injury and continue for about 3 months and include the following (Fig. 2.1.25).

Axis cylinder. Axis cylinder becomes swollen and irregular in shape within a few hours of injury. After a few days, it breaks up into small fragments; the neurofibrils within it break down into granular debris and are seen in the space occupied by axis cylinder.

Myelin sheath shows slow disintegration which starts on the 8th day and continues up to the 32nd to 35th days. In fact,

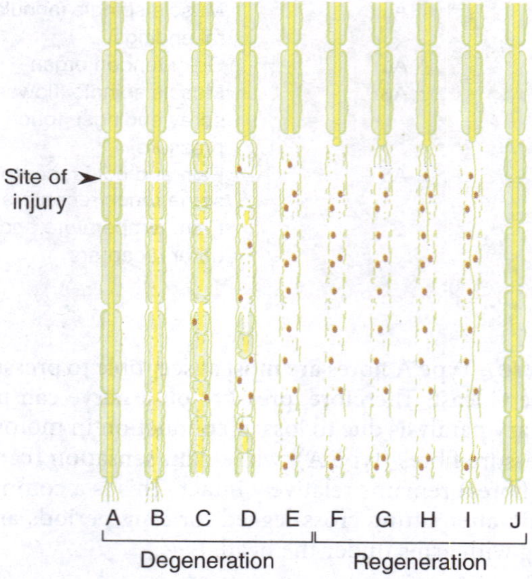

Fig. 2.1.25 Degenerative changes (Wallerian degeneration) in distal part of a nerve fibre after injury **A–E,** and subsequent regenerative changes **F–J.**

Table 2.1.6 Sunderland versus Seddon classification of nerve injury

	Damage				
	Myelination	**Axonal damage**	**Axon and endoneurium**	**Axon + endoneurium − perineurium**	**Axon + endoneurium + perineurium**
Sunderland (1951)	I	II	III	IV	V
Seddon (1942)	Neurapraxia	Axonotmesis, lesion in continuity	Neurotmesis (division of nerve)		

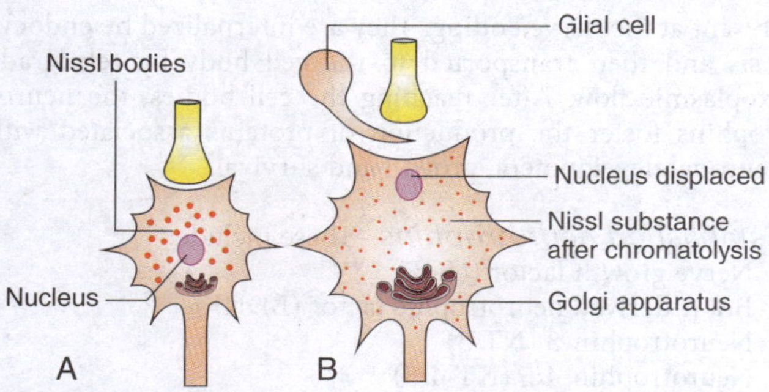

Fig. 2.1.26 Changes in cell body of a neuron after injury **B,** and normal cell body of a neuron **A**.

myelin sheath is converted into fat droplets containing cholesterol esters.

Neurilemmal sheath is usually unaffected but the Schwann cells start multiplying rapidly.

Macrophages invade the region and remove degenerating axons, myelin and cellular debris and thus the neurilemmal tube becomes empty (ghost tubes).

Schwann cell's cytoplasm proliferates rapidly and fills up the empty neurilemmal tube. These cells produce a large series of membranes that help to form numerous tubes which play a vital role in the regeneration of nerve fibres.

Changes in the Cell Body of Neuron

Changes in the cell body of the injured neuron start within 48 hours and continue up to 15–20 days. The changes are as follows (Fig. 2.1.26):

Nissl substances undergo disintegration and dissolution (*chromatolysis*). The process of chromatolysis starts around the nucleus and spreads in the periphery.

Golgi apparatus, mitochondria and neurofibrils are fragmented and eventually disappear.

Cell body draws in more fluid, enlarges and becomes spherical.

Nucleus is displaced to the periphery (towards cell membrane). Sometimes, the nucleus is extruded out of the cell, in which case the neuron atrophies and finally disappears completely.

Severity of degenerative changes in the cell body. Severity of degenerative changes in the cell body is variable. The changes are more severe when the injury to the axon is near the cell body, and when the injury is caused by a forcible tear rather than a sharp cut. In some cases, the chromatolysis ends in cell death followed by degeneration of all its processes. If the cell survives, the changes described above are reversed after a period of time.

Changes in the Part of Axon Proximal to Injury

Changes in the part of axon proximal to injury occur only up to the first or second node of Ranvier near the injury and are similar to the changes seen in the distal part of the axon. Changes seen in the proximal part of axon along with those seen in the cell body of neuron constitute the *retrograde degeneration*.

Transneuronal degeneration. It is sometimes observed that changes resulting from axonal injury are not confined to the injured neuron, but extend to other neurons with which the injured neuron synapses. This phenomenon is referred to as *transneuronal degeneration*. The degeneration can extend through several synapses (as demonstrated in the visual pathway).

STAGE OF REGENERATION

The stage of degeneration is followed by stage of regeneration under favourable circumstances (listed below). It starts within 4 days of injury but becomes more active after 30 days and may take several months to 1 year for complete recovery.

Factors Affecting Regeneration

- Regeneration occurs more rapidly when a nerve is crushed than when it is severed and the cut ends are separated.
- Chances of regeneration of a cut nerve are considerably increased if the two cut ends are near each other (gap does not exceed 3 mm), and if scar tissue does not intervene between them.
- Chances of regeneration are more if the two cut ends remain in the same line, and are not moved away from each other.
- Presence of neurilemma is a must for regeneration to occur. Therefore, axons in CNS once degenerated never regenerate as these nerve fibres have no neurilemma.
- Presence of nucleus in the neuron cell body is also a must for regeneration to occur. If it is extruded, the neuron is atrophied and the regeneration does not occur.

Regenerative Changes

Anatomical Regeneration

1. Changes in the axon occur in stages:

Stage of fibre formation Axis cylinder from the proximal cut end of the axon elongates and gives out fibrils up to 100 in number in all directions. These branches grow into the connective tissue at the site of injury in an effort to reach the distal cut end of the nerve fibre (Fig. 2.1.25F and G).

Stage of entry of fibrils into endoneural tube. Strands of Schwann cells from the distal cut end of axon guide the regenerating fibrils to enter their axon endoneural tube and once the fibril enters the endoneural tube, it grows rapidly within it. The rate of growth which is initially low (0.25 mm/day) increases rapidly once the regenerating axon enters the endoneural tube (3–4 mm/day). The axonal fibrils that fail to enter any one of the tubes degenerate. It often happens that more than one fibril (1–25) enters the same tube. Under such circumstances, the largest fibril survives and the rest degenerate.

Stage of active growth. The axonal fibril growing through the endoneural tube enlarges and establishes contact with an appropriate peripheral end organ. The new axon formed in this way is devoid of myelin sheath (Fig. 2.1.25H and I). The process of regeneration up to this stage takes about 3 months.

Stage of myelination. The myelin sheath is then formed by the cells of Schwann slowly. The myelination is completed in 1 year. Thus, there occurs a progressive increase in the thickness of nerve fibre. The regenerated nerve fibre, however, obtains only 80% of the original diameter.

2. Changes in the cell body of neuron occur as:

- Nissl granules followed by Golgi apparatus appear in the cell body.
- The cell loses excess fluid and regains its normal size.
- The nucleus occupies the central position.

The above-mentioned changes in some of the neurons start within 20 days of injury and are completed in 80 days. Regenerative changes in the cell body may occur, even when the axon does not regenerate.

Functional Regeneration

The above-described regenerative changes constitute anatomical regeneration. The functional (physiological) recovery, however, occurs after a long period.

Important Notes

Axonal regeneration is promoted by growth-promoting factor secreted by Schwann cell and adhesion molecules of immunoglobulin family neural cell adenosonian molecules (NCAMs).

- In CNS, the neurons do not require a growth-promoting factor for regeneration.
- Events such as astrocyte proliferation, microglial activation, scar formation and inflammatory reaction following CNS injury are unfavourable for regeneration.

COMPLICATIONS FOLLOWING NERVE INJURY

1. ***Complete atrophy*** of the nerve fibre occurs in severe injuries where regeneration does not occur due to absence of favourable circumstances.
2. ***Functional complications*** in the form of misinterpretation of sensations occur when the fibrils do not enter the appropriate tubes and thus there are faulty connections.
3. ***Neuroma formation*** occurs if during regeneration, the gap between two cut ends is too large and the nerve fibrils growing from the proximal cut end of axon do not find their way. Under such circumstances, the fibrils turn around in search of the endoneural tube in a whorl-like mass known as *neuroma*, which may be quite painful.

Phantom limb. is a feeling sometimes perceived by a patient following amputation of the limb. Neuroma, developed at the site of amputation, when excited, causes the patient to feel like the lost limb is present (a feeling of phantom limb).

FACTORS PROMOTING NEURONAL GROWTH

Various factors affecting neuronal development, growth and survival have been isolated and studied. These can be broadly arranged into two groups:

- Neurotrophins
- Other factors affecting neuronal growth

NEUROTROPHINS

Neurotrophins are the proteins which provide trophic support to the neurons, i.e. they promote nerve growth and survival. They also have a role in neuronal plasticity.

Production. The neurotrophins are produced by the muscles or other structures, especially the glands that the neurons innervate. Some of the neurotrophins are produced by the astrocytes.

Transport. The neurotrophins produced by various structures innervated by a particular neuron bind to the receptors present at the nerve ending. They are internalized by endocytosis and then transported to the cell body by retrograde axoplasmic flow. After reaching the cell bodies, the neurotrophins foster the production of proteins associated with neuronal development, growth and survival.

Established neurotrophins. These include:

- Nerve growth factor (NGF)
- Brain-derived neurotrophic factor (BDNF)
- Neurotrophin-3 (NT-3)
- Neurotrophin-4/5 (NT-4/5)

1. ***Nerve growth factor***. NGF is probably the first neurotrophin recognized. It promotes the growth of *sympathetic nerves and* some sensory nerves.
   - It is found in various tissues in human beings and many species of animals. NGF is particularly found in high concentration in the submaxillary salivary glands of the male mice.
   - NGF is made up of 2α, 2β and 2γ subunits.
     - The α subunits have trypsin-like activity.
     - The β subunits are similar in structure to insulin and possess all the nerve growth–promoting activities.
     - The γ subunits are serine proteases. Their functions are unknown.
   - Receptor of NGF is TrkA (tyrosine kinase activity A).
   - A low-affinity NGF receptor called $P75^{NTR}$ forms a heterodimer with TrkA receptors, and increases the affinity and specificity for NGF. However, in the absence of Trk receptors, it forms homodimer, which causes apoptosis.
   - NGF is also present in the brain and appears to be responsible for the growth and maintenance of cholinergic neurons in the basal forebrain and striatum.
   - Immunosympathectomy, i.e. complete destruction of the sympathetic ganglia, is produced when antiserum against NGF is injected in a newborn animal.
2. ***Brain-derived neurotrophic factor***
   - It has a growth-promoting role for peripheral sensory nerves, since it has been seen that BDNF-deficient mice lose peripheral sensory nerves and have severe degenerative changes in their vestibular ganglia.
   - Receptor for BDNF is TrkB.
3. ***Neurotrophin-3***
   - The NT-3 plays a growth-promoting role in cutaneous mechanoreceptors, since its disruption by gene knockout gives rise to marked loss of these receptors.
   - Receptors for NT-3 are TrkC (mainly) and TrkA and B (to some extent).
4. ***Neurotrophin-4/5***
   NT-4/5 is important for growth of neurons that innervate the hair follicles.
   - Receptor for NT-4/5 is TrkB.

OTHER GROWTH-PROMOTING FACTORS

Factors, other than neurotrophins, which promote nerve growth include:

Ciliary neurotrophic factor (CNTF). It is produced by Schwann cells and astrocytes and plays a growth-promoting role in lesioned and embryonic spinal cord neurons. It is believed that it may be of some value in treating human diseases in which motor neurons degenerate are the following:

Leukaemia inhibitory factor (LIF)
Insulin-like growth factor-I (IGF-I)

Transforming growth factor (TGF)
Fibroblast growth factor (FGF)
Platelet-derived growth factor (PDGF)

MECHANISM AND PHYSIOLOGICAL SIGNIFICANCE OF GROWTH-PROMOTING FACTORS

The growth factors exert their growth-stimulating role by activating signalling molecules that control cellular responses through binding of transmembrane receptors on the target cells. For details, see page 656.

Important Note

Most of the growth factors have stimulating effect on cell division, differentiation and growth; however, some cytokines have negative effect and signal apoptosis (cellular death), e.g. Fas ligand.

Self-Assessment

1. Describe the structure and types of neuron.
2. Discuss the property of excitability and its ionic basis in a neuron.
3. How is the nerve impulse conducted in myelinated and nonmyelinated nerve fibres?
4. Mention the significance of the following:
   - Strength duration curve
   - All-or-none response
   - Property of refractory period
   - Infatiguability
5. Write notes on the following:
   - Compound action potential
   - Basis of classification of nerve fibres
   - Wallerian degeneration
   - Phases of action potential
   - Nerve growth factor

Clinical Cases

Case 1

A 46-year-old male patient came in the hospital with complaint of pain in the back of eyes on head movements, and muscle weakness. The patient is thoroughly examined and investigated by carrying out blood tests, nerve conduction velocity measurements and MRI, and diagnosed a case of multiple sclerosis (MS).

Q1. Explain the underlined pathophysiology of this condition.

Case 2

A young boy met an accident. For treatment, his right leg was amputated, and after few months there was formation of neuroma on the stump. Now he complains of pain sensation on movement in the part which is not present.

Q1. What is this condition?
Q2. What is the cause of false sensations?

Case 3

A 10-year-old boy brought to the emergency with a gaping wound on the thigh. The doctor sutured the wound after giving local anaesthesia.

Q1. What is the mechanism of action of local anaesthesia?
Q2. What type of nerve fibres are blocked by local anaesthesia?

Case 4

A 38-year-old male consumed alcohol in the night party and slept with his right arm hanging by the side of the couch. Next morning, he had numbness in the right upper limb and extending towards wrist and fingers.

Q1. What is this condition?
Q2. What is the synonym of this condition?
Q3. According to Seddon classification of nerve injury, this condition belongs to which form?

2.2 Neuromuscular Junction

CHAPTER OUTLINE

STRUCTURE OF NEUROMUSCULAR JUNCTION

Neuromuscular junction refers to the intimate contact of the nerve endings with the muscle fibre to which they innervate. Characteristics of the nerve and muscle fibre at and near the neuromuscular junction are given in Fig. 2.2.1.

Terminal button The axon of a neuron supplying a skeletal muscle loses its myelin sheath and divides into a number of fine branches that end in small swellings (knobs) called *terminal buttons* or end feet, which form a neuromuscular junction at the centre of muscle fibre (Fig. 2.2.1A). The nerve terminal or the so-called synaptic knob contains a large number of vesicles (about 3 lakh) containing acetylcholine (ACh). Mitochondria are also present in the nerve terminal. The ACh is synthesized by the mitochondria and is stored in the vesicles (Fig. 2.2.1B). The mitochondria contain adenosine triphosphate (ATP) which is the source of energy for synthesis of ACh.

Presynaptic membrane This refers to the axonal membrane lining the *terminal buttons* of the nerve endings.

Synaptic cleft It is a 50- to 100-nm-wide space between the presynaptic membrane and the postsynaptic membrane. It is filled by extracellular fluid with reticular fibres forming the matrix.

Postsynaptic membrane (Fig. 2.2.1B) This is the name given to the muscle fibre membrane (sarcolemma) in the region of neuromuscular junction. The muscle membrane in this region is thickened and depressed to form the *synaptic trough* in which the terminal button fits. This thickened portion of the muscle membrane is also called *motor endplate*. On each endplate, only one nerve fibre ends (like other synapses, there is no convergence of multiple inputs). Furthermore, the postsynaptic membrane is thrown into a large number of folds called *subneural clefts* or palisades. These increase the surface area. The postsynaptic membrane, near the junction folds, contains *receptor sites* for ACh called the *nicotinic–ACh receptors* (AChRs). The matrix of subneural cleft contains the enzyme cholinesterase which can degrade ACh.

NEUROMUSCULAR TRANSMISSION

The skeletal muscle is stimulated only through its nerve. The neuromuscular junction transmits the impulses from the nerve to muscle. The *sequence of events* which causes transmission of impulse through neuromuscular junction is as follows:

- Release of ACh by the nerve terminals
- Effect of ACh on postsynaptic membrane
- Development of endplate potential (EPP)
- Miniature EPP
- Removal of ACh by cholinesterase
- Initiation of the action potential in muscle fibre

Release of acetylcholine by the nerve terminals

When the nerve impulse (action potential) travelling in the nerve fibre (axon) reaches the terminal buttons, the voltage-gated Ca^{2+} channels present on the presynaptic membrane open up, increasing its permeability to Ca^{2+} ions. Consequently, the Ca^{2+} ions present in the ECF of synaptic cleft enter the terminal buttons.

The elevated Ca^{2+} levels in the cytosol of terminal buttons bring about a fusion of vesicles (containing ACh) with the presynaptic membrane and trigger a marked increase in exocytosis of vesicles releasing ACh in the synaptic cleft. Each vesicle contains about 10,000 molecules of ACh, and at a time about 125 vesicles burst by exocytosis (Fig. 2.2.2). Voltage-gated Ca^{2+} channels are present on the nerve terminal membrane.

Effect of acetylcholine on the postsynaptic membrane The ACh so released diffuses in the synaptic cleft and binds to the nicotinic–ACh receptors located mainly on the junctional folds of the motor endplate (postsynaptic membrane).

Each receptor is actually *an ACh-gated ion channel* (Fig. 2.2.3) made up of a protein complex having molecular weight of 275,000 and is composed of five subunits (two alpha and one each of beta, delta and gamma). This protein complex penetrates all the way through the membrane forming a tubular channel which is kept closed (Fig. 2.2.4A).

When two molecules of ACh get attached to the binding site of the receptors (i.e. two alpha units), there occurs a conformational change in the protein complex leading to opening up of the tubular channels (Fig. 2.2.4B). In other words, conductance to Na^{+} and Ca^{2+} ions is increased at the motor endplate.

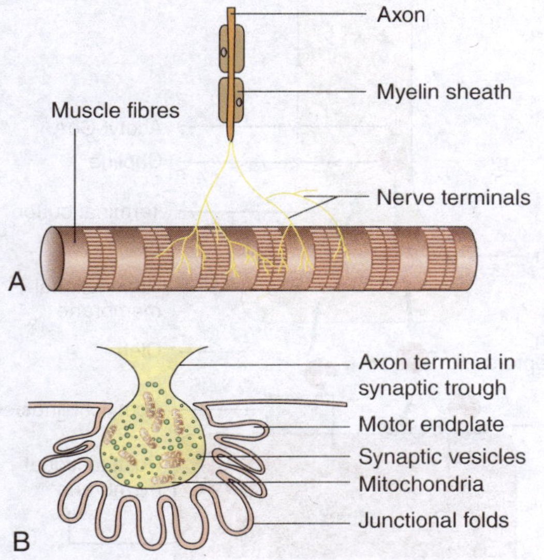

Fig. 2.2.1 Structure of neuromuscular junction: **A**, the axon of the neuron loses its myelin sheath and divides into fine branches; and **B**, structure of terminal button and motor endplate.

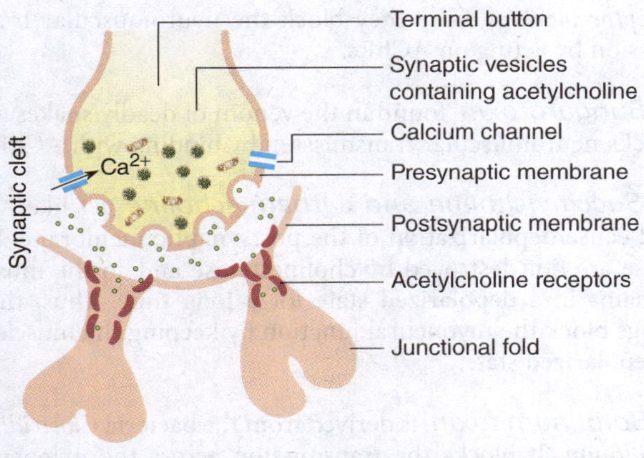

Fig. 2.2.2 Detailed structure of neuromuscular junction showing Ca^{2+} channels on presynaptic membrane and ACh receptors on postsynaptic membrane.

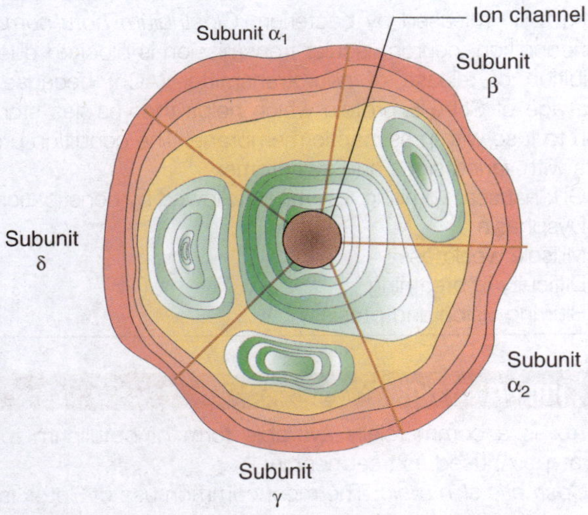

Fig. 2.2.3 Structure of acetylcholine receptor from below.

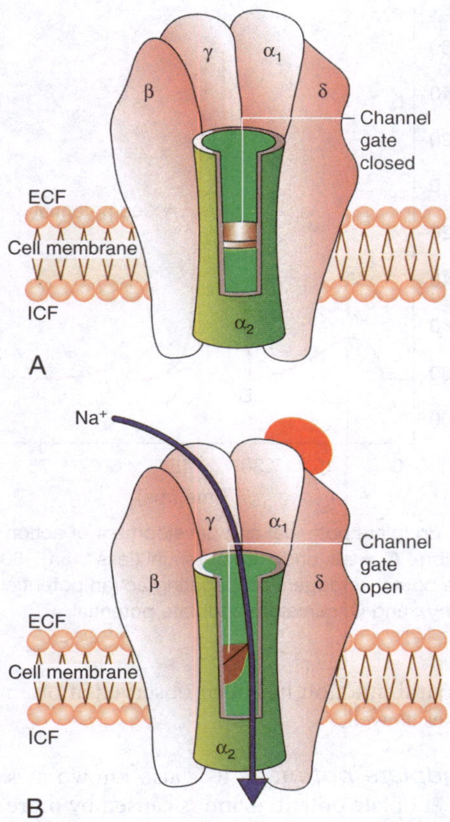

Fig. 2.2.4 Acetylcholine-gated ion channels: **A**, closed state; and **B**, open state (conformational change occurred due to binding of two molecules of ACh to the binding sites).

Development of endplate potential Due to opening of the ACh-gated channels in the endplate membrane, a large number of Na^+ ions from the ECF enter inside the muscle fibre following the electrochemical gradient.

The resting membrane potential at the postsynaptic membrane is about −80 to −90 mV. When sodium ions enter inside carrying with them large numbers of positive charges, there occurs depolarization causing a local positive potential change inside the muscle fibre membrane called the *EPP*.

Endplate potential It is not the action potential. It is localized and nonpropagated, does not obey the all-or-none law and decays exponentially away from the plate.

The EPP is nonpropagative, but when a critical level of −60 mV is reached, it triggers the development of action potential in the muscle fibre (Fig. 2.2.5). The action potentials are generated on either side of the endplate and are conducted away from the endplate in both the directions along the muscle fibres, thus causing muscle contraction.

Miniature endplate potential Even at rest, small quanta of ACh are released randomly from the nerve terminal. Each quantum of ACh produces a weak EPP of about 0.5 mV in magnitude. This is called *miniature EPP*. The size of the quanta of ACh released in this way varies directly with the Ca^{2+} concentration and inversely with the Mg^{2+} concentration at the endplate. The miniature EPP similar to that seen at

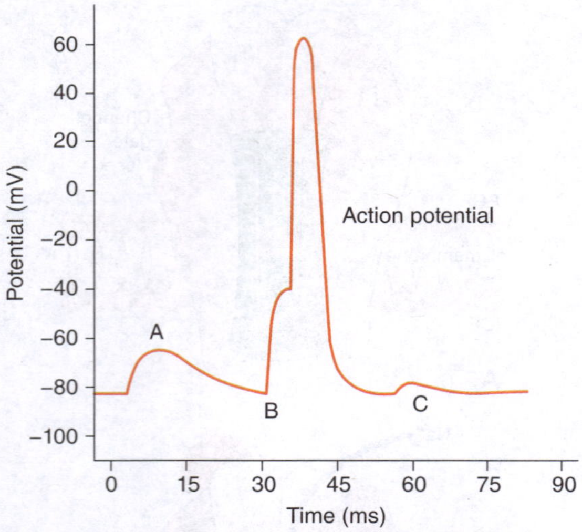

Fig. 2.2.5 Endplate potential and development of action potential in muscle fibre: **A**, weak endplate potential (less than −60 mV); **B**, endplate potential triggers propagating action potential (more than −60 mV); and **C**, miniature endplate potential.

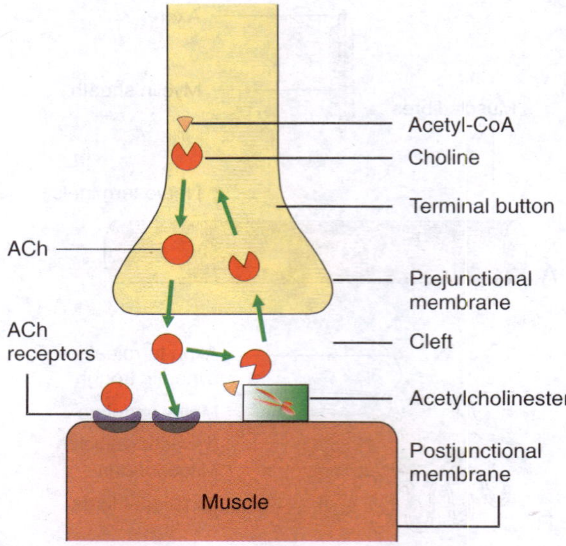

Fig. 2.2.6 Removal of acetylcholine from the synaptic cleft of neuromuscular junction.

the myoneural junction has been observed at other cholinergic synapses as well.

Giant endplate potential It is also known as slow-rising miniature endplate potential and is caused by more release of ACh. The endplate potential rises up to 12 mV, yet not sufficient to generate action potential, which is known as *giant endplate potential*.

Removal of acetylcholine ACh released in the synaptic cleft is removed within 1 millisecond by two means (Fig. 2.2.6):

- Most of the ACh is destroyed by the enzyme acetylcholinesterase which is present in the matrix of synaptic cleft.
- A small amount of the ACh diffuses out of the synaptic space and is then no longer available to act on the muscle fibre membrane.

The ACh is so potent that its stay in the synaptic space even for this short period of 1 millisecond is sufficient to excite the muscle fibre.

Important Note

It is important to note that the rapid removal of ACh prevents the repeated excitation of muscle fibre.

DRUGS AFFECTING NEUROMUSCULAR JUNCTION

Neuromuscular Blockers

Neuromuscular blockers are the drugs that block transmission at the neuromuscular junction. Some of the common neuromuscular blockers, which are commonly used, in clinical practice and in research are as follows:

1. Curare or the active principle of d-tubocurarine prevents the neuromuscular transmission by combining with AChRs. The ACh released thus cannot combine with the receptors and so the EPP does not develop. The curariform drugs are called *receptor blockers* since they block the neuromuscular transmission by acting on AChRs.

2. Bungarotoxin found in the venom of deadly snakes also blocks neuromuscular transmission by binding with AChRs.

3. Succinylcholine and carbamylcholine act like ACh and cause depolarization of the postsynaptic membrane. But these are not destroyed by cholinesterase and so the muscle remains in a depolarized state for a long time. Thus, these drugs block the myoneural junction by keeping the muscle in a depolarized state.

4. Botulinum toxin is derived from the bacteria *Clostridium botulinum*. It blocks the transmission across the myoneural junction by preventing the release of ACh from the terminal buttons of the nerve endings.

Applied Aspects

Botulism is a food-borne disease which occurs due to botulinum toxin released by bacterium *Clostridium botulinum*. In this condition, neuromuscular transmission is blocked due to inhibition of release of neurotransmitter (ACh) because of cleavage of SNARE protein which helps the vesicles storing ACh to fuse with presynaptic membrane. The condition presents with varied signs and symptoms:

- GIT: nausea, vomiting, diarrhoea followed by constipation
- Dysphasia
- Muscle weakness
- Difficulty in breathing
- Blurring vision and ptosis

Important Note

Botox is a commercially available form of botulinum toxin (serotype A) used as treatment in:

- *Cosmetic skin clinic:* The most common use of Botox is to minimize face wrinkles.

- *Neurology:* It is used for treatment of spasticity in patients suffering with multiple sclerosis.
- *Ophthalmology:* The most common oculoplastic application of Botox include blepharospasm (eye twitching) and strabismus/squint (disorder in which both eyes do not line up in same direction).

Neuromuscular stimulators

Drugs having acetylcholine-like action The drugs methacholine, carbachol and nicotine act like ACh and produce EPP exciting the muscle fibre. However, these drugs are either not destroyed or destroyed very slowly by the enzyme acetylcholinesterase. Hence, they cause repeated stimulation and continuous action of muscle, thereby causing a state of muscle spasm.

Drugs that inactivate the enzyme cholinesterase (anticholinesterase) The drugs like neostigmine, physostigmine and diisopropylfluorophosphate (DFP) stimulate the neuromuscular junction by inactivating the enzyme acetylcholinesterase. Once this enzyme is inactivated, the ACh released at the nerve terminal cannot be hydrolysed; this leads to repeated stimulation and continuous action of muscle.

The effect of neostigmine and physostigmine lasts for several hours while that of DFP lasts for several weeks. The DFP is thus a lethal poison which can cause death due to laryngeal spasm.

Black widow spider venom Its bite can be dangerous because the venom contains *α-latrotoxin, which* is a presynaptic neurotoxin. It exerts toxic effect by stimulating uncontrolled exocytosis of neurotransmitter from nerve terminals by increasing Ca^{2+} uptake.

Applied Aspects

Disorders of Neuromuscular Junction

Myasthenia Gravis

Myasthenia gravis (MG) is a disorder in which the myoneural junction is unable to transmit signals from the nerve fibre to muscle fibres, thereby causing paralysis of the involved muscles. The worldwide incidence of this disease is 25–125 of 100 million people. The disease is more common in women than men. Myasthenia is probably an autoimmune disease.

Pathophysiology. In this disease, 85% of the patients of MG have autoantibodies against ACh receptors (ACH are voltage-gated channels present on the motor endplate), which are destroyed by these antibodies. Thus, the ACh released at the nerve terminal is not able to produce adequate EPP to excite the muscle fibre. Depending on the presence/absence of antibodies against AChRs, there are two groups of patients with myasthenia: seropositive MG group and seronegative MG (SNMG) group.

- In SNMG, though antibodies against AChR are absent, in 70% of SNMG cases, IgG antibodies to muscle-specific kinase (MuSK) have been identified.
- In severe cases of MG, thymus may play a role by supplying helper T cells sensitized against thymic protein that cross-react with nicotinic–AChRs and destroy them. Studies show that the number of receptors on motor endplates of affected muscle is reduced by 70%–90%.

Clinical Features. The main clinical feature of the disease is muscle fatigue with sustained or repeated activity. It is usually presented in the following forms:

- In one form, mainly extraocular muscles are involved, and in the other form there is generalized weakness of skeletal muscles.
- If the disease is intense enough, then patient dies due to paralysis of respiratory muscles.

The characteristic features are as follows:

- Difficulty in talking, swallowing and breathing
- Problem in walking up the stairs
- Facial paralysis, hoarse voice
- Drooping of eyelids (ptosis) and double vision (diplopia)

Treatment Weakness of the muscles improves after a period of rest or administration of drugs.

i. ***Commonly used drugs are:***
   - *Acetylcholinesterase inhibitors.* Commonly recommended ACh esterase inhibitors are neostigmine and pyridostigmine
   - *Immunosuppressants* such as corticosteroids
   - *Non-immunosuppressants* like azathioprine, methotrexate and cyclosporine

   Note: These medications do not cure the disease but help to improve the symptoms.
ii. ***Surgical removal of thymus*** (thymectomy) may also improve the symptoms.
iii. ***Plasmapheresis*** to remove antibodies.

Lambert–Eaton myasthenic syndrome (LEMS)

It is a rare neuromuscular disorder. In this disease, antibodies are produced against the calcium channels present on the presynaptic membrane, which destroy the channels. Consequently, Ca^{2+} influx into the nerve terminal is markedly decreased and thereby release of ACh is also reduced. Scanty amount of ACh is not able to produce adequate EPP to excite muscle fibres, producing muscular weakness. It is most often seen in people with small-cell lung cancer. A similar type of syndrome can also occur after the use of aminoglycoside antibiotics which impair the functioning of Ca^{2+} at nerve terminals.

Sign and symptoms. LEMS can affect many muscles but usually it causes weakness of proximal muscles of lower limbs. Weakness is often relieved temporarily after exercise or exertion. The characteristic features of LEMS include the following:

- Difficulty in walking
- Tingling sensations in the hands or feet
- Drooping eyelids
- Fatigue
- Dry mouth
- Difficulty in speaking and swallowing
- Bladder and bowel changes
- Erectile dysfunction

Treatment

- The initial therapy is with agents that increase the release of ACh across the neuromuscular junction or by decreasing the action of ACh esterase (e.g. pyridostigmine).
- Anti-inflammatory drugs.
- Immunosuppressive medication (steroids).
- Aminopyridine increases the number of nerve impulses by increasing relief of ACh.
- If the disease is associated with cancer, direct treatment of cancer relieves the symptoms of LFMS.

- Physiotherapy and yoga exercises.
- Plasmapheresis – to filter the blood to remove antibodies.
- Intravenous administration of immunoglobulins.

Guillain–Barré syndrome

It is a rare disorder in which a person's own immune system attacks the peripheral nerves. This condition usually occurs after some bacterial/viral infection and manifests as:

- Pain in muscles
- Muscle weakness (mainly in the arms and legs)
- Abnormal walking
- Problem with coordination, speaking and swallowing
- Abnormal heart rhythm and high blood pressure
- Shortness of breath
- Slowness of reflexes
- Burning sensations and urinary retention

Treatment. No specific treatment is there; however, following measures are recommended:

- *Medication*
  Immunoglobulin therapy by injecting IgG antibodies
  Plasma exchange to remove antibodies which are affecting the cells
- *Supportive care*
  Intubation and mechanical ventilation to facilitate breathing
- *Physiotherapy* in the form of different exercises to prevent muscular atrophy

Self-Assessment

1. Draw a well-labelled diagram of the structure of neuromuscular junction and neuromuscular transmission.
2. Describe:
   - Neuromuscular disorders
   - Drugs affecting neuromuscular junction
3. Write short notes on:
   - Endplate potential
   - Giant potential
   - Acetylcholine receptors

Clinical Cases

Case 1

A 30-year-old female was presented in the eye OPD with drooping of eyelids and double vision. She also had difficulty in talking, swallowing and breathing.

Q1. What are the probable diagnosis and the cause?
Q2. What is the underlying pathophysiology of this condition?
Q3. What is the most commonly used drug in this case for treatment?

Case 2

A 12-year-old girl developed diarrhoea, nausea and vomiting, blurred vision and drooping of eyelids after 24 hours of eating mushroom pizza. On examination, it is found that her pulse rate was 100/min; low volume; and pupils were dilated and not responding to light.

Q1. What is the provisional diagnosis?
Q2. Which toxin is involved in this case?

Case 3

A 45-year-old woman is administered Botox to smooth out frown lines on her forehead by a dermatologist.

Q1. What is the mechanism of action of Botox?
Q2. For which condition, botulinum toxin was used for first time?
Q3. What are the side effects of Botox?

Case 4

A fully treated lung cancer patient developed muscle weakness, had difficulty in walking, tingling sensations and drooping of eyelids. The patient was diagnosed a case of myasthenia gravis and treated with drug neostigmine but there was no improvement. The case was further investigated and diagnosed as a case of Lambert–Eaton myasthenic syndrome (LEMS).

Q1. What specific test was performed for final diagnosis?
Q2. What are the different modes of treatment of this disease?

Case 5

A 5-year-old male child was admitted in the emergency department of medical college of Gujrat with the following complaints:

- Excessive salivation and lacrimation
- Tachycardia
- Tremors

The mother stated that while the child was playing in the garden, he was bitten by some insect. The sting site was red and swollen.

Q1. What is the probable diagnosis?
Q2. What is the best treatment for this condition?

Skeletal Muscle 2.3

CHAPTER OUTLINE

INTRODUCTION

The muscle cell, like the neuron, is an excitable tissue, i.e. an action potential (AP) is generated when it is stimulated chemically, electrically or mechanically. Furthermore, the muscle is a contractile tissue with a chemically stored energy which can be transformed into mechanical energy.

There are three different types of muscles in the body: skeletal muscles, cardiac muscles and smooth muscles. Based on certain distinctive features, the muscles can be grouped as follows.

Striated versus nonstriated muscles *Striated muscle* cells show a large number of cross-striations at regular intervals when seen under a light microscope. Skeletal and cardiac muscles are striated.

Nonstriated muscle cells do not show any striations. Smooth muscles or the so-called plain muscles are nonstriated.

Voluntary versus involuntary muscles *Voluntary muscles* can be made to contract under our will to perform the movements we desire. All skeletal muscles are voluntary muscles. These are supplied by somatic motor nerves.

Involuntary muscle's activities cannot be controlled at will. Cardiac and all smooth muscles are involuntary muscles. These are innervated by autonomic nerves.

Skeletal muscles The skeletal muscles, as the name indicates, are attached with the bones of the body skeleton and their contraction results in the body movements. They constitute about 40% of the total body mass.

FUNCTIONAL ANATOMY AND ORGANIZATION

STRUCTURAL ORGANIZATION OF MUSCLE

Structurally, the skeletal muscle consists of a large number of muscle fibres and a connective tissue framework organized as follows (Figs 2.3.1 and 2.3.2):

- Each *muscle fibre* is surrounded by delicate connective tissue called *endomysium* which contains large quantity of elastic tissue arranged longitudinally.
- The muscle fibres are grouped into a number of bundles called *fasciculi*. Each fasciculus is surrounded by a stronger sheath of connective tissue called *perimysium*.
- All the fasciculi collectively form the *muscle belly*. The connective tissue that surrounds the entire muscle belly is called *epimysium*.
- At the junction of the muscle with its tendon, the fibres of endomysium, perimysium and epimysium become continuous with the fibres of the tendon.

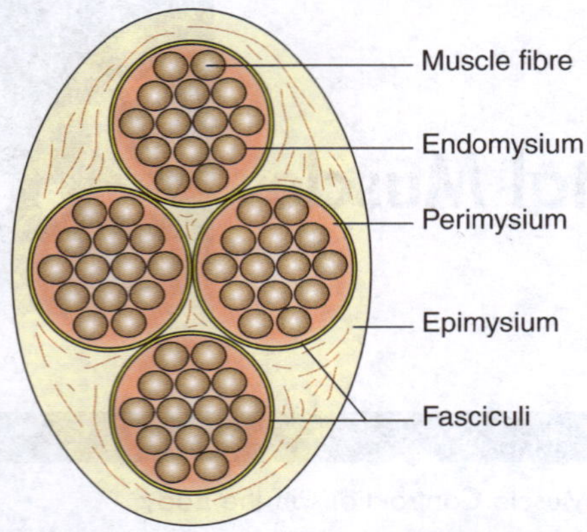

Fig. 2.3.1 Transverse section of skeletal muscle seen under light microscope.

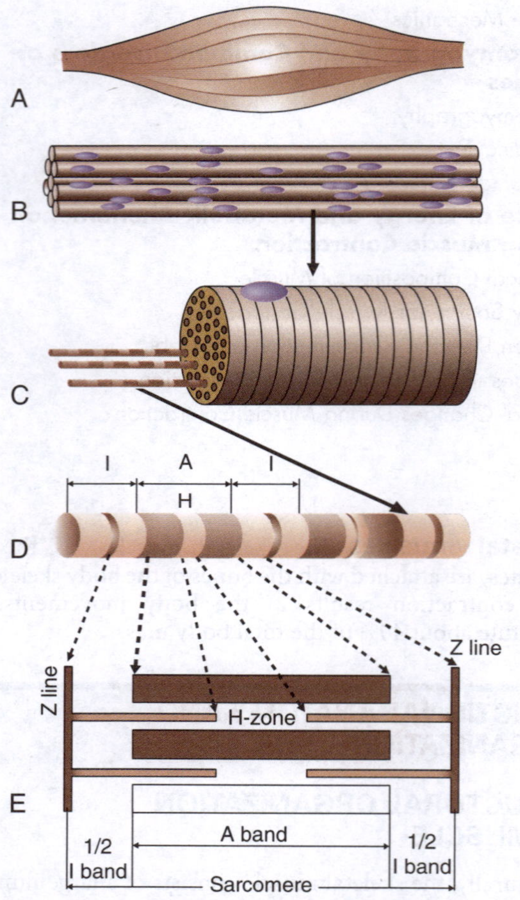

Fig. 2.3.2 Schematic diagram showing structural organization of skeletal muscle: **A**, muscle belly; **B**, muscle fibres grouped into fasciculi; **C**, muscle fibre; **D**, myofibril; and **E**, arrangement of thick and thin filaments.

- *Tendons* are fibrous terminal ends of the muscles made up of collagen fibres.

STRUCTURE OF A MUSCLE FIBRE

Each muscle fibre is basically a long (1–4 cm), cylindrical (10–100 μm in diameter), multinucleated cell. Its cell membrane is called *sarcolemma* and the cytoplasm is called *sarcoplasm*. Like any other cell, many structures are embedded in the sarcoplasm, such as the nuclei, Golgi apparatus, mitochondria, sarcoplasmic reticulum, ribosomes and glycogen and occasional lipid droplets. In addition, the sarcoplasm mainly contains a number of *myofibrils* which form the main structure of a muscle fibre. The sarcolemma along with the sarcoplasmic reticulum forms the so-called *sarcotubular system* which will be described in detail later.

Myofibril

Each muscle fibre consists of a large number of myofibrils which are arranged parallel to each other and run along the entire length of the muscle fibre. Myofibril is about 1–2 μm in diameter and 1–4 cm in length depending on the length of the muscle fibre.

Each myofibril consists of many thick and thin filaments (myofilaments) made up of a number of contractile proteins. Thick filaments are made up of myosin and are about 1500, while thin filaments are made of actin and about 3000 in number in each myofibril. The peculiar arrangement of these myofilaments when seen under a *light microscope* gives an appearance of alternate dark and light bands (striations) as described in the subsequent text.

Striations of Muscle Fibres

The dark and light bands result from a difference in the refractive index of its different parts. The arrangement is as follows (Fig. 2.3.2D):

- The dark band is called *A band* (anisometropic to polarized light). It is 1.5 μm in length. In the area of A band, the thick (myosin) filaments line up the thin filaments.
- In the centre of each A band, there is a lighter H-zone where thin filaments do not overlap the thick filaments (the word H represents the discoverer, Henson, or the hell which in German means light).
- In the centre of each H-zone is seen an M line, which is more pronounced during muscle contraction.
- The light band is called *I band* because it is isotropic to polarized light. It is about 1 μm in length. This area contains only thin (actin) filaments.
- Each I band is bisected by a narrow dark *Z line* (the word Z has been taken from Zwischenscheibe which in German means between discs).
- The portion of myofibril between two successive Z lines is called a *sarcomere*. Thus, a sarcomere includes 1/2 I band + A band + 1/2 I band and is about 2.5 μm in length at rest. The sarcomere is the structural and functional unit of the muscle fibre. During muscle contraction, the sarcomere reduces in length to 1.5 μm and during stretching of the muscle it increases in length to 3.5 μm.

Thick and Thin Filaments

The thick and thin filaments (Fig. 2.3.2E) form the *contractile apparatus* of a striated muscle. These are made up of three types of proteins:

- *Contractile proteins* are *myosin* and *actin* which interact to generate the contractile force in a muscle.
- *Regulatory proteins*, also called relaxation proteins, include *tropomyosin and troponin.* These regulate the interaction between the myosin and actin.
- *Anchoring proteins*, as the name indicates, anchor the different proteins to each other as well as to the sarcolemma and the extracellular matrix. These include α-actinin, titin, nebulin and *dystrophin*.

The detailed structure of thick and thin filaments forming the myofibril as revealed by *electron microscopy* is described as follows.

Thick filament Thick filaments are about twice the diameter of thin filaments. Each thick filament is surrounded by six thin filaments arranged in a regular hexagonal manner. A thick filament is made up of hundreds of molecules of a complex actin-binding contractile protein called *myosin*.

Structure of myosin molecule. The myosin molecule has a molecular weight of 480,000 and is made up of six polypeptide chains, two heavy chains (each having molecular weight 200,000) and four light chains (each having molecular weight 20,000). The two heavy chains wrap around each other to form a double helix, which constitutes the *tail and body* of the myosin molecule (Fig. 2.3.3A). The light chains combine with the terminal part of the heavy chains to form the globular *head* of myosin molecule. The myosin molecule present in the skeletal muscle has two heads and is called *myosin-II* (Fig. 2.3.3B) (single-headed myosin present in some other cells of the body is called myosin-I). These heads contain an *actin-binding site* and a *catalytic site* that hydrolyses ATP. During muscle contraction, the head forms the *cross-bridging* (described later). Digestion with trypsin generates two fragments of myosin molecules (Fig. 2.3.4):

Light meromyosin (LMM) comes from the tail part of the myosin. It does not have any ATPase activity or actin-binding ability (Fig. 2.3.4B).

Heavy meromyosin (HMM) contains the globular head as well as part of the tail (Fig. 2.3.4B). HMM can be further split by papain into two parts (Fig. 2.3.4C): the *globular HMM-SI*, which has all the ATPase activity and actin-binding ability, and the fibrous, HMM-S2, which has none of it.

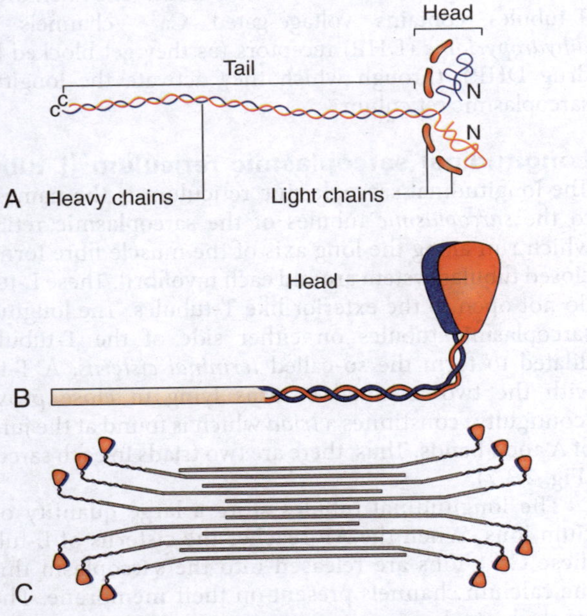

Fig. 2.3.3 Myosin molecules: **A**, structure of myosin molecule; **B**, molecule of myosin-II (with two heads); and **C**, arrangement of myosin molecules in thick filament.

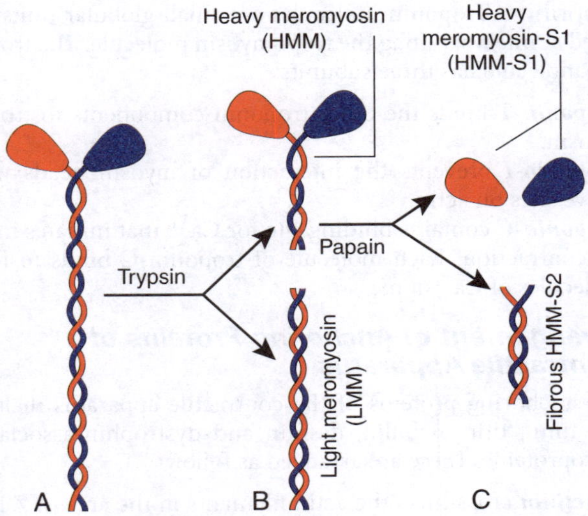

Fig. 2.3.4 Myosin molecule after digestion with trypsin and papain: **A**, before digestion with trypsin; **B**, after digestion with trypsin (forms two fragments LMM and HMM); and **C**, heavy meromyosin fragment after digestion with papain.

Arrangement of myosin molecules in a thick filament. In a thick filament, half of the myosin molecules are oriented with their heads in one direction and the remaining half in the opposite direction (Fig. 2.3.3C). Because of this arrangement, the central portion of a thick filament is devoid of the head portions of the myosin molecules. This accounts for the comparatively lighter H-zone seen in the centre of dark A band. The central overlapping of the myosin molecules of each side creates a central bulge in each of thick filaments which accounts for the M line seen on light microscopy.

Thin filament The thin filament has a head end (which extends into the A band) and a tail end that is anchored to the Z line (through a protein called α-actinin). Each thin filament is made up of contractile protein molecules (actin) and two types of regulatory protein molecules (tropomyosin and troponin) (Fig. 2.3.5).

Actin. About 300–400 actin molecules are present in each thin filament. The actin molecules form a long double helix consisting of two chains of globular units. The globular molecules are *G-actin*, and the chain formed by them is designated as *F-actin*.

Tropomyosin. About 40–60 tropomyosin molecules are present in each thin filament. Tropomyosin is made up of long filaments that lie in the groove between the two chains of actin molecules. It covers the binding site of actin where the myosin head comes in contact with actin. Thus, it is a regulatory protein that prevents the interaction between actin and myosin filaments.

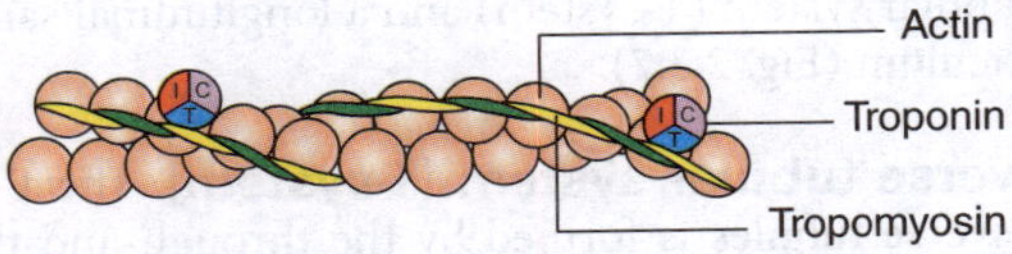

Fig. 2.3.5 Structure of a thin filament.

Troponin. Troponin molecules are small globular units located at intervals along the tropomyosin molecule. The troponin molecule has three subunits:

Troponin-T binds the other troponin components to tropomyosin.

Troponin-I prevents the interaction of myosin heads with active sites on actin.

Troponin-C contains binding site for Ca^{2+} that initiates muscle contraction. Each molecule of troponin-C binds to four molecules of Ca^{2+} ions.

Arrangement of Anchoring Proteins of Contractile Apparatus

The anchoring proteins of the contractile apparatus include α-actinin, titin, nebulin, desmin and dystrophin-associated glycoproteins. These are arranged as follows:

α-Actinin cross-links the actin filaments in the area of Z line (Fig. 2.3.6A).

Titin, earlier called *connectin* or gap filament, is a large elastic filament which connects the Z lines to M line in the sarcomere. It forms the *series elastic components* (SECs) of the muscle.

Nebulin is an inextensible filament which is connected at one end to the α-actinin in the area of Z line and at another end to the tropomyosin–troponin complex of thin filaments at regular intervals. It binds to about 200 actin monomers.

Desmin is a muscle-specific type III intermediate filament that integrates the sarcomere Z line and nuclear membrane in a sarcomere and regulates sarcomere architecture.

Dystrophin–glycoprotein complex. The dystrophin–glycoprotein complex (Fig. 2.3.6B) forms the best known anchor protein complex, which provides structural support and strength to myofibril. As shown in Fig. 2.3.6B, the *dystrophin* molecule forms a rod that connects the thin actin filament to the two proteins (α- and β-dystroglycan) present in the sarcolemma which in turn are connected to the merosin subunit of *laminin* molecule present in the basal lamina matrix. The dystroglycans in turn are associated with transmembrane glycoprotein complex made up of α, β, γ and δ sarcoglycans.

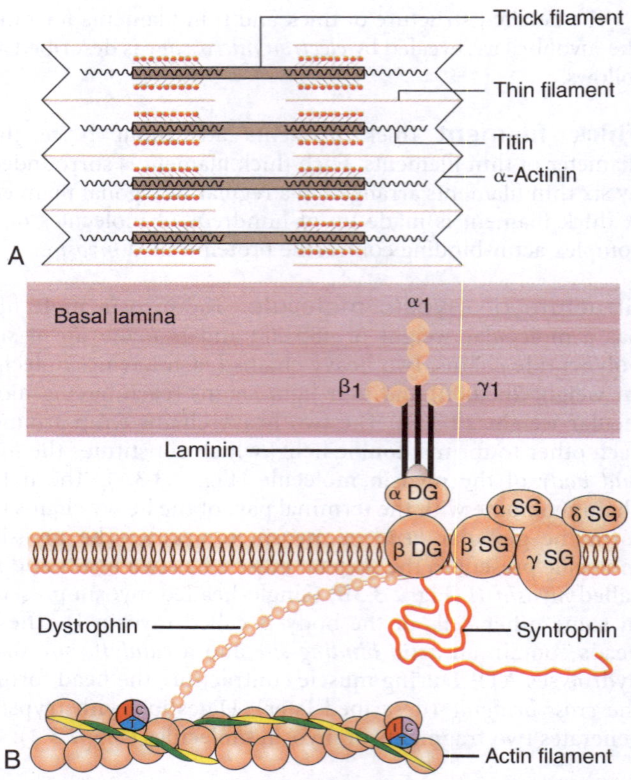

Fig. 2.3.6 Arrangement of anchoring proteins of the contractile apparatus: **A**, α-actinin (which cross-links the thin filament in area of Z lines) and titin (interconnects two Z lines); and **B**, dystrophin–glycoprotein (DG) complex associated with sarcoglycan (SG) complex of four glycoproteins α, β, γ and δ.

> **Important Note**
>
> The dystrophin–glycoprotein complex is of special importance because genetic defects in dystrophin lead to absence/deficiency of all associated proteins and result in Duchenne muscular dystrophy (DMD).

SARCOTUBULAR SYSTEM

The sarcolemma (cell membrane of muscle cell) along with the sarcoplasmic reticulum (the endoplasmic reticulum of muscle cell) forms a highly specialized system called sarcotubular system. This plays an important role in the internal conduction of depolarization within the muscle fibre. The sarcotubular system (which under an electron microscope appears as vesicles and tubules) is primarily formed by a transverse tubular system (T-system) and a longitudinal sarcoplasmic reticulum (Fig. 2.3.7).

Transverse tubular system (T-system) The T-system of transverse tubules is formed by the through-and-through invagination of sarcolemma into the muscle fibre in the region of junction of A and I bands (Fig. 2.3.7). Since the T-tubules are formed by the invagination of sarcolemma, their lumen contains ECF which surrounds the muscle cell. These T-tubules facilitate the rapid transmission of the impulse in the form of AP from sarcolemma to the myofibrils. The membrane of T-tubules contains voltage-gated Ca^{2+} channels called *dihydropyridine* (DHP) receptors (as they get blocked by the drug DHP), through which they activate the longitudinal sarcoplasmic reticulum.

Longitudinal sarcoplasmic reticulum (L-tubules) The longitudinal sarcoplasmic reticulum is the name given to the *sarcoplasmic* tubules of the sarcoplasmic reticulum which run along the long axis of the muscle fibre forming a closed tubular system around each myofibril. These L-tubules do not open to the exterior like T-tubules. The longitudinal sarcoplasmic tubules on either side of the T-tubule are dilated to form the so-called *terminal cisterns.* A T-tubule with the two terminal cisterns lying in close proximity (contiguity) constitutes a *triad* which is found at the junction of A and I bands. Thus, there are two triads in each sarcomere (Fig. 2.3.7).

The longitudinal tubules store a large quantity of calcium ions. When the AP reaches the cisterns of L-tubules, these Ca^{2+} ions are released into the sarcoplasm through the calcium channels present on their membrane. The calcium channels are not voltage gated. These are called *ryanodine receptors* (RYRs), as they are kept in open position by ryanodine alkaloid.

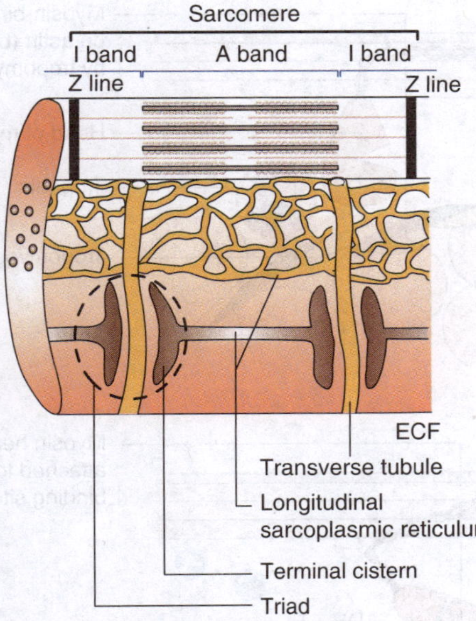

Fig. 2.3.7 Sarcotubular system showing transverse tubules and longitudinal sarcoplasmic reticulum.

PROCESS OF MUSCLE EXCITABILITY AND CONTRACTILITY

As we know, the muscle is an excitable tissue, i.e. when stimulated an AP is produced (*electrical phenomenon*). The skeletal muscle responds to stimulus by contracting (*mechanical phenomenon*). The events that link the electrical phenomenon with the mechanical phenomenon are called *excitation–contraction coupling phenomena*. The three phenomena which mark the excitability and contractility of the muscle when stimulated by the nerve innervating it are discussed.

PROCESS OF MUSCLE EXCITATION

It refers to electrical phenomenon and ionic fluxes in skeletal muscle fibres. As discussed in the transmission across neuromuscular junction (page 76), an endplate potential (EPP) is developed at the motor endplate by the nerve impulse travelling across the innervating axon. The EPP, as discussed earlier (page 77), is localized and nonpropagated. However, when EPP reaches a threshold level, it produces an *AP* which propagates over muscle fibre surface and into the muscle fibre along the transverse tubules.

Essential features of electrical phenomena Essential features of electrical phenomena which occur in the muscle fibre (resting membrane potential [RMP] and AP) are similar to those occurring in a nerve fibre. These have been described on page 59 (students are advised to revise them). However, there are some quantitative differences between the electrical phenomenon occurring in a skeletal muscle fibre and in a nerve fibre which are summarized as follows:

1. RMP in a skeletal muscle fibre is about −90 mV, while in a nerve fibre it is about −70 mV.
2. Initial excitation threshold level for a muscle fibre is 30–40 mV, while that for a nerve fibre is about 15 mV.

Table 2.3.1 Equilibrium potential of different ions in skeletal muscle fibre and nerve fibre

	Equilibrium potential (mV)	
Ion	**Skeletal muscle fibre**	**Nerve fibre**
Na^+	+65	+60
K^+	−95	−90
H^+	−32	−25
Cl^-	−90	−70
HCO_3^-	−32	−25

3. Magnitude of AP produced in a muscle fibre is about 120–130 mV while that produced in the nerve fibre is about 100–105 mV.
4. Duration of spike potential is longer in a muscle fibre (5 milliseconds) than in a nerve fibre (0.4–2 milliseconds).
5. Absolute refractory period (ARP) is also longer in a muscle fibre (1–3 milliseconds) than in a nerve fibre (0.4–2 milliseconds).
6. The maximum number of impulses which can pass through a muscle fibre is much less (100–200/s) than that through the nerve fibre (1000/s).
7. The excitability of the muscle is far less than that of the neuron, that is, *chronaxie* in a muscle fibre is longer while in a nerve fibre it is shorter.
8. Conduction velocity of APs in a skeletal muscle fibre is low, 3–5 m/s. In a nerve fibre, the conduction velocity of an AP is variable, being directly proportional to its diameter. In a myelinated nerve fibre, the conduction velocity can be as high as 120 m/s.
9. Equilibrium potential for different ions in a skeletal muscle fibre and a nerve fibre is as shown in Table 2.3.1.

PROCESS OF EXCITATION–CONTRACTION COUPLING

The process by which depolarization of a muscle fibre initiates contraction is called excitation–contraction coupling. The sequence of events by which an AP in the plasma membrane of a muscle fibre leads to cross-bridge activity (excitation–contraction coupling) is as follows:

- AP initiated in the plasma membrane of a muscle fibre spreads rapidly on the surface as well as into the interior of the muscle fibre through the T-tubules.
- When the AP reaches the tip of the T-tubule, it activates the voltage-gated channels called DHP receptors which are located in the T-tubule membrane (Fig. 2.3.8).
- Activated DHP receptors in turn trigger the opening of Ca^{2+}-release channels located on the terminal cisterns, the so-called *RYR*. This is possible because the lateral cisterns are located very close to the tips of T-tubules and the protein channels of the cisterns (DHP and RYR) are mechanically interlocked. Thus, in short, when the DHP is activated by the depolarization of T-tubules, it undergoes conformational changes which result in the opening of RYR (being actually pulled open).
- Due to opening of calcium-release channels (RYR), calcium ions diffuse into the cytoplasm. The concentration of Ca^{2+} in the ICF is increased by approximately 2000 times, i.e. from 10^{-7} to 2×10^{-4} moles/L.

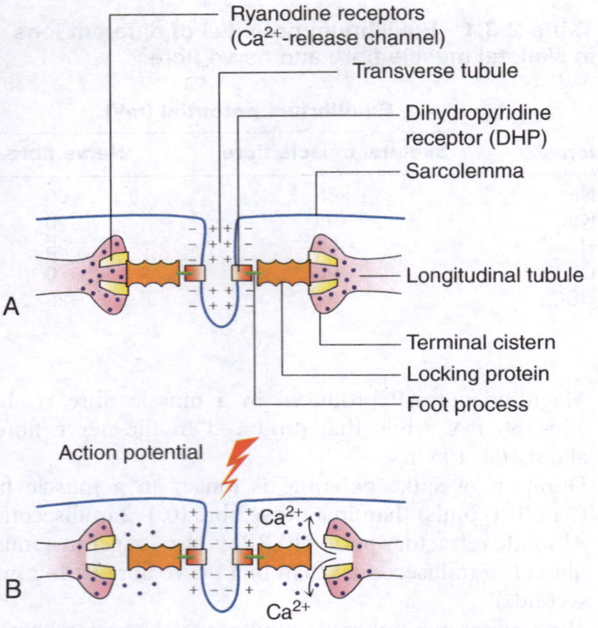

Fig. 2.3.8 Mechanism of release of calcium ions from terminal cistern of longitudinal tubules: **A**, in resting state Ca^{2+}-release channels (RYR) remain closed due to mechanical interlocking between DHP and RYR; and **B**, during activation state (depolarization of T-tubule). Conformational change in DHP results in opening of RYR and release of Ca^{2+}.

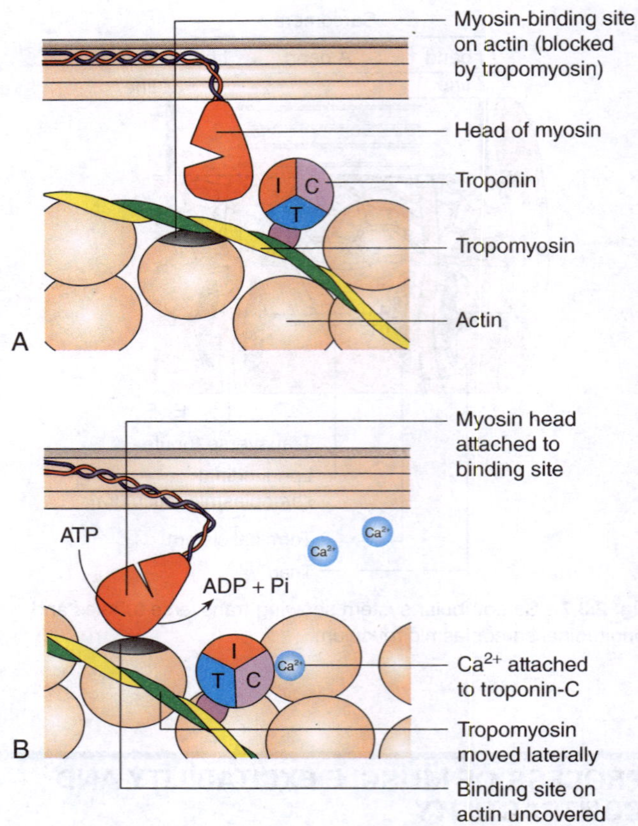

Fig. 2.3.9 Initiation of cross-bridge cycling: **A**, resting state (myosin-binding site on actin is covered by troponin–tropomyosin complex); and **B**, on activation, Ca^{2+} binds to troponin-C subunit and this results in conformational change and lateral displacement of tropomyosin causing uncovering of binding site for myosin (head of myosin) on actin (initiation of cross-bridge cycle).

- The Ca^{2+} ions get attached to troponin-C and start a chain of events (discussed in the subsequent text) which produces contraction. Thus, the calcium ions act as a linking or coupling material between the excitation and the contraction of the muscle. Hence, the calcium ions are said to form the basis of excitation–contraction coupling.

PROCESS OF MUSCLE CONTRACTION

Molecular Basis of Muscle Contraction

The process of muscle contraction is initiated by the calcium ions as discussed above. The molecular basis of muscle contraction describes the role that contractile molecules myosin and actin play in the process of muscle contraction. A.F. Huxley and H.E. Huxley in 1954 put forward the *sliding theory* or *ratchet theory* to explain how the actin filaments slide over myosin filaments forming the actin–myosin complex during muscular contraction. This theory is called *walk-along theory* or the modern theory of muscular contraction. This theory explains that the sliding of filaments is brought about by a repeated cycle of formation of the *cross-bridges* between the head of myosin and actin molecules.

Steps of cross-bridge cycling

1. Initiation of cross-bridge cycling. During the resting stage, troponin-I is lightly bound to actin and the tropomyosin molecules are located in the groove between the strands of actin filaments in such a way that they block the myosin-binding sites on actin. Thus, during resting stage, no actin–myosin cross-bridges are formed. Thus, the *troponin–tropomyosin complex*, so-called *relaxing proteins*, inhibits the interaction between actin and myosin (Fig. 2.3.9A). When activation takes place, the Ca^{2+} ions released into the cytosol from the terminal cisterns of the sarcoplasmic reticulum get attached to *troponin-C* subunit of the protein troponin. It results in a conformation change which causes the tropomyosin molecule to move laterally, uncovering the binding sites on the actin molecules for head of the myosin molecules. Seven myosin-binding sites on the actin filament are uncovered for each molecule of troponin that binds a Ca^{2+} ion. Thus, the cross-bridge cycle is switched on (initiated) by the lateral movement of tropomyosin (Fig. 2.3.9B).

Note: Myosin molecules present in skeletal muscle are dimers having two heads but only one head binds to actin at any given time.

2. Formation of actin–myosin complex (i.e. attachment of myosin head to active site of actin filament). The head of myosin molecule binds with ATP. The ATPase activity of myosin head immediately causes breaking of ATP to ADP and Pi cleavage products which remain bound to myosin head. The head of myosin therefore becomes energized. The activated myosin head extends perpendicularly (at 90° conformation) towards the actin filament and gets attached to the actin filament (Fig. 2.3.10) (Stages I and II). The reaction occurs as follows:

$$A + M.ADP.Pi \xrightarrow{\text{actin binding}} A\text{-}M\text{-}ADP.Pi$$

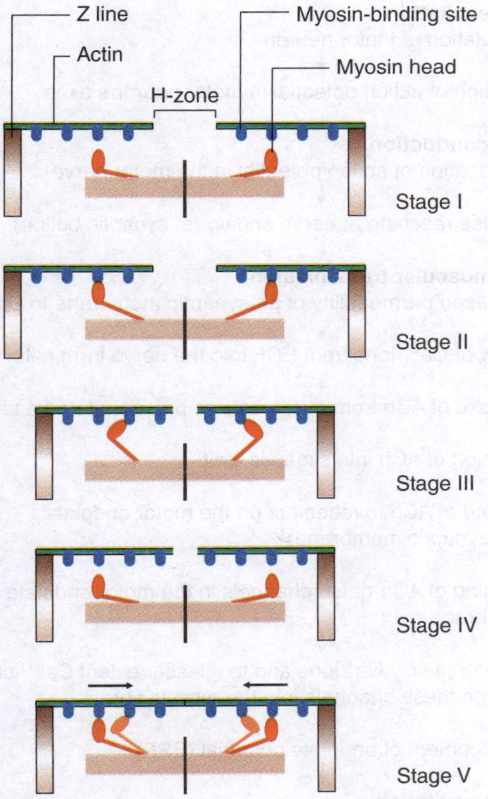

Fig. 2.3.10 Stages of cross-bridge cycling (for details, see text).

3. The power stroke. Formation of the *actin–myosin–ADP Pi* complex triggers simultaneously the following two events:

- Release of the Pi and ADP from the complex.
- A conformational change in the myosin head causing it to flex towards the arm of the cross-bridge. The flexion of the myosin head from the high-energy 90° conformation to low-energy 45° conformation generates mechanical force (the power stroke). The power stroke has either or both of the following effects:
- *If the load on the muscle is small*, then the actin filament slides over the myosin filament, producing muscle shortening (Fig. 2.3.10) (Stage III).
- *If the load on muscle is large*, then the actin filaments are unable to slide over the myosin filament; under such circumstances, the flexion of the myosin head will produce stretching of the elastic neck of myosin molecule.

Thus, the energy stored in head of myosin cross-bridge is utilized for the power stroke. The reaction occurs as follows:

$$\text{A-M-ADP.Pi} \xrightarrow{\textit{bridge movement}} \text{A-M.} + \text{ADP} + \text{Pi}$$

Myosin head still remains attached to active site of actin filament at 45° position but stops sliding.

4. Detachment of head of a cross-bridge from active site of actin filament. The release of ADP and Pi allows a fresh ATP molecule to bind to the myosin head. The *myosin–ATP complex* has a low affinity for actin, and, therefore, it results in the dissociation of myosin head from the actin filament (Fig. 2.3.10) (Stage IV). The reaction is as follows:

$$\text{A-M.} + \text{ATP.} \rightarrow \text{A} + \text{M.ATP}$$

5. Reactivation of myosin head. The freshly bound ATP molecule splits again, and the myosin head is reactivated for the next cycle to begin. The energized head extends perpendicularly towards the actin filament and gets attached to the new active site for repeating the cycle. This reaction occurs as follows:

$$\text{M.ATP} \xrightarrow{\textit{energized cross-bridge}} \text{M.ADP. Pi}$$

Thus, with each cross-bridge cycle, there is movement of the actin filament towards the centre of myosin to a small degree. Repeated cross-bridge cycling causes the movement of actin filaments of either side towards the centre of myosin filament of the sarcomere leading to muscle contraction (Fig. 2.3.10) (Stage V).

Note: During each power stroke, sarcomere shortens by 10 nm. It has been estimated that during rapid contraction, the rate of power stroke cycle is five times per second.

Steps in Muscle Relaxation

Within a few milliseconds of the AP, sarcoplasmic/endoplasmic reticulum Ca^{2+}–ATPase (SERCA) pump transports Ca^{2+} ions present in sarcoplasm during contraction back into the longitudinal portion of the sarcoplasmic reticulum, from where the Ca^{2+} ions are discharged into the terminal cistern for storage (Fig. 2.3.11).

Removal of calcium from troponin restores blocking action of troponin–tropomyosin complex. Myosin cross-bridge cycle closes and muscle relaxes.

Functions of ATP in skeletal muscle contraction and relaxation

1. Hydrolysis of ATP by myosin energizes the cross-bridges providing the energy for force generation.

2. Binding of ATP to myosin causes dissociation of cross-bridges, allowing the bridges to repeat their cycle of activity.

3. Hydrolysis of ATP by Ca^{2+}–ATPase in the sarcoplasmic reticulum (SERCA) provides the energy for active transport of calcium back into the cisternae, lowering cytoplasmic calcium, ending the contraction and allowing muscle fibre to relax.

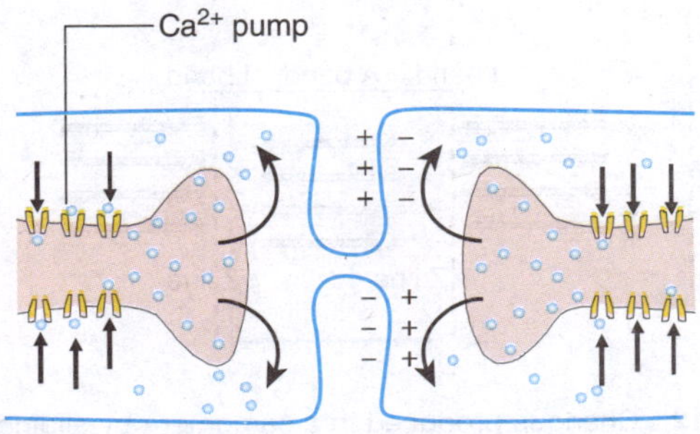

Fig. 2.3.11 Transport of Ca^{2+} from sarcoplasm into longitudinal tubules by Ca^{2+} pump.

Applied Aspect

Rigor mortis refers to shortening and rigidity of all the body muscles which occurs some hours after death. The rigidity occurs because of fixation of cross-bridges of myosin head to actin filaments in an abnormal and resistant manner due to loss of all the ATP (which is normally required for detachment of cross-bridges of myosin heads from the actin filaments causing relaxation). Depending on the environmental temperature and other factors, the rigidity disappears after some hours due to destruction of the muscle proteins by enzymes released from cellular lysosomes. The appearance and disappearance of rigor mortis is used by the forensic experts in fixing the time of death.

Changes produced by sliding of thin filaments over thick filaments during muscle contraction

Fig. 2.3.12 shows the following changes produced by sliding of thin filaments over thick filaments during muscle contraction:

1. The width of A band remains constant.
2. H-zone disappears.
3. I bandwidth decreases.
4. The Z lines move closer.
5. The sarcomere shortens.
6. The actin filaments from the opposite end of the sarcomere approach each other, and when the muscle shortening is marked, these filaments apparently overlap.

Sequence of events during muscle contraction and relaxation when stimulated by a nerve

The events that occur during contraction and relaxation in a skeletal muscle when excited by a nerve are summarized sequence-wise as follows.

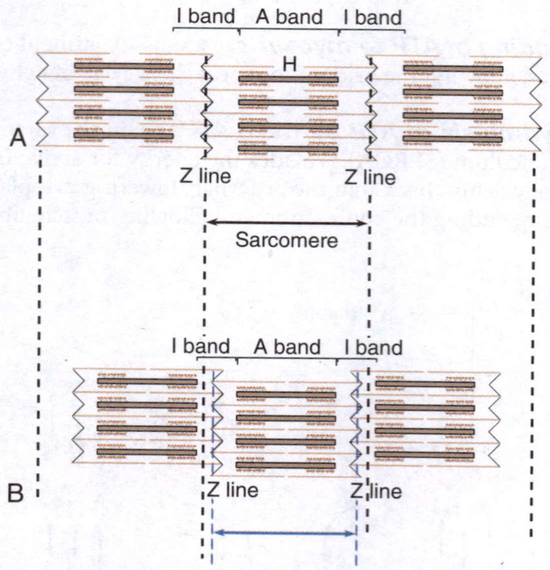

Fig. 2.3.12 Changes produced in a sarcomere by sliding of thin filament (actin) over thick filament (myosin) during muscle contraction: **A**, relaxed state; and **B**, contracted state.

Nerve excitation
- Stimulation of motor neuron
↓
- Initiation of action potential in motor neuron's axon
↓

Nerve conduction
- Propagation of action potential in the motor nerve
↓
- Impulse reaching at nerve ending (at synaptic button)
↓

Neuromuscular transmission
- Increased permeability of presynaptic membrane to Ca^{2+} ions
↓
- Inflow of Ca^{2+} ions from ECF into the nerve terminals
↓
- Release of ACh from microvesicles present at nerve terminal
↓
- Diffusion of ACh into synaptic cleft
↓
- Binding of ACh to receptors on the motor endplate (postsynaptic membrane)
↓
- Opening of ACh-gated channels in the motor endplate membrane
↓
- Entry of mainly Na^+ ions and to a lesser extent Ca^{2+} ions through these channels into the muscle fibre
↓
- Development of endplate potential (EPP)
↓

Muscle excitation
- Local EPP when reaches a threshold magnitude, voltage-gated Na^+ channels are opened up at the site
↓
- Generation of action potential (AP) in the muscle fibre by endplate depolarization
↓
- Propagation of AP in muscle fibre along the surface and into the fibre along the T-tubules
↓

Excitation–contraction coupling
- Release of Ca^{2+} ions from terminal cistern
↓
- Diffusion of Ca^{2+} ions into the sarcoplasm
↓
- Binding of Ca^{2+} ions to troponin-C
↓

Muscle contraction (molecular theory)
- Uncovering of binding sites for myosin on actin
↓
- Cross-bridge formation between myosin head and actin
↓
- Angular movement of cross-bridges (power stroke)
↓
- Sliding of thin filaments over thick filaments
↓
- Initiation of muscle contraction
↓

Muscle relaxation
- Active transport of Ca^{2+} into sarcoplasmic reticulum
↓
- Decreased concentration of Ca^{2+} in sarcoplasm
↓
- Removal of Ca^{2+} ions from troponin-C
↓
- Cessation of cross-bridge cycling
↓
- Relaxation of muscle fibre

CHARACTERISTICS OF MUSCLE EXCITABILITY AND CONTRACTILITY

EXCITABILITY

Excitability is the property by which tissues respond to stimuli. The skeletal muscles respond by undergoing depolarization (development of AP).

Characteristics of Electrical Phenomenon in a Skeletal Muscle

The essential features of the RMP and AP of skeletal muscles are similar to those of a nerve (see page 58). The quantitative differences between the electrical phenomenon occurring in a skeletal muscle fibre and in a nerve fibre are summarized on page 88.

Characteristics of Skeletal Muscle Fibre Excitability vis-à-vis Characteristics of the Stimulus

The skeletal muscle fibres exhibit some peculiar characteristics of the excitability depending on the strength and duration of the stimulus used and the electrogenic state of the muscle fibre when stimulus is applied. Some of the important excitability characteristics are described as follows.

Strength–duration curve The essential features of strength–duration curve plotted for a skeletal muscle are similar to that plotted for a nerve (see page 63), except that the chronaxie value of skeletal muscle fibre is longer than that of nerve fibre (Fig. 2.1.13A and B).

- Chronaxie value in frog's skeletal muscle is about 3 milliseconds.
- Normal value of chronaxie in human skeletal muscles varies from 0.08 to 0.32 millisecond.
- Chronaxie is 10 times more in skeletal muscles of infants than in those of adults.

CONTRACTILITY

To understand contractile response and its characteristics after discussing the process of muscle excitability and contraction, it is essential to have a knowledge about the following elementary aspects in relation to skeletal muscle:

- Contractile and elastic components of a muscle
- Concept about muscle length
- Motor unit

Contractile and Elastic Components of a Muscle

To understand certain facts associated with muscle contraction such as shortening, contraction without shortening and effect of passive stretch, a *three-component model* has been proposed. According to this model, the skeletal muscle as a whole consists of three components (Fig. 2.3.13A):

- Contractile component (CC)
- SEC
- Parallel elastic component (PEC)

1. Contractile component The CC represents the thick (myosin) and thin (actin) filaments present in the myofibrils. It is considered to be viscous in nature, i.e. it offers no resistance to stretch and is unable to return to its original length after it has shortened. The CC comprises 60% (three-fifth) of the total muscle proteins.

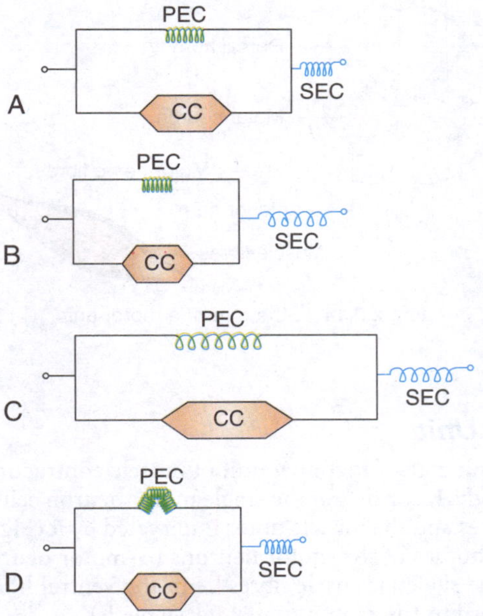

Fig. 2.3.13 Three-component model of skeletal muscle consisting of contractile component (CC), series elastic component (SEC) and parallel elastic component (PEC): **A**, when muscle is at normal length; **B**, during isometric contraction; **C**, when muscle is passively stretched; and **D**, in isotonic contraction.

2. Series elastic component The SEC refers to that elastic tissue of the muscle which is present in series with the CC of the muscle. It consists of the elastic tendon of the muscle. In resting condition, the SEC offers resistance to passive stretch and explains how muscle is able to contract even when its external length does not change, i.e. isometric contraction (Fig. 2.3.13B). It also explains how the muscle regains its original length after contracting isometrically.

3. Parallel elastic component The PEC refers to the elastic tissue of the muscle which is attached parallel to the CC. It is represented by the structural elastic tissue of the muscle such as connective tissue sheaths of the muscle, sarcolemma and gap filaments. Presence of this component explains why the muscle regains its original length after it is passively stretched (Fig. 2.3.13C and D). In an isotonic contraction, this component gets folded up. It also offers some resistance to passive stretch.

The SEC and PEC combinedly form 40% (two-fifth) of total muscle proteins.

Concepts About Muscle Length

The following concepts about muscle length will be useful in understanding certain characteristics about muscle contraction:

Optimum length refers to that length of the muscle at which it will develop *maximum active tension*.

Resting length of a muscle represents the length of the muscle during relaxed state under natural conditions in the body. The resting length of many muscles in the body is optimum length.

Equilibrium length refers to the length of a relaxed muscle cut free from its bony attachments.

Initial length is the length of the muscle before it contracts.

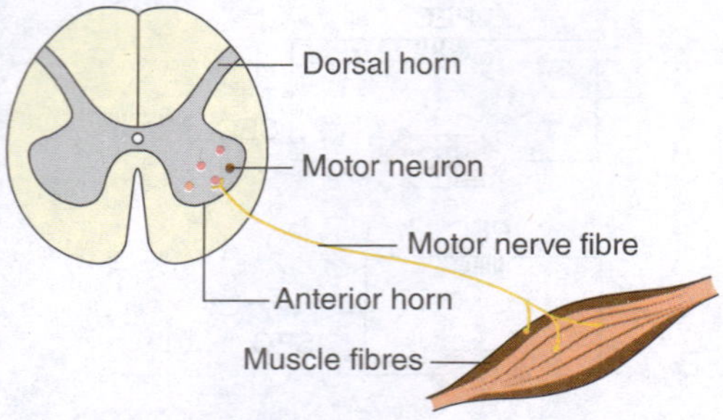

Fig. 2.3.14 Structure of a motor unit.

Motor Unit

Motor unit is the functional unit of muscle contraction in the intact body. It consists of the single motor neuron cell body, its axon fibres and the muscle fibres innervated by it (Fig. 2.3.14). The cell bodies of the motor neurons (α-motor neuron) supplying the skeletal muscle fibres lie in the ventral horn of the spinal cord or the motor cranial nerve nuclei.

Characteristic features of motor unit are:

Innervation ratio. The number of muscle fibres supplied by single neuron constitutes the innervation ratio or the size of the motor unit. The innervation ratio of a motor unit varies with the precision of the movement to be produced by the muscle supplied. For example, in extraocular muscles (concerned with the eye movements) and hand muscles (for fine movements), the innervation ratio is only 3–6 muscle fibres per motor unit, whereas in gastrocnemius muscle and in muscles of the back (concerned with posture maintenance), the innervation ratio is up to 2000 muscle fibres per motor unit.

Motor neuron pool. All the motor neurons for a given muscle make up the motor neuron pool.

Recruitment of motor units. The force of contraction is graded by recruitment of additional motor units (size principle). The *size principle* states that as additional motor units are recruited, more motor neurons are involved and more tension is generated.

Motor unit territory. The motor unit territory is the term used for the area occupied by a single motor unit in a transverse section of a muscle. For example, in biceps muscle, the motor unit territory ranges from 2 to 5 mm in diameter. The muscle fibres of each motor unit are not bunched together in the muscle, but are scattered and overlap with other motor units. In other words, there is overlapping of motor unit territories (Fig. 2.3.15). The intermingling of motor fibres from different motor units results in smooth muscle movements. The importance of overlapping of motor units will be discussed later in detail.

Type of motor units. Each motor neuron innervates only one type of muscle fibre. In other words, in a single motor unit, the muscle fibres supplied by it are of the same type. Therefore, depending on the type of muscle fibres, the (fast or slow type) motor units are also of two types:

- ***Type I*** (red or slow) motor units
- ***Type II*** (white or fast) motor units

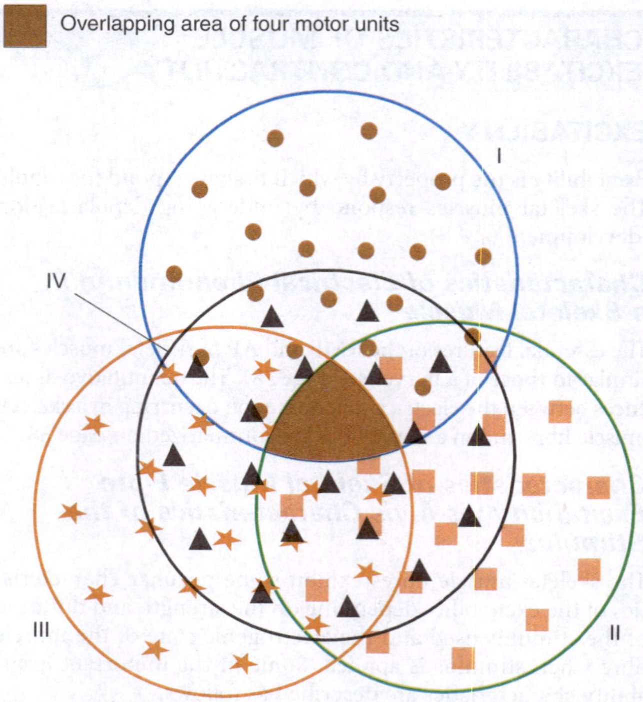

Fig. 2.3.15 Motor unit territory of four motor units (I–IV) along with their central overlapping area seen in a schematic cross-section.

The characteristic features of each type of motor units are given in Table 2.3.2. The difference between different types of motor units depends on activity.

Contractile Response

Contractile response is the characteristic feature of a skeletal muscle. When stimulated, an AP is developed in the muscle fibres, which is followed by the muscle contraction. The muscle contraction is manifested by either shortening (*isotonic contraction*) or development of tension (*isometric contraction*) or both. The contractile response can be studied in an *isolated* nerve–muscle preparation. In experimental studies, frog's gastrocnemius–sciatic nerve preparation is used to demonstrate the different characteristics of the contractile response. The contractile response of a muscle to a single stimulus through its nerve can be recorded using a suitable lever system on kymograph or physiograph.

A typical contractile response consists of a brief contraction followed by relaxation, and is referred to as *single muscle twitch*. The contractile response of a skeletal muscle can be discussed under the following headings:

- Isometric versus isotonic contraction
- Single muscle twitch
- Factors affecting force of contraction

Isometric versus isotonic contraction

Isometric contraction. As the name indicates (iso = same, metric = measure, i.e. length), in this type of contraction, the length of muscle remains same but tension is developed in the muscle. Thus, there is no movement of the object. Since work done is the product of *force × distance*, therefore, in isometric contraction *no external work is done.*

How the muscle length remains same in isometric contraction is depicted in Fig. 2.3.13B. As shown in this figure, the

Table 2.3.2 Characteristic features of type I and type II motor units

Characteristics	Motor unit type I	Motor unit type II
1. Muscle fibre type	The muscle fibres of type I motor unit are slow, red and involved in tonic activity	The muscle fibres of type II motor units are fast, white and involved in phasic activity
2. Motor unit innervation ratio	High (120–160 muscle fibres/axon), e.g. postural muscles	Low (<6 muscle fibres/axon), e.g. extraocular muscles
3. Metabolism	Aerobic, low glycolytic and high oxidative capacity	Anaerobic, high glycolytic and low oxidative capacity
• Mitochondria number	High	Low
• Glycogen contents	Low	High
• Capillary density	High	Low
• Blood supply	High	Normal
• Myoglobin content	High	Low
• Enzymes:	High	Low
NADH dehydrogenase		
Phosphorylase activity	Low	High
Myosin ATPase activity	Low	High
4. Axon diameter	Small	Large
5. Axon conduction velocity	Slow	Fast
6. Twitch duration of the muscle	Long	Brief
7. Tetanic tension	Small	Large
8. Type of movements	These are adapted for tonic contraction, i.e. for posture maintenance and are first to be recruited during muscle contraction	These are adapted for phasic contractions, e.g. fine and skilled movements, and these remain inactive during contraction and are recruited only when brief and powerful contraction is required
9. Fatiguability	Fatigue resistant	Easily fatiguable
10. Further types	–	Type II motor units are further of four types: IIa, IIb, IIc and IIm IIa: Are fast, fatigue resistant and glycolytic IIb: Are fast, fatiguable and glycolytic IIc: Contain muscle fibres found in fetal stage IIm: Are superfast, having unique myosin structure and present mainly in the jaw muscles

shortening produced by *CC* of the muscle is compensated by the stretching of the SEC.

Examples of isometric. muscle contraction:

- Contraction of muscles which help in maintaining posture against gravity
- Contraction of arm muscles when trying to push a wall

Isotonic contraction. As the name indicates (iso = same, and tonic = tone or tension), in this type of contraction, the tension in the muscle remains same, whereas its length decreases. Since the muscle length is shortened, so the *external work is done* in isotonic contraction. As shown in Fig. 2.3.13D, in isotonic contraction, the CC and PEC are shortened, but the SEC does not stretch further, producing a visible shortening of the muscle.

Examples of isotonic muscle contraction:

- Contraction of leg muscles during walking and running
- Contraction of muscles while lifting a weight
- Contraction of muscles during flexion of arm

Single Muscle Twitch

As mentioned earlier, the single muscle twitch, also known as the simple muscle twitch, refers to the typical contractile response of a skeletal muscle to the single stimulus.

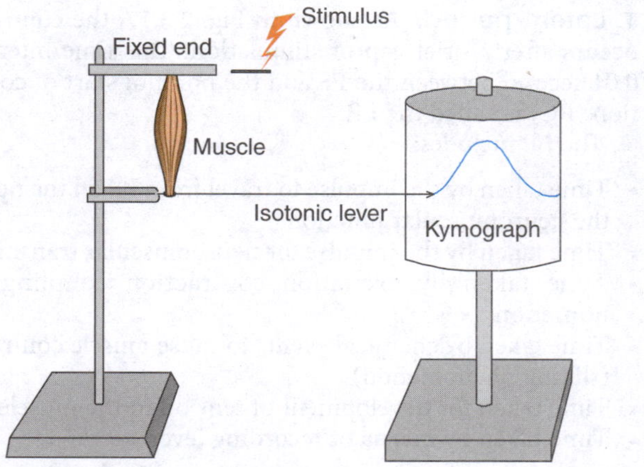

Fig. 2.3.16 Arrangement for recording isotonic contraction.

Recording of Single Muscle Twitch.

For experimental demonstration, the single muscle twitch is recorded using frog's *gastrocnemius–sciatic nerve preparation*. Ideally, the single muscle twitch should be recorded in isotonic conditions. Technically speaking, to get a perfect isotonic contraction is impossible, but practically near-isotonic contraction can be recorded by using a very light isotonic lever. Fig. 2.3.16 shows the arrangement for recording the

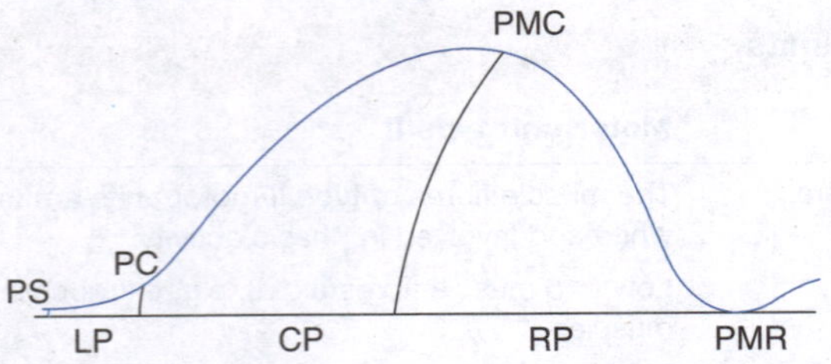

Fig. 2.3.17 Typical single muscle curve recorded from frog's gastrocnemius–sciatic nerve preparation. CP, contraction period; PC, point of start of contraction; PMC, point of maximum contraction; PMR, point of maximum relaxation; PS, point of stimulation; RP, relaxation period.

isotonic contraction. In this, one end of the muscle is tied and the other end is kept free to allow shortening and is connected to the isotonic lever which is moved easily by the muscle.

Phases of single muscle twitch. A single muscle twitch recorded under isotonic conditions from a frog's gastrocnemius–sciatic preparation shows (Fig. 2.3.17):

- *Point of stimulation (PS)* denotes the time when the stimulus is applied.
- *Point of contraction (PC)* refers to the starting point of muscle contraction.
- *Point of maximum contraction (PMC)* denotes the highest point of muscle contraction.
- *Point of maximum relaxation (PMR)* refers to the point where relaxation is completed.

The total duration of the muscle twitch is 0.1 second and it shows three phases: latent period (LP), contraction phase (CP) and relaxation phase.

1. Latent period. As shown in Fig. 2.3.17, the contraction occurs after a brief gap of stimulation. This time interval of 0.01 second between the PS and the point of start of contraction (PC) is called the LP.

The LP includes:

- Time taken by the impulse to travel from PS on the nerve to the neuromuscular junction
- Time taken by the impulse for neuromuscular transmission
- Time taken by excitation–contraction coupling phenomenon
- Time taken by chemical events to cause muscle contraction (sliding phenomenon)
- Time taken for development of tension in the muscle
- Time taken by inertia of recording lever

Factors affecting latent period are:

- LP is longer when the distance between the PS on nerve and the neuromuscular junction is more and vice versa.
- LP is more if the load on muscle is heavier.
- It decreases with increase in temperature and vice versa.

2. Contraction phase. CP of about 0.04 second extends from the PC to the PMC and is recorded as upward movement of the lever. During this phase, the muscle shortens by about 20% of its resting length. The magnitude of contraction is affected by many factors.

3. Relaxation phase. The CP is followed by the relaxation phase of about 0.05 second during which the muscle is stretched back to its original length by the dead weight suspended from the recording lever. It is recorded as downward movement of the recording lever system. The relaxation period is prolonged when the dead weight is lighter. In general, the relaxation phase is longer than the CP.

Duration of twitch. The total duration of twitch (*contraction time*) varies with the *type of muscle fibres*:

- *Fast (white) muscle fibres* (e.g. extraocular muscles and muscle of hands for fine movements) have shorter contraction time (about 0.025 second).
- *Slow (red) muscle fibres* (e.g. back muscles) have longer contraction time (0.1 second).

The total duration of twitch also varies from species to species. In human skeletal muscle, the duration of twitch is 30–50 milliseconds in comparison to 100 milliseconds in frog's (amphibian's) muscle.

Relation between electrical and mechanical events of single muscle twitch. Fig. 2.3.18 shows the electrical events (AP) and mechanical response (simple muscle twitch curve) plotted on the same time scale after being recorded separately. From this relationship graph, it can be concluded that:

- The twitch starts about 2 milliseconds after the start of depolarization of the membrane but always before the repolarization is completed.
- The refractory period (ARP) is very short and lies in the first half of the LP of the single muscle twitch.

Factors Affecting Contractile Response

The factors that can affect the contractile response (force of contraction) of a skeletal muscle are as follows:

- Strength of stimulus
- Frequency of stimulus
- Load on the muscle (preload and after-load)

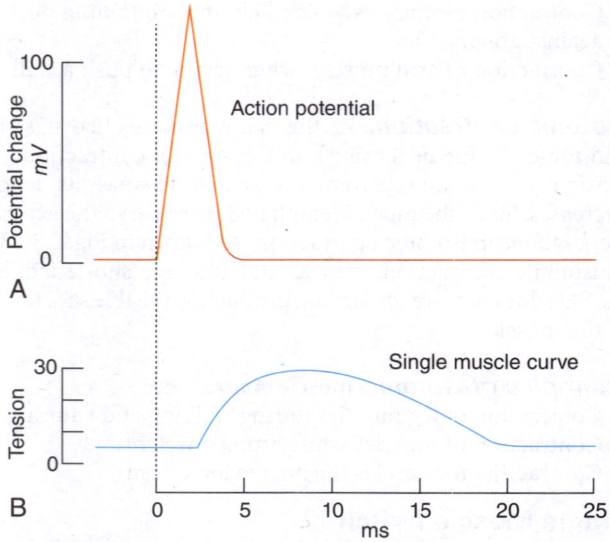

Fig. 2.3.18 Electrical **A**, and mechanical **B**, responses of mammalian skeletal muscle fibre to a single maximum stimulus plotted on same time scale.

- Initial length of muscle
- Temperature

1. Strength of stimulus ***A single muscle fibre*** obeys the all-or-none law, i.e.:

- A subthreshold stimulus evokes no response.
- With threshold, maximal and supramaximal stimuli, the contractile response remains constant.

The whole muscle, however, when stimulated with different-intensity stimuli, the response obtained (force of contraction) is a graded one. This fact can be well demonstrated in an isolated nerve–muscle preparation.

In the isolated nerve–muscle preparation. The graded response is obtained when stimuli of different intensities were applied through the nerve in a nerve–muscle preparation (Fig. 2.3.19). The whole muscle responds to the stimuli as follows:

Subthreshold stimuli do not evoke any response.
Threshold stimulus, i.e. a stimulus just sufficient to elicit response and produce minimal contraction.
Suprathreshold stimuli produce a graded response (i.e. the force of contraction goes on increasing with the increase in strength of stimulus till a maximum limit is reached). This is because, as the strength of stimuli is increased, more and more muscle fibres are recruited into activity. This phenomenon is called *quantal* or *multifibre summation*. The graded response achieved by suprathreshold stimuli is called *submaximal response*.
Maximal stimulus is that stimulus which produces the maximal response (i.e. the maximal stimulus excites all the motor units).
Supramaximal stimulus refers to the stimulus which exceeds the maximal value. Supramaximal stimuli do not increase the response beyond the maximal response. This is because, at the maximal stimulus, all the motor units are already contracting to their maximum extent and thus any further increase in the strength of stimuli (supramaximal stimulus) has no effect in increasing the force of contraction.

In the intact body. In the intact body, the whole muscle gets stimulus from the activity of anterior horn cells through their axons to the muscle fibres supplied by that particular neuron, i.e. by *recruitment of motor units.* With minimum activity, only a few motor units are recruited for activity. With increasing activity, more and more motor units (from the motor neuron pool of a muscle) are recruited into activity. This phenomenon is called *multiple motor unit summation.*

Thus, in an intact body, the relationship between the number of motor units recruited and the mechanical response achieved in terms of type of stimulus can be interpreted as follows:

At subthreshold stimulus, no motor units are recruited and hence no response is achieved.
At threshold stimulus, the minimum number of motor units (say one or two) are recruited which are just sufficient to excite minimal response.
At suprathreshold stimuli, more and more motor units are recruited producing progressively increasing response.
At maximal stimulus, all the motor units are recruited producing the maximal response.
At supramaximal stimuli, no further motor units are left to be recruited, and hence the response achieved is not more than the maximal response.

2. Frequency of stimulus The effect of repeated stimuli on the contractile response of a skeletal muscle depends on the number of stimuli (frequency). The effect of number of stimuli can be better understood by keeping the strength of stimuli constant and varying the time interval between the successive stimuli.

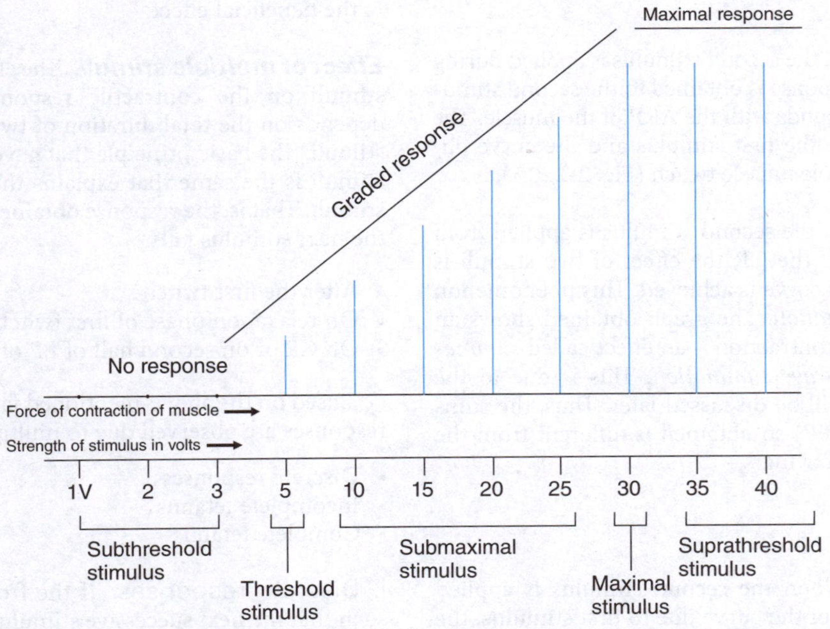

Fig. 2.3.19 Effect of strength (intensity) of stimulus on an isolated nerve–muscle preparation of frog.

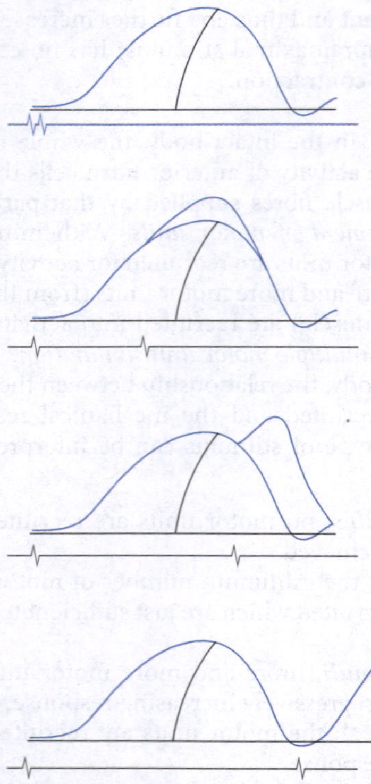

Fig. 2.3.20 Effect of two successive stimuli in an isolated gastrocnemius–sciatic nerve preparation: **A**, no response (when second stimulus applied in absolute refractory period of the first response); **B**, summation effect; **C**, superposition (incomplete summation); and **D**, beneficial effect.

Effect of two successive stimuli. Depending on the length of interval between the two successive stimuli, the following types of effects are observed:

- No response
- Summation
- Superposition
- Beneficial effect

i. No response. When the second stimulus is applied during first half of the LP, no response is obtained to the second stimulus as this period corresponds with the ARP of the muscle. The muscle responds only to the first stimulus and the curve obtained is similar to a simple muscle twitch (Fig. 2.3.20A).

ii. Summation. When the second stimulus is applied from second half of the LP to the CP, the effect of two stimuli is summed up and a single curve is achieved. This phenomenon is called *complete summation*. The graph obtained shows an increase in the force of contraction – an effect called *summation of contractions* or *wave summation*. This is due to the *beneficial effect* which will be discussed later. Thus, the summation curve (Fig. 2.3.20B) so obtained is different from the simple muscle curve by having:

- A greater amplitude
- A broader base

iii. Superposition. When the second stimulus is applied during relaxation phase of the curve due to first stimulus, the relaxation phase is cut short and another contraction occurs. The second curve is superimposed over the first curve (Fig. 2.3.20C). This is called phenomenon of *superposition* or *incomplete summation* of waves. The amplitude of the second curve is more than that of the first curve. This is also due to the beneficial effect, which is explained below.

iv. Two separate curves with beneficial effect. When the second stimulus is applied soon after the relaxation phase of the curve due to first stimulus, another complete curve is obtained. However, the force of second contraction is greater than that of the first contraction (Fig. 2.3.20D). The increase in the force of contraction of second curve is due to the beneficial effect.

Beneficial effect and its causes. As discussed above, when second stimulus is applied at any stage after the first half of the LP (i.e. at any time after the ARP), the force of second contraction is more than that of the first one. In other words, the contraction produced by first stimulus proves beneficial for the second one. This is called *beneficial effect*.
Causes of beneficial effect are as follows:

- Some of the *calcium ions* released from the terminal cisterns into the sarcoplasm during first contraction are also available in addition to those released by the second stimulus when the two stimuli are applied successively. These additional Ca^{2+} ions increase the duration of active state of second stimulus. The prolonged active state in turn increases the amount of stretch on the SEC of the muscle and so more force is transmitted to the recording lever (or to the bones in the intact body), thus increasing the height of the curve.
- *Viscosity of the muscle* and thus the elastic inertia of the muscle is decreased to some extent by the first contraction, which contributes to the beneficial effect for the second contraction.
- *Increase in H^+* ion concentration due to the first contraction also adds to the beneficial effect for the second contraction.
- *Increase in the temperature* due to first contraction decreases the viscosity of the muscle and thus contributes to the beneficial effect.

Effect of multiple stimuli. The effect of multiple successive stimuli on the contractile response of a skeletal muscle depends on the total duration of twitch and the frequency of stimuli. The basic principle that governs the effect of multiple stimuli is the same that explains the effect of two successive stimuli. That is, the response obtained will depend on whether the next stimulus falls:

- After the first twitch
- On relaxation phase of first twitch
- On CP or on second half of LP of first twitch

Based on the above-mentioned facts, the following types of responses are observed due to multiple stimuli:

- Discrete responses
- Incomplete tetanus
- Complete tetanus

i. Discrete responses. If the frequency of stimulation is such that the next successive stimulus falls after completion of

relaxation phase of the previous twitch, then the succeeding contractions obtained, with brief intervals between them, are complete individual twitches (with contraction and relaxation phases). Such a response is called a *discrete response*. Furthermore, each successive twitch has increased force of contraction (due to beneficial effect of previous twitch) till a maximal beneficial effect is achieved (Fig. 2.3.21A). This phenomenon is called the *staircase effect* or *treppe* (a German word for staircase).
Thus, if the total duration of a twitch is 100 milliseconds, then frequencies less than 10/s (i.e. each stimulus coming after every 100 milliseconds) will produce discrete responses with a staircase effect.

ii. Incomplete tetanus or clonus. When the frequency of multiple stimuli is such that the next successive stimulus falls on the relaxation phase of the previous twitch, the succeeding contraction obtained will be superposed over the previous twitch due to incomplete summation of waves. The record so obtained shows a progressive increase in amplitude up to a certain level beyond which there is no further increase. This phenomenon, as already mentioned, is called *staircase effect* or *treppe*. On stoppage of stimulation, the lever returns to normal (Fig. 2.3.21B). The series of jerky contractions of the muscle, with period of incomplete relaxation in between, so obtained is referred to as state of *subtetanus* or *incomplete tetanus* or *clonus*.

Thus, when the total duration of a twitch is 100 milliseconds, frequencies between 10 and 20/s (i.e. each stimulus coming after every 50 milliseconds but before 100 milliseconds) will fall on the relaxation phase of previous twitch and produce incomplete tetanus.

iii. Complete tetanus. When the frequency of multiple stimuli is such that the next successive stimulus falls on the second half of LP to the CP of the previous twitch (i.e. before relaxation begins), due to complete summation effect, the muscle will remain in a state of sustained, smooth and forceful contraction called *tetanus* or tetanic contraction (Fig. 2.3.21C). The graph shows an increasing slope of the uninterrupted tracing, which exceeds the peaks of single twitches. When the stimulation is stopped, the muscle relaxes immediately. However, if the stimulation is continued further, a plateau is maintained until the muscle begins to fatigue, after which it relaxes gradually. During complete tetanus, the tension developed in the muscle is four times greater than that developed during the individual muscle twitch.

Thus, when the total duration of twitch is 100 milliseconds, frequencies more than 20/s (i.e. each stimulus coming before 50 milliseconds) will fall on the CP of previous twitch and produce complete tetanus. The rate of stimulation at which there is complete fusion of individual contraction to produce tetanus is called the *tetanizing* or *fusion* frequency.

Ionic basis of tetanus. The Ca^{2+} ions released in sarcoplasm during single twitch are removed quickly and relaxation occurs. When the muscle is stimulated in rapid succession, a progressive accumulation of Ca^{2+} ions occurs in the sarcoplasm. The longer stay of Ca^{2+} ions in the sarcoplasm increases the duration of active state (due to continuous recycling of myosin heads). This increases the amount of stretch on the SEC and the tension developed rises to tetanic levels.

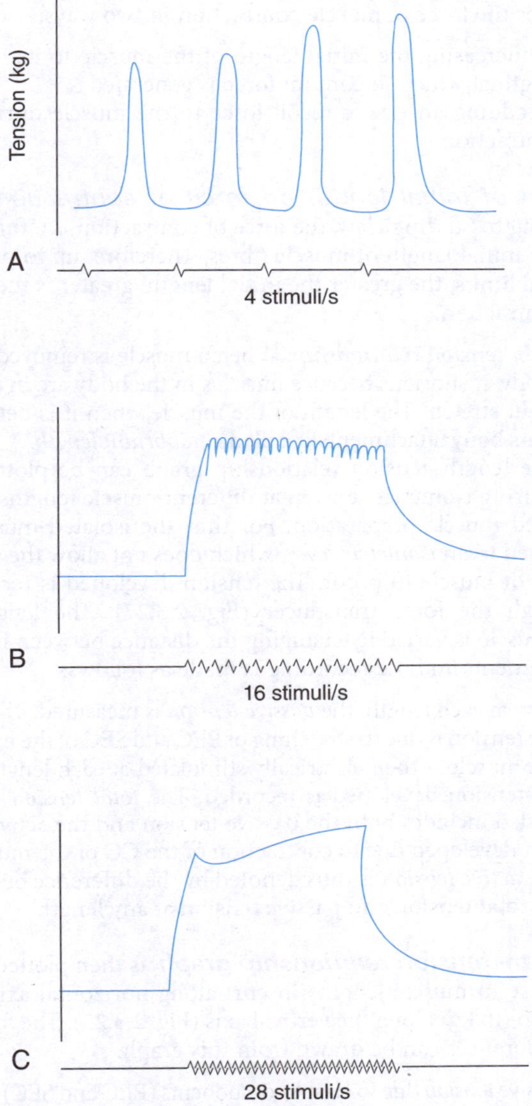

Fig. 2.3.21 Effect of multiple stimuli in an isolated gastrocnemius–sciatic nerve preparation: **A**, discrete responses; **B**, incomplete tetanus (clonus); and **C**, complete tetanus (sustained contraction).

3. Effect of load *Load* is the force exerted by the weight of an object on the muscle. The force exerted by the contracting muscle on the object is known as *muscle tension*. Thus, muscle load and muscle tension are two opposing forces. The load acting on the muscle is of two types: free load (or preload) and after-load.

Effect of free load. A load that starts acting on a muscle before it starts to contract is called free load (or preload). Example of a free load on the muscles in an intact body is filling water from a tap by holding a bucket in the hand. The free load increases the force of contraction and work efficiency of the muscle. It stretches the muscle passively producing a *passive tension* across the muscle. This passive tension increases the force of muscle contraction in two ways:

- By increasing the initial length of the muscle to its resting length at which maximum force is generated
- By adding an elastic recoil force to the muscle during its contraction

Effect of initial length on force of contraction.

According to Starling's law, the force of contraction is a function of the initial length of muscle fibres. Therefore, up to physiological limits, the greater the initial length, greater is the force of contraction.

Length–tension relationship. When a muscle is removed from the body, it shortens because muscles in the body are in a state of slight stretch. The length of the muscle when it is detached from its bony attachments is called *equilibrium length.*

The length–tension relationship graph can be plotted by measuring isometric tension at different muscle lengths in an isolated muscle preparation. For this, the isolated muscle is attached to an *isometric lever*, which does not allow the shortening of muscle to occur. The tension developed is recorded through the force transducer (Fig. 2.3.22). The length of the muscle is varied by changing the distance between its two attachments and the recording is made as follows:

- First, at each length, the *passive tension* is measured. The passive tension is due to stretching of PEC and SEC of the muscle.
- The muscle is then electrically stimulated at each length and the tension developed is recorded. The *total tension* so recorded includes both the passive tension and the active tension developed due to contraction of the CC of the muscle.
- The *active tension* is thus denoted by the difference between the total tension and passive tension at any length.

Length–tension relationship graph is then plotted with increase in muscle length (in cm) along horizontal axis and tension (in kg) along the vertical axis (Fig. 2.3.23). The following inferences can be drawn from this graph:

- *Passive tension* due to elastic components (PEC and SEC) of the muscle increases with the passively increased muscle length.

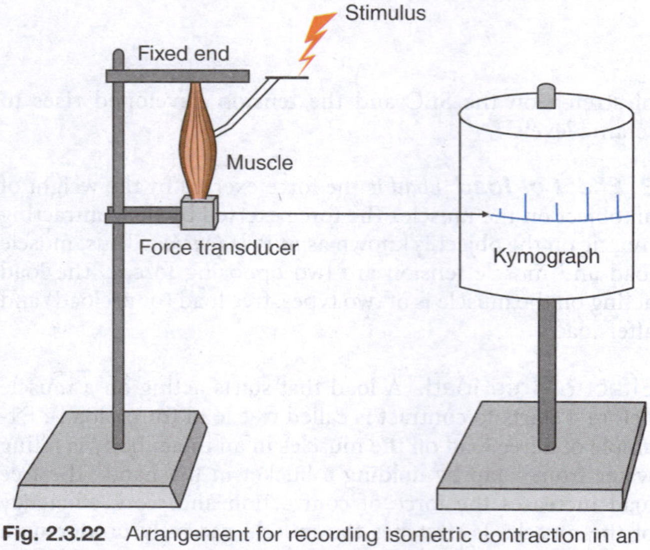

Fig. 2.3.22 Arrangement for recording isometric contraction in an isolated nerve–muscle preparation.

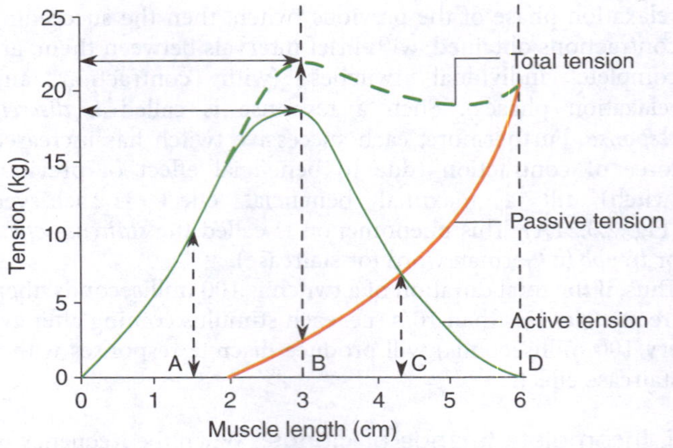

Fig. 2.3.23 Length–tension relationship graph.

- *Active tension* developed is maximum at the *optimum length* of the muscle (position B in Fig. 2.3.23) which is equivalent to the *resting length* in intact body.
- *Total tension* is contributed by active tension and passive tension at different muscle lengths as follows:
  At muscle length less than optimal level, the total tension is mainly due to active tension (position A in Fig. 2.3.23) because at such a lower initial length, there is no stretch on the muscle and so passive tension fails to develop.
  At a muscle length twice the optimal length, the total tension is mainly due to passive tension (position D in Fig. 2.3.23) because at this muscle length, the contractile tissue cannot contract and so the active tension is at zero level.
  At a muscle length 1.5 times the optimal length, the total tension is equally contributed by the active and passive tension (position C in Fig. 2.3.23).

Molecular basis of length–tension relationship. During isometric contraction, the tension developed in the muscle is proportional to the cross-bridges formed between actin and myosin filaments. The effect of muscle length on the tension produced during contraction can be explained by the sliding filament theory of muscle contraction as follows:

- *At optimum length* (position B in Fig. 2.3.24), there is optimum overlapping between the actin and myosin filaments, so maximum cross-bridges are formed between them.
- *At muscle length shorter than optimum* length (at position A in Fig. 2.3.24), the thin filaments overlap each other and thus reduce the cross-bridges between actin and myosin filaments and so the active tension produced is less.
- *When the muscle is overstretched* (position C in Fig. 2.3.24), the Z lines are pulled apart and the overlapping between the actin and myosin filaments is markedly reduced and so no active tension is developed at this level.

Effect of after-load.

After-load refers to the load which acts on the muscle after the beginning of muscular contraction. Thus, the after-load opposes the force produced by muscle contraction. The work done by an after-loaded muscle is less than that by a free-loaded muscle. An example of after-load in an intact body is lifting any object from the ground. The load acts on the muscles of arm only after lifting the object off the ground, i.e. only after beginning of the muscular contraction.

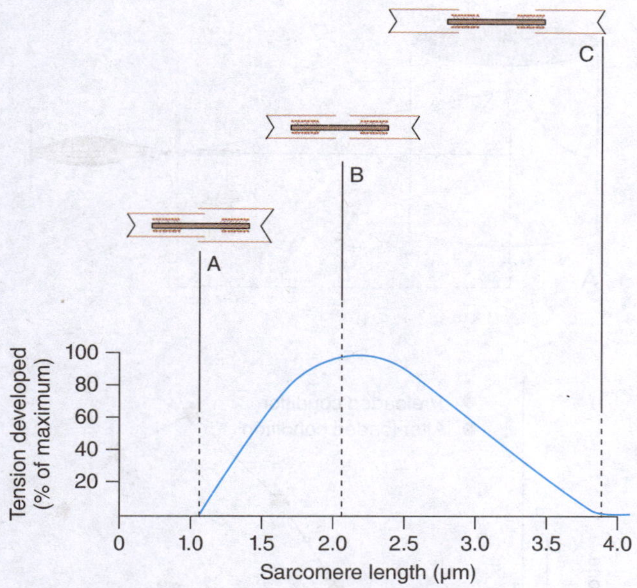

Fig. 2.3.24 Molecular basis of length–tension relationship.

Phases of muscle contraction with after-load. *Experimentally*, the effect of after-load can be studied by subjecting the muscle to *after-load preparation*; when a muscle contracts against a load, it shows three phases:

i. Initial isometric CP. In this phase of muscular contraction, as the name indicates, there occurs no shortening of the muscle. The contraction of CCs stretches the SEC and there occurs a rise in the tension (Fig. 2.3.25B). The rise in tension continues till it equals the load. This is the end point of isometric phase.

ii. Intermediate isotonic CP. This starts when the muscle tension exceeds the load and load starts moving. There occurs shortening of the muscle without further stretching of SEC (Fig. 2.3.25C).

iii. Terminal isometric phase. After the muscle becomes shorter than the resting length, any further shortening is associated with a decrease in the tension. When the tension generated equals the load, the muscle once again starts contracting isometrically.

Effect of increasing load in after-loaded condition. Fig. 2.3.26 is the graph depicting effect of progressively increasing weight in after-loaded muscle preparation. It shows that:

- As the load increases, the LP increases due to lever inertia.
- The amplitude of contraction decreases progressively as the muscle has to lift greater load.
- Contraction period decreases due to decrease in the duration of active state.
- Relaxation period also decreases, since the load hastens the return of the lever to the baseline.

Comparison of the muscle curves recorded in an isolated nerve–muscle preparation in preloaded and after-loaded conditions (Fig. 2.3.27) depicts the following differences:

- *LP* is less in preloaded as compared to that in after-loaded condition.
- *Height of contraction* is more in preloaded as compared with that in after-loaded curve.
- *Duration of twitch* is less in preloaded and more in after-loaded condition.

Force–velocity relationship. The force–velocity curve (Fig. 2.3.28) is plotted by noting the velocity of shortening of muscle with progressively increasing load on the muscle. The following inferences can be drawn from the force–velocity curve:

- When load is zero, the muscle contracts rapidly and the velocity of muscle shortening is maximum (V_{max}).
- As the load increases, the velocity of shortening decreases. With further increase in the load, a stage comes when the muscle is unable to lift the load. At this point, the muscle contracts isometrically.
- Between the two extremes of zero load and immovable load, all contractions have variable durations of isometric and isotonic contractions.
- In the force–velocity curve, mt is the point of maximum efficiency of the muscle. It lies about one-third from the abscissa and one-third from the ordinate.

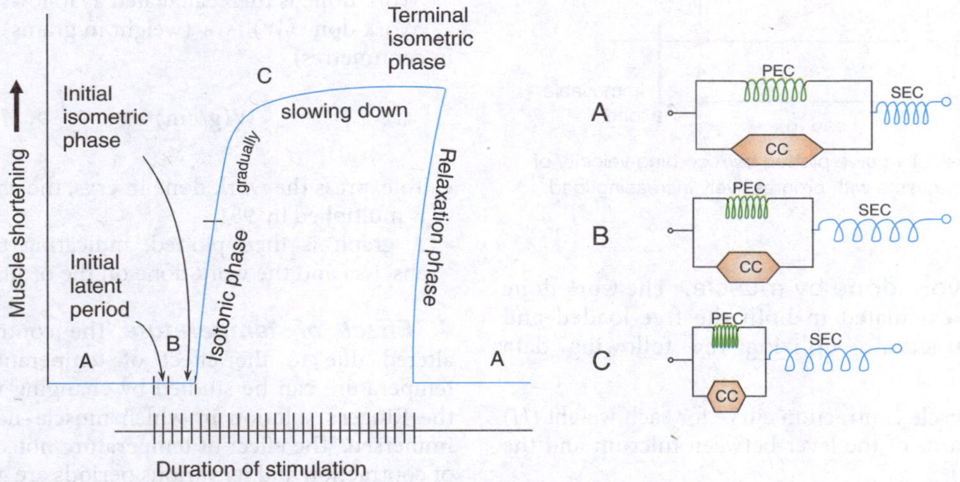

Fig. 2.3.25 Phases of muscle contraction in after-loaded condition: **A**, resting state; **B**, initial isometric contraction; and **C**, intermediate isotonic contraction which gradually slows down and tension decreases and becomes equal to load and no further shortening (terminal isometric phase).

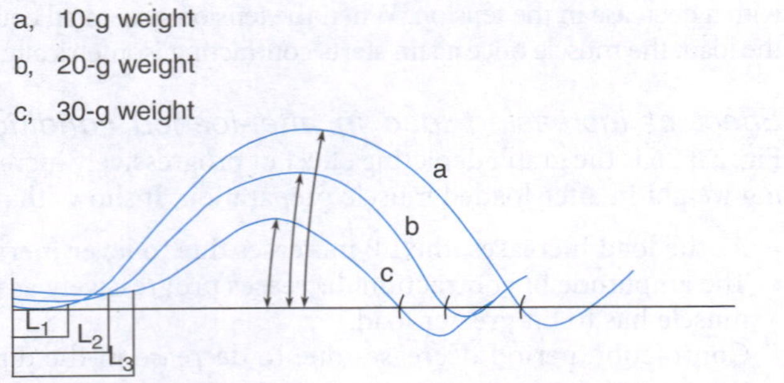

Fig. 2.3.26 Effect of increasing load in after-loaded condition in an isolated muscle–nerve preparation.

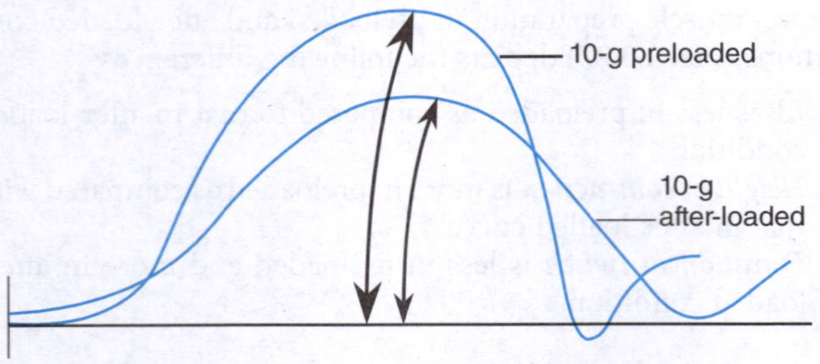

Fig. 2.3.27 Comparison of muscle curves recorded during preloaded and after-loaded conditions using 10 g weight.

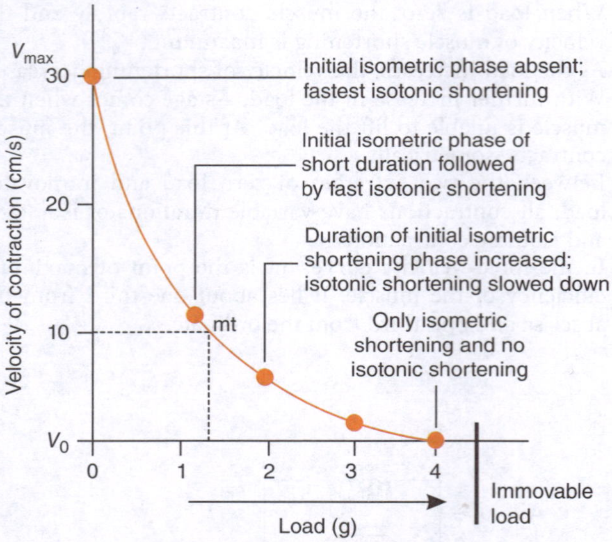

Fig. 2.3.28 Force–velocity curve plotted by recording velocity of shortening of skeletal muscle with progressively increasing load.

Calculation of work done by muscle. The work done by the muscle is calculated in both the free-loaded and after-loaded contractions, utilizing the following data (Fig. 2.3.29A):

- Height of the muscle contraction curve for each weight (H)
- Length of long arm of the lever between fulcrum and the writing point (L)
- Length of short arm of the lever between fulcrum and point where weight is added (l)
- Actual height up to which the weight is lifted (h)

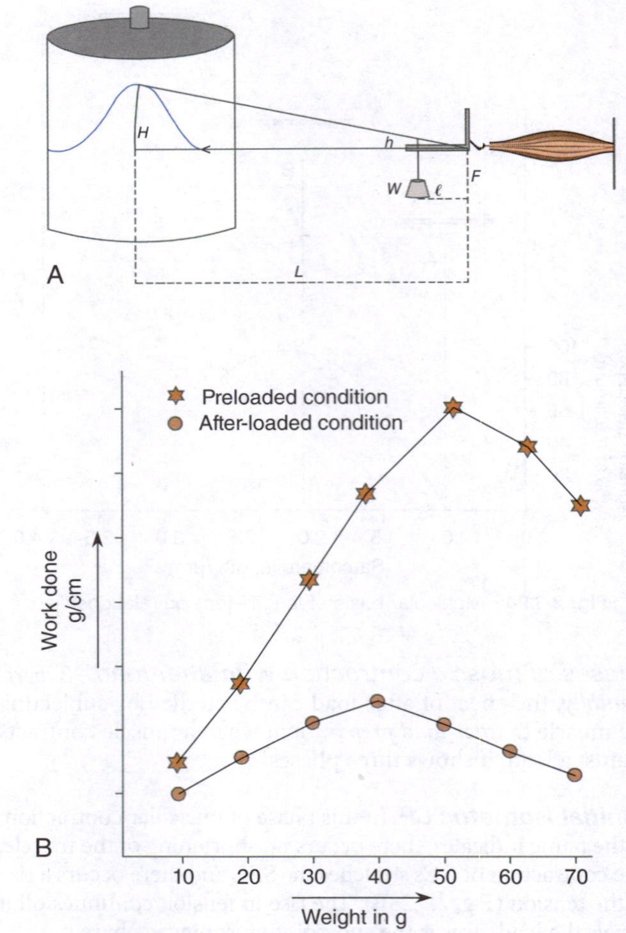

Fig. 2.3.29 Work done by the muscle: **A**, calculation of work done by finding actual height of contraction; and **B**, graphical representation of work done by the muscle in preloaded and after-loaded conditions.

Calculations. Actual height (h) is calculated taking into consideration the magnification factor (which is equal to L/l):

$$\frac{h}{H} = \frac{l}{L},\ h = H \times \frac{l}{L}$$

Work done is then calculated as follows:
Work done (W) = w (weight in grams) × h (actual height in centimetres)

$$W(\text{g/cm}) = w \times \frac{l}{L} \times H$$

- To express the work done in ergs, the above-stated reading is multiplied by 981.
- A graph is then plotted, indicating the weight on the abscissa and the work done on the ordinate (Fig. 2.3.29B).

4. Effect of temperature The contractile response is altered due to the effect of temperature. The effect of temperature can be studied by changing the temperature of the Ringer's solution in which muscle–nerve preparation is immersed. The effect of temperature noted on the amplitude of contraction and its various periods are given as follows:

At room temperature, a normal simple muscle is recorded as shown in Fig. 2.3.30A.

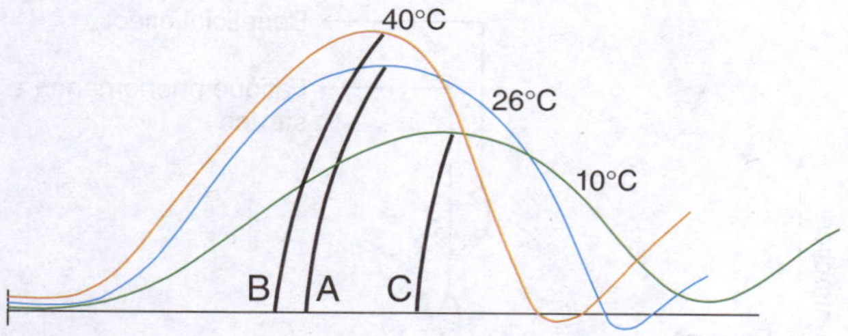

Fig. 2.3.30 Effect of temperature in an isolated nerve–muscle preparation: **A,** at room temperature (26°C); **B,** at moderately high temperature (40°C); and **C,** at cold temperature (10°C).

At moderately high temperature (say 40°C), there occurs: Faster diffusion of Ca^{2+} ions from sarcoplasmic reticulum to sarcoplasm leading to:

- An increase in the muscle excitability
- Acceleration of the chemical processes involved in muscle contraction
- A decrease in muscle viscosity

Because of the above-mentioned effects of temperature, the following changes are noted in an isotonic muscle twitch (Fig. 2.3.30B):

- Total duration of the twitch is decreased with shortening of all the periods.
- Speed of contraction increases, as is evident from the steep slope of CP.
- Relaxation is also faster.
- An increase in amplitude of muscle curve occurs due to increase in isotonic shortening of muscle. This occurs due to decrease in the internal viscoelastic resistance.

At low temperature (say 5–10°C), the reverse changes occur, i.e.:

- A decrease in the muscle excitability
- Slowing down of chemical processes involved in muscle contraction
- An increase in the muscle viscosity

The above-mentioned effects of cold, result in (Fig. 2.3.30C):

- A decrease in the force of contraction
- Prolongation of all the periods

However, the effects of cold are reversible. So, if the muscle is gradually rewarmed, excitability is regained.

At high temperature (above 50–60°C), there occurs coagulation of the muscle proteins leading to stiffness and shortening of the muscle fibres. This condition is called *heat rigor.* It is an irreversible phenomenon.

Important Note

Some other types of rigors (other than the heat rigor) are also described here because of the similar changes:

- *Cold rigor.* It occurs following exposure to severe cold. It is a reversible phenomenon.
- *Calcium rigor.* It occurs due to increased calcium content. It is also a reversible phenomenon.
- *Rigor mortis* (see page 88).

SOME CHARACTERISTICS OF THE SKELETAL MUSCLES IN THE INTACT BODY

- Muscle tone
- Nature of muscle contraction in the intact body
- Gradation of muscular activity
- Muscle fatigue
- Mechanics of muscles

MUSCLE TONE

Muscle tone is the state of slight contraction with certain degree of vigour and tension. All the skeletal muscles exhibit muscle tone. However, it is more marked in the antigravity muscles, i.e. extensors of the lower limbs, trunk muscles and muscles of the neck.

Maintenance of muscle tone. Muscle tone is a state of partial tetanus of the muscle maintained by asynchronous discharge of impulses from gamma motor neurons in the anterior grey horn of the spinal cord concerned with the motor nerve supply of the muscles. The gamma motor neurons in turn are controlled by some higher centres in the brain (see page 910).

Applied Aspects

Abnormalities of the muscle tone include:

- *Hypertonic state* or the spastic paralysis of the skeletal muscles that occurs in upper motor neuron lesions. Spasticity results due to exaggerated activity of lower motor neurons following or loss of inhibitional activity of upper motor neurons.
- *Hypotonic state* or the flaccid paralysis of the muscles that occurs in lower motor neuron lesions. The tone of the affected muscles is decreased or totally lost and ultimately the muscles undergo wasting.

NATURE OF MUSCLE CONTRACTIONS IN THE BODY

A simple muscle twitch is not a physiological event. Basically, all contractions in the body are tetanic in nature. Weak contractions result from low frequency of firing (5–10/s) of the motor units. The expected jerkiness and the disadvantage of incomplete tetanus are overcome by the asynchronous discharge (out of step firing) of groups of motor units. When one group is firing, the others are silent, and vice versa. Algebraic summation occurs, the individual variations are evened out and a smooth contraction results. The degree to which the motor neuron discharge is asynchronous is related to both the force and duration of contraction. (In a subtetanus experiment, the muscle fibres contract and relax at the same time in response to the low-frequency stimulation.) Such a situation does not occur in the body.

With increasing firing rates and, of course, with more recruitment of motor units, contractions become stronger until, at and beyond the tetanizing rate, sustained and powerful contractions result.

GRADATION OF FORCE OF MUSCLE CONTRACTION IN THE INTACT BODY

For performing different kinds of work, e.g. picking up a pen from the table or lifting a 10-kg weight, same muscles are involved but in these different situations, muscles can generate different degree of power. This property of skeletal muscles is known as gradation of force of contraction. Gradation of muscle power in muscles is made possible by certain factors which affect the force of contraction. These are as follows:

1. ***Recruitment of motor units.*** The force of contraction produced in a muscle depends on the number of motor units recruited. When minimal activity is required, only a few motor units are recruited. With increasing effort, more and more motor units from the *motor neuron pool* of a muscle are recruited into activity. This phenomenon is called multiple motor unit summation.
2. ***Frequency of nerve impulses.*** The motor control system in the brain can vary the force of contraction by varying the frequency of nerve impulses stimulating the muscle. As the impulse frequency increases, its effects are summated (*wave summation*) and the muscle tension increases.
3. ***Synchronization of impulses.*** At any one time, the motor units are in different phases of activity, i.e. some are contracting and others are relaxing. Due to algebraic summation, the muscle gives a steady but weak pull. With increasing synchronization of the motor units, the force of contraction increases.
4. ***Effect of initial length of muscle fibre.*** According to Starling's law, up to an optimal limit, the greater the initial length of the muscle fibres, greater is the force of contraction. This, however, is not the usual method of varying the force of contraction in the intact body.
5. ***Warming up.*** Warming up is the term used in the parlour of sportspersons for the exercises performed before actually participating in any game event. This pregame 'warm-up' due to beneficial effects of the exercise increases the muscle performance when the person takes part in the actual event.

MUSCLE FATIGUE

Failure of a muscle to maintain tension as a result of previous contractile activity is known as muscle fatigue. If the muscle is allowed to rest after the onset of fatigue, it recovers its ability to contract. Muscle fatigue is discussed under two separate situations:

- Fatigue in an isolated muscle
- General fatigue

Fatigue in Isolated Nerve–Muscle Preparation

In an isolated nerve–muscle preparation, when the muscle is repeatedly stimulated through its nerve, the graph (Fig. 2.3.31) obtained shows the following features:

- The first few contractions increase in amplitude due to beneficial effect.
- As stimulation is continued, there occurs a progressive increase in the LP, and a decrease in the amplitude. The rise of tension becomes slower, relaxation becomes more gradual and incomplete, and finally the muscle fails to contract altogether, and the recording lever does not return to the

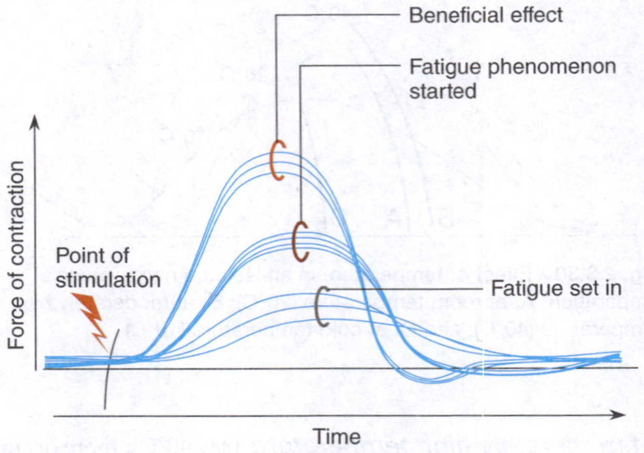

Fig. 2.3.31 Phenomenon of fatigue in an isolated muscle–nerve preparation.

baseline, i.e. the muscle remains in a state of partial contraction called *contraction remainder or contracture.* This failure of response, after repeated stimuli, is called fatigue.

Site and cause of fatigue. The site of fatigue, when the muscle has undergone fatigue through stimulation of its nerve, is *neuromuscular junction,* because the muscle responds briskly on direct stimulation. The *cause of fatigue* is depletion of acetylcholine from the motor nerve endings and interference with neuromuscular transmission by substances like pyruvic and lactic acids, and breakdown products of ATP.

The repeated stimulation of muscle itself leads to actual muscle fatigue and is due to depletion of muscle glycogen.

General Fatigue

General fatigue refers to the fatigue of most of the muscles that develops after prolonged general exercise such as marathon running and competitive football match playing.

Onset and recovery of fatigue depends on:

- Intensity and duration of exercise.
- Type of muscle fibres. Fast glycolytic fibres fatigue early and also recover rapidly from fatigue. Slow oxidative fibres do not fatigue early but they also require longer time of rest (up to 24 hours) for complete recovery.

Site, causes and mechanism of fatigue. In the human body, the sites of fatigue are in the following order:

- Fatigue of *synapses of central nervous* system due to slight hypoxia occurs first of all. It is particularly of very high intensity in short-duration exercises.
- The second site of fatigue is *motor neurons* (anterior grey horn cells) of spinal cord.
- *Motor endplate* in the neuromuscular junction may also be fatigued.
- Changes in muscles also contribute to development of fatigue:
  - In short-duration high-intensity exercises such as weight lifting and short distance running, there occurs increased acidity in the muscle cells which accompanies rise in lactic acid (formed due to anaerobic glycolysis). H^+ ion concentration directly inhibits cross-bridge cycles and therefore force generated by them. The second cause is

decrease in release of Ca^{2+} ions from the sarcoplasmic reticulum.
- In long-duration low-intensity exercises such as marathon race, depletion of muscle glycogen is an important contributing factor.

Psychological Fatigue

Lack of motivation due to failure of cerebral cortex to send excitatory signals to motor neurons causes an individual to stop exercising. The psychological fatigue (feeling of weariness) is different from *physiological fatigue* of the muscles. The muscles are actually not fatigued (therefore, it is not a true muscle fatigue). An athlete's performance, therefore, depends on not only the physical status of appropriate muscle but also psychological fatigue.

MUSCLE MECHANICS

Common Terms Used in Muscle Mechanics

Strength of the muscle. Strength of the muscle can be defined as the maximal contractile force produced per square centimetre of the cross-sectional area of the skeletal muscle. On an average, the normal force produced by a muscle is about 3–4 kg/cm^2 area of the muscle. Thus, strength of a muscle is directly proportional to the size of the muscle. The size of the muscle can be increased by regular exercise.

The strength of the muscle is of two types:

1. ***Contractile strength*** of the muscle is exhibited during actual shortening (isotonic contraction) of the muscle. For example, the strength developed in the leg muscles during taking off the body from the ground while jumping is the contractile strength.
2. ***Holding strength*** refers to the force produced while stretching the contracted muscles. For example, the force developed in the leg muscles while landing after jumping is the holding force. The holding strength of a muscle is greater than the contractile strength.

Power of the muscle. Power of the muscle refers to the amount of work done by the muscle in a given unit of time. It is expressed in kilogram metre per minute (kg-m/min). Thus, the muscle power is the product of strength and speed. The power output of a muscle is determined by the energy input per second and its mechanical efficiency.

Endurance of the muscle. Endurance of the muscle refers to its capacity to withstand the power produced during activity. In other words, it is the ability of the muscle to contract repeatedly over time. The muscle endurance depends mostly on the nutrition to the muscle.

Muscle tension and excursion When a muscle contracts, the external work done is observable as the force generated by the muscle, which is known as *muscle tension*, and/or a change in the muscle length, which is known as *muscle excursion*. Muscle length usually shortens during isotonic contraction. However, due to simultaneous passive stretching, the muscle length may increase under certain circumstances. In such situations, the work done is negative.

Muscle action. When a muscle or group of muscle contracts, a movement is produced in the associated part of the skeletal lever system of the body; such a resultant movement is referred to as the action of that muscle. For example, flexion or extension produced at some joint in the body is the action of the concerned muscles.

Certain Facts About Muscle Mechanics

Certain facts about the muscle mechanics in human body are as follows:

1. ***Skeletal lever system.*** In our body, the muscle, bones and joints form a system of lever. At most places in the body, the anatomical system provides third-class levers. According to principles of physics, with third-class levers, much greater force is required to lift the same load, although the speed of lifting is faster. Therefore, speed of action with human muscle is fast but requires greater force.
2. ***Advantage of resting length.*** Attachments of most of the muscles in the body are such that many of them are normally at or near their resting length when they start to contract, and thus force of contraction produced is more.
3. ***Situations for isometric contractions.*** In muscles that extend over more than one joint, movement at one joint may compensate for movement at another in such a way that relatively little shortening of the muscle occurs during contraction. Such situations, for nearly isometric contraction, permit development of maximal tension per contraction. For example, in the case of hamstrings muscles which extend over the hip as well as knee joint, the lengthening of the muscles across the hip joint compensates the shortening across the knee joint.
4. ***Peculiar integration of momentum and balance into the body movements.*** This makes a possible maximal motion with minimal muscular exertion. Due to such integration, the stress put on the tendon and bones is rarely over 50% of their failure strength, protecting them from damage. For example, during walking, each limb passes rhythmically through two phases: the support or *stance phase* (when the foot is on the ground) and the *swing phase* (when the foot is off the ground). The support phases of the two legs overlap, so that there are two periods of double support during each cycle. There is a brief burst of activity in the leg flexors at the start of each step, and then the leg is swung forward with little more active muscular contraction. Thus, in this way, the muscles are active for only a fraction of each step. Therefore, walking for long periods causes relatively little fatigue.
5. ***Integrated muscle action.*** The muscles may play a functional role as an agonist, antagonist or synergist during a particular movement. These relationships are not absolute, but vary with the activity, position of the body and the direction of the resistance that the muscle must overcome.
   - *Agonist* refers to a muscle (or group of muscles) which on contraction acts as the principal muscle producing a joint motion.
   - *Antagonists* refer to those muscles which have actions opposite to the agonist. They do not contract during a particular movement, but passively elongate or shorten to permit the motion to occur.
   - *Synergists* refer to those muscles which contract along with the agonist to produce a motion. The synergist may act as an assistant mover, neutralizer or a stabilizer.
   - *Assistant mover* is the muscle which aids the prime mover (agonist) in performing a particular motion.

- *Neutralizers* are the muscles which neutralize the action of those muscles which prevent the agonist to produce a particular movement. For example, the extensors of the wrist neutralize the wrist flexors and these allow the long flexors of the fingers to contract and close the fist.
- *Stabilizers* refer to those muscles which stabilize a proximal joint so that another muscle may act effectively at a distal joint. For example, the wrist extensors stabilize the wrist joint, so that the hand can be used effectively.

6. ***Active and passive insufficiency.*** This phenomenon is seen in muscles which extend over two joints. Failure to produce a tight fist by the finger flexors when the wrist is in flexion is an example of active insufficiency. Passive insufficiency of rectus femoris occurs due to excessive stretching when there is knee flexion with hip extension.

ELECTROMYOGRAPHY AND COMMON DISORDERS OF MUSCLES

ELECTROMYOGRAPHY

Electromyography (EMG) refers to the technique of recording the total electrical activity of the motor nerve and the muscle under study. The machine used to record the said electrical activity is called *electromyograph* and the record obtained is called the *electromyogram*.

Recording Technique

The basic recording unit of the electromyograph is a cathode ray oscilloscope. The EMG can be recorded using two types of electrodes:

1. ***Surface electrodes*** or skin electrodes are placed on the skin above the surface of the muscle to be studied. They are convenient but are not precise, so they are not commonly used.
2. ***Needle electrodes*** are inserted into the muscle under study. The commonest inserted electrode used in EMG is the *bipolar concentric needle electrode*. It consists of an insulated stainless steel hypodermic needle which contains an insulated fine wire in its barrel: the wire and the needle have bared tips. With needle electrodes, it is usually possible to pick up the activity of a single muscle fibre.

Protocol for Recording EMG

For recording of EMG, the patient is made to lie comfortably in a quiet room. The needle electrode is inserted into the muscle and a ground lead is attached to the same limb to which the muscle under study belongs. The recordings are then taken as follows:

At rest, the muscle is explored systematically for the presence of any *spontaneous activity*.

During slight muscle contraction, the recording is made from different sites to assess the size and duration of activity of different motor units (*motor unit potentials* [MUPs]).

During maximal muscle contraction (against resistance) to record the *interference pattern*, which helps in determining the abnormal recruitment of motor units, if any. Observations made help in differentiating whether the problem is myogenic or neurogenic.

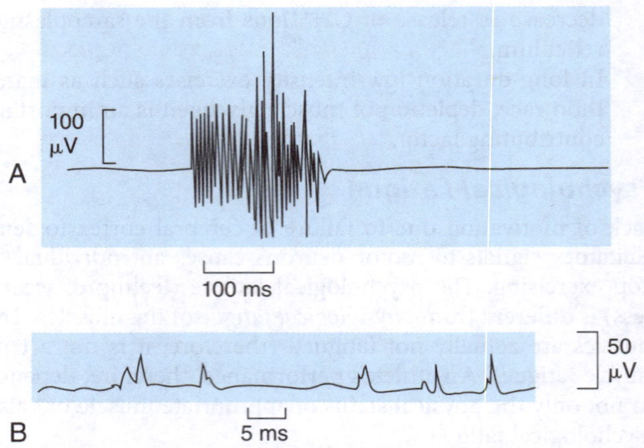

Fig. 2.3.32 Electromyogram showing spontaneous activity at rest: **A**, complete silence followed by insertion activity; and **B**, endplate potential noise.

Electromyogram

Components of a normal electromyogram along with the common abnormalities which can be detected are given as follows.

Spontaneous activity at rest. Normally, at rest, there is complete electrical silence and no spontaneous activity is recorded, except for:

1. ***The insertion activity.*** When a needle electrode is inserted into a muscle, it evokes a discharge of APs (due to mechanical stimulus). These potentials are of short duration and small amplitude (Fig. 2.3.32A). The insertion activity is
   - Prolonged in denervated muscle
   - Absent when muscle tissue is not viable
2. ***Endplate noise.*** After the cessation of insertion activity, no other spontaneous activity is seen but for a monophasic negative potential in the endplate region called *endplate noise* (Fig. 2.3.32B). These potentials correspond to the miniature endplate potential (MEP) of the neuromuscular junction.

Voluntary activity during muscle contraction. The potential change recorded during muscle contraction is called *MUP*. The MUP is the compound potential which represents the sum of the individual APs generated in the few muscle fibres of the motor unit that are within the pick-up range of the recording electrode. Since fibres of several motor units intermingle singly, each EMG electrode records the activity of more than one motor unit. MUPs are usually biphasic or triphasic in shape; however, if more than four phases are recorded, they are denoted as polyphasic. The characteristic features of a typical MUP are as follows (Fig. 2.3.33).

Amplitude of MUP is usually between 200 μV and 3 mV and is determined largely by the distance between the recording electrode and the active fibres that are closest to it. In the record, it is measured as peak-to-peak distance.

Duration of each spike of MUP normally varies between 2 and 15 milliseconds and is related to the anatomic scatter of endplates of these muscle fibres in the motor units that are within the pick-up zone of the recording electrode.

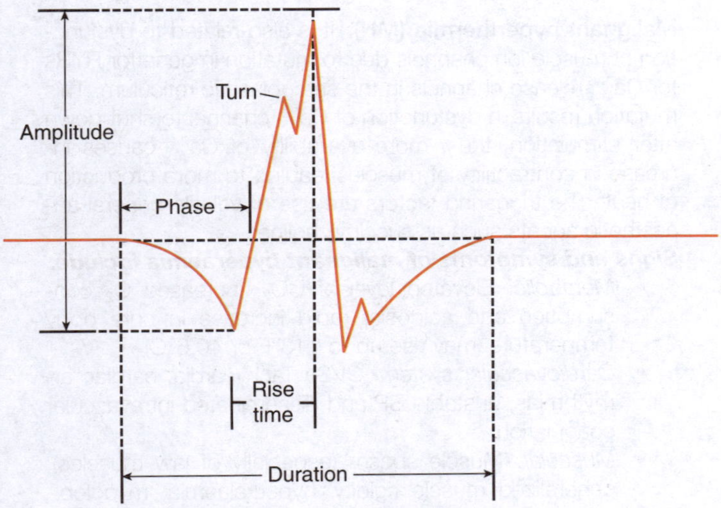

Fig. 2.3.33 Motor unit potential (MUP).

Duration of MUP is measured from the beginning of phase to return to the baseline.

Significance. Increased duration of MUP occurs in lower motor neuron lesion (LMNL), neuropathy and reduced muscle temperature, whereas decreases myelopathy and myasthenia gravis.

Phases and turns. In MUP, record phase is defined as peak after crossing over the baseline and turn is labelled as peak before crossing over the baseline.

Rise time is duration from initial positive peak to next negative peak. The average rise time is 500 μs.

The electromyographic records obtained *during different grades of muscle* contraction have the following characteristics:

1. ***On minimal voluntary contraction***, only a single or two smaller motor units in the vicinity of needle electrode give off electrical discharge (Fig. 2.3.34A).
   - It has a regular rhythmic fashion.
   - Frequency is low (5–10/s).
2. ***With the progressive increase in the voluntary contraction***, the firing rate of small units increases until it reaches a certain frequency, when larger units are recruited. Fig. 2.3.34B shows the recruitment pattern with moderate force of contraction.
3. ***During maximal contraction***, many motor units are recruited and thus the many rhythmically recurring MUPs become so superimposed on one another on the oscilloscope screen that it is impossible to determine their individual characteristics. The resulting appearance of the EMG is designated as *normal interference pattern* (Fig. 2.3.34C).

Interpretation of EMG record taken during muscle contraction.

Features to be noted while analysing the EMG record taken during voluntary muscle contraction include:

Onset frequency, i.e. the frequency when the MUPs first appear

Recruitment frequency, i.e. the frequency at which a particular unit must fire before another is recruited

Density of the interference pattern, i.e. the frequency of MUPs at maximal contraction

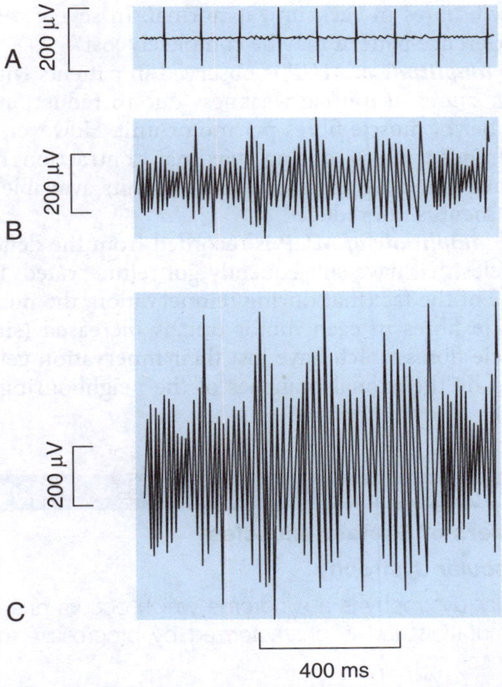

Fig. 2.3.34 Electromyogram during voluntary muscle activity: **A**, on minimal contraction; **B**, on moderate contraction (recruitment pattern); and **C**, on maximum contraction (normal interference pattern).

Abnormal spontaneous activities.

Abnormal spontaneous activities which can be recorded during resting phase are as follows:

1. ***Fasciculation potentials*** resemble MUPs and represent the involuntary contraction of muscle fibres of a single motor unit. The fasciculation (jerky, visible twitching of a group of muscle fibres) occurs in patients with chronic partial denervation especially due to spinal cord lesions.
2. ***Fibrillation potentials*** are of very short duration (0.5–2 milliseconds) and low amplitude (25 and 100 μV). They occur at a regular rhythm (2–10/s) and always have an initial positive phase and a secondary negative phase (Fig. 2.3.35).

The fibrillation potentials are produced due to involuntary contraction of the single muscle cells which have been dissociated from nervous control following denervation.

Abnormalities during voluntary activity.

Abnormalities of MUP frequency and amplitude detected during voluntary activity are as follows:

1. ***Decrease in the density of the interference*** or the so-called *sparse interference pattern* is seen in patients with *neurogenic weakness* of the muscle when the number of functional motor units is reduced and thus the MUP frequency during maximal contraction is decreased. The amplitude of MUP record is however normal, since the number of

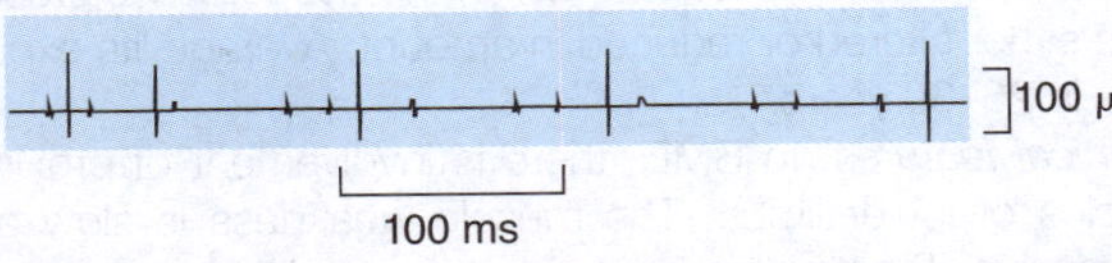

Fig. 2.3.35 Fibrillation potential recorded from denervated muscle.

muscle fibres in each unit is normal. In severe cases, the interference pattern may be completely lost.

2. ***Low amplitude of MUP*** is observed in patients with *myogenic causes* of muscle weakness due to reduction in the number of muscle fibres per motor unit. However, the interference pattern during maximal contraction remains normal since the number of motor units available for recruitment is not reduced.
3. ***High amplitude of MUP*** is recorded from the denervated muscles that have subsequently got reinnervated. It is because of the fact that during reinnervation, the number of muscle fibres in each motor unit is increased (since the muscle fibres which have lost their innervation get innervated by the axonal branches of the neighbouring motor unit).

Applied Aspects

Disorders of Skeletal Muscles

1. Muscular dystrophy

Muscular dystrophy is a syndrome which occurs due to genetic mutation and is characterized by progressive muscle weakness.

Duchenne muscular dystrophy (DMD). It is caused by mutations of the dystrophic gene that cause dystrophin to be absent from the muscles. It is an X-linked disorder occurring in about 1 of every 5000 male infants. It causes great disability and eventually proves fatal by the age of 30 years.

Signs and symptoms. The symptoms usually appear before the age of 6 years. The main symptom of DMD is progressive muscle weakness associated with muscle wasting, the voluntary muscles being first affected, especially of lower limbs. The other physical symptoms include awkward types of walking, stepping as running because of adaptation to knee extensor weakness, frequent falls and fatigue.

Difficulty with motor skill (running, hopping and jumping).

Diagnosis of DMD is carried out by the following:

- Genetic testing at birth will help in diagnosis
- EMG depicts polyphasic MUPs of reduced duration
- Muscle biopsies and immunohistochemistry

Treatment. Although there is no specific cure, physiotherapy and other measures can help in relieving the symptoms which includes:

1. *Corrective surgery* may help with some symptoms.
2. *Assisted ventilation* when there is weakness of breathing muscles.
3. *Medication* includes:
   - Steroids to slow the muscle degeneration
   - Anticonvulsants to control seizures
   - Immunosuppressants to delay damage
4. *Gene therapy* in early stages may be quite useful.

Becker muscular dystrophy (BMD). It is the most common type of muscular dystrophy. It is an autosomal recessive disorder occurring due to a mutation in the gene for sarcoglycan or other components of dystrophin–glycoprotein complex. It is a milder form of the disease in which the dystrophin is present but is either altered or reduced in amount. Average life expectancy is 26–30 years.

Clinical features. In BMD, there is involvement of proximal muscles of lower limbs. The muscle weakness is slow and progressive. Toe walking is seen in this condition.

Malignant hyperthermia (MH). It is also related to dysfunction of muscle ion channels due to mutation in gene for RYRs for Ca^{2+}-release channels in the sarcoplasmic reticulum. This mutation results in dysfunction of Ca^{2+} channel to shut down after stimulation; thus, more availability of Ca^{2+} causes increase in contractility of muscles leading to more production of heat. The triggering factors are use of volatile general anaesthetic agents such as succinylcholine.

Signs and symptoms of malignant hyperaemia include:

- *Metabolic*: Elevated level of CO_2, increased O_2 consumption and acidosis, rapid increase in core body temperature (may rise up to 113°F or 40.6°C)
- *Cardiovascular system (CVS):* Tachycardia, cardiac arrhythmias, unstable BP and disseminated intravascular coagulation
- *Muscular:* Muscle spasm (especially of jaw muscles), generalized muscle rigidity, hyperkalaemia, myoglobinaemia and myoglobinuria

Treatment. No specific treatment for MH is recommended

For hyperthermia: The following measures can be taken to relieve hyperthermia:

- Intravenous administration of 2–3 L of chilled (4°C) 0.9% saline.
- Surface cooling by wet cold sheets under fan or by ice packs; cooling should be stopped if temperature comes down to 38.5°C.

For hyperkalaemia – use of

- 50 mL 5% dextrose, with 50 IU of insulin.
- $CaCl_2$: 10 mL $CaCl_2$ for 70-kg adult, and sometimes dialysis may be required.

For acidosis

- Ask the patient to hyperventilate.
- Intravenous administration of Na_2HCO_3 if pH is <7.2.

For arrhythmia

- β-Blockers, e.g. propranolol, if tachycardia persists.
- Maintain urinary output >2 mL/kg/h by use of diuretics (furosemide).

Central core disease (CCD). It is also called central core myopathy and is an autosomal dominant inherited muscular disorder present from birth. It occurs due to mutation of RYR1 gene. The common symptoms include the following:

- Hypotonia (low muscle tone)
- Muscle weakness
- Delayed milestones
- Breathing and swallowing difficulty

2. Myotonia

Myotonia is a disorder that occurs due to abnormalities of the sodium and chloride channels caused by abnormal genes on chromosomes 7, 17 or 19. It is characterized by an abnormally prolonged muscle relaxation after voluntary contraction.

3. Myasthenia gravis

It is a disorder of the neuromuscular junction, characterized by a grave weakness of the muscles (see page 79).

4. Abnormal muscle tone

The normal muscle tone of a muscle may be increased or decreased constituting an abnormal muscle tone (see page 99).

5. Metabolic myopathies

Metabolic myopathies occur due to mutation of genes that code enzymes involved in carbohydrate and protein metabolism of the muscles for the production of ATP (McArdle syndrome). Metabolic myopathies usually present as intolerance to exercise.

6. Fibrillation and denervation hypersensitivity

The denervation of skeletal muscles in lower motor neuron lesions causes flaccid paralysis of the muscle, fibrillation and denervation hypersensitivity.

Fibrillation. Skeletal muscle fibrillation refers to small, local, muscular contractions that occur in response to spontaneous activation of single muscle fibre which then contracts independently of surrounding fibres.

Denervation hypersensitivity refers to sharp increase of sensitivity of postsynaptic membrane to the chemical neurotransmitter after denervation.

It is suggested that two factors interact to produce denervation hypersensitivity: the pressure of degenerative nerve tissue and concomitant cellular change, leading to changes in muscle fibre membrane to become hypersensitive.

SOURCE OF ENERGY AND METABOLIC PHENOMENON DURING MUSCLE CONTRACTION

- Chemical composition of muscle
- Energy source for muscle contraction
- Oxygen demand, consumption and debt
- Changes in pH during muscle contraction
- Thermal changes during muscle contraction

CHEMICAL COMPOSITION OF MUSCLE

Chemical composition of a skeletal muscle is as follows:

1. ***Water*** constitutes the major bulk of (75%) the muscle weight.
2. ***Muscle proteins*** form 20% of the muscle mass. These include the contractile proteins (actin, myosin, troponin and tropomyosin), myogen and myoglobin. Myoglobin is a conjugated protein. Like haemoglobin, its main function is to carry oxygen.
3. ***Organic substances other than proteins*** present in the muscle fibre include:
   - *Carbohydrates:* glycogen and hexaphosphate
   - *Lipids:* neutral fat, cholesterol, lecithin and steroids
   - *Nitrogenous substances:* ATP, adenylic acid, creatine, phosphocreatine, urea, uric acid, xanthine and hypoxanthine
4. ***Inorganic substances*** present in the muscle are as follows:
   - *Cations:* potassium, sodium, calcium, magnesium
   - *Anions:* chloride, phosphate and sulphate

ENERGY SOURCE FOR MUSCLE CONTRACTION

The muscle contraction requires lot of energy. In fact, the muscle has been labelled as a *machine for converting chemical energy into mechanical work.* The immediate source of energy is ATP and the ultimate source is the intermediary metabolism of carbohydrate and lipids.

Hydrolysis of ATP The hydrolysis of ATP provides energy for muscle contraction (for details, see the section 'Molecular Basis of Muscle Contraction', page 86). ATP stored in the muscle initiates the contractile activity but is consumed after a few twitches. In about 3 seconds, all the ATP stored in the muscle cell is depleted. Thus, there is need for resynthesis of ATP.

Resynthesis of ATP There are three ways in which a muscle fibre can resynthesize ATP from ADP during contractile activity.

1. Phosphorylation of ADP by creatine phosphate. Immediately after the depletion of ATP stores of the muscle, ATP is regenerated using the energy released by the dephosphorylation of creatine phosphate reserves of the muscle fibre.

$$\text{Creatine phosphate} + \text{ADP}^{\text{TM}} \Leftrightarrow \text{creatine} + \text{ATP}$$

The above reaction, known as *Lohmann reaction,* is rapid and requires only single enzyme. It is reversible and obeys law of mass action. Since the amount of creatine phosphate is limited, the amount of ATP formed by this mechanism is only sufficient for contraction of the muscle for next about 5 seconds. Therefore, the next mechanism comes into play immediately.

(At rest, the muscle contains large quantities of ATP; therefore, the reaction proceeds from right to left forming creatine phosphate, and thus the store is built up.)

2. Glycolysis. After depletion of creatine phosphate reserves, the next important source of energy which is used to reconstitute both ATP and phosphocreatine is glycogen (previously stored in the muscle cell) by the process of glycolysis which can sustain muscle contraction for about 1 minute. As shown in Fig. 2.3.36, each molecule of glycogen after glycolysis produces two molecules of pyruvic acid and two molecules of ATP. Further changes in pyruvic acid depend on the availability of oxygen.

- In the absence of oxygen, the pyruvic acid is converted into lactic acid which is released into the blood. From the blood, lactic acid is taken up by the kidney and liver where it is reconverted into glucose and released back into circulation (Cori cycle).
- If oxygen is available, the pyruvic acid enters *Krebs cycle.*

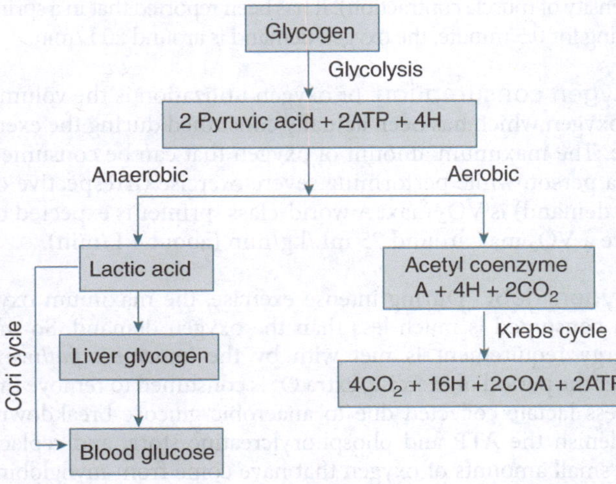

Fig. 2.3.36 Schematic diagram showing breakdown of glycogen stored in a muscle cell.

A total of 38 ATP molecules are formed during breakdown of each glycogen molecule as follows:

- Two molecules of ATP are formed during glycolysis.
- Two molecules of ATP are formed during Krebs cycle.
- Thirty-four molecules of ATP are formed utilizing the hydrogen ions produced during breakdown of a glycogen molecule.

Importance of glycolysis is twofold:

- First, the glycolytic reactions occur even in the absence of oxygen, so that muscle contraction can be sustained for a short time even when oxygen is not available.
- Second, the rate of formation of ATP by glycolysis process is about 2.5 times as rapid as ATP formation when the cellular foodstuffs react with oxygen.

3. Oxidative metabolism. Oxidative metabolism, i.e. combining of oxygen with various cellular foodstuffs to liberate ATP, is the final source of energy during muscle contraction. This source contributes more than 95% of all energy used by the muscles for sustained long-term contraction. Foodstuffs used in oxidative metabolism include fats, carbohydrates and proteins as:

- *Fatty acids* are used for resynthesis of most of the ATP during prolonged muscle contraction lasting over a period of many hours.
- *Glycogen* contributes about half of the energy required for muscle contraction lasting for 2–4 hours.

Important Notes

- During intense but short-lasting exercise, e.g. in a 100-m race that takes 10 seconds, 85% of the energy consumed is derived anaerobically.
- During moderate-intensity exercise, e.g. in a 3-km race that takes 16 minutes, 20% of the energy consumed is derived anaerobically.
- During mild-intensity prolonged exercise, e.g. in a long-distance race that takes about an hour, only 5% of the energy comes from anaerobic metabolism.

OXYGEN DEMAND, CONSUMPTION AND DEBT

Oxygen demand increases with the intensity of exercise (i.e. intensity of muscle contraction). It has been reported that in a sprint lasting for 0.5 minute, the oxygen demand is around 20 L/min.

Oxygen consumption or oxygen utilization is the volume of oxygen which has been actually consumed during the exercise. The maximum amount of oxygen that can be consumed by a person while performing severe exercise (irrespective of the demand) is VO_2 max. A world-class sprinter is expected to have a VO_2 max around 75 mL/kg/min (about 4 L/min).

Oxygen debt. During intense exercise, the maximum oxygen consumed is much less than the oxygen demand. So the energy requirement is met with by the *anaerobic pathway*. After the period of exercise, extra O_2 is consumed to remove the excess lactate collected due to anaerobic glucose breakdown, replenish the ATP and phosphorylcreatine store, and replace the small amounts of oxygen that have come from myoglobin. This amount of extra oxygen consumed is called O_2 debt and is proportionate to the extent to which energy demands during exercise exceeded the capacity of aerobic synthesis of energy store, i.e. extent to which *oxygen deficit occurred* during exercise. Oxygen debt can be measured experimentally by determining oxygen consumption after exercise until constant basal consumption is reached and then subtracting the basal oxygen consumption from total oxygen consumed during this period (Fig. 2.3.37).

Applied Aspects

To avoid excessive O_2 debt early in the race, the experienced long-distance runners begin the race very slowly to allow the cardiorespiratory system to gear up to the energy demands of muscular activity; once a steady state is attained due to cardiorespiratory readjustment, the oxygen supply balances the oxygen requirements of the muscles. This state of oxidative metabolism to provide energy for the muscles can continue for several hours without producing excessive oxygen debt. This prevents too much anaerobic metabolism and accumulation of lactic acid which hamper the efficiency.

Mechanical efficiency of muscle During contraction, the efficiency of muscle is about 25%. Mechanical efficiency is equal to output/input. Therefore, mechanical efficiency is equal to:

$$\frac{\text{Work done by the muscle } (W)}{\text{Oxygen consumption } (VO_2)}$$

Or

$$\frac{W \text{ (kilopond metre/min/426.7)}}{VO_2 \text{(L/min)} \times 5}$$

(since 426.7 kilopond m/min = 1 kcal, and 1 L/min VO_2 at STPD produces 5 kcal of energy; STPD means standard temperature [0°C] and pressure [760 mm Hg] and dry.)

- Therefore, mechanical efficiency in isotonic contraction is approximately 25% of the energy expenditure and rest 75% is degraded as heat.
- During isometric contraction, as no external work is done, mechanical efficiency is nil and 100% energy expenditure disappears as heat.

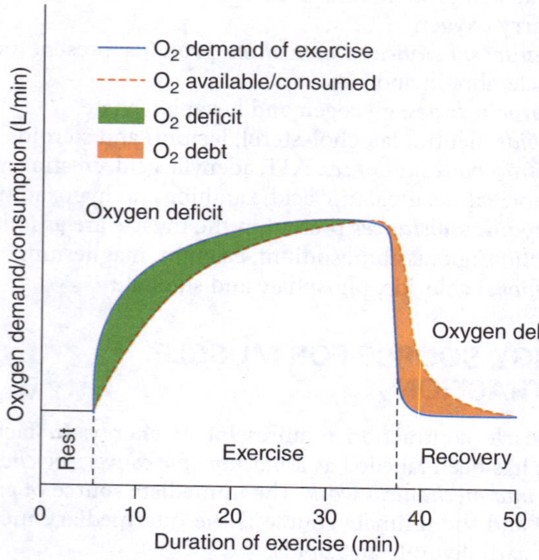

Fig. 2.3.37 Oxygen debt.

CHANGES IN pH DURING MUSCLE CONTRACTION

Changes occurring in the pH and reaction of the muscle during contraction are as follows:

During resting condition, the reaction of muscle is alkaline with a pH of 7.3.

During onset of muscle contraction, due to dephosphorylation of ATP to ADP, the pH of muscles becomes acidic.

During later part of muscle contraction, due to resynthesis of ATP from creatine phosphate, the muscle reaction again becomes alkaline.

At the end of muscle contraction, due to formation of pyruvic acid and/or lactic acid, the muscle reaction once again becomes acidic.

THERMAL CHANGES DURING MUSCLE CONTRACTION

Thermal changes in the muscle during contraction can be accurately measured using suitable thermocouple. The different phases of heat production during muscle contraction are as follows:

1. Resting heat. Resting heat is the heat generated when the muscle is at rest, i.e. not contracting. It is the external manifestation of the basal metabolic process of the muscle.

2. Initial heat. Initial heat refers to the heat generated in excess of resting heat during muscular contraction. It is made up of the following components:

Activation heat. refers to initial rapid liberation of energy before the actual contraction of the muscle. It is mostly due to the heat liberated while calcium ions are released from the L-tubules of sarcoplasmic reticulum and the myosin ATPase is activated.

Shortening heat. is produced when the muscle contracts isotonically. It is produced due to various structural changes in the muscle fibre like movement of cross-bridges and myosin heads and breakdown of glycogen. It is absent during isometric contraction.

Maintenance heat. is generated during isometric contraction when no actual shortening of the muscle fibre takes place. Its cause is complicated and mostly obscure.

3. Recovery heat. Recovery heat refers to the heat produced in excess of resting heat, following muscle contraction. It continues for about 30 minutes after the cessation of muscle contraction. This heat is generated by the metabolic processes that restore the muscle to its precontraction state. These include calcium ATPase activity which pumps back calcium into the sarcoplasmic reticulum and also regeneration of ATP and other energy substrates. The recovery heat is approximately equal to initial heat (heat produced during contraction).

4. Relaxation heat. This is the extra heat, in addition to the recovery heat, which is produced during relaxation of the isotonically contracted muscle. It is the external manifestation of the extra work done on the muscle to stretch it back to its original length.

Important Note

Fenn effect

Fenn effect states that the heat produced is directly proportional to the work done. When the work done is more, the expenditure of ATP will also be more; therefore, Fenn effect can be considered to state that more work done causes more expenditure of energy.

Self-Assessment

1. Discuss the process of muscle excitability and contractability.
2. Discuss electromyography and its significance.
3. Describe:
   - Energy requirement during muscle contraction
   - Molecular basis of length-tension relationship
4. Write notes on:
   - Muscular dystrophy
   - Oxygen debt
   - Mechanical efficiency of muscle

Clinical Cases

Case 1

Under volatile anaesthesia, a 32-year-old woman was undergoing surgery for appendicitis.

During surgery, her temperature raised to 46°C.

Q1. What is this condition known as?
Q2. What is the reason for raised temperature during surgery?
Q3. What is the pathophysiology of this?

Case 2

An unclaimed dead body was brought by the police in the mortuary for postmortem. The body was very stiff.

Q1. What is this condition called?
Q2. What is the physiological basis of stiffness after death?
Q3. Discuss the medicolegal significance related to this condition.

Case 3

A 4-year-old male child is brought to paediatric OPD with complaint of progressive weakness of muscles of lower limb and not able to stand and walk properly. On examination, the calf muscles show hypertrophy and weakness of shoulder girdle. The provisional diagnosis of muscular dystrophy was made. On further investigations, the following were noted:

- EMG findings reveal polyphasic MUPs of increased frequency, reduced amplitude and duration.
- Biochemical tests show increased level of creatine phosphokinase

Q1. What is the final diagnosis?
Q2. How does this disease transmit?
Q3. What is the pathophysiology?

Case 4

A 9-year-old male child with leg braces brought with complains of progressive increase in muscular weakness. On detailed history, it was found that the disease started at the age of 5 years with palpitation and later involved the hip and thigh region. On the basis of EMG and biochemical findings, it was diagnosed as a case of Becker muscular dystrophy (BMD).

Q1. Which type of disease is BMD?
Q2. How is it transmitted?
Q3. Which specific biochemical test is used to detect this disease?

2.4 Smooth Muscle and Cardiac Muscle

CHAPTER OUTLINE

SMOOTH MUSCLE

FUNCTIONAL ANATOMY AND ORGANIZATION

Smooth muscles (nonstriated muscles), as the name indicates, are characterized by the absence of the typical cross-striated patterns seen in skeletal muscles. Because of their spontaneous activity or activity through the autonomic nervous system, they are also called *involuntary muscles*.

The smooth muscle cells are long fusiform in shape and are aggregated to form bundles or *fasciculi*. The fasciculi are aggregated to form layers of variable thickness. Thus, smooth muscles exist in either sheet or bundles of fibres. In each layer, the cells are so arranged that the thick central part of one cell is opposite the thin tapering ends of adjoining cells (Fig. 2.4.1).

TYPES OF SMOOTH MUSCLES

Smooth muscles are of two types: single-unit or unitary and multiunit smooth muscles.

1. Single-unit (unitary) smooth muscles Single-unit smooth muscles are also called *visceral smooth muscles* since they are present in the walls of hollow viscera such as gastrointestinal tract, uterus, ureters, urinary bladder and respiratory tract.

Salient features of single-unit smooth muscles are:

- These are arranged in the form of large sheets and have low-resistance bridges between individual muscle cells and function in a *syncytial fashion* and that is why they are called single-unit muscles (Fig. 2.4.2). The low-resistance intercellular bridges or the so-called *gap junctions* are in abundance and have high conductance for the ions. Therefore, the syncytium contracts as a single unit in many large areas.
- These muscles have their own rhythmic contractility *myogenic tone* that is independent of the nerve supply. The rate of contraction may be determined by the *pacemaker regions* present within the muscles. The nervous influence only modulates their activity, i.e. the role of the nerves is to increase or decrease the rate of rhythmic contraction.
- Contraction of this kind of smooth muscles is also stimulated by *stretching*. The muscles of smaller blood vessels are mainly of this kind and their contraction in response to stretch is involved in autoregulation of blood flow.
- In addition to the autonomic nervous system, their contractile activity is also influenced by some non-neural stimuli, e.g. hormones and local tissue factors (such as temperature and pH).

2. Multiunit smooth muscles Multiunit smooth muscles, as the name indicates, are made up of multiple individual units without interconnecting bridges, i.e. *nonsyncytial in* character (Fig. 2.4.1). These are *located* in most blood vessels, epididymis, vas deferens, iris, ciliary body and piloerector muscles.

Salient features of multiunit smooth muscles are:

- These muscles are made up of multiple individual units of muscle fibres, each innervated by a single nerve ending.
- Each muscle fibre has an outer membrane made up of glycoproteins which help to insulate and separate the muscle fibres from each other. These muscles contract when an appropriate nerve stimulus reaches, i.e. contraction is *neurogenic*. Here, a single stimulus to the nerve causes repeated firing of action potential which produces *irregular tetanic contraction* (rather than a single muscle twitch produced by a single action potential as seen in skeletal muscle).
- These fibres do not exhibit spontaneous contraction, i.e. *no pacemaker activity*.
- Since the *gap junctions* are not present, the excitation remains localized within the motor unit.
- These muscles do not respond to stretch.

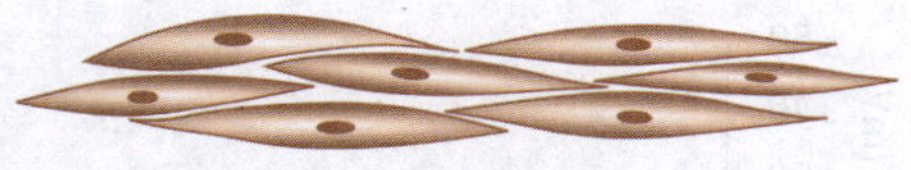

Fig. 2.4.1 Arrangement of smooth muscle fibres.

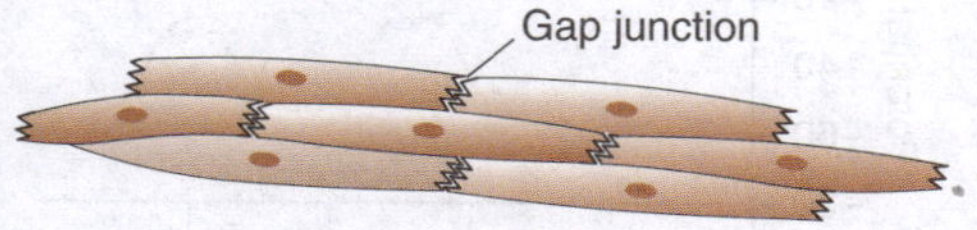

Fig. 2.4.2 Single-unit smooth muscle fibre showing gap junctions between two adjacent cells.

INNERVATION AND NEUROMUSCULAR JUNCTION OF SMOOTH MUSCLES

Nerve supply Smooth muscles are innervated by autonomic nerves, both sympathetic and parasympathetic. The two have opposite effects. In some organs, sympathetic stimulation causes contraction and parasympathetic stimulation causes relaxation of smooth muscles. In contrast, in some other organs, a reverse action is seen. The autonomic nerves supplying the smooth muscles emerge out as *preganglionic fibres* which relay in a ganglion. Postganglionic fibres run along the length of muscle fibres and groove them.

Neuromuscular junction The postganglionic nerve fibres approach the smooth muscles, branch extensively and come in close contact with a large number of smooth muscle fibres (Fig. 2.4.3). The neuronal network so formed has a beaded appearance due to the large enlargements called *varicosities* (Fig. 2.4.4). These varicosities contain the chemical neurotransmitter (acetylcholine or norepinephrine).

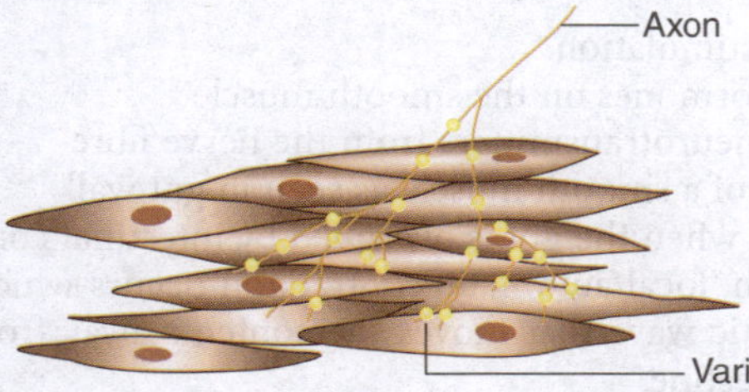

Fig. 2.4.3 The nerve supplying to smooth muscle showing varicosities (beaded appearance).

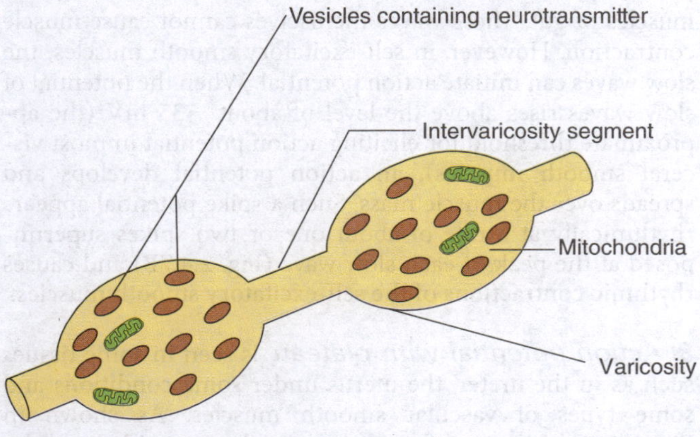

Fig. 2.4.4 Detailed structure of postganglionic nerve ending innervating smooth muscle cells.

In the smooth muscle, the nerve fibres are not ending in *motor endplates* (as seen in skeletal muscles), i.e. the nerve fibres do not make any direct contact with the muscle fibres. Instead, the nerve fibres release their neurotransmitter from each varicosity into the interstitial fluid close to the muscle fibres. The neurotransmitter so released diffuses into a large number of cells and causes activation of all muscle fibres up to where it is forming a syncytium. Therefore, here a single stimulus does not cause stimulation of all muscle fibres in the whole organ. Thus, repeated stimuli are needed to cause release of more chemical transmitter to stimulate the remaining cells. Furthermore, in a sheet of smooth muscle cells, often only the cells on the surface are innervated. The deeper cells are stimulated by spread of action potentials through the gap junctions.

Excitatory junctional potential (EJP) or inhibitory junctional potential (IJP), i.e. either a depolarizing or a hyperpolarizing response, may be recorded from a smooth muscle, in response to an appropriate nerve stimulus. These potentials summate with repeated stimuli. The EJP and IJP are *local responses* like those seen in a synapse (excitatory postsynaptic potential [EPSP] and inhibitory postsynaptic potential [IPSP]).

STRUCTURE OF SMOOTH MUSCLE FIBRE

Each smooth muscle fibre is a long spindle-shaped cell (myocyte) having a broad central part and tapering ends (Fig. 2.4.5A). The length of smooth muscle fibre is highly variable (15–500 μm) depending on the organ in which it is present. For example:

- *Digestive tract* fibres are 30–40 μm long and 5 μm in diameter.
- Fibres in *blood vessels* are 15–20 μm long and 2–3 μm in diameter.
- Fibres in *uterus* are 300 μm long and 10 μm in diameter.

Salient Features of Structure of a Smooth Muscle Fibre

Plasma membrane which binds the smooth muscle is surrounded by an external lamina. Adjacent smooth muscle cells communicate through gap junctions.

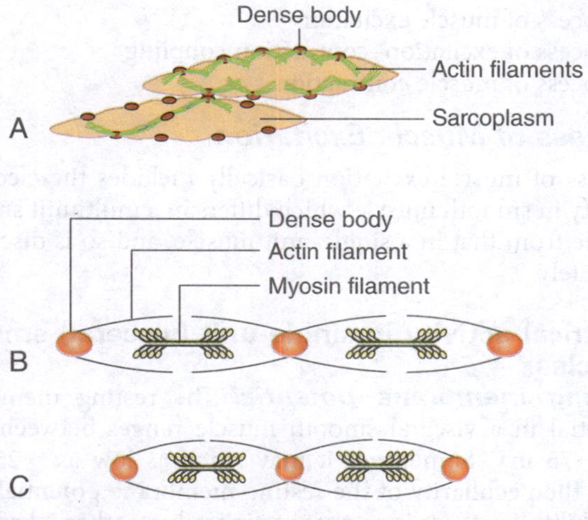

Fig. 2.4.5 Structure of smooth muscle: **A,** arrangement of thin (actin filaments attached to dense bodies) and thick (myosin) filaments; **B,** position of dense bodies in relaxed state; and **C,** the dense bodies are drawn closer to each other in contracted state.

Nucleus is oval or elongated and lies in the central part of the cell.

Sarcoplasm, in addition to a single nucleus, contains other cell organelles like mitochondria (source of energy), a Golgi complex, some granular endoplasmic reticulum and free ribosomes. Apart from these, it also contains myofibrils and intermediate filaments.

Sarcoplasmic reticulum similar to that in skeletal muscle is present, but is not as developed.

Myofibrils are made up of contractile proteins, myosin and actin filaments. The *longitudinal striations* seen on light microscopy are due to these myofibrils. Since the thick and thin filaments do not have the highly ordered arrangement as seen in striated muscles, no cross-striations are seen. Other salient differences from the skeletal muscle are as follows:

- The *sarcotubular system* and *triads* encountered in striated muscles are not well developed in smooth muscles.
- Smooth muscles contain relatively less *thick filaments* and more *thin filaments*.
- Z line is not well defined in smooth muscles.
- *Myosin-II* present in smooth muscle is chemically different from that seen in skeletal muscles. It binds to actin only if its light chain is phosphorylated. Thus, phosphorylation of myosin is necessary for the contraction of smooth muscles.
- *Thin actin filaments* are also different from those in skeletal muscle due to absence of the troponin protein molecules.
- *Dense bodies* are bound by α-actinin (Fig. 2.4.5B), and attached to the cell membrane through α-actinin. The actin filaments are attached to these dense bodies. The thick myosin filaments are situated in between actin filaments. There are cross-bridges between actin and myosin, which help in the sliding mechanism of muscle contraction. When the muscle contracts, the points on the cell membrane where dense bodies are attached are drawn closer to each other. This converts an oblongated smooth muscle into one that is oval (Fig. 2.4.5C).

PROCESS OF EXCITABILITY AND CONTRACTILITY

- Process of muscle excitation
- Process of excitation–contraction coupling
- Process of muscle contraction

Process of Muscle Excitation

Process of muscle excitation basically includes the electrical activity in smooth muscle which differs in a multiunit smooth muscle from that in a single-unit muscle, and so is discussed separately.

Electrical activity in single-unit (visceral) smooth muscles

Resting membrane potential The resting membrane potential in a visceral smooth muscle ranges between −50 and −75 mV. Sometimes it may reach as low as −25 mV. Thus, the peculiarity of the resting membrane potential is its *unstability*, i.e. there is no true resting value, rather it keeps on oscillating between −55 and −35 mV (Fig. 2.4.6). These oscillations in the RMP occur due to superimposition by the *pacemaker potentials* which in turn occur due to rhythmic changes in either Ca^{2+} channel permeability or the activity of Na^+–K^+ pump.

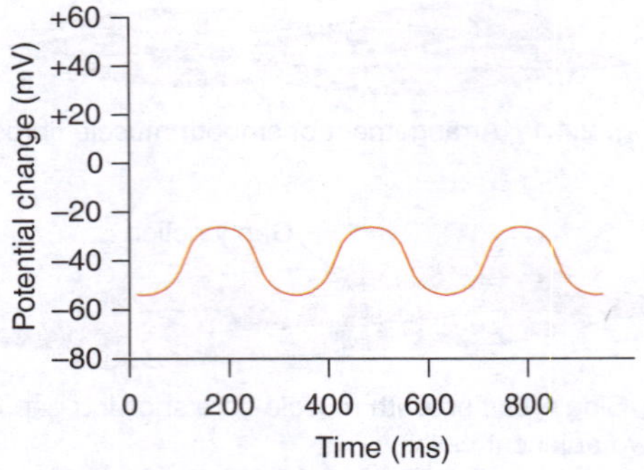

Fig. 2.4.6 Resting membrane potential (fluctuating type) in visceral smooth muscle.

Action potential When depolarization reaches threshold potential, an action potential is generated, which is transmitted to the adjacent muscle cells through the gap junction. Three types of action potentials are known to occur in the visceral smooth muscle fibres, i.e. spike potential, spike potential superimposed over pacemaker potential and action potential with plateau.

1. Spike potential. A typical spike potential, similar to that seen in skeletal muscles, is also observed in most, if not all, single-unit smooth muscles. However, it differs from the spike potential of skeletal muscle in many ways: (i) its average duration varies between 10 and 50 milliseconds; (ii) its amplitude is very low; and (iii) it does not reach the isoelectric base (Fig. 2.4.7A). The spike action potential, in a smooth muscle, can occur due to following modes of stimulations:

- Electrical stimulation
- Effect of hormones on the smooth muscle
- Action of neurotransmitters from the nerve fibre
- By stretch of a smooth muscle as seen in gut wall

For example, when the gut is overfilled by intestinal contents, due to stretch, local automatic contraction occurs which sets up a peristaltic wave that moves the contents away from the overfilled intestine.

2. Spike potential superimposed over slow wave potentials. The slow wave rhythms, also called pacemaker waves, are seen in many visceral smooth muscles such as muscles of gut. These waves themselves cannot cause muscle contraction. However, in self-excitatory smooth muscles, the slow waves can initiate action potential. When the potential of slow waves rises above the level of about −35 mV (the approximate threshold for eliciting action potential in most visceral smooth muscles), an action potential develops and spreads over the muscle mass. Such a spike potential appears rhythmically at a rate of about one or two spikes superimposed at the peak of each slow wave (Fig. 2.4.7B) and causes rhythmic contractions of the self-excitatory smooth muscles.

3. Action potential with plateau is seen in some tissues such as in the ureter, the uterus under some conditions and some types of vascular smooth muscles. As shown in Fig. 2.4.7C, this type of action potential starts with rapid depolarization as is seen in the skeletal muscles. However, like

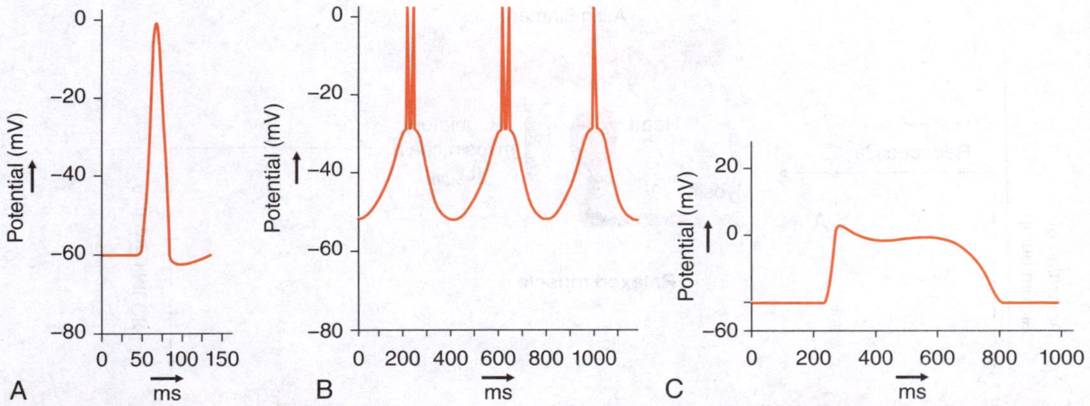

Fig. 2.4.7 Three types of action potentials recorded from smooth muscles: **A,** spike potential; **B,** spike potential superimposed over slow wave potentials; and **C,** action potential with plateau.

skeletal muscles, the repolarization does not occur immediately, but is delayed by 100–1000 milliseconds. This prolonged depolarization accounts for the sustained contraction of certain smooth muscle fibres.

Ionic basis of action potential In smooth muscles, the depolarization occurs due to entry of Ca^{2+} ions from ECF to the inside of the cell rather than Na^{+} ions (as seen in skeletal muscles). The smooth cell membrane has far more *voltage-gated calcium channels* than does skeletal muscle but few voltage-gated sodium channels. Unlike sodium channels, the calcium channels open and close slowly. This accounts for the prolonged action potential observed in smooth muscles. The calcium ions, in addition to causing depolarization, also produce contraction of smooth muscles by directly acting on the contractile mechanism.

Electrical activity in multiunit smooth muscles

The multiunit smooth muscles (such as the muscles of iris and piloerector muscles) usually respond to nerve stimuli. The nerve endings secrete the neurotransmitter (acetylcholine or norepinephrine), which causes depolarization of the smooth muscle membrane. Since fibres are too small, they do not generate an action potential. The local depolarization is called the *EJP*. However, the EJP spreads electrotonically over the entire fibre and is sufficient to cause the muscle contraction.

Process of Excitation–Contraction Coupling

Excitation–contraction coupling refers to the sequence of events by which an excited plasma membrane of a muscle fibre leads to cross-bridge activity by increasing cytosolic (sarcoplasmic) calcium concentration. Since a smooth muscle can be excited by so many possible ways, there are different ways of excitation–contraction coupling as well. Three different mechanisms of excitation–contraction coupling known in smooth muscles are described as follows:

1. Electromechanical coupling occurs when the smooth muscle is excited through sarcolemmal depolarization. Due to depolarization of the membrane, the *voltage-gated* Ca^{2+} channels present on it are opened and the Ca^{2+} ions from the ECF move into the sarcoplasm. These Ca^{2+} ions in turn stimulate the release of more Ca^{2+} from the sarcoplasmic reticulum. This process is called Ca^{2+}-induced Ca^{2+} release (CICR). The raised sarcoplasmic Ca^{2+} level brings about the excitation–contraction coupling.

2. Pharmacomechanical coupling occurs when the smooth muscle is excited by some chemical agent and not by membrane depolarization. Two mechanisms of pharmacomechanical coupling known are as follows:

- The chemical agents (neurotransmitters and hormones) bind to the *ligand-gated* Ca^{2+} channels present on the sarcolemma and open them up resulting in influx of Ca^{2+} from the ECF.
- The chemical agents bind to the *membrane receptors* and activate the second messenger system of G-protein → generation of inositol triphosphate (IP_3) from the membrane phospholipids → release of calcium ions from the *intracellular* Ca^{2+} stores, i.e. from the sarcoplasmic reticulum.

3. Mechanomechanical coupling occurs when the muscle is excited by stretch. Due to stretching, the *stretch-sensitive* Ca^{2+} channels present on the sarcolemma open up resulting in influx of Ca^{2+} from the ECF.

The excitation–contraction coupling in smooth muscle is a slow process. Calcium initiates this process by binding with calmodulin. The *calcium–calmodulin complex* so formed triggers muscle contraction by a sequence of events discussed as follows.

Process of Smooth Muscle Contraction

The molecular mechanism of smooth muscle contraction by cross-bridge cycling and sliding of filaments is similar to that of the skeletal muscle. However, since the smooth muscle does not contain the regulatory proteins tropomyosin and troponin, its regulation is different. In a smooth muscle, one of the light chains of the myosin filament located in the neck region serves the function of tropomyosin and thus is called the *regulatory chain of myosin.* Similarly, the Ca^{2+}-binding protein *calmodulin* plays the role of troponin.

Steps of Cross-Bridge Cycling

Steps of cross-bridge cycling in a smooth muscle are summarized (Fig. 2.4.8) as follows.

1. Activation of the enzyme myosin light chain kinase (MLCK) The enzyme MLCK is activated by the Ca^{2+}–calmodulin complex.

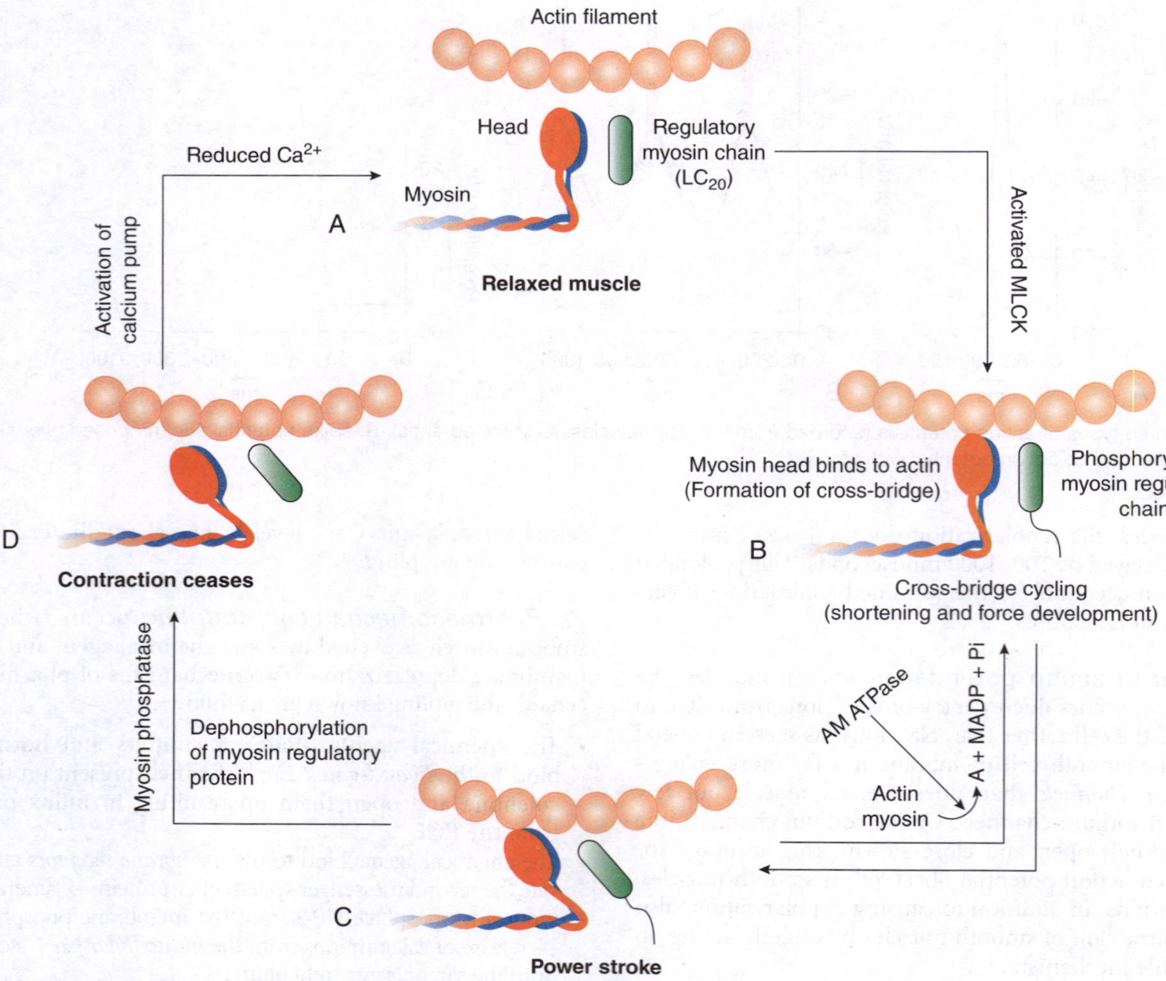

Fig. 2.4.8 Steps of cross-bridge cycling in smooth muscle: **A,** relaxed muscle; **B,** activation of myosin light chain kinase (MLCK) catalyses phosphorylation of myosin regulatory chain and initiates cross-bridging between myosin head and actin filament; **C,** power stroke, triggered by conformational change in myosin head due to formation of actin–myosin ADP-Pi complex; and **D,** dephosphorylation of myosin regulatory protein resulting in cessation of cross-bridging.

2. Phosphorylation of the myosin regulatory chain The activated enzyme MLCK uses ATP to phosphorylate the myosin regulatory chain.

3. Cross-bridging When the myosin regulatory chain is phosphorylated, the head of myosin filament acquires the capability to bind with actin filament to form the cross-bridge (Fig. 2.4.8B).

4. Power stroke Formation of the actin–myosin ADP-Pi complex triggers a conformational change in the myosin head causing it to flex towards the arm of the cross-bridge. The flexion of the myosin head generates mechanical force (*the power stroke*) (Fig. 2.4.8C).

Due to power stroke, the actin filament slides over the myosin filament producing contraction. As shown in Fig. 2.4.5C, the *dense bodies* play a role in the contraction of a smooth muscle fibre. In fact, the dense bodies of smooth muscles serve the same role as the Z disc (Z line) in skeletal muscle.

5. Relaxation of smooth muscle To cause relaxation of the smooth muscle contraction, it is necessary to remove the calcium ions from the sarcoplasm. This is accomplished by the calcium pump which pumps the calcium from ICF to ECF and also from ICF into the sarcoplasmic reticulum. When the cytoplasmic Ca^{2+} falls to the resting level, the processes involved in the contraction of smooth muscle automatically reverse except for the phosphorylation of the myosin head. Reversal of this occurs when the enzyme *myosin phosphatase* causes dephosphorylation of the myosin regulatory chain. After this, the cross-bridge cycling stops and the contraction ceases (Fig. 2.4.8D). The time required for relaxation of contracted muscle, therefore, is determined to a great extent by the amount of active myosin phosphatase in the cell.

The calcium pumps operating in the smooth muscles are slow acting in comparison with the fast-acting sarcoplasmic reticulum pump in skeletal muscles. Therefore, the duration of smooth muscle contraction is prolonged (in seconds) as compared to that of skeletal muscles (from 1/100th to 1/10th of a second).

CHARACTERISTICS OF SMOOTH MUSCLE EXCITATION AND CONTRACTION

Certain characteristic features of smooth muscle excitation and contraction are as follows:

1. Slow excitation–contraction coupling As shown in Fig. 2.4.9, a smooth muscle starts contracting approximately 200 milliseconds after the start of the spike potential (i.e.

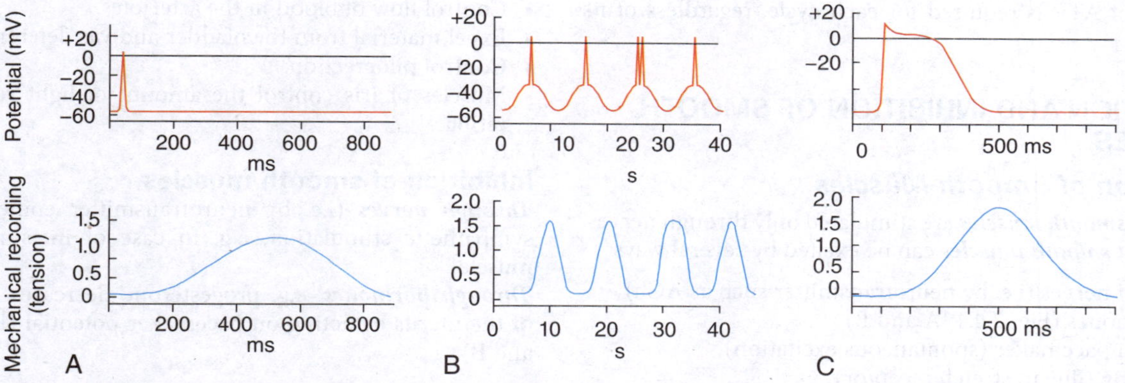

Fig. 2.4.9 Record of mechanical activity of smooth muscle following various types of potential: **A,** spike potential; **B,** spike potential superimposed over slow wave potential; and **C,** action potential with plateau.

150 milliseconds after the spike is over). The peak of contraction is reached after 500 milliseconds of the spike. Thus, the excitation–contraction coupling is very slow in smooth muscles compared with that in the skeletal muscles.

2. Plasticity A smooth muscle exhibits the property of plasticity, i.e. it can readjust its resting length (the length at which a muscle generates maximum active tension). Thus, the smooth muscle defies the usual *length–tension relationship* that is valid for striated muscles (skeletal as well as cardiac muscles); when a smooth muscle is passively stretched, it first exerts increased tension, which gradually reduces to prestretch level (even when the stretch is maintained). Therefore, the *length–tension relationship curve* in a smooth muscle is not a smooth curve but a jagged line (Fig. 2.4.10).

It has been explained by the observation that at longer fibre lengths, the thick filaments are disposed in series (Fig. 2.4.11A) while at shorter length, the thick filaments are disposed in *parallel* (Fig. 2.4.11B).

3. Latch phenomenon Latch phenomenon is another characteristic exhibited by smooth muscles. It refers to the mechanism by which a smooth muscle can maintain a high tension without actively contracting. This phenomenon allows long-term maintenance of tone in many smooth muscle organs. In such a state, the muscle cannot generate active tension but can effectively resist passive stretching. This phenomenon appropriately suits the function of smooth muscles, since in most instances, they have to resist stretch rather than actively move a load. These smooth muscles are mostly found in the walls of hollow viscera that must resist excessive stretching. The latch phenomenon can be explained by the fact that when both the myosin kinase and myosin phosphatase enzyme are strongly activated, the cycling frequency of the myosin heads and the velocity of contraction are great. Then, as the activation of the enzymes decreases, the cycling frequency decreases, but at the same time, the lower activation of the enzymes causes the myosin heads to remain attached to the actin filaments for a larger and longer proportion of the cycling period. Therefore, the number of heads attached to the thin filament at any given time remains large. Because the number of heads attached to the actin determines the static force of contraction, tension is maintained, yet little energy is used by the muscle, because ATP is not degraded to ADP.

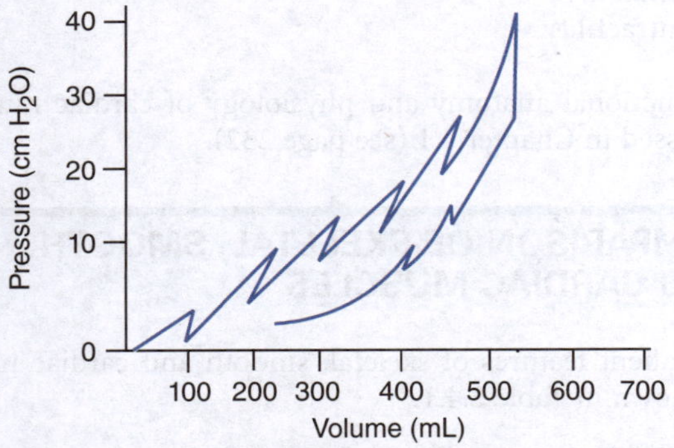

Fig. 2.4.10 Plasticity in smooth muscle fibre.

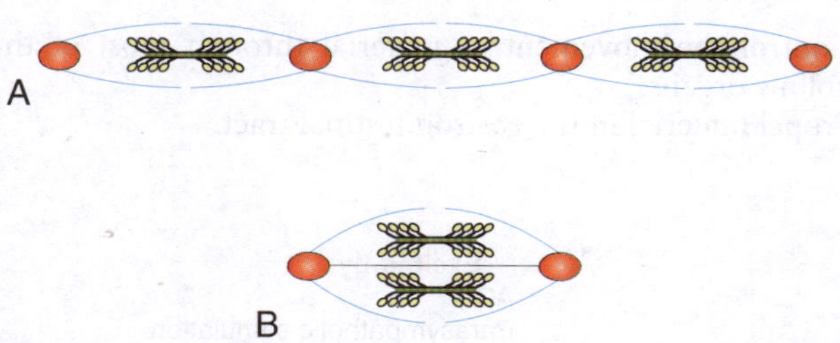

Fig. 2.4.11 **A,** at longer fibre length, myosin filaments are disposed in series; and **B,** at shorter fibre length, thick filaments are disposed in parallel.

4. Marked shortening of smooth muscle during contraction Marked shortening of smooth muscle during contraction is another characteristic of smooth muscle that makes it different from the skeletal muscle. A smooth muscle can contract more than two-thirds its stretched length, while a skeletal muscle can contract up to one-third its stretched length. This property allows the smooth muscle to perform especially important functions in the hollow viscera, allowing the gut, bladder, blood vessels and other internal bodily structures to change their lumen diameters from very large down to almost zero.

5. Energy required to sustain smooth muscle contraction Energy required to sustain smooth muscle contraction is much less than that required by a skeletal muscle. It is because of the fact that the attachment cycling of the cross-bridges is slow in smooth muscles and that only one molecule of ATP is required for each cycle, regardless of its duration.

EXCITATION AND INHIBITION OF SMOOTH MUSCLES

Excitation of Smooth Muscles

Multiunit smooth muscles are stimulated only through nerves. ***Single-unit smooth muscles*** can be excited by several ways:

- Through nerves (i.e. by neurotransmitter such as ACh)
- By hormones (Fig. 2.4.12A and B)
- Through pacemaker (spontaneous excitation)
- Stretching (due to stretch receptor)
- Cold temperature

Functions After excitations, smooth muscles perform the following functions:

- Control the movement of material through most of the hollow organs.
- Propel material in the gastrointestinal tract.
- Control flow of blood in the arterioles.
- Expel material from the bladder and vas deferens.
- Control piloerection.
- Muscles of iris control the amount of light reaching the retina.

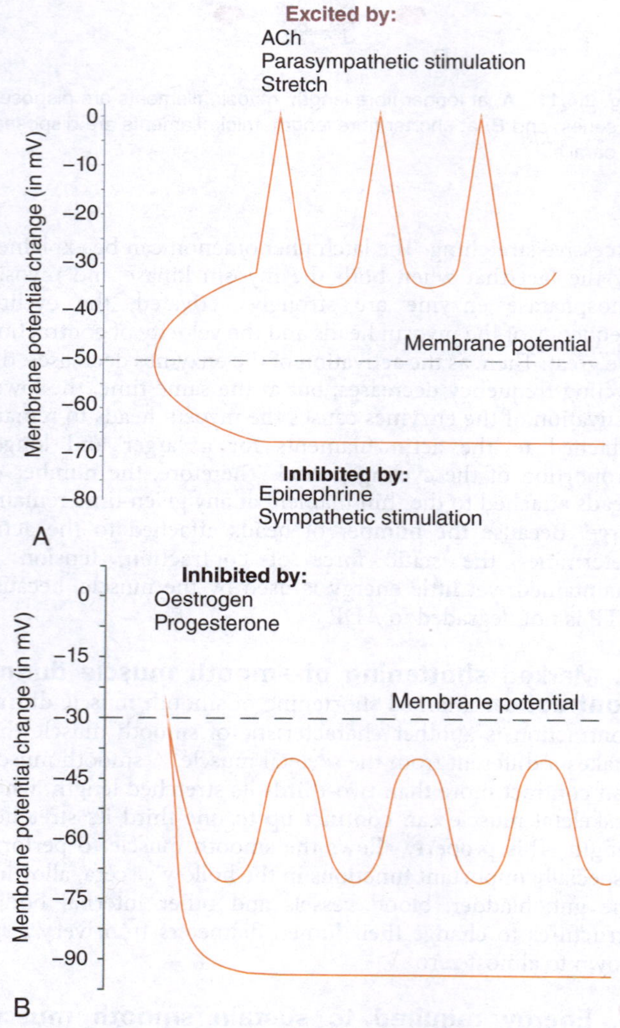

Fig. 2.4.12 Effect of various agents on the membrane potential of smooth muscles: **A,** intestinal wall; and **B,** uterus.

Inhibition of smooth muscles

Through nerves (i.e. by neurotransmitter epinephrine) by sympathetic stimulation, e.g. in case of intestinal smooth muscle

Through hormones, e.g. progesterone decreases the activity of the uterus by acting on pacemaker potential (Fig. 2.4.12A and B)

> **Applied Aspects**
>
> ***In bronchial asthma,*** overexcitation of airway's smooth muscles leads to bronchial constriction; therefore, for quick relief, inhalers are commonly used because they deliver β-adrenergic agonist (e.g. vilanterol, albuterol and salmeterol).
>
> ***To increase blood flow, nitric oxide (NO)*** is a natural molecule that relaxes smooth muscles of the blood vessels. Its mechanism of action through enzyme phosphodiesterase (PDE), which transforms cyclic guanosine monophosphate (cGMP) into GMP. The specific inhibitors of PDE V (an isoform found in corpora cavernosa of penis) like sildenafil, tadalafil and vardenafil are used for increasing blood flow to offset erectile dysfunction. For details, see page 340.

CARDIAC MUSCLE

Functional anatomy

- Structural organization of cardiac muscle
- Structure of a cardiac muscle fibre
- Sarcotubular system

Process of excitability and contractility

- Electrical potentials in cardiac muscle
- Excitation–contraction coupling phenomenon
- Process of cardiac muscle contraction

Properties of cardiac muscle

- Automaticity
- Rhythmicity
- Conductivity
- Excitability
- Contractility

Functional anatomy and physiology of cardiac muscle is discussed in Chapter 4.1 (see page 232).

COMPARISON OF SKELETAL, SMOOTH AND CARDIAC MUSCLES

The salient features of skeletal, smooth and cardiac muscles are shown in Table 2.4.1.

Table 2.4.1 Comparison of skeletal, smooth and cardiac muscles

Features	Skeletal muscle	Cardiac muscle	Smooth muscle
Structural features			
• Striations	Present	Present	Absent
• Size of fibres			
• *Length*	1–40 mm	80–100 µm	50–500 µm
• *Diameter*	50–500 µm	15 µm	2–10 µm
• Shape of the muscle fibre	Cylindrical	Cylindrical	Spindle shaped
• Branching of fibres	Absent	Present	Absent
• Connection between fibres	Absent	Functional connections present forming functional syncytium	In single-unit muscle, functional connections are present; in multiunit muscles, no connections
• Nucleus	Single or multiple at periphery	Single, central with many nuclei	Single
• Sarcoplasmic reticulum (SR)	Very well developed	Well developed but not as in skeletal muscles	Moderately developed
• Sarcotubular system	Well developed, two triads present at A–I junction	Present, one triad per sarcomere, T-tubule present at Z line	Present, but not well developed
• Thick and thin filaments	Arranged regularly	Arranged regularly	Not arranged regularly
• Sarcomere	Present	Present	Not present
• Regulating protein	Troponin	Troponin	Calmodulin
• Calcium store and calcium pump in SR	High	Moderate	Low
• Sodium channels in the membrane	Fast voltage-gated Na^+ channels	Fast voltage-gated Na^+ channels with slow voltage-gated Na^+–Ca^{2+} channels	Mainly slow voltage-gated Na^+–Ca^{2+} channels; very few fast voltage-gated Na^+ channels
• Mitochondria	Few	Many	Few
Nerve supply and control			
• Nerve supply	Somatic nerves	Autonomic nerves • Sympathetic: excitatory (transmitter – norepinephrine) • Parasympathetic: inhibitory (transmitter – acetylcholine)	Autonomic nerves • Sympathetic: inhibitory • Parasympathetic: excitatory
• Control	Voluntary	Involuntary	Involuntary
Electrical features			
• Action potential shape and duration	−90 mV Spike potential of 5 ms	−90 mV Plateau potential of 100–300 ms	−55 mV • Single-unit muscle: variable, plateau potential of 100–1000 ms and spike potential also seen of 10- to 50-ms duration • Multiunit muscle: spike potential
• Stimulated by	Somatic nerves	Autonomic nerves	Autonomic nerves, hormones and local tissue factors
• Excitability	High	Moderate	Low
• Conductivity	Fast	Slow	Slow
• Absolute refractory period	1–3 ms	180–200 ms	Not defined
• Autorhythmicity	Not present	Present	Present in single-unit muscle
Excitation–contraction coupling			
• Speed of phenomenon	Rapid	Very rapid	Very slow
• Site of calcium attachment	Troponin	Troponin	Myosin
• Mechanism of Ca^{2+} mobilization	T-tubule is depolarized	Ca^{2+}-induced Ca^{2+} release	Inositol triphosphate increases release of Ca^{2+}
• Dependence on concentration of ECF calcium concentration	Not dependent	Partly dependent	Almost totally dependent

(Continued on following page)

Table 2.4.1 Comparison of skeletal, smooth and cardiac muscles—(Continued)

Features	Skeletal muscle	Cardiac muscle	Smooth muscle
Contractility characteristics			
• Rate of contraction	Fast	Fast	Slow
• Rate of relaxation	Fast	Fast	Slow
• Duration of muscle twitch	• In fast fibres: 7.5 ms • In slow fibres: 100 ms	1.5 times the total duration of action potential	About 1000 ms
• All-or-none law	Obeyed by single muscle fibre	Obeyed by whole muscle	• Single-unit muscle: obeyed by whole muscle • Multiunit muscle: obeyed by single muscle fibre
• Multiple fibre (quantal) summations	Possible	Not possible, as it is a functional syncytium	Not possible
• Tetanus (wave summation)	Possible	Not possible due to long refractory period	Not possible, as the process of contraction is long
• Fatigue	Possible	None, since long refractory period ensures recovery and also due to presence of more blood supply	Possible but difficult to demonstrate
• Length–tension relationship	Maximum tension is developed at optimal length	Maximum tension developed at optimal length	Shows property of plasticity
Chemical composition, blood supply, oxygen consumption and muscle energetics			
• Protein	Maximum	Less	Less
• Glycogen	Less	More	Less
• ATP and phosphagen	Present	Present	Present
• Fats	Mainly neutral fats	More phospholipids and cholesterol than others	Mainly neutral fats
• Blood supply	840 mL/min (3–4 mL/100 g/min)	Abundant, 250 mL/min (80 mL/100 g/min)	350 mL/min (1.4 mL/100 g/min)
• Oxygen consumption	Moderate	High	Low
Energy utilization under basal state by			
• Fats	20%	60%	Mainly
• Carbohydrates	60%	35%	Very few
• Proteins	20%	5%	Very few

Self-Assessment

1. Discuss the process of excitability and contraction in smooth muscle and its characteristics.
2. Write notes on:
   a. Excitatory junctional potential
   b. Property of latch phenomenon
   c. Plasticity in smooth muscle

Clinical Case

Case 1

A 64-year-old male patient was admitted in the hospital with oedema and congestive heart failure. On examination and laboratory tests, it was found to be a case of diastolic dysfunction (inadequate ventricular filling during diastole) due to decreased vascular compliance.

Q1. Which muscle protein is responsible for decreased vascular compliance?

BLOOD AND IMMUNE SYSTEM

SECTION 3

SECTION OUTLINE

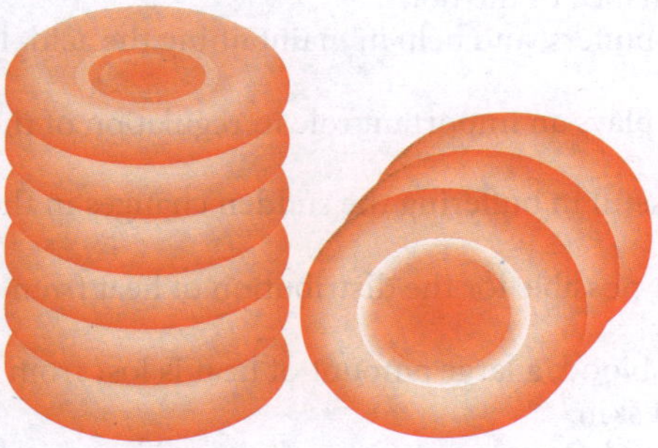

INTRODUCTION

Blood is a fluid connective tissue which transports substances from one part of the body to another. It provides nutrients and hormones to the tissues and removes their waste products. Blood, confined in the cardiovascular system, constitutes a major part of the extracellular fluid of the body.

Some of the important physical characteristics of blood are as follows:

Colour of blood is opaque red due to the pigment haemoglobin in the RBCs. The arterial blood is bright red and venous blood is dark red in colour.
Volume of blood in an average adult is about 5–6 L (8% of the body weight or 80 mL/kg body weight).
Viscosity of blood is five times more than that of water.
Specific gravity of blood is 1.050–1.060. Specific gravity of RBC is greater (1.090) than that of plasma (1.030).
pH of blood is about 7.4 (ranges from 7.38 to 7.42), i.e. it is alkaline in nature. In acidosis, pH of blood falls below 7.38 and in alkalosis pH is more than 7.42.

Blood is composed of two main components, plasma and cellular elements.

Plasma constitutes about 55% of the blood volume. It is a clear straw-coloured fluid portion of blood.

- *Plasma proteins*, an important constituent of plasma, form about 7% of its volume.

Cellular elements of blood are about 45% of the total blood volume and constitute the so-called packed cell volume (PCV).

Blood cells are
- Erythrocytes or red blood cells (5 million/mm^3).
- Leucocytes or white blood cells (4000–11,000/mm^3).
- Platelets or thrombocytes (1.5–4 lakh/mm^3).

FUNCTIONS OF BLOOD

1. ***Nutritive function:*** Blood carries the nutritive substances like glucose, amino acids, fatty acids, vitamins, electrolytes and others, from the gut to the tissues where they are utilized.
2. ***Respiratory functions:*** Blood picks up oxygen from the lungs and delivers it to the various tissues. The most important function of blood is the uninterrupted delivery of O_2 to the heart and brain. It also carries away CO_2 from the tissues to the lungs, from where it is expelled out in the expired air.
3. ***Excretory function:*** Blood transports various metabolic waste products, such as urea, uric acid and creatinine, to the excretory organs (kidney, skin, intestine and lungs) for their disposal.
4. ***Transport function:*** The various hormones produced by the endocrine glands, the biological enzymes and antibodies are transported by the blood to the target tissue, to modulate metabolic process.
5. ***Protective function:*** Blood plays an important role in the defence mechanism of the body:
   - Neutrophils and monocytes engulf the microorganisms entering the body by phagocytosis.
   - Lymphocytes and gamma globulins initiate an immune response.
   - Eosinophils accomplish detoxification, disintegration and removal of foreign proteins.
6. ***Homeostatic function:*** Blood plays an important role in maintaining the internal environment of the body (homeostatic function):
   - The water content of blood is freely interchangeable with the interstitial fluid and helps in maintaining the water and electrolyte balance of the body.
   - Plasma proteins and haemoglobin act as buffers, and help in maintaining the acid–base balance and pH of the body fluids.
7. ***Maintenance of body temperature:*** Blood plays an important role in regulation of the body temperature, as described below:
   - *Specific heat* of blood is high, which is useful in buffering the sudden changes in the body temperature.
   - *High heat conductivity of blood* renders it possible for the distribution of heat from deep organs to the skin and lungs for dissipation.
   - Due to *high latent heat of evaporation* of blood, a large amount of heat is lost from the body by evaporation of water from the lungs and skin.
8. ***Storage function:*** Blood serves as a readymade source of substances stored in it (such as glucose, water, proteins and electrolytes for use in emergency conditions like starvation, fluid loss and electrolyte loss).
9. Maintenance of osmotic pressure and osmolality by plasma proteins.

IMMUNE SYSTEM

The immune system that constitutes the body's defence system consists of immunological cells distributed in two main components: mononuclear phagocytic system and lymphoid component. The immune system of the body responds to an antigen by two ways:

- ***Humoral or antibody-mediated immunity (AMI)*** which is mediated by antibodies produced by plasma cells
- ***Cell-mediated immunity (CMI)*** which is mediated directly by the sensitized lymphocytes

Plasma and Plasma Proteins

3.1

CHAPTER OUTLINE

PLASMA

Plasma is the clear straw-coloured fluid (with dissolved solid substances) portion of the blood minus its cellular elements. It constitutes about 55% of the blood volume.

COMPOSITION

Plasma contains the following constituents:

Water. Water is the main constituent of plasma, forming 91% of it.

Solids. The solids dissolved in the plasma constitute a total of 9% of the plasma. The solid constituents of the plasma are given as follows:

Plasma proteins Form 7% of the solids in plasma. Their normal value ranges from 6.4 to 8.3 g/dL. They include albumin, globulins, fibrinogen and others.

Other organic molecules which form 1% of the solids include the following:

- *Carbohydrates,* mainly glucose (100–120 mg/dL).
- *Fats* are neutral fats (30–150 mg/dL), phospholipids (150–300 mg/dL) and cholesterol (150–240 mg/dL).
- *Nonprotein nitrogenous (NPN) substances* (28–40 mg/dL) are ammonia (traces), amino acids, creatine (1–2 mg/dL), creatinine (0.6–1.2 mg/dL), xanthine (traces), hypoxanthine (traces), urea (20–40 mg/dL) and uric acid (2–4 mg/dL).
- *Hormones, enzymes and antibodies.*

Inorganic substances which constitute 1% of the solids in plasma include sodium, potassium, calcium, magnesium, chloride, iodide, iron, phosphates and copper.

Gases. Gases present in the plasma are oxygen, carbon dioxide and nitrogen.

Serum Plasma from which fibrinogen and clotting factors (II, V and VIII) have been removed is called serum. Serum is formed when the blood is allowed to clot in a test tube and clot is retracted. Serum has a higher serotonin (5-HT) content because of the breakdown of platelets during clotting.

PLASMA PROTEINS

CLASSIFICATION OF PLASMA PROTEINS

Plasma proteins form the major solid constituent of the plasma. The total plasma protein concentration is 7.4 g/dL (ranges from 6.4 to 8.3 g/dL). The major forms of plasma proteins are albumin, globulins and fibrinogen. Since serum is plasma minus clotting protein (fibrinogen), the albumin and globulins are usually referred to as serum albumin and serum globulins. Presently, more than 100 types of plasma proteins have been identified. The original classification is based on the classical method of precipitation of salts as described by Howe (1922). By electrophoretic techniques, the globulins have been further subclassified. Based on these, the important fractions of plasma proteins are given as follows:

Albumin (4.8 g/dL)

Globulins (2.3 g/dL) include:

Alpha-1 (α_1) globulin comprises:

- α_1 Antitrypsin
- Transcortin (corticosteroid binding globulin)
- Thyroxin binding protein

Alpha-2 (α_2) globulin comprises:

- Haptoglobin
- Ceruloplasmin

Beta (β) globulin further consists of:

- β Lipoprotein
- Plasminogen
- Transferrin

Gamma (γ) globulin forms immunoglobulins

Fibrinogen (0.3 g/dL)

METHODS OF SEPARATION OF PLASMA PROTEINS

1. Precipitation by salting out Different fractions of the plasma proteins are precipitated out by using different concentrations of the salts as described below.

Sodium sulphate solution was used by Howe in 1922. He fractionized the plasma proteins in three major fractions:

Fibrinogen is removed with clot converting plasma into serum.
Globulins are precipitated out by 22% sodium sulphate solution from the serum.
Albumin remains in the serum.

Ammonium sulphate solution is utilized to precipitate the plasma protein fractions in different strengths:

Albumin is precipitated by full saturation.
Globulins are precipitated by half saturation. Among the globulins, there is a fraction which can be precipitated by one-third saturation with ammonium sulphate and is termed *euglobulin*. The rest is called *pseudoglobulin*.
Fibrinogen is separated by one-fifth saturation with ammonium sulphate.

2. Cohn's fractional precipitation method Varying concentrations of *ethanol* solution are used at low temperature to fractionalize the plasma proteins. Each fraction, so obtained, though being a mixture of proteins, contains one of the proteins predominantly as given below:

- *Fraction I* is rich in fibrinogen.
- *Fraction II* mainly contains gamma globulins.
- *Fraction III* contains alpha and beta globulins, including isoagglutinins and prothrombin.
- *Fraction IV* mainly consists of alpha and beta globulins.
- *Fraction V* is rich in albumin.

3. Electrophoresis separation of protein fractions The electrophoresis method separates the plasma proteins into different fractions, depending on the electric charge of each fraction due to a difference in their migration rates. Serum should be used for electrophoresis, as the fibrinogen of plasma gives a discrete band which can easily be mistaken for a paraprotein.

Technique. Various techniques of electrophoresis have been developed. Depending on the support medium used, following are the common methods:

Tiselius or free-boundary electrophoresis
Paper electrophoresis
Cellulose acetate strip electrophoresis
Agarose gel electrophoresis

Electrophoretic protein patterns. Mostly in clinical laboratories, cellulose acetate is used as a supporting medium. After resolution and staining, five bands of plasma proteins are identified. The amount of these bands can be quantified using densitometric staining techniques. On the basis of paper electrophoresis, the following classes of serum proteins (Fig. 3.1.1) are identified:

Albumin (55%)
Alpha-1 globulins (5%)
Alpha-2 globulins (9%)
Beta globulins (13%)
Gamma globulins (11%)

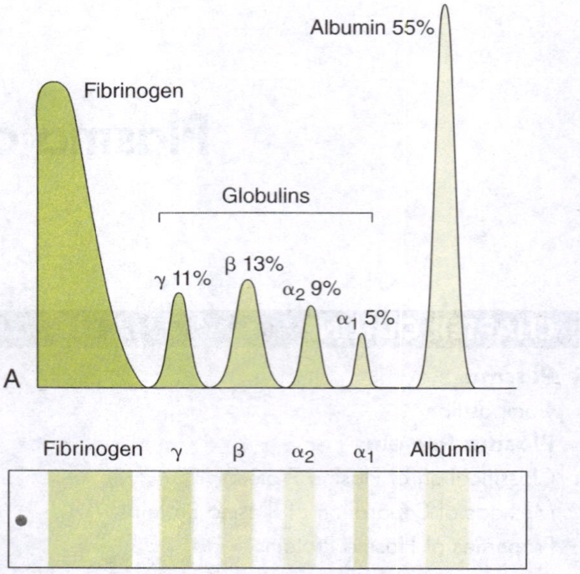

Fig. 3.1.1 Paper electrophoresis showing: **A,** relative amount of plasma proteins; **B,** bands of different plasma proteins.

Clinical use. Electrophoretic separation is very useful in clinical diagnosis. It helps in knowing:

The change in relative concentration of different proteins
The presence of abnormal proteins
The absence of normal proteins

4. Immunoelectrophoresis technique This technique makes use of the antigenicity and electric charge of protein to separate them. The proteins are separated on the basis of electrophoretic patterns formed by precipitation at the site of antigen–antibody reaction. This technique is more specific and the number of fractions obtained is much more than that in the ordinary electrophoresis.

5. Ultracentrifugation technique In this technique, a suitable preparation of plasma in buffered solution is centrifuged at a speed up to 60,000 rpm and a force up to 160,000 *g*. The proteins are separated into fractions depending on their *sedimentation constant*, which is the property of weight, shape and density of the protein molecules.

Three different sediments, albumin, globulin and fibrinogen, are formed. This method is also useful in determining the molecular weight of these proteins.

PROPERTIES OF PLASMA PROTEINS

1. Molecular weight. Plasma proteins are large molecules with the following molecular weight:

- Albumin: 69,000
- Globulins: 90,000–156,000
- Fibrinogen: 500,000

Thus, fibrinogen has the highest molecular weight. Relative size and shape of different plasma proteins are shown in Fig. 3.1.2.

2. Osmotic pressure. The plasma proteins exert an oncotic pressure of about 25 mm Hg.

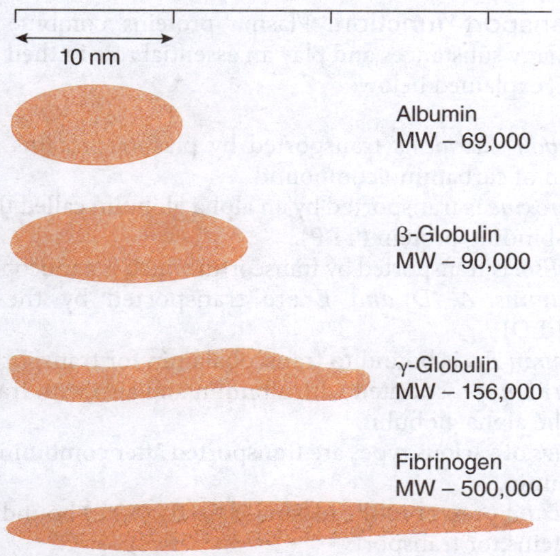

Fig. 3.1.2 Relative dimensions, molecular weights and shapes of different plasma proteins.

3. *Specific gravity.* The specific gravity of the plasma proteins is 1.026.

4. *Isoelectric point.* Proteins can ionize either as acids or as bases owing to the fact that the side chains of their constituent amino acids contain a selection of amino group (NH_2) and carboxyl groups (–COOH). At an intermediate pH (specific for each protein), the protein molecules carry an equal number of positive and negative charges and, hence, have a zero net charge. This pH value for electrical neutrality of the molecule is known as the *isoelectric point*.

5. *Electrophoretic mobility.* Proteins act as *anions* in alkaline solutions and as *cations* in acidic solutions. Because of this property, they possess electrophoretic mobility.

6. *Precipitation by salts.* Proteins can be precipitated by different concentrations of salts. This property of proteins is utilized for their separation by the precipitation method.

7. *Water solubility.* Protein molecules are soluble in water because of the presence of polar residues like NH_2 and COOH.

8. *Amphoteric nature.* Protein molecules are amphoteric in nature because of the presence of NH_2 and COOH groups. By virtue of their amphoteric nature, the plasma proteins act as efficient buffers.

FEATURES OF INDIVIDUAL FRACTIONS OF PLASMA PROTEINS

1. Albumin

Plasma levels are 4.8 g/dL (range 3–5 g/dL).
Molecular weight of prealbumin is 60,000 and that of albumin is 69,000.
Synthesized in liver.
Half-life is about 10 days.

2. Globulins

Plasma levels are 2.3 g/dL (range 2–3 g/dL).
Molecular weight varies from 90,000 to 15,600.
Types include alpha-1, alpha-2, beta-1, beta-2 and gamma globulins.
Forms of globulins: The forms of globulin are described as follows:

i. *Glycoproteins* consist of carbohydrates and protein.
ii. *Lipoproteins* consist of alpha-2 globulin and lipids. They have the following subtypes:
- *High-density lipoproteins (HDL):* These are alpha lipoproteins which contain 50% protein with large amount of cholesterol and phospholipids.
- *Low-density lipoproteins (LDL):* These are beta lipoproteins and contain large amount of glycerides.
- *Very low density lipoproteins (VLDL):* These are also beta lipoproteins and have higher proportion of fat in the form of triglycerides or cholesterol.
- *Chylomicron (CM)* contains 98% triglycerides. It is synthesized in the intestine following a meal.

Important Note

The HDL level is decreased by smoking, sedentary habits and obesity, whereas exercise and moderate intake of alcohol increase the level of HDL.

iii. *Transferrin* is an alpha-2–beta globulin having a molecular weight of 90,000. It has the specific property of iron binding, and thus helps in its transport and storage. Each molecule of transferrin binds two atoms of ferric iron.
iv. *Haptoglobin (Hb–Hp)* is an alpha-2 globulin having a molecular weight of 90,000. It forms stable complexes with free haemoglobin. However, the Hb–Hp complex is too large to pass through glomerulus; thus, the function of Hb–Hp is to prevent the loss of free Hb into the urine, thereby conserving valuable iron present in the haemoglobin.
Haptoglobin is an acute phase protein and its level is elevated in many inflammatory states.
v. *Ceruloplasmin* is an alpha-2–beta globulin having a molecular weight of 16,000. It binds with copper and helps in its transport and storage.

Applied Aspects

Wilson disease (hepatolenticular degeneration), a disease caused due to abnormal copper metabolism due to deficiency of ceruloplasmin in which the liver and brain are damaged due to high levels of free copper.
Menkes disease is another disorder of copper metabolism that occurs due to mutation in the gene for copper binding P-type of ATPase. It is a sex-linked disease, which affects only the male infants, mainly involves the nervous system, connective tissue and vasculature, and is usually fatal in infancy. This disease is also called '*kinky or steely hair disease*'.

vi. *Fetuin* is a growth-promoting protein seen in infants and newborns.
vii. *Immunoglobulins* are gamma globulins which play a role in immunity.
viii. *Angiotensinogen* is an alpha-2 globulin.
ix. *Haemagglutinins* are antibodies against the red blood cell antigens.

3. Fibrinogen

- ***Plasma levels*** are 0.3 g/dL.
- ***Molecular weight*** varies from 400,000 to 500,000.
- ***Synthesized*** in the liver.
- ***Chemical structure:*** Protein part of the molecule is made up of six polypeptide chains (α_2, β_2 and γ_2) joined by disulphide bonds.
- ***Functions*** as a clotting protein.

4. Prothrombin

- ***Plasma levels*** are 40 mg/dL.
- ***Molecular weight*** is 68,000.
- ***Synthesized*** in the liver. Synthesis is promoted by vitamin K.

FUNCTIONS OF PLASMA PROTEINS

1. Exert osmotic pressure. Protein molecules are unable to pass across the capillary membrane and consequently exert colloid osmotic pressure of about 25 mm Hg on the capillary membrane. About 70%–80% of the osmotic pressure is contributed by the albumin fraction. The colloid osmotic pressure plays an important role in the exchange of water between the blood and tissue fluid as explained below:

- At the *arterial end of capillaries,* due to higher hydrostatic pressure than the colloid osmotic pressure, filtration of fluid occurs from vessels to tissue spaces.
- At the *venous end of capillaries,* due to lower hydrostatic pressure than the colloid osmotic pressure, absorption of fluid from the tissue spaces into the vessels occurs (see page 309).

2. Contribution to blood viscosity. Plasma proteins, owing to their size and particularly their shape, greatly contribute to the blood viscosity. Fibrinogen and globulins are significant contributors to blood viscosity because of their asymmetrical shape. The blood viscosity plays an important role in the maintenance of blood pressure by providing resistance to the flow of blood in blood vessels.

3. Role in coagulation of blood. Fibrinogen, prothrombin and other coagulation proteins present in the plasma play an important role in the coagulation of blood. Whenever there is injury to the blood vessels, fibrinogen is converted into fibrin which forms a blood clot. For details, see page 202.

4. Role in defence mechanism of the body. The gamma globulins are antibodies which play an important role in the immune system meant for defence of the body against microorganisms. For details, see page 182.

5. Role in maintaining acid–base balance of the body. Plasma proteins act as buffers and contribute for about 15% of the buffering capacity of blood. Because of their amphoteric nature, plasma proteins can combine with acids and bases as explained below:

- *In acidic pH,* the NH_2 group of the proteins acts as a base and accepts proton and is converted to NH_4.
- *In alkaline pH,* the COOH group of the proteins acts as an acid and can donate a proton and thus becomes COO^-.
- *At normal pH* of blood, proteins act as acids and combine with cations (mainly sodium).

6. Transport function. Plasma proteins combine easily with many substances and play an essential role in their transport as explained below:

- *Carbon dioxide* is transported by plasma proteins in the form of carbamino compound.
- *Thyroxine* is transported by an alpha globulin called thyroxine-binding protein (TBP).
- *Cortisol* is transported by transcortin which is a mucoprotein.
- *Vitamins A, D and E* are transported by the HDL and LDL.
- *Vitamin B_{12}* is bound to transcobalamin for transport.
- *Bilirubin* is associated with albumin and also with fractions of the alpha globulin.
- *Drugs* of various types are transported after combining with albumin.
- *Calcium* present in the plasma is partly (50%) bound to the proteins for transport.
- *Copper* is bound to ceruloplasmin (alpha-2 globulin) for transport.
- *Free haemoglobin* in the vessels is bound by haptoglobin and carried to the reticuloendothelial system.

7. Role as reserve proteins. Plasma proteins serve as reserve proteins and are utilized by the body tissues during conditions like:

- Fasting
- Inadequate protein intake
- Excessive catabolism of body proteins

8. Role in the suspension stability of the red blood cells. Suspension stability refers to the property of red blood cells by the virtue of which they remain uniformly suspended in the blood. Globulins and fibrinogen accelerate this property.

9. Fibrinolytic function. The enzymes of the fibrinolytic system digest the intravascular clot (thrombus) and thus save from the disastrous effects of thrombosis.

10. Role of nourishment of tissue cells. Plasma proteins are utilized by the leucocytes to produce substances known as *trephones* or *carrel,* which are essential for the nourishment of tissue cells.

11. Role in genetic information. Many plasma proteins exhibit *polymorphism.* Polymorphism is a Mendelian trait that exists in the population with differing prevalence. Plasma proteins serve as a valuable tool for the studies of population genetics. Plasma proteins that show polymorphism are haptoglobin, transferrin, ceruloplasmin and immunoglobulins.

12. Antiprotease action. Proteases are enzymes which can digest connective tissue elements.

Alpha-1 antitrypsin (α_1AT) and alpha-2 macroglobulin (α_2M) act as antiprotease and are able to inactivate enormous varieties of proteinases.

SYNTHESIS OF PLASMA PROTEINS

Site of Synthesis

In an embryo, plasma proteins are synthesized by the mesenchymal cells through a process of secretion or dissolution of their substances. First, albumin is produced and then other proteins are synthesized.

In adults, plasma proteins are synthesized as described below:

- Albumin and fibrinogen are synthesized mostly by reticuloendothelial cells of the liver.
- Alpha and beta globulins are synthesized by the liver, spleen and bone marrow.
- Gamma globulins are synthesized by B lymphocytes.

Plasma proteins are generally synthesized on the membrane-bound polyribosomes. They traverse the major secretory route in the cell (rough ER membrane → smooth ER membrane → Golgi apparatus → secretory vesicle) before entering the plasma. Thus, most plasma proteins are synthesized as preprotein form.

Factors Affecting Synthesis of Plasma Proteins

1. Dietary proteins. Dietary proteins play the most essential role in the synthesis of plasma proteins. The relation of plasma proteins with diet was studied in plasma protein-depleted dogs first by George H. Whipple in 1956 by *plasmapheresis*.

Plasmapheresis. In this experiment, the dog is rendered hypoproteinaemic by repeatedly withdrawing whole blood and injecting back the cellular elements of the blood (suspended in Ringer–Locke solution). This process is repeated daily till the level of plasma proteins falls to 4 g/dL. Thereafter, different standard diets are given and their effects on protein synthesis are studied. Following conclusions have been drawn from these experiments:

- *Dietary proteins* are essential for the synthesis of plasma proteins.
- *Chemical resemblance* of food protein amino acid with those of the plasma proteins to be synthesized determines their efficacy to synthesize a particular protein.
- *Essential amino acids* must be present in the diet for the satisfactory synthesis of plasma proteins.
- *Dietary proteins of animal origin* favour albumin synthesis.
- *Dietary proteins of plant origin* favour globulin synthesis.
- *Regeneration period:* Regeneration of plasma proteins occurs within 14 days.
- *Rate of regeneration* of plasma proteins is very fast, within first 24 hours.

2. Other factors. Other factors which affect plasma protein synthesis in the body are as follows:

- *Presence of infection* in the body reduces plasma protein synthesis.
- *Exposure to some antigen* stimulates formation of antibodies.
- *Inflammatory conditions* promote the synthesis of a number of other proteins.
- *Variation in colloid oncotic pressure* influences the albumin synthesis.
- *Interleukin-1*, a material released by the activated macrophages in the body, stimulates the synthesis of many acute phase proteins in the liver.
- *Prostaglandins* are also reported to increase the synthesis of acute phase proteins, possibly through stimulation of macrophage release of interleukin-1.

CHANGES IN PLASMA PROTEINS IN HEALTH AND DISEASE

Normal Levels

- *Total proteins:* 7.4 g/dL (range 6.4–8.3 g/dL)
- *Albumin:* 4.8 g/dL (range 3.5–5.5 g/dL)
- *Globulin:* 2.3 g/dL (range 2–3.5 g/dL)
- *Albumin–globulin ratio (A/G ratio):* 1.7:1

Physiological Variations

- *In infants*, the total protein level is low (about 5.5 g/dL) due to low gamma globulins.
- *In old age*, there is a tendency for the albumin level to fall and the total globulin level to rise.
- *In pregnancy*, during first 6 months, the albumin and globulin levels decrease while the fibrinogen level increases.

Applied Aspects

Abnormalities of Plasma Protein Levels

Hypoproteinaemia

Hypoproteinaemia refers to generalized decrease in the levels of plasma proteins.

Causes of hypoproteinaemia. These include the following:

Dietary deficiency and starvation are associated with hypoproteinaemia after the body's reserve proteins are depleted.

Malabsorption syndrome due to intestinal diseases, such as sprue, is associated with hypoproteinaemia.

Liver diseases like hepatitis and cirrhosis cause hypoproteinaemia due to reduced synthesis of proteins in the liver.

Renal diseases like nephrotic syndrome cause hypoproteinaemia due to more loss of proteins in the urine.

Haemorrhage and extensive burns are associated with acute hypoproteinaemia.

Hereditary analbuminaemia is an inborn defect in the genetic level, where there is no synthesis of albumin.

Congenital afibrinogenaemia is a rare condition characterized by defective blood clotting.

Effects of hypoproteinaemia. Low levels of plasma proteins are associated with a decrease in the plasma osmotic pressure, which causes water retention and oedema of the body tissue.

Hyperproteinaemia

Hyperproteinaemia, i.e. increase in the plasma protein levels, is seen in the following conditions:

Acute inflammatory conditions are associated with increased synthesis of the so-called *acute phase proteins*, which include C-reactive proteins, alpha antitrypsin, haptoglobin, fibrinogen and ceruloplasmin.

Acute tissue destruction as in myocardial infarction is also associated with raised levels of acute phase proteins.

Chronic inflammation and malignancies are also associated with raised levels of C-reactive proteins.

Multiple myeloma is associated with the increased levels of the so-called *Bence–Jones* proteins and myeloma globulin due to their abnormal formation in the bone marrow.

Reversal of normal A/G ratio

The normal A/G ratio (1.7:1) is reversed in the following conditions:

- When albumin synthesis is decreased as it occurs in liver diseases (globulin levels being normal because many globulins are synthesized by B lymphocytes)
- When globulin levels are increased (as occurs in most of the conditions) associated with hyperproteinaemia

Important Note

C-reactive protein levels are used as diagnostic marker of inflammatory conditions.

Self-Assessment

1. Discuss the different types of plasma proteins, their characteristics and functions.
2. Discuss briefly the sites and factors affecting the synthesis of plasma proteins.
3. Write notes on:
   - Plasma pharesis
   - Electrophoretic mobility
   - Hypoprotenemia

Clinical Cases

Case 1

A 9-year-old male child presents in the paediatric OPD with swelling in the legs and face, loss of muscle mass, dry skin, hair brittle and scanty, nails cracked and pitted. The parents reported history of frequent fever and generalized weakness.

Q.1 What is the probable diagnosis?

Q.2 What laboratory investigations should be advised for final diagnosis?

Q.3 What is the main cause for presenting features?

Case 2

A 40-year-old male patient presented with abdominal pain, fatigue and loss of weight. On physical examination, tremors, excessive salivation and difficulty in speech were observed. Provisional diagnosis was Wilson disease.

Q.1 What is the main cause of presenting signs and symptoms?

Q.2 What is the most specific test to reach the final diagnosis?

3.2 Red Blood Cells and Anaemias

CHAPTER OUTLINE

CHARACTERISTIC FEATURES OF RED BLOOD CELLS

FUNCTIONAL MORPHOLOGY

The red blood cells (RBCs; mature erythrocytes) form one of the important constituents of the cellular elements of the blood. Each RBC, like any other cell in the body, is bound by a *cell membrane* but is *non-nucleated* and lacks the usual cell organelles. The cytoplasm of the RBC contains a special pigmented protein called the *haemoglobin* (Hb) which forms 90% of the weight of the erythrocyte. The red colour of the RBCs, and thus of the blood, is due to the presence of Hb.

Normal Size, Shape and Counts of RBCs (Erythropoisis)

Normal Size

- *Diameter* of each RBC is 7.2 μm (range: 6.9–7.4 μm).
- *Thickness* in the periphery is 2 μm and in the centre 1 μm.
- *Surface area* of each RBC is about 120–140 μm^2.
- *Volume* is about 80 μm^3 (range: 78–86 μm^3).

Normal Shape

The RBCs are circular, biconcave discs (Fig. 3.2.1).

Advantages of biconcave shape are as follows:

- It renders the red cells quite flexible so that they can pass through capillaries whose minimum diameter is 3.5 μm (Fig. 3.2.2).
- The biconcavity provides greater surface area as compared to volume which allows considerable alterations in the cell volume. Thus, the RBC can withstand considerable changes of osmotic pressure or minimum tension is offered on the membrane when changes in volume of cells occur. In this way, the RBCs can resist haemolysis to a certain extent when placed in hypotonic solutions.
- Greater surface area allows easy exchange of O_2 and CO_2 and rapid diffusion of other substances.

Normal Counts

- *At birth*, normal RBC count is 6–7 million/mm^3.
- *In children,* it varies from 4.6 to 4.8 million/mm^3.
- *In adult males*, the normal count varies from 5 to 6.5 million/mm^3 (average 5.5 million/mm^3).

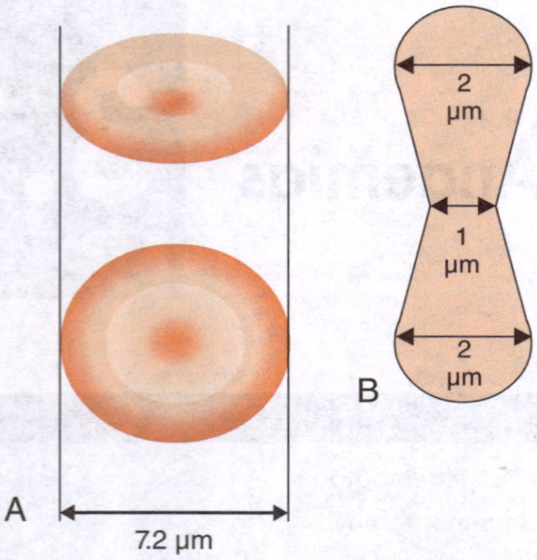

Fig. 3.2.1 Size and shape of a normal red blood cell: **A,** biconcave disc (diameter 7.2 µm); and **B,** thickness (2 µm at the periphery and 1 µm in the centre).

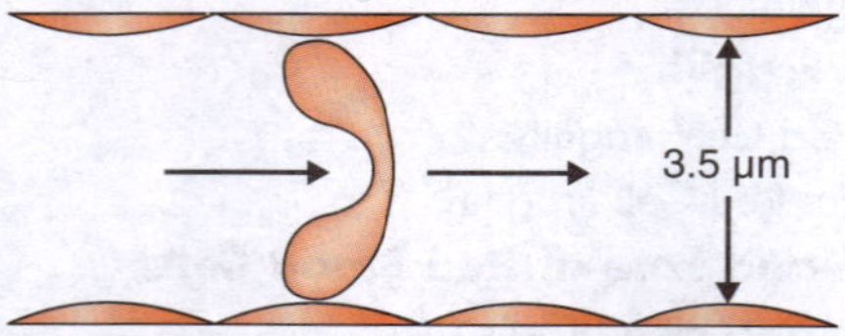

Fig. 3.2.2 Showing how flexibility of red blood cell allows it to pass through smaller capillaries (diameter 3.5 µm).

- *In females,* it varies from 4.5 to 5.5 million/mm^3 (average 4.8 million/mm^3).
- *Clinically,* a count of 5 million/mm^3 is considered as 100%.

Variations in Size, Shape and Counts of RBCs

Variations in size Variation in size is called anisocytosis:

Microcytosis, i.e. decrease in the size of RBCs, occurs:
- In iron-deficiency anaemia
- During prolonged forced breathing
- When osmotic pressure of blood is increased

Macrocytosis, i.e. increase in the size of RBCs, occurs:
- In megaloblastic anaemia
- During muscular exercise
- When osmotic pressure of blood is decreased

Variations in shape Variation in shape is called *poikilocytosis*. Abnormal shapes of the RBCs are (Fig. 3.2.3) given as follows:

Crenation or shrinkage of RBCs is seen when they are suspended in hypertonic solution. This occurs because of the outward diffusion of water from the RBCs.

Spherocyte is a globular-shaped RBC. It is seen in a hereditary disease called spherocytosis. These cells are more fragile. Similar changes in the shape of RBCs are observed when they are suspended in hypotonic solutions.

Elliptocytes, i.e. elliptical-shaped RBCs, are seen in certain anaemias.

Sickle cell, i.e. crescent shape of the RBCs, occurs in sickle cell anaemia because of the presence of abnormal Hb (haemoglobin S [HbS]). For details, see page 140.

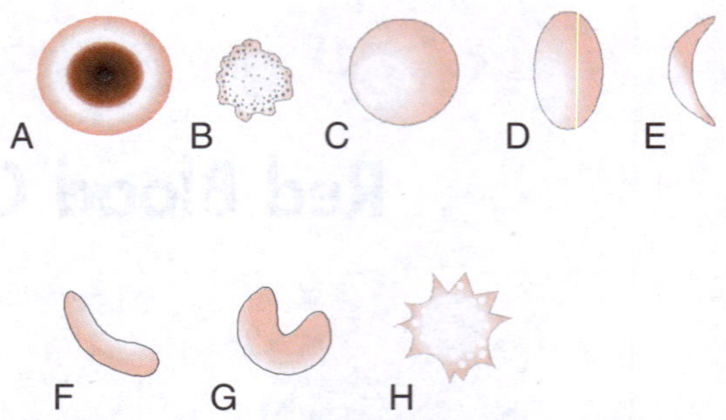

Fig. 3.2.3 Variations in the shapes of red blood cells: **A,** normal; **B,** crenation; **C,** spherocyte; **D,** elliptocyte; **E,** sickle cell; **F,** discocyte; **G,** stomatocyte; and **H,** echinocyte.

Poikilocytes, i.e. unusual shapes of RBCs such as flask-shaped, hammer-shaped or other abnormal shapes, occur due to deformed cell membrane.

Variations in counts ***Physiological increase in the RBC count*** (physiological polycythaemia) is seen in the following circumstances:

Age. At birth, the RBC count is 6–7 million/mm^3 of blood. After about 10 days of birth, the count decreases due to destruction of cells. This is the cause of *physiological jaundice* in the newborns. In infants, the RBC count is slightly more than that in the adults.

Sex. RBC count in adult females (average 4.8 million/mm^3) is lower than adult males (average 5.5 million/mm^3).

High altitude. RBC count of the individuals residing in high-altitude areas (above 10,000 feet from the sea level) is high (7 million/mm^3) because of hypoxic stimulation of erythropoiesis.

Excessive exercise. Mild hypoxia and spleen contraction cause temporary increase in the RBC count.

Emotional conditions like anxiety are associated with temporary increase in the RBC count due to sympathetic stimulation.

Increase in atmospheric temperature causes a temporary elevation of RBC count.

After meals, the RBC count is raised slightly.

Relative polycythaemia or apparent polycythaemia occurs when plasma volume decreases and mass of RBCs remains normal, for example in dehydration.

Polycythaemia can also occur in normal infants because of delay in umbilical cord clamping during childbirth leading to transfer of RBCs from the placenta.

Applied Aspects

Polycythaemia

Pathological increase in RBC count (above 7 million/mm^3) is of two types:

Primary polycythaemia or polycythaemia vera (PV) is also called erythema, and occurs in myeloproliferative disorders, like malignancies of the bone marrow. The RBC count is persistently above 14 million/mm^3 and is always associated with high WBC count.

Secondary polycythaemia occurs due to certain conditions producing a state of chronic hypoxia in the body, such as:
- Congenital heart disease
- Chronic respiratory disorders like emphysema

- Repeated mild haemorrhages
- Phosphorus and arsenic poisoning

Pathophysiology of polycythaemia. In 95% of cases, PV occurs due to mutation of gene JAK2V617F, which needs to enhanced activities of Janus kinase (*JAK2*). This gene controls the production of a protein that helps in formation of RBCs.

Diagnosis of PV. *Diagnosis of PV is mainly based on complete blood count (CBC).* In polycythaemia, haematocrit may be raised up to 60%–70% and total blood volume also increases. As a result, there is engorgement of the entire vascular system. Blood viscosity also increases (three times as that of normal).

Effects of polycythaemia. Greater increase in blood viscosity due to polycythaemia is responsible for:

i. *Thrombosis:* The incidence of thrombosis increases because the blood flow through peripheral vessels becomes sluggish.
ii. *Increase in arterial pressure* due to rise in total peripheral resistance.
iii. *Ruddy complexion:* A person with PV has a ruddy complexion due to increased RBC count with a bluish tint (cyanotic) to the skin due to increased deoxygenated Hb, as a result of the sluggish blood flow through the skin capillaries.

Treatment. *In low-risk patients, PV is a chronic condition that does not have any specific cure; however, treatment can help to manage its symptoms and to prevent complications. To prevent blood clotting, medications involved are as follows:*

- *Aspirin* in low dose is recommended, which affects platelets, thus decreasing the risk of blood clot formation.
- *Hydroxyurea (Droxia)* is a cancer drug that prevents formation of too many RBCs.
- *Interferon-alpha* helps the immune system and fights off overactive bone marrow.
- *Busulfan (Myleran)* is used for treating leukaemia.
- *Ruxolitinib (Jakafi)* acts by inhibiting growth factor which is responsible for formation of RBCs.

Phlebotomy, i.e. taking out small amount of blood from the veins once a week (this procedure reduces blood cell count) and then once in a month until haematocrit levels are nearly closer to normal values

To relieve itching, antihistaminics (i.e. selective serotonin reuptake inhibitors)

Phototherapy

- Narrow-band (UVB) phototherapy is useful in treating pruritis associated with PV.

Complications of PV. Myelofibrosis, heart attack due to ischaemia, deep vein thrombosis and pulmonary embolism.

Physiological decrease in RBC count *resulting in anaemia which is seen in the following conditions:*

- *At high barometric pressure,* the RBC count is decreased slightly due to high O_2 tension of the blood.
- *After sleep,* the RBC count is decreased slightly.
- *In pregnancy,* there occurs relative reduction in RBC count due to haemodilution caused by increase in the plasma volume.

Anaemia In anaemia, there may occur marked reduction in the RBC count, or the Hb level, or both (see page 149).

Packed Cell Volume and Red Cell Indices

The red cell indices or absolute values (blood standards) include the entities mean corpuscular volume (MCV), mean corpuscular haemoglobin (MCH) and the mean corpuscular haemoglobin concentration (MCHC). These indices are quite helpful in diagnosing the type of anaemia. These indices are calculated from the values of packed cell volume (PCV), the Hb concentration and the red cell count.

Packed Cell Volume

PCV refers to the percentage of the cellular elements (RBCs, WBCs and platelets) in the whole blood. Since the volume of WBCs and platelets is very less, so for all practical purposes, the PCV is considered equivalent to the volume of packed red cells (VPRC), or the so-called *haematocrit value*. However, in conditions where the number of WBCs is markedly increased, the values of PCV differ from those of the VPRC (haematocrit values). The normal values of PCV in males are about 45% (47% ± 5%) and in females about 42% (42% ± 5%). The VPRC is increased in polycythaemia and decreased in anaemia.

Determination of PCV. The blood is mixed with anticoagulant oxalate and is centrifuged in a graduated tube called the *haematocrit tube* or the Wintrobe tube (Fig. 3.2.4) at a speed of 3000 rpm for about 30 minutes. The heavier RBCs settle at the bottom leaving clear plasma above. The white blood cells and platelets which constitute only about 1% of the volume of blood are seen as a thin white layer called *buffy coat* on the top of the red cell mass.

- *Observed haematocrit* is the value of haematocrit obtained by the above-described method.

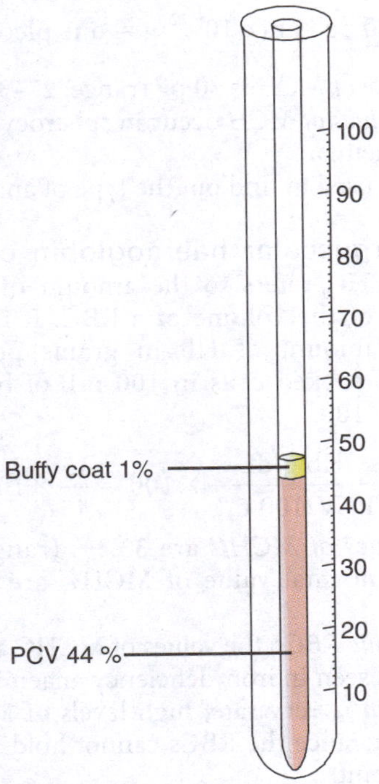

Fig. 3.2.4 Wintrobe tube showing packed cell volume.

- *True haematocrit* is calculated by multiplying observed haematocrit by 0.98. It is calculated because even if the red cells are fully packed, about 2% of plasma is trapped in between the cells.
- *Body haematocrit* is present in large and small blood vessels. It is calculated by multiplying the observed haematocrit with 0.87. It is calculated because the haematocrit is estimated from the venous blood whose haematocrit is greater than that of the whole body. In general, haematocrit in larger vessels is more than in the smaller vessels.

Red Cell Indices

The red cell indices defined in the subsequent text are calculated taking normal values of RBC count 5 million/mm³, PCV 45% and Hb level of 15 g/dL.

1. Mean corpuscular volume. The MCV refers to the average volume of a single RBC. It is calculated by dividing the PCV by the red cell count.

$$MCV = \frac{\text{PCV in 1000 mL of blood, i.e. (PCV} \times 10)}{\text{RBC count/mm}^3}$$
$$= \frac{45 \times 10}{5} = 90\ \mu m^3$$

- One μm^3 is equal to 1 fL.
- Normal value of MCV is 90 μm^3 (range: 78–94 μm^3); when the MCV value is normal, it is referred to as *normocytosis.*
- Decreased value of MCV occurs in *microcytosis.*
- Increased value of MCV occurs in *macrocytosis.*

2. Mean corpuscular haemoglobin (MCH). MCH refers to the average mass of Hb contained in each RBC. It is calculated by dividing the amount of Hb in 1 L of blood by the red cell count in 1 L of blood.

$$MCH = \frac{\text{Hb g/L}}{\text{RBC count/L}} = \frac{\text{Hb g/dL} \times 10}{\text{RBC count/mm}^3 \times 10^{12}}$$
$$= \frac{15 \times 10}{5 \times 10^{12}} = 30 \times 10^{-12}\ g$$
$$= 30\ pg\ [\text{since } 10^{-12}\ g = \text{one picogram (pg)}]$$

- *Normal value of MCH* is 30 pg (range: 27–33 pg).
- *Increased values of MCH* occur in spherocytosis and megaloblastic anaemia.
- MCH is not used to find out the type of anaemia.

3. Mean corpuscular haemoglobin concentration (MCHC). MCHC refers to the amount of Hb expressed as percentage of the volume of a RBC. It is calculated by dividing the amount of Hb in grams per decilitre by the volume of packed cells in 100 mL of blood and then multiplying by 100.

$$MCHC = \frac{\text{Hb g/dL}}{\text{PCV/100 mL}} \times 100 = \frac{15}{45} \times 100 = 33.3\%$$

- *Normal values of MCHC* are 33.3% (range: 30%–38%). RBCs with normal value of MCHC are called *normochromic.*
- *In hypochromic RBCs,* the values of MCHC are less than the normal, as is seen in iron-deficiency anaemia.
- *Hyperchromia* is very rare; high levels of MCHC (>38%) cannot occur, since the RBCs cannot hold Hb beyond the saturation point.
- Since MCHC is independent of RBC count and size of RBCs, it is considered to be of greater clinical significance compared with other absolute values.

4. Red cell distribution width (RDW) It is a measurement derived from the RBC distribution curve generated on automated haematology analyser, and is an indicator of variation in RBC size within a blood sample. RDW is used along with the indices (MCV, MCH, MCHC) to describe population of RBCs. The RDW measures deviation of the RBC width and not the actual width or size of individual cell. The value of RDW can be calculated by two methods:

- Red cell distribution width coefficient of variation (RDW-CV)
- Red cell distribution width standard variation (RDW-SD)

RDW-CV is calculated in percentage using the following formula: standard deviation of mean RBC size divided by MCV multiplied by 100:

$$\frac{\text{SD of mean cell size}}{\text{MCV}} \times 100$$

Normal range is 11%–15%, if there is

- A homogenous population of RBCs with narrow distribution curve and low MCV, then value of RDW-CV, may be elevated
- A heterogonous population of RBCs with broad distribution curve and high MCV, then value of RDW-CV may be normal

RDW-SD is an actual measurement in femtolitres. The width of distribution curve is measured at the point that is 20% above the baseline. Since RDW-SD is not influenced by MCV, so it more accurately reflects the RBC size variation as shown in Fig. 3.2.5.

Normal range of RDW-SD for adults is 40–50 fL.

5. Colour index. The colour index (CI) refers to the ratio of Hb to RBC. For calculating CI, Hb of 14.8 g/dL is taken as 100% and RBC count of 5 million/mm³ is taken as 100%.

$$CI = \frac{\text{Percentage of normal Hb}}{\text{Percentage of normal RBC count}} = \frac{100}{100} = 1$$

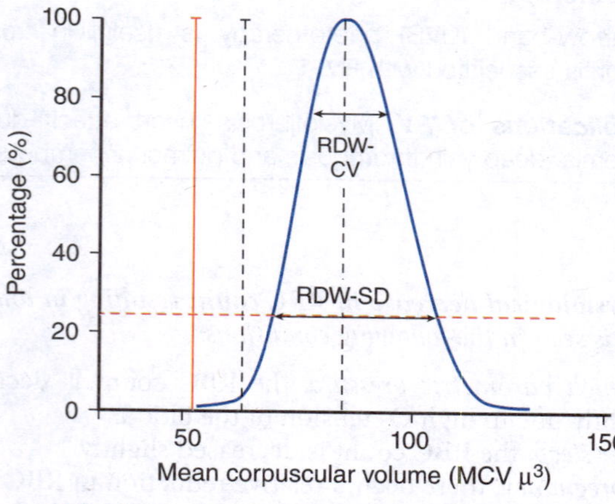

Fig. 3.2.5 Red cell width distribution curve.

For example, if the Hb level is 14.8 g/dL, i.e. 100% of normal values, and RBC count is 4.5 million, i.e. $4.5 \times 100 = 90\%$ of the normal values, then

$$CI = 100/90 = 1.11$$

Normal values of CI vary from 0.85 to 1.15.

- CI is insignificant because normal range of RBC is very wide. Therefore, it has been long abandoned and is not used for any diagnostic purposes.

Rouleaux Formation and Erythrocyte Sedimentation Rate

Rouleaux Formation

- Rouleaux formation refers to the tendency of RBCs to pile up one over the other like a pile of coins (Fig. 3.2.6). The discoid shape and protein coating of red cells play a major role in rouleaux formation. Rouleaux formation does not occur in normal circulation under physiological conditions, as the moving cells show little or no tendency to adhere. However, within a blood vessel, in the absence of significant flow and when the blood is taken out, the red cells tend to form rouleaux.
- This is a reversible phenomenon, but it promotes sedimentation of RBCs. It should not be confused with agglutination where the cells are irreversibly clumped.
- Albumin decreases the rouleaux formation, while fibrinogen, globulin and other products of tissue destruction increase rouleaux formation.

Erythrocyte Sedimentation Rate

Erythrocyte sedimentation rate (ESR) is the rate at which the RBCs sediment (settle down) when the blood containing an anticoagulant is allowed to stand in a vertically placed tube. It is expressed in millimetre at the end of the first hour.

Methods of determination of erythrocyte sedimentation rate are:

1. Westergren method. A total of 1.6 mL of blood diluted with 0.4 mL of 3.8% sodium citrate (making a total of 2 mL) is loaded in the Westergren pipette which is then fitted to stand vertically. The reading is taken after 1 hour. The Westergren tube is 30 cm long and is open at both the ends (Fig. 3.2.7A).

2. Wintrobe method. About 1 mL of blood mixed with anticoagulant EDTA is loaded in a Wintrobe tube up to '0' mark and the reading is taken after 1 hour. The Wintrobe tube is 11 cm long and is open only at one end (Fig. 3.2.7B).

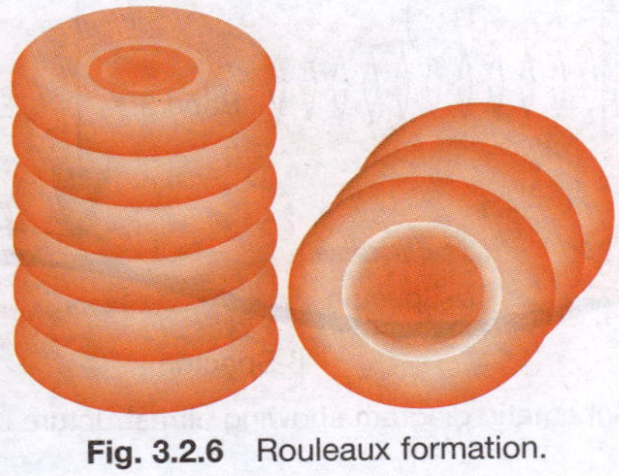

Fig. 3.2.6 Rouleaux formation.

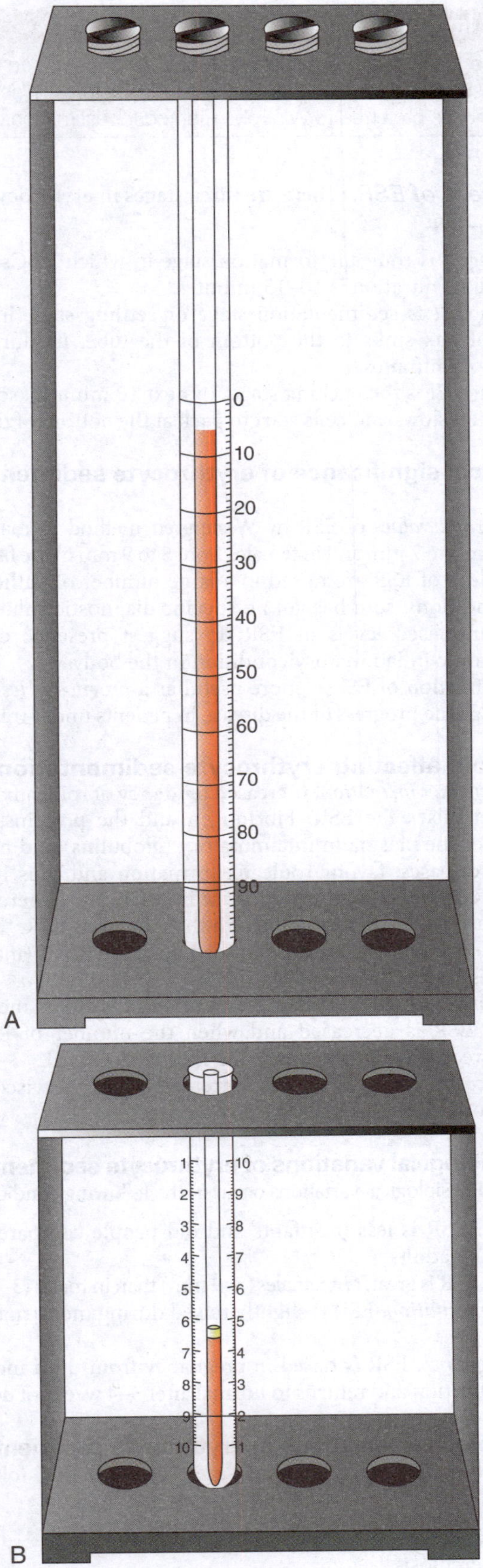

Fig. 3.2.7 **A,** Westergren pipette and **B,** Wintrobe tube, used for determining erythrocyte sedimentation rate (ESR).

Important Note

Since the Westergren pipette is longer, chances of an error in measurement of ESR is reduced. Therefore, Westergren method is preferred to Wintrobe method for estimation of ESR.

Process of ESR. There are three stages in erythrocyte sedimentation:

- *Stage I* is rouleaux formation stage in which RBCs pile up and its duration is 10–15 minutes.
- *Stage II* is sedimentation stage or settling stage in which rouleaux sinks to the bottom of the tube. Its duration is 40–45 minutes.
- *Stage III* is the packing stage. In next 10 minutes, sedimentation slows and cells start to pack at the bottom of the tube.

Clinical significance of erythrocyte sedimentation rate

- *Normal values* of ESR by Westergren method in males vary from 3 to 7 mm and in females from 5 to 9 mm in the first hour.
- Values of ESR are raised in a large number of pathological conditions, so it has got no specific diagnostic value. However, raised levels of ESR do suggest presence of some chronic inflammatory condition in the body.
- Estimation of ESR is more useful as a *prognostic test*, i.e. to judge the progress of the disease in patients under treatment.

Factors affecting erythrocyte sedimentation rate

- *Rouleaux formation.* Increased tendency of rouleaux formation raises the ESR. Fibrinogen and the proteins, which enter the plasma in inflammatory (globulins) and neoplastic diseases, favour rouleaux formation and thus increase ESR. Increase in MCV, decrease in MCH and spherocytosis retard rouleaux formation and thus decrease ESR.
- *Size of the RBCs.* Increase in the size of the RBCs (macrocytosis) raises the ESR.
- *Number of RBCs.* When the number of RBCs is increased, the ESR is decreased and when the number of RBCs is decreased (as in anaemia), the ESR is increased.
- *Viscosity of blood.* ESR is increased when the viscosity of blood is decreased and vice versa.

Physiological variations of erythrocyte sedimentation rate

Physiological variations occur in the following conditions:

- *Age.* ESR is less in infants and old people compared with young adults.
- *Sex.* ESR is greater in females (5–9 mm) than in males (3–7 mm).
- *Menstruation.* ESR is slightly raised during menstruation in females.
- *Pregnancy.* ESR is raised in pregnancy from third month to parturition and returns to normal after 3–4 weeks of delivery.

Pathological variations in erythrocyte sedimentation rate

Pathological variations are seen in the following conditions:

Increase in ESR occurs in:

- Tuberculosis
- Malignant diseases
- Collagen diseases
- All anaemias except sickle cell anaemia
- Chronic infections

Decrease in ESR occurs in the following pathological conditions:

- Polycythaemia
- Decreased fibrinogen levels
- Sickle cell anaemia
- Allergic conditions
- Peptone shock

RED CELL MEMBRANE, COMPOSITION AND METABOLISM OF RED BLOOD CELLS

Red Cell Membrane

Structure Red cell membrane is a *trilaminar structure* having a bimolecular lipid layer interposed between the two layers of proteins (Fig. 3.2.8; see also Fig. 1.2.2).

Important lipids of the cell membrane are glycolipids, phospholipids and cholesterol.

Proteins in the cell membrane are present as peripheral proteins and integral proteins spanning the whole membrane.

The outer peripheral protein surface is rich in *lecithin and sphingomyelin.*

The important membrane-spanning integral proteins include an anion exchange protein (*band 3*) and *glycophorins* which contain a number of polysaccharide *blood group antigens.*

- *Band 3* is an anion transport protein, also known as anion exchanger 1 (AE_1), transmembrane glycoprotein with its carboxyl terminal end (towards external surface) and its amino terminal end (towards cytoplasmic surface), extending across the bilayer at least 10 times, therefore, also called multipass membrane protein. It forms a tunnel permitting exchange of Cl^- for HCO_3^- (chloride shift). The cytoplasmic amino acid terminal binds many proteins (4.1, 4.2, ankyrin, several glycolytic enzymes and also Hb).
- *Glycophorins A, B and C* are single-pass type at transmembrane proteins. The amino acid terminal extrudes out from the surface of RBCs which contain polysaccharides (blood group antigens). The carboxyl terminal end extends into the cytosol and binds to protein 4.1, which in turn binds to spectrin.
- The inner surface of the cell membrane contains more phosphatidylserine and phosphatidylethanolamine. The peripheral proteins like spectrin, ankyrin and actin

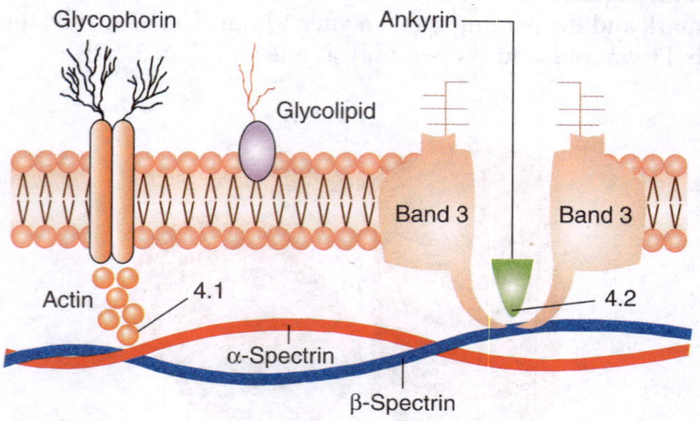

Fig. 3.2.8 Schematic diagram showing ultrastructure of red cell membrane.

present on the inner surface of the membrane help in maintaining the shape and flexibility of the RBC. *Spectrin* is the major protein of the cytoskeleton; protein 4.1 binds to both spectrin and actin and also interacts with certain phospholipids (thereby connecting the cytoskeleton to the lipid layer).

Applied Aspects

Abnormalities in the amount or structure of spectrin cause hereditary spherocytosis or elliptocytosis.

Hereditary spherocytosis is a genetic disease transmitted as an autosomal dominant trait, which affects about 1:5000 North Americans. It is characterized by spherocytes (spherical RBCs with low surface area to volume ratio) in the peripheral blood. The spherocytes are nondeformable structures susceptible to osmotic lysis. Their lifespan is shorter than that of normal RBCs.

Hereditary elliptocytosis is also a genetic disorder similar to hereditary spherocytosis. In this condition, red cells assume an elliptical or disc-like shape. It also occurs due to abnormality of spectrin, protein 4.1 or glycophorin C.

Permeability. The red cell membrane is a *semipermeable membrane*, allowing some substances to pass through and preventing some:

- *Impermeable* to sodium, calcium and barium ions, to fats and sugars
- *Slightly impermeable* to amino acids
- *Freely permeable* to all anions like Cl^-, SO_4^- and HCO_3^-, and to urea, ammonia, aldehyde, alcohol and bile salts

Composition of Red Blood Cells

The body of RBCs bound by the cell membrane contains a sponge-like stroma which is composed of the following structures:

- *Water* constitutes 60% of the wet weight of RBC.
- *Hb*, held in the meshes of stroma, constitutes 35% of the wet weight and 90% of the dry weight of RBC.
- *Lipids* form the major constituents of the rest of 5% of stroma. These include cephalin, lecithin and cholesterol.
- *Proteins* include glutathiones and an albumin-like insoluble protein. These act as reducing agents preventing damage to the Hb.
- *Lipoproteins.* Almost half of the lipids are bound to the protein forming a lipoprotein complex known as *elenin (Calvin).*
- *Enzymes* of the glycolytic system, catalase, carbonic anhydrase and other enzymes and inorganic salts are also present in the RBC.
- *Glucose and amino acids* are present in small amounts.
- *Ions.* Anions of the plasma (Cl^-, PO_4^-, HCO_3^-) are present often in large amounts. The cations Na^+ and Ca^{2+} either are present in very small amount or are absent. Cation K^+ is present in sufficient amount inside the RBC.
- *Nonprotein nitrogenous (NPN) substances.* Urea, NH_4, creatine and uric acid have a higher concentration inside the RBC than in the plasma.

Metabolism of Red Blood Cells

Glucose, taken up by facilitated diffusion, is the only fuel utilized by the RBC. The mature RBC has a low respiratory quotient and consumes very little oxygen. The glucose metabolism and its special significance in RBC are described below:

Embden–Meyerhof pathway It is responsible for 90% of the glycolysis. Two molecules of ATP are generated from each molecule of glucose. Special significance of this pathway is given below.

2,3-Biphosphoglycerate (2,3-BPG) synthesized in a side reaction in this pathway influences the oxygen affinity of Hb and thus plays an important role in the red cell physiology. Factors affecting 2,3-BPG concentration in RBC include the following:

- *Acidaemia* hinders glycolysis and thereby decreases 2,3-BPG synthesis.
- *Hypoxia* prevents Krebs cycle and thereby increases 2,3-BPG synthesis.
- *Thyroid hormone,* androgens and growth hormone increase 2,3-BPG concentration.

Hexose monophosphate (HMP) shunt It oxidizes about 10% of glucose. Special significance of this pathway in RBC metabolism is given as follows:

- *NADPH* generated by this pathway keeps the glutathione in reduced form. Reduced glutathione, in turn, protects sulphydryl groups in Hb and RBC membrane from oxidation by peroxides, superoxide, drugs and toxins.
- *Glucose-6-phosphate dehydrogenase (G6PD)* is the key enzyme in the HMP shunt. Inherited deficiency of this enzyme leads to compromise of RBC function and viability in the face of such oxidant stress, thus causing a number of disorders characterized by susceptibility to haemolysis (see page 144).

Utilization of ATP A major portion of ATP obtained through glycolysis is utilized in maintaining the Na^+/K^+-ATPase pump.

- Some of the energy is utilized in maintaining the integrity of the red cell membrane.
- Some of the energy is spent in maintaining the Hb iron in reduced form (Fe^{2+}).

FORMATION OF RED BLOOD CELLS

Formation of RBCs is a part of the process of development of blood cells (RBCs, WBCs and platelets) called *haemopoiesis* which includes:

- Erythropoiesis, i.e. development of RBCs
- Leucopoiesis, i.e. development of WBCs
- Thrombopoiesis or megakaryocytopoiesis, i.e. development of platelets

SITES OF HAEMOPOIESIS

In the first 2 months of gestation, the *yolk sac* is the main site of haemopoiesis (*mesoblastic* stage) (Fig. 3.2.9).

From the third month of gestation, the liver and spleen become the main sites of blood formation and continue to do so till birth. The spleen makes a small contribution as compared to the liver *(hepatic stage)*.

From the 20th week of gestation, haemopoiesis begins in the bone marrow and by the 7th or 8th month, it becomes the main site *(myeloid stage)*.

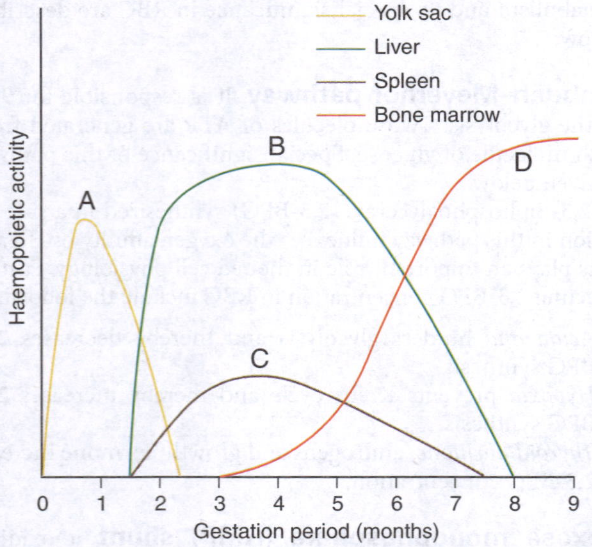

Fig. 3.2.9 Sites of haemopoiesis during different periods in human life: **A,** yolk sac; **B,** liver; **C,** spleen; and (D) bone marrow.

At birth (in normal full-term), almost whole of the haemopoiesis occurs in the bone marrow.

In young children, active haemopoietic bone marrow is found in both axial skeleton and bones of extremities. The active haemopoietic bone marrow is red in colour due to marked cellularity and hence is called *red bone marrow*. However, during this period, there occurs a progressive fatty replacement throughout the long bones converting red bone marrow into the so-called *yellow bone marrow*.

In adults, therefore, haemopoietic (red) bone marrow is confined to *axial skeleton* (skull, vertebrae, sternum, ribs, sacrum and pelvis) and *proximal ends of long bones* (humerus, femur and tibia). Even in these haemopoietic areas, about 50% of the bone marrow consists of fat. The differences between red and yellow bone marrow are summarized in Table 3.2.1.

In adults, during pathological conditions, when there is an increased demand of blood cells, the nonhaematopoietic (yellow) marrow is capable of reverting back to active haematopoietic.

Table 3.2.1 Differentiating features of red and yellow bone marrow

Red bone marrow	Yellow bone marrow
1. Red bone marrow is red in colour and is an active haemopoietic tissue	1. Yellow bone marrow is yellowish in colour and is inactive
2. Cellularity is marked; it contains different stages of all types of developing blood cells	2. Cellularity is very less and replaced by fatty tissue
3. Red bone marrow is present in axial skeleton (skull, vertebrae, sacrum, sternum and pelvis) and long bones in children	3. In adults, except ends of long bones and axial skeleton, all other bones contain yellow bone marrow
4. Known as active bone marrow	4. Known as inactive bone marrow

During pathological conditions, when the increased demand of blood cells cannot be met by the hyperactivity of bone marrow alone, even the liver and spleen resume their fetal role of haemopoiesis, as the stem cell retains its potential haemopoietic activity. Such a situation is referred to as extramedullary haemopoiesis.

BLOOD CELL PRECURSORS

The stem cells The *monophyletic theory* of haemopoiesis is now widely accepted, according to which all blood cells originate from a single ancestral cell called pluripotent or multipotent stem cell or haematopoietic stem cell (HSC). The stem cells have the appearance of small- or intermediate-sized lymphocytes. Stem cells possess two *fundamental properties*:

- *Self-replication*, i.e. stem cells are capable of cell division to give rise to more stem cells
- *Differentiation and commitment*, i.e. the stem cells have the ability to differentiate into specialized cells called *progenitor cells* (committed stem cell)

Progenitor cells The stem cells, after a series of divisions, differentiate into progenitor cells:

Pluripotent progenitor cells which can give rise to any type of blood cells

Lymphoid (immune system) stem cells which ultimately develop into lymphocytes

Myeloid (trilineage) stem cells which later differentiate into three types of cell lines:

- *Granulocyte–monocyte progenitors* which produce all leucocytes except the lymphocytes
- *Erythroid progenitors* which produce RBCs
- Megakaryocyte progenitors which produce platelets

Features of progenitor cells. Morphologically, the progenitor cells present in the bone marrow cannot be differentiated from the stem cells, as both of them look alike. However, they can be differentiated by immunological techniques, taking advantage of the different types of molecules present on their cell membrane.

Progenitor cells possess ability to give rise to clones (group of cells), so they are also called colony-forming cells (CFCs) or colony-forming units (CFUs). The three types of progenitor cells are given as follows:

Colony-forming unit–granulocyte, erythroid, megakaryocyte, macrophage (CFU-GEMM) refers to a multipotent progenitor cell, i.e. *myeloid progenitor cells*.

Colony-forming unit–erythroid (***CFU-E***) develops into erythrocytes.

- *Ba-CFU* refers to basophil CFUs.
- *Eo-CFU* are eosinophil CFUs.
- *M-CFU* refers to monocyte CFUs.
- *G-CFU* are neutrophil-forming units.

The broad outlines of haemopoiesis discussed above are summarized in Fig. 3.2.10. Further details of erythropoiesis are discussed in this chapter and details of development of other blood cells are discussed in the relevant chapters.

Bone Marrow Examination

The red bone marrow contains the stem cells, progenitor cells, CFCs and various types of blood cells in different stages of

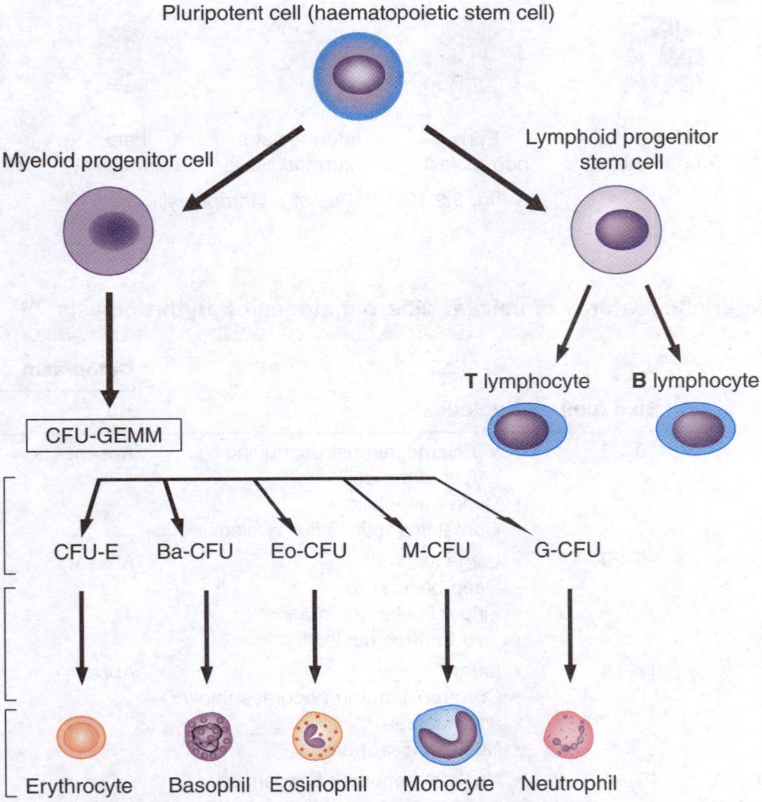

Fig. 3.2.10 Schematic broad outline of haemopoiesis.

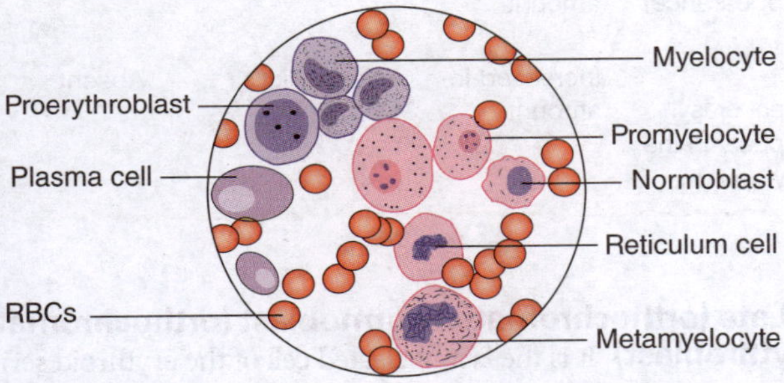

Fig. 3.2.11 Smear from red bone marrow showing various types of cells at different stages of development.

development, which can be observed in a stained smear of red marrow obtained from the iliac bone or sternum (Fig. 3.2.11). Normally, in the red marrow, the haemopoietic stem cells comprise only 0.01%–0.5% of the total marrow population. About 75% of the cells are immature white cells and about 25% of the cells are immature red cells, thus forming a ratio of 3:1, while in peripheral blood the ratio of white and red cells is 1:600. This vast difference is because the lifespan of red cells is far greater than that of the white cells.

CONTROL OF HAEMOPOIESIS

The growth of different blood cells from the stem cells is controlled and regulated by the haemopoietic growth factors, which in general are called *cytokines*. Cytokine is a general term used to denote the proteins released by cells that act as intercellular mediators. The cytokines which control the formation of different types of blood cells are called *colony-stimulating factors (CSFs)*, which are given as follows:

- *G-CSF* stimulates granulocytic precursors.
- *M-CSF* stimulates monocytic precursors.
- *GM-CSF* stimulates both the granulocytic and monocytic precursors.
- *Interleukins (IL)* refer to the cytokine-stimulating lymphocytic precursor, for example, IL-1 and IL-3.
- *Erythropoietin* (EPO) refers to the cytokine stimulating the erythroid series of cells along with IL-3 and IL-6.

Stages of Erythropoiesis

The RBCs develop from colony-forming unit–erythrocyte (CFU-E) which are derived from the committed progenitor cells.

The well-defined and readily recognizable lineages of nucleated red cells (erythroid series) which form different stages of erythropoiesis (Fig. 3.2.12; Table 3.2.2) are as follows:

1. Pronormoblast or proerythroblast It is the earliest recognizable cell of the erythroid series seen in the red bone marrow. Its features are as follows:

- *Size* is large with a diameter of 15–20 μm.
- *Cytoplasm* is scanty and deeply basophilic. The deep blue colour of cytoplasm is due to high content of RNA which is associated with active protein synthesis.
- *Nucleus* is large, central with a fine reticular chromatin and contains many nucleoli.
- *Hb* is absent at this stage.
- *Mitosis* is seen in these cells.

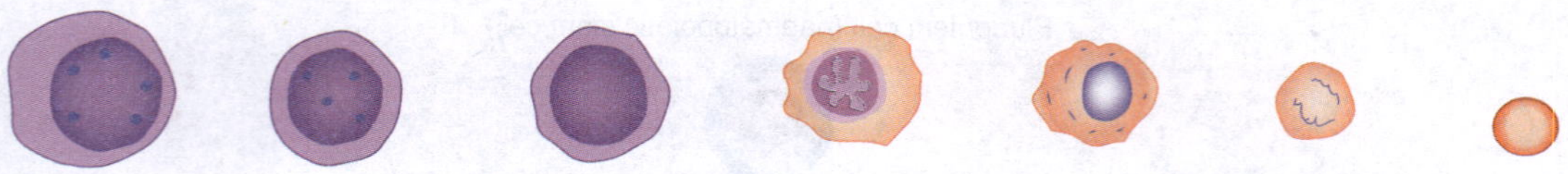

Fig. 3.2.12 Stages of erythropoiesis.

Table 3.2.2 Characteristic features of cells at different stages of erythropoiesis

Stage	Size (μm)	Nucleus	Cytoplasm		Mitosis
			Hb	Staining	
1. Haemocytoblast (stem cell)	19–23	• Very large (almost occupying whole of the cell) • Deep basophilic • Containing four to five nucleoli	Absent	Deep basophilic	Present ++
2. Pronormoblast (proerythroblast)	15–20	• Large (central) • Deep basophilic • Fine reticular chromatin • Two to three nucleoli	Absent	Scanty and deep basophilic	++
3. Early normoblast	12–16	• Large • Chromatin strand becomes thicker and coarser • Nucleoli disappears	Absent	Still basophilic	++
4. Intermediate normoblast (polychromatic normoblast)	10–14	• Nucleus becomes condensed, coarse and basophilic • Nucleoli absent	Appears	Acidophilic with basophilic hue (polychromatic)	+
5. Late normoblast (orthochromatic normoblast)	8–10	• Nucleus small, pyknotic with dark chromatin (cart-wheel appearance) • Nucleoli absent	Increased in amount	Acidophilic	Absent
6. Reticulocyte	7–7.5	• Nucleus absent • With supravital stain (brilliant cresyl blue), remnants of RNA appear in the form of reticulum in the cytoplasm	Increased in amount	Acidophilic	Absent

2. Early (basophilic) normoblast (basophilic early erythroblast) The pronormoblast progresses into the early normoblast, which is a round cell having the following features:

- *Size* is large with a diameter of 12–16 μm.
- *Cytoplasm* is scanty and still basophilic.
- *Nucleus* is large, chromatin strands are thicker and coarse and nucleoli have disappeared.
- *Hb* is not present.
- *Mitosis* is seen. The basophilic normoblasts undergo rapid proliferation.

3. Intermediate (polychromatic) normoblast (polychromatic erythroblast) It is the next maturation stage in the erythroid series. Its features are as follows:

- *Size* is about 10–14 μm.
- *Cytoplasm* becomes polychromatic, i.e. contains admixture of basophilic RNA and acidophilic Hb.
- *Nucleus* becomes condensed, coarse and deeply basophilic with no nucleoli.
- *Hb* appears.
- *Mitosis* is still present.

4. Late (orthochromatic) normoblast (orthochromatic erythroblast) It is the last nucleated cell of the erythroid series. Its features are as follows:

- *Size* is reduced to 8–10 μm.
- *Cytoplasm* is characteristically acidophilic with diffuse basophilic hue.
- *Nucleus* at this stage is small, pyknotic with dark chromatin.
- *Hb* increases in amount.
- *Mitosis* is absent at this stage.

5. Reticulocyte It is the last stage in the formation of erythrocytes, and is also called young red cell. Its features are as follows:

- *Size and shape.* The reticulocyte is flat, disc-shaped, slightly larger (7–7.5 μm) than the mature erythrocytes.
- *Cytoplasm* still contains small amounts of RNA. With supervital stain such as brilliant cresyl blue, the RNA appears in the form of a reticulum (net-like structure) and because of this character the cell is called a reticulocyte. With Romanowsky stain, the cytoplasm gives a faint polychromatic tint.
- *Nucleus* is absent; the reticulocyte results when the nucleus is extruded from the late normoblast within the marrow.

- *Hb* increases in amount equal to that present in a mature erythrocyte.
- *Mitosis* is absent.

Maturation of reticulocyte into erythrocyte The reticulocytes are juvenile red cells devoid of nucleus but contain ribosomal RNA so that they are still able to synthesize Hb. A reticulocyte spends 1–2 days in marrow and circulates for 1–2 days in the peripheral blood before maturing to become a biconcave red cell. The mature red cell has lost its nucleus, as well as the ribosomes and mitochondria. It thus cannot synthesize Hb and any other protein. The immature cells in various stages of development are found outside (around) the blood sinusoids of the bone marrow. The reticulocytes are also found normally in the peripheral blood. Normal range of reticulocytes in healthy adults is 0.5%–2% and in infants is 2%–6%. Abnormal increase in circulating reticulocytes is called *reticulocytosis*. This is seen when the rate of erythropoiesis is very high, as occurs in haemolytic anaemia and following the treatment of deficiency anaemias.

The reticulocytes in the peripheral blood are distinguished from mature red cells by a slightly basophilic hue in the cytoplasm, similar to that of an orthochromatic normoblast. Reticulocytes can be counted in the laboratory by vital staining with dyes, such as new methylene blue or brilliant cresyl blue and Romanowsky stain.

Summary of Changes Occurring in Cells of Erythroid Series During Maturation

It takes 7 days for the formation and maturation of RBCs. Till the reticulocyte stage, it takes 5 days and to become a matured red cell from the reticulocyte, it takes 2 days. Various changes which occur during maturation from the pronormoblast to the erythrocyte stage are summarized as follows:

Size of the cell (from 15 to 20 µm of pronormoblast) goes on decreasing with subsequent stages till it reaches about 7 µm.
Nucleus first condenses, then becomes pyknotic and finally disappears at the stage of reticulocyte formation.
Hb synthesis starts at the stage of intermediate normoblast and then its content increases progressively.
Cytoplasm staining. Initially, before the appearance of Hb, the cytoplasm is basophilic. When Hb starts appearing, cytoplasm becomes polychromatic, i.e. stained by both acidic and basic dyes. In the stage of late normoblast when Hb synthesis is almost completed, cytoplasm is stained by acidic dye.
Mitosis is seen up to the stage of intermediate normoblast. During these stages, three to five cell divisions occur. In this way, each pronormoblast gives rise to 8–320 late normoblasts. From the stage of late normoblast onwards, the mitosis ceases and the cell only matures.

Regulation of Erythropoiesis

Erythropoietin (EPO)

EPO is also known as haematopoietin or haemopoietin, a hormone which regulates the process of erythropoiesis. It is a glycoprotein cytokine having a molecular weight of 34,000.

Site of formation. EPO is mainly (85%) produced by the juxtaglomerular apparatus of the kidney. Extrarenal sources like the liver and spleen persisting residual cells and cells of the tissue macrophage system produce about 15% of *EPO*, especially when hypoxia is marked.

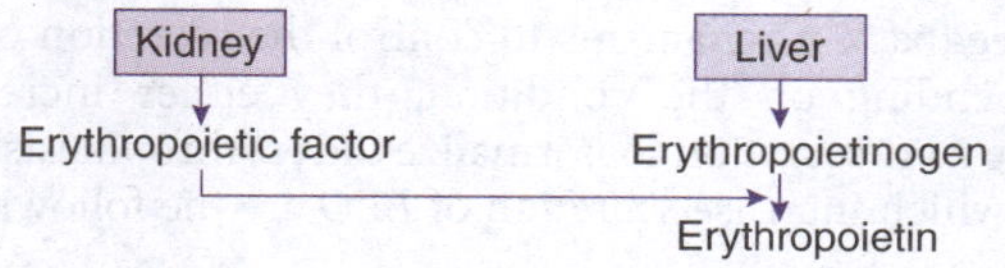

Fig. 3.2.13 Mechanism of erythropoietin secretion.

Stimulus for secretion. A certain basal level of the hormone is necessary for the normal rate of erythropoiesis. The main function of the RBCs is to supply oxygen to the tissues. Therefore, whenever there is hypoxia or a decrease in the number of RBCs (e.g. after haemorrhage or in haemolytic anaemia), there occurs a release of renal erythropoietic factor from juxtaglomerular cells (interstitial fibroblast of the kidney), which acts on the plasma alpha-globulin called erythropoietinogen to form the *EPO* (Fig. 3.2.13). Thus, the levels of *EPO* vary with degree of hypoxia and the number of circulating RBCs. This explains how polycythaemia (increased RBC count) is observed in hypoxic states such as in normal individuals residing at high altitude or in patients suffering from cardiopulmonary disorder. On the other hand, if the number of RBCs in circulation is more, e.g. after transfusion of blood in a normal person, the *EPO* formation is decreased. For details, see page 779.

Applied Aspect

In chronic renal failure, associated anaemia is due to lack of EPO production.

Actions of erythropoietin. EPO increases erythropoiesis by acting at the site of erythropoiesis (it may be yolk sac, liver, spleen and bone marrow depending on the age). *EPO*, along with cooperation of other factors (e.g. IL-3 and insulin-like growth factor), promotes erythropoiesis because of its following actions:

- *EPO* exerts its chief effect on the stem cells causing them to differentiate into colony-forming units (CFU-E).
- It promotes Hb synthesis by increasing globin synthesis and potentiating δ-aminolaevulinic acid synthetase.
- It also promotes every stage of maturation from pronormoblast to the mature red cells.
- *EPO* also promotes release of RBCs from bone marrow into the peripheral circulation.

Other actions of EPO. Besides stimulation of erythropoiesis, EPO has other important actions such as:

- Protective role for kidney, heart and retina.
- Promotes angiogenesis and protects vascular bed.
- Promotes wound healing.
- Stimulates erythropoiesis, angiogenesis and development of brain tissue in the fetus.

Mechanism of action. EPO acts by binding to specific receptors present on the surface of erythroid precursor cells. For further details, see page 779.

Factors increasing erythropoietin secretion. The degree of oxygenation and the number of RBCs in circulation act as feedback mechanisms to control the secretion of *EPO*, i.e. depending on the condition, they either increase or decrease *EPO* secretion to normalize the erythropoiesis. Other factors which increase secretion of *EPO* are the following:

1. Hormones Following hormones increase *EPO* secretion:

- *Androgens* (male sex hormones) enhance *EPO* secretion. This explains the greater RBC counts in males compared with that in females.
- *Thyroxine* also promotes erythropoiesis. This explains the occurrence of polycythaemia in hyperthyroidism.
- *Other hormones* which increase *EPO* secretion are growth hormone, prolactin, ACTH and adrenocortical steroids.

2. Haemolysates These are the products released following RBC destruction, which increase *EPO* secretion.

3. Nucleotides These enhance *EPO* secretion and include cAMP, NAD and NADP.

4. Vasoconstrictor drugs These produce renal hypoxia, which in turn increases *EPO* secretion.

Factors decreasing erythropoietin secretion. These are the following:

Adenosine antagonists Example includes theophylline.

Oestrogen This decreases *EPO* secretion by:

Decreasing synthesis of globin in liver
Depressing the erythropoietic response to hypoxia

Important Notes

For therapeutic purpose (in anaemic state due to renal failure), recombinant erythropoietin (rEPO) is available as epoetin α and β.

- EPO is used mainly to treat anaemia secondary to conditions such as renal failure, cancers, HIV and pre-/postsurgery to reduce the need for blood transfusion.
- EPO is most commonly used by athletes for endurance, as higher RBC count means better oxygen transportation and so higher rate of aerobic respiration. However, this is included as blood doping.

Side effects of erythropoietin include increased blood viscosity, fever, nausea, headache and anxiety.

Factors Necessary for Erythropoiesis

Factors necessary for erythropoiesis can be divided into three groups:

- General factors
- Special maturation factors
- Factors necessary for haemoglobinization

I. General Factors

The main general factors necessary for the process of erythropoiesis are optimum level of the hormone *EPO* and the efficient feedback mechanism controlling the secretion of *EPO*.

All the factors (including hypoxia) affecting EPO and feedback mechanism have been discussed in the section 'Regulation of Erythropoiesis'.

II. Special Maturation Factors

Special factors which are essential for maturation of an RBC include vitamin B_{12}, intrinsic factor of Castle and folic acid.

Vitamin B_{12} Vitamin B_{12} (cyanocobalamin), also known as extrinsic factor, is essential for maturation of red cells.

Daily requirement of vitamin B_{12} in adults is 1–2 μg. Since its deficiency causes pernicious anaemia, it is also called antipernicious factor.

Sources of vitamin B_{12}. There is no plant source for vitamin B_{12}. Dietary sources of vitamin B_{12} are milk, meat and liver of animals. It is present in the normal diet and is also synthesized by the bacterial flora of the colon. The colonic cobalamins are unabsorbable in humans.

Absorption of vitamin B_{12}. It is not possible in the absence of the intrinsic factor. The *intrinsic factor of Castle* is a glycoprotein secreted by the parietal cells of gastric mucosa. It combines with dietary vitamin B_{12} present in the stomach to form the intrinsic factor–cyanocobalamin complex which then becomes bound to specific receptors in the ileum and is absorbed by endocytosis (Fig. 3.2.14).

Transport of vitamin B_{12}. Inside the mucosal cells, the cobalamin is transferred from the intrinsic factor to transcobalamin II, another binding protein which transports vitamin B_{12} in the blood (Fig. 3.2.14).

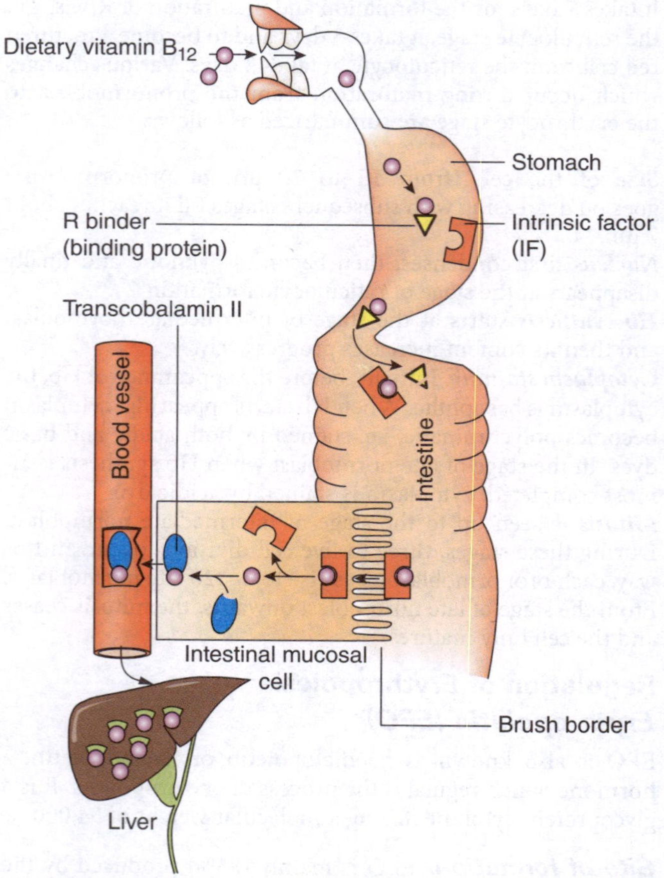

Fig. 3.2.14 Schematic diagram showing absorption and transport of vitamin B_{12}.

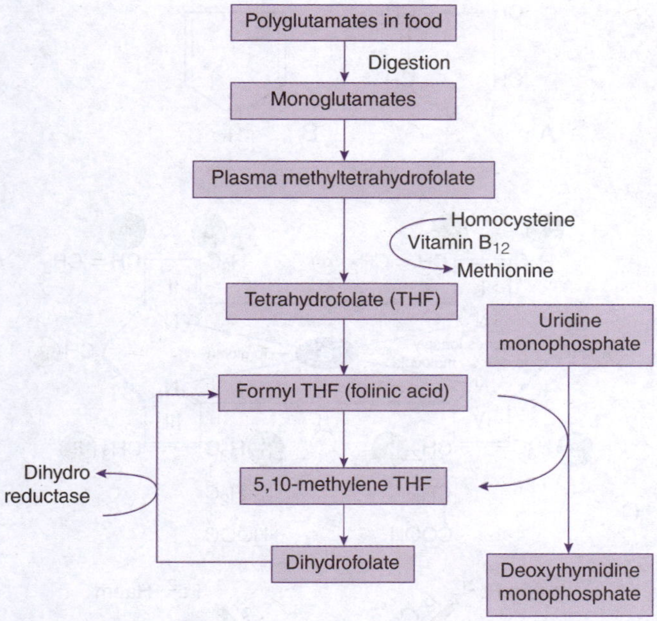

Fig. 3.2.15 Metabolic pathway showing interaction of vitamin B_{12} and folate in the synthesis of DNA.

Storage of vitamin B_{12}. It is stored in large amounts in liver (there may be up to 3 years' supply) and also to some extent in the muscles. Whenever required, it is transported from the liver into the bone marrow.

Role of vitamin B_{12}. It is required for the synthesis of DNA and maturation of nucleus and cell. Its interaction with folic acid is shown in Fig. 3.2.15. Deficiency of vitamin B_{12} leads to:

- Failure of maturation of nucleus.
- Cells remain large (megaloblasts) and become more fragile. Normally, during maturation, cell size decreases progressively.
- There occurs a reduction in the cell division.

Folic acid Folic acid (pteroylglutamic acid) and related compounds are known as folates – play an important role in the synthesis of DNA.

Daily requirement of folates for a normal healthy adult is 100 μg.

Sources of folates are leafy vegetables, yeasts, pulses and liver. The body obtains folates by the breakdown of food polyglutamates to monoglutamates in the small intestine or mucosal cells. Folic acid, as such, is available only as a medicinal compound.

Role of folic acid in DNA synthesis. In the plasma, folate appears as methyltetrahydrofolate, which is changed to tetrahydrofolate (THF) by a pathway for which vitamin B_{12} is essential (Fig. 3.2.15). Without this, active folate coenzymes are poorly formed. For synthesis of DNA, 5,10-methylene THF is the essential form. Dihydrofolate from this step is reconverted to the THF by dihydrofolate reductase, an enzyme inhibited by the folate antagonist (methotrexate).

> **Important Note**
>
> Formyl THF (folinic acid) will bypass both the metabolic blocks created by vitamin B_{12} deficiency and methotrexate and acts as an antidote to this drug.
>
> ***Folate deficiency*** causes megaloblastic anaemia (see page 155).

Role of calcium in erythropoiesis

- Intracellular Ca^{2+} concentration plays an important role in differentiation of erythroid progenitor cells.
- Erythropoietin induces increase in concentration of Ca^{2+} in erythroid progenitor cells and mediate signals for differentiation and proliferation.

Role of reduced glutathione

- Reduced glutathione increases absorption of nonhaem and haem iron.
- Glutathione peroxidase 4 (GPX4) also causes erythroid enucleation.

III. Factors Necessary for Haemoglobinization

Various factors necessary for Hb formation in the RBCs are described on page 143.

HAEMOGLOBIN

The cytoplasm of erythrocytes (RBCs) contains an *oxygen-binding protein* called Hb. Erythrocyte precursors synthesize Hb, while the mature erythrocytes lose the property of synthesizing Hb. The inclusion of Hb within the erythrocytes is most effective for functional purposes, since it avoids the following *disadvantages* which would have occurred if the Hb was present in the plasma as free Hb:

- Increase in blood viscosity causing a rise in blood pressure
- Increase in the osmotic pressure
- Rapid destruction of Hb by the reticuloendothelial system
- Excretion of Hb by kidney (Hb urea)

In pathological states, e.g. acute haemolytic disorder, Hb appears in the plasma and may lead to above-mentioned consequences.

NORMAL BLOOD HAEMOGLOBIN

The normal blood Hb concentration at different ages is given as follows (Fig. 3.2.16):

In fetus just before birth, the Hb concentration of blood from the umbilical cord ranges from 16.5 to 18.5 g/dL.

After birth. The Hb concentration increases rapidly and may reach up to 23 g/dL. This occurs due to:

The transfusion of cells from the placenta to infant
Haemoconcentration by reduction of plasma volume

At the end of 3 months. After 2 days of birth, the Hb levels start falling and stabilize at the end of 3 months to 10.5 g/dL.

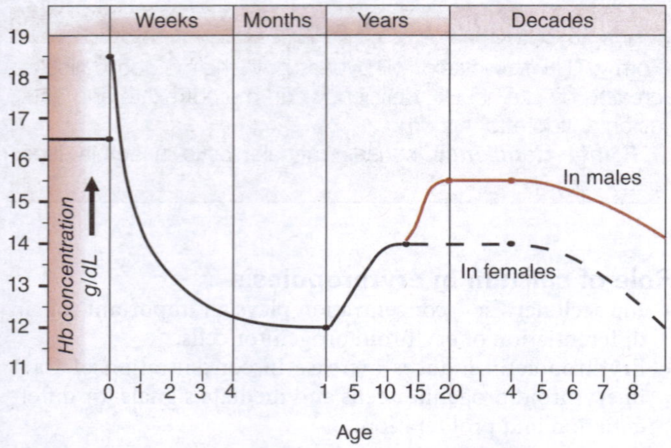

Fig. 3.2.16 Normal blood haemoglobin concentration at different ages.

At 1 year of age. The concentration then rises gradually to reach 12 g/dL.

In adult males The mean blood Hb concentration is 15.5 g/dL (range: 14–18 g/dL).

In adult females The mean Hb concentration is 14 g/dL (range: 12–15.5 g/dL).

Important Notes

- The normal haemoglobin becomes 100% saturated when blood is equilibrated with 100% oxygen (PO_2, 760 mm Hg).
- One gram of haemoglobin when fully saturated combines with 1.34 mL oxygen. Thus, Hb concentration is an index of oxygen-carrying capacity of blood. Thus, normal value of oxygen-carrying capacity in males is 1.34 × 15.5 = about 21 mL/dL, and in females is 1.34 × 14 = about 18.5 mL/dL.
- *Clinically*, irrespective of the age, a level of 14.8 g/dL is considered as 100% haemoglobin.

STRUCTURE OF HAEMOGLOBIN

Hb is a globular molecule having a molecular weight of 68,000. It consists of the protein *globin* combined with iron-containing pigment called *haem*.

Structure of Globin

The protein globin, present in the Hb, is made up of four polypeptide chains. The polypeptide chains are of different types (described in types of haemoglobin, page 139). The globin of the common type of adult haemoglobin, called ***haemoglobin A*** (HbA), consists of the following four polypeptide chains:

- *Two α-chains*, each containing 141 amino acid residues
- *Two β-chains*, each containing 146 amino acid residues

Therefore, the normal adult HbA is written as HbA ($\alpha^2\beta^2$).

Structure of Haem

The haem is an iron–porphyrin complex called *iron–protoporphyrin IX*, i.e. it consists of a porphyrin nucleus and iron. The structural characteristics of the haem (iron–protoporphyrin IX) are given below (Fig. 3.2.17A–C).

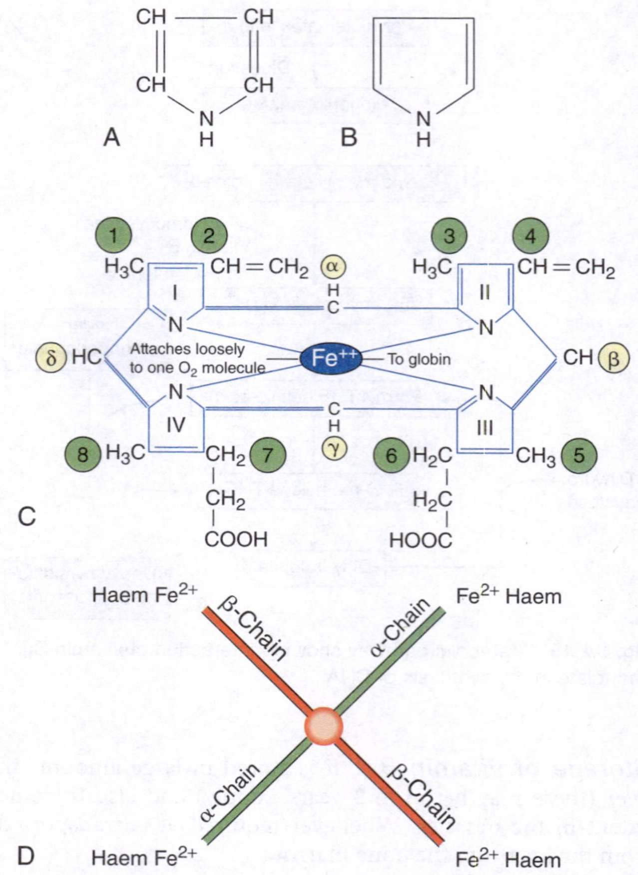

Fig. 3.2.17 Chemistry of haemoglobin: **A**, structure of a pyrrole ring; **B**, conventional outline of a pyrrole ring; **C**, arrangement of pyrrole rings in one unit of haem (iron protoporphyrin X); and **D**, arrangement of four units of haem in one molecule of haemoglobin.

Porphyrin Nucleus

Porphyrin nucleus consists of four *pyrrole rings* numbered I, II, III and IV, i.e. porphyrins are tetrapyrroles.

The *pyrrole rings* are joined together by four *methine bridges* (=CH–). The carbon atoms of methine bridges are labelled α, β, γ and δ.

Eight side chains are attached to the pyrrole ring at positions labelled 1–8. These are as follows:

- Four methyl (H_3C) side chains at positions 1, 3, 5 and 8
- Two vinyl ($CH \bullet CH_2$) side chains at positions 2 and 4
- Two propionic acid (CH_2CH_2COOH) side chains at positions 6 and 7

Iron

- The iron in the haem is in *ferrous* (Fe^{2+}) form.
- The iron is attached to the nitrogen atom of each pyrrole ring.
- On the iron (Fe^{2+}), a bond is available for loose union, where:
  In ***oxyhaemoglobin,*** O_2 is attached.
  In ***carboxyhaemoglobin,*** CO is attached, and so on (Derivatives of Haemoglobin, see page 142).

Attachment of haem to globin. One molecule of Hb contains four units of haem, each attached to one of the four polypeptide chains constituting globin (Fig. 3.2.17D). As there are four units of haem in one molecule of Hb, so there are four iron atoms in one molecule of Hb which can carry four molecules (eight atoms) of oxygen.

FUNCTIONS OF HAEMOGLOBIN

1. Transport of O_2 from Lungs to Tissues

- In the lungs, one molecule of O_2 is attached loosely and reversibly at the sixth covalent bond of each iron atom of the Hb to form *oxyhaemoglobin* represented as HbO_2:

Hb	+	O_2	→	HbO_2
Deoxygenated (reduced) haemoglobin				Oxygenated haemoglobin

- Oxygenation of the first haem molecule in the Hb increases the affinity of the second haem for oxygen, which in turn increases the affinity of the third haem, and so on. In this way, affinity of Hb for the fourth oxygen molecule is many times that for the first molecule. Because of this:
  - Hb reacts with oxygen very rapidly taking less than 0.01 second. Similarly, deoxygenation of Hb is also very rapid.
  - The oxygen–Hb dissociation curve becomes sigmoid shaped (see page 420).
- The affinity of Hb for oxygen is influenced by pH, temperature and concentration of 2,3-biphosphoglycerate or 2,3-BPG (a product of metabolism of glucose) in the RBCs.
- As the concentration of 2,3-BPG rises, the affinity of Hb for oxygen falls and the oxygen–Hb dissociation curve is shifted to the right (see page 422) and as a result more oxygen is released by blood to the tissues.

Important Notes

It is important to note that:
At high altitude *(e.g. 5000 m above the sea level), 2,3-BPG concentration in red cells increases by 50% and thus more oxygen is available to the tissues.*
As 2,3-BPG accumulates*, it depresses hexokinase and 2, 3-BPG mutase activity by negative feedback control. Glucose metabolism in this way is related to oxygen transport via intracorpuscular 2,3-BPG concentration.*
Stored blood loses *its 2,3-BPG concentration and oxygen affinity increases resulting in less release of oxygen. The addition of inosine and adenosine to stored blood increases 2,3-BPG formation and restores the normal affinity of haemoglobin for oxygen.*

2. Transport of CO_2 from the Tissues to the Lungs

Hb also transports CO_2 from the tissues to the lungs.

- It is important to note that CO_2 from the tissues is transported by combining with amino acids of the globin part as shown below and not in combination with Fe^{2+} atom like O_2:

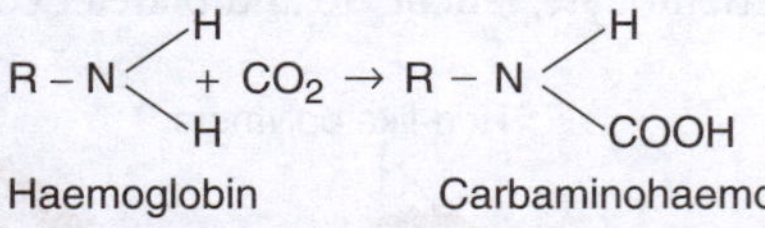

- Deoxygenated Hb forms carbaminohaemoglobin more readily than oxygenated Hb. That is why venous blood becomes more suitable for transport of CO_2 from the tissues to the lungs.

3. Control of pH of the Blood

The Hb constitutes the most important acid–base buffer system of blood. Although the concentration of Hb is roughly twice the concentration of plasma proteins, Hb has six times the buffering capacity compared with plasma proteins.

DEVELOPMENT OF HAEMOGLOBIN

- The human Hb first appears at about 6 weeks after gestation. The red cells contain embryonic Hb Portland ($\zeta_2\gamma_2$), Hb Gower I ($\zeta_2\varepsilon_2$) and Hb Gower II ($\alpha_2\varepsilon 2$) (Fig. 3.2.18).
- At about 10–11 weeks, fetal Hb (haemoglobin F [HbF] [$\alpha_2\gamma_2$]) becomes prominent.
- At about 38 weeks, there is synthesis of adult Hb (HbA [$\alpha_2\beta_2$]); a small amount of HbF is produced during postnatal life because few red cell clones called F cells (small pool of immature committed erythrocyte precursor) retain the ability to produce HbF.

Important Notes

The human haemoglobin is encoded by gene clusters (α and β). The α-like gene clusters are located on chromosome 16 and β-like on chromosome 11. The locus control region (LCR) element is located in the upstream control expression of each cluster. Therefore, normal red blood cell differentiation requires coordinated expression of the globin genes, genes responsible for *haem and Fe metabolism*.

VARIETIES OF HAEMOGLOBIN

Apart from species differences, several varieties of Hb occur in human beings. In all varieties of Hb, the haem moiety remains the same. It is the composition of polypeptide chains of the globin part of the Hb which differs in various varieties of Hb. Various varieties of Hb can be grouped as follows:

- Physiological varieties of Hb
- Haemoglobinopathies

Physiological Varieties of Haemoglobin

Adult haemoglobin. Adult haemoglobin is of two types:

i. ***HbA*** ($\alpha_2\beta_2$). It is the main form of normal adult haemoglobin. As described on page 138, its globin part consists of two alpha- and two beta-polypeptide chains. It is a spheroidal molecule with a molecular weight of 68,000.
ii. ***Haemoglobin A2*** (*HbA*$_2$ [$\alpha_2\delta_2$]). It is a minor component (about 2.5% of the total Hb) in normal adults. Its globin part consists of two alpha- and two delta-polypeptide chains. Delta-chains have slightly different amino acid

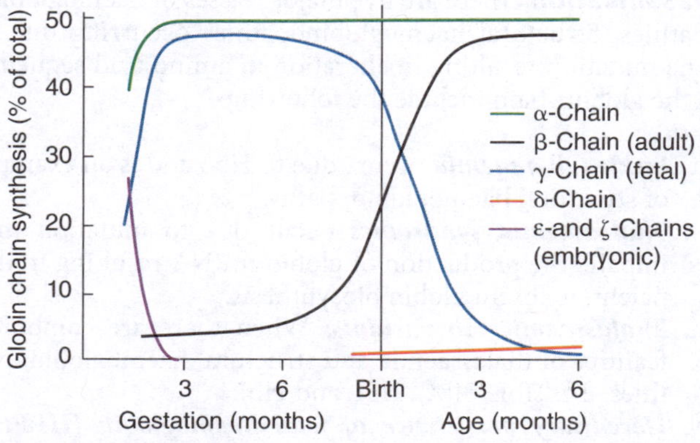

Fig. 3.2.18 Development of human haemoglobin chains.

Table 3.2.3 Amount of HbF and HbA at various stages in human beings

Stage	HbF (%)	HbA (%)
• At 20 weeks of intrauterine	94	6
• At birth	80	20
• At 2 months after birth	50	50
• At 4 months after birth	10	90
• At more than 1 year after birth	<1	>99

composition (out of 146, 10 amino acids are different) compared with β-chains.

Fetal haemoglobin. Fetal Hb, or HbF ($\alpha_2\gamma_2$) as the name indicates, refers to the Hb present in the fetal RBCs and gradually disappears 2–3 months after birth.

Amount of HbF and HbA The amount of these present at various stages is as given in Table 3.2.3.

Structure of HbF It is similar to that of HbA, except that its globin part consists of two alpha- and two gamma-polypeptide chains (in place of beta-chains). Gamma-chains also have 146 amino acids, but its 37 amino acids are different than those of beta-chains.

Special features The special features of RBC with HbF are given as follows:

- *Affinity for oxygen* in case of HbF is more than that of with HbA, i.e. it can take more oxygen than HbA at low oxygen pressure. It is owing to poor binding of 2,3-BPG by the gamma-polypeptide chain. Because of this, movement of oxygen from maternal to fetal circulation is facilitated. At PO_2 20 mm Hg, HbF is 70% saturated while HbA is only 30%–35% saturated. For details, see page 422.
- *Resistance to action of alkalies* is more in HbF than in HbA. This property is used in a photoelectric colorimetric method to estimate HbF in the presence of HbA.
- *Lifespan* of HbF is much less (1–2 weeks) compared with that of HbA (120 days).

Haemoglobinopathies

Haemoglobinopathy, i.e. abnormal formation of Hb, occurs due to disorders of globin synthesis, haem synthesis being normal.

Classification There are five major classes of haemoglobinopathies. Structural haemoglobinopathies occurring due to gene mutation resulting in alteration in amino acid sequence in the globin chain include the following:

i. ***Sickle cell anaemia*** occurs due to HbS and is an example of structural haemoglobinopathy.
ii. ***Thalassaemia syndromes*** occur due to mutation that impairs the production of globin mRNA resulting in deficient or absent globin biosynthesis.
iii. ***Thalassaemic Hb variants:*** When there are combined features of thalassaemia and structural haemoglobinopathies, e.g. HbE, HbC, HbL and HbJ.
iv. ***Hereditary persistence of fetal haemoglobin (HPFH):*** Due to increased levels of fetal Hb in adult life.
v. ***Acquired haemoglobinopathies*** occur due to modification of Hb molecule by toxins, e.g. methaemoglobin, sulphaemoglobin, carboxyhaemoglobin and HbH in leukaemia.

1. Sickle Cell Anaemia or Sickle Cell Haemoglobin (HbS)

1. Sickle cell Hb or HbS. HbS is the most important haemoglobinopathy. It primarily occurs in African-dependent and Hispanics of Caribbean ancestry.

- It occurs in 10%–20% of Africans–Americans. Sickle cell gene originated in the black population in Africa.
- HbS is formed due to substitution of valine for glutamic acid at position 6 in the beta-chain of HbA.
- When HbS is reduced (e.g. in low O_2 tension or when pH at tissue level is low), it becomes much less soluble and precipitates into crystals within the RBCs. The crystals elongate producing changes in shape of the cells from biconcave to sickle-shaped cells (sickling) (Fig. 3.2.19).
- The cells containing HbS are less flexible compared with RBCs containing HbA, hence leading to blockade of microcirculation.
- Sickle-shaped cells greatly increase blood viscosity, thereby decreasing the blood flow to tissues.
- Sickle-shaped cells are more fragile and are very liable to undergo haemolysis producing the so-called sickle cell anaemia.
- Sickle cell disease is caused by a mutation in beta-chain of Hb molecule, resulting in polymerization of Hb when deoxygenated.
- Sickle trait is inherited as Mendelian dominant, but the full-blown disease is autosomally recessive. A heterozygous individual with sickle cell trait rarely has severe symptoms, but a homozygous individual develops full-blown disease.
- The individual with the sickle cell trait has resistance to malaria caused by falciparum.

Pathophysiology of sickle cell crisis *has been depicted in* Fig. 3.2.20. Signs and symptoms of sickle cell anaemia These vary from person to person and include:

- *Anaemia* – leading to the fatigue.
- *Pain* – periodic episodes of pain in SCD are the major symptom. Pain develops due to blockage of tiny blood vessels by sickled RBCs, causing painful swelling of hands and feet.
- *Infection* – sickle cells can damage the spleen; therefore, infection rate increases.
- *Delayed growth and development* due to lack of oxygen availability.
- *Visual problems* due to involvement of retinal tiny blood vessels.
- *Heart problem.*

Diagnosis of sickle cell anaemia

- Peripheral blood smear shows sickle-shaped cells
- Increase in reticulocyte, leucocyte and platelet count

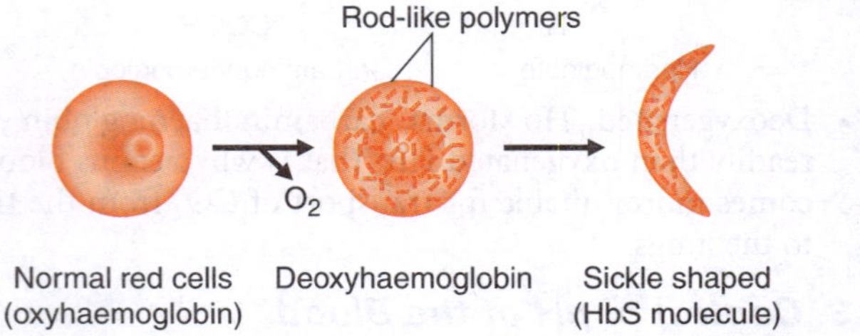

Fig. 3.2.19 Mechanism of sickling of red blood cell containing haemoglobin S (HbS).

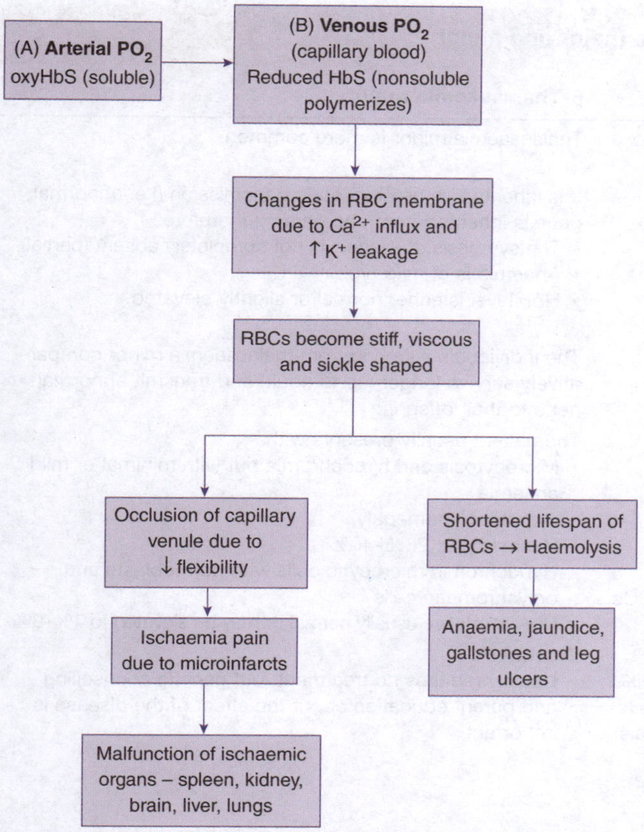

Fig. 3.2.20 Pathophysiology of sickle cell crisis.

- Red cell indices show normocytic normochromic anaemia
- Hb electrophoresis; high performance liquid chromatography identifies HbS

Treatment of sickle cell anaemia The treatment includes medication, blood transfusion and bone marrow transplantation rarely.

- Presence of HbF in RBCs decreases the polymerization of deoxygenated HbS. There are two drugs: *5-azacytidine* and *hydroxyurea*, which lead to formation of HbF in children and adults. These drugs have been tried in patients with sickle cell anaemia and have shown good preliminary results.
- Bone marrow transplantation has cured the disease in some cases.

2. Thalassaemia

Thalassaemia or Mediterranean anaemia is a haemoglobinopathy characterized by the following features:

Causes Thalassaemia results due to defect in the synthesis of polypeptide chain α and β of HbA.

Types Depending on whether α- or β-chains are not synthesized, α-thalassaemia or β-thalassaemia may occur, respectively.

α-Thalassaemia syndrome may present in the following forms depending on deletion of α-globin loci:

- *α-Thalassaemia trait.* When two of the alpha-chains are deleted, it may be a symptomatic or silent carrier state or may resemble β-thalassaemia minor.
- *α-Thalassaemia trait (carrier).* When one of the alpha-chains is deleted.
- *Hb Barts hydrops fetalis – homozygous state of α-thalassaemia.* In this condition, there is excess of γ-globin form, i.e. Hb Barts (γ_4), which has very high oxygen affinity. Hence, there is no delivery of the oxygen to fetal tissues leading to asphyxia, oedema (hydrops fetalis), congestive heart failure and death in utero.

Diagnosis:

- Hb is usually <6 g/dL (severe anaemia).
- Peripheral blood smear shows anisopoikilocytosis, hypochromic microcytic cells, polychromasia basophilic stippling, target cell and normoblasts.
- Serum bilirubin levels are increased.

β-Thalassaemia is more common and is further of two types: thalassaemia major and thalassaemia minor.

Clinical features of thalassaemia:

- Retarded growth, pathological fractures are common.
- Overgrowth of maxillary bone and frontal bossing (chipmunk facies), crow-cut appearance due to wide skull pole (Fig. 3.2.21).
- These patients also suffer from liver cirrhosis, infections and thrombosis.

Differentiating features of thalassaemia major and minor are depicted in Table 3.2.4.

3. Thalassaemic Hb Variants

Hb variants include:

i. Haemoglobin E (HbE), i.e. $\alpha_2\beta_2{}^{26\ \mathrm{glu\ lys}}$ is the most common variant of Hb detected in the United States. In HbE, abnormality lies in the β-chain in which at 26th position glutamate is substituted with lysin. HbE homozygous are asymptomatic.

Blood picture shows microcytosis, hypochromia and Hb levels are rarely less than 10 g/dL.

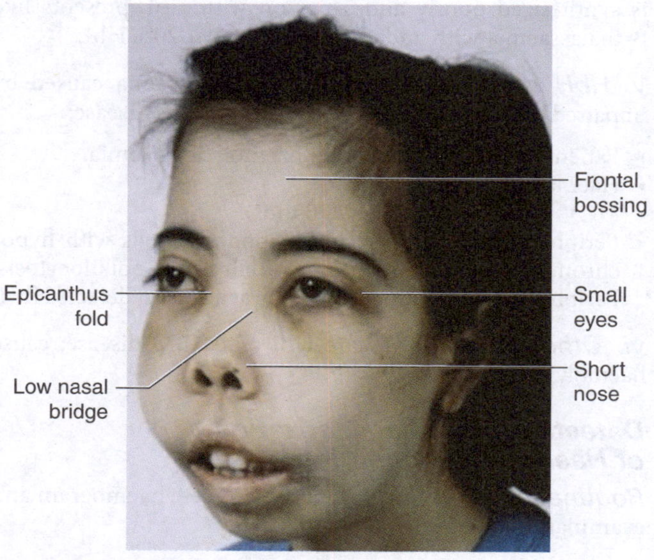

Fig. 3.2.21 Photograph showing facial features face (chipmunk face) in thalassaemia.

Table 3.2.4 Main differentiating features of β-thalassaemia major and minor

S. no.	β-Thalassaemia major	β-Thalassaemia minor
1.	β-Thalassaemia major is also called *Mediterranean anaemia or Cooley anaemia*, and is less common	Thalassaemia minor is more common
2.	It is inherited as homozygous transmission (i.e. abnormal genes are inherited from both the parents); therefore: • There is complete absence of β-chain synthesis • Absence of β-chain synthesis results in moderate to severe anaemia • HbF level is markedly increased	It is inherited as heterozygous transmission (i.e. abnormal gene is inherited from one parent); therefore: • The synthesis of β-chain is not completely absent (partial) • Anaemia is of mild type • HbF level is either normal or slightly elevated
3.	The individual suffering from thalassaemia major has short lifespan, i.e. dies young (17–18 years)	The individuals suffering from thalassaemia minor comparatively survive longer (up to adult) and transmit abnormal gene to their offspring
4.	The patient presents with: • Severe anaemia • Very low haematocrit • Ineffective erythropoiesis Peripheral blood smear shows: • Microcytic hypochromia, anisopoikilocytosis, target cells, Howell–Jolly bodies, basophilic stippling and nucleated RBCs • Elevated levels of HbF and HbA_2	The patient usually presents with: • Microcytosis and hypochromia but with minimal or mild anaemia • Hepatosplenomegaly • Haematocrit: 28%–40% • Hypochromic microcytic cells with normoblasts and polychromatic cells • HbA_2 levels are usually normal or may be elevated to 4%–8%
5.	**Treatment:** • Blood transfusion maintains haematocrit at least 27%–30% • Allogenic bone marrow transplantation • Fe-chelating agents (deferoxamine to avoid haemosiderosis) • Folic acid supplements • Splenectomy increases the volume of RBCs per kilogram body weight to more than 50% • Employ treatment of Fe-deficiency anaemia	**Treatment:** • Usually requires no treatment, but genetic counselling and parent education about the effect of the disease is important

ii. Haemoglobin C (HbC). HbC, like HbS, is formed by substitution of lysine for glutamic acid at β-6 position. In HbC type of variant, there is no sickling of RBCs, but HbC may precipitate in polymer formation in association with HbS. Homozygous HbC disease presents with mild haemolytic anaemia, splenomegaly, mild jaundice and pigment gallstones (Ca-bilirubinate stones).

iii. Haemoglobin D (HbD). In HbD variant, glutamic acid is substituted by glutamine at position 121 of β-chain.

iv. Haemoglobin lepore (HbL, i.e. $\alpha_2(\delta\beta_2)$). In HbL, globin is synthesized poorly and a person with HbL presents like β-thalassaemia with added presence of 2%–20% HbL.

v. HbH disease: It is form of α-thalassemia caused by impaired production of *α-globin chain*. In this disease:

- Patients present with marked haemolytic anaemia.
- Haematocrit is 22%–32%.
- MCV is markedly low (60–70 μm^3).
- Peripheral blood smear shows abnormal cells with hypochromia, microcytosis, target cells and poikilocytosis. Peripheral smear stained with supravital stain detects HbH.

vi. Other Hb variants are HbJ and HbM disease; cause haemolytic anaemia.

Detection and Characterization of Haemoglobinopathies

Routine investigations include complete haemogram and examination of peripheral blood smear.

Screening and quantification can be done by Hb electrophoresis and also by using specialized technique like isoelectric focusing and high-pressure liquid chromatography (HPLC).

Function assays for HbS include sickling test, solubility test, precipitation test and oxygen affinity (P_{50}) to detect low/high affinity of oxygen.

Spectrophotometry to detect percentage of abnormal Hb, e.g. methaemoglobin and carboxyhaemoglobin.

For complete characterization of haemoglobinopathy, the following tests should be done:

- Amino acid sequencing
- Polymerase chain reaction (PCR)
- Allele-specific oligomer hybridization, automated DNA hybridization
- Automated DNA sequencing

Derivatives of Haemoglobin (Reactions of Haemoglobin)

Hb has the property to readily react with any gas or other substance to form the so-called derivatives of Hb. These include:

1. Oxyhaemoglobin. As described on page 139, Hb reacts readily with oxygen to form oxyhaemoglobin which is an unstable and reversible compound, i.e. oxygen can be released from this compound. In this compound, iron remains in ferrous state.

2. Reduced Hb or deoxygenated Hb is formed when oxygen is released from the oxyhaemoglobin.

$$HbO_2 \text{ (Oxyhaemoglobin)} \rightarrow Hb \text{ (Reduced haemoglobin)} + O_2$$

3. Carbaminohaemoglobin is a compound of Hb with carbon dioxide:

$$HbNH_2 + CO_2 \rightarrow HbNHCOOH$$

4. Carboxyhaemoglobin or carbon monoxy haemoglobin is a compound of Hb with carbon monoxide (CO):

$$Hb + CO \rightarrow COHb$$

The affinity of Hb for CO is much more (200–250 times) than its affinity for oxygen. Because of this, the CO displaces oxygen from Hb, thereby reducing the oxygen-carrying capacity of blood. For details, see page 423.

5. Methaemoglobin (HbM). When reduced or oxygenated Hb is treated with an oxidizing agent, e.g. potassium ferricyanide, the ferrous (Fe^{2+}) is oxidized to ferric (Fe^{3+}); the sixth bond is attached to OH to form the compound methaemoglobin. Methaemoglobin is represented as HbOH.

Disadvantages of methaemoglobin are as follows:

- It cannot unite reversibly with gaseous oxygen; the O_2 of the attached OH is not given off in a vacuum.
- When present in large amount, it produces blue colour of skin (cyanosis) because of its dark colour.

Normally, some oxidation of Hb to methaemoglobin (HbOH) does occur, but the methaemoglobin formed is soon converted back to Hb by the enzyme NADH methaemoglobin reductase present in the RBCs. Hereditary methaemoglobinaemia *may result due to congenital absence of this enzyme.*

6. Sulphaemoglobin is formed by a combination of Hb with hydrogen sulphide (H_2S).

7. Nitrous oxide Hb is formed when Hb combines with nitrous oxide.

8. Glycosylated Hb is a derivative of HbA present in very small amounts, e.g. *haemoglobin A_{1C}* (HbA_{1C}), in which glucose is attached to terminal valine in the β-chains. The level of glycosylated Hb in the blood increases in poorly controlled patients of diabetes mellitus.

Important Note

Normally, the fraction of Hb glycosylated is approximately 5% and is proportionate with blood glucose level. Since half-life of an erythrocyte is 60 days (lifespan 120 days), level of HbA_{1C} reflects the mean blood glucose concentration over preceding 6–8 weeks. Therefore, estimation of HbA_{1C} provides valuable information about management of diabetes mellitus.

- Normal HbA_{1C}: ranges from 4% to 5.6%
- In prediabetics: 5.7% to 6.4%
- In diabetics: >6.5%
- Normal HbA_{1C}: 5.7%

Derived Products of Haemoglobin

Derived products of Hb are of two types: iron containing and iron free.

1. Iron-containing derived products of Hb are:

- *Acid haematin* or *alkali haematin* is formed by the action of acid or alkali with Hb.
- *Haemochromogen* is obtained by reduction of alkali haematin.
- *Cathaemoglobin* is a compound of Hb containing ferric ion with denatured globin.
- *Haem.*

2. Iron-free derived products of Hb are:

- Haematoporphyrin
- Haem pyrrole
- Haematoidin
- Bilirubin

SYNTHESIS OF HAEMOGLOBIN

Hb is synthesized in the cytoplasm of intermediate normoblasts. Minute amount of haemoglobin is synthesized in reticulocytes as they contain ribosomes. The steps of haemoglobin synthesis include the following.

Synthesis of Haem

Haem is synthesized in the mitochondria. Steps of synthesis are as follows (Fig. 3.2.22):

- Succinyl-CoA (derived from the citric acid cycle in mitochondria) and glycine are the starting substances in the synthesis of haem. These condense to form α-amino-β-ketoadipic acid. The condensation requires pyridoxal phosphate for activation of glycine.
- The α-amino-β-ketoadipic acid gets rapidly decarboxylated to δ-aminolaevulinic acid (ALA) in the presence of enzyme ALA synthetase in the mitochondria.
- The protoporphyrin IX is then formed after a series of reactions promoted by other enzymes.
- Finally, ferrous ion is introduced into the protoporphyrin IX molecule to form haem in a reaction catalysed by the enzyme haem synthetase.

Synthesis of Globin

Globin, the protein part of the Hb, is synthesized in ribosomes.

Factors Controlling Haemoglobin Formation

Whipple's standard anaemic dog studies show that both iron and dietary proteins play a very important role in the synthesis of Hb. In addition, certain other minerals and vitamins also control the Hb formation.

1. Role of proteins. First-class proteins provide amino acids required for synthesis of globin part of the Hb. A low protein

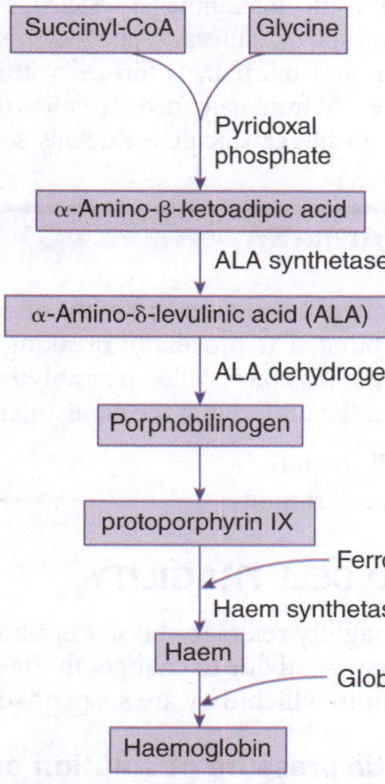

Fig. 3.2.22 Steps of synthesis of haemoglobin.

intake retards Hb regeneration even in the presence of excess iron, the limiting factor being lack of globin. The relative values of various foods in providing the required amino acids are as follows:

- *Most valuable* food is of animal origin and consists of liver, spleen, kidney and heart.
- *Foodstuffs of intermediate value* are again of animal origin and include the muscles.
- *Foodstuffs of least* value include bread and other cereals, dairy products, most vegetables and fruits and salmon.

2. Role of iron. Iron is necessary for formation of haem part of Hb. In addition to dietary iron, the iron released by degradation of RBCs is also reused for synthesis of Hb. Various aspects of iron metabolism are discussed on page 150.

3. Role of other metals

Copper. Copper is essential for Hb synthesis, as it promotes the absorption, mobilization and utilization of iron. Usually, copper deficiency seldom occurs, since requirement of copper is very little and it occurs in adequate amounts in the diet and most iron preparations contain traces of copper.

Cobalt. Cobalt is required for synthesis of vitamin B_{12} by bacterial action in the lumen of gut of sheep and other cattle. However, its role in humans is not evidenced. Furthermore, in some species, cobalt increases the production of *EPO* which in turn stimulates RBC formation.

Calcium. Calcium is reported to help indirectly by conserving iron and its subsequent utilization.

4. Role of vitamins. Vitamin B_{12}, folic acid and vitamin C help in synthesis of nucleic acid which, in turn, is required for the development of RBCs. Vitamin C also helps in absorption of iron from the gut.

5. Role of bile salts. Presence of bile salts in the intestine is necessary for proper absorption of metals like copper and nickel, which in turn are essential factors for synthesis of Hb.

Degradation of Haemoglobin

Tissue macrophages (reticuloendothelial system), especially those lining the hepatic and splenic sinusoids, phagocytize the old RBCs. Hb is broken down and bilirubin is formed within the macrophages. The iron released from degraded Hb enters the plasma and the bilirubin enters the bile canaliculi. For details, see page 146.

RED CELL FRAGILITY

Red cell fragility refers to the susceptibility of red cell membrane to break or burst. The process of breaking of RBCs and release of Hb into the plasma is called haemolysis. Red cell fragility, depending on the underlying mechanism, is of two types:

- Osmotic red cell fragility
- Mechanical red cell fragility

OSMOTIC RED CELL FRAGILITY

Osmotic red cell fragility refers to the susceptibility of the red cell membrane to get lysed due to changes in the osmotic pressure of the solution in which they are suspended.

Effect of osmotic pressure of solution on the RBCs

Isotonic solutions have tonicity as that of plasma. These include 0.9% NaCl, 5% glucose, 10% mannitol and 20% urea. When RBCs are placed in these solutions, they remain suspended in them, i.e. neither swell nor shrink. This is because the osmotic pressure of the isotonic solutions is equal to the osmotic pressure within the RBCs.

Hypertonic solutions (e.g. >0.9% NaCl, 20% mannitol) have osmotic pressure more than the osmotic pressure within the RBCs. Therefore, when the RBCs are placed in such solutions, fluid goes out of the cells and they shrink.

Hypotonic solutions (e.g. <0.9% NaCl) have osmotic pressure less than the osmotic pressure within the RBCs. Therefore, when the RBCs are placed in such solutions, they swell up by absorbing water from outside and finally burst, i.e. get haemolysed.

Osmotic Red Cell Fragility Test To perform the osmotic red cell fragility test, the NaCl solutions of different concentrations (from 0.2% to 0.9%) are taken in series of Cohn's tubes. One or two drops of blood are added in each tube, mixed gently and left undisturbed for 1 hour. Following observations may be made:

No haemolysis. The RBCs settle down as red dots at the bottom of the tube with clear saline solution above.

Onset of haemolysis. A few RBCs rupture and the saline is tinged red with the released Hb. The RBCs which have not ruptured are seen as red dots at the bottom of tube with red-tinged saline solution above.

Completion of haemolysis. All the RBCs rupture and make the whole saline solution uniformly red with no red dots at the bottom of the tube.

Normal values (index of fragility) is as under:

Onset of haemolysis (fragility) in normal RBCs occurs in 0.48% NaCl.

Completion of haemolysis (ending of fragility) occurs in 0.35% NaCl.

Explanation Normally, only the older red cells with comparative fragile membrane are haemolysed in around 0.48% of NaCl solution, since these cells cannot withstand this hypotonicity. But younger cells are not affected. In 0.35% NaCl, even the youngest cells are haemolysed and so haemolysis is completed.

Applied Aspects

Abnormal osmotic fragility

Increase in osmotic fragility index occurs in the following conditions:

Congenital spherocytosis, i.e. when the RBCs are spherical. In this condition, the onset of haemolysis occurs at 0.7% NaCl and it is completed at 0.45% NaCl solution.

Autoimmune haemolytic anaemia in which the autoantibodies damage the structure proteins and render the red cells more fragile.

Deficiency of G6PD increases the tendency of red cells to get haemolysed by antimalarial drugs and other agents.

Venom of cobra and other insects contains lecithinase, which dissolves lecithin from red cell membranes making them more fragile.

Decrease in osmotic fragility index occurs when the RBCs become slender, e.g. in iron-deficiency anaemia. In this condition, the onset of haemolysis occurs at 0.36% NaCl and is completed at 0.24% NaCl solution.

MECHANICAL RED CELL FRAGILITY

The red cells are subjected to mechanical stress and trauma as they pass through the capillaries and trabeculae of the spleen approximately 300,000 times during their lifespan of 120 days. They are made more brittle due to unusual mechanical stress. The red cells can become more rigid as a result of pathological changes in the membrane or in the cell contents caused by a number of red cell disorders. The cells thus become mechanically more fragile, i.e. less liable to tolerate deforming stresses, than the normal healthy red cell.

A normal or less osmotic fragility does not rule out the possibility of high mechanical fragility. For example, in sickle cell anaemia, the RBCs are sickle-shaped and have a high mechanical fragility, but the osmotic fragility of the sickled cells is normal or even low.

Mechanical fragility test. Mechanical fragility test can be performed by placing blood in a flask containing glass beads, and vigorously rotating the flask. The Hb concentration of the supernatant is then measured, which provides an idea about the degree of haemolysis.

LIFESPAN AND FATE OF RED BLOOD CELLS

LIFESPAN OF RED BLOOD CELLS

Normally, the average lifespan of RBCs is 120 days.

Determination of Lifespan of Red Blood Cells

1. Differential agglutination method. In this method, an individual is transfused with RBCs of a different but compatible group. For example, 'O' group blood is transfused to an 'A' group individual. About 1 L of blood should be transfused so that substantial number of donor cells can be obtained to count. Then, a small quantity of blood is withdrawn from the recipient. The red cells are separated and treated with anti-A serum. The 'A' cells agglutinate and 'O' cells remain dispersed, which are counted. The procedure is repeated every day till the group 'O' cells are seen. The experiments show that some of the transfused cells can be seen surviving for about 120 days.

2. Radioactive isotope method. In this method, about 15–20 mL of blood is withdrawn from an individual and then RBCs are tagged with radioactive substances like radioactive iron or radioactive chromium (^{51}Cr). These RBCs are injected back into the same individual. Blood samples are then collected from the individual every day and radioactivity is determined. The isotope survival curve is plotted by plotting the radioactivity of blood as a function of time and the mean lifespan of RBCs is calculated. If the curve for loss of radioactivity is suitably corrected, it is found to be almost linear, falling to zero at about 120 days. The half-life of the cells (50% destruction) being about 60 days, the curve gives the maximum survival time of the youngest cells, the mean survival time and the average destruction of the cells in a heterogeneous sample. The disadvantage is that ^{51}Cr cannot be used due to radioactivity and should be avoided in pregnant women and children.

3. Nonradioactive covalent (biotin) method. In this method, washed RBCs are reacted with *N*-hydroxysuccinimide (NHS)–biotin, or with sulpho-NHS–biotin (covalently labelled membrane proteins with biotin) and retransfused. Then the RBCs of post-transfusional blood samples are reacted with fluorescently conjugated streptavidin, and the biotin-labelled RBCs are quantitated as percentage of the total RBC by flowmetry.

Note: The nonradioactive (biotin-label) method is used in newborns to determine RBC volume and the lifespan.

4. Other methods Metabolic precursors like carbon monoxide method and label glycine method.

Applied Aspects

Causes of Reduction in the Lifespan of Red Blood Cells

I. Defects in red blood cells (corpuscular defects)

1. Hereditary spherocytosis It is an autosomal dominant disorder characterized by small and spherical RBCs. These cells cannot be compressed; therefore, they get easily ruptured while passing through pulp of spleen. They show increased osmotic fragility so that haemolysis may commence at 0.7% NaCl and be completed at 0.4% NaCl solution; lifespan of such RBCs is reduced to 15–20 days. In this condition, the spleen is enlarged and serum bilirubin level may be raised to 20–50 mmol/L.

2. Sickle cell anaemia In this condition, RBCs contain abnormal Hb, called HbS. The cell membrane of sickle-shaped RBCs is more fragile and gets easily haemolysed and their lifespan is reduced. For details, see page 140.

3. Thalassaemias In this condition, the RBCs are abnormal in having reduced amount of HbA, to compensate for which there are increased amounts of HbA_2 ($\alpha_2\delta_2$) and HbF ($\alpha_2\gamma_2$). The red cells are rapidly haemolysed and thus their lifespan is reduced. Children with thalassaemia get hypochromic anaemia, fail to thrive and die young. For details, see page 141.

4. Deficiency of red cell enzymes The RBCs deficient in certain enzymes become more susceptible to haemolysis and their lifespan is decreased. Some of such conditions are as follows:

Glucose-6-phosphate dehydrogenase (G6PD) deficiency It is inherited as sex-linked character. G6PD catalyses the reaction in pentose phosphate pathway and produces nicotinamide adenine dinucleotide phosphate (NADPH). NADPH plays a key role as a reducing agent in RBCs and other cells.

NADPH in RBCs serves as a cofactor for glutathione reductase in generating reduced glutathione, which detoxifies hydrogen peroxide (H_2O_2). In absence of reduced glutathione, Hb is oxidized and gets denatured and forms precipitates called *Heinz* bodies, which causes membrane damage. Therefore, deficiency of G6PD results in oxidative damage to RBCs due to impaired production of NADPH (Fig. 3.2.23).

Pyruvate kinase deficiency may also produce haemolytic anaemia with reduction in lifespan of RBCs.

5. Paroxysmal nocturnal Hb urea It is a rare condition in which red cells are hypersensitive to lysis by complement.

II. Extracorpuscular defects

1. Transfusion of mismatched blood. It produces haemolysis, drastically reducing lifespan of RBCs.

2. Autoimmune haemolytic disorders. In such conditions, antibodies are formed against the patient's own RBCs. These autoantibodies may be of IgG or IgM class and they may be bound to red cell membrane or occur in serum. Some react maximally at 37°C (warm type) and others at 20°C (cold type).

3. Hypersplenism Hypersplenism due to any cause, may enhance destruction of RBCs, leucocytes and platelets.

FATE OF HAEMOGLOBIN

The cell membrane of old RBCs (after about 120 days) becomes more fragile due to decreased NADPH activity. The younger RBCs can easily pass through the capillaries which have a diameter smaller than the red cells. The older cells with fragile membranes are destroyed while trying to squeeze through the capillaries. The destruction of red cells occurs mostly in the capillaries of spleen because they have very thin lumen. Because of this, the spleen is also called the graveyard of RBCs. The Hb released after haemolysis of red cells is taken up by the tissue macrophages.

The tissue macrophage system (reticuloendothelial system) includes the following phagocytic cells:

- *In the bone marrow*, these cells form part of the lining of the blood sinuses (littoral cells).
- *In the liver*, they lie at intervals along the vascular capillaries (Kupffer cells).

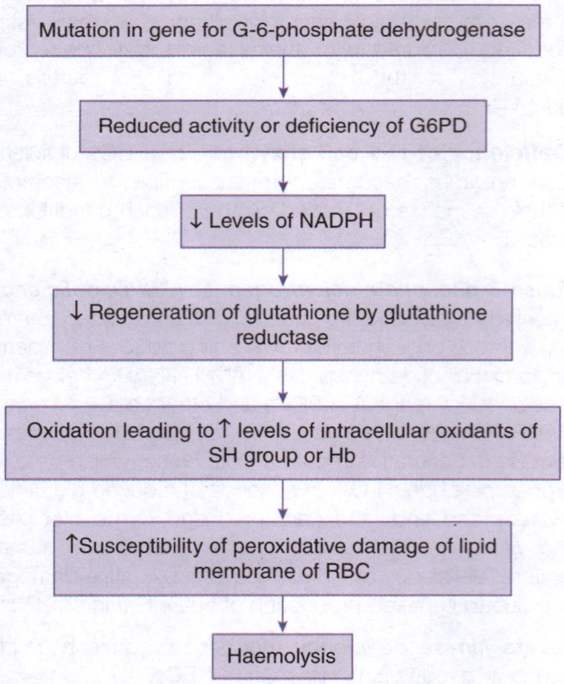

Fig. 3.2.23 Flow diagram depicting effects of deficiency of G-6-phosphate dehydrogenase.

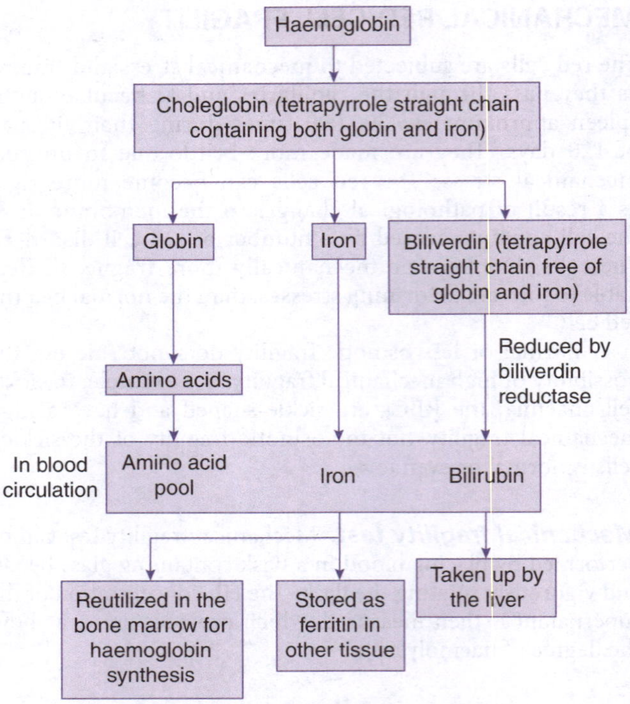

Fig. 3.2.24 Fate of haemoglobin.

- *In the spleen*, they are found in the pulp.
- *In the lymph nodes*, they line the lymphatic paths.

Fate of haemoglobin (Fig. 3.2.24)

- In the macrophages, the haem part of the Hb molecule is altered by oxidation of one of its methine (=CH) bridges. The tetrapyrrole ring structure is thus broken and four pyrrole groups become arranged as a straight chain. As a result of this chemical change, the green iron-containing compound *choleglobin is formed*. As the name implies, the choleglobin molecule still contains the original globin.
- Next, the *choleglobin splits off* into globin, iron and biliverdin (tetrapyrrole straight chain free from globin and iron).
- *Globin* is degraded into amino acids and joins the amino acid pool of plasma and is released.
- *Iron* released into the circulation:
  - Is carried into the bone marrow for reutilization
  - Combines with apoferritin in the other tissues to form the ferritin (storage form of iron)
- *Biliverdin* (tetrapyrrole straight chain free from globin and iron) is converted into bilirubin (by the enzyme biliverdin reductase) and is released into the blood.

BILIRUBIN AND JAUNDICE

BILIRUBIN FORMATION AND ITS FATE

As discussed above, the bilirubin is formed in the macrophages after degradation of Hb. It undergoes the following changes (Fig. 3.2.25).

1. Uptake of bilirubin. Macrophages release the bilirubin into circulation. This bilirubin is called free or *unconjugated*

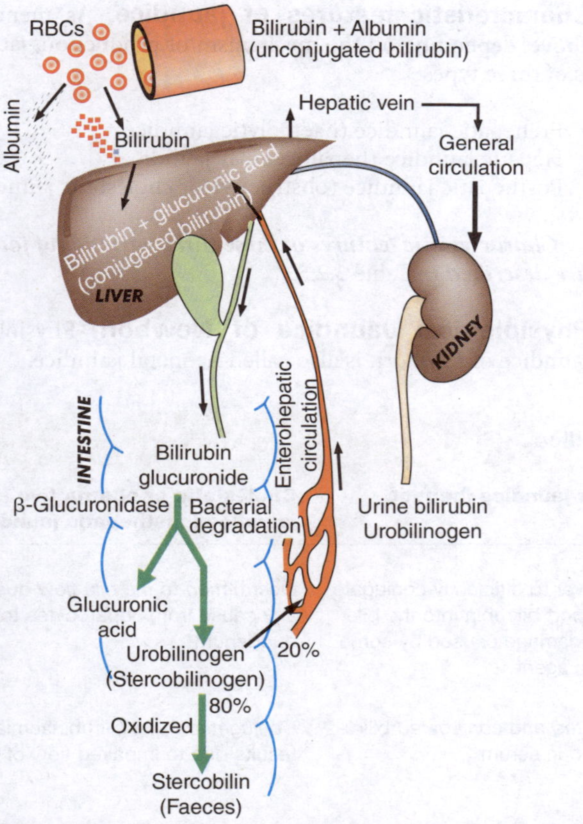

Fig. 3.2.25 Formation of bilirubin in the body (details in the text).

bilirubin. It is lipid soluble and in the plasma it is bound to the albumin (protein-conjugated). It is this protein conjugation of bilirubin which is responsible for solubility of the bilirubin complex in the plasma and which prevents its excretion by the kidneys.

2. Conjugation of bilirubin. The unconjugated bilirubin (bound to albumin) from the circulation is taken up by the liver.

In the liver, the bilirubin is removed from the albumin and taken up at sinusoidal surface of hepatocytes by a member of organic anion-transporting polypeptide (OATP).

- Once bilirubin enters the hepatocytes, it binds to certain cytosolic proteins (ligandin and protein Y). These proteins help to keep the bilirubin in solubilized form before conjugation, and also prevent efflux of bilirubin back into bloodstream.
- In the hepatic cells, it is conjugated with uridine diphosphate glucuronic acid (UDP-glucuronic acid) making it a water-soluble conjugated *bilirubin*. The reaction is catalysed by the enzyme *glucuronyl transferase* present in the hepatic microsomes (smooth endoplasmic reticulum of liver cells). The reaction occurs in two stages:

$$\text{Bilirubin + UDP – glucuronic acid} \xrightarrow{\text{UDP–glucuronyl transferase}} \text{Bilirubin monoglucuronide + UDP}$$

$$\text{Bilirubin monoglucuronide + UDP – glucuronic acid} \xrightarrow{\text{UDP–glucuronyl transferase}} \text{Bilirubin diglucuronide + UDP}$$

3. Excretion of bilirubin. The conjugated bilirubin from the hepatic cells is excreted into the bile canaliculi through active transport, i.e. it is excreted against a concentration gradient into the bile canaliculi. This active transport is the rate-limiting step in the entire process of bilirubin excretion and needs energy. The protein involved is multidrug resistance-like protein 2 (MRP-2), also called multispecific organic anion transporter (MOAT). ATP-dependent transporters located on the plasma membrane of bile canaliculi help in excretion of conjugated bilirubin into the bile canaliculi.

Most of the conjugated bilirubin is excreted into the bile and enters the intestine. Some of it escapes into general circulation and is excreted by the kidneys in urine as *urine bilirubin*.

4. Formation and excretion of urobilinogen. The conjugated bilirubin which enters the intestine with the bile is degraded by the intestinal bacteria in the terminal ileum and the large intestine. The bacterial enzyme β-glucuronidase splits off the glucuronide and converts bilirubin into the *urobilinogen* (stercobilinogen), which is a colourless compound.

- Some urobilinogen (20%) from the intestine is reabsorbed and goes via the portal system to the liver. From the liver, some urobilinogen escapes into general circulation and some gets re-excreted into the bile (enterohepatic circulation).
- From general circulation, the urobilinogen is filtered off by the kidney and is excreted in the urine.

Bilirubin

The normal serum bilirubin level ranges from 0.3 to 1.0 mg/dL. The total serum bilirubin includes conjugated as well as unconjugated bilirubin. The van den Bergh test described in the subsequent text is helpful in determining the type of bilirubin present in the serum.

Van den Bergh test. It is used for quantitative estimation of bilirubin contents in the serum.

Van den Bergh test is performed using the diazo reagent (mixture of sulphanilic acid, hydrochloric acid and sodium nitrite). It is of two types.

Direct van den Bergh reaction. When diazo reagent is added to the serum containing conjugated bilirubin (water soluble), a reddish-brown colouration is obtained within 30 seconds. This is called direct positive van den Bergh reaction.

Indirect van den Bergh reaction. When diazo reagent is added to the serum mainly containing unconjugated bilirubin (water insoluble), no colour is obtained. However, if some solvent like methanol (which dissolves the unconjugated bilirubin) is added, the reddish-brown colouration is obtained. This is called indirect positive van den Bergh reaction.

Jaundice (Hyperbilirubinaemia)

Jaundice (icterus) refers to the yellow appearance of the skin, sclera and mucous membranes resulting from an increased bilirubin concentration (*hyperbilirubinaemia*) in the body fluids. Clinically, jaundice is detectable when the plasma bilirubin exceeds 2–3 mg/dL. Internal tissues and body fluids are coloured yellow, but not the brain, as bilirubin does not cross the blood–brain barrier other than in the immediate neonatal period.

Mechanisms producing jaundice. Hyperbilirubinaemia producing jaundice can result from the following mechanisms:

1. Excessive breakdown (haemolysis) of RBCs. It produces the so-called haemolytic jaundice or prehepatic jaundice or retention hyperbilirubinaemia due to overproduction.

2. Damage to the liver cells (infective or toxic). It produces the so-called hepatic or hepatocellular jaundice.

3. Obstruction to bile ducts. It produces the obstructive or posthepatic or cholestatic jaundice or regurgitation hyperbilirubinaemia (due to reflux into bloodstream).

Characteristic features of jaundice. As mentioned above, depending on the mechanism of production, jaundice is of three types:

- Prehepatic jaundice (haemolytic jaundice)
- Hepatic jaundice (hepatocellular jaundice)
- Posthepatic jaundice (obstructive or cholestatic jaundice)

Characteristic features of these three varieties of jaundice are described in Table 3.2.5.

Physiological Jaundice of Newborn Physiological jaundice of newborn is also called neonatal jaundice.

TABLE 3.2.5 Characteristic features of three types of jaundice

Haemolytic jaundice (prehepatic jaundice)	Hepatocellular jaundice (hepatic jaundice)	Cholestatic or obstructive jaundice (posthepatic jaundice)
1. Mechanism of production		
Excessive breakdown of RBCs producing unconjugated bilirubin in amounts more than the healthy liver can conjugate and excrete	*Inability of the liver* to efficiently conjugate as well as transport bilirubin into the bile due to liver cell damage caused by some infective or toxic agent	*Obstruction to the bile flow* due to any cause from hepatocytes to duodenum
2. Types of serum bilirubin accumulated		
Unconjugated hyperbilirubinaemia occurs since it is being produced in excess of what can be conjugated by the liver	*Both unconjugated* and *conjugated* bilirubin are increased in serum	*Conjugated hyper*bilirubinaemia results due to impaired flow of bile
3. Van den Bergh test		
Indirect positive reaction (because unconjugated bilirubin is present in blood)	*Biphasic reaction* (because conjugated and unconjugated bilirubin are present)	*Direct positive reaction* (because only conjugated bilirubin is present)
4. Urine bilirubin		
Absent Unconjugated bilirubin is insoluble in water; it is transported in plasma in bound form with albumin; since albumin is not filtered into urine, unconjugated bilirubin too is not filtered in urine; because of this, haemolytic jaundice is also called *acholuric jaundice* (no bile pigment in urine)	Present Conjugated bilirubin is water soluble and is present in plasma in dissolved form; it gets easily filtered in urine; this type of jaundice is also called *choluric jaundice*, i.e. bile pigment present in urine	Present Since conjugated bilirubin is filtered in urine
5. Urine urobilinogen		
Increases (because liver is excreting lot of conjugated bilirubin in the intestine with the bile, so more urobilinogen is formed; part of it is reabsorbed and goes to general circulation and thus urine urobilinogen is increased)	Decreases (because damaged liver cells are producing and excreting less of conjugated bilirubin and thus less urobilinogen is formed)	Markedly decreased or absent (because of obstruction, the conjugated bilirubin is not released into the intestine and thus no urobilinogen is formed)
6. Faecal stercobilinogen (normal, 25–250 mg/day)		
• *Markedly increased* (because of more formation as described above) • So faeces are *dark brown* in colour	• *Reduced* (because of less formation as described above) • So stools are *pale* in colour	• *Absent* (when obstruction is complete) • So stools are *clay* coloured
7. Faecal fat level		
Normal, i.e. 5%–6% of total intake per day (as bile is present in gut for normal digestion of fats)	*Increased* up to 40%–50% (because of deficiency of bile in the intestine, emulsification and absorption of fat is inadequate; this produces bulky, pale, greasy and foul-smelling faeces, called steatorrhoea)	*Increased*
8. Specific blood tests		
• *Peripheral blood film* shows signs of haemolysis, i.e. anaemia, reticulocytosis and abnormal RBCs	• Normal	• Normal
• *Plasma albumin, globulin and A/G ratio:* Normal	• Albumin is decreased due to less synthesis by damaged liver, globulin increases and A/G ratio decreases	• Normal
• *Serum alkaline phosphatase:* Normal, i.e. 5–13 KA units/100 mL (because excreted in bile)	• Increased (because less excretion in bile)	• Markedly increased (because not excreted in bile)
• *Liver function tests: Normal* (as liver is healthy)	• *Impaired* (as liver is damaged)	• *Normal or* mildly impaired

Mechanism of production. A hyperbilirubinaemia producing jaundice may be seen normally in the newborn. It appears within 2–5 days of birth and usually disappears in 2 weeks. Its mechanism of production includes the following:

Excessive destruction of RBCs It occurs in first few days after birth causing increase in serum bilirubin.

Hepatic immaturity It also contributes to increased serum bilirubin in the first few (7–10) days after birth. In the fetus, bilirubin is removed from circulation by the placenta. Immediately after birth, the liver has to take up this work which takes 7–10 days to mature and fully conjugate the bilirubin.

Prevention. Neonatal jaundice can be prevented by administration of hepatic microsomal enzyme inducers (e.g. phenobarbital) to the pregnant mother or newborn. The microsomal enzyme inducers increase the activity of glucuronyl transferase in liver.

Treatment. Normal jaundice can be effectively treated by *phototherapy*. Exposure of the skin to white light causes photoisomerization of bilirubin to water-soluble *lumirubin* which can be rapidly excreted in bile without requiring any conjugation. Thus, phototherapy is of value in treating infants with jaundice, irrespective of its cause.

Applied Aspects

Kernicterus. Unconjugated bilirubin because of its hydrophobic property can cross the blood–brain barrier. When concentration of unconjugated bilirubin in plasma exceeds that which can be tightly bound to albumin (20–25 mg/dL), it enters the central nervous system and thus results in kernicterus or encephalopathy. The basal ganglia of CNS are mainly affected. For details, see page 922.

Congenital nonhaemolytic jaundice. (Crigler–Najjar syndrome types I and II):

Crigler–Najjar syndrome type I is a rare autosomal recessive disorder which occurs due to mutation of gene encoding bilirubin UGT activity. The disease is characterized by raised serum bilirubin levels (usually exceed 20 mg/dL). The disease is fatal and phenobarbital has no effect on formation of bilirubin. Liver transplantation is the only treatment.

Crigler–Najjar syndrome type II. In this, some activity of the enzyme is retained; therefore, in these patients, serum bilirubin level does not exceed 20 mg/dL and responds to phototherapy and phenobarbital.

Gilbert syndrome is also caused by mutation in genes encoding bilirubin-UGT, but 30% enzyme activity persists. Therefore, there are no harmful effects.

Dubin–Johnson syndrome is a benign autosomal recessive disorder with conjugated hyperbilirubinaemia either in childhood or in adulthood. It occurs due to mutation in the gene encoding MRP-2 (the protein involved in secretion of bilirubin in the bile).

Rotor syndrome is a rare benign condition which may be occurring due to abnormality in hepatic storage of bilirubin, characterized by chronic conjugate hyperbilirubinaemia.

Toxic hyperbilirubinaemia occurs due to toxin-induced liver dysfunctions, caused by chloroform, acetaminophen, viral hepatitis and mushroom poisoning.

ANAEMIAS

DEFINITION AND CLASSIFICATION

Definition

Anaemia is not a single disease but a group of disorders in which Hb concentration of blood is below the normal range for the age and sex of the subject. Therefore, anaemia is labelled when Hb concentration is less than:

- 13 g/dL in adult males
- 11.5 g/dL in adult females
- 15 g/dL in newborn
- 9.5 g/dL at 3 months of age

Low RBC count (less than 4 million/mm^3) is usually, but not always, associated with low Hb levels in anaemia.

Grading of anaemia, depending on the level of Hb, has somewhat arbitrarily been made as follows:

- Mild anaemia: Hb 8–10 g/dL
- Moderate anaemia: Hb 6–8 g/dL
- Severe anaemia: Hb less than 6 g/dL

Classification

Aetiological (Whitby's) Classification

Types of anaemia depending on the causative mechanism are given as follows.

A. Deficiency anaemias include:

- Iron-deficiency anaemia.
- Megaloblastic anaemia (pernicious anaemia) due to deficiency of vitamin B_{12}.
- Megaloblastic anaemia due to deficiency of folic acid.
- Protein and vitamin C deficiency can also cause anaemia.

B. Blood loss anaemias. Blood loss anaemias or haemorrhagic anaemias are commonly known and can be:

- *Acute posthaemorrhagic anaemia* as in accidents
- *Chronic posthaemorrhagic anaemia*

C. Haemolytic anaemias. These are relatively uncommon and occur in conditions associated with increased destruction of RBCs. These can be:

1. Hereditary haemolytic anaemias For example, as seen in:

- Thalassaemia (see page 141)
- Sickle cell anaemia (see page 140)
- Hereditary spherocytosis (see page 145)
- G6PD deficiency (see page 145)

2. Acquired haemolytic anaemias For example, immunohaemolytic anaemia (due to antibodies against RBCs)

- Microangiopathic haemolytic anaemia (due to mechanical damage to RBCs)
- Haemolytic anaemia due to direct toxic effects (e.g. in malaria, snake venom, toxic effects of drugs and chemicals)
- Haemolytic anaemia in splenomegaly

- Haemolytic anaemia in paroxysmal nocturnal haemoglobinuria (PNH)

D. Aplastic anaemia. It occurs due to failure of bone marrow to produce RBCs. It is of two main types:

- Primary aplastic anaemia
- Secondary aplastic anaemia

E. Anaemia due to chronic diseases. It is seen in tuberculosis, chronic infections, malignancies and chronic lung diseases. The mechanism of causation of anaemia is complex. The tissue macrophages are believed to become activated so that RBCs are removed from the blood faster than they can be formed in bone marrow.

Morphological (Wintrobe) Classification

Based on the mean corpuscular volume (MCV), i.e. cell size, and the MCHC, i.e. Hb saturation of RBCs, the anaemias can be classified as follows.

1. Normocytic normochromic anaemias. These are characterized by normal MCV (78–94 μm^3) and normal MCHC (30%–38%). Such a morphological picture is seen in:

- Acute posthaemorrhagic anaemia
- Haemolytic anaemias
- Aplastic anaemias

2. Microcytic hypochromic anaemias. These are characterized by reduced MCV (<78 μm^3) and reduced MCHC (<30%). Examples of such anaemias are as follows:

- Iron-deficiency anaemia
- Chronic posthaemorrhagic anaemia
- Sideroblastic anaemia
- Thalassaemia

3. Macrocytic normochromic anaemia. It is characterized by increased MCV (>94 μm^3) and normal MCHC (30%–38%). Examples are as follows:

- Megaloblastic anaemia (pernicious anaemia) is due to deficiency of vitamin B_{12}.
- Megaloblastic anaemia is due to deficiency of folic acid.

GENERAL CLINICAL FEATURES OF ANAEMIA

Anaemic hypoxia It results due to decreased O_2-carrying capacity of blood in anaemia owing to reduced Hb concentration. The hypoxia brings about several cardiorespiratory compensatory responses. So, general clinical features (symptoms and signs) in patients with anaemia are due to those caused by:

- Resulting tissue hypoxia
- Resulting compensatory mechanisms

Hb level at which symptoms and signs of anaemia develop depends on three main factors:

- *Speed of onset of anaemia.* Rapidly progressive anaemia causes more symptoms than anaemia of slow onset.
- *Severity of anaemia.* Mild anaemia usually produces no symptoms. Severe anaemia (Hb < 6 g/dL) of rapid onset produces significant clinical features.
- *Age of the patient.* Young patients tolerate anaemia quite well vis-à-vis elderly patients and develop less marked features.

General clinical manifestations of anaemia which occur either due to tissue hypoxia or due to compensatory mechanisms are as follows:

Generalized muscular weakness, tiredness and easy fatigability occur due to muscle hypoxia.

Pallorness of skin and mucous membranes (buccal and pharyngeal mucous membrane, conjunctiva, lips, earlobes, palm and nail bed) occurs due to deficiency of red-coloured Hb in the blood.

Respiratory symptoms such as breathlessness with increased rate and force of respiration occur due to compensatory stimulation of respiratory centre.

Cardiovascular manifestations such as palpitation, tachycardia and cardiac murmurs occur as a result of compensatory mechanisms increasing the cardiac output. In very severe cases of anaemia, features of cardiac failure and angina pectoris may also occur.

Central nervous system (CNS) manifestations due to cerebral hypoxia include lethargy, headache, faintness especially on exertion, tinnitus, restlessness, confusion and drowsiness.

Ocular manifestations include visual disturbances and retinal haemorrhages and cotton wool spots.

Gastrointestinal system symptoms include anorexia, flatulence, nausea and constipation. In pernicious anaemia, atrophy of papillae on the tongue occurs.

Reproductive system involvement occurs in females in the form of menstrual disturbances such as amenorrhoea and menorrhagia and loss of libido.

Renal system involvement may occur in severe anaemia causing disturbances of renal function and albumin urea.

Basal metabolic rate (BMR) is increased in severe anaemia.

DESCRIPTION OF DIFFERENT TYPES OF ANAEMIAS

Deficiency Anaemias

Deficiency anaemias are quite common and occur due to deficiency of factors necessary for erythropoiesis. These include the following:

- Iron-deficiency anaemia
- Megaloblastic anaemia due to vitamin B_{12} deficiency (pernicious anaemia)
- Megaloblastic anaemia due to folic acid deficiency
- Anaemia due to protein deficiency
- Anaemia due to vitamin C deficiency

A. Iron-deficiency Anaemia

Iron-deficiency anaemia is the commonest nutritional deficiency disorder present throughout the world, but its prevalence is higher in the developing countries. In India, iron deficiency is the commonest cause of anaemia. Iron-deficiency anaemia is much more common:

- In women between 20 and 45 years than in men
- At periods of active growth in infancy, childhood and adolescence

Before discussing the different aspects of iron-deficiency anaemia, it will be worthwhile to discuss about normal iron metabolism.

Iron metabolism Iron is one of the most important metals present in the human body. The body of a healthy adult contains 4–5 g (72–90 mmol) of iron in the following forms:

- *Hb* contains about 70% of the total body iron (2.5 g or 45 mmol).
- *Storage iron* amounts to about 20%–23% of total body iron (1.5 g, i.e. 18–27 mmol). Two-third of the iron is stored as ferritin and one-third as haemosiderin.
- *Myoglobin* (myohaemoglobin) present in the red muscles contains about 5% of the total body iron (0.2 g or 3.6 mmol).
- *Intracellular enzymes* account for less than 0.1 g (1.8 mmol), i.e. about 2%–3% of total body iron. The iron-containing enzymes include cytochrome oxidase, catalase and peroxidase cytochrome.

Daily requirement and dietary sources of iron

Daily requirement. Only 10% of the dietary intake of iron is absorbed. Therefore, daily requirement in adult males is 5–10 mg/day and in females is 20 mg/day (to compensate the menstrual loss). Pregnant and lactating women require about 40 mg of iron per day.

Dietary sources. Foodstuffs vary in both their iron content and availability of iron for absorption into the body. The dietary sources of iron are meat, liver, egg, leafy vegetables, whole wheat and jaggery. The iron in foods of animal origin is better absorbed than iron in foods of vegetable origin.

Absorption of iron. Absorption occurs mainly in the duodenum and upper jejunum.

- Normally, about 10% of the 15–20 mg iron ingested each day is actually absorbed in healthy adult male. This absorption is more in menstruating women.

Mechanism of iron absorption. Mechanism of iron absorption for the purpose of understanding can be described under three headings:

Transport of iron across the brush border of enterocyte
Fate of iron in the enterocyte
Transport of iron in the plasma

A. Transport of iron across brush border of enterocyte. In the diet, iron may be present as haem (derived from meat) or nonhaem iron.

1. ***Absorption of haem iron.*** Haem iron is the iron present in myoglobin, Hb and related compounds. From these compounds, the haem is released by proteolytic enzymes in the gut. From the lumen, the haem is transported inside the enterocyte across the brush border membrane by an unidentified *haem transport* protein. Inside the cell, the ferrous iron (Fe^{2+}) is released from the haem by the enzyme haemoxygenase. The fate of Fe^{2+} so released is as that of nonhaem Fe^{2+} as given in Fig. 3.2.26. Haem iron absorption is not affected by other dietary constituents.
2. ***Absorption of nonhaem iron.*** Most of the dietary nonhaem iron is present in ferric form (Fe^{3+}), whereas iron can be absorbed more efficiently in ferrous form (Fe^{2+}).
   - Iron has got tendency to form insoluble complexes with dietary phytates, phosphates and dietary fibres. These complexes are more soluble at low pH. Gastric HCl tends to break insoluble iron complex apart and thus facilitates iron absorption. This explains the occurrence of iron-deficiency anaemia in patients with deficient gastric acid secretion (achlorhydria).
   - Ascorbic acid and other reducing agents promote iron absorption by reducing ferric iron to ferrous form and also by preventing iron from forming insoluble iron complexes within the chyme.
   - Ferrous iron (Fe^{2+}) is transported across the brush border by the *iron transport protein*, i.e. proton-coupled divalent metal transporter (DMT-1) present on the cell membrane (Fig. 3.2.26). This protein is not specific for iron, as it can transport a large variety of divalent cations. Once inside the enterocyte, the fate of nonhaem ferrous iron is the same as that of haem iron.

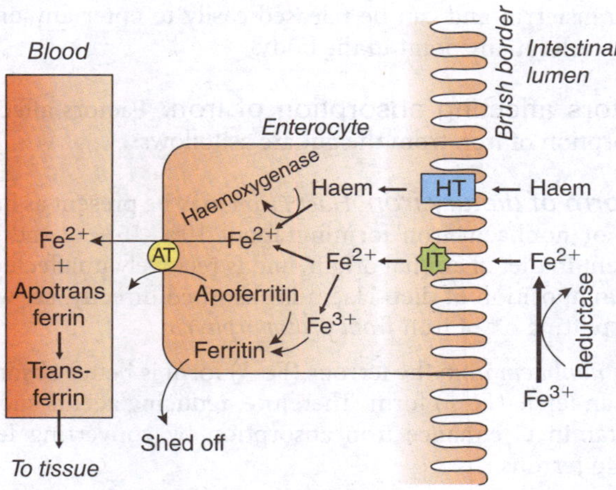

Fig. 3.2.26 Absorption of iron. Haem is carried across brush border of enterocyte by a haem transport protein (HT), and Fe^{2+} of nonhaem iron by iron transport protein (IT). Inside the enterocyte, some iron binds to ferritin and some crosses the basolateral membrane by active transport (AT) process. In the blood, iron binds to the transport protein transferrin (TF).

B. Fate of iron in the enterocyte. As shown in Fig. 3.2.26, in the cytosol of enterocyte, the free ferrous iron (Fe^{2+}) has two fates:

- A part of Fe^{2+}, depending on the body's requirement, is actively transported across the basolateral membranes of the enterocytes into the interstitium, from where it enters the blood. Across the basolateral membrane of enterocytes, the transport is carried out by two components: a copper-containing iron oxidase known as hephaestin and another protein called iron-regulatory protein-I (IRP-I).
- Rest of the ferrous iron is oxidized to ferric form and bound to apoferritin forming ferritin. It is difficult to release iron from this storage form, and in general the ferritin stays in the enterocyte until the cell is sloughed off at the tip of villus.

C. Transport of iron in the blood. Normally, the iron absorbed into the blood binds with a beta-globulin (apotransferrin) to form the transferrin and is transported in this form in the plasma. Iron combines loosely in the globulin apotransferrin and can be released easily to enter any of the tissue cells at any point in the body.

Factors affecting absorption of iron. Factors affecting absorption of iron from the gut are as follows:

1. Form of dietary iron *Haem iron* may be present as haem iron or nonhaem iron forming about 10%–15% of the iron present in diet of animal origin, and is relatively unaffected by the composition of diet. Haem is absorbed directly, i.e. without splitting off of iron *from protoporphyrin*.

- In *nonhaem iron*, the ferrous (Fe^{2+}) form is better absorbed than ferric (Fe^{3+}) form. Therefore, reducing agents such as vitamin C enhance iron absorption by converting ferric into ferrous.

2. Meat and fish in the diet considerably enhance absorption of nonhaem iron. The exact mechanism is, however, unknown.

3. Human breast milk improves the iron absorption.

4. The acid gastric juice (HCl from stomach) favours absorption of nonhaem iron by causing its solubilization and reduction. Therefore, absorption of ferric iron is impaired in subjects with gastrectomy or achlorhydria.

5. Dietary factors inhibiting nonhaem iron absorption are as follows:

- *Phytates* in foods (cereals) reduce iron absorption by forming insoluble iron salts.
- *Phosphates*, calcium, egg white and bovine milk proteins inhibit iron absorption.
- *Phenols* present in legumes, tea, coffee and wine cause poor absorption of iron.

6. Iron stores in the body affect iron absorption as:

- *Decrease* in iron store of the body (e.g. in iron-deficiency anaemia or when erythropoiesis is increased due to hypoxia) enhances iron absorption.
- *An increase in iron storage* in the body reduces iron absorption by the gut mucosa.

Storage of Iron in the Body

In the body, iron is stored in two forms, the ferritin and the haemosiderin.

Storage of iron as ferritin. The iron released into the tissues by apotransferrin combines with the protein apoferritin to form the *ferritin*. Thus, iron is stored as ferritin in the cells of the body. Maximum amount of iron is stored in the hepatocytes of liver and cells of reticuloendothelial system. In other cells of the body, only a small amount of iron is stored.

Storage of iron as haemosiderin. When the intake of iron in the diet is in extremely large quantities, some amount of iron is also stored as a compound *haemosiderin* in reticuloendothelial cells. The haemosiderin is highly insoluble and thus represents a more stable form of storage iron than the ferritin. Therefore, iron exchanges mostly with the ferritin, since exchange with haemosiderin is very slow.

Regulation of body iron

Regulation of body iron, i.e. iron balance in the body, is unique in that it is achieved by control of absorption rather than by control of excretion. Regulation of mucosal absorption has been explained by mucosal block theory.

Mucosal block theory of absorption. This theory states that:

- Iron absorption is increased when body iron stores are depleted or when erythropoiesis is increased, and decreased under the reverse conditions.
- As compared to normal conditions (Fig. 3.2.27A), in iron-deficiency states, a larger percentage of dietary iron enters the circulation and a smaller amount forms ferritin in the epithelial cells (Fig. 3.2.27B).
- In the presence of iron overload, more ferritin is formed in the enterocytes and shed with these cells in the stools (Fig. 3.2.27C).

The details of the regulatory processes involved remain obscure. However, the following views have been put forward to explain the mucosal block theory:

1. Saturation of apoferritin and apotransferrin. Most of the iron in the body is stored as ferritin, which is formed by a combination of iron with the protein apoferritin present in the

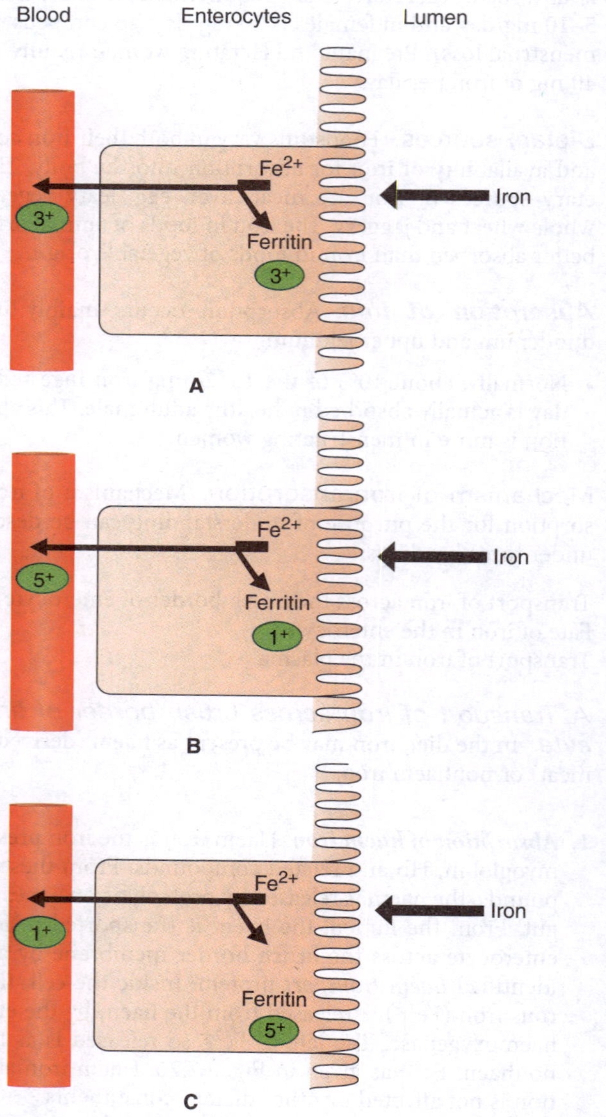

Fig. 3.2.27 Mucosal block theory of regulation of iron absorption: **A,** normally (e.g. equal amount [3⁺] of iron is bound to form ferritin and enters the blood across basolateral membrane); **B,** in iron-deficiency states, less iron forms ferritin (e.g. 1⁺) and more enters the blood, e.g. 5⁺; and **C,** in iron overload, more ferritin is formed (5⁺) and less enters the blood 1⁺.

cytoplasm of the body cells. When essentially all apoferritin in the body is saturated with iron, it becomes difficult for the transferrin to release its iron to the tissue cells. Consequently, the whole of the apotransferrin is saturated with iron and thus the mucosal cells are loaded with the transferrin. Because of the unavailability of the apotransferrin, the mucosal cells are not able to take up any more luminal iron. Mucosal cells have a lifespan of 3–4 days, at the end of which they get sloughed off into the intestine. Mucosal transferrin (containing iron) is also lost with it and the body gets rid of excess of iron.

2. Decreased rate of apoferritin synthesis. When body has excess of iron, due to feedback mechanism, the rate of apoferritin synthesis in the liver is also decreased and thus less iron is absorbed by the intestinal cells.

3. Role of specific iron receptors in the brush border. Recently it has been proposed that the absorption of iron by the enterocytes is determined by the presence of receptors on the brush border. Iron receptors in brush border preparations of the small intestine are inversely related to the level of body iron stores. Iron-deficient animals show an increase in the number of receptor population, which can be reversed by iron loading.

4. Role of iron regulatory proteins (IRPs). IRPs play an important role in regulation of iron metabolism. IRP controls the expression of DMT-1, mRNA and protein which is a limiting intestinal iron importer.

IRP deficiency impairs iron absorption and promotes mucosal iron retention via ferritin-mediated mucosal blocks.

Conclusion. The current understanding of the regulation of body iron is still in a state of fix with the following conclusions:

- The control seems to reside primarily in the need-based transfer of iron from the enterocyte to the portal blood.
- Some control is also exerted at the level of uptake of iron from the intestinal lumen.
- In cases of iron overload, some iron can be transported from the plasma to the enterocytes. This iron is lost when the enterocytes are shed into the lumen. In this way, the intestine serves to excrete excess iron in a bid to prevent accumulation of excessive iron in the body. Thus, the statement that iron content of the body is regulated only by absorption is also true, only to a limited extent.

The iron cycle The iron cycle refers to the continuous exchange of iron between the plasma and RBCs. The steps of iron cycles are as follows (Fig. 3.2.28):

- From the plasma, the iron is transported into bone marrow as transferrin.
- In the bone marrow, the transferrin binds to the specific transferrin receptors present on the surface of intermediate normoblasts.
- In the intermediate normoblasts, the iron is incorporated into the Hb. The mature RBCs containing Hb are then released into the plasma.
- RBCs, after their death (on completion of lifespan), are engulfed by macrophages.
- After phagocytosis, the red cell membrane is lysed and haem is released from the Hb. By the haemoxygenase reaction, iron is liberated from the haem.
- Macrophages lining the sinuses of liver and spleen release iron back into the plasma where it binds with the apotransferrin to form transferrin, thus completing the iron cycle.

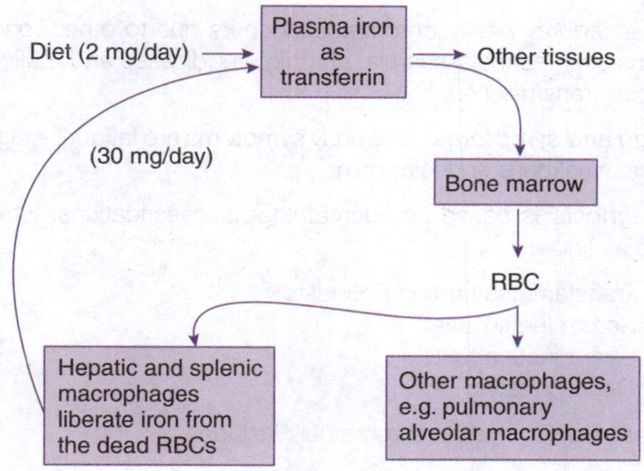

Fig. 3.2.28 Iron cycle.

Each day, about 30 mg of iron goes through this cycle. In addition, about 2 mg iron enters the plasma from the diet also.

Role of iron in the body. Iron is utilized in the synthesis of:

- *Hb* in the RBCs (main role)
- *Myoglobin* in the muscles
- *Cytochromes*, the intracellular enzymes

Uptake of the iron by tissues

RBCs are the main takers of iron (about 30 mg/day). Other tissues take up about less than 2 mg iron each day as follows:

- *Liver.* Out of the tissues other than RBCs, liver takes up the largest amount of iron.
- *Intestinal mucosal cells.* Iron is stored as transferrin in the intestinal mucosal cells which regulate the iron absorption as discussed above.
- *Skeletal muscles.* Iron is utilized to produce myoglobin by the muscles.
- *Proliferating cells of the body.* Iron is utilized for synthesis of enzymes cytochrome and catalases, which are required in excess by the proliferating cells of the body.

Applied Aspect

Iron deficiency results in iron-deficiency anaemia.

Iron excess. Iron overload may occur when its absorption exceeds its excretion. Such a condition occurs due to:

- *Excessive intake* of iron
- *Idiopathic* or congenital failure of mucosal feedback mechanism controlling iron absorption
- *Excessive destruction* of erythrocytes may also be associated with siderosis.

The excess of iron in the body results in accumulation of haemosiderin in the tissues producing the so-called haemosiderosis. Excess of haemosiderin damages the tissues and produces the condition of haemochromatosis.

Haemochromatosis may be hereditary or acquired.

The *hereditary or primary* haemochromatosis occurs due to mutation of *HFE* gene located on chromosome 6. Two common mutations in *HFE* gene are $C_2$82Y and H63D. The individual with homogeneous mutated *HFE* gene absorbs excess amounts of iron because normally the *HFE* gene inhibits expression of the transporter responsible for iron intake.

Secondary haemochromatosis occurs due to other conditions such as thalassaemia, chronic liver disease and multiple blood transfusions.

Sign and symptoms. The early symptoms are fatigue, weight loss, weakness and joint pain.

Diagnosis is based on haematological investigations, which are as follows:

- Transferrin saturation (TS) test
- Serum ferritin levels
- Liver function tests
- Genetic testing

Treatment of haemochromatosis includes:

- Therapeutic phlebotomy – in this procedure, about 1 L of blood is removed once or twice in a week till blood iron levels come to normal.
- Iron chelation therapy, i.e. use of drugs which remove excess of iron from the body.
- Dietary changes – avoid iron, limited use of vitamin C (because vitamin C helps in iron absorption) and avoid alcohol intake (because alcohol increases risk of liver diseases).

Causes of Iron-deficiency Anaemia

The causes vary with age, sex and country of residence of patient. In general, the causes of iron-deficiency anaemia can be grouped as:

1. Inadequate dietary intake of iron For example, in:

- Milk-fed infants
- Poor economic status individuals
- Anorexia, e.g. in pregnancy
- Elderly individuals due to atrophy and poor dentition

2. Increased loss of iron (as blood loss) from the body For example:

- *Uterine bleeding in females* in the form of excessive menstruation, repeated miscarriages, postmenopausal bleeding, etc.
- *Gastrointestinal bleeding* due to peptic ulcer, haemorrhoids, ulcerative colitis, etc.
- *Renal tract bleeding*, e.g. haematuria
- *Nasal bleeding*, i.e. repeated epistaxis
- *Bleeding from lungs* as in haemoptysis

3. Increased demand of iron For example, in:

- Infancy, childhood and adolescence
- Menstruating females
- Pregnant females

4. Decreased absorption of iron As seen in:

- Partial or total gastrectomy
- Achlorhydria
- Intestinal malabsorption diseases

Clinical Features, Laboratory Findings and Treatment

Clinical features of anaemia are:

1. General features of anaemia
See page 150.

2. Characteristic features of iron-deficiency anaemia are in the form of following epithelial tissue changes (Fig. 3.2.29):

- *Nails* become dry, soft and spoon shaped (koilonychia).
- *Tongue* becomes angry red (atrophic glossitis).
- *Mouth* may show angular stomatitis.
- *Oesophagus* may develop its membranous webs at the postcricoid area leading to dysphagia (Plummer–Vinson syndrome).

Laboratory findings of iron-deficiency anaemias are:

1. Blood picture and red cell indices These show the following:

- *Hb* concentration is decreased.
- RBCs are hypochromic (deficient in Hb) and microcytic (smaller in size). They show anisocytosis and poikilocytosis.
- *Red cell indices* like MCV, MCH and MCHC are decreased.

2. Bone marrow findings. These are as follows:

- Marrow cellularity: Erythroid hyperplasia
- Erythropoiesis: Normoblastic
- Marrow iron: Deficient reticuloendothelial iron stores and absence of siderotic iron granules

3. Biochemical findings These show the following:

- Serum iron decreases, often less than 50 µg/dL (normal, 60–160 µg/dL).

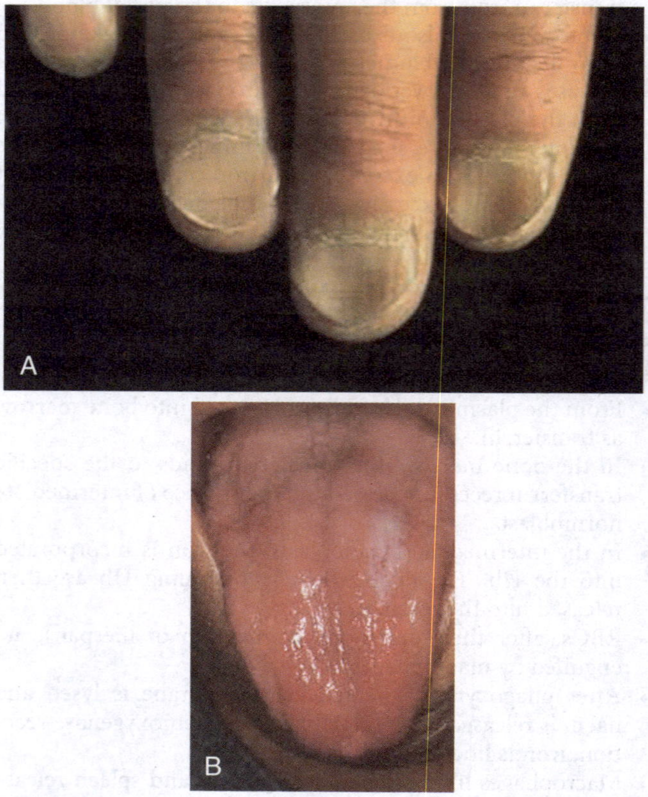

Fig. 3.2.29 Clinical features of iron-deficiency anaemia; **A,** spoon-shaped nails (koilonychia); and **B,** angry red tongue (atrophic glossitis).

- Serum bilirubin is less than 0.4 mg/dL.
- Serum ferritin is less than 30 μg/dL indicating poor tissue iron stores.
- Total iron-binding capacity (TIBC) is increased.
- *Transferrin saturation.* The percentage of total iron-binding capacity (TIBC) expresses the amount of iron bound to the transferrin.
- *Red cell distribution width (RDW)* measures the variation in diameter of RBCs. In iron-deficiency anaemia, the value of RDW increases.

Treatment Depending on the cause, treatment of iron-deficiency anaemia consists of medications such as:

- Iron supplements in the form of:
  - Oral/parental (iron dextran and iron sorbitol)
  - Diet: Consumption of iron-rich diet, e.g. green leafy vegetables, meat, liver, jaggery; food should be cooked in iron utensils

Blood transfusion in severe anaemia, preferably fresh blood should be transfused.
  - Oral administration of Fe^{2+} salts
  - *Correction of causative* factor if possible

B. Megaloblastic Anaemia

Megaloblastic anaemias are characterized by abnormally large cells of erythrocyte series. These are caused by defective DNA synthesis due to deficiency of vitamin B_{12} and/or folic acid (folate); therefore, aetiologically megaloblastic anaemia is of two types:

I. Megaloblastic anaemia due to vitamin B_{12} deficiency Salient features of vitamin B_{12} and intrinsic factor of Castle should be understood before discussing other aspects of anaemia due to vitamin B_{12} deficiency (see page 136).

Causes of vitamin B_{12} deficiency are:
1. ***Inadequate dietary intake*** may occur in:
   - Strict vegetarians
   - Breast-fed infants
2. ***Malabsorption of vitamin B_{12}*** is more often the cause of deficiency and may be due to:
   - *Gastric causes* leading to deficiency of intrinsic factors such as an autoimmune cause of failure of secretion of intrinsic factor (Addisonian pernicious anaemia), gastrectomy and congenital lack of intrinsic factor.
   - *Intestinal causes* which are associated with decreased vitamin B_{12} absorption are tropical sprue, ileal resection, Crohn disease, fish tapeworm infestation and intestinal blind loop syndrome.

Addisonian Pernicious Anaemia Addisonian pernicious anaemia is the term which is used specifically for the megaloblastic anaemia due to vitamin B_{12} deficiency occurring as a result of failure of secretion of intrinsic factor by the stomach owing to an autoimmune atrophy of gastric mucosa. Thus, pernicious anaemia is an autoimmune disease and in about 50% of patients, antibodies to intrinsic factor can be demonstrated. The disease is rare before the age of 30 years, occurs mainly between 45 and 65 years and affects females more frequently than males.

Features of pernicious anaemia include:

Features of megaloblastic anaemia
Specific features of pernicious anaemia:

- Anti-intrinsic factor antibodies in serum (present in 50% of cases)
- Abnormal vitamin B_{12} absorption test corrected by addition of intrinsic factor (Schilling test)

Treatment. For pernicious anaemia, the treatment involves regular administration of vitamin B_{12} by intramuscular route.

II. Megaloblastic anaemia due to folate deficiency
Salient features of folic acid and its role in erythropoiesis (see page 137)

Causes of folate deficiency are:

1. ***Inadequate dietary*** *intake* due to poor intake of vegetables as seen in poor people, infants and alcoholics
2. ***Malabsorption***, e.g. in coeliac disease, tropical sprue and Crohn disease
3. ***Increased demand*** as occurs in:
   - Physiological conditions such as pregnancy, lactation and infancy
   - Pathological conditions of cell proliferation, such as increased haematopoiesis (as in haemolysis) and malignancies
4. ***Effect of drugs*** such as certain anticonvulsants (e.g. phenytoin), contraceptive pills and certain cytotoxic drugs (e.g. methotrexate)
5. ***Excess urinary folate loss***, e.g. in active liver disease and congestive heart failure

Features of folate deficiency anaemia are:

- *Features of megaloblastic anaemia*
- *Specific features of folate deficiency*
  - Low serum folate levels
- Low red cell folate levels

Treatment of pernicious anaemia due to folic acid deficiency consists of:

- Diet supplementation
- Oral folic acid tablets

Important Note

Use of folic acid is contraindicated in anaemia when cause is not known because folic acid restores only cell counts but does not prevent development of subacute combined degeneration in pernicious anaemia, rather accelerates neurological manifestations in vitamin B_{12}–deficiency situations.

Clinical features of megaloblastic anaemia

General features of anaemia. See page 150.

Characteristic features of megaloblastic anaemia are:
Gastrointestinal manifestations include:
- Atrophic glossitis
- Angular stomatitis
- Painful ulcers in the mouth
- Gingivitis

- Gastric atrophy
- Achlorhydria
- Loss of appetite

Neural manifestations occur as:

- Headache
- Lethargy
- Sensory ataxia
- Peripheral neuropathy
- Psychosis
- In advanced stage: Subacute combined degeneration of spinal cord causing tingling sensations due to involvement of dorsal and lateral column pathways

Diagnosis

1. Blood picture and red cell indices

- *Hb* level is low.
- RBCs are larger in size (macrocytosis) but contain a normal concentration of Hb (normochromia).
- *MCV* increases to 95–160 μm³ (normal, 78–94 μm³).
- *MCH* increases to 50 pg (normal, 28–32 pg).
- *MCHC* usually normal (35% ± 3%) because both MCV and MCH increase. In late stages, MCHC may decrease.
- *Peripheral smear* shows nucleated RBCs with marked anisocytosis and poikilocytosis.
- *Reticulocyte count* increases to more than 5% (normal less than 1%).
- *Lifespan of RBCs* is decreased.
- *WBCs and platelets* decrease because of encroachment of megaloblastic tissue.

2. Bone marrow picture

It shows *megaloblastic hyperplasia* characterized by presence of:

- Seventy per cent proerythroblasts and early normoblasts (normal, 30%)
- Thirty per cent intermediate and late normoblasts (normal, 70%)

Marrow iron. Prussian blue staining for iron in the marrow shows an increase in the number and size of iron granules in the erythroid precursors.

3. Biochemical findings

- *Serum bilirubin* increases more than 1 mg/dL (normal, 0.2–0.8 mg/dL) due to excessive destruction of RBCs in spleen, liver and bone marrow.
- *Urine urobilinogen* excretion may increase due to increased serum bilirubin.
- *Serum iron and* ferritin levels are usually increased because iron is not utilized by immature RBCs.
- *Serum vitamin B_{12}* levels are decreased (normal, 150–350 pg/mL) in patients with megaloblastic anaemia due to vitamin B_{12} deficiency.
- *Serum folate levels* are decreased in patients with megaloblastic anaemia due to folic acid deficiency.
- *Red cell folate levels* are a more reliable indicator of tissue stores of folate than serum. In folic acid deficiency, red cell folate levels are decreased.

4. Schilling test.

It is performed in two stages:

In the first stage, a large intramuscular dose of vitamin B_{12} is given to saturate the plasma transport protein. Thereafter, radiolabelled vitamin B_{12} is administered orally, and 24-hour urine samples are collected to detect vitamin B_{12}. Normally, more than 7% of the dose is present in the urine and patients with impaired absorption will have less than 3% of the dose.

The second stage of Schilling test is performed to detect pernicious anaemia due to lack of intrinsic factor. Radiolabelled vitamin B_{12} along with intrinsic factor is administered. Combined use of vitamin B_{12} and intrinsic factor should correct abnormally low absorption due to lack of intrinsic factor. Therefore, urine vitamin B_{12} level will be improved.

Self-Assessment

1. Describe the stages of erythropoiesis and its regulation.
2. Describe the characteristics features of different phases of erythropoiesis and factors necessary for erythropoiesis.
3. What is the role of vitamin B_{12} and folic acid in erythropoiesis?
4. Describe the functions of haemoglobin and factors controlling the formation of haemoglobin.
5. What are the lifespan and fate of RBCs?
6. Write a short note on:
   - RBC indices
   - Erythropoietin
   - Van den Bergh test
   - Pernicious anaemia
   - Bilirubin
   - Osmotic fragility
   - Thalassaemia
   - Sickle cell haemoglobin

Clinical Cases

Case 1

A 12-year-old boy complained of fatigue and generalized weakness, loss of weight and loss of appetite.

On examination, the paediatrician observed pallor, jaundice, tachycardia, cardiac murmur and enlarged spleen.

Laboratory tests showed the following:

- Hb: 6 g/dL
- Red cell morphology: Microcytic cells and many small spherocytes
- MCV 92 fL; MCH 30 pg; and MCHC 38%
- Bilirubin: 3.5 mg/dL
- Reticulocyte count: 5%
- Osmotic fragility test positive (completed at 45% NaCl solution)

Q1. What is the probable diagnosis?
Q2. What is the cause of the disease?
Q3. What treatment could be advised?

Case 2

A 35-year-old male patient attended the medicine OPD with complaints of abdominal pain, change of skin colour, dark colour urine, loss of appetite, weight loss and feeling sick.

Q1. What is the probable diagnosis?
Q2. What laboratory tests should be done for the final diagnosis?

Case 3

A 30-year-old woman having two children aged 3 and 2 years presented with history of lethargy, giddiness, breathlessness and

Clinical Cases—(Continued)

palpitation on exertion and difficulty in swallowing. Examination findings revealed pallor of skin and mucus membrane; tachycardia; dry, brittle and spoon-shaped nails; smooth and angry red tongue. Investigation findings were as follows: Hb, 6 g/dL; ESR, 50 mm in first hour; peripheral blood smear showed microcytic hypochromic RBCs; red cell indices: MCV, MCH and MCHC decreased.

Q1. What is the provisional diagnosis?

Q2. What are the further tests required to decide the final diagnosis? What would be the treatment?

Case 4

An 18-year-old girl student from South Africa brought to hospital emergency with severe joint pain and chest pain. She was thoroughly examined and investigated.

Laboratory findings:

- CBC findings
  - Hb decreased
  - Blood smear: RBCs microcytic hypochromic, many small irregular red cells and also nucleated cells present
  - Reticulocyte count: 12%
- TLC: 12,000/mm^3; DLC within normal range
- Platelet count: Normal

Q1. What is the probable diagnosis?

Q2. Name two more tests to reach the definitive diagnosis.

Q3. What is the main cause for acute chest pain?

Case 5

A 2-year-old male child presented to paediatrics OPD with fatigue, weakness, deformed facial bones, stunted growth as per his age, abdominal swelling and pallor. On physical examination the doctor observed jaundice, splenomegaly, bony enlargement and tachycardia.

Laboratory tests revealed decreased Hb. Blood smear showed microcytic hypochromic picture with large number of nucleated RBCs.

Q1. What is the provisional diagnosis?

Q2. What are the further investigations to confirm the diagnosis?

Q3. If not treated, then what complications may occur?

Case 6

A 55-year-old female suffered with breast carcinoma and had treatment in the form of chemotherapy and radiation therapy. After 2 weeks, she developed generalized weakness and pallor; bleeding from nose; lot of bruises over the body; and frequent infection. There was no history of trauma/injury.

Q1. What is the cause of signs and symptoms?

Q2. What is the probable diagnosis?

Q3. What is the blood picture in this case?

Case 7

A 45-year-old female was suffering with off and on fever, generalized weakness, breathlessness and palpitation on exertion and tingling sensations in hands and feet.

On examination, it was found that she had anaemia and jaundice. Haematological investigations revealed the following:

- Hb: 5 g/dL
- Blood smear: Macrocytic hypochromic picture of RBCs
- Bilirubin level: Increased
- Shilling test: Positive

Treatment advised was vitamin B_{12} and folic acid orally, but no improvement occurred in the condition.

Q1. What is the cause of signs and symptoms in this case?

Q2. What are the further investigations required to find the cause?

3.3 White Blood Cells

CHAPTER OUTLINE

WHITE BLOOD CELL TYPES AND THEIR COUNTS

White blood cells (WBCs) or leucocytes are so named since they are colourless in contrast to the red colour of the RBCs. These are nucleated cells which play an important role in the defence mechanism of the body.

The leucocytes of the peripheral blood are of two main varieties, distinguished by the presence or absence of granules. These are granulocytes and nongranulocytes.

TYPES OF WHITE BLOOD CELLS

Granulocytes WBCs with granules in their cytoplasm are called granulocytes. Depending on the colour of granules, granulocytes are further divided into three types.

Neutrophils. They contain granules which take both acidic and basic stains.

Eosinophils They contain granules which take acidic stain.

Basophils They contain granules which take basic stain.

Agranulocytes WBCs that do not contain granules in their cytoplasm are called agranulocytes. These are of two types:

- Lymphocytes
- Monocytes

NORMAL WBC COUNTS

Total leucocyte count Total leucocyte count (TLC) varies with age as follows:

Adults: 4000–11,000/mm^3 of blood
At birth, in full-term infants: 10,000–25,000/mm^3 of blood
Infants up to 1 year of age: 6000–16,000/mm^3 of blood
Children, 4–7 years of age: 5000–15,000/mm^3 of blood
Children, 8–12 years of age: 4500–13,500/mm^3 of blood

Differential and absolute leucocyte count Differential leucocyte count (DLC) and absolute count in normal adults are shown in Table 3.3.1.

Clinical significance of differential and absolute counts DLC tells us whether there is an increase or decrease in a particular type of leucocyte, because in different diseases, one or the other type of cells shows an increase or decrease in its numbers. The differential count is done in 100–200 cells, and tells only a relative increase or decrease in a particular variety of cells, with a corresponding decrease or increase in the other types of cells. For example, an increase in the percentage of neutrophils would be associated with a decrease in the percentage of lymphocytes, thus giving an impression of lymphocytopenia. But if the TLC is taken into account, the absolute lymphocyte count could be within a normal range. Therefore, DLC alone is not of much importance and so is never done as an isolated test, but always it is part of full blood counts, including TLC and then calculating absolute count.

Table 3.3.1 Differential leucocyte count and absolute count in normal adults

WBCs	Differential count (%)	Absolute count (per mm³)
Granulocytes		
• Neutrophils	40–75	2000–7500
• Eosinophils	1–6	40–440
• Basophils	0–1	0–100
Agranulocytes		
• Lymphocytes	20–40	1500–4000
• Monocytes	2–10	500–800

VARIATIONS IN WBC COUNT

Leucocytosis

Leucocytosis refers to increase in total WBC count above 11,000/mm^3.

Physiological causes of leucocytosis are:

Age: In newborn babies up to the age of 1 year, the WBC count is higher. At birth, the WBC count is about 18,000/mm^3, which drops gradually to the adult level.

Exercise: The WBC count is increased after exercise.

After food intake, the WBC count is raised.

Mental stress and emotional conditions like anxiety are associated with raised WBC count.

Pregnancy: At full-term pregnancy, the WBC count is 12,000–15,000 mm^3.

Exposure to low temperature also causes leucocytosis.

Pathological causes of leucocytosis are:

Acute bacterial infections, especially by pyogenic organisms

Acute haemorrhage

Burns

Postoperative period

Tuberculosis

Glandular fever

Leucopenia

Leucopenia refers to decrease in the total WBC count below 4000/mm^3.

Causes of leucopenia are:

Infections by nonpyogenic bacteria, especially typhoid fever and paratyphoid fever

- *Viral infections* such as influenza, smallpox, mumps
- *Protozoal infections*

Starvation and malnutrition

Aplasia of bone marrow. Bone marrow depression due to:

- Drugs such as Chloromycetin and cytotoxic drugs used in malignant diseases
- Repeated exposure to X-rays or radiations
- Chemical poisons like arsenic, dinitrophenol and antimony

Leukaemia

Leukaemia is a malignant disease of the blood in which there occurs an increase in the total WBC count associated with the presence of immature WBCs in the peripheral blood. Total WBC count is usually above 50,000/mm^3, and may be as high as 100,000–300,000/mm^3 (see page 170).

FORMATION OF WHITE BLOOD CELLS

The process of development and maturation of WBCs (leucocytes), called *leucopoiesis*, is a part of haemopoiesis (formation of blood cells). All the blood cells develop from the so-called pluripotent *haemopoietic* stem cells (PHSCs). The stem cells after a series of divisions differentiate into *progenitor* cells, which are also called colony-forming units (CFU) (for details, see page 132).

Leucopoiesis can be discussed under two headings:

- Formation of granulocytes (granulopoiesis) and monocytes
- Formation of lymphocytes (lymphopoiesis)

FORMATION OF GRANULOCYTES AND MONOCYTES

The granulocytes and monocytes are formed in the bone marrow from the colony-forming unit granulocytes and monocytes (CFU-GM); the progenitor cells (CFU-GM) forming different cells are further named as follows:

- CFU-G are neutrophil-forming units.
- CFU-EO refers to eosinophil-forming units.
- CFU-Ba are basophil-forming units.
- CFU-M refers to monocyte-forming units.

The development of granulocytes through various stages is called *myeloid series* and development of monocytes through various stages is called *monocyte–macrophage series.*

Myeloid Series

Some facts about granulopoiesis

- The cells of myeloid series include myeloblast (most primitive precursor), promyelocytes, myelocytes, metamyelocytes, band forms and segmented granulocyte (mature form). These cells can be grouped together in two pools:
  - Proliferative or mitotic pool is formed by the myeloblast, promyelocyte and myelocyte.
  - Mature or postmitotic pool includes the metamyelocytes, band forms and segmented granulocytes.
- The process of granulopoiesis takes about 12 days.
- Granulocytes are formed and stored in the bone marrow. When need arises, they are released in circulation. Normally, about three times as many granulocytes are stored in the bone marrow as circulated in the peripheral blood.

Features of the cells of myeloid series (Fig. 3.3.1)

1. Myeloblast Myeloblast is the earliest recognizable cell of the granulocyte series. Myeloblasts form about 2% of the total marrow cells. Its features are as follows:

Size: Myeloblast varies in diameter from 16 to 20 µm.

Cytoplasm is basophilic, present as thin rim around the nucleus, and is devoid of granules.

Nucleus is large (nearly filling the cells), round to oval, has fine chromatin and contains two to five well-defined pale nucleoli.

Mitosis is marked (+++).

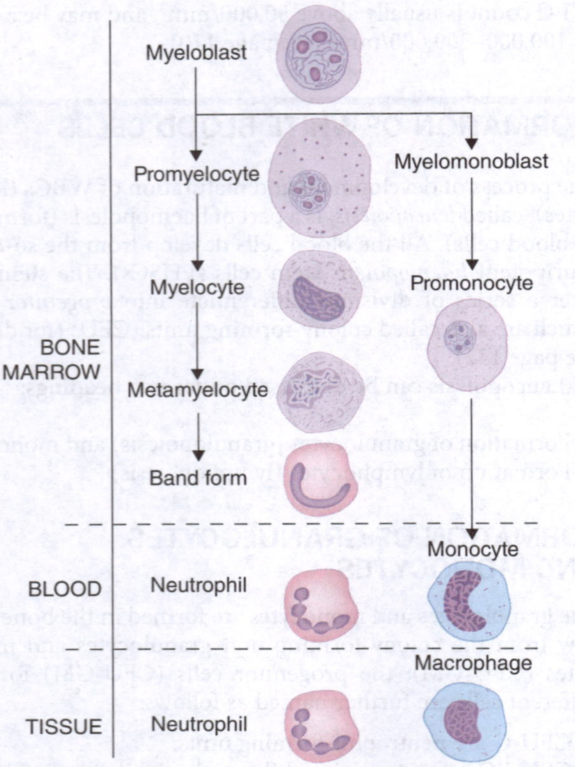

Fig. 3.3.1 Granulopoiesis and features of the cells of myeloid series and monocyte–macrophage series.

2. Promyelocytes. Myeloblasts progress into the promyelocyte which has the following features:

Size varies from 14 to 18 μm.
Cytoplasm increases in amount and is characterized by the presence of *azurophil granules.* These granules are also called *primary nonspecific granules* and these give a positive reaction with the peroxidase stain.
Nucleus is round or oval, slightly small than the nucleus of myeloblast and having fine chromatin, which is condensed. The nucleoli are present but are less prominent and fewer than those in the myeloblast.
Mitosis is a characteristic feature (+++).

3. Myelocyte Myelocyte, also called myelocyte proper, is the next cell in myeloid series. Its features are as follows:

Size varies from 12 to 16 μm.
Cytoplasm is characterized by the presence of *specific (secondary) granules* and accordingly the cell can be identified at this stage as:

- Neutrophil myelocyte
- Eosinophil myelocyte
- Basophil myelocyte

The primary granules are also present at this stage but their formation is stopped.

Nucleus is eccentric, round to oval, having coarse nuclear chromatin and no nucleoli.
Mitosis continues up to this stage. Multiplication of these cells is maximum.

4. Metamyelocyte. It has the following features:

Size varies from 10 to 14 μm.
Cytoplasm increases in amount and becomes more liquid. Both primary and secondary granules are present. Depending on the features of secondary granules, the metamyelocytes are distinguished as:

- Neutrophil metamyelocyte
- Eosinophil metamyelocyte
- Basophil metamyelocyte

Nucleus decreases in size, and becomes indented and lobed (horseshoe shape). The nuclear chromatin is dense and clumped. Nucleoli are absent.
Mitosis stops at this stage.

5. Band or stab form. It refers to juvenile granulocytes which have the following features:

Size is slightly smaller than metamyelocyte.
Cytoplasm is pink and contains fine evenly distributed granules.
Nucleus is characterized by further condensation of chromatin and transformation of nucleus shape into a band configuration (deeply indented V-shaped) of uniform thickness which may be twisted.

6. Mature granulocytes Mature granulocytes ultimately formed are neutrophils, eosinophils and basophils. Their morphological features are described on page 161.

Monocyte–Macrophage Series (Fig. 3.3.1)

The series of cells basically form a part of myeloid series along with the granulocytes and are thus formed in the bone marrow. These are described separately because of the different morphological stages which include monoblast, promonocyte and monocyte.

1. Monoblast. It is a large cell similar in structure to the myeloblast from which it cannot be distinguished on morphological grounds alone. Therefore, it is preferable to call the earliest precursor of granulocytic series *myelomonoblast.*

2. Promonocyte. It has following features:

Size: It is a young monocyte about 20 μm in diameter.
Nucleus is large, indented (often kidney shaped) and contains one nucleolus. The nuclear chromatin is arranged in a loose network.
Cytoplasm is basophilic and contains *no azurophilic granules,* but may have fine granules which are larger than those in mature monocyte.

3. Monocyte. Morphological features of a mature monocyte are described on page 169. These resemble metamyelocytes and are best distinguished by the presence of fine chromatin. In metamyelocytes, the chromatin is dense and clumped.

From the bone marrow, the monocytes migrate into the spleen and the lymphoid tissues in considerable numbers. The transformed stages of these cells in various tissues are called tissue macrophages and form a part of tissue–macrophage system, which was previously known as reticuloendothelial system.

FORMATION OF LYMPHOCYTES

Lymphocytes are formed from the *lymphocyte stem cells*, which are formed from PHSCs in the bone marrow (Fig. 3.2.10). The lymphocyte stem cells migrate into the thymus and peripheral lymphoid tissues, where they proliferate and mature into lymphocytes. In humans, the bone marrow and thymus form the primary lymphopoietic *organs*, where lymphoid stem cells undergo spontaneous division independent of antigenic stimulation. The tissues that actively produce lymphocytes from the germinal centres of lymphoid follicles as a response to antigenic stimulation constitute the so-called *secondary or reactive lymphoid tissue*. It is composed of

- Lymph nodes
- Spleen
- Gut-associated lymphoid tissue (GALT)

Lymphoid Series

The maturation stages of lymphoid series are given in Fig. 3.3.2.

1. Lymphoblast. It is the earliest recognizable cell of the lymphoid series. It is an actively dividing cell and resembles the myeloblast morphologically, except for the following minor differences:

- The nucleus contains fewer nucleoli (one to two) compared with the myeloblast (two to five).
- Nuclear chromatin is slightly clumped and stippled compared with fine meshwork in myeloblast.
- Nuclear membrane is fairly dense compared with that of the myeloblast.

2. Prolymphocyte. It is the intermediate stage between the lymphoblast and mature lymphocyte. Its features are as follows:

Diameter is 9–18 μm.
Nucleus is round to indented, with slightly stippled or coarse chromatin, and may have zero to one nucleolus.
Cytoplasm is scanty and nongranular.

3. Lymphocytes. Prolymphocytes mature successively into large lymphocyte and small lymphocyte, both of which are found in the circulation.

- Then some lymphocytes enter thymus, where they are processed and come out as T lymphocytes. In thymus, a factor called *thymosin* plays an important role in the processing.
- Some lymphocytes are processed in the liver (in fetal life) and bone marrow (after birth). These come out as B *lymphocytes*. The word B comes from 'bursa of Fabricius', which is the site of B-cell processing in birds. Morphological features of large and small lymphocytes are described on page 168.

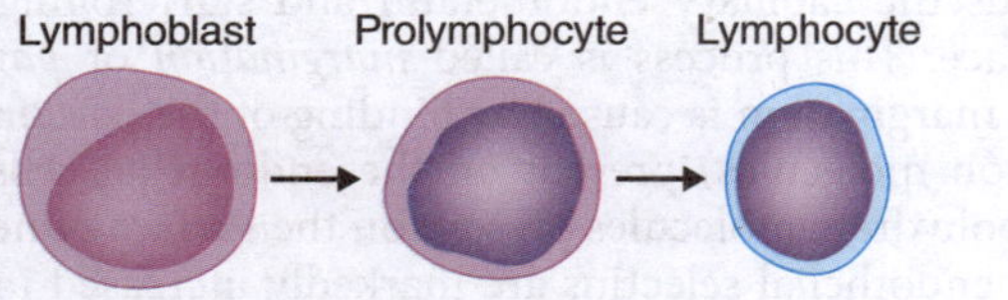

Fig. 3.3.2 Formation of lymphoid series cells.

REGULATION OF LEUCOPOIESIS

The constancy of leucocyte count suggests an efficient feedback mechanism to control their production and release (Fig. 3.3.3). During tissue injury and inflammation, bacterial toxins, products of injury, etc. cause a great increase in the rate of production and release of leucocytes. Thus, unlike erythropoiesis, the products of dead and dying white cells themselves control leucopoiesis. The substances that stimulate or inhibit the process of leucopoiesis are complex and include the following.

Role of cytokines The cytokines that control the formation of different types of granulocytes are called *colony-stimulating factors (CSFs)*. The CSFs are glycoproteins formed by monocytes and T lymphocytes and include:

- *G-CSF* which stimulates granulocyte precursors
- *M-CSF* which stimulates monocytic precursors
- *GM-CSF* which stimulates both the granulocyte and monocytic precursors

The cytokines that control lymphocyte formation are called *interleukins*, e.g. IL-1 and IL-3. Interleukins are formed by monocytes, macrophages and endothelial cells (see page 188).

Role of prostaglandins Prostaglandins formed by monocytes, *lactoferrin* and possibly some other agents also play a role in control of leucopoiesis.

MORPHOLOGY, FUNCTIONS, LIFESPAN AND VARIATIONS IN COUNTS OF WBCS

Morphological features of various types of WBCs, as studied under microscope with Leishman staining and haematoxylin-eosin stain (Fig. 3.3.4), are summarized next along with their functions and variations in their counts.

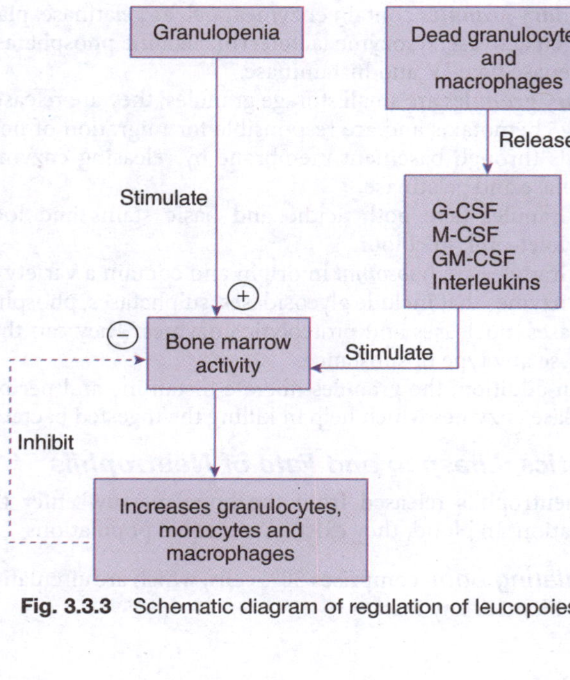

Fig. 3.3.3 Schematic diagram of regulation of leucopoiesis.

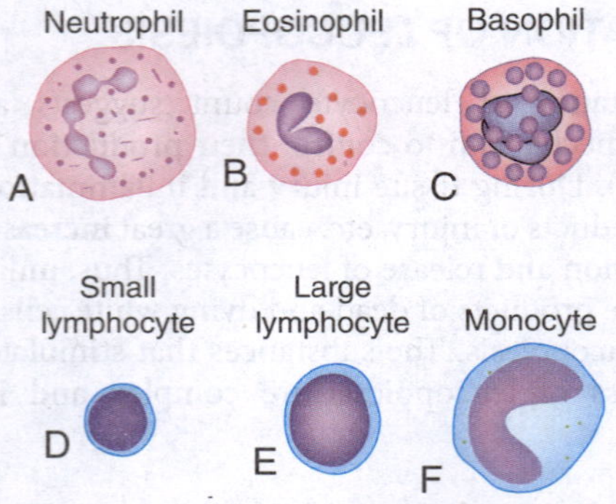

Fig. 3.3.4 Morphological features of white blood cells: **A,** neutrophil; **B,** eosinophil; **C,** basophil; **D,** small lymphocyte; **E,** large lymphocyte; and **F,** monocyte.

NEUTROPHILS

Morphological Features

The polymorphonuclear neutrophils, commonly called polymorphs or neutrophils, have the following morphological features (Fig. 3.3.4A):

Diameter. Diameter of a neutrophil varies from 10 to 14 μm.

Nucleus. A young neutrophil has a single horseshoe-shaped nucleus, which becomes lobed as the cell grows. Nucleus of a mature neutrophil is purple in colour and multilobed (two to six lobes); that is why a neutrophil is also called polymorphonuclear leucocyte. The lobes of the nucleus are connected by chromatin filaments, seen clearly through the cytoplasm.

Cytoplasm. Cytoplasm of neutrophil is pale bluish in colour and full of fine (pinpoint) granules. The cytoplasm of neutrophils contains three types of granules:

Primary granules or azurophilic granules or antimicrobial granules, containing bactericidal permeability-increasing protein (BP1), cathepsin G, acid hydrolase and myeloperoxidase (MPO).

Secondary granules contain enzymes such as gelatinase, plasminogen activase, lysozyme lactoferrin, alkaline phosphatase, collagenase type IV and histaminase.

Tertiary granules are small storage granules; they are released during chemotaxis and are responsible for migration of neutrophils through basement membrane by releasing enzymes proteinase and gelatinase.

- Granules take both acidic and basic stains and look violet-pink in colour.
- Granules are *lysosomal* in origin and contain a variety of enzymes that include glycosidases, sulphatases, phosphatases, nucleases and proteolytic enzymes. They can thus lyse any type of substance.
- In addition, the granules liberate histamine and peroxidase enzymes which help in killing the ingested bacteria.

Kinetics, Lifespan and Fate of Neutrophils

The neutrophils released from the bone marrow enter the circulation. In blood, they exist in two equal populations:

Circulating pool comprises 50% cells, which are circulating in the blood at any instant.

Marginal pool is constituted by the rest of 50% of cells, which remain marginated or sidelined, i.e., sticking to the endothelial cells of closed capillaries, venules, small veins and sinusoids.

There is a rapid exchange between the two pools.

- For every neutrophil in blood, there are about 100 mature neutrophils held in the bone marrow as reserve. These are released in the circulation when required. The stimulus for their release comes from the dead leucocytes, which release a granulocyte-inducing factor, and also by the hormone cortisol.
- Following their release from the bone marrow, granulocytes remain in circulating blood for 8–10 hours and then they enter the tissues. After migration into tissues, they never return to the bloodstream. In the tissues, they are either destroyed during phagocytosis or die due to senescence after 4–5 days. The dead neutrophils are taken up by the macrophages. In cases of severe infection, lifespan of neutrophils may become as short as few hours.
- A huge number of neutrophils is also eliminated daily, mainly into the intestine and out via faeces and to some extent into the respiratory secretions.
- Old senile neutrophils are characterized by:
  - Loss of motility
  - Poorly stained granules
  - Increased nuclear lobulation
  - Easy breakability while making blood smear

Functions

The neutrophils along with monocytes constitute the first line of defence against microorganisms, viruses and other injurious agents that enter the body. Neutrophils subserve this role by the following mechanisms:

Phagocytosis: The neutrophils engulf dead tissue (but sparing the normal tissue), the foreign particles or bacteria, digest them and ultimately may kill them by a process called phagocytosis.

Reaction of inflammation: The neutrophils also release leucotrienes, prostaglandins, thromboxanes, etc. that bring about the reactions of inflammation like vasodilatation and oedema.

Febrile response: The neutrophils contain a fever-producing substance called endogenous pyrogen, which is an important mediator of febrile response to the bacterial pyrogens.

Phagocytosis Phagocytosis (cell eating) refers to the process of engulfment and destruction of solid particulate material by the cells. The cells performing this function are called phagocytes. In addition to neutrophils, the monocytes and fixed tissue macrophages also work as phagocytes. The process of phagocytosis involves the following steps.

1. Margination The normal axial blood flow consists of central stream of cells (leucocytes and RBCs) and peripheral cell-free layer of plasma close to vessel walls. In the area of infection, the neutrophils get *marginated*, i.e. get attached towards the capillary endothelium and start rolling along its surface. This process is called *margination* or *pavementing*. The margination is caused by binding of the *selectins* (cell adhesion molecules) present on the endothelial cells with the carbohydrate molecules present on the surface of neutrophils. The endothelial selectins are markedly increased in the areas where there is inflammation (Fig. 3.3.5A).

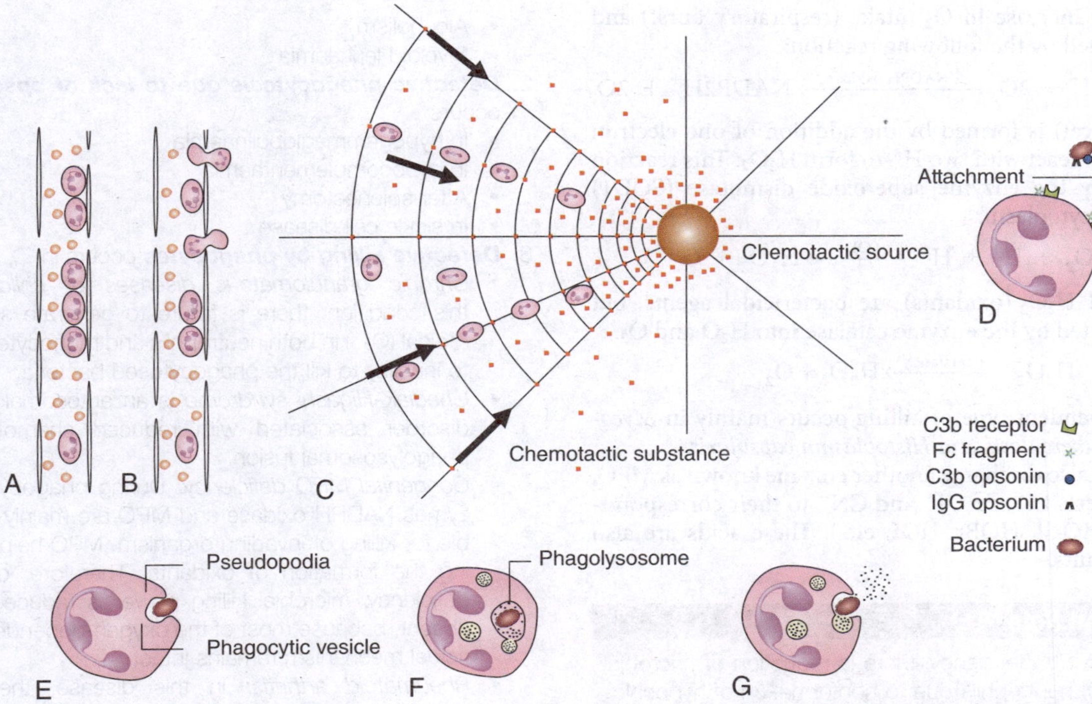

Fig. 3.3.5 Stages of phagocytosis: **A,** margination; **B,** diapedesis; **C,** chemotaxis; **D,** opsonization; **E,** engulfment; **F,** formation of phagolysosome; and **G,** degranulation.

2. Emigration and diapedesis The marginated neutrophils are emigrated in a large number from the blood at the site of *infection* caused by the foreign microorganism. They are motile and move by diapedesis into the tissues by passing through the junction between the endothelial cells of the blood vessels (Fig. 3.3.5B). The diapedesis of neutrophils is brought about by microtubules, microfilaments and interaction of actin with myosin-I on the inner side of the cell membrane.

3. Chemotaxis Chemotaxis refers to the process by which the neutrophils are attracted towards bacteria at the site of inflammation. The process of chemotaxis is mediated by the chemotactic agents called *chemokines*, which are released at the infected area. There are various types of chemokines, which include:

- Leukotriene B_4 (LTB_4)
- Components of the complement system (C5a) and cytokines (polypeptides from lymphocytes and monocytes)

The chemoattractants increase the adhesive nature of neutrophils, which form clumps surrounding the infected area (Fig. 3.3.5C).

4. Opsonization (attachment stage) Opsonization refers to the process of coating of bacteria by the *opsonins* by which bacteria become tasty to the phagocytes. The principal opsonins are naturally acting factors in the plasma and include:

- IgG opsonin
- C3b opsonin (a product of complement cascade)
- Lectin (carbohydrate-binding protein)
- Opsonin fragment of complement protein

As shown in Fig. 3.3.5D, the opsonized bacteria are easily bound to the surface of phagocyte (attachment stage). This process triggers G protein–mediated responses and increases motor activity of the cell, exocytosis and respiratory bursts.

5. Engulfment stage The increased motor activity of neutrophils leads to prompt ingestion of bacteria by endocytosis. The neutrophils project *pseudopodia* in all directions around the opsonized particle, which is bound to the surface of neutrophil (Fig. 3.3.5E). This occurs due to activation of actin filaments present underneath the cell membrane. Pseudopodia meet each other on opposite side and fuse. This creates an enclosed chamber with engulfed material. It breaks away from the membrane forming a *phagocytic vesicle*. Then the lysosomes of the cell fuse with the phagocytic vesicle to form a *phagolysosome* or phagosome (Fig. 3.3.5F).

6. Secretion (degranulation) stage Once the bacteria are engulfed, the granules of phagocytes get discharged in the phagosomes and also in interstitial space (Fig. 3.3.5G). This process is called degranulation. There are large numbers of proteolytic enzymes, especially geared up for digesting the bacteria. In addition, there is release of interleukins; IL-2, IL-6, tumour necrotic factor (TNF), arachidonic acid, leukotrienes, and oxygen metabolites. Lysosomes of macrophages also contain lipases which can digest the thick lipid membranes possessed by certain bacteria.

7. Killing or degradation stage The neutrophils and macrophages contain *bactericidal agents* (defensins α and β), which can kill most of the bacteria even when lysosomal enzymes fail to digest them. The bactericidal substance accomplishes the killing process by the following mechanisms:

Oxygen-dependent bactericidal mechanism, which is mediated by oxidizing agents (superoxides, H_2O_2, etc.) formed by the membrane-bound enzyme NADPH oxidase which leads to sharp increase in O_2 intake (respiratory burst) and O_2^-, is generated by the following reaction:

$$NADPH + H^+ + 2O_2 \xrightarrow{\text{NADPH oxidase}} NADP2H^+ + 2O_2^-$$

O_2^- (free radical) is formed by the addition of one electron to O_2. Two O_2^- react with two H^+ to form H_2O_2. This reaction is catalysed by the enzyme superoxide dismutase (SOD1) present in the cytoplasm.

$$O_2^- + O_2^- + H^+ + H^+ \xrightarrow{\text{SOD1}} H_2O_2 + O_2$$

Both O_2^- and H_2O_2 (oxidants) are bactericidal agents, but H_2O_2 is converted by the enzyme catalase into H_2O and O_2.

$$H_2O_2^- \xrightarrow{\text{catalase}} H_2O + O_2$$

- Oxygen dependent type of killing occurs mainly in *Mycobacterium tuberculosis* and *Histoplasma capsularis.*
- Neutrophils also discharge another enzyme known as MPO, which converts Cl^-, Br^-, I^- and CN^- to their corresponding acids (HOCl, HOBr, HOI, etc.). These acids are also potent oxidants.

Important Note

In congenital MPO deficiency, there is reduction of microbial killing power of neutrophils due to nonformation of hypochlorous acid.

Oxygen-independent bactericidal mechanism works through lysosomal hydrolases, defensins and cationic protein. Elastases and metalloproteinases directly attack the collagen, and other proteinases destroy the membrane of invading bacteria.

Nitric oxide (NO)–dependent killing: The macrophages also produce nitric oxide, which also plays role in killing and inflammatory process.

Important Notes

Respiratory burst reaction is the process by which phagocytic cells consume a large amount of oxygen and generate oxygen-containing compounds. It is a crucial reaction in which there is rapid release of reactive oxygen such as superoxide and H_2O_2.

- Phagocytosis is completed after the stage of killing is over.
- A neutrophil can usually phagocytose 5–20 bacteria, before it itself becomes inactivated or dead.
- Neutrophils are not capable of phagocytosing particles much larger than bacteria.
- Neutrophils killed by the toxins released from the bacteria are collected in the centre of infected area. These are called pus cells and together with plasma leaked from the blood vessels, liquefied tissue cells and red blood cells escaped from the damaged capillaries constitute the pus.

Applied Aspects

Defective phagocytic functions

Defective phagocytic functions make the patients prone to recurrent infections. The following abnormalities may be associated with defective phagocytic functions:

1. ***Defective chemotaxis*** occurs in the following conditions:
   - Lazy leucocyte syndrome, a rare congenital abnormality
   - Corticosteroid therapy
   - Aspirin ingestion
   - Alcoholism
   - Myeloid leukaemia
2. ***Defective phagocytosis due to lack of opsonization*** occurs:
   - In hypogammaglobulinaemia
   - In hypocomplementaemia
   - After splenectomy
   - In sickle cell disease
3. ***Defective killing by phagocytes*** occurs in:
   - *Chronic granulomatous diseases of childhood:* In this condition, there is failure to generate superoxide radical (O_2^-) in both neutrophils and monocytes, leading to inability to kill the phagocytosed bacteria.
   - *Chediak–Higashi syndrome* is an autosomal recessive disorder associated with reduced chemotaxis and phagolysosomal fusion.
   - *Congenital MPO deficiency:* During phagocytosis, enzymes NADPH oxidase and MPO are mainly responsible for killing of invading organism. MPO helps catalysing the formation of oxidants. Therefore, due to its deficiency, microbial killing power is reduced but not absent, because most of the oxygen-dependent bactericidal mechanism remains intact.
   - *Rheumatoid arthritis:* In this disease, the enzyme NADPH in the neutrophils may cause local destruction of the host tissue.
   - *Severe congenital glucose-6-phosphate deficiency* leads to failure in NADPH production, and thus O_2^- generation. Multiple infections occur in this condition due to defective killing of organisms.
   - *Amyotrophic lateral sclerosis,* mutation of SOD-encoding gene, results in defective absence of SOD. In this disease, there is accumulation of O_2^- molecule in motor neurons which destroys them.
4. ***Neutrophil hypomotility*** is associated with decreased phagocytosis. In this condition, actin present in the neutrophils does not polymerize normally; therefore, neutrophils move slowly.

Inflammation

Inflammation is a protective tissue reaction or tissue change complex brought about by the substances released from the injured tissue or in response to foreign substances such as bacteria.

Cardinal signs or characteristics of inflammation are redness, swelling, tenderness or pain and local rise in the temperature.

Types of inflammations are acute inflammation and chronic inflammation.

Acute inflammation refers to initial body response towards harmful stimulus. It can be divided into the following phases:

Vascular phase – in this phase (Fig. 3.3.6):

- Vasodilatation of local blood vessels occurs.
- Leakage of large quantity of fluid into the interstitial spaces (due to increased capillary permeability and its clotting due to leakage of fibrinogen and other clotting factors) occurs.
- Nitrous oxide plays an important role.

Cellular phase – in this phase:

- Migration of large number of granulocytes and monocytes into the tissue occurs.
- Swelling of the tissue occurs.

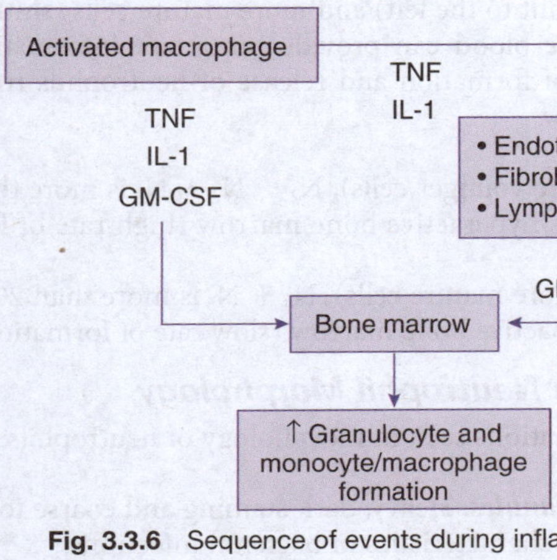

Fig. 3.3.6 Sequence of events during inflammation.

The substances released from the injured tissues include histamine, serotonin, prostaglandins, lymphokines, reaction products of complement and clotting system.

Events during inflammation In inflammation, tissue macrophages are the first line of defence against infection. Within an hour or so, neutrophils from the blood invade the inflamed area. Therefore:

- Within few hours, there is an acute increase in neutrophil count (neutrophilia) that may go up to 4000–5000/µL.
- Along with neutrophils, monocytes also enter inflamed tissue and enlarge to become macrophages. As mentioned earlier, macrophages can phagocytize about five times more bacteria and larger particles (including even neutrophil and necrotic tissue).
- The next reaction is increased production of granulocytes and monocytes in the bone marrow as a result of stimulation of GM-progenitor cells, due to the release of CSFs (GM-CSF). A powerful feedback mechanism to remove the cause of inflammation is provided by GM-CSF, along with TNF and IL-1.

Walling-off effect of inflammation is to wall off the area of injury from remaining tissue. This effect is brought about by blockage of tissue spaces and lymphatics by clotting of tissue fluid by fibrinogen. The walling-off process is important for delaying the spread of infection.

Chronic inflammation occurs when there is failure to eradicate the cause of acute inflammation; it is a long-term inflammation that lasts for months to years, e.g. tuberculosis and leprosy.

Depending on the defence mechanism of body, the outcome of the inflammation is depicted in Fig. 3.3.7.

Important Note

- **Nuclear factor-κB** (NF-κB) is a transcription factor that plays a key role in the inflammatory response. NF-κB normally exists as bound form to IκBα (inactive state) in the cytoplasm of the cell. The stimuli such as cytokines, oxidants and viruses separate NF-κB from IκBα. Free NF-κB enters the nucleus and gets bound to DNA of genes, responsible for inflammatory mediators and causing increase in their production and secretion.
- **Glucocorticoids:** *The anti-inflammatory action of* glucocorticoids is by increasing the production of IκBα to inhibit NF-κB activity.

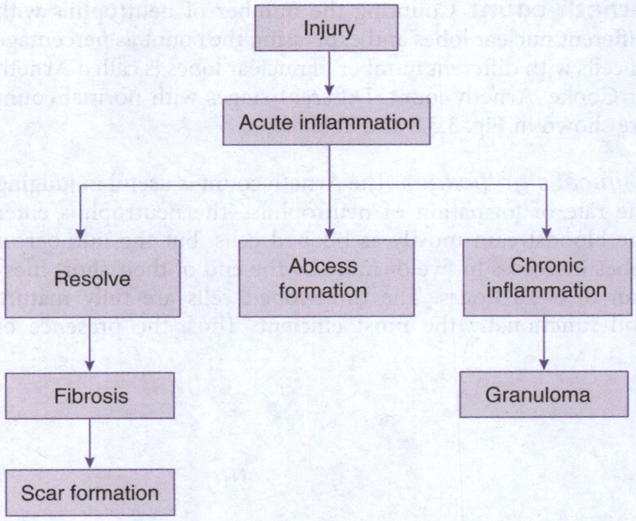

Fig. 3.3.7 Flow diagram showing outcome of inflammatory reaction.

Variations in Counts

Neutrophilia Neutrophilia refers to increase in the circulating neutrophil counts (absolute count >10,000/mm^3). It is the commonest cause of leucocytosis.

Physiological causes of neutrophilia:

- Newborn babies
- After exercise
- After meals
- Pregnancy
- Menstruation
- Parturition
- Lactation
- Mental stress and emotional stress
- After injection of epinephrine

Pathological causes of neutrophilia:

- Acute pyogenic bacterial infections
- Noninfective inflammatory conditions like gout and acute rheumatic fever
- Acute tissue destruction as in:
  Burns
  Postoperatively
  Myocardial infarction
- Acute haemorrhage
- Myeloproliferative disorders like polycythaemia vera
- Poisoning by chemicals and drugs like lead and mercury
- Poisoning by insect venom
- Intoxicating conditions like uraemia and diabetic ketoacidosis

Neutropenia Decrease in neutrophil count is known as neutropenia (absolute count <2500/mm^3).

Causes of neutropenia:

- Typhoid and paratyphoid fever
- Malaria
- Aplasia of bone marrow
- Bone marrow depression due to:
  - *Drugs* such as Chloromycetin and cytotoxic drugs used in malignant diseases
  - *Repeated exposure* to X-rays and radiations
  - *Chemical poisons* like arsenic

Arneth count Counting the number of neutrophils with different nuclear lobes and expressing the count as percentage of cells with different number of nuclear lobes is called Arneth or Cooke–Arneth count. Different stages with normal count are shown in Fig. 3.3.8 and Table 3.3.2.

Clinical significance The Arneth count is useful in judging the rate of formation of neutrophils. The neutrophils enter the bloodstream mostly as bilobed cells, but the number of lobes increases to five or more by the end of their short lifespan of 8–10 hours. The three-lobed cells are fully mature and functionally the most efficient. Thus, the presence of younger cells (shift to the left) and more mature cells (shift to the right) in the blood can provide important information about the rate of formation and release of neutrophils from the bone marrow.

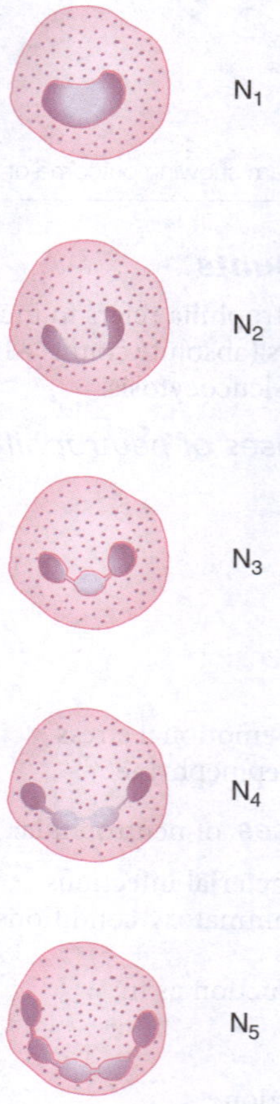

Fig. 3.3.8 Stages of Cooke–Arneth count.

Table 3.3.2 Cooke–Arneth count

Stage	Nuclear lobes	Normal count (%)
• Stage I (N_1)	1 (the nucleus is C-shaped)	5–10
• Stage II (N_2)	2 lobes are connected by a filament	20–30
• Stage III (N_3)	3 lobes connected by chromatin filament	40–50
• Stage IV (N_4)	4 lobes connected by chromatin filament	10–15
• Stage V (N_5)	5 lobes or more	3–5

In left shift (more younger cells), $N_1 + N_2 + N_3$ is more than 80%. It indicates hyperactive bone marrow (high rate of formation).
In right shift (more mature cells), $N_4 + N_5$ is more than 20%. It indicates hypoactive bone marrow (slow rate of formation).

Variations in Neutrophil Morphology

Some of the variations seen in morphology of neutrophils:

Variations in granules: Heavy, dark staining and coarse toxic granules are the characteristics of bacterial infections.
Formation of vacuoles in cytoplasm: Cytoplasmic vacuolation may develop in bacterial infections such as in septicaemia.
Formation of Dohle bodies in cytoplasm: Dohle bodies are small, round or oval patches, 2–3 µm in size seen in the cytoplasm of neutrophils (Fig. 3.3.9A) in patients with bacterial infections.
Presence of sex chromatin with nuclear lobes: Sex chromatin is a normal finding seen in 2%–3% of neutrophils in females. It consists of a drumstick appendage of chromatin about 1 µm across, and attached to one of the nuclear lobes by a thin chromatin strand (Fig. 3.3.9B). Its presence is indicative of 2X chromosomes.
Hypersegmented neutrophils: Presence of hypersegmented (more than five nuclear lobes) neutrophils in the peripheral blood (Fig. 3.3.9C) is called a *shift-to-right*. It is indicative of a hypoactive bone marrow, as seen in megaloblastic anaemia and uraemia.
Band and star form neutrophil: Presence of band and star form neutrophils, i.e. premature neutrophils with decreased nuclear lobes (Fig. 3.3.1), in the peripheral blood is called *shift-to-left*. It is indicative of hyperactive bone marrow, as seen in severe infections and leukaemias.
Pelger–Huet anomaly: It is an inherited disorder in which majority of the neutrophils have decreased number of nuclear segments (one to two) and coarsely staining chromatin. The nuclei appear rod like, dumbbell like or spectacle like (Fig. 3.3.9D).

EOSINOPHILS

Morphological Features

Morphological features of eosinophils (Fig. 3.3.4B) are as follows:

Diameter: Diameter of eosinophils is similar to that of neutrophils, i.e. 10–14 µm.

Nucleus: Nucleus is purple in colour and is bilobed in 85% of the cells. The two lobes are connected by the chromatin strands and thus looked spectacle shaped. The remaining 15% of the eosinophils have trilobed nucleus.

Cytoplasm: Cytoplasm is acidophilic and appears bright pink in colour. It contains coarse, deep red-staining granules which do not cover the nucleus.

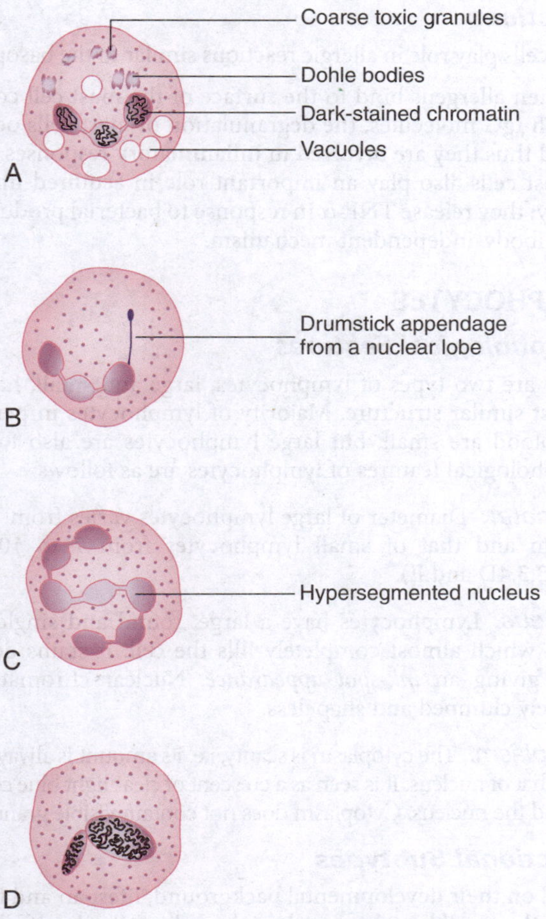

Fig. 3.3.9 Some variations in neutrophil morphology: **A,** Dohle bodies; **B,** female sex chromatin; **C,** hypersegmented neutrophil; and **D,** hereditary Pelger–Huet anomaly.

The granules of eosinophil are as follows:

- *Azurophilic granules* are primary granules containing acid hydrolase and other enzymes.
- *Specific granules.*

The granules in eosinophils contain basic protein and stain more intensely for peroxidase than granules in the neutrophils.

The granules contain histamine, lysosomal enzymes eosinophil chemotactic factor of anaphylaxis (ECF-A).

Functions of Eosinophils

1. Mild phagocytosis. Eosinophils are not very motile and thus have very mild phagocytic activity. Like neutrophils, eosinophils are attracted towards the endothelial cells by selectins and enter the tissue by diapedesis.

2. Role in parasitic infestations. Eosinophils play an important role in the defence mechanism of body, especially in *parasitic infestations.* Eosinophils get attached to the larvae of parasites and helminths coated with immunoglobulin and release the granules the following lethal substances present in their granules:

Major basic protein (MBP) makes up about 50% of the mass of large granules. It is a highly *larvicidal* polypeptide. Because of this, eosinophils are able to damage the parasitic *larvae,* which are large to be engulfed by phagocytosis.

Eosinophil cationic protein (ECP) is a potent bactericidal and major destroyer of helminths. It is about 10 times more potent than MBP in destroying helminths by means of complete disintegration. It is also a neurotoxin.

Eosinophil peroxidase is capable of destroying helminths, bacteria and tumour cells.

Eosinophil-derived neurotoxin is capable of destroying the nerve fibres.

3. Role in allergic reaction. The eosinophils increase in number in allergic conditions like bronchial asthma and hay fever.

- They are capable of *detoxifying* inflammation-inducing substances (released by mast cells and basophils) like histamine and bradykinin.
- They inhibit mast cell degranulation.
- They phagocytose and destroy antigen–antibody complexes and thus prevent spread of local inflammatory process.
- *Arylsulphatase B,* present in the fine granules of eosinophils, has the ability of inactivating sulphur-containing leukotrienes that tissue mast cells liberate in immediate hypersensitivity reactions.
- *Lysophospholipase* is an unusual membrane-bound protein present in the eosinophils, which forms crystals called *Charcot–Leyden crystals* in the pulmonary secretions of patients with bronchial asthma.

4. Role in immunity. The eosinophils are present in abundance in the mucosa of respiratory tract, gastrointestinal tract and urinary tract, where they probably provide mucosal immunity.

Variation in Counts

Eosinophilia Eosinophilia refers to increase in the eosinophil count (absolute count $>500/mm^3$).

Causes of eosinophilia:

- Allergic conditions like bronchial asthma and hay fever
- Tropical pulmonary eosinophilia
- Parasitic infestation, e.g. intestinal worms like hookworm, roundworm and tapeworm
- Skin diseases like urticaria
- Scarlet fever

Eosinopenia Eosinopenia is the decrease in eosinophil count (absolute count $<50/mm^3$).

Causes of eosinopenia:

- ACTH and steroid therapy
- Stressful conditions
- Acute pyogenic infections

BASOPHILS

Morphological Features (Fig. 3.3.4C)

Diameter: Diameter of a basophil is similar to that of neutrophil and eosinophil, i.e. 10–14 μm.

Nucleus: Nucleus of basophils is irregular, may be bilobed or trilobed, and its boundary is not clearly defined because of overcrowding with coarse granules.

Cytoplasm: Cytoplasm of basophils is slightly basophilic and appears blue. It is full of granules.

- Granules of basophils are very coarse and stain deep purple or blue with basic (methylene) dye.
- Granules are in plenty and completely fill the cell and overload the nucleus.
- The granules of basophils contain heparin, histamine and 5-HT (5-hydroxytryptamine).

Functions

1. Mild phagocytosis. Basophils have very mild phagocytic function.

2. Role in allergic reaction. Basophils also enter the tissue and release cytokine and inflammatory mediators such as histamine, bradykinin, slow-reacting substances of anaphylaxis (SRS-A) and serotonin (5-HT). These substances, in turn, cause local vascular and tissue reactions that cause allergic manifestations by binding of specific antigen to cell-fixed IgE molecules (for details, see pages 182 and 193).

3. Role in preventing spread of allergic inflammatory process. Basophils also release eosinophil chemotactic factor that causes eosinophils to migrate towards the inflamed allergic tissue. Eosinophils then phagocytose and destroy the antigen–antibody complexes and prevent spread of local inflammatory process.

Important Note

Although eosinophils and basophils play opposite roles during allergic condition, they act in a balanced way to manage the condition.

4. Release of heparin. Basophils release heparin in the blood, which:

- Prevents clotting of the blood.
- Activates the enzyme lipoprotein lipase which removes fat particles from the blood after a fatty meal.

Variation in Counts

Basophilia Basophilia refers to increase in the basophil count (absolute count $>100/\text{mm}^3$).

Causes of basophilia:

- Viral infections, e.g. influenza, smallpox and chickenpox
- Allergic diseases
- Chronic myeloid leukaemia (CML)

Basopenia Decrease in basophil count is called basopenia.

Causes of basopenia:

- Corticosteroid therapy
- Drug-induced reactions
- Acute pyogenic infections

MAST CELLS

Mast cells are large tissue cells resembling the basophils. These are present in bone marrow and immediately outside the capillaries in the skin. Mast cells are granulated cells of connective tissue; their granules contain proteoglycans, histamine and many proteases.

Functions

Mast cells play role in allergic reactions similar to the basophils.

- When allergens bind to the surface of the mast cell coated with IgG molecules, the degranulation of mast cells occurs and thus they are involved in inflammatory responses.
- Mast cells also play an important role in acquired immunity; they release TNF-α in response to bacterial product by antibody-independent mechanism.

LYMPHOCYTES

Morphological Features

There are two types of lymphocytes, large and small, having almost similar structure. Majority of lymphocytes in peripheral blood are small, but large lymphocytes are also found. Morphological features of lymphocytes are as follows:

Diameter: Diameter of large lymphocytes varies from 12 to 16 μm and that of small lymphocytes from 7 to 10 μm (Fig. 3.3.4D and E).

Nucleus: Lymphocytes have a large, round and single nucleus, which almost completely fills the cell. It stains deeply blue, giving an *ink-spot appearance*. Nuclear chromatin is coarsely clumped and shapeless.

Cytoplasm: The cytoplasm is scanty, i.e. its amount is always less than that of nucleus. It is seen as a crescent of clear light blue colour around the nucleus. Cytoplasm does not contain visible granules.

Functional Subtypes

Based on their developmental background, lifespan and functions, the small lymphocytes have been broadly classified into three subtypes (Fig. 3.3.10):

1. B lymphocytes, which are processed in the bone marrow, are concerned with the humoral immunity.

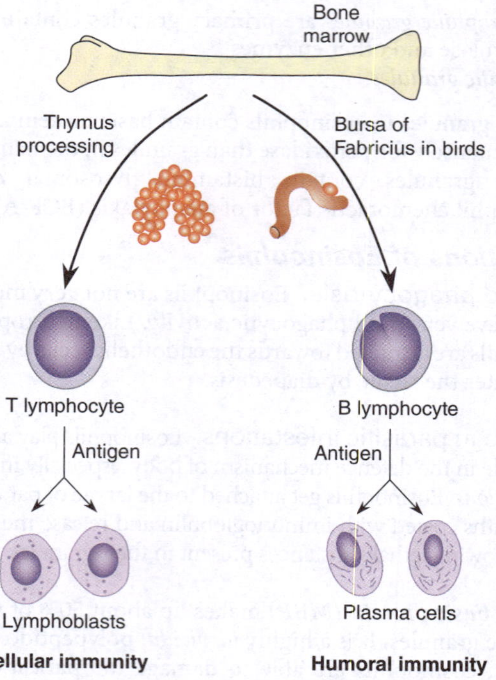

Fig. 3.3.10 Processing of stem cells in thymus and bone marrow to become immunocompetent T and B lymphocytes.

2. T lymphocytes, which are processed in the thymus, are concerned with the cellular immunity.

3. Natural killer (NK) cells are lymphocyte-like cells that nonspecifically kill any cell that is coated with immunoglobulin IgG. This phenomenon is called *antigen-dependent cell-mediated cytotoxicity (ADCC)*. Thus, NK cells provide *innate immunity*. They are highly cytotoxic against tumour cells and virus-infected cells.

The aforementioned functional subtypes of lymphocytes are not morphologically distinguishable, but they have distinctive surface molecules that are identifiable by immunochemical methods. The NK cells lack identifying surface markers.

Kinetics, Lifespan and Fate of Lymphocytes

- After processing, the T lymphocytes (processed in the thymus) and B lymphocytes (processed in the bone marrow; B stands for 'bursa of Fabricius', the site of B-cell processing in birds) enter the circulation where they are present in an approximately 70:30 ratio.
- Many of the lymphocytes remain in circulation for a few hours, and then leak out through the venules and settle in the *peripheral lymphoid tissues*, which include lymph nodes and spleen.
- GALT and lymphoid tissue are associated with respiratory and urinary tracts. At any given time, only about 2% of the body lymphocytes are in the peripheral lymphoid tissue.
- Some of the lymphocytes re-enter the blood circulation through the lymphatics, draining the peripheral lymphoid tissues. In this manner, they recirculate for months or years. Thus, the lymphocytes have a lifespan of months or a year depending on body's need for these cells.

Functions

Lymphocytes play an important role in immunity. *Immunity* is the capacity of human body to resist all types of microorganisms and toxins that tend to damage the tissue or organ. Functionally, the lymphocytes are classified into two types – B lymphocytes and T lymphocytes.

Functions of B lymphocytes. B lymphocytes as well as their derivatives, the plasma cells, are responsible for the development of *humoral immunity*, also called antibody-mediated immunity (AMI). B lymphocytes produce antibodies (gamma globulins) which circulate in the blood and constitute the humoral immunity. Humoral immunity is the major mechanism of defence against the invading organisms, especially the bacteria. Antibodies fight against the invading organisms:

- By direct action.
- By making them inactive by agglutination, precipitation, neutralization or lysis.
- Through complement system.

Functions of T lymphocytes. T lymphocytes are responsible for the development of *cellular immunity*, also called cell-mediated immunity (CMI) or T-cell immunity. CMI plays an important defensive role against:

- Viral infections.
- Some bacterial infections.
- Tumour cells.

T lymphocytes are associated primarily with two main functions in immune mechanism:

1. ***Cellular immune reactions and hypersensitivity reactions:***
   - Cellular immune reactions are mediated by the T lymphocytes such as cytotoxic or killer T cells ($CD3^+$) and $CD8^+$ T cells.
   - Hypersensitivity reaction is mediated by $CD4^+$ T cells.
2. ***Immunoregulatory function:*** The $CD4^+$ helper cells regulate the immune mechanism by regulating the function of other T cells, B cells and haemopoietic stem cells.

For details of the role of lymphocytes in immunity, see page 183.

Variations in Count

Lymphocytosis Lymphocytosis refers to increase in the lymphocyte count (absolute count >4000/mm^3).

Physiological causes of lymphocytosis:

- *In healthy infants and young children*, the lymphocyte count is usually high (about 60% in DLC) while the TLC is normal (relative lymphocytosis).
- *In females*, during menstruation, lymphocytes are increased.

Pathological causes of lymphocytosis:

- Chronic infections like tuberculosis, hepatitis and whooping cough
- Viral infections like chickenpox
- Autoimmune diseases like thyrotoxicosis
- Infectious mononucleosis
- Lymphatic leukaemia (most common cause of lymphocytes; >10,000/mm^3)

Lymphopenia Lymphopenia or lymphocytopenia refers to decrease in the lymphocyte count (absolute count less than 1500/mm^3).

Causes of lymphopenia:

- Patients on corticosteroid and immunosuppressive therapy
- Hypoplastic bone marrow
- Widespread irradiation
- Acquired immunodeficiency syndrome (AIDS; see page 195)

MONOCYTES

Morphological Features (Fig. 3.3.4F)

Diameter: Monocyte is the largest mature leucocyte in the peripheral blood measuring approximately 12–20 μm in diameter.

Nucleus: The nucleus of monocyte is large, single and eccentric in position, i.e. present on one side of the cell. It may be notched or indented, i.e. horseshoe or kidney shaped. It may appear oval or rounded in side view. Nucleus has characteristically fine reticulated chromatin network.

Cytoplasm: The cytoplasm is abundant, pale blue and usually clear (no granules); sometimes, it may contain fine purple, dust-like granules called *azur granules* which may be few or numerous.

Kinetics, Lifespan and Fate of Monocytes

- The kinetics of monocytes is less well understood than that of granulocytes.
- After release from the bone marrow, the monocytes remain in circulation for 10–20 to over 40 hours and then they leave the blood to enter the extravascular tissues.

- In the tissues, the monocytes get converted to macrophages and form the part of so-called *tissue macrophage system* (reticuloendothelial system). In the tissues, they can live for months or even years unless destroyed while performing the phagocytic function.

Functions

1. Role in defence mechanism Monocytes along with neutrophils play important role in the body's defence mechanism. Their main function is *phagocytosis*. Monocytes after entering the tissue get converted to macrophages. These are more powerful phagocytes than neutrophils and are capable of phagocytosing as many as 100 bacteria. They also have the ability to engulf large particles such as red blood cells and malarial parasites.

The process of phagocytosis by monocytes is similar to that described in neutrophils (see page 162).

2. Precursor of tissue macrophages Monocytes are the precursors of tissue macrophages. The mature monocytes stay in the blood only for few (10–20) hours. Then they leave the blood to enter the extravascular tissue and get converted into tissue macrophages (for details, see page 173).

3. Role in tumour immunity Monocytes may also kill tumour cells after sensitization by lymphocytes.

4. Synthesis of biological substances. Monocytes synthesize complement and other biologically important substances.

Variations in Count

Monocytosis A rise in the blood monocytes above 800/mm^3 is termed monocytosis.

Causes of monocytosis:

- *Certain bacterial infections* such as tuberculosis, syphilis and subacute bacterial endocarditis
- *Infectious mononucleosis* or the so-called glandular fever
- *Viral infections*
- *Protozoal* and rickettsial infections, e.g. malaria and kala-azar
- *Haemopoietic disorders* like monocytic leukaemia and myeloproliferative disorders
- *Collagen vascular disorder*

Monocytopenia Monocytopenia refers to decrease in the monocyte count.

Causes: Monocytopenia is rare. It may be seen in hypoplastic bone marrow.

Applied Aspects

Leukaemoid reactions

Leukaemoid reaction refers to a reactive excessive leukocytosis in the peripheral blood resembling that of leukaemia in a subject who does not have leukaemia. In spite of confusing blood picture, the leukaemoid reactions are characterized by:

- Absence of the clinical features of leukaemia such as splenomegaly, lymphadenopathy and haemorrhages.
- Presence of the features of underlying disorders causing leukaemoid reaction, such as infections, intoxication and malignant diseases.
- Leucocyte alkaline phosphate enzyme is increased in leukaemoid reaction but not in leukaemia.

Types of leukaemoid reactions Leukaemoid reaction may be myeloid or lymphoid.

1. ***Myeloid leukaemoid reaction*** is characterized by *leucocytosis*, usually moderate, not exceeding 100,000/mm^3. In majority of the cases, the granulocyte series is involved.
2. ***Lymphoid leukaemoid reaction*** is also characterized by moderate leucocytosis. TLC usually does not exceed 100,000/mm^3. DLC reveals mostly mature lymphocytes simulating the blood picture seen in chronic lymphoid leukaemia.

Leukaemias

Leukaemias constitute a group of malignant diseases of the blood in which there occurs an increase in the total WBC count associated with the presence of immature WBCs in the peripheral blood. The total WBC count is usually above 50,000/mm^3 and may be as high as 100,000–300,000/mm^3.

- The proliferation of leukaemic cells takes place primarily in the bone marrow and in certain form in the lymphoid tissues.
- There are associated features of:
  - Bone marrow failure (e.g. anaemia and thrombocytopenia).
  - Involvement of other organs (e.g. liver, spleen, lymph nodes, meninges, brain, skin).

Types of leukaemias Leukaemias account for 4% of all cancer deaths. They are classified on the basis of cell types predominantly into *myeloid* (involving cells derived from the myeloid stem cells) and *lymphoid* (involving the cells derived from lymphoid stem cells). On the basis of natural history of disease, each variety can be divided into *acute* and *chronic* types. In this way, the main types of leukaemias are as follows:

Acute myeloid leukaemia (AML) is a type of cancer in which there is rapid and abnormal growth of myeloid line of cells in the bone marrow.

Causes: The exact cause of most childhood leukaemias is not known but certain changes in the DNA inside the bone marrow cells can cause them to become leukaemia cells. Common type of DNA change that can lead to leukaemia is chromosome translocation.

Chronic myeloid leukaemia (CML) is a blood cancer in which bone marrow produces too many white cells (i.e. granulocytes). The cells gradually crowd the bone marrow interfering with normal blood cell production.

Acute lymphoblastic leukaemia (ALL) is a type of cancer in which there is formation of rapid and enormous growth of lymphoid line of cells characterised by a large number of immature lymphocytes.

Chronic lymphocytic leukaemia (CLL) is a cancer that affects lymphocytes. CLL usually grows slowly; therefore, symptoms may not appear for years. CLL results in build-up of B lymphocytes in the bone marrow, lymph nodes and blood. These cells do not function properly and crowd over the normal healthy blood cells.

Causes. CLL is caused by multiple genetic mutations and epigenetic changes. CLL is divided into two main types – hose with mutated *IgHV* gene and those without. It can spread to lymph node and other organs such as liver and spleen.

Signs and symptoms of leukaemia Many patients with slow-growing types of leukaemia do not have symptoms. But rapidly growing types of leukaemia may cause symptoms that include:

- Fever or chills
- Persistent fatigue and weakness
- Frequent infections
- Weight loss
- Swollen lymph nodes, enlarged liver or spleen
- Easy bleeding or bruising and petechiae

Diagnosis The diagnosis of leukaemia is based on the following:

- Abnormal WBC count
- Complete blood count (CBC)
- Bone marrow examination
- Blood chemistry
- Bleeding and clotting factors
- To confirm and to identify specific type of leukaemia, a needle biopsy and aspiration of bone marrow is done for testing leukaemia cells
- Cytochemistry
- Immunophenotyping
- Cytogenic and molecular studies (e.g. DNA markers and chromosomal changes)

Treatment Treatment for leukaemia is highly variable and depends on severity. For slow-growing leukaemia, treatment may include monitoring and that for aggressive state; treatment includes chemotherapy that sometimes is followed by radiations and stem cell transplant.

Chemotherapy kills the cells which are growing or multiplying at faster rate.

Blood transfusion: Blood components are administered to replace the deficiencies in the bloodstream.

Medical procedures include haemopoietic stem cell transplantation.

Surgical: Surgical removal of spleen if there is enlargement of spleen.

Self-Assessment

1. Discuss the different types of leucocytes and their characteristic features.
2. Describe the regulation of leucopoiesis.
3. Describe the process of phagocytosis.
4. Write short notes on:
   - Variations of leucocyte counts
   - Functions of eosinophils
   - Inflammation
   - Functions of monocyte

Clinical Cases

Case 1

A 50-year-old male patient complains of; shortness of breath, chest tightness, wheezing sounds during exhalation and coughing particularly during harvesting season (March and April).

Investigations reveal X-ray chest normal.

Blood tests show increased eosinophil count (absolute and DLC).

Q1. What is the probable diagnosis?

Q2. What is the role of eosinophils in this condition?

Case 2

A 30-year-old male patient presents with history of frequent episodes of fever and infection, Bone pain, lethargy, fatigue, pale skin, easy bruising and bleeding from nose and gums.

Haematological investigations reveal:

- Decrease in Hb, RBC and platelet count
- Abnormal high WBC count
- Bone marrow biopsy shows cancerous cells

Q1. What is the probable diagnosis?

Q2. What are further tests to be done to conclude final diagnosis?

3.4 Immune Mechanisms

CHAPTER OUTLINE

INTRODUCTION

Immunity refers to resistance of the body to pathogens and their toxic products. Various aspects in relation to the immune mechanisms which need detailed discussion are introduced briefly.

Types of immunity Immunity primarily is of two types: innate immunity which is present by birth, and acquired or adaptive immunity which is achieved during the lifetime by the individual.

Antigens Antigens are substances that can stimulate an immune response in the body.

Antibodies Antibodies or immunoglobulins (Igs) are gamma globulins which are produced in response to antigenic stimulation.

Immune system The immune system that constitutes the body's defence system consists of lymphoid organs, reticulo-endothelial components and the various types of immunological cells distributed throughout the body.

Immune response The immune system of the body responds to an antigen by two ways:

- *Humoral or antibody-mediated immunity (AMI)* which is mediated by antibodies produced by plasma cells
- *Cell-mediated immunity (CMI)* which is mediated directly by the sensitized lymphocytes

Immune tolerance Immune tolerance refers to the inability of a host to express a specific immunological response to an antigen.

Autoimmunity It refers to the condition when the body's immune response gets directed towards its own tissues which are normally exempted as self.

Immunomodulation It refers to the process of modifying the body's immune response. It may be in the form of:

- *Immunoenhancement (immunopotentiation)*, i.e. to enhance the antibody- or cell-mediated immune response against an antigen
- *Immunosuppression*, i.e. to reduce the body's immune response against the antigens

Hypersensitivity It refers to an abnormal immune response which produces physiological or histopathological damage in the host.

ARCHITECTURE (COMPONENTS) OF IMMUNE SYSTEM

The immune system which constitutes the body's defence system consists of immunological cells distributed into two main components:

1. Mononuclear phagocytic system (MPS)
2. Lymphoid component

MONONUCLEAR PHAGOCYTIC SYSTEM

MPS, also known as *tissue macrophage system*, is the new name given to the system previously called *reticuloendothelial system* (*RES*).

Formation of mononuclear phagocytic system The monocytes enter the blood from the bone marrow and circulate for about 3 days. From the blood, the monocytes migrate into the tissue where they attain maturity, i.e. they increase in size and a large number of lysosomes and mitochondria develop in their cytoplasm. In this way, they acquire the ability to phagocytose and thus get converted to macrophages. The macrophages wander through tissues (*mobile macrophages*) and perform scavenger functions of eliminating microorganisms and other foreign particles that invade the tissues. Some of these macrophages become attached to certain tissues in the body (*fixed macrophages*) and remain there for several months. These tissue macrophages scattered in different parts of the body combinedly constitute the *tissue macrophage system* or the so-called *MPS*. The tissue macrophage system includes the macrophages present at the following sites in the body:

- Macrophages lining the sinusoids of liver (Kupffer cells)
- Spleen
- Bone marrow (littoral cells)
- Lymph nodes
- Lungs (pulmonary alveolar macrophages [PAM], also called dust cells)
- Connective tissue (histiocytes)
- Pleura and peritoneum
- Subcutaneous tissue
- Bones (osteoclasts)
- Central nervous system (microglial cells)

Constituent cells of mononuclear phagocytic system The term MPS was coined in 1960 to include the following constituents:

- Precursor cells of the monocyte series from bone marrow
- Promonocytes from the bone marrow
- Monocytes from the bone marrow and blood
- Tissue macrophages present in the above-cited sites in the body

The MPS does not include the following cells which were included in the RES:

- Reticulum cells of the spleen and lymph nodes
- Endothelial cells
- Fibroblasts

Functions of mononuclear phagocytic system The MPS functions as a physiological unit, i.e. if any part of it is put out of action, the rest of the system undergoes compensatory hypertrophy and makes up the deficiency. The MPS plays the following roles in the body.

1. Role in inflammation and healing The cells of MPS ingest cell debris, broken-down RBCs, fibrin and bacteria from the inflamed area and promote healing process.

2. Role in defence against the bacteria invading the body tissues These cells ingest the invading bacteria and are thus concerned with the defence of the body against the bacteria. During infection, these cells rapidly increase in number resulting in enlargement of the organs which are rich in these cells, e.g. spleen and lymph nodes.

3. Role in the immune response Role in the immune response played by MPS:

- The cells of MPS ingest and process the antigen entering the body. The processing of antigen is essential before an antigen can evoke CMI or stimulate antibody formation in plasma cells.
- The cells of MPS have receptors for Igs and complements, so these are very efficient in phagocytosing the antigen–antibody complement complexes.

4. Role in removal of old RBCs The aged RBCs or those damaged by the action of antibodies are removed by the cells of MPS in different organs like spleen, bone marrow and liver.

5. Role in removal of old WBCs and platelets Like RBCs, WBCs and platelets are also removed by the cells of MPS system.

6. Storage function The cells of MPS store excess lipids and mucoprotein and become swollen.

LYMPHOID ORGANS

The lymphoid component of the immune system consists of a network of lymphoid organs, tissues and cells and the product of these cells. Lymphoid organs can be classified into:

A. ***Central or primary lymphoid organs***, which include:
   I. Thymus
   II. Bursa equivalent (fetal liver and bone marrow)

B. ***Peripheral lymphoid organs***, which include:
   I. Lymph nodes
   II. Spleen
   III. Mucosa-associated lymphoid tissues (MALT)

Primary (Central) Lymphoid Tissues

Thymus

The thymus gland is a complex lymphoreticular organ located in mediastinum just above the heart. It consists of two (right and left) encapsulated lobes joined together by a fibrous connective tissue. Each lobe is divided into many lobules. Histologically, each lobule consists of outer *cortex* and inner *medulla*. Both cortex and medulla consist of two types of cells:

Epithelial cells. These cells form a network in which thymocytes and macrophages are found.

Thymocytes refer to the immature lymphocytes predominantly present in the cortex and mature lymphocytes mainly present in the medulla. Lymphocytes produced in the thymus are called thymus-derived lymphocytes or T lymphocytes or simply T cells. Lymphocyte proliferation in thymus is not dependent on antigenic stimulation.

Role of thymus in the immune system The main function of the thymus is development of CMI. The stem cells destined to form T lymphocytes leave the bone marrow and migrate to the thymus where they further differentiate.

- The thymus confers immunological competence on the lymphocytes during their stay in the organ. In the thymus, T lymphocytes are educated so that they become capable of mounting a cell-mediated immune response against an appropriate antigen. This is affected under the influence of the thymic microenvironment and several hormones, such as *thymosin* and *thymopoietin*, produced by the thymic epithelium.
- The *immunologically competent lymphocytes* migrate from thymus into peripheral lymphoid organs as mature T lymphocytes which are precommitted to their function and antigen specificity. These are selectively seeded into paracortical areas of peripheral lymph nodes and into the white pulp of the spleen around the central arterioles. These regions are known as *thymus-dependent* areas.

Applied Aspects

Effects of thymectomy

1. ***Thymectomy in newborn animals*** produces:
   - Lymphopenia and atrophy of peripheral lymphoid tissue
   - Suppression of delayed hypersensitivity reactions
   - Failure to reject foreign tissue grafts
   - Markedly increased susceptibility to infections
2. ***Thymectomy in adult animals*** produces immune deficiency after a few months, i.e. after the existing pool of immunologically competent lymphocytes is depleted.

   The above observations 1 and 2 prove that:
   - The thymus is responsible for development of immunologically competent T lymphocytes.
   - The thymus is also responsible for maintenance of an adequate pool of T lymphocytes in adult life.

Bursa Equivalent

In humans, the fetal liver and bone marrow appear to be the equivalent of avian bursa of Fabricius. *Bursa of Fabricius* in birds is also a site of lymphocytic proliferation and differentiation. Immunocompetent lymphocytes produced in the bursa are called bursa lymphocytes or B lymphocytes or B cells. The mature B cells migrate from the bursa into outer or superficial cortex of the germinal follicles and medullary cords of lymph nodes and lymphoid follicles of spleen. These sites are known as *bursa-dependent* or *thymus-independent* areas. Following appropriate antigenic stimulation, B lymphocytes transform into plasma cells and secrete antibodies which constitute the *humoral immunity* or *AMI*. Surgical removal of bursa (bursectomy) from newly hatched birds destroys their subsequent ability to produce antibodies but does not affect their ability to produce CMI.

Since fetal liver and bone marrow appear to be the mammalian equivalent of the avian bursa of Fabricius, the bone marrow is the site of not only haemopoiesis but also initial differentiation of stem cells to B lymphocytes.

Peripheral Lymphoid Organs

Lymph Nodes

The lymph nodes are small bean-shaped or oval structures which form part of the lymphatic network distributed throughout the body.

Structural characteristics of lymph node (Fig. 3.4.1)

Capsule of connective tissue covers each lymph node. From the capsule, trabeculae penetrate into the lymph node.

Afferent lymphatics enter each lymph node at its convex surface and drain into the peripheral subcapsular sinus.

Efferent lymphatics leave the lymph node at the concavity (hilum) as a single large lymph vessel.

Microscopically, the lymph node consists of two parts – peripheral cortex and central medulla.

- *Cortex* of the lymph node consists of several rounded aggregates of lymphocytes called *lymphoid follicles*. Each follicle has a pale-staining germinal centre surrounded by small dark-staining area of lymphocytes representing *B-cell area* of the node. Besides proliferating lymphocytes, the follicles contain dendritic macrophages which capture and process the antigens.

  Paracortex is the deeper part of cortex, i.e. the zone between the peripheral cortex and the inner medulla, and represents the *T-cell area (the bursa-independent area)*.
- *Medulla* is predominantly composed of cords of plasma cells and some lymphocytes *(medullary cords)*. The medullary cords contain B lymphocytes and along with the lymphoid follicles constitute the *bursa-dependent areas* of the lymph node.

Functions of lymph nodes

1. To mount immune response in the body. It is the main function of lymph nodes. A bulk of antigens is processed and antibody production occurs in the lymphoid follicles (for details, see page 183).

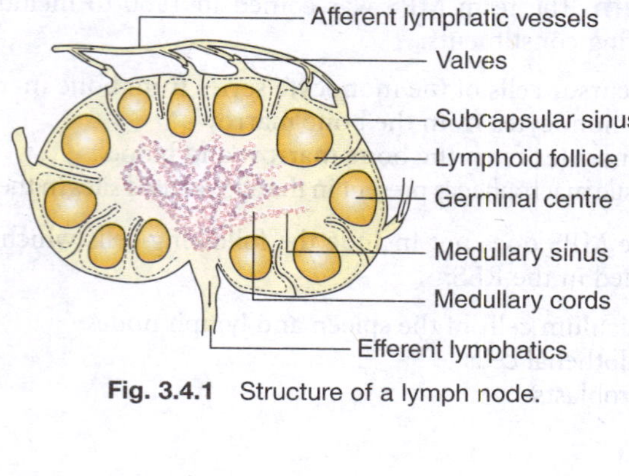

Fig. 3.4.1 Structure of a lymph node.

2. To perform the function of active phagocytosis for particulate material is another main function of the lymph nodes. The lymph nodes constitute a series of inline filters. Lymph must pass through at least one lymph node before mixing with the bloodstream. Over 99% of the lymph passes through the lymph sinuses, and only 1% penetrates the lymphoid follicles.

Spleen

The spleen is the largest lymphoid organ of the body. Under normal conditions, the average weight of the spleen is about 150 g.

Structural characteristics (Fig. 3.4.2) ***Capsule*** of connective tissue surrounds the spleen. From the capsule extend connective tissue *trabeculae* into the pulp of the organ and serve as a supportive network. Unlike some animals like cats and dogs, the capsule of human spleen contains very few smooth muscle fibres; hence, it is not capable of marked contraction.

Grossly on a cut section, the spleen consists of a homogeneous, soft, dark red mass called *red pulp*. In the red pulp, scattered white nodules called *white pulp* (Malpighian bodies) are seen.

Microscopically, the structural characteristics are as follows:

Red pulp consists of the thin-walled *blood sinuses* with *splenic cords* between them. The splenic cords consist of a collection of lymphocytes and macrophages arranged in cords in the fine network of reticular cells and fibres. This finer network forms a filtering bed that filters out red cells, white cells and platelets passing through the red pulp.

White pulp consists of lymphocytes surrounding an eccentrically placed central artery. These periarteriolar lymphocytes are mainly *T lymphocytes*. In addition, the white pulp also contains the lymphoid follicles composed principally of *B lymphocytes*.

Blood circulation. Blood enters the spleen by the *splenic artery* which divides into branches that penetrate the splenic tissue via trabeculae. From the trabeculae, small branches called *central arteries* arise. Each central artery gives off a number of *penicillar arterioles* which open into large, thin-walled blood *sinusoids*. From the sinusoids, the blood is drained into the venous channels. This pattern of circulation is called the *closed circulation*. According to another view, the spleen has an open circulation, i.e. the penicillar arterioles open into the fine network of red pulp. Ultimately, blood is drained into sinusoids and venous channels.

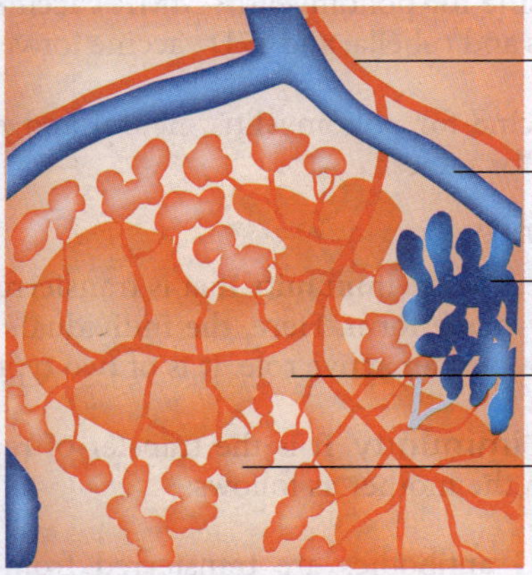

Fig. 3.4.2 Structure of spleen.

Functions of spleen are:

1. Role in immune response. The spleen constitutes an important component of the defence system. It is an active site for production of T and B lymphocytes and antibodies. Blood-borne antigens entering the spleen are phagocytosed and processed by macrophages and fixed phagocytic mononuclear cells. Presentation of antigens, on the surface of such cells, to the splenic lymphocytes results in the formation of secondary follicles containing germinal centres of dividing and differentiating B cells which ultimately form antibodies.

Important Note

After splenectomy, antibody production continues to occur in other lymphoid organs but the antibody response is delayed and the antibody titre does not rise as high as in normal individuals.

2. Role in removal of old RBCs, WBCs and platelets. Tissue macrophages present in the spleen like other components of the *MPS* play an important role in the removal of old RBCs, WBCs and platelets. The spleen seems to possess a special capability of trapping even mildly damaged erythrocytes. This ability has been attributed to the uniquely slow circulation of RBCs along the splenic cords where RBCs come in close contact with the splenic macrophages. This ability of spleen to detect and destroy abnormal type of blood cells is called *cutting action of spleen*.

3. Role in haematopoiesis. During the fourth and fifth months of fetal life, erythropoiesis occurs in spleen. In postnatal life, under pathological conditions when the entire bone marrow is exhausted, the spleen may become the site of *extramedullary erythropoiesis*.

4. Role in iron metabolism. Spleen macrophages have a special ability to recycle iron liberated from the phagocytosed RBCs, for synthesis of fresh haemoglobin in the bone marrow. Other tissue macrophages have this ability much less, and the lung macrophages (PAM) do not have this ability at all.

5. Role as a reservoir. Spleen serves as a reservoir for mobilization of RBCs in some animals like cats and dogs. In humans, this function is not important since the splenic capsule lacks smooth muscles and thus cannot contract to any significant degree. However, spleen serves as reservoir for *platelets*. About 30% of the total circulating platelets may be present in the spleen adhering to the reticular cells in the red pulp or endothelial cells of the sinusoids.

6. Role in regulating portal blood flow. The vasculature of spleen also plays a role in regulating the portal blood flow.

Mucosa-Associated Lymphoid Tissue

Mucosa-associated lymphoid tissue (MALT) refers to the lymphoid tissue distributed along the mucosa lining the alimentary, respiratory, genitourinary and other surfaces which are constantly exposed to numerous antigens. Tonsils, adenoids and Peyer patches of small intestine are known as gut-associated lymphoid tissue (GALT). Peyer patches are small patches of organized lymphoid tissue along the intestine containing B lymphocytes (in germinal centre) and T lymphocytes. They play a primary role in defence against infectious organisms entering via the gastrointestinal tract (GIT).

IMMUNITY

Immunity refers to resistance of the body to pathogens and their toxic products. It can be classified as:

I. *Innate immunity*
- Nonspecific
- Specific innate immunity

II. *Acquired (adaptive) immunity*
- Active acquired (adaptive) immunity
- Passive acquired (adaptive) immunity

INNATE IMMUNITY

Innate or natural immunity is the inborn capacity of the body to offer resistance to pathogens and their toxic products. It is due to genetic and constitutional makeup of an individual. It may be *specific* (against a particular organism) or *nonspecific*. Innate immunity may be:

Species immunity, i.e. resistance to a pathogen shown by all members of a species

Racial immunity, i.e. resistance to a pathogen shown by only a particular race within a species

Individual immunity, i.e. resistance to a pathogen shown by a particular individual within a race

Mechanisms of Innate Immunity

1. Mechanical barrier This barrier against invading microorganisms is provided by the intact skin and mucosa in the body.

2. Surface secretions These constitute one of the important mechanisms of innate immunity. These include:

Secretions from the sebaceous glands of skin, which contain both saturated and unsaturated fatty acids that kill many bacteria and fungi.

Saliva, constantly produced in the mouth cavity, has an inhibitory effect on many microorganisms.

Gastric juice and highly acidic environment of stomach may hydrolyse microbial invaders.

Tears poured in the conjunctival sac mechanically wash away the particles and a hydrolytic enzyme lysozyme, present in the tears, can destroy most of the microorganisms.

3. Humoral defence mechanisms These provide innate immunity by the nonspecific microbicidal substances present in the body fluids. A few examples are as follows:

Lysozyme is found in high concentration in most tissue fluids except colony-stimulating factor (CSF), sweat and urine. It is a mucolytic enzyme which kills microorganisms by splitting sugars of the structural mucopeptide of their cell wall.

Basic polypeptides containing nonspecific microbicidal activity include leukins, arginine- and lysine-containing proteins protamine and histone.

Complements have lytic and several other effects on foreign substances (see page 185).

Interferons (IFNs) are antiviral substances produced by the cells stimulated by live or killed viruses. IFN-α and -β are part of innate immunity.

4. Cellular mechanisms of defence Cellular mechanisms of defence which provide nonspecific innate immunity are as follows:

Phagocytes, i.e. neutrophils and the monocyte–macrophage system cells, constitute the most important nonspecific cellular defence against the invading microorganisms (see page 162).

Eosinophil granules contain enzymes and toxic molecules that act against larvae of helminths (see page 167).

Natural killer (NK) cells refer to a subpopulation of lymphocytes which provide nonspecific cellular defence against viruses, tumour cells and other infected cells (see page 169).

ACQUIRED (ADAPTIVE) IMMUNITY

The resistance that an individual acquires during his/her lifetime is known as acquired or adaptive immunity. It is antigen specific and may be antibody or cell mediated. It is of two types: active and passive.

1. Active Immunity

Active immunity is acquired by the synthesis of antibodies (humoral immunity) and production of immunocompetent cells (CMI) by the individual's own immune system in response to an antigenic stimulation. Active immunity can be induced naturally or artificially.

i. Natural active immunity Natural active immunity results from either a subclinical or clinical infection. For example, a large majority of adults in the developing countries possess natural active immunity to poliomyelitis due to repeated subclinical infections with poliovirus during childhood.

ii. Artificial active immunity Artificially, active immunity is induced by introducing antigens in the body in the form of vaccines and this process is called *active immunization*. The vaccines are preparations of live or killed microorganisms or their products. Examples of vaccines are as follows:

Bacterial vaccines
- Live: BCG vaccine for tuberculosis
- Killed: TAB vaccine for typhoid

Bacterial product vaccines
- Tetanus toxoid
- Diphtheria toxoid

Viral vaccines
- Live: Sabin vaccine for poliomyelitis; MMR vaccine for measles, mumps and rubella; and 17D vaccine for yellow fever
- Killed: Salk vaccine for poliomyelitis, neural and nonneural vaccines for rabies

2. Passive Immunity

Passive immunity refers to the immunity that is transferred to a recipient in a ready-made form. Here, the individual's immune system does not play an active role. It is of two types:

i. Natural passive immunity It is the transfer of readymade antibodies from the mother as follows:

- In a fetus, the IgG antibodies are transferred from the mother through the placenta.

- After birth, Igs are passed to the newborn through breast milk. Human colostrum is rich in IgA antibodies which are resistant to digestion in stomach and small intestine.

Passively transferred antibodies are generally against all common infectious diseases in the locality. These confer immunity on the neonate up to 3 months of age. Therefore, most paediatric infections are more common after the age of 3 months when maternal Igs disappear.

Important Note

By active immunization of mother during pregnancy, the immune status of the neonate can be improved. Therefore, immunization of pregnant women with tetanus toxoid is recommended in countries where neonatal tetanus is common.

ii. Artificial passive immunity Artificially, passive immunity can be transferred to the recipients by injecting ready-made antibodies. This is done by administration of hyperimmune sera of humans or animals.

Examples of artificial passive immunity include injection of:

- Antitetanus serum (ATS)
- Antidiphtheric serum (ADS)
- Antigas gangrene serum (AGS)

After first administration, the passively administered antibodies are removed by metabolism and immune elimination. Therefore, immunity conferred is short lived.

Differences Between Active and Passive Immunity

Differences between active and passive immunity are summarized in Table 3.4.1.

ANTIGENS

DEFINITION

Antigen. Antigens are substances that can stimulate an immune response in the body. Most antigens are proteins, but some are carbohydrates, lipids and nucleic acids. The specificity of an antigen is due to specific areas of its molecule called *determinant sites* or *epitopes*. The epitopes can bind to specific binding sites called *paratopes* of the antibody molecule (Fig. 3.4.3). A pure protein can have several epitopes and thus can stimulate formation of many distinct antibodies.

Hapten or incomplete antigen is a chemical substance of low molecular weight that cannot induce an immune response by itself. Nevertheless, haptens can produce the immune response when combined with larger molecules (usually proteins), which serve as carriers. For example, the atropine molecule is a hapten and does not produce an immune response, but when it combines with tear proteins, it can excite immune response.

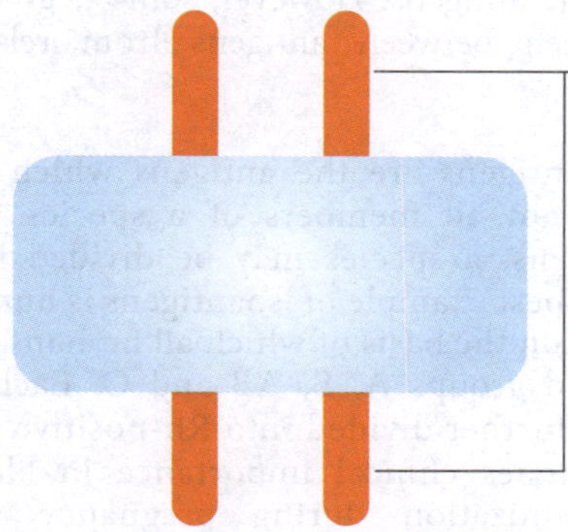

Fig. 3.4.3 Structure of an antigen.

Table 3.4.1 Differences between active and passive immunity

Active immunity	Passive immunity
1. **Production** Antibodies are produced by the body's own immune system in response to antigens introduced naturally or artificially in the body	Received passively by the host; no participation of host's immune system; it is conferred by administration of ready-made antibodies naturally or artificially in the body
2. **Negative phase** Negative phase is present in development of active immunity during which the immunity is transiently lowered; this is due to an antigen combining with the pre-existing antibodies and lowering their level	There is no negative phase in passive immunity, as antigens are not injected
3. **Latent period** Active immunity develops after a latent period varying from 4 days to 4 weeks; this is the time required for generation of antibodies and immunocompetent cells	There is no latent period; passive immunity is effective immediately
4. **Secondary response** Due to immunological memory, the secondary response, i.e. response to antigen introduced second time, is more enhanced	There is no immunological memory; rather, subsequent administration of antibodies is less effective due to immune elimination
5. **Duration** Active immunity is long lasting	Passive immunity is short lasting
6. **Effectivity** Active immunity is more effective and confers better protection	Passive immunity is less effective and provides inferior immunity
7. **Applicability in immunodeficient individuals** Active immunity is not applicable in immunodeficient individuals	Passive immunity is applicable in immunodeficient hosts

In contrast to complete antigens, haptens contain a single epitope.

SOME FACTS ABOUT ANTIGENICITY

Immunogenicity It is the ability of an antigen to stimulate an immune response, and is determined by:

- Size of molecule
- Foreignness of molecule
- Chemical structure of molecule
- Susceptibility of the substance to the tissue enzymes
- Genetic constitution of the host
- Dosage, route and timing of administration

Antigen specificity It is determined by chemical grouping and acid radicals. The antigen specificity is not absolute, i.e. some cross-reactions can occur between antigens which bear stereochemical similarities.

Species specificity Tissues of all individuals in a species contain species-specific antigens. However, some degree of cross-reactivity is seen between antigens from related species.

Isospecificity Isoantigens are the antigens which are found in some but not all members of a species. On the basis of isoantigens, a species may be divided into different groups. The best example of isoantigens is human blood group antigens on the basis of which all humans can be divided into blood groups A, B, AB and O. Each of these groups may be further divided into Rh-positive and Rh-negative. This carries clinical importance in blood transfusion, isoimmunization during pregnancy and disputed paternity.

HISTOCOMPATIBILITY ANTIGENS

Histocompatibility antigens refer to the antigens present on the plasma membrane of cells of each individual of a species. These antigens are encoded by genes known as histocompatibility genes which collectively constitute the major histocompatibility complex (MHC). These genes are located on the short arm of chromosome 6. In human, it contains more than 200 genes and called human leucocyte antigen or HLA genes as they were first discovered through antigenic difference between white cells from different individuals.

These have been studied extensively in organ transplantation. The major histocompatibility antigens in humans and mouse are known as HLA and H_2, respectively. No two persons, except identical twins, have the same MHC proteins. No two persons can have the same MHC proteins on plasma membranes of their cells.

Classes of MHC genes. There are three subclasses of MHC genes: classes I, II and III.

- *MHC class I* molecules: The genes coding α-chain of MHC class I molecules and α- and β-chains of MHC class II molecules are linked within the complex, and found on the surface of virtually all the cells of the body excluding red blood cells. The MHC class I refers to the products of HLA-A, HLA-B and HLA-C loci (Fig. 3.4.4A).

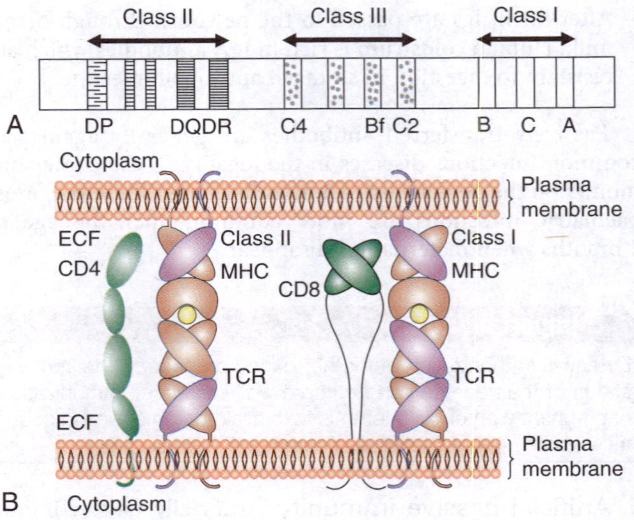

Fig. 3.4.4 HLA complex: **A,** showing the location of MHC class I, II and III antigen proteins in HLA complex; and **B,** structure of MHC proteins and their relation to CD4 and CD8.

- *MHC class II* antigens: These are encoded by the HLA-DP, HLA-DQ and HLA-DR loci, all of which reside within HLA-D region of HLA complex (Fig. 3.4.4A). In humans, MHC class II antigens are found only on immunologically reactive cells such as B lymphocytes, macrophages, monocytes and activated T lymphocytes.
- *MHC class III:* The genes coding for the complement components of the classical (C_2 and C_4) and the alternative (properdin factor B) pathways also reside in the MHC gene complex located between MHC class I and class II regions (Fig. 3.4.4A).

STRUCTURE OF MAJOR HISTOCOMPATIBILITY COMPLEX

- MHC class I molecules are heterodimers that consist of two polypeptide chains α and β_2 microglobulin (β_2M). The two chains are linked noncovalently via interaction of β_2M and α_3 domain (plasma membrane spanning and interacts with CD8 co-receptors of T cells). The α_3-CD8 interaction holds the MHC-I in place while the T-cell receptors (TCRs) on the surface of cytotoxic T cells bind to α_1 and α_2 heterodimer ligand (Fig. 3.4.4B).
- MHC-II class molecules are also heterodimers consisting of an α- and β-polypeptide chains. MHC-II class molecules interact mainly with immune cells like T-helper cells (CD4) Fig. 3.4.4B)

HLA tissue typing Histocompatibility typing or the so-called HLA tissue typing refers to detection of MHC class I and MHC class II antigens. HLA typing is used:

- To determine HLA compatibility prior to organ/tissue transplantation from one individual to another within a species
- For paternity testing
- For anthropologic studies
- For establishing HLA disease association

ANTIBODIES

Antibodies or Igs are gamma globulins which are produced in response to antigenic stimulation. These react specifically with the antigens which stimulated their production. All antibodies are Igs but all Igs are not antibodies. Igs have been divided into five distinct classes or isotypes, namely IgG, IgA, IgM, IgD and IgE.

STRUCTURE OF ANTIBODY

IgG has been studied extensively and serves as a model of basic structural unit of all Igs. An Ig is a Y-shaped molecule made of four polypeptide chains: two heavy (H) and two light (L). These are held together by disulphide bonds (Fig. 3.4.5).

Heavy Chains

- H chains have a molecular weight of 50,000 Da.
- H chains are structurally and antigenically distinct for each class of Ig and are named as follows:
  α (alpha) in IgA
  δ (delta) in IgD
  ε (epsilon) in IgE
  γ (gamma) in IgG
  μ (mu) in IgM
- The NH_2 terminal half of each chain has a variable sequence of amino acids and is called the *variable region*. In the H chain, it is designated as VH.
- The COOH terminal of each chain has a relatively constant sequence and is called the *constant region*. In the H chain, it is designated as CH.
- Two H chains are always identical in a given molecule. In IgG, each H chain contains 440 amino acids.
- Intrachain sulphide bonds fold each chain into incomplete loops. In the H chains, there are four loops of 110 amino acids, and each loop forms a globular domain. One domain designated as VH lies in the variable region and CH_1, CH_2 and CH_3 lie in the constant region (Fig. 3.4.5).

Light Chains

- Molecular weight of L chains is 25,000 Da.
- L chains are of two types: κ (kappa) and λ (lambda). A molecule of Ig may have either κ or λ chains but never both together. κ and λ chains occur in a ratio of about 2:1 in human serum.
- Similar to H chains, the variable region of L chains is designated as VL and constant region is designated as CL.

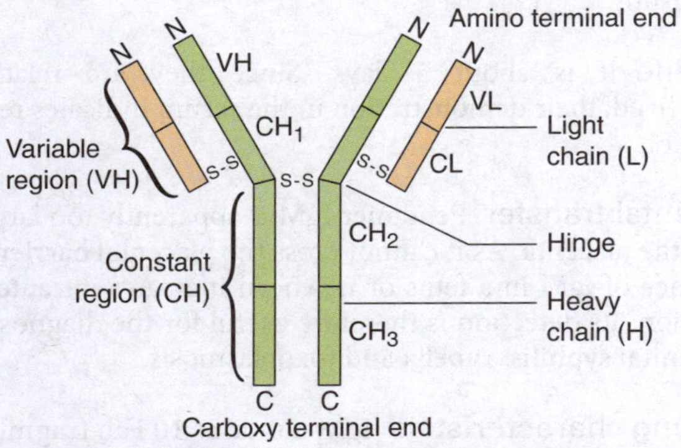

Fig. 3.4.5 Basic structure of an antibody showing the arrangement of heavy and light chains and its variable and constant domains.

- Like H chains, the L chains are also always identical in a given molecule. In IgG, each L chain contains 220 amino acids.
- In the L chain, there are two loops each containing 110 amino acids. Each loop forms a globular domain. One domain in variable region is designated as VL and the other in the constant region is designated as CL (Fig. 3.4.5).

Fragments of Immunoglobulins

1. When treated with enzyme papain Each Ig splits into three fragments (Fig. 3.4.6A):

Fab (fragment antigen binding) are two identical fragments. Each Fab bears all the variable regions and thus possesses the antigen-binding sites. The portion of the H chains present in the Fab is called Fd piece.

Fc (fragment crystallizable) is the third fragment having a molecular weight of 5000 Da. As the name indicates, it can be crystallized. It lacks the ability to bind to antigen and it serves the following functions:

- Binds complements leading to complement fixation.
- Binds to cell receptors (Fc receptors [FcRs]).
- Determines placental transfer of Ig.
- Determines skin fixation and catabolic rate.
- Antigenic determinants that distinguish one class of antibody from another are also located on Fc.

2. Treatment of Ig with enzyme pepsin Enzyme pepsin cleaves H chains on the carboxy terminal side of the interchain disulphide bonds of the hinge region. Therefore, two Fab fragments remain united. This fragment is designated as $F(ab)_2$ with two antigen-binding sites. It is about 10% larger than the two Fab fragments obtained from the papain digestion of Ig (Fig. 3.4.6B).

- Pepsin also degrades part of the Fc portion to small peptides and leaves a dimer of the carboxy terminal quarter of the chain, termed pFc (Fig. 3.4.6B).

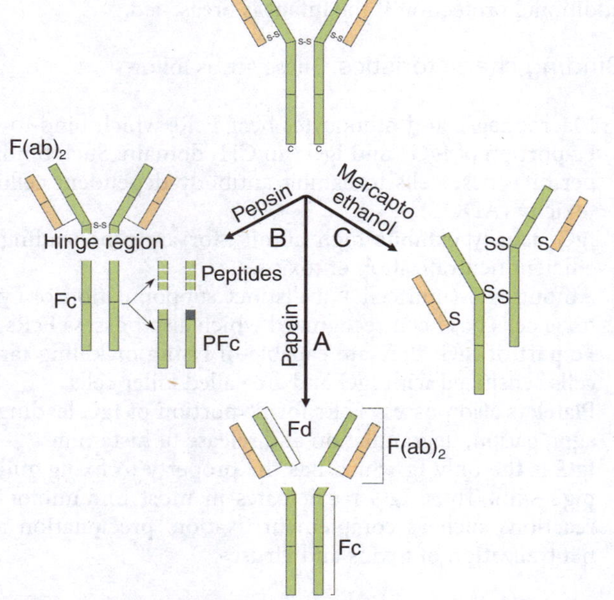

Fig. 3.4.6 Various fragments of an antibody when treated with: **A,** enzyme papain; **B,** enzyme pepsin; and **C,** a reducing agent (mercaptoethanol).

3. Treatment of Ig with reducing agent Treatment of Ig with reducing agent such as mercaptoethanol, in the presence of urea, reduces disulphide bonds releasing the four peptide chains, two heavy and two light (Fig. 3.4.6C).

Types of Immunoglobulins

On the basis of physiochemical and antigenic structure, five distinct classes of Igs are identified in human serum. These are IgG, IgA, IgM, IgD and IgE.

IgG

Distribution IgG is the most abundant class of Ig in the body, constituting approximately 75% of the total body Igs. It is distributed equally between the intravascular and extravascular pools. It is also found in milk, saliva, nasal and bronchial secretions.

Production A little IgG is produced during the early stage of primary response to antigen. But it is the major form of antibody produced during secondary response in which the initial IgM production gives way to IgG production (class switch).

Molecular weight IgG is a glycoprotein with a molecular weight of 150,000 Da.

Serum concentration Its serum concentration is normally about 12 ng/mL.

Half-life It is 21 days.

Subclasses There are four subclasses of human IgG: IgG1, IgG2, IgG3 and IgG4, possessing distinct types of H chains known as γ_1, γ_2, γ_3 and γ_4, respectively.

Placental transfer IgG is the only class of Igs that can cross the placenta and is responsible for protection of the infant during the first few months of life. It is also found along with IgA in milk during the first few weeks after birth, providing additional protection if the infant is breast-fed.

Binding characteristics These are as follows:

- Macrophages and monocytes bear FcRs which bind to the Fc portion of IgG1 and IgG3 in CH_3 domain. Such binding permits these cells to exhibit antibody-dependent cellular toxicity (ADCT).
- IgG usually exhibits high affinity for antigens leading to efficient neutralization of toxins.
- Among NK (null cells), a distinct subpopulation of cytotoxic cells has been recognized which also possess FcRs for Fc part of IgG; they are capable of lysing or killing target cells sensitized with IgG and are called killer cells.
- Platelets also possess FcRs for Fc portion of IgG leading to aggregation, degranulation and release of histamine.
- IgG is the only Ig which has the property to fixing guinea pig's skin. Thus, IgG participates in most immunological reactions such as complement fixation, precipitation and neutralization of toxins and viruses.

Catabolism The catabolism of IgG is unique in that it varies with its serum concentration, that is, when its level is raised, catabolism is rapid.

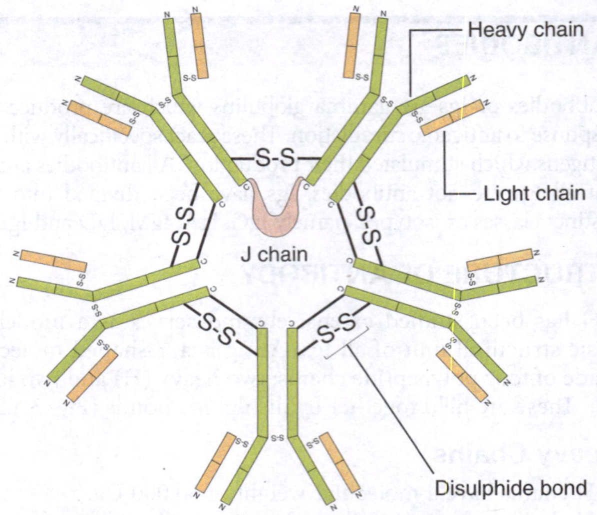

Fig. 3.4.7 Structure of IgM immunoglobulin.

IgM

Distribution IgM constitutes about 10% of the total serum Igs. In contrast to IgG, IgM, because of its large size, remains almost exclusively in the serum and is not usually found extravascularly in body cavities or secretions.

Production Phylogenetically, IgM is the oldest Ig class. It is the only Ig which is produced before birth. It is the predominant Ig produced during primary response. It appears early in the secondary response but its level does not rise significantly thereafter.

Structure IgM normally exists as a pentamer consisting of five Ig subunits (Fig. 3.4.7).

- Its H chain is μ type and L chain is κ or λ.
- The Hμ chain has four CH domains rather than three as seen in H chains of IgG.
- H chains are held together by disulphide bonds between CH_3 domains.
- There is an additional peptide chain called the joining (J) chain. The J chain may be largely responsible for the polymerization process, which occurs shortly before the molecule is secreted by plasma cells.

Molecular weight IgM is a glycoprotein with a molecular weight of 9,000,000 Da. Serum concentration of IgM is 1.2 ng/mL.

Half-life It is about 5 days. Since they are relatively short-lived, their demonstration in the serum indicates recent infection.

Placental transfer Pentamer IgM is apparently too large to cross the placenta. As it cannot cross the placental barrier, the presence of IgM in a fetus or newborn indicates intrauterine infection. Its detection is therefore useful for the diagnosis of congenital syphilis, rubella and toxoplasmosis.

Binding characteristics IgM contains 10 Fab fragments, and thus 10 antigen-binding sites. Therefore, theoretically, it can bind to 10 antigen molecules. However, practically,

IgM is capable of binding to as few as five molecules of antigen.

- IgM is much more efficient than IgG in its ability to fix complement by the classical pathway promoting lysis and death of most Gram-negative bacteria. This greater efficiency is due to the fact that the complement may bind to several Fc regions of pentameric IgM simultaneously, thus initiating a complement cascade and target cell lysis with a single molecule.
- IgM causes effective agglutination but its opsonizing power is rather weak.

IgA

Distribution IgA is the second-most abundant class constituting about 15% of human serum Igs where it exists as a *monomeric* Ig. Its more important form is the *dimeric* form, known as *secretory* IgA (SIgA). It is the predominant class of Igs in secretions such as milk, tears, nasal secretions, saliva, lung secretions, genitourinary and gastrointestinal fluids.

Production SIgA is synthesized by plasma cells in the subepithelial tissues of the body.

Structure The basic structure of IgA is similar to that of IgG. It contains two identical L chains (either κ or λ) and two heavy α-chains.

- SIgA is a dimer containing four H chains, four L chains and one J chain which is similar to J chain found in pentameric IgM (Fig. 3.4.8). It also possesses an additional structural unit called secretory component (SC) which is attached to the Fc portions of IgA molecules. Due to this SC, the SIgA is relatively resistant to digestive enzymes.
- In the intestinal mucosa, the M cells take up the bacterial and viral antigens and pass them onto Peyer patches (underlying the aggregate lymphoid tissue) and activate B-cell lymphocytes, and then the lymphocytes infiltrate into the mucosa of gastrointestinal, respiratory, genitourinary and female reproductive tracts and also the breast tissue. There these B cells secrete Ig as when exposed to an antigen that initially activates them. The Sc component of IgA antibodies is secreted by epithelial cells that acts as a receptor for binding to IgA. This thus provides secretory immunity.

Molecular weight It is 160,000 Da, while that of SIgA is 385,000 Da.

Serum concentration It is 2 ng/mL.

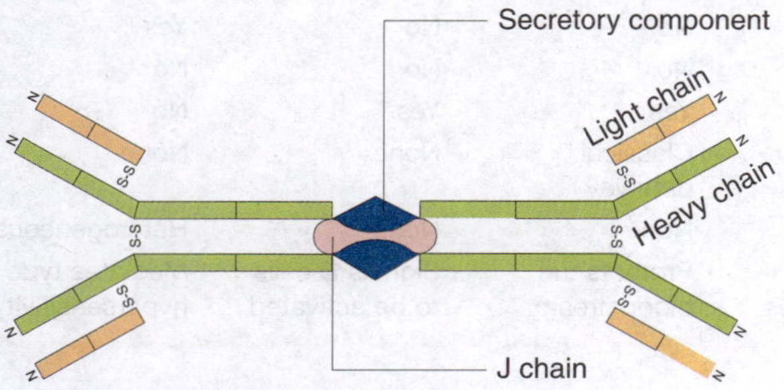

Fig. 3.4.8 Structure of secretory IgA molecule.

Half-life It is about 6 days.

Binding characteristics IgA does not fix complement in the classical pathway but can activate the alternative pathway. It promotes phagocytosis and intracellular killing of microorganisms.

> **Important Note**
>
> - SIgA coats the microbes and inhibits their adherence to the mucosal cells, thereby preventing the entry into the body tissues. *Neisseria gonorrhoeae* which produces IgA protease can penetrate the mucosal barrier even in an immune person.

IgD

Structure Like other monomeric antibodies, IgD is composed of two L chains (either κ or λ) and two H chains designated as δ chains.

Molecular weight It is 180,000 Da.

Distribution IgD is present on the surface of B lymphocytes (which are destined to differentiate into antibody-producing plasma cells) and is known to act as antigen receptor for the B cells.

Serum concentration It is 0.03 ng/mL.

Half-life It is about 3 days.

Placental transfer It does not cross the placenta.

Binding characteristics IgD does not bind complement. Since it is present on the surface of B lymphocytes, it is involved in antigen recognition. Reaction of an antigen with surface Ig may lead to cell differentiation and antibody synthesis.

IgE

Structure Structure of IgE is similar to that of IgG. It consists of two L chains (either κ or λ) and two H chains designated as δ chain.

Molecular weight It is 190,000 Da.

Production IgE is chiefly produced in the lining of the respiratory and intestinal tracts.

Distribution and serum concentration Mostly a person's IgE is fixed to the surface of mast cells and basophils. It is present in extremely low concentration (0.00004 ng/mL) in the serum. However, the serum IgE levels are raised in atopic (type I hypersensitivity) conditions like asthma and hay fever.

Half-life It is about 2 days.

Heat stability In contrast to other Igs, IgE is heat labile and gets inactivated by heating at 56°C for 30 minutes.

Placental transfer It does not cross the placental barrier.

Binding characteristics It does not fix complement.

- The Fc portion of IgE binds to the FcRs present on the surface of mast cells and basophils leaving antigen-binding sites free to react with specific antigen. When a specific antigen binds with such IgE, the reaction results in the degranulation of mast or basophil cells with the release of pharmacologically active substances such as histamine, slow-reacting substances of anaphylaxis (SRS-A), mast cell chemotactic factor and eosinophil chemotactic factor.
- IgE production is particularly known to be stimulated in parasitic infestation. It has been suggested that mast cell–bound IgE reacts with antigens on the parasite followed by release of histamine. This results in increased vascular permeability followed by influx of plasma and cells (particularly eosinophils) and destruction of parasite.

Summary of Characteristic Features and Functions of Immunoglobulins

The characteristic differentiating features of various Igs are summarized in Table 3.4.2

From the available information, the specific functions of various Igs appear as follows:

- *IgG* protects the body fluids.
- *IgA* protects the body surfaces.
- *IgM* protects the bloodstream.
- *IgE* mediates type I hypersensitivity.
- *IgD* signals B cells to get activated.

DEVELOPMENT OF IMMUNE RESPONSE

Development of an immune response implies *development of acquired active immunity* in the body. The immune system of the body responds to an antigen by two ways:

- Humoral or antibody-mediated immunity (AMI)
- Cell-mediated immunity (CMI)

DEVELOPMENT OF HUMORAL IMMUNITY

The humoral immunity is mediated by antibodies and so is also called AMI. The antibodies are produced by plasma cells which in turn are produced by B lymphocytes.

Role of Humoral Immunity

- The humoral immunity provides defence against most extracellular bacterial pathogens and viruses that infect through the respiratory and intestinal tracts.
- It participates in immediate hypersensitivity reactions of types I, II and III.
- Humoral immunity is also associated with certain autoimmune diseases.

Types of Humoral Immune Responses

The antibody response to stimulation by an antigen is of two types (Fig. 3.4.9):

- Primary humoral response
- Secondary humoral response

Primary response It refers to the response of the body's immune system to an antigen which is introduced into the body for the first time. Always there is a latent period varying from 4 days to 4 weeks before the primary response in the form of a rise in the serum antibodies titre can be detected.

Secondary response It refers to the response of the body's immune system to an antigen which is introduced into the body on a second occasion. Such a response occurs more quickly and more abundantly. This is because of the fact that the immune system is liable to retain the memory of a prior antigenic exposure for long periods (immunological memory) and produce enhanced response when encountered with the same antigen for the second time.

Table 3.4.2 Characteristic differentiating features of various immunoglobulins

Feature	IgG	IgA	IgM	IgD	IgE
Structure characteristics					
• Structural unit	Monomer	SIgA is dimer	Pentamer	Monomer	Monomer
• Heavy-chain class	γ_1, γ_2, γ_3, γ_4	α_1, α_2	μ	δ	ϵ
• Light-chain class	κ or λ	κ or λ	κ or λ	κ or λ	–
Additional chain	–	J, SC	J	–	–
Molecular weight (kDa)	150	160–385	900	180	190
Carbohydrate content (%)	3	8	12	13	12
Serum concentration (ng/mL)	12	2	1.2	0.03	0.00004
Half-life (days)	21	6	5	3	2
Secretion from serous membranes	No	Yes (SIgA)	No	No	Yes
Placental transfer	Yes	No	No	No	No
Heat stability (56°C)	Yes	Yes	Yes	Yes	No
Complement fixation	Classical pathway	Alternative pathway	Classical pathway	None	None
Binding to tissue	Heterogeneous	None	None	None	Heterogeneous
Role in the body	Protects the body fluids	Protects the body surfaces	Protects the bloodstream	Signals B cells to be activated	Mediates type I hypersensitivity

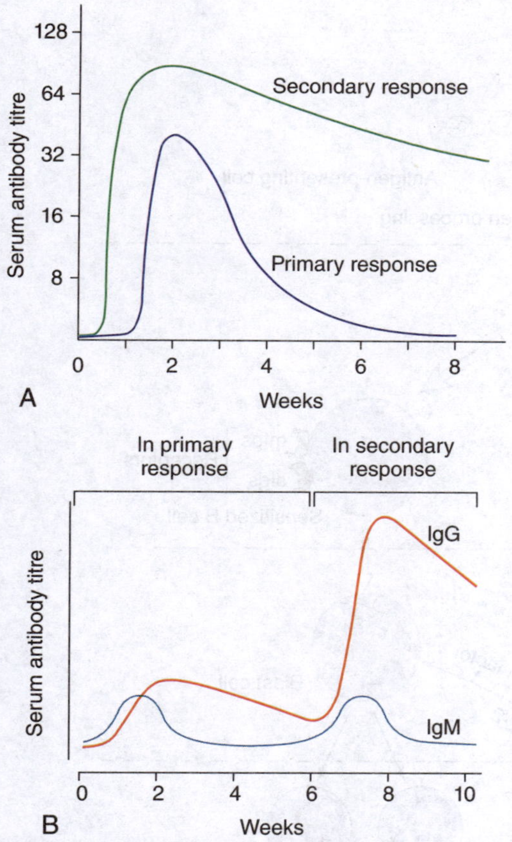

Fig. 3.4.9 Response of body's immune system to an antigen: **A,** time course of antibody production in primary versus secondary response; and **B,** serum levels of IgM and IgG antibodies in primary and secondary response.

PHASES OF HUMORAL IMMUNE RESPONSE (FIGS 3.4.10 AND 3.4.13)

1. Antigen processing and presentation Once the antigen enters the body, it is phagocytosed by the macrophages (nonspecific response). Phagocytosed material is broken down into polypeptide fragments. The antigen polypeptide fragments then combine with the MHC-II present in the macrophages and move to the cell surface. This is called *processing of antigen*. The processed antigen is then presented to immunocompetent lymphocytes by the macrophages. So, the macrophages are also called *antigen-presenting cells (APCs)*. Other APCs which can process and present the antigen to lymphocytes are as follows:

- B lymphocytes themselves
- Dendritic cells present in the skin (Langerhans cells), thymus (medulla), lymph nodes (cortex and paracortex), spleen and other secondary lymphoid organs

2. Recognition of antigen by lymphocytes The lymphocytes possess the antigen recognition receptors. These include the membrane-bound (surface) immunoglobulins (mIgs or sIgs) in B lymphocytes and T-cell receptors (TCRs) in the T lymphocytes. These receptors serve as specific surface receptors, recognizing and interacting with only a single antigenic determinant on the antigen presented to the lymphocytes. This process of binding of processed antigen to specific receptors on the surface of lymphocytes in technical terms is called *recognition of antigen by lymphocytes*. Thus, many million different T and B lymphocytes, each with the ability to respond to particular antigen, are present in the body.

> **Important Note**
>
> The receptors on circulating T cell (T-cell receptors [TCRs]) are mainly made of α- and β-polypeptide units, hence called α- and β-T cells. About 10% of TCRs have γ- and δ-polypeptide units, and they are designated as γδ T cells.

3. Lymphocyte activation The lymphocytes that have combined with antigen are activated, i.e. the lymphocytes become larger and look like a lymphoblast. This is known as *blast transformation*. Activated B lymphocytes and helper T cells (T_H cells; CD4 cells) play a major role in humoral immunity. The macrophages liberate interleukin-1 (IL-1) and cause further activation of B lymphocytes and helper (CD4 T) cells.

Activation of T lymphocytes Activation of T_H cells by the processed antigen complex is essential for humoral immunity. The activated T_H cells secrete two substances: IL-2 and B-cell growth factor, which further promote proliferation of B lymphocytes and their transformation into plasma cells. This phenomenon is called *T–B cooperation* (Fig. 3.4.13).

Activation of B lymphocytes After receiving cooperation from T-helper cells (T–B cooperation), B lymphoblasts proliferate forming clones of cells that respond to this antigen (*clonal selection*). A clone is the population of cells descended by asexual reproduction from a single cell. The B lymphocytes proliferate and transform into two types:

- Plasma cells
- Memory B cells

Role of plasma cells. When a B lymphocyte is converted to a plasma cell, its cytoplasm expands. It is filled with granular endoplasmic reticulum. The plasma cells secrete antibodies.

Role of memory B cells. A small portion of the activated B lymphocytes do not enlarge or undergo blast transformation. Instead, they only proliferate and transform into small-sized memory B cells, which occupy the lymphoid tissue throughout the body. Memory B cells have a long lifespan and remain inactive. When the body is exposed to the same antigen for the second time, the memory B cells are able to recognize it and become active, i.e. they are responsible for secondary response of antibodies.

4. Production of antibodies The plasma cells so formed secrete antibodies which are also called Igs. Igs are actually secreted form of antigen-binding receptors. For structure and class of Igs, see page 179. The rate of antibody production is very high, i.e. each plasma cell produces about 2000 molecules of antibodies per second. A plasma cell secretes an antibody of

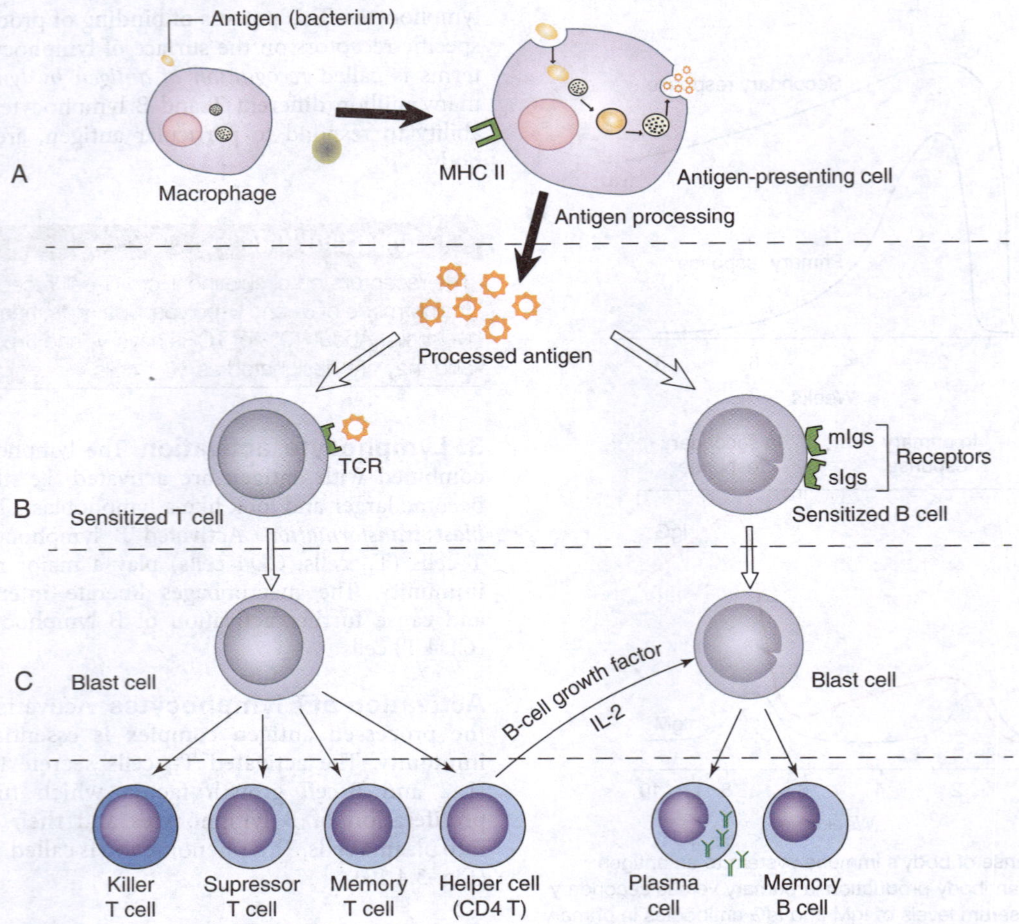

Fig. 3.4.10 Broad outline of development of humoral immune response: **A,** antigen processing and presentation to immunocompetent cells; **B,** recognition of antigen by the lymphocytes; and **C,** activation of lymphocytes (blast transformation).

a single specificity of a single antibody class and a single L chain type. However, in a primary antibody response, a plasma cell produces IgM initially and later it may switch onto IgG production.

Theories of antibody production The antibody produced in response to an antigen is highly specific, i.e. it reacts only with the antigen which has evoked its production. How this is possible is not known exactly. Various theories have been put forward to explain this immune specificity. ***Clonal selection theory*** put forward by Burne in 1957 is more widely accepted than other theories.

- According to this theory, during immunological development, a large number of B lymphocytes capable of reacting with different antigens are formed. Each specific B cell multiplies and establishes a population of genetically and immunologically identical B cells called a *clone*. An antigen has only to select and stimulate its specific clone. That is why this theory is named clonal selection theory.
- This theory also states that cells with immunological reactivity with self-antigens are eliminated during embryonic life. Such clones are known as *forbidden clones*. Their persistence or development in the later life leads to autoimmunity.
- The diversity for production of a large number of different types of Igs by human B cells has a genetic basis.
- The Ig molecules possess two types of L chains and eight types of H chains. In the H chain, there are variable regions (V, D and J segments). The gene responsible for V segment has several hundred coding regions, about 20 for D segment and 4 for J segment. During B-cell proliferation, one coding region for each (V, D and J segments) is randomly selected; therefore, about 10^{15} different Ig molecules are permitted by this mechanism. Similar mechanisms operate for diversity in TCR production.

5. Inactivation of antigen or attack phase or effector phase of immune response This is the last phase of immune response and involves the inactivation of antigen by the antibodies. Antibodies act on the invading antigen in two ways.

(i) Direct attack on the invading agents Because of the bivalent nature of antibody and multiple antigen sites on most of the invading agents, antibodies can inactivate the invading agent by the following reactions:

Agglutination. By this reaction, a large number of particles (bacteria or red cells) with antigens on their surface are bound together to form a clump. Clumping increases the susceptibility to phagocytosis.

Precipitation. In this reaction, the antigen–antibody complex forms an insoluble precipitate.

Neutralization. Antibodies cover the toxic sites of antigen and neutralize them.

Cytolysis. Antibodies attach to the membranes of cellular agents, thereby causing rupture of cells.

(ii) Attack on the antigen through complement system The complement system includes 11 enzymatic proteins which are named C1–C9, B and D. All these are present in the blood as plasma proteins. These are also present in the tissue fluid. The complement system acts in three ways (Fig. 3.4.11).

(a) Classical pathway This is activated by an antigen–antibody reaction. When an antibody binds with an antigen, a specific reactive site on the constant portion of the antibody becomes uncovered where the protein C1 binds and thus gets activated. The activated C1 in turn activates the other complements in a series of cascade reactions. The products of complement activation cause the following effects:

Opsonization. Opsonization is the coating of antigen by antibody and complement. It helps the neutrophils and macrophages to phagocytose the antigen. The activated C3a product acts as an opsonin.

Bacterialysis, i.e. destruction of bacteria by rupturing the cell membrane. A membrane attack complex is formed by C5b–C6–C7–C8–C9. The cell lysis is brought about by the complement system by inserting proteins called *perforins* into the cell membrane. Perforins make holes in the cell membranes, resulting in free flow of ions and disrupting membrane permeability.

Agglutination, i.e. clumping of bacteria and RBCs.

Chemotaxis, i.e. attraction of leucocytes to the site of antigen–antibody reaction. Chemotaxis is enhanced by C5b–C6–C7 complex.

Neutralization, i.e. covering the toxic sites of antigenic products.

Activation and degranulation of mast cells and basophils are caused by C4b. This releases factors like histamine and heparin which cause hypersensitivity reaction and producing vasodilatation and chemotaxis. Vasodilatation increases capillary

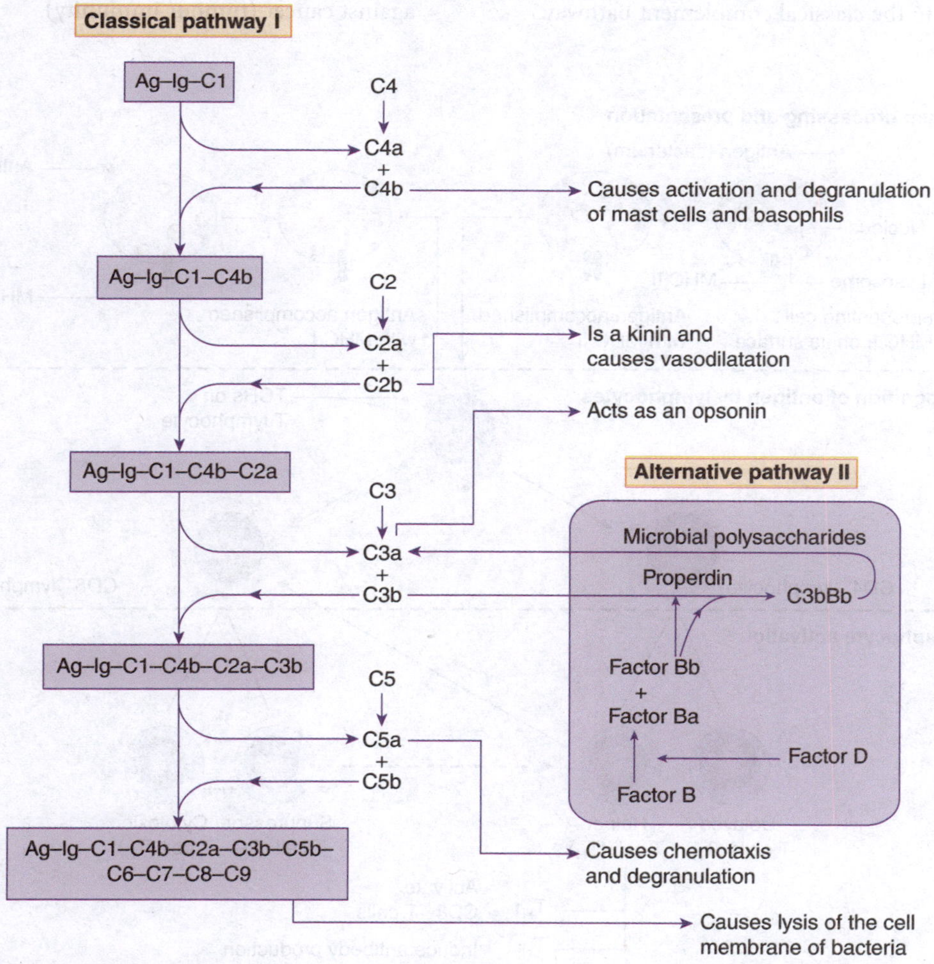

Fig. 3.4.11 Broad outline of classical and alternative pathway of complement system.

permeability; therefore, plasma proteins enter the tissues and antigenic products are inactivated.

Amplification of inflammation response. The products of complement system C2b lead to increase in blood flow due to vasodilation, increase capillary permeability and leakage of plasma proteins into tissue fluid thus causes amplification of inflammatory response.

The antibodies which can fix and thereby activate complements are IgM and IgG. IgA also fixes complements but does so by the *alternative pathway* and not by the *classical pathway*.

(b) Alternative pathway In the alternative pathway, the complement system is activated without an antigen–antibody reaction. The alternative or properdin pathway is initiated by binding of the factor I (a protein in circulation) with polysaccharide present in the cell wall of invading organism, i.e. bacteria (endotoxin) and yeast cell wall (zymogen). This binding triggers reactions that activate C3 and C5 which ultimately attack the antigenic products of invading organisms. *Properdin* (a circulating protein) stabilizes the activating enzyme complex; that is why the alternative pathway is also called properdin pathway. Because this pathway does not involve an antigen–antibody reaction, it is one of the first lines of defence against invading organisms.

(c) Mannose-binding lectin pathway The lectin pathway is a type of cascade reaction in the complement system similar in structure to the classical complement pathway.

After activation, it proceeds through the action of C4 and C2 to produce activated complement proteins further down cascade to form C3 convertase (C4b–C2a) on the surface of pathogen and further acts as classical pathway. The mannose-binding lectin pathway is triggered when lectin binds to mannose groups in bacteria.

In this pathway, mannose-binding lectin (MBL) binds to mannose, glucose or other sugars of surface membrane component of the bacterial cell wall and forms a complex with mannose as MBL-associated serine protease 1 to 3 ($MAsP_1$ to $MAsP_3$).

DEVELOPMENT OF CELLULAR IMMUNE RESPONSE

The cellular immunity refers to specific acquired immunity which is accomplished by effector T cells and macrophages (Figs 3.4.12 and 3.4.13). It is also called CMI.

Role of Cellular Immunity

- Cellular immunity protects the host against fungi, most of the viruses and intracellular bacterial pathogens like *Mycobacterium tuberculosis, M. leprae* and *Brucella*.
- It participates in allograft rejection and graft versus host reaction.
- CMI participates in delayed hypersensitivity reaction.
- CMI is also associated with certain autoimmune diseases.
- It provides immunological surveillance and immunity against cancer (tumour immunity).

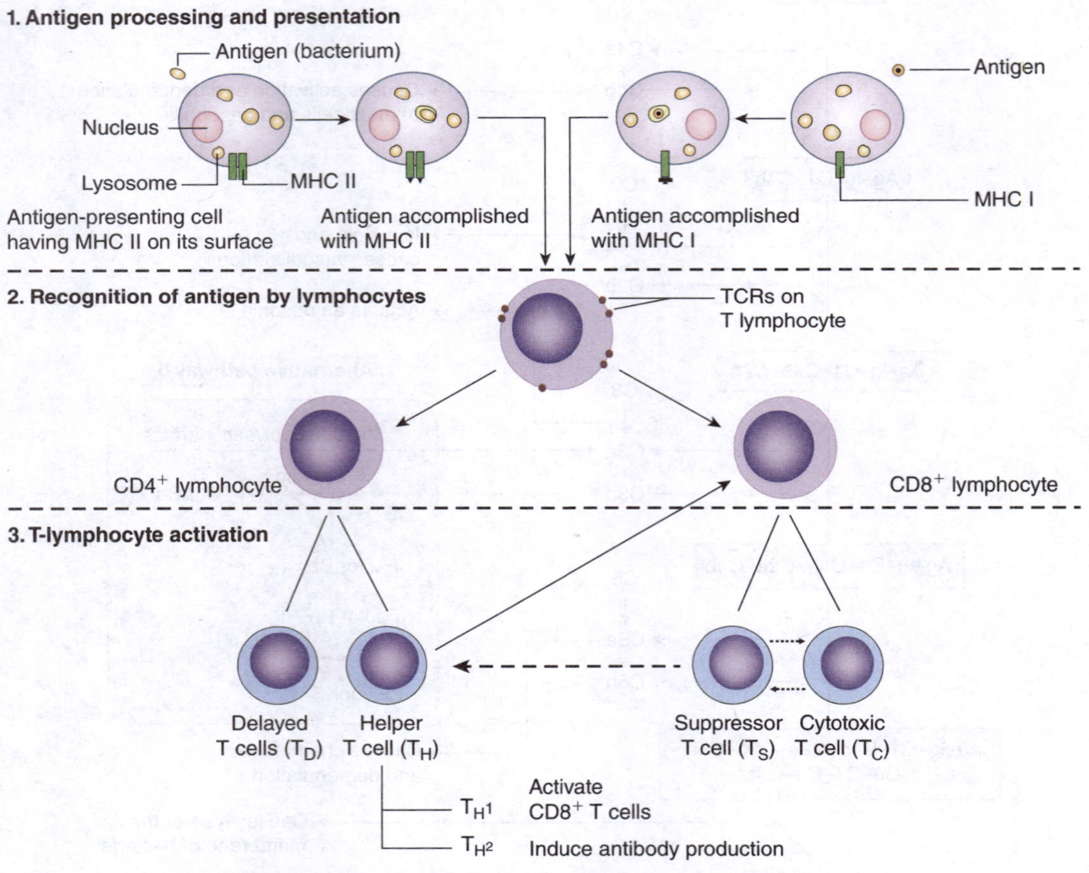

Fig. 3.4.12 Development of cellular immune response.

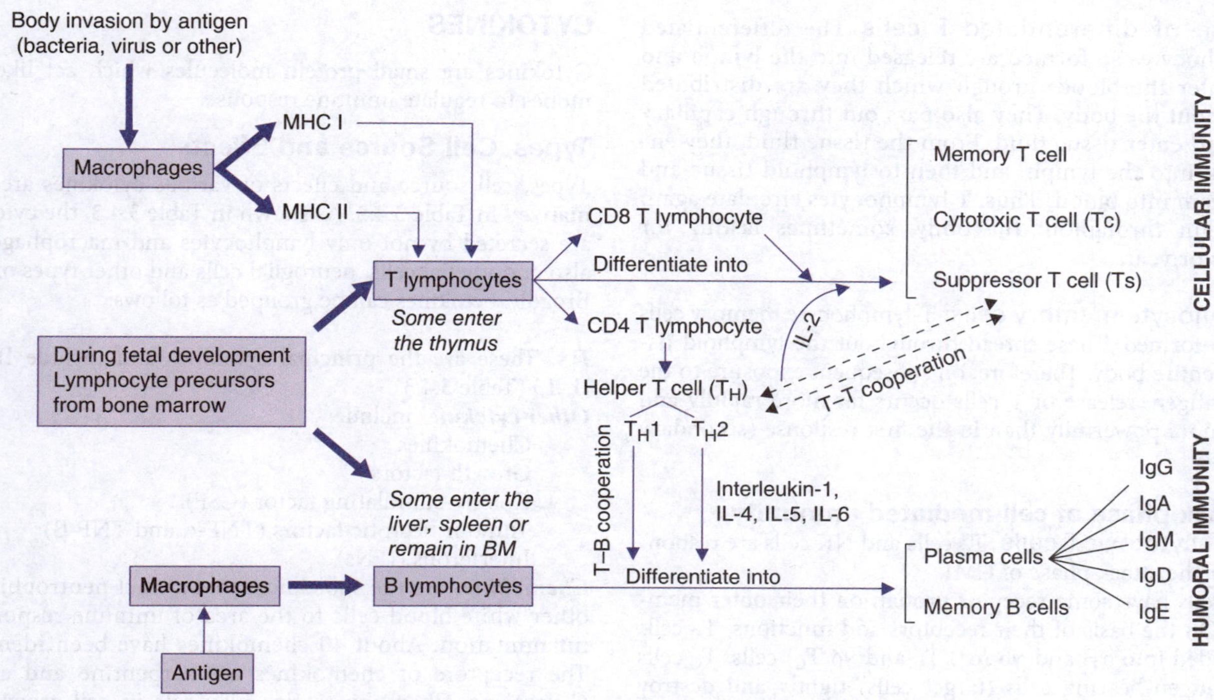

Fig. 3.4.13 Summary of immune response.

Types of Cellular Immune Response

Like humoral immune response, the cellular immune response is also of two types:

Primary cellular response which is produced by initial contact with a foreign antigen.
Secondary cellular response which is produced when the host is subsequently exposed to the same antigen. The secondary cell-mediated immune response is usually more pronounced and occurs more rapidly. Furthermore, because of the availability of specific memory cells, an increased number of effector cells are produced in secondary response.

PHASES OF CELLULAR IMMUNE RESPONSE

The development of cellular immune response can be subdivided, using the concept of immune response arch, into the following phases.

1. Antigen processing and presentation An antigen entering the host body is phagocytosed and degraded into polypeptide fragments by the antigen-processing or -presenting cells (APCs) which include macrophages and dendritic cells present in the peripheral lymphoid tissue. The antigen polypeptide fragments then become associated with MHC antigen and are expressed on the surface of APC. Two modes of antigen processing are known:

Processing of phagocytosed material, e.g. bacterial antigen, is accomplished by combining with MHC-II molecules.
Processing of antigen derived within the cell, e.g. viral antigens synthesized in infected cell, is accomplished by combining with MHC-I molecules (probably in the endoplasmic reticulum).

2. Recognition of antigen by lymphocytes T lymphocytes possess the antigenic recognition receptors known as *TCRs*. These receptors serve as specific surface receptors recognizing and interacting with only single antigenic determinant on the antigen presented to lymphocytes. Furthermore, the mature T lymphocytes can be differentiated into two antigenic subtypes depending on the ensemble of their surface antigens: $CD4^+$ cells and $CD8^+$ cells.

- $CD8^+$ cells recognize the combination of foreign antigen and MHC class I antigen.
- $CD4^+$ cells recognize the combination of foreign antigen and MHC class II antigen.

3. T-lymphocyte differentiation (activation)
$CD8^+$ type of T lymphocytes After combining with foreign antigen–MHC-I complex are activated and differentiate into:

- Cytotoxic T cells (T_C cells)
- Suppressor T cells (T_S cells)

$CD4^+$ type of T lymphocytes After combining with foreign antigen–MHC-II complex are activated and differentiate into:

- T_H cells
- Delayed-type hypersensitivity T cells (T_D cells)

T–T cooperation. The differentiation of T lymphocytes into T_H, T_C, T_S and T_D cells is interdependent. This interdependence is called T–T cooperation.

Release of differentiated T cells The differentiated T lymphocytes so formed are released into the lymph and then enter the blood through which they are distributed throughout the body. They also pass out through capillary walls and enter tissue fluid. From the tissue fluid, they enter back into the lymph, and then to lymphoid tissue and once again into blood. Thus, T lymphocytes circulate again and again throughout the body, sometimes lasting for months or years.

T-lymphocyte memory cells T-lymphocyte memory cells are also formed. These spread throughout the lymphoid tissues of entire body. Therefore, on subsequent exposure to the same antigen, release of T cells occurs far more rapidly and much more powerfully than in the first response (secondary response).

4. Attack phase of cell-mediated immunity

Role of cytotoxic T cells T_C cells and NK cells are responsible for the attack phase of CMI.

T_C cells have some receptor protein on their outer membrane. On the basis of their receptors and functions, T_C cells are divided into $\alpha\beta$ and $\gamma\delta$ ($\alpha\beta$ T_C and $\gamma\delta$ T_C) cells. T_C cells bind antigen-bearing cells (target cells) tightly and destroy them by the following mechanisms:

i. ***Perforin-mediated killing.*** The T_C cells after binding with the target cell secrete a hole-forming protein called *perforin*. The perforins literally punch round holes in the membrane of target cells in the presence of extracellular calcium (calcium-dependent lysis). The pores so formed cause cell death by disrupting cell homeostasis.
ii. ***Lysis through cytotoxic substances.*** After binding with target cells, the T_C cells enlarge and release cytotoxic substances.
iii. ***Induction of apoptosis.*** T_C cells secrete tumour necrosis factor-β (TNF-β) which increases the Ca^{2+} permeability of antigen-bearing cell. The increased intracellular calcium activates enzymes that cause degradation of nucleus producing apoptosis.

Role of helper T cells T_H cells are of two types: helper T^1 (T_H^1) and helper T^2 (T_H^2).

i. T_H^1 cells play their roles by secreting three cytokines:
   - *IL-2* secreted by T_H^1 cells activates the $CD8^+$ cells to differentiate into T_C cells and T_S cells (T–T cooperation).
   - *Interferon-γ* (IFN-γ) has the direct ability to kill antigen-bearing cells.
   - *TNF-β* can induce apoptosis in antigen-bearing cells.
ii. T_H^2 cells secrete IL-4, IL-5, IL-6, IL-10 and IL-13 and primarily with activation of B lymphocytes produce antibodies (T–B cooperation).

Role of suppressor T lymphocytes (T_S cells) T_S cells regulate the activity of T_C cells. Thus, the cellular immune response is a balance between T_C cells and T_S cells.

- T_S cells also play an important role in preventing the T_C cells from destroying the body's own tissue along with the invading organism.
- T_S cells also suppress the activities of T_H cells.

CYTOKINES

Cytokines are small protein molecules which act like hormones to regulate immune response.

Types, Cell Source and Effects

Types, cell source and effects of various cytokines are summarized in Table 3.4.3. As shown in Table 3.4.3, the cytokines are secreted by not only lymphocytes and macrophages but also endothelial cells, neuroglial cells and other types of cells. Broadly, cytokines can be grouped as follows:

ILs. These are the principal cytokines and include IL-1 to IL-13 (Table 3.4.3).
Other cytokines include:
- Chemokines
- Growth factors
- Colony-stimulating factor (CSF)
- Tumour necrotic factors (TNF-α and TNF-β)
- Interferons (IFNs)

Chemokines are the substances that attract neutrophils and other white blood cells to the area of immune response or inflammation. About 40 chemokines have been identified. The receptors of chemokines are serpentine and act via G proteins. Chemokines also play role in cell growth and angiogenesis.

Mechanism of action

1. Local effects Cytokines act in an *autocrine* (i.e. on the cell that produced them) or *paracrine* (i.e. on the cell close by) manner through their specific receptors.
Receptors of cytokines have been grouped under the superfamily. The *superfamily* includes receptors of:

- Cytokines
- Haematopoietic growth factors
- Prolactin
- Growth hormone

The superfamily of receptors has been divided into three *subfamilies*:

- *Subfamily type I* includes receptors for IL-4, IL-7, erythropoietin, growth hormone prolactin and colonies stimulating factor-G (CSF-G).
- *Subfamily type II* includes receptors for IL-3, IL-5, IL-6, IL-11, ciliary neurotrophic factor, oncostatin and leukaemia inhibitory factor (LIF).
- *Subfamily type III* includes receptors for IL-2, IL-4, IL-9, IL-19 and other cytokines and related proteins, e.g. IL-2R and Tac antigen.

Systemic effects IL-1 affects the various body systems:
Central nervous system effect. It causes fever, slow-wave sleep, secretion of corticotropic hormone (CRH) and anorexia.
Metabolic effects. It increases hepatic protein synthesis and excretion of sodium, and decreases plasma zinc and iron level and also cytochrome P_{450}. It also causes lactic acidosis.
Haematological effects. It increases the number of circulating neutrophils, CSF and nonspecific resistance.
Vascular system effect. It stimulates leucocyte adherence to the vessel wall, increases synthesis of prostaglandins, releases platelet-activating factor and increases the capillary permeability.

Table 3.4.3 Main characteristics of human interleukins and other immunoregulatory cytokines

Type of cytokine	Cell source	Effects
I. Interleukins (IL)		
IL-1 a and b	Macrophages and other antigen-processing cells (APCs)	i. B-cell proliferation ii. Ig production iii. Stimulation of T cells iv. Inflammation, fever
IL-2	Activated helper cells (T_H^1), cytotoxic cells (T_C) and natural killer (NK) cells	i. Proliferation of activated T cell ii. B-cell proliferation, Ig expression
IL-3	T lymphocytes	Growth of early progenitor cell
IL-4	T_H^2 and mast cells	i. Eosinophil growth and its function ii. B-cell proliferation iii. Ig expression iv. MHC class II expression v. Proliferation of T_H^2 and T_C cells vi. Inhibition of production of inflammatory cytokines
IL-5	T_H^2 and mast cells	Growth of eosinophil and its function
IL-6	Activated T_H^2 cells, APC and other somatic cells	i. Act with IL-I and TNF to stimulate T cells ii. Proliferation of B cells and Ig production iii. Stimulates thrombopoiesis
IL-7	Thymic and bone marrow stromal cells	Lymphopoiesis (T and B cells)
IL-8	Macrophages	Stimulates neutrophil activity and promotes their accumulation
IL-9	From cultured T cells	Stimulates haematopoietic and thymopoietic factors
IL-10	Activated helper cells (T_H^2), CD8$^+$, B lymphocyte and macrophages	i. Inhibition of cytokine production ii. Stimulates B cells and antibody production and its functions iii. Suppresses cell-mediated immunity iv. Causes growth of mast cells Stimulates haematopoiesis and thrombopoiesis
IL-11	Stroma cells	Stimulates proliferation of cytotoxic T cells and killer cells (T_C and NK)
IL-12	Macrophages and B cells	Promotes cell-mediated immune response
IL-13	T_H^2 cells	i. B-cell proliferation, IgG expression, MHC class II expression ii. Proliferation of T_H^2, T_C cells and their function iii. Inhibition of production of inflammatory cytokines
II. Other cytokines		
TNF-α	Activated macrophages	i. IL-I–type effects ii. Causes vascular thrombosis and necrosis of tumour cells
TNF-β	Activated T_H^1 cells	Vascular thrombosis and tumour cell necrosis
Interferon (IFN-α and -β)	Macrophages, neutrophils and other somatic cells	i. Antiviral effects ii. Stimulates MHC class II cells iii. Activation of macrophages and NK cells
IFN-γ	Activated T_H^1 and NK cells	i. Antiviral effect ii. Activation of MHC class I cells and MHC class II cells iii. Promotes cell-mediated immunity
TGF-β	Activated T lymphocytes, platelets, macrophages and somatic cells	i. Anti-inflammatory effect by suppressing cytokine production and MHC-II cells ii. Inhibits proliferation of macrophages and lymphocytes iii. Proliferation of B cells iv. Healing (by stimulating fibroblast cells)

OTHER IMMUNE MECHANISM–RELATED ASPECTS

Some other aspects related to immune mechanisms which need to be elaborated are as follows:

- Immune tolerance
- Immune modulation
- Autoimmunity
- Hypersensitivity
- Immunodeficiency diseases

IMMUNE TOLERANCE

Types of Immune Tolerance

Immune tolerance may be defined as a state of unresponsiveness to an antigen. It occurs in two forms: natural and acquired.

1. Natural immune tolerance It refers to nonresponsiveness to a self-antigen. During embryonic development, when the immune system is immature, any antigen which comes in contact with the immature immune system is recognized as self-antigen. Therefore, it does not evoke any response in later life when body is exposed to the same antigen.

2. Acquired immune tolerance It means unresponsiveness to a potential antigen. It is of further two types: general and specific.

(i) ***General immunological tolerance*** results due to impairment of the immune system; hence, there is lack of responsiveness to potential antigens.

(ii) ***Specific immunological tolerance*** arises when a potential antigen induces a state of unresponsiveness to itself and not to other antigens. This happens when an antigen becomes tolerogenic (tolerogen).

- In some instances, when an antigen is presented at particular concentration, it might induce specific immunological tolerance or unresponsiveness, whereas when presented at some other concentration, it promotes immunity. Therefore, an antigen that induces tolerance is referred to as *tolerogen*.
- Specific acquired tolerance has consequences for the host defences. Presence of tolerogenic epitopes on the pathogens compromises with the ability of the body to resist infections.

Mechanism of Immune Tolerance

Immunotolerance can arise by three possible mechanisms:

- Clonal deletion
- Clonal anergy
- Suppression

1. Clonal deletion During embryonic life, clones of B and T cells are formed. These B and T cells possess receptors which recognize the antigens and are selectively deleted or eliminated and, therefore, not available to respond on subsequent exposure to that antigen in later life.

2. Clonal anergy Clones of B-cell receptors and TCRs which recognize self-antigen might remain, but cannot be activated. This is referred to as clonal anergy.

3. Suppression Clones of B and T cells expressing receptors that recognize self-antigen are preserved and capable for recognition of an antigen when activated. However, an immune response might be inhibited through active suppression.

Factors Influencing Induction of Tolerance

A number of factors influence induction of immunological tolerance. These are species, competency of the host, antigen and age of the host.

1. Species Immunological tolerance varies from species to species. For example, species like rabbits and mice can be rendered tolerant more rapidly as compared to guinea pigs and chickens.

2. Immunological competency of the host It also affects induction of tolerance. If degree of immunological competency of the host is high, then induction of tolerance is very difficult. On the other hand, newborns and embryos are particularly susceptible for induction of tolerance because their immune system is immature and not very competent.

3. Antigen Induction of tolerance also depends on the antigen (i.e. its physical nature, dose and its route of administration).

i. ***Physical nature of an antigen*** refers to the form of an antigen, i.e.:
   - Aggregated form
   - Soluble (free form)

   For example, human gamma globulin is *heat aggregated* and it is highly immunogenic in mice. But when deaggregated, it becomes tolerogenic. This is probably due to the fact that antigens in the aggregated form are easily phagocytosed by the macrophages and then presented to antibody-forming cells. On the other hand, soluble antigens or deaggregated antigens or free antigens escape phagocytization by the macrophages; therefore, they are not so easily processed and are tolerogenic.

ii. ***Dose.*** The induction of tolerance is also dose dependent. It has been observed that high doses of antigen tolerize the B cells and minute doses of an antigen when introduced repeatedly tolerize the T cells, but a moderate dose of the same antigen is immunogenic. Dose-dependent tolerance occurs by two ways:
   - *Immune paralysis* or *high-zone tolerance* occurs when high doses of antigen are introduced. It may be because of depletion of specific clone cells.
   - *Low-zone tolerance* occurs when a subimmunogenic dose of some thymus-dependent antigen is repeatedly introduced.

iii. ***Route of administration*** of an antigen also affects the induction of tolerance. An antigen when introduced intravenously, can cause tolerance. This is due to the fact that the antigen has a fast contact with more number of cells and also reaches the spleen, to which the suppressor cells (T_S) migrate leading to tolerance.

4. Age of the host As mentioned above, the immune system competency is related to the age of the host. Therefore, embryo and newborns can develop immune tolerance easily.

Tolerance to Fetus

Fetus is genetically different from the mother and thus it should evoke an immune response in the mother. However, it usually never happens and it is considered to be the best example of immune tolerance. Various factors which prevent an immunological response in a mother against its fetus are described next.

1. Placenta Placenta plays an important role by different ways:

- Immediately after implantation, the trophoblast cells lose their immunogenic capacity due to decrease in MHC antigen density.
- There is formation of mucoprotein coating on the cell surface.
- Anti-MHC antibodies which are produced in the mother get absorbed into the placenta and their entry into fetal circulation is prevented. Thereby, the placenta acts as a shield against the immunological response.
- Placental trophoblasts cells do not express class I and II MHC, rather express HLA-G, a nonpolymorphic gene (which otherwise recognize fetal HLA-A and HLA-B molecule as foreign antigens). During pregnancy, HLG-G plays

immune tolerance role by inhibiting the cytotoxicity of T cells and NK cells.

Therefore, antibodies against fetal protein do not develop.

2. Alpha-fetoprotein During embryonic development, α-fetoprotein (AFP) is produced which acts as an immunosuppressive agent.

3. Progesterone During pregnancy, high levels of progesterone have an immunosuppressive effect.

4. Fetal T cells Fetal T cells get activated when the fetus is exposed to mother T cells through the placenta and suppress the mother's T cells.

5. Fas ligand Fas ligand of placenta also causes apoptosis of immunogenic T cells.

Immune Modulation

Immune modulation refers to modification of the immunological response. It can be either enhanced or suppressed.

Immune enhancement Immune enhancement means that there is increase in the response in terms of rate, intensity, duration and even induction of response to substances which were earlier nonimmunogenic.

Immunological response can be potentiated by use of certain substances referred to as adjuvants.

Adjuvants Adjuvants are the compounds which when introduced along with or mixed with an antigen nonspecifically enhance or modify the immune response to that antigen. The first adjuvant was discovered by Freund, hence known as Freund's adjuvant. Their contribution in enhancement of response is basically achieved by two ways:

i. *More and prolonged production* of antibodies
ii. *Increasing the number of effector* cells

Mechanism of action. Adjuvants act by the following ways:

- They alter the distribution and persistence of an antigen in the host.
- They stimulate lymphocyte number nonspecifically.
- They activate macrophages.

Types. Adjuvants are of two main types:

i. *Incomplete adjuvants.* Substances like aluminium hydroxide, aluminium phosphate and certain mineral oils (lanolin oil) act as incomplete adjuvants. When an aqueous solution of an antigen is mixed with mineral oil, an emulsion is formed, which serves as a depot for that antigen causing slow and prolonged release of the antigen.
ii. *Complete adjuvant.* The cell walls of certain bacteria like tubercular bacilli and Gram-negative bacilli (e.g. diphtheria and whooping cough) act as complete adjuvants because the constituents of the cell wall convert the soluble antigen into insoluble and particulate form which can be easily phagocytosed by macrophages. A typical example of a complete adjuvant is *killed Mycobacterium bacilli.*

Adverse effects of adjuvants are delayed hypersensitivity reactions in human beings (see page 194) and formation of local granuloma (inflammatory reaction, at the site of inoculation).

Immune suppression Immune suppression refers to reduction in the immunological response. It is of two types.

1. Specific immune suppression or immune tolerance See page 189.

2. Nonspecific immune suppression It is caused by immunosuppressive agents which inhibit the immune response of macrophages and B and T cells leading to either lowered phagocytosing capacity of the macrophages or production of antibodies and lymphokines.

Immunosuppressive Agents

These refer to methods or substances causing immunosuppression. These have been grouped as physical, chemical and biological agents.

A. Physical Immunosuppressive Agents (methods)

1. Irradiations. This is the most common method for prolonged survival of transplants. Irradiations cause breakage in the nucleic acid chains of replicating cells.

2. Surgical procedures like thymectomy, splenectomy and thoracic duct drainage:

Thymectomy. Removal of fetal thymus gland ensures absolute depletion of mature T cells but the effect of thymectomy decreases with age. Therefore, this method is not usually applicable.

Splenectomy. Though most of the antibodies are formed in the spleen, splenectomy has little effect in adult life (because other peripheral organs – lymph nodes – can compensate for absence of spleen).

Thoracic duct drainage is another method of immune suppression first used in humans during heart transplant. In this, the thoracic duct is cannulated and lymph is drained for many days, leading to decrease in size and weight of lymph node and depletion of lymphocyte (lymphopenia).

B. Chemical Methods

Chemical methods are nonspecific suppressants and have limited effectiveness. This group includes the following drugs:

Corticosteroids suppress the immune response by the following ways:

- They impair the maturation of activated cells.
- They suppress the production of antibodies.
- They have an anti-inflammatory effect and diminish the responsiveness of B and T lymphocytes.
- They also inhibit production of IL-1 and IL-2.

Corticoids, though commonly used, have limited effectiveness due to their side effects, as prolonged use leads to hypertension, bone necrosis, cataract and mental disturbances.

Cyclosporine or tacrolimus (FK-506) has been widely used as an immunosuppressive drug in organ transplants. This acts by inhibiting the production of IL-2. Normally, activation of TCR increases intracellular calcium (Ca^{2+}) that activates calcineurin via calmodulin. Calcineurin in turn dephosphorylates the transcription factor NF-AT that moves into the nucleus and increases the gene coding activity for IL-2. The drugs cyclosporin (Csp) and tacrolimus (Tcl) prevent dephosphorylation of NF-AT (Fig. 3.4.14). They also have adverse effects on the liver and kidney.

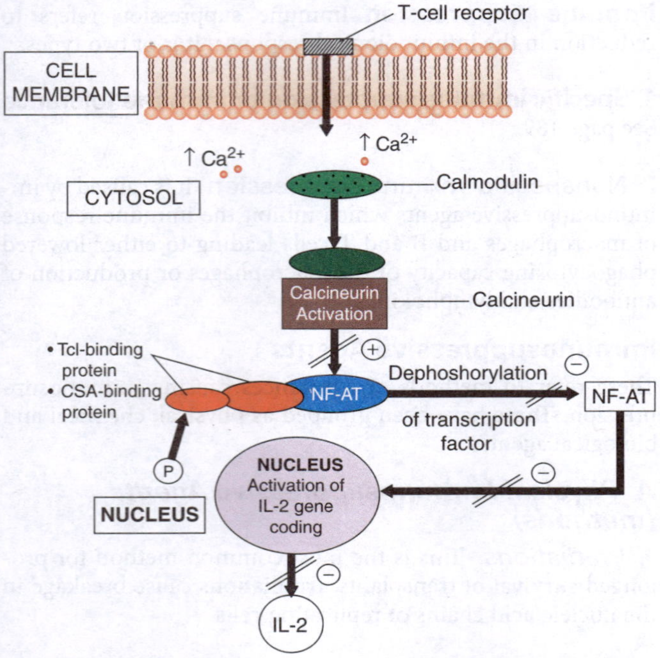

Fig. 3.4.14 Mechanism of action of cyclosporine C and tacrolimus in T lymphocytes.

Cytotoxic drugs such as *azathioprine* and *cyclophosphamide* act on various stages of nucleic acid synthesis and thus prevent replication of lymphocyte. *Methotrexate*, an antagonist of folic acid, produces competitive inhibition of an enzyme reductase (essential for synthesis of DNA). This drug is a known anticancer drug.

Antilymphocyte globulin (ALG) is an infusion of animal antibodies against human T cells. It is available as brand name *Atgam*. It is used with other medication to prevent or treat rejection of kidney transplant.

C. Biological Methods

1. Antigen-induced suppression. This method is used for desensitization against an allergen. In this method, if the body is exposed to small doses of antigen for long time, then it can develop resistance to that antigen.

2. Antibody-induced suppression. This method of immunosuppression is used in pregnant mothers (Rh −ve) to prevent sensitization against Rh antigen (from fetus) by injecting anti-D after expulsion of placenta.

3. Antilymphocytic serum is used for depletion of T-cell population. In this method, antilymphocytic serum is prepared from horse by injecting human lymphocytes. The antibodies present in the horse serum destroy body T-cell pool, but antibody production remains normal. The main drawback of this method is that the ability to fight against viral infection is tremendously decreased.

TISSUE TRANSPLANTATION

Tissue transplantation refers to the transplant of a tissue or whole organ from one part of an individual to another part of the same individual or to another individual. When tissues such as skin and kidney are transplanted from a donor to a recipient of the same species, the transplant is usually taken up for some time, but then becomes necrotic and is rejected. The grafts are rejected because the recipient produces an immune reaction against the grafted tissue (foreign tissue).

Types of grafts Different types of grafts are as follows:

Autografts. When a graft tissue is taken from one part of the body and transplanted to another part of the body of same individual

Isograft. When transplanted tissue is taken from the identical twins

Allograft. When transplanted tissue is taken from an individual and grafted to another person of same species

Xenograft. When the transplanted tissue is taken from an individual of a different species (i.e. taken from an animal and grafted to human)

Rejection of grafts In autografts and isografts, the antigens are of the same type as in recipients; therefore, the transplanted tissue is taken up easily if blood supply is adequate. On the other hand, in xenografts, an immune response always occurs and within few weeks the graft is rejected. The organs or tissue like skin, kidney, liver, heart, bone marrow and lung transplanted as allografts are taken up safely if proper matching is done and after transplantation proper immunosuppressive therapy is carried out.

Tissue typing The HLA complex is mainly responsible for graft rejection. Six of these antigens are present on the cell membrane of each person. There are more than a trillion possible combinations. Therefore, development of significant immunity against any one of these antigens can cause graft rejection. The tissue type matching between siblings and parents of a recipient is more successful for transplantation.

Techniques involved for tissue typing histocompatibility testing involve various methods of assays for HLA differences. Most commonly used method is polymerase chain reaction to compare the DNA of the person, organ or graft being tested with known pieces of genes encoding MHC antigens.

Graft versus host reaction Graft versus host disease (GVHD) is a condition that might occur following the receipt of transplanted tissues from a genetically different person. The white blood cells present within the transplanted tissue attack the recipient body's cells which leads to GVHD. GVHD occurs in two forms: acute GVHD and chronic GVHD.

Acute GVHD is normally observed within first few days (post-transplant). The characteristic features varied and depend on the involvement of body organ system.

- *Liver:* damage
- *Skin:* rash
- *GIT:* diarrhoea, abdominal pain, nausea and vomiting

It also involves:

- *Immune system*, haemopoietic tissue, bone marrow and thymus
- *Lungs:* pneumonitis

Chronic GVHD occurs normally after 100 days. It also affects all the organ systems as in acute condition, but over its long term causes damage to the connective tissue and exocrine glands.

Prevention of graft rejection Prevention of graft rejection can be achieved by suppressing the immune system of the recipient. For details, see page 191.

AUTOIMMUNITY

During fetal life, when many antigens are presented to the immune system, they are recognized as self-antigens and antibodies and T_C cells are not produced.

Therefore, tolerance to self-antigen is produced. However, sometimes body starts producing antibodies or T cells against self-antigen (own cells or tissue) leading to an autoimmune disease. Therefore, autoimmunity may be defined as immune response to self-antigen.

Mechanism of autoimmunity The possible mechanisms involved in development of autoimmunity are given next.

1. Forbidden clones According to clonal selection theory, antibody-forming lymphocytes are formed against different antigens. In fetal life, lymphocytes are also formed against self-antigens, but get depleted. The clones of these cells are called forbidden clones and hence an immune response does not occur against self-antigen. However, persistence of these clones or their development in later life by some mutations leads to autoimmunity.

2. Hidden antigen or sequestrated antigen Certain self-antigens are present in the close system and never exposed to the immune system during fetal life. These are known as hidden antigens or sequestrated antigens, e.g. *lens protein* being enclosed by its capsule does not come in contact with blood; therefore, immunological tolerance against such antigens does not develop. When such antigens in later life are somehow exposed to the immune system (accidental leak of lens protein during cataract surgery), this leads to an immune response and damages the other eye also. Another example of a hidden antigen is *sperm antigen*. Injury to testes or viral infections (mumps) leads to leakage of sperm proteins into the circulation and thus evokes an immune response against one's own testes and orchitis occurs.

3. Neoantigen or altered antigen Certain cells of the body undergo alterations due to exposure to irradiations, drugs, sunlight, etc., and start producing an immune response.

4. Cross-reacting antigen Although antibodies are highly specific for a particular antigen, in some cases they cross-react with other cells or body tissue. This phenomenon is called *molecular mimicry* and these antigens are called cross-reacting antigens. For example, in rheumatic heart disease, the heart is damaged by antibodies formed against streptococci.

5. Mutations The body's immune system becomes competent for self-antigen by certain mutations.

6. Unbalanced activity of helper and suppressor T cells It has been observed that optimum antibody response always depends on the balanced activity of T_H and T_S cells. If somehow the activity of these cells is altered, i.e. overactivity of T_H cells and underactivity of T_S cells, then it may result in autoimmunity.

Bystander activation of autoreactive CD4$^+$ cells Autoimmunity is sometimes associated with infections. Though the exact pathway is not clearly understood, it is speculated that activation of CD4 T cells occurs via cytokines and is T-Cr or antigen independent of link between infection and autoimmunity.

Autoimmune diseases Common autoimmune diseases include:

1. ***Autoimmune anaemia.*** For example:
   - Haemolytic anaemia. Antibodies react with one's own RBCs.
   - Pernicious anaemia. Antibodies react against gastric mucosa.
2. ***Thrombocytopenic purpura.*** Autoantibodies react with self-platelets.
3. ***Graves disease.*** Autoantibodies bind to thyroid cells and stimulate them.
4. ***Hashimoto disease.*** T cells react against the antigen on the thyroid cells.
5. ***Insulin-dependent diabetes mellitus.*** Antibodies damage the β-cells (insulin-producing cells) of the pancreas.
6. ***Rheumatoid arthritis.*** Antibodies damage the joints.
7. ***Rheumatic fever.*** Antibodies cross-react with valves of the heart.

HYPERSENSITIVITY

Hypersensitivity is an abnormal response which produces physiological or histopathological damage in the host. There are five types of hypersensitivity reactions:

- Type I (anaphylaxis or IgE mediated)
- Type II (antibody-mediated cytotoxicity)
- Type III (immune complex–mediated disorders)
- Type IV (delayed-type or T-cell–mediated hypersensitivity)
- Type V (stimulatory)

The characteristic features of type I–IV hypersensitivity reaction are given in Table 3.4.4.

Type I hypersensitivity or anaphylaxis Type I hypersensitivity or anaphylaxis is an allergic reaction that occurs within minutes, in which B cells are stimulated by CD4$^+$ T_H2 cells to produce IgE antibodies specific to an antigen.

It is mediated by IgE antibodies and occurs due to mast cell degranulation resulting in release of histamine and many other vasoactive substances. Type I reaction (anaphylaxis) depends on the amount of histamine release and route of stimulating antigen. It occurs in two forms: local anaphylaxis and generalized anaphylaxis.

Local anaphylaxis occurs when an antigen called allergen is administered locally in smaller dose. Examples of local anaphylaxis are asthma and hay fever.

Systemic or generalized anaphylaxis is a shock-like condition. It occurs in individuals who are intensely allergic and when an antigen is administered in large amount or through systemic route.

Mechanism of type I hypersensitivity In type I hypersensitivity reaction, the individual first comes in contact with an antigen and antibodies (IgE) are produced which get bound to mast cells or to fixed basophils. The specific IgE antibodies are fixed to mast cell surface by its Fc portion. After

Table 3.4.4 Characteristics of hypersensitivity reactions

Characteristics	Type I	Type II	Type III	Type IV
1. Time of onset of reaction	0.5–8 hours	5–12 hours	3–8 hours (peak 48–72 hours)	24–48 hours
2. Reaction mediators	IgE, histamine, serotonin, SRS-A, etc.	IgG, IgM and complement	IgG, IgM, neutrophils, eosinophils, lysosomal enzymes	T lymphocytes, macrophages and lymphokines
3. Response to intradermal injection of antigen (allergen)	Wheal and flare	–	Erythema and oedema	Erythema and induration
4. Passive transfer with	Serum	Serum	Serum	T cells
5. Examples	• Anaphylaxis • Asthma • Hay fever • Allergic with food and insect bite	• Transfusion reactions (incompatibility reaction) • Haemolytic disease of newborn • Drug-induced allergies	• Arthus reaction • Serum sickness	• Tuberculin test • Contact dermatitis • Graft rejection

second exposure, the allergen passes on to these sensitized cells (IgE-fixed mast cells) and gets attached onto the Fab site of IgE molecule attached to mast cell. Antigen–antibody binding triggers the degranulation of mast cells and releases pharmacologically active chemicals (histamine, serotonin, bradykinin and SRS-A) causing vasodilatation, sensory nerve ending stimulation, etc. The individuals susceptible to type I hypersensitivity reaction are called *atopic* and reaction is known as *atopy*. Examples of type I hypersensitivity include allergic rhinitis and atopic dermatitis.

Type II hypersensitivity or antibody-mediated autotoxicity It is an immediate reaction involving antibody-mediated destruction of cells. In this, specific antibodies (IgG or IgM) bind to the cell surface antigen and destroy the cell, such as circulating red blood cells.

The mechanism involved in this reaction is either complement- or antibody-mediated cytotoxicity.

Examples Type II hypersensitivity is most commonly seen in:

- Incompatible blood transfusion.
- Autoimmune haemolytic anaemia.
- Haemolytic disease of the newborn. When antibodies react with the cells on which these antigens are present, i.e. RBCs get damaged.

Type III hypersensitivity (immune complex–mediated hypersensitivity) Monocytes and macrophages are efficient in binding and removal of antigen–antibody complexes. When the body is exposed repeatedly to an antigen, which is not cell bound (free, small and soluble), the body faces great difficulty, because the antigen–antibody complex formation occurs in the serum and subsequently gets deposited in the normal body tissue. The damaging inflammatory reaction is triggered by large insoluble immune complex with IgM or IgG antibodies in the circulation.

There is overproduction of immunoglobulins IgG and IgM to a foreign or self-antigen. Complement system is also activated (particularly C3a and C5a), which is cytotoxic for monocytes, macrophages and even nearby normal tissue where the antigen–antibody complexes are deposited. *Glomerulonephritis* is the best example of type III hypersensitivity reaction.

Type IV or delayed hypersensitivity Delayed hypersensitivity is the cell-mediated reaction in tissues of a sensitized individual. The reaction is due to sensitization of T lymphocytes and not by antibodies or by B lymphocytes. The reaction starts after several hours (48–72 hours). Two types of delayed hypersensitivity reactions are recognized: tuberculin (infection) type and contact dermatitis.

Tuberculin test In this test, a small dose of tuberculin, or purified protein derivative from *M. tuberculosis*, is injected intradermally in an individual sensitized earlier by tubercular protein by infection or by immunization.

Within 48–72 hours, an inflammatory reaction of 5 mm diameter appears at the site of injection. The inflammatory reaction is recognized by erythema (increased blood flow) and induration (due to infiltration with a large number of T lymphocytes and macrophages).

Contact dermatitis It is type IV hypersensitivity reaction. Hypersensitivity against various chemicals in the forms of ointments, dyes, cosmetics, etc., is tested by *patch test*.

Patch test. In this test, a patch of an allergen is applied to the skin under a dressing. If itching occurs within 4–5 hours and local reaction in the form of redness and induration appears within 24 hours, then the test is positive.

Type V or stimulatory hypersensitivity Over the past few years, type V hypersensitivity has been added to the original four types. In this reaction, an antibiotic can act as a stimulant to target cell or organ. An example is long-acting thyrostimulatory (LATS) antibody, a feature of Graves disease. The LATS antibody is directed towards a portion of TSH receptor in the thyroid and mimics the function of thyroid stimulatory hormone.

IMMUNODEFICIENCY DISEASES

Immunodeficiency diseases occur when the defence mechanisms of body are impaired. The defect may lie in one or more of the following components of the immune system:

- Lymphocytes (B and T) and NK cells
- Phagocytic cells
- Complement proteins

Immunodeficiency diseases may be classified as primary or secondary.

Primary immunodeficiency Primary immunodeficiency occurs due to defect in the development of the immune system. Various primary immunodeficiency syndromes are given as follows.

1. Humoral immune deficiency Humoral immune deficiency occurs due to B-cell deficiency defect and may manifest as:

X-linked agammaglobulinaemia is the first immune deficiency disorder recognized by Bruton in 1952, hence also known as Bruton disease. It is seen in males but sporadic cases are found in females. The basic defect in this disorder is failure of premature B cells to differentiate into mature B cells. The disease is characterized by the following:

- Recurrent infections with pyogenic bacteria.
- Tonsils and adenoids are atrophied.
- Lymph node biopsy reveals depletion of bursa-dependent areas.
- B cells are either absent or remarkably decreased.
- Serum Igs (all the five classes) are absent.

2. Cellular immunodeficiencies Cellular immunodeficiencies occur due to defect in T cells and manifest as:

- Thymic hypoplasia (DiGeorge syndrome)
- Purine nucleoside phosphorylase (PNP) deficiency

i. ***Thymic hypoplasia or DiGeorge syndrome*** results due to a congenital malformation affecting third and fourth pharyngeal pouches from where thymus develops. Defective or nondevelopment of thymus T cells are deficient or absent in circulation. The disease is characterized by the following:
   - Thymus is hypoplastic.
   - In lymph nodes and in spleen, thymus-dependent areas are absent.
   - Infants with this defect are susceptible to viral and intracellular bacterial infections.
   - B cells are normal.
   - Ig levels are normal.

ii. ***Purine nucleoside phosphorylase (PNP) deficiency.*** Due to gene defect in chromosome 14, PNP enzyme is lacking resulting in defective metabolism of cytosine and inosine to purine which is essential for T-cell proliferation. Therefore, a patient with this disorder shows decreased CMI.

3. Combined immunodeficiencies Combined immunodeficiencies occur due to defect in both B and T cells. This defect may manifest as *severe combined immunodeficiency diseases* (SCID). Many distinct patterns have been described:

- Agammaglobulinaemia
- Adenosine deaminase deficiency
- Reticular dysgenesis

4. Complement immune deficiency disorder In this disorder, complement proteins are deficient due to genetic defect resulting in lack of various complement functions like phagocytosis, antibody killing of bacteria, lysis of virus, tumour cells and histamine release by mast cells.

5. Phagocytic disorders Phagocytic disorders lead to increased susceptibility to infections.

Secondary immunodeficiency disease Acquired deficiencies of immunological response mechanisms can occur secondarily to a number of diseases. Secondary immunodeficiency is more common than the primary immunodeficiency. Acquired immune deficiency syndrome (AIDS) is the most important.

AIDS is characterized by reduction in the number of T_H cells because of infection by human immunodeficiency virus (HIV). It was first detected in the United States in 1981. HIV is of two types, HIV-1 and HIV-2.

Spread of disease AIDS is a major worldwide life-threatening disease spreading rapidly. Daily about 8500 persons get infected with HIV. The high-risk groups include sex workers, drug addicts, homosexual males, persons with extramarital relations and recipients of unscreened blood transfusion.

Transmission There are mainly three routes of transmission:

1. ***Parenteral route*** is through blood contact involving:
   - Unscreened blood transfusion
   - Tattooing
   - Use of infected razors, syringes, needles, etc.
   - Use of poorly sterilized dental instruments
   - Organ transplants
2. ***Sexual route*** accounts for about 85% of HIV infection due to multiple sex partners, sex workers, homosexuality and artificial insemination. The virus is present in sufficient concentration in the semen and vaginal secretions of the infected person.
3. ***Transplacental route.*** Infection can be transmitted from infected mother to her fetus (vertical transmission) across the placenta and also to the infant through breast milk (perinatal transmission).

AIDS does not spread through mosquito bites, hugging, kissing and sharing meals.

Structure of HIV HIV is a retrovirus having rounded outline and consists of the following (Fig. 3.4.15):

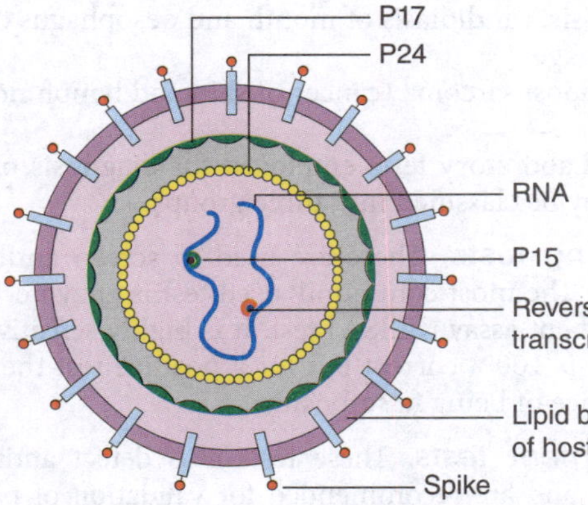

Fig. 3.4.15 Schematic diagram of structure of HIV.

The core has two single strands of genomic RNA, enzyme reverse transcriptase and protein P15 associated with genomic RNA. Genomic RNA is surrounded by two coverings:

- Inner covering is cone shaped, consisting of P24.
- Outer covering of P17.

Genome has two types of genes – overlapping and split genes (eight in HIV-1 and nine in HIV-II). Virus is surrounded by *host-derived envelop with spikes containing* protein components complementary to CD4 or T_H receptors present on the surface of T_H cells, monocytes, macrophages and some other nerve cells.

Virus multiplication When virus comes in contact with the cells having receptors of T_H antigen (T_H cells, monocytes, macrophages and some nerve cells), it sticks to the receptor site and then passes into the cell. Then free genomic RNA synthesizes a copy DNA with help of enzyme reverse transcriptase and biochemicals of the host.

- The copy DNA forms complement strand and the duplex attaches to the host DNA in the form of *provirus*. Provirus may multiply with host cell and ultimately forms *genomic RNA* and messenger RNA.
- The messenger RNA synthesizes viral proteins. Then genomic RNA and viral proteins are packed to form virions and these bud off from the host cell, get covered by an envelope and attack a new host cell.
- The infected host cell ultimately gets killed leading to reduction in the number of cells belonging to the immune system.

Incubation period It varies from 2 to 10 years (commonly 27–28 months). The first 2–6 months are called *window period* because in this period tests are negative. Then onwards, HIV positivity increases, which is indicated by:

- Presence of P_{24}
- Antiviral antibodies
- Reduction in the number of T cells

Signs and symptoms These are mostly of opportunistic infections due to decreased immunity, and include:

- Repeated episodes of diarrhoea
- Unexplained weight loss
- Prolonged cough, night sweating, continuous fever for more than 1 month
- Tuberculosis, candidiasis of mouth and oesophagus
- Brain damage
- Ulcers, Kaposi sarcoma (cancer of skin and lymph nodes)

HIV tests Laboratory tests employed for diagnosis of HIV infection may be classified into three groups:

A. Screening tests. These are used to screen antibodies against HIV. The most commonly used test is enzyme-linked immune sorbent assay (ELISA) test. It is highly sensitive. For negativity, it is 100% correct but for a positive test there is a 5%–6% chance of being false-positive.

B. Supplement tests. These tests also detect antibodies against HIV and are recommended for validation of positive tests on screening. The commonly employed test is *western blot*.

Western blot test separates the blood proteins and detects the specific proteins (HIV antibodies), which indicates HIV infection. It is used to confirm a positive ELISA and combined test is 99.9% positive. It is a highly sensitive and specific assay for culturing blood and testing plasma for virus.

C. Confirmatory tests. These tests confirm HIV infection in an individual who is seropositive. These tests include:

Virus isolation. Nucleic acid test (NAT) detects HIV virus in **the blood** of infected person. This test is also called HIV virus load test. The NAT can detect HIV sooner than other tests.

Detection of P_{24}. The P_{24} antigen test can detect the P_{24} protein within 10–14 days after infection with HIV-2, -3, -11 and -12. The main drawback is that the peak of P_{24} protein reaches around 3–4 weeks after exposure to HIV and is usually not detected for 5–6 weeks.

Rapid HIV test is immune-chromatographic technique in which blood/plasma/serum reacts with HIV antigen–coated particles in the test strip. The mixture then migrates upwards on the membrane chromatographically by capillary action with recombinant HIV antigen. This test is usually done with blood from finger stick or oral fluid and results are obtain within 20 minutes.

Treatment Treatment consists of HIV antivirals. No cure exists for AIDS, but strict adherence to antiviral regimen (ARVs) can slow the disease process as well as prevent secondary infections and complications. Highly active antiviral therapy (HAART) is the most effective treatment for HIV. The cocktail of antiviral drugs included in HAART is as follows:

Nucleoside reverse transcriptase inhibitors (NRTIs) – prevent virus replication, such as zidovudine and lamivudine.

Non-nucleoside reverse transcription inhibitors (NNRTIs), nevirapine. These inhibitors disable the key protein that HIV requires to replicate.

- Protease inhibitors (PIs) such as ritonavir and indinavir inhibit the protease.
- Entry or fusion inhibitors – block the virus entry into the body CD4 cells.
- Integrase inhibitors (INSTIs) – these inhibitors block the ability of virus to insert genetic material into the cell.

Prevention Preventive measures against HIV infection include:

Education. The National AIDS Control Organization (NACO) has been set up under the Ministry of Health and Family Welfare. Awareness is being imparted through all means of publicity and by NGOs in schools, colleges, factories, farms, etc.

Screening is compulsorily carried out in case of blood donors, organ donors, semen donors, foreigners and sex workers.

AIDS-positive persons are advised to prevent sexual contacts and pregnancy.

Ban on prostitution.

Safer sex with single partner, use of condoms and barrier creams.

Use of disposable syringes, needles, blood bags and i.v. sets.

Proper sterilization of razors, blades and dental equipment by using 70% alcohol, 35% sodium hypochlorite, 5% formaldehyde, boiling for 15 minutes or autoclaving.

Self-Assessment

1. Describe the role of thymus in the immune system.
2. Describe the cellular immune response.
3. Describe the humoral immune response.
4. Write notes on:
   - Histocompatibility antigen
   - Structure of IgG antibody
   - Functions of immunoglobulins
   - Cytokines
   - Autoimmunity and immune tolerance
   - Complement system
5. Differentiate between:
   - Active and passive immunity
   - Humoral immunity and CMI
   - Classical and alternative pathways of the complement system
   - Primary and secondary responses of the immune system

Clinical Cases

Case 1

A 45-year-old male patient suffering with renal failure, not responding to dialysis was advised kidney transplantation. A donor from the family is ready to donate his one kidney.

Q1. What measures should be taken before and after the transplantation to prevent rejection?

Case 2

A booster dose of vaccination was given orally to an 18-month-old child. Within 6 hours, the child developed swelling in leg, pain on the side of vaccination and inability to walk.

On examination, the vitals were as follows: Temperature, 38.8°C; tachycardia; and tachypnoea.

Clinical findings: Swelling of right thigh with redness and pain; no swelling noted on the left thigh; no generalized oedema.

Q1. What is the probable diagnosis?

Q2. What treatment should be advised?

3.5 Platelets, Haemostasis and Blood Coagulation

CHAPTER OUTLINE

PLATELETS

STRUCTURE AND COMPOSITION

Platelets (small plates), also known as thrombocytes (thrombo, clot; cytes, cells), are the third types of blood cells having the following features:

Size. Platelets are the smallest blood cells varying in diameter from 2 to 4 μm, with an average volume of 5.8 μm^3.
Shape and colour. Platelets are colourless, spherical or oval discoid structures.
Leishman staining shows that a platelet consists of a faint bluish cytoplasm containing reddish-purple granules.
Nucleus is absent in the platelets, and, therefore, these cannot reproduce.

Electron microscopic structure Under an electron microscope, a platelet shows the following structural and compositional characteristics (Fig. 3.5.1).

1. Cell membrane. Each platelet is enclosed in a 6-nm-thick trilaminar membrane identical to plasma membrane of tissue cells. It consists of lipids (phospholipids, cholesterol and glycolipids), carbohydrates, proteins and glycoproteins. Its salient features are as follows:

Glycoproteins forming the surface coat of the platelet membrane prevent adherence of platelets to normal endothelium, but accelerate the adherence of platelets to collagen and damaged endothelium in injured blood vessels.
Phospholipids of the platelet membrane contain platelet factor 3 (PF-3), which plays an activating role at several points in the blood clotting process.
Invagination of the surface membrane forms the so-called *canalicular system* or the *surface connecting system*.
Receptors present on the platelet membrane are meant for combining with specific substances like collagen, fibrinogen ADP and the von Willebrand factor (VWF) in vessel walls.
Precursors of various substances like thromboxane A_2, prostaglandins, leukotrienes and PF-3, thrombopoietin (TPO) and platelet factor 4 (PF-4) are also present in the platelet membrane.

2. Microtubules. Microtubules are made up of polymerized proteins called tubulins. These form a compact bundle which is present immediately beneath the platelet membrane and encircles the whole cytoplasm. These are responsible for maintenance of the discoid shape of circulating platelets.

3. Cytoplasm. Cytoplasm of the platelets contains Golgi apparatus, endoplasmic reticulum, few mitochondria, microtubules, microvesicles, filaments, granules, glycogen, lysosomes, proteins, enzymes and hormonal substances. The role of some of the active factors is described as follows:

Endoplasmic reticulum and Golgi apparatus. These structures synthesize various enzymes and store large quantities of calcium.

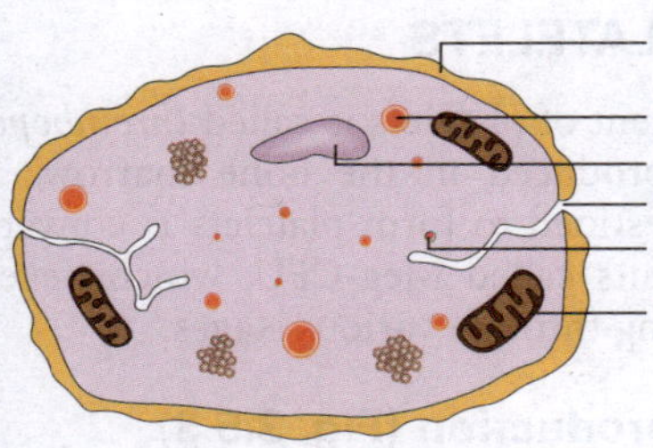

Fig. 3.5.1 Ultrastructure of a platelet.

Mitochondria. These are capable of forming ATP and ADP.

Contractile proteins include actin, myosin and thrombosthenin. Actin and myosin molecules are similar to those of contractile proteins of the muscles. Contractile proteins can cause the platelet to contract and are thus responsible for the clot retraction.

Other proteins present in the cytoplasm are as follows:
Fibrin-stabilizing factor. It is an important protein having a role in blood coagulation.
Platelet-derived growth factor (PDGF). It causes growth of vascular endothelial cells, vascular smooth muscle cells and fibroblasts, and thus is involved in the repair of damaged blood vessels.

Granules. Two types of granules are present in the cytoplasm of platelets:
Dense granules: Under electron microscope, they appear dense and are present as 3–8 granules/cell. They contain substances like phospholipids, triglycerides and cholesterol); ATP; ADP; and serotonin (5-HT). Platelets cannot synthesize 5-HT, so they obtain their 5-HT while passing through GIT.
α-Granules: These contain secreted proteins such as clotting factors and PDGF, platelet factor 4 (PF-4), fibronectin and thrombosthenin.
Lysosomal granules are very less.

Enzymes present in the cytoplasm of platelets include adenosine triphosphatase and the enzyme necessary for synthesis of prostaglandins. Prostaglandins act as local hormones and have local vascular and tissue reactions.

PROPERTIES AND FUNCTIONS

Properties of platelets (Fig. 3.5.2)

1. Adhesiveness. Platelets possess the property of adhesiveness, i.e. when they come in contact with any wet or rough surface, they are activated and stick to the surface. Factors responsible for adhesiveness are collagen, thrombin, ADP, thromboxane A_2, calcium ions and the VWF. Whenever there is injury to the vessel wall, platelets adhere to the exposed collagen and the VWF, to their receptors present on the platelet membrane. VWF forms a connecting link between collagen and platelets.

2. Aggregation. Platelets have the property to aggregate, i.e. they stick to each other. This is due to ADP and thromboxane A_2. Platelet binding causes their activation which results in release of contents of the granules. The released ADP acts on ADP receptors on the platelet membrane and produces further accumulation of platelets (platelet aggregation). Platelet aggregation is also fostered by the platelet-activating factor (PAF), cytokines (secreted by

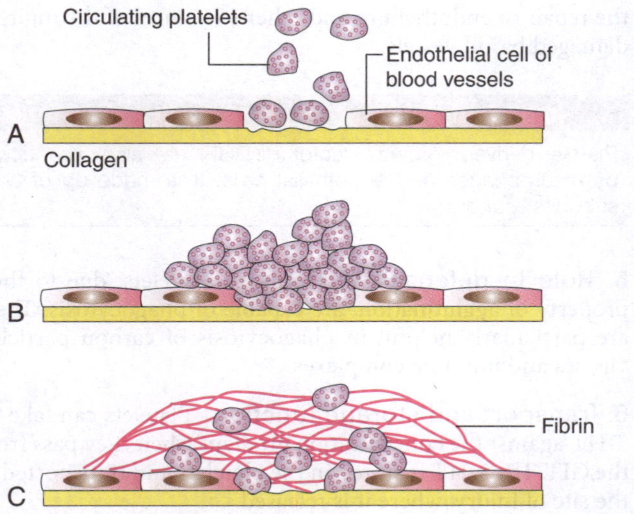

Fig. 3.5.2 Properties of platelets: **A**, adhesiveness; **B**, aggregation; and **C**, formation of haemostatic plug.

platelets), neutrophils and monocytes. The PAF acts via a G protein–coupled receptor (GPCR).

> **Important Note**
>
> In human beings, there are different types of ADP receptors (P_2Y_1, P_2Y_2 and P_2X_1).
>
> The drugs used as treatment of stroke/myocardial infarction (MI) act by inhibitory effect on these receptors.

3. Agglutination. Clumping together of platelets is called agglutination. This occurs due to the action of some platelet agglutinins.

Functions of Platelets

Platelets when activated, perform the following functions.

1. Role in haemostasis. Haemostasis refers to spontaneous arrest of bleeding from an injured blood vessel. Process of haemostasis is discussed in detail on page 201. Platelets play the following roles in haemostasis:

Vasoconstriction is induced by the serotonin (5-HT) and other vasoconstrictors secreted by the platelets.
Temporary haemostatic plug is formed by the platelets due to their properties of adhesiveness and aggregation.
Definitive haemostatic plug formation process is also initiated by platelets.

2. Role in clot formation. Process of clot formation involves a complex series of events (described on page 203). Platelets play an important role in the formation of the intrinsic prothrombin activator which is responsible for the onset of blood clotting.

3. Role in clot retraction. Process of clot retraction is described on page 205. Contractions of contractile proteins (actin, myosin and thrombosthenin) present in the platelets play an important role in clot retraction.

4. Role in repair of injured blood vessels. The PDGF present in the cytoplasm of platelets plays an important role in the repair of endothelium and other structures of the injured/damaged blood vessels.

> **Important Note**
>
> Platelet-derived growth factor (PDGF) is also produced by macrophages and endothelial cells. It is made up of two subunits α and β.

5. Role in defence mechanism. Platelets, due to their property of agglutination, are capable of phagocytosis. These are particularly helpful in phagocytosis of carbon particles, viruses and immune complexes.

6. Transport and storage function. Platelets can take up 5-HT against the concentration gradient when they pass from the GIT. The 5-HT is stored in the platelets and transported to the site of injury, where it is released.

NORMAL COUNT AND VARIATIONS

Normal Count

Normal platelet count ranges from 1.5 to 4.5 lakh/μL with an average count of 2.5 lakh/μL.

Physiological variations

1. ***Age.*** Platelet count is less in infants (1–2 lakh/μL). Adult levels are reached by the third month after birth.
2. ***Sex.*** Normally, there is no difference in the platelet counts of males and females. However, during menstruation, the count is reduced in females.
3. ***After meals***, the platelet count is slightly increased.
4. ***After strenuous muscular exercise***, platelets may increase.
5. ***At high altitude***, the platelet count increases.

Pathological variations

A. Thrombocytosis. An increase in the number of platelets more than 4.5 lakh/μL is called thrombocytosis.

Causes of thrombocytosis. Platelet count is increased:

1. ***After splenectomy***
2. ***After haemorrhage***, severe injury, major surgical operation and parturition.
3. ***In myeloproliferative disorders*** such as chronic myeloid leukaemia, polycythaemia vera and myelofibrosis.

B. Thrombocytopenia. Decrease in the number of platelets below 1.5 lakh/μL is called thrombocytopenia.

Causes of thrombocytopenia:

1. *Idiopathic thrombocytopenic purpura*
2. *Bone marrow depression* due to:
   - Effects of various cytotoxic drugs
   - Whole-body irradiation
   - Hypoplastic and aplastic anaemia
3. *Acute leukaemia* or secondary deposits of malignancy in the bone marrow
4. *Infections* like smallpox, chickenpox, scarlet fever, typhoid and dengue fever
5. *Hypersplenism* and drugs that cause increased destruction of platelets, e.g. thiazide and oestrogen
6. *Toxaemia*, septicaemia and uraemia

FORMATION OF PLATELETS

Formation or development of platelets is called *thrombopoiesis*. The platelets are produced in the bone marrow. The pluripotent stem cell destined to form platelets is converted into colony-forming units called Meg-CFU, which develop into platelets after passing through various stages.

Stages in platelet production (Fig. 3.5.3)

1. Megakaryoblast. The earliest recognizable precursor of platelets in the bone marrow is megakaryoblast. It arises from Meg-CFU by a process of differentiation.

- *Diameter* of megakaryoblast is about 20–30 μm.
- *Cytoplasm* is small, blue and nongranular.
- *Nucleus* is large, oval or kidney-shaped with several nucleoli.

2. Promegakaryocyte. Promegakaryocyte is formed from the megakaryoblast. A megakaryoblast undergoes endoreduplication of nuclear chromatin, i.e. nuclear chromatin replicates repeatedly in multiples of two without division of the cell. Ultimately, a large cell containing up to 32 times the normal diploid content of nuclear DNA is formed when further nuclear replication ceases and the cytoplasm becomes granular. The granules are intensely basophilic.

3. Megakaryocyte. A promegakaryocyte matures into a megakaryocyte with the following features:

- *Diameter.* Mature megakaryocyte is a large cell, 30–90 μm in diameter.
- *Nucleus.* Megakaryocyte has single multilobed (4–16 lobes) nucleus with coarsely clumped chromatin.
- *Cytoplasm.* It is abundant, light blue in colour and contains red-purple granules.
- *Cell margin.* It is irregular and shows many pseudopodia. Platelets are formed from pseudopodia of megakaryocyte cytoplasm which get detached into the bloodstream. Each megakaryocyte may form up to 4000 platelets. The formation of platelets from the stem cell takes about 10 days.

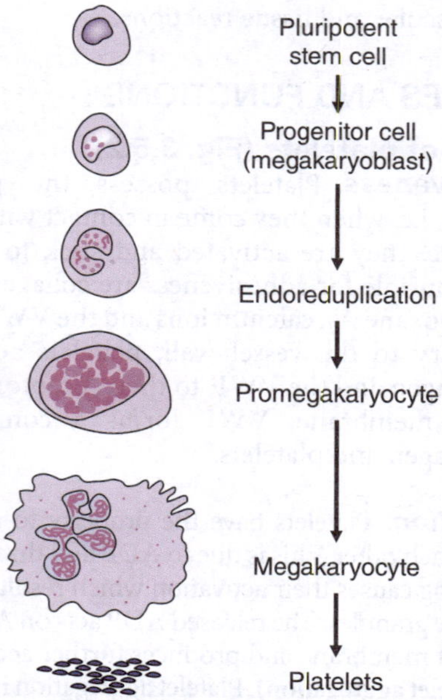

Fig. 3.5.3 Stages of thrombopoiesis.

Control of Thrombopoiesis

Thrombopoiesis seems to be regulated by the following humoral factors:

- Thrombopoietin
- Megakaryocyte colony–stimulating factor (Meg-CSF)

Thrombopoietin. It promotes maturation of megakaryocytes and is a circulating protein produced by the liver and kidney. Thrombopoietin acts through its receptors present on platelets and controls the platelet production by feedback mechanism, i.e. when the number of platelet count is low, less will bind to the platelets and more will be available for platelet production. On the other hand, when the number of platelets is high, more will bind to the receptors and less will be available for stimulation of platelet production.

Megakaryocyte colony–stimulating factor. It controls the production of megakaryocytes. Thrombosthenin is produced by liver and kidney and it plays main role in maturation of platelets.

LIFESPAN AND FATE OF PLATELETS

Lifespan of platelets varies from 8 to 12 days with an average of 10 days. Platelets are destroyed by the tissue macrophage system in the spleen. Therefore:

- *Splenomegaly* causes reduction in the platelet count.
- *Splenectomy* is followed by an increase in platelet count.

HAEMOSTASIS

Haemostasis refers to spontaneous arrest or prevention of bleeding from injured/damaged vessels by the physiological process. The process of haemostasis is initiated immediately following an injury/damage to the blood vessel. It involves three main steps (Fig. 3.5.4):

- Vasoconstriction
- Formation of temporary haemostatic plug
- Formation of the definitive haemostatic clot

1. Vasoconstriction Vasoconstriction plays an important role in the process of haemostasis. It is induced as follows.

Initial vasoconstriction. It affects several centimetres in both the directions from the site of injury and occurs immediately following injury to the vessels. The degree of spasm is proportionate to the degree of trauma to the blood vessel. The vasoconstriction may be intense enough to stop the bleeding from small vessels. Initial vasoconstriction is caused by the direct effect of injury on the vascular smooth muscles. It is transient and is maintained for several minutes or even hours by humoral facilitation.

Humoral facilitation of vasoconstriction. Following an injury/damage to the wall of blood vessel, the platelets get adhered to the damaged endothelium and exposed collagen. These platelets immediately release 5-HT and other

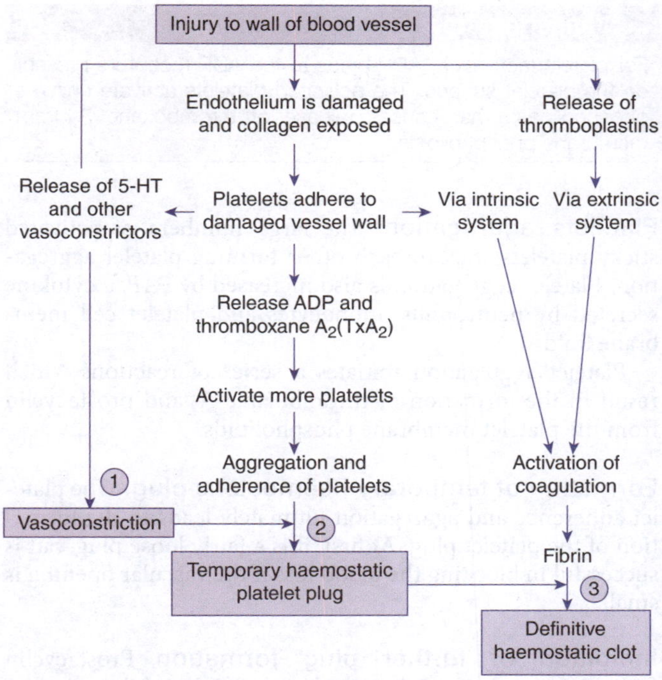

Fig. 3.5.4 Steps of haemostasis.

vasoconstrictors which augment the initial vasoconstriction. The vasoconstriction so induced is, thus, purely a local phenomenon. Usually arterioles and small arteries respond by vasoconstriction and decrease the loss of blood from the damaged blood vessel.

Thromboxane A_2 (TxA_2) is a potent vasoconstrictor produced by endothelial cells and macrophages. It also plays an important role.

2. Formation of temporary haemostatic plug Formation of a temporary haemostatic plug by the platelets at the site of injury involves the following steps.

Platelet adhesion. Following injury, platelets come in contact with damaged collagen fibres and endothelial cells of the vessel wall and change their characteristics. That is, they begin to swell and assume irregular forms with large numbers of pseudopodia protruding from the surface. The contractile proteins of the platelets contract forcibly and cause release of granules that contain multiple factors. They become sticky and therefore adhere to the collagen of damaged cell walls and to the damaged endothelium.

> **Important Note**
>
> von Willebrand factor (VWF) acts as a connecting link between collagen and platelets because platelets have receptor for VWF on the surface.

Platelets activation. The platelets secrete large quantities of ADP and thromboxane A_2 (T_XA_2) which act on the nearby platelets and cause their activation. Stickiness of these additional platelets causes them to adhere to originally activated platelets. In this way, a vicious cycle is initiated which leads to activation and adherence of a large number of platelets.

Important Note

For platelet activation, ADP binds to the ADP receptors present on the platelet surface. The activated platelets activate enzyme phospholipase that causes release of thromboxane A_2 from membrane phospholipids.

Platelets aggregation. The large numbers of activated sticky platelets stick to each other forming platelet aggregation. Platelet aggregation is also increased by *PAF*, a cytokine secreted by neutrophils, monocytes and platelet cell membrane lipids.

Platelet aggregation initiates a series of reactions which result in the formation of thromboxane A_2 and prostacyclin from the platelet membrane phospholipids.

Formation of temporary haemostatic plug. The platelet adherence and aggregation ultimately leads to the formation of the platelet plug. At first, it is a fairly loose plug, but is successful in blocking the blood loss if the vascular opening is small.

Inhibition of further plug formation. Prostacyclin formed from the membrane phospholipids inhibits thromboxane formation, and thus curtails the process of further plug formation. This reaction keeps the platelet plug localized, i.e. prevents intravascular spread of plug.

3. Formation of definitive haemostatic plug The temporary platelet plug is converted into the definitive haemostatic plug by the process of clot formation (blood coagulation), which involves a complex series of events (see page 203). Platelets play an important role in the formation of the intrinsic prothrombin activator which is responsible for initiating the process of clot formation (page 204). The blood clot formed at the site of injury results in a tight unyielding seal or the so-called definitive haemostatic plug.

BLOOD COAGULATION

Blood remains in a fluid condition within the blood vessels throughout life. But when the blood is shed from the blood vessels or collected in a container, it loses its fluidity within a few minutes and gets converted into a jelly-like mass, which is called a *clot*. This phenomenon is called *coagulation* or clotting of blood. Both of these properties of blood are essential for life:

Fluidity is essential for circulation.
Coagulation provides an indispensable defence against excessive bleeding from the wounds. Thus, coagulation of the blood is one of the mechanisms involved in the process of haemostasis (prevention of blood loss).

The process of blood coagulation consists of a complex cascade of reactions. The final step in the process of coagulation is transformation of plasma protein *fibrinogen* into *fibrin* forming a sort of network within which the cellular elements of the blood are arrested. Before discussing the mechanism of blood coagulation in detail, it will be worthwhile to study the essential features of the various clotting factors involved in this process.

CLOTTING FACTORS

The process of coagulation essentially involves a stepwise activation of certain substances, mostly proteins, present in the blood and/or tissue fluids. These substances are called clotting factors and have been given Roman numerals:

- Factor I (fibrinogen)
- Factor II (prothrombin)
- Factor III (thromboplastin)
- Factor IV (calcium)
- Factor V (labile factor or proaccelerin or accelerator globulin)
- Factor VI (nonexistent)
- Factor VII (stable factor or proconvertin or autoprothrombin I)
- Factor VIII (antihaemophilic factor A [AHF] or antihaemophilic globulin [AHG])
- Factor IX (Christmas factor or plasma thromboplastin component [PTC or antihaemophilic factor B])
- Factor X (Stuart–Prower factor)
- Factor XI (plasma thromboplastin antecedent [PTA] or antihaemophilic factor C)
- Factor XII (Hageman factor or glass factor or contact factor)
- Factor XIII (fibrin-stabilizing factor or fibrinase or Laki–Lorand factor)
- High-molecular-weight kininogen (HMW-K or Fitzgerald factor)
- Prekallikrein (pre-Ka or Fletcher factor)
- Kallikrein (Ka)
- Platelet phospholipid (PL)

Factor I (fibrinogen). It is a soluble plasma protein globulin in nature. Its molecular weight is 340,000 Da and is synthesized in the liver. It has six polypeptide chains, with its plasma concentration about 0.3 g/dL. It is converted into fibrin in the presence of the enzyme thrombin.

Factor II (prothrombin). It is an inactive precursor of thrombin. Its features are described on page 204.

Factor III (thromboplastin). It is also called tissue factor (TF) or tissue thromboplastins. It is released in the extrinsic pathway of formation of prothrombin activator (see page 203).

Factor IV (calcium). Ionic calcium is essential for blood coagulation. Its role in coagulation is described on page 205.

Factor V (labile factor). It is also called proaccelerin. It is a protein and, as the name indicates, it is the labile or unstable factor of the plasma. It is required for the formation of the prothrombin activator and thus conversion of prothrombin to thrombin in both extrinsic and intrinsic mechanisms of blood coagulation. Factor V is consumed during clotting and is therefore absent from serum. Its deficiency occasionally occurs as a congenital anomaly simulating haemophilia.

Factor VII (stable factor or autoprothrombin I). It is a stable protein synthesized in liver in the presence of vitamin K. It is required for activation of factor X in the extrinsic pathway. It is not consumed during clotting and therefore is present in serum, as well as in plasma. Deficiency of factor VII is a rare natural occurrence, but is frequently induced by oral anticoagulant drugs of the coumarin type, overdosage of which may lead to bleeding.

Factor VIII (antihaemophilic globulin). It is a protein of β_2-globulin type synthesized in the liver. It is required for the activation of factor X, and thus formation of the prothrombin activator in intrinsic pathway. It is consumed during clotting and is therefore absent from the serum. Its congenital deficiency causes classical haemophilia (haemophilia A), which is an inherited disease in which the clotting time (CT) is prolonged.

Factor IX (Christmas factor). It is also called plasma thromboplastin component (PTC) or autoprothrombin II. It is a protein synthesized in the liver independent of vitamin K. It is activated by the active factor XI in the presence of Ca^{2+}, and is essential for the formation of prothrombin activator in the intrinsic pathway. Its absence or deficiency causes haemophilia B, which is an inherited disease and is similar to haemophilia A. This disease was first discovered in a patient named Christmas and hence the factor was termed *Christmas factor*.

Factor X (Stuart–Prower factor). It is a protein present in plasma and is synthesized in the liver. It is activated by active factor IX in the presence of factor VIII, Ca^{2+} and phospholipids. Activated factor X, along with active factor V, Ca^{2+} and phospholipids, forms a complex which is called *prothrombin activator*, in both extrinsic and intrinsic pathways.

Factor XI (plasma thromboplastin antecedent). It is activated by active factor XII. It is required for the activation of factor IX in the presence of Ca^{2+} in intrinsic pathway. Its deficiency causes a haemorrhagic state.

Factor XII (Hageman factor). Factor XII is activated to XIIa when it comes in contact with negatively charged surfaces, foreign substances or rough surfaces. Its activation in the blood initiates intrinsic pathway by activating factor XI (PTA) to XIa. Activated factor XII also activates prekallikrein to activated kallikrenin (pre-Ka to KA), which in turn activates XII to XIIa (*feedback activations*). In deficiency of factor XII, blood clots very slowly in glass but there is no haemorrhagic state.

Factor XIII (fibrin-stabilizing factor). This is a plasma protein which is required for stabilization of fibrin polymers in the presence of Ca^{2+}.

High-molecular-weight kininogen. It is responsible for attracting pre-Ka and factor XI to the site of reaction with factor XII. This is possible because HMW-K, like factor XII, is attracted towards the negatively charged surfaces which provide the site of reactions.

Prekallikrein and kallikrein. Pre-Ka is activated to KA by XIIa, which in turn activates XII to XIIa. This phenomenon is called feedback activation of XII and is shown as follows.

Platelet phospholipids (PPL). Platelets contain phospholipids which are essential for clotting in the absence of tissue extract, i.e. in intrinsic pathway of coagulation. *Arabic* numerals are sometimes used for platelet activities affecting blood coagulation. For example, the term:

- *PF-3* is used for platelet phospholipid procoagulant activity.
- *PF-4* is used for heparin neutralizing activity of platelets.

MECHANISM OF COAGULATION

Normally, blood circulates in the blood vessels and does not clot spontaneously. Factors responsible for this will be discussed later. Clot formation is initiated under the following situations:

- Trauma to the vascular wall and adjacent tissues
- Trauma to blood
- Contact of blood with damaged endothelial cells or collagen or other tissue elements outside the vessel

The process of coagulation involves a *cascade* of reactions in which activation of one factor leads to activation of the next clotting factor (Fig. 3.5.5). This enzyme cascade reaction is also called waterfall *sequence*. It is important to note that each factor activates (compared to its own amount) a huge quantity of the other factor, i.e. at each stage, amplification of result is obtained. Thus, the process can be viewed as a *bio-amplifier*. The process of coagulation can be divided into three main steps:

A. Formation of prothrombin activator
B. Conversion of prothrombin to thrombin
C. Conversion of fibrinogen into fibrin

A. Formation of Prothrombin Activator

Process of coagulation is initiated by formation of a complex substance called prothrombin activator. Two different mechanisms involved in the formation of the prothrombin activator are as follows:

1. Extrinsic pathway
2. Intrinsic pathway

Extrinsic Pathway

The extrinsic pathway of formation of prothrombin activator begins with trauma to the vascular wall or the tissues outside the blood vessel. It includes the three basic steps given next (Fig. 3.5.5).

1. Release of tissue thromboplastins. The traumatized tissues release several substances which are together known as *tissue thromboplastin (factor III)*. This includes phospholipids of cell membranes of the tissues and lipoprotein complex containing glycoprotein which acts as an enzyme.

2. Activation of factor X to form activated factor X. Tissue thromboplastin combines with factor VII (stable factor) to form the tissue thromboplastin factor VII complex, which in the presence of Ca^{2+} activates factor X to form activated factor X (Xa).

3. Effect of activated factor X to form prothrombin activator. The activated factor X, along with tissue phospholipids or phospholipids released from platelets, factor V (labile factor) and Ca^{2+}, forms a complex which is called prothrombin activator.

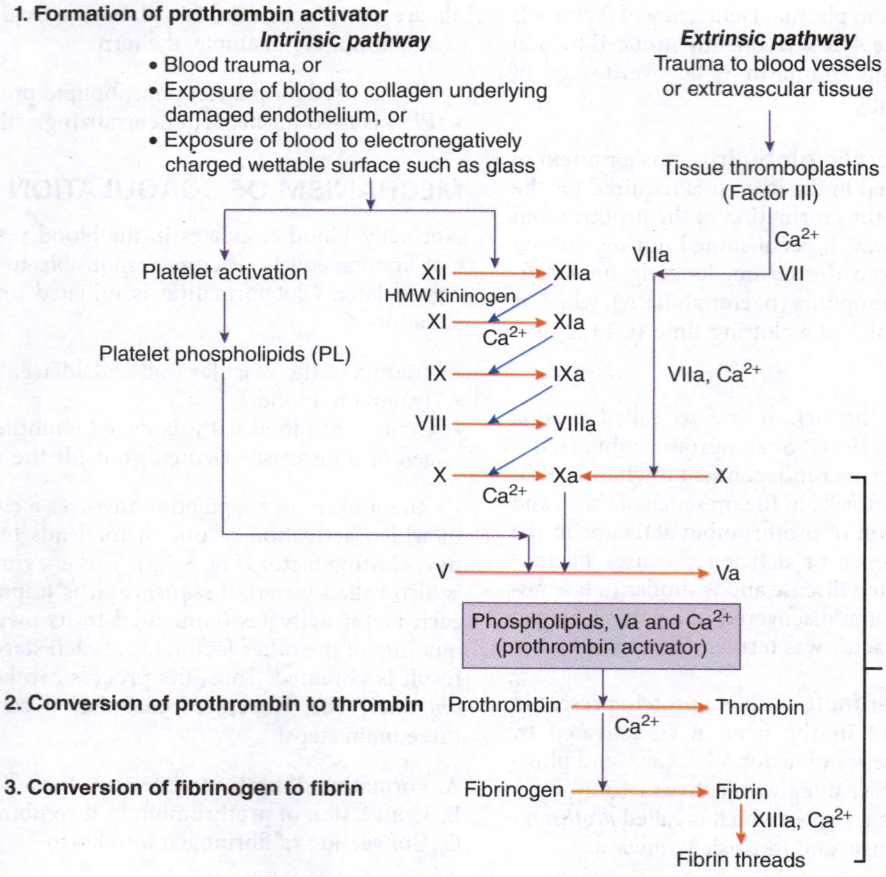

Fig. 3.5.5 Mechanism of blood coagulation.

Intrinsic Pathway

The intrinsic pathway of formation of prothrombin activator begins in the blood itself following trauma to the blood or exposure of blood to collagen in a traumatized vascular wall. The steps of intrinsic pathway are summarized in Fig. 3.5.5.

Activation of factor XII. Trauma to blood or exposure to collagen fibres underlying damaged vascular endothelium (or electronegatively charged wettable surface such as glass, in vitro) activates plasma factor XII to form XIIa and initiates the intrinsic pathway. Platelets are also activated.

Activation of factor XI Activation of factor XI to form XIa is caused by the activated factor XII. HMW-K and prekallikrein accelerate this reaction.

Activation of factor IX Activation of factor IX to form IXa is in turn caused by the activated factor XI in the presence of Ca^{2+}.

Activation of factor X. Factor IXa in the presence of activated factor VIII, Ca^{2+} and phospholipids (released by activated platelets) activate factor X to form Xa. In thrombocytopenia and deficiency of factor VIII (classical haemophilia), this reaction is deficient.

Formation of prothrombin activator. The activated factor X, along with the phospholipids released by activated platelets, activated factor V and Ca^{2+}, forms a complex which is called prothrombin activator.

Extrinsic versus intrinsic pathway

- Extrinsic pathway begins with trauma to the vascular wall or the tissue outside the vessel wall, while intrinsic pathway begins in the blood itself.
- Extrinsic pathway is explosive in nature, with severe tissue trauma clotting occurring in as little as 15 seconds, while intrinsic pathway is much slower to proceed, usually requiring 2–6 minutes to cause clotting.
- The extrinsic and intrinsic pathways are initiated by different factors, though both converge at factor X and then follow the same common pathway (Fig. 3.5.5).

B. Conversion of Prothrombin to Thrombin

Prothrombin

Prothrombin (factor II) is a plasma protein (an α_2 globulin) with the following features:

- It is the inactive precursor of enzyme thrombin (which is not present normally in the circulating blood).
- Its molecular weight is about 69,000 Da.
- It is synthesized in liver in the presence of vitamin K. (***Note:*** Hepatic synthesis of factors VII, IX and X is also dependent on the presence of vitamin K.)
- Its concentration in plasma of an adult is 40 mg/dL which falls in liver diseases. In a newborn baby, plasma concentration of prothrombin is lower.

Conversion of prothrombin to thrombin. It is caused by the prothrombin activator in the presence of Ca^{2+}. This occurs on the surface of platelets which form the platelet plug at the site of injury. Thus, clot formation starts at the site of injury. The rate of formation of thrombin is directly proportional to the quantity of prothrombin activator available, which in turn is proportional to degree of trauma to the vessel wall or to the blood.

Thrombin

Thrombin so formed acts as proteolytic enzyme. Its molecular weight is 34,000 Da, exactly half of prothrombin. The amount of thrombin produced is in excess of the need. It has been estimated that the amount of thrombin produced during clotting of only 1 mL of blood is sufficient to coagulate 3 L of blood. Thus, this presents a dangerous possibility of extensive intravascular clotting whenever the haemorrhage mechanism is in operation (even in a trivial cut). However, practically it does not occur so, since there exist adequate mechanisms in the body to prevent it (see page 208).

Roles played by thrombin are:

Conversion of fibrinogen to fibrin (discussed below).
Positive feedback role of thrombin. It accelerates the rate of formation of prothrombin activator by activating factors VIII, V and XIII. The cascade mechanism of enzyme activation acts in such a way that small amounts of activated factor XII ultimately generate large amounts of prothrombin activator. In this way, thrombin itself can cause further conversion of prothrombin into thrombin (amplification effect).
Activation of protein C (which is an anticoagulant).

C. Conversion of Fibrinogen to Fibrin

Fibrinogen

Fibrinogen (factor I) is a soluble plasma protein globulin in nature.

- Its molecular weight is 340,000.
- It is synthesized in the liver.
- It has six polypeptide chains each having 450 amino acids.
- Its plasma concentration is about 0.3 g/dL.

Conversion of fibrinogen into fibrin. Conversion of fibrinogen into fibrin involves three reactions (Fig. 3.5.6).

1. Proteolysis. Thrombin acting as proteolytic enzyme removes four low-molecular-weight peptide chains from each molecule of fibrinogen to convert it into fibrin monomer.

2. Polymerization. Fibrin monomer polymerizes with another monomer to form *long fibrin* threads which form reticulum of the clot. Initially, the clot is weak because the fibrin threads are not cross-linked with each other.

3. Stabilization of fibrin polymers. Fibrin-stabilizing factor (factor XIII), which is normally present in the plasma and also released from the activated platelets, is activated by the thrombin to form XIIIa, but XIIIa in the presence of Ca^{2+} causes formation of covalent cross-linkages between fibrin threads, thus adding tremendous strength to the fibrin meshwork. The fibrin meshwork traps the remaining

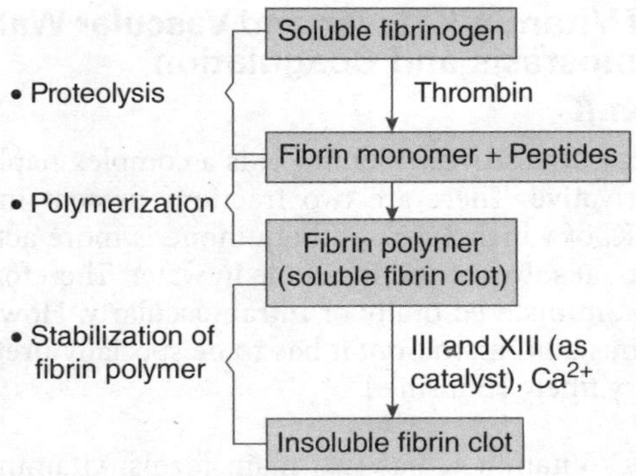

Fig. 3.5.6 Types of reactions involved in conversion of soluble fibrinogen into insoluble fibrin clot.

components of plasma and blood cells to form a solid mass called clot.

BLOOD CLOT RETRACTION

The blood clot formed at the end of the coagulation process is composed of a meshwork of fibrin threads running in all directions along with the entrapped blood cells, platelets and plasma. The fibrin threads adhere to the damaged surface of blood vessels.

At this juncture, it is important to note that *coagulation is the property of plasma alone*. The RBCs and WBCs do not take part in it. They only become caught up in the meshwork of the clot.

- Within a few minutes after a clot is formed, it begins to contract and usually squeezes out most of the fluid called *serum* (plasma without fibrinogen and other clotting factors) within 30–60 minutes.
- *Platelets are essential* for clot retraction. They are attached to fibrin fibres of the clot in such a way that they actually bind different fibres together. The contractile proteins (platelet thrombosthenin, actin and myosin) present in the cytoplasm of platelets cause strong contraction of platelet spicules attached to fibrin fibres. This helps to compress the fibrin meshwork, i.e. cause clot contraction. This contraction is activated by thrombin and calcium ions. The process of contraction of blood clot and oozing of serum is called *clot retraction*.
- If a blood clot is kept for several hours, the clot retracts to about 40% of its original volume.
- Clot retraction is impaired if blood platelets have been removed.

Role of Calcium in Blood Coagulation

From the study of mechanism of blood coagulation, it is quite clear that except for the first two steps in the intrinsic pathway, calcium ions are required for promotion of all the reactions. Therefore, in the absence of calcium ions, blood clotting will not occur. Thus, coagulation of blood can be prevented in vitro (e.g. for storage in the blood bank or for separation of plasma) by removal of calcium ions. The use of oxalates and citrates as in vitro anticoagulants is based on this principle. However, in vivo, the degree of hypocalcaemia (e.g. due to deficiency of vitamin D or hypoparathyroidism) is compatible with life and does not cause bleeding disorder.

Role of Vitamin K, Liver and Vascular Wall in Haemostasis and Coagulation

Vitamin K

Chemical structure. Vitamin K is a complex naphthoquinone derivative. There are two fractions present in natural vitamin K, of which 1,4-naphthoquinone is more active. It is soluble in fat solvents and insoluble in water. Therefore, it can only be administered orally or intramuscularly. However, for intravenous administration, it has to be specially prepared by being very finely emulsified.

Sources. Vitamin K has two main forms: vitamin K_1 and vitamin K_2. Vitamin K_1 (phylloquinone) is present in plant food like green leafy vegetables, whereas vitamin K_2 (menaquinone) is found in fermented food and animal products and also produced by gut bacteria.

Vitamin K is obtained from food, as well as synthesized by bacterial flora in the gut.

Dietary vitamin K and that synthesized by the bacterial flora is absorbed from the gut and reaches the liver. Its absorption from the small intestine occurs only in the presence of adequate amounts of bile salts. In the liver, synthesis of the following factors is dependent on vitamin K:

- Prothrombin
- Factors VII, IX and X
- Circulatory anticoagulant proteins

Applied Aspects

Vitamin K deficiency

Effects. In the deficiency of vitamin K, prothrombin time and blood CT is prolonged and serious haemorrhages may occur.
Causes. As mentioned above, vitamin K deficiency is unlikely to develop in dietary deficiency alone. Deficiency of vitamin K is seen in the following clinical conditions:

1. *Obstructive jaundice.* In this condition, bile salts do not reach the gut and thus vitamin K cannot be absorbed.
2. *Newborn babies* are likely to develop vitamin K deficiency and thus haemorrhagic disorders because gut bacterial flora which synthesizes vitamin K is not developed satisfactorily in the early infancy. Therefore, it is recommended that the newborn babies should be routinely given injection of vitamin K to prevent its deficiency.
3. *Chronic diarrhoea.* The syndrome of vitamin K deficiency has been reported in chronic diarrhoea. The cause may be failure of absorption or an abnormal state of the intestinal bacteria leading to defective synthesis of vitamin K. This syndrome may also occur with defective fat absorption in sprue.
4. *Side effect of antibiotics.* Vitamin K deficiency has also been reported in morbid patients living on glucose–saline transfusion and receiving heavy amounts of broad-spectrum antibiotics, particularly *cephalosporin*. Antibiotics kill the bacterial flora of the gut leading to deficient synthesis of vitamin K.

Role of Liver

Liver plays the following significant roles in the coagulation mechanism:

1. ***Synthesis of procoagulants.*** It is the site of synthesis of factors V, VII, IX and X, prothrombin and fibrinogen.
2. ***Removal of activated procoagulants.*** Liver also removes the activated procoagulants from the blood.
3. ***Synthesis of anticoagulants.*** Liver also synthesizes anticoagulants like heparin, antithrombin III and protein C.

Applied Aspects

Liver failure can cause

- *Bleeding disorders* due to hypocoagulability of the blood.
- *Uncontrolled extensive clotting* inside the blood vessels where clotting is not only unwanted but also dangerous.

Role of Blood Vessels

Role played by endothelium, subendothelial tissue and smooth muscles of the media of the blood vessels in coagulation and haemostasis mechanisms is summarized next.

Endothelium. Endothelium plays both an anticoagulatory and a coagulatory role.

Anticoagulatory roles played by endothelium are:

- It acts as a barrier between the thrombogenic subendothelial tissue and the blood.
- It produces heparin and α_2-macroglobulin which are coagulation inhibitors.
- Smoothness of uninjured endothelial cells prevents platelet aggregation.
- Endothelial cells produce PGI_2 (a prostaglandin), which opposes platelet aggregation.

Roles in clotting mechanism are:

- Endothelium secretes VWF. The plasma VWF acts as a connecting bridge between the platelets and the subendothelial tissue (exposed after injury) and thus initiates platelet aggregation and haemostasis.
- TF is released by endothelial cells following trauma. It initiates the process of extrinsic pathway of clotting mechanism.
- Plasminogen activator which activates plasminogen to plasmin is also released by endothelial cells.

Subendothelial tissue. Subendothelial tissue, which chiefly consists of collagen fibres, plays the following roles in coagulation:

- *Platelet aggregation* is initiated when blood comes in contact with the subendothelial collagenous tissue.
- *Intrinsic coagulation pathway* is initiated when factor XII is activated following contact of blood with subendothelial collagenous tissue.

Vascular smooth muscle. Smooth muscles of the vascular wall play a role in haemostasis by causing vasoconstriction. Vasoconstriction is initiated by mechanical injury to muscles and is later facilitated by the vasoconstrictors such as serotonin, prostaglandins and noradrenaline released by the platelets which adhere at the site of injury.

Why circulating blood does not clot We all know that blood circulating in the blood vessels does not clot and that fluidity of the blood is essential for life. By now we have discussed most of the factors responsible for fluidity of the blood. They are summarized as follows.

1. Velocity of circulation Blood is pumped into the vessels and circulated at a constant velocity which contributes to its fluidity. That is why a decrease in circulation velocity in certain conditions is associated with intravascular clotting.

2. Surface effects of endothelium Smoothness of endothelial lining inhibits platelet adhesion and thus prevents initiation of intrinsic clotting mechanism.

- A layer of glycocalyx (mucopolysaccharide) adsorbed to the inner surface of endothelium being negatively charged repels clotting factors (anion proteins) and platelets and thereby prevents clotting.
- Intact endothelium acts as a barrier between the thrombogenic subendothelial collagenous tissue and the blood.
- Endothelial cells also produce thrombin-binding protein (thrombomodulin), which slows the process of clotting by removing thrombin (see page 341).

3. Circulatory anticoagulants Circulatory anticoagulants or the so-called natural anticoagulants present in the blood, which prevent clotting, are as follows:

- Heparin
- Antithrombin III
- α_2-Macroglobulin
- Protein C (for details, see page 209).

4. Fibrinolytic mechanism Protein C is a naturally occurring anticoagulant which inactivates factors V and VIII, and also inactivates an inhibitor of tissue plasminogen activator (TPA) increasing the formation of plasmin which acts fibrinolytic.

- Further, whenever there is trauma, along with activation of clotting mechanism, the fibrinolytic system is also activated, which prevents spread of intravascular clotting.

5. Removal of activated clotting factors Liver plays a role in preventing the intravascular clotting by removing activated clotting factors in the event of onset of spontaneous clot formation.

Applied Aspects

Thrombosis

We have studied that physiologically, under normal conditions, the circulating blood does not clot and that clotting of blood occurs only extravascularly when a vessel has been injured and bleeding has occurred. However, under certain pathological conditions, intravascular clotting may occur. The intravascular clotting is called *thrombosis*, and the clot so formed is called thrombus. Thus, *thrombus* may be defined as a solid mass formed in the living heart or blood vessels from the constituents of blood. Intravascular thrombosis can be distinguished from extravascular clotting or clotting in wounds, and also from clotting which occurs in blood vessels after death.

Predisposing factors

Virchow described three primary events which predispose to thrombus formation (*Virchow's* triad). These are as follows:

1. **Endothelial injury** We have studied how an intact endothelium prevents coagulation (page 206). Endothelial injury may occur in many conditions, of which a few important ones are as follows: ulcerated plaques in advanced atherosclerosis, haemodynamic stress in hypertension, arterial disease, diabetes mellitus and hypercholesterolaemia.
2. **Alterations in flow of blood** In both turbulence and stasis of blood, normal axial flow of blood is disturbed and platelets come in contact with endothelium initiating thrombus formation. Stasis of blood is commonly associated with venous thrombosis especially in leg veins after major operations on the abdomen (postoperative thrombosis), or otherwise bedridden patients in whom muscular contraction in legs and trunk (responsible for normal venous blood flow) is decreased.
3. **Hypercoagulability of blood** Hypercoagulability of blood which predisposes to thrombosis may occur due to:
   - Increase in coagulation factors such as fibrinogen, prothrombin, and factors VIa, VIIa and Xa
   - Increase in platelet count and their adhesiveness
   - Decreased levels of coagulation inhibitors such as antithrombin III and fibrinogen degradation products

Sequence of Events in Thrombogenesis

Sequence of events which lead to the formation of a thrombus is as follows.

Adherence of platelets. Adherence of platelets to endothelium (in the individuals having any of the above-listed predisposing factors) is the first step in thrombogenesis. The mass of platelets grows by adhesion of other platelets as they pass by. The laminae of platelets (which fuse together and lose their identity) stand out as layers running transversely to the bloodstream. Passing leucocytes adhere to their borders (like flies on sheets of sticky flypaper).

Activation of coagulation system. The platelets liberate thromboplastin and activate coagulation system; thus, filaments of fibrin spread out from them on all sides. Fibrin filaments from one lamella meet with filaments from the next lamella. The lamellae of platelets are thus braced together by fibrin filaments.

Entanglement of red blood cells and white blood cells. The entanglement occurs in the fibrin network, and finally a solid mass of a peculiarly constructed clot called thrombus is formed. The red cells disintegrate and lose their haemoglobin; the initial red thrombus as it ages becomes yellowish-grey, but newly formed thrombi added to it will be red.

Types of Thrombi

Grossly, there are three types of thrombi.

Red thrombi. Venous thrombi are usually red and occlusive. Red thrombi are soft, red and gelatinous. They closely resemble blood clots in vitro.

White thrombi. Arterial thrombi usually tend to be white and mural, whereas white thrombi are pale and firm.

Mixed or laminated thrombi. These are also common and consist of alternate white and red layers called *lines of Zahn*.

Effects of Thrombi

Intravascular thrombi may cause variable effects (may be even life-threatening) depending on their size and site. Thrombi cause harmful effects by one of the following mechanisms:

1. **Ischaemia and infarction** Thrombi may decrease or stop the blood supply to part of an organ and cause ischaemia, which may subsequently result in infarction. *Arterial thrombi* usually produce ischaemia and infarction. For example, thrombus formation in coronary arteries may cause myocardial ischaemia and infarction.
2. **Thromboembolism** The thrombus or its part may get dislodged and be carried along in the bloodstream as *embolus* to lodge in a distant vessel. Cardiac and venous thrombi produce emboli more frequently than arterial thrombi. Examples of emboli formation are as follows:
   - *Pulmonary embolism*, i.e. blockage of pulmonary artery, may be caused by an embolus arising from the calf veins.
   - *Cerebral embolism*, i.e. blockage of cerebral artery, may be caused by an embolus arising from the heart or carotid artery.

Prevention of Thrombi

Formation and/or extension of a thrombus can be prevented by administration of:

- *Drugs which decrease platelet adhesiveness* such as aspirin, dextran or dipyridamole
- *Anticoagulants* such as low doses of heparin and dicoumarol
- *Intermittent compression* or electrical stimulation of the calf muscles is necessary in addition to above-mentioned drugs for preventing postoperative venous thrombosis.

ANTIHAEMOSTATIC MECHANISMS

The factors which balance the tendency of the blood to clot in vivo constitute the *antihaemostatic factors*. These can be grouped as:

- Factors preventing platelet aggregation
- Factors preventing coagulation (circulatory anticoagulants)
- Factors causing fibrinolysis (fibrinolytic mechanism)
- Anticoagulants

FACTORS PREVENTING PLATELET AGGREGATION

Prostacyclin Prostacyclin is a prostaglandin 12, member of eicosanoid family of lipid molecules produced by vascular smooth muscle and endothelium which prevents platelet aggregation by inhibiting the thromboxane A_2 formation (which promotes platelet aggregation). Normally, there is a delicate balance between thromboxane A_2 (by irreversibly inhibiting cyclo-oxygenase enzyme, which is required for the formation of precursors of thromboxane A_2 within platelets) and prostacyclin, which keeps the platelet plug localized, i.e. prevents intravascular spread of plug. For details, see page 783.

Applied Aspects

The drug *aspirin* also inhibits the formation of thromboxane A_2 and thus can prevent platelet plug formation. This makes aspirin a valuable drug for the prevention of thrombosis in patients prone to myocardial infraction and stroke.

CIRCULATORY ANTICOAGULANTS

The natural anticoagulants circulating in the blood constitute the anticoagulant mechanism of the body. These include:

- Heparin
- Antithrombin III or heparin cofactor II
- Protein C

1. Heparin

Heparin is a powerful, naturally acting anticoagulant since it was first isolated from the liver, and so it is named heparin (hepar, liver). However, it is also present in many other organs. It is a polysaccharide (glycosaminoglycan) containing many sulphate groups. Its molecular weight is 15,000–18,000 Da.

Secretion. Heparin is secreted by the basophils and mast cells (present in various tissues such as liver, lungs and tissues rich in connective tissue).

Destruction. Heparin is destroyed by the enzyme *heparinase* present in the liver.

Functions. Heparin is one of the factors which maintains fluidity of the circulating blood and prevents spread of intravascular thrombosis postoperatively and after trauma to vessels. It is also used before surgery to reduce the risk of blood clot.

Mechanism of action. Heparin is present on the luminal surface of vascular endothelium. Heparin by itself has little or no anticoagulant properties, but it acts as cofactor with antithrombin III (antithrombin–heparin cofactor) and increases the effectiveness of antithrombin III by hundredfold for removing thrombin. During clot formation, most of the thrombin formed from prothrombin gets adsorbed onto fibrin threads; heparins thus prevent further excessive spreading of the clot. The remaining thrombin that does not get adsorbed on fibrin soon combines with antithrombin III and blocks the effect of thrombin on fibrinogen. Therefore, heparin acts as an anticoagulant by the following mechanisms:

- Prevents activation of prothrombin to thrombin
- Inhibits the action of thrombin on fibrinogen
- Facilitates the action of antithrombin III, i.e. acts as its cofactor and thereby inhibits the active forms of clotting factors IX, X, XI and XII

Important Note

Heparin acts as anticoagulant both in vivo and in vitro. It is mainly used in the following conditions:

- Prevention and treatment of angina and myocardial infarction.
- Thrombolytic prophylaxis after major surgeries like joint replacement and open-heart surgery.

Heparin antagonists (antidote). Protamine sulphate forms irreversible complex with heparin, therefore used as an antidote to prevent heparin toxicity.

2. Antithrombin III Antithrombin III is present in plasma as well as vascular endothelium. It is a protease inhibitor, which inactivates a number of coagulation factors (active form of factors IX, X, XI and XII) including thrombin. Its action is greatly facilitated by heparin as mentioned above.

3. Protein C Protein C is a plasma protein synthesized in liver. It, along with thrombomodulin and protein S, constitutes an important negative feedback pathway that keeps the coagulatory process under control. The steps of protein C pathway are given in Fig. 3.5.7.

Thrombomodulin It is a thrombin-binding protein produced by all endothelial cells except those in the cerebral microcirculation. It converts thrombin into *protein C* activator.

Protein C It is activated by the protein C activator. For the formation of activated protein C (APC), a cofactor protein S is required.

Activated protein C It inactivates factors VIIIa and Va and thus inhibits the clotting mechanism. It also increases fibrinolysis by promoting plasmin formation.

FIBRINOLYTIC MECHANISM

Fibrinolysis refers to the process that brings about the dissolution of fibrin. The important component of the fibrinolytic system is *plasmin* or fibrinolysin, which is present in the blood in an inactive form called *plasminogen* or profibrinolysin. The fibrinolytic or the so-called plasmin system causes lysis of blood clot allowing slow cleaning of extraneous blood clots in the tissue. It also allows reopening of clotted blood vessels. Especially, it removes minute clots which are formed in many tiny peripheral vessels, which would eventually occlude if there was no plasmin system.

Plasminogen Plasminogen is a β-globulin produced by the liver. Structurally, human plasminogen consists of a heavy chain of 560 amino acids and a light chain of 241 amino acids. The heavy chain at its amino terminal is folded into five loops, which are held together by disulphide bonds. These loops are called kringles. The kringles are the binding sites by which the molecule attaches to fibrin and to other clotting proteins (clotting factors) and also to prothrombin. During clotting or purification of fibrinogen, it is associated closely with the fibrinogen molecule. It is extremely difficult to prepare fibrinogen free of plasminogen. A normal clot usually contains sufficient amounts of plasminogen to ensure clot dissolution if it is activated. Plasminogen is activated by plasminogen activator systems to produce plasmin.

The receptors of plasminogen are located mainly on the surface of endothelial cells and also on different types of cells. When plasminogen binds to its receptors, it gets activated.

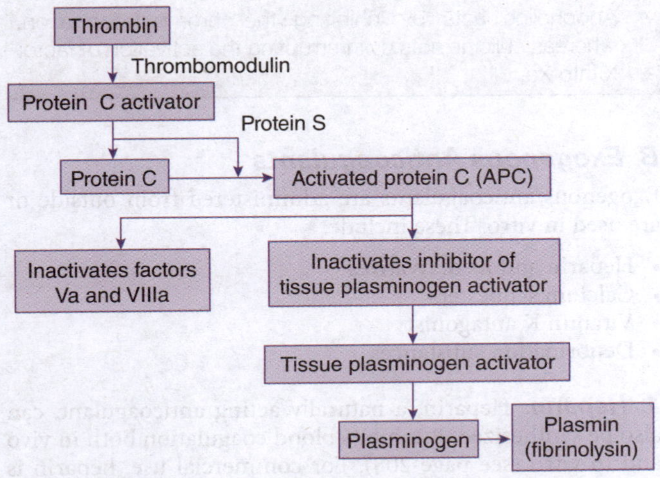

Fig. 3.5.7 Steps of protein C pathway in inhibiting coagulation and promoting fibrinolysis.

Plasmin Plasmin is a powerful protease formed from its precursor, the plasminogen. It lyses fibrin and fibrinogen into fragments known as *fibrin degradation products (FDP)* that inhibit thrombin. Thus, there is a negative feedback which controls plasmin generation. There are two plasminogen activator systems in the body: intrinsic and extrinsic.

Extrinsic plasminogen activator system It seems to be the predominant mechanism of plasminogen activation since, in its absence, there is extensive spontaneous fibrin deposition.

The extrinsic activator system (Fig. 3.5.8) operates through the following agents.

1. Tissue plasminogen activator TPA, also called vascular plasminogen activator, is released from the vascular endothelium. The release of TPA from the vessel wall depends on the release of serotonin from platelets and also release of adrenaline. When there is physical/mental stress or exercise or liberation of adrenaline on sympathetic stimulation, the TPA is released vigorously and thus removes fibrin so that bleeding tends to prolong. In violent deaths (e.g. of a soldier in the battlefield), the blood is fluid and incoagulable due to fibrinolysis. This is due to a large amount of adrenaline released into the blood before death. The adrenaline causes rapid release of TPA from endothelial cells causing massive fibrinolysis. Another factor which regulates release of TPA is fibrin itself (autoinactivation).

Mechanism of action: TPA binds to fibrin via lysine-binding sites and activates plasminogen to plasmin.

> **Important Note**
>
> It is important to note that TPA is now produced by recombinant DNA techniques and is available for clinical use. It lyses clots in the coronary arteries if given to patients soon after the onset of myocardial infarction (MI).

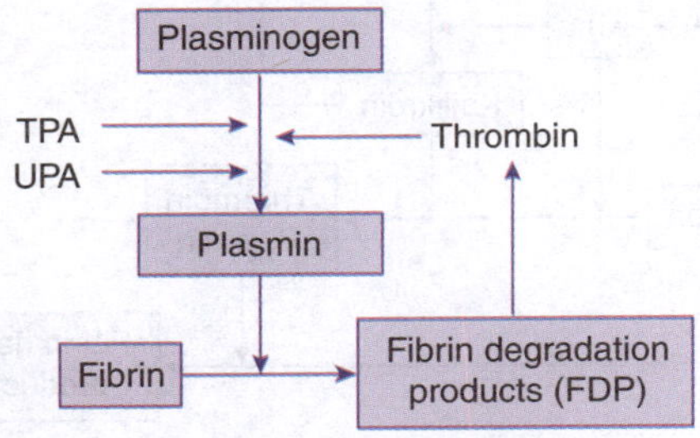

Fig. 3.5.8 Fibrinolytic mechanism operating through extrinsic plasminogen activator system.

2. Urokinase-type plasminogen activator. The urokinase-type plasminogen activator (UPA) is found in a number of tissues including endothelial cells, renal cells and tumour cells. Urokinase is isolated from cultured human kidney cells and induces a systemic lytic state like TPA.

Note: *Streptokinase and staphylokinase* are bacterial enzymes known to produce activation of plasmin-like TPA and UPA. Streptokinase (Streptase) is a protein produced by β-haemolytic streptococci. It forms streptokinase–plasminogen complex which produces a conformational change that exposes active sites on plasminogen molecule and lyse to form plasmin. Therefore, they are used in the treatment of early MI to lyse thrombi.

Intrinsic plasminogen activator system Contact factors (factor XIIa and KA) that initiate clotting mechanism also stimulate the dissolution of clots by activating plasminogen and constitute the intrinsic plasminogen activator system (Fig. 3.5.9).

Fibrinolysis inhibitors The rate of fibrinolysis is influenced by the promoters (i.e. plasminogen activators) and inhibitors. Fibrinolysis inhibitors are present in plasma, blood cells, tissues and extracellular matrix. These can inhibit plasmin (antiplasmin) or prevent the activation of plasminogen. The various inhibitors are as follows:

- *Antiplasmins* such as α_2-antiplasmin
- *Aprotinin* (a trypsin inhibitor)
- *Epsilon-aminocaproic acid* (EACA)

Physiological Role of Fibrinolysis System

Plasmin of the fibrinolysis system plays the following physiological roles.

1. Cleaning the minute clots of tiny vessels. It has been suggested that in physiological conditions, the clotting system of the plasma is continually forming small amounts of fibrin, which are deposited to form a thin layer on vascular endothelium, and that the fibrinolytic system is constantly in action to prevent excessive fibrin formation.

2. Promote normal healing process. Lysis of clot formed as a result of tissue injury helps to promote normal healing process.

3. Liquefaction of menstrual clot. Liquefaction of menstrual clot in the vagina is carried out by fibrinolytic system.

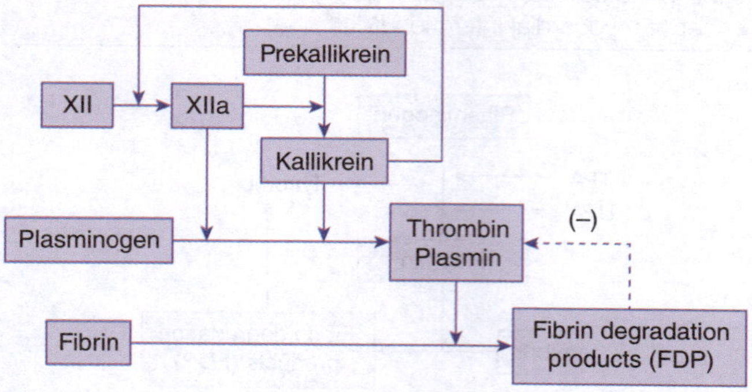

Fig. 3.5.9 Fibrinolytic mechanism operating through intrinsic plasminogen activator system.

4. Liquefaction of sperms in the epididymis. Liquefaction of sperms in the epididymis when seminal ejaculation does not occur is caused by the fibrinolysin system.

5. Role in inflammatory response. In addition to its fibrinolytic activity, plasmin can form plasma kinins (bradykinins and kallidin) and thus contribute to the vascular and sensory features (pain) of the inflammatory response to injury.

ANTICOAGULANTS

Anticoagulants refer to the substances which delay or prevent the process of coagulation of blood. In vitro, blood clotting can be prevented by substances which sequester calcium, e.g. sodium citrate or oxalate and sodium edetate (ethylenediaminetetraacetic acid [EDTA]).

In vivo, the tendency of thrombosis can be inhibited by:

- Antagonizing clotting factors (e.g. heparin)
- Destruction of the key substance fibrinogen
- Inhibiting the synthesis of factors II, VII, IX and X (vitamin K antagonists)

Types. Anticoagulants may be divided into endogenous and exogenous anticoagulants.

A. Endogenous Anticoagulants

Endogenous anticoagulants are those which are present inside the blood naturally:

- Heparin
- Antithrombin III
- Protein C (for details, see page 209)

> **Important Note**
>
> **Salivary gland anticoagulants.** The saliva of mosquitoes contains anticoagulants to prevent formation of blood clots. After biting its victim, a female mosquito injects saliva; the anticoagulant present in the saliva neutralizes the platelets in the blood so it remains in fluid form and does not block the mouth parts of the vector.
>
> - There are two types of salivary gland anticoagulants: anopheline and culicine.
> - Anopheline acts by inhibiting the thrombin formation, whereas culicine acts by interrupting the activation of factor X into Xa.

B. Exogenous Anticoagulants

Exogenous anticoagulants are administered from outside or are used in vitro. These include:

- Heparin and its derivatives
- Calcium sequesters
- Vitamin K antagonist
- Defibrination substances

1. Heparin. Heparin, a naturally acting anticoagulant, can also be synthesized. It inhibits blood coagulation both in vivo and in vitro (see page 208). For commercial use, heparin is extracted from certain animal tissues, and is prepared in pure form. Synthesized form has longer life; therefore, its action lasts for 4–5 hours. It mainly inhibits activated factors of intrinsic and common pathway including thrombin and factors Xa and IXa. This effect results in prolongation of platelet thromboplastin time (PTT) and thrombin time (TT). See page 216.

Clinical use: Due to its rapid action, heparin can be used:

- To treat thrombosis and pulmonary emboli
- In initial management of patient with unstable angina, acute MI and during cardiac bypass surgery
- In selected patients with disseminated intravascular coagulation (DIC)
- ***Danaparoid*** is a mixture of nonheparin glycosamine glycan isolated from porcine intestinal mucosa cells (84% heparin, 12% dermatan sulphate and 4% chondroitin sulphate). It mainly causes inhibition of factor Xa by antithrombin, but does not prolong PTT.
- ***Lepirudin*** is a recombinant derivative of hirudin present in salivary gland secretion of medicinal leech. It is a direct inhibitor of thrombin.

2. Calcium sequesters or decalcifying agents. In vitro, blood clotting can be prevented by substances which sequester (remove) calcium from the blood. These include two types of agents:

Substances which form insoluble salts with calcium such as sodium citrate and sodium oxalate.

Double oxalate (ammonium oxalate and potassium oxalate in ratio of 3:2) is mainly used in estimation of ESR. Note: Ammonium oxalate increases the volume of RBCs and potassium oxalate causes shrinkage of RBCs.

Citrates. Potassium, sodium and ammonium citrate (trisodium citrate) in concentration of 2–3 mg/mL blood is used for estimation of ESR by Westergren's method in ratio of 4:1(blood:citrate).

Sodium fluoride. It inhibits glycolytic enzymes. It is used for:

- Collection of blood sample for estimation of blood glucose levels.
- Preservation of blood sample at room temperature for 24 hours.
- Preservation of blood sample in refrigerator for 5–6 days.

Ethylenediaminetetraacetic acid (EDTA). It inhibits conversion of fibrinogen to fibrin.

Calcium chelators, such as EDTA, which bind calcium.

3. Vitamin K antagonists. These are used orally and thus can prevent coagulation in vivo effectively. These agents occupy vitamin K receptor sites in the liver and prevent vitamin K from carrying out its normal physiological function, hence the name vitamin K antagonists. Thus, these substances inhibit synthesis of vitamin K–dependent factors, i.e. factors VII, IX and X. These include coumarin derivatives (e.g. dicoumarol), warfarin, phenindione and nicoumalone.

i. Dicoumarol. It is the first original oral anticoagulant isolated for clinical use, but because of its slow and erratic absorption, it is seldom used.

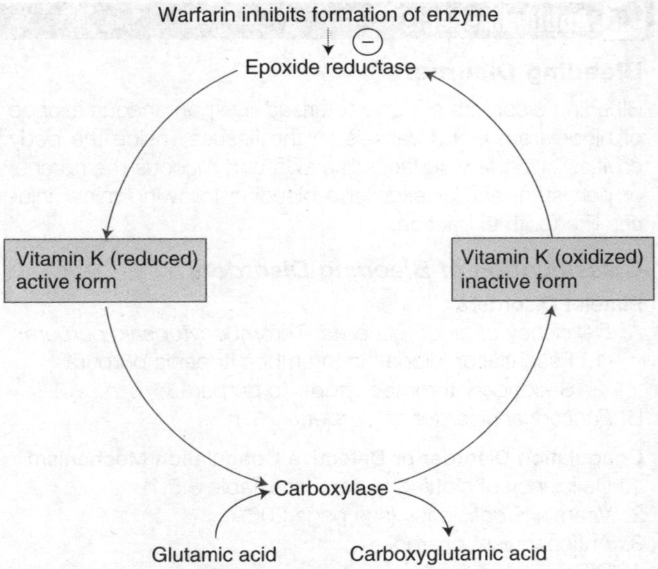

Fig. 3.5.10 Vitamin K cycle.

ii. Warfarin. For synthesis of vitamin K–dependent coagulation factors, vitamin K acts as cofactor for formation of γ-carboxyglutamic acid residues on the coagulation factors. The enzyme γ-glutamyl carboxylase and epoxide reductase are responsible for formation and metabolism of vitamin K. Warfarin acts by inhibiting enzyme epoxide reductase complex-1 (VKOR-1). This enzyme converts inactive (oxidized) form of vitamin K into active (reduced) form (Fig. 3.5.10). The anticoagulant function of warfarin begins after 24 hours and lasts longer.

4. Thrombolytic drugs. These include TPA, streptokinase and urokinase. For details, see page 209.

5. Antiplatelet drugs. Antiplatelet drugs like aspirin prevent platelet plug formation (for details, see page 208).

6. Defibrination substances. Defibrination substances are those which cause destruction of fibrinogen. These include:

Malaysian pit viper venom. It is a type of snake venom which in vivo acts as anticoagulant by causing defibrination and also by stimulating the fibrinolytic system. In vitro, it has a direct anticoagulant effect on fibrinogen by forming imperfect fibrin polymer.

Arvin or ancord. It is a purified preparation of snake venom. It is glycoprotein in nature and is administered by injection. It acts as an anticoagulant by causing defibrination and thus producing fibrinogenopenia.

7. Cold. Keeping blood cold (at 5–10°C) can retard the process of coagulation but cannot absolutely prevent it. Because of this reason, blood is stored in blood banks at low temperature but some anticoagulant agent is always used. Furthermore, it looks paradoxical that whenever bleeding occurs, ice is applied to arrest the haemorrhage (while cold delays coagulation); in fact, when ice is applied on the surface, it prevents bleeding by inducing reflex vasoconstriction.

Applied Aspects

Bleeding Disorders

Bleeding disorders are characterized by spontaneous escape of blood from blood vessels (in the tissues, inside the body cavities or on few surfaces like skin and mucous membrane) or persistent and/or excessive bleeding following minor injuries like tooth extraction.

Classification of Bleeding Disorders

Platelet Disorders

A. *Deficiency of blood platelets. Thrombocytopenic purpura:*
 1. Essential or idiopathic thrombocytopenic purpura
 2. Secondary thrombocytopenic purpura

B. *Functional disorder of platelets*

Coagulation Disorder or Defective Coagulation Mechanism

1. Deficiency of clotting factors (see Table 3.5.1)
2. Vitamin K deficiency (see page 206)
3. Anticoagulant overdose
4. DIC

Vascular Disorders: Damage of Capillary Endothelium (Nonthrombocytopenic Purpura)

- Due to infection by bacteria and their toxins
- Due to toxic effects of drugs and chemicals
- Due to avitaminosis C
- Allergic purpura
- Connective tissue diseases

Only a few important bleeding disorders are described briefly.

Purpura

Purpura is a group of bleeding disorders occurring due to various causes. The term purpura is derived from purple-coloured petechial haemorrhages and bruises in the skin. The blood that leaks out changes colour from red to blue to dark blue and green over a period of time.

Causes and types of purpura

I. Platelet disorders. Platelets play an important role in haemostasis and coagulation (see the section 'Functions of Platelets', page 199); therefore, platelet disorders are associated with bleeding disorders. Platelet disorders include:

1. Deficiency of platelets (thrombocytopenic purpura). Normal platelet count ranges from 1.5 to 4.5 lakh/μL, with average count of 2.5 lakh/μL. Decrease in the platelet count below 1.5 lakh/μL is called thrombocytopenia. Thrombocytopenic purpura may be:

Primary thrombocytopenic purpura (idiopathic, cause not known). In many of the idiopathic cases, antibodies develop against platelets (immune thrombocytopenic purpura [ITP]).

Secondary causes of platelet deficiency (secondary thrombocytopenic purpura):

- Bone marrow depression due to effects of various cytotoxic drugs; whole-body irradiation and hypoplastic and aplastic anaemia.
- Leukaemia and secondary deposits of malignancies in the bone marrow.
- Acute septicaemia, toxaemia, uraemia.
- Hypersplenism.

Relation between platelet count and bleeding

• Above 100,000/μL	No clinical symptoms; bleeding is rare
• From 50,000 to 100,000/μL	Bleeding may occur after major surgery
• From 20,000 to 50,000/μL	Bleeding occurs with minor trauma in everyday life
• Below 20,000/μL	Spontaneous haemorrhage in urinary tract, GI tract, nosebleeds, etc.
• At very low counts	Fatal haemorrhage may occur in the brain

Treatment

- In thrombocytopenic purpura, bleeding can be effectively stopped for few days by transfusing either fresh blood or platelets only.
- Splenectomy is also helpful because the spleen removes large numbers of platelets from the blood.

2. Functional disorders of platelets (thrombocytopenic purpura). Functional disorders of platelets (defects in platelet adhesion or aggregation) are characterized by prolonged bleeding time (BT) with normal platelet counts. Functional disorders of platelets include the following:

- ***Drug-induced defects*** occur with aspirin, large doses of penicillin and other drugs.

Table 3.5.1 Deficiency of clotting factors

Deficiency of factor	Clinical syndrome	Cause
• Factor I	Fibrinogenopenia Afibrinogenaemia	Depletion during pregnancy with premature separation of placenta Congenital (rare)
• Factor II	Hypoprothrombinaemia (haemorrhagic tendency in liver disease)	Decreased hepatic synthesis, usually secondary to vitamin K deficiency
• Factor V	Parahaemophilia	Congenital
• Factor VII	Hypoconvertinaemia	Congenital
• Factor VIII	Haemophilia A or classical haemophilia	Congenital defect due to abnormal gene on X chromosome
• Factor IX	Haemophilia B or Christmas disease	Congenital
• Factor X	Stuart–Prower factor deficiency	Congenital
• Factor XI	PTA deficiency	Congenital
• Factor XII	Hageman trait (does not produce bleeding)	Congenital
• von Willebrand factor	von Willebrand disease	Congenital

- ***von Willebrand disease (VWD).*** It is inherited as an autosomal dominant trait. This condition is associated with a deficiency of factor VIII–related antigen (VIII R:Ag), also called VWF. This factor acts as a carrier of factor VIII, so its deficiency results in diminished adherence of platelets to collagen fibres in a damaged vessel.

Types: Three main types of VWD are type 1, type 2 and type 3.

Type 1: It is the most common type of von Willebrand disease; it is of a mild type and patient is usually asymptomatic and may experience mild bleeding problems, but is able to live a normal life.

Type 2: In type 2 VWD, the level of VWF is normal but due to structural and functional defect will not work properly. The type 2 VWD is further divided into four subtypes: 2A, 2B, 2M and 2N.

Type 3: VWD is most severe and dangerous type. There is absence of VWF due to nonproduction; as a result, the platelets are not able to clot the blood.

Treatment. von Willebrand disease can be treated by injecting 1-deamino-8-D-arginine vasopressin (DDAVP) or desmopressin intravenously. DDAVP releases VWF and factor VIII from endothelial stores.

Antifibrinolytic agents like eamino caproic acid (EACA) or tranexamic acid are an important therapy either alone or with DDAVP, particularly during dental procedures (e.g. tooth extraction).

Other diseases in which platelet functions become defective are uraemia, cirrhosis and leukaemia.

II. Vascular disorders. Bleeding tendencies seen in patients with vascular disorders (damage to capillary endothelium) are referred to as *nonthrombocytopenic purpura*. In all cases of purpura due to vessel wall defects, the platelet counts are normal, but BT is prolonged and capillary fragility test is positive.

Causes of nonthrombocytopenic purpura are:

1. ***Drug-induced damage to capillary wall*** is seen in patients with prolonged treatment with corticosteroids, penicillin, sulpha drugs and aspirin.
2. ***Deficiency of vitamin C (scurvy)*** causes failure of collagen formation and is associated with impaired hydroxyproline synthesis. Petechiae and bleeding from gums occur due to decreased intercellular substance and less stable capillary basement membrane.
3. ***Allergic purpura*** occurs due to damage to capillary walls by antibodies.
4. ***Infections*** such as typhus, bacterial endocarditis and haemolytic *Streptococcus* may be associated with capillary wall damage.
5. ***Senile purpura*** refers to purpuric haemorrhagic spots seen on the back of hands and forearms due to prolonged pressure or mild trauma. Small vessels in old age rupture due to increased mobility of skin resulting from loss of elastic and connective tissues around the blood vessels.
6. ***Connective tissue diseases*** are also sometimes associated with damage to capillary walls and purpuric haemorrhages.
7. ***Thrombasthenic purpura*** is a rare autosomal recessive bleeding disorder. The molecular basis is linked to quantitative/qualitative abnormalities of integrin, resulting in lack of aggregation of platelets. However, the platelet count remains normal.
8. ***Henoch–Schönlein purpura (HSP)*** also called spring fever. HSP is a disorder causing inflammation and bleeding in small blood vessels, mainly affects the vessels of skin, joints, intestines and kidney. It is more common in children of 2–6 years. It is characterized by:
   - Reddish purple spots or rashes resembling bruises on hips, feet, arms, trunk and on the face.
   - Depending on the body part involved, there is swollen joints (usually knee and ankle joints), abdominal pain, vomiting, blood in the stools and haematuria.

Haemophilia

Haemophilia is the name given to a group of disorders occurring due to *hereditary deficiency of coagulation* and characterized by bleeding tendencies hardly distinguishable from one another, associated with increased clotting time (CT). The haemophilia includes:

- Haemophilia A (83% of cases)
- Haemophilia B (15% of cases)
- Haemophilia C (2% of cases)

1. Haemophilia A

- Haemophilia A, also known as true or classical haemophilia, occurs due to *deficiency of factor VIII, i.e.* AHG.
- It is the most common hereditary coagulation disorder. Being a sex-linked recessive disease, it affects males exclusively and females act as carriers (Fig. 3.5.11). The carrier female shows no symptoms due to the presence of the X chromosome, which is dominant over recessive chromosome (X*) X. Only mating of a haemophilic male with a carrier female will produce a haemophilic female, which is a very rare occurrence.

The majority of patients with haemophilia A have blood levels of factor VIII below 5%, and so usually bleed severely on

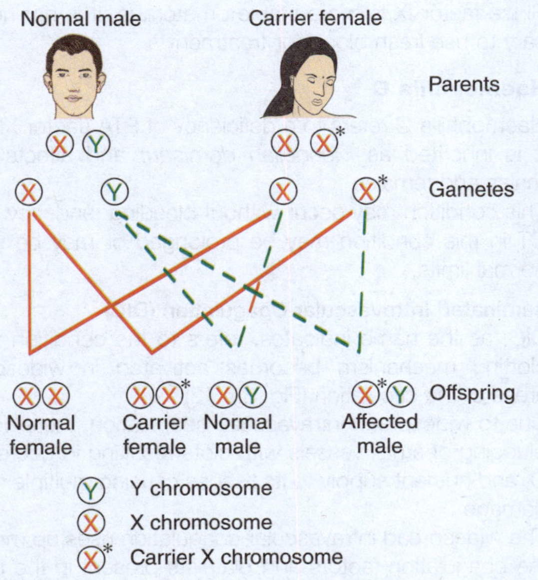

Fig. 3.5.11 Sex-linked inheritance of haemophilia A.

minor trauma. Relationships of levels of factor VIII with status of haemostasis are as follows:

Factor VIII activity	Status of haemostasis
>50%	Normal haemostasis
25%–50%	Excessive bleeding after severe trauma
5%–25%	Excessive bleeding after minor trauma
1%–5%	Severe bleeding on minor trauma
<1%	Spontaneous bleeding

Clinical features (bleeding tendency) are not apparent since birth but generally start early in life (within first 3 years).

- People with haemophilia have the tendency to bleed into soft tissues, muscles, joints, GI tract and urinary tract, and from the nose.
- Joints of patients with haemophilia become severely damaged due to repeated joint haemorrhage.
- Haemorrhage into the soft tissue around the floor of the mouth may cause respiratory obstruction and death by suffocation.
- People with haemophilia have normal BT, platelet count and prothrombin time (PT). Coagulation time (CT) is increased and typically, the patients have prolonged partial thromboplastin time (PTT).

Treatment. Haemophilia A can be treated by transfusion of:

- Repeated, small-volume, fresh blood, within 30 minutes of collection (because factor VIII is lost rapidly on storage)
- Fresh plasma
- Factor VIII concentrate commercially available as cryoprecipitated antihaemophilic factor for intravenous infusion

2. Haemophilia B (Christmas Disease)

- Haemophilia B is also known as *Christmas disease because it was first* discovered in a family with the surname Christmas. It occurs due to deficiency of factor IX (Christmas factor or PTC).
- Like haemophilia A, haemophilia B is also a recessive X-linked disease that occurs in males and is transmitted by females.
- The clinical features of haemophilia B are same as of haemophilia A.
- Since factor IX is more stable on storage, it is not necessary to use fresh blood for treatment.

3. Haemophilia C

- Haemophilia C refers to a deficiency of PTA (factor XI).
- It is inherited as *Mendelian dominant* and affects both males and females.
- This condition may occur without bleeding tendency.
- CT in this condition may be prolonged or may be within normal limits.

Disseminated Intravascular Coagulation (DIC)

- DIC, as the name indicates, refers to the condition when clotting mechanism becomes activated in widespread areas of the circulation (Fig. 3.5.12).
- Due to widespread intravascular coagulation, there occurs plugging of small vessels with clots resulting in decreased O_2 and nutrient supply to its tissues causing multiple organ damage.
- The widespread intravascular coagulation uses up most of the coagulation factors and platelets present in the blood resulting in failure of haemostatic mechanism. The patient thus develops bleeding tendencies and, hence, the condition is also called *consumption coagulopathy*.

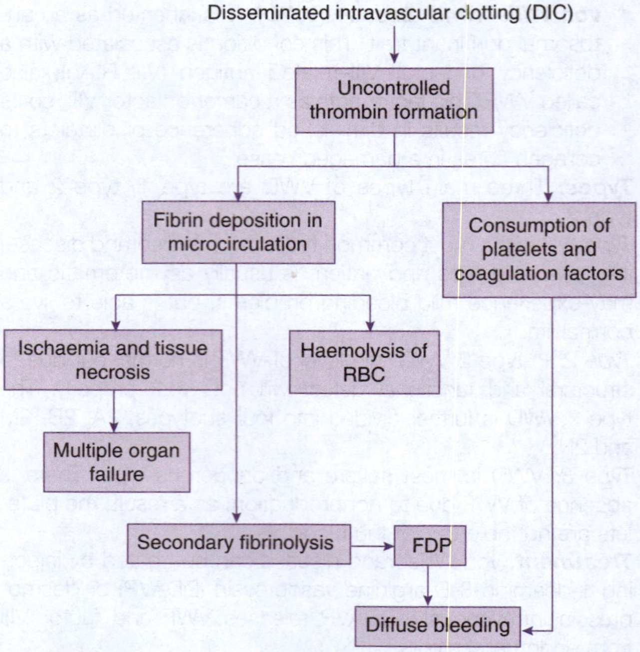

Fig. 3.5.12 Interaction between coagulation and fibrinolytic pathway results in thrombosis and bleeding in disseminated intravascular coagulation.

- The FDP that are formed as a result of fibrinolysis of the clot have antihaemostatic effect and further aggravate the bleeding tendency.
- DIC is thus a grave condition. It can result as a consequence of an adverse condition in which large amounts of traumatized or dying tissue occur in the body, which release thromboplastin, or toxins accumulate in the body, which stimulate many coagulation factors. DIC is associated with conditions like septicaemic shock, metastatic malignancies, prolonged postpartum haemorrhage and snake bite.

Treatment: The main basis of DIC treatment is

- To control or eliminate underlying primary cause
- To manage haemorrhagic symptoms due to thrombocytopenia by platelet concentrate (dose 1–2 units/kg body weight
- Drugs to control coagulation, such as heparin, antithrombin III or fibrinolytic agents (EACA or tranexamic acid in low doses)

Laboratory Tests in Bleeding Disorders

1. Bleeding Time

Bleeding occurs from the skin when it is pricked with a needle, which normally stops of its own within a few minutes. The time lapse between the skin prick and the arrest of bleeding is called *BT*.

Procedure. BT can be estimated by the following methods:

(i) Duke's method. To estimate BT, the tip of a finger or earlobe is pricked with a sharp needle. A stopwatch is run and

blood is wiped away with a clean filter paper every 15 seconds till bleeding stops. The time taken for the arrest of bleeding is BT. ***Normal BT by Duke's method*** varies from 1 to 6 minutes. Normal BT indicates that platelet count and their function, as well as health of capillaries, are normal.

(ii) Ivy's method. In this method, a pressure of 40 mm Hg is applied to the upper arm with a blood pressure cuff and then a skin-deep prick is made on the anterior surface of the forearm. Rest of procedure is same as above.

Normal BT by Ivy's method is 3–6 minutes at 37°C.

Important Note

BT depends on the depth of the prick. Specified depth of prick in Duke's method for earlobe is 4 mm and for Ivy's method for forearm is 2.5 mm.

Prolonged BT occurs in purpura, while it is normal in haemophilia.

Important Notes

- A clean or straight cut with a blade or knife bleeds longer than an irregular injury. In an irregular cut, bleeding time is less because collagen gets exposed and a rough surface available for platelet aggregation and factor XII can get activated.
- Bleeding time depends on:
  Size of the wound
  Functioning of platelets
  Temperature (low temperature decreases bleeding time due to vasoconstriction and rise in temperature increases bleeding time)

2. Capillary Fragility Test of Hess or Tourniquet Test

Tourniquet test is performed to assess the mechanical fragility of the capillaries by raising pressure within them. It may demonstrate latent purpura.

Procedure. A circle of 1-inch diameter is marked on the front of the forearm. Any purple spots present in the circle are marked with blue ink. Then a pressure midway between systolic and diastolic blood pressure is applied on the upper arm for 15 minutes using the blood pressure cuff. Appearance of 10 or more new petechiae is a positive test. *Positive tourniquet test* occurs in various types of purpura and vessel wall defects.

3. Platelet Count

Normal platelet count. It varies from 1.5 to 4.5 lakh/μL with an average 2.5 lakh/μL. Platelet count is decreased in primary and secondary thrombocytopenic purpura (page 212).

Procedure It involves two methods:

(i) ***Direct method.*** Fresh blood should be diluted in a RBC pipette with Rees–Ecker fluid and the stained platelets should then be counted in a haemocytometer.

(ii) ***Indirect method.*** In this method, platelet count is calculated from the RBC count and platelet:RBC ratio. Normally, there is 1 platelet to 16–18 red cells.

4. Coagulation Time

Definition. CT refers to the time taken by the fresh fluid blood to get coagulated (demonstrated by formation of fibrin threads). It is an insensitive measure in the assessment of coagulation defects and is abnormally prolonged when the coagulation factors are seriously deficient.

Procedure. Coagulation time is tested by:

(i) Capillary tube method. In this method, a capillary tube is filled with fresh blood from the finger prick and 1-cm bits of the tube are broken from one end every 30 seconds. The end point is reached when fibrin threads span a gap of 5 mm between the broken ends (*rope formation*). *Normal CT* by capillary method is 3–6 minutes.

Comments. It is important to note that clotting of blood with this method involves both the intrinsic and extrinsic systems, as there is injury to the blood, as well as to the tissue.

(ii) Modified Lee-White test tube method (whole-blood CT). Presently, this method is considered the standard method to estimate CT.

Principle of this method is to collect blood with a clean non-traumatic venipuncture and put it in an 8-mm-diameter test tube at 37°C and see how long it takes to clot. The end point is reached when test tube can be tilted through an angle greater than 90° without spilling the blood.

Normal value of CT by Lee–White method is 8–12 minutes for a glass tube and 20–60 minutes for a siliconized tube. CT is more because siliconized tubes are smooth surfaced, and, therefore, activation of factor XII becomes slow or difficult.

Comments. This method tests the intrinsic system of blood clotting as there is no admixture of blood with tissue fluid. Therefore, this method is considered more reliable than the capillary tube method.

Importance of clotting time. The CT is prolonged in haemophilia and other clotting disorders, because thrombin cannot be normally generated; however, the BT, which reflects vasoconstriction and platelet plug formation independently of clot formation, is normal since CT can increase due to deficiency of any of the factors so it is a nonspecific test. More specific tests include *PT, PTT, thromboplastin generation test (TGT), TT,* etc. Specific tests can pinpoint the particular deficient factor.

- *Physiologically,* CT is reduced during menstruation and before and during parturition.
- *Pathologically, CT is prolonged in* haemophilia, liver diseases, afibrinogenaemia, Christmas disease, vitamin K deficiency and DIC.

5. Prothrombin Time

Procedure *Quick's one-stage method* now is the standard method to measure PT. In this method, tissue factor or tissue thromboplastin (commercially available) and calcium chloride solution (to provide calcium ion) are added to the oxalated or citrated plasma of the patient, and the mixture is incubated at 37°C. The end point is conversion of fluid plasma into a gel (due to formation of fibrin).

Normal PT is 11–16 seconds.

Prothrombin ratio (PTR). Plasma from a normal person is used as a control and the result is expressed as prothrombin ratio (PTR). Normal PTR varies from 0.9 to 1.2.

Note:
Prothrombin – international normalized ratio (INR). PT may vary even in the same individual depending on the difference in the TF activity and analytical system. INR is devised for standardized measurement of PT. For each type and batch of TF, the manufacturing company assigns an international sensitivity index (ISI), which indicates the TF activity with the standardized sample. The INR is the ratio of PT of person to normal control sample raised to the power of ISI:

$$\text{INR} = [\text{PT test/PT control}]^{\text{ISI}}$$

The normal range of INR is 0.9–1.3.
Prothrombin concentration curve. PT is predictive of low plasma prothrombin concentration.

Short PT or low INR (e.g. 0.5) is mainly determined by prothrombin concentration. The curve relating PT to prothrombin concentration is used to quantify the concentration of prothrombin in the blood (Fig. 3.5.13).

Comments. Intrinsic system is not involved in this test since plasma does not contain platelets. Obviously it is extrinsic system which is tested. In this test, calcium nullifies the effect of oxalate or citrate and tissue thromboplastin acts as the prothrombin activator, i.e. it initiates extrinsic pathway. Though originally introduced as a test for prothrombin activity (hence its name), it is also sensitive to deficiency of factors I, V, VII and X.

Importance of PT during different conditions:
PT is increased in patients on oral anticoagulants, liver failure, vitamin K deficiency, abnormally low fibrinogen concentration, and deficiency of factors II, V, VII and X.
PT is normal in haemophilia and Christmas disease. It is used to monitor patients receiving anticoagulant therapy (e.g. warfarin) to adjust its dose.

6. Partial Thromboplastin Time

PTT, also known as kaolin cephalin clotting time (KCCT), detects coagulation defects too small to lead to prolongation of the whole blood CT.

Procedure. To the oxalated or citrated plasma of the patient, kaolin (to provide surface contact), cephalin (to provide phospholipids) and calcium chloride (to provide calcium ions) are added, and the mixture is incubated at 37°C. The end point is formation of plasma gel. Normal PTT is about 40 seconds.

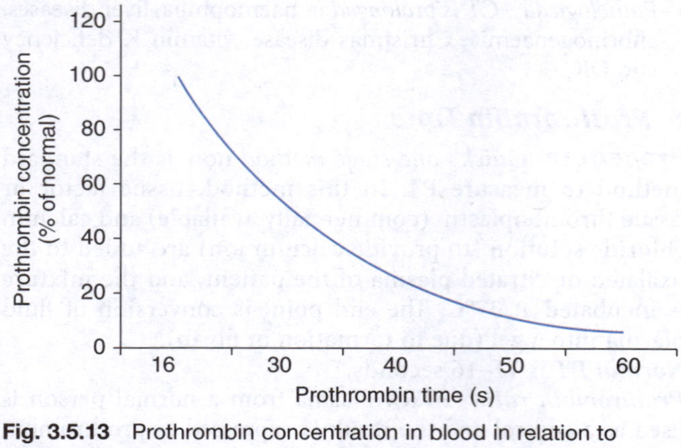

Fig. 3.5.13 Prothrombin concentration in blood in relation to prothrombin time.

Comments. Since the mixture so formed lacks tissue thromboplastins, extrinsic pathway is not involved in this test. Thus, it measures the intrinsic pathway, i.e. factors XII, XI, X, IX, VIII, V, II and I.

Importance of PTT. It is used to monitor the heparin therapy.

PTT is prolonged in haemophilia, von Willebrand disease, liver failure, deficiency of contact factor XII, anticoagulant therapy and intravascular clotting.

7. Thromboplastin Generation Test

This test measures generation of thromboplastin, i.e. the efficiency of a part of the intrinsic mechanism of coagulation.

Normal value of TGT is 12 seconds or less.
Prolonged TGT indicates deficiency of factors needed to form prothrombin activator by the intrinsic mechanism, i.e. factors VIII, IX, X and V.

Comments. From values of PT and TGT, the following inferences can be drawn:

- In haemophilia, PT is normal but TGT is prolonged.
- In pure factor VII deficiency, PT is prolonged, but TGT will remain normal.
- In factor X deficiency, both PT and TGT will be abnormal.

8. Thrombin Time (TT)

This test measures the final step in coagulation, i.e. functional fibrinogen available. In this test, thrombin is added to plasma, which will convert fibrinogen present in the plasma to fibrin. Normally, a clot is formed in about 10 seconds, which is the end point.

TT is prolonged in hypofibrinogenaemia, dysfibrinogenaemia, DIC and heparin treatment.

9. Clot Retraction Test

Clot retraction test measures time needed for contraction of an undisturbed clot. It indicates the function and number of platelets. Normally, clot retraction begins within 2 hours and is completed within 24 hours.

- *Clot retraction is retarded* in thrombocytopenia.
- Clot is small and soft in thrombasthenia, i.e. functional disturbance of platelets.

Self-Assessment

1. Describe the structure of thrombocyte, its composition and functions of its constituents.
2. Describe the process of formation of thrombocytes.
3. Describe the mechanism of coagulation.
5. Write notes on:
   - Haemostasis
   - Role of calcium in blood coagulation
   - Thrombosis
   - Heparin
   - Significance of fibrinolytic mechanism
   - Calcium sequester
   - Purpura
   - Haemophilia
   - Disseminated intravascular coagulation
   - von Willebrand factor
   - Clot retraction

Clinical Cases

Case 1

A young 25-year-old female came to medicine OPD with complaints of red small spots on the skin of lower limbs (legs and ankles), heavy menstrual bleeding during periods which continues for 10–12 days.

On examination, the following were observed: petechial haemorrhages on lower parts of the legs; pallor; no jaundice; temperature, pulse and BP – normal.

Q1. What is the provisional diagnosis?
Q2. What investigations should be advised to confirm the final diagnosis?

Case 2

A 5-year-old male child accompanied his mother to the paediatric OPD. He had bruises all over the body. There was history of cut on the finger with blade, which bled for long time. The mother mentioned about the same type of history in maternal uncle of the child. Presently, there is no history of trauma/injury.

Haematological tests revealed the following:

- Hb, RBC counts, red cell indices, WBCs (absolute and differential) and platelets – normal range
- Bleeding time – normal
- Clotting time – increased
- Prothrombin time – increased

Q1. What is the probable diagnosis?
Q2. What is the hereditary genetics of this condition?
Q3. What is the treatment basis?

Case 3

A 36-year-old male patient presented with chronic diarrhoea, multiple bruises on the body. There was no history of trauma/injury. The patient was a chronic alcoholic. On examination, hepatomegaly was observed.

Haematological investigations revealed the following:

- Hb, RBC, WBC, platelet counts – normal range
- PCV – 42%
- Bleeding time – normal
- Clotting and prothrombin time – increased

Q1. What is the cause of bruises in this condition?
Q2. What is the probable diagnosis?

Case 4

A 65-year-old male had fracture of right femur and underwent surgery. After a week, he suffered from swelling of leg, pain and cramps, which mainly started in the calf muscle.

On examination, it was diagnosed as a case of deep vein thrombosis.

Q1. What is the basic pathophysiology?
Q2. What is the specific treatment for this condition?
Q3. What are the preventive measures?

Case 5

A 34-year-old female patient had a minor cut on the finger while doing household chores in the kitchen. The bleeding was profuse and did not stop for a long period. The patient was taking drug aspirin for the last 3 years (as advised by the cardiologist). She also had heavy menstrual bleeding during periods that would continue for 10–12 days. For this, she had consulted a gynaecologist, and no abnormal findings were observed on ultrasound.

Haematological tests revealed the following:

- Hb, 10 g/dL; RBC count, 3.86 million/mm^3; WBC and platelet counts, within normal range
- Bleeding time – increased
- Clotting time and PTT – normal

Q1. What is the cause for profuse bleeding?
Q2. What is the mechanism of action of drug?

3.6 Blood Groups and Blood Transfusion

CHAPTER OUTLINE

BLOOD GROUPS

INTRODUCTION

Agglutinogens and Agglutinins

Agglutinogens refer to the antigens present on the cell membranes of RBCs. A variety of antigens are present on the cell membrane, but only a few of them are of practical significance.
Agglutinins refer to the antibodies against the agglutinogens. These are present in the plasma.
Agglutination of RBCs can be caused by the antigens present on their cell membrane in the presence of suitable agglutinins (antibodies). That is why, these antigens are called agglutinogens.

Blood Grouping Systems

Depending on the type of agglutinogen present or absent on the red cell membranes, various blood grouping systems are known, which can be classified as follows:

Major blood group systems are based on the presence of agglutinogens which are widely prevalent in the population and are known to cause the worst transfusion reactions. These include:

- The classical ABO blood grouping system
- Rh (CDE) blood grouping system

Minor blood group systems are based on the presence of agglutinogens which are found only in a small proportion of the population and occasionally produce mild transfusion reactions. These include:

- MNS blood group system
- P blood group system

Familial blood group systems are based on the presence of agglutinogens which are found only in a few families. Examples of familial blood group systems are Kell, Duffy, Lutheran, Lewis, Diego, Kidd and many others.

Note: From a clinical point of view, only major blood group systems, i.e. classical ABO and Rh (CDE) blood grouping systems, are important and so will be discussed in detail.

Landsteiner law Karl Landsteiner, in 1900, framed a law in relation to agglutinogens and agglutinins, which states that:

1. ***If an agglutinogen is present*** on the red cell membrane of an individual, the corresponding agglutinin must be absent in the plasma.
2. ***If an agglutinogen is absent*** from the cell membrane of RBCs of an individual, the corresponding agglutinin must be present in the plasma.

Important Note

It is important to note that:

- The Landsteiner law is applicable to ABO blood group system only.
- The law is not applicable to other blood group systems, because there are no naturally occurring agglutinins in these systems.

CLASSICAL ABO BLOOD GROUPING SYSTEM

A and B Agglutinogens

- The classical ABO blood grouping system is based on the presence of antigens called A and B agglutinogens on the cell membrane of RBCs.

- A and B agglutinogens are complex oligosaccharides differing in their terminal sugars. In antigen A, the terminal sugar is *N*-acetylgalactosamine while in B antigen, the terminal sugar is galactose. Basically, these antigens are carbohydrates present on the backbone of the cell membrane of RBCs, as either glycosphingolipids or glycoproteins, and are secreted into plasma and body fluids as glycoproteins. H substance is the precursor on which A and B antigens are added, and H substance is formed by addition of fructose to glycoprotein or glycolipid backbone. Then, addition of *N*-acetylgalactosamine produces A antigen and of galactose the B antigen.
- The A and B antigens present on the membranes of RBCs are also present in many other tissues, like salivary glands, pancreas, kidney, liver, lungs and testis, and also in body fluids like saliva, semen and amniotic fluid. The antigens on RBC membrane are glycolipids, while in the tissues and body fluids they are soluble glycoproteins.
- In addition to A and B antigens, H antigen is also present usually in all individuals. H antigen is not antigenic, so there is no corresponding antibody (Fig. 3.6.1).

Anti-A and Anti-B Agglutinins

All individuals produce antibodies to ABH carbohydrate antigen that they lack; thus, A blood group individual produces anti-B, 'B' blood group anti-A, 'AB' blood group neither A nor B and O blood group produces both anti-A and anti-B.

- The individuals with rare *Bombay blood group* produce antibodies to H substance as well as to A and B antigens.

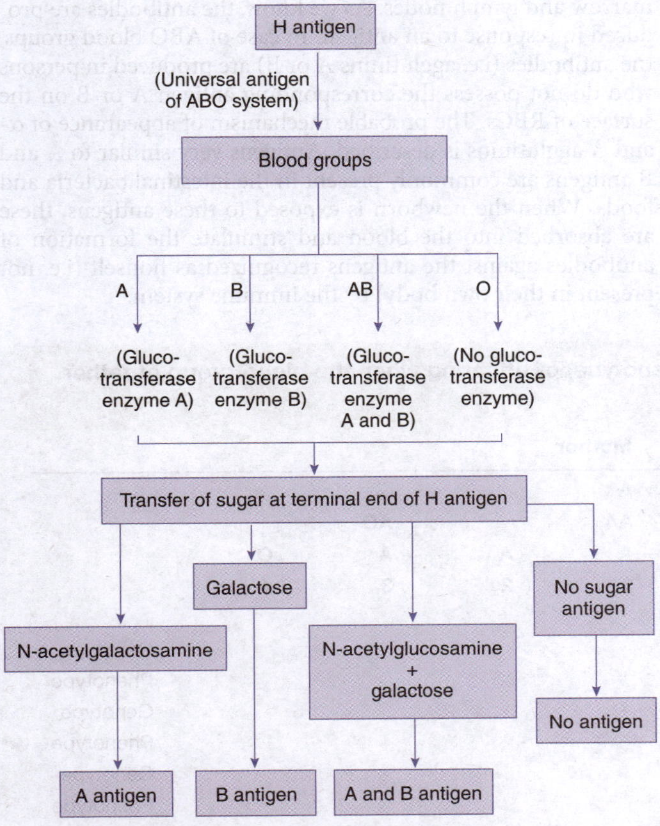

Fig 3.6.1 Role of H antigen in ABO blood group system.

- The naturally occurring antibodies are termed isoagglutinins and demonstrable agglutinins are present in 50% of newborns only that have been filtered across the placenta.
- The specific agglutinins start appearing at 10 days; reach a peak at 10 years and then decline.
- Anti-A (or α) agglutinin and anti-B (or β) agglutinin refer to the antibody, i.e. which reacts with or acts on antigen A and antigen B, respectively.
- The α- and β-agglutinins are globulins of the IgM type and *cannot cross the placenta*.
- There are two types of α-agglutinins: the α_1- and α-proper.
- Presence or absence of α- and β-agglutinins is determined by Landsteiner law as described above.
- The α- and β-agglutinins act best at low temperature (5–20°C) and are therefore also called cold antibodies.

However, the production of anti-A and anti-B has been explained by the fact that the blood group substance (antigen) has similarity with substances present in food and bacterial antigens. They enter the body along with food, bacteria and other ways. The bacterial antigens that belong to intestinal flora get absorbed and induce antibody production, because they are recognized as nonself antigens.

Types of ABO Blood Groups

Depending on the presence or absence of A and B agglutinogens and α- and β-agglutinins, there are four types of blood groups.

Blood group A It is characterized by:

- Presence of A agglutinogen and absence of B agglutinogen on the cell membrane of RBCs
- Presence of anti-B (or β) agglutinin and absence of anti-A (or α) agglutinin from the plasma

Group A has two subgroups: A_1 and A_2. The α_1-agglutinin agglutinates with subgroup A_1 only, while α-proper agglutinin agglutinates with both A_1 and A_2 subgroups.

Blood group B It is characterized by:

- Presence of B agglutinogen and absence of A agglutinogen on the membrane of RBCs
- Presence of anti-A (or α) agglutinin and absence of anti-B (β) agglutinin from the plasma

Blood group AB It is characterized by:

- Presence of both A and B agglutinogens on the cell membrane of RBCs
- Absence of both anti-A (or α) and anti-B or (β) agglutinins from the plasma

Blood group AB has two subgroups, namely A_1B and A_2B.

Blood group O It is characterized by:

- Absence of both A and B agglutinogens on the red cell membrane
- Presence of both anti-A and anti-B agglutinins in the plasma

Population Distribution of ABO Blood Groups (Table 3.6.1)

Population distribution of ABO blood groups in India versus Britain is depicted in Table 3.6.1.

Table 3.6.1 Population distribution of ABO blood groups in India vis-à-vis in Britain

Blood group	India (%)	Britain (%)
A	20	42
B	40	9
AB	8	3
O	32	46

Inheritance of ABO Blood Groups

Agglutinogens A and B or the nonantigenic substances which determine the blood groups are genetically inherited as Mendelian dominant in the classical Mendelian pattern.

- The genes that determine A and B phenotypes are located on chromosome 9P. The enzymes glycosyltransferases are the gene products which confer enzymatic ability for addition of specific antigenic carbohydrates. Therefore, individuals who lack 'A' and 'B' transferases are 'O' type, while those who inherit both 'A' and 'B' transferases are 'AB' type.
- Individuals who lack the H gene (responsible for coding fructose transferase) cannot produce H substance. Such individuals are homozygous for silent h allele (hh) and are known as Bombay phenotype, i.e. (Oh), but are rare. The ABO phenotype and possible genotype have been listed in Table 3.6.2.

If the blood group of the father is B and that of the mother is A, then the blood group of the offspring will be as shown in Table 3.6.3.

The various possibilities of inheritance of antigen A, B or nonantigenic substance O from the mother and father will determine the blood group of the offspring as shown in Table 3.6.4.

- If both parents have AB blood group, then offspring can have A, B or AB blood group. However, the probability will be A, 25%; AB, 50%; and B, 25%.
- If both parents have blood group O, then offspring can have blood group O but never have A, B or AB.
- If one of the parents has blood group A with genotype AA and other has blood group B of genotype BB, then the offspring can have blood group AB but not A, B or O.
- If the father has blood group A with genotype AO and the mother has blood group B with genotype BO, then the offspring can have blood group AB, A, B or O with probability of 25% each.

Table 3.6.2 The ABO phenotypes and possible genotypes

Phenotype	Genotypes
Blood group A	AA, AO
Blood group B	BB, BO
Blood group AB	AB
Blood group O	OO

Agglutinogens A and B first appear in the sixth week of fetal life.

Their concentration at birth is one-fifth of adult level and it progressively rises during puberty and adolescence.

Important Note

ABO agglutinogens are stable, therefore can be detected in the dried blood, blood stains and even in other body fluids, hence carries forensic serology importance.

Anti-A (or α) and anti-B (or β) agglutinins.

Anti-A (or α) and anti-B (or β) agglutinins (specific blood group antibodies) are absent at birth, but they appear 10–15 days after birth and reach a maximum concentration by the age of 10 years.

Origin of agglutinins.

Agglutinins A and B are of gamma globulins (mainly IgM and IgG types) produced by the bone marrow and lymph nodes. As we know, the antibodies are produced in response to an antigen. In case of ABO blood groups, the antibodies (i.e. agglutinins A or B) are produced in persons who do not possess the corresponding antigen A or B on the surface of RBCs. The probable mechanism of appearance of α- and β-agglutinins is described. Antigens very similar to A and B antigens are commonly present in the intestinal bacteria and foods. When the newborn is exposed to these antigens, these are absorbed into the blood and stimulate the formation of antibodies against the antigens recognized as nonself (i.e. not present in their own body) by the immune system.

Table 3.6.3 The possible blood groups (genotype and phenotype) of offspring when the blood group of father is B and that of mother is A

	Father				Mother				
Phenotype	B				A				
Genotype	BB		BO		AA		AO		
Inherited gene	B	B	B	O	A	A	A	O	
	I	II	III	IV	1	2	3	4	
Offspring	1	2	3	4					
I	AB	AB	AB	BO					Genotype
	AB	AB	AB	B					Phenotype
II	AB	AB	AB	BO					Genotype
	AB	AB	AB	B					Phenotype
III	AB	AB	AB	BO					Genotype
	AB	AB	AB	B					Phenotype
IV	AO	AO	AO	OO					Genotype
	A	A	A	O					Phenotype

Table 3.6.4 Possible blood groups of offspring depending on the blood group of father and mother

Mother		Father					
Phenotype →	Genotype →	A	B		AB	O	
↓	↓	AA	AO	BB	BO	AB	OO
A	AA AO	A, O	AB, B, A, O			B, AB O	B, O
B	BB BO	A, B, AB, O		B, O		A, B, AB	B, O
AB	AB	A, B, AB		A, B, AB		A, B, AB	A, B
O	OO	A, O		B, O		A, B	O

Important Note

The gut of an infant is relatively permeable to larger protein molecules compared with adults; therefore, the bacterial antigens get absorbed intact from the gut and induce antibody production.

Agglutinin titre. The quantity of agglutinin is practically nil immediately after birth. The titre of agglutinin starts rising after 2 months as the infant begins to produce agglutinins and maximum titre is attained by the age of 8–10 years and then starts declining throughout the life (Fig. 3.6.2). The relative concentration of agglutinins in saliva and semen is 600, amniotic fluid 175, tears 5, urine 3, cerebrospinal fluid 0 and red plasma 832 after diluting.

Note: The figures indicate the dilution factor before losing the agglutinating potency.

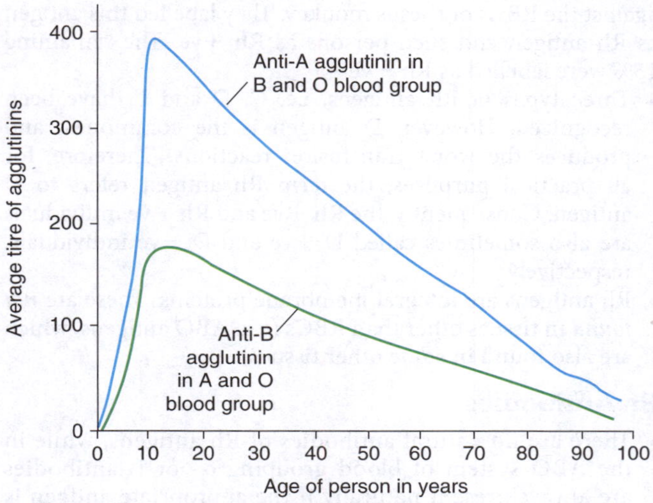

Fig. 3.6.2 Titre of agglutinins with age. The figure indicates the dilution factor before losing its agglutinating potency.

Determination of ABO Blood Groups

The ABO blood group of an individual can be determined by mixing one drop of suspension of his/her red cells (in isotonic saline) with a drop each of antiserum A (containing α-agglutinins) and antiserum B (containing β-agglutinins) separately on a glass slide. The antiserum A will cause agglutination (clumping of RBCs having A antigens and antiserum B will cause agglutination of RBCs having B antigens). The blood group of the individual will be shown by the presence of agglutination with one, both or none of the sera (Table 3.6.5; Fig. 3.6.3).

Note: The antisera A and B are available commercially. For a quick identification, the anti-A serum is tinted blue and anti-B serum is tinted yellow.

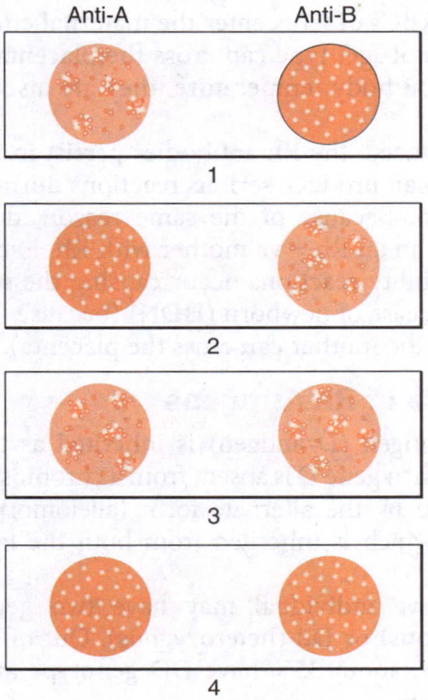

Fig. 3.6.3 Determination of blood groups – the RBCs showing agglutination with antisera are 1, of blood group 'A' with antisera A; 2, of blood group B with antisera B; 3, of blood group 'AB' with antisera A and B (both); and 4, of blood group 'O' with none.

Table 3.6.5 Determination of blood group of an individual

	Agglutination with	
Blood group of RBC suspension	Antiserum A (containing α-agglutinins)	Antiserum B (containing β-agglutinins)
A	+	–
B	–	+
AB	+	+
O	–	–

RH (RHESUS) BLOOD GROUPING SYSTEM

Rh Antigens

- The antigens responsible for this blood grouping system are called Rh antigens or Rh agglutinogens or Rh factor because these were first discovered in the RBCs of rhesus monkeys. Based on the presence of Rh antigen, two types of blood groups are described:
  - ***Rh +ve blood group***
  - ***Rh −ve blood group***

The Rh antigens were discovered by Landsteiner and Weiner in 1940. They noticed that when RBCs of the rhesus monkey (monkey with red ischial callosity) were injected into a rabbit, antibodies were formed against these RBCs. When this rabbit's serum was tested against human red cells, agglutination occurred in 85% of the cases, i.e. the RBCs of this person contained antigens which reacted with antibodies formed against the RBCs of rhesus monkey. They labelled this antigen as Rh antigen and such persons as Rh +ve. The remaining 15% were labelled as Rh −ve.

- Three types of Rh antigens, i.e. C, D and E, have been recognized. However, D antigen is the commonest and produces the worst transfusion reactions. Therefore, for all practical purposes, the term Rh antigen refers to D antigen. Consequently, the Rh +ve and Rh −ve individuals are also sometimes called D +ve and D −ve individuals, respectively.
- Rh antigens are integral membrane proteins. These are *not found* in tissues other than RBCs (e.g. ABO antigens, which are also found in some other tissues).

Rh Antibodies

- There are no natural antibodies of Rh antigens, while in the ABO system of blood grouping α- or β-antibodies are always present naturally if the appropriate antigen is absent.
- Rh antibodies (also called anti-D) are produced only when an Rh −ve individual is transfused with Rh +ve blood or when an Rh −ve mother gives birth to an Rh +ve baby (Rh +ve RBCs of fetus enter the maternal circulation); Rh antibodies of IgG type can cross the placenta. Since these react best at body temperature, they are also called warm antibodies.
- Once produced, the Rh antibodies persist in the blood for years and can produce serious reactions during the second transfusion. Because of the same reason, during second pregnancy in an Rh −ve mother with Rh +ve fetus, severe incompatibility reactions occur causing the so-called haemolytic disease of newborn (HDN) (because Rh antibodies present in the mother can cross the placenta).

Inheritance of Rh Antigens

- The Rh antigen (D antigen) is inherited as the dominant gene *D*. When gene *D* is absent from a chromosome, its place is occupied by the alternate form (allelomorph) called '*d*' Rh gene, which is inherited from both the father and the mother.
- An Rh +ve individual may have two genotypes, DD (homozygous) or Dd (heterozygous). Out of 85% Rh +ve individuals, about 35% have DD genotype and 50% have Dd genotype.
- The genotype of Rh −ve individuals is dd.

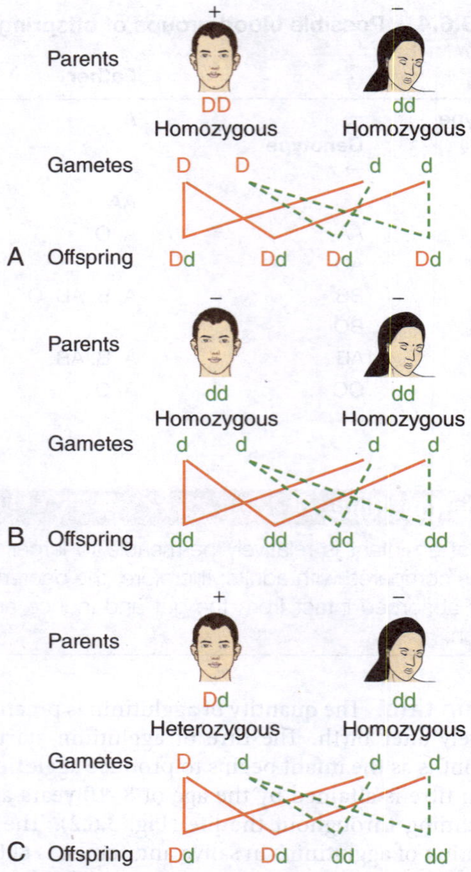

Fig. 3.6.4 Inheritance of Rh antigen: **A,** when father is homozygous Rh +ve and mother is homozygous Rh −ve, all the offspring are heterozygous Rh +ve; **B,** when both father and mother are homozygous Rh −ve, all the offspring are homozygous Rh −ve; and **C,** when father is heterozygous Rh +ve and mother is homozygous Rh −ve, 50% of offspring are Rh +ve (heterozygous) and other 50% are Rh −ve (homozygous).

- Therefore, the genotype (gene composition) of the offspring will be:
  - *DD when gene D is carried by both sperm and ovum*
  - *Dd when one gamete carries D and the other d*
  - *dd when both the gametes carry gene d*

  Inheritance of Rh antigen is summarized in Fig. 3.6.4.

Applied Aspects

Haemolytic Disease of Newborn (HDN)

HDN occurs as a result of incompatibility of Rh blood groups between the mother and fetus. The mechanism is described in the subsequent text. It is important to note that incompatibility of ABO blood groups between the mother and fetus is very common, but there is seldom any complication because the α- and β-agglutinins, i.e. antibodies against antigens A and B, are of IgM type, which cannot cross the placental barrier.

Mechanism of Haemolytic Disease of Newborn in Rh Incompatibility

Mechanism of development of HDN can be described under the following steps:

1. Entrance of Rh +ve fetal RBCs into Rh −ve mother's circulation during first pregnancy.

When an Rh −ve mother (genotype dd) bears an Rh +ve child (genotype Dd) with father being Rh +ve (genotype DD or Dd), at the time of delivery, the fetal RBCs enter maternal circulation because of severance of umbilical cord. Before delivery, usually the fetal and maternal circulation do not mix. Since the Rh +ve RBCs enter maternal circulation during delivery, the first child is usually normal.

2. Production of Rh antibodies (anti-D) in mother.
   During postpartum period, i.e. within a month after delivery, the mother develops Rh antibodies in her blood. As mentioned earlier, the Rh antibodies are of IgG type and are able to cross the placental barrier. Once formed, the Rh antibodies persist for a long period in the mother's blood.
3. Rh incompatibility reaction during second pregnancy.
   When the Rh −ve mother in the second pregnancy also bears an Rh +ve child, the Rh antibodies present in the mother's blood enter the fetal circulation by crossing the placental barrier and cause agglutination of fetal RBCs leading to HDN.

Manifestations of Haemolytic Disease of Newborn

Depending on the severity, the HDN may manifest as:

- Erythroblastosis fetalis
- Icterus gravis neonatorum
- Kernicterus
- Hydrops fetalis

1. ***Erythroblastosis fetalis*** is characterized by:
   - *Erythroblastosis*, i.e. appearance of a large number of erythroblasts in peripheral blood occurs as the haemopoietic tissue of the baby attempts to rapidly replace the haemolysed RBCs.
   - *Anaemia* occurs due to excessive haemolysis of RBCs by Rh antibodies. Infant may even die of severe anaemia.
2. ***Icterus gravis neonatorum***
   - *Jaundice* may occur within 24 hours of birth due to excessive formation of bilirubin as a result of excessive haemolysis of RBCs.
   - *Liver and spleen* are enlarged.
3. ***Kernicterus***. It is a neurological syndrome occurring in newborns with severe haemolysis. The excessive bilirubin formed may enter the brain tissue as the blood–brain barrier is not well developed in infants and cause damage. The bilirubin mostly affects the basal ganglia, producing disturbance of motor activities. It usually develops when the serum bilirubin level exceeds 18 mg/dL.
4. ***Hydrops fetalis***, i.e. the fetus is grossly oedematous. It occurs when haemolysis is very severe. Usually, intrauterine death of fetus occurs, or if born prematurely or even at term, the infant dies within a few hours.

Prevention

Screening for HDN in pregnancy.

At 12–16 weeks, every pregnant woman should be tested for ABO and Rh group, and for red cell alloantibodies that maybe directed against paternal blood group antigens.

Anti-D immunoglobulin prophylaxis.

In a mother who is Rh −ve and has not been sensitized, Rh immunoglobulin available as trade name RhoGAM is infused. This medicine can stop antibodies from reacting with fetal Rh +ve RBCs.

Prevention for Haemolytic Disease of Newborn

HDN during second pregnancy can be prevented by injecting a single dose of Rh antibodies (anti-D) in the form of Rh immunoglobulin to the mother soon after the first childbirth within 72 hours of delivery. These antibodies will destroy the Rh +ve RBCs of the fetus which have gained access to maternal circulation. In this way, active antibodies will not be formed by the mother.

Note: Maternal blood sample is checked for remaining fetal RBCs and extra anti-D should be given if indicated.

Treatment of Haemolytic Disease of Newborn

Treatment of HDN is replacement of baby's Rh +ve blood with Rh −ve blood. The baby's own blood is removed slowly with the help of a polyethylene catheter into the inferior vena cava along the umbilical vein, and is replaced by an equal amount of Rh −ve blood. This is called exchange transfusion.

About 400 mL of Rh −ve blood is infused in 1.5–2 hours. The procedure may be repeated many times during the few weeks of neonatal period to maintain low levels of bilirubin to prevent kernicterus.

By this time (6–18 weeks), the infant's own Rh +ve RBCs replace the Rh −ve infused RBCs, the time required for formation of RBCs (erythropoiesis).

CLINICAL APPLICATIONS OF BLOOD GROUPING

1. In blood transfusion.
For details, see page 224.

2. In preventing haemolytic disease. Blood grouping helps in preventing haemolytic disease in HDN due to Rh incompatibility (as discussed above).

3. In paternity disputes. The ABO, Rh and MNS blood grouping is helpful in settling cases of disputed paternity. Antigens A and B are dominant, whereas O is recessive. It is possible to prove that a person could not have been the father, but not that he was or is father, e.g.:

- If the child's blood group is O, whatever be the blood group of the mother, a person with blood group AB cannot be the father.
- If the child's blood group is AB, whatever be the blood group of the mother, a person with blood group O cannot be the father (Table 3.6.6). The predictive value of such a test is strengthened further if several blood group systems are considered. DNA fingerprinting can prove or disprove fatherhood with 100% certainty.

4. In medicolegal cases. Any red stain on a clothing may be claimed to be blood by a supposed victim. Therefore, it is first confirmed that it really is blood by preparing haemin crystals from the stain extract. Blood grouping of the extracted sample can then prove or disprove the claims of victim.

Table 3.6.6 Predictive blood groups of parents in paternity disputes

Blood group of child	Parents must have given blood group	Mother's blood group	Father not have been of blood group
O	O + O	No matter which	AB
AB	A + B	No matter which	O
A	A + O or A + A	B or O	B or O
B	B + O or B + B	A or O	A or O

Note: The child's true ABO typing may not be set until 1 year of age.

5. In knowing susceptibility to diseases. The incidence of certain diseases is related to blood groups, e.g.:

- Individuals with blood group O (nonsecretors) are said to be more susceptible to duodenal ulcer (peptic ulcer) than the individuals with blood group A and B (secretors).
- Individuals with blood group A are more susceptible to carcinoma of stomach, pancreas and salivary glands.
- To some extent, incidence of diabetes mellitus is more in individuals with blood group A.

OTHER BLOOD GROUP SYSTEMS

More than 100 blood group systems are recognized, which are composed of more than 500 antigens. These include:

Lewis system (Le): In this system, carbohydrate antigen is not the integral part of the red cell membrane but is adsorbed on RBC membrane from the plasma. Lewis system consists of two antigens; Le^a and Le^b. The Le antigens are also present in lymph and other body secretions. The antibodies to Lewis are IgM type and cannot cross the placenta.

I system: In this system, the antigens are oligosaccharides related to H, A, B and Le, but differ in their branching system. The antibodies produced are cold agglutinins, and their binding is low at body temperature.

P system is another blood group in which the carbohydrate antigen is controlled by specific glycotransferases, and its clinical significance is in rare cases.

MNSsU system. MNS system has three antigens M, N and S expressed on the surface of RBCs, and endothelial cells of renal capillaries are regulated by genes located on chromosome 4. M and N are determinants of an RBC membrane protein i.e., glycophorin A_1 and Ss are of glycophorin B.

Kell blood group system is complex and contains antigens which are K, k, KP^a, Js^a and Js^b that are highly immunogenic. The antigens are third most potent for triggering an immune reaction, after the A, B, O and Rh blood groups.

Duffy system has highly immunogenic glycoprotein antigens present on the surface of RBCs. The antigens are FY^a and FY^{ab}.
Note. The persons with Duffy blood group are resistant to malaria caused by *Plasmodium vivax*.

Bombay blood group. The Bombay blood group is h/Oh blood group. It occurs due to deficiency of H antigen. The phenotype of this blood group is first discovered in Bombay by Dr Y M Bhende in 1952. Bombay blood group is characterized by the absence of A, B and H antigens. It occurs rarely (1 per 10,000), especially in tribal population of India.

EMM blood group. Recently EMM-negative blood group is detected in a 65-year-old heart patient in Gujrat by Dr Sammukh Joshi. It is a rare blood group (only 9 persons globally registered). The EMM antigens are antibodies that develop naturally in the human body.

BLOOD TRANSFUSION

INDICATIONS

Blood transfusion is a life-saving measure and should be carried out when it is absolutely essential. Common situations in which blood transfusion is indicated are as follows.

1. Blood loss. Severe blood loss is the most important indication for blood transfusion. It may occur in:

- Accidents
- Major operations
- Ruptured peptic ulcer
- Ruptured aortic aneurysm
- Ruptured ectopic pregnancy

2. For quick restoration of haemoglobin. In patients with severe anaemia, it is required in situations like pregnancy and emergency surgery.

3. Exchange transfusion. Exchange transfusion is required in HDN.

4. Blood diseases. Blood diseases like aplastic anaemia, agranulocytosis, leukaemias, haemophilia, purpura and clotting defects may require blood transfusion.

5. Acute poisoning. Blood transfusion is required in case of acute poisoning, e.g. carbon monoxide poisoning.

DONOR AND RECIPIENT

Donor. Donor refers to a person who donates the blood and the person who receives blood is a recipient.

Precautions to be taken while selecting a donor are as follows:

- Donor should be healthy, and aged between 18 and 60 years.
- Pregnant and lactating mothers preferably should not donate blood.
- Donor should be screened to exclude the diseases which are spread through blood such as AIDS, viral hepatitis, malaria and syphilis.
- Haemoglobin and PCV of the donor should be within normal range.

Universal donor. Blood of the individuals with blood group O does not contain any agglutinogen. So, when this blood is transfused to a person with any blood group (A, B, AB or O), theoretically its RBCs will not be agglutinated. Because of this fact, an individual with blood group O is called universal donor. However, practically this term is no longer valid, as it ignores the complications produced by existence of the Rh factor and other blood group systems.

Universal recipient. Blood of an individual with blood group AB does not contain any agglutinins. So, theoretically when such an individual receives blood from an individual with any blood group (A, B, AB or O), there should be no transfusion reaction. Because of this fact, an individual with AB blood group is called universal recipient. However, practically this term is also no more valid because it ignores the complications produced by the existence of Rh factor and other blood group systems.

PRECAUTIONS TO BE OBSERVED DURING BLOOD TRANSFUSION

1. Absolute indication. Absolute indication should always be there for the transfusion of blood.

2. Cross-matching. Cross-matching should always be done before the blood transfusion. For it, blood is collected from donor as well as recipient. Plasma and RBCs are separated in each. The cross-matching involves two steps: major and minor cross-matching.

Major cross-matching (direct cross-matching) will reveal the presence of anti-ABO agglutinin in the serum of recipient and also complete anti-D. Major cross-matching involves mixing of donor's cells with recipient's plasma. This is called major cross-matching because of the fact that when mismatched blood is transfused in a recipient, the donor cells get agglutinated as against their agglutinogen there is sufficiently high concentration of agglutinins in the recipient's plasma.

Minor cross-matching. It involves mixing of recipient's cells with donor's plasma. This is called a minor cross-match due to the fact that reaction of donor's plasma and recipient's cells usually does not occur or is very mild on giving mismatched blood transfusion because:

- First, the donor's plasma in the transfusion (about 250 mL) is usually so diluted by the much larger volume of recipient's blood (about 5 L) that it rarely causes agglutination even when the titre of agglutinins against the recipient's cell is high.
- Second, donor's agglutinins are also neutralized by soluble agglutinogens which are found free in the recipient's body fluid.

Coombs test. Coombs test is also known as antiglobulin test due to detection of antibodies against circulating RBCs in the body, which induce haemolysis. There are two types of Coomb tests: detects incomplete anti-D. It is carried out in two stages:

Direct Coombs test: The direct Coombs test detects the presence of antibodies (IgG and IgM) that are sticked to the RBCs.

Procedure. In direct Coombs test, the RBCs of the donor washed and suspended in the 5% isotonic solution are tested against recipient's plasma. Presence of agglutination indicates direct positive Coombs test.

When tested against the recipient's plasma, direct Coombs test reveals presence of incomplete antibodies present on the RBCs.

Indirect Coombs test: This test is supplemented on washed red blood cells and recipient plasma to detect incomplete antibodies, which are not present on the RBCs. Indirect Coombs test is a two-stage test.

Procedure

- In stage one, the RBCs are incubated at 37°C with serum, then
- The RBCs are washed with saline to remove the globulins, then
- Anti-human globulins (Coombs serum) are added to the washed RBCs.

Interpretation. Agglutination of RBCs indicates that the original serum has antibodies which are coated on the RBCs.

Important Notes

- *For all practical purposes*, if there is no agglutination in either of the cases (major as well as minor cross-matching) described above, only then the recipient can safely receive donor's blood.
- *In extreme emergencies* like war casualties and massive train accidents, where time does not permit the grouping and cross-matching, O Rh −ve blood (universal donor) may be used.

3. Rh +ve blood should never be transfused to Rh −ve person. It is particularly a must for females at any age before menopause, because once she is sensitized by the Rh antigen, the anti-D antibodies are formed and she will not be able to bear an Rh +ve fetus. In other words, Rh +ve transfusion may make a woman permanently childless.

4. Donor's blood should always be screened. Donor's blood should always be screened for diseases which are spread through blood such as AIDS, hepatitis B, malaria and syphilis.

5. Blood bag/bottle should be checked. Blood bag/bottle should be checked for the name of recipient and blood group on the label before starting the blood transfusion.

6. Blood transfusion should be given at slow rate. Blood transfusion should be given at slow rate (not more than 20 drops/min). If rapid transfusion is given, citrate present in stored blood may cause chelation of calcium ions leading to decreased serum calcium level and tetany.

7. Proper aseptic measures. Proper aseptic measures must be taken during transfusion of blood.

8. Careful watch on recipient's condition. Careful watch on recipient's condition is a must for the first 10–15 minutes of starting the transfusion, and from time to time, later. The transfusion must be stopped if there is a rapid rise of temperature (>40°C), or any other reaction.

HAZARDS OF BLOOD TRANSFUSION

1. Mismatched transfusion reactions. Mismatched transfusion reaction is the most serious and potentially fatal hazard of blood transfusion. It is characterized by:

Agglutination of donor's red blood cells in the recipient's circulation. For occurrence of agglutination, the concentrations of agglutination and agglutinogen should be same (i.e. zone phenomenon).

Tissue ischaemia occurs due to blockage of certain vessels by agglutinated cells. Soon, the patient complains of violent pain in the back or elsewhere and tightness of chest.

Haemolysis of agglutinated red cells occurs rapidly releasing large amounts of haemoglobin in circulation (haemoglobinaemia).

Haemolytic jaundice may occur due to excessive formation of bilirubin from haemoglobin released by haemolysed RBCs.

Renal vasoconstriction is caused by toxic substances released from the haemolysed RBCs.

Circulatory shock occurs due to loss of circulating red cells and release of toxic substances leading to fall in arterial blood pressure and decreased renal blood flow.

Haemoglobinuria occurs when total free haemoglobin becomes more than that can bind with haptoglobin (plasma protein binding haemoglobin). The extra free haemoglobin leaks through glomerular membrane and is passed in urine producing haemoglobinuria.

Renal tubular damage. If urine is acidic and glomerular filtration is slow, the free haemoglobin passing through glomeruli is precipitated in the tubules as acid haematin. This obstructs the lumen of tubules producing renal tubular damage.

Acute renal shutdown (anuria) sets in ultimately due to the combined effects of renal vasoconstriction, circulatory shock, hypotension and renal tubular damage. Acute renal shutdown usually occurs within a few minutes to few hours after transfusion of mismatched blood and continues.

Uraemia (increased nitrogenous substances and potassium in the body) results due to acute renal failure, soon producing coma and death.

Transfusion-related acute lung injury (TRALI). Acute respiratory distress syndrome may occur within 6 hours of transfusion, characterized by:

- Tachypnoea
- Dyspnoea
- Hypotension
- Cyanosis
- Fever

2. Circulatory overload. Circulatory overload due to hypervolaemia may occur following blood transfusion when the transfusion is rapid, especially in patients with cardiac diseases, chronic anaemia and kidney diseases. The rate of transfusion should be 2 mL/min (120 mL/h) for first 15 minutes, then increase the rate to 5–10 mL/min for next 1–2 hours; however, the blood transfusion should not exceed >4 hours.

- In neonates and paediatric age group, the blood transfusion rate should be 5 mL/kg for 1–2 hours. It should not exceed 1 mL/kg body weight per hour.

3. Transmission of blood-borne infections. Blood-borne infections such as AIDS, viral hepatitis, malaria and syphilis may be transmitted to recipient from the infected donor.

4. Pyrogenic reaction. Pyrogenic reaction characterized by fever and chills may occur probably due to destruction of leucocytes and platelets by antibodies against them.

5. Allergic reactions. Allergic reactions such as skin rashes and asthma may occur if donor blood contains substances to which patient is allergic.

6. Hyperkalaemia. Hyperkalaemia may occur after excessive transfusion because K^+ concentration in stored blood is high owing to leakage of K^+ from the RBCs into the plasma.

7. Hypocalcaemia. Hypocalcaemia producing tetany may occur following massive transfusion of citrated blood. Following rapid and massive transfusion, the citrate cannot be metabolized fully. The extra citrate chelates calcium ions leading to decreased serum calcium levels and tetany. That is why, intravenous calcium gluconate is given with citrated blood transfusion.

8. Reduced tissue oxygenation. Reduced tissue oxygenation may occur in patients receiving large amounts of transfusion. Red cells in stored blood have very low amounts of 2,3-BPG in them and thus have high affinity for O_2 and consequently tend to give off less O_2 to the tissues. The reduced release of O_2 to tissues can cause serious problems.

9. Haemosiderosis. Haemosiderosis due to iron overload may occur following repeated transfusions, as in thalassaemic patients. The excessive iron is deposited in liver, heart and endocrine organs and produces damage.

10. Thrombophlebitis. Thrombophlebitis at the venepuncture site may develop if the needle remains in the same site for many hours.

11. Air embolism. Air embolism, i.e. entry of air into the blood, is much less likely to occur because of the use of plastic bags which collapse down as they empty out of blood.

AUTOLOGOUS BLOOD TRANSFUSION

Autologous blood transfusion refers to transfusion of an individual's own blood which has been withdrawn and stored. Autologous transfusion is done under the following situations:

For elective surgery A self-predonation is a common practice in some hospitals. After starting a course of iron tablets, 2 units of blood are collected, one 16 days and another 8 days before surgery. This practice avoids the hazards of transfusion of blood donated by some other individual.

During surgery The cell-saver machine when used sucks up blood from the wound, recycles it and returns it to the patient's body. This is known as intraoperative blood salvage.

Some sportspersons are also known to use autologous transfusion a few days before an important event to improve the athletic performance. The red cells are collected from the athlete's blood, stored for few weeks and then re-injected in two to three spells few days before the event.

Important Note

Autologous blood transfusion in sportspersons is considered blood doping nowadays and has been declared illegal and banned by the sports committees.

STORAGE OF BLOOD FOR TRANSFUSION

In the blood banks, storage of blood is done to preserve the blood for long time. The main aim of blood storage is to provide viable and functional blood components to the patients.

Some facts about the storage of donated blood are as follows:

One unit of blood (420 mL) can be collected from a donor at a time under all aseptic measures. An individual can safely donate 1 unit of blood every 6 months. ACD mixture (120 mL) is added to the blood and stored in a sterile container.

Contents of ACD mixture:

- Acid citrate (monohydrous), 0.48 g
- Trisodium citrate, 1.32 g
- Dextrose, 1.47 g
- Distilled water, 100 mL

Dextrose (glucose) present in ACD mixture provides energy for maintenance of sodium–potassium pump activity. The pump activity is essential for maintaining the size of cells. Therefore, if the glucose is not added to stored blood, the RBCs swell up and haemolyse rapidly. Furthermore, glucose liberates lactic acid, which by decreasing the pH helps in survival of RBCs, both in vitro and in vivo.

Anticoagulant activity is provided by the citrates present in the ACD mixture, which also decreases the pH of blood.

- Up to 21 days, the blood can be stored under the above-mentioned conditions.

The changes which occur in stored blood are as follows:

The RBCs in the stored blood swell up due to the following changes as a result of decreased cell metabolism in cold storage:

- *Loss of intracellular* K^+, which increases plasma K^+ concentration from 4–5 to 20–30 mEq/L
- *Increase in intracellular* Na^+ from 12 to 30–40 mEq/L
- *Increase in intracellular water content.* Because of the above-mentioned changes, the RBCs become more spherocytic and their haemoglobin in hypotonic solution increases. Such cells may rupture in vitro even in 0.8% NaCl solution. With reference to Na^+ and K^+ content, volume, shape and saline fragility, the RBCs become normal within 48 hours of transfusion.

WBCs and platelets in stored blood are virtually absent after 24 hours of storage. Therefore, stored blood is not a suitable medium for transferring WBCs and platelets to a recipient.

After transfusion of stored blood, 80% RBCs survive for 24 hours, and, thereafter, surviving cells are destroyed at a rate of 1% per day.

BLOOD COMPONENTS

The whole blood is routinely collected for transfusion. The most donated blood is processed into its various components:

- Packed red blood cells (PRBCs)
- Platelets
- Fresh frozen plasma (FFP)
- Cryoprecipitates
- Plasma derivatives
- WBC concentrates

Whole blood. The whole blood provides oxygen-carrying capacity and volume expansion. Therefore, it is an ideal for patients with acute haemorrhage (>25% of total volume loss).

The whole blood is separated into RBCs and platelet-rich plasma by slow centrifugation. The platelet-rich plasma is then centrifuged at high speed to yield 1 unit of platelets and 1 unit of FFP. The cryoprecipitate is produced by thawing FFP to precipitate the plasma proteins and then separated by centrifugation.

Apheresis is technology which is used to separate particular constituent from the blood and the remaining part returned to the circulation.

1. PRBCs increase the oxygen-carrying capacity. Therefore, they are used in severely anaemic patients to maintain adequate oxygenation (especially hypoplastic and haemolytic anaemia).

Advantages of PRBC over whole blood are the following:

a) Circulatory overloading is prevented.
b) Extra burden of sodium, potassium and other electrolytes on the body system can be prevented.
c) Plasma can be used for other patients (e.g. burns).

2. Platelets are collected either as pools prepared from five to eight random donors (RDs) or as single-donor apheresis (SDAPs). These are transfused in patients with thrombocytopenia to reduce the incidence of bleeding. The threshold for prophylactic platelet concentrate transfusion is 5000/μL. Other indications for platelet concentrate transfusion are as follows:

- Prolonged surgical procedure in which patients' platelets are consumed to stop bleeding
- Massive blood transfusions of stored blood (platelets and leucocytes have short life)
- Leukaemia and lymphoma, because of less production of platelets
- Patients receiving chemotherapy/radiotherapy as a treatment for malignancy because anticancer drugs suppress the bone marrow activity

Important Note

Grouping and cross-matching should be done because platelet concentrate is not absolutely free from RBCs.

3. FFP contains plasma proteins (fibrinogen, albumin, protein C, protein S and antithrombin) and stable factors. Therefore, indications for FFP may be used as plasma for replacement therapy to expand blood volume in conditions where fluid lost from the body (e.g. burns) is massive. The indications for FFP are as follows:

- For correction of coagulation disorders
- In cases of deficient plasma proteins (hypoalbuminaemia)
- Reversal of warfarin effects
- Treatment for thrombotic thrombocytopenic purpura

4. Cryoprecipitate. Cryoprecipitate is an ideal source of fibrinogen, factor VIII, and von Willebrand factor (VWF).

5. Plasma derivatives. Pooled plasma from multiple donors provides specific protein derivatives:

- Albumin solution is used as a plasma substitute for replacing fluid volume. Also, it acts as volume expander because it stays longer in the circulation due to its high molecular weight.
- Immunoglobulin preparations are used in:
  - Immunodeficient patients to prevent infections
  - Anti-D immunoglobulins to prevent the development of endogenous response to Rh antigen (see page 223)

- Antisera containing immunoglobulins against hepatitis B, C, etc.

6. WBC concentrates. WBC concentrate is prepared from fresh whole blood by leukapheresis. It is used in patients with granulocytopenia and immunodeficiency (occurs due to chemotherapy and radiotherapy) or any other cause where infection becomes unresponsive to antibiotic therapy.

Self-Assessment

1. Discuss the basis of classification of blood groups.
2. Discuss the inheritance of ABO blood groups.
3. Describe:
   - Rh blood group system and significant
   - Haemolytic disease of newborn
4. Write notes on:
   - Landsteiner law
   - Rh incompatibility
   - Kernicterus
   - Hydrops fetalis
   - Autologous blood transfusion
   - Cross-matching
   - Precautions during blood transfusion
   - Blood components
   - Storage of blood
   - Hazards of blood transfusion

Clinical Cases

Case 1

A 25-year-old female with blood group A Rh −ve was married to O Rh +ve male. The first delivery was uneventful; however, during second delivery she had stillbirth and fetus was grossly oedematous.

Q1. What is the cause of stillbirth?

Q2. How it can be prevented?

Case 2

In a severely anaemic female with blood group B Rh +ve, blood transfusion was started. Within 15 minutes, she complained of pain in the back, tightness in the chest, redness of face and fever. The transfusion was stopped immediately.

Q1. What is reason for these symptoms?

Q2. What precautions should be followed before transfusion?

Q3. What are the complications that could have occurred if the transfusion would have continued?

Case 3

A normal healthy 25-year-old male had a road accident and had massive blood loss and was alert. He received blood transfusion with 3 units of compatible blood; during the transfusion of 4th unit, he developed cramps in legs, arrhythmia and the temperature decreased to 35.8°C.

Q1. What is the cause for these signs and symptoms?

CARDIOVASCULAR SYSTEM

SECTION 4

SECTION OUTLINE

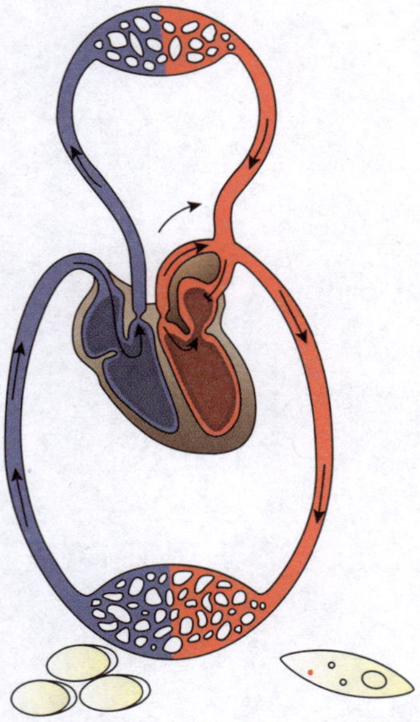

INTRODUCTION

The cardiovascular system (CVS) consists of the heart and the blood vessels. The *heart* acts as a system of two pumps working in series and forms the driving force for blood flow. The blood vessels that take blood from the heart to various tissues are called *arteries*. The smallest arteries are called *arterioles*. Arterioles open into a network of *capillaries*, which constitute the microcirculation. The most important function of blood vessels, i.e. the rapid exchange of materials between the blood and the extracellular fluid, bathing the tissue cells is served by the capillaries. In other words, capillaries serve as the *exchange region*. In some situations, capillaries are replaced by slightly different vessels called *sinusoids*. Blood from capillaries (or from sinusoids) is collected by small *venules* which join to form *veins*. Veins serve as the blood reservoir and return the collected blood to the heart.

FUNCTIONS OF CVS

Primary functions of the CVS as a transport system are carried out by *convection* (i.e. the mass movement of fluid caused by a difference in pressure between two points). These functions are as follows:

- Distribution of nutrients and oxygen (O_2) to all body cells
- Collection of waste products and CO_2 from different body cells and carrying them to excretory organs for excretion

Secondary functions that are subserved by the CVS are as follows:

1. Thermoregulation by control of blood flow to the skin and extremities to enhance or retard heat loss
2. Distribution of hormones to the target tissues
3. Delivery of antibodies, platelets and leucocytes to aid body defence mechanism

PHYSIOLOGY OF CVS

Physiology of CVS includes various aspects of physiology of the heart as a pump and physiology of two main divisions of blood circulation – the pulmonary and systemic circulation.

- The heart consists of two pumps in series (right and left halves) that are connected by pulmonary and systemic circulation.
- In systemic circulation, the various systemic organs receive blood through parallel distribution channels. The parallel arrangement of vessels supplies the body organs with blood of the same arterial composition (i.e. same O_2 and CO_2 tension, pH, glucose level) and essentially the same arterial pressure.
- Since the pulmonary and systemic circulation divisions are arranged in series, both ventricles must pump the same amount of blood over any significant time period. Such a balanced output is achieved by an intrinsic property of the cardiac muscle known as *Frank–Starling mechanism*.

4.1

Functional Anatomy of Heart and Physiology of Cardiac Muscle

FUNCTIONAL ANATOMY OF HEART

The heart is a muscular pump designed to ensure the circulation of blood through the tissues of the body. The human heart weighs approximately 300 g and it consists of two halves, right and left, both structurally and functionally. The right half circulates blood through the lungs for the purpose of oxygenation (i.e. through pulmonary circulation). The left heart circulates blood to tissues of the entire body (i.e. through the systemic circulation).

CHAMBERS OF HEART

Each half of the heart consists of an inflow chamber called the *atrium* and an outflow chamber called the *ventricle* (Fig. 4.1.1). Thus, there are four chambers in the heart.

Atria

Interatrial septum separates the right and left atria which are thin-walled chambers.

Right atrium receives deoxygenated blood from tissues of the entire body through the *superior and inferior venae cavae.* This blood passes into the right ventricle through the right *atrioventricular (AV) orifice* which is guarded by *tricuspid valve.* The right atrium has the pacemaker known as *sinoatrial node* that produces cardiac impulses and the *AV* node that conducts these impulses to the ventricles.

Left atrium receives oxygenated blood from the lungs through the four *pulmonary veins* (two right veins and two left veins). This blood passes into the left ventricle through the *left AV orifice* which is guarded by the mitral valve.

Ventricles

Interventricular septum separates the right ventricle from the left ventricle.

Interior of each ventricle has an inflow part and an outflow part. The inflow part of each ventricle is a rough inner surface because of the presence of numerous bundles of cardiac muscles called *trabeculae carneae. Papillary muscles* are finger-like processes attached to the ventricular wall at one end, but free at the other. They are functionally related to the AV valves.

Right ventricle receives blood from the right atrium and pumps through the pulmonary trunk (which divides into right and left pulmonary arteries) into the lungs. The *pulmonary valve* is present at the junction of right ventricle and pulmonary trunk.

Left ventricle receives blood from the left atrium and pumps out into systemic circulation through the aorta. *Aortic* valve is present at the junction of the left ventricle and the *ascending aorta.*

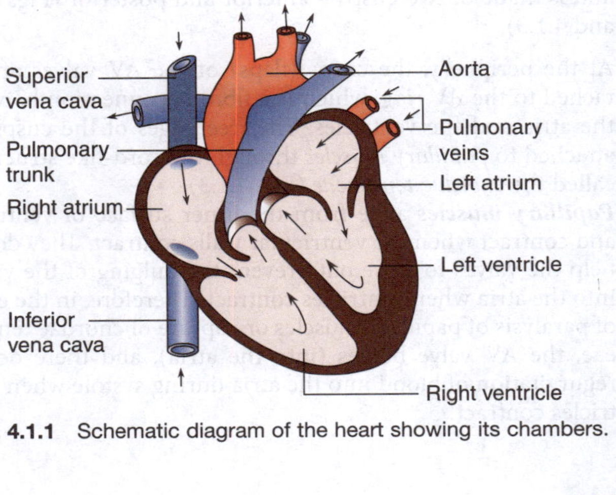

Fig. 4.1.1 Schematic diagram of the heart showing its chambers.

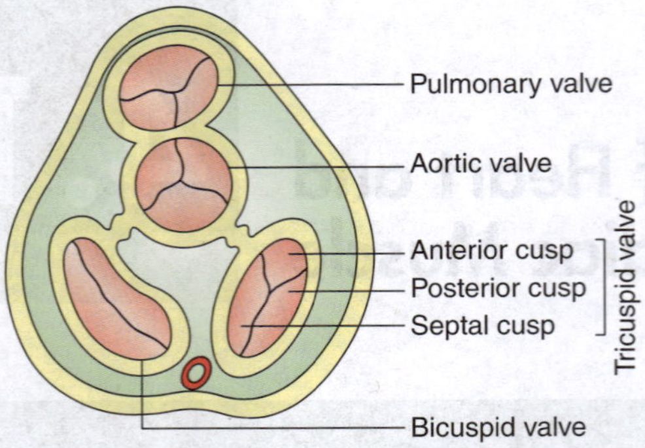

Fig. 4.1.2 Valves of the heart.

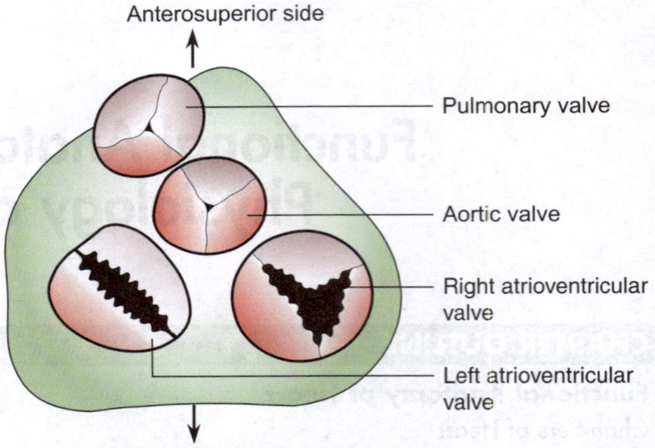

Fig. 4.1.4 Semilunar valves and atrioventricular valves viewed from the posterosuperior aspect after removing the atria.

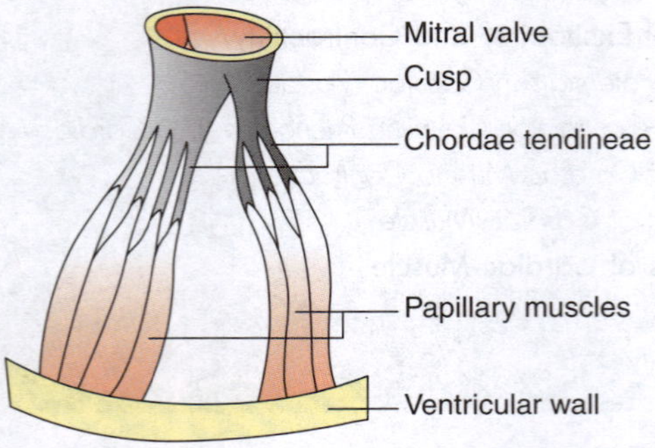

Fig. 4.1.3 Bicuspid valve attached with papillary muscles and chordae tendineae.

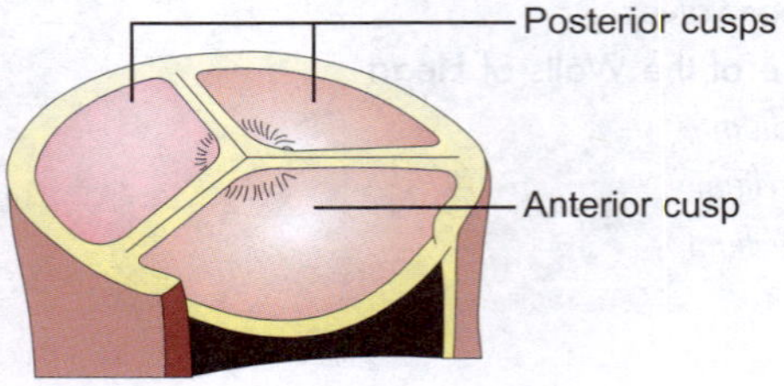

Fig. 4.1.5 Aortic valve.

VALVES OF HEART

There are four valves in the human heart – two AV valves and two semilunar valves. Valves allow unidirectional flow of blood.

Atrioventricular Valves

The AV valves open towards the ventricles and close towards the atria. They allow blood to flow from atria to ventricles. But when ventricles contract, they are closed, and thus prevent backflow of blood from ventricles to atria.

Right AV valve is known as *tricuspid valve* and is made of three cusps – anterior, posterior and septal (Fig. 4.1.2).

The left AV valve is called *mitral valve* or *bicuspid valve* and is made of two cusps – anterior and posterior (Figs 4.1.2 and 4.1.3).

At the periphery, the cusps (flaps) of the AV valves are attached to the *AV ring*, which is a fibrous connection between the atria and the ventricles. The free edges of the cusps are attached to *papillary muscles* through the cord-like structures called the *chordae tendineae* (Fig. 4.1.3).

Papillary muscles arise from the inner surface of ventricles and contract when the ventricular walls contract. They do not help the valves to close but prevent the bulging of the valves into the atria when ventricles contract. Therefore, in the event of paralysis of papillary muscles or rupture of chordae tendineae, the AV valve bulges (into the atria), and there occurs regurgitation of blood into the atria during systole when ventricles contract.

Semilunar Valves

The semilunar valves are named so because these valves have half-moon-shaped cusps. These valves allow the blood to flow from the ventricles during ventricular contraction (systole). The two semilunar valves are the following:

Aortic valve is the semilunar valve present at the opening of aorta in left ventricle. It is made of three semilunar cusps – one anterior and two posterior (Figs 4.1.4 and 4.1.5).

Pulmonary valve is the semilunar valve present at the opening of pulmonary trunk into the right ventricle. It is also made of three semilunar cusps – one posterior and two anterior (Fig. 4.1.4).

- *Semilunar valves open* away from the ventricles and close towards the ventricles. These valves open when ventricles contract, allowing the blood to flow from left ventricle to aorta and from right ventricle to pulmonary trunk.
- *Semilunar valves close* when ventricles relax, thus preventing backflow of blood from the aorta or pulmonary trunk into the ventricles.

STRUCTURE OF THE WALLS OF HEART

Walls of the heart are composed of a thick layer of cardiac muscles, the *myocardium* (see page 234), covered externally by the epicardium and lined internally by the *endocardium*.

- Walls of the atrial portion of the heart are thin.
- Walls of the ventricular portion of the heart are thick.

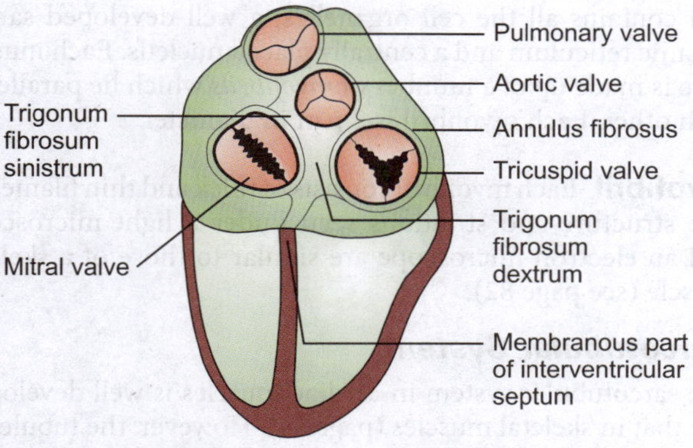

Fig. 4.1.6 Skeleton of the heart.

Skeleton of the heart (Fig. 4.1.6) consists of fibrous rings that surround the AV, pulmonary and aortic orifices and are continuous with the membranous part of the ventricular septum. The fibrous rings around the AV orifices separate the muscular walls of the atria from those of the ventricles but provide attachment for the muscle fibres. The fibrous rings support the bases of the valve cusps and prevent the valves from stretching and becoming incompetent.

Pericardium

The heart and roots of the great vessels are enclosed by a fibroserous sac called pericardium. Its function is to restrict excessive movements of the heart as a whole and to serve as a lubricated container in which different parts of the heart can contract. Pericardium consists of two layers – outer fibrous and inner serous (Fig. 4.1.7A and B).

Fibrous pericardium surrounds the heart like a bag and is attached with the surrounding structures.

Serous pericardium has parietal and visceral layers. The *parietal layer* of serous pericardium lines the fibrous pericardium and is reflected around the roots of the great vessels to become continuous with the *visceral layer of serous pericardium* that closely covers the heart and is often called the *epicardium*. The slit-like space between the parietal and visceral layers of the serous pericardium is called *pericardial cavity* which contains small amount of *pericardial fluid* that acts as a lubricant to facilitate the movement of the heart.

Myocardium

The myocardium (muscular tissue of the heart) is the main tissue constituting the walls of the heart. It consists of three types of muscle fibres:

- *Cardiac muscles* forming the walls of the atria and ventricles – contractile unit of the heart
- Muscle fibres forming the *pacemaker* which is the site of origin of cardiac impulse (see page 244)
- Muscle fibres forming the conducting system which transmits the impulse to the various parts of the heart (see page 242)

Important Notes

- The ventricular muscle bundles are spirally coiled around the ventricular champers in three well-defined layers; outer layer runs in clockwise direction, middle layer in horizontal direction and inner layer in clockwise direction. This arrangement of myocardial muscles facilitates squeezing of blood from the ventricles during ventricular contraction.
- During contraction, the heart slightly rotates towards the right, causing apex of the heart being slightly pushed towards chest wall, therefore palpated as apex beat in left fifth intercostal space.

Endocardium

Endocardium is a thin, smooth and glistening membrane lining the myocardium internally. It consists of a single layer of endothelial cells. The endocardium continues as the endothelium of great vessels opening in the heart.

PHYSIOLOGY OF CARDIAC MUSCLE

FUNCTIONAL ANATOMY

The myocardium consists of three types of muscle fibres:

- Cardiac muscles forming the walls of atria and ventricles (contractile unit of the heart)
- Muscle fibres forming the *pacemaker* which is the site of origin of cardiac impulse

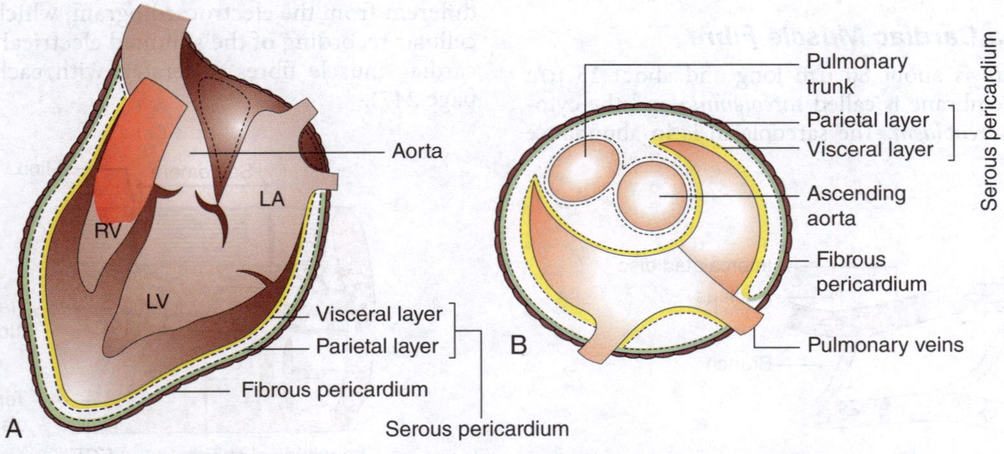

Fig. 4.1.7 Schematic sagittal section of the heart showing fibrous and serous pericardium **A** and transverse section through upper part of the heart and pericardium **B**.

- Muscle fibres forming the *conductive system* which transmits the impulse to the various parts of the heart

This chapter is mainly devoted to physiology of cardiac muscles forming the walls of atria and ventricles.

Structural Organization of Cardiac Muscle

- The cardiac muscle fibres are *striated* and resemble skeletal muscle fibres quite a lot in structure. However, unlike the skeletal muscles, the cardiac muscles are *involuntary* (like smooth muscles). Thus, cardiac muscles share some characteristics with skeletal muscles and some with smooth muscles.
- The cardiac muscle fibres are *ribbon-like* rather than cylindrical. These are *branched* and interdigitate freely with each other, but each fibre is a complete separate unit. The branches from the neighbouring fibres join together. At the point of contact of two muscle fibres, the membranes of both muscle fibres are fused together and thrown into extensive infolding forming the so-called *intercalated disc* (Fig. 4.1.8). These discs form tight junctions between the muscle fibres and do not allow the ions to pass through. However, the intercalated discs provide a strong union between fibres and thus play an important role during contraction of muscle fibres by transmitting the pull of one contractile unit along its axis to the next, thereby increasing the force of contraction.
- Along the sides near the outer border of intercalated disc, the two adjacent muscle fibres are connected with each other through the *gap junctions*. Although there is no anatomical connection between different cardiac muscle fibres, from functional point of view, the action potential passes from one cardiac muscle cell to the other through gap junctions which provide *low-resistance bridges* and thus the cardiac muscle acts as a *functional syncytium* of many cardiac cells. In this way, the cardiac impulse spreads throughout the muscle mass quickly resulting in a coordinated contraction of the whole tissue. In the heart, the cardiac muscle forms two separate syncytia - the *atrial syncytium* (walls of the two atria) and the *ventricular syncytium* (walls of the two ventricles). Action potential is conducted from the atrial syncytium to the ventricular syncytium by way of specialized conducting system. Each syncytium obeys all-or-none law. Because atrial and ventricular syncytia are two separate syncytia, therefore, atria contract a short time ahead of ventricular contraction.
- The cardiac muscle fibres are supplied richly by the capillaries (one capillary/fibre).

Structure of a Cardiac Muscle Fibre

Each muscle fibre is about 80 μm long and about 15 μm broad. Its cell membrane is called *sarcolemma* and the cytoplasm is called *sarcoplasm*. The sarcoplasm is in abundance and contains all the cell organelles, a well-developed sarcoplasmic reticulum and a centrally placed nucleus. Each muscle fibre is made up of a number of *myofibrils* which lie parallel to each other. Each myofibril is 2 μm in diameter.

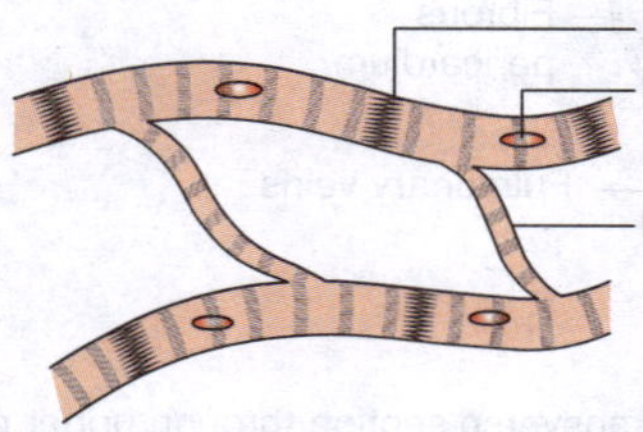

Fig. 4.1.8 Structure of cardiac muscle.

Myofibril Each myofibril consists of thick and thin filaments. The structure and striations seen under a light microscope and an electron microscope are similar to those of a skeletal muscle (see page 82).

Sarcotubular System

The sarcotubular system in cardiac muscles is well developed like that in skeletal muscles (page 84). However, the tubules of the T-system penetrate the sarcomere at Z-line (Fig. 4.1.9) and not at the junction of A and I bands (as in skeletal muscles). Therefore, in cardiac muscles, there is only one triad per sarcomere as compared with two in skeletal muscles (page 84). Furthermore, the tubules are much wider than in skeletal muscles and typical triads are not always present. They are often replaced by dyads having one T-tubule and one cistern of the sarcoplasmic reticulum (L-tubule).

PROCESS OF EXCITABILITY AND CONTRACTILITY

The cardiac muscle being an excitable tissue produces an action potential (*electrical phenomenon*) when stimulated and responds by contracting (*mechanical phenomenon*). The events which link the electrical phenomenon with mechanical phenomenon constitute the *excitation–contraction coupling phenomenon*. These three phenomena are discussed separately. As discussed earlier, the cardiac muscles comprise working myocardial cells or the contractile myocardial cells (CMC), pacemaker and conducting tissue. The present discussion is limited to activities in the CMC.

Electrical Potentials in Cardiac Muscle

Resting Membrane Potential

The resting membrane potential (RMP) of a normal cardiac muscle fibre is −85 to −95 mV (negative interior with reference to exterior).

Action Potential

When stimulated, each cardiac muscle fibre shows an electrical activity known as propagated action potential. It is different from the electrocardiogram, which refers to extracellular recording of the summed electrical events of all the cardiac muscle fibres generated with each heartbeat (see page 247).

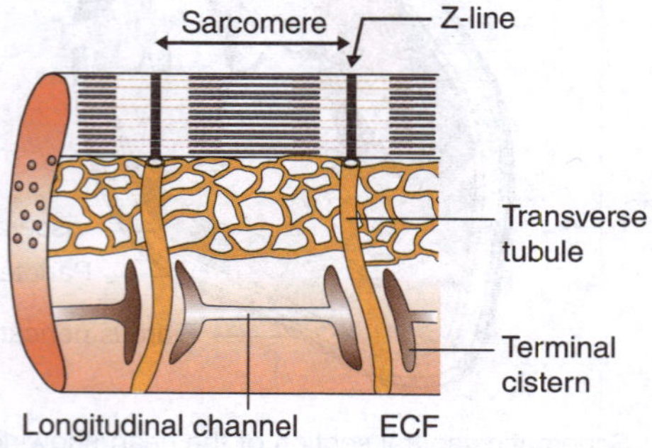

Fig. 4.1.9 Sarcotubular system in the cardiac muscle.

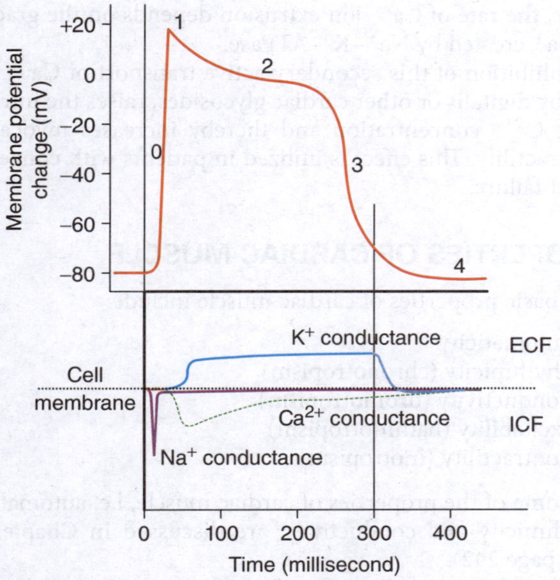

Fig. 4.1.10 Various phases of action potential and ion conductance: phase 0, depolarization; phase 1, rapid repolarization; phase 2, plateau phase; phase 3, late rapid repolarization; and phase 4, resting potential.

Phases of cardiac action potential are: The action potential recorded from a single cardiac muscle fibre is unusually long and can be divided into five distinct phases (Fig. 4.1.10) as given next.

Phase 0: Rapid depolarization The phase 0 (upstroke) is characterized by the depolarization which proceeds rapidly; an overshoot is present, as in skeletal muscle and nerve. In the mammalian heart, depolarization lasts about 2 milliseconds. In this phase, amplitude of potential reaches up to +20 to +30 mV (positive interior with reference to exterior).

Ionic basis: The initial rapid depolarization and the overshoot are due to the rapid opening of voltage-gated Na^+ channels and rapid influx of Na^+ ions similar to that occurring in nerve and skeletal muscle.

At −30 to −40 mV membrane potential, the calcium channels also open up and influx of Ca^{2+} ions also contributes in this phase. ***Note:*** Tetrodotoxin (TT_X) is a specific blocker of sodium channels, and acts as a very potent poison, because it blocks the influx of sodium ions; hence, there is no excitation of cardiac muscle fibres and, therefore, no contraction.

Phase 1: Initial rapid repolarization Rapid depolarization is followed by a very short-lived slight rapid repolarization. The membrane potential reaches from +30 to −10 mV during this phase.

Ionic basis: The initial rapid repolarization is due to closure of Na^+ channels and opening of K^+ channels resulting in transient outward current.

Phase 2: Plateau During plateau phase, the cardiac muscle fibre remains in the depolarized state. The membrane potential falls very slowly only to 240 mV during this phase. The plateau lasts for about 100–200 milliseconds. This plateau in action potential explains the 5–15 times longer contraction time of the cardiac muscle as compared with that of the skeletal muscle.

Ionic basis: Very slow repolarization during the plateau phase is due to:

- Slow influx of Ca^{2+} ions resulting from opening of sarcolemmal *L-type* Ca^{2+} channels
- Closure of a distinct set of K^+ channels called the inward-rectifying K^+ channels

Phase 3: Repolarization During this phase, complete repolarization occurs and the membrane potential falls to the approximate resting value of −80 mV. This phase lasts for about 50 milliseconds.

Ionic basis: The slow repolarization results from closing of Ca^{2+} channels and opening of the following two types of K^+ channels:

- *Delayed outward rectifying* K^+ *channels*, which are voltage-gated and are activated slowly
- Ca^{2+}*-activated* channels which are activated by the elevated sarcoplasmic Ca^{2+} levels

Phase 4: Resting potential In this phase of RMP (also called polarized state), the potential is maintained at −90 mV.

Ionic basis: The RMP is maintained by a resting K^+ current, the largest contributor to which is the inward rectifying K^+ current.

And ultimately membrane potential is restored by Na^+–K^+-ATPase.

Duration of Action Potential The duration of action potential (primarily repolarization) is about 250 milliseconds at a heart rate of 75 beats/min. It decreases with increased heart rate (150 milliseconds at a heart rate of 200 beats/min). It is shorter in the atrial muscle. This type of action potential found in CMCs of the ventricles is referred to as *fast response*.

Spread of Action Potential Through Cardiac Muscles As discussed in the section 'Functional Anatomy of Heart', the cardiac muscle acts as a physiological syncytium due to the presence of gap junctions among the cardiac muscle fibres. Because of this, the action potential spreads through the cardiac muscles very rapidly. Furthermore, as there are two syncytia (the atrial and the ventricular) in the heart, the action potential is transmitted from atria to ventricles only through the fibres of specialized conductive system.

Excitation–Contraction Coupling Phenomenon in Cardiac Muscles

Excitation–contraction coupling refers to the sequence of events by which an excited plasma membrane of a muscle fibre leads to cross-bridge activity by increasing sarcoplasmic calcium concentration.

The sequence of events during excitation–contraction coupling in the cardiac muscles is similar to that observed in a skeletal muscle (see page 85), with the following exception: In cardiac muscles (as against that in skeletal muscles), extra calcium ions diffuse into the sarcoplasm from T-tubules without which the contraction strength would be considerably reduced. The T-tubules of cardiac muscle contain mucopolysaccharides which are negatively charged and bind an abundant store of calcium ions. The T-tubules open directly to the exterior and, therefore, Ca^{2+} ions in them directly come from extracellular fluid. These Ca^{2+} ions diffuse into the sarcoplasm when action potential propagates along the T-tubules (Fig. 4.1.11A and B). Because of this, strength of cardiac muscle contraction depends to a great extent on Ca^{2+} concentration in ECF, whereas skeletal muscle contraction is hardly affected by the calcium concentration in ECF.

Process of Cardiac Muscle Contraction

The molecular mechanism of cardiac muscle contraction by cross-bridge cycling and sliding of filaments is primarily similar to that of skeletal muscle contraction (page 86) and smooth muscle contraction (page 111). However, its regulation shows features of both the skeletal and smooth muscles.

- Troponin–tropomyosin complex controls the onset and offset of cross-bridge cycling, similar to that in the skeletal muscles.
- Like smooth muscles, the contractility of cardiac muscle is sensitive to *phosphorylation*.

Relaxation of Cardiac Muscle

Relaxation of cardiac muscle (diastole) occurs when levels of Ca^{2+} ions fall in the cardiac muscle fibres. During diastole, the Ca^{2+} ions are extruded out of the cardiac muscle fibre by a carrier system operating at the sarcolemma in which two Na^+ ions are exchanged for each Ca^{2+} ion extruded (Fig. 4.1.11C).

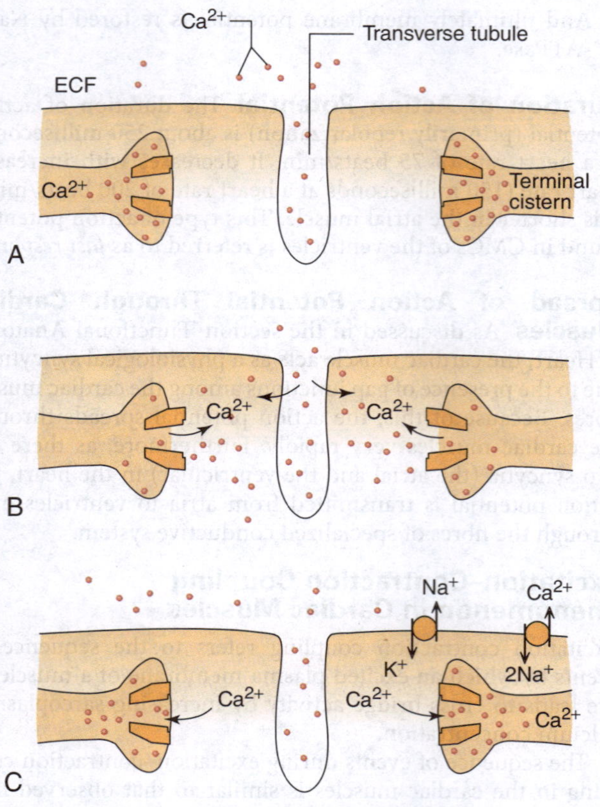

Fig. 4.1.11 Dynamics of Ca^{2+} during excitation–contraction coupling phenomenon and relaxation in cardiac muscle: **A**, in resting state; **B**, calcium-induced calcium release during excitation and contraction state; and **C**, during relaxation state.

Thus, the rate of Ca^{2+} ion extrusion depends on the gradient of Na^+ created by Na^+–K^+-ATPase.

Inhibition of this secondary active transport of Ca^{2+} ions, e.g. by digitalis or other cardiac glycosides, raises the intracellular Ca^{2+} concentration and thereby increases myocardial contractility. This effect is utilized in patients with congestive heart failure.

PROPERTIES OF CARDIAC MUSCLE

The basic properties of cardiac muscle include:

- Automaticity
- Rhythmicity (chronotropism)
- Conductivity (dromotropism)
- Excitability (bathmotropism)
- Contractility (inotropism)

Some of the properties of cardiac muscle, i.e. automaticity, rhythmicity and conductivity, are discussed in Chapter 4.2 (see page 242).

The characteristics of excitability and contractility are described here.

Excitability

Excitability (bathmotropism) is the property by which tissues respond to stimuli. The cardiac muscle responds by depolarization (development of action potential). The essential features of the RMP and action potential of cardiac muscle are discussed on page 244.

One of the characteristics of cardiac muscle excitability which needs a special emphasis is its refractory period.

Refractory Period

Refractory period refers to the period following action potential during which the cardiac muscle does not respond to a stimulus. Cardiac muscle has a long refractory period (250–300 milliseconds in ventricles and about 150 milliseconds in atria). It is of two types.

Absolute and relative refractory periods

1. Absolute refractory period (ARP) During this period, the cardiac muscle does not show any response at all. It extends from phase 0 to half of phase 3 of action potential, the second stimulus even when the intensity of stimulus is much higher than that of the first one, i.e. until the membrane potential reaches approximately −50 mV during repolarization (Fig. 4.1.12). Normal duration of ARP in ventricles is about 180–200 milliseconds.

2. Relative refractory period (RRP) During this period, the muscle shows response if the strength of stimulus is increased to maximum. It extends from second half of phase 3 to phase 4 of the action potential. Normal duration of RRP in ventricles is about 50 milliseconds.

Significance of long refractory period in cardiac muscle. As shown in Fig. 4.1.12, the cardiac muscle is refractory to any stimulus during the contraction phase (systole); therefore, the complete summation of contractions and thus tetanus cannot be produced in the cardiac muscle. This property is very useful. Since the heart has to function as a pump, it must relax, get filled up with blood and then contract to pump out the blood. A tetanized heart would be useless as a pump.

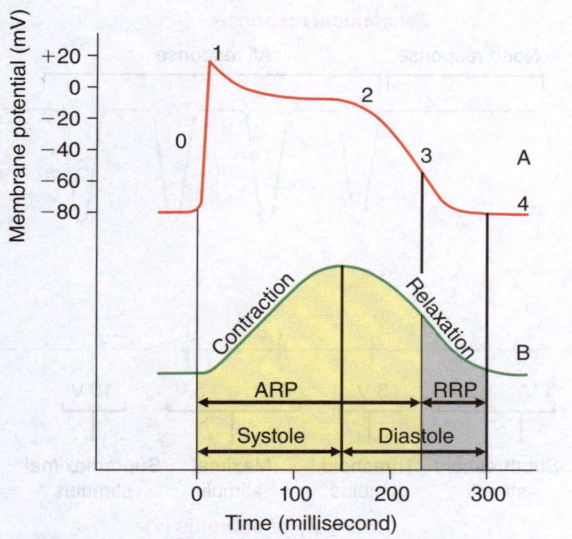

Fig. 4.1.12 Record of action potential **A**, and mechanical response **B**, from the cardiac muscle fibre shown on same time scale depicting the significance of long refractory period. ARP, absolute refractory period; RRP, relative refractory period.

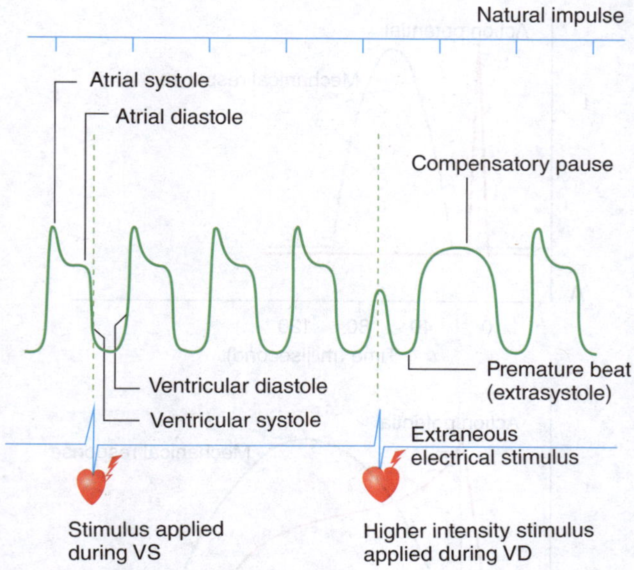

Fig. 4.1.13 Demonstration of refractory period in beating heart of a frog. VD, ventricular diastole; VS, ventricular systole.

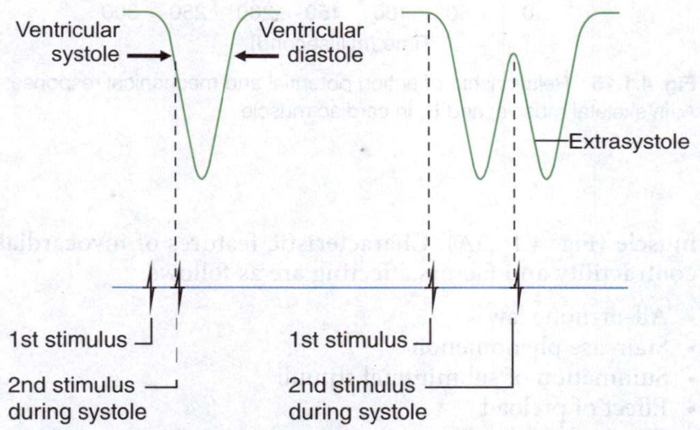

Fig. 4.1.14 Refractory period in quiescent heart of a frog.

Experimental Demonstration of Refractory Period in Heart

Experimental demonstration of refractory period in the heart can be done both in a beating heart and in a quiescent heart.

Refractory period in a beating heart

The refractory period in a beating heart of a pithed frog can be demonstrated during recording of a cardiogram as shown in Fig. 4.1.13.

When the electrical stimulus is applied to the base of ventricle during systole, no response is seen, depicting thereby that the heart is in ARP during systole.

When the stimulus is applied during diastole, the heart responds by premature contraction producing *extrasystole* followed by a *compensatory pause*. The total duration of the extrasystole and the compensatory pause is equivalent to the duration of two cardiac cycles. These events can be explained as:

- When the stimulus is applied during diastole, the premature contraction occurs since the heart is in the phase of *RRP*.
- The natural impulse from the sinus venosus arrives at the time of premature contraction (ARP) and cannot produce contraction and thus the heart has to wait for the arrival of the next natural impulse. The heart stops during this period in relaxation, producing the so-called *compensatory pause*.

Refractory period in a quiescent heart

The refractory period in a quiescent heart can be demonstrated as:

- The heart is made quiescent by applying the first *Stannius ligature* between the sinus venosus and the right auricle.
- An electrical stimulus is applied at the base of the ventricle to stimulate the heart which starts contracting. When another stimulus is applied immediately after the first (i.e. during systole phase), the heart does not show any response, indicating that during contraction (systole), the heart is in ARP (Fig. 4.1.14).
- When the second stimulus is applied during diastole, the heart responds producing extrasystole and the compensatory pause (Fig. 4.1.14), indicating that the heart is in the state of *RRP* during diastole.

Contractility

Contractility is the ability of the cardiac muscle to actively generate force to shorten and thicken to do work when sufficient stimulus is applied. Process of myocardial contractility is discussed on page 236.

Mechanical response in cardiac muscle fibre begins just after the start of depolarization and lasts about 1.5 times as long as the action potential (Fig. 4.1.15B). Thus, the mechanical response (300 milliseconds) overlaps the electrical response (200 milliseconds) for the whole period. This is in contrast to skeletal muscle, where the mechanical response begins a few milliseconds after the end of repolarization and lasts for 30–50 milliseconds in mammalian skeletal muscle and 100 milliseconds in amphibian skeletal

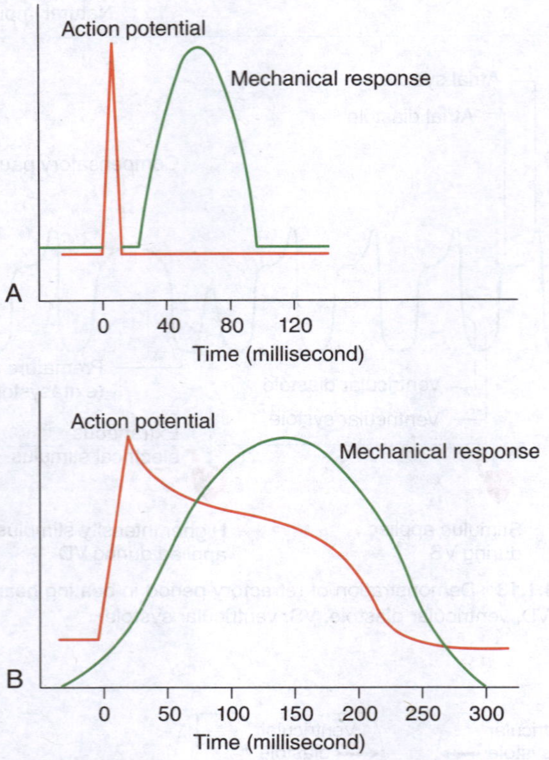

Fig. 4.1.15 Relationship of action potential and mechanical response: **A**, in skeletal muscle; and **B**, in cardiac muscle.

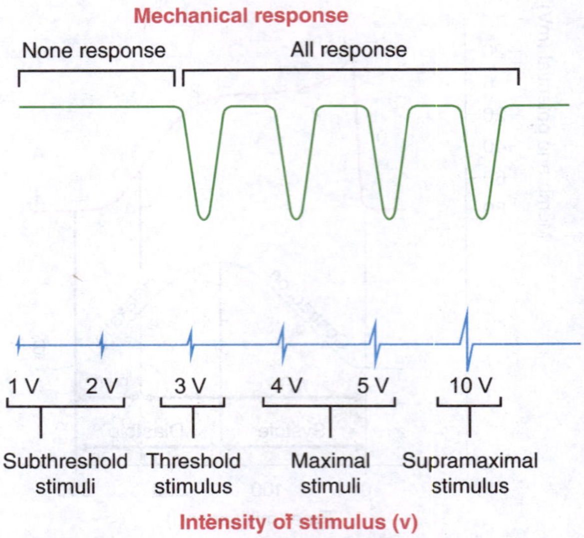

Fig. 4.1.16 Demonstration of all-or-none law in quiescent heart of a frog.

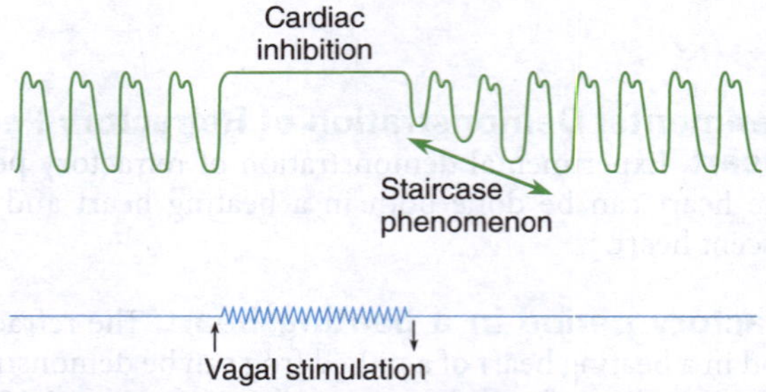

Fig. 4.1.17 Staircase phenomenon (treppe) in cardiac muscle after vagal stimulation in frog.

muscle (Fig. 4.1.15A). Characteristic features of myocardial contractility and factors affecting are as follows:

- All-or-none law
- Staircase phenomenon
- Summation of subminimal stimuli
- Effect of preload
- Effect of afterload
- Effect of ions (see page 265)

1. All-or-none Law The response of the cardiac muscle to a stimulus is all or none in character, i.e. when a stimulus is applied, the heart either does not contract at all (none response) or contracts to its maximum ability (all response). This is because of the syncytial arrangement of the cardiac muscle fibres. Therefore, the 'all-or-none' law in the heart is applicable to the whole functional syncytial unit, i.e. the entire atria or entire ventricle. In contrast, in skeletal muscles, it is applicable only to a single muscle fibre.

Demonstration of 'all-or-none' law It can be done in the quiescent heart of frog as:

- *Quiescent heart* is made by applying the first Stannius ligature between sinus venosus and atrium.
- When *subthreshold stimulus* is applied to the ventricle, no response is obtained.
- When *threshold stimulus* is applied to the ventricle, a contraction is recorded.
- *Maximal and supramaximal* strength of stimuli produce contractions of amplitude similar to those produced by the threshold stimulus (Fig. 4.1.16), proving 'all-or-none law' property of the cardiac muscle.

2. Staircase Phenomenon (Treppe) Staircase phenomenon or effect refers to the successive increase in the force of cardiac contractions in the first few (four to five) contractions after the quiescent heart starts beating, e.g. as seen after vagal stimulation (Fig. 4.1.17). This is because of the beneficial effect.

Cause of beneficial effect When the heart stops, there occurs an increase in Na^+ and a decrease in K^+ concentration inside the cell, which increases Ca^{2+} influx. Thus, there occurs a progressive increase in the Ca^{2+} concentration in sarcoplasm due to the increase in Ca^{2+} influx with each action potential. This produces a progressive increase in the strength of the few (four to five) cardiac muscle contractions.

Demonstration of staircase phenomenon The demonstration of staircase phenomenon can be done in the quiescent heart of frog as:

- *Quiescent heart* is made by applying the first Stannius ligature between sinus venosus and atria.
- *Ventricle is stimulated* repeatedly at intervals of 2 seconds without changing the strength of the stimulus.
- *Graph obtained* (Fig. 4.1.18) will show that in the first few contractions, the force of contraction is increased and then

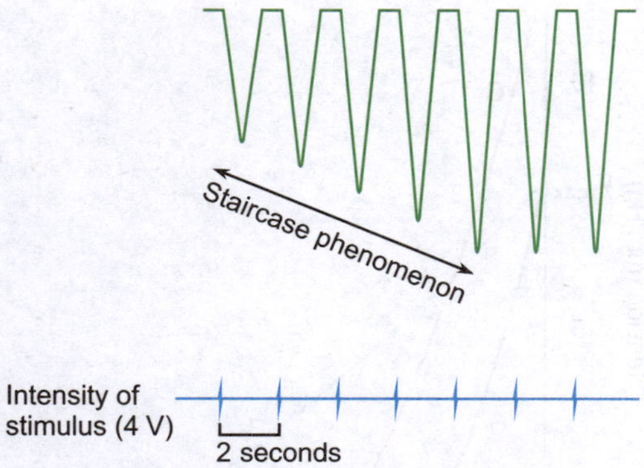

Fig. 4.1.18 Demonstration of staircase phenomenon in quiescent heart of a frog.

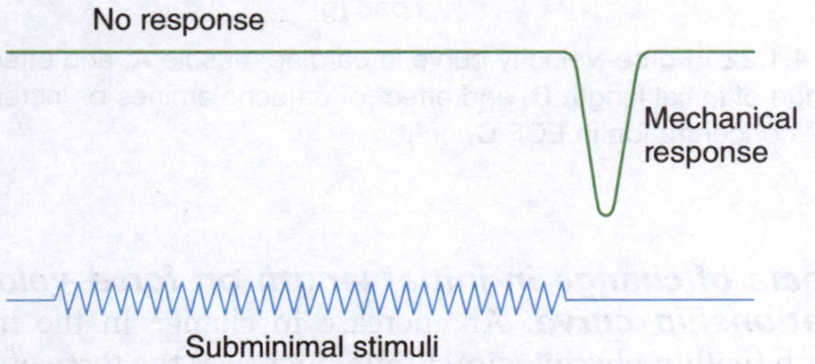

Fig. 4.1.19 Temporal summation of subminimal stimuli in quiescent heart of a frog.

it remains constant. This is called staircase phenomenon or treppe (German word for staircase).

3. Summation of Subminimal Stimuli When a subthreshold stimulus is applied to the quiescent heart, there occurs no response. However, when subthreshold stimuli are applied repeatedly at an interval of 0.5–1 second, there occurs a contraction of the heart after about 10–20 stimuli. This phenomenon is called *temporal summation* of subminimal stimuli (Fig. 4.1.19).

4. Effect of Preload A load which starts acting on a muscle before it starts to contract is called *preload*. The preload increases the initial length of the muscle. According to Starling law, the force of contraction is the function of the initial length of the muscle fibres, and up to physiological limits, the greater the initial length, the greater is the force of contraction. In the case of heart muscles, the end-diastolic volume forms the preload. The effect of changing end-diastolic volume on force of cardiac contraction has been studied by Frank and Starling in 1910. *The Frank–Starling law of the heart* states that within physiological limits, the force of cardiac contraction is proportional to its end-diastolic volume.

Length–tension relationship Length–tension relationship, i.e. the relation between initial fibre length and total tension in cardiac muscle, is basically similar to that in skeletal muscle (see page 96). In cardiac muscles, the length–tension relationship graph is plotted with the end-diastolic volume in millilitre (representing initial length) along the horizontal axis and the pressure developed in the ventricle in millimetre of mercury (representing tension) along the vertical axis

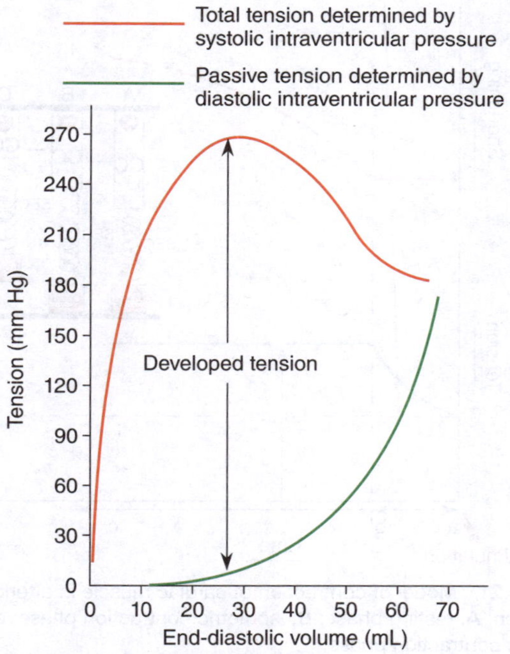

Fig. 4.1.20 Length–tension relationship in cardiac muscle.

(Fig. 4.1.20). The following inferences can be drawn from this graph (Starling curve):

Diastolic intraventricular pressure represents the passive tension and it increases with the increase in end-diastolic volume (i.e. with the passively increased muscle length). It is important to note that the pressure–volume curve for ventricles in diastole is initially quite flat, indicating that large increase in volume can be accommodated with only small increase in pressure.

Systolic ventricular pressure represents the active tension developed (isometric tension) which is proportionate to the degree of diastolic filling of the heart (initial length of muscle fibres). The graph (Fig. 4.1.20) shows that the developed tension increases as the diastolic volume increases until it reaches a maximum (ascending limb of Starling curve), and then tends to decrease (descending limb of Starling curve). However, unlike skeletal muscle, the decrease in developed tension at high degrees of stretch is not due to decreased number of cross-bridges between actin and myosin, because even severely dilated hearts are not stretched to this degree. The descending limb is instead due to beginning of disruption of the myocardial fibres.

Clinical significance of Frank–Starling law of heart

The clinical significance of Frank–Starling law of the heart and its role in control of cardiac output are discussed in Chapter 4.3 (see page 283).

5. Effect of Afterload Afterload refers to the load which acts on the muscle after the beginning of muscular contraction. The afterload affecting the force of contraction of the cardiac muscle is represented by the resistance against which the ventricles pump the blood. The afterload (resistance) for right ventricle is low in pulmonary artery due to its intrathoracic location. The afterload (resistance) for left ventricle is high in the aorta due to the resistance to blood flow through

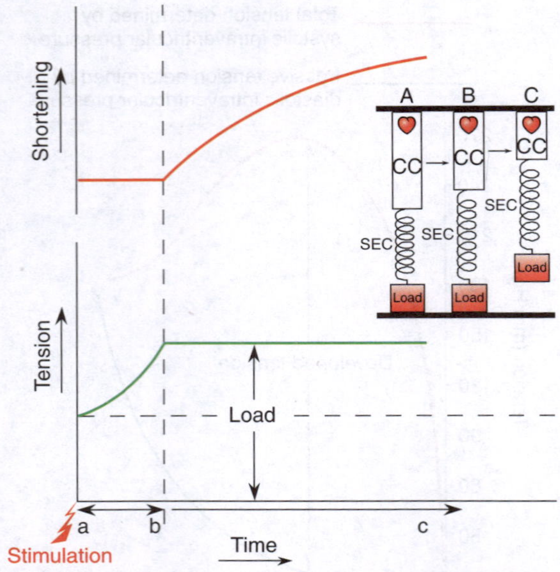

Fig. 4.1.21 Model of contraction of cardiac muscle in afterloaded condition: **A**, resting phase; **B**, isometric contraction phase; and **C**, isotonic contraction phase.

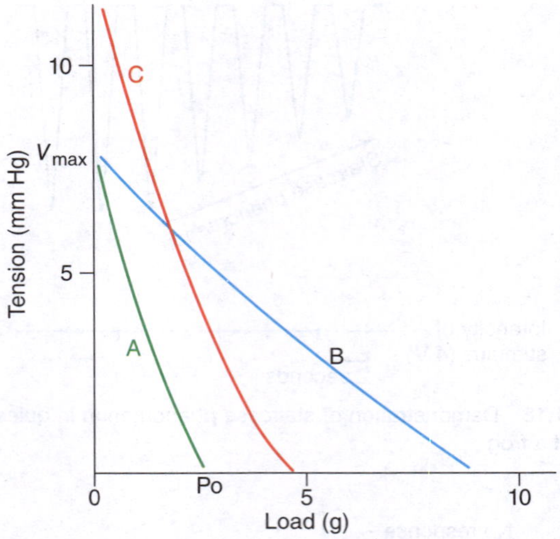

Fig. 4.1.22 Force–velocity curve in cardiac muscle **A**, and effect of change of initial length **B**, and effect of catecholamines or increased Ca^{2+} concentration in ECF **C**, on it.

the aortic valves and systemic blood vessels, called *peripheral resistance*.

Cardiac muscle contraction with afterload The model for contraction with afterload in cardiac muscle is shown in Fig. 4.1.21. It shows two phases given as follows:

Isometric contraction phase: In this phase, the muscle contracts but there occurs no shortening of the muscle. The contraction of contractile component (CC) of the muscle stretches the series elastic component (SEC) and there occurs a rise in tension (Fig. 4.1.21B). The rise in tension continues till it equals the load. This is the end point of isometric contraction.

Isotonic contraction phase: It starts when the muscle tension exceeds and the load starts moving. There occurs shortening of the muscle without further stretching of SEC (Fig. 4.1.21C). The performance of CC is given by the force–velocity relationship.

Force–velocity relationship The force–velocity curve is plotted by noting the velocity of muscle contraction with progressively increasing the load on the muscle. In the heart, the load is represented by the resistance against which the ventricles pump the blood and velocity of muscle contraction is represented by the stroke output. The following inferences can be drawn from the force–velocity curve (Fig. 4.1.22A):

- When the load is zero, the muscle contracts rapidly and the velocity of muscle shortening is maximum (V_{max}).
- As the load increases progressively, the velocity of shortening decreases till it reaches zero. At this point, the force developed is called maximum isometric force and is represented by Po. Therefore, during muscle contraction, the velocity of shortening and force developed are inversely related. The force–velocity relationship curve is influenced by change in initial length of the muscle and the effect of catecholamines.

Effects of change in initial length on force–velocity relationship curve. An increase in change in the initial length (within physiological limits) increases the force of contraction (Po) without changing the velocity (V_{max}), i.e. the relationship shifts to the right (Fig. 4.1.22B).

Effect of catecholamines or increased calcium concentration in ECF. The catecholamines or increased Ca^{2+} concentration in ECF causes an increase in both Po and V_{max} (Fig. 4.1.22C).

Clinical implication of force–velocity relationship The cardiac muscle can alter its work and power (rate of working) at any given load and muscle length by nature of its changing force–velocity relationship in different chemical environment as:

- When the pressure against which the heart is pumping the blood is raised, the heart strokes out less blood than it receives for several beats. Consequently, blood accumulates in the ventricle increasing the end-diastolic volume which increases the initial length of muscle fibres (i.e. size of the heart). The distended heart beats more forcefully and output returns to its previous level, i.e. by an increase in the initial length of cardiac muscle, the Po is increased and the V_{max} is achieved.
- Conversely, when the pressure against which the heart is pumping the blood is reduced, the stroke output rises transiently but the size of the heart decreases and the stroke output falls to the previous constant level.

Self-Assessment

1. Discuss the significance of the following properties of cardiac muscle in the intact body:
   - Refractory period
   - All-or-none law
   - Length–tension relationship
   - Velocity–tension relationship
2. Discuss the Starling law of the heart and its clinical significance.

Clinical Cases

Case 1

A 70-year-old woman presented with fatigue and shortness of breath. The doctor examined the patient and administered dopamine. Immediately, the condition of the patient improved due to inotropic effect.

Q1. What is the mechanism of action of drug on the heart?

Case 2

While preparing for physical examination to get entry into the army services, a young boy who was undergoing exercise developed tachycardia and hypertension, which normalized sometime after the stoppage of exercise.

Q1. What is the cause for tachycardia and hypertension?

Q2. What is the mechanism of action?

4.2 Origin and Spread of Cardiac Impulse and Electrocardiography

CHAPTER OUTLINE

ORIGIN AND SPREAD OF CARDIAC IMPULSE

INTRODUCTION

The cardiac muscle possesses special properties which include autorhythmicity, conductivity, excitability and contractility. The heart is able to perform its action as a unique pump because of these properties interacting in the same sequence as enumerated above.

Autorhythmicity refers to the property of cardiac muscle which enables the heart to initiate its own impulse at constant rhythmical intervals. Because of this property, the heart continues to beat even after all nerves to it are sectioned or even if the heart is cut into pieces, the pieces continue to beat. This is one of the earliest properties manifested during development even before the muscle fibres acquire the typical histological features. This is because of the presence of the specialized *pacemaker tissue* in the heart that can initiate repetitive action potentials. The pacemaker tissue makes a *conduction system* that normally spreads impulses through the heart.

ANATOMIC CONSIDERATION

Conducting System of the Heart

The conducting system of the heart consists of specialized fibres of the heart muscle present as the sinoatrial (SA) node, the interatrial tract, internodal tracts, the atrioventricular (AV) node, the AV bundle of His and its right and left terminal branches, and the subendocardial plexuses of Purkinje fibres (Fig. 4.2.1).

1. Sinoatrial Node

SA node is an oval-shaped structure about 10–30 mm long, 5–7 mm wide and 1–2 mm thick.

SA node is located in the wall of right atrium, just to the right of the opening of superior vena cava. Spontaneous rhythmical electrical impulses arise from the SA node and spread in all directions to:

- Cardiac muscles of atria
- Interatrial tract to left atrium
- Internodal tracts to AV node

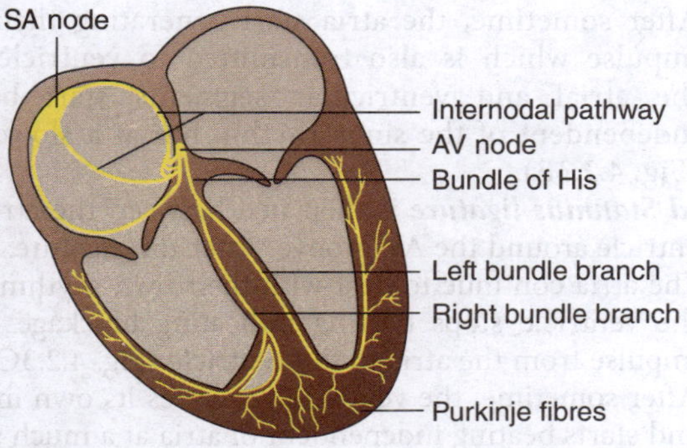

Fig. 4.2.1 Specialized conducting tissues of the heart.

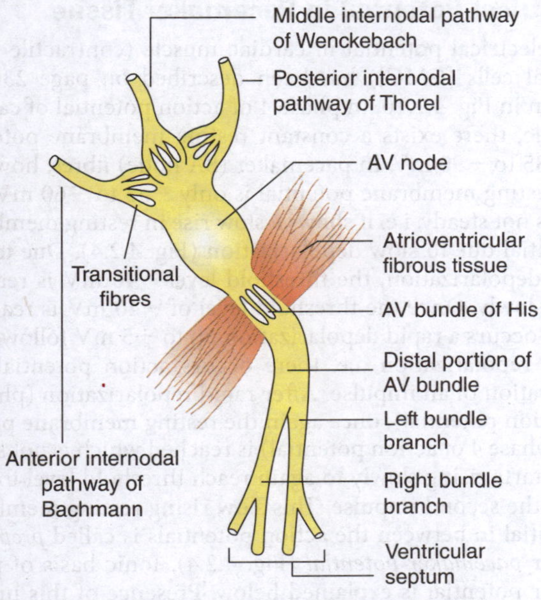

Fig. 4.2.2 Internodal conduction pathways.

2. Interatrial Tract (Bachmann Bundle)

It is a band of specialized muscle fibres that run from SA node to left atrium. It causes simultaneous depolarization of the atria, since the velocity of conduction of impulse in this tract is faster than in the rest of the atrial muscles.

3. Internodal Conduction Pathway

Impulses from the SA node have been shown to travel to the AV node more rapidly than they can travel by passing along the ordinary myocardium. This phenomenon has been explained by the description of special pathways in the atrial wall (Fig. 4.2.2), having a structure consisting of a mixture of Purkinje fibres and ordinary cardiac muscle cells. Three internodal conduction paths have been described:

Anterior internodal pathway of Bachmann leaves the anterior end of SA node and passes anterior to the superior vena cava opening. It then descends on the atrial septum and ends in the AV node.

Middle internodal pathway of Wenckebach leaves the posterior end of SA node and passes posterior to superior vena cava opening. It then descends on the atrial septum to end in the AV node.

Posterior internodal pathway of Thorel leaves the posterior part of the SA node and descends through the crista terminalis and the valve of inferior vena cava to the AV node.

4. AV Node

The AV node is strategically located just beneath the endocardium on the right side of lower part of atrial septum, near the tricuspid valve. It is stimulated by the excitation wave that travels through internodal tracts and atrial myocardium. From it, the cardiac impulse is conducted to ventricles by the AV bundle.

5. AV Bundle of His

The AV bundle of His is an elongated segment. It arises from the AV node, descends through the fibrous skeleton of the heart and divides into right bundle branch (RBB) for the right ventricle and left bundle branch (LBB) for the left ventricle. It is approximately 1.8 cm long in an adult heart and primarily located within deep connective tissue.

Note: Bundle of His is named after the Swiss cardiologist *Wilhelm His*, who discovered the specialized muscle fibres in the heart in 1893.

The branches break up and become continuous with the plexus of Purkinje fibres.

6. Purkinje Fibres

These are spread out deep to the endocardium and reach all parts of the ventricles, including the bases of papillary muscles.

Characteristic Histological Features of Conducting System

- The conduction system of the heart is composed of modified cardiac muscle that has *fewer striations* and *indistinct boundaries*.
- The SA node, and to a lesser extent the AV node, also contains *small round cells* with few organelles, which are connected by *gap junctions*. These are probably the actual pacemaker cells, and therefore they are called *P cells*.
- The atrial muscle fibres are separated from those of the ventricles by a fibrous ring. Normally, the AV bundle is the only pathway of cardiac muscle that connects the myocardium of the atria and myocardium of ventricles and is thus the only route along which the cardiac impulse can travel from the atria to the ventricles.

Innervational Characteristics of Heart

- Both SA node and AV node are richly supplied by the sympathetic as well as parasympathetic nerves. Parasympathetic fibres come from the vagus nerve and most sympathetic fibres come from the stellate ganglion.
- SA node develops from the structures on the right side of the embryo and that is why it is supplied by right vagus and right-sided sympathetic nerves.
- AV node develops from the structures on the left side of the embryo and that is why it is supplied by left vagus and left-sided sympathetic nerves.
- Noradrenergic fibres are epicardial, whereas the vagal fibres are endocardial.
- Connections exist for reciprocal inhibitory effects of sympathetic and parasympathetic innervation of the heart on each. Thus, acetylcholine acts presynaptically to reduce norepinephrine release from the sympathetic nerves, and conversely, neuropeptide Y released from the noradrenergic endings may inhibit the release of acetylcholine.

MECHANISM OF ORIGIN OF RHYTHMIC CARDIAC IMPULSE

Pacemaker

The part of the heart from which rhythmic impulses for heartbeat are produced is called *pacemaker*. In a mammalian heart, although the other parts of the heart like AV node, atria and ventricle can also produce the impulse, *SA node acts as a pacemaker* because the rate of impulse generation by SA node is the highest. However, when there occurs blockage of transmission of impulse from SA node to AV node, the pacemaker activity may shift from SA node to other sites, e.g. AV node. When pacemaker is other than SA node, it is called *ectopic pacemaker*. Ectopic pacemaker causes abnormal sequence of contraction of different parts of the heart.

Rate of production of rhythmic impulses by different parts of the heart is as follows:

- SA node: 70–80/min
- AV node: 40–60/min
- Atrial muscle: 40–60/min
- Ventricular muscles: 20–40/min

Experimental evidence to prove that SA node acts as a pacemaker in mammalian heart is as follows:

- SA node becomes electrically negative before any other part of the atria, thereby indicating that it is the first region to become active.
- Stimulation of SA node accelerates the heart rate.
- Local cooling of SA node reduces the heart rate and warming increases the heart rate.
- When SA node is destroyed artificially, there occurs immediate stoppage of the heart followed by an altered rhythm of heartbeats (due to ectopic pacemaker taking over the function).

Pacemaker in Amphibian Heart

In an amphibian heart, *sinus venosus* acts as pacemaker; however, other parts of the heart can also produce rhythmic impulses. These facts can be proved by blocking the conduction mechanically by applying *Stannius ligatures*.

First Stannius ligature when tied between the *sinus venosus and atria*:

- The heart stops beating while the sinus continues to beat, indicating blockage of impulse from sinus to atria (Fig. 4.2.3A).
- After sometime, the atria start generating their own impulse which is also transmitted to ventricles and the atrial and ventricular segments start beating independent of the sinus rhythm but at a slower rate (Fig. 4.2.3B).

Second Stannius ligature is then tied between the atria and the ventricle around the AV groove. After this ligature:

- The atria continue to beat with their own rhythm while the ventricle stops beating indicating blockage of the impulse from the atria to the ventricle (Fig. 4.2.3C).
- After sometime, the ventricle generates its own impulse and starts beating independent of atria at a much slower rate than the atrial rate. This is referred to as idioventricular rhythm (Fig. 4.2.3D).

Electrical Potential in Pacemaker Tissue

The electrical potential in cardiac muscle (contractile myocardial cells [CMC]) has been described on page 234. As shown in Fig. 4.1.10, in phase 4 of action potential of cardiac muscle, there exists a constant resting membrane potential of −85 to −90 mV. In pacemaker (SA node) fibres, however, the resting membrane potential is only −55 to −60 mV, and this is not steady, i.e. it shows a slow rise in resting membrane potential due to slow depolarization (Fig. 4.2.4). Due to this slow depolarization, the threshold level −40 mV is reached very slowly. Once the threshold level of −40 mV is reached, there occurs a rapid depolarization up to +5 mV followed by rapid repolarization, i.e. there occurs action potential and generation of an impulse. After rapid repolarization (phase 3 of action potential), once again the resting membrane potential (phase 4 of action potential) is reached which is not stable and starts rising slowly to again reach threshold level to produce the second impulse. This slow rising resting membrane potential in between the action potentials is called *prepotential* or *pacemaker potential* (Fig. 4.2.4). Ionic basis of pacemaker potential is explained below. Presence of this unique feature in the cells of pacemaker tissue is the underlying mechanism responsible for self-generation of rhythmic impulses (autorhythmicity).

Ionic Basis of Pacemaker Potential and Action Potential in SA Node

The myocardial cells present in the SA node and AV node are called *slow fibres* and the other myocardial cells are called *fast fibres* depending on the membrane potential and the shape and conduction velocity of the action potential (Fig. 4.2.5).

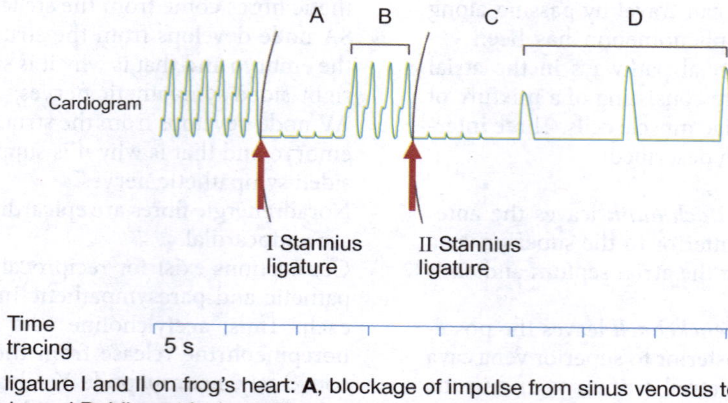

Fig. 4.2.3 Effect of Stannius ligature I and II on frog's heart: **A**, blockage of impulse from sinus venosus to atria; **B**, atrial rhythm; **C**, blockage of impulse from atria to ventricle; and **D**, idioventricular rhythm.

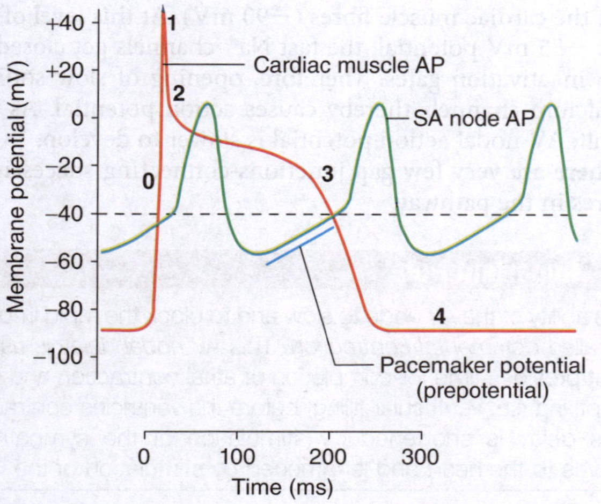

Fig. 4.2.4 Phases of action potential in cardiac muscle fibre (0, 1, 2, 3, 4) and SA node showing pacemaker potential. AP, action potential; SA, sinoatrial.

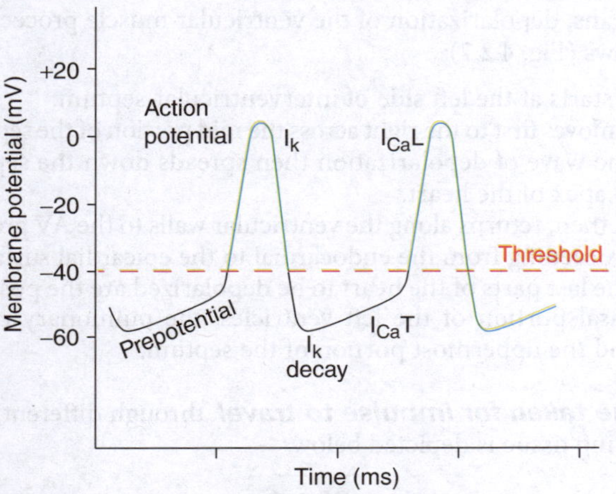

Fig. 4.2.5 Pacemaker potential and its ionic basis. IcaL, Ca^{2+} conductance through long-lasting channels; IcaT, Ca^{2+} conductance through transient calcium channels; Ik, potassium conductance.

- The slow fibres of the pacemaker tissue have a unique feature, i.e. leakage of resting membrane for sodium (while the resting membrane of fast fibres is relatively impermeable to Na^+). This causes *slow diffusion of Na^+ into the SA nodal fibres under resting condition. This slow entry of Na^+ in the cells slowly raises the potential to −55 mV* (i.e. causes slow depolarization) due to the presence of nonselective channels. This slow depolarization forms the initial part of pacemaker potential (Fig. 4.2.5). Nodal tissues also possess certain funny (f) channels because of their unusual activation following hyperpolarization, associated with increased permeability to both sodium and potassium, but dominant effect is that of sodium conductance. These channels are also called 'h' channels, because of their activation during hyperpolarization of the membrane (−40 to −60 mV).
- Then the transient ('T') calcium channels open up and there is slow influx of Ca^{2+} causing further depolarization in the same at slower rate till a threshold level of −40 mV is reached. Thus, calcium current (Ica) due to the opening of 'T calcium channels' forms the later part of pacemaker potential.
- At the threshold level (−40 mV), the 'long-lasting calcium channels' open up and the action potential starts with rapid depolarization due to influx of Ca^{2+}. Thus, it is important to note that the depolarization in SA node is mainly due to influx of Ca^{2+} rather than that of Na^+. Consequently, the depolarization is not as sharp as in the other myocardial fibres.
- At the end of depolarization, potassium channels open up and calcium channels close. This causes K^+ to diffuse out of the fibres resulting in rapid repolarization to −55 to −60 mV.
- Again, due to the unique feature of slow fibres of the SA node (i.e. *leakage of resting membrane to Na^+*), the resting potential does not become stable but slow depolarization starts due to slow influx of Na^+ making initial part of prepotential. Ultimately, due to repetition of the above-described steps, another action potential is initiated. In this way, impulses are generated at regular intervals of time (*autorhythmicity*).

Role of Autonomic Nervous System in Controlling Heart Rhythm

Vagal Tone

SA node is richly innervated by parasympathetic fibres from the right vagus. Normal activity of vagus liberates acetylcholine from its nerve endings which increases the permeability of SA nodal fibres for potassium producing hyperpolarization (due to rapid efflux of K^+). This hyperpolarization slows the firing rate of SA node from its automatic rate of 90–120 impulses/min to the actual heart rate of about 72 beats/min. The normal vagal activity is called vagal tone.

Effect of Parasympathetic Stimulation

Parasympathetic stimulation causes release of acetylcholine at vagal nerve endings and by the above-described mechanism causes (Fig. 4.2.6A):

- Decrease in heart rate by decrease in the rate of sinus rhythm. The acetylcholine released at the cholinergic nerve endings to nodal tissue causes hyperpolarization of the membrane by increasing permeability to K^+. The increase in conductance (efflux) of K^+ decreases the slope of prepotential.

Mechanism of action: This action of ACh is mediated by M_2 receptors via βγ-subunit of G protein, which opens the special set of K^+ channels and slows the depolarizing effect of Na^+ channels (I_h).

Activation of M_2 receptors also decreases cyclic adenosine 3′,5′-monophosphate in the pacemaker cells and slows the Ca^{2+} channels opening, thus decreasing the firing rate.

- Decrease in the rate of transmission of impulses to ventricles is due to decreased excitation of the conducting system. Strong parasympathetic stimulation may even completely block the transmission and ventricles may stop beating for 4–10 seconds. If it happens, Purkinje system initiates the rhythm causing ventricular contraction at a rate of 15–40/min. This phenomenon is called *vagal escape*.

Effect of Sympathetic Stimulation

Stimulation of sympathetic nerves causes release of norepinephrine at the nerve endings. Probably this increases permeability of cardiac muscle fibres to calcium by opening up 'L calcium channels'. This increases the rate of sinus rhythm and rate of conduction of impulse as well as excitability in all the portions of the heart. Force of contraction of atria and ventricles also increases greatly (Fig. 4.2.6B).

Mechanism of action: Norepinephrine released acts by binding to $β_1$-receptors on the nodal tissue and increases

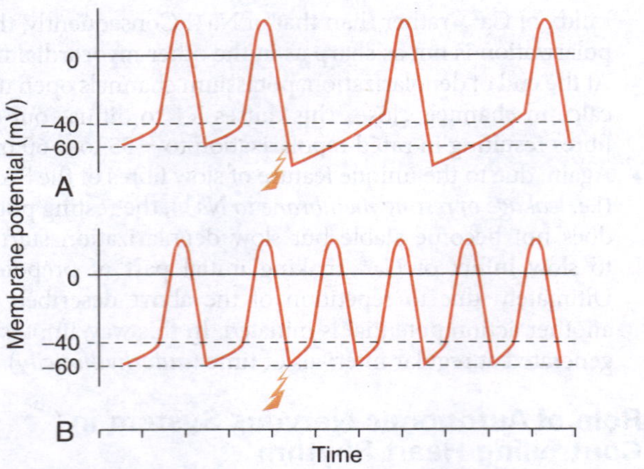

Fig. 4.2.6 Effect of parasympathetic (**A**) and sympathetic (**B**) stimulations on pacemaker potential.

intracellular cAMP, which facilitates the opening of long-lasting Ca^{2+} channels.

SPREAD OF CARDIAC IMPULSE

The cardiac impulse which originates in the SA node in the form of action potential spreads throughout the heart through the conduction system (properties of which are summarized in Table 4.2.1) in the sequence given as follows:

SA node and atria: The impulse travels over the muscle fibres of atria with which the ends of SA nodal fibres are fused, and through the interatrial tract to the left atrium. Conduction through these fibres causes simultaneous depolarization of both the atria. Atrial depolarization is completed in about 0.1 second. Through the internodal tracts (anterior, middle and posterior), the impulse reaches AV node from SA node within 0.03 second after its origin.

AV node: Conduction through AV node is slow; there is a delay of about 0.1 second. *The causes of AV nodal delay are as follows:*

- Transitional fibres connecting internodal tracts and AV node are very small and conduct the impulse at a very slow rate, i.e. 0.02–0.05 m/s. AV nodal fibres also conduct the impulse at a very slow rate (0.02–0.05 m/s).
- Resting membrane potential of transitional fibres and AV nodal fibres (−50 mV) is much less negative than that of rest of the cardiac muscle fibres (−90 mV). At this level of −50 to −55 mV potential, the fast Na^+ channels get closed due to inactivation gates. Therefore, opening of slow sodium-calcium channels thereby causes action potential. As a result, AV nodal action potential is slower to develop.
- There are very few gap junctions connecting successive fibres in the pathway.

Table 4.2.1 Properties of the conduction system

Tissue	Fibre diameter (μm)	Resting membrane potential (mV)	Conduction velocity (m/s)
SA node	–	−40 to −50	0.05
Atrial muscle	8–10	−70 to −80	0.3–0.5
Interatrial and internodal tract	15–20	−80 to −90	1.0
AV node	Variable	−50	0.02–0.05
Purkinje fibres	70–80	−70	2.0–4.0
Ventricular muscle	10–16	−80	<1.0

AV, atrioventricular; SA, sinoatrial.

Important Note

The ability of the AV node to slow and to block the rapid impulse is called *detrimental contraction*. This *AV nodal delay is useful*, for it provides time for completion of atrial contraction and their emptying (i.e. ventricular filling) before the ventricles contract. This delay is shortened by stimulation of the sympathetic nerves to the heart and lengthened by stimulation of the vagi.

Ventricular conduction: The impulses conducted through the AV node are distributed to ventricles through bundle of His, its branches and Purkinje fibres in 0.08–0.15 second. In humans, depolarization of the ventricular muscle proceeds as follows (Fig. 4.2.7):

- It starts at the left side of interventricular septum.
- It moves first to the right across the mid portion of the septum.
- The wave of depolarization then spreads down the septum to apex of the heart.
- It, then, returns along the ventricular walls to the AV groove, proceeding from the endocardial to the epicardial surface.
- The last parts of the heart to be depolarized are the posterobasal portion of the left ventricles, the pulmonary conus and the uppermost portion of the septum.

Time taken for impulse to travel through different conducting tissue is depicted below.

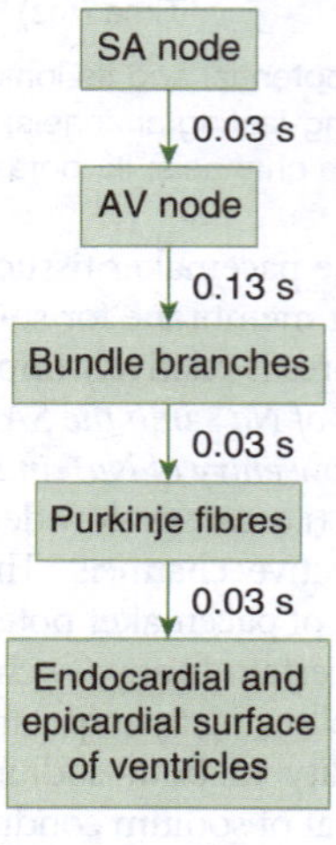

Thus, total time required for conduction from SA node to endocardial surface is 0.22 second.

Important Note

The AV bundle is the only connecting tissue between atria and ventricles. Therefore, if there is destruction of the AV node, then atria and ventricles beat independent of one another, i.e. atria at the rate of 72 beats/min and ventricles at a slower rate (30–40 beats/min). There is a complete dissociation of atrial and ventricular beating and is called *idioventricular rhythm*.

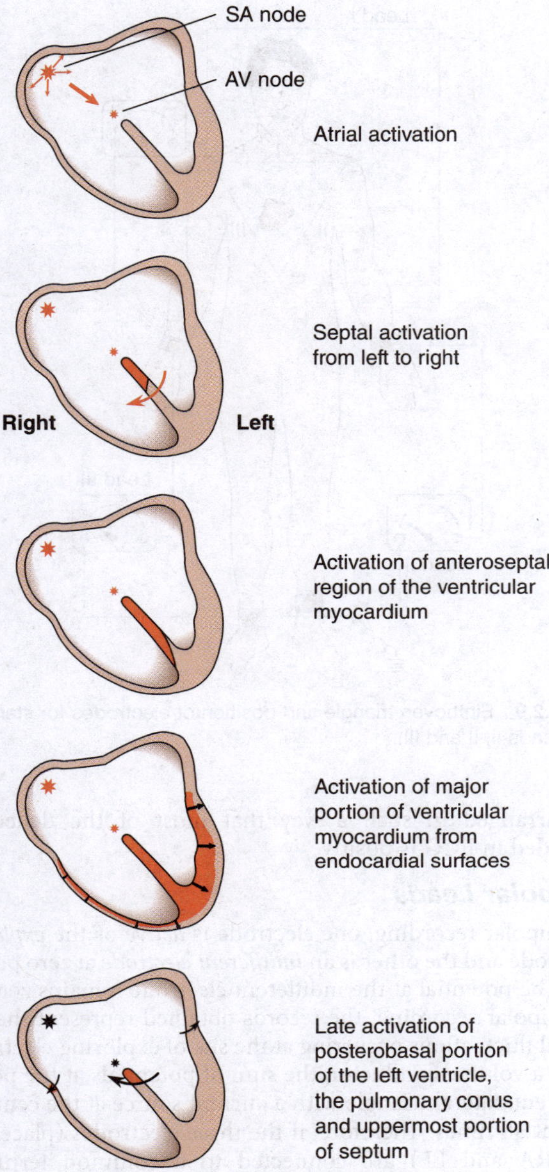

Fig. 4.2.7 Spread of cardiac impulse.

HEART RATE

The normal heart rate in an adult male is 70–80 beats/min.

Factors Affecting Heart Rate

The factors that affect heart rate are given as follows:

1. ***Age:*** Heart rate varies with age, i.e. it decreases as the age increases due to increase in the degree of vagal tone. The normal range of heart rate with different age groups is shown in Table 4.2.2.
2. ***Sex:*** In females, the resting heart rate is comparatively higher than in males of same age group.
3. ***Temperature:*** Heart rate increases with rise in body temperature. For each 1°F rise in body temperature, the heart rate increases by 10 beats/min.
4. ***Blood pressure:*** Heart rate is inversely related to the arterial pressure; this is referred to as *Marey's law*.
5. ***Emotions:*** Tachycardia occurs in emotions such as anxiety, anger and fear. Bradycardia is associated with sudden shock and grief. The emotional effects on heart rate are mediated through corticohypothalamic pathways.
6. ***Exercise:*** During muscular exercise, heart rate increases. For details, see page 1173.
7. ***Painful stimuli***
   - *Superficial pain* causes tachycardia and hypertension (rise in blood pressure).
   - *Deep pain* (visceral pain) is associated with bradycardia and hypotension (fall in blood pressure).
8. ***Respiration:*** Heart rate varies with phases of respiration; it increases with inspiration and decreases during expiration. This phenomenon is referred to as *sinus arrhythmia*. It is quite common in infants and children during normal breathing but is observed in adults only during deep breathing.

Table 4.2.2 Heart rate values in relation to age

Age	Heart rate (beats/min)
Birth	140–150
1 month	130–140
1 year	110–115
5 years	105–110
10 years	95–100
15 years	80–85
Adults	70–80
Old age	Up to 100

Regulation of Heart Rate

Heart rate is mainly controlled by two mechanisms – cardiac innervations.

It consists of two divisions of autonomic nervous system, such as parasympathetic and sympathetic, as described on page 245.

ELECTROCARDIOGRAPHY

INTRODUCTION

William Einthoven, a Dutch physiologist, originally developed the technique of electrocardiography (ECG). He was awarded the Nobel Prize in 1924 for his contribution and is called the father of modern ECG.

ECG refers to extracellular recording of the summed-up electrical events of all the cardiac muscle fibres generated with each heartbeat. Electrically, the heart behaves as a *dipole*, i.e. a two-terminal battery in which the excited part (depolarized segment) forms a negative pole and the nonexcited part forms the positive pole (Fig. 4.2.8). Thus, ECG is nothing but the surface recording of the potential difference between the two poles of the heart dipole at a given time. The record of the potential fluctuations during the cardiac cycle is called the *ECG*. The machine used to record these potential fluctuations is called *electrocardiograph*, which is essentially a sensitive galvanometer.

RECORDING OF ECG

ECG Leads

ECG leads refer to the two electrodes which are placed on the body surface and connected to ECG machine for measuring the potential fluctuations between only two points. ECG is

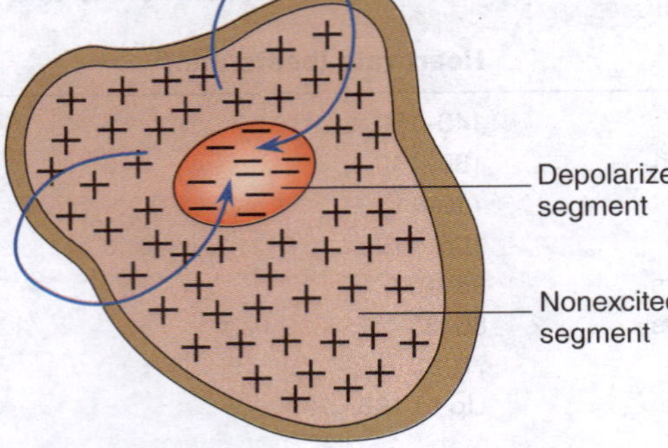

Fig. 4.2.8 The heart as a dipole.

recorded using two types of leads – the bipolar and unipolar leads.

Bipolar Leads

In bipolar recording, *both the electrodes are active* and one of the active electrodes is connected to the negative terminal of the ECG machine and the other to the positive terminal. Three standard limb leads used in bipolar recording are based on Einthoven's assumption that the body is like an electrically homogeneous plate in which the right and left shoulders and the pubic region form the corners of an equilateral triangle with the heart in its centre (Einthoven triangle) and that two active electrodes need to be placed at the two corners of this triangle (Fig. 4.2.9). However, for convenience, the electrodes are connected to the left arm (LA), right arm (RA) and left foot (LF) instead of the shoulders and the pubic region (Fig. 4.2.9). Practically, it does not make any difference whether the electrodes are placed in proximal or distal part of the extremities, because the current flows in the body fluids and so the records obtained are similar.

In three standard limb leads, the two active electrodes are connected as:

Lead I (LI) In LI, the two active electrodes are connected to LA and RA.

- LA electrode is connected to the positive terminal.
- RA electrode is connected to the negative terminal of the ECG machine.

Lead II (LII) In LII, the electrodes are connected to RA and LF.

- LF electrode is connected to the *positive* terminal.
- RA electrode is connected to the *negative* terminal of the ECG machine.

Lead III (LIII) In LIII, the electrodes are connected to LA and LF.

- LF electrode is connected to the positive terminal.
- LA electrode is connected to the negative terminal of the ECG machine.

The position of electrodes in bipolar standard limb leads has been shown in Fig. 4.2.9. The direction in which positive electrode points is called the axis of the lead. The direction of the lead axis is same in which the current flows in the heart and recorded deflection is upwards (positive). The electrodes are arranged in such a way that most of the deflection recorded in ECG is positive.

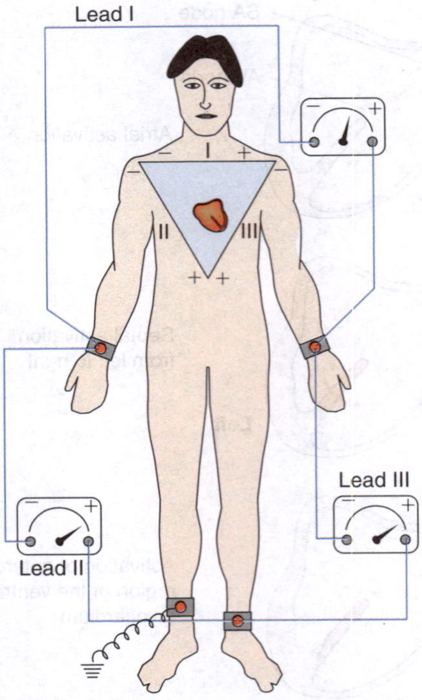

Fig. 4.2.9 Einthoven triangle and position of electrodes for standard limb leads (I, II and III).

Unipolar Leads

In unipolar recording, one electrode is *active* or the *exploring* electrode and the other is an *indifferent electrode* at zero potential. The potential at the indifferent electrode remains zero, so in unipolar recording, the records obtained represent the potential fluctuations occurring at the site of exploring electrode.

In a volume conductor, the sum of potentials at the points of an equilateral triangle with a current source at the centre is zero at all times. Therefore, if the three electrodes (placed on LA, RA and LF) are connected to a common terminal, through a resistance, an indifferent electrode that stays near zero potential is obtained. In clinical ECG, two types of unipolar leads are used.

Unipolar chest leads There are six unipolar chest leads (precordial leads) designated V_1–V_6. The indifferent electrode is obtained as described above and the active electrode is placed on six points on the chest given as follows (Fig. 4.2.10):

- *Lead V_1*: In the right fourth intercostal space, just near the sternum
- *Lead V_2*: In the left fourth intercostal space, just near the sternum
- *Lead V_3*: Halfway between V_2 and V_4
- *Lead V_4*: In the left fifth intercostal space at midclavicular line
- *Lead V_5*: In the left fifth intercostal space at anterior axillary line
- *Lead V_6*: In the left fifth intercostal space at midaxillary line

Unipolar limb leads These include lead VL, VF and VR. In unipolar limb leads, one *exploring* (active) *electrode* is

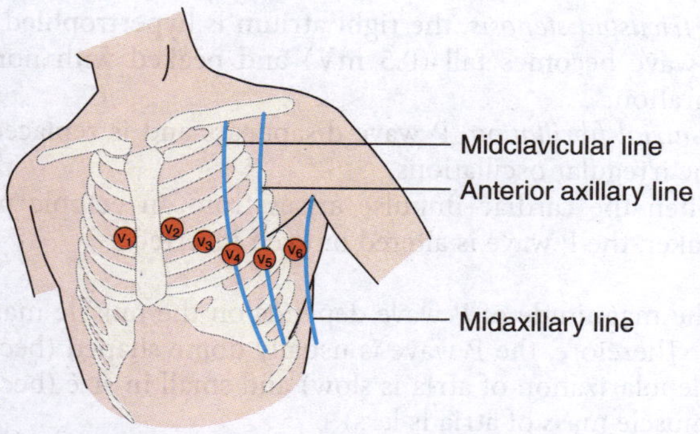

Fig. 4.2.10 Position of electrodes for chest leads (V_1–V_6).

placed over a limb (in lead VL over the LA, in VF over the LF and in lead VR over the RA), and is connected to the positive terminal of the electrocardiograph. The *indifferent electrode* is obtained as described above and is connected to the negative terminal of the electrocardiograph. These leads are not used and have been replaced by augmented limb leads.

Augmented unipolar limb leads Generally, augmented unipolar limb leads designated as aVR, aVL and aVF are used. In augmented leads, the size of potential is increased by 50% without any change in the configuration from the nonaugmented record. The *active electrode* is from one of the limbs, and the indifferent electrode is obtained by connecting the other two limbs through 5000 Ω resistance as:

- Lead aVR: Active electrode is from RA and indifferent electrode is from LA + LF.
- Lead aVL: Active electrode is from LA and indifferent electrode is from RA + LF.
- Lead aVF: Active electrode is from LF and indifferent electrode is from RA + LA.

Why these leads are called augmented leads is explained below.

Suppose in nonaugmented unipolar limb leads, the potential at LA (VL) = the potential at RA (VR) = the potential at LF (VF).

Then,

$$aVF = VL - \frac{VR + VF}{2}$$

Or

$$2\,aVF = 2VL - (VR + VF) \qquad (I)$$

In Einthoven triangle, if electrodes are connected to three limbs through a high resistance, then

$$VL + VR + VF = 0$$

Or

$$VL = -(VR \quad VF) \qquad (II)$$

Substituting value of $-(VR + VF)$ in equation (I):

$$2aVL = 2VL + VL$$

Or

$$aVL = \frac{3}{2}VL$$

Thus, potential recorded in aVL is 1.5 times as that recorded in VL.

Electrocardiograph

The electrocardiograph (ECG machine) is essentially a sophisticated string galvanometer. A modern electrocardiograph amplifies and records the potential fluctuations on a moving strip of paper. The following recording mechanisms are used:

- Some machines have a writing ink pen that records directly on the moving sheet of paper.
- In other machines, instead of ink pen, special paper is used which turns black on exposure to heat. The stylus (recording pen) is made hot by electrical current flowing through its tip.

Calibration of Time and Voltage on ECG Paper

- The special ECG paper having 1- and 5-mm squares (Fig. 4.2.11) is used. The tracing is usually made at a standard recording speed of 25 mm/s.
- On horizontal axis, therefore, each millimetre represents 0.04 second (1/25).
- The sensitivity of electrocardiograph is adjusted in such a way that a potential fluctuation of 1 mV causes a vertical deflection of 1 cm. Thus, on vertical axis, each millimetre represents 0.1 mV magnitude of potential.

Monitoring For ECG monitoring, the following methods are used:

- In coronary care units (CCU), ECG monitoring is done continuously; the monitors also have alarm system to sound at the onset of life-threatening arrhythmia.
- Holter monitor is a small portable tape recorder used for recording ECG in ambulatory individuals during their normal routine activity.
- The ECG record obtained with monitor is very useful in diagnosis of arrhythmia and planning of treatment.

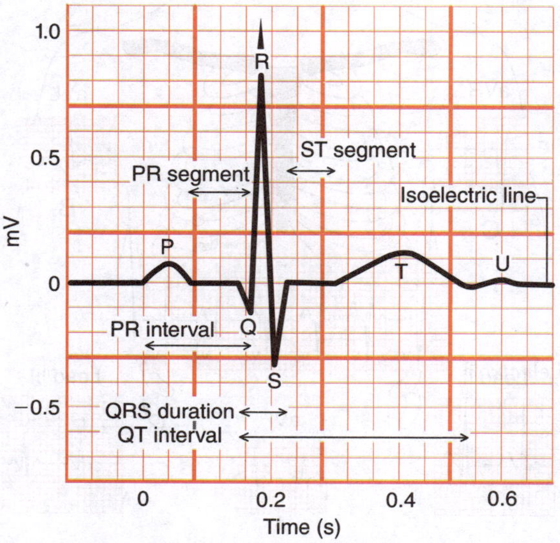

Fig. 4.2.11 Calibration of time and voltage (amplitude) on special ECG paper. ECG, electrocardiography.

NORMAL ELECTROCARDIOGRAM

Electrocardiogram (ECG) refers to the record of the potential fluctuations during the cardiac cycle. As a result of sequential spread of the excitation in the atria, the interventricular septum and the ventricular walls (Fig. 4.2.7) and finally repolarization of the myocardium, a series of positive and negative waves designated as P, Q, R, S and T is recorded during each cardiac cycle. Depolarization moving towards an active electrode in a volume conductor produces a positive deflection, whereas depolarization moving in the opposite direction produces a negative deflection.

Therefore, the shape and polarity of P, Q, R, S and T waves will vary in different leads due to differences in the orientation of each lead with respect to the heart (Fig. 4.2.12). Configuration of a typical ECG from a bipolar limb LII is described below (Fig. 4.2.11).

Waves of ECG

P Wave

Configuration P wave is the positive (upright) rounded deflection.

Cause It is produced by the depolarization of atrial musculature so also called atrial complex.

Duration Duration of P wave is not more than 0.1 second.

Amplitude Amplitude of P wave is from 0.1 to 0.12 mV.

Clinical significance Magnitude of P wave is a guide to the functional activity of atria.

- *In mitral stenosis*, the left atrium is hypertrophied and P wave becomes larger and prolonged.

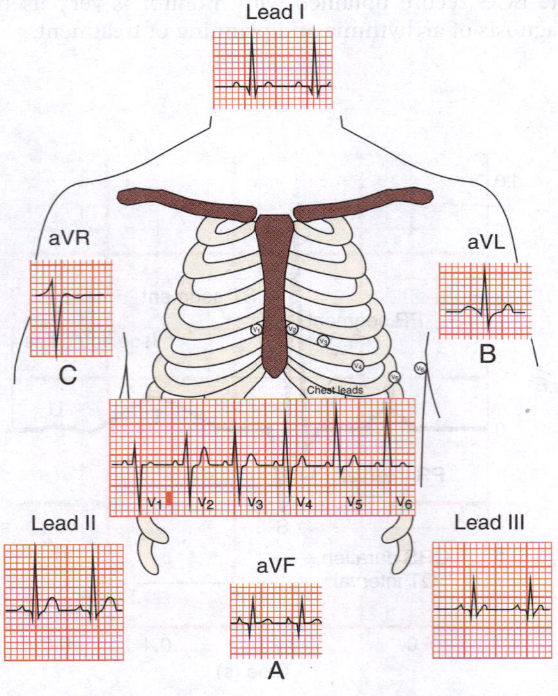

Fig. 4.2.12 The electrocardiographic complexes recorded from different leads.

- *In tricuspid stenosis*, the right atrium is hypertrophied and P wave becomes tall (0.5 mV) and peaked with normal duration.
- *In atrial fibrillation*, P wave disappears and is replaced by fine irregular oscillations.
- When the cardiac impulse arises from an ectopic pacemaker, the P wave is altered or even inverted.

The magnitude of P wave depends on the muscle mass of atria. Therefore, the P wave is usually dome shaped (because the depolarization of atria is slow) and small in size (because the muscle mass of atria is less)

QRS Complex

Configuration QRS complex consists of three consecutive waves. Q wave is a small negative wave which may be absent normally quite often. It is continued as a tall positive R wave which is followed by a small negative S wave.

Cause The QRS complex is caused by ventricular depolarization.

Duration Duration of QRS complex is normally less than 0.08 second. It is a measure of intraventricular conduction time.

Magnitude. The magnitude of Waves of QRS Complex are:

Q wave: Amplitude of the Q wave is 0.1–0.2 mV, that of R wave is 1.0 mV and that of S wave is 0.4 mV (total 1.5–1.6 mV).

- Due to passage of wave of depolarization from left to right of interventricular septum, the apex of the heart becomes more negative in comparison to the base of the heart. This produces small negative deflection of Q wave.
  The amplitude of Q wave is 0.1–0.2 mV. The P wave is best studied in LII and lead V_1.
  R wave: As the wave of depolarization progresses from subendocardium to epicardial surface, it produces tall sharp positive deflection as R wave. The amplitude of R wave is 1.0 mV. The higher amplitude of R wave is due to more muscle mass of the left ventricle as compared with that of the right ventricle (three times higher).
  S wave: Small negative wave occurs when wave of depolarization passes through the posterobasal part of the left ventricle, pulmonary conus and uppermost part of interventricular septum; as a result, the apex becomes more negative than the base part of the heart.
  The amplitude of S wave is 0.4 mV.
  The total amplitude of QRS complex is 1.5–1.6 mV.

Clinical significance QRS complex from precordial leads is more important than limb leads.

- Deep Q wave (more than 0.2 mV) along with other changes is an important sign of myocardial infarction (MI).
- Tall R wave (more than 1.3 mV) is seen in ventricular hypertrophy.
- Low-voltage QRS complex (total sum less than 1.5 mV) is seen in hypothyroidism and pericardial effusion.
- QRS complex is prolonged in bundle branch block. Prolonged QRS complex is seen when one or both the ventricles are hypertrophied or dilated.

- In blockage of Purkinje system, the QRS complex is abnormally prolonged (>0.12 second) due to decrease in impulse conduction.
- Bizarre pattern of QRS complex is caused by destruction of cardiac muscle in ventricular region and local blockages in the Purkinje system resulting in irregular impulse conduction, rapid shifts in voltages and axis deviations.

T wave

Configuration T wave is the last, positive, dome-shaped deflection. Normally, it is in the same direction as QRS complex, because ventricular repolarization follows a path opposite to depolarization.

Part that depolarizes last repolarizes first (epicardium towards endocardium).

Cause T wave represents ventricular repolarization.

Duration Duration of T wave is approximately 0.27 second.

Amplitude Amplitude of T wave is about 0.3 mV.

Clinical significance Clinical significance of T wave is as follows:

- In old age, T wave is flattened.
- Exercise increases its amplitude in healthy hearts.
- Inverted T wave is an important sign of myocardial ischaemia or infarction. It is physiologically also seen in young children and sometimes during deep inspiration and after heavy exercise.
- Tall and peaked T wave occurs in hyperkalaemia.

> **Important Note**
>
> ***Digitalis toxicity:*** Digitalis is a drug used for increasing the strength of cardiac muscle (glycoside). Nonspecific changes in T wave (inversion of T wave, biphasic T wave) may occur; biphasic T wave is the earliest sign of digitalis toxicity.

U Wave

Configuration It is a small, round, positive wave.

Cause It occurs due to slow repolarization of papillary muscle.

Duration Duration of U wave when present is 0.08 second.

Amplitude Amplitude of U wave is about 0.2 mV.

Significance It is rarely seen normally. It becomes prominent in hypokalaemia.

Note: Since atrial repolarization coincides with ventricular depolarization, it is merged with QRS complex and thus not normally recorded as a separate wave.

Intervals and Segments of ECG

PR Interval

It is measured from the onset of P wave to the onset of the QRS complex. Actually, it is PQ interval but Q wave is frequently absent; therefore, it is called PR interval.

- It measures the *AV conduction time*, including the AV nodal delay.
- Its *duration* varies from 0.12 to 0.21 second depending on the heart rate.
- *Clinical significance:* Prolonged PR interval indicates AV conduction block. First-degree block is produced when PR interval is between 0.2 and 0.3 second and second-degree block is produced when PR interval is increased (0.3–0.45 second).

J Point

J point refers to the point on ECG which coincides with the end of depolarization and start of repolarization of ventricles, i.e. it occurs at the end of QRS complex. At this point, since all parts of the ventricles are depolarized, no current flows around the heart. Therefore, at J point, the potential of ECG is exactly zero voltage.

QT Interval

It is the time from the start of the QRS complex to the end of T wave.

- It indicates total *systolic time of ventricles*, i.e. ventricular depolarization and repolarization.
- *Duration* of QT interval is about 0.4 second (QRS duration and ST-segment duration).

Clinical significance: Ischaemia and any ventricular conduction defects prolong the QT interval. In hypocalcaemia also, QT interval is prolonged.

TP Interval

It is measured from the end of T wave to the beginning of P wave.

- It measures the *diastolic period* of the heart.
- Variable TP interval indicates AV dissociation.

PP Interval

PP interval is the interval between two successive P waves. Equal PP intervals indicate rhythmic depolarization of the atria.

ST Segment

It is an isoelectric period between the end of QRS complex and the beginning of T wave.

- Its *duration* is about 0.32 second.
- It corresponds with *ventricular repolarization*.
- *Clinical significance:* ST segment is elevated in patients with MI. In fact, whenever there is current of injury, the TP segment shifts away from the zero and so it does not remain at the same potential level as ST segment. However, since in ECG, TP is considered as reference potential level, so whenever a current of injury is evident in ECG, it is called ST-segment shift.

Characteristic Features of ECG Complex in Unipolar Chest Leads

The ECG complex produced in unipolar chest leads (V_1–V_6) represents the electrical activity of the part of the heart which lies nearest to the active electrode (Fig. 4.2.13).

P Wave

P wave is positive in all the leads because the excitation wave moves from SA node to AV node, i.e. posterior to anterior.

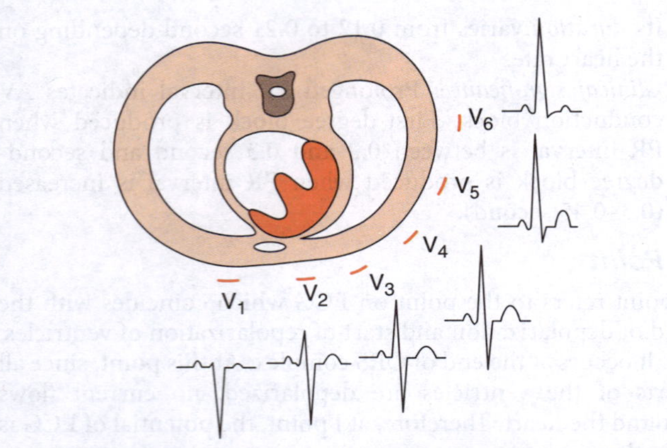

Fig. 4.2.13 Pattern of QRS complex in chest leads (V_1–V_6).

QRS Complex

QRS complex represents the electrical activity of ventricles and so its configuration changes in different leads are as follows:

- *In V_1 and V_2* (which reflect right ventricular activity), the main QRS complex is *negative*.
- *In V_3 and V_4* (which reflect activity of both ventricles including interventricular septum), the main QRS complex is *biphasic*.
- *In V_5 and V_6* (which reflect left ventricular activity), mainly the main QRS complex is *positive*.

Thus, as shown in Fig. 4.2.13:

R Wave

R wave gradually increases in size from V_1 to V_6 leads. In lead V_1, R wave represents activity of right ventricle and in lead V_6 that of left ventricle.

S Wave

S wave gradually decreases in size from lead V_1 to V_6. In lead V_1, S wave represents activity of left ventricle and in lead V_6 that of right ventricle.

Characteristic Features of ECG Complex in Unipolar Limb Leads and Augmented Limb Leads

The ECG complex in unipolar limb leads and augmented limb leads is characterized by the electrical activity of that part of the heart which faces the active electrode of that particular unipolar limb lead as:

Leads VF and aVF

These leads reflect the electrical activity of inferior surface of the heart which is formed by parts of both right and left ventricles and interventricular septum. Therefore, QRS complex in these leads is like that in V_3 and V_4 (predominantly *biphasic*; Fig. 4.2.12A).

Leads VL and aVL

These leads reflect the electrical activity of left outer side of the heart which is mainly formed by the left ventricle. Therefore, QRS complex in these leads, like that in V_6, is predominantly *positive* (Fig. 4.2.12B).

Leads VR and aVR

These leads reflect the activity of the cavity of the ventricles, irrespective of the position of the heart. Therefore, *P wave, QRS complex and T wave* all are *negative deflection* (Fig. 4.2.12C).

VECTORIAL ANALYSIS OF ELECTROCARDIOGRAM AND VECTOR CARDIOGRAPHY

In the discussion until this point, we have studied the configuration of various positive and negative waves of the ECG complex and their clinical significance. In addition to the information gained from the changes in the configuration of various waves, the vectorial analysis of the ECG also provides useful information pertaining to cardiac abnormalities. The concept of cardiac vector, methods of vector analysis and their clinical significance are discussed.

Concept of Cardiac Vectors

- During cardiac cycle (depolarization and repolarization of the heart), current flows in the heart at every instant. The magnitude and direction of the potential generated can be represented in the form of an arrow which is called a vector. By convention, the arrowhead points towards the direction and the length of the arrow is drawn proportional to the voltage of the potential.
- During most of the cycle of ventricular depolarization, direction of electrical potential (negative to positive) is from the base of ventricles towards the apex. This preponderant direction of potential during depolarization is called the *mean QRS vector* (mean electrical axis [MEA] of the heart) and is drawn through the centre of the ventricles in a direction from the base of the heart towards the apex (Fig. 4.2.14).
- The *instant vector*, however, represents the magnitude and direction of potential at a particular instant during the cardiac cycle. The instantaneous vectors of five different instants during the process of ventricular depolarization are shown in Fig. 4.2.15.

Calculating the MEA from Standard Lead Electrocardiogram

As discussed earlier, the MEA refers to the *mean vector* produced during a cardiac cycle (i.e. by P, QRS and TP, ECG complex).

- In the frontal plane, MEA can be calculated from any two standard (i.e. bipolar) limb leads (using Einthoven triangle or triaxial reference system) or any two augmented limb leads (using hexaxial reference system).

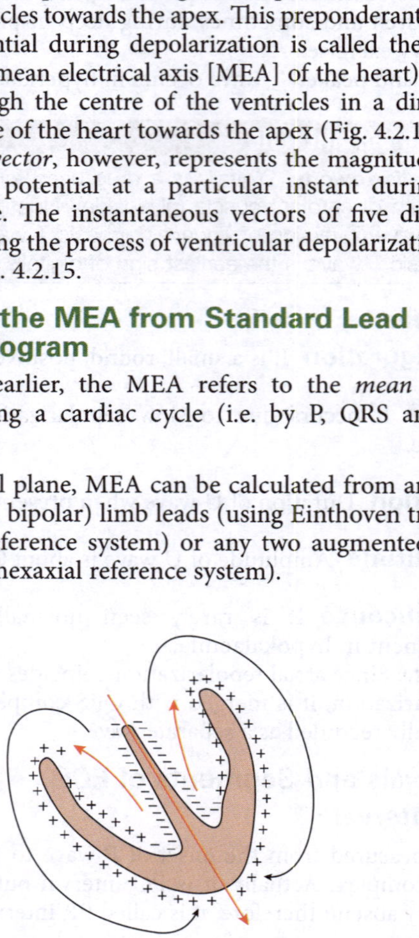

Fig. 4.2.14 Instantaneous mean vector during ventricular depolarization.

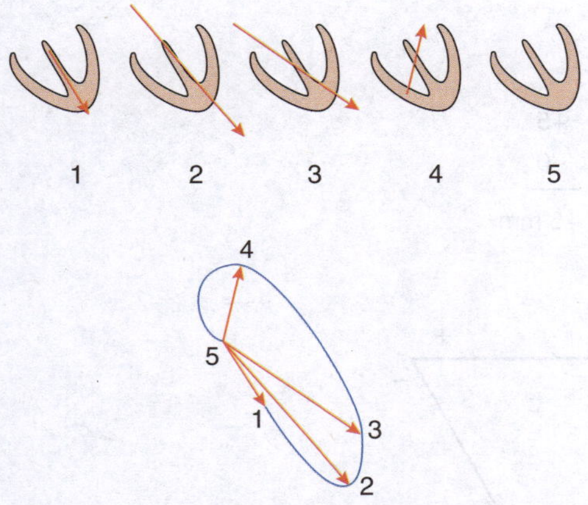

Fig. 4.2.15 The instantaneous mean vector of five different instants during process of ventricular depolarization and construction of QRS vector cardiogram.

- The MEA in the horizontal plane is derived using the precordial (chest) leads.

Triaxial Reference System

The triaxial reference system involves moving the sides of Einthoven triangle so that they intersect at the centre of triangle. LI then divides the system into an upper (negative) and a lower (positive) hemisphere. The triaxial system of representation reveals that (Fig. 4.2.16B):

- The axis of LI is 0°, because the electrodes lie in the horizontal direction with positive electrode to the left.
- The axis of LII is about 60°, because the electrodes are placed on the RA (negative) and LF (positive).
- The axis of LIII is about 120°, because the electrodes are placed on the LA (negative) and LF (positive).

Hexaxial Reference System

The hexaxial reference system involves superimposition of the axis of augmented limb leads on the triaxial system. The hexaxial system of vector representation reveals that (Fig. 4.2.16C):

- The axis of lead aVF is +90°.
- The axis of lead aVR is −150°.
- The axis of lead aVL is −30°.

Clinically, the frontal MEA of the QRS complex is more useful and is determined from the two standard limb leads as follows:

- The Q and S waves (negative values) are added algebraically to the R wave (positive value) for each of two leads. The result gives the magnitude and the direction of the QRS vector (+ or −) in each lead. For example:
  - *In LI*, the algebraic sum of Q(0), R(+5), S(0) = 0 + 5 − 0 = 5 mV.
  - *In LII*, the algebraic sum of Q(−1), R(+16), S(0) = −1 + 16 − 0 = 15 mV.
  - *In LIII*, the algebraic sum of Q(−1), R(+11), S(0) = −1 + 11 − 0 = 10 mV.
- The QRS magnitude is plotted along the respective leads from the zero point towards the appropriate polarity with the arrow pointing towards the correct pole (positive or negative) using the Einthoven triangle (Fig. 4.2.17) or the triaxial reference system.

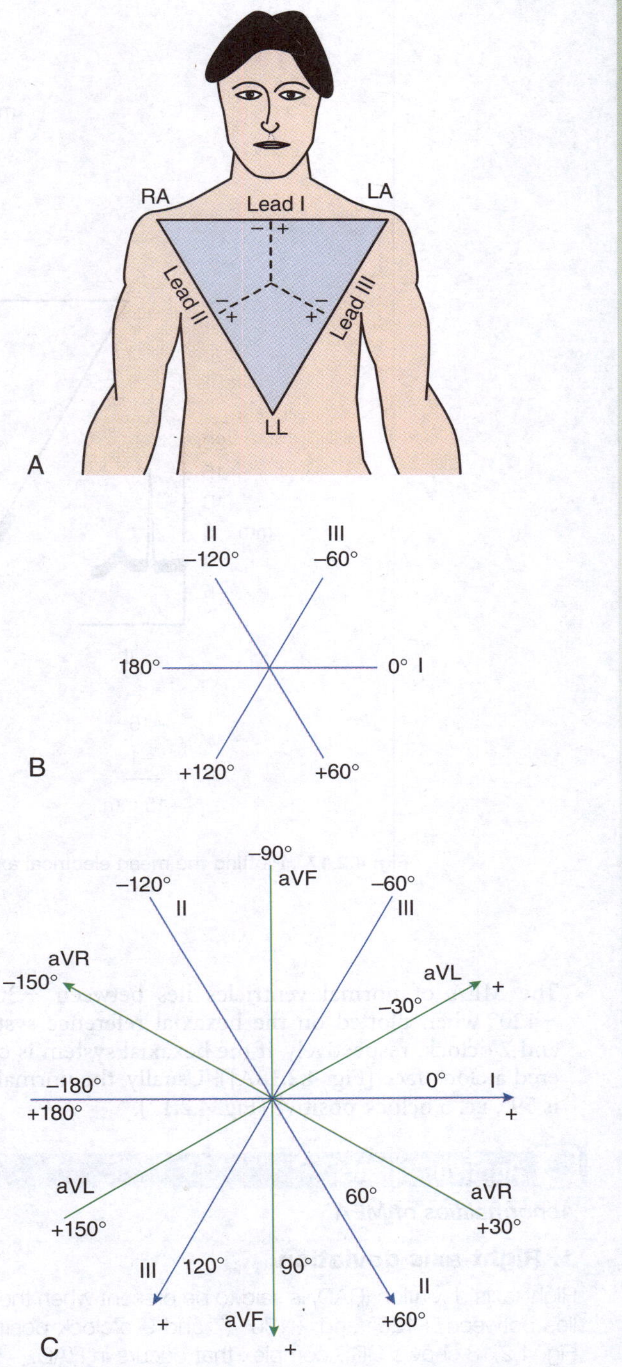

Fig. 4.2.16 Schematic drawing for calculating the mean electrical axis (MEA): **A**, Einthoven triangle and connections of bipolar limb leads; **B**, the triaxial reference system in which leads I, II and III collapsed into their respective zero points; and **C**, the hexaxial reference system obtained by adding augmented unipolar limb leads (aVR, aVL and aVF) to triaxial system.

- Perpendiculars are then drawn from the leads of the two vectors until they intersect.
- The intersection marks the head of the mean electrical vector. The MEA is then drawn from the centre of the triangle (electrical zero for the system) to the perpendiculars' intersection. The length of this arrow represents the magnitude of the MEA, and its direction in degrees represents the electrical axis in the frontal plane.

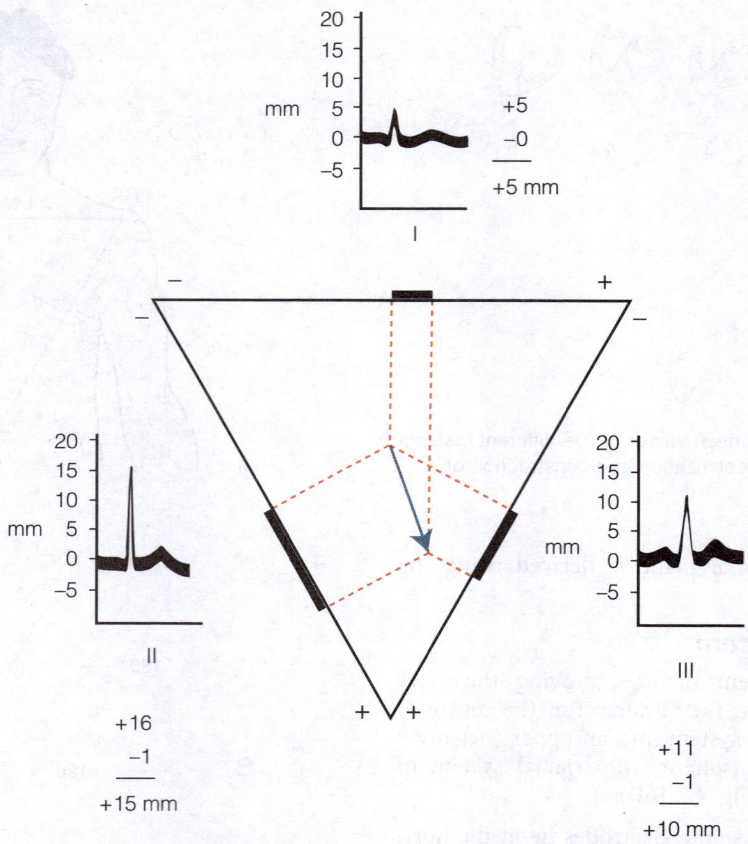

Fig. 4.2.17 Plotting the mean electrical axis (MEA) of the ventricles from two electrocardiographic leads.

- The MEA of normal ventricles lies between −30° and +120° when plotted on the hexaxial reference system (2 and 7 o'clock, respectively, if the hexaxial system is considered a clock face [Fig. 4.2.18A]). Usually, the normal MEA is 59°, i.e. 5 o'clock positive (Fig. 4.2.17).

Applied Aspects

Abnormalities of MEA

1. Right-axis deviation

Right-axis deviation (RAD) is said to be present when the MEA lies between +120° and +180° (7 and 9 o'clock positions). Fig. 4.2.18 shows QRS complex that occurs in RAD.

Causes of RAD include:

- Right ventricular hypertrophy (RVH) secondary to chronic lung disease or pulmonary valve stenosis
- RBB block causing delayed activation of the right ventricle
- Posterior (or inferior) MI

2. Left-axis deviation

Left-axis deviation (LAD) is said to be present when the MEA lies between −30° and −90° (or 2 and 12 o'clock positions). Fig. 4.2.18 shows typical QRS complex that occurs in LAD.

Causes of LAD are as follows:

- Left ventricular hypertrophy
- Obesity
- Left bundle branch block (LBBB)
- Anterolateral MI

Vector Cardiography

As discussed earlier, the vector of current flow through the heart changes rapidly as the impulse spreads through the myocardium. The vector changes into two aspects:

- Increases or decreases in length corresponding to change in voltage (magnitude)
- Changes its direction because of changes in the average direction of the electrical potential of the heart

Figs 4.2.15 and 4.2.19 show the instant vectors of eight different successive instants during the process of ventricular depolarization (i.e. in a normal QRS complex). On joining the positive ends of the vectors, a loop is obtained which is called *vector cardiogram*.

A continuous record of all the vectors is made using an *oscilloscope*. The procedure is called vector cardiography and the record obtained in the form of a loop is called vector cardiogram (similar to P, QRS and T described above). Three loops can be recorded during one cardiac cycle (Fig. 4.2.20). Atrial depolarization cannot be recorded with standard technique of vector cardiography because of the prolonged time course and small voltages involved.

1. P Loop

It is caused by atrial depolarization. It is small and is directed leftward and inferiorly, resulting in a positive P wave in three bipolar limb leads.

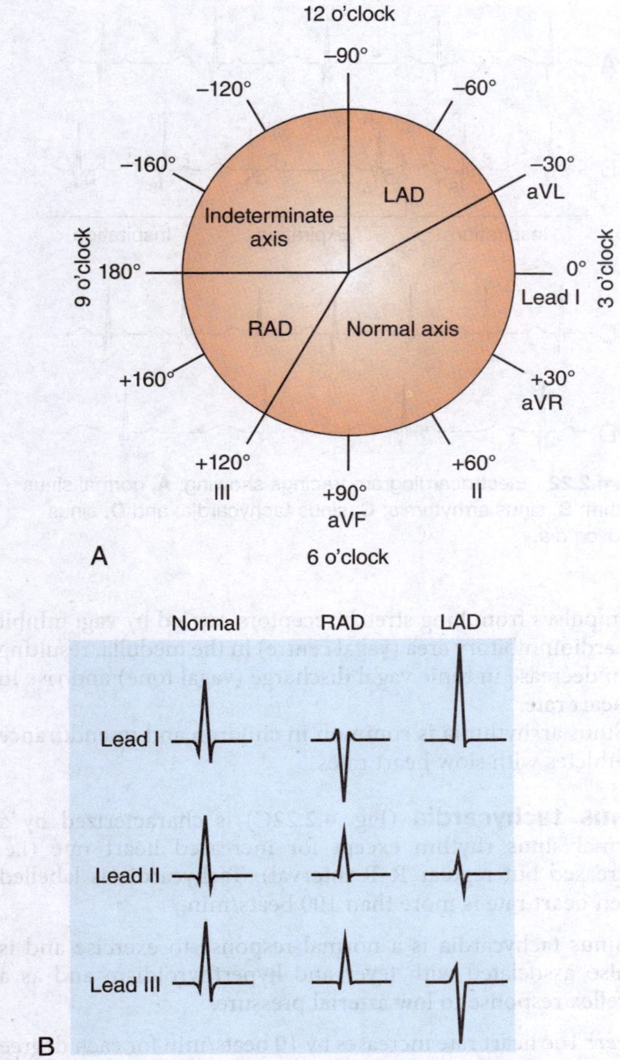

Fig. 4.2.18 **A**, Mean electrical axis (MEA) in the frontal plane (using hexaxial system) showing normal axis, right-axis deviation (RAD) and left-axis deviation (LAD); and **B**, QRS complexes (normal in RAD and in LAD) seen in leads I, II and III.

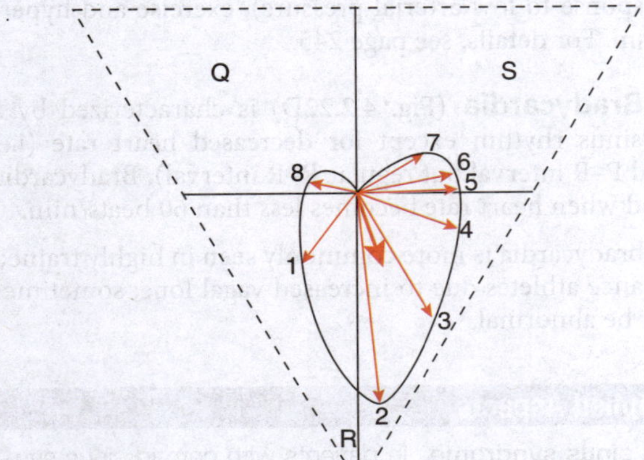

Fig. 4.2.19 Instant vector of eight arbitrary stages of ventricular depolarization and reconstruction of QRS complex from QRS loop for three bipolar limb leads. Arrows indicate the direction of loop recording.

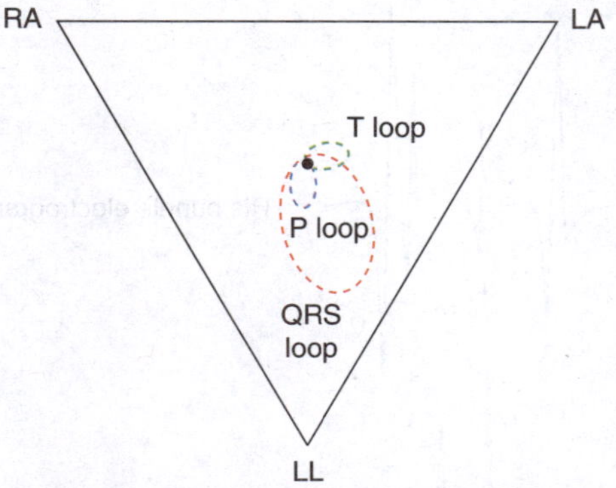

Fig. 4.2.20 The vector cardiographic loops P, QRS and T.

2. QRS Loop

It is caused by ventricular depolarization. The normal QRS loop is inscribed counterclockwise and is directed leftward, inferior and posterior. Fig. 4.2.19 shows how the QRS loop generates the QRS complex in three limb leads.

3. T loop

It results from ventricular repolarization, which is roughly opposite in direction to the depolarization. This reversal of direction results in T wave that normally is in the same direction as the QRS complex.

HIS BUNDLE ELECTROGRAM

- His bundle electrogram (HBE) refers to recording the electrical activity of the heart obtained through the intracardiac ring electrodes placed near the tricuspid valve.
- It is accomplished with a catheter containing ring electrodes at its tip that is passed through a vein to the right side of the heart and manipulated into a position close to the tricuspid valve. Three or more standard electrocardiographic leads are recorded simultaneously.
- Normal HBE shows the following deflections (Fig. 4.2.21):
  A deflection corresponds to activation of AV node.
  H spike is due to transmission of impulse through the His bundle.
  V deflection is produced during ventricular depolarization.

Uses of HBE

It is especially useful in patients with heart blocks. From the HBE and ECG from standard leads, it is possible to accurately time the following three intervals:

PA Interval

PA interval is measured from the P wave of ECG record to the A wave of HBE.

It is the time from the first appearance of atrial depolarization to the A wave in HBE. It represents conduction time from the SA node to the AV node. Normal value of PA interval is 27 milliseconds.

AH Interval

It is the time from the A wave to the start of H spike in HBE. It represents the AV nodal conduction time. Normal value of AH interval is 92 milliseconds; the higher value of AH interval shows relative slowness of conduction in the AV node.

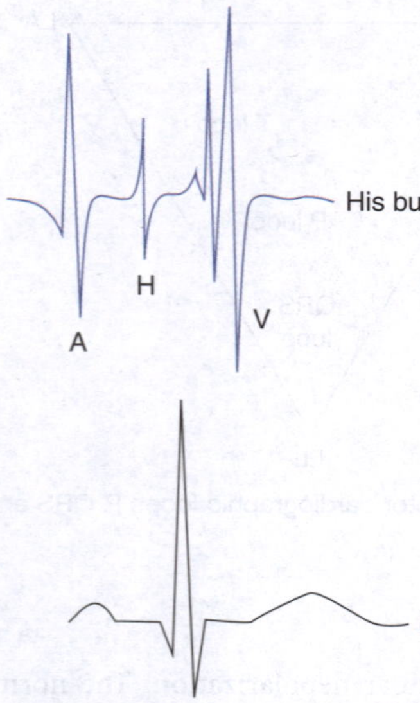

Fig. 4.2.21 Normal His bundle electrogram (HBE) with simultaneously recorded ECG. ECG, electrocardiography.

HV Interval

It is the time from the start of the H spike in HBE to the start of QRS complex deflection in the ECG. It represents conduction in the bundle of His and the bundle branches. Normal value of HV interval is 43 milliseconds.

CLINICAL APPLICATIONS OF ELECTROCARDIOGRAPHY

ECG is an indispensable tool in the diagnosis, prognosis and planning treatment in most of the cardiac disorders. The important applied aspects which need special mention are as follows:

- Cardiac arrhythmias
- Myocardial infarction (MI)
- Hypertrophy of various cardiac chambers
- Effects on ECG of changes in the ionic composition of blood

Cardiac Arrhythmias

Cardiac arrhythmia refers to disruption of the normal cardiac rhythm. The normal cardiac rhythm implies a regular sinus rhythm with a normal cardiac rate, between 60 and 100 beats/min (average 72 beats/min). *Sinus rhythm* is said to be present when the SA node is pacemaker, and each P wave is followed by a normal QRS complex, the PR and QT intervals are normal, (Fig. 4.2.22A), and RR interval is regular. Cardiac arrhythmias may be discussed as:

- Abnormal sinus rhythm
- Conduction disturbances (heart blocks)
- Ectopic cardiac rhythm

Abnormal Sinus Rhythm

Sinus arrhythmia (Fig. 4.2.22B) is characterized by a normal sinus rhythm except for the R–R interval (cardiac rate) which varies in a set pattern.

- Sinus arrhythmia is usually, but not always, synchronized with respiration. Usually, heart rate increases during inspiration and decreases during expiration, as a result of variations in vagal tone that affect the SA node. During inspiration, impulses from lung stretch receptors carried by vagi inhibit cardioinhibitory area (vagal centre) in the medulla, resulting in decrease in tonic vagal discharge (vagal tone) and rise in heart rate.
- Sinus arrhythmia is common in children and in endurance athletes with slow heart rates.

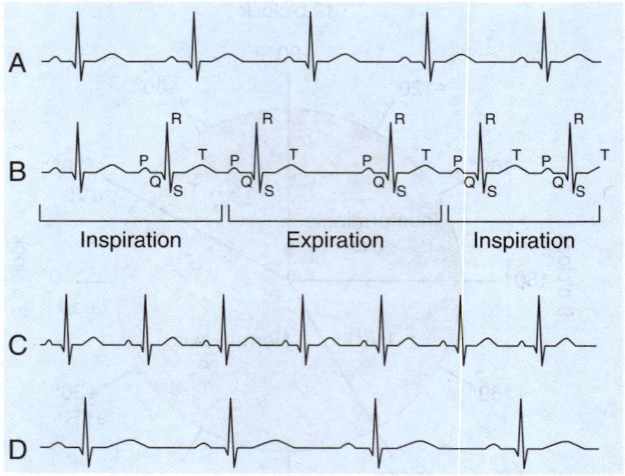

Fig. 4.2.22 Electrocardiogram tracings showing: **A**, normal sinus rhythm; **B**, sinus arrhythmia; **C**, sinus tachycardia; and **D**, sinus bradycardia.

Sinus tachycardia (Fig. 4.2.22C) is characterized by a normal sinus rhythm except for increased heart rate (i.e. decreased but regular R–R interval). Tachycardia is labelled when heart rate is more than 100 beats/min.

- Sinus tachycardia is a normal response to exercise and is also associated with fever and hyperthyroidism and as a reflex response to low arterial pressure.

Fever: The heart rate increases by 10 beats/min for each degree Fahrenheit or 18 beats/min for each degree Celsius rise in body temperature up to 105°F (40.5°C); with further rise in body temperature, heart rate may decrease due to debility of heart muscle. Tachycardia in fever occurs due to increase in metabolic rate of SA node which directly increases its excitability.
Sympathetic activity: Factors which increase sympathetic activity also lead to tachycardia, e.g. hypovolaemic shock (as a reflex response to low arterial pressure), exercise and hyperthyroidism. For details, see page 245.

Sinus Bradycardia (Fig. 4.2.22D) is characterized by a normal sinus rhythm except for decreased heart rate (i.e. increased P–R interval but regular R–R interval). Bradycardia is labelled when heart rate becomes less than 60 beats/min.

- Sinus bradycardia is more commonly seen in highly trained endurance athletes due to increased vagal lone; sometimes it may be abnormal.

Applied Aspects

Carotid sinus syndrome. In patients with carotid sinus syndrome, the baroreceptors present in carotid sinus are very sensitive; even mild pressure on the neck elicits strong baroreceptor reflex to cause bradycardia; sometimes the heart may stop for 5–10 seconds. For baroreceptor reflex details, see page 330.

Applied Aspects—cont'd

Sick sinus syndrome. Sick sinus syndrome refers to a condition characterized by marked bradycardia accompanied by dizziness and syncope.

Causes. Causes of sick sinus syndrome include:

- Sinus bradycardia that does not improve with sympathetic stimulation or vagal inhibition
- SA nodal block (see below)
- Sinus arrest, i.e. complete stoppage of sinus discharge

Treatment. When the condition causes severe symptoms, implantation of artificial pacemaker. Sinus node dysfunction accounts for over half of the pacemaker implants.

- *Pacemakers* are the electronic devices that sense and pace the activity of the chambers of the heart by programming in most physiological way to maintain the cardiac output. The artificial pacemakers are the stimulators planted underneath the skin and electrodes are usually connected to right ventricles to provide rhythmical impulses to ventricles.

Conduction Disturbances (Heart Blocks)

Heart blocks refer to slowing down or blockage of cardiac impulse (generated from SA node) along the cardiac conductive pathway. Conduction blockage may occur as:

- SA nodal block
- AV nodal block
- Bundle branch block

SA nodal block or the so-called SA block is characterized by the blockage of impulse conduction from SA node to atria.

- It occurs in the elderly and in patients recovering from coronary artery occlusion.
- It occurs suddenly, and initially the heart stops (i.e. neither atria nor ventricles contract for a while). After an interval of approximately two cardiac cycles, the AV node becomes the pacemaker, and the heart starts functioning again. This is called *AV nodal rhythm*.
- SA block may manifest as *sick sinus syndrome* (described above).
- AV nodal rhythm, also called *junctional rhythm* (Fig. 4.2.23), is characterized by inverted P wave and normal QRS complex, and the rate is slower than that of sinus rhythm.

AV nodal block AV nodal blockage may occur as *incomplete heart* block (which includes first-degree and second-degree heart blocks) or complete heart block (third-degree heart block). AV nodal blockages are associated with the following conditions:

- *Coronary insufficiency* can cause AV nodal ischaemia.
- *Compression of AV node* by scar tissue or by calcification can cause AV nodal ischaemia.

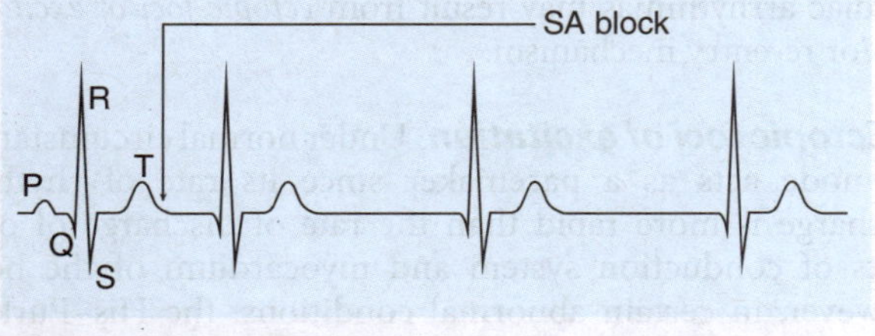

Fig. 4.2.23 AV nodal rhythm seen in SA node blockage. AV, atrioventricular; SA, sinoatrial.

- *Inflammation of AV node* results in depression of conduction of impulse from atria to ventricles.
- *Vagal excitation* results due to strong stimulation of baroreceptors as in carotid sinus syndrome.

First-degree AV nodal block First-degree AV nodal (or heart) block is characterized by slowing of conduction at the level of AV node. Although all the atrial impulses reach the ventricles, the PR interval is abnormally long, i.e. more than 0.21 second (Fig. 4.2.24B), but seldom increases more than 0.30 second.

Second-degree AV nodal block In second-degree AV nodal block (Fig. 4.2.24C and D), not all atrial impulses are conducted to ventricles. It is usually associated with organic heart diseases. Consequently, there may be one ventricular contraction after every two, three or four atrial contractions producing the so-called 2:1, 3:1 or 4:1 block (*constant block*). Other forms of second-degree heart blocks are as follows:

Wenckebach phenomenon (Mobitz type I block) It is characterized by a progressive lengthening of the P–R interval in successive beats and finally a failure of one impulse to be transmitted.

Periodic block (Mobitz type II block) It is characterized by an occasional failure of conduction that results in an atrial to ventricular rate of, e.g. 6:5 or 8:7. The P–R interval is constant.

Third-degree (complete) AV nodal block. In third-degree complete AV block, no impulse from atria can pass to the ventricles.

- The ventricles start beating at their own rhythm (about 40 beats/min) called idioventricular rhythm.
- The atria, however, continue to beat at the normal sinus rhythm of about 72 beats/min. Thus, ECG shows that there is complete dissociation between P waves and QRS complexes called *AV dissociation* (Fig. 4.2.24E).
- Third-degree block is *caused* by organic heart diseases, septal MI and damage to bundle of His during surgical repair of congenital interventricular septal defects.
- Third-degree block may be associated with prolonged ventricular standstill (asystole) until a ventricular focus begins firing.

Important Note

The asystole, lasting for 1 minute, may result in cerebral ischaemia producing dizziness and fainting (syncope); the condition is termed *Stokes–Adams syndrome*. Even death may also occur due to prolonged cerebral ischaemia.

Treatment Mostly these patients are provided with artificial pacemakers.

Bundle branch block refers to conduction blocks in one or more branches of the bundle of His.

- In this condition, excitation passes normally down the bundle on the intact side and then sweeps back through the muscle to activate the ventricle on the blocked side.
- Therefore, the ventricular rate is normal, but the QRS complexes are prolonged (beyond 0.12 second) and deformed

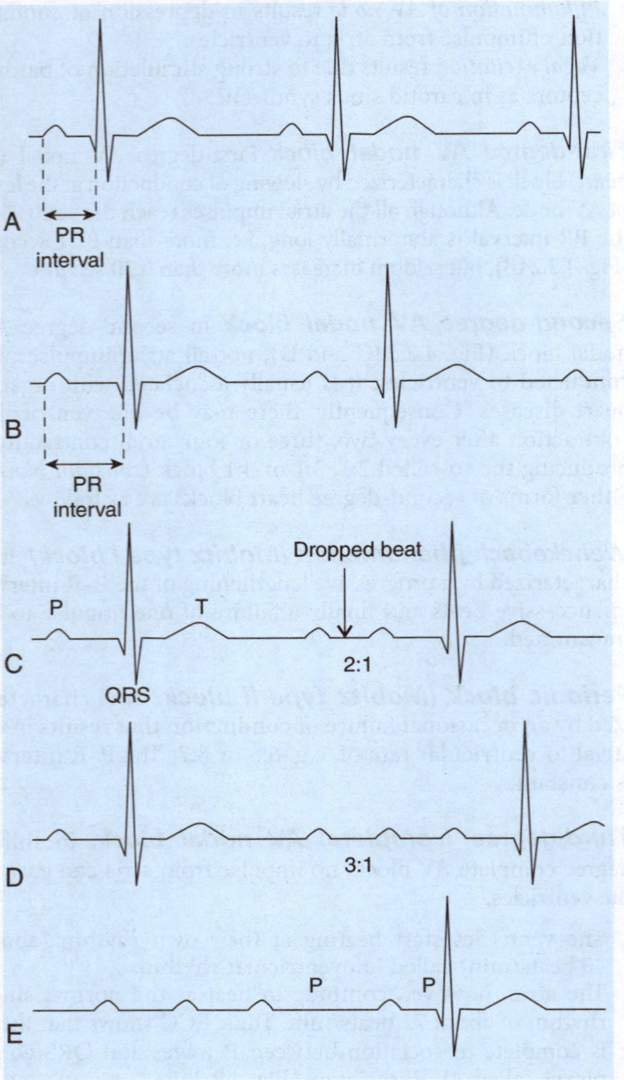

Fig. 4.2.24 Various types of AV nodal blocks: **A**, normal sinus rhythm; **B**, first-degree AV block; **C**, second-degree AV block (2:1); **D**, 3:1 block; and **E**, complete AV block (third degree). AV, atrioventricular.

(Fig. 4.2.25). The characteristic features of the branch involved are as follows:

Right bundle branch block Right bundle branch block (RBBB) may occur in otherwise healthy individuals or secondary to chronic pulmonary disease. The activation of right ventricle is delayed and ECG may show features of right-axis deviation (RAD; Fig. 4.2.25A).

Left bundle branch block LBB block is usually associated with organic heart disease. It is best diagnosed using left precordial leads (Fig. 4.2.25B).

Hemiblock or fascicular block Hemiblock or fascicular block refers to block in either anterior or posterior fascicle of LBB. Left anterior hemiblock (LAH) produces abnormal left-axis deviation (LAD) in ECG, whereas left posterior hemiblock (LPH) produces abnormal RAD (for detail see page 254).

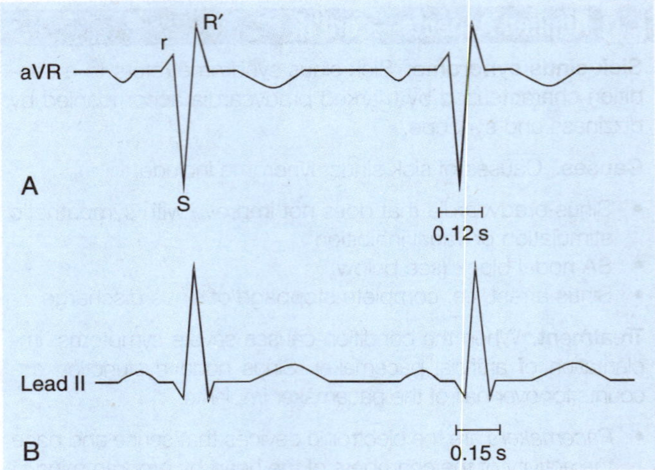

Fig. 4.2.25 Electrocardiogram characteristics in bundle branch blocks: **A**, right bundle branch block; and **B**, left bundle branch block.

Bifascicular block The term bifascicular block refers to:

- Conduction disturbances below AV node, in which the RBB and one or two fascicles (anterior or posterior) of the LBB are involved. Bifascicular block presents with the following ECG patterns:
  - RBBB with left anterior fascicular block (LAFB) manifests as LAD.
  - RBBB with left posterior fascicular block (LPFB) manifests as RAD.

Note: HBE is useful for detailed analysis of the site of block when there is a defect in the conduction system.

Ectopic Cardiac Rhythm

Ectopic cardiac rhythm refers to abnormal cardiac excitation produced by either an ectopic focus or a re-entry phenomenon. Ectopic cardiac rhythm includes the following conditions:

A. Atrial arrhythmias Atrial arrhythmias are as follows:

1. Atrial extrasystole
2. Paroxysmal atrial tachycardia (PAT)
3. Atrial flutter
4. Atrial fibrillation

B. Ventricular arrhythmias Ventricular arrhythmias are as follows:

1. Ventricular extrasystole
2. Paroxysmal ventricular tachycardia
3. Ventricular fibrillation

Mechanisms of development of cardiac arrhythmias

Cardiac arrhythmias may result from *ectopic foci of excitation* and/or re-entry mechanism.

1. Ectopic foci of excitation Under normal circumstances, SA node acts as a pacemaker since its rate of rhythmic discharge is more rapid than the rate of discharge of other parts of conduction system and myocardium of the heart. However, in certain abnormal conditions, the His–Purkinje fibres or the myocardial fibres become hyperexcitable and discharge spontaneously. In these conditions, increased automaticity of the heart is said to be present. The site in the heart which becomes hyperexcitable is called an *ectopic focus* which may behave as:

Single discharge: When the irritable ectopic focus discharges once, an *extrasystole* or *premature* beat is caused before the next normal beat. Depending on the site of ectopic focus, the premature beat may be atrial, nodal or ventricular.

Repetitive discharge: If the ectopic focus discharges impulses repeatedly at a rate higher than that of SA node, tachycardia with very high rate (tachyarrhythmia) results. Depending on the rate and rhythm and the site of ectopic focus, the tachyarrhythmias are named as:

- Paroxysmal tachycardia (atrial, nodal and ventricular)
- Atrial flutter
- Atrial fibrillation
- Ventricular fibrillation

2. Re-entry mechanism Re-entry mechanism or the circus movement refers to a phenomenon in which the wave of excitation propagates repeatedly (continuously) within a closed circuit. It is a more common cause of tachyarrhythmias. Re-entry of excitation wave is known to occur under two situations: (1) in the presence of transient block in the conduction pathway and (2) in the presence of an abnormal extra bundle of conducting tissue called bundle of Kent.

Re-entry due to transient block in the conduction system Normally, during depolarization of a ring of cardiac tissue, the impulse spreads in both directions of the ring (Fig. 4.2.26A) and the tissue behind each branch of the impulse is refractory and thus the impulse cannot go down the other side.

- When there is a transient block on one side, the impulse can go down on the other side of ring (Fig. 4.2.26B), because this portion is not depolarized and so not refractory.
- If the transient block is worn off, the impulse from retrograde direction is conducted through this (previously blocked) area and then continues to circle indefinitely. This phenomenon is called circus movement or re-entry phenomenon (Fig. 4.2.26C).
- The site of re-entry keeps on producing impulses continuously. If the re-entry is in AV node, the re-entrant activity depolarizes the atrium and the resulting atrial beat is called an *echo beat*. In addition, the re-entrant activity in the node propagates back down to ventricles producing paroxysmal nodal tachycardia. The re-entrant activity can also become established in atrial muscle fibres (producing atrial tachycardias, flutter or fibrillation) and in ventricular muscle fibres (producing ventricular tachycardia or ventricular fibrillation).

Re-entrant activity in the presence of bundle of Kent Bundle of Kent is an abnormal extra bundle of conducting tissues present in some individuals. This bundle connects the atria and ventricles directly, so the conduction is very rapid than through the regular conductive system.

- If a transient block develops in the normal conductive system, the impulse from SA node reaches the ventricle through the bundle of Kent and produces excitation. If the blockage in the normal conduction system wears off, the excitation wave from the ventricle travels in the opposite direction and re-enters the AV node and a circus movement is established (Fig. 4.2.27).
- This re-entrant activity produces echo beat in atria and nodal paroxysmal tachycardia or the so-called supraventricular tachycardia.
- The nodal paroxysmal tachycardia occurring in patients with bundle of Kent is called *Wolff–Parkinson–White syndrome*, producing short PR interval and prolonged slurred QRS deflection but normal PJ interval (start of P wave to end of QRS complex).

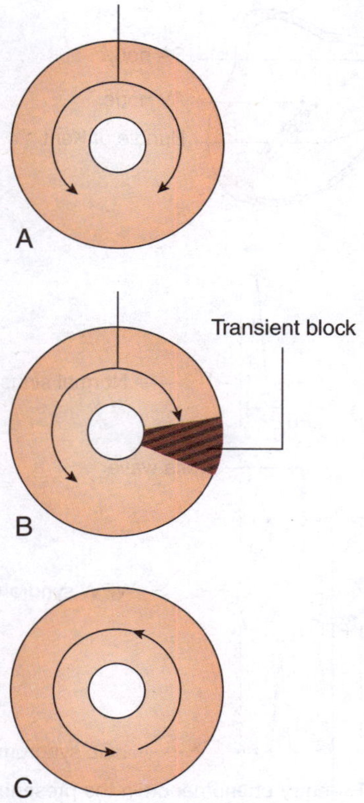

Fig. 4.2.26 Re-entry phenomenon or circus movements, a cause of cardiac arrhythmias: **A**, normal depolarization of a ring cardiac tissue; **B**, spread of wave of excitation in presence of transient block; and **C**, circus movement.

Salient Features of Cardiac Arrhythmias

Extrasystole Extrasystole (premature beat, premature contraction or ectopic beat) refers to the contraction of the heart prior to the time that normal contraction would have been expected. It is caused by some ectopic focus in the atria or ventricles and thus the premature beat may be atrial or ventricular.

Causes of extrasystole: The main cause of ectopic foci is mechanical irritation, which occurs due to ischaemia of local area of the heart, calcified plaques, cardiac catheterization and local toxic irritation caused by drugs, nicotine, caffeine, etc.

Atrial extrasystole (premature beat) Atrial premature beat is caused by an ectopic focus in the atrium which becomes pacemaker for one beat. Atrial premature beats may

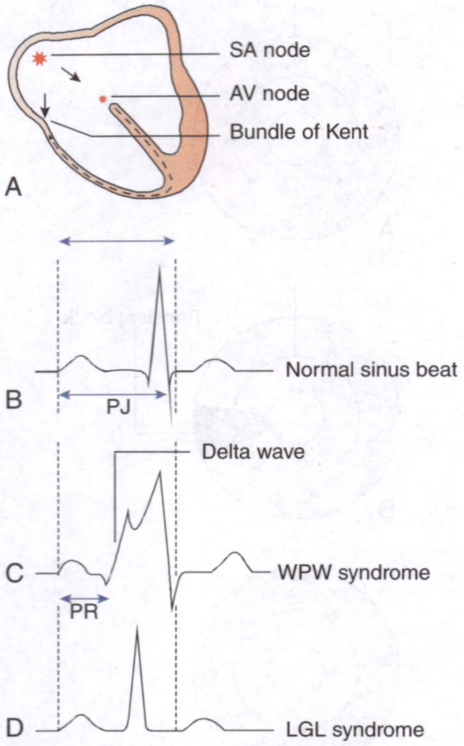

Fig. 4.2.27 **A**, Re-entry phenomenon in the presence of bundle of Kent; **B**, normal electrocardiogram; **C**, record in a patient with bundle of Kent showing short PR interval, wide and slurred QRS complex with normal PJ interval (Wolff–Parkinson–White [WPW] syndrome); and **D**, Lown–Ganong–Levine (LGL) syndrome.

occur frequently in healthy persons; due to lack of sleep, increased consumption of coffee and smoking.

ECG appearance (Fig. 4.2.28B) of atrial premature beat is characterized by:

- A premature P wave occurs early and has an aberrant configuration and an abnormal short PR interval because of the different path of atrial depolarization.
- QRS complex and T wave are normal.
- Interval between premature beat and next succeeding beat is slightly prolonged called compensatory pause.
- The subsequent cardiac rhythm is shifted and reset, because the premature beat discharges the SA node, which then repolarizes and fires after the normal interval.

Significance: Since atrial extrasystole occurs normally, the patient may or may not be aware of an occasional irregularity in the cardiac rhythm.

Ventricular extrasystole can arise from any portion of the ventricular myocardium and occasionally occur in otherwise healthy individuals. Frequently ventricular premature beats occur with many forms of heart disease, especially coronary artery disease (because ischaemia increases the irritability of the myocardium).

ECG appearance of ventricular premature beat is characterized by (Fig. 4.2.28C):

- P wave preceding the QRS complex is absent.
- QRS complex is prolonged and bizarre shaped because of the slow spread of the impulse from the ectopic focus through the ventricular muscle to the rest of the ventricle.

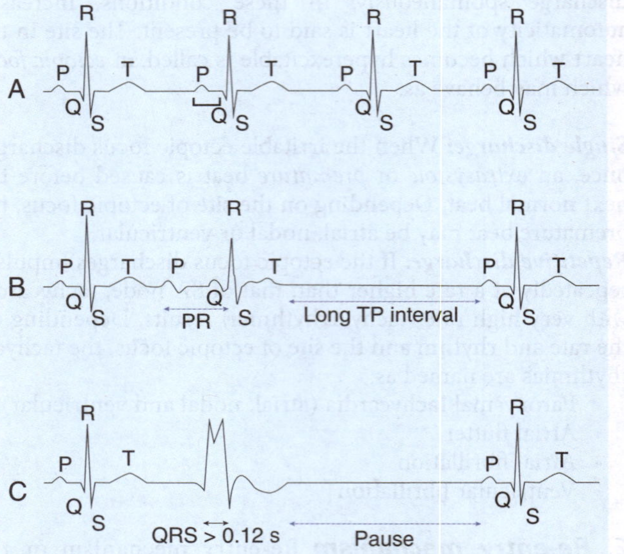

Fig. 4.2.28 Electrocardiographic record in extrasystole: **A**, normal ECG; **B**, ECG with atrial premature beat (atrial extrasystole); and **C**, ECG with ventricular premature beat. ECG, electrocardiography.

- T wave is usually appositely directed from the QRS complex.
- Compensatory pause is often long. Since retrograde transmission of depolarization to the atria usually does not occur with premature ventricular beat, so, the atrial rate remains unaltered. The atrial depolarization that follows the premature ventricular beat arrives while the AV node is still refractory and, therefore, it is not conducted to the ventricles, creating a pause in the ventricular rhythm. This pause is usually fully compensatory so that R–R interval of the beat preceding the premature ventricular beat interval together equals two normal cycle lengths. Thus, the ventricular premature beats do not interrupt the regular discharge of the SA node, whereas atrial premature beats often interrupt and 'reset' the normal rhythm.

Important Note

Beat following ventricular premature beat: It is usually stronger than the normal because of the added stroke volume and thus usually detected by the patient.

Interpolated beats: When the patient's sinus rhythm is slow, a premature ventricular beat may occur without altering the normal R–R interval. Such a premature ventricular beat is termed an interpolated beat.

Pulse deficit Ventricles contract ahead of time in atrial and ventricular premature beats. Sometimes by that time, ventricles are not filled with blood and stroke volume output during the contraction is therefore decreased or even absent. During such a contraction, pulse wave passing to periphery may be so weak that it is not felt at the radial artery. A deficit in the number of pulses felt in the radial pulse in relation to the number of contraction in the heart is called pulse deficit.

Atrial arrhythmias

Atrial tachycardia Atrial tachycardia (Fig. 4.2.29A) occurs when an atrial site (outside the SA node) becomes the dominant pacemaker. It is characterized by very regular rates ranging from 140 to 220 beats/min. Atrial tachycardia may be caused by overindulgence in caffeine, nicotine or alcohol and may also occur during anxiety attack.

Paroxysmal atrial tachycardia PAT, as the name indicates, occurs in paroxysms, which usually begin suddenly, and lasts for few seconds. It may result from discharge of a single *ectopic site* or a *re-entry phenomenon* (described on page 259).

ECG appearance of PAT is characterized by an inverted P wave before each QRS complex, and this P wave is partially superimposed onto the normal T wave of the preceding beat (Fig. 4.2.29B).

Atrial flutter Atrial flutter is said to occur with atrial rates of 220–350 beats/min. During atrial flutter, AV node is unable to transmit all of the atrial impulses and therefore the ventricular rate may be half, one-third or one-fourth of the atrial rates. Like atrial tachycardia, atrial flutter may result from either a single ectopic focus or a re-entry phenomenon.

ECG appearance in atrial flutter: The P wave is strong and QRS–T complex follows once after two P waves or three P waves (2:1 or 3:1 rhythm).

Atrial fibrillation Atrial fibrillation (Fig. 4.2.29C) is characterized by a totally irregular, rapid rate (350–500 beats/min). In it, there occurs contraction of only small portion of the atrial musculature at one time because large portion of the atria is still in refractory period. *Ventricular rate* is completely irregular because only a fraction of the atrial impulses that reach the AV node are transmitted to the ventricles.

ECG appearance is characterized by:

- Small irregular oscillations called F waves are present. There are no recognizable P waves.

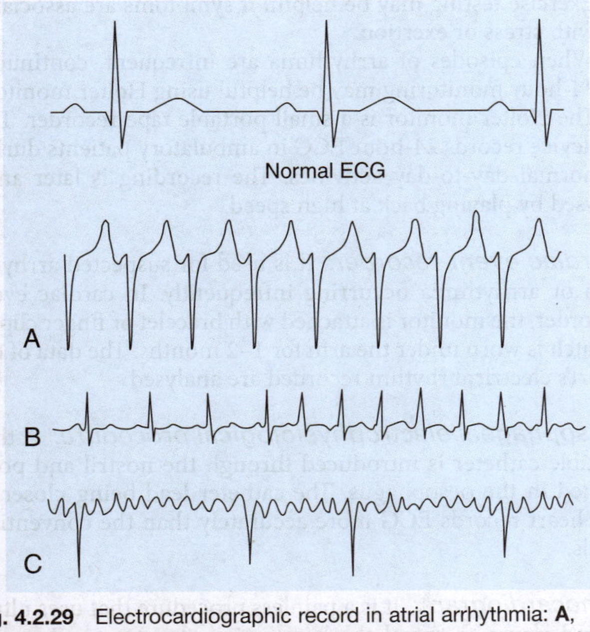

Fig. 4.2.29 Electrocardiographic record in atrial arrhythmia: **A**, atrial tachycardia; **B**, paroxysmal atrial tachycardia – onset in middle of record (lead I); and **C**, atrial fibrillation.

- R-R interval is irregularly irregular.
- QRS complex and T wave are normal because the impulses that are transmitted through the AV node are conducted normally through the ventricles.

Causes: Atrial fibrillations are frequently associated with enlarged atria secondary to AV valve diseases.

Treatment: The treatment includes medication, electric shock therapy to set heart rhythm, catheter procedure (cardioversion) and invasive surgery in the form of ablation.

- *Medication* include β-blockers, calcium channel blockers, antiarrhythmic drugs and anticoagulants.
- *Procedure* includes cardioversion.
- *Surgery/catheter procedure* includes ablation of AV node.

Atrial fibrillations can be converted back to normal rhythm by cardioversion/defibrillation. A strong single electric shock of alternating current is passed through the heart for a fraction of a second. All action potentials stop and the heart remains quiescent for few seconds (3–5 seconds) or refractoriness of the heart occurs. After that, the heart begins to beat with normal rhythm.

Complications: Long-term fibrillation is associated with *thrombi* in the atrial appendages.

Nodal arrhythmia include:

Nodal paroxysmal tachycardia Nodal paroxysmal tachycardia is similar to atrial tachycardia and may be indistinguishable on ECG. It is called *supraventricular tachycardia*.

Signs and symptoms include palpitation, pain in the chest, sweating, shortness of breath and fatigue.

ECG appearance: Almost normal QRS–T complexes are present, but P wave is either totally missing or obscured; nodal paroxysmal tachycardia can be distinguished from the paroxysmal ventricular tachycardia by HBE. In supraventricular tachycardia, there is a His bundle (H) deflection, whereas in ventricular tachycardia, there is none.

Treatment includes:

- For sudden episodes of SVT, vagal manoeuvres such as bearing down, coughing or holding the breath
- Medication such as antiarrhythmic drugs, β-blockers and calcium channel blockers
- Catheter ablation (in symptomatic patients, first line of treatment is catheter ablation because this is less invasive procedure than surgical ablation)

Wolff–Parkinson–White syndrome Wolff–Parkinson–White syndrome (LGL; Fig. 4.2.27C), also known as accelerated AV conduction, refers to occurrence of repeated attacks of nodal paroxysmal tachycardia due to presence of bundle of Kent. The *bundle of Kent* is aberrant musculature or nodal tissue which connects the atria and ventricles directly. This bundle conducts more rapidly than the slowly conducting AV node, and one ventricle is excited early. The presence of *bundle of Kent* rapidly establishes re-entry phenomenon (circus movement) in prone patients (see page 259).

Lown–Ganong–Levine syndrome Lown–Ganong–Levine (LGL) syndrome (Fig. 4.2.27D) is characterized by attacks of paroxysmal supraventricular tachycardia, usually nodal tachycardia in individuals with short PR intervals and normal

QRS complexes. In this condition, depolarization presumably passes from the atria to the ventricles via an *aberrant bundle* that bypasses the AV node but enters the intraventricular conducting system distal to node.

Signs and symptoms are as follows:

- Patients with LGL syndrome usually have long history of palpitation, which begins in early adulthood and becomes less frequent with age.
- Palpitation usually accompanied by angina pectoris, dizziness, light-headedness and shortness of breath is present.

Treatment mainly consists of medication to prevent tachyarrhythmia.

Ventricular arrhythmias include

Paroxysmal ventricular tachycardia Paroxysmal ventricular tachycardia occurs when a ventricular site discharges rapidly and repetitively, usually as a result of *re-entry phenomenon*. Alterations in vagal tone (by carotid sinus massage or Valsalva manoeuvre) do not affect ventricular tachycardia because the ventricles do not receive any efferent vagal innervation.

Causes: Ventricular tachycardias are usually associated with serious heart disease or drug toxicity.

ECG appearance is characterized by (Fig. 4.2.30B):

- Wide, bizarre QRS complexes that occur at rapid rate
- Usually indistinguishable P waves

Significance: Ventricular tachycardia is more serious because cardiac output is decreased; sustained ventricular tachycardia can be life-threatening when it degenerates into ventricular fibrillation.

Ventricular fibrillation Ventricular fibrillation occurs when small segments of ventricular myocardium show rapid, irregular ineffective contractions. In this condition, cardiac output is zero and so the peripheral pulse is absent. ECG is must to differentiate ventricular fibrillation from the cardiac standstill.

Causes: Ventricular fibrillation is very common during electric shock and during ischaemia of conductive system. Other

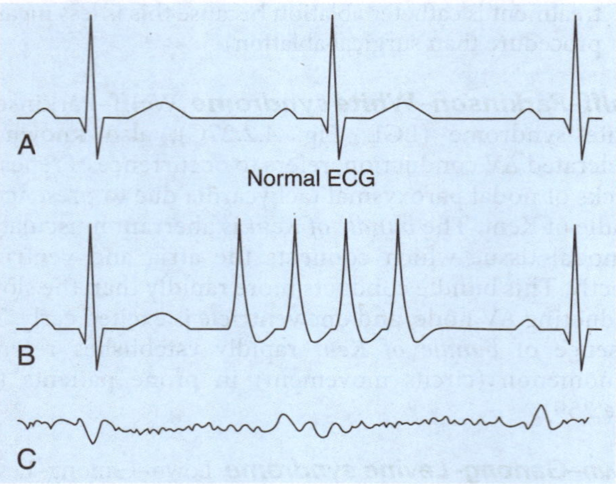

Fig. 4.2.30 Electrocardiographic record in ventricular arrhythmias: **A**, normal; **B**, paroxysmal ventricular tachycardia; and **C**, ventricular fibrillation.

causes are coronary occlusion, trauma to the heart, chloroform anaesthesia and improper handling of the heart during cardiac surgery.

ECG appearance (Fig. 4.2.30C) is characterized by:

- Undulating waves of varying frequency and amplitude. The voltage of the ECG waves in ventricular fibrillation is about 0.2–0.5 mV or less.
- Ventricular premature beats are usually seen as the precipitating cause, one of which falls on the *vulnerable period* of the T wave (i.e. the interval near the peak of the T wave when the ventricle is partially repolarized). A premature beat during the vulnerable period produces fibrillation because the chances of re-entry occurring are more.

Significance: Ventricular fibrillation is the most common cause of sudden death in patients with myocardial infarcts.

Treatment: Cardiopulmonary resuscitation must be started immediately to prevent tissue death. For details, see page 461.

Immediate electric or electronic defibrillation (cardioversion) should be performed.

- The cardioversion/defibrillation is done by applying electrodes directly to two sides of the heart or on the chest wall using 110 V of 60 cycles at alternating current for 0.1 second or 1000 V of direct current for thousandth of a second.

Techniques for Evaluation of Arrhythmia

1. Electrocardiographic monitoring Electrocardiographic monitoring is the ideal way of establishing a correlation between symptoms and a rhythm disturbance, but this is not always easy because symptoms are usually sporadic.

Stress ECG: In this test, a person walks or runs on the treadmill and continuous ECG is recorded. Gradually the speed is increased till the patient is exhausted or predictive heart rate is achieved. Any significant change in the ECG pattern (especially ST segment) is suggestive of ischaemia.

- Exercise testing may be helpful if symptoms are associated with stress or exertion.
  When episodes of arrhythmia are infrequent, continuous 24-hour monitoring may be helpful using Holter monitor. The Holter monitor is a small portable tape recorder. This device records 24-hour ECG in ambulatory patients during normal day-to-day activities. The recording is later analysed by playing back at high speed.

Cardiac event recorder: It is used for suspected arrhythmia or arrhythmia occurring infrequently. In cardiac event recorder, the monitor is attached with bracelet or finger clip or a patch is worn under the arm for 1–2 months. The data of the heart's electrical rhythm recorded are analysed.

Oesophageal electrophysiological procedure: A thin flexible catheter is introduced through the nostril and positioned in the oesophagus. The catheter lead being closer to the heart records ECG more accurately than the convention leads.

Echocardiogram: It is a painless procedure that uses ultrasound waves to reveal the heart's size, structure and movements and provides useful information.

2. Heart rate variability Heart rate variability (HRV) refers to beat-to-beat variation of heart rate. The R–R interval variations during resting condition represent a fine tuning of beat-to-beat control mechanisms. HRV reflects fluctuations rather than absolute levels of sympathetic and parasympathetic impulse. The analysis of beat-to-beat variation in heart rate is used to investigate sympathovagal imbalance, i.e. integrity of autonomic activity and vulnerability to various cardiovascular disorders resulting from autonomic imbalance. HRV is recorded by ECG LII on Polyrite D system and its time domain and frequency domain variables are analysed. Details of HRV are beyond the scope of the book.

3. Electrophysiological testing Electrophysiological testing is intracardiac; electrocardiographic recordings are useful in diagnosis and management of complex arrhythmia.

In this procedure, under local anaesthesia, temporary electrode catheters are introduced through peripheral vein into the heart using fluoroscope. These electrodes are then positioned in the atria/ventricles or both. They record the heart's electrical signals and map the path of electrical rhythm.

4. Autonomic testing Autonomic testing is an important component of evaluation in patients with recurrent syncope. It can be done by simple head-up tilt (HUT) test, also called tilt table test.

Tilt table testing Tilt table testing is based on the fact that in upright posture, there is venous pooling in lower limbs that reflexly increases heart rate and vasoconstriction (compensatory mechanism). HUT testing can identify the syncope due to vasovagal/autonomic imbalance.

Treatment of Arrhythmia

1. Mechanical measures Mechanical measures are used to interrupt the attack. These include Valsalva manoeuvre and carotid sinus massage. These manoeuvres stimulate the vagus nerve, delay A–V conduction and block the re-entry mechanism, and ultimately terminate arrhythmia.

2. Antiarrhythmic drugs Antiarrhythmic drugs have limited efficiency due to frequent side effects. Broadly, antiarrhythmic drugs are divided into four classes based on their electropharmacological actions:

Class I agents block membrane sodium channels, thus slowing conduction and prolonging the refractoriness. These include quinine and procainamide.
Class II agents are β-adrenergic blockers, which decrease automaticity and prolong AV conduction. Examples are propranolol and metoprolol.
Class III agents block K^+ channels and prolong repolarization and QT interval.
Class IV agents are calcium channel blockers, which decrease automaticity and A–V conduction, e.g. verapamil.

3. Radiofrequency ablation Cardiac catheter with electrodes attached to its tip is passed into the chambers of the heart, and exact location of ectopic focus or accessory bundle responsible for arrhythmia is identified. The ablation can be done by applying radiofrequency band (300–3000 kHz) with catheter tip. Radiofrequency is particularly useful in conditions that cause supraventricular tachycardias, Wolff–Parkinson–White syndrome and atrial flutter.

The radiofrequency generates energy for biomedical applications like coagulation and cauterization of the tissue.

Myocardial Infarction (MI)

MI refers to the ischaemic necrosis of a part of myocardium which occurs when coronary blood flow ceases or is reached below a critical level (see page 348). The ECG is very useful for diagnosing and localizing areas of MI.

ECG appearance

The ECG undergoes a series of changes following the MI. These changes must be recorded daily with ECG tracing for diagnostic purpose. The hallmark of acute MI is as follows:

- *Elevation of ST segment* (Fig. 4.2.31, LI) in the leads overlying the area of infarct
- *Depression of ST segment* (Fig. 4.2.31, LII) in the leads on the opposite side of area of infarct

ECG appearance in old cases of myocardial infarct is characterized by:

- Return of ST segment to normal
- Appearance of Q wave (Fig. 4.2.31, LI and LII) in some of the leads in which it was not previously present
- An increase in the size of normal Q wave in some of the other leads

Physiological basis of ECG changes in acute myocardial infarction The alterations in ECG pattern seen in acute MI are attributed to *injury current* which flows from the affected to the unaffected part of myocardium. This happens because of the fact that the affected part of myocardium gets depolarized partly or completely but does not get repolarized rapidly. The three major abnormalities that cause ECG changes (ST-segment elevation) in acute MI are as follows:

1. Decline in resting membrane potential The ischaemic necrosis of the myocardial fibres results in breakdown of cell membrane producing increased K^+ efflux and increased Na^+ influx. Therefore, inside of the infarcted cells becomes less negative as compared with the unaffected area. Therefore, during ventricular diastole, the *current flows into the infarct* from the unaffected area (Fig. 4.2.32B). This results in a depression of TQ segment of the ECG in the leads

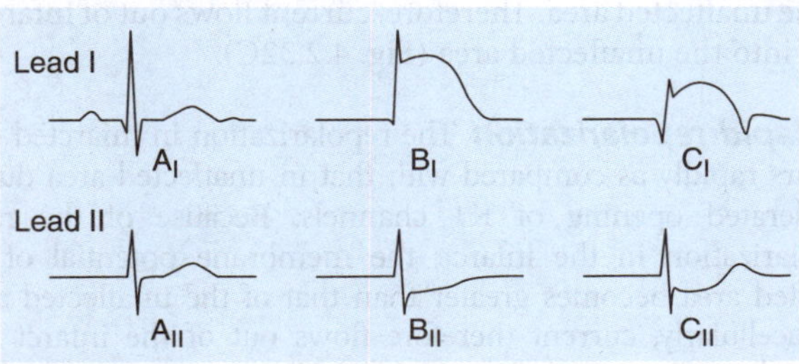

Fig. 4.2.31 Electrocardiographic record in anterior wall ischaemia in lead I and lead II, respectively: A_I and A_{II}, normal ECG; B_I and B_{II}, ECG within few hours of ischaemia, note ST-segment elevation in lead I and depression in lead II (reciprocal); and C_I and C_{II}, ECG after several weeks, note that ST segment returns to normal and Q wave appears. ECG, electrocardiography.

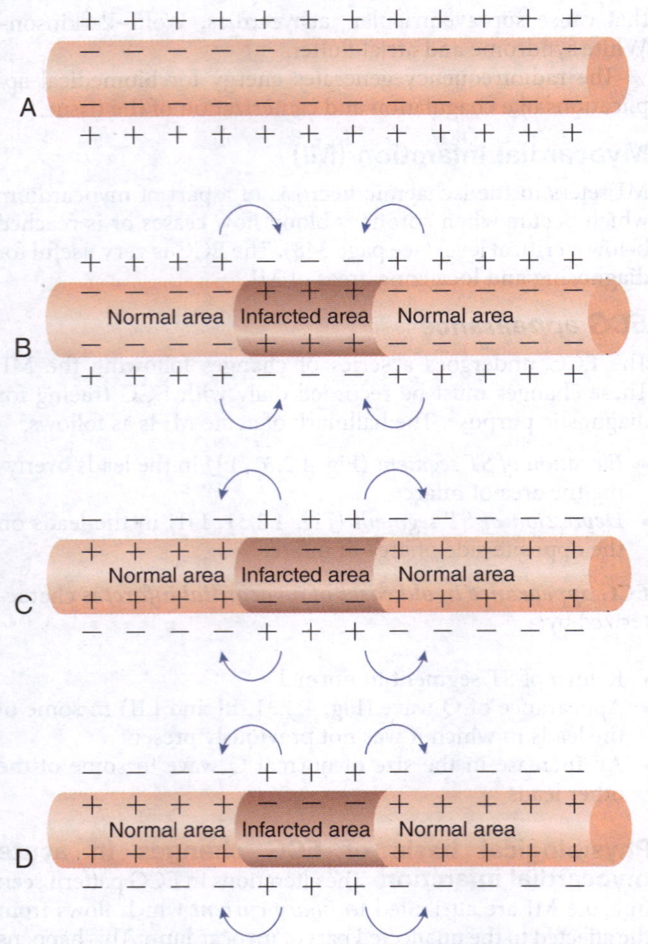

Fig. 4.2.32 Physiological basis of ECG changes (ST-segment elevation) in acute myocardial infarction: **A**, normal resting state; **B**, decline in resting membrane potential in infarct area as compared with that in normal neighbouring (unaffected) region; **C**, delayed depolarization of infarct area as compared with that of neighbouring areas; and **D**, rapid repolarization of infarct area in comparison to that of normal neighbouring areas. ECG, electrocardiography.

overlying the infarcted area. However, the electronic arrangement in electrocardiographic recorders is such that TQ segment depression is recorded as ST-segment elevation.

2. Delayed depolarization Delayed depolarization of infarcted cells causes the infarcted area to be positive relative to the unaffected area. Therefore, current flows out of infarcted area into the unaffected area (Fig. 4.2.32C).

3. Rapid repolarization The repolarization in infarcted cells occurs rapidly as compared with that in unaffected area due to accelerated opening of K^+ channels. Because of the rapid repolarization in the infarct, the membrane potential of the affected area becomes greater than that of the unaffected area. Extracellularly, current therefore flows out of the infarct into normal unaffected area (Fig. 4.2.32D). This current flows towards electrodes over the injured area, causing increased positivity between the S and T waves of ECG. Consequently, leads on the opposite side of the heart show ST-segment depression.

Physiological basis of ECG changes in old cases of myocardial infarction After some days or weeks of infarction, the dead myocardium and scar tissue become electrically silent. Therefore, the affected area becomes negative relative to the unaffected normal myocardium during systole, and it fails to contribute its share of positivity to the electrocardiographic complexes. The occurrence of Q wave in some leads (which normally lack) and deepening of Q wave in other leads is one of the manifestations of this negativity.

Localization of area of myocardial infarction

Anterior MI

- Leads showing changes of MI are LI, aVL and V_3–V_5.
- Leads showing reciprocal changes are LII, LIII and aVF.

Posterior (inferior) MI

- Leads showing changes of MI include LII, LIII and aVF.
- Leads showing reciprocal changes are LI, aVR, aVL and V_1–V_6.

Lateral MI

- Leads showing changes of MI include LI, aVL and V_6.
- Leads showing reciprocal change are LII, LIII, aVF and V_1.

Septal MI

- Leads showing changes of MI are V_1–V_3.

Complications Complications of MI are ventricular arrhythmias which mainly occur due to re-entrant activity during the first 30 minutes of infarction and increased automaticity after 12 hours.

Important Notes

- The infarcts which affect epicardial part of myocardium damage the sympathetic nerves resulting in denervation hypersensitivity to catecholamines in the area beyond the infarct.
- On the other hand, endocardial lesions interrupt vagal activity; therefore, unopposed sympathetic fibres activity results.

Ventricular Hypertrophy

Ventricular hypertrophy occurs when the work of the ventricle is increased sufficiently. In ventricular hypertrophy, the number of myocardial cells remains the same, but the diameter of the individual cells increases, raising the diffusion distance for O_2 and other metabolites.

Left Ventricular Hypertrophy

Left ventricular hypertrophy (LVH) occurs in patients with systemic hypertension or aortic valve stenosis. Right ventricular hypertrophy (RVH) occurs in patients with pulmonary hypertension, pulmonary valve stenosis and some congenital heart disease.

ECG appearance ECG appearance is characterized by (Fig. 4.2.18B) the following:

R wave: There is direct correlation between the thickness of ventricular wall and the height of R wave in the overlying leads. Therefore:

- In LVH, the R wave is tall in leads I, aVL, V_5 and V_6.
- In RVH, the R wave is tall in leads III, aVR, V_1 and V_2. For detail see page 250.

QRS duration is increased slightly due to the increased muscle mass. It is usually less than 0.12 second, but occasionally may exceed this value.

MEA shows (Fig. 4.2.18A):

- LAD in LVH
- RAD in RVH

Effect of Changes in the Ionic Composition of Blood on Electrical Activity of Heart

The electrical activity of the heart depends on the distribution of ions like Na^+, K^+ and Ca^{2+} in the ECF. Therefore, changes in the ECF concentration of these ions will affect the potentials of myocardial fibres and produce changes in the ECG described as follows:

Plasma Levels of Sodium Low plasma (ECF) levels of Na^+ may be associated with low-voltage ECG complexes.

Plasma Levels of Potassium Depending on the levels of plasma K^+, the following ECG changes are seen:

With Normal Plasma Levels of K^+ (4–5.5 mEq/L)

The normal ECG tracings (Fig. 4.2.33A) are produced with PR interval = 0.16 second, QRS interval = 0.06 second and QT interval = 0.4 second.

Hyperkalaemia Hyperkalaemia, i.e. increase in plasma K^+, is a very dangerous and potentially lethal condition because of its effects on the heart.

In hyperkalaemia with plasma K^+ ± 7.0 mEq/L, the PR and QRS intervals are within normal limits. The T wave become tall and peaked (Fig. 4.2.33B), which is a manifestation of altered repolarization.

In hyperkalaemia with plasma K^+ levels 8.5 mEq/L, the ECG shows (Fig. 4.2.33C):

- Broad and slurred QRS complex with a QRS interval of 0.2 second occurs due to paralysis of atria.

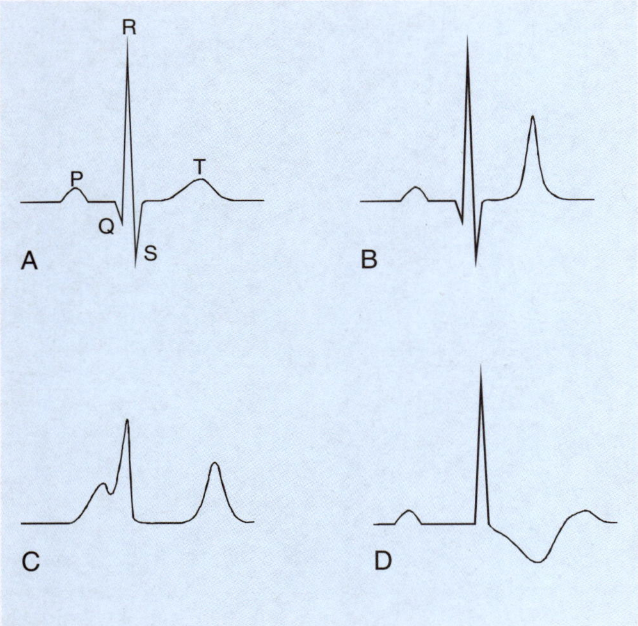

Fig. 4.2.33 Electrocardiographic changes in relation to plasma levels of potassium: **A**, normal tracing (plasma K^+ 4–5.5 mEq/L); **B**, hyperkalaemia (plasma K^+ 7.0 mEq/L); **C**, hyperkalaemia (plasma K^+ 8.0 mEq/L); and **D**, hypokalaemia (plasma K^+ 2.5–3.5 mEq/L).

- T wave remains tall and slender.

  A further increase in plasma K^+ levels may result in ventricular tachycardia and ventricular fibrillation.

  As the extracellular K^+ concentration increases, the resting membrane potential of the muscle fibres decreases. Eventually the fibres become unexcitable, and the heart stops in diastole.

Hypokalaemia Hypokalaemia, i.e. decrease in the plasma levels of potassium, is a serious condition but it is not as rapidly fatal as hyperkalaemia. It produces the following changes in ECG (Fig. 4.2.33D):

- PR interval is prolonged.
- U waves become prominent.
- ST segment is depressed.
- Late T-wave inversion may occur in the precordial leads.
- If the T and U waves merge, the apparent QT interval is often prolonged, but if the T and U waves are separated, the true QT interval is of normal duration.

Long QT syndrome Long QT syndrome occurs due to genetic abnormality which blocks one type of K^+ channels $KVLQT_1$, resulting in slow K^+ efflux, prolonging cardiac action potential and hence QT interval. The incidence of ventricular arrhythmia and sudden death is more with prolonged QT interval.

Normally this K^+ channel (protein) in the heart is responsible for normal QT interval, and in the stria vascularis for maintaining the high concentration of K^+ in the endolymph.

Mutation of $KVLQT_1$ results in long QT interval syndrome. In this syndrome, patients are deaf and also predispose to ventricular arrhythmia (because vulnerability of the heart for irregular repolarization is high). This syndrome is also caused by certain drugs and electrolyte abnormality.

Plasma Levels of Calcium effect the ECG

Hypercalcaemia Hypercalcaemia, i.e. increase in extracellular Ca^{2+}, clinically is rare if ever high enough to affect the heart. However, when large amounts of calcium are infused into experimental animals, the heart relaxes less during diastole and eventually stops in systole (*calcium rigor*).

Hypocalcaemia Hypocalcaemia, i.e. decreased plasma level of Ca^{2+}, produces prolongation of the ST segment and consequently the QT interval is also increased.

Self-Assessment

1. Discuss about pacemaker tissue of the heart, its innervations and effects of stimulation, and pacemaker potential and its ionic basis.
2. Discuss the following:
   - Physiological basis of ECG in myocardial infarction
   - Mechanism of development of cardiac arrhythmia
   - Concepts of cardiac vector and its clinical significance
3. Write notes on:
   - His bundle electrogram
   - Sick sinus syndrome
   - ECG changes in hyperkalaemia
   - Long QT syndrome
   - Heart blocks

Clinical Cases

Case 1

A 65-year-old male patient visited the cardiologist with complaint of palpitation and dizziness. On examination, pulse rate was 100 beats/min and BP 90/58 mm Hg, and ECG findings revealed ventricular fibrillations and long QT interval.

Q1. What is the probable diagnosis?

Q2. Is there any other cause for long QT interval?

Case 2

A cardiac patient on drug digitalis is having headache, malaise, insomnia, nausea and vomiting, and visual change in colour vision. The probable diagnosis made is digitalis toxicity.

Q1. What is the earliest sign observed in ECG pattern for this condition?

Case 3

A 45-year-old woman is brought to the emergency in a state of syncope.

On examination, pallor is present, pulse rate is 36 beats/min and BP is very low.

ECG findings reveal sinus bradycardia and increased PR interval; diagnosis made is sick sinus syndrome.

Q1. What is the main cause of this condition?

Q2. If the symptoms do not improve with medication, what should be the next line of treatment?

Case 4

A 12-lead ECG of a patient shows:

- R wave >12 mm in aVL
- S wave (in lead V_1) + Q wave (in lead V_6) >36 mm
- MEA −90°

Q1. On ECG findings, what is the probable diagnosis?

Case 5

A 70-year-old man suddenly developed severe chest pain, shortness of breath and sweating.

Q1. What is the probable diagnosis?

Q2. To confirm the diagnosis, what further tests are required?

Case 6

A 30-year-old athlete became alarmed when he noticed series of palpitations after several hours of finishing exercise in the gym. He approached the physician.

On examination:

- Vitals were normal.
- ECG findings showed normal sinus rhythm with occasional premature ventricular complexes (PVCs).

Q1. What is the most common cause for PVCs?

Q2. For PVCs, what is the site for initiation of heartbeat?

Q3. What is the pattern of ECG in this condition?

Case 7

A 42-year-old female with diabetes presented in the hospital with complaints of palpitation, shortness of breath and vomiting. Physical examination and laboratory findings revealed very high levels potassium.

Q1. What is the main ECG change expected in this condition?

4.3

Heart as a Pump: Cardiac Cycle, Cardiac Output and Venous Return

CHAPTER OUTLINE

CARDIAC CYCLE

INTRODUCTION

The heart as a pump can be considered actually comprising two separate pumps in the series: a *right heart* that pumps the blood through the lungs and a *left heart* that pumps the blood through the peripheral organs. Furthermore, each pump consists of an atrium and a ventricle. The atria act as *primary pumps* for the ventricles, helping to move the blood into the ventricles. The ventricles in turn provide the major force that propels the blood through pulmonary and systemic circulations. To act as a pump, the heart contracts and relaxes rhythmically. The terms *systole* (contractile phase) and *diastole* (relaxation phase) usually refer to ventricular events but may be prefixed by 'atrial' to refer to atrial contraction and relaxation, respectively. The heart has an *intrinsic contraction rate* because it contains its own pacemaker normally located in the SA node. As discussed in Chapter 4.2, the cardiac impulse arising from the SA node spreads in the whole heart. The electrocardiogram records the *electrical events* that precede and initiate the corresponding *mechanical events* as:

- P wave is caused by spread of depolarization through the atria, and this is followed by *atrial contraction.*
- QRS waves which appear 0.16 second after the onset of P wave are caused by depolarization of the ventricles, which initiates *contraction of the ventricles.*
- *T wave* represents the repolarization of the ventricles while the ventricular muscle fibres begin to relax. Therefore, T wave occurs slightly before the end of ventricular contraction.

The cardiac cycle thus includes both electrical and mechanical events that occur from the beginning of one heartbeat to the beginning of the next.

Cardiodynamics is the study of the mechanical events associated with the contraction and relaxation of the heart. These include:

- Pressure changes in the ventricles.
- Pressure changes in the atria.
- Pressure changes in the aorta.
- Pressure changes in pulmonary artery
- Volume changes in the ventricles.
- Valvular events, i.e. production of heart sounds.

PHASES OF CARDIAC CYCLE

Duration of each cardiac cycle at a normal heart rate of 75 beats/min is 60/75 = 0.8 second.

During each cardiac cycle, both atria contract (*atrial systole*) and relax (*atrial diastole*) and both ventricles contract (*ventricular systole*) and relax (*ventricular diastole*).

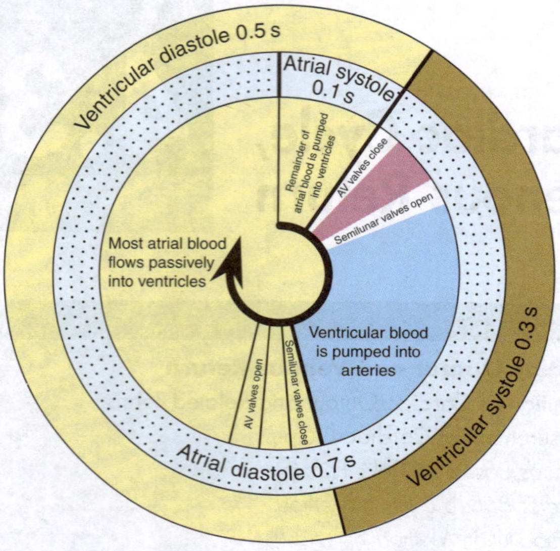

Fig. 4.3.1 Duration of phases of cardiac cycle.

Therefore, each cardiac cycle can be considered to consist of simultaneously occurring atrial and ventricular cycles with the following phases (Figs 4.3.1 and 4.3.2).

Atrial cycle consists of:

1. ***Atrial systole*** or atrial contraction phase (0.1 second)
2. ***Atrial diastole*** (0.7 second)

Ventricular cycle consists of:

Ventricular systole (0.3 second) consisting of:

1. Isovolumic (isometric) contraction phase (0.05 second).
2. Phase of ventricular ejection which can be further divided into rapid ejection phase (0.1 second) and slow ejection phase (0.15 second).

Ventricular diastole (0.5 second) consisting of:

1. Protodiastole (0.04 second).
2. Isovolumic (isometric) relaxation phase (0.06 second).
3. Rapid passive filling phase (0.11 second).
4. Reduced filling phase or diastasis (0.19 second).
5. Last rapid filling phase which coincides with the atrial systole (0.1 second).

Atrial Cycle

Atrial Systole

Atrial systole or the atrial contraction phase lasts for 0.1 second and coincides with the last rapid filling phase of ventricular diastole (Figs 4.3.1 and 4.3.2).

- Before the beginning of atrial systole, the ventricles are relaxing, atrioventricular (AV) valves are open and blood is flowing from the great veins into the atria and from the atria into the ventricles. Thus, the atria and ventricles are forming a continuous cavity.
- When the atrial contraction begins, approximately 75% of the blood has already flown into the ventricles. Thus, atrial contraction usually causes an additional 25% filling of the ventricles. Therefore, even if the atria fail to function, it is unlikely to be noticed unless a person exercises.

The contraction of atria causes:

Increase in intra-atrial pressure by 4–6 mm Hg in right atrium and 7–8 mm Hg in left atrium. The pressure rise in right atrium is reflected into the veins and is recorded as a wave from the jugular vein.

Increase in the ventricular pressure occurs slightly due to pumping of blood in the ventricles.

Narrowing of great veins at the origin (inferior vena cava and superior vena cava opening in right atrium and pulmonary veins opening in left atrium) decreasing venous return to the heart. Some regurgitation of the blood occurs into the great veins as no valves are present at their entrance into the atria.

Atrial Diastole

After the atrial systole, there occurs atrial diastole (0.7 second). This period coincides with the ventricular systole and most of the ventricular diastole (Fig. 4.3.1).

- During atrial diastole, atrial muscles relax and there occurs gradual filling of the atria due to continuous venous return, and the pressure gradually increases in the atria and drops down to almost zero with the opening of AV valves (Fig. 4.3.3). Then the pressure again rises and follows the ventricular pressure during the rest of atrial diastole.

Ventricular Cycle

Ventricular Systole

After the atrial contraction phase is over, the ventricles get excited by the impulse travelling along the conduction system and the ventricles start contracting. The ventricular systole lasts to 0.3 second, and has the following phases.

1. Phase of isovolumic (isometric) contraction With the beginning of ventricular contraction, the ventricular pressure exceeds atrial pressure very rapidly causing closure of AV valves (this event is responsible for production of first heart sound).

- Since the AV valves have closed and semilunar valves have not opened, the ventricles contract as a closed chamber and the pressure inside the ventricles rises rapidly.
- As the ventricles contract, the volume of blood in the ventricles does not change; hence, this phase is called *isovolumic contraction phase.*

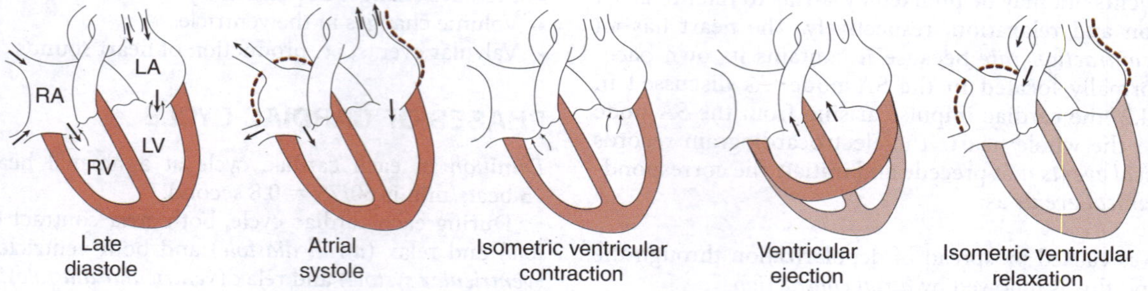

Fig. 4.3.2 Phases of cardiac cycle.

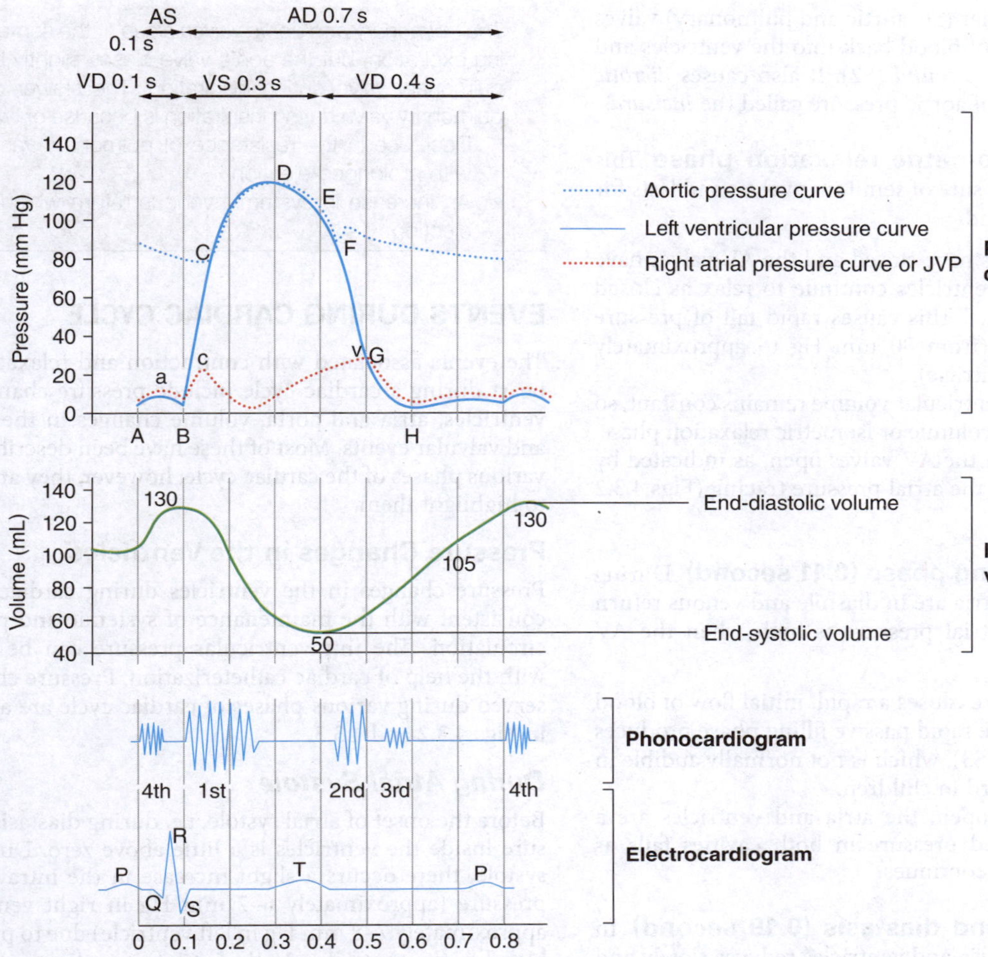

Fig. 4.3.3 Phases and events during cardiac cycle.

- During this phase, due to sharp rise in ventricular pressure, there occurs bulging of AV valves into the atria producing a small but sharp rise in intra-atrial pressure called c wave.
- This phase lasts for 0.05 second, until the pressure in the left and right ventricles exceeds the pressure in the aorta (80 mm Hg) and pulmonary artery (10 mm Hg) and the aortic and pulmonary valves open.

2. Phase of ventricular ejection The ventricular ejection phase begins with the opening of semilunar valves and lasts for approximately 0.25 second. It can be further divided into two phases.

Rapid ejection phase As soon as the semilunar valves open, the blood is rapidly ejected out for approximately 0.1 second. Approximately two-thirds of the stroke volume is ejected in this rapid ejection phase. Pressure rises to 120 mm Hg in the left ventricle and to 25 mm Hg in the right ventricle. The right ventricular ejection begins before that of left and continues even after left ventricular ejection is complete. As both the ventricles eject almost the same volume of blood, the velocity of right ventricular ejection is less than that of the left ventricle.

Slow ejection phase It refers to the latter two-thirds of systole (approximately 0.15 second) during which rate of ejection declines. Approximately one-third of the stroke volume is ejected during this phase. The intraventricular pressure starts declining and falls to a value slightly lower than that in aorta, but for a short period momentum keeps the blood flowing forward.

Volume changes. At the end of each diastole, the ventricular volume is approximately 130 mL. This is called end-diastolic volume.

- Approximately 80 mL of blood is ejected out by each ventricle during each systole. This is called *stroke volume.*
- Thus, approximately 50 mL of the blood is left in each ventricle at the end of systole. This is called *end-systolic volume.*

Ventricular Diastole

Ventricular diastole consists of the following phases:

1. Protodiastole When the ventricular systole ends, the ventricles start relaxing and intraventricular pressure falls rapidly. This phase lasts for 0.04 second. During this phase, the elevated pressure in the distended arteries (aorta and pulmonary artery) immediately pushes the blood back towards the ventricles which snaps the semilunar valves to close. Closure of semilunar (i.e. aortic and pulmonary) valves prevents the movement of blood back into the ventricles and produces the *second heart sound* (S2). It also causes *dicrotic notch* in the downslope of aortic pressure called the *incisura*.

2. Isovolumic or isometric relaxation phase This phase begins with the closure of semilunar valves and lasts for approximately 0.06 second.

- Since semilunar valves have closed and the AV valves have not yet opened, the ventricles continue to relax as closed chambers in this phase. This causes rapid fall of pressure inside the ventricles (from 80 mm Hg to approximately 2–3 mm Hg in left ventricle).
- As in this phase, the ventricular volume remains constant, so this phase is called isovolumic or isometric relaxation phase.
- This phase ends when the AV valves open, as indicated by the peak of *v wave* on the atrial pressure tracing (Figs 4.3.2 and 4.3.3).

3. Rapid passive filling phase (0.11 second) During ventricular systole, the atria are in diastole and venous return continues so that the atrial pressure is high when the AV valves open.

- The high atrial pressure causes a rapid, initial flow of blood into the ventricles. The rapid passive filling phase produces the *third heart sound* (S3), which is not normally audible in adults but may be heard in children.
- Once the AV valves open, the atria and ventricles are a common chamber and pressure in both cavities falls as ventricular relaxation continues.

4. Reduced filling and diastasis (0.19 second) In this phase, pressure in atria and ventricles reduces slowly and remains little above zero. This decreases the rate of blood flow from atria to ventricle causing a very slow filling or virtually cessation of ventricular filling called *diastasis*.

> **Important Note**
>
> It is important to note that approximately 75% blood passes from atria to ventricles during rapid filling and reduced filling phases of ventricular diastole.

5. Last rapid filling phase (0.1 second) The last rapid filling phase of ventricular diastole coincides with the atrial systole.

- As described in the beginning, the atrial systole brings about the last rapid filling phase and pushes the additional 25% blood in the ventricles. With this phase, the ventricular cycle is completed.

> **Important Notes**
>
> **Cardiac Cycle: Right Versus Left Heart**
>
> Both ventricles pump the same volume of blood over any significant time period; therefore, by and large, events on the two sides of the heart are similar. However, there exists a minor asynchronicity between the two sides as:
>
> - *Right atrial systole precedes left atrial systole*, but right ventricle starts contracting after the left ventricle. However, right ventricular ejection begins before the left ventricular ejection because the pulmonary arterial pressure is lower than the aortic pressure.
> - *The pulmonary and aortic valves close* at the same time during expiration, but the aortic valve closes slightly before the pulmonary valve during inspiration. The slower closure of pulmonary valve during inspiration is because of two factors:
>   - Decrease in the resistance of pulmonary vascular tree with prolonged ejection
>   - An increase in systemic venous return which prolongs ejection

EVENTS DURING CARDIAC CYCLE

The events associated with contraction and relaxation of the heart during a cardiac cycle include pressure changes in the ventricles, atria and aorta, volume changes in the ventricles and valvular events. Most of these have been described during various phases of the cardiac cycle; however, they are repeated to highlight them.

Pressure Changes in the Ventricles

Pressure changes in the ventricles during cardiac cycle are consistent with the maintenance of systemic and pulmonary circulation. The intraventricular pressure can be measured with the help of cardiac catheterization. Pressure changes observed during various phases of cardiac cycle are as depicted in Figs 4.3.2 and 4.3.3.

During Atrial Systole

Before the onset of atrial systole, i.e. during diastasis the pressure inside the ventricles is a little above zero. During atrial systole, there occurs a slight increase in the intraventricular pressure (approximately 6–7 mm Hg in right ventricle and approximately 7–8 mm Hg in left ventricle) due to pumping of blood in the ventricles. In the intraventricular pressure curve (Fig. 4.3.3), the segment AB represents the pressure changes during atrial systole. The point A denotes the onset of atrial systole and the point B denotes the closure of AV valve.

During Ventricular Systole

The ventricular pressure changes during various phases of ventricular systole are as follows:

During phase of isovolumic (isometric) contraction Since the AV valves have closed and semilunar valves have not opened, the ventricles contract as a closed chamber and pressure inside them rises rapidly to a high level. In the intraventricular pressure curve (Fig. 4.3.3), this phase is represented by the segment BC. Point C denotes the opening of semilunar valves and commencement of ventricular ejection phase.

During rapid ejection phase The ventricles contract at a rate greater than the rate at which blood is ejected, so a great rise in the pressure occurs. Pressure rises to maximum of 120 mm Hg in the left ventricle and 25 mm Hg in the right ventricle. The maximum pressure in the left ventricle is four to five times more than that in the right ventricle. This is because of the thick wall of the left ventricle. In the intraventricular pressure curve (Fig. 4.3.3), this phase is denoted by the segment CD. Point D denotes the peak point of intraventricular pressure after which it starts declining.

During slow ejection phase There is no further ventricular contraction and the pressure starts declining (Fig. 4.3.3, segment DE).

During Ventricular Diastole

The ventricular pressure changes during various phases of ventricular diastole are as follows:

During protodiastole The intraventricular pressure drops rapidly as the ventricles start relaxing. When the intraventricular pressure falls below that of aorta and pulmonary artery, the semilunar valves are closed due to backflow of blood. In the intraventricular pressure curve (Fig. 4.3.3), this phase is represented by segment EF; point F denoted the closure of semilunar valves.

During isovolumic (isometric) relaxation phase Since the semilunar valves have closed and AV valves have not yet opened up, the ventricles relax as closed chamber and there occurs a rapid fall in the intraventricular pressure (from 80 mm Hg to approximately 2–3 mm Hg in left ventricle). When the pressure inside the ventricles fall below the pressure in atria, the AV valves open up and the phase of rapid passive filling commences. In the intraventricular pressure curve (Fig. 4.3.3), the segment FG represents this phase; point G coincides with the opening of AV valve.

During rapid passive filling phase The intraventricular pressure further falls, since the ventricles are relaxing though blood is being filled in them (Fig. 4.3.3, segment GH).

During reduced passive filling phase There is no turbulence and the blood flows very slowly and smoothly, and virtually there occurs cessation of ventricular filling (*diastasis*). The ventricular pressure remains a little above zero.

Pressure Changes in the Atria

The intra-atrial pressure can be studied by recording with the help of intracardiac catheterization. The left atrial pressure can also be determined indirectly by measuring the pulmonary capillary wedge pressure. The tracing of the jugular venous pulse is also similar to the intra-atrial pressure curve, and it has three positive waves called a, c and v and two descents namely x and y (Fig. 4.3.3). Relationship of intra-atrial pressure changes with the phases of cardiac cycle.

During Atrial Systole

Before the onset of atrial systole, the intra-atrial pressure is slightly above zero and is slightly greater than the ventricular pressure. During atrial systole, a sharp rise in intra-atrial pressure (by 4–6 mm Hg in right atrium and by 7–8 mm Hg in left atrium) occurs and causes a pressure wave recorded as a wave from the jugular vein ('a' stands for atrial systole). Immediately after atrial systole, the intra-atrial pressure falls due to start of atrial relaxation in atrial diastole. 'a' wave becomes prominent during inspiration due to decreased intrathoracic pressure (Fig. 4.3.3).

During Ventricular Systole

Atrial pressure changes during different phases of ventricular systole are as follows:

During phase of isovolumic (isometric) contraction Due to sharp rise in intraventricular pressure, AV valves bulge into the atria producing a small but sharp rise in atrial pressure producing the so-called *c wave* ('c' stands for contraction of the ventricle).

During ventricular ejection phase The intra-atrial pressure drops sharply in rapid ejection phase. This happens so because the papillary muscles (attached to the cusps of AV valves by chordae tendineae) contract when the ventricular walls contract and pull down the fibrous AV ring causing enlargement of atrial lumen, thus decreasing the intra-atrial pressure. This drop in the intra-atrial pressure produces the 'x' descent. The 'x' descent occurs due to both relaxation of atria and downward pull of tricuspid valve during ventricular systole (ejection phase). Therefore, as the ventricles contract, the atria get slowly filled with blood flowing in from the great veins and the atrial pressure starts rising.

During Ventricular Diastole

During isovolumic (isometric) relaxation phase The atrial pressure continues to rise as long as AV valves remain closed, i.e. till the end of isovolumic relaxation. This results in the third positive wave called v wave ('v' stands for venous filling). This shows a gradual increase in atrial pressure.

During rapid passive filling phase The AV valves open allowing rapid flow of blood from atria to ventricles. So, the atrial pressure drops sharply to a little above zero level and remains so till the beginning of next atrial systole. This fall in atrial pressure produces the 'y' descent.

Important Notes

Clinical Significance of Jugular Vein Pulsations

A careful inspection of the pulsations of jugular vein may give useful information in the following clinical conditions:

- Large 'a' wave occurs in tricuspid stenosis.
- *Giant* 'a' wave (cannon wave) may be observed in patients with complete heart block.
- Differentiation between atrial and ventricular premature beats may be made by inspection of jugular pulse. It will show 'a' wave in atrial premature beats and not in ventricular premature beats.
- 'a' wave is absent in atrial fibrillations.
- Prominent 'v' wave is observed in tricuspid regurgitation.

Pressure Changes in the Aorta

Pressure in the aorta varies between 80 and 120 mm Hg during the cardiac cycle and can be recorded by using a catheter. Aortic pressure changes during various phases of cardiac cycle (Fig. 4.3.3) are explained as follows:

During Atrial Systole

The pressure in the aorta is approximately 80 mm Hg.

During Ventricular Systole

The intraventricular pressure rises and reaches above that of the aorta during beginning of the ventricular ejection phase when the aortic semilunar valve opens and blood starts flowing from the left ventricle into the aorta. Hence, the aortic pressure starts rising along with the intraventricular pressure during rapid ejection phase and reaches maximum (120 mm Hg) at the end of rapid ejection phase. It is important to note that during most of the rapid ejection phase, the aortic pressure remains slightly lesser than the ventricular pressure during reduced ejection phase and the aortic pressure starts falling along with the ventricular pressure.

During Ventricular Diastole

Aortic pressure changes during different phases of ventricular diastole are as follows

During protodiastole Aortic pressure is slightly higher than that in the left ventricle. This causes backward flow of blood and closure of aortic semilunar valve. Due to sudden closure of semilunar valve, the backflowing blood collides against the closed aortic valve. This collision causes a small but sharp rise in aortic pressure. This small rise produces a notch called incisura. This sharp pressure rise is recordable even from peripheral arteries and is called dicrotic notch.

During rest of the diastole The aortic pressure smoothly declines. By the time, the aortic pressure declines to approximately 80 mm Hg, another ventricular systole boosts the aortic pressure again.

Pressure Changes in Pulmonary Artery

Pressure curve in the pulmonary artery is similar to that of aorta but pressures are low (approximately one-sixth of that in aorta). Pulmonary artery systolic pressure averages 15–18 mm Hg and its pressure during diastole is 8–10 mm Hg.

Volume Changes in the Ventricles During Cardiac Cycle

During Atrial Systole

Atrial systole coincides with the last rapid filling phase of ventricular diastole. When the atrial contraction begins, approximately 105 mL (75%) of the blood has already entered into the ventricles. The atrial contraction causes additional 25 mL (25%) filling of the ventricles (Fig. 4.3.3). In the ventricular volume curve, this phase is represented by the AB segment. Thus, at the end of atrial systole, i.e. at the end of ventricular diastole, the ventricular volume is approximately 130 mL. This is called end-diastolic volume.

During Ventricular Systole

Volume changes in ventricles during different phases of ventricular systole are as follows:

During isovolumic contraction phase As the name suggests, there occurs no change in the ventricular volume (Fig. 4.3.3, segment BC).

During ventricular ejection phase Approximately 80 mL of the blood is ejected out by each ventricle. This is called stroke volume (Fig. 4.3.3, segment CD). The percentage of the end-diastolic volume that is ejected out with each stroke during systole (approximately 65%) is called ejection fraction. Thus, approximately 50 mL of the blood in each ventricle at the end of ventricular systole is called end-systolic volume.

During protodiastole and phase of isovolumic relaxation No change occurs in the ventricular volume.

During rapid filling phase and slow filling phase The ventricular volume changes rapidly and then slowly. Approximately 75% of the ventricular filling (105 mL of blood) occurs during these phases.

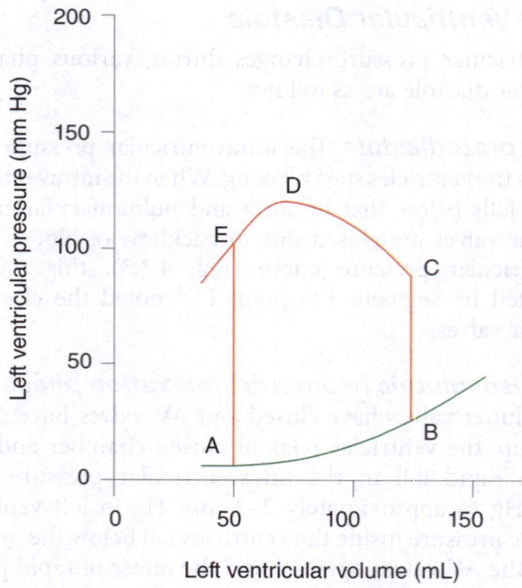

Fig. 4.3.4 Pressure–volume loop of left ventricle.

Pressure–volume loop Ventricular pressure–volume loop refers to the graph obtained in the form of a loop by plotting pressure along the ordinate and volume along the abscissa at various stages of cardiac cycle. Thus, the pressure–volume loop is an alternate method of representing the cardiac cycle. Normal ventricular pressure–volume loop is shown in Fig. 4.3.4.

Segment AB represents the rapid, passive filling phase, reduced filling phase and last rapid filling phase (atrial systole) of the ventricular diastole. This segment reveals that

- Ventricular volume at the end of diastole (at point B) is approximately 130 mL (end-diastolic volume). Point B marks the closure of AV valves.
- Ventricular pressure rises from 2–3 mm Hg point A to approximately 6–7 mm Hg at point B (end of atrial systole).

Segment BC represents the isovolumic contraction phase of ventricular systole. This segment reveals that during this phase

- Volume remains same, i.e. approximately 130 mL, but the pressure rises from 6–7 mm Hg to approximately 80 mm Hg.

Segment CE represents the ventricular ejection phase of ventricular systole. Point C marks the opening of semilunar valves. Segment CD represents the rapid ejection phase and segment DE represents the *slow ejection phase.* The segment CE reveals that

- During rapid ejection phase (segment CD), the ventricular pressure increases rapidly up to a maximum of 120 mm Hg and then falls during slow ejection phase (segment DE) to approximately 80 mm Hg.
- During ventricular ejection phase (segment CE), the ventricular volume decreases from approximately 130 mL to approximately 50 mL, called *end-systolic volume.*

Segment EA of the pressure–volume loop represents the phase of *isovolumic relaxation.* Point E marks the closure of semilunar valves. This segment reveals that

- Ventricular pressure falls rapidly from approximately 80 mm Hg to approximately 2–3 mm Hg.
- Ventricular volume remains unchanged.

Disadvantage of pressure–volume loop In this, the time dimension is eliminated and therefore it is not possible to tell from this loop how fast the events are occurring.

Advantage of pressure–volume loop The work done by the heart is instantly apparent from the area enclosed by the loop.

Clinical significance of pressure volume loop:

Shift to right: In systolic dysfunction of ventricles, the pressure–volume loop shifts to the right.

Shift to left: In diastolic dysfunction of ventricles, the pressure–volume loop shifts to the left.

The pressure–volume loop can be utilized in changed haemodynamic states like exercise and heart failure to understand pressure–volume events during cardiac cycle.

Valvular Events (Heart Sounds)

A total of four heart sounds (first, second, third and fourth) are produced by certain mechanical activities during each cardiac cycle. The study of heart sounds has important diagnostic value in many heart diseases. There are three methods to study the heart sounds:

Auscultation with stethoscope: The first and second heart sounds can be heard normally with the help of a stethoscope. By using microphone, the amplified heart sounds (first, second and third) can be heard using a loudspeaker.
Phonocardiogram is the graphical record of all the four heart sounds. This is achieved by placing an electronic sound transducer over the chest and connecting it to a recording device like polygraph. The four heart sounds are described as follows.

First Heart Sound (HS_1)

Cause The first heart sound is produced by vibrations set up by the sudden closure of AV valves at the start of ventricular systole, during phase of isovolumic contraction (Fig. 4.3.3).

Characteristics The first heart sound is long and soft when heart rate is low, and loud when the heart rate is high. Its duration is approximately 0.15 second and frequency is 25–45 Hz. It sounds like the spoken word 'LUBB'.

Site for auscultation It can be heard by auscultation of the chest with stethoscope. It is best heard over mitral and tricuspid areas. *Mitral area* is located in the fifth intercostal space just internal to mid-clavicular line. *Tricuspid area* is located in the fifth intercostal space near the sternum (Fig. 4.3.5).

In phonocardiogram the first heart sound is recorded as a single group of 9–13 waves. The amplitude of the waves is small to start with but later rapidly rises to fall to form *crescendo and diminuendo* series of waves (Fig. 4.3.3).

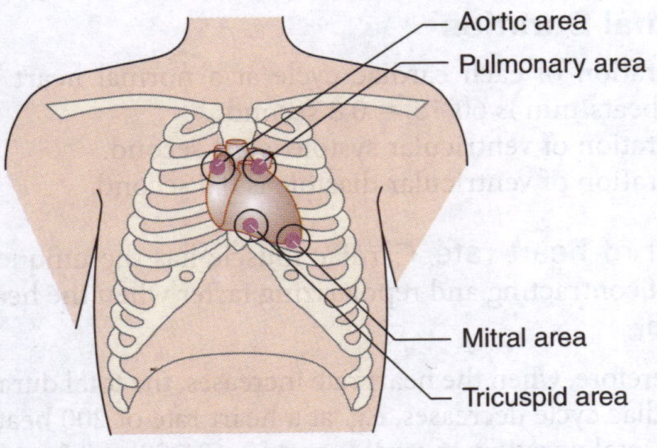

Fig. 4.3.5 Auscultatory areas over the chest.

Correlation with ECG First heart sound coincides with peak of R wave in ECG (Fig. 4.3.3).

Second Heart Sound (HS_2)

Cause It is caused by vibrations associated with closure of the semilunar valves just at the onset of ventricular diastole.

Characteristics The second heart sound is a short, loud and high-pitched sound. Its duration is 0.12 second and frequency is 50 Hz. It sounds like the spoken word 'DUBB'.

Site for auscultation It can be heard by auscultation of the chest with a stethoscope. It is best heard over the aortic and pulmonary areas. *Aortic area* lies in the right second intercostal space near the sternum, *pulmonary area* is in the left second intercostal space close to sternum (Fig. 4.3.5).

In phonocardiogram The second heart sound is recorded as a single group of 4–6 waves having same amplitude (Fig. 4.3.3).

Correlation with ECG The second heart sound usually coincides with end of T wave in ECG (Fig. 4.3.3).

Note: During inspiration, time interval between closure of aortic and pulmonary valve is prolonged. Therefore, the second heart sound is to be reduplicated, which is called *physiological splitting of second heart sound.*

Applied Aspect

Pathological splitting of second heart sound occurs in the following conditions:

- Bundle branch block
- Atrial septal defect
- Pulmonary stenosis
- Advanced aortic stenosis
- Right ventricular hypertrophy

Third Heart Sound (HS_3)

Cause The third heart sound is caused by vibrations set up in the cardiac wall by the inrush of blood during *rapid filling phase* of ventricular diastole.

Characteristics The third heart sound is a short, soft and low-pitched sound. Its duration is 0.1 second. Normally, it cannot be heard by auscultation with stethoscope.

In phonocardiogram The third heart sound is found with only 1–4 waves grouped together (Fig. 4.3.3).

Correlation with ECG The third heart sound appears between T and P waves of ECG (Fig. 4.3.3).

Note: Gallop rhythm refers to the cardiac rhythm when three heart sounds are clearly heard during each heartbeat.

Fourth Heart Sound (HS_4)

Cause It is caused by vibrations set up during atrial systole which coincides with last rapid filling phase of ventricular diastole.

Characteristics It is normally not audible. Sometimes, it can be heard immediately before the first sound when atrial pressure is high or when ventricle is stiff in condition such as ventricular hypertrophy. It is a short and low-pitched sound. Its duration is approximately 0.03 second and frequency approximately 3 Hz.

In phonocardiogram The fourth heart sound merges with first heart sound many times. When it appears as a separate entity, it has 1–2 waves with very low amplitude (Fig. 4.3.3).

Correlation with ECG The fourth heart sound coincides with the interval between the end of P wave and onset of Q wave.

Note: Heart sounds HS_3 and HS_4 are comparatively less important because normally they are inaudible.

Applied Aspects

Cardiac Murmurs

Cardiac murmurs are the abnormal heart sounds produced during the cardiac cycle.

Mechanism of Production

Cardiac murmurs are produced by a turbulent blood flow or by change in the direction of blood flow. Normally, the blood flows through the heart and blood vessels as *laminar flow* which is streamlined and silent. The *turbulent flow,* on the other hand, produces vibrations in the tissues that are heard as murmurs.

Causes

Murmurs are caused in the following conditions:

Valvular stenosis, i.e. narrowing of any of the cardiac valves (mitral, tricuspid, aortic or pulmonary valve).

Valvular insufficiency, i.e. regurgitation of any of the cardiac valves.

Ventricular septal defect (VSD), i.e. a congenital hole in the ventricular septum.

Atrial septal defect (ASD), i.e. a congenital hole in the interatrial septum.

Coarctation of aorta, i.e. congenital narrowing of systemic aorta.

Patent ductus arteriosus (PDA), i.e. a congenital disorder in which there is backward flow of blood from aorta into the pulmonary artery.

Types

Depending on the timing of appearance, these have been classified as follows (Fig. 4.3.6):

- *Systolic murmur,* which is produced during systole.
- *Diastolic murmur,* which is produced during diastole.
- *Continuous murmur,* which is produced continuously.

The types of murmur produced depend on the site and type of abnormality (Table 4.3.1).

Site of Auscultation

The murmurs are best heard by placing the stethoscope on the chest wall closest to their origin, e.g. aortic area, pulmonary area, mitral area and tricuspid area.

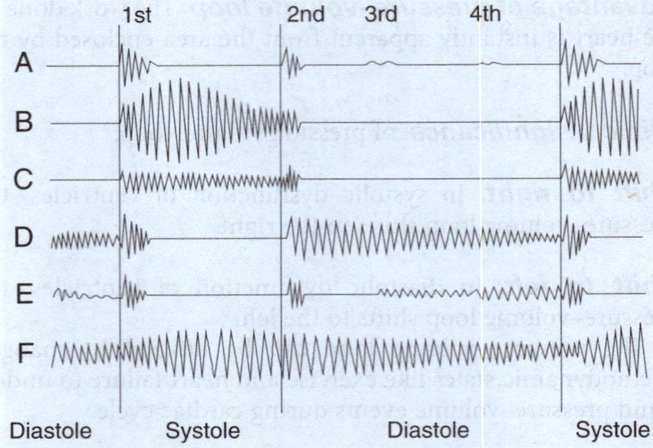

Fig. 4.3.6 Cardiac murmurs on phonocardiography: **A,** normal phonocardiogram; **B,** systolic murmur (in aortic stenosis); **C,** systolic murmur (in mitral regurgitation); **D,** diastolic murmur (in aortic regurgitation); **E,** diastolic murmur (in mitral stenosis); **F,** continuous murmur (in patent ductus arteriosus).

Note: Abnormal vascular sounds heard over blood vessels are called *bruit*. Bruits can be heard in the following conditions:

- In case of highly vascular goitre.
- In atherosclerosis, bruit can be heard over carotid artery when its lumen gets narrowed or distorted.
- Over an aneurysm (dilation of a large artery).

Table 4.3.1 Types of murmurs depending on site and type of abnormality

Site of abnormality	Type of abnormality	Type of murmur
• Aortic or pulmonary valve	Stenosis Insufficiency	Systolic Diastolic
• Mitral or tricuspid valve	Stenosis Insufficiency	Diastolic Systolic
• Interventricular septum	Congenital hole	Systolic
• Aorta	Coarctation	Systolic
• Ductus arteriosus	Patent	Continuous
• Blood	Anaemia	Systolic

DURATION OF SYSTOLE AND DIASTOLE VIS-À-VIS HEART RATE

Normal Duration

- Duration of each cardiac cycle at a normal heart rate of 75 beats/min is 60/75 = 0.8 second.
- Duration of ventricular systole is 0.3 second.
- Duration of ventricular diastole is 0.5 second.

Effect of heart rate Cardiac muscle has the unique property of contracting and repolarizing faster when the heart rate is high.

- Therefore, when the heart rate increases, the total duration of cardiac cycle decreases, e.g. at a heart rate of 200 beats/min, the total duration of cardiac cycle is 60/200 = 0.3 second.

Table 4.3.2 Change in duration of various events of cardiac cycle with increase in heart rate

	Duration in seconds	
Event	**At heart rate of 75 beats/min**	**At heart rate of 200 beats/min**
Cardiac cycle	0.8	0.3
Systole	0.3	0.16
Diastole	0.5	0.14

- It is important to note that though the duration of all phases of the cardiac cycle decreases at high heart rate, the *duration of diastole* decreases much more than the duration of systole. For example, when the heart rate increases from 75 to 200 beats/min, the duration of systole decreases from 0.3 to 0.16 second, while that of diastole decreases from 0.5 to 0.14 second (Table 4.3.2).

This fact has the following important physiologic and *clinical implications:*

- It is during diastole that the heart muscle rests, and coronary blood flow to the subendocardial portion of the left ventricle occurs only during diastole. Therefore, at very high rate, reduction in cardiac perfusion occurs and there are chances of myocardial ischaemia.
- Furthermore, most of the ventricular filling occurs in diastole. At a heart rate up to 180 beats/min, filling is adequate as long as there is ample venous return and cardiac output per minute is increased by an increase in heart rate. However, at very high heart rate, filling may be compromised to such a degree that cardiac output per minute falls and symptoms of heart failure develop.

Clinical Indices

Information about the duration of isovolumic ventricular contraction is of considerable clinical importance in many cardiac disorders. However, exact measurement of the duration of isovolumic ventricular contraction is difficult in clinical situations. Therefore, certain other indices have been evolved from which indirectly required information can be obtained. These indices given below are relatively easy to measure from the recording of ECG, phonocardiogram and carotid pulse simultaneously (Fig. 4.3.7).

Total electromechanical systole (QS_2) is the period from the onset of QRS complex to the closure of the aortic valve, as determined by the onset of second heart sound.
Left ventricular ejection time (LVET) is the period from the beginning of the carotid pressure rise to the dicrotic notch.
Pre-ejection period (PEP) is the difference between QS_2 and LVET and represents the time for the electrical as well as the mechanical events that precede systolic ejection.
Ratio of PEP/LVET is normally approximately 0.35, and it increases without a change in QS_2, when left ventricular performance is compromised in many cardiac diseases.

ARTERIAL PULSE

Arterial pulse is also an event related to cardiac cycle. The blood forced into the aorta during systole not only moves the blood in the vessels forward but also sets up a pressure wave

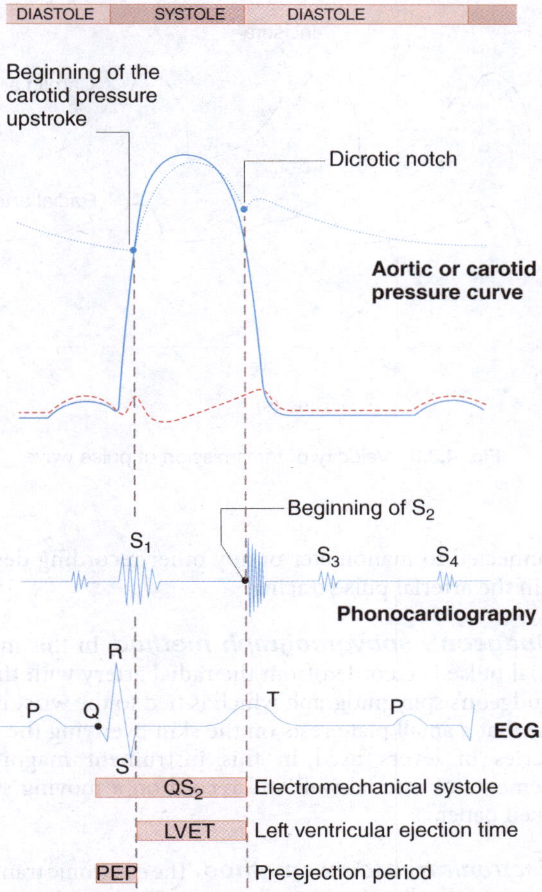

Fig. 4.3.7 Durations of systolic time interval. LVET, left ventricular ejection time; PEP, pre-ejection period.

that is transmitted along the *arteries to the* periphery. The pressure wave expands the arterial walls as it travels, and expansion is palpable as the *pulse.*

Velocity of transmission of pulse wave Velocity of transmission of pulse wave is independent of and much higher than the velocity of blood flow, the maximum value of which in larger arteries is only 50 cm/s. The rate of travel of pulse wave is about

- 4 m/s in the aorta and its branches.
- 8 m/s in the large arteries.
- 16 m/s in the small arteries of young adults.

Consequently, the pulse is felt at the arteries after short interval of the peak of systolic ejection into the aorta (Fig. 4.3.8). This interval can be measured accurately by recording and is directly proportional to the distance of artery from the heart. For the common carotid artery, this period is approximately 0.02 second, whereas for the radial artery at the wrist, it is approximately 0.1 second. With the advancing age, the arteries become more rigid and the pulse wave moves faster.

Methods of recording arterial pulse The tracings of arterial pulse can be made by the following techniques of recording:

1. Manometric technique It is used in animals. In this technique, a cannula is inserted into the dissected artery and

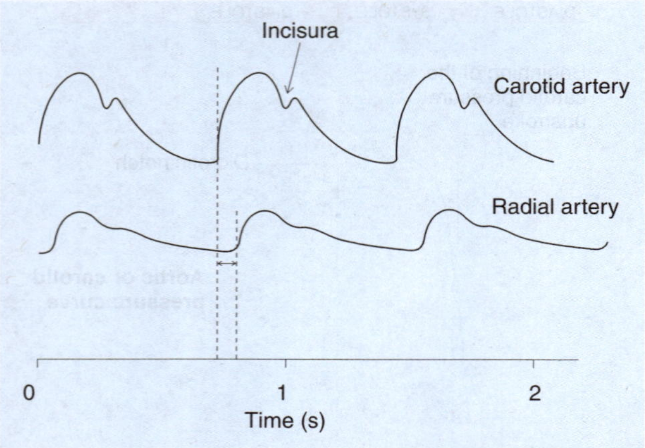

Fig. 4.3.8 Velocity of transmission of pulse wave.

is connected to manometer or any other recording device to obtain the arterial pulse tracing.

2. Dudgeon's sphygmograph method In this method, arterial pulse is recorded from the radial artery with the help of Dudgeon's sphygmograph which is tied to the wrist in such a way that a small plate rests on the skin overlying the artery. A series of levers used in this instrument magnify the movements of arterial wall and record on a moving strip of smoked paper.

3. Electronic transducer method The electronic transducer is placed on the skin overlying any artery. The transducer throws light on the artery and the light reflected from the flowing blood is deducted by the sensor of the transducer. The alterations in the frequency of reflected light rays are amplified and the arterial pulse is recorded by connecting the transducer to a recording device like polygraph.

Interpretation of arterial pulse tracing The pulse tracing recorded from the carotid artery shows the following characteristics (Fig. 4.3.9):

Ascending limb, also known as *anacrotic limb* or primary limb, is due to the rise in pressure during systole.
Descending limb, also known as *catacrotic limb* represents the fall in pressure during diastole.
Percussion wave (P) corresponds to ejection phase of ventricular systole.
Tidal wave (T) is due to falling blood column during slow ejection phase.
Dicrotic notch (N) is due to closure of aortic valve and marks end of ventricular systole.

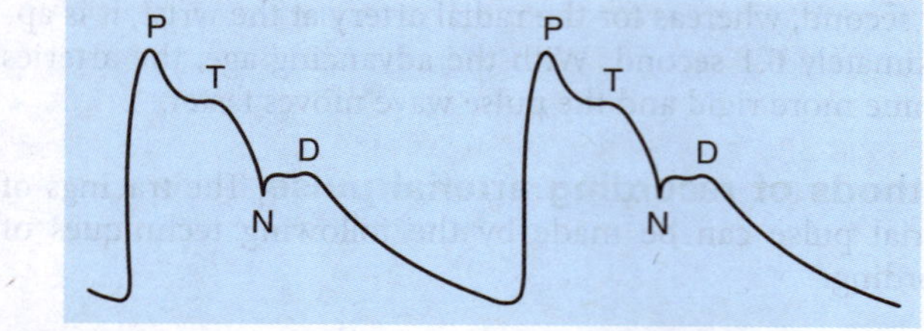

Fig. 4.3.9 Record of arterial pulse from carotid artery. P, percussion wave; T, tidal wave; N, dicrotic notch; D, dicrotic wave.

- *Dicrotic wave (D)* is due to rebound of blood column from closed aortic valve.

When the record is taken from peripheral arteries at a distant place from the heart, e.g. femoral or radial arteries, the contour or shape of record changes. In arterioles and capillaries, the waves disappear.

Examination of arterial pulse Examination of the arterial pulse is an essential feature of clinical examination. Arterial pulse can be palpated from any superficial artery, e.g. radial, femoral, dorsalis pedis, carotid. Most frequently, pulse is examined from the radial artery because it is conveniently approached without exposing the body, and can be easily palpated as it is placed superficially against the bone.

Examination of the pulse should include the following aspects:

1. Pulse rate It refers to the number of pulses per minute. It is a convenient method for determining heart rate.

Normal pulse rate varies with age, being 150–180/min in fetus, 130–140/min at birth, approximately 90/min at the age of 10 years and approximately 72/min in adults.
Increased pulse rate represents tachycardia and occurs during exercise, in anxiety, in fever, in hyperthyroidism and in atrial and ventricular tachycardias.
Decreased pulse rate represents bradycardia and is seen in hypothyroidism, athlete, during meditation and incomplete heart blocks.

Applied Aspects

Pulse deficit refers to pulse rate less than the heart rate. It is determined by simultaneous auscultation of heart rate at the apex and palpation at any peripheral artery (radial artery).

- Pulse deficit is best calculated by counting apex beat and radial pulse for full 1 minute. Then, subtract radial pulse from the apex beat.
- Pulse deficit is usually observed in atrial fibrillation.
- Pulse deficit also occurs when heart is weak and unable to pump enough blood to produce palpable pulse.

2. Volume of pulse also known as strength of arterial pulse or amplitude or impact can be felt. It represents stroke volume or the pulse pressure (i.e. systolic–diastolic pressure). Pulse pressure is mainly affected by stroke output, by compliance (distensibility) of the arterial tree and to some extent by the character of ejection of blood from the heart. Therefore, pulse pressure is determined by the ratio of stroke output to compliance of arterial tree. For details, see page 370.
Rapid and thready pulse occurs in hypovolaemia as in severe haemorrhage and there is marked reflex vasoconstriction.
Increased volume pulse is seen during exercise and in ventricular hypertrophy.

3. Rhythm of pulse It is noted as regular or irregular. Under normal conditions and during sinus bradycardia or sinus tachycardia, pulse appears at regular intervals.

Irregular pulse rhythm is a feature of extrasystole, atrial fibrillation and other cardiac arrhythmias; type of arrhythmia is confirmed only on ECG (see page 256). The irregular pulse rhythm may be regularly irregular or irregularly irregular.

4. Character of pulse It is felt on palpation. It denotes the tension and waves in the pulse. Feeling of different characters of the pulse can be learnt by subjective experience.

Normal character (Fig. 4.3.10A) of the pulse is sinuous on examination, i.e. an upstroke is followed by downstroke. Normally, it is not possible to feel the different waves of the pulse or slight variations in the character. However, in certain heart diseases and valvular defects, the normal character is altered and can be easily felt while palpating the peripheral arterial pulse.

Applied Aspects

A few *abnormal characters* of the pulse are:

Watson's Water hammer pulse (Fig. 4.3.10B), also known as collapsing pulse or Corrigan pulse is characterized by a sudden upstroke followed by a sudden downstroke without incisura. It is best felt by raising the patient's arm and holding it by grasping the wrist with palm of the observer. Sometimes the upstroke is so strong that it leads to head nodding with each heartbeat, called Corrigan sign or Corrigan pulse.

Cause of water hammer pulse is aortic insufficiency or regurgitation.

Mechanism of water hammer pulse in aortic regurgitation is as follows:

- When the aortic valve closes, blood regurgitates from the aorta into the left ventricle. So, aorta empties earlier and this is the cause of sudden downstroke.
- Due to regurgitation of blood from aorta into left ventricle, the end-diastolic volume is increased. So the next beat is forceful (due to Frank–Starling mechanism), and this is the cause of sudden upstroke of next beat.

Anacrotic pulse (Fig. 4.3.10C): Normally, there is a single upstroke in the arterial pulse. In anacrotic pulse, there are two upstrokes. It occurs in patients with aortic stenosis. First upstroke in anacrotic pulse is due to slow rise in ventricular systole owing to aortic stenosis and second is due to dicrotic wave which normally occurs on the downstroke.

Bisferiens pulse (Fig. 4.3.10E): This is a combination of anacrotic and collapsing pulses; both can be felt distinctly. It is found in conditions when aortic stenosis and incompetency are combined.

Pulsus alternans (Fig. 4.3.10D): In this condition, every normal pulse alternates with a weak pulse. This is because of alternate variation in the force of ventricular contraction. The rhythm and rate of pulse is normal. It occurs in severe myocardial diseases.

Pulsus paradoxus (Fig. 4.3.10F): The pulse becomes smaller or even disappears at the end of inspiration when the patient breathes deeply, but heart sounds may be heard on auscultation. It occurs in pericardial effusion and in constrictive pericarditis.

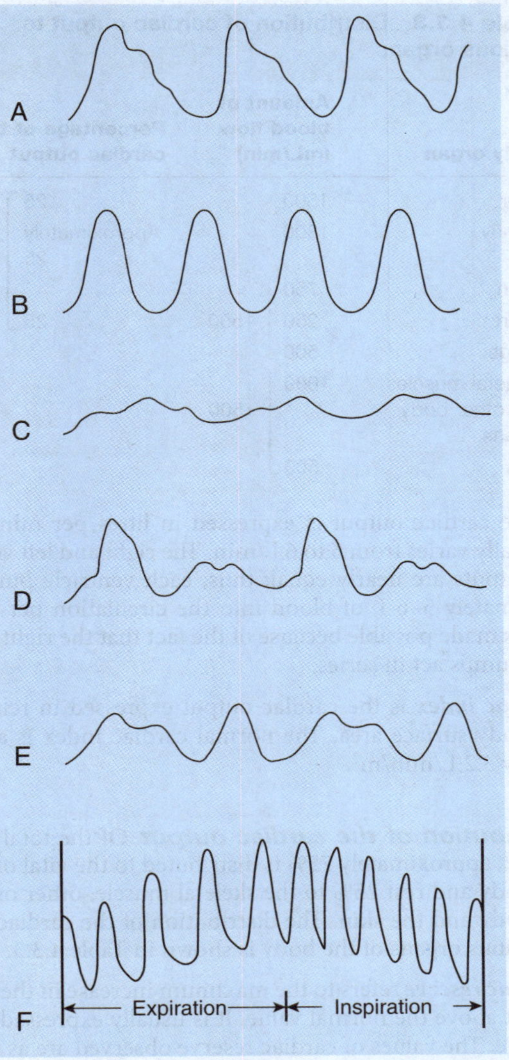

Fig. 4.3.10 Character of arterial pulse: **A,** normal character; **B,** water hammer pulse; **C,** anacrotic pulse; **D,** pulsus alternans; **E,** pulsus bisferiens; and **F,** pulsus paradoxa.

CARDIAC OUTPUT AND VENOUS RETURN

DEFINITION OF CARDIAC OUTPUT AND RELATED TERMS

The main function of the heart is to pump blood to meet the metabolic needs of the body. The measure of the heart's ability to pump blood is cardiac output. The *cardiac output* refers to the amount of blood ejected by each ventricle per minute. The *stroke volume* is the amount of blood pumped out by each ventricle per beat or per contraction. Therefore, cardiac output (CO) can be calculated by multiplying the stroke volume (SV) by the heart rate (HR):

$$CO = SV \times HR$$

Under normal conditions, the average heart rate is approximately 70 beats/min and stroke volume is approximately 80 mL; thus, the cardiac output is $80 \times 70 = 5.6$ L/min.

Table 4.3.3 Distribution of cardiac output to various organs

Body organ	Amount of blood flow (mL/min)		Percentage of total cardiac output	
Liver	1500		25	
Kidney	1300		Approximately	75
			25	
Brain	750			
Heart	250	1500	25	
Lungs	500			
Skeletal muscles and other body organs	1000	1500		
Skin	500			

The cardiac output is expressed in litres per minute and normally varies from 5 to 6 L/min. The right and left ventricular outputs are nearly equal; thus, each ventricle pumps approximately 5–6 L of blood into the circulation per minute. This is made possible because of the fact that the right and left side pumps act in series.

Cardiac index is the cardiac output expressed in relation to the body surface area. The normal cardiac index is approximately 3.2 L/min/m^2.

Distribution of the cardiac output Of the total cardiac output, approximately 75% is distributed to the vital organs of the body and rest 25% to the skeletal muscle, other organs of the body and the skin. The distribution of the cardiac output to various organs of the body is shown in Table 4.3.3.

Cardiac reserve refers to the maximum increase in the cardiac output above the normal value. It is usually expressed in percentage. The values of cardiac reserve observed are as follows:

- In healthy young adults: 300%–400%
- In old age: 200%–250%
- In athletes: 500%–600%

The cardiac reserve is

- Maximum during heavy exercise.
- Minimum or nil in cardiac diseases.

MEASUREMENT OF CARDIAC OUTPUT

Cardiac output, in experimental animals, can be measured directly with the help of an electromagnetic flowmeter placed on the ascending aorta. However, in human, only indirect methods are possible, which include:

- Methods based on Fick's principle.
- Indicator or dye dilution method.
- Thermodilution method.
- Method employing inhalation of inert gases.
- Physical methods such as:
  Doppler technique echocardiography
  Ballistocardiography
  Cineradiographic technique

Methods Based on Fick's Principle

1. Fick's principle It states that the amount of a substance taken up by an organ (or by the whole body) per unit of time (Q) is equal to the arterial level of the substance (A) minus the venous level (V) times the blood flow (F), i.e.

$$Q = (A - V)F$$

or

$$F = \frac{Q}{(A - V)}$$

This principle is applicable only in situations in which the arterial blood is the sole source of the substance taken up. The Fick's principle can be used to measure cardiac output by two methods:

- Fick's principle – direct method
- Fick's principle – indirect method

Fick's Principle (Direct Method)

In this method (Fig. 4.3.11), cardiac output is determined by measuring the pulmonary blood flow. As we know:

- Pulmonary blood flow/min = right ventricular output
- Right ventricular output (5 L/min) = left ventricular output (cardiac output)

Measurement of pulmonary blood flow can be made by measuring the amount of O_2 taken by the blood from the lungs, O_2 concentration of the venous blood from pulmonary artery (PAO_2) and O_2 concentration of the arterial blood from the pulmonary vein (PVO_2).

- Amount of O_2 uptake per minute is determined with the help of a spirometer.
- PAO_2 is measured from the venous blood sample taken from the pulmonary artery directly with the help of a cardiac catheter. The cardiac catheter is inserted into a vein at the forearm and is then guided up under fluoroscopic control through the venous channels into the right atrium, right ventricle and pulmonary artery.
- PVO_2, because of practical difficulty in taking sample from pulmonary vein, is measured from the arterial blood sample taken from any peripheral artery, e.g. brachial artery (the O_2 content of all the major arteries is same as that of pulmonary veins). According to Fick's principle:

$$\text{Pulmonary blood flow} = \frac{\text{Amount of } O_2 \text{ taken by the lungs per minute}}{PVO_2 - PAO_2}$$

or

$$\text{Cardiac output} = \frac{O_2 \text{ taken by the lungs per minute}}{PVO_2 - PAO_2}$$

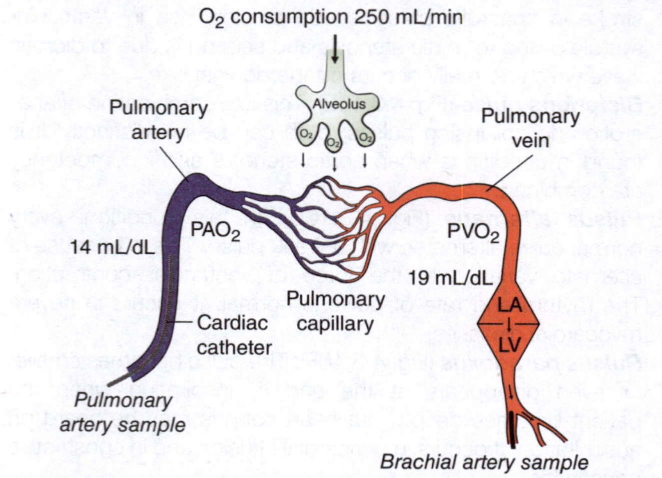

Fig. 4.3.11 Estimation of cardiac output by Fick's principle. PAO_2, oxygen content of pulmonary artery blood; PVO_2, oxygen content of pulmonary vein blood.

For example, if O_2 uptake is 250 mL/min, PVO_2 is 19 mL/100 mL and PAO_2 is 14 mL/100 mL, then

$$\begin{aligned} &= \frac{250 \times 100}{19 - 14} \\ \text{Cardiac output} &= \frac{25{,}000 \text{ mL/min}}{5} \\ &= 5000 \text{ mL/min} \\ &= 5 \text{l/min} \end{aligned}$$

Disadvantages of Fick's principle (direct method) are as follows:

- It is an invasive technique, so there are risks of infection and haemorrhage.
- The cardiac output estimated may be somewhat higher than normal as the patient becomes conscious of the whole technique.
- A fatal complication like ventricular fibrillation may occur if the indwelling catheter irritates the ventricular walls, especially when the cardiac output is being measured during heavy exercises.

Fick's Principle (Indirect Method)

In this method, arterial puncture and right heart catheterization are avoided and CO_2 excretion by the lungs is used instead of O_2 uptake.

- CO_2 excretion by the lungs is measured by spirometry.
- Arterial CO_2 ($PACO_2$) is estimated from alveolar air.
- Mixed venous blood CO_2 ($PVCO_2$) is estimated by rebreathing into a closed bag. With rebreathing, the CO_2 in the bag will come into equilibrium with the venous blood in lungs. The breathing should be done in an interrupted manner so that the blood level of CO_2 is not increased.

According to Fick's principle:

$$\text{Cardiac output} = \frac{CO_2 \text{ output per minute}}{PACO_2 - PVCO_2}$$

Indicator or Dye Dilution Method

Principle

In this method, a known amount of the dye is injected into a large vein or preferably into right atrium by cardiac catheterization. By its passage through heart and pulmonary circulation, it will be evenly distributed in the bloodstream. Its mean concentration during the first passage through an artery can be determined from successive samples of blood taken from artery. The blood flow in litres per minute (*F*) is given by the following formula:

$$F = \frac{Q}{Ct}, \text{ where:}$$

Q = Quantity of the dye injected
C = Mean concentration of dye
t = Time duration in seconds of the first passage of dye through the artery

Prerequisites for an Ideal Indicator

The indicator (dye) used should have the following characteristics:

- It should be nontoxic.
- It must mix evenly in the blood.
- It should be relatively easy to measure its concentration.
- It should not alter the cardiac output or haemodynamics of blood flow.
- Either it must not be changed by the body during mixing period or the amount changed must be known.
- The dye commonly used in humans for determining the cardiac output is *Evans blue* (T-1824) or radioactive isotopes.

Procedure

Injection of dye A few millilitres of venous blood is withdrawn from the antecubital vein and it is mixed with 5 mg Evans blue dye. The blood containing dye is then injected rapidly into the vein.

Estimation of duration of first passage of dye (t) and mean concentration (C) of dye in arterial blood Serial samples of arterial blood from the brachial artery are taken every 2 seconds and the dye concentration is determined.

- When the dye concentration is plotted as a function of time, a curve as shown in Fig. 4.3.12 (A, B, C and D) is obtained. The curve shows that the dye concentration reaches a peak and then steadily declines only to rise again (CD part of the curve) owing to recirculation of the dye.
- *Time duration of first passage of dye through the artery (t)* is determined by extrapolation of the descending limb (BC) of the curve to time scale axis. The point (E) on the time scale where the extrapolated limb meets it, tells the time (AE) of first circulation of dye in seconds.
- *The mean concentration (C)* of the dye is determined by representing the triangle area ABE as a rectangle AEFG with same area and one of its arm being AE. The height of the rectangle (AG) tells the mean concentration (*C*) of dye.
- *Calculation of cardiac output* is then made using the formula described above. For example, when:
  - Amount of dye injected (*Q*) is 5 mg
  - Time duration for first circulation is 40 seconds
  - Mean concentration of dye (*C*) = 15 mg/L, then

$$\text{Cardiac output} = \frac{Q \times 60}{C \times t} = \frac{5 \times 60}{1.5 \times 40} = \frac{300}{60} = 5\text{L/min}$$

Earlier the dye curves were used for investigating cardiac septal defects, but nowadays due to availability of sophisticated noninvasive techniques, this method is not usually used.

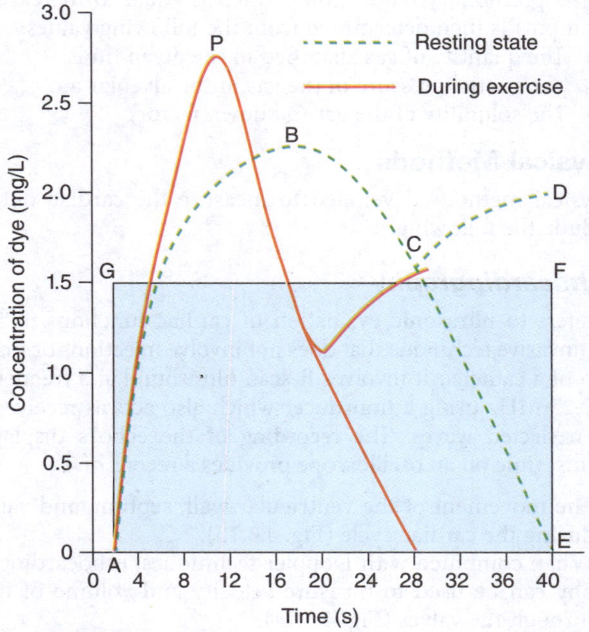

Fig. 4.3.12 Estimation of cardiac output by indicator (dye) dilution method.

Thermodilution Method

Principle It is also an indicator dilution technique in which instead of a dye, 'cold saline' is used as an indicator. The cardiac output is measured by determining the resultant change in the blood temperature in pulmonary artery.

Procedure In this technique, two thermistors, one each in the inferior vena cava and pulmonary artery are placed with the help of cardiac catheter.

- A known volume of sterile cold saline is then injected into the inferior vena cava.
- Temperature of the blood entering the heart from inferior vena cava and that of the blood leaving the heart via pulmonary artery is determined by the thermistors.
- The cardiac output is then measured from the values of temperature by applying the principle of indicator dilution technique.

$$F = V_I \times (T_B - T_I)/\Delta T_B \times t$$

where:

F = blood flow in litres per second
V_I = volume of the injectate
T_B and T_I = temperature of blood and injectate, respectively
ΔT_B = mean change in the pulmonary artery blood
t = duration of first passage of injectate in seconds

Note: The advantage of thermal dilution over dye dilution method is that withdrawal of blood for sampling is not required. Therefore, this method is useful for estimating cardiac output in infants and small children in whom the blood volume is limited.

Method Employing Inhalation of Inert Gases

- In this technique, an inert gas which dissolves in plasma but does not combine with Hb or other constituents of the blood is used as an indicator. Such gases include nitrous oxide and acetylene; the last one gives more accurate results.
- The pulmonary blood flow (which is equal to the cardiac output) is then determined from the following values:
  - The quantity of gas absorbed in the given time
  - The partial pressure of the gas in the alveolar air
  - The solubility of the gas (a known factor)

Physical Methods

Physical methods developed to measure the cardiac output include the following:

Echocardiography

It refers to ultrasonic evaluation of cardiac functions. It is a noninvasive technique that does not involve injections or insertion of a catheter. It involves B-scan ultrasound at a frequency of 2.25 MHz using a transducer which also acts as receiver of the reflected waves. The recording of the echoes displayed against time on an oscilloscope provides a record of:

- The movement of the ventricular wall, septum, and valves during the cardiac cycle (Fig. 4.3.13).
- When combined with Doppler techniques, echocardiography can be used to measure velocity and volume of flow through the valves (Fig. 4.3.14).

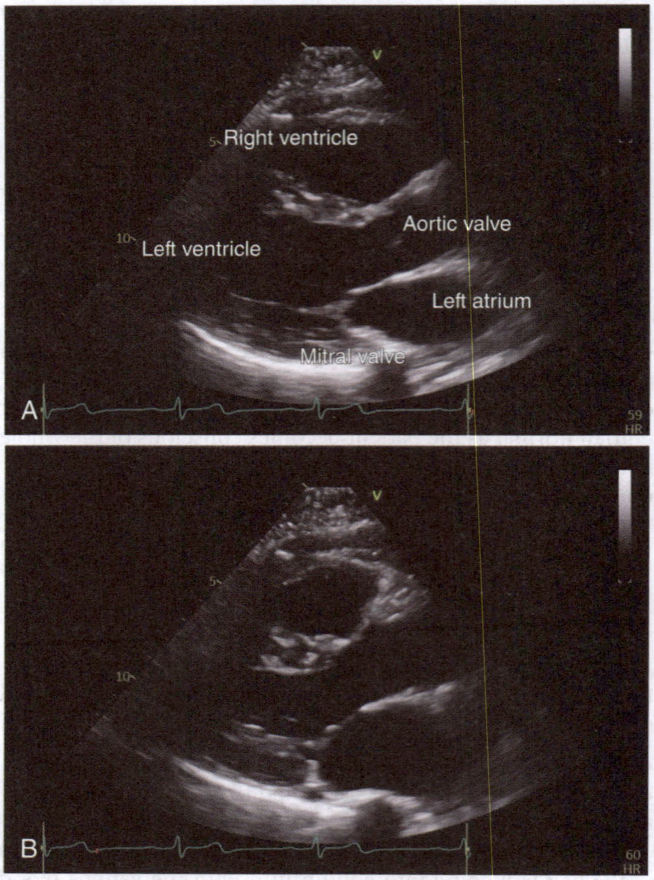

Fig. 4.3.13 Parasternal long-axis view of the heart showing **A,** the inflow of the left ventricle from the left atrium via mitral valve, and **B,** outflow of the left ventricle into the aorta via aortic valve.

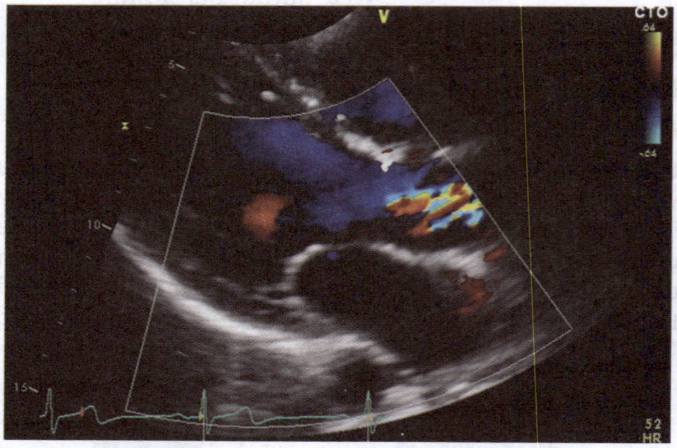

Fig. 4.3.14 Parasternal long-axis view of the heart with colour Doppler showing red flow (coming towards the echo probe) from the left atrium to the left ventricle, and the blue flow (away from the echo probe) from the left ventricle to the aorta.

- Thus, echocardiography is particularly useful in evaluating the end-diastolic volume, end-systolic volume, cardiac output and valvular defects.

Ballistocardiography Method

This method is not used practically. Ballistocardiography refers to graphical record of the pulsations created due to ballistic recoil of the pumping heart. The ballistic recoil occurs in accordance with Newton's third law of motion, i.e. when heart pumps blood into aorta and pulmonary artery, recoil is given to the heart and the body in the opposite direction. This is similar to that of ballistic recoil when a bullet is fired from the rifle.

The ballistic recoil pulsations can be recorded graphically by making the subject to lie on a suspended bed movable in the long axis of the body. The cardiac output is determined by analysing the graph obtained.

VARIATIONS IN CARDIAC OUTPUT

Physiological Causes of Variations in Cardiac Output

Age: Because of less body surface area, children have more cardiac index than adults.

Sex: Since the body surface area is less in females, they have higher cardiac index than the males.

Diurnal variation: In the early morning, cardiac output is low, which increases in the day time depending on the basal condition of the individual.

Environmental temperature: Moderate change in environmental temperature does not cause any change in cardiac output. A high environmental temperature is associated with an increase in the cardiac output.

Anxiety and excitement: These are reported to increase the cardiac output by 50%–100%.

Eating: It is associated with an increase in cardiac output approximately by 30%.

Exercise: It may increase the cardiac output up to 700% depending on the vigorousness of exercise.

Pregnancy: An increase in cardiac output to the tune of 45%–60% is reported during the later months of the pregnancy.

High altitude: The cardiac output is increased at high altitude due to release of adrenaline as a consequence to hypoxia.

Posture change: Sitting or standing from lying down position may decrease the cardiac output by 20%–30% because of pooling of blood in lower limbs.

Pathological Causes of Variations in Cardiac Output

Increase in cardiac output is seen in the following conditions:

- *Fever,* due to increased oxidative processes
- *Anaemia,* due to hypoxia
- *Hyperthyroidism,* due to increased metabolism

Decrease in cardiac output may occur in the following conditions:

- *Rapid arrhythmias,* due to incomplete filling
- *Congestive cardiac failure,* due to weak contractions of heart
- *Cardiac shock,* due to poor pumping and circulation
- *Incomplete heart block,* owing to defective pumping action of the heart
- *Haemorrhage,* because of decreased blood volume
- *Hypothyroidism,* due to decreased basal metabolism

REGULATION OF CARDIAC OUTPUT

The cardiac output increases or decreases in various physiological and pathological conditions as described above. The variations in the cardiac output are brought out by certain factors operating through certain mechanisms by an integrated role.

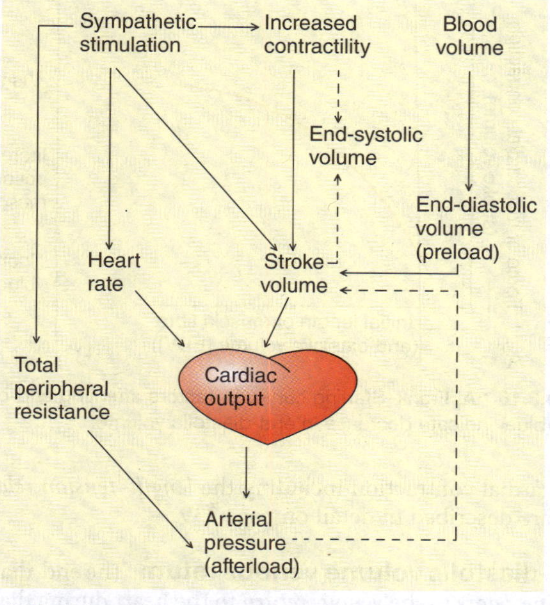

Fig. 4.3.15 Interaction between the factors that regulate cardiac output and arterial pressure. Solid lines indicate increase and dotted lines indicate a decrease.

The cardiac output (CO), as we know, is the product of stroke volume (SV) and heart rate (HR), i.e. $CO = SV \times HR$. Therefore, variations in the cardiac output can be produced by the factors that change stroke volume or heart rate, or both. The main factors affecting cardiac output are venous return, myocardial contractility, peripheral resistance and heart rate (Fig. 4.3.15).

Cardiac Output Control Mechanisms

The cardiac output is regulated by two mechanisms: intrinsic and extrinsic.

1. Intrinsic Regulation (Frank–Starling Mechanism)

The force of contraction of cardiac muscle fibres like that of skeletal muscle fibres depends on its preload. The preload determines the initial length (resting length) of the muscle fibres.

- According to *Frank–Starling law* of heart, 'within physiological limits' the force of contraction of *cardiac muscle* is proportionate to the initial length of muscle fibres.
- In the heart, end-diastolic volume forms the preload. Thus, the stretching of the cardiac muscle fibres to increase their initial length depends on the end-diastolic volume. Therefore, precisely, the Frank–Starling law of heart can be stated as, within physiological limits the force of cardiac contraction is proportional to its end-diastolic volume. This fact was demonstrated approximately a century ago by Frank and Starling on the heart–lung preparation in a dog, described on page 286. Since, in this intrinsic regulation mechanism, cardiac muscle fibres are stretched to increase their initial length, it is also termed as *heterometric mechanism.*

The relationship between ventricular stroke volume and end-diastolic volume is called the *Frank–Starling curve* (Fig. 4.3.16). Details of the effect of preload on force of

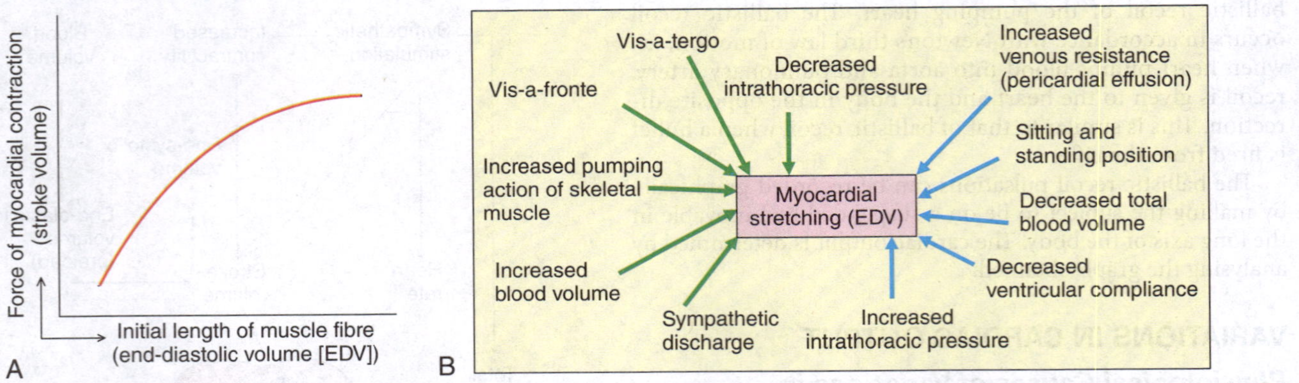

Fig. 4.3.16 **A,** Frank–Starling curve. **B,** factors affecting end-diastolic volume. Arrows on the left (green) indicate increase and arrows on right (blue) indicate decrease in end-diastolic volume.

myocardial contraction including the *length–tension relationship* are described in detail on page 239.

End-diastolic volume venous return The end-diastolic volume refers to the *venous return* to the heart during diastole. Therefore, the factors that normally operate to regulate end-diastolic volume, i.e. the degree to which cardiac muscle is stretched are the same which affect the venous return.

Up to physiological limits, the cardiac output is directly proportional to the venous return. Thus, over any significant period of time, venous return must equal cardiac output. For an individual at rest, the cardiac output and venous return are approximately 5 L/min. A complicated interaction of neural, humoural and physical factors determine the flow rate. Factors affecting venous return (Fig. 4.3.16):

Factors affecting end diastolic volume (venous return)

The following factors increase/decrease the venomous return:

1. Respiratory pump Normally the intrapleural (intrathoracic) pressure at the end of expiration is approximately −2 mm Hg. During inspiration, the intrathoracic pressure becomes more negative (approximately −5 mm Hg) due to which the diameter of inferior vena cava is increased and pressure inside it is reduced; and there occurs descent of diaphragm which increases the intra-abdominal pressure. The decreased pressure inside the inferior vena cava coupled with increased intra-abdominal pressure during inspiration results in increased flow of blood into the right atrium. This mechanism of increased blood flow during inspiration is called *respiratory pump.* This respiratory pump operates strongly in forced respiration and in severe muscular exercise, increasing the venous return.

2. Cardiac pump The cardiac pump influences the venous return by two kinds of forces: 'vis-a-tergo' and 'vis-a-fronte'.

Vis-a-tergo refers to the forward push from behind, i.e. the propelling force which pushes the blood from veins into the right atrium. Vis-a-tergo results from the myocardial contraction during systole and is supplemented by the elastic recoil of the arterial wall (Windkessel effect, see page 305).

Vis-a-fronte refers to the suction force acting from the front which basically pulls the blood from the great veins into the right atrium. This suction force is created by ventricular contraction and has the following two components:

- *Ventricular systolic suction* results from pulling down of the fibrous AV ring causing enlargement of atrial lumen and thus decreasing the intra-atrial pressure which sucks blood from the inferior vena cava and superior vena cava. The fibrous AV ring is pulled down due to contraction of papillary muscles.
- *Ventricular diastolic suction* results from the opening of AV valves allowing rapid flow of blood from atria to ventricles. The sudden decrease in atrial pressure in turn sucks blood from the great veins.

  So, a decrease in ventricular compliance, i.e. an increase in the ventricular stiffness produced by myocardial infarction, infiltrative diseases and other abnormalities will decrease the venous return.

3. Muscle pump The muscle pump mechanism is responsible for flow of blood from the veins of the limbs to the heart. Therefore, increased pumping action of skeletal muscles will increase the venous return and decreased pumping of skeletal muscles will decrease the venous return.

Working of muscle pump is now explained. Two types of veins are present in the limbs: superficial and deep veins. Blood flows from the superficial veins into deep veins through communicating veins. Due to the presence of valves in the limb veins, the blood flows in one direction, i.e. from the periphery towards the heart and not in the reverse direction.

- *When the skeletal muscles contract*, the deep veins present in between the muscles are compressed, and due to increased pressure, the valve present proximal to the contracting muscle is opened up while the valve present on distal end is tightly closed and in this way the blood is propelled up towards the heart (Fig. 4.3.17A).
- *When the skeletal muscle relaxes*, a negative pressure is created in the segment of veins. So, due to backflow the proximal valve is closed and the distal valve is opened and blood is sucked up (Fig. 4.3.17B).
- *With rhythmic contractions of skeletal muscles* in this way, the blood is squeezed out of the limbs towards the heart.

Applied Aspect

In certain professions (e.g. nurses, traffic police), the individuals have to keep standing for a long time of a day. In such persons, sometimes the excessive venous pressure stretches the veins of the legs to such an extent that their diameter increases and the venous valves become incompetent. The venous pressure further increases and gradually the veins of lower limbs become large, tortuous and bulbous. This condition is called *varicose veins*.

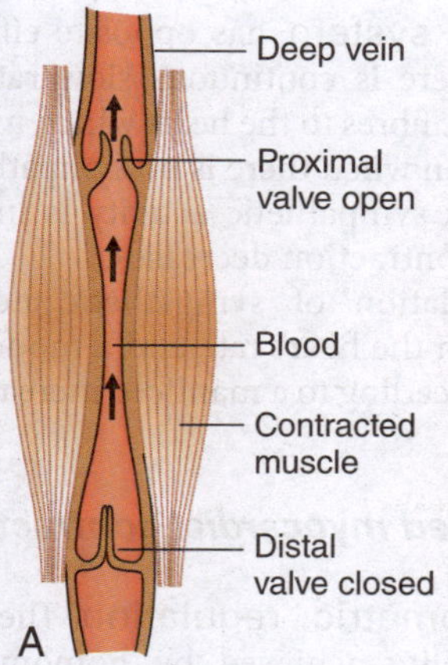

Fig. 4.3.17 Mechanism of muscle pump: **A,** during contraction of muscles; **B,** during relaxation of muscles.

4. *Blood volume* The mean circulating filling pressure (MCFP), which is equivalent to mean systemic filling pressure (MSFP), refers to the equilibrated pressure measured everywhere as a result of stoppage of blood flow in systemic circulation when heart stops pumping. The level of MSFP influences the venous return. Greater the MSFP, more the venous return; lower the MSFP, lesser the venous return (Fig. 4.3.18).

The MCFP in turn depends on the level of blood volume. When relationship of blood volume and MCFP is plotted, the graph (Fig. 4.3.19) shows the following:

- At blood volume of 4 L, the MCFP is nearly zero because the veins are unstressed.
- At blood volume of 5 L, the MCFP raises to 7 mm Hg.
- At higher blood volume, there is linear increase in MCFP.

Thus, the increased blood volume increases the venous return and a decreased blood volume decreases the venous return.

5. *Sympathetic discharge* On sympathetic stimulation, there occurs increase in the venous tone which decreases the capacity of the venous system (veins are capacitance vessels). Due to decrease in the venous capacity, the MCFP rises which increases the venous return. At normal blood volume, a strong sympathetic stimulation raises the MCFP from 7 to 17 mm Hg. Inhibition of sympathetics decreases the MCFP from 7 to

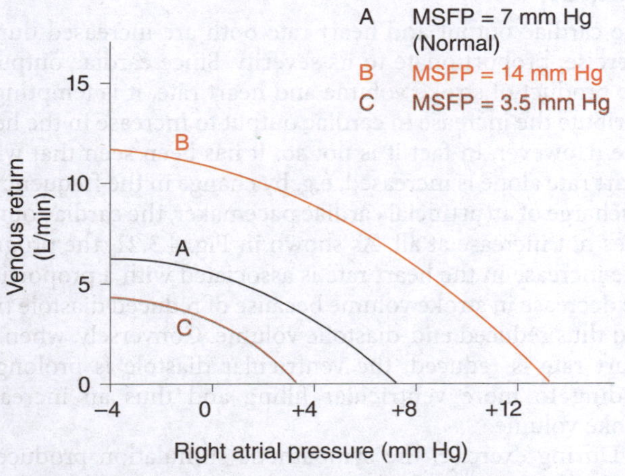

Fig. 4.3.18 Venous return curve showing relationship with mean systemic filling pressure.

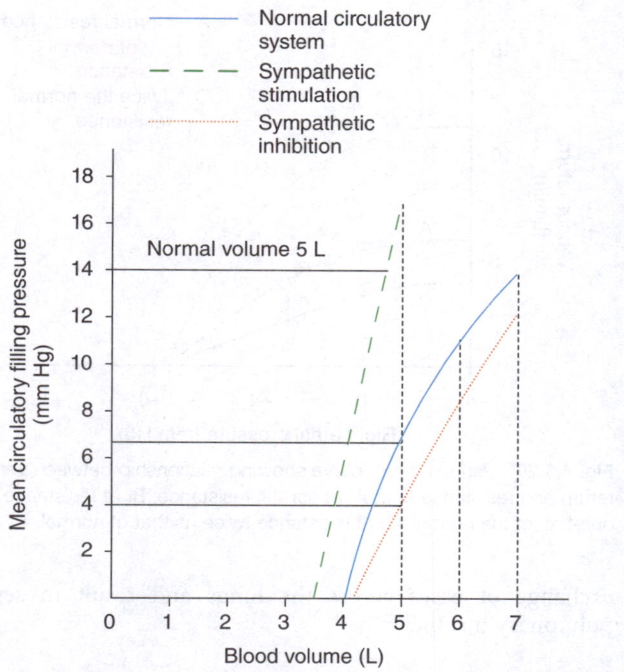

Fig. 4.3.19 Relationship between mean circulatory filling pressure and blood volume.

4 mm Hg (due to venous dilatation) and thus decreases the venous return (Fig. 4.3.19).

6. *Standing body position* It is associated with a decreased venous return due to peripheral pooling of the blood.

7. *Resistance to venous return* Normally, two-third resistance to venous flow is offered by veins and one-third by the arteries. Resistance decreases the venous return. The venous resistance is considered to be more important regarding venous return, as the veins being capacitance vessels, rise in the venous pressure is less effective to push the blood towards the heart. On the other hand, as with increased resistance in arterioles or small arteries, with little accumulation of blood in the arteries there is great increase in the pressure (30 times as compared to veins), which overcomes the effect of increase in resistance. As shown in Fig. 4.3.20, decrease in the resistance to venous return to one-half of the normal increases the venous return two times and rotates the curve upwards (Fig. 4.3.20B), whereas an increase in the resistance to venous flow twice the normal decreases the venous return to half and rotates the curve downwards (Fig. 4.3.20C).

Clinical significance of frank–starling mechanism

For small, momentary adjustments necessary for keeping the outputs of two ventricles equal and adjusting them to match the venous return, the intrinsic regulation works continuously. For example, if the output of the right ventricle increases momentarily, the venous return to left heart will increase, which in turn increases the output of the right ventricle. The accuracy with which this adjustment is made can be understood by considering what would happen if the right ventricular output exceeds left ventricular output by as little as 0.1 mL/beat, i.e. 7 mL/min. Then, in a period of 3 hours, the pulmonary blood volume will be increased by more than 1 L ($7 \times 60 \times 3 = 1260$ mL). This will prevent the optimal

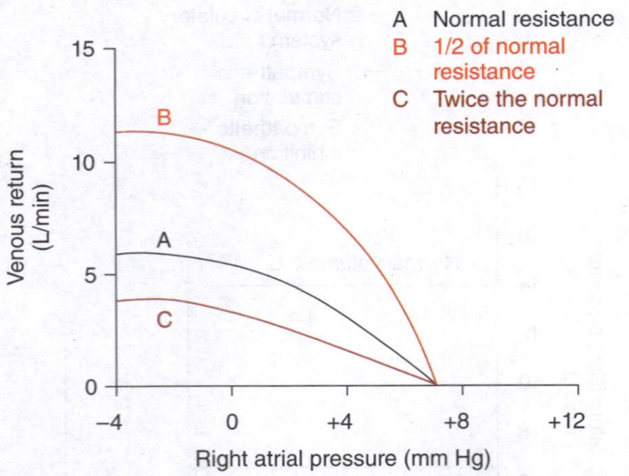

Fig. 4.3.20 Venous return curve showing relationship between venous return and resistance to it: **A,** at normal resistance; **B,** at resistance one-half of the normal; **C,** at resistance twice as that of normal.

exchange of gases across the lungs and result in severe pulmonary insufficiency.

Maintenance of constant stroke volume when the peripheral resistance is increased is carried out by intrinsic mechanism When the peripheral resistance (blood pressure) is increased, initially the heart is unable to pump all the blood it normally does. The accumulated blood in the ventricle stretches the muscle fibres leading to great force of contraction; thus, the stroke volume is restored to normal in spite of greater resistance to the outflow.

Intrinsic control mechanism serves as a life-saving device in cardiac failure Left ventricular failure causes accumulation of blood within left ventricle, thereby decreasing blood supply to vital organs. Soon, accumulation of blood in the left ventricle increases the initial length of muscle fibres, leading to greater cardiac output according to Frank–Starling mechanism. However, when accumulation of blood is too great, the Frank–Starling law will fail to operate leading to decrease in blood supply to the vital organs and ultimately death may occur.

2. Extrinsic Regulation (Autonomic Neural Mechanism)

In this mechanism, stroke volume increases due to *increased myocardial contractility* without any increase in the initial muscle length. Therefore, it is also called *homometric mechanism*. The homometric regulation is governed by autonomic neural mechanism.

Stimulation of the sympathetic nerves to the heart results in increased myocardial contractility and is known as *positive inotropic effect*. The positive inotropic effect of the norepinephrine liberated at the sympathetic nerve endings is augmented by circulating norepinephrine.

Positive inotropic effect can also be defined as an increase in the *maximal velocity* of shortening (V'_{max}) when it is plotted as a function of afterload. For the ventricles, the afterload is the arterial pressure during the ejection phase. During any muscle contraction, the velocity of shortening and the force developed are inversely related. For details of the effect of afterload and the *force velocity curve*, see page 240.

Inhibition of sympathetic system has opposite effects. Under normal conditions, there is continuous slow rate of discharge through sympathetic fibres to the heart which maintains pumping 30% above (even when there is no sympathetic stimulation). Therefore, when sympathetic activity is inhibited, the ventricular force of contraction decreases.

In intact animals, stimulation of sympathetic nerves produces a marked increase in the heart rate and a moderate increase in the stroke volume leading to a manifold increase in the cardiac output.

Characteristics of increased myocardial contractility are:

Characteristics of homometric regulation The increased myocardial contractility achieved by homometric regulation differs from the increase in force of contraction of myocardium achieved by heterometric regulation. Its characteristic features are as follows:

- The ventricles contract more forcefully and more rapidly, i.e. velocity of shortening of muscle is increased. As a result, the ventricles are able to do more work per stroke, i.e. ejection fraction increases at the same end-diastolic volume (without increase in venous return).
- Due to more complete emptying of ventricles during each systole, the *end-systolic volume is decreased.*
- Due to increased stroke output, *arterial pressure is increased.*

Mechanism of effects of sympathetic stimulation Sympathetic stimulation increases the myocardial contractility by causing *activation of* β_1-adrenergic receptors and Gs. Activation of β_1-receptors results in activation of adenylyl cyclase and increased intracellular cyclic AMP, which in turn

- Increases the concentration of Ca^{2+} within the myocardial cells causing a more rapid and forceful contraction.
- Protein kinase causes more rapid intake of Ca^{2+} by sarcoplasmic reticulum (SR), which shortens the duration of both the action potential and contraction.

Parasympathetic activity There is a negative inotropic effect of parasympathetic (vagal) stimulation. This effect, however, is not much because vagal fibres are mainly distributed to the atria and not much to the ventricles.

Role of Heart Rate in Control of Cardiac Output

The cardiac output and heart rate both are increased during exercise, proportionate to its severity. Since cardiac output is the product of stroke volume and heart rate, it is tempting to attribute the increase in cardiac output to increase in the heart rate. However, in fact it is not so. It has been seen that when heart rate alone is increased, e.g. by change in the frequency of discharge of an artificial cardiac pacemaker, the cardiac output does not increase at all. As shown in Fig. 4.3.21, the progressive increase in the heart rate is associated with a proportionate decrease in stroke volume because of reduced diastole time and thus reduced end-diastolic volume. Conversely, when the heart rate is reduced, the ventricular diastole is prolonged, leading to more ventricular filling and thus an increased stroke volume.

During exercise, the sympathetic stimulation produces a marked increase in the heart rate (200%–300%) due to positive chronotropism and moderate increase (50%–60%) in the

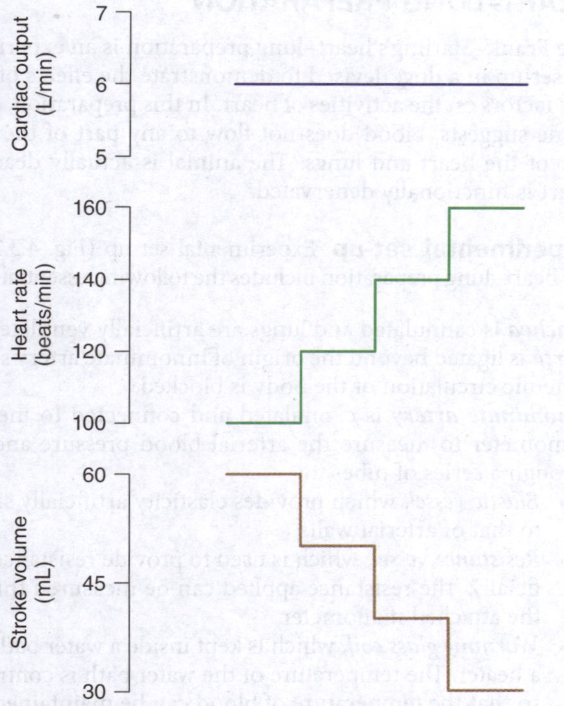

Fig. 4.3.21 Effect of increase in heart rate through an artificial pacemaker on stroke volume and cardiac output.

stroke volume due to positive inotropism, leading to manifold increase in cardiac output.

Integrated Control of Cardiac Output

In intact animals and humans, the intrinsic and extrinsic mechanisms described above operate simultaneously in an integrated way to maintain cardiac output. Therefore, in a given situation, depending on the status of end-diastolic volume and status of myocardial contractility, the individual will have one of the curves from the 'family of Frank–Starling curves'.

Interaction of Frank–Starling Mechanism and Myocardial Contractility

Factors causing increased myocardial contractility

shift the Frank–Starling curve to the left (Fig. 4.3.22). Increased contractility (positive inotropism) refers to greater contraction force at a given preload or end-diastolic volume. Factors increasing myocardial contractility:

1. ***Sympathetic stimulation*** increases myocardial contractility by causing activation of β_1-adrenergic receptors, as discussed above.
2. ***Catecholamines*** also exert their positive inotropic effect via their action on cardiac β_1-adrenergic receptors by a mechanism similar to that of sympathetic stimulation.
3. ***Xanthines*** such as caffeine and theophylline exert their positive inotropic effect by inhibiting the breakdown of cyclic AMP.
4. ***Glucagon*** causes positive inotropic effect by increasing the formation of cyclic AMP.
5. ***Digitalis and related drugs*** exert their positive inotropic effect by their inhibitory effect on Na^+–K^+ ATPase in the myocardium. The inhibition causes an increase in intracellular Na^+, which in turn increases the availability of Ca^{2+} in the cell. Digitalis, which was initially prepared from the plant *Digitalis purpurea,* has been used for centuries to treat heart failure.

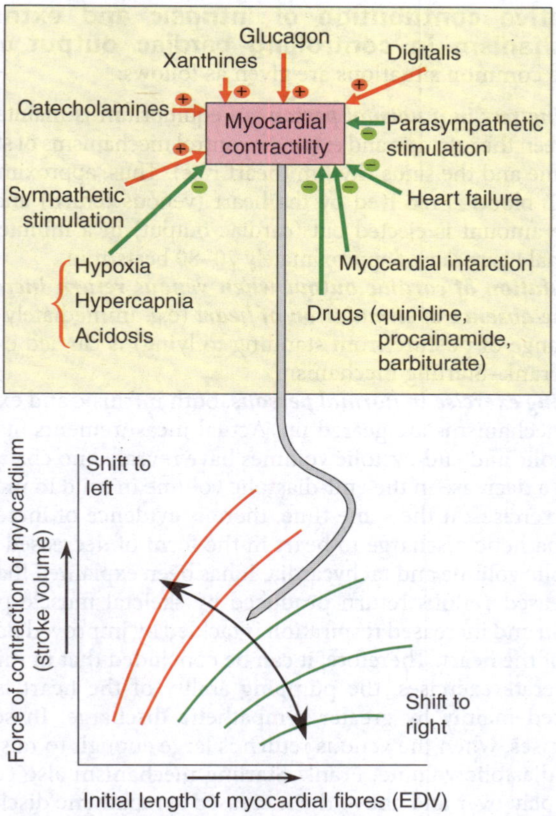

Fig. 4.3.22 Effect of changes in myocardial contractility on Frank–Starling curve. The factors which increase the contractility shift the curve to left and those decrease the contractility shift the curve to right. EDV, end-diastolic volume.

Factors causing decreased myocardial contractility

These factors shift the Frank–Starling curve to the right (Fig. 4.3.22). The decreased contractility (negative inotropism) represents a decrease in the force of contraction at any fibre length or ventricular volume. Its causes are as follows:

1. ***Parasympathetic (vagal) stimulation:*** Since the vagal fibres are distributed mainly to atria and not to ventricles, vagal stimulation causes negative inotropic effect on the atrial muscles and indirectly mild negative inotropic effect on the ventricles, reducing strength of heart contraction by 20%–30%.
2. ***Heart failure*** is also associated with reduced myocardial contractility due to intrinsic depression. The cause of this depression is not known.
3. ***Myocardial infarction*** may result in fibrotic and nonfunctional area in myocardium, resulting in reduction of total ventricular performance.
4. ***Hypercapnia, hypoxia and acidosis*** produce negative inotropic effect by causing a decrease in the formation of cyclic AMP.
5. ***Drugs*** such as quinidine, procainamide and barbiturates depress myocardial contractility.

Relative contribution of intrinsic and extrinsic mechanism in controlling cardiac output under some common situations are given as follows:

During rest in a normal person, an equilibrium is maintained between the intrinsic and extrinsic control mechanisms of stroke volume and the sinus rhythm (heart rate). Thus, approximately 5–6 L blood is received by the heart (venous return) and the same amount is ejected out (cardiac output) in a minute at a normal heart rate of approximately 70–80 beats/min.

Regulation of cardiac output when venous return increases in the absence of stimulation of heart (e.g. immediately after a change of posture from standing to lying) is carried out by the Frank–Starling mechanism.

During exercise in normal persons, both intrinsic and extrinsic mechanisms are geared up. Actual measurements of end-diastolic and end-systolic volumes have revealed no change or even a decrease in the end-diastolic volume in mild to moderate exercise. At the same time, there is evidence of increased sympathetic discharge to heart in the form of decreased end-systolic volume and tachycardia. It has been explained that the increased venous return produced by skeletal muscle pump action and increased respiration is tackled by improved pumping of the heart. Therefore, it can be concluded that in mild to moderate exercises, the pumping ability of the heart is enhanced mainly by greater sympathetic discharge. In severe exercises, when the venous return is large enough to raise the end-diastolic volume, Frank–Starling mechanism also comes into play over and above the increased sympathetic discharge thus result in very high cardiac output.

In patients with transplanted hearts, Frank–Starling mechanism is practically the only mechanism regulating the cardiac output, since there is absence of cardiac innervation (Fig. 4.3.23). During exercise, the increase in cardiac output seen in these patients is not so rapid, and their maximal increase is smaller than that in normal individuals but is appreciable.

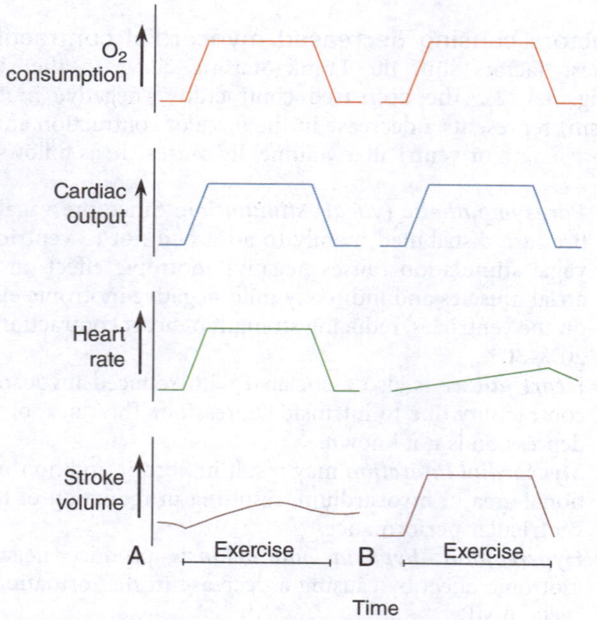

Fig. 4.3.23 Cardiac response to moderate exercise: **A,** in normal human; **B,** in patients with transplanted heart.

HEART–LUNG PREPARATION

The Frank–Starling's heart–lung preparation is an experimental set-up in a dog, devised to demonstrate the effects of various factors on the activities of heart. In this preparation, as the name suggests, blood does not flow to any part of the body except the heart and lungs. The animal is actually dead and heart is functionally denervated.

Experimental set-up Experimental set up (Fig. 4.3.24) of the heart–lung preparation includes the following essential steps:

Trachea is cannulated and lungs are artificially ventilated.

Aorta is ligated beyond the origin of innominate artery so that systemic circulation of the body is blocked.

Innominate artery is cannulated and connected to mercury manometer to measure the arterial blood pressure and also through a series of tubes to:

- *Elastic vessel,* which provides elasticity artificially similar to that of arterial wall.
- *Resistance vessel,* which is used to provide resistance artificially. The resistance applied can be measured through the attached manometer.
- *Warming glass coil,* which is kept inside a water bath with a heater. The temperature of the water bath is controlled, so that the temperature of blood can be maintained.
- *Flowmeter,* which determines the amount of blood flowing through it (cardiac output).
- *Venous reservoir,* which represents the peripheral venous system. It is connected through a tube to the superior vena cava. A screw-type clamp is fitted to the rubber tube. It is used to adjust the amount of blood returning to heart (venous return).

Thus, the blood ejected from the left ventricle after passing through the above attachment ultimately reaches the right atrium. From there, the blood flows to the right ventricle, pulmonary artery, lungs and back to heart through the pulmonary veins.

Inferior vena cava is attached to manometer to record the right atrial pressure.

Bell's cardiometer is fitted to the ventricle for measuring the stroke volume of the heart. The recording is made through *Marey's tambour* connected to the cardiometer.

Uses of heart–lung preparation In the heart–lung preparation, heart works as an isolated organ. It can be used to demonstrate the effect of various factors on the heart's activities as:

1. Effect of venous return on stroke volume (Frank–Starling mechanism)

Venous return to the heart is changed through the venous reservoir and stroke volume at different levels of venous return is recorded through the cardiometer. The record shows:

- An increase in stroke volume with increase in venous return (Fig. 4.3.25).
- A decrease in stroke volume with decrease in venous return.

These observations demonstrate the Frank–Starling's law (intrinsic mechanism controlling stroke volume).

2. Effect of sympathetic stimulation on stroke volume

When the stellate ganglion (cardiosympathetic nerve) is stimulated without any change in the venous return, the stroke volume is increased but with lower end-systolic

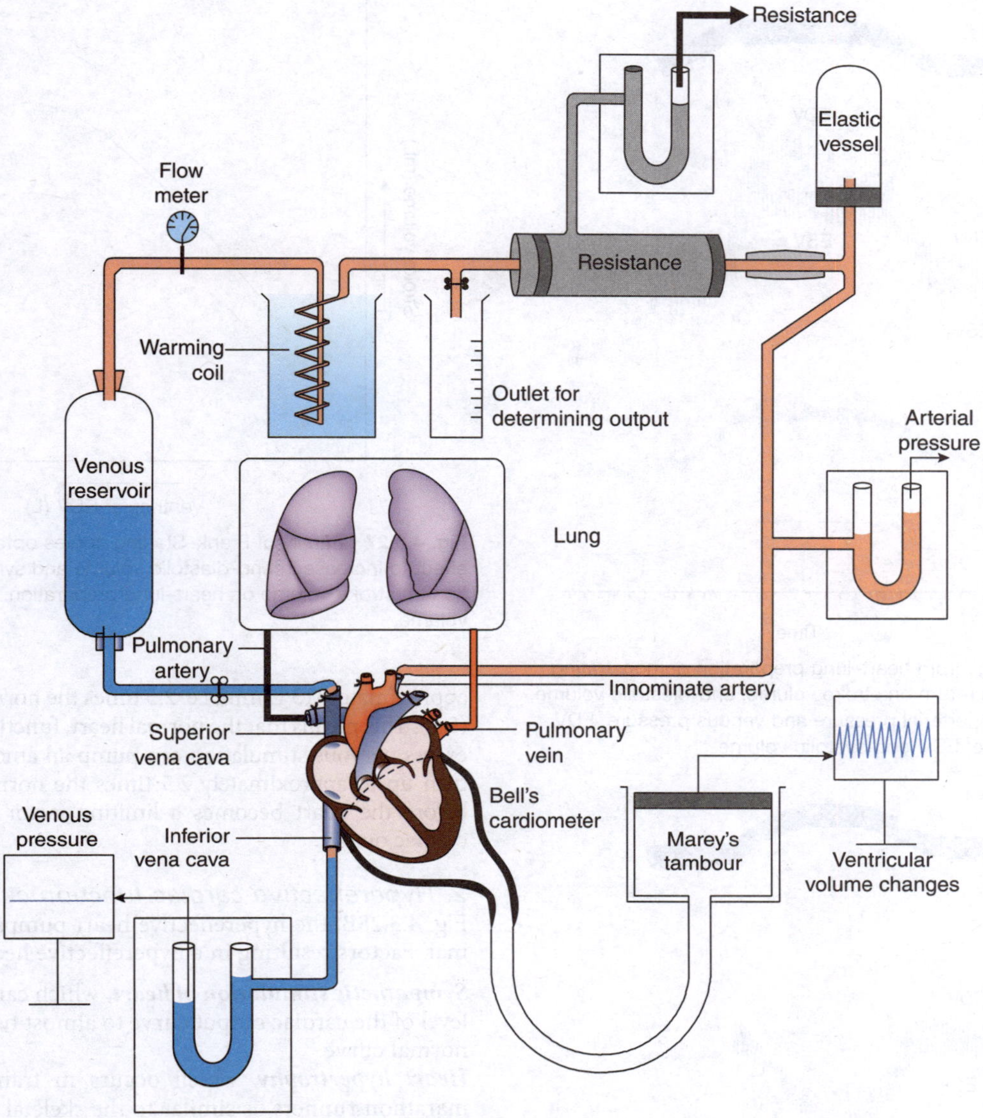

Fig. 4.3.24 Heart–lung preparation.

and end-diastolic volume (Fig. 4.3.26). This activity demonstrates the extrinsic control mechanism of stroke volume. Right atrial pressure is also reduced. It is due to increased suction of blood from the atria by the vigorously contracting ventricle.

3. Combined effect of increase in end-diastolic volume and sympathetic stimulation on stroke volume At a given rate of sympathetic stimulation, the end-diastolic volume is gradually increased and the resulting stroke volume is plotted against the end-diastolic volume to give a Frank–Starling curve; with different rates of sympathetic stimulation (0/S–10/S), a family of such curves is obtained (Fig. 4.3.27). From these curves, it can be inferred that even during sympathetic stimulation, an increase in end-diastolic volume increases the stroke volume of heart.

4. To demonstrate the effect of peripheral resistance on cardiac output Resistance is increased through the resistance vessel and its effect on cardiac output is recorded:

- With increase in the peripheral resistance, cardiac output is increased.
- With decrease in the peripheral resistance, the cardiac output is decreased.

5. Cardiac function curves These curves can also be recorded using a heart–lung preparation. These include:

- The cardiac output curves
- The venous return curves
- The cardiovascular curves

Cardiac and Vascular Function Curves

The cardiac and vascular function curves provide the graphic analysis of cardiac output, capacity of the ventricles to pump and relationship between cardiac output and central venous pressure (CVP). Such a graphical analysis provides useful information in patients with cardiac failure. Most of the curves are obtained from animal experiments by using heart–lung preparation. However, they do represent the function of ventricles in human heart. These curves include:

- Cardiac function curves
- Vascular function curves
- Cardiovascular function curves

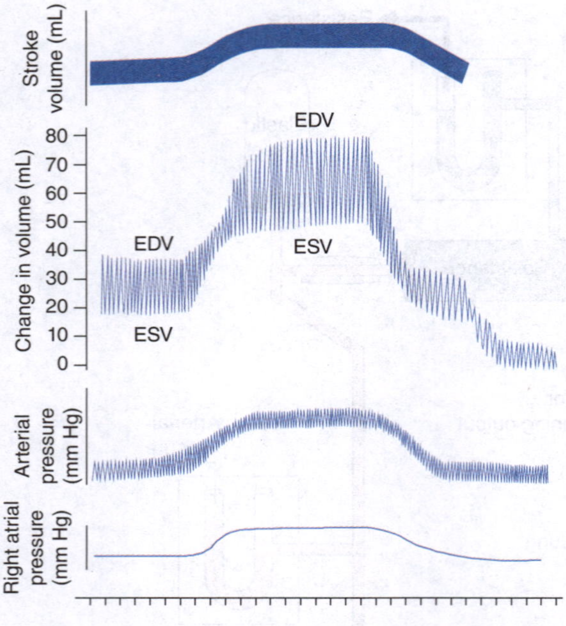

Fig. 4.3.25 Tracings from heart–lung preparation demonstrating the effect of venous return on stroke volume, end-diastolic volume, end-systolic volume, arterial pressure and venous pressure. EDV, end-diastolic volume; ESV, end-systolic volume.

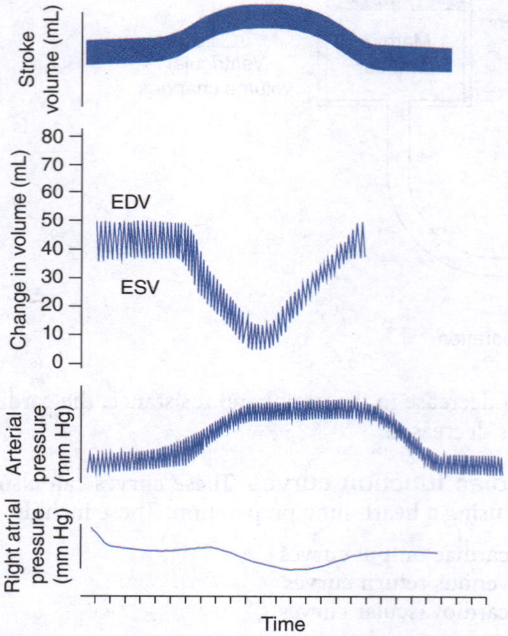

Fig. 4.3.26 Tracings from heart–lung preparation demonstrating the effect of sympathetic nerve stimulation on stroke volume, end-diastolic volume, end-systolic volume, arterial pressure and venous pressure. EDV, end-diastolic volume; ESV, end-systolic volume.

Cardiac function curves The cardiac function curves reflect the relationship between CVP, i.e. right atrial pressure, and the cardiac output (Frank–Starling curve). There are three types of cardiac function curves.

1. Normal cardiac function curve As shown in Fig. 4.3.28A, the plateau level of normal cardiac function curve is

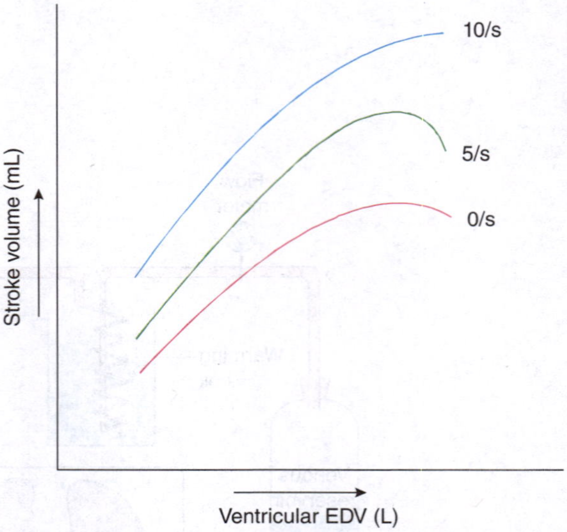

Fig. 4.3.27 Family of Frank–Starling curves obtained by combined effect to increase in end-diastolic volume and sympathetic stimulation on stroke volume on heart–lung preparation. EDV, end-diastolic volume.

approximately 13 L/min, i.e. 2.5 times the normal cardiac output (5 L). This means that the normal heart, functioning without any excess nervous stimulation can pump an amount of venous return up to approximately 2.5 times the normal venous return before the heart becomes a limiting factor in the control of cardiac output.

2. Hypereffective cardiac function curve As shown in Fig. 4.3.28B, the hypereffective heart pumps better than normal. Factors resulting in a hypereffective heart:

Sympathetic stimulation of heart, which can raise the plateau level of the cardiac output curve to almost twice the plateau of normal curve.
Heart hypertrophy, which occurs in trained athletes, e.g. marathon runners, is similar to the skeletal muscle hypertrophy occurring due to heavy exercise. This increases the plateau level of cardiac output curve, sometimes 50%–100%, and therefore allows the heart to pump much greater than the usual amount of cardiac output. When combined with sympathetic excitation, the effect can allow the heart to pump 30–40 L/min. This increased level of pumping is one of the most important factors in determining the runner running time.

3. Hypoeffective cardiac function curve This curve (Fig. 4.3.28C) results due to the factors that decrease the heart's ability to pump blood. These factors include:

- Reduced sympathetic discharge
- Decreased ventricular compliance as in myocardial infarction, myocarditis
- Insufficient pumping as in valvular or septal defects of the heart
- Reduced ventricular filling as in pericardial effusion or cardiac tamponade
- Increased load on the heart, as in hypertension

Vascular function curves The vascular function curves reflect the relationship between venous return and venous pressure. Normal vascular function curve and the factors

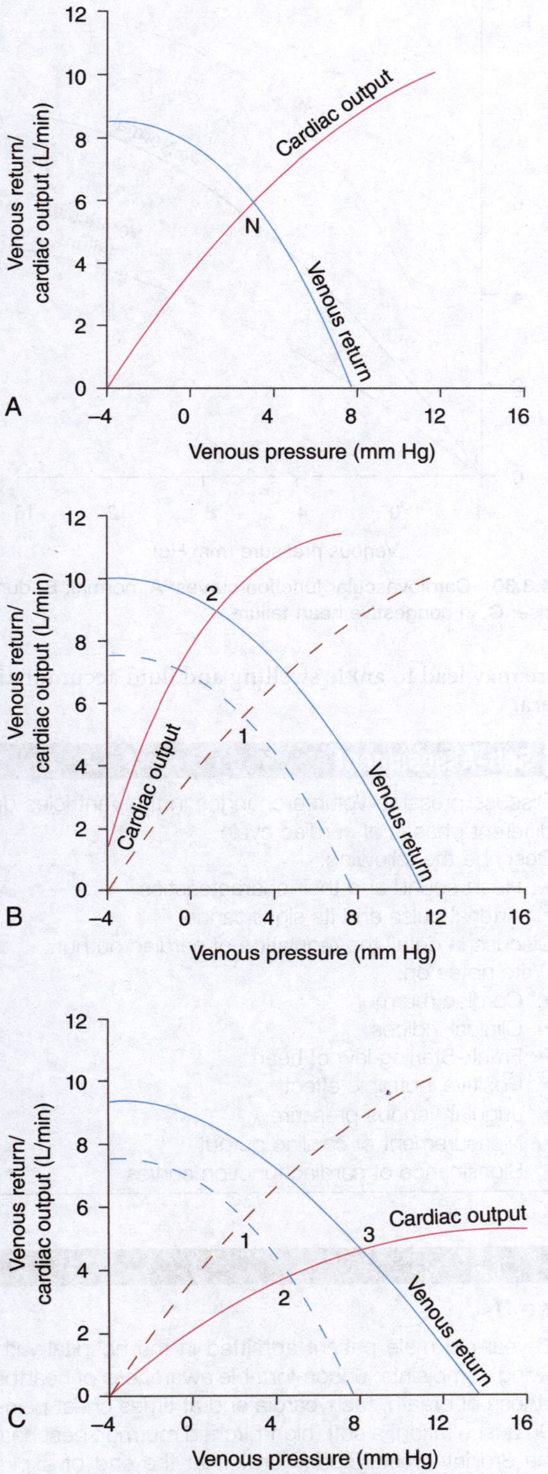

Fig. 4.3.28 Cardiac function curve: **A,** normal; **B,** hypereffective; **C,** hypoeffective.

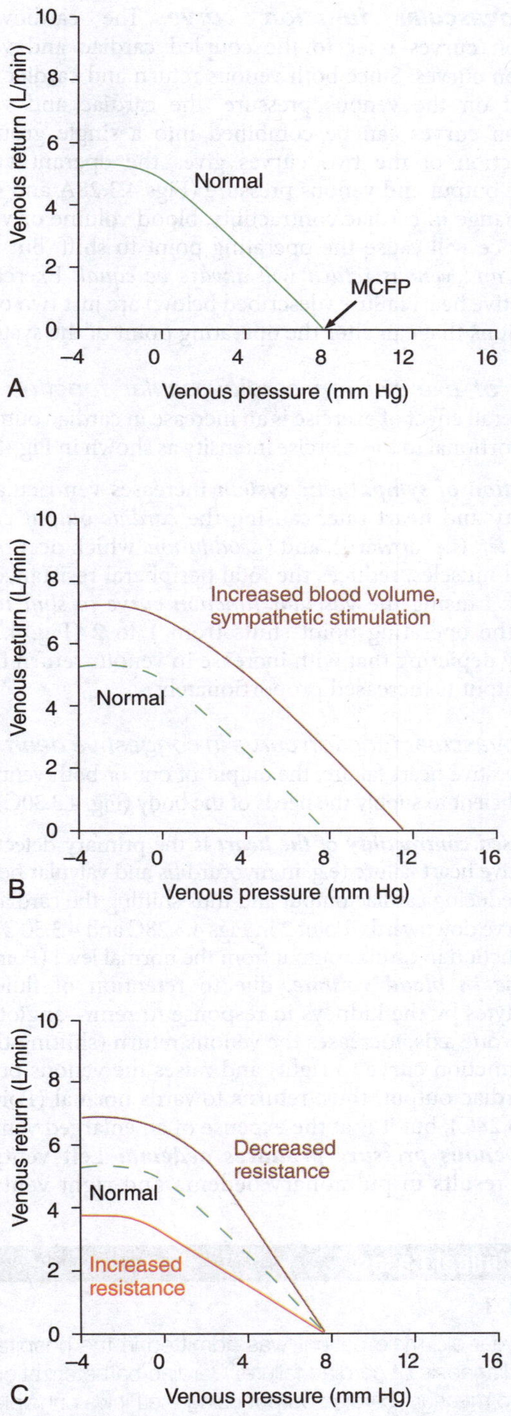

Fig. 4.3.29 Vascular function curves: **A,** normal; **B,** effect of increased blood volume and sympathetic stimulation; **C,** effect of change in arterial resistance.

affecting are depicted in Fig. 4.3.29, which can be interpreted as follows:

- As shown in Fig. 4.3.29A, in a *normal curve,* the venous pressure decreases as venous return increases because the transfer of blood from the venous to the arterial system increases. When venous return is zero, venous pressure is maximum and is referred to as the mean circulatory filling pressure (MCFP).
- The MCFP increases with increase in blood volume (Fig. 4.3.19) and with increase in sympathetic stimulation (which increases venous tone). These factors, which increase the MCFP, cause the vascular function curve to shift to the right (Fig. 4.3.29B).
- *Changes in arteriolar resistance* alter the slope of the vascular function curve. An increased resistance reduces the cardiac output (venous return) and a decreased resistance increases the venous return (Fig. 4.3.29C).

Cardiovascular function curves The cardiovascular function curves refer to the coupled cardiac and vascular function curves. Since both venous return and cardiac output depend on the venous pressure, the cardiac and vascular function curves can be combined into a single group. The intersection of the two curves gives the operant value of cardiac output and venous pressure (Figs 4.3.28A and 4.3.30). Any change in cardiac contractility, blood volume or vascular resistance will cause the operating point to shift, but *cardiac output and venous return will always be equal.* Exercise and congestive heart failure (described below) are just two of many conditions that can alter the operating point of the system.

Effect of exercise on cardiovascular function curve

The overall effect of exercise is an increase in cardiac output that is proportional to the exercise intensity as shown in Fig. 4.3.30B.

Activation of sympathetic system increases ventricular contractility and heart rate, causing the *cardiac output curve to shift to left* (i.e. upward), and *vasodilation,* which occurs in the skeletal muscles, reduces the total peripheral resistance or afterload, causing the *vascular function curve to shift to right.* Thus, the operating point shifts from 1 to 2 (Fig. 4.3.28B), thereby depicting that with increase in venous return the cardiac output is increased proportionately.

Cardiovascular function curve in congestive heart failure

In congestive heart failure, the output of one or both ventricles is not sufficient to supply the needs of the body (Fig. 4.3.30C).

Decreased contractility of the heart is the primary defect in the congestive heart failure (e.g. in myocarditis and valvular heart disease), reducing cardiac output and thus shifting the cardiac function curve downwards. Point 2 in Figs 4.3.28C and 4.3.30C reflects the reduction in cardiac output from the normal level (Point 1).
Increase in blood volume, due to retention of fluids and electrolytes by the kidneys in response to renin–angiotensin-aldosterone axis, increases the venous return (shifting the vascular function curve to right) and raises the venous pressure. The cardiac output, thus, returns towards normal (Point 3 in Fig. 4.3.28C), but it is at the expense of an enlarged ventricle.
High venous pressure produces oedema: Left ventricular failure results in pulmonary oedema and right ventricular failure may lead to ankle swelling and fluid accumulation in viscera.

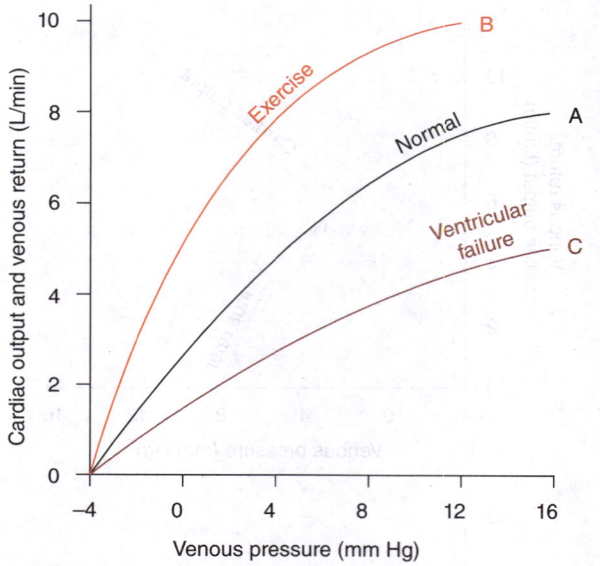

Fig. 4.3.30 Cardiovascular function curves: **A,** normal; **B,** during exercise; **C,** in congestive heart failure.

Self-Assessment

1. Discuss pressure volume changes in the ventricles during different phases of cardiac cycle.
2. Describe the following:
   - Heart sound and their characteristics
   - Arterial pulse and its significance
3. Discuss in detail the regulation of cardiac output.
4. Write notes on:
   - Cardiac murmur
   - Clinical indices
   - Frank-Starling law of heart
   - Positive inotropic effect
   - Jugular venous pressure
   - Measurement of cardiac output
   - Significance of cardiac function curves

Clinical Cases

Case 1

A 35-year-old male patient was admitted in the hospital with initial diagnosis of cardiac failure. Cardiac catheterization was done to measure cardiac output using the Fick's principle. The data obtained were as follows:
PAO_2 = 20 mL/dL
PVO_2 = 12 mL/dL
Oxygen consumption = 280 mL/min
Q1. How much is the cardiac output in this case?

Case 2

A patient presents to the emergency with intermittent chest pain. ECG and blood tests were performed to exclude the myocardial infarction. Echocardiogram shows thickening of left ventricular muscles and narrowing of aortic valves.
Q1. What is the diagnosis?
Q2. To decrease afterload, which medication should be advised?
Q3. How should the effectiveness of the drug be judged?

Case 3

A 66-year-old male patient admitted in the hospital with the following complaints: uncomfortable awareness of heartbeats, shortness of breath, tachycardia and at times chest pain.
- On auscultation, a soft, high-pitched murmur, best heard in the 3rd intercostal space on left at the end of expiration was observed.
- Pulse pressure was very high

Q1. What is the diagnosis?
Q2. What is the cause of murmur?
Q3. What is the reason for high pulse pressure?

Case 4

During routine examination of a 50-year-old female patient, third heart sound was heard on auscultation.
Q1. What is the most common condition in which the third heart sound is heard, and what are its signs and symptoms?

Case 5

A 67-year-old male patient presented to the physician with a complaint of difficulty in breathing when he exercises.

On auscultation, the doctor heard systolic murmur between apex and left sternal border.

Q1. What is the cause of systolic murmur?

Case 6

A 36-year-old female complained of intermittent chest discomfort that occurred frequently when she drinks lot of coffee to meet the deadline at work. On the basis of history and examination, a probable diagnosis of angina was made, and a stress test was advised to rule out ischaemia.

Q1. What is stress test?

Q2. What are the observations of stress test in this case?

Case 7

A 25-year-old female visited the physician with complains of generalized weakness and fatigue. On examination, it was found that she had pallor and breathlessness. On auscultation, systolic murmur was heard, and a probable diagnosis of severe anaemia was made.

Q1. What is cause of systolic murmur in this case?

Q2. What is the pathophysiology of systolic murmur in this case?

4.4 Dynamics of Circulation: Pressure and Flow of Blood and Lymph

CHAPTER OUTLINE

INTRODUCTION

Dynamics of circulation is concerned with flow of blood and lymph and also the pressure in the various segments of the vascular system of the body. For descriptive purposes, the 'dynamics of circulation' is discussed under the following headings:

- Functional organization and structure of vascular system
- Haemodynamics
- Blood flow and pressure in different segments of circulatory system
- Blood pressure (BP)

FUNCTIONAL ORGANIZATION AND STRUCTURE OF VASCULAR SYSTEM

ORGANIZATION OF VASCULAR SYSTEM

The vascular system, which consists of different types of blood vessels, constitutes the transport system of the body whose *primary functions* are as follows: (i) distribution of nutrients and oxygen to all body cells, and (ii) collection of waste products and CO_2 from different body cells and carrying them to excretory organs for excretion.

Secondary functions subserved by the vascular system are thermoregulation, distribution of hormones to the target tissues and distribution of antibodies and cells concerned with defence mechanism to various parts of the body.

To perform the above-mentioned functions, the vascular system is organized into two separate circulations, systemic and pulmonary, arranged in series (Fig. 4.4.1). In addition, parallel to the circulation of blood is the disposed circulation of lymph which helps the blood circulation to perform its various functions.

Systemic circulation Systemic circulation supplies blood to various systemic organs through parallel distribution channels (Fig. 4.4.1). This parallel arrangement of vessels ensures the supply of blood of the same arterial composition (i.e. same O_2 and CO_2 tension, pH, glucose level and essentially the same arterial pressure) to various body organs. In systemic circulation, from the left ventricle, blood is pumped through the arteries and arterioles to the capillaries, where it equilibrates with the interstitial fluid. The capillaries drain through the venules into the veins and ultimately to the right atrium.

Pulmonary circulation Pulmonary circulation is meant for oxygenation of blood. Since pulmonary circulation is arranged in series with systemic circulation, it receives the same amount of blood over any significant time period. Such a balanced output is achieved by the intrinsic property of the cardiac muscle known as Frank–Starling mechanism which has been described in Chapter 4.3 (page 401). In pulmonary circulation, from the right ventricle, blood is pumped through the pulmonary arteries to the pulmonary capillaries. In the pulmonary capillaries, the blood equilibrates with the O_2 and CO_2 of alveolar air. The capillaries then drain the oxygenated blood through venules and then through pulmonary veins into the left atrium.

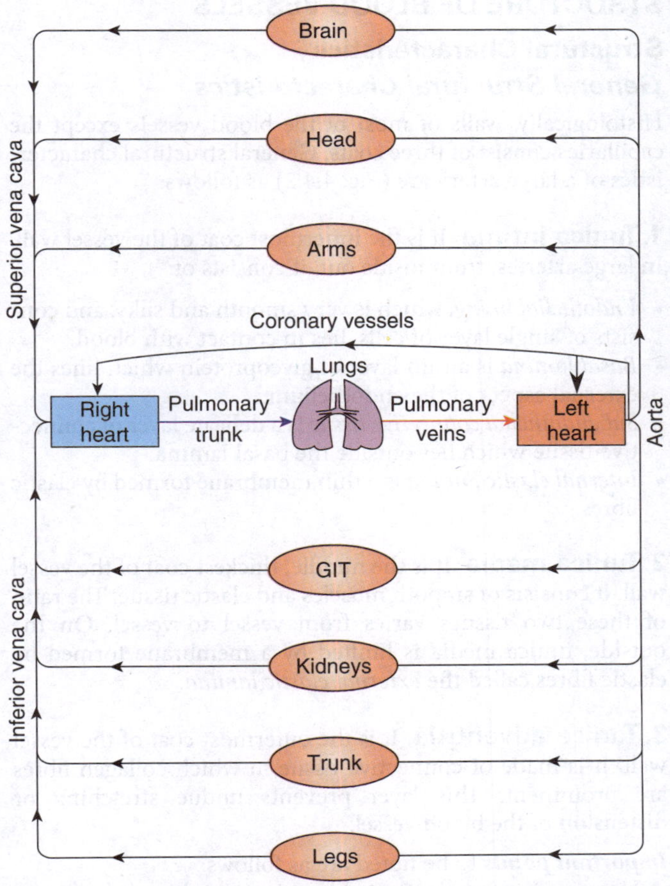

Fig. 4.4.1 A schematic illustration of the organization of cardiovascular system depicting the series arrangement of pulmonary and systemic circulation and parallel arrangement of vessels supplying blood to organs.

Lymphatic circulation Lymphatic circulation which is disposed in parallel to the circulation of blood can be considered a third type of circulation. Some tissue fluid enters the lymphatic channels as lymph, which is ultimately drained into the venous system via the thoracic lymphatic duct and the right lymphatic duct.

Systemic Vascular Tree

The arrangement of systemic circulation permits wide variations in regional distribution of blood. For descriptive purposes and from a functional point of view, the systemic vascular tree can be divided into the following types of blood vessels:

- *Large elastic arteries* (Windkessel vessels) which include aorta and its main branches such as carotid, iliac and axillary arteries
- *Large muscular* arteries (distribution vessels) which include most of the arteries of the body, e.g. arteries like radial, ulnar and popliteal arteries
- *Arterioles and precapillary sphincters* (resistance vessels)
- *Meta-arterioles and capillaries* (exchange vessels)
- *Venules* (postcapillary resistance vessels)
- *Veins* (capacitance vessels)
- *Arteriovenous anastomoses* (shunt or thoroughfare vessels)

STRUCTURE OF BLOOD VESSELS

Structural Characteristics

General Structural Characteristics

Histologically, walls of most of the blood vessels except the capillaries consist of three coats. General structural characteristics of a large artery are (Fig. 4.4.2) as follows:

1. Tunica intima It is the innermost coat of the vessel wall. In large arteries, from inside out, it consists of:

- *Endothelial lining*, which is very smooth and silky, and consists of single layer of cells, lies in contact with blood.
- *Basal lamina* is a thin layer of glycoprotein which lines the external aspect of the endothelium.
- *Subendothelial connective tissue* is a delicate layer of connective tissue which lies outside the basal lamina.
- *Internal elastic lamina* is a thin membrane formed by elastic fibres.

2. Tunica media It is the middle, thickest coat of the vessel wall. It consists of smooth muscles and elastic tissue. The ratio of these two tissues varies from vessel to vessel. On the outside, tunica media is limited by a membrane formed by elastic fibres called the *external elastic lamina*.

3. Tunica adventitia It is the outermost coat of the vessel wall. It is made of connective tissue in which collagen fibres are prominent. This layer prevents undue stretching or distension of the blood vessel.

Important points to be noted are as follows:
- Fibrous elements in the adventitia (mainly collagen) run longitudinally (i.e. along the length of the vessel).
- Elastic tissue and smooth muscles forming tunica media run circularly.
- Elastic fibres forming internal and external elastic laminae are often in the form of fenestrated sheets.

Specific Structural Characteristics

Large (elastic) arteries, in their tunica media, have dominant elastic tissue which provides them property of distensibility and elastic recoil.
Medium-sized arteries: In these arteries, the elastic tissue, in both intima and media, is much less and thus the proportion of smooth muscles increases.
Arterioles have characteristically no elastic tissue. Their media consists of a thick layer of smooth muscles and they have a *relatively narrow lumen*. Because of their structural characteristics, they act as resistance vessels.

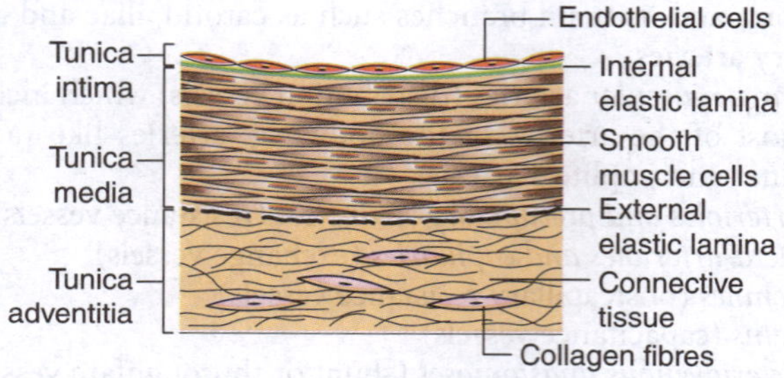

Fig. 4.4.2 Histological structure of an artery.

Meta-arterioles are relatively high-resistance conduits between arterioles and veins.
Capillaries arise directly from arterioles or meta-arterioles. A cuff of smooth muscle cells called the *precapillary sphincter* surrounds the origin of capillaries in some region. The capillary wall does not contain any tunica media and adventitia. It is formed essentially by endothelial cells which are lined on the outside by a basal lamina (glycoproteins), branching perivascular cells called *pericytes*. Further details of capillaries are described in 'Microcirculation' (see page 307).
Postcapillary venules, which measure 20–60 µm in diameter, are the *most permeable part* of microcirculation.
Veins are relatively thin-walled structures that contain very small amount of elastic tissue and smooth muscles compared with arteries. These are highly distensible part of the vascular system and that is why also form the so-called *reservoir vessels*.

Essential Characteristics

Essential characteristics of blood vessels like lumen diameter, wall thickness, approximate total cross-sectional area (TA) and percentage of blood volume contained are shown in Table 4.4.1.

VASCULAR SMOOTH MUSCLE

Vascular smooth muscle (VSM) is a key structure in the physiology of vascular system and thus needs special emphasis.

Arrangement in Tunica Media of the Vessels

VSM is found in all segments of vascular tree, except the capillaries. Arrangement of VSMs, however, varies in different segments:

- *In the Windkessel vessels*, they are disposed in a spiral fashion.
- *In the arterioles*, they are arranged more circularly and so on contraction may cause complete obliteration of the lumen.

Types of VSM

From a functional point of view, VSM is of two types – single unit (visceral type) and multiunit. The visceral-type VSM fibres have inherent property of myogenic activity to stretch and are mainly present in small arteries, arterioles and meta-arterioles. The multiunit smooth muscle fibres are not excited by stretch.

Table 4.4.1 Essential characteristics of various types of blood vessels

Types of blood vessels	Lumen diameter	Cross-sectional area (cm²)	Velocity of blood flow	Pressure as cumulative blood volume (%)
Aorta	2.5 cm	4.5	20 cm/s	2
Arteries	0.4 cm	20	4 cm/s	8
Arterioles	30 µm	400	2 mm/s	1
Capillaries	05 µm	4500	0.2 mm/s	5
Venules	20 µm	4000	0.2 mm/s	54
Vein	0.5 cm	40	2 cm/s	
Vena cava	3 cm	18	4.5 cm/s	

Innervational Characteristics

- Smooth muscles of the blood vessels are innervated by sympathetic fibres. These muscles contain α-adrenergic receptors. Therefore, noradrenaline causes contraction of muscle fibres leading to vasoconstriction.
- Sympathetic fibres exert tonic effect even at rest, resulting in the existence of vasomotor tone in the blood vessels.
- Stimulation of sympathetics increases the vasomotor tone; as a result, the vessels are constricted and narrowed.
- Inhibition of sympathetic discharge results in decreased vasomotor tone and hence vasodilation.
- Besides α-adrenergic receptors, smooth muscles of the blood vessels are also stimulated by other agents like O_2 tension and lactic acid, which are described in local control (page 339).

Important Note

Skeletal muscle arterioles also contain β_2-receptors in addition to the α-receptors; therefore, adrenaline causes dilation of these vessels.

Excitation and Contraction Characteristics of VSM

- *Resting membrane potential (RMP)* is rather low in VSM compared with in cardiac and skeletal muscles.
- *Typical action potential (AP)* is absent in VSM; nevertheless, with activity, some changes in membrane potential, resembling AP, are seen.
- *Cause of development of AP* in VSM is entry of Ca^{2+} from ECF to ICF; therefore, calcium channel blockers like *nifedipine* powerfully prevent VSM contraction. That is why these drugs are extremely popular in the treatment of hypertension (HT).
- *Contraction*, once developed in the VSM, takes long time to relax again, i.e. there occurs *sustained contraction*. Thus, sympathetic stimulation elevates BP which tends to stay for some time.

HAEMODYNAMICS

Haemodynamics, which refers to study of blood flow in various segments of the vascular system, can be discussed under the following headings:

- General principles governing (factors affecting) blood flow
- Circulation time
- Types of blood flow
- Measurement of blood flow
- Distribution of blood flow to various regions of the body
- Regulation of blood flow in different situations

GENERAL PRINCIPLES GOVERNING (FACTORS AFFECTING) BLOOD FLOW

Flow–Pressure–Resistance Relationship

Relationship between flow of a fluid and the pressure and resistance offered to it through a rigid tube was first studied by a French physiologist Poiseuille in 1842. Hagen, a contemporary of Poiseuille, worked further with the problem and found out the mathematical expression. Poiseuille's results (and their mathematical expression) were based on the measurement of the flow of a Newtonian fluid, i.e. a fluid that showed a viscosity which was unaffected by flow rate, through rigid tubes under the influence of steady head of pressure. The relationship studied is known as Poiseuille's law or Poiseuille–Hagen law.

Poiseuille's Law

Poiseuille's law expressing the relation between the flow (Q) and the pressure gradient (ΔP) in a long narrow tube of length (L), viscosity of fluid (η) and radius (r) of the tube is as follows:

$$Q = \frac{\Delta P \pi r^4}{8\eta L}$$

Thus, according to Poiseuille's law, the flow (Q) of a Newtonian fluid through a rigid tube is determined by:

1. Pressure gradient (Δp) Pressure gradient (Δp), is the difference in the pressure between the two ends of the tube. In other words, fluid always flows from an area of high pressure (P_1) to one of lower pressure (P_2), and rate of flow (Q) is determined by the pressure gradient ($P_1 - P_2$), i.e. $Q \propto P$ or ($P_1 - P_2$).

2. Radius of tube The flow of fluid varies directly as the fourth power of radius (r^4). Thus, if the radius is halved, the flow will decrease by 16 times and vice versa. Thus, this factor is very important for flow of blood through the blood vessels.

3. Viscosity of fluid (η) The flow of fluid varies inversely with the viscosity of fluid, i.e. greater the viscosity, lesser the flow and vice versa.

4. Length of the tube (L) The flow is inversely proportional to the length of the tube. This is easily understandable, as every segment of the tube is offering resistance to the flow; therefore, longer the length, greater will be the total resistance offered.

5. Resistance (R) According to mathematical calculation in principles of physics, resistance (R) is represented by $8L\eta/\pi r^4$. By replacing $8L\eta/\pi r^4$ with R in Poiseuille's law, it becomes:

$$Q = \frac{\Delta P}{R}$$

Thus, Poiseuille's law can be considered analogous to Ohm's law of current in which:

$$\text{Current (flow)} = \frac{\text{Voltage (pressure gradient)}}{\text{Resistance}}$$

Hence, the rate of flow (Q) is inversely proportional to the resistance (R).

Important Note

The Poiseuille's law is valid for straight rigid tubes with Newtonian fluid flowing through them. Since blood vessels are not rigid tubes and blood is not a Newtonian fluid, strictly speaking, the Poiseuille's law does not apply to flow of blood through the vascular system.

Nevertheless, the important principles relating flow, pressure gradient and resistance remain applicable, so they are discussed in relation to blood flow as:

- Blood flow and pressure gradient relationship
- Blood flow and resistance relationship

Blood Flow and Pressure Gradient Relationship

According to Poiseuille's law, fluid always moves from an area of higher pressure to one of lower pressure. This downhill movement of blood (i.e. along the pressure gradient) occurs in the vascular system. Fig. 4.4.3 depicts the mean lateral pressure and blood flow in various components of the cardiovascular system (represented as cumulative blood volume in per cent). In systemic circulation, pressure at the beginning of aorta is about 100 mm Hg and near the terminal portion of inferior vena cava it is nearly zero. Therefore, $P_1 - P_2 = (100 - 0) = 100$ mm Hg. Note the progressive decrease in pressure from the left ventricle through the systemic circulation until blood enters the right ventricle.

Important Note

It is important to note that the greatest pressure drop occurs in the arterioles, which represent the highest resistance segment of the systemic circulation.

Furthermore, according to Poiseuille's law, at constant length and radius of a tube and viscosity of the fluid, the relationship between pressure and flow through a rigid tube is linear, i.e. as pressure increases, flow of fluid also increases (Fig. 4.4.4A). The relationship between flow of blood and pressure in the blood vessels is however not linear:

In distensible vessels (e.g. aorta), the increase in flow as a result of a rising pressure head is initially less than that occurring in rigid tube, as due to elastic recoil they are slightly collapsed. However, later the flow in such vessels is greater than that in the rigid tubes (Fig. 4.4.4B), as they distend. At further higher pressure, the flow becomes linear as the vessels cannot distend any more due to the presence of fibrous tissue in the adventitia.

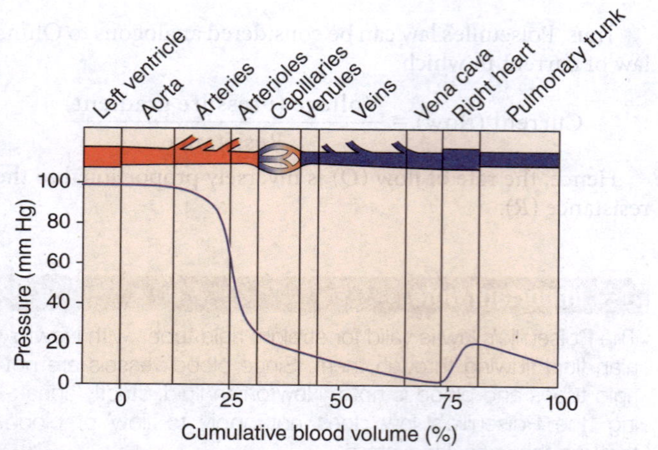

Fig. 4.4.3 Mean lateral pressure in various components of vascular system and cumulative blood volume.

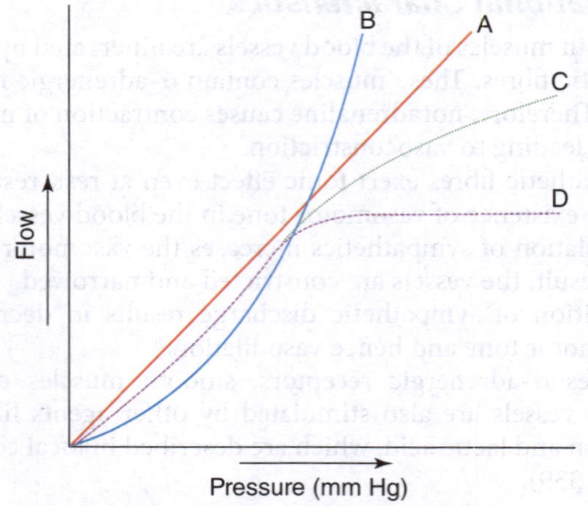

Fig. 4.4.4 Relationship of pressure with flow: **A**, in a rigid tube; **B**, in a distensible blood vessel (aorta); **C**, in a distensible blood vessel containing active myogenic contractile element, whose contraction affects the distensible effects of raised pressure; and **D**, in a distensible vessel containing myogenic contractile element, which serves to stabilize flow over a wide range of pressure (80–200 mm Hg), such vessels would show autoregulation.

In resistance vessels, i.e. arterioles, the distension in the absence of other influences, at a given pressure head, would increase their internal radius and would correspondingly cause a raised flow at the pressure. However, in real life, it does not occur so because smooth muscles present in the media of arterioles when distended react actively to stretch by contracting. This myogenic contractile response to stretch offsets the elastic effect and so the flow in these vessels becomes less than the rigid tubes, i.e. the curve becomes concave to the pressure axis (Fig. 4.4.4C).

In the arterioles where the myogenic contractile response exceeds even the elastic effect of raised pressure, the blood flow is maintained and does not increase with the further increase in the pressure (Fig. 4.4.4D). Thus, as shown in Fig. 4.4.4D, such arterioles serve to stabilize the blood flow over a wide range of pressure (80–200 mm Hg). This phenomenon is called *autoregulation*.

Critical Closing Pressure

Since the flow–pressure relationship in a rigid tube is linear, the flow will cease only if the pressure is zero (Fig. 4.4.5A). However, in a blood vessel, the flow ceases when the BP is 20 mm Hg or even more (Fig. 4.4.5B). The pressure value at which the vessel collapses, its lumen closes and flow ceases is called *critical closing pressure (CCP)*. The blood flow ceases when the BP falls below the CCP because:

- Certain amount of intramural pressure is essentially required to push the RBCs (with average diameter of 7.5 μm) through the capillaries (average diameter 5 μm).
- Furthermore, the tissue pressure exerted over the vessels also causes their collapse. So, a certain amount of intramural pressure is a must to counteract the tissue pressure and thus to keep the vessels patent and to maintain the blood flow.

  The values of critical closing pressure are:
  - When whole blood is flowing through the vessels, the average value of CCP is 20 mm Hg (Fig. 4.4.5B).
  - When plasma is flowing, the value of CCP is about 5–10 mm Hg.

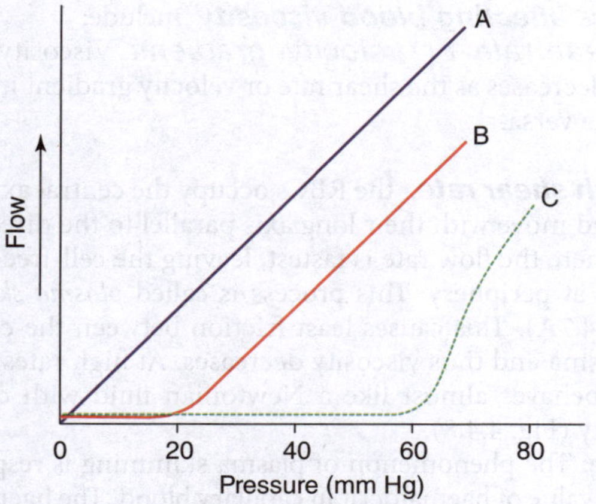

Fig. 4.4.5 Relationship of critical closing pressure (CCP) with flow in a rigid tube **A**, and in a blood vessel **B**, and with sympathetic stimulation **C**.

- On sympathetic stimulation, the value of CCP increases to 60 mm Hg (Fig. 4.4.5C).
- On sympathetic inhibition, the value of CCP falls to 0 mm Hg.

Equilibrium of Factors at Critical Closing Pressure

In general, vasomotor tone of the blood vessels tries to constrict the vessels. This tone is increased by sympathetic stimulation and decreased by sympathetic inhibition.

- Intramural pressure tries to dilate the blood vessels up to a certain limit. At the point where the intramural pressure (*P*) is not able to maintain an equilibrium with tension (*T*) in the vessel wall, the blood vessel closes and the pressure at which it occurs is called CCP. Law of Laplace described below helps to explain this equilibrium relationship.

Law of Laplace

Law of Laplace governs relation between the distending pressure and the tension in the wall of a distensible viscus including blood vessels (Fig. 4.4.6). According to this law, the distending pressure (*P*) in a distensible hollow object is equal at equilibrium to the tension in wall (*T*) divided by the two principal radii of curvature of the object (r_1 and r_2):

$$P = T\left(\frac{1}{r_1} + \frac{1}{r_2}\right), \text{ where}$$

T is expressed in dynes per centimetre, r_1 and r_2 are in centimetre, and so *P* is expressed in dynes per square centimetre.

- *In a sphere*, $r_1 = r_2$. Therefore,

$$P = \frac{T}{r}$$

- *In a cylinder* such as a blood vessel, one radius is infinite. Therefore,

$$P = \frac{T}{r}$$

Physiological applications of law of laplace This law applies to all the hollow viscous structures in the body. Some of its important applications are as follows:

In vascular system As described above, for blood vessels, Laplace equation is $P = T/r$. This equation shows that smaller the radius of a blood vessel, lesser is the tension (*T*) on the walls of the blood vessel required to balance the distending pressure or force (*P*). For example:

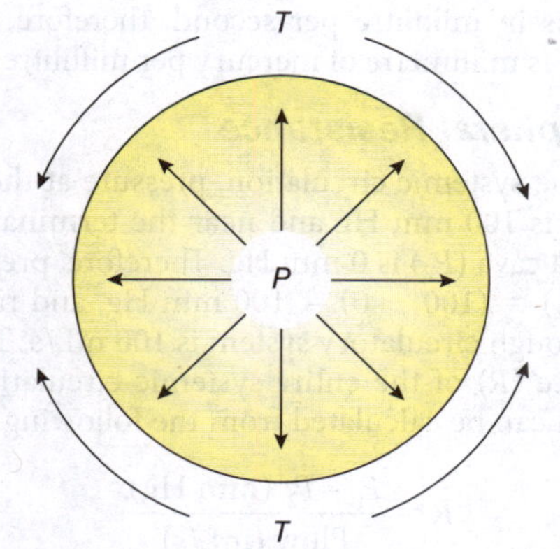

Fig. 4.4.6 Relationship between distending pressure (*P*) and wall tension (*T*) in a hollow viscus.

- In aorta, the tension at normal pressure is 170,000 dynes/cm.
- In inferior vena cava, it is about 21,000 dynes/cm.
- But in the capillaries, it is approximately 16 dynes/cm. This explains why capillaries being so thin walled and delicate are not prone to rupture.

In heart *Law of Laplace also explains* the disadvantage faced by a dilated heart. When the radius of a cardiac chamber is increased, a greater tension must be developed in the myocardium to produce any given pressure; consequently, a dilated heart must do more work than a nondilated heart.

In lungs The radii of curvature of the alveoli become smaller during expiration, and these structures would tend to collapse because of the pull of surface tension if the tension were not reduced by the surface tension–lowering agents (surfactants).

In urinary bladder For application of law of Laplace, see page 550.

BLOOD FLOW AND RESISTANCE RELATIONSHIP

Peripheral Resistance

From Poiseuille's law, it can be derived that flow is inversely proportional to the resistance, i.e. $Q \propto 1/R$, and that resistance is represented by $8L\eta/\pi r^4$, i.e. resistance depends on the length (*L*) and fourth power of radius (r^4) of the tube and viscosity of the fluid (η). Before discussing the effect of these factors on the blood flow, it will be worthwhile to know about the *peripheral resistance unit* (PRU), i.e. unit of peripheral resistance (PR) in vascular system, and concept of total peripheral resistance (TPR) in the body.

Peripheral Resistance Unit

As discussed above, Poiseuille's law can be considered analogous to Ohm's law, so:

$$\text{Flow, i.e. } Q\ (\text{mL/s}) = \frac{P_1 - P_2\ (\text{mm Hg})}{\text{Resistance } (R)}$$

$$\text{Thus, } R = \frac{P_1 - P_2\ (\text{mm Hg})}{Q\ (\text{mL/s})}$$

As flow is in millilitre per second, therefore, in vascular system, *PRU* is millimetre of mercury per millilitre per second.

Total Peripheral Resistance

At rest, in the systemic circulation, pressure at the beginning of aorta (P) is 100 mm Hg and near the terminal portion of inferior vena cava (P_2) is 0 mm Hg. Therefore, pressure gradient ($P_1 - P_2$) = (100 − 0) = 100 mm Hg, and rate of blood flow (Q) through circulatory system is 100 mL/s. Thus, at rest, the resistance (R) of the entire systemic circulation is called 'TPR', which can be calculated from the following formula:

$$R = \frac{P_1 - P_2 \text{ (mm Hg)}}{\text{Flow (mL/s)}}$$

$$\text{TPR at rest} = \frac{100 \text{ mm Hg}}{100 \text{ mL/s}} = 1 \text{ mm Hg/mL/s} = 1 \text{ PRU}$$

- TPR during maximum vasoconstriction may increase to 4 PRU.
- TPR during maximum vasodilation may decrease to 0.2 PRU.
- Pulmonary vascular resistance is about 0.1–0.2 PRU.

Factors that Affect Resistance to Blood Flow

According to Poiseuille's law, resistance (R) depends on the length of tube (L), fourth power of radius of tube (r^4) and viscosity of the fluid (η). Since in an intact body the length of the blood vessels does not change, i.e. remains constant, the major factors that determine the resistance to flood flow are as follows:

i. The viscosity of blood
ii. The radius of vessels

Blood Viscosity and Resistance

Resistance (R) to Blood Flow is Directly Proportional to Viscosity (η) of Blood.

Definition and unit of viscosity *Viscosity* was described by Isaac Newton in 1713 as internal friction to flow in a fluid or lack of slipperiness. These terms emphasize that when a fluid moves along a tube, laminae in the fluid slip on one another and move at different speeds, thereby causing a velocity gradient in a direction perpendicular to the wall of the tube. This velocity gradient is called the *rate of shear*. A simple viscous fluid known as *Newtonian fluid* is defined as one whose viscosity does not vary with the rate of shear and remains constant at different rates of laminar flow. Therefore, resistance met by the fluid moving through a tube in a streamlined flow is due to the friction between adjacent laminae and not due to the friction between vessel wall and fluid. Thus, greater the internal friction, greater is the difference in velocity (shear rate) between two laminae and greater is the coefficient of viscosity.

Unit of viscosity is *poise* (P; after Poiseuille). A fluid of 1 P viscosity has a force of 1 dyne/cm^2 of contact between layers when flowing with a velocity gradient of 1 cm/s. One poise consists of 100 cP. *Viscosity of water* at 21°C is 0.01 P or 1 cP. *Relative viscosity* is a more often used term, and refers to the viscosity of a fluid relative to the viscosity of water at body temperature (37°C).

- Water has a viscosity of 0.695 cP at body temperature.
- Plasma, which has a viscosity of 1.2 cP at 37°C, thus has a relative viscosity of 1.7.
- Blood (plasma plus cells), which has a viscosity of 2.8–3 cP at 37°C, thus has a relative viscosity of about 4–5.

Factors affecting blood viscosity include:

1. Shear rate or velocity gradient: Viscosity of the blood decreases as the shear rate or velocity gradient increases and vice versa.

At high shear rate, the RBCs occupy the central axis of the tube and move with their long axis parallel to the direction of flow where the flow rate is fastest, leaving the cell-free zone of plasma at periphery. This process is called *plasma skimming* (Fig. 4.4.7A). This causes least friction between the cells and the plasma and thus viscosity decreases. At high rates of flow, blood behaves almost like a Newtonian fluid with constant viscosity (Fig. 4.4.8).

Note: The phenomenon of plasma skimming is responsible for low value of haematocrit in capillary blood. The haematocrit of capillary blood is about 25% lower than that of venous blood.

When shear rate is low (at low flow rate), tendency of RBCs to occupy central axis decreases (Fig. 4.4.7B). The suspended RBCs in plasma increase internal friction due to collision among these suspended particles. So, with slow shear rate, the viscosity increases.

2. Haematocrit: In general, variation in the haematocrit is the major factor that changes the viscosity of blood. An increase in haematocrit tends to reduce flow rate because of increased viscosity. The normal haematocrit for men is 40%–45%, whereas the normal value for premenopausal women is 35%–40%. Viscosity of blood with a haematocrit of 40% is approximately three times that of water.

In vitro, the relative viscosity of blood increases proportionally with increase in haematocrit (above 45%).
In vivo, the effect of increased haematocrit on viscosity is affected by the diameter of the vessels, discussed as follows:

- In large vessels, increase in haematocrit causes appreciable increase in the viscosity. However, in small vessels (<10 μm diameter), i.e. arterioles, capillaries and venules, change in viscosity per unit change in haematocrit is much less compared with in large vessels (Fig. 4.4.9). How it happens is explained here.

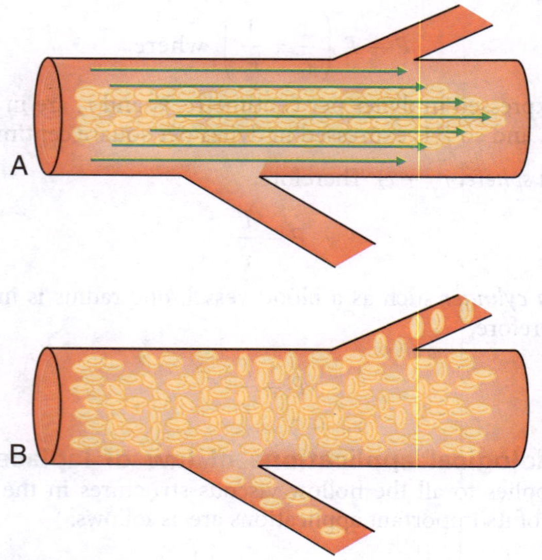

Fig. 4.4.7 Features of streamlined flow at high flow rate **A**, and at slow flow rate **B**.

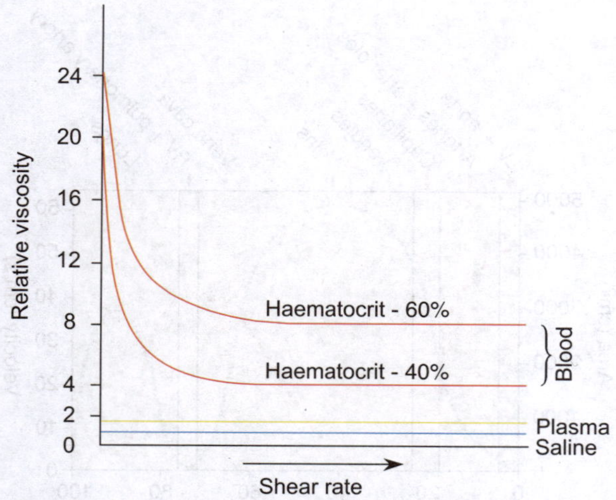

Fig. 4.4.8 Effect of shear rate on relative viscosity of blood. Note that, at higher shear rate, the viscosity of blood becomes constant and it behaves like a Newtonian fluid such as plasma or saline.

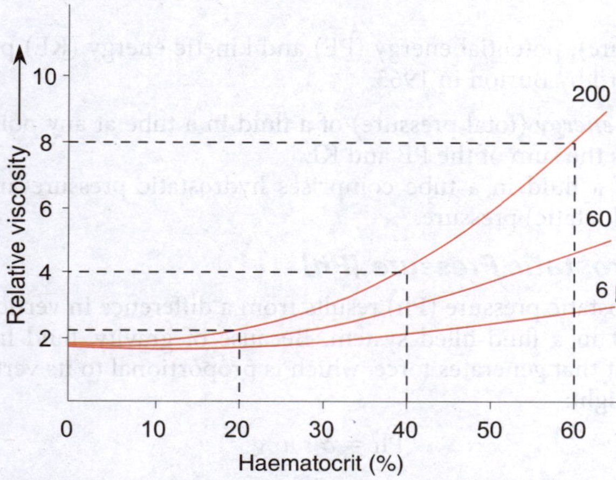

Fig. 4.4.9 Relationship between the haematocrit and the relative viscosity when blood flows through a tube of diameter 200, 60 and 6 μm.

3. Diameter of blood vessels: The relationship between viscosity and diameter of the vessels is expressed as *Fahraeus–Lindqvist effect* after the name of the workers. According to their experimental observations, the viscosity of blood in vessels with smaller diameter is less than the viscosity of blood in larger-diameter vessels. These workers reported that in a tube of 40 μm diameter, the relative viscosity of blood was only 70% of that through a tube of 150 μm diameter. Furthermore, studies have also shown that in a tube of 14 μm diameter, the viscosity was only 47% of that through a tube of 150 μm diameter.

Explanation for Fahraeus–Lindqvist effect: This effect was observed only when the experiments were performed using blood and not when studied with water and plasma. Factors responsible for this effect are as follows:

- The RBCs present in the blood are deformable in nature, so that apparent viscosity of blood does not change while passing through a tube of smaller diameter.
- Due to the phenomenon of plasma skimming in large- and moderate-sized vessels, blood that enters the small vessels such as capillaries is of lesser haematocrit (25% less than the whole blood haematocrit). The width of cell-free zone at the periphery is constant whatever may be the tube diameter and correspondingly occupies a bigger proportion in narrow tubes. As a result, the total relative viscosity is less in smaller-diameter vessels. Because of this effect, a satisfactory flow rate exists even in the blood vessels whose diameters are small.
- In addition, there is a suggestion that capillary endothelial cells secrete a substance (mucopolysaccharide) which further helps to lower the viscosity of the blood in the capillaries.

Applied Aspects

Applied aspect of Fahraeus–Lindqvist effect: Because of this effect, haematocrit changes have relatively little effect on the *resistance* except when the changes are large.

4. Temperature: Cooling increases the viscosity of blood. In an intact body, although there is no variation in the body temperature normally, the cutaneous and subcutaneous vessels and even those of deeper regions in the limbs are subjected to considerable alteration of temperature due to atmospheric temperature. Thus, when the hand is kept in ice water, regional viscosity of the blood shows a threefold increase.

Applied Aspects

Pathological conditions associated with high blood viscosity are as follows:

- Severe polycythaemia
- Abnormally shaped RBCs (congenital spherocytosis)
- Abnormally high immunoglobulin level
- Lowered body temperature (in frost bite)

To summarize: Viscosity of blood is inversely proportional to:

- Flow rate (shear rate)
- Temperature within limit

Viscosity of blood is directly proportional to:

- Haematocrit, i.e. packed cell volume (PCV)
- Concentration of plasma proteins, especially immunoglobulins
- Diameter of vessel wall

Radius of Blood Vessels and Resistance

As mentioned earlier, the rate of flow is proportional to the fourth power of the radius (r^4) of the blood vessels. Thus, even a small change in the calibre of the blood vessels will produce a marked change in blood flow. For example, at a pressure head of 100 mm Hg, the change in flow rate with change in the radius is as follows:

Radius (mm)	*Flow rate (mL/min)*
1	1
2	16
4	256

Among the blood vessels, in aorta and large arteries, there is little resistance. Arterioles are the major seat of vascular resistance because of the following facts:

- These are small bored vessels (30 μm in diameter).

- A large amount of smooth muscles is present in their wall. Thus, constriction of arterioles increases the resistance and decreases blood flow, whereas dilation of arterioles decreases the resistance and increases the blood flow.

Control of blood flow to organs or tissues is thus regulated primarily by altering the radius of the arterioles. Because the arterioles control the flow to various vascular beds, they are considered the *stopcocks* of the circulation. In our body, arterioles are in large bulk in splanchnic region and skeletal muscles, and constitute the major site of PR. Because of their characteristics, arterioles play an important role in the following functions:

- Control of blood flow during alteration in arterial BP, i.e. autoregulation (see page 306)
- Control of blood flow following occlusive ischaemia, i.e. reactive hyperaemia (see page 307)
- Control of blood flow during exercise (see page 357)
- Conversion of pulsatile flow from the heart to a steady flow, in association with elastic vessels (see page 305)

VELOCITY OF BLOOD FLOW

The velocity of blood flow refers to displacement of blood per unit time, i.e. centimetre per second, whereas the rate of blood flow is the amount of blood flowing per unit time, i.e. cubic centimetre per second. The physiologically important aspects to be considered in relation to velocity of blood flow are as follows:

- Velocity and cross-sectional area relationship
- Velocity–pressure relationship

Velocity and Cross-Sectional Area Relationship

- The relationship between velocity (*V*), quantity of blood flow (*Q*) and cross-sectional area (*A*) of the blood vessel is as follows:

$$V = \frac{Q}{A}$$

- Thus, if quantity of blood flow (*Q*) remains constant and the cross-sectional area (*A*) increases, then the velocity of blood flow will decrease.
- Since cross-sectional area of capillaries is 1000 times as that of aorta, the velocity of blood flow in capillaries is approximately 1 mm/s as compared with 40 cm/s in aorta.
- The total cross-sectional area (TA) of various types of blood vessels, the velocity of blood flow and pressure in the various segments of the cardiovascular system plotted as a function of the cumulative blood volume are shown in Fig. 4.4.10 and Table 4.4.1.

Thus, Fig. 4.4.10 depicts that to keep the flow rate equal, the velocity of flow must vary inversely with the cross-sectional area of each vascular segment. This is in accordance with the continuity principle, according to which in any system arranged in series, the flow through each vascular segment must be equal to the flow through every other, unless one segment becomes progressively distended.

Velocity–Pressure Relationship

To understand the effect of velocity of blood flow on pressure, it is important to understand the concept of total energy (total

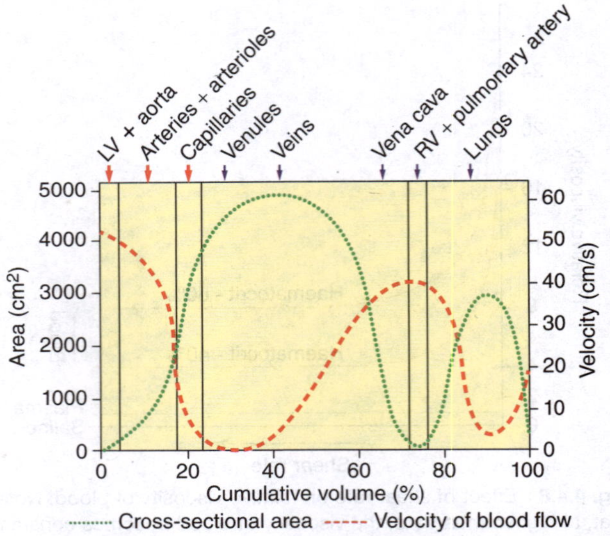

Fig. 4.4.10 Relationship between cross-sectional area, velocity of blood flow and pressure as a function of cumulative blood volume.

pressure), potential energy (PE) and kinetic energy (KE) put forward by Burton in 1965.

Total energy (total pressure) of a fluid in a tube at any point equals the sum of the PE and KE.

PE of a fluid in a tube comprises hydrostatic pressure and lateral (static) pressure.

Hydrostatic Pressure (Ph)

Hydrostatic pressure (Ph) results from a difference in vertical height in a fluid-filled system. Because of gravity, fluid has weight that generates force, which is proportional to its vertical height:

$$\text{Ph} = \delta \cdot h \cdot g$$

where δ is the fluid density, *h* is the height of fluid column above or below a reference level and *g* is the gravitational constant.

Some facts about effects of hydrostatic pressure on human vascular system are as follows:

- The reference point is at the right atrium, so vascular segments higher than reference point will have negative gravitational effect and vascular segments below reference point will have positive gravitational effect.
- Both arteries and veins at any given horizontal level are affected by the same hydrostatic pressure of blood so that the pressure gradient between arteries and veins is same (about 100 mm Hg), i.e. it is not altered (Fig. 4.4.11).
- As shown in Fig. 4.4.11, in an upright person, assuming that the foot is 100 cm below the heart, the pressure in the vessels (arteries as well as veins) of the foot is 100 cm H_2O (approx 80 mm Hg) higher than the pressure at the root of aorta.
- In a supine position, the hydrostatic effect is eliminated because the entire cardiovascular system is essentially at the same horizontal level.

Lateral (Static) Pressure

Lateral (static) pressure represents the pressure in the cardiovascular system that is usually measured with a strain gauge or transducer after eliminating the hydrostatic pressure effect.

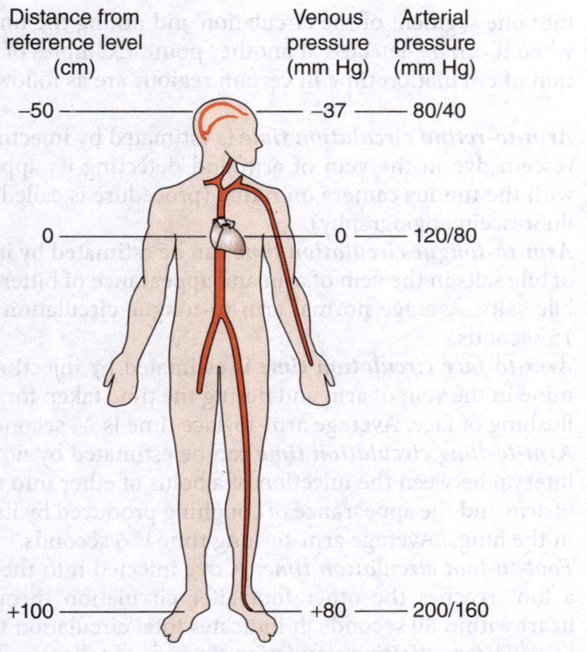

Fig. 4.4.11 Effect of hydrostatic pressure of blood on arterial and venous pressure in an upright position.

To eliminate hydrostatic pressure effect, it is essential to place the gauge or the sphygmomanometer cuff at the *zero reference* (phlebostatic) level, which is equivalent to the level of right atrium.

Kinetic Energy (KE)

KE is the momentum that blood gains because of its mass and velocity:

$$KE = \frac{mV^2}{2}$$

where m is the mass and V is the velocity.
Thus, when velocity of flow is very low, KE is negligible.

Total Energy (Total Pressure)

As stated above according to Burton, at any point equals the sum of the PE and the KE. Therefore, when velocity of flow is very low (i.e. with negligible KE), the magnitude of total energy (i.e. total pressure or perfusion pressure) is almost equal to the lateral pressure. However, when the velocity of flow is high, the lateral pressure exerted by the flowing fluid is much less than the total pressure exerted. This is because of the fact that at high velocity of flow, some PE is *converted into KE*. The effect of velocity of flow on total pressure exerted is expressed mathematically by:

Bernoulli's principle Bernoulli's principle states that in a supine position (i.e. when the effect of gravity or hydrostatic pressure effect is removed), the total energy or pressure (E) of flowing blood in a vessel is as follows:

$$E = P + \tfrac{1}{2}\rho V^2$$

where P is the lateral pressure, ρ is the density of blood and V is the velocity of blood in the vessel.

Experimental demonstration of velocity–pressure relationship The velocity–pressure relationship expressed above in *Bernoulli's principle* can be demonstrated experimentally by a system of pilot tubes (Fig. 4.4.12) as follows:

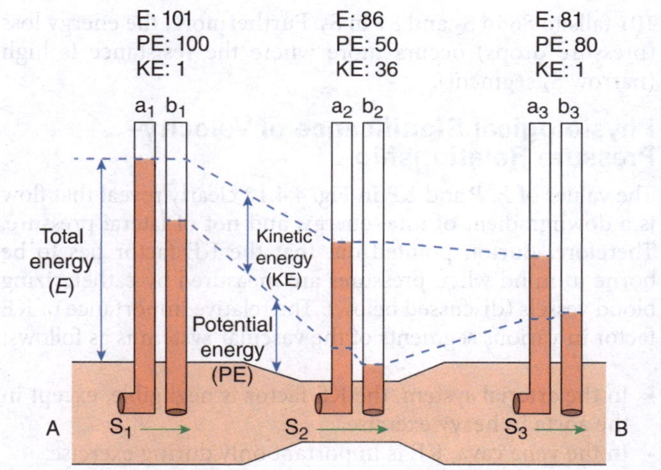

Fig. 4.4.12 Experimental set-up demonstrating the effect of velocity on pressure and also effect of resistance on pressure (for explanation, see text).

- AB is a tube through which fluid is flowing from direction A to B.
- The tube AB has central narrow segment S_2 where velocity of flow is higher. On each side of the narrow segment are wide segments S_1 and S_3, where velocity of flow is low. The length of arrows represents relative velocity of flow.
- Six tubes (a_1, a_2, a_3, b_1, b_2 and b_3) are inserted in the tube AB. Lower ends of tubes a_1, a_2 and a_3 are so constructed that they face upstream and hence record the total energy (total pressure), whereas tubes b_1, b_2 and b_3 record lateral pressure only.
- *In segment S_1* of the tube AB, where velocity of the flow is low (because the diameter is big), there is little difference in the height of fluid level in a_1 (representing total energy) and b_1 (representing lateral pressure).
- *In segment S_2* of the tube AB, where velocity of the flow is very high (due to smaller diameter), there is marked difference in the height of fluid level in a_2 (representing total energy) and b_2 (representing lateral pressure). This shows that when velocity of flow is high, PE is converted into KE and the PE (lateral pressure) becomes much less than the total pressure (PE plus KE).
- *In segment S_3 of the tube AB*, where velocity of the flow slows again (due to bigger diameter), part of the KE is transformed into PE and consequently lateral pressure is increased, and the difference between the height of fluid level in a_3 (representing total energy) and b_3 (representing lateral pressure) decreases.

Conversion of energy and loss of energy Considering the values of total pressure (E), lateral pressure (P) and KE in tubes a_1, a_2, a_3 and b_1, b_2, b_3, the following conclusions can be drawn:

Energy can be converted between PE and KE ($P \Leftrightarrow$ KE), as:

- In segment S_1, P is 100 and KE is 1.
- In segment S_2, P falls to 50 and KE increases to 36.
- In segment S_3, P increases to 80 and KE falls to 1.

Energy in a moving fluid is progressively lost due to resistance offered by the walls of the tubes as E which in segment S_1 is

101 falls to 86 in S_2 and 81 in S_3. Furthermore, the energy loss (pressure drops) occurs more where the resistance is high (narrow S_2 segment).

Physiological Significance of Velocity–Pressure Relationship

The values of *E*, *P* and KE in Fig. 4.4.12 clearly reveal that flow is a downgradient of total energy, and not of lateral pressure. Therefore, Burton pointed out that the KE factor has to be borne in mind when pressures are measured by catheterizing blood vessels (discussed below). The relative importance of KE factor in various segments of the vascular system is as follows:

- In the arterial system, the KE factor is negligible, except in the aorta in heavy exercise.
- In the vena cava, KE is important only during exercise.
- In the atria and pulmonary artery, KE is not inconsiderable at rest and is very important when the CO is increased.
- It has been calculated (Burton, 1965) that the KE factor is 50%–55% of the total energy in the venae cavae, atria and pulmonary artery.
- Thus, in the circulation at rest, the KE factor is of little importance on the systemic arterial side and of only moderate significance in the systemic veins. Flow, therefore, can be regarded as occurring between the root of aorta and the right atrium by virtue of a pressure gradient ($P_1 - P_2$).

Significance of Kinetic Energy Factor While Measuring Pressure by Catheterizing Blood Vessels

- When measuring pressure, unless the tip of the catheter has its opening at right angles to the stream (Fig. 4.4.13A) (measuring 'side pressure'), the pressure recorded is not accurate at that point. If the catheter faces the oncoming bloodstream or if an end cannula is tied into the artery, the flow of blood is prevented and the manometer registers a pressure higher than that by the factor $1/2\rho V^2$ (Fig. 4.4.13B).
- If the catheter opening faces downstream (Fig. 4.4.13C), the pressure recorded is slightly lower than the pressure recorded in the fluid by the factor $1/2\rho V^2$ (flow is distorted by streaming around the catheter tip and this reduces the correction required). Such a catheter placement is the accepted technique for recording of pulmonary arterial pressure.

Circulation Time

Circulation time refers to the time taken by the particles in blood in reaching from one point to another. It measures average linear velocity of blood. Calculation of circulation time in different regions of the body has clinical importance in circulation disorders of that particular region. The circulation time between two points can be estimated by injecting a substance

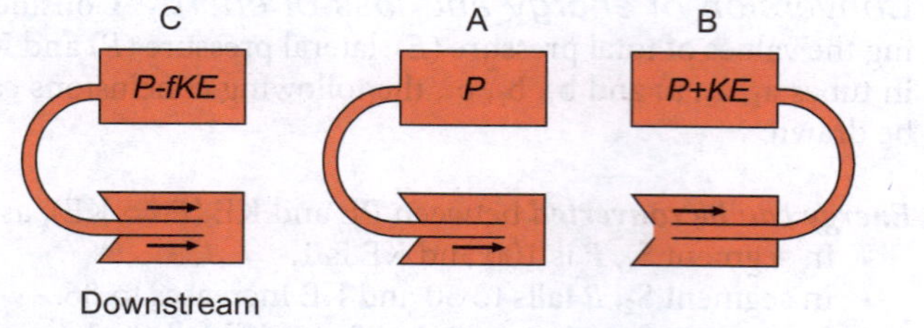

Fig. 4.4.13 Experimental set-up demonstrating significance of kinetic energy factor while measuring pressure by catheterizing a blood vessel.

into one segment of the circulation and noting the time lapse when it can be detected at another point. Examples of estimation of circulation time in certain regions are as follows:

Arm-to-retina circulation time is estimated by injecting fluorescein dye in the vein of arm and detecting its appearance with the fundus camera on retina (procedure is called fundus fluorescein angiography).

Arm-to-tongue circulation time can be estimated by injection of bile salts in the vein of arm and appearance of bitter taste of bile salts. Average normal arm-to-tongue circulation time is 15 seconds.

Arm-to-face circulation time is estimated by injecting histamine in the vein of arm and noting the time taken for causing flushing of face. Average arm-to-face time is 24 seconds.

Arm-to-lung circulation time can be estimated by noting the interval between the injection of a bolus of ether into the vein of arm and the appearance of coughing produced by its arrival in the lungs. Average arm-to-lung time is 6 seconds.

Foot-to-foot circulation time: A dye injected into the vein of a foot reaches the other foot after circulation through the heart within 80 seconds. It indicates total circulation time.

- *Factors affecting circulation time* are as follows:
  - Increased CO
  - Exercise
  - Excitement
  - Adrenaline
  - Basal metabolic rate

BLOOD FLOW: TYPES, MEASUREMENT AND DISTRIBUTION

Types of Blood Flow

Blood flow in the vascular system is of two types:

- Laminar blood flow
- Turbulent blood flow

Laminar Blood Flow

Blood flow in the blood vessels is normally in streamline, like the flow of liquids in narrow rigid tubes. Such a blood flow is called laminar blood flow and is considered to consist of a series of thin laminae slipping over one another.

- The outermost lamina, i.e. an infinitely thin layer of blood in contact with the wall of the blood vessel, does not move and the next lamina has some velocity. The subsequent inner layers have progressively increasing velocity, and thus the innermost lamina, i.e. the core of the bloodstream, has the maximum velocity (Fig. 4.4.14).
- The laminar blood flow being streamlined is noiseless and within physiological limits shows a linear relationship with pressure.

Turbulent Blood Flow

The above-described laminar blood flow occurs up to a certain velocity, at or above which the blood flow becomes turbulent. The velocity of flow at which blood flow becomes turbulent is called critical velocity.

- In turbulent blood flow, the blood moves in irregular varying paths continuously mixing within the vessel and colliding with the vessel wall. This causes a greater energy loss compared with that in laminar flow.

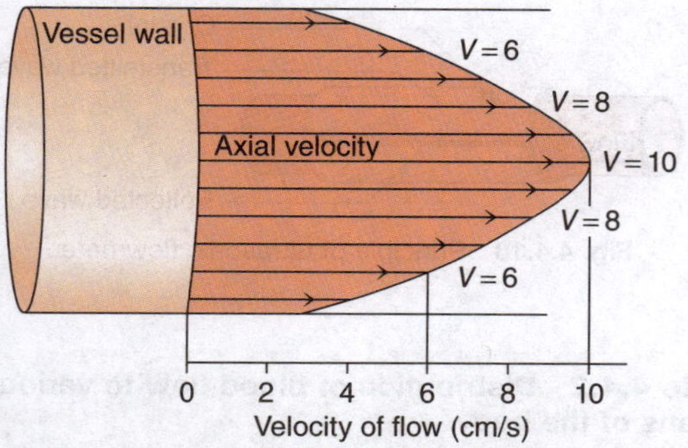

Fig. 4.4.14 Laminar blood flow showing different velocities of the different laminae resulting in parabolic distribution of velocities. Note that the central core of bloodstream has greatest velocity.

- Turbulent blood flow is noisy and does not show a typical linear relationship with the pressure.
- Normally, none of the small vessels show turbulent flow. In humans, the critical velocity sometimes exceeds in the aorta at the peak of systole.

Probability of turbulence The chances of blood flow becoming turbulent are determined by the *probability of turbulence*, which is denoted as *Re* (Reynolds number), named for the man who described it. According to Reynold, the probability of turbulence (*Re*) is:

- *Directly proportional to:*
  - Density of blood (ρ) equal to 1
  - Diameter of the vessel (*D*) in centimetre
  - Velocity of blood flow (*V*) in centimetre per second
- *Indirectly proportional to:*
  - Viscosity of the blood (η) in poises:

$$\text{Thus, } Re = \frac{\rho DV}{\eta}$$

- Blood flow is usually not turbulent when *Re* is less than 2000.
- Chances of blood flow becoming turbulent are increased when *Re* exceeds 2000. When *Re* is more than 3000, turbulence is almost always present.

Conditions associated with turbulent blood flow include:

Constriction of the artery by an atherosclerotic plaque (Fig. 4.4.15) or by any other cause, e.g. application of external pressure while measuring the BP with sphygmomanometer, is associated with a blood flow velocity which exceeds critical velocity and thus causes the turbulent blood flow. The turbulent flow generates vibrations (sounds) which can be heard over the artery by a stethoscope, e.g. *Korotkoff sounds* heard while recording the BP or the *murmur* heard over a constricted artery.

Anaemia is frequently associated with turbulence, because of *lowered blood viscosity*. This may be the explanation of the systolic murmurs that are common in anaemia.

Large-diameter vessels, e.g. ascending aorta, as mentioned above, may have turbulent flow at the peak of systolic ejection which may cause *ejection systolic murmur*.

Shear stress: Force exerted by flowing blood on the vascular endothelium is known as shear stress, which is parallel to the long axis of the blood vessel. Shear stress (γ) depends on viscosity of the blood and shear rate as follows:

$$\text{Shear stress } (\gamma) = \text{viscosity } (\eta) \times \text{shear rate } (dy/dr)$$

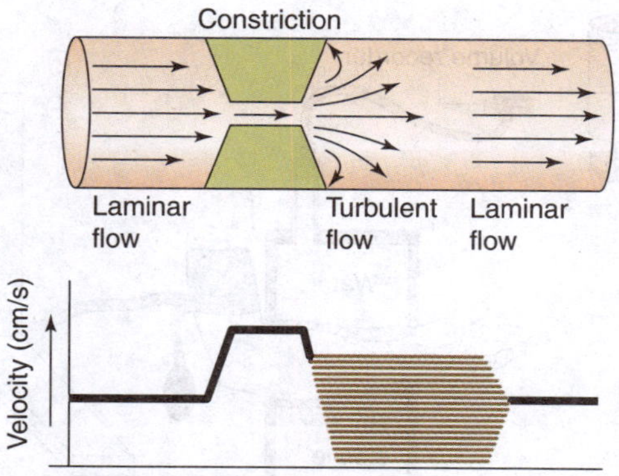

Fig. 4.4.15 Turbulent blood flow caused by constriction of the lumen of blood vessel.

Applied Aspects

The shear rate or velocity gradient increases from wall of blood vessel towards the central part of the bloodstream.

In endothelium, the shear stress plays an important role in formation of atherosclerotic plaques in atherosusceptible region (branches and curvatures of arterial tree) by gene activation and the transcription factors such as:

- Early growth response protein-1 (erp-1)
- Activator protein-1 (AP-1)
- Nuclear factor (NF-κB)
- Specificity protein-1 (sP-1)
- Shear stress responsive element (SSRE)

Measurement of Blood Flow

The following methods are known for measurement of blood flow in various parts of the body:

1. Methods based on Fick's principle Methods based on Fick's principle can be used to measure blood flow through some of the organs like the lungs, the heart and the brain. The methods are similar to those described for measurement of CO (page 278).

2. Para-aminohippuric acid clearance method *para*-Aminohippuric acid clearance method is used to determine the renal blood flow and thus study the renal physiology (see page 542).

3. Venous occlusion plethysmography Venous occlusion plethysmography is a simple but crude method of measuring blood flow through the limbs.

Principle It is based on the principle that if venous return of a region (part) is suddenly obstructed, that part increases in size due to arterial flow. The increase in size is equivalent to the blood flow to that part.

Procedure To measure blood flow through a limb (say a forearm), the part is enclosed in a watertight chamber (plethysmograph) connected to a volume recorder. The venous drainage from the limb is occluded for a few seconds by inflating the sphygmomanometer cuff to 60 mm Hg. The increase in the size of the arm will displace the water in the plethysmograph, which will be recorded with a volume

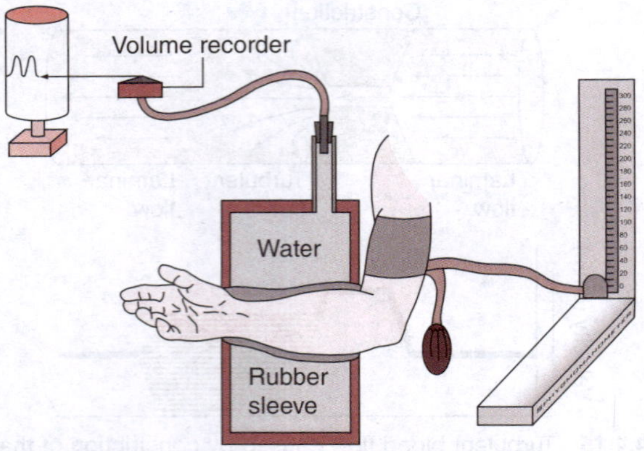

Fig. 4.4.16 Plethysmography showing measurement of blood flow in forearm.

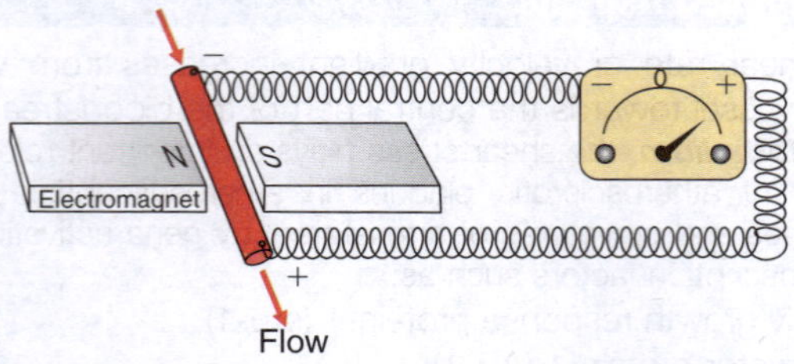

Fig. 4.4.17 Principle of electromagnetic flowmeter.

recorder (Fig. 4.4.16). The displacement is equal to the blood flow to the part during that period.

4. Electromagnetic flowmeter The electromagnetic flowmeter is based on the principle that when a vessel containing blood (a conductor) is placed between the two poles of a magnet, voltage is generated in the blood flowing through the magnetic field. The magnitude of the voltage is proportionate to the volume of flow and can be measured with an appropriately placed electrode on the surface of the vessel (Fig. 4.4.17).

5. Doppler flowmeter (ultrasonic flowmeter) Ultrasonic flowmeter is based on the principle of Doppler effect. In this instrument, ultrasonic waves are sent into a vessel diagonally from one crystal, and the waves reflected from the red and white blood cells are picked up by a second downstream crystal (Fig. 4.4.18). The frequency of the reflected waves is higher by an amount that is proportionate to the rate of flow towards the second crystal because of the Doppler effect.

Distribution of Blood Flow to Various Regions of the Body

At rest, about 5 L of blood enters aorta per minute. In terms of tissue weight, blood flow to the liver, brain and heart is very high. The kidney has high blood flow because it is related to excretory function rather than to metabolic requirement. The distribution of blood flow to various organs and regions of the body during resting conditions and during maximum activity conditions is shown in Table 4.4.2.

- At rest, at least 50% of the circulating blood volume is in the systemic veins, 12% is in the heart cavities and 18% in the lower pressure pulmonary circulation; only 2% is in the aorta, 8% in the arteries, 1% in the arterioles and 5% in the capillaries.
- When extra blood is administered by transfusion, less than 1% of it is distributed in the arterial system (the high-pressure system) and all the rest in the systemic veins, pulmonary circulation and heart chambers other than the left ventricle (the 'low-pressure system').

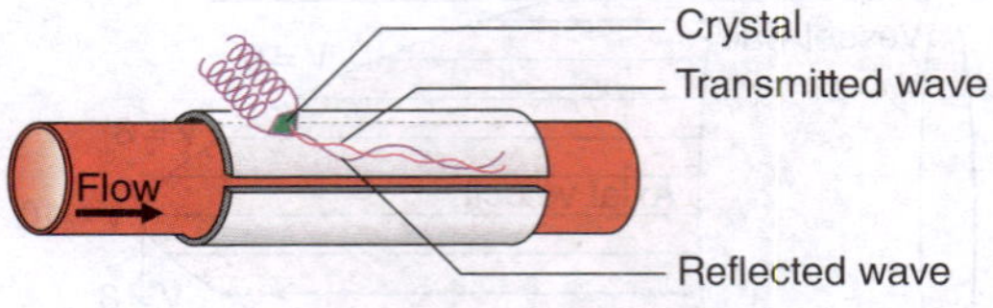

Fig. 4.4.18 Principle of ultrasonic flowmeter.

Table 4.4.2 Distribution of blood flow to various organs of the body

Organs	Blood flow per organ (mL/min) At rest	Blood flow per organ (mL/min) During maximum activity	Blood flow (mL/100 g/min) At rest	Blood flow (mL/100 g/min) During maximum activity
Heart	250	1200	80	400
Brain	750	2100	55	150
Liver	1500	3000	58	120
Skeletal muscles	150	1800	04	70
Kidney	1200	1400	400	450
Skin	200	3500	08	150

PRESSURE AND FLOW IN VARIOUS FUNCTIONAL SEGMENTS OF SYSTEMIC VASCULAR TREE

Pressure and velocity of flow of blood in the various parts of systemic circulation along with the pulmonary circulation summarized in Table 4.4.1 and Fig. 4.4.19 show that:

Pressure in the left ventricle, aorta and large arteries is *pulsatile* (i.e. rises to a peak value during systole and decreases to minimum during diastole) and becomes continuous in the capillaries. Based on the pressure changes, the whole of the vascular system is broadly divided into:

High-pressure system includes left ventricle, arteries and arterioles. This system controls the BP and blood flow in the body.

Low-pressure system includes capillaries, venules, veins, right atrium, pulmonary vessels and left atrium. It is responsible for the control of blood volume and venous return.

Velocity of blood flow in proximal part of aorta averages 40 cm/s. However, the flow in aorta is phasic, and velocity ranges from 120 cm/s during systole to even a negative value at the time of transient backflow before the aortic valve closes in diastole.

Total cross-sectional area (TA) of the vessels increases from 4.5 cm^2 in the aorta to 4500 cm^2 in the capillaries.

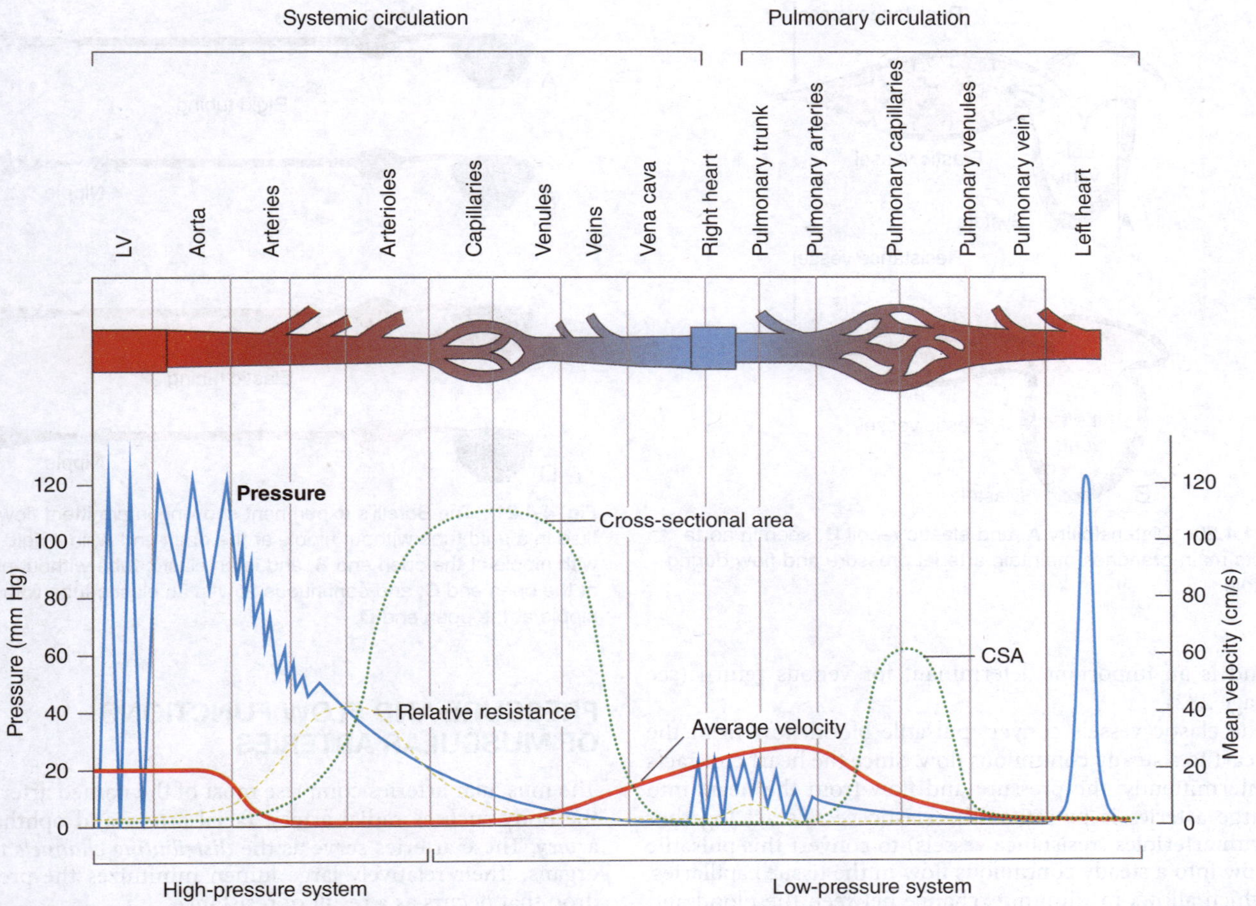

Fig. 4.4.19 Diagram showing pressure changes, velocity of blood flow through systemic circulation, total cross-sectional area of the blood vessels and relative resistance in the vessels (which is highest in the arterioles).

Relative resistance (RR) is the highest in the arterioles. As mentioned in the beginning of the chapter, from functional point of view, the systemic vascular tree has been divided into various functional segments. Pressure and flow functions of the following functional segments of systemic vascular tree are given next:

- Elastic arteries
- Muscular arteries
- Arterioles
- Microcirculation
- Venous circulation
- Lymphatic circulation

PRESSURE AND FLOW FUNCTIONS OF ELASTIC ARTERIES

The large elastic arteries (Windkessel vessels) include aorta and its main branches such as carotid, iliac and axillary arteries. These vessels contain elastic tissue in their walls in abundance which provides them two properties of distensibility and elastic recoil. The effect of these two properties of the elastic arteries on pressure and flow of blood is distensibility and elastic recoil.

Distensibility

As we know, the heart acts as a pump and ejects about 70 mL of blood into the aorta with each systole. The distensibility (compliance) of the elastic arteries allows them to accommodate the stroke volume of the heart with only a moderate increase in pressure (from 80 to 120 mm Hg) (Fig. 4.4.20A). Due to distension of these vessels, a part of energy released from the heart is stored as PE in the wall of aorta.

Elastic recoil

During diastole, the stretched elastic wall of the aorta recoils and the PE stored in the wall is released into the blood. This causes the blood to flow during diastole also; in this way, the pressure in the aorta does not fall below 80 mm Hg (Fig. 4.4.20B). In other words, the elastic recoil of big arteries acts as a subsidiary pump for a continuous blood flow. This recoil effect is called *Windkessel effect*. Windkessel is a German word meaning elastic reservoir.

Functions of elastic vessels

1. They reduce velocity of blood flow to some extent during ventricular contraction (systole) due to property of distensibility.
2. They cause increase in velocity of blood flow to some extent during ventricular diastole by elastic recoil. Thus, the Windkessel effect reduces the energy expenditure of the heart.
3. Pumping action of the heart along with elastic recoil of aorta constitutes a driving force for blood to move forward (towards periphery). This force is called *vis-a-tergo force*,

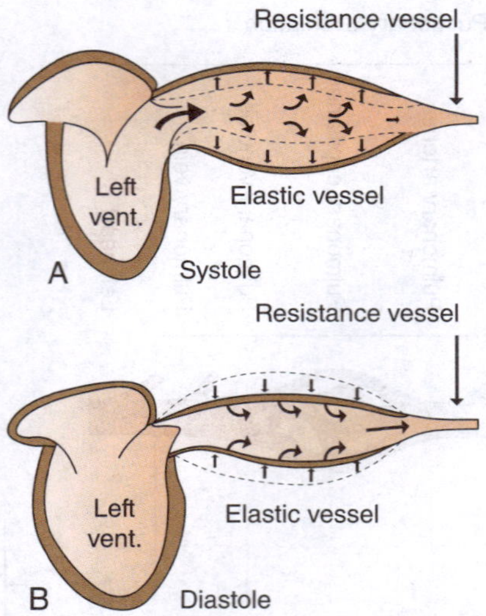

Fig. 4.4.20 Distensibility **A**, and elastic recoil **B**, seen in aorta and its main branches maintain arterial pressure and flow during diastole.

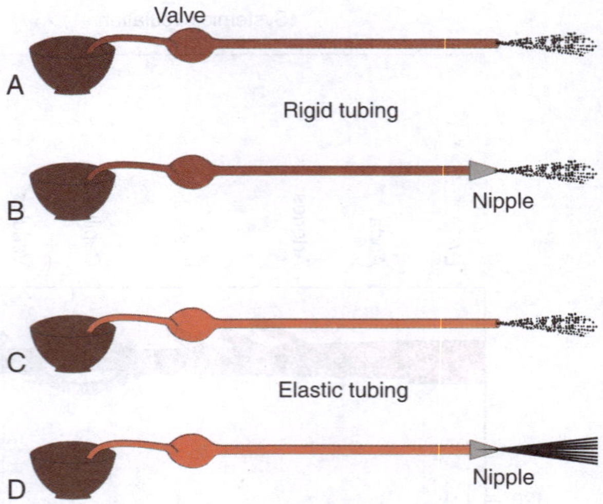

Fig. 4.4.21 The Borelli's experiment showing intermittent flow of fluid in a rigid tube without nipple at the open end **A**, in a rigid tube with nipple at the open end **B**, and in an elastic tube without nipple at the open end **C**, and continuous flow in an elastic tube with nipple at the open end **D**.

and is an important determinant for venous return (see page 282).

4. The elastic vessels convert pulsatile blood flow from the heart to a steady continuous flow. Since the heart contracts intermittently, the pressure and flow from the heart into large arteries is pulsatile. The elastic vessels act together with arterioles (resistance vessels) to convert this pulsatile flow into a steady continuous flow in the tissue capillaries, which allows maximum exchange between the blood and the tissues. This role of elastic vessels and the arterioles can be explained by a simple experiment performed by Borelli.

Borelli's experiment

In this experiment, one end of a rubber bulb having a one-way valve is dipped into a beaker of pure water and its other end is attached to a tube (Fig. 4.4.21). When the bulb is squeezed repeatedly, the water flow in different situations is as follows:

Intermittent flow is seen when the tube is rigid whether without (Fig. 4.4.21A) or with (Fig. 4.4.21B) a narrow nipple attached to the outlet (open end), and also when the tube is elastic but without a narrow nipple attached (Fig. 4.4.21C).

Continuous flow is, however, seen when a narrow nipple is attached to the outlet of an elastic tube (Fig. 4.4.21D). This set-up can be compared with combined effect of the aorta (elastic tubes) and arterioles (narrow nipples producing resistance) which produce a continuous and streamlined flow of blood.

Applied Aspects

Due to age-related degenerative changes, the elasticity of large vessels is decreased and so is the Windkessel effect. Therefore, in old age, systolic BP increases due to loss of distensibility and diastolic BP decreases (due to loss of elastic recoil). Thus, in a normal healthy individual aged about 70 years, typical BP is 160/70 mm Hg. That is, there occurs *systolic HT* with *increased pulse pressure (PP)*.

Atherosclerotic changes in small blood vessels are also common in old age. These produce *essential HT*, i.e. an increase in systolic pressure as well as diastolic BP.

PRESSURE AND FLOW FUNCTIONS OF MUSCULAR ARTERIES

The muscular arteries comprise most of the named arteries in the body such as radial artery, facial artery and ophthalmic artery. These arteries serve as the *distributing channels* to the organs. Their relatively large lumen minimizes the pressure drop that occurs as a result of resistance.

PRESSURE AND FLOW FUNCTIONS OF ARTERIOLES

Structural Characteristics

Each arteriole is only a few millimetres long and branches many a times to supply about 10–100 capillaries. The characteristic features of arterioles are as follows:

- They have a thick muscular wall having profuse vasomotor (sympathetic) innervation.
- They have a relatively narrow lumen (30 μm), because of which these vessels are considered the major site of PR. The arterial pressure drops by about 50 mm Hg while passing through few-millimetre-long arterioles (Fig. 4.4.19).

Functions of Arterioles

1. Control of Blood Flow to the Organs

The arterioles play a major role in the control of blood flow to organs or tissues. So, they are considered *stopcocks (valves) of circulation*. The constriction of arterioles increases the resistance and decreases the blood flow, whereas dilation of arterioles decreases the resistance and increases the blood flow. Thus, blood flow is primarily regulated by altering the radius of arterioles, since according to Poiseuille's law rate of flow, it is proportional to the fourth power of the radius, i.e. r^4 (see page 299). The arterioles control blood flow to organs by the following two mechanisms:

Control of blood flow during alterations in blood pressure (autoregulation) It is the ability of an organ or

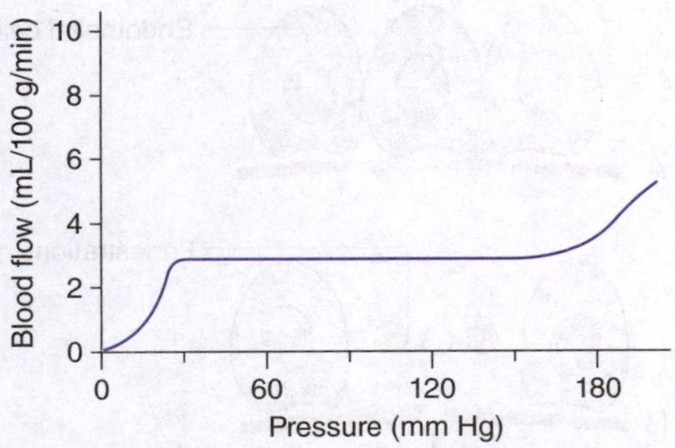

Fig. 4.4.22 Autoregulation of blood flow. Note that the blood flow remains relatively constant over a wide range of arterial pressure. This is accomplished by change in resistance proportionate to change in arterial pressure.

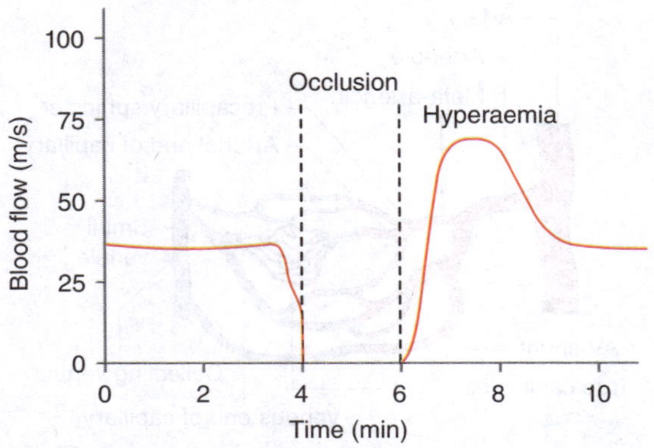

Fig. 4.4.23 Phenomenon of reactive hyperaemia, which increases blood flow after a period of ischaemia.

tissue to adjust its vascular resistance and maintain a relatively constant blood flow over a wide range of arterial pressure (Fig. 4.4.22). This is accomplished by a change in the resistance (due to change in lumen as above) proportionate to change in the arterial pressure. Autoregulation is well developed in the kidney, brain, heart, skeletal muscle and mesentery. Two theories have been put forward to explain the phenomenon of autoregulation.

Metabolic theory proposed that an increased arterial BP initially increases blood flow to a tissue or organ. This increased blood flow washes out the vasodilator substances such as CO_2, H^+, nitric oxide, adenosine, prostaglandins, K^+, phosphate ions and low oxygen levels in the area. As a result, the arterioles constrict, vascular resistance increases and blood flow returns to normal. However, it has been reported that changes in the concentration of any of the above-mentioned substances cannot explain autoregulation.

Myogenic theory: According to this theory, the VSM responds to wall tension, which is a function of pressure and wall radius according to the law of Laplace (see page 297). An increase in arterial pressure initially stretches the smooth muscle fibres, in response to which the VSM contracts and returns the wall tension to control levels that can be achieved only with vessels of smaller radius. The narrowed lumen increases the resistance and compensates for the higher arterial pressure, returning the blood flow to control levels.

Control of blood flow after occlusive ischaemia (reactive hyperaemia) Reactive hyperaemia is a phenomenon by which the vessels control blood flow to the organ after a period of ischaemia following occlusion of the artery to an organ or tissue. Due to this phenomenon, the blood flow exceeds the control level when the occlusion is resolved. The magnitude and duration of reactive hyperaemia depends on the duration of occlusion (Fig. 4.4.23). It has been proposed that reactive hyperaemia occurs due to a metabolic mechanism that controls blood flow to tissues.

Control of blood flow during exercise The arteriolar smooth muscles respond not only to sympathetic discharge but also to products of local metabolism. So, by these two mechanisms, regional blood flow is controlled in such a way that it is almost exactly proportional to the metabolic requirements of the tissues. For example, during muscular exercise, strong sympathetic discharge causes constriction of arterioles of the splanchnic region (where blood is not immediately required). Also, in the skeletal muscles, metabolites like CO_2, H^+ and lactic acid cause marked arteriolar dilation and consequently blood flow is diverted from the splanchnic region to the skeletal muscles and heart to meet the elevated demand due to metabolic activity.

2. Conversion of Pulsatile Flow from Heart to a Steady Continuous Flow

As described in 'Functions of Elastic Vessels', the arterioles along with the elastic vessels convert the pulsatile flow in the arteries to a steady flow in capillaries. For explanation, see Borelli's experiment (see page 306).

MICROCIRCULATION

Architecture of Microcirculation

The microcirculation involves a meshwork of vessels less than 100 μm in diameter. These include small arterioles, meta-arterioles, capillaries, postcapillary venules and arteriovenous shunts (Fig. 4.4.24):

Meta-arterioles: The arterioles divide into smaller muscle-walled vessels, sometimes called meta-arterioles, and these in turn feed into capillaries.

Precapillary sphincters refer to a cuff of smooth muscle cells that surround the origin of capillaries. These determine the size of capillary exchange area at one particular moment in the tissue. For example, increase in the sphincter patency increases the number of open capillaries. It is unsettled whether the meta-arterioles are innervated, and it appears that the precapillary sphincters are not. However, they can of course respond to local or circulating vasoconstrictor substances.

Capillaries arise directly from arterioles or meta-arterioles. These vessels allow easy exchange of gases and nutritive substances across them and so are also called *exchange vessels*. Capillaries constitute the most important segment of the circulatory system. Their structure and functions will be discussed in detail.

Postcapillary venules, which measure 20–60 μm in diameter, are the *most permeable part* of the microcirculation.

Arteriovenous anastomoses (shunt or thoroughfare vessels) are short, low-resistance connections between the arterioles and veins, bypassing the capillaries. These are abundantly

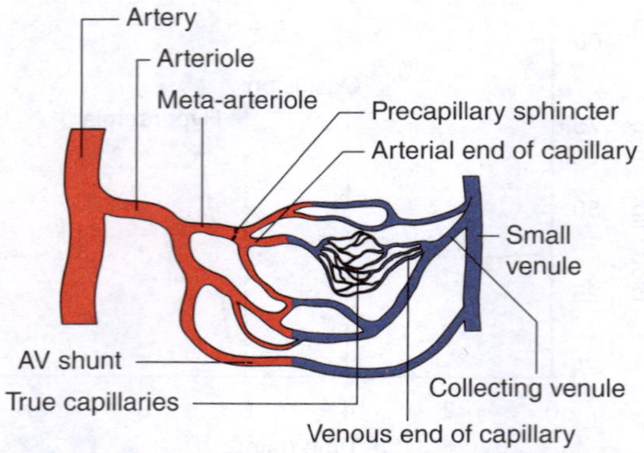

Fig. 4.4.24 Architecture of microcirculation.

innervated by vasomotor sympathetic fibres. These vessels are especially found in the skin of fingers, toes and earlobes, where they are involved in the regulation of body temperature.

Structural Characteristics of Capillaries

Each capillary has an average diameter of 5 μm, length of 50 μm, wall thickness of 1 μm and cross-sectional area of 40 μm^2.

The capillary wall essentially consists of a single layer of endothelial cells which are lined on the outside by a basal lamina (glycoprotein); overlying the basal lamina, there may be isolated branching perivascular cells called *pericytes*.

The endothelial structure of capillaries varies in different organs depending on the function of the particular tissue. Under electron microscope, three types of capillaries have been identified – continuous or nonfenestrated capillaries, fenestrated capillaries and discontinuous capillaries or sinusoids.

1. Continuous capillaries Continuous capillaries are characterized by a single layer of endothelial cells which are almost continuous, except for small clefts of 6–7 nm in size in between the cells. It is believed that most of water-soluble ions (Fig. 4.4.25A) and molecules pass across the capillary through these clefts (or *slit pores*). These are the most common type of capillaries and are found in most of the body tissues, e.g. skeletal muscle, adipose tissue, connective tissue and pulmonary circulation.

Note: The junctions between endothelial cells of capillaries of the brain and retina are tight and possess a complete basement membrane that retards or prevents the transfer of many substances and constitutes the so-called *blood–brain barrier and blood–retinal barrier*, respectively.

2. Fenestrated capillaries Fenestrated capillaries consist of thin endothelial cells with large fenestrations (20–100 nm in diameter) in between which are bridged by a thin basement membrane which surrounds the endothelial cells (Fig. 4.4.25B). The fenestrations permit the passage of relatively large molecules and make the capillaries porous. Fenestrated capillaries are found in organs where transport of fluid is paramount, e.g. renal glomeruli, intestinal villi, most endocrinal glands, ciliary processes in the eye and choroid plexus.

3. Discontinuous capillaries Discontinuous capillaries are characterized by large gaps (600–3000 nm in diameter) between endothelial cells that are not closed by basement membrane (Fig. 4.4.25C). Through these gaps, even formed

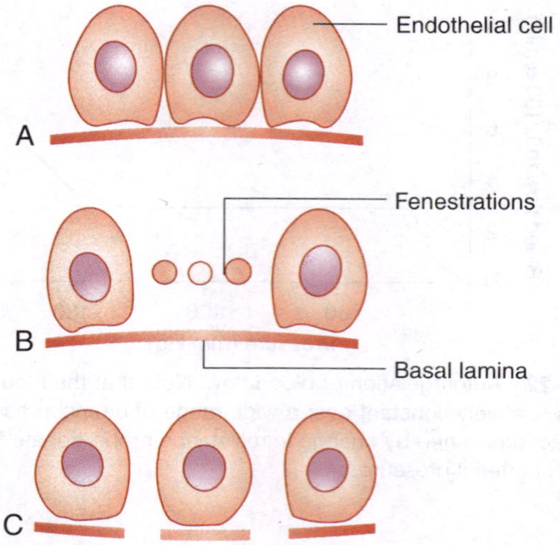

Fig. 4.4.25 Structure of different types of capillaries: **A**, continuous; **B**, fenestrated; and **C**, discontinuous.

elements of blood can pass freely. Such capillaries are also called sinusoids and are found in the bone marrow, liver and spleen.

Functional Characteristics of Capillaries

The primary function of circulation is to transport nutrients to the tissues and remove waste products – occurs in the capillaries. About 10 billion capillaries, which have a total surface area of 500–700 m^2, provide this function for the body. The cross-sectional area of capillary bed when fully patent is 2800 times that of aorta.

Active and Inactive Capillaries

In resting tissues In resting tissues, most of the capillaries (75%) are collapsed (inactive capillaries) and blood bypasses them to flow through the *thoroughfare vessels* connecting arterioles to the venules.

In active tissues In active tissues, the meta-arterioles and the precapillary sphincters dilate. The intracapillary pressure rises, overcoming the CCP, and blood flows through all the capillaries (active capillaries).

The opening and closing of the precapillary sphincters is controlled mostly by the local metabolic vasodilators and possibly also through sympathetic innervation.

Capillary Pressure and Flow

Capillary pressure Capillary pressure varies considerably; therefore, it is difficult to describe a generalized picture of capillary pressure and flow. However, typical values in human nail bed capillaries are 35 mm Hg at the arteriolar end and 15 mm Hg at the venous end, and thus vary over the length of capillary (average being 25 mm Hg). The pulse pressure (PP) is approximately 5 mm Hg at the arteriolar end and 0 mm Hg at the venous end. Average capillary pressure is less than 10 mm Hg in pulmonary capillaries and hepatic sinusoids.

Blood flow velocity The capillaries are short, but blood moves slowly (average velocity being 0.3–0.4 mm/s) because of a large cross-sectional area. The velocity varies widely – within short periods of time; it can range from 0 to 1 mm/s within the same capillary. The transit time of blood between the arteriolar end and the venular end of an average-sized capillary is 1–2 seconds.

Blood flow Blood flows into the capillaries intermittently because of the phenomenon of vasomotion, i.e. intermittent contraction of meta-arterioles and precapillary sphincters. This in turn is mainly controlled by concentration of oxygen and waste products of tissue metabolism.

Transcapillary exchange

The capillary blood brings oxygen, electrolytes and nutrients to the tissues and removes the waste products of cellular metabolism. The exchange of these substances occurs across the thin membrane formed by the endothelial cells. Before discussing the chief mechanism of transcapillary exchange, it will be worthwhile to know about interstitium and interstitial fluid.

Interstitium and interstitial fluid. The spaces in between the cells in the body are collectively known as *interstitium*, which constitutes about one-sixth of the body. The fluid present in the interstitium is called *interstitial fluid*. The interstitium also contains two major types of solid structures – collagen fibre bundles and proteoglycan filaments. Collagen fibres are strong and therefore they provide most of the tensional strength to the tissues.

Proteoglycan filaments Consist of 98% hyaluronic acid and 2% protein, and form fine reticular filaments described as *brush file*.

Most of the interstitial fluid is entrapped in the proteoglycan filaments and the two combinedly constitute the *tissue gel*. Rest of the interstitial fluid (<1%) forms the *free fluid*. Free fluid and gel are continuously interchanging with each other. Fluid can pass through the tissue gel very slowly but diffusion can occur through it as rapidly as in free fluid. Gases, nutrients and cellular waste products diffuse through the tissue gel very freely.

Important Note

Oedema results due to increased free fluid in the tissues.

Mechanisms of transcapillary exchange Exchange of substances occurs primarily in the capillaries and postcapillary venules. The major mechanisms of exchange are diffusion and filtration (bulk flow). Some substances also pass through the cells by *vesicular transport*.

Diffusion across microvascular endothelium Diffusion is the principal mechanism of microvascular exchange of materials between the plasma and the interstitial fluid against their concentration gradient.

Lipid-soluble substances like O_2 and CO_2 diffuse most freely across the cell membrane.

Water and water-soluble micromolecules (molecular weight less than 69,000) like Na^+, Cl^-, K^+, glucose and urea diffuse almost freely through the intercellular clefts and intracellular pores in the capillary membrane.

Large molecules (molecular weight more than 69,000) such as albumin and other plasma proteins cannot cross the endothelial barrier. However, some amount of albumin does enter the interstitial fluid.

Factors affecting rate of diffusion The factors affecting rate of diffusion across the capillary wall thus are the pore size of the capillary, molecular size of the diffusing substance and concentration difference of the substances between two sides of the membrane.

For details about the 'diffusion', see page 19.

Filtration and reabsorption across microvascular endothelium The backflow or ultrafiltration of protein-free plasma determines the distribution of fluid across the capillaries. The rate of filtration and absorption at any point along the capillary wall depends on the balance of forces known as *Starling forces*. According to Starling's hypothesis, the filtration absorption is expressed as follows:

$$K(P_c + \pi_c) - (P_i + \pi_c)$$

where

K = the permeability–surface area coefficient
P_c = the hydrostatic capillary pressure
P_i = the hydrostatic interstitial pressure
π_c = oncotic pressure of blood
π_i = oncotic pressure of the interstitium

Thus, $P_c - P_i$ represents the hydrostatic pressure gradient, and $\pi_c - \pi_i$ represents the oncotic pressure gradient.

Starling forces are defined next.

1. Hydrostatic capillary pressure (P_c) Hydrostatic capillary pressure (P_c) tends to force the fluid out through the capillary membrane. The values of hydrostatic capillary pressure in most of the tissues are as follows:

- At the arterial end, 30–40 mm Hg
- At the venous end, 10–15 mm Hg
- In the middle, 25 mm Hg

It is important to note that in the kidneys, the glomerular capillary pressure is 45 mm Hg (see page 483). The hydrostatic capillary pressure depends on:

- The arterial BP
- Precapillary and postcapillary resistance
- Venous pressure (most important)

2. Hydrostatic interstitial pressure (P_i) Hydrostatic interstitial pressure (P_i) tends to force fluid inward through the capillary membrane. It is about −2 mm Hg in subcutaneous tissue but is positive in the liver and kidneys, and as high as +6 mm Hg in the brain.

3. Oncotic pressure of blood or plasma colloid osmotic pressure (π_c) Oncotic pressure of blood or plasma colloid osmotic pressure (π_c) results from the osmotic pressure of plasma proteins. It tends to pull fluid inward through the capillary membrane. It is about 25–27 mm Hg.

4. Oncotic pressure of the interstitium (π_i) Oncotic pressure of the interstitium (π_i) is due to the presence of proteins in the interstitial space. It tends to pull fluid out of the capillary membrane. The effective oncotic pressure in the interstitium is estimated to range between 5 and 10 mm Hg (average 8 mm Hg).

Calculation of net filtration at the capillaries From the above-mentioned description, the net forces acting on the

Table 4.4.3 Calculation of net filtration force at the capillaries

	At the arteriolar end (mm Hg)	At the venous end (mm Hg)
Forces tending to move fluid outward		
• Capillary hydrostatic pressure (P_c)	35	10
• Interstitial oncotic pressure (π_i)	3	3
Total outward **force** ($P_c + \pi_i$)	38	13
Forces tending to move fluid inward		
• Oncotic pressure of blood (π_c)	25	25
• Interstitial hydrostatic pressure (P_i)	−2	−2
Total outward force ($\pi_c + P_i$)	23	23
Filtering force	38 − 23 = 15	13 − 23 = −10
Net filtering force of the whole capillary	15 − 10 = 5	

fluid at the arteriolar and venous ends of a typical muscle *capillary* can be calculated (Table 4.4.3):

- Thus, at arteriolar end, the filtering force of 15 mm Hg moves the fluid out of capillary (filtration) into the interstitium, whereas at venous end, the filtering force of −10 mm Hg moves the fluid into the capillary (reabsorption) from the interstitium.
- The net filtering force for the whole capillary is 5 mm Hg.

In the example given above, we have studied the balance of Starling forces at the arteriolar and venous ends of the capillary only. However, over the length of the capillary, the hydrostatic pressure gradually declines to zero near the middle of the capillary. From here, the inward forces become dominant and reabsorption process starts to reach its maximum at the venular end (Fig. 4.4.26).

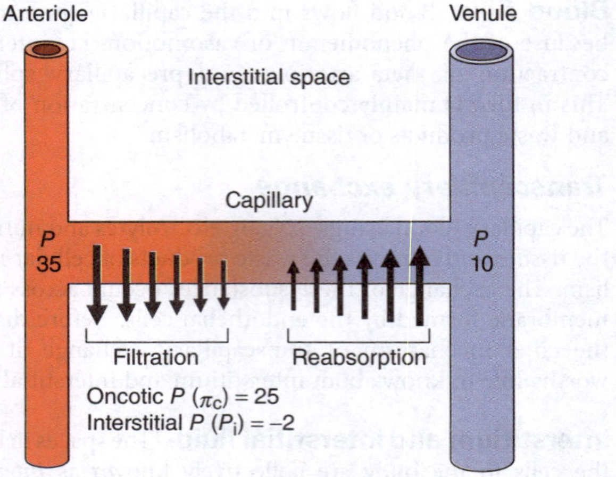

Fig. 4.4.26 Filtration and reabsorption in a capillary due to balance of Starling forces.

Capillary filtration and reabsorption in different tissues

In the above-mentioned example, we have calculated *net filtration forces*. However, the net filtration in the capillaries varies in the different tissues not only by the balance of Starling forces (net filtration force) but also by the capillary filtration coefficient (*K*).

Capillary filtration coefficient Capillary filtration coefficient or the so-called permeability–surface area coefficient (*K*) of a tissue depends on the number of capillaries receiving blood flow and the permeability of capillaries (i.e. type of capillaries). Because of the extreme difference in the permeabilities and surface areas of the capillary systems in different tissues, the capillary filtration coefficient (*K*) may vary more than 100-fold among the different tissues. For example:

In subcutaneous tissues, '*K*' is −0.01 mL/min/mm Hg/100 g tissue.

In kidney, '*K*' is −4.2 mL/min/mm Hg/100 g tissues, which is almost 400 times as great as '*K*' of many other tissues.

This obviously causes a much greater rate of filtration in the glomerular capillaries of the kidney.

Thus, depending on the balance of Starling forces and capillary filtration coefficient (*K*), the capillary exchange in some important tissues is as follows:

- *In renal glomerular capillaries,* fluid moves out of almost the entire length of the capillaries.
- *In interstitial capillaries,* fluid moves out of the capillaries from the arteriolar end up to the middle part and then moves into the capillaries.
- *In pulmonary capillaries,* filtration does not occur at all.

Flow-limited and diffusion-limited capillary exchange

Flow-limited exchange It is worth noting that small molecules often equilibrate with the interstitial fluid of the tissues near the arteriolar end of each capillary. In such situations, the total diffusion can be increased by increasing the blood flow. Therefore, exchange of such substances is called flow limited (Fig. 4.4.27).

Diffusion-limited exchange The transfer of substances that do not reach equilibrium with the tissues during their passage through the capillaries is called diffusion-limited exchange (Fig. 4.4.27). Therefore, exchange of such substances cannot be increased by increasing the blood flow.

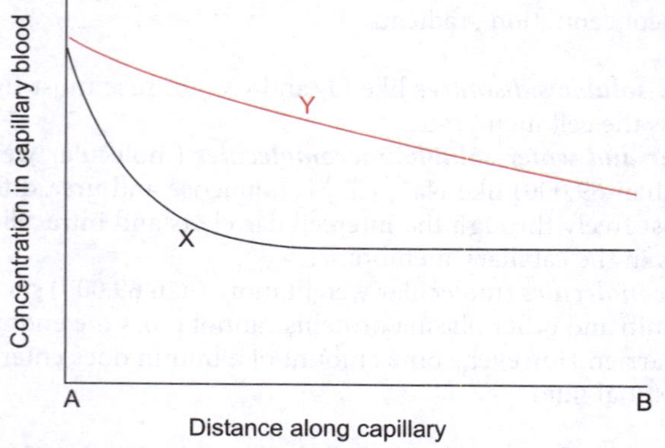

Fig. 4.4.27 Flow-limited (X) and diffusion-limited (Y) capillary exchange. **A** and **B**, arteriolar and venous ends of the capillary.

Exudate versus transudate

Exudate Exudate refers to the protein-rich fluid that comes out of the capillaries with marked increase in their permeability under conditions of inflammation due to any cause.

Transudate Transudate refers to the fluid that enters the interstitial fluid through normal capillaries. It does not have appreciable amount of proteins.

Total capillary exchange in the body It has been observed that in the whole body (leaving aside the glomerular capillary filtration), approximately 24 L of fluid is transferred per day from the capillaries to the interstitial spaces of the body. Of this, about 85%–90% is reabsorbed back to the capillaries and the rest is returned to the circulation via the lymphatics. Since the capillaries are said to be impermeable to plasma proteins, the filtered fluid should contain all the constituents of plasma except proteins. However, a small amount of albumin does pass out of the capillary membrane. And practically whole of it is returned to the circulation through the lymphatics.

LYMPHATIC CIRCULATION

Lymph: Formation and Composition

Formation As discussed in capillary exchange, most (90%) of the fluid filtered at arterial end of the capillary is reabsorbed at its venous end, and the remaining 10% enters the circulation through lymphatics and is called lymph. Thus, the lymph is a transudate formed from blood in the tissue spaces, i.e. it is derived from the interstitial fluid.

Composition Composition of lymph is similar to that of plasma except that its protein content is usually lower than that of plasma.

Protein content of the lymph varies with the region it drains:

- In most of the tissues, protein concentration of the interstitial fluid is 2 g/100 mL, so lymph also has the same content of protein.
- Lymph from the liver has protein concentration of 6 g/100 mL and that from the intestine has protein concentration of 3–4 g/100 mL.
- Since about two-thirds of the lymph is derived from the liver and intestine, the thoracic duct lymph (mixture of lymph from different areas) has usually a protein content of 3–5 g/100 mL.

Fat content: Since the lymphatic system also provides a route of absorption of long-chained fatty acids and cholesterol from the intestine (in the form of *chylomicrons*), the lymph from the intestine contains these large molecules of fat. After a fatty meal, these fat globules may be so numerous that the lymph becomes milky and is then called *chyle*.

Cellular content: Suspended in the lymph are cells that are chiefly lymphocytes. Most of these lymphocytes are added to the lymph as it passes through lymph nodes, but some are derived from the tissues drained by the nodes.

Lymphatic Vessels

The lymphatic system constitutes an accessory route for the removal of interstitial fluid. The small lymph vessels are called lymph capillaries and the large lymph vessels are called lymphatic trunks and the largest lymph vessel is thoracic duct.

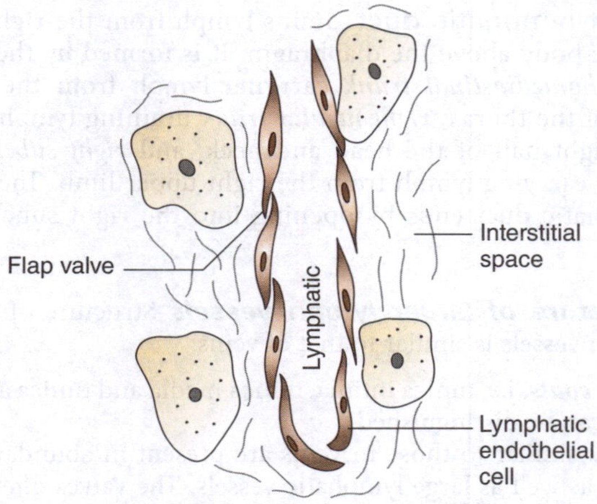

Fig. 4.4.28 Structure of lymphatic capillary.

Lymph capillaries The lymph capillaries *originate* as closed endothelial tubes that are permeable to fluid and high-molecular-weight compounds.

Structure of lymph capillaries (Fig. 4.4.28) is basically similar to that of blood capillaries with the following differences:

- The basal lamina around the endothelial cells is absent or poorly developed.
- Pericytes or connective tissue is not present around the lymph capillaries.
- There are no visible fenestrations in the endothelium.
- The junctions between endothelial cells are open, with no tight intercellular connections. In fact, the edges of the endothelial cells overlap in such a way that they form minute flap valves. So, through the lymph capillary, the substances that can pass are larger molecules such as proteins, fat droplets and particulate matter like bacteria. But once inside, the fluid particles cannot move out of capillary wall, since the tendency to backflow closes the flap valve (Fig. 4.4.28).

Important Note

The lymph capillaries are *present* in most tissues of the body except the brain, cartilage, splenic pulp, bone marrow and avascular structures (e.g. cornea and nails).

Larger lymph vessels The lymphatic capillaries join to form larger lymph vessels which ultimately form lymphatic trunks and lymphatic ducts as follows:

Thoracic duct is the largest lymph vessel in the body. It carries lymph from both sides of the body below the diaphragm and from the left side above the diaphragm. Near its termination, it receives the *left subclavian lymphatic trunks* carrying lymph from left upper limb, the *left jugular lymphatic trunk* carrying lymph from left half of the head and neck, and sometimes the *left bronchomediastinal lymphatic trunk* carrying lymph from left half of the thorax (usually this trunk enters the subclavian vein independently).

The thoracic duct ends by opening into the junction of the left subclavian vein and the internal jugular vein.

Right lymphatic duct drains lymph from the right half of the body above the diaphragm. It is formed by the *right bronchomediastinal trunk* carrying lymph from the right half of the thorax, *right jugular trunk* draining lymph from the right half of the head and neck, and *right subclavian trunk* carrying lymph from the right upper limb. The right lymphatic duct ends by opening into the right subclavian vein.

Structure of larger lymph vessels Structure of larger lymph vessels is similar to that of veins:

Three coats, i.e. tunica intima, tunica media and tunica adventitia, can be distinguished.

Valves similar to those in veins are present in abundance in small as well as large lymphatic vessels. The valves often give lymph vessels a beaded appearance.

Lymph Flow

Functions of Lymph Flow

1. Returns proteins from tissue spaces to blood Lymph flow represents the only mechanism for returning albumin and other interstitial macromolecules to the circulatory system. The lymphatic system recovers approximately 200 g of protein daily that has been lost from the microcirculation. In addition, excess fluid is removed from the interstitium to maintain a gel state.

2. Absorption of nutrients Lymph flow helps in absorption of nutrients, especially fats from the gastrointestinal tract.

3. Acts as transport mechanism Lymph flow acts as transport mechanism to remove red blood cells that have lost into the tissues as a result of haemorrhage.

4. Supplies nutrients and oxygen Lymph flow supplies nutrients and oxygen to those parts where blood cannot reach.

5. Role in defence mechanism Lymph nodes associated with lymphatic system act as efficient filters. They have sinuses lined with phagocytic cells that engulf bacteria, red cells and other particulate material.

Mechanism of Lymph Flow

1. Intrinsic lymphatic pump Lymph is pumped out of the tissues by the lymphatic vessels which have valves and smooth muscles in their walls. They contract in a peristaltic fashion, propelling the lymph along the vessels. The extensive system of one-way valves present in the lymphatics maintains lymph flow towards the heart.

2. Pumping by external compression of the lymphatics Although the contractions of lymphatics are the principal factor propelling the lymph, the lymph is also pumped by the external compression of the lymphatics by:

- Contraction of the skeletal muscles
- Movements of different body parts
- Arterial pulsations
- Compression of tissue by objects outside the body

3. Negative intrathoracic pressure Negative intrathoracic pressure during inspiration increases the rate of lymph flow.

4. Suction effect of high-velocity blood flow Suction effect of high-velocity blood flow in the veins in which the lymphatics terminate also promotes lymph flow.

5. Interstitial fluid pressure An increase in the interstitial fluid pressure increases the lymph flow up to a certain limit.

6. Increase in capillary surface area Increase in capillary surface area by capillary distension is associated with increased lymph flow under the following conditions:

- Increased capillary pressure
- Increase in local temperature
- Infusion of fluid

7. Increase in capillary permeability Increase in capillary permeability under the following conditions is also associated with increased lymph flow:

- Increase in temperature
- Effect of toxins
- Decreased oxygen (hypoxia)

8. Increase in functional activity of the tissue Increase in functional activity of the tissue also increases the lymph flow.

Normal Lymph Flow

Normal lymph flow is 2–4 L/day (80–150 mL/h) for the entire body.

Rate of lymph flow Rate of lymph flow varies in different organs and is highest in the gastrointestinal tract and the liver.

In lymphatics In lymphatics, rate of lymph flow is 100 mL/h through thoracic duct and about 20 mL/h through other lymphatic channels.

Rate of formation of lymph is somewhat accelerated by regional venous obstruction (which leads to decreased absorption of tissue fluids into blood capillaries) and also by arteriolar dilations (which leads to increased tissue fluid formation).

Applied Aspects

Lymph oedema refers to tissue swelling caused by accumulation of protein-rich fluid which is mainly drained by lymphatics. It mainly occurs due to obstruction of lymphatics; the common cause of lymph oedema is cancer because cancer cells block the lymph vessels after removal of lymph nodes during surgery.

The signs and symptoms of lymph oedema are as follows:

- Swelling in the arms or legs that may be accompanied by pain or discomfort
- Dimpled skin which gives orange peel appearance
- Frequent skin infection of the affected extremity
- Swollen lymph nodes

Treatment consists of use of devices and therapy.

- Devices include those in the form of elastic bandage and compression stockings.
- Therapy includes physical exercise, especially stretching exercises, self-care and use of moisturizers.

VENOUS CIRCULATION

Structural Characteristics of veins

Walls Walls of veins, compared with those of arteries, at equivalent levels in the vascular tree are thin and contain small amount of elastic tissue and smooth muscle, and have larger lumen. Because of their structural characteristics, they are more distensible and collapsible.

Lumen Lumen of the veins is larger than that of the equivalent arteries. In comparable vessels, the veins provide a larger cross-sectional area than the arteries.

Valves Valves are present in the veins of the dependent parts of the body (Fig. 4.3.17) that prevent the backflow of venous blood. They also support the column of blood so that increase in capillary pressure in the dependent parts of the body (caused by hydrostatic pressure) is minimized.

Functions of the Veins

1. Blood Reservoirs

Because of their feature of *distensibility and collapsibility*, the veins serve as blood reservoirs. About 60%–70% of the circulating blood is present in the venous system. When their blood content decreases, the veins assume an elliptical profile because of their *collapsibility*. As the venous blood content increases, they assume more and more circular profile to accommodate progressively greater amount of blood per unit length. Further increase in the volume of blood is accommodated by distension of the walls without any significant increase in venous pressure. In other words, small changes in pressure can cause large changes in volume (Fig. 4.4.29). Due to this property, veins are also called *capacitance vessels*.

> **Important Note**
>
> Certain portions of the circulatory system are highly compliant and are especially important as blood reservoirs. These include:
> ***Spleen*** can sometimes decrease in size and release as much as 100 mL of blood into the reservoir of circulation.
> ***Liver*** sinuses can also release several hundred millilitres of blood into the rest of circulation.
> ***Large abdominal veins*** can contribute as much as 300 mL.
> ***Venous plexuses beneath the skin*** can also contribute several hundred millilitres of blood.

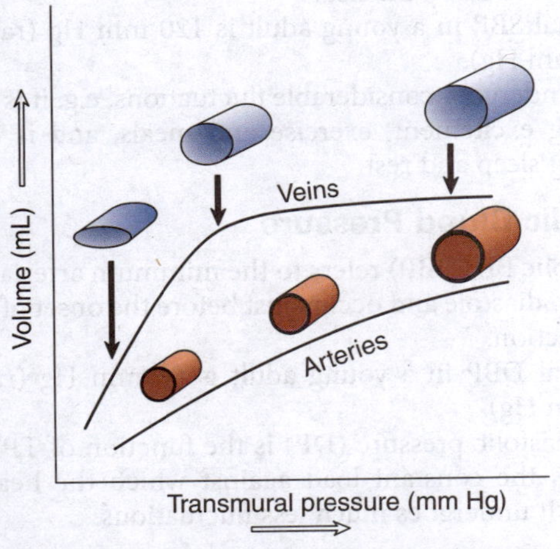

Fig. 4.4.29 Pressure–volume relationship of arteries and veins. The slope of each line at any point represents compliance (distensibility). Note that the veins are much more compliant than the arteries at low pressure because veins are not completely distended at these pressures.

2. Conduits

The systemic veins carry blood from the tissues to the right atrium, and the pulmonary veins collect blood from the lungs and return it to the left atrium.

3. Maintenance of Cardiac Output

Veins help to maintain the CO whenever there is loss of blood. After blood loss from an external or internal injury, reflex increase in sympathetic discharge produces contraction of the smooth muscles in the walls of the veins. As a result of venular contraction, there occurs a decrease in their capacity leading to increased venous return to the heart. In this way, veins help to maintain CO by maintaining normal venous return in spite of blood loss.

Venous Pressure and Flow

The venous system is a low-resistance, low-pressure and highly distensible part of the vascular system. At normal pressures, the veins are approximately 20 times more compliant than the arteries.

Central Venous Pressure

Central venous pressure refers to the pressure in the right atrium because all the systemic veins open into the right atrium. The normal right atrial pressure is about 0 mm Hg (i.e. equal to atmospheric pressure), but it can rise to as high as 20–30 mm Hg under abnormal conditions such as heart failure and massive blood transfusion. The right atrial pressure can decrease to as low as −3 to −5 mm Hg when the heart (right atrium) is pumping with vigour or when venous return is greatly depressed.

Peripheral Venous Pressure

The pressure in the venules is about 10 mm Hg. As the veins approach the heart, there is a gradual decrease in the venous pressure. In the great veins, near the heart, venous pressure is approximately 5 mm Hg. Large veins do not offer any resistance when they are distended. However, many of the large veins entering the thorax are compressed by the surrounding tissues, so they are at least partially collapsed or collapsed to an ovoid state. This impedes the blood flow. Therefore, large veins do offer considerable resistance to blood flow and thus pressure in the peripheral veins is usually greater (4–7 mm Hg) than the right atrial pressure. This produces a pressure gradient which propels the venous blood towards the heart (venous return).

Factors affecting peripheral venous pressure are:

1. Effect of gravitational pressure Gravitational *hydrostatic pressure* occurs in the vascular system because of the weight of the blood in the vessels. Peripheral venous pressure, like arterial pressure, is affected by this gravitational hydrostatic pressure. When an adult person stands absolutely still, the pressure in the body veins because of the effect of hydrostatic pressure is as follows (Fig. 4.4.11):

- At the level of the heart, it is 0 mm Hg.
- At the level of the ankles, it is approximately +80 mm Hg.
- At other levels in the body, from the heart to the feet, the venous pressure varies between 0 and 80 mm Hg. It increases by 0.77 mm Hg for each centimetre below the right atrium. Therefore, if the venous valves are incompetent, as in *varicose veins*, it results in venous pooling, i.e. accumulation of blood in the lower parts of the body.

- Pressure in the veins above the right atrium decreases by 0.77 mm Hg for each centimetre. Therefore, *neck veins* completely collapse due to atmospheric pressure on the outside of the neck, and pressure inside the vein almost remains zero.

Applied Aspects

Due to gravitational effect, *subdural venous sinuses in the skull* cannot collapse because of the tough noncollapsible nature of dura mater; therefore, a negative hydrostatic pressure (−10 mm Hg) exists in them. Because of this reason, if a dural sinus is opened during a neurosurgical procedure with the patient seated, air is sucked into the sinus, resulting in *air embolism*.

2. Effect of venous resistance Increased venous resistance can raise peripheral venous pressure to some extent. Like arterioles, myogenic tone of the veins induced by sympathetic constrictor nerves helps to adjust the capacity of vascular system. This is especially useful in postural changes. For example, sudden change of posture from lying down to standing position results in peripheral pooling of the blood in veins of legs and feet due to effect of gravity. Therefore, venous return to the heart decreases and systemic BP falls which may cause dizziness. However, normally, the compensatory mechanism operated via baroreceptor reflex prevents any fall in BP (see page 330). Increase in venous resistance due to compression of peripheral veins within or without causes an increase in peripheral venous pressure.

3. Effect of central venous pressure Peripheral venous pressure, to a great extent, depends on the central venous pressure. Therefore, any factor that increases central venous pressure (i.e. right atrial pressure) will also increase the peripheral venous pressure. *Common causes associated with rise in right atrial pressure are as follows:*

- Increased blood volume e.g. in massive blood transfusion
- Heart failure
- Arteriolar dilation which decreases PR, causing rapid flow of blood from arterioles, and thus increasing the central venous pressure

4. Effect of venous valves and venous pump The venous pressure in feet is approximately +90 mm Hg in a standing position because of hydrostatic pressure effect. However, movements of legs and muscle contractions (*muscle pump or venous pump*) squeeze the blood out of veins; the *valves* in the veins are arranged in such a way that the direction of blood can only be towards the heart. Thus, the pressure in the veins is lowered. Therefore, in walking adults, venous pressure remains less than 25 mm Hg due to combined effect of 'venous pump' and venous valves.

Measurement of peripheral and central venous pressure Clinical assessment of venous pressure is made by observing the degree of distension of neck veins. When right atrial pressure is increased up to 10 mm Hg, the lower neck veins begin to protrude in sitting position (in normal person, in this position, the neck veins are never distended).

Peripheral venous pressure measurement with a manometer can be made easily by connecting it to cannula inserted into a superficial vein.

Central venous pressure measurement using a cardiac catheter whose tip is led up to superior vena cava through a superficial vein can be made accurately. The other end of the catheter is connected to a pressure transducer.

Venous Flow and Venous Return

As we know, the blood flows in the veins towards the heart due to a pressure gradient which exists between the right atrial pressure (0 mm Hg) and the peripheral veins (6–7 mm Hg). The *velocity of blood flow* in the veins increases with increase in the size of vein. In inferior vena cava, the average velocity of blood flow is 10 cm/s.

Venous return has been discussed in detail on page 282.

BLOOD PRESSURE

DEFINITIONS (TERMINOLOGY)

Blood Pressure (BP)

BP is the lateral pressure exerted by the flowing blood on the walls of the vessels. It is usually measured in millimetres of mercury. Without any further qualification, the term BP denotes the *arterial pressure*. While describing the pressure exerted by the blood column in other types of blood vessels, the type of vessels is also mentioned, e.g. *capillary pressure* and *venous pressure*.

As described in *Bernoulli's experiment* (page 301), the lateral pressure exerted on the vessel wall by the flowing blood represents the *PE* and the *end on pressure* (perfusion pressure) represents the total energy, i.e. KE plus PE. KE depends on the velocity of blood flow. Therefore, with velocity of flowing blood remaining constant, a rise in lateral pressure (PE) indicates a rise in perfusion pressure (total energy) and vice versa.

Systolic Blood Pressure

- The arterial pressure varies with phases of cardiac cycle. The maximum arterial pressure during systole is called *systolic BP (SBP)*, and occurs during ventricular ejection.
- The SBP is a function of the CO, i.e. it represents the extent of work done by the heart.
- Normal SBP in a young adult is 120 mm Hg (range: 105–135 mm Hg).
- SBP undergoes considerable fluctuations, e.g. it is increased during excitement, exercise and meals, and is decreased during sleep and rest.

Diastolic Blood Pressure

- Diastolic BP (DBP) refers to the minimum arterial pressure during diastole and occurs just before the onset of ventricular ejection.
- Normal DBP in a young adult is 80 mm Hg (range: 60–90 mm Hg).
- The diastolic pressure (DP) is the function of TPR and indicates the constant load against which the heart has to work. It undergoes much less fluctuations.

Conventional Expression of Blood Pressure

Conventionally, SBP and DBP are denoted as numerator and denominator, respectively. For example, BP of a normal person is written as 120/80 mm Hg.

Pulse Pressure (PP)

- PP is the arithmetic difference between SBP and DBP.
- Normally, average PP is 40 mm Hg.
- It determines the pulse volume.
- It depends on three factors – arterial volume, stroke volume and arterial elastic constant. Thus, according to Young's elastic modulus:

$$PP = \frac{\Delta V}{V} - \frac{1}{Ka}, \text{ where}$$

  - ΔV is arterial uptake volume (approximately equal to but not less than the stroke volume).
  - V is arterial volume (proportional to the mean arterial pressure [MAP]).
  - Ka is arterial elastic constant.
- The high PP is indicative of systolic HT and indirectly determines decrease in elasticity of blood vessels.

Mean Arterial Pressure

- MAP is the average of all pressure measured millisecond by millisecond throughout the cardiac cycle.
- Since the duration of systole (0.3 second) is shorter than the duration of diastole (0.5 second), the MAP is not equal to the algebraic mean of the SBP and DBP, i.e. it is not equal to ([systolic pressure] + [DP])/2.
- A mathematically precise method for finding out MAP is to find the area under the arterial pressure curve and divide it by the duration of curve (Fig. 4.4.30). However, it is a time-consuming and cumbersome method.
- Practically, MAP is roughly equal to DP plus one-third of PP, i.e.:

$$DBP + \frac{1}{3}PP$$

- MAP, in fact, equals TPR divided by CO, i.e.:

$$MAP = \frac{TPR}{CO}$$

- MAP is same for each organ and determines the pressure head. Thus, regional blood flow through an organ depends on it.
- Normal value of MAP is 93 mm Hg (range: 90–100 mm Hg).

Note: All cardiovascular reflexes are sensitive to MAP.

DETERMINANTS OF (FACTORS AFFECTING) ARTERIAL BLOOD PRESSURE

- The arterial BP is a function of the product of CO and TPR, i.e.:

$$\text{Arterial BP} = CO \times PR$$

- Therefore, arterial BP is affected by conditions that affect either CO or PR.
- Changes in CO affect the systolic pressure more than DP, whereas changes in PR affect DP more than the systolic pressure.
- As discussed in Chapter 4.3 (page 281), the CO is a function of *heart rate* and *stroke volume*, so these two are important determinants of the BP.
- The PR (page 297) depends on the viscosity of blood, elasticity of the vessel wall and velocity of the blood flow. Thus, these factors are also important determinants of the BP.

Effect of some of the important determinants of the BP is shown in Fig. 4.3.15 (page 281) and described here briefly.

1. Heart rate An increase in heart rate usually increases the CO and decreases the duration of cardiac cycle and thus raises the BP. The increase in CO due to increase in heart rate increases DP more than the systolic pressure (because increased heart rate duration of diastole decreases more than systole and the tendency of fall in pressure during diastole decreases).

After an increase in heart rate, the arterial pressure rises, increasing the driving pressure for flow, until the amount of blood exiting the arterial system equals the amount entering. At this time, the transfer of blood from the venous to the arterial system has raised the arterial pressure and lowered the venous pressure.

Conversely, reduction in heart rate decreases the arterial BP.

2. Stroke volume An increase in stroke volume increases the CO and raises the arterial pressure, and the reverse effect

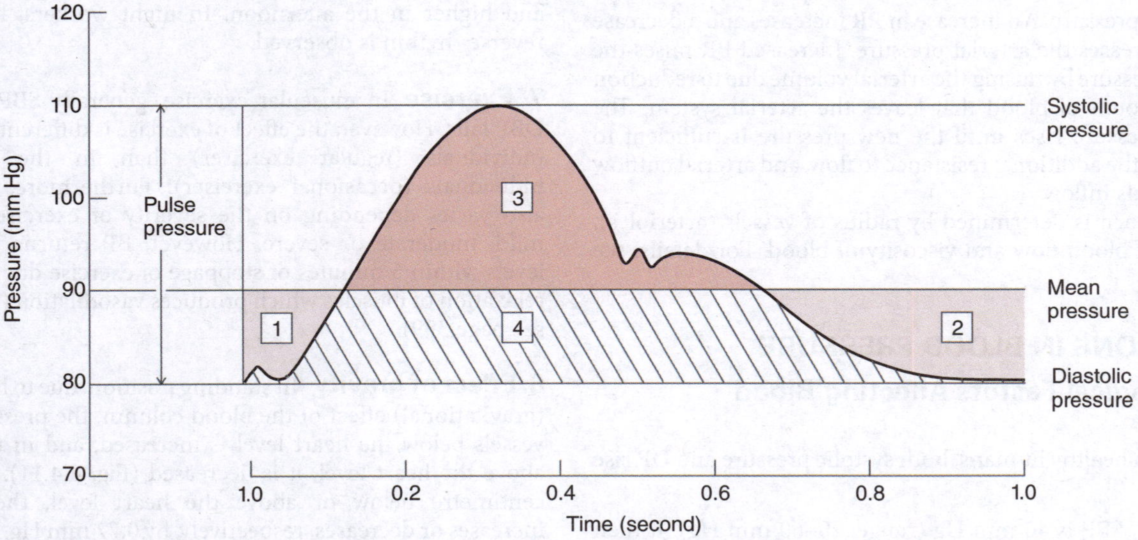

Fig. 4.4.30 Arterial pressure curve. The line for MAP is drawn in a way indicating that area (1 + 2) = area 3. MAP, mean arterial pressure.

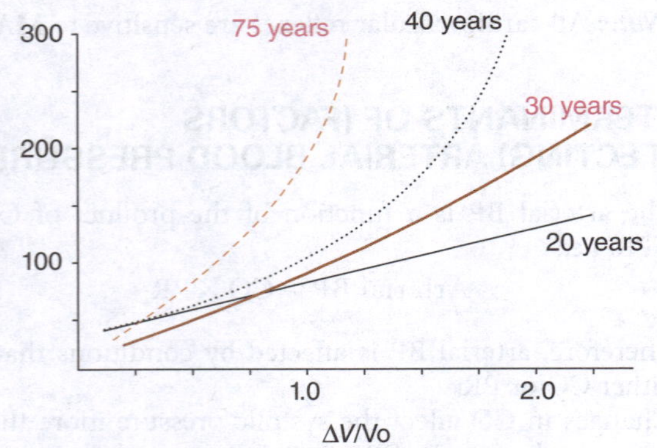

Fig. 4.4.31 The average pressure–volume relationship of arterial system in 20-, 30- and 40-year-old individuals. Note the increasing elastance (decreased distensibility) that occurs with ageing. ΔV, volume change; Vo, unstressed arterial volume.

occurs due to decrease in the stroke volume. When increase in CO is primarily due to increase in stroke volume, it mainly increases SBP. In contrast, an increase in CO due to increase in both the stroke volume and the heart rate increases systolic pressure as well as DP.

3. Arterial elastic constant It refers to stiffness of the arterial system which progressively increases from birth to death (Fig. 4.4.31). An increase in arterial elastic constant (or loss of elasticity of vessel wall) with advancing age results in decreased stretching of the elastic vessels during systole. This results in increased pressure during systole (*systolic HT*) with normal DBP. It is characterized by high PP. When stiffness occurs in small vessels, the DBP is also increased.

4. Arterial blood volume An increase in total blood volume increases both SBP and DBP by increased quantity of blood in the arterial system and greater stretching of the vessel wall.

Conversely, *haemorrhage* and *blood pooling* reduces the arterial pressure by reducing the circulating blood volume. Gravity or marked vasodilation by neural, chemical or mechanical factors may lead to blood pooling in dependent portions of the body and decrease circulating blood volume.

5. Peripheral resistance PR is an important determinant of arterial pressure. An increase in PR increases and a decrease in PR decreases the arterial pressure. Increased PR raises the arterial pressure by raising the arterial volume due to reduction in the amount of blood that leaves the arterial system. The arterial pressure rises until the new pressure is sufficient to overcome the additional resistance to flow, and arterial outflow again equals inflow.

PR in turn is determined by radius of vessels (arterioles), velocity of blood flow and viscosity of blood. For details, see page 298.

VARIATIONS IN BLOOD PRESSURE

Physiological Factors Affecting Blood Pressure

1. Age In healthy humans, both systolic pressure and DP rise with age.

- *At birth*, SBP is 40 mm Hg (range: 20–60 mm Hg). It then rises rapidly up to 1 month of age.
- *At 1 month* of age, the SBP becomes about 80 mm Hg and then rises slowly.
- *At about 17 years* of age, normal adult level of BP 120/80 mm Hg is reached, which remains almost constant up to 40 years of age and then very slowly rises.
- *At about 70 years of age*, the normal value of BP is 160/90 mm Hg. The increase in BP associated with advancing age is due to increase in rigidity of vessel wall owing to arterio-sclerotic changes.
- *A convenient empirical formula* as to what should be considered as normal BP at various ages (after 10 years of age) is as follows:
  - SBP: 110 + 3/5 of age in years
  - DBP: 70 + 2/5 of age in years

2. Sex *Before menopause*, females have little lower (4–6 mm Hg) SBP than in males of corresponding age. This may be because of effect of oestrogen. In contrast, *after menopause*, SBP in females is little higher (4–6 mm Hg) than in males of same age group.

3. Effect of meals SBP increases by 4–6 mm Hg after meals and this effect lasts for about 1 hour. This occurs due to two reasons:

- *Increase in heart rate* due to pressure over the heart by distended abdomen
- *Increased epinephrine release* from adrenal medulla

DBP either remains unchanged or decreases slightly due to vasodilation in splanchnic vessels.

4. Emotions Increased sympathetic activity during emotional situations such as excitement, fear and worry leads to increase in SBP due to increase in the CO.

5. Climatic temperature *Exposure to cold* produces rise in the BP by increase in PR due to cutaneous vasoconstriction through hypothalamic stimulation. Conversely, *exposure to hot temperature* lowers the BP by decreasing PR due to cutaneous vasodilation, again through hypothalamic pathway.

6. Diurnal variation SBP shows a diurnal variation of about 6–10 mm Hg, the values being lower in the morning and higher in the afternoon. In night workers, however, a reverse rhythm is observed.

7. Exercise In muscular exercise, generally SBP rises and DBP falls. However, the effect of exercise is different in trained individuals (regular exerciser) than in the untrained individuals (occasional exerciser). Furthermore, the effect also varies depending on the severity of exercise, whether mild, moderate or severe. However, BP returns to normal levels within 5 minutes of stoppage of exercise due to sudden relaxation of muscles which produces vasodilation (for details, see page 339).

8. Effect of gravity In standing position, due to hydrostatic (gravitational) effect of the blood column, the pressure in the vessels below the heart level is increased, and in the vessels above the heart level, it is decreased (Fig. 4.4.11). For every centimetre below or above the heart level, the pressure increases or decreases, respectively, by 0.77 mm Hg. Therefore, in an individual having 120/80 mm Hg BP in the brachial artery, the BP in the dorsalis pedis artery (which is about 100 cm below the heart level) will be about 200/160 mm Hg, i.e. about 80 mm Hg more ($0.77 \times 100 = 77$ mm Hg = about 80 mm Hg). Therefore, for clinical recording, BP should always be checked at the heart level.

9. Effect of change in posture Sudden change in posture from lying down to standing initiates some momentary changes in BP which in normal humans are immediately rectified by baroreceptor reflexes, and practically such changes are not experienced. However, in patients with autonomic disturbances, these changes become symptomatic. A chain of physiological changes in BP during change of posture is as follows:

- *Immediately on standing*, there occurs peripheral pooling of blood in dependent parts leading to decreased venous return and decreased CO, and momentary fall in SBP. Fall in systolic pressure immediately decreases baroreceptor discharge via vasomotor centre leading to increased *DBP*. On standing, there also occurs an increase in PR and momentary increase in DBP.

Thus, immediately after standing from lying down posture, a rise in DBP can be recorded for about 30–60 seconds. Later on, due to decrease in baroreceptor discharge, BP comes back to normal and no symptoms are experienced by the normal individuals.

10. Sleep In completely relaxed state, during early hours of sleep, there occurs general vasodilation leading to fall in BP up to 15–20 mm Hg. However, in disturbed sleep, BP increases due to increased sympathetic discharge.

11. Body built SBP is slightly higher in obese individuals compared with in thin-built individuals. Furthermore, falsely higher values are obtained in obese individuals while testing brachial artery BP using standard arm cuff. This occurs because there is more tissue between the cuff and the artery and so, some of the cuff pressure is dissipated. Therefore, use of a cuff that is wider than the standard arm cuff is recommended for accurate record of BP in obese individuals.

MEASUREMENT OF BLOOD PRESSURE

Direct Method

Direct method of measuring BP is used in experimental studies. In it, a cannula or T-tube is inserted into an artery and connected to either of the following:

Mercury manometer in which pressure is recorded on the kymograph

Pressure transducer (strain gauge) which in turn is connected to Polyrite for recording

The record will show fluctuations as depicted in Fig. 4.4.32, upper level of which indicates SBP and lower level indicates DBP.

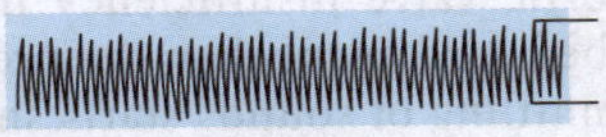

Fig. 4.4.32 Record of arterial blood pressure obtained by direct arterial cannulation method.

Indirect Method

In humans, BP is measured indirectly by using a sphygmomanometer.

Sphygmomanometer

Commonly called BP apparatus, a sphygmomanometer is the instrument used to measure BP. It consists of the following parts:

1. Manometer Two types of manometers are used:

Aneroid manometer (Fig. 4.4.33) in which metal bellows, mechanical rings and a dial replace the glass tube mercury manometer. It is also very commonly used nowadays. However, it needs calibration against a mercury manometer from time to time.

Mercury manometer has been the gold standard for office BP measurement for several decades.

It is commonly used in a classical sphygmomanometer (Fig. 4.4.34). It consists of a *graduated narrow glass tube* having markings 0–300. Upper end of the tube is closed and lower end is connected to lower end of a wide-lumen *mercury reservoir*. Upper end of the mercury reservoir is connected to an inflatable rubber bag through a rubber tube. However mercury devices are no longer being used due to environmental concerns about mercury.

2. The cuff The BP apparatus cuff, also known as 'armlet' or 'Riva-Rocci cuff' (after the name of discoverer), consists of an inflatable rubber bag which is enclosed in a cotton bag having

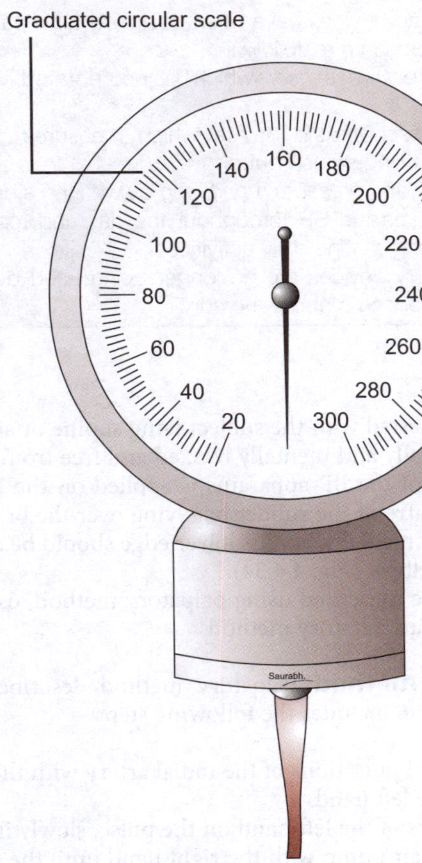

Fig. 4.4.33 Aneroid sphygmomanometer.

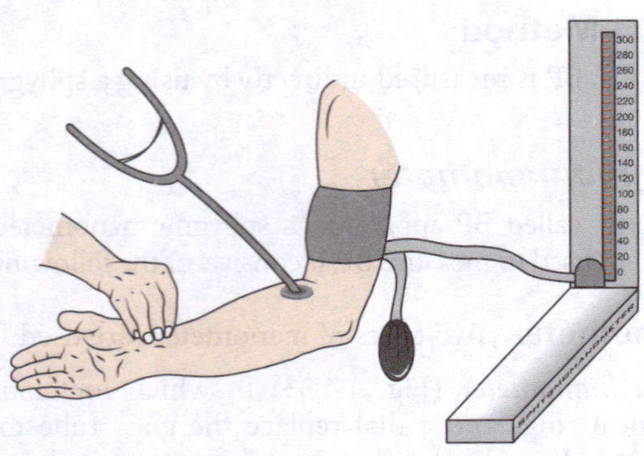

Fig. 4.4.34 Procedure of recording blood pressure by auscultatory method.

a long strip of inelastic cloth. The dimensions of the commonly used rubber bag are 24 × 12 cm. It should be at least as wide as half the upper arm's circumference. The bag width (12 cm) should be more for obese adults, about 4–5 cm for children and 2–3 cm for the newborns.

3. Air pump It is a rubber bulb with a one-way valve at its free end, and a 'leaky valve' and a knurled screw at the other end where the rubber tube leading to the cuff is attached. The cuff can be inflated by turning the leak-valve screw clockwise and alternately compressing and releasing the bulb. Deflation is achieved by turning the screw anticlockwise.

Important Note

Many manometric devices have been designed for measurement of blood pressure as follows:

- *Electronic pressure sensor* which is incorporated within the cuff
- *Automated oscillometric* device which measures blood pressure with single push button
- *Ambulatory blood pressure monitoring* by wearing a device which measures the BP throughout the day and records changes during routine daily activities

However, mercury devices are no longer being used due to environmental concerns about mercury.

Procedure

The BP may be tested with the subject lying supine or sitting, but being physically and mentally relaxed and free from excitation. The cuff of the BP apparatus is applied on the upper arm with the centre of the rubber bag lying over the brachial artery which lies medially, and its lower edge should be about 3 cm above the elbow (Fig. 4.4.34).

The BP can be measured using palpatory method, oscillatory method or auscultatory method.

1. Palpatory method Palpatory method described by Riva-Rocci in 1896 includes the following steps:

- Palpate and feel pulsations of the radial artery with the tips of finger of the left hand.
- Keeping fingers of the left hand on the pulse, slowly inflate the cuff using air pump with the right hand until the pulse disappears. Then raise the pressure further by 30–40 mm Hg in the manometer.
- Open the leak valve of air pump and control it so that the pressure gradually falls in steps of 2–4 mm Hg. Note the reading at which pulse just reappears. This reading corresponds to *SBP*. After this, deflate the cuff quickly to zero pressure.
- Take three readings in each arm, fully deflating the cuff a few minutes between each reading. Mean of the three readings should be taken as SBP. The actual pressure is usually 4–6 mm Hg higher than the recorded value, since initial two to three beats are often missed while feeling the pulse.
- *Disadvantage* of the palpatory method is that the DBP cannot be measured by this method.

2. Auscultatory method Auscultatory method, described by Korotkoff in 1905, is the most useful technique.

- Initial steps up to raising the pressure in the cuff by 30–40 mm Hg above the level where the radial artery pulse disappears are similar to those in the palpatory method. However, before inflating the cuff, the point just before the brachial artery bifurcating the cubital space, just medial to the tendon of biceps muscle, is marked.
- Then the diaphragm of stethoscope is placed on the mark in cubital space and is kept in position with the help of the thumb and fingers of the left hand.
- Pressure in the cuff is lowered slowly by opening the leak valve of the air pump with the right hand. While doing so, initially no sound is heard. However, when mercury column is lowered further, a tap sound is heard. The character and quality of sound go on changing while further lowering the mercury column by deflating the cuff, and ultimately the sound disappears. These sounds are called Korotkoff sounds and from these the levels of SBP and DBP are noted as described in the subsequent text. When the sounds disappear, the cuff should be deflated quickly.

Korotkoff sounds Depending on the characteristic features, the Korotkoff sounds have been described in five phases (Fig. 4.4.35):

Phase I sounds start with a *clear tap* which indicates the *SBP*. The clear, tapping and sharp sounds last for 10–12 mm Hg fall in mercury column.

Phase II sounds are *murmurish*, i.e. soft and swishing, and last for next 14–15 mm Hg fall in mercury column.

Phase III sounds are clear, knocking and banging in character and last for next 14–15 mm Hg fall in mercury column.

Phase IV sounds start with *sudden muffling* and mark the *DBP*. The muffled sounds are indistinct, dull and faint, as if coming from a distance, and last for next 4–5 mm Hg fall in mercury column.

Phase V is labelled when no sound is heard. Since the beginners may not appreciate beginning of muffling of sounds, disappearance of the sound may be considered as a mark of DP. However, in some clinical situations such as hyperthyroidism and aortic valve insufficiency in which the sounds continue to be heard even when the pressure is low, the level at which muffling of sounds starts should be taken as DBP.

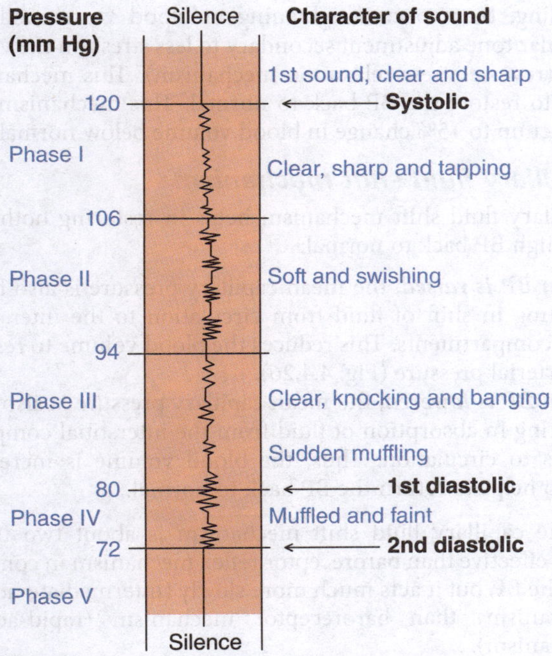

Fig. 4.4.35 Phases of Korotkoff sounds.

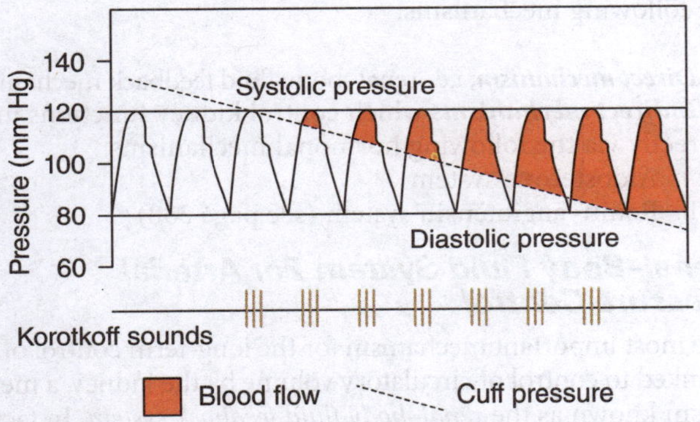

Fig. 4.4.36 Change in blood flow and production of Korotkoff sounds with change in cuff pressure.

Mechanism of korotkoff sounds Normally, the blood flow through the arteries is streamlined or laminar, and no sounds are heard over them when auscultated.

- As shown in Fig. 4.4.36, while testing BP, when the cuff pressure is raised above the expected systolic pressure level, the blood flow in the brachial artery completely ceases and no sounds are heard. When the cuff pressure is reduced gradually, a time comes when, at the peak of each systole, the intra-arterial pressure just exceeds the cuff (extra-arterial) pressure. The small amounts of blood that are ejected at high velocity (exceeding the critical velocity) through the partially narrowed artery result in *intermittent turbulence* which produces the sounds. Also, the blood column in the distal part of the artery, i.e. below the cuff, is set into vibrations by the jets of blood striking against it, which contributes to the sounds. These sounds are called *Korotkoff sounds.*
- When the cuff pressure nears the DP level, the artery is still partially constricted, but the turbulent flow is now continuous and the sounds have a *muffled quality* (phase IV).
- As the cuff pressure falls further, the blood flow becomes laminar once again and the sounds disappear (phase V).
- The change in character of sounds from phase I to phase IV is related to the degree of turbulence.
- In aortic regurgitation, there occurs a continuous turbulent flow so the muffled sounds continue and do not disappear at all. Therefore, as mentioned earlier, in such cases, the start of muffling of sounds should be considered a mark of DP. In fact, in this condition, a slight pressure with a stethoscope alone (without the cuff) may produce clear, sharp, snapping sounds, called the *pistol-shot sounds.*

Auscultatory gap: In some patients with HT, there may be a gap in the Korotkoff sounds. As the mercury is lowered, a few faint sounds are heard which soon disappear only to reappear once again at a much lower pressure. This brief interruption in the sounds is called the *auscultatory or silent gap.* If the mercury column is raised to this gap only, one may miss the first appearance of sounds, which indicates systolic pressure, and thus record a false low systolic pressure. To avoid this mistake, the mercury column must always be raised 50–60 mm Hg above the level at which the radial pulse disappears. One can then be sure that the cuff pressure is well above the systolic level.

Mechanism of auscultatory gap: The mechanism of auscultatory gap is uncertain, but may be associated with reduced peripheral blood flow due to increased stiffness of the arterial wall.

Precautions to be taken while recording blood pressure Basal arterial pressure should always be recorded in the lying down (recumbent) position. This will avoid effect of gravity on BP (page 300) and for this reason the arterial pressure will be same if recorded from any artery.

- The position of the arm and sphygmomanometer should be at the heart level, again to avoid the effect of gravity.
- The cuff size should always be appropriate for accurate measurement of BP (see page 318).
- The palpatory method must always be used first to avoid auscultatory gap.
- The cuff pressure should never be kept high for any length of time because the discomfort may cause generalized reflex vasoconstriction, thus raising the BP.
- It is a good practice to compare the pressure in the two arms when measuring the pressure for the first time.
- Last but not the least, the subject should be physically relaxed and free from tension and anxiety.

Note: The SBP as measured by sphygmomanometer is usually 10–20 mm Hg lower and the DP is higher by about 8 mm Hg than those measured by direct arterial cannulation method.

REGULATION OF BLOOD PRESSURE

Arterial BP is controlled by several mechanisms which under physiological conditions maintain the normal MAP within a narrow range of 95–100 mm Hg. The different mechanisms concerned with regulation of BP have been discussed in detail in Chapter 4.5 (page 324) and have been briefed here just for orientation about control of BP. Each mechanism performs a specific function. Various mechanisms controlling arterial pressure can be grouped as follows:

A. Rapid BP control mechanism
B. Intermediate BP control mechanisms
C. Long-term BP control mechanisms

Rapid Blood Pressure Control Mechanism (Nervous Regulating Mechanism)

Rapid BP control mechanism or the so-called short-term control mechanism primarily includes the following three nervous reflexes:

1. Baroreceptor reflexes (see page 330)
2. Central nervous system ischaemic response (see page 336)
3. Chemoreceptor reflexes (see page 335)

Salient features The nervous reflexes that rapidly control the BP are described in detail in Chapter 4.5. Their salient features are as follows:

- These *act very rapidly*, i.e. within seconds to few minutes of alterations in the BP.
- These are *short-term mechanisms*, i.e. these act for few hours to few days, and are thus insignificant in long-term regulation of BP.
- These are useful in preventing *acute decreases in BP* (e.g. during severe haemorrhage) as well as in preventing *excessive increases in BP* (e.g. as might occur in response to excessive blood transfusion).

Intermediate Blood Pressure Control Mechanisms

The intermediate BP control mechanisms that are important in BP control after several minutes of acute pressure changes are as follows:

1. Renin–angiotensin vasoconstrictor mechanism (for details, see page 338)
2. Stress relaxation and reverse stress relaxation mechanism
3. Capillary fluid shift mechanism

Salient features Salient features of intermediate BP control mechanisms are as follows:

- These mechanisms come into play after several minutes of acute pressure changes and reach full function within a few hours.
- These mechanisms play their role from few days to few weeks.
- All these mechanisms basically try to control the alterations in BP by altering the blood volume.

Stress Relaxation and Reverse Stress Relaxation Mechanisms

Stress relaxation mechanism Stress relaxation mechanism refers to vasodilation occurring due to stress on the VSMs. When pressure in the vessels becomes too high (e.g. following massive slow intravenous transfusion), the vessels become stretched and continue to stretch for minutes or hours. This causes relaxation of blood vessels simply by vascular tone adjustment. This leads to an increase in the capacity of the arterial system with a concomitant fall in BP.

Reverse stress relaxation mechanism Reverse stress relaxation mechanism operates when the BP is low due to less stress on the vessel walls and the body tries to restore it back to normal. For example, when BP falls due to prolonged slow bleeding, there occurs tightening of blood vessel walls by vascular tone adjustment secondary to less stress on the vessel wall (reverse stress relaxation mechanism). This mechanism tries to restore the BP back to normal. This mechanism can correct up to 15% change in blood volume below normal.

Capillary fluid shift mechanism

Capillary fluid shift mechanism helps in restoring both low and high BP back to normal:

When BP is raised, the mean capillary pressure is also high, resulting in shift of fluid from circulation to the interstitial fluid compartments. This reduces the blood volume to restore the arterial pressure (Fig. 4.4.26).

When BP is lowered, the mean capillary pressure is also low, resulting in absorption of fluid from the interstitial compartments to circulation. Thus, the blood volume is increased which helps to return the BP back to normal.

The capillary fluid shift mechanism is about two times more effective than baroreceptor reflex mechanism in controlling the BP, but it acts much more slowly (intermediate-acting mechanism) than baroreceptor mechanism (rapid-acting mechanism).

Long-term Blood Pressure Control Mechanisms

The kidneys play main role in the long-term control of BP by the following mechanisms:

1. ***Direct mechanism***, i.e. 'renal–body fluid feedback mechanism'
2. ***Indirect mechanisms*** which control kidney functions indirectly via the following hormonal mechanisms:
   i. Aldosterone system
   ii. Renin–angiotensin system (see page 338)

Renal–Body Fluid System For Arterial Pressure Control

The most important mechanism for the long-term control of BP is linked to control of circulatory volume by the kidney, a mechanism known as the *renal–body fluid feedback system.* In fact, it is similar to the capillary fluid shift mechanism except that only the renal glomerular capillaries are involved in the process.

Modes of operation of renal–body fluid feedback system The renal–body fluid system corrects BP by causing appropriate changes in blood volume through *diuresis* and *natriuresis*:

When BP rises too high, the kidneys excrete increased quantities of sodium and water because of *pressure natriuresis* and *pressure diuresis*, respectively. As a result of increased renal excretion, both the extracellular fluid volume and the blood volume decrease until BP returns to normal and the kidneys excrete normal amounts of sodium and water.

When the BP falls too low, the kidneys reduce the rate of sodium and water excretion, and over a period of hours to days, if the person drinks enough water and eats enough salt to increase blood volume, the BP will return to its previous level. This mechanism being very slow to act is not of major importance in the acute control of arterial pressure. However, it is by far the most potent of all long-term arterial pressure controllers.

The sequence of events in order of occurrence during control of BP by this mechanism is summarized as follows:

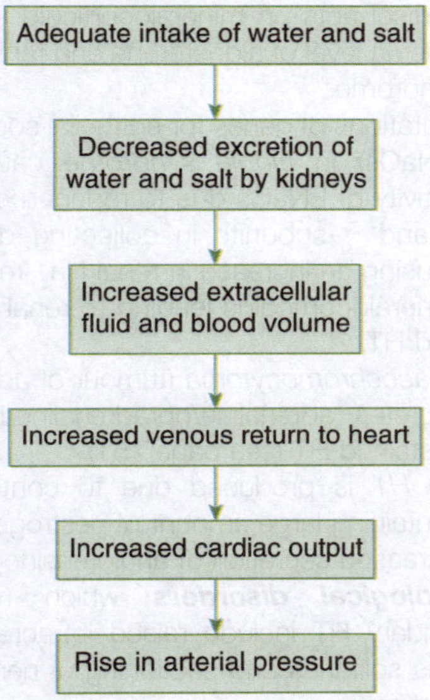

Determinants of the renal–body fluid feedback mechanism The two factors that determine the long-term control of arterial pressure by renal–body fluid mechanism are renal output curve for salt and water and level of salt and water intake. As long as these two factors remain constant, the MAP will also remain exactly at the normal level of 100 mm Hg. For arterial pressure to deviate from the normal level for long periods of time, one of these two factors must be altered.

Fig. 4.4.37 shows the effect of different arterial pressures on urine volume output by an isolated kidney. The figure demonstrates that:

- As arterial pressure rises, there occurs a marked increase in the output of volume (pressure diuresis) and sodium (pressure natriuresis).
- As long as the arterial pressure will remain above the normal equilibrium point, renal output will exceed the intake of salt and water resulting in a progressive decline in extracellular fluid volume.

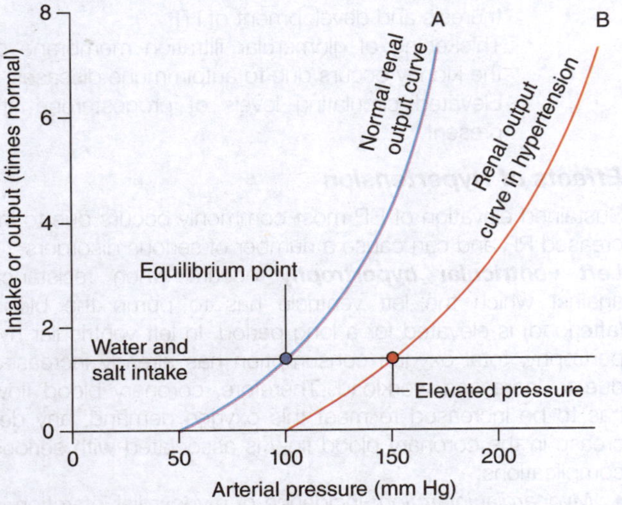

Fig. 4.4.37 Analysis of arterial blood pressure regulation by equating the renal output curve with salt and water intake. The equilibrium point describes the level at which arterial pressure will be regulated.

- When BP falls below the equilibrium point, the renal output of water and salt will be lower than the intake resulting in a progressive increase in extracellular volume.
- At the normal arterial pressure, a balance between renal output and intake of salt and water occurs at the so-called *equilibrium point*.
- As shown in Fig. 4.4.37 (B), due to an abnormality of the kidney, the renal output curve is shifted and the equilibrium point is obtained at a level of high BP (150 mm Hg).
- The renal output and salt and water intake demonstrate that theoretically arterial pressure will be raised with increase in salt and water intake. However, in reality, the BP does not rise every time the sodium intake is increased. This is accomplished mainly by decreasing the formation of angiotensin II and aldosterone, which increases the ability of kidney to excrete salt and water, and results in compensatory *left shift of the pressure natriuresis curve.*

Salient features of renal–body fluid feedback mechanism The salient features of the renal–body fluid feedback mechanism can be summarized as follows:

- The renal–body fluid feedback mechanism takes several hours to show any significant response.
- These mechanisms operate very powerfully to control arterial pressure over days, weeks and months.
- The effectiveness of these mechanisms becomes steadily greater with time.
- These mechanisms, if given sufficient time, control arterial pressure at the level that provides normal output of salt and water by the kidneys.
- As long as kidney function is unaltered, these mechanisms overcome the disturbances that tend to alter arterial pressure such as increased TPR over a long period and thus are able to control the BP.

Conclusion To conclude, it can be stated that *rapid control* of arterial pressure begins with life-saving measures of the *nervous reflexes*, continues with sustaining characteristics of the *intermediate pressure controls* and finally is stabilized at the *long-term pressure level by the renal–body fluid feedback mechanism.*

Applied Aspects

Pathological Variations in Blood Pressure

Hypertension

Definition Hypertension (HT) refers to a condition in which value of systolic BP is persistently more than 140 mm Hg and/or that of diastolic BP is above 90 mm Hg. If there is an increase only in systolic BP, it is called systolic HT in which the PP is raised.

Types of Hypertension It is of two types – primary and secondary HT.

1. **Primary HT**, also known as *essential HT*, is characterized by a raised BP without any underlying disease. Risk factors for primary HT include heredity, obesity, mental tension and smoking. BP is raised due to increased PR. Primary HT presents in two clinical forms:
   - *Benign HT*, in which BP is moderately raised. Untreated HT over the years may cause cardiac, vascular and renal complications.

- *Malignant HT* or accelerated HT refers to a sudden marked rise in BP (e.g. systolic up to 250 mm Hg and diastolic up to 150 mm Hg). It is an emergency and may sometimes be even fatal.

2. **Secondary HT** refers to a condition in which BP is raised due to some other underlying disease. Common causes of secondary HT are as follows:

Cardiovascular diseases producing secondary HT are atherosclerosis and coarctation of aorta.

Renal diseases causing secondary HT are stenosis of renal artery, glomerulonephritis and tumour of juxtaglomerular cells leading to formation of excess of angiotensin II.

(i) ***Goldblatt HT***, also known as renovascular HT, refers to the HT due to compression of renal artery or its branches. It can be of two types:

- *One-kidney Goldblatt HT:* This happens when one kidney is already removed and the renal artery of other kidney is constricted due to any reason.
- *Two-kidney Goldblatt HT:* This occurs when the artery to one kidney is constricted while the artery to other kidney is normal.

Mechanism: Due to occlusion of renal artery, there occurs renal ischaemia, which triggers release of renin causing rapid elevation of BP for the first hour or so. This is followed by a slower additional rise in BP during next several days. This happens because the hyperreninaemia increases angiotensin II levels (for details, see causing severe vasoconstriction and aldosterone release leading to sodium and water retention).

(ii) ***Endocrinal disorder*** associated with secondary HT is Cushing syndrome (excessive secretion of glucocorticoids from adrenal cortex).

Hyperaldosteronism (excessive secretion of aldosterone or other mineralocorticoids from adrenal cortex) causes renal Na^+ and water retention, consequently leading to expansion of ECF volume, and BP rises. It occurs due to mutations in a number of genes. In humans, different gene mutations have been identified which are responsible for HT.

- HT caused by mutation of a single gene is referred to as monogenic HT that is a rare entity (Ô°ú1%).
- A hybrid gene encodes adrenocorticotropic-sensitive aldosterone synthetase enzyme that causes hyperaldosteronism; this condition is known as *glucocorticoid-remediable hyperaldosteronism (GRA)*. Normally, glucocorticoids do not suppress aldosterone secretion, but in this autosomal dominant disorder, HT can be remedied by administering glucocorticoids that suppress ACTH secretion.
- The genes coding aldosterone synthase and 11β-hydroxylase are identical and close to each other on chromosome 8. Therefore, mutation of hybrid gene in GRA also results in 11β-hydroxylase deficiency, which causes HT by increasing the secretion of deoxycorticosterone.
- In deficiency of 11β-hydroxysteroid type 2 enzyme due to gene mutation, the cortisol has marked mineralocorticoid effect and the syndrome is known as *apparent mineralocorticoid excess (AMI)*. In this condition, there is loss of specificity for mineraloreceptors. Therefore, clinical picture resembles that of hyperaldosteronism because cortisol acts on mineralocorticoid receptors. The plasma level of aldosterone and renin is low in this syndrome.
- Mutations of genes for epithelial sodium channels (ENaCs) in *Liddle syndrome* cause increased activity of ENaCs due to reduced degradation of β and γ subunits in collecting ducts, thereby causing an increase in renal Na^+ reabsorption by mineralocorticoids leading to renal Na^+ retention and HT.
- *Phaeochromocytoma* (tumour of adrenal medulla) secretes adrenaline/noradrenaline/both, causing sustained HT (see page 751).
- *Pill HT* is produced due to contraceptive pills containing large amount of oestrogen that causes increased secretion of angiotensinogen.

(iii) ***Neurological disorders*** which may produce secondary HT include raised intracranial pressure, tractus solitarius and sectioning of nerve fibres from carotid sinus.

(iv) ***Pregnancy-induced hypertension (PIH)*** is noticed in some of the pregnant women. Its exact cause is not known. It may be because of some autoimmune processes during pregnancy or the release of some vasoconstrictor agents from placenta or due to excessive secretion of hormones causing rise in BP.

HT in preeclampsia (toxaemia of pregnancy): Preeclampsia or toxaemia of pregnancy is a syndrome that occurs in approximately 5%–10% of expectant mothers. HT is one of the major manifestations of this syndrome. The precise cause is not clearly known, but ischaemia of placenta and subsequently release of toxic factors are believed to play role in manifestations of preeclampsia.

- HT occurs due to endothelial dysfunction of vasculature resulting in decreased release of nitrous oxide and other substances causing vasoconstriction, decreased GFR, impaired renal pressure natriuresis and development of HT.
- Thickening of glomerular filtration membrane of the kidney occurs due to autoimmune diseases.
- Elevated circulating levels of progesterone are present.

Effects of Hypertension

Sustained elevation of BP most commonly occurs due to increased PR and can cause a number of serious disorders.

Left ventricular hypertrophy occurs when resistance against which the left ventricle has to pump the blood (afterload) is elevated for a long period. In left ventricular hypertrophy, total oxygen consumption has already increased due to increased workload. Therefore, coronary blood flow has to be increased to meet this oxygen demand; any decrease in the coronary blood flow is associated with serious complications:

- *Myocardial infarction:* Incidence of myocardial infarction is higher in individuals with HT. For details, see page 349.

- *Atherosclerosis:* The incidence of atherosclerosis increases in individuals with HT.
- *Thrombosis:* Individuals with HT are predisposed to cerebral thrombosis resulting in stroke and haemorrhage.
- *Renal failure* is an additional complication of HT.
- *Heart failure* occurs due to increase in the afterload. For details, see page 373.

Treatment

The incidence of heart failure, stroke and renal failure can be avoided by active treatment. BP can be lowered effectively by use of the following drugs:

- α-Adrenergic receptor blockers
- β-Adrenergic receptor blockers
- Inhibitors of angiotensin-converting enzyme
- Calcium channel blockers

Details of treatment are beyond the scope of this book. Therefore, for mechanism of action, doses, etc., students are advised to consult pharmacology and medicine books.

Hypotension

Hypotension refers to a condition in which values of BP are below the normal range. Clinically, when the systolic BP is less than 90 mm Hg, it is considered hypotension. It is of the following types:

Primary hypotension, also known as essential hypotension, is a disorder of unknown aetiology.

Secondary hypotension, as the name indicates, occurs secondary to some other underlying diseases such as myocardial infarction, neurogenic shock, haemorrhagic shock, hypoactivity of pituitary gland and hypoactivity of adrenal glands.

Postural hypotension refers to sudden fall in BP when patients stand up from lying down posture. It occurs due to some dysfunction of autonomic nervous system.

Self-Assessment

1. Discuss about peripheral resistance, its significance and factors affecting it.
2. Discuss the regulatory mechanism of blood pressure.
3. Discuss the haemodynamics in reference to different type of blood vessels of systemic arterial system.
4. Write notes on:
   - Transcapillary exchange
   - Mechanism of Korotkoff sounds
   - Renal fluid feedback system
   - Pathophysiology of hypertension
   - Orthostatic hypotension
   - Windkessel effect and its significance

Clinical Cases

Case 1

In a patient with hypertension, injection captopril was given, and the patient was advised to take low-sodium diet. In follow-up visit, the blood pressure recorded was normal.

Q1. What is the mechanism of action of the drug in this case?

Q2. How does low-sodium diet help in lowering the blood pressure?

Case 2

A young male patient is brought to the hospital emergency with severe headache, blurring of vision and confused state. There is no history of head injury, but the patient is a case of hypertension. The probable diagnosis made is brain haemorrhage. On examination, pulse rate is 34/min and BP 200/112 mm Hg.

Q1. What further test should be carried out to confirm the diagnosis?

Q2. What is reason for bradycardia in this case?

4.5 Cardiovascular Regulation

CHAPTER OUTLINE

INTRODUCTION

Cardiovascular control makes *circulatory adjustments* which are essential to cope with the timely needs of each and every organ of the body and is thus of fundamental importance for survival.

NEED FOR CARDIOVASCULAR CONTROL

Functions served by cardiovascular control are as follows:

- *To increase the blood supply* to active tissues, e.g. during exercise to skeletal and cardiac muscles
- *Redistribution of blood* to increase or decrease the heat loss from the body as per requirements
- *Circulatory adjustments* during routine cardiovascular stresses like change in posture, hours of excitement, fear, anxiety, meals and sleep
- *Maintenance of adequate flow to vital organs* such as the brain, heart and kidney at all the times including emergencies such as shock and haemorrhage, even at the expense of the circulation to the rest of the body, as the vital organs may develop irreversible changes in no time (e.g. the brain is irreversibly damaged within 3 minutes of ischaemia, whereas the skin, skeletal muscle and gastrointestinal tract can tolerate reduction of blood for longer duration; the earlier-described functions subserved by the cardiovascular control system, in other words, qualify the need for cardiovascular control)

CIRCULATORY ADJUSTMENTS

Circulatory adjustments which ensure that all of the organs receive sufficient blood flow are as follows: (1) control of blood volume and (2) control of arterial pressure. These circulatory adjustments are made by the cardiovascular control mechanisms primarily by regulating the following parameters:

A. Regulation of cardiac performance

Regulation of cardiac performance, i.e. alterations in the activities of the heart, includes:

1. ***Chronotropic action***, i.e. effect on heart rate which may be in the form of:
   - Increased heart rate (tachycardia) or positive chronotropic effect
   - Decreased heart rate (bradycardia) or negative chronotropic effect
2. ***Inotropic action***, i.e. effect on force of contraction which may be in the form of:
   - Increase in the force of contraction (positive inotropic effect) or
   - Decrease in the force of contraction (negative inotropic effect)
3. ***Dromotropic action***, i.e. effect on conduction of impulse through the heart, which may be in the form of:
   - Increase in the velocity of impulse conduction (positive dromotropic effect) or
   - Decrease in the velocity of impulse conduction (negative dromotropic effect)
4. ***Bathmotropic action***, i.e. effect on the excitability of the cardiac muscle, which may be in the form of:
   - Increased excitability of cardiac muscle (positive bathmotropic effect) or
   - Decreased excitability of cardiac muscle (negative bathmotropic effect)

B. Regulation of performance of blood vessels

Regulation of performance of blood vessels primarily includes:

1. ***Alterations in diameter of arterioles*** which change the peripheral resistance and also the hydrostatic pressure in the capillaries
2. ***Alteration in diameter of veins*** which changes the venous pressure and thus venous return and the cardiac output

Cardiovascular Control Mechanisms

The cardiovascular control mechanisms which play their role in making circulatory adjustments during the routine and emergency cardiovascular stresses can be grouped as:

- Neural control mechanism
- Humoral control mechanism
- Local control mechanisms

NEURAL CONTROL MECHANISM

Neural regulation of circulation is of fundamental importance since it responds within seconds. However, neural mechanism has little to do with local adjustments of blood flow to the tissues, except for certain tissues such as the skin.

The nervous regulation mainly controls systemic functions of the circulatory system (whenever required) such as:

- Redistribution of blood flow to different parts of the body
- Increasing pumping activity of the heart
- Rapid control of arterial pressure

Components of neural control mechanism

The neural cardiovascular regulating mechanism consists of:

A. **Medullary cardiovascular control centres:** These are the prime centres concerned with neural control of circulation. These include:
   - Medullary sympathetic centre (vasomotor centre [VMC])
   - Medullary parasympathetic centre (nucleus ambiguus)
   - Medullary relay centre for cardiorespiratory and afferents (nucleus of tractus solitarius [NTS])

B. **Autonomic nervous system (ANS) supplying the heart and blood vessels:** The regulation of circulation by medullary control centres is exerted almost entirely through the ANS. The sympathetic component of ANS is most important for controlling circulation, and the parasympathetic component mainly contributes to regulation of heart functions.

C. **Afferent impulses to medullary centres:** VMC is influenced by afferent impulses from the higher centres and a large number of other areas.

D. **Role of skeletal nerves and muscles in controlling blood pressure**

A. MEDULLARY CARDIOVASCULAR CONTROL CENTRES

1. Vasomotor Centre

Although popularly known as VMC, more appropriately it should be called *medullary sympathetic centre*. It is the primary cardiovascular regulatory centre located in the medulla oblongata of brainstem. It consists of groups of neurons situated bilaterally in the reticular substance of medulla at the floor of fourth ventricle. The medullary cardiovascular centre is constituted by the following different areas (Fig. 4.5.1):

Pressor Area

Pressor area is located in the rostral ventrolateral medulla (RVLM). It contains glutaminergic neurons which exert *excitatory* effect on thoracolumbar spinal sympathetic neurons.

Continuous sympathetic vasoconstrictor tone: Normally, the neurons forming the pressor area of the VMC show *inherent tonic activity*, i.e. they discharge rhythmically (at a rate of about 1 impulse/s) in a tonic fashion to excite sympathetic preganglionic neurons present in the intermediolateral (IML) grey column of the spinal cord. In this way, the continuous signals are passed to the sympathetic vasoconstrictor nerves

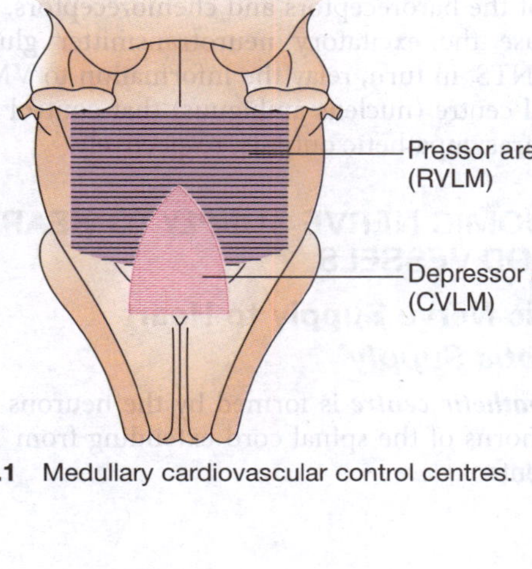

Fig. 4.5.1 Medullary cardiovascular control centres.

fibres over the entire body. This *sympathetic vasoconstrictor tone* maintains a partial state of contraction of blood vessels. When this tone is blocked, e.g. by spinal anaesthesia, the blood vessels throughout the body dilate and arterial pressure may fall to as low as 50 mm Hg.

Stimulation of pressor area produces:

- *Arteriolar constriction* which increases the systemic blood pressure
- *Venoconstriction* which decreases blood stored in the venous reservoir and increases venous return
- *Increase in heart rate* or positive chronotropic effect
- *Increase in force of contraction* or positive inotropic effect

Important Note

Cases of essential hypertension are associated with neurovascular compression of RVLM. Magnetic resonance angiography (MRA) in patients with schwannoma or meningiomas lying nearer to RVLM has indicated higher incidence of coexistence of hypertension and neurovascular compression due to increased sympathetic activity. For details of hypertension, see page 321.

Depressor Area

Depressor area is situated bilaterally in the *caudal ventrolateral medulla* (CVLM). Stimulation of neurons forming the depressor area produces decrease in the sympathetic activity due to inhibition of the tonically discharging impulses of the pressor area causing:

- *Arteriolar dilation* which decreases systemic blood pressure
- *Venodilatation* which increases storage of blood in venous reservoir and decreases venous return and cardiac output
- *Decrease in the heart rate* or negative chronotropic effect
- *Decrease in force of contraction* or negative inotropic effect

2. Medullary Parasympathetic Centre

Medullary parasympathetic centre or *cardiac vagal centre* (earlier also called cardioinhibitory centre) is now called by its specific name, i.e. the *nucleus ambiguus.* It is located lateral to the medullary reticular formation (the neurons located in this centre are not tonically active). Nucleus ambiguus receives afferents via NTS and in turn sends inhibitory pathway in the form of vagal fibres to the *heart* to decrease heart rate and force of cardiac contraction.

3. Medullary Relay Station for Cardiorespiratory Afferents

NTS of the vagus nerve forms the so-called medullary relay station for cardiorespiratory afferents. It receives afferents from most of the baroreceptors and chemoreceptors. The afferents release the excitatory neurotransmitter glutamate. Cells of the NTS, in turn, relay the information to VMC and cardiac vagal centre (nucleus ambiguus) that control sympathetic and parasympathetic outputs, respectively.

B. AUTONOMIC NERVE SUPPLY TO HEART AND BLOOD VESSELS

Autonomic Nerve Supply to Heart

Sympathetic Supply

Spinal sympathetic centre is formed by the neurons located in the IML horns of the spinal cord extending from T_1 to L_2 spinal segments.

The IML cells are neurons from which the sympathetic fibres actually originate.

Preganglionic sympathetic fibres (small, myelinated) supplying the heart arise from the neurons lying in the IML horns of the T_1 to T_5 *spinal segments* and pass into the sympathetic trunk to superior, middle and inferior cervical ganglia and upper thoracic ganglia where they synapse (Fig. 4.5.2).

Postganglionic fibres (long, unmyelinated) leave the ganglia and pass via superior, middle and inferior *cardiac sympathetic nerves* and supply to nodal tissues (sinoatrial [SA] node and atrioventricular [AV] node) and cardiac muscles (of atria and ventricles; Fig. 4.5.2).

Important Note

It is important to note that:

- Sympathetics from right side are primarily distributed to SA node.
- Sympathetics from left side are primarily distributed to AV node.

Stimulation of cardiac sympathetic nerves Stimulation of cardiac sympathetic nerves causes:

- *Increased heart rate* (positive chronotropic effect) by increasing rhythmicity of SA node (see page 245)
- *Increase in the conduction of impulse* through the heart (positive dromotropic action, see page 245)
- *Increase in the excitability* of myocardium (positive bathmotropic effect)
- *Increase in the force of contraction* of myocardium (positive inotropic effect, see page 284)

Parasympathetic Supply

Parasympathetic fibres to the heart are carried through two vagi (Fig. 4.5.3).

Preganglionic fibres (long, myelinated) arise from the *nucleus ambiguous* located in the medulla and travel along the vagi to reach the heart through their cardiac branches to synapse in the *ganglia* located within the superficial and deep cardiac plexuses and also in the walls of atria.

Postganglionic fibres (small, unmyelinated) are distributed to the atria, SA node, AV node and AV bundle. It is important to note that:

- The right vagus is distributed mainly to SA node.
- The left vagus is distributed mainly to AV node.
- No vagal motor fibres are distributed to the ventricles.
- Parasympathetic fibres to the heart are *endocardiac.*

Stimulation of parasympathetic fibres Stimulation of parasympathetic fibres to the heart causes:

- *Decrease in heart rate* by decreasing rate of impulse generation by SA node (negative chronotropic effect; for details, see page 245)
- *Decrease in conduction of impulse* through the conduction tissue (negative dromotropic effect)
- *Decrease in the excitability of atria* only (negative bathmotropic effect; see page 245)
- *Decrease in the force of contraction* of atria only (negative inotropic effect; there is no effect on force of contraction of ventricles)

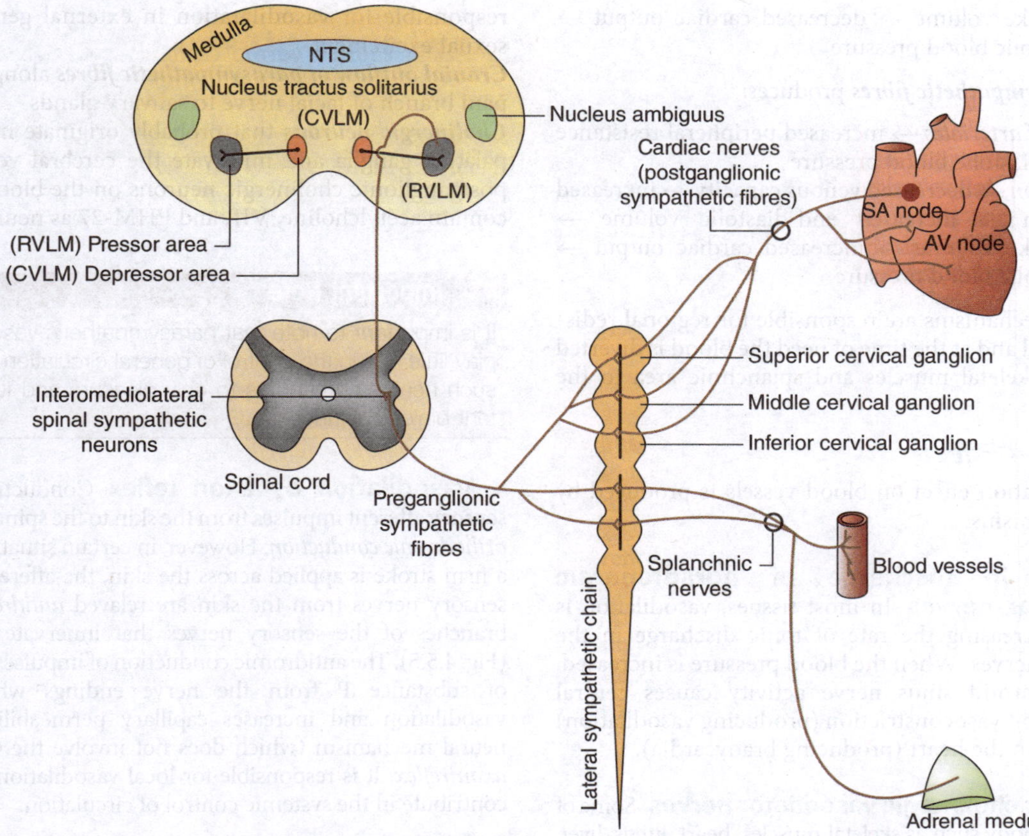

Fig. 4.5.2 Sympathetic innervation to heart and blood vessels.

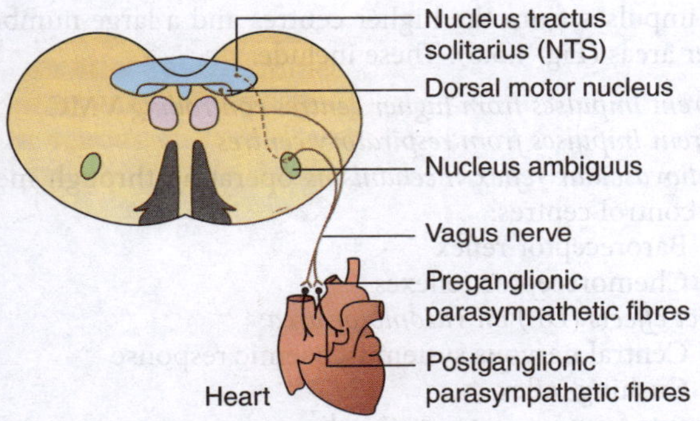

Fig. 4.5.3 Parasympathetic innervation of the heart.

Vagal tone There is a moderate amount of tonic discharge in the cardiac sympathetic nerves at rest, but there is a good deal of tonic vagal discharge, called the *vagal tone*, in humans and other large animals. Therefore, when vagi are cut in the experimental animals, the heart rate rises. Similarly, in adult humans, the resting heart rate which is about 72 beats/min rises to 150–180 beats/min after the administration of vagolytic drugs such as atropine, because of the unopposed sympathetic tone. When both adrenergic and cholinergic systems are blocked in humans, the heart rate is approximately 100 beats/min. Since the resting heart rate is about 72/min, it confirms that at rest, the vagal tone is greater than the sympathetic tone (see page 245).

Autonomic Nerve Supply to Blood Vessels

The autonomic efferents supplying the blood vessels produce two types of effects:

- Vasoconstriction
- Vasodilatation

Vasoconstriction Effect

Vasoconstriction effect is produced by the sympathetic fibres supplying the blood vessels which originate from the IML horns in T_1 to L_2 spinal segments.

Vasoconstrictor fibres have norepinephrine and sometimes neuropeptide Y as neurotransmitter and are called *noradrenergic fibres.*

These noradrenergic fibres innervate all the blood vessels of the body except the *true capillaries* and cerebral regional circulation. The small arteries and arterioles are more richly innervated as compared with large vessels. Furthermore, arterioles of the skin, skeletal muscles and splanchnic arterioles have more supply as compared with those of the brain and myocardium.

Sympathetic vasoconstrictor fibres show tonic (i.e. continuous) discharge at the rate of about 1 impulse/s.

When the sympathetic nerves are cut (sympathectomy), there occurs:

- *Vasodilatation* (of arterioles) → decreased peripheral resistance → decreased diastolic blood pressure; and *venodilatation* → increased venous capacity → decreased venous return → decreased end-diastolic volume →

decreased stroke volume → decreased cardiac output → decreased systolic blood pressure

Stimulation of sympathetic fibres produces:

- *Constriction of arterioles* → increased peripheral resistance → increased diastolic blood pressure
- *Venoconstriction* → decreased venous capacity → increased venous return → increased end-diastolic volume → increased stroke volume → increased cardiac output → increased systolic blood pressure

Both these mechanisms are responsible for regional redistribution of blood and at the time of need the blood is diverted from the skin, skeletal muscles and splanchnic area to the heart and brain.

Vasodilatation Effect

Neural vasodilatation effect on blood vessels is produced by following mechanisms:

1. Decrease in discharge of noradrenergic vasoconstrictor nerves In most tissues, vasodilation is produced by decreasing the rate of tonic discharge in the vasoconstrictor nerves. When the blood pressure is increased, the increased carotid sinus nerve activity causes central reflexes that inhibit vasoconstriction (producing vasodilation) and tonic effect on the heart (producing bradycardia).

2. Sympathetic cholinergic vasodilator nerves Some of the organs of the body such as skeletal muscles, heart, lungs, liver, kidney and uterus in addition to adrenergic vasoconstrictor sympathetic fibres also receive innervation by *cholinergic vasodilator sympathetic* fibres having acetylcholine and vasoinhibitory peptide (VIP) as neurotransmitter. These fibres originate from the cerebral cortex, relay in the hypothalamus and midbrain, and pass through the medulla (without relay in the VMC) to the sympathetic neurons located in the IML grey column of the spinal cord (Fig. 4.5.4). These fibres are not *tonically active*, and get activated only in biological stresses, e.g. during exercise and childbirth, and help in increasing the blood flow.

3. Parasympathetic vasodilator nerves Blood vessels, in general, do not have parasympathetic innervation with the following exceptions:

Sacral outflow parasympathetic fibres represented by ***nervi erigentes*** which supply sexual erectile tissue and are responsible for vasodilatation in external genitalia during sexual excitement

Cranial outflow of parasympathetic fibres along chorda tympani branch of facial nerve to salivary glands

Cholinergic neurons that probably originate in the sphenopalatine ganglia and innervate the cerebral vessels and the postganglionic cholinergic neurons on the blood vessels that contain acetylcholine, VIP, and PHM-27 as neurotransmitters

> **Important Note**
>
> It is important to note that parasympathetic vasodilator fibres play little role in the control of general circulation. Activation of such nerves contributes to only pleasure and fulfilling important biological functions.

4. Vasodilation by axon reflex Conduction of normal sensory afferent impulses from the skin to the spinal cord is called *orthodromic conduction*. However, in certain situations, e.g. when a firm stroke is applied across the skin, the afferent impulses in sensory nerves from the skin are relayed *antidromically* down branches of the sensory nerves that innervate blood vessels (Fig. 4.5.5). The antidromic conduction of impulses causes release of substance P from the nerve endings which produces vasodilation and increases capillary permeability. This local neural mechanism (which does not involve the CNS) is called *axon reflex*. It is responsible for local vasodilation and does not contribute in the systemic control of circulation.

C. AFFERENT IMPULSES TO MEDULLARY CARDIOVASCULAR CONTROL CENTRES

The medullary control centres are influenced by afferent control impulses from the higher centres and a large number of other areas (Fig. 4.5.6). These include:

Afferent impulses from higher centres controlling VMC

Afferent impulses from respiratory centres

Cardiovascular reflex mechanisms operating through medullary control centres:

- Baroreceptor reflex
- Chemoreceptor reflexes

Direct effects (DE) on vasomotor area:

- Central nervous system ischaemic response
- Cushing reflex

Afferents from nociceptive stimuli

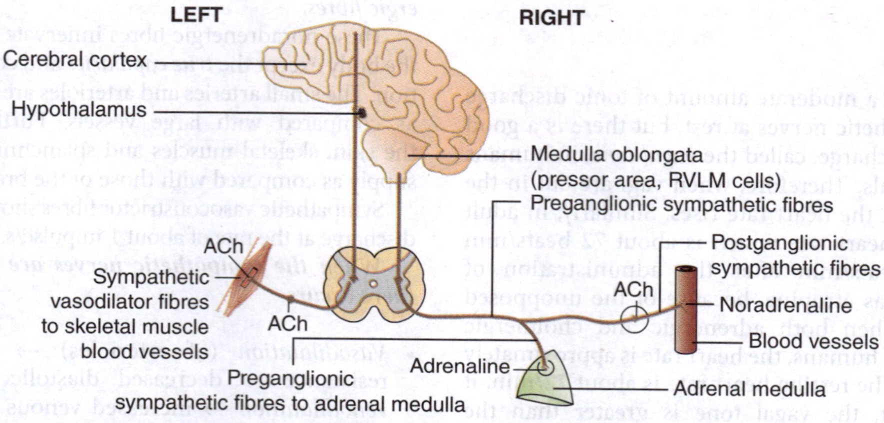

Fig. 4.5.4 Pathway of sympathetic vasodilator fibres (on left side) and sympathetic vasoconstrictor system (on right side).

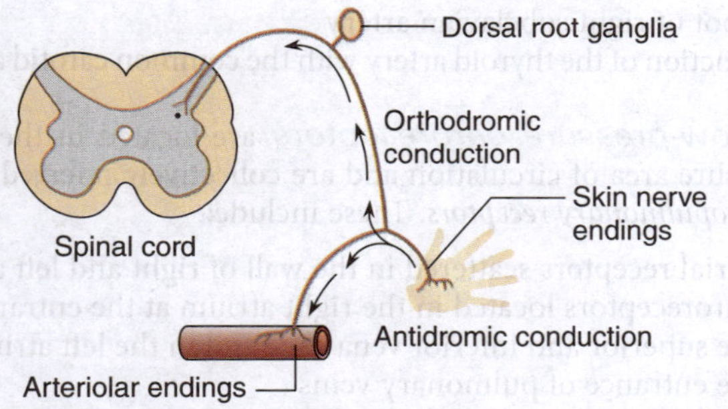

Fig. 4.5.5 Pathway of axon reflex.

(a) Afferent Impulses from Higher Centres Controlling Vasomotor Centre and Cardiac Vagal Centre

Cerebral Cortex

Stimulation of various areas of motor cortex leads to complex motor responses that include appropriate cardiovascular adjustments. There are descending tracts to the vasomotor area from the cerebral cortex (particularly the limbic cortex) that relay in the hypothalamus. Some examples of the influence of limbic system on the VMC are as follows:

Tachycardia and hypertension produced by emotions such as sexual excitement and anger

Bradycardia and fainting occurring during sudden emotional shock

Fight or flight response which is a complex set of responses which increases cardiac output and raises blood pressure in anticipation of flight or physical defence

Hypothalamus

The connections between the hypothalamus and the vasomotor area are reciprocal, with afferents from the brainstem closing the loop. The hypothalamus serves to integrate many somatic and autonomic responses. Examples are as follows:

Temperature regulation: The effect of temperature changes on the hypothalamic centres is relayed to the medulla, which causes the vessels of skin to constrict (heat conservation) or to dilate (heat dissipation).

Emotional stresses influence the heart rate and blood pressure by impulses relayed from hypothalamus to stimulate or inhibit the medullary centres.

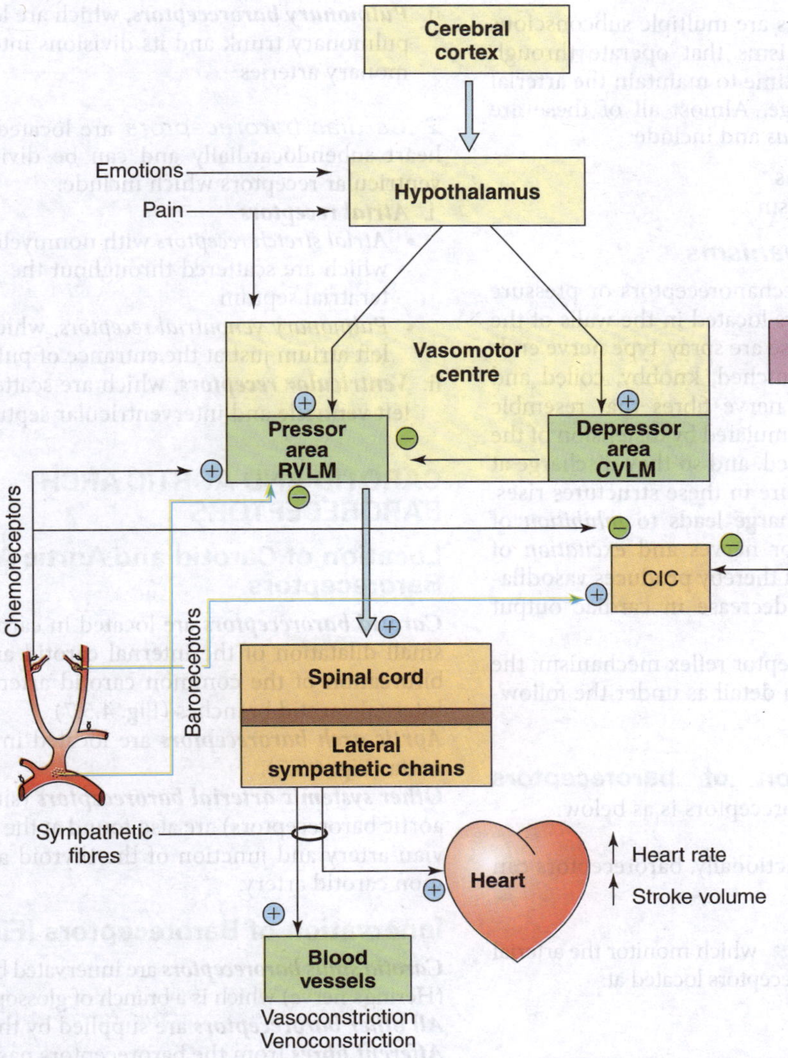

Fig. 4.5.6 Scheme to show afferent impulses affecting medullary cardiovascular control centres.

Reticular Formation

Reticular formation of pons, mesencephalon and diencephalon also influences the vasomotor area, e.g.:

- Pain usually causes rise in blood pressure via afferent impulses in the reticular formation converging on the vasomotor area. However, prolonged severe pain may cause vasodilation and fainting.

(b) Afferent Impulses from Respiratory Centres

Impulses arising from the respiratory centres affect the heart rate by changing the vagal tone and the alterations produced are known as *sinus arrhythmia* which occurs during forced breathing. Sinus arrhythmia is common in some children and in some adults even during quiet breathing.

During inspiration, the impulses arising from the respiratory centres during inspiration inhibit the cardiac vagal centre causing reduced vagal tone and *sinus tachycardia*.

During expiration, the respiratory centres stop sending inhibitory impulses to the cardiac vagal centre causing increased vagal tone and sinus bradycardia.

(c) Cardiovascular Reflex Mechanisms Affecting Medullary Control Centres

Cardiovascular reflex mechanisms are multiple subconscious special nervous control mechanisms that operate through medullary control centres all the time to maintain the arterial pressure within the normal range. Almost all of these are *negative feedback reflex mechanisms* and include:

- Baroreceptor reflex mechanisms
- Chemoreceptor reflex mechanism

Baroreceptor Reflex Mechanisms

Baroreceptors, also known as mechanoreceptors or pressure receptors, are the stretch receptors located in the walls of the heart and large blood vessels. These are spray-type nerve endings, i.e. they are extensively branched, knobby, coiled and intertwined ends of myelinated nerve fibres that resemble Golgi tendon organs. These are stimulated by distension of the structures in which they are located, and so they discharge at an increased rate when the pressure in these structures rises. The increased baroreceptor discharge leads to *inhibition* of tonic discharge of vasoconstrictor nerves and *excitation* of vagal innervation of the heart and thereby produces vasodilation, venodilation, bradycardia, decrease in cardiac output and decrease in blood pressure.

With this definition of baroreceptor reflex mechanism, the baroreceptors will be discussed in detail as under the following headings:

Classification and location of baroreceptors Classification and location of baroreceptors is as below:

Functional classification Functionally, baroreceptors can be grouped as:

1. High-pressure baroreceptors, which monitor the arterial circulation. These include the baroreceptors located at:

- Carotid sinus
- Aortic arch
- Wall of left ventricle
- Root of right subclavian artery
- Junction of the thyroid artery with the common carotid artery

2. Low-pressure baroreceptors are located in the low-pressure area of circulation and are collectively referred to as *cardiopulmonary receptors*. These include:

- Atrial receptors scattered in the wall of right and left atria
- Baroreceptors located in the right atrium at the entrance of the superior and inferior vena cave and in the left atrium at the entrance of pulmonary veins
- Pulmonary receptors located in the wall of pulmonary trunk and its divisions into right and left pulmonary arteries

Anatomical classification Anatomically, baroreceptors can be grouped as:

1. Arterial baroreceptors, which are located in the walls of the arteries, distributed mainly in adventitial layer. These can be further divided into two groups:

i. ***Systemic arterial baroreceptors*** which are located at:
   - Carotid sinus
   - Aortic arch
   - Root of right subclavian artery
   - Junction of thyroid artery and common carotid artery

ii. ***Pulmonary baroreceptors,*** which are located in the wall of pulmonary trunk and its divisions into right and left pulmonary arteries

2. Cardiac baroreceptors are located in the walls of the heart subendocardially and can be divided into atrial and ventricular receptors which include:

i. ***Atrial receptors***
   - *Atrial stretch receptors* with nonmyelinated afferent fibres which are scattered throughout the wall of atria and interatrial septum
   - *Pulmonary venoatrial receptors,* which are located in the left atrium just at the entrance of pulmonary veins

ii. ***Ventricular receptors,*** which are scattered throughout the left ventricle and interventricular septum

CAROTID AND AORTIC ARCH BARORECEPTORS

Location of Carotid and Aortic Arch Baroreceptors

Carotid baroreceptors are located in carotid sinus which is a small dilatation of the internal carotid artery just above the bifurcation of the common carotid artery into external and internal carotid branches (Fig. 4.5.7).

Aortic arch baroreceptors are located in the wall of arch of aorta (Fig. 4.5.7).

Other systemic arterial baroreceptors (similar to carotid and aortic baroreceptors) are also found at the root of right subclavian artery and junction of the thyroid artery and the common carotid artery.

Innervation of Baroreceptors (Fig. 4.5.8)

Carotid sinus baroreceptors are innervated by carotid sinus nerve (Hering's nerve) which is a branch of glossopharyngeal nerve.

All other baroreceptors are supplied by the vagus nerve.

Afferent fibres from the baroreceptors pass via the glossopharyngeal and vagus nerves to the medulla. Most of them end in

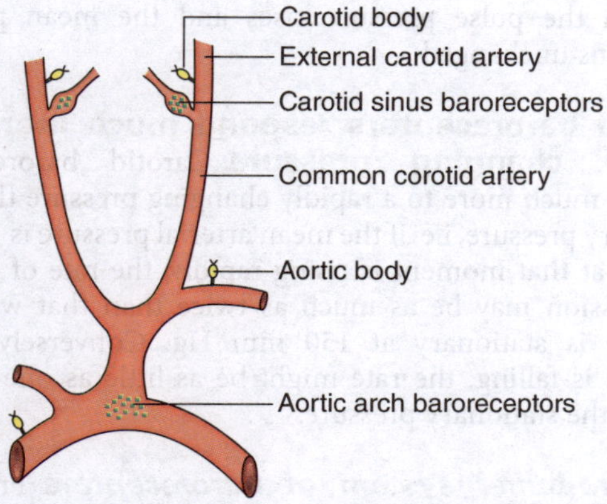

Fig. 4.5.7 Location of baroreceptors (carotid sinus and aortic arch) and chemorecepters (carotid bodies and aortic bodies).

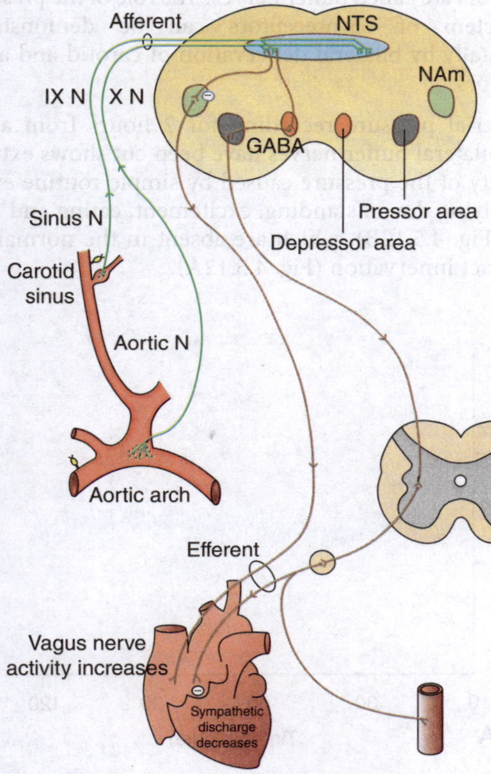

Fig. 4.5.8 Neural pathway of baroreceptor reflex.

the NTS, where they secrete an excitatory transmitter, presumably glutamate.

Buffer nerves: The carotid sinus nerve and vagal fibres from the carotid sinus and aortic arch baroreceptors, respectively, are commonly called buffer nerves, as these are involved in buffering the blood pressure, i.e. preventing sudden rise and fall in blood pressure.

Projections from NTS (excitatory glutaminergic projections) terminate onto the:

Depressor area of VMC (CVLM), where they stimulate Gamma-aminobutyric acid (GABA), secreting inhibitory neurons, which produce decrease in the sympathetic activity by inhibiting the tonically discharging impulses from the pressor area of VMC, and *sympathetic preganglionic neurons* of spinal cord and decrease sympathetic activity

- *Cardiac vagal centre* (nucleus ambiguus), receives the impulses from NTS and *sends inhibitory impulses* along the vagus nerve to the *heart* through cardiac branches of the vagus nerve to decrease heart rate and force of contraction.

Response of Carotid and Aortic Baroreceptors to Pressure

Response from carotid baroreceptors has been studied in detail and that from aortic receptors has not been studied in such great deal. However, there is no reason to believe that responses of aortic receptors differ significantly from those of the carotid receptors. Salient features of these receptor responses to pressure are as follows:

Baroreceptor Response

At normal blood pressure levels, the fibres of the buffer nerves discharge at a low rate which increases when the pressure in the carotid sinus and aortic arch rises, and declines when the pressure falls (Figs 4.5.9 and 4.5.10).

The effect of different arterial pressure levels on the discharge rate The effect of different arterial pressure levels on the discharge rate in carotid sinus nerve shown in Fig. 4.5.10 depicts that:

- From 0 to 50 mm Hg levels of mean arterial pressure, carotid baroreceptors are not stimulated at all. The minimum pressure about 50 mm Hg at which carotid baroreceptors are stimulated is called *threshold of baroreceptor reflex.*
- Above threshold level, the baroreceptors respond progressively more rapidly till the discharge rate reaches a *plateau*, at 180–200 mm Hg, i.e. there is no further increase in response. Thus, the carotid baroreceptors exhibit a great sensitivity as they respond to pressure that varies from approximately 50 to 200 mm Hg.
- In the normal operating rate at 95–100 mm Hg, even a slight change in pressure causes a strong change in the

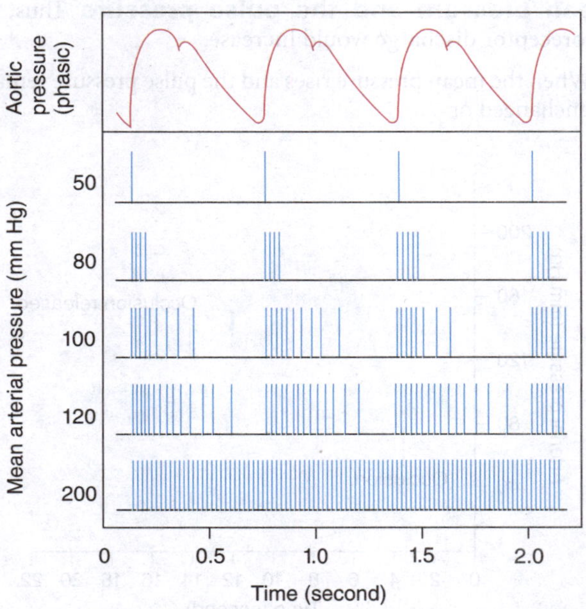

Fig. 4.5.9 Discharges (vertical lines) in a single afferent nerve fibre from carotid sinus at various levels of mean arterial pressure, plotted against changes in aortic pressure with time.

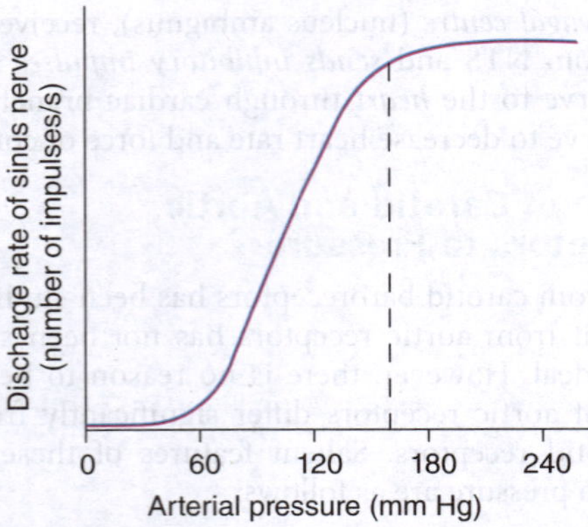

Fig. 4.5.10 Response of carotid baroreceptors at different levels of arterial pressure.

baroreceptor reflex signals to readjust the arterial pressure back towards the normal. Thus, the baroreceptor feedback mechanism functions most effectively in the pressure range where it is most needed.

- When pressure decreases below normal levels, the baroreceptor discharge decreases and reflexly brings the pressure to normal. Conversely, when pressure increases above normal, the baroreceptor discharge also increases and reflexly brings the pressure to normal. The effect of carotid receptors response to change in arterial pressure can be demonstrated experimentally as:
Bilateral occlusion of common carotid arteries at their origin reduces the carotid sinus pressure; as a result, the carotid baroreceptors become inactive and lose their inhibitory effect on the VMC and the blood pressure is raised. Because aortic and cardiac baroreceptors respond to raised pressure, the occlusion of both carotid arteries causes only a moderate pressure response. When the common carotid occlusion is removed, the arterial pressure returns to normal (Fig. 4.5.11).

The carotid baroreceptors respond to both the mean pressure and the pulse pressure Thus, the baroreceptor discharge would increase:

- When the mean pressure rises and the pulse pressure remains unchanged or

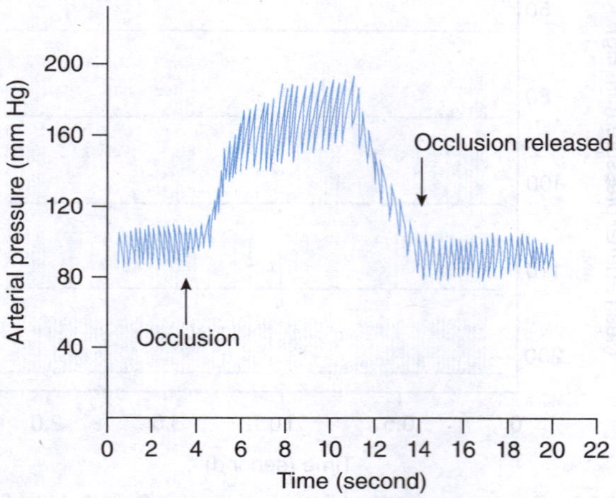

Fig. 4.5.11 Effect of occlusion of both common carotid arteries on arterial pressure in dog.

- When the pulse pressure rises and the mean pressure remains unchanged

Carotid baroreceptors respond much more to a rapidly changing pressure Carotid baroreceptors respond much more to a rapidly changing pressure than to a stationary pressure, i.e. if the mean arterial pressure is 150 mm Hg and at that moment is rising rapidly, the rate of impulse transmission may be as much as twice than that when the pressure is stationary at 150 mm Hg. Conversely, if the pressure is falling, the rate might be as little as one-quarter that for the stationary pressure.

Pressure-buffer system of baroreceptors From the above description, it is clear that baroreceptor system opposes both increase and decrease in arterial pressure. Therefore, it is called a *pressure-buffer system*, and the nerves from the baroreceptors are called buffer nerves. The role of the pressure-buffer system of baroreceptors can be demonstrated experimentally by bilateral denervation of carotid and aortic baroreceptors.

- The arterial pressure recording for 2 hours from a dog whose bilateral buffer nerves have been cut shows extreme variability of the pressure caused by simple routine events such as lying down, standing, excitement, eating and defecation (Fig. 4.5.12B), which are absent in the normal dog with intact innervation (Fig. 4.5.12A).

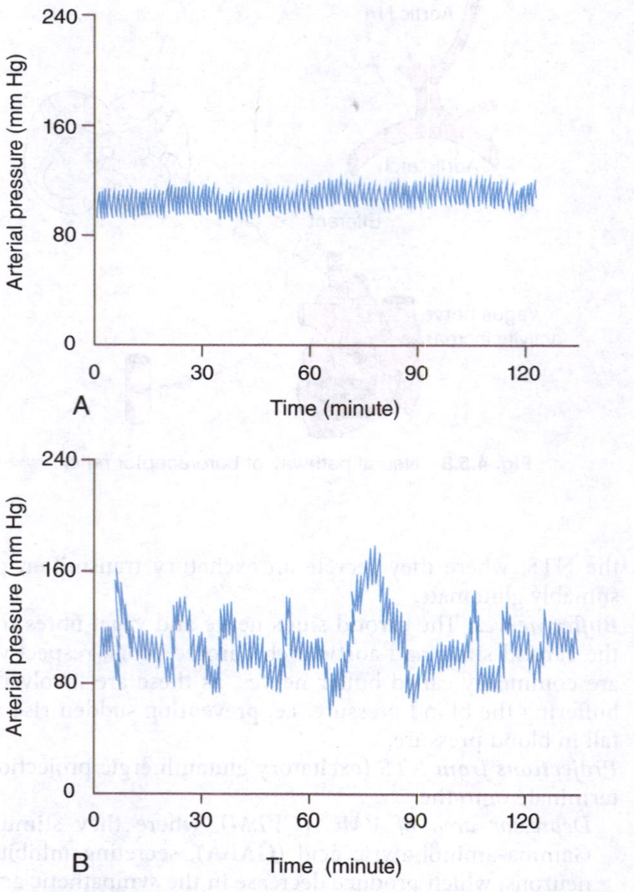

Fig. 4.5.12 **A**, Two-hour record of arterial pressure in a normal dog with intact innervation; and **B**, in same dog after several weeks after denervation of baroreceptors.

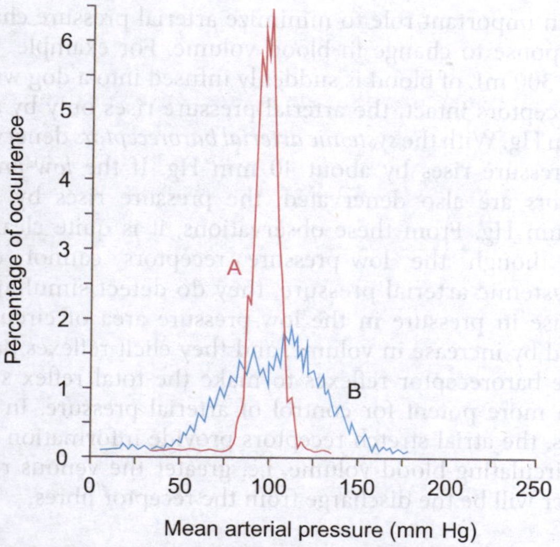

Fig. 4.5.13 Frequency distribution curve of the arterial pressure for 24-hour period: **A**, in a normal dog; and **B**, in the same dog several weeks after denervation of baroreceptors.

- The frequency distribution curve of mean arterial pressure recorded for 24 hours from a normal dog shows that during most of the day with all routine activities, the arterial pressure wave is maintained at 95–105 mm Hg (Fig. 4.5.13A), whereas that from a dog whose baroreceptors have been denervated shows that the arterial pressure varies extremely from 50 to 160 mm Hg (Fig. 4.5.13B).
- From the above experiment, it can be confirmed that baroreceptors serve as *pressure-buffer system* and reduce the minute-by-minute variation in the arterial pressure occurring with daily routine activities.

Baroreceptor resetting Baroreceptors possess a property to reset themselves in 1–2 days to whatever pressure they are exposed. Therefore, in chronic hypertension, the baroreceptor reflex mechanism resets to maintain an elevated rather than a normal arterial pressure. This fact can be demonstrated by perfusion studies on hypertensive experimental animals (Fig. 4.5.14). Little is known about how and why this occurs, but resetting occurs rapidly in experimental animals. It is also rapidly reversible, both in experimental animals and in clinical situations. Because of this property, the *baroreceptor system has no role to play for long-term regulation of the mean arterial pressure*. Thus, the baroreceptor reflex mechanism plays important role only in preventing the extreme variations in blood pressure which occur for a short term and prolonged regulation of mean arterial pressure requires other control system, principally, the *renal–body fluid–pressure control system* along with its associated hormonal mechanisms (see page 320).

Transmission of Baroreceptor Response

Receptor potential The systemic arterial baroreceptors generate a receptor potential in response to pressure-induced distension of the vascular walls. The receptor potential so generated has two components:

- *Dynamic receptor response* is the initial receptor potential, which is proportional to the rate of change in arterial pressure.

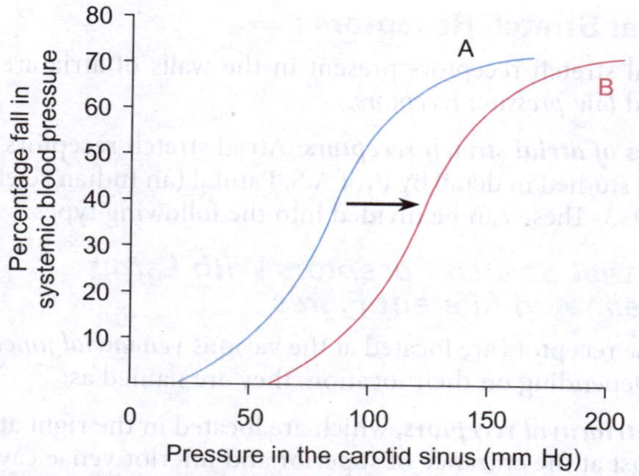

Fig. 4.5.14 Percentage fall in systemic blood pressure produced by raising the pressure in the isolated carotid sinus: **A**, in a normal monkey; and **B**, in a hypertensive monkey. Note the graphs obtained are similar (due to resetting of baroreceptors to raised pressure).

- *Static receptor response* is proportional to the new steady pressure and continues without adaptation as long as the pressure is maintained.

Afferent action potentials Afferent action potentials (APs) are generated by the receptor potentials and are carried over the sinus and aortic nerves in response to increasing arterial blood pressure. The *AP frequency* is linearly related to the increase in arterial pressure over a wide range.

Applied Aspects

Carotid sinus massage is used clinically to interrupt paroxysmal atrial tachycardia by inducing a vagally mediated slowing of the heart.

Stokes–Adams syndrome refers to an increased sensitivity of the carotid sinus seen in some elderly individuals who experience syncope as a result of vagally mediated sinus arrest, which causes a prolonged period of ventricular systole.

Effect of Carotid Clamping and Bilateral Vagotomy

- Bilateral clamping of the carotid arteries proximal to the carotid sinus lowers the pressure in the sinuses which is followed by a decline in discharge rate from the carotid baroreceptors leading to rise in blood pressure and heart rate.
- When along with bilateral occlusion of the common carotid arteries, bilateral vagotomy is also performed, the blood pressure rises to 300/200 mm Hg or higher and is unstable.
- Bilateral destruction of NTS, the site of termination of the baroreceptor afferents, also causes a marked pressure response producing severe hypertension which can be even fatal.
- These forms of experimentally induced hypertension due to neurogenic lesions are called *neurogenic hypertension*.

CARDIAC BARORECEPTORS

Cardiac baroreceptors are located in the walls of the heart subendocardially. All cardiac receptors are innervated by vagus nerve. These include:

- Atrial stretch receptors
- Ventricular receptors

Atrial Stretch Receptors

Atrial stretch receptors present in the walls of atria are also called *low-pressure receptors.*

Types of atrial stretch receptors: Atrial stretch receptors have been studied in detail by Prof A.S. Paintal (an Indian scientist) in 1953. These can be divided into the following types:

1. Atrial Stretch Receptors With Large Myelinated Afferent Fibres

These receptors are located at the various *venoatrial junctions.* Depending on their location, they are named as:

i. ***Atriocaval receptors***, which are located in the right atrium just at the entrance of superior and inferior venae cavae
ii. ***Pulmonary venoatrial receptors***, which are located in the left atrium just at the entrance of pulmonary vein

Depending on the discharge pattern, the atrial stretch receptors with large myelinated afferents fibres are of three types:

i. ***Type A receptors*** discharge during atrial systole only and their impulse activity occurs in the PR interval of the electrocardiogram (Fig. 4.5.15).
ii. ***Type B receptors*** discharge in the later part of atrial diastole when the atria are distended with blood. That is, these receptors discharge just before the onset of atrial contraction and reach peak after T wave of the electrocardiogram (Fig. 4.5.15). Type B receptor discharge increases when the venous return is increased.
iii. ***Intermediate-type receptors*** discharge during both atrial systole and diastole. Therefore, their discharge pattern is characterized by type A receptor discharge followed by type B receptor discharge.

2. Atrial Stretch Receptors with Nonmyelinated Afferent Fibres

These receptors are scattered throughout the atria and the interatrial septum. Their discharge is sparse (1 impulse/sec) and irregular.

Role of atrial stretch receptors The atrial stretch receptors have been associated with the following roles in the cardiovascular control:

1. As low-pressure receptors The atrial stretch receptors (especially type B receptors) along with pulmonary receptors play an important role to minimize arterial pressure changes in response to change in blood volume. For example, when about 300 mL of blood is suddenly infused into a dog with all the receptors intact, the arterial pressure rises only by about 15 mm Hg. With the *systemic arterial baroreceptors* denervated, the pressure rises by about 40 mm Hg. If the *low-pressure receptors* are also denervated, the pressure rises by about 100 mm Hg. From these observations, it is quite clear that even though the low-pressure receptors cannot detect the systemic arterial pressure, they do detect simultaneous increase in pressure in the low-pressure area of circulation caused by increase in volume, and they elicit reflexes parallel to the baroreceptor reflexes to make the total reflex system much more potent for control of arterial pressure. In other words, the atrial stretch receptors provide information about the circulating blood volume, i.e. greater the venous return, greater will be the discharge from the receptor fibres.

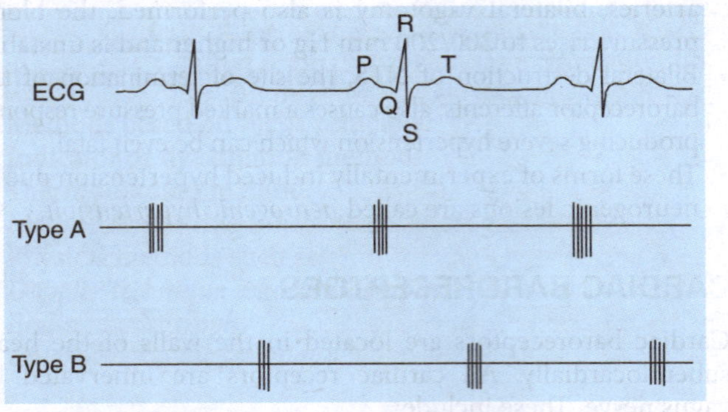

Fig. 4.5.15 Discharge pattern of type **A** and type **B** atrial stretch receptors as recorded from vagus nerve and their correlation with electrocardiogram recording.

2. Atrial reflex control of heart rate (bainbridge reflex) Francis Arthur Bainbridge noted that sudden rise in atrial pressure after rapid infusion of saline or blood (increased venous pressure) in anaesthetized animals produced tachycardia, if the initial heart rate was low. This effect is described as Bainbridge reflex. Atrial stretch receptors of both the sides may be responsible for this reflex. The afferent signals from these receptors pass through the vagus nerves to the medulla of the brain. The efferent signals are transmitted back through both the vagal and the sympathetic nerves to increase the heart rate and force of contraction. Thus, this reflex helps to prevent damming of blood in the veins, atria and pulmonary circulation. This reflex has a different purpose from that of controlling arterial pressure.

3. Atrial reflex control of blood volume (volume reflex) When there is volume overload, the atrial stretch receptors help to return the blood volume back towards normal by the following mechanisms, which collectively are called volume reflex:

Stretch of the atria causes very significant reflex dilatation of the afferent arterioles in the kidney leading to rise in glomerular capillary pressure, with resultant increase in filtration of fluid into the kidney tubules.

Stretch of the atria also transmits signals to the hypothalamus to decrease the secretion of antidiuretic hormone (ADH), which diminishes the reabsorption of water from tubules (see page 523).

The mechanisms (1) and (2) reduce the increased blood volume back towards normal.

Stretch of the atria also causes release of a chemical called *atrial natriuretic peptide* (ANP) which causes powerful diuresis and thus adds still further to the loss of fluid in the urine and return of blood volume back to normal. For details, see page 524.

The above-described mechanisms (1, 2 and 3), which combinedly constitute volume reflex, act as volume controller and thus indirectly act as *pressure controller* as well, because excess volume increases the cardiac output and thus the arterial pressure as well.

Ventricular Receptors

The ventricular baroreceptors are scattered throughout the left ventricle and interventricular septum. They discharge irregularly. These receptors exhibit the following responses:

Response to Increased Left Ventricular Pressure

When the left ventricle is distended in experimental animals, there occurs bradycardia and hypotension. The distension required to produce these effects is so high that no physiological significance can be attached to these receptors. However, left ventricular stretch receptors may play a role in the maintenance of the vagal tone that keeps the heart rate low at rest.

von Bezold–Jarisch reflex or coronary chemoreflex

von Bezold–Jarisch reflex or coronary chemoreflex refers to reflex apnoea followed by rapid breathing, hypotension and bradycardia which occur following injection of certain drugs like capsaicin, phenyl guanide, serotonin, veratridine or nicotine into the coronary arteries supplying the left ventricle (injection into the right coronary artery is ineffective) in experimental animals. This reflex is probably produced by the chemical stimulation of left ventricular stretch receptors. The receptors are probably C fibre endings, and the afferents are vagal. A similar response is produced by stimulation of C fibre endings in the lungs (pulmonary chemoreceptors). The reflex has been named after the person who first reported this response pattern.

Physiological significance of this reflex is uncertain, but it has been speculated that the persistent hypotension in some patients with acute myocardial infarction may be due to stimulation of ventricular receptors by substances released from the necrotic cardiac tissue.

Defence against chemical toxic pollutants and temperature is also provided by activation of cardiopulmonary reflexes.

Vasovagal syncope, i.e. syndrome of cardiac slowing and hypertension, has also been attributed to activation of this reflex.

PULMONARY BARORECEPTORS

Pulmonary baroreceptors are located in the walls of pulmonary trunk and its divisions, the right and left pulmonary arteries. The pulmonary receptors along with atrial receptors constitute the so-called *low-pressure receptors or cardiopulmonary receptors* and play an important role to minimize arterial pressure changes in response to change in blood volume as discussed above (see page 523).

Role of Chemoreceptor Reflexes in Cardiovascular Control

Chemoreceptors are chemosensitive cells that respond to the following changes in blood:

- Oxygen lack (decreased PO_2)
- Carbon dioxide excess (increased pCO_2)
- Hydrogen ion excess (decreased pH)

Location of Chemoreceptor

The peripheral chemoreceptors are present in (Fig. 4.5.7):

1. ***Carotid bodies*** are 1–2 mm in size and are located in the bifurcation of each common carotid artery. These are innervated by carotid sinus nerve which is a branch of glossopharyngeal nerve.
2. ***Aortic bodies*** are one to three in number, located adjacent to arch of aorta. These are innervated by aortic nerve (branch of vagus nerve).

Functions of Chemoreceptors

1. Respiratory control Chemoreceptors are primarily concerned with the regulation of pulmonary ventilation and are discussed in much more detail in Chapter 5.6, page 436.

2. Cardiovascular control In physiological conditions, i.e. in healthy individuals breathing normal air, there is very little discharge from the chemoreceptors and there is no contribution to the regulation of the cardiovascular system. The chemoreceptors exert their role in cardiovascular regulation under the following conditions:

In hypoxia, there occurs increased chemoreceptor discharge, which not only produces hyperventilation but also excites the VMC leading to peripheral vasoconstriction and increase in arterial blood pressure. Thus, unlike the inhibitory action of arterial baroreceptors, the chemoreceptors have an excitatory effect on the VMC.

In hypotension due to severe haemorrhage, the increased chemoreceptor discharge may help to raise the arterial blood pressure. The role of chemoreceptors in severe hypotension can be demonstrated experimentally. Bilateral section of sinus and aortic nerves in animals which have been bled severely to produce hypotension causes further fall in blood pressure. Since in such animals the baroreceptor discharge is already absent, the section of sinus and aortic nerves abolishes the chemoreceptor drive as well. Thus, further fall in blood pressure in such animals indicates that chemoreceptors were contributing to some extent to the maintenance of blood pressure.

Chemoreceptor discharge may contribute to Mayer waves. Mayer waves are observed as slow, regular oscillations in arterial pressure recordings at the rate of about 1/20–40 seconds, during hypotension (produced by haemorrhage in experimental animals). Hypoxia under these conditions stimulates chemoreceptors leading to rise in arterial pressure which improves the blood flow to chemoreceptors and, therefore, there is an elimination of stimulus to the chemoreceptors. The BP again falls and a new cycle of chemoreceptor stimulation gets activated and again rise in pressure occurs (Fig. 4.5.16).

Important Notes

It is important to note that the chemoreceptor reflex is not a powerful arterial pressure controller in the normal arterial pressure range because the chemoreceptors themselves are not stimulated strongly until the arterial pressure falls below 60 mm Hg. Therefore, it is at lower pressures that this reflex becomes important and helps to prevent still further fall in pressure.

Mayer waves should not be confused with Traube–Hering waves, which are fluctuations in blood pressure recordings synchronizing with phases of respiration.

Traube–Hering waves

During inspiration in early phase, due to inflation of lungs, there is vasodilation and fall in blood pressure, but in later part of inspiration, blood volume increases due to increase in end-diastolic volume due to decrease in intrathoracic pressure and rise in intra-abdominal pressure. This response is mediated via vagal afferents from the lungs that inhibit vasomotor discharge. *During expiration*, first there is rise and further fall in blood pressure occurs due to opposite effects (Fig. 4.5.16).

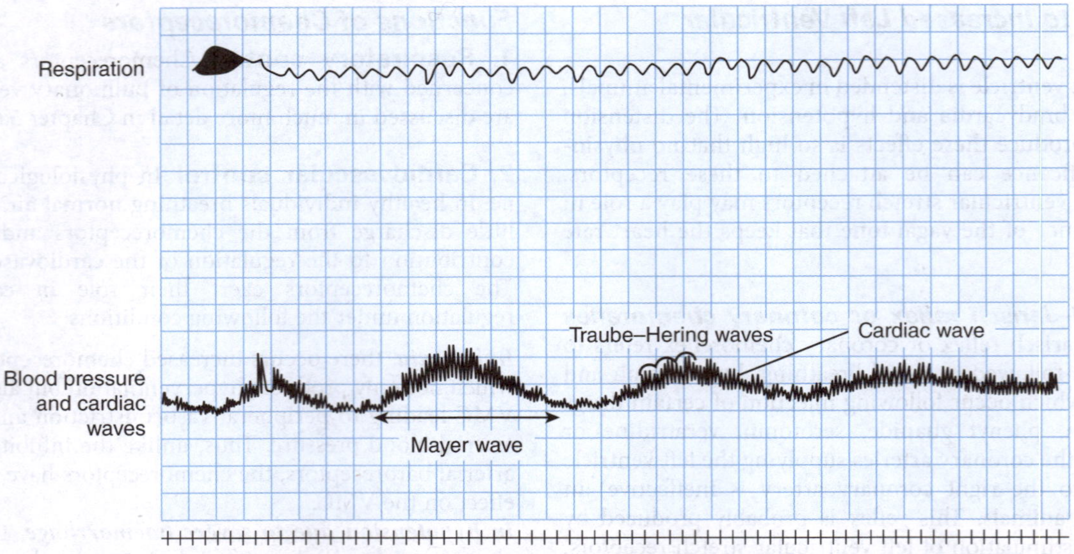

Fig. 4.5.16 Mayer waves recorded on polygraph while observing the effect of haemorrhage in rabbit.

(d) Direct Effects on Vasomotor Area

The VMC is directly affected by locally produced hypoxia and hypercapnia. Examples of DE are central nervous system ischaemic response and Cushing reflex.

1. Central Nervous System Ischaemic Response

- When blood pressure falls below 60 mm Hg, the blood flow to the vasomotor area in the brainstem is decreased enough to cause CNS ischaemia.
- As a result of CNS ischaemia, the CO_2/lactic acid is accumulated locally near the VMC and excites the neurons of VMC strongly.
- Excitation of VMC causes strong sympathetic stimulation leading to vasoconstriction. Peripheral vessels become totally occluded at certain areas, e.g. kidney. There occurs immediate increase in the blood pressure. This most powerful response that activates sympathetic vasoconstrictor system strongly is called *CNS ischaemic response*. This acts as an emergency arterial pressure control system. If rise of pressure does not relieve CNS ischaemia, neural cells begin to suffer and within 3–10 minutes become totally inactive.

2. Cushing Reflex

When intracranial pressure is increased and becomes equal to the arterial pressure, it compresses the arteries in the brain and blood supply to the vasomotor area is compromised. The hypoxia and hypercapnia produced locally increase the discharge from VMC. The resultant rise in systemic pressure tends to restore the blood supply to medulla. This effect, which protects the vital centres in the brain, is called *Cushing reflex*. The resultant increase in blood pressure also causes reflex bradycardia via baroreceptor response. Thus, bradycardia is an important feature of raised intracranial pressure.

Important Note

A rise in arterial pCO_2 activates RVLM, but direct peripheral effect of hypercapnia is vasodilation. The peripheral and direct effects of hypercapnia cancel each other; therefore, there is little change in blood pressure, but exposure to high concentration of CO_2 causes cerebral vasodilation (the effect is mediated via increase in H^+ concentration in the CSF) and vasoconstriction of splanchnic and cutaneous vessels through activation of peripheral chemoreceptors; hence, there is slow rise in blood pressure.

(e) Afferents from Nociceptive Stimuli

Afferents carrying pain sensations also affect VMC and evoke either pressor or depressor reflex effect as:

Pressor effect in the form of increase in the blood pressure and tachycardia is caused due to sympathetic activity by *somatic pain afferents*, i.e. unmyelinated C fibres which stimulate the pressor area of VMC (RVLM).

Depressor effect in the form of hypotension and bradycardia is produced by *visceral pain afferents*, i.e. thin myelinated fibres which synapse with depressor area of VMC (CVLM) and cause inhibition of sympathetic activity.

D. ROLE OF SKELETAL NERVES AND MUSCLES IN CONTROLLING BLOOD PRESSURE

Although ANS plays the main role in control of circulation, the skeletal muscles and nerves also contribute as:

1. Abdominal Compression Reflex

Whenever VMC is stimulated, e.g. by baroreceptor reflex or chemoreceptor reflex, other areas of reticular formation of brainstem are also stimulated along with. They send simultaneous impulses through skeletal nerves to skeletal muscles of the body, especially abdominal muscles. The contraction of abdominal muscles compresses the abdominal venous reservoirs increasing the venous return to the heart and thereby the cardiac output. This response as a whole is called abdominal compression reflex.

2. Role of Skeletal Muscles During Exercise

During exercise, the skeletal muscles, especially those of limbs, contract and compress the venous reservoirs.

This causes translocation of large quantities of blood from the peripheral vessels into the heart and lungs. This increases the cardiac output.

HUMORAL CONTROL MECHANISMS

Humoral regulation of circulation refers to the regulation by substances secreted into or absorbed into body fluids, e.g. hormones and ions. Most important humoral factors affecting circulation are as follows:

1. Circulating vasodilators
2. Circulating vasoconstrictors
3. Ions and other chemical factors

CIRCULATING VASODILATORS

The circulating vasodilators include kinins, VIP (see page 617) and ANP (see pages 524 and 777).

Kinins

Kinins are peptides which cause vasodilation. Two forms of kinins with similar action found are as follows:

Bradykinin is nonapeptide found in the plasma.

Lysyl-bradykinin or kallidin is a decapeptide found in body tissues.

Synthesis and Secretion

- The kinins are formed from high-molecular-weight kininogen (HMWK) and low-molecular-weight kininogen (LMWK) by the action of plasma and tissue kallikreins:

$$\text{HMWK} \xrightarrow{\text{Plasma kallikrein}} \text{Bradykinin}$$
$$\text{LMWK} \xrightarrow{\text{Plasma Kallikrein}} \text{Lysyl-bradykinin}$$

- Lysyl-bradykinin can be converted to bradykinin by aminopeptidase.

$$\text{Lysyl-bradykinin} \xrightarrow{\text{Aminopeptidase}} \text{Bradykinin}$$

- Kinins are metabolized to inactive fragments by the enzymes kininase I and II and angiotensin-converting enzyme (ACE).

$$\text{Kinins} \xrightarrow[\text{ACE}]{\text{Kinase I and II}} \text{Inactive peptides}$$

- Kinin release is inhibited by glucocorticoids.

Note: Kininase II is the same enzyme as ACE, which removes histidine and leucine from the terminal carboxyl end of angiotensin I.

Functions of Kinins

- They cause *vasodilation* by relaxing vascular smooth muscle (VSM) via nitric oxide (NO) and increase *capillary permeability*.
- Kinins play role in regulating blood flow especially to the skin, salivary glands and GIT glands. Therefore, they are formed during active secretion in sweat glands and salivary glands, and in exocrine portion of the pancreas.
- By regulating blood flow to the skin, the kinins probably play a role in thermoregulatory vascular adjustments.
- Kinins appear to be responsible for some episodes of vasodilation in patients with carcinoid tumours.
- Kinins are responsible for inflammation because of their following actions:
  - *Increase in vascular permeability*, especially of venules and capillaries, leading to escape of plasma proteins into tissues
- *Excitation of sensory nerve endings and production* of pain (which is enhanced by 5-HT)
  - Attraction and migration of leucocytes from blood to tissues
- Kinins cause contraction of visceral smooth muscles of the ileum, uterus and bronchioles (leading to bronchoconstriction in patients with asthma).

Mechanism of Action

The actions of kinins are mainly paracrine and quite similar to those of histamine. Kinins act through their receptors. Two types of bradykinin receptors have been identified (B_1 and B_2); both types of receptors are coupled with G protein. The B_1 receptors mediate pain-producing effect of kinins, and the B_2 receptors have homology to histamine (H_2) receptors.

CIRCULATING VASOCONSTRICTORS

The circulating vasoconstrictors include catecholamines, angiotensin II and vasopressin.

Catecholamines

Catecholamines are released on sympathetic stimulation and include epinephrine and norepinephrine. The effects of epinephrine and norepinephrine are brought about by action on α- and β-adrenergic receptors, which are further subdivided into α_1 and α_2 subtypes and β_1, β_2 and β_3 subtypes, respectively.

Epinephrine It stimulates both α- and β-adrenergic receptors:

- *Stimulation of α-receptors* results in vasoconstriction in the skin and splanchnic areas.
- *Stimulation of β-receptors* results in dilation of the vessels in the skeletal muscles, liver and coronary arteries.
- The β-receptor-induced vasodilation is more dominant than α-receptor-induced vasoconstriction. So, the net effect is slight lowering of peripheral resistance producing slight fall in diastolic blood pressure.
- The β-receptor-induced increase in stroke volume and heart rate results in higher cardiac output, a rise in systolic blood pressure and widening of pulse pressure.

Norepinephrine Norepinephrine has a generalized vasoconstrictor action as it has much greater effect on α- than on β-receptors.

- Therefore, it increases peripheral resistance and raises the diastolic blood pressure.
- Since it has negligible effect on β-receptors, direct cardiac stimulation is insignificant. Rather, there occurs reflex cardiac inhibition due to the rise in diastolic blood pressure.

Renin–Angiotensin System

The renin–angiotensin system has important roles in the regulation of blood pressure and in the regulation of extracellular fluid volume.

Renin Secretion and Angiotensin Formation

- *Renin*, a protease enzyme, is secreted by *juxtaglomerular cells* of the kidney into the blood. Its secretion is stimulated by a decrease in the blood pressure.
- Renin catalyses the conversion of *angiotensinogen* (α_2-globulin substrate present in the plasma) to angiotensin I.
- *Angiotensin I* is converted into angiotensin II by the action of ACE present in the endothelium of blood vessels throughout the body, especially in the lungs and kidneys.
- *Angiotensin II* persists in the blood until it is rapidly inactivated by multiple blood and tissue enzymes collectively called *angiotensinases*.

$$\text{Angiotensinogen} \xrightarrow{\text{Renin}} \text{Angiotensin I}$$
$$\text{Angiotensin I} \xrightarrow{\text{ACE}} \text{Angiotensin II}$$

Effects of Angiotensin II

Angiotensin II has three principal effects by which it can elevate the arterial pressure:

1. Vasoconstriction Angiotensin II is the most potent pressor substance, being four to eight times more potent than norepinephrine. By producing generalized vasoconstriction of arterioles and veins throughout the body, it raises both systolic and diastolic pressure. This effect of angiotensin II is important in intermediate blood pressure control during circumstances such as acute haemorrhage.

Mechanism: For vasoconstrictor effect, angiotensin II binds to the receptors and activates G protein, which further activates phospholipase C and increases Ip_3 and formation of diacylglycerol (DAG) resulting in increased influx of Ca^{2+} leading to vasoconstriction.

2. Decrease in salt and water excretion by kidney This action slowly increases extracellular fluid volume, which increases arterial pressure over a period of hours and days. Thus, this effect of angiotensin II plays important role in the long-term control of arterial pressure.

Angiotensin II causes salt and water retention by the kidney in two ways:

By direct actions on the kidneys:

- Angiotensin II constricts the efferent arterioles, which diminishes blood flow through the peritubular capillaries, allowing rapid osmotic reabsorption from the tubules.
- Angiotension II directly stimulates the epithelial cells of renal tubules to increase reabsorption of sodium and water.

By stimulating secretion of aldosterone: Angiotensin II stimulates the adrenal glands to secrete aldosterone which in turn increases salt and water reabsorption by the epithelial cells of the renal tubules.

3. Stimulation of thirst Angiotensin II is a powerful stimulator of thirst. It leads to consumption of large volumes of water, leading to a rise in blood volume. This mechanism also plays some role in long-term control of blood pressure.

Other functions of angiotensin II on CVS Angiotensin II has a significant role as a growth factor in the heart and blood vessels. Therefore, use of ACE inhibitors and angiotensin receptor antagonists (losartan) is recommended for treatment of heart failure, as these drugs inhibit growth effects of angiotensin II.

Vasopressin

Vasopressin or ADH is a powerful vasoconstrictor, but it is secreted in minute quantities and therefore mainly affects water reabsorption in renal tubules. However, after a severe haemorrhage, its concentration rises to a high level and then it has vasoconstrictor effect. Its role in blood pressure regulation is discussed on page 524.

Urotensin II

Urotensin II is a potent vasoconstrictor present in cardiac and vascular tissue. It is a polypeptide first isolated from the spinal cord of fish.

Applied Aspects

In patients with hypertension and heart failure, the levels of urotensin II and its receptors have been shown to be elevated, therefore may be the markers of the disease.

Ions and Other Chemical Factors

The increased concentration of many different ions and chemical factors can also alter local blood flow by causing vasodilation or vasoconstriction.

- Calcium ions cause vasoconstriction.
- Potassium ions cause vasodilatation.
- Hydrogen ions (decreased pH) cause vasodilation.
- Carbon dioxide causes vasodilation in most tissues and marked vasodilation in the brain.
- Glucose or other vasoactive substances, when increased in quantities, raise the osmolarity of blood and cause vasodilation.

LOCAL CONTROL MECHANISMS

NEED OF LOCAL CONTROL MECHANISMS

Local cardiovascular control mechanisms are primarily concerned with the control of blood flow to the tissues locally. The ability of the tissues to regulate their own blood flow locally serves many *functions*; a few examples are as follows:

1. Local control of blood flow permits the tissues to maintain adequate nutrition and perform necessary functions in maintaining homeostasis. In general, the blood flow to the tissues is related to rate of metabolism of the organ; greater the rate of metabolism, greater is the blood flow.
2. These mechanisms help in temporarily curtailing blood flow to some organs so as to divert more blood to a metabolically active organ.
3. Control of blood flow to the skin helps in control of body temperature.
4. Control of blood flow to the kidney allows them to rapidly excrete the waste products of the body.

CLASSIFICATION OF LOCAL CONTROL MECHANISMS

A. ***Mechanisms involved in acute control of blood flow:***
   1. General mechanisms
   2. Special mechanisms

B. ***Mechanisms involved in long-term blood flow regulation***

Mechanisms Involved in Acute Control of Blood Flow

Acute control occurs within seconds to minutes through constriction or dilation of arterioles, meta-arterioles and precapillary sphincters. The mechanisms involved in acute control of blood flow include the following:

I. General Mechanisms

These are the mechanisms that are present in most tissues of the body and are as follows:

1. Autoregulation, i.e. control of flow during changes in arterial pressure
2. Role of local vasodilator metabolites and factors
3. Role of local vasoconstrictors
4. Role of substances secreted by endothelial cells

1. Autoregulation (control of flow during changes in arterial pressure) Autoregulation is the ability of an organ or tissue to adjust its vascular resistance and maintain a relatively constant blood flow over a wide range of arterial pressure. For details, see page 306.

2. Role of local vasodilator metabolites The accumulation of local vasodilator metabolites increases local blood flow. The greater the rate of metabolism in the tissue, the greater is the rate of production of tissue metabolites.

Metabolic changes that produce vasodilation are as follows:

Decrease in O_2 tension and pH causes vasodilation in most tissues. These changes cause relaxation of the arterioles and precapillary sphincters. Decrease in O_2 tension occurs either due to decreased O_2 availability such as high altitude and in pneumonia or due to increased O_2 demand during increased tissue activity.

A local fall in pO_2 produces a hypoxia-inducible factor-1α (HIF-1α) that causes expression of a vasodilatory gene.

Increase in pCO_2 and osmolality also dilates the vessels. The direct dilation action of CO_2 is most pronounced in the skin and brain.

Rise in temperature exerts a direct vasodilator effect, and the temperature rise in active tissues (due to the heat of metabolism) may contribute to vasodilation.

Potassium (K^+) and lactate ions are other substances that accumulate locally and play role in vasodilation, especially in skeletal muscles. The vasodilation effect of K^+ is produced by hyperpolarization of VSMs.

Histamine released from damaged cells in injured tissues increases capillary permeability.

Adenosine may play a vasodilator role in cardiac muscles but not in skeletal muscles. It also inhibits the release of norepinephrine.

Active hyperaemia Active hyperaemia refers to the vasodilation which occurs when the tissue metabolic rate increases. The dilation of local blood vessels helps the tissues to receive the additional nutrients required to sustain its new level.

Metabolic theory of autoregulation Metabolic theory of autoregulation states that any vasodilator metabolites which accumulate in the tissues during active metabolism will produce autoregulation. When blood flow decreases, they accumulate and the vessels dilate; when blood flow increases, they are washed away.

Reactive hyperaemia Reactive hyperaemia is a phenomenon by which the local blood flow to the organ is controlled after a period of ischaemia (also see page 307). This phenomenon also appears to be a manifestation of local metabolic blood flow regulation mechanisms. After vascular occlusion, there occurs accumulation of tissue vasodilator metabolites and the development of oxygen deficiency in the tissues. The extra blood flow during reactive hyperaemia lasts long enough to almost exactly repay the tissue oxygen deficiency and to wash out accumulated vasodilator metabolites.

3. Role of local vasoconstrictors is as:

Serotonin released from platelets in the injured tissue is responsible in part for the vasoconstriction which occurs in haemostasis.

Decrease in tissue temperature causes vasoconstriction, and this local response to cold plays a part in temperature regulation (see page 316).

4. Role of substances released by endothelium Vascular endothelial cells make up a large and important organ. These cells secrete many growth factors and vasoactive substances which play important role in the local control of blood flow. The vasoactive substances include:

- Prostaglandins and thromboxane A_2
- Endothelium-derived relaxing factor (EDRF)
- Endothelins (ETs)

i. Prostaglandins and thromboxane A_2

Prostacyclin is prostaglandin produced by endothelial cells from arachidonic acid via cyclooxygenase pathway. It inhibits platelet aggregation and promotes vasodilation.

Thromboxane A_2 is produced by platelets also from arachidonic acid. It promotes platelet aggregation and vasoconstriction.

Balance between prostacyclin and thromboxane A_2 fosters localized platelet aggregation and consequent clot formation while preventing excessive extension of clot and maintaining blood flow around it.

Important Note

The prostacyclin–thromboxane A_2 balance can be shifted towards prostacyclin by administering low doses of aspirin. Aspirin produces irreversible inhibition of cyclooxygenase. Obviously, this reduces production of both prostacyclin and thromboxane A_2. However, endothelial cells produce new cyclooxygenase in a matter of hours, whereas platelets cannot manufacture the enzyme, and the level rises only as new platelets enter the circulation. This is slow process because platelets have a half-life of about 4 days. Therefore, administration of small amounts of aspirin for prolonged periods reduces clot formation and has been shown to be of value in preventing myocardial infarction, unstable angina, transient ischaemic attacks and stroke.

ii. Endothelium-derived relaxing factor EDRF is the name given to a substance which is released by vascular endothelial cells and produces vasodilation. Later on, it was identified to be *NO* in chemical structure.

Synthesis of NO It is synthesized from arginine (Fig. 4.5.17) in a reaction catalysed by *nitric oxide synthase (NOS).* NOS is a very complex enzyme, using cofactors like NADPH, FAD, FMN and tetrahydrobiopterin. Three isoforms of NOS have been identified:

- NOS-1 is found in the nervous tissue.
- NOS-2 is found in macrophages and other immune cells.
- NOS-3 is found in endothelial cells.

NOS-1 and NOS-3 are activated by agents that increase intracellular Ca^{2+} concentration, including the vasodilators acetylcholine and bradykinin, whereas NOS-2 is activated by cytokinase.

Inactivation of NO NO has a very short life (3–5 seconds), as it is highly reactive. It is inactivated by haemoglobin. NO and its products are inactivated through oxidation into nitrite (NO_2^-) and nitrate (NO_3^-) which are excreted in urine. The plasma and urine concentration of NO_3^- and cyclic GMP (cGMP) are useful indicators for NO production rate.

Mechanism of vasodilation by NO The NO that is synthesized in the endothelium diffuses to smooth muscle cells, where it activates soluble guanylyl cyclase, producing cGMP (Fig. 4.5.17), which in turn mediates the relaxation of VSM by decreasing intracellular Ca^{2+} concentration.

Functions of NO It has been recognized by direct and indirect evidence that NO performs many functions in the body which include:

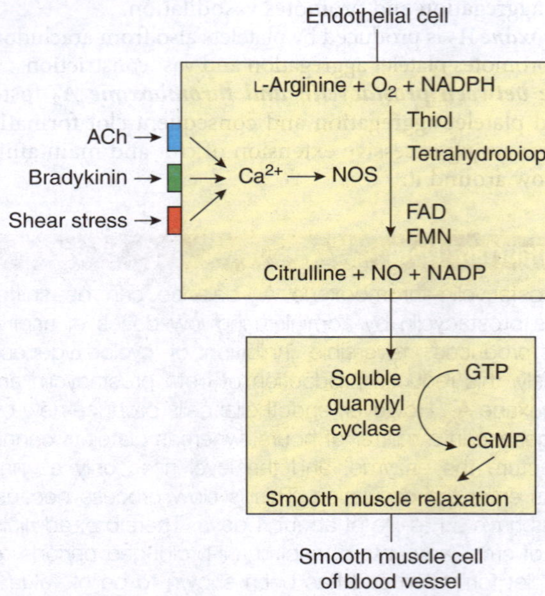

Fig. 4.5.17 Synthesis and mechanism of action of endothelium-derived relaxing factor (EDRF).

1. Relaxation of VSM produced by NO. It serves various functions in different circumstances:

Flow-induced vasodilation is thought to occur due to local release of NO. When flow to a tissue is suddenly increased by arteriolar dilation, the large arteries to the tissue also dilate.

- *Poststenotic vasodilation* is an example of flow-induced vasodilation. Any narrowing of arterial vessels increases the local blood flow velocity which stimulates NO release and results in poststenotic vasodilation.
- *Vasodilation during physical exercise* is also supposed to be flow induced. It is evidenced by an increase in urinary NO_3^- and cGMP excretion rates after submaximal exercise in healthy subjects. Exercise-induced NO release may explain the beneficial effects of endurance training on the cardiovascular system.

Tonic release of NO under basal physiological conditions is necessary to maintain normal blood pressure. This is evidenced by the observation that when various derivatives of arginine that inhibit NOS are administered to experimental animals, there is prompt rise in blood pressure. Nitroglycerin and other nitrovasodilators that are of great value in the treatment of angina act by stimulating guanylyl cyclase in the same manner as NO does.

Penile erection which is consequent to vasodilation and engorgement of corpora cavernosa is also thought to be produced by release of NO. The drug *sildenafil* (Viagra), a selective inhibitor of GMP-specific phosphodiesterase, acts by inhibiting the inactivation of NO.

Modulation of effect of vasoconstrictor and vasodilator substances. Adenosine, ANP and histamine via H_2 receptors produce relaxation of VSM that is independent of endothelium. However, acetylcholine, bradykinin, VIP, substance P and some other polypeptides act via the endothelium. Various vasoconstrictors that act directly on VSM would produce much greater constriction if they did not simultaneously cause the release of NO. Conversely, the vasodilators that have direct actions of VSM produce greater vasodilation by triggering the simultaneous release of NO.

Many of these substances are products of platelet aggregation and cause release of NO, and thus resulting vasodilation helps to keep blood vessels patent with an intact endothelium. This is in contrast to injured blood vessels, where the endothelium is damaged at the site of injury and platelets therefore aggregate and produce vasoconstriction. NO interferes with the secretion and action of ET, a potent vasoconstrictor. There seems to be a balance between endothelium-derived vasoconstrictor and vasodilators.

2. Inhibition of platelet adhesion and aggregation caused by NO is somewhat complementary to its vasodilator effect, both of which are extremely important for the maintenance of normal blood flow.

3. Antiatherosclerotic effect: NO decreases LDL oxygenation and inhibits superoxide anion (O_2^-) production by inhibiting NADPH reductase activity. These actions are related to the strong antiatherosclerotic effect exerted by NO.

4. Role of NO in vascular remodelling and angiogenesis is also suggested. NO may also be involved in pathogenesis of atherosclerosis. It is interesting in this regard that some patients with heart transplants develop an accelerated form of atherosclerosis in the vessels of the transplant, and there is reason to believe that this is triggered by endothelial damage.

5. NO plays role in cytotoxic activity of macrophages, including their ability to kill cancer cells.

6. NO acts as a mediator of inflammatory response; therefore, its production is increased in inflammatory disease. NO inhibits leucocyte adhesion and migration.

7. In GIT, NO produces smooth muscle relaxation.

iii. Endothelins ETs are family of three similar polypeptides: ET-1, ET-2 and ET-3. ET-1 produced by endothelial cells is one of the most potent vasoconstrictor agents yet isolated. The structure of ET is similar to that of polypeptide sarafotoxin, found in venom of a type of snake.

Synthesis and secretion In endothelial cells, the product of ET-1 gene is processed to a 39–amino acid prohormone, called *big ET-1*, which is cleaved to form ET-1 by ET-converting enzyme. Small amounts of big ET-1 and ET-1 are secreted into the blood, but most of the ET-1 is secreted into the tunica media of the blood vessels and acts in a paracrine fashion.

Factors affecting endothelin-1 secretion *Stimulators* of ET-1 secretion are angiotensin II, catecholamines, growth factors, hypoxia, insulin, oxidized LDL, HDL, shear stress and thrombin. *Inhibitors* of ET-1 secretion include NO, ANP, PGE and prostacyclin.

Mechanism of action ET-1 exerts its vasoconstrictor effect through the ET_A receptor which is found predominantly on VSM. ET_B receptor is found on endothelial cells and responds to all the three ET (ET-1, ET-2 and ET-3). When activated, ET_B receptor stimulates release of NO and thus favours vasodilation.

Biological actions of endothelins Biological actions of ETs include the following:

Effect on cardiovascular system: ET-1 is primarily a local paracrine regulator of vascular tone. Veins are possibly more sensitive than arteries.

- ETs increase the heart rate and force of contraction of myocardium.
- ETs play a role in closing the ductus arteriosus at birth.

Effect on central nervous system: In the brain, ETs play a role in regulating transport across the blood–brain barrier and across the synapses.
Effect on kidneys: In the renal glomerulus, ET causes contraction of mesangial cells, decreases glomerular filtration rate (GFR) and renal blood flow, and regulates Na^+ reabsorption.
Effect on endocrines: ETs increase plasma levels of renin, aldosterone, catecholamines and ANP.
Effect on lungs: ETs produce bronchospasm.
Effect on GIT: ETs enhance glucogenesis and regulate gastrointestinal blood flow. Megacolon (Hirschsprung disease) occurs when cells that form myenteric plexus fail to migrate to the distal colon; it has also been associated with ET-1 gene.

Promitogenic effects: ET also induces mitogenesis and thus stimulates cell growth in numerous cell lines. The gasotransmitters such as carbon monoxide, hydrogen sulphide and NO present in cardiovascular tissue also regulate vascular tone, but their relative role is yet to be established.

II. Special Mechanisms

In addition to the above-described general mechanisms, there are special mechanisms that control blood flow in special areas. These are discussed in relation to specific organs, but the following two are notable mechanisms:

1. Tubuloglomerular feedback mechanism in kidneys In the kidneys, blood flow control is vested, in part, in a mechanism called *tubuloglomerular feedback*, in which the composition of fluid in the early distal tubule is detected by the macula densa, which is located where the tubule abuts the afferent and efferent arterioles at the juxtaglomerular apparatus. When too much fluid filters from the blood through the glomerulus into the tubular system, feedback signals from the macula densa cause constriction of the afferent arterioles, thereby reducing renal blood flow and GFR back towards normal (see page 478 for further details).

2. Role of concentration of CO_2 and hydrogen controlling blood flow to brain In the brain, the concentrations of CO_2 and H^+ play prominent roles in local blood flow control. An increase in CO_2 and H^+ dilates the cerebral blood vessels, which allows rapid washout of the excess CO_2 and H^+ ions.

Long-Term Blood Flow Regulation

The long-term blood flow regulation develops over a period of days to months to match the metabolic needs of the tissues. It is required by:

- Ischaemic tissues
- Tissues that are growing rapidly
- Tissues that become chronically hyperactive

The long-term blood flow regulation is brought by an increase in the physiological size of the vessels in a tissue, and in certain circumstances even by an increase in the number of blood vessels. One of the major factors that stimulate the increased vascularity of the tissues is a low oxygen concentration. The growth of the new vessels is called angiogenesis.

Angiogenic factors

These are the substances which are responsible for angiogenesis. Three of the best characterized angiogenic factors which have been isolated from tumours or from other tissues that are rapidly growing or have inadequate blood supply are as follows:

- Vascular endothelial growth factor (VEGF)
- Fibroblast growth factor (FGF)
- Angiogenin

Mechanism of Angiogenesis

Essentially all of the angiogenic factors promote new vessel growth by causing the vessels to sprout from small venules or, occasionally, from capillaries. The basement membrane of endothelial cells is dissolved, followed by the rapid production of new endothelial cells that stream out of the vessel in extended cords directed towards the source of angiogenic factor. The cells continue to divide and eventually fold over into a tube. The tube then connects with another tube budding from another donor vessel and forms a capillary loop through which blood begins to flow. If the flow is sufficiently great, smooth muscle cells eventually invade the wall so that some of these vessels grow to be small arterioles and venules, or perhaps even larger vessels.

Development of Collateral Blood Vessels

Collateral blood vessels refer to those new vessels which develop around a blocked artery or vein and allow the affected tissue to be at least partially resupplied with blood. An important example is the development of collateral blood vessels after thrombosis of one of the coronary arteries in old people.

Self-Assessment

1. Discuss the role of baroreceptors in cardiovascular regulation.
2. Discuss the role of endothelium in regulation of blood flow.
3. Describe:
   - Role of atrial stretch receptors in cardiovascular regulation.
   - Role of local vasodilators and vasoconstrictors in acute control of blood flow.
4. Write notes on:
   - Atrial stretch reflex
   - Pressure buffer system
   - Central nervous system ischaemic response
   - Reactive hyperaemia
   - Mode of action of renin–angiotensin system
   - Angiogenesis
   - Significance of Mayer waves

Clinical Cases

Case 1

A 45-year-old male patient complains of erectile dysfunction, for which the doctor prescribed the drug sildenafil. During follow-up visit, he mentioned improvement in erection.

Q1. What is the mechanism of action of the drug in improving erectile dysfunction?

Case 2

In a postgraduate seminar, the resident who was presenting the topic is feeling uncomfortable, and having palpitation, weakness, dizziness and chest pain. The chairperson (physician) immediately gave him carotid sinus massage and symptoms got relieved.

Q1. What is the mechanism underlying the relief of symptoms?

Q2. What is the probable diagnosis?

Q3. What are the further tests required to rule out myocardial ischaemia?

Case 3

A well-dressed executive visited the cardiologist with complaints of repeated episodes of loss of consciousness for brief period. The doctor advised for ECG recording by Holter monitoring. ECG findings did not reveal any AV block or any other heart disease. The probable diagnosis made was Stokes–Adams syndrome.

Q1. What is the probable cause of this condition?

Regional Circulation 4.6

CHAPTER OUTLINE

INTRODUCTION

After discussing the 'dynamics of circulation' and 'cardiovascular regulation mechanisms', it will be worthwhile to know how these basic principles apply to circulation in various regions of the body. This chapter includes:

- Coronary circulation
- Cerebral circulation
- Cutaneous circulation
- Skeletal muscle circulation
- Splanchnic circulation

Circulation to other regions, such as pulmonary circulation, renal circulation and fetal circulation, has been described in the concerned sections.

CORONARY CIRCULATION

CORONARY BLOOD VESSELS

Coronary Arteries

Two coronary arteries (right and left) arise from the root of ascending aorta and supply blood to the myocardium.

Right coronary artery (RCA) supplies blood to the right ventricle, right atrium, the posterior part of left ventricle, posterior part of interventricular septum and major portion of the conducting system of heart including SA node.

Left coronary artery (LCA) thus supplies blood mainly to the anterior part of left ventricle, left atrium, anterior part of the interventricular septum and a part of the left branch of bundle of His.

Predominant supply by RCA described above is seen in approximately 50% of individuals. In 20% of individuals, the predominant supply to m0yocardium is by LCA. In 30% of individuals, it is the balanced supply, i.e. equal supply by the two arteries.

Major Coronary Arteries

These (i.e. RCA and its main branch – posterior interventricular branch; and LCA and its main branches – the circumflex artery and anterior interventricular artery) travel in the epicardium of the heart and are superficial vessels (Fig. 4.6.1) which divide and subdivide, sending *penetrating branches* through the myocardium. The penetrating branches subdivide into arcades that distribute blood to the myocardium.

End Arteries

Normally, the coronary arteries appear to function as *end arteries*. However, the presence of an arterial plaque or occlusion allows the *anastomoses* present between vessels to become functional. These anastomoses are of two types.

Cardiac anastomoses These are present between branches of two coronary arteries and between the branches of coronary artery and deep venous system.

Extracardiac anastomoses These include those present between the branches of coronary arteries and vessels lying near the heart such as vasa vasorum of aorta, vasa vasorum of pulmonary arteries, intrathoracic arteries, bronchial arteries and phrenic arteries.

Coronary Veins

Coronary Sinus

It is a wide vein, approximately 2-cm long, which drains most of the venous blood from the myocardium (mainly left ventricle) into the right atrium. Its tributaries are the *great cardiac vein*, the *small cardiac vein*, the *posterior vein of left ventricle* and the *oblique vein of left ventricle* (Fig. 4.6.2).

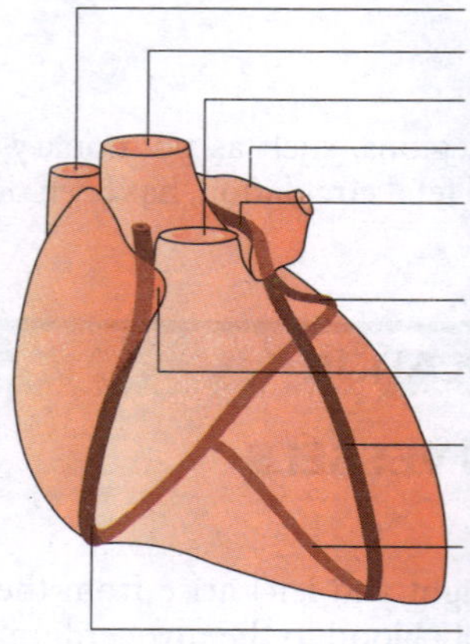

Fig. 4.6.1 Major coronary arteries and their branches.

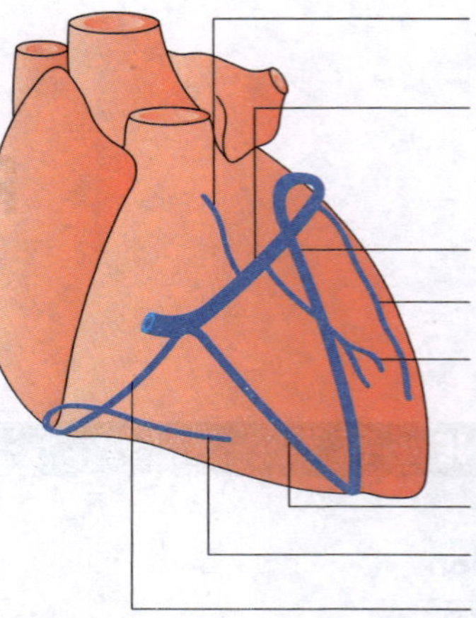

Fig. 4.6.2 Coronary sinus and its tributaries.

Anterior Cardiac Vein

It drains venous blood mainly from the right ventricle and opens directly into the right atrium.

Thebesian Veins

Thebesian veins and *coronary-luminal vessels* (connections between the coronary vessels and the lumen of heart) constitute the deep venous system. These vessels drain only less than 10% of the venous blood from myocardium directly into the various cardiac chambers, contributing to an *anatomic shunt effect*. The coronary luminal connections carry a larger proportion of the flow in the right ventricle than in the left ventricle.

CORONARY BLOOD FLOW: CHARACTERISTIC FEATURES

Normal Coronary Blood Flow and Oxygen Demand

A continuous flow of blood to the heart is essential to maintain an adequate supply of O_2 and nutrients.

Normal coronary blood flow (CBF) at rest is approximately 250 mL (70 mL/100 g tissue/min), i.e. approximately 5% of the resting cardiac output (5 L). Three- to sixfold increase in the CBF may occur during exercise. Blood flow to the left ventricle (80 mL/100 g/min) is twice the flow to right ventricle. Atrial blood flow is approximately one-fourth of the ventricular flow.

Oxygen consumption by the myocardium It is very high (8 mL/min/100 g at rest). Because of this, even at rest, 70%–80% of the oxygen is extracted from each unit of the coronary blood compared with the whole body (average of 25%) oxygen extraction at rest. The increased oxygen demand of the myocardium during exercise is met with by almost total (nearly 100%) extraction of oxygen and by manifold increase in the CBF. Oxygen supply and utilization by myocardium vis-à-vis rest of the body (average) is shown in Table 4.6.1.

Phasic Changes in Coronary Blood Flow

The CBF shows changes during phases of cardiac cycle. The blood flow is determined by the balance between *pressure head* (i.e. aortic pressure) and the resistance (i.e. extravascular pressure exerted by the myocardium on the coronary vessels)

Table 4.6.1 Oxygen supply and consumption by myocardium vis-à-vis rest of the body (average)

Parameter	Rest of the body (average)	Myocardium
Oxygen content		
• Arterial blood	19 mL%	19 mL%
• Venous blood	14 mL%	6 mL%
A–V O_2 difference	5 mL%	13 mL%
Coefficient of O_2 utilization	5/19 × 100 = 26%	13/19 × 100 = 70%
Oxygen saturation of venous blood	14/19 × 100 = 74% with PO_2 40 mm Hg	6/19 × 100 = 32% with $PO_2 < 20$ mm Hg

Table 4.6.2 Pressure gradients between ventricles and aorta during systole and diastole

Phase of cardiac cycle	Pressure (mm Hg)			Pressure gradient (mm Hg) between aorta and ventricle	
	Right ventricle	Left ventricle	Aorta	Right ventricle	Left ventricle
Systole	25	121	120	95	−1
Diastole	0	0	80	80	80

offered to blood flow during various phases of cardiac cycle, and is shown in Table 4.6.2 and Fig. 4.6.3 and described here.

Blood Flow to Left Ventricle

During systole The tension developed in the left ventricle is so high that it has throttling effect on the branches of coronary arteries penetrating through them. As a result, the average blood flow through the capillaries of left ventricles falls to the extent that during some moments of the isometric contraction phase, the blood flow to the left ventricle practically ceases, i.e. becomes zero. This is particularly true for the subendocardial region of the left ventricle. However, the epicardial parts of the left ventricle do receive some flow of blood during systole as the effect of intraventricular pressure is sufficiently dampened in these parts.

During diastole The cardiac muscles relax and blood flow increases. *Maximal flow in the left coronary vessels usually occurs during isovolumic relaxation phase*, while the arterial pressure is still relatively high and the myocardium is relaxed. Thus, most of the CBF (over 70%) occurs during diastole (Fig. 4.6.3). In severe tachycardia, the duration of diastole is drastically reduced. This tends to reduce the CBF during diastole as well, but due to local metabolic regulation, the blood flow to the myocardium is not seriously affected.

Blood Flow to Right Ventricle and Atria

Blood passing through coronary capillaries of right ventricle also shows phasic changes similar to that passing through left ventricle. However, the changes in right ventricular flow are far less because force of contraction of the right ventricle is much less (Table 4.6.2). Thus, the blood flow to the right ventricle and atria occurs both during systole and diastole.

Blood Flow Through Coronary Sinus

As shown in Fig. 4.6.3, in the coronary sinus, the inflow of blood gradually rises from the *isovolumic ventricular contraction phase* and reaches its peak during *protodiastole phase* and then gradually falls.

Applied Aspects

Clinical Importance of Phasic Coronary Blood Supply

1. Subendocardial region of left ventricle receives no blood supply during systole so this region is particularly vulnerable to ischaemia and is the *most common site of myocardial infarction* (MI). This is true in spite of the fact that this region has been provided with the following *compensatory (protective) mechanisms*:

Capillary density in subendocardial region of left ventricle is much higher (1100 capillaries/mm^2) than in the epicardial region (750 capillaries/mm^2). Therefore, during diastole, flow to the subendocardial region of the left ventricle is considerably higher.

Minimum diffusion distance between the capillaries and myocardial cells is 20% shorter in subendocardial region of left ventricle (16.5 μm) compared with in epicardial region (20.5 μm).

Myoglobin content (O_2 storage pigment) is higher in the subendocardial region than in the epicardial region of the left ventricle.

2. In aortic stenosis, pressure in the left ventricle is much higher than that in aorta, because the ventricle has to force the blood against a narrow aortic orifice. This leads to severe compression of coronary vessels during systole and thus chances of MI are increased in such cases.

3. In congestive heart failure (CHF), increase in venous pressure decreases aortic diastolic pressure. As a result, the effective coronary perfusion pressure falls and CBF decreases.

MEASUREMENT OF CORONARY BLOOD FLOW

1. Nitrous Oxide Method (Kety Method)

Principle Nitrous oxide method is the most common method used for measuring CBF. It gives almost accurate value and is based on the Fick's principle (see page 278).

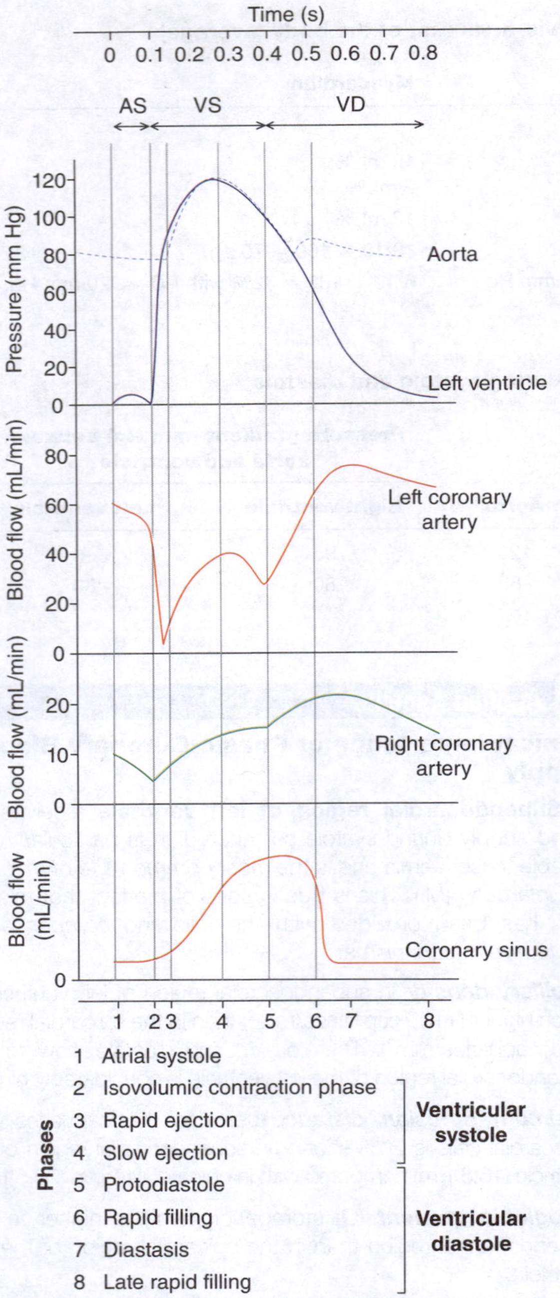

Fig. 4.6.3 Blood flow in right and left coronary arteries and coronary sinus during different phases of cardiac cycle. AS, atrial systole; VD, ventricular diastole; VS, ventricular systole.

Procedure The individual is made to inhale a mixture of 15% nitrous oxide and air for 10 minutes.

- During inhalation of gases, serial samples of arterial and coronary sinus venous blood (through a catheter introduced) are taken at fixed intervals for 10 minutes.
- The CBF is then determined from the amount of nitrous oxide taken up per minute and the difference of nitrous oxide content of arterial (A) and venous (V) blood, i.e.

$$\text{CBF} = \frac{\text{N}_2\text{O taken up/min}}{\text{A}-\text{V}}$$

2. Radionuclide Utilization Technique

Principle The radioactive tracers are pumped into cardiac muscle cells by the enzymes Na^+–K^+-ATPase and equilibrate with the intracellular K^+ pool. Distribution of radioactive tracers is directly proportional to myocardial blood flow and this forms the basis of this technique.

Procedure Radionuclide such as thallium-201 (^{201}Tl) is injected intravenously. After 10 minutes, the amount of ^{201}Tl taken up by the myocardial cells is then measured with the help of gamma-scintillation camera over the chest. The amount of CBF is calculated from these values. Areas of ischaemia are detected by their low uptake. Some radiotracers such as technetium-99m stannous pyrophosphate (^{99m}Tc-PYP) are selectively taken up by the infarcted tissues only by an unknown mechanism. These substances are used to detect areas of myocardial infarcts which stand out as *hot spots* on the scintiscans of the chest.

3. Coronary Angiographic Technique

Coronary angiography, when combined with measurement of ^{133}Xe washout using a multiple-crystal scintillation camera, provides detailed analysis of CBF (Fig. 4.6.4).

4. Electromagnetic Flowmeter Technique

- This technique is employed in animals to measure the CBF. The main advantages of this technique are that it tells the phasic flow and the flow per minute.
- In this technique, blood flow through the left ventricle is determined with the help of electromagnetic flowmeter implanted around the main LCA or around its circumflex branch. The arterial and venous (with the help of a catheter passed into coronary sinus) blood samples are analysed for O_2 content. From the measured flow, and the difference of O_2 content of arterial and venous blood, the myocardial consumption of O_2 is then determined directly.

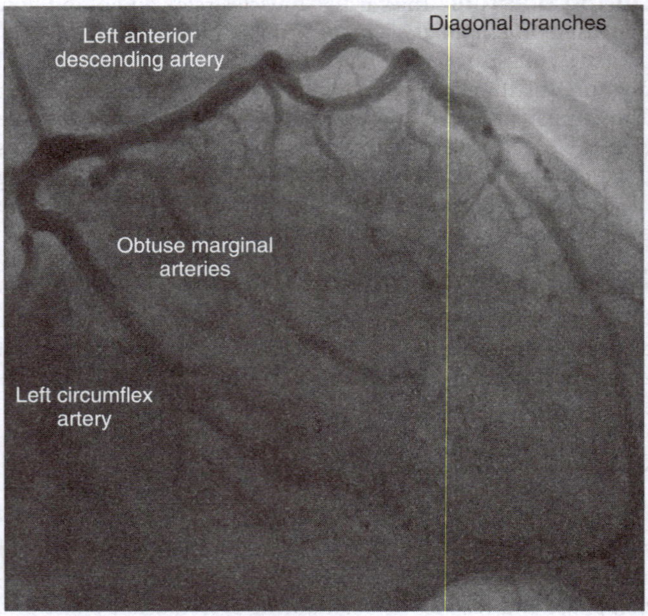

Fig. 4.6.4 Coronary angiography.

REGULATION OF CORONARY BLOOD FLOW

I. Local Control Mechanism

1. Autoregulation

Like other vital organs of the body, coronary circulation shows well-developed phenomenon of autoregulation. As described in detail on page 306, autoregulation refers to the ability of an organ/tissue to adjust its vascular resistance and maintain a relatively constant blood flow over a wide range of arterial blood pressure. However, this phenomenon of autoregulation of CBF fails when blood pressure falls below 70 mm Hg and coronary perfusion is seriously compromised.

2. Role of Local Metabolites

Metabolic local factors are the most important factors which regulate the CBF and, therefore, they override even the effect of nervous stimulation.

It is important to note that under resting state, approximately 50%–70% of O_2 is released to the myocardium from the haemoglobin of arterial blood (in contrast, haemoglobin releases approximately 25% of its O_2 content for the body as a whole). Therefore, not much additional oxygen can be provided to myocardium unless the blood flow increases. Consequently, a direct and almost linear correlation is observed between the CBF and myocardial O_2 consumption (Fig. 4.6.5). How the O_2 consumption regulates the coronary vascular resistance is not known exactly. Probably the following mechanisms are involved:

Role of adenosine (Berne's hypothesis) Adenosine is considered the major factor in production of coronary vasodilation during hypoxic states. In myocardial ischaemia, due to generalized hypoxia or due to increased myocardial metabolism, the intracellular myocardial *adenine nucleotides* are degraded to *adenosine*. The adenosine is capable of crossing myocardial cell membrane and thus comes out in the ECF and gains access to the resistance vessels, including the precapillary sphincters of the coronary system, producing an extremely strong vasodilator response (Fig. 4.6.6). The adenosine is then reabsorbed back into the cardiac cells to be reused.

Direct effect of O_2 It has been proposed that a decrease in the tissue PO_2 could also act directly on the arterioles and cause vasodilation.

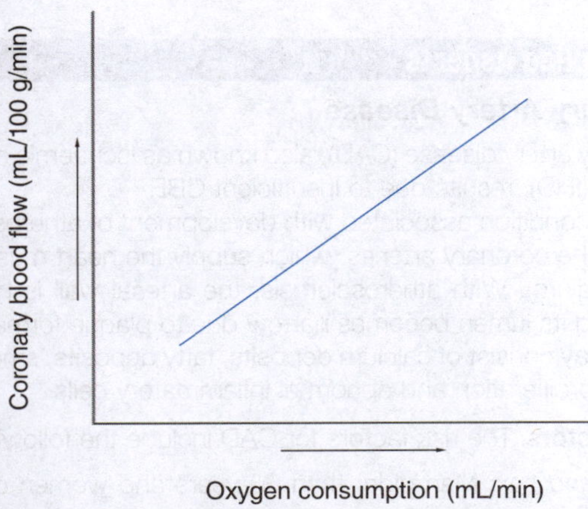

Fig. 4.6.5 Relation between coronary blood flow and myocardial oxygen consumption.

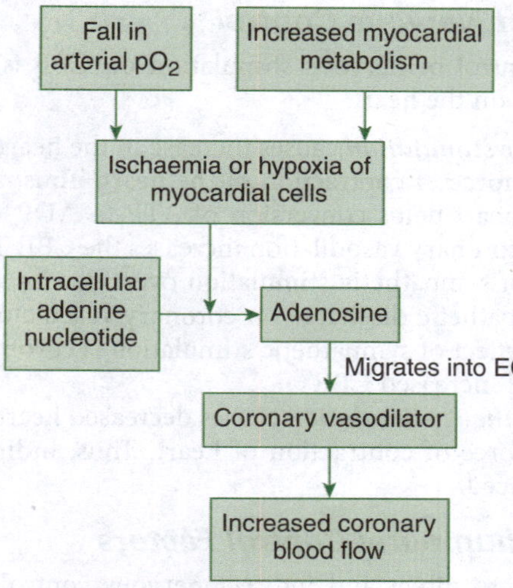

Fig. 4.6.6 Berne's hypothesis (adenosine mechanism) of increase in coronary blood flow.

Role of other local metabolites Hydrogen ions, bradykinin, CO_2 and prostaglandins are the other suggested vasodilator substances.

3. Role of Endothelial Cells

- Endothelial cells release several *vasodilator* autacoids that contribute to the physiological regulation of coronary vasomotor tone. These include endothelium-derived relaxing factor (EDRF), prostacyclin (PGI_2) and endothelium-derived hyperpolarizing factor (EDHF).
- Endothelial cells also release *vasoconstrictor autacoids* that may have a pathological role, such as endothelin-1 (ET-1), angiotensin II and endothelium-derived contracting factors (EDCF).

II. Nervous Control Mechanism

Autonomic nerves control the CBF directly as well as indirectly.

1. Direct Nervous Control

Direct nervous control on coronary circulation is exerted through sympathetic and parasympathetic nerve supply to the coronary vessels.

Parasympathetic nerve fibres These nerve fibres to coronary vessels through vagus are so less that parasympathetic stimulation has very little direct effect, causing vasodilation.

Sympathetic nerve fibres These fibres extensively innervate the coronary vessels. The transmitters released at their nerve endings are epinephrine and norepinephrine. The coronary vessels contain both α- and β-receptors.

- Norepinephrine acts on α-receptors and causes vasoconstriction. Epicardial vessels have preponderance of α-receptor.
- Epinephrine acts on β-receptors of coronary vessels, causing vasodilation. Intramuscular arteries have preponderance of β-receptors.
- The net result of direct effect of sympathetic stimulation is vasoconstriction.

2. Indirect Nervous Control

Indirect control of nervous stimulation on CBF is through their action on the heart.

Sympathetic stimulation causes increase in the heart rate and increase of force of contraction of the heart. Thus, increased activity of heart helps conversion of ATP to ADP which by producing coronary vasodilation increases the CBF. This indirect effect of sympathetic stimulation overrides the direct effect of sympathetic discharge on coronary vasculature. Thus, the overall effect of sympathetic stimulation is coronary vasodilation and increased CBF.

Parasympathetic stimulation causes decreased heart rate and decreased force of contraction of heart. Thus, indirectly the CBF is reduced.

3. Neurohumoural Control Factors

In addition to direct and indirect nervous control through sympathetic and parasympathetic neurotransmitters, several nonadrenergic–noncholinergic neurotransmitters also play a modulatory role:

ATP (purine) It is co-released with norepinephrine from nerve terminals and produces vasoconstriction through P_1 receptors and vasodilation through P_2 receptors present on vascular smooth muscles.

Neuropeptide Y (NPY) It is released with norepinephrine during sympathetic stimulation and causes severe vasoconstriction.

Calcitonin gene–related peptide (CGRP) The most powerful coronary vasodilator. The CGRP is present in heart, lungs, GIT and parafollicular C cells of thyroid gland.

Mechanism of action: CGRP acts through G protein–coupled receptors (GPCR).

Functions: The main physiological functions of CGRP are as follows:

- Potent vasodilator of coronaries.
- Involvement in pathogenesis of pain.
- Helps in satiety promotion.
- Plays significant role in descent of testis.

Applied Aspects

CGRP receptor blocker (galcanezumab) is used as treatment of migraine as CGRP is released from trigeminal nerve endings.

Substance P, which is also found in cardiac nerves, causes release of EDRF and produces maximal dilation of epicardial coronary arteries.

FACTORS AFFECTING CORONARY BLOOD FLOW

1. Mean aortic pressure This is the force for driving blood into the coronary arteries. Rise in mean aortic pressure increases the blood flow and vice versa. But if pressure remains high for a long time, because of increased workload on the heart, it will lead to CHF.

2. Muscular exercise Normal CBF at rest is approximately 70 mL/100 g tissue/min. During exercise, CBF increases approximately four times because of sympathetic stimulation by the following mechanisms:

- Increased activity of heart
- Increased cardiac output (≥fivefold)
- Increase in mean arterial pressure

3. Emotional excitement During emotional excitement states such as fright, auditory and olfactory stimuli, the CBF is increased due to increased sympathetic discharge.

4. Hypotension There occurs reflex increase in noradrenergic discharge during hypotension, which produces coronary vasodilation to increase CBF. This effect is observed secondary to the metabolic changes in myocardium at a time when there occurs vasoconstriction of splanchnic, renal and cutaneous vessels.

5. Hormones Hormones affecting CBF are as follows:

- *Thyroid hormones* increase CBF because of increase in metabolism.
- *Adrenaline and noradrenaline* cause increase in CBF as already explained, indirectly by acting on β-receptors in heart.
- *Acetylcholine* may increase CBF by its action on heart similar to parasympathetic stimulation.
- *Pitressin* is known to decrease CBF by increasing coronary resistance.
- *Nicotine* is reported to increase CBF through the liberation of norepinephrine.

6. Heart rate When heart rate is increased, stroke volume decreases; therefore, phasic CBF and O_2 consumption per beat also decreases.

7. Effect of ions Potassium ions (K^+) in low concentration cause dilation of coronary vessels increasing CBF, whereas high K^+ ion concentration causes constriction of coronary vessels decreasing CBF.

8. Metabolic factors Increased metabolism of the heart increases O_2 consumption leading to relative hypoxia. Hypoxia causes vasodilation due to direct effect and also due to release of adenosine leading to increased CBF.

9. Temperature Hyperthermia increases metabolism and so causes increase in CBF while hypothermia decreases metabolic rate and thus decreases CBF as well.

Applied Aspects

Coronary Artery Disease

Coronary artery disease (CAD), also known as ischaemic heart disease (IHD), results due to insufficient CBF.

It is a condition associated with development of atherosclerosis in the coronary arteries, which supply the heart muscles (myocardium). With atherosclerosis, the arterial wall is hardened and its lumen becomes narrow due to plaque formation which may consist of calcium deposits, fatty deposits, smooth muscle proliferation and abnormal inflammatory cells.

Risk Factors The risk factors for CAD include the following:

- *Age and sex:* Men older than 60 years and women older than 65 years are more prone.
- *Family history:* It is a predisposing factor.

- *Diseases:* Diabetes, hypercholesterolaemia and hypertension are proven risk factors.
- *Smoking:* It is a big risk factor.
- *Obesity*
- *Diet:* Diet rich in saturated fats and low in antioxidants.
- *Lifestyle:* Sedentary worker with lack of exercise.

Pathophysiology and Manifestations of Coronary Artery Disease Coronary artery atherosclerosis per se or with superadded arterial spasm or thrombus leads to limitation of blood flow to the heart muscle causing ischaemia (cell starvation due to a lack of oxygen) of the myocardial cells. Myocardial ischaemia clinically may manifest as:

1. Angina pectoris
2. Acute coronary syndrome: MI

Angina Pectoris

Angina pectoris refers to a transient form of myocardial ischaemia, especially occurring during increased oxygen demand (e.g. during exercise) in patients with CAD having approximately 60%–70% narrowing of coronary arteries. Superadded thrombus formation causing incomplete coronary occlusion results in an unstable angina.

Characteristic features Typically, the angina is described as a feeling of uncomfortable pressure, fullness, squeezing or pain in the substernal region, which may be localized or may be referred to the inner border of left arm, neck or jaw. Pain occurs due to accumulation of anoxic myocardial metabolites and *factor P*, which stimulates pain nerve endings.

Types Angina is of two types: stable and unstable.

Stable angina, also known as effort angina, refers to the occurrence of above-described features of angina precipitated by some activity (walking, running, exercise, etc.) with minimal or nonexistent symptoms at rest.

Unstable angina occurs at rest and usually lasts for more than 10 minutes. Attacks are frequent.

Diagnosis The diagnosis of angina is based on:

1. ***Electrocardiography:*** The characteristic ECG changes observed during angina episode are as follows:
   - ST-segment depression that reverses after disappearance of ischaemia.
   - T-wave flattening/inversion may also occur.
   - Stress test/exercise electrocardiography is most useful for detecting ischaemia that is not present at rest but precipitated by exercise (stress). Exercise testing can be done on motorized treadmill or with bicycle ergometer. The speed of treadmill is increased every 3 minutes until limited by symptoms.
2. ***Laboratory testing:*** It includes serum lipid levels.

Treatment The treatment consists of the following:

Nitroglycerine: Sublingual nitroglycerine is the drug of choice. Nitrates decrease arteriolar and venous tone, reduce preload and afterload, and lower the oxygen demand.

Nitrates also improve myocardial blood flow by dilating collaterals and in the presence of increased vasomotor tone.

Prevention of further angina attacks includes:

- Aggravating factors like hypertension, strenuous activity, emotional stress and cold temperature should be identified and treated or avoided.
- Nitroglycerine: Use of nitroglycerine sublingually/translingually by spray; or long-acting nitrates should be taken before any strenuous activity.
- Beta-blockers prevent angina by reducing myocardial oxygen requirement during exertion or stress. This effect is accomplished by reducing the heart rate, myocardial contractility and blood pressure.
- Calcium channel–blocking agents like verapamil, diltiazem and dihydropyridine prevent angina by reducing myocardial oxygen requirements.

Myocardial Infarction

MI or acute myocardial infarction (AMI), commonly known as a 'heart attack', refers to a degree of myocardial ischaemia (due to interruption of blood supply) that causes irreversible changes (necrosis, i.e. cell death or infarction) in the myocardium. Commonly, MI occurs when partially occluded coronary artery is constricted further by vasospasm or plaque (most common cause), which triggers formation of thrombus and occludes coronary artery.

Causes These include the following:

- Atherosclerosis of coronary arteries
- Thrombus formation
- Embolus coming from other areas
- Spasm of coronary vessels

Since atheromatous coronary artery stenosis is the commonest cause, it has become synonymous with CAD.

Signs and symptoms These include the following:

- Sudden severe chest pain is a classical symptom of MI. Pain lasts for more than 30 minutes and typically may radiate to left arm and left side of neck. Pain occurs due to the anoxic metabolites and necrotic tissue products.
- Associated symptoms often complained with pain are shortness of breath, nausea, vomiting, palpitation, sweating and anxiety (often described as a sense of impending doom).

Note

Approximately 25% of all MI are 'silent', i.e. without chest pain or other symptoms. Silent MI usually occurs in diabetics with associated autonomic neuropathy in elderly and also in patients with heart transplants.

Diagnosis Diagnosis of MI is made by:

- Typical signs and symptoms associated with
- ECG changes seen on serial tracings
- Changes in serum levels of certain enzymes and proteins (cardiac biomarkers)

ECG changes in myocardial infarction These are very important to diagnose, localize the area of infarction and to know the duration of infarction. Typical ECG changes (hallmark) seen in MI include:

- Elevation of ST segment in the leads overlying the infarct area
- Depression of ST segments in the reciprocal leads

For details, see page 263.

Measurement of serum enzymes and proteins related to myocardial infarction Certain enzymes and proteins called cardiobiomarkers leak into the circulation from the damaged myocardial cells. These include the following:

Troponin-T and troponin-I are cardiac specific proteins, released 2–4 hours after MI. Peak levels are seen after 12 hours and persist up to 7 days. These are the most sensitive and specific for MI.

Creatine kinase (CK-MB) levels increase within 4–6 hours and last for 2–3 days. They are relatively specific when skeletal muscle damage is not present.

Lipoprotein(a) [Lp(a)]: There is a relation between atherosclerosis and circulating levels of Lp(a). Lp(a) interferes with the fibrinolysis by decreasing plasmin generation.

Lactate dehydrogenase (LDH) levels peak within 72 hours. LDH is not specific as troponin.

Homocysteine: This substance damages endothelial cells of coronary vessels. There is a strong positive correlation of circulating levels of homocysteine I and MI.

Note
Homocysteine is converted into nontoxic substance (methionine) by vitamin B_{12} and folic acid. Therefore, supplements of folate and vitamin B_{12} lower the incidence of MI.

Highly sensitive C-reactive protein and other inflammatory markers are correlated with the presence of inflammatory cells in the atherosclerotic lesion. Therefore, estimation of plasma C-reactive protein is also helpful in diagnosis.

Glycogen phosphorylase isoenzyme BB (GPBB) is one of the new cardiobiomarkers. A rapid rise in blood levels can be seen in MI and unstable angina within 3 hours after process of ischaemia and peak levels are seen within 7 hours. It has a high sensitivity and specificity, if estimated early after chest pain.

Serum transaminases (AST/ALT): These are nonspecific cardiac biomarkers as they exist in other tissues, namely liver skin, RBC, etc. However, the levels of serum transaminases with characteristic symptoms and ECG changes can be used as a marker.

For localization of the infarct and to decide further management, other investigations are as follows:

Echocardiography provides assessment of left ventricular and regional functioning, and can help in diagnosis and management of infraction.

Doppler echocardiography is the most convenient procedure for diagnosing postinfarction damage.

Scintigraphic studies with technetium-99m stannous pyrophosphate and thallium-201 identify the regions of ischaemia. For more details, see page 345.

Radionuclide angiography demonstrates akinesis in the area of infraction and also measures ejection fraction (Fig. 4.6.7).

Treatment In MI, treatment should be started immediately to avoid irreversible changes. Therefore, main aim is to restore blood flow to the affected area.

A. ***General measures:*** Coronary care unit monitoring should be instituted as early as possible.
B. ***Drug therapy*** includes:

1. Aspirin (for mechanism of action, see page 209) *Analgesia:* To relieve pain, sublingual nitroglycerine should be attempted

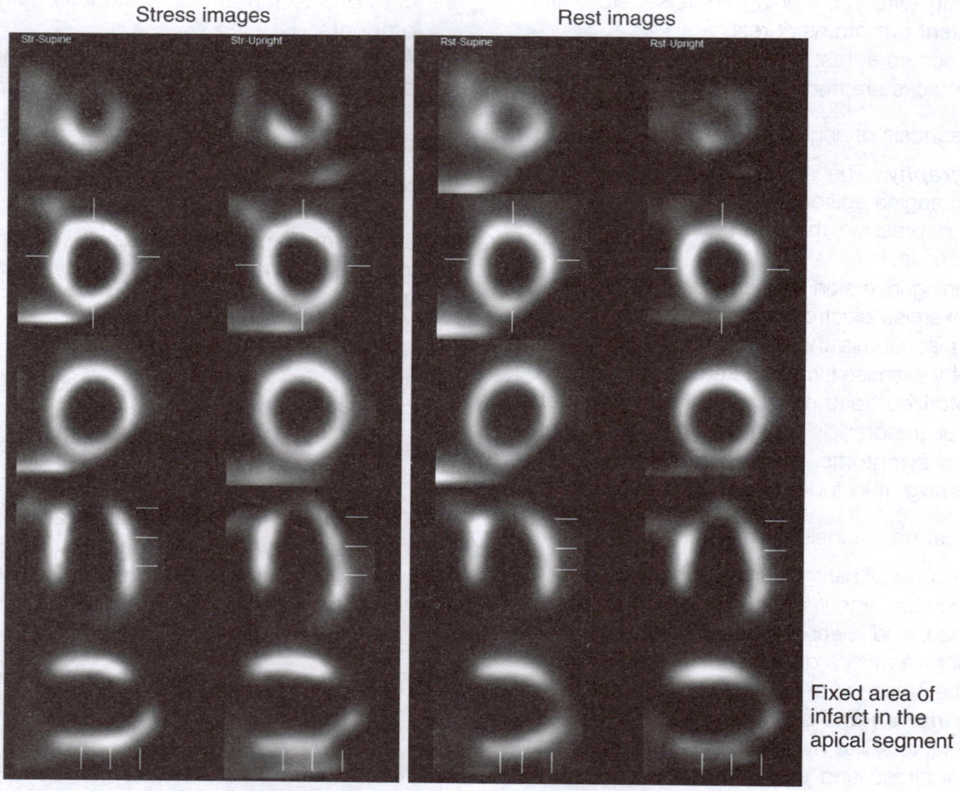

Fig. 4.6.7 Radionuclide angiography.

first; if no relief, then intravenous opioids provide effective and rapid analgesia.

2. *Thrombolytic therapy* reduces mortality and limits the infarct size. The greatest benefit occurs if treatment is initiated within first 3 hours. Thrombolytic agents commonly used are as follows:

- *Streptokinase,* the first thrombolytic agent, is less clot specific and less effective, and causes hypotension and allergic reaction, therefore not generally administered.
- *Anistreplase* (anisoylated plasminogen streptokinase activator complex [APSAC]) is injected as a bolus and provides continued thrombolytic activity.
- *Alteplase* (recombinant tissue plasminogen activator [tPA]) is a naturally occurring thrombolytic agent. Two additional clot-specific agents available are reteplase (closely related to tPA) and tenecteplase (TNK-tPA).
- *Heparin-post-thrombolytic management* should be done by anticoagulation therapy with intravenous heparin (60 units/kg bolus followed by 12 units/kg/min to maintain a PTT of 50–75 seconds).

3. *Beta-adrenergic agents* (see page 1198)

4. *Angiotensin-converting enzyme (ACE) inhibitors* (see page 323)

5. *Calcium channel blockers*

C. ***Surgical treatment*** includes the following:

- *Aortic coronary bypass surgery* is performed to remove discrete points of blockage due to atherosclerosis. In this procedure, a section of subcutaneous vein from either arm or leg is removed and then grafting is done from root of aorta to the peripheral artery (beyond the blockage point).
- *Coronary angioplasty* is used to open partially blocked coronary vessels. A small balloon-tipped catheter, approximately 1 mm in diameter, is passed under radiographic guidance into the coronary system and pushed through partially occluded vessel till balloon reaches the blocked point. Then, the balloon is inflated under pressure, which stretches the diseased artery. After the procedure, blood flow increases by three- to fourfold and 75% of patients are relieved of ischaemic symptoms.
- *Stents* are small stainless steel mesh tubes, which are placed inside the coronary artery (dilated by angioplasty) to keep the artery open and prevent restenosis. The endothelin usually grows over the stents and allows smooth blood flow through the stent. Drug-eluting stents are usually preferred because these slowly release the drugs, which prevent the excessive growth of scar tissue and decrease the incidence of restenosis.
- *Laser beam coronary artery catheterization* is a new procedure alternative to thrombolysis.

Complications A variety of complications can occur even when treatment is initiated promptly in MI. These include the following:

- *Postinfarction angina:* Approximately 30% of patients will have postinfarction angina.
- *Arrhythmia:* Abnormalities of rhythm and conduction are common in MI (for details, see page 256).
- *Myocardial dysfunction:* The severity of myocardial dysfunction is proportionate to the extent of myocardial necrosis. Acute left heart failure, hypotension and shock are common myocardial dysfunctions.
- *Mechanical defects:* Mechanical defects in the form of partial or complete rupture of papillary muscle or of interventricular septum or myocardial rupture may occur in less than 1% of AMI.
- *Left ventricular aneurysm:* It may develop in 10%–20% of patients surviving AMI.
- *Pericarditis and post-MI syndrome (Dressler syndrome):* It occurs in less than 5% of patients. This is an autoimmune phenomenon and presents as pericarditis, associated with fever, leucocytosis and pericardial/pleural effusion.
- *Mural thrombosis:* Mural thrombi are also common, and can be detected by echocardiography or CT scan.

CEREBRAL CIRCULATION

CEREBRAL BLOOD VESSELS

Arteries of the Brain

The arteries which supply the brain are derived from two internal carotid arteries and the basilar artery (formed by union of the right and left vertebral arteries). Branches of the internal carotid arteries and of basilar artery anastomose on the inferior surface of the brain to form the circulus arteriosus (circle of Willis).

The *circle of Willis* (Fig. 4.6.8) is thus basically a free anastomosis between the two internal carotid arteries and the two vertebral arteries, which equalize pressure on the arteries of the two sides. In this way, the circulus arteriosus allows blood that enters by either internal carotid or vertebral artery to be distributed to any part of both cerebral hemispheres.

Six large arteries, taking part in formation of circle of Willis, supply blood by their central and cortical branches to the brain substance.

Anatomical peculiarities of cerebral capillaries and their role in *blood–brain barrier* are discussed on page 352.

Venous Drainage of the Brain

The cerebral hemisphere has two sets of veins: the superficial and deep. The veins draining the brain open into the various dural venous sinuses. Ultimately, the blood from all these sinuses reaches the sigmoid sinuses which become continuous

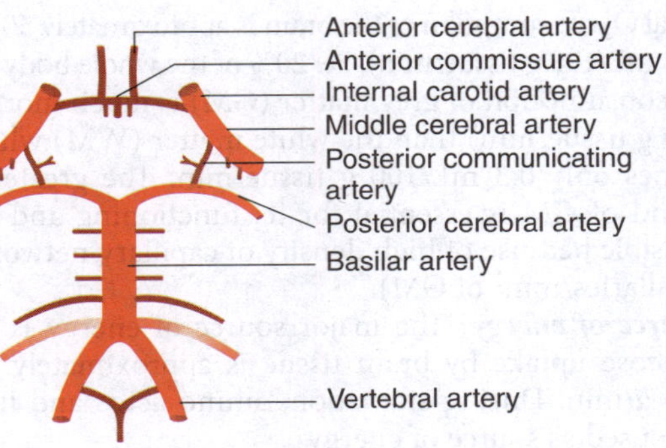

Fig. 4.6.8 The circle of Willis.

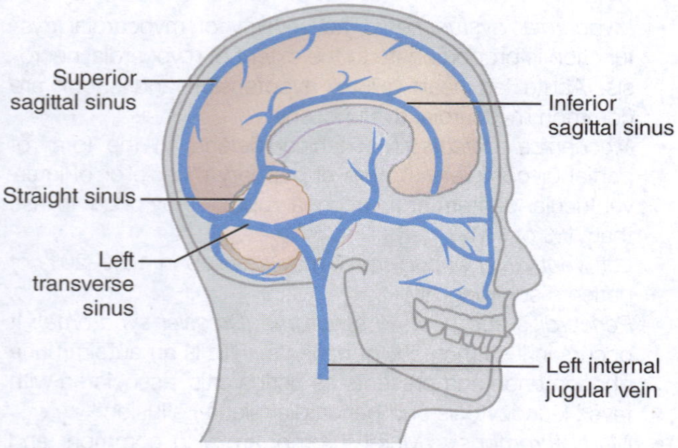

Fig. 4.6.9 Veins of the cerebral hemisphere.

with the two internal jugular veins. The venous drainage of individual part of the brain is as follows (Fig. 4.6.8).

Veins of the Cerebral Hemisphere (Fig. 4.6.9)

- The veins of the cerebral hemisphere consist of two sets: superficial and deep veins.
- *Superficial veins* drain into neighbouring venous sinuses.
- *Deep veins* of the cerebral hemisphere are two internal cerebral veins and two basal veins. The internal cerebral veins join to *great cerebral veins.* Basal veins end in the great cerebral vein which in turn ends in straight sinus.

CEREBRAL BLOOD FLOW: CHARACTERISTIC FEATURES

Normal Blood Flow

- Brain relies on a continuous blood flow for adequate function. It is most susceptible to ischaemia. Interruption of blood flow for only 5–10 seconds causes a loss of consciousness, and circulatory arrest for only 3–4 minutes results in irreversible brain damage. The vegetative structures in brainstem are more resistant to hypoxia than cerebral cortex.
- Brain has a very rich blood supply. Normal blood flow to brain (which forms <2% of the body weight) represents approximately 15% of the resting cardiac output (75 mL/min), or approximately 50-55 mL blood/100 g tissue/min. The average weight of brain is 1400 g; therefore, blood flow to brain is approximately 750 mL/min.
- When cerebral blood flow falls below 18 mL/100 g tissue/min (*critical flow level*), there occurs unconsciousness.

Normal O_2 Consumption

- Total O_2 consumption of the brain is approximately 50 mL/min (3.3 mL/100 g tissue/min), i.e. 20% of the whole body at rest.
- O_2 consumption of grey matter (GM) is much more (3 mL/100 g tissue/min) than the white matter (WM) which consumes only 0.3 mL/100 g tissue/min. The greater O_2 demand of GM is essential for its functioning and is made possible because of high density of capillary network (4000 capillaries/mm^2 of GM).

  Source of energy: The major source of energy is glucose. Glucose uptake by brain tissue is approximately 5.5 mg/100 g/min. During starvation, amino acids and lipids are also used as source of energy.

  Respiratory quotient: It ranges between 0.95 and 0.99.

Distribution of Blood

Major cerebral arteries are not end arteries as they anastomose at circle of Willis. Because of this, blood flows adequately to different parts of the brain. However, under normal circumstances, blood from each carotid artery is distributed largely to the same side of the brain and very little mixing occurs between the two circulations because a pressure gradient is normally not present due to equal blood pressure on the two sides. The major cerebral arteries supply the brain tissue through their central and cortical branches.

Central branches of the cerebral arteries are end arteries, i.e. they do not anastomose with each other. Therefore, thrombosis or rupture of any of them invariably causes infarction.

Cortical branches of the anterior, middle and posterior cerebral arteries supplying the surfaces of hemispheres overlap, forming border zones between the areas supplied by these arteries. However, these border zones susceptible to ischaemic damage and under condition of inadequate perfusion develop the so-called *watershed infarcts.*

Applied Aspects

Anterior watershed infarct results due to inadequate perfusion of the border zone between supply of anterior and middle cerebral arteries and is characterized by development of contralateral hemiparesis of the leg and expressive language or behavioural changes.

Posterior watershed infarct results due to inadequate perfusion of the border zone between supply of middle and posterior cerebral arteries and commonly produces a partial visual loss accompanied by a variety of language problems.

Measurement of Cerebral Blood Flow

1. Kety Method

Principle It is based on Fick's principle (see page 278).

Procedure In this method, subject is made to breathe a mixture of 15% nitrous oxide and air for 10 minutes. During this period, serial samples are taken every minute from the internal jugular vein (representing venous blood from brain) and a peripheral artery. The cerebral blood flow then is calculated as:

$$\text{Cerebral blood flow} = \frac{N_2O \text{ taken up by brain tissue per minute}}{A-V \text{ difference of } N_2O \text{ concentration}}$$

Disadvantages The disadvantages of this technique are as follows:

- It gives an average value but no information about regional differences in the blood flow. For example, a reduction in flow to one part of the brain may be completely compensated by an increase in flow to other part so that total blood flow remains unchanged in spite of the fact that a region may be damaged.
- It measures the blood flow to only perfused areas of brain.
- It can be used only in steady state and not for the measurement of rapidly changing blood flow.

2. By Using Radioactive Substances, i.e. Single-photon Emission Computed Tomography (SPECT)

Principle In this technique, blood flow to a region of brain is measured from the clearance curve of an inert radioactive tracer.

Procedure Commonly used radioactive substance in this method is radioactive xenon (^{133}Xe or ^{123}Xe). A known amount of ^{133}Xe gas dissolved in saline is injected within 1–2 seconds in the internal carotid artery with the help of a thin catheter. The arrival and clearance of the tracers is detected for 10 minutes by multiple collimated scintillation detectors built into a helmet that fits over the cranium. Each detector is collimated to scan approximately 1 cm^2 of brain surface. The output from the detectors is processed in computer and displayed on coloured television screen. The colour is proportional to amount of blood flow. Resolution can be improved by computerized tomographic reconstruction. The mean cerebral blood flow in millilitre per gram per minute is calculated from the following equation:

$$\text{Cerebral blood flow} = \frac{\lambda b\left(H_{max} - sH_{10}\right)}{A_{10}}$$

λb = Brain–blood partition coefficient
H_{max} = Maximal height of clearance
H_{10} = Clearance height at 10 minutes
A_{10} = Area under clearance curve

Advantage The advantage of this technique is that blood flow to different regions of the cerebral cortex can be measured in conscious humans.

3. Positron Emission Tomography (PET)

It can also be employed to measure regional cerebral blood flow. As blood flow is coupled to brain metabolism, a short-half-life radioisotope such as ^{18}F, ^{11}O or ^{15}O is labelled to a compound such as 2-deoxyglucose and compound is injected.

The arrival and clearance of the tracer is detected by scintillation detector placed over the head. The local uptake of 2-deoxyglucose is a good index of blood flow and its concentration in different parts can be easily monitored.

4. Magnetic Resonance Imaging (MRI)

In this technique, regional concentration of individual metabolites is measured and changes in local O_2 utilization are mapped from which regional cerebral blood flow is studied.

This technique is based on detecting signals from different tissues in a magnetic field. Functional magnetic resonance imaging (fMRI) measures the amount of blood flow in a tissue area. During activity, the local blood flow and oxygen utilization by the tissue increases; therefore, when neural activity increases, there is an increase in discharge activity that changes field potentials. The fMRI detects increase in oxygenated blood.

Advantages of fMRI: As fMRI does not involve the use of radioisotope activity, it can be used at frequent intervals to detect regional brain blood flow changes in same individual during different types of activity (e.g. awake state, during sleep and involvement in specific activity like solving mathematical problems).

Applied Aspects

Certain brain diseases are associated with regional/general changes in cerebral blood flow, which are detected by fMRI. A few conditions are as follows:

- *In epileptic seizure*, blood flow to ectopic foci increases, whereas it reduces to other parts of brain.
- *In Alzheimer disease*, first change noticed is decreased metabolic activity and reduced blood flow to superior parietal cortex than to frontal cortex.
- *In Huntington disease*, there is reduction in blood flow to caudate nuclei.
- *In manic depressive disorder*, there is generalized reduction of blood flow.
- *In schizophrenia*, evidence suggests reduction of blood flow to frontal and temporal lobes, and to basal ganglia.

Regulation of Cerebral Blood Flow

The perfusion pressure which determines cerebral blood flow is the difference between the mean arterial pressure at the head level and the internal jugular pressure (cerebral venous pressure). Therefore, the factors which affect the cerebral blood flow are as follows:

- Arterial blood pressure
- Intracranial pressure
- Resistance, i.e. viscosity of the blood
- Diameter of the cerebral blood vessels

The cerebral blood flow is regulated by the following mechanisms.

1. Metabolic Regulation

Measurement of local cerebral blood flow has revealed that blood flow in individual segments of the brain changes within seconds in response to local neuronal activity. For example, the act of making a fist with the hand causes an immediate increase in blood flow in the motor cortex of the opposite cerebral hemisphere; similarly, the act of reading elevates the blood flow in the occipital cortex and in the language perception area of temporal cortex.

This change in blood flow with the neuronal activity of the particular area of the brain is related to the level of metabolism. The important metabolic factors which play important role are as follows.

i. Carbon dioxide Physiologically, pCO_2 is the most potent vasodilator of cerebral blood vessels. With increase in pCO_2, there occurs a linear increase in the cerebral blood flow (Fig. 4.6.10A). However, when arterial pCO_2 increases above 80 mm Hg, no further increase in cerebral blood flow occurs due to maximal dilation of blood vessels. Similarly, when arterial pCO_2 falls below 20 mm Hg, there occurs no further decrease in cerebral blood flow due to cerebral venoconstriction.

It has been observed that a maintained increase of arterial pCO_2 of 1 mm Hg above its normal range increases cerebral

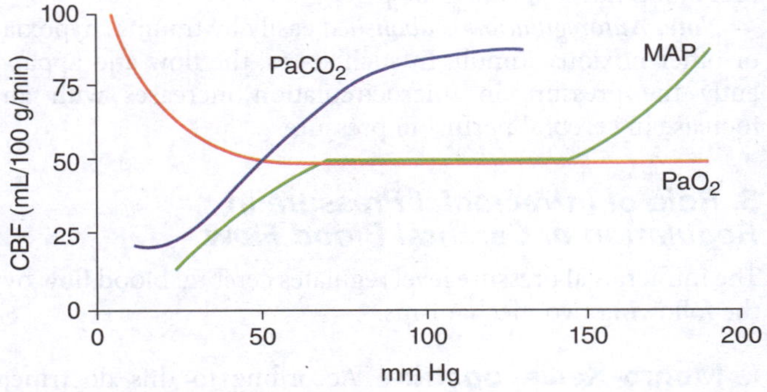

Fig. 4.6.10 Effect of pCO_2 on cerebral blood flow and autoregulation of cerebral blood flow.

blood flow by 3 mL/100 g/min, while a maintained decrease in arterial pCO_2 of 1 mm Hg below its normal range decreases cerebral blood flow by 1.5 mL/100 g/min. This is an important factor in the production of cerebral symptoms during hyperventilation.

Effect of CO2 is mediated via change in pH as described: A rise in pCO_2 is associated with a rise in H^+ concentration. Carbon dioxide easily diffuses through the blood–brain barrier and reaches the CSF. In the CSF, CO_2 combines with water to form carbonic acid, which partially dissociates to form H^+ ions. The H^+ ions induce cerebral vasodilation in proportion to their concentration. The H^+ ions, however, do not cross the blood–brain barrier. Therefore, any substance that increases the acidity of brain and, therefore, the H^+ ion concentration will increase cerebral blood flow; such substances include lactic acid, pyruvic acid or other acidic compounds that are formed during the course of metabolism.

ii. pO_2 Slight fall in pO_2 causes vasodilation and produces increase in cerebral blood flow (Fig. 4.6.10B). Any stimulus, which either reduces the O_2 supply to the brain or increases the O_2 need of the brain, results in rapid formation of *adenosine*, which is potent dilator of pial arterioles.

Inhalation of hyperbaric O_2 causes cerebral vasoconstriction and thus cerebral blood flow decreases. High cerebral pO_2 disrupts neuronal metabolism producing convulsions, coma and death.

iii. K^+ ions An increase in K^+ concentration in the CSF following hypoxia, electrical stimulation of brain and seizures causes rapid increase in cerebral blood flow. However, increase in K^+ is not sustained throughout the period of stimulation. Hence, only the initial increase in cerebral blood flow is attributable to the release of K^+ ions.

2. Autoregulation of Cerebral Blood Flow

Like other vital organs of the body, cerebral circulation also shows phenomenon of autoregulation (for details, see page 306). Due to autoregulation, cerebral blood flow remains nearly constant between 60 and 140 mm Hg of blood pressure (Fig. 4.6.10C). When blood pressure falls below 60 mm Hg, the cerebral blood flow becomes extremely compromised, and syncope may result. When blood pressure rises above 140 mm Hg, there may occur disruption of blood–brain barrier due to stretching and cerebral oedema or cerebral haemorrhage may result.

Mechanism of autoregulation: Both metabolic and myogenic theories of autoregulation are considered (see details on page 307). In metabolic theory, main regulating substance of cerebral blood flow appears to be pCO_2.

Note. *Autoregulation is abolished* easily by trauma, hypoxia or other noxious stimuli. In such states, the flow and apparently the pressure in microcirculation increases with an increase in cerebral perfusion pressure.

3. Role of Intracranial Pressure in Regulation of Cerebral Blood Flow

The intracranial pressure level regulates cerebral blood flow by the following two mechanisms.

i. Monro–Kellie doctrine According to this doctrine, the brain, CSF and blood in the cerebral vessels are three elements enclosed in a rigid cranial cavity, and when any of them increases, it is at the expense of other two. This relationship helps to maintain the cerebral blood flow when changes in the arterial blood pressure occur at the level of head as explained:

When the body is accelerated upwards (positive g), blood moves towards the feet and the arterial pressure at the level of head decreases, and theoretically the cerebral blood flow should be severely compromised. However, practically it does not occur so because due to gravity, the venous pressure and intracranial pressure are also decreased, and so the pressure on the vessels is decreased. Thus, the blood flow is less severely affected.

When the body is accelerated downwards (negative g), the reverse occurs, i.e. the arterial pressure at the level of head increases and theoretically the cerebral vessels could have ruptured. However, practically it does not occur so, because due to negative 'g', intracranial pressure also rises, which supports the vessels and prevents them for rupturing. The Monro–Kellie doctrine also explains the maintenance of normal cerebral blood flow during posture changes, coughing and Valsalva manoeuvre.

ii. Cushing reflex When intracranial pressure is increased and becomes equal to the arterial pressure, it compresses the arteries in the brain and blood supply to vasomotor area is compromised. The hypoxia and hypercapnia produced locally increases the discharge from VMC. The resultant rise in systemic pressure tends to restore the cerebral blood flow. The rise in blood pressure is proportionate to rise in intracranial pressure up to a certain limit, beyond which cerebral circulation ceases. This effect which protects the vital centres in brain is called Cushing reflex. The resultant increase in blood pressure also causes reflex bradycardia via baroreceptor response. Thus, bradycardia is an important feature of raised intracranial pressure.

4. Nervous Regulation of Cerebral Blood Flow

The cerebral blood vessels are innervated by noradrenergic vasoconstrictor fibres and cholinergic vasodilator fibres. The precise role of these fibres in regulation of cerebral blood flow is still a matter of debate. However, under normal conditions, vasomotor nerves do not regulate the cerebral blood flow. These nerves may act indirectly by release of substances from the astrocytes which act paracranially and regulate vasomotor tone.

In severe hypertension, the noradrenergic sympathetic nerves cause vasoconstriction reducing cerebral blood flow. This prevents cerebral vascular haemorrhage and stroke and also protects the integrity of blood–brain barrier, which gets disrupted at high blood pressure.

In severe hypotension, the cholinergic sympathetic vasodilator nerves play role in maintaining the cerebral blood flow.

Applied Aspects

Syncope

Syncope refers to transient fainting, i.e. transient loss of consciousness due to momentary but significant decrease in cerebral blood flow. It may be cardiogenic or noncardiogenic.

Cardiogenic syncope occurs in the following cardiac conditions:

- *Obstruction to cardiac output*, e.g. in aortic stenosis. It usually occurs due to exertion and is also called effort syncope.

- *Cardiac arrhythmias*, such as sinus arrest, heart blocks and Stokes–Adams syndrome.
- *Myocardial infarction.*

Noncardiogenic syncope occurs in the following forms:

- *Vasovagal syncope* occurs due to vasovagal reflex causing sudden hypotension and bradycardia.
- *Postural syncope* results due to inadequate vasomotor response to postural changes in blood pressure.
- *Carotid sinus syncope* or the carotid sinus syndrome results due to excessive sensitivity of the carotid sinus to compression, e.g. as by a tight collar.
- *Valsalva manoeuvre syncope* is associated with increased intrathoracic pressure in the following situations:
  - Micturition (micturition syncope)
  - Defecation (defecation syncope)
  - Coughing (tussive syncope)

- ***Metabolic syncope*** occurs in the following situations:
  - *Hyperventilation* leads to hypocapnia, which causes cerebral vasoconstriction.
  - *Hypoglycaemia* impairs the activity of vasomotor centre.

CUTANEOUS CIRCULATION

CUTANEOUS BLOOD VESSELS (FIG. 4.6.11)

Cutaneous arterioles These form a dense network just under the dermis layer of the skin.

Meta-arterioles, which arise from the arterioles, are relatively high-resistance conduits present between the arterioles and capillaries.

Cutaneous capillaries: The meta-arterioles subdivide into capillary loops, which provide a large surface area for heat exchange.

Venules form an extensive subpapillary venous plexus, which hold large quantity of blood and lie parallel to the surface of skin and play important role in maintaining the body temperature.

Arteriovenous anastomoses (A-V) are located in the distal parts of the extremities (hands and feet), the nose, lips and ear lobules. These vessels are wide, low-resistance connections that serve as shunts and allow blood to bypass the superficial capillary loops and play major role during control of body temperature.

CUTANEOUS BLOOD FLOW: CHARACTERISTIC FEATURES

Main function of cutaneous circulation is to aid in the regulation of body temperature. The metabolic rate of the skin is relatively small so that a minimal amount of blood flow to the skin can supply the nutritive function.

Resting cutaneous blood flow, i.e. the flow when a person is at thermal equilibrium with the environment (at approximately 27°C atmospheric temperature), is approximately 10–15 mL/min/100 g of skin tissue.

During exposure to cold, when sweating is minimal, the cutaneous blood flow falls to approximately one-tenth of resting blood flow, i.e. approximately 1 mL/min/100 g tissue.

During exposure to heat, when sweating is maximum, the cutaneous blood flow may increase 10 times of resting blood flow, i.e. approximately 150 mL/min/100 g tissue. Maximum cutaneous blood flow that occurs on heat exposure imposes a heavy circulatory load on the heart. That is why persons working under maximal heat loads may simply collapse with circulatory failure unless supervised adequately.

Regional variation in cutaneous blood flow exists due to presence of A-V anastomoses in abundance in certain area such as hands, feet, nose and ear lobules. During heat stress, the blood flow to the area with rich A-V anastomoses increases much more (approximately 75 mL/100 g/min) compared with to the rest of the skin (approximately 25 mL/min/100 g tissue).

Cutaneous blood flow and skin colour: The colour of skin is basically determined by the pigment present; however, the amount of blood and degree of oxygenation also affect the skin colour tinge which may be reddish, bluish or some shade in between.

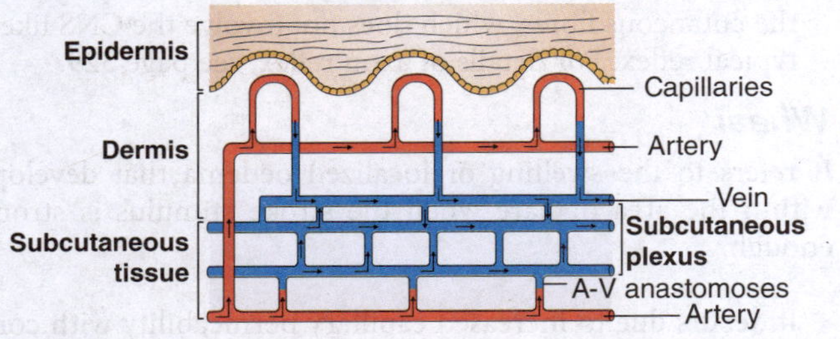

Fig. 4.6.11 Arrangement of blood vessels in subcutaneous region.

REGULATION OF CUTANEOUS BLOOD FLOW

The skin has very little metabolic activity. Consequently, it has little O_2 consumption, i.e. only 0.3 mL/min/100 g compared with 3.3 mL/min/100 g in brain and 9.7 mL/min/100 g in cardiac muscles. Therefore, in contrast to most other tissues, the cutaneous blood flow is predominantly regulated by the nervous control instead of metabolic control.

Nerve Supply of Cutaneous Vessels

Sympathetic vasoconstrictor nerves supplying the cutaneous vessels exhibit a sympathetic constrictor discharge under resting condition. The sympathetic tonic discharge is more marked on A-V anastomosis vessels than the other vessels.

Parasympathetic vasodilator nerves do not supply the cutaneous blood vessels. Vasodilation of cutaneous vessels results due to:

- Reduction of sympathetic vasoconstrictor effect
- Local production of bradykinin (a potent vasodilator polypeptide) in sweat glands
- Production of other local vasodilator substances (see page 339)

Neural Control Mechanisms

The cutaneous blood flow is regulated by the following neural control mechanisms.

1. Hypothalamic Control Mechanism

The reflex increase or decrease in sympathetic discharge to cutaneous vessels during thermoregulation is mediated through the temperature regulation centres of the hypothalamus as:

Under resting conditions, i.e. when the person is at thermal equilibrium with the environment (at approximately 27°C atmospheric temperature), the sympathetic vasoconstrictor fibres have a mild tonic discharge. The tonic sympathetic discharge normally keeps the A-V anastomoses closed.

During exposure to heat stress, the tonic sympathetic discharge is reflexly abolished by a hypothalamic mechanism. Thus, the blood flow to skin is increased by the following responses in a chronological sequence:

- First of all, A-V anastomoses of hands, feet and ear lobules dilate due to reduction in the sympathetic tonic discharge.
- Second, rest of the cutaneous vessels dilate due to progressive withdrawal of sympathetic vasoconstrictor activity.
- Finally, sweat glands get activated due to cholinergic sympathetic discharge. The *bradykinin* produced by the secretory activity of the sweat glands acts locally as a powerful vasodilator and increases blood flow to skin.

All the above-mentioned mechanisms combinedly may increase the cutaneous blood flow to as high as 150 mL/min/100 g tissue. Thus, total cutaneous blood flow during heat stress may be over 3 L/min. The increased blood flow carries heat to the surface of the body, where it is dissipated by *radiation, evaporation* and *conduction* to the environment. If the environmental temperature is higher than the body temperature, heat can be dissipated only by means of evaporation of sweat; under these conditions, radiation and conduction would cause the body to gain heat.

During exposure to cold stress, via hypothalamic mechanism, there occurs widespread cutaneous vasoconstriction due to increased sympathetic discharge. Consequently, cutaneous blood flow is markedly decreased to as low as 1 mL/min/100 g. Thus, total blood flow to skin during exposure to cold stress may be even less than 50 mL/min. In this way, *heat conservation* is accomplished by markedly diminishing the rate of blood flow to skin. Body heat is preserved because less heat is dissipated to the environment.

For details of temperature regulation, see page 1198.

2. Baroreceptor-Mediated Reflex

Cutaneous blood vessels participate in baroreceptor-mediated reflexes during conditions of circulatory stress such as exercise and haemorrhage. They exhibit considerable vasoconstriction and act as compensatory mechanism to divert blood from periphery to the central pool.

3. Cortical Control Mechanism

The *emotions* affect the cutaneous circulation through corticohypothalamic pathway. The impulses are relayed from the corticohypothalamic centres to the thoracolumbar sympathetic cell bodies and thence to the skin vessels. The effects of emotions on cutaneous circulation manifest in the following forms:

Blanching of skin during situations of fear (pale with fear) occurs due to vasoconstriction mediated through cortical mechanism.

Phenomenon of blushing, i.e. emotional embarrassment, occurs due to vasodilation of vessels. It is supposed to be the result of bradykinin (a potent vasodilator) release, secondary to a brief corticohypothalamically controlled discharge of sympathetic cholinergic fibres to the sweat glands.

CUTANEOUS VASCULAR RESPONSES

Certain peculiar cutaneous vascular responses are as follows:

- White reaction
- Triple response
- Dermatographia
- Axon reflex
- Reactive hyperaemia
- Cold vasodilation
- Cold vasoconstriction

White Reaction

White reaction refers to appearance of a pale stroke line when a pointed object is drawn lightly over the skin. This occurs due to the fact that the mechanical stimulus initiates contraction of the precapillary sphincter, and blood drains out of the capillaries and small veins. This response appears in approximately 15 seconds.

Triple Response

Triple response is three-part response, consisting of the red reaction, wheal and flare, which occurs as a normal reaction to the skin which is more in intensity than that which simply causes white reaction. In other words, even when the skin is stroked more firmly with a pointed instrument, instead of white reaction, there occurs triple response.

The Red Reaction

It refers to the red line which appears at the site of injury in approximately 10 seconds.

- It occurs due to dilation of the precapillary sphincters in the injured area.
  The dilation of the precapillary sphincters is not mediated by nerves but is produced by histamine and/or some polypeptides such as bradykinin released from the damaged skin.
- Since it is not neurally mediated, local anaesthesia of skin does not prevent the red reaction.

The Flare

It refers to the diffusely spreading and irregularly outlined redness of the skin surrounding the red line.

- It occurs after a few minutes of the appearance of red line.
- It occurs due to the dilation of the arteriole and precapillary sphincters. An arteriole supplies blood to the capillaries in an irregularly outlined area. This explains the irregular outline of flare.
- The dilation of the arteriole increases local blood flow.
- The dilation of arteriole is mediated by nerves, since it is abolished by the local anaesthetic agents.
- Since the blockade of the concerned afferent nerve fibres away from the site of injury does not abolish the response, it is believed that the flare is mediated by the *axon reflex* in the cutaneous fibres, which does not involve the CNS like a typical reflex. For details of axon reflex, see page 329.

Wheal

It refers to the swelling or localized oedema that develops within the area of flare when the stroke stimulus is strong enough.

- It occurs due to increased capillary permeability with consequent extravasation of fluid.

- The increase in capillary permeability responsible for wheal formation is produced in part by histamine or histamine-like substance released from local mast cells and mediated via H_1 receptors, in part by P substance and CGRP, the transmitter released at the central termination of the sensory fibre neurons. Thus, there is histaminergic as well as a peptidergic component of the wheal.

Note. The use of effective nonpeptide antagonist to substance P reduces extravasation of the fluid, thus preventing wheal formation.

Axon Reflex

For details, see page 329.

Dermatographia

Dermatographia refers to striking triple response that occurs as an unusual reaction in some individuals. Thus, in the prone individuals, anything drawn on the skin even with a blunt point becomes conspicuous within a few minutes. The exact cause of dermatographia is not known. Possibly, it is due to excessive release of the histamine from the involved skin area (Fig. 4.6.12).

Reactive Hyperaemia

Reactive hyperaemia is a phenomenon by which the vessels control blood flow to the organ after a period of *ischaemia* following occlusion of the artery to an organ or tissue. This response of the blood vessels occurs in many organs but is visible in the skin. Due to this phenomenon, the blood flow exceeds the control level when the occlusion is removed. For example, when the blood supply to a limb is occluded, the cutaneous arterioles below the occlusion dilate. When the circulation is re-established, blood flowing into the dilated vessels makes the skin fiery red. Oxygen diffuses a short distance through the skin, and reactive hyperaemia is prevented if the circulation of the limb is occluded in an atmosphere of 100% O_2. Therefore, it has been proposed that the arteriolar dilation is apparently due to local effect of hypoxia. The magnitude and duration of reactive hyperaemia depends on the duration of occlusion.

Cold Vasodilation

As discussed above, normally during exposure to cold stress, there occurs widespread cutaneous vasoconstriction via hypothalamic mechanism. However, prolonged and severe vasoconstriction may lead to tissue damage known as *frostbite*. This usually occurs when skin temperature falls below 10°C. The tissue injury so produced is painful and associated with the release of histamine and/or some other polypeptide, which excites the sensory terminals and produces *vasodilation* due to *axon reflex* operating particularly on A-V anastomoses. In addition, exposure to severe cold promotes the formation of *plasma kinins*, which also produce vasodilation; cold vasodilation is the cause of ruddy cheeks seen in fair-complexioned individuals on a cold day.

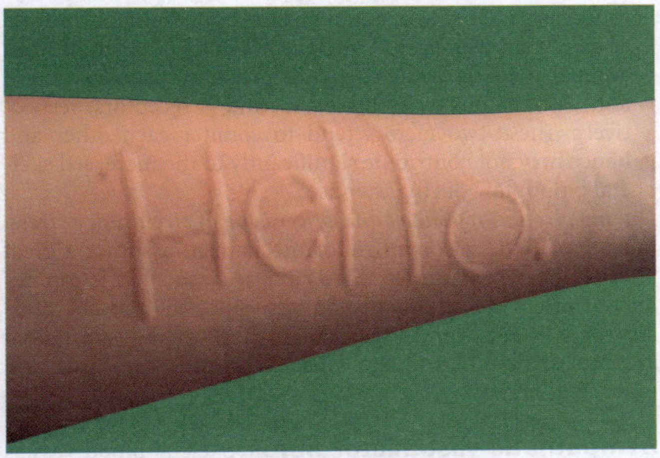

Fig. 4.6.12 Dermatographia.

Cold Vasoconstriction

Exposure to cold causes vasoconstriction via hypothalamic mechanism. Cutaneous vasoconstriction results in decrease in nutrient supply to the skin and also decreases metabolic rate of the tissue. Due to decreased metabolism, the metabolite accumulation is very slow so, unlike in muscles, the local metabolites of the skin are not able to produce local vasodilation and oppose (escape) the sympathetic vasoconstriction. As a result, the maximal vasoconstrictor discharge to the precapillary resistance vessels of the skin is well sustained. So, prolonged cold-induced vasoconstriction especially in damp conditions results in cutaneous ischaemia-producing lesions such as *trench foot*.

SKELETAL MUSCLE CIRCULATION

SKELETAL MUSCLE BLOOD FLOW: CHARACTERISTIC FEATURES

At rest The blood flow to the skeletal muscle is approximately 2–4 mL/min/100 g of muscle tissue.

- Since the whole-body skeletal muscle weight is approximately 30 kg in adults, the total blood flow to the body muscle mass is approximately 750–800 mL/min.
- At rest, only 20%–25% of muscle capillaries have flowing blood.

During exercise During strenuous exercise, muscle blood flow can increase up to 20 times, i.e. approximately 50–80 mL/min/100 g muscle tissue or over 20 L/min to the whole-body skeletal mass. This is called exercise hyperaemia.

- The tremendous increase in muscle blood flow mainly occurs due to local metabolite-induced vasodilation. During exercise, there occurs dilation of the arterioles and precapillary sphincters, and all the dormant capillaries open up, greatly increasing the surface area and the rate of blood flow to the skeletal muscles.
- During exercise, the blood flow to the muscle is intermittent because during each contraction muscle fibres squeeze the blood vessels passing through them and thus the blood flow decreases or even stops (Fig. 4.6.13). During relaxation period, muscle blood flow increases and myoglobin acts as an O_2 acceptor and it yields its O_2 to the myofibrils during the subsequent muscle contraction.
- Sustained and severe contractions lasting more than 10 seconds lead to cessation of blood flow; myoglobin supply of O_2 is exhausted and anaerobic metabolites accumulate causing fatigue and ischaemic pain.

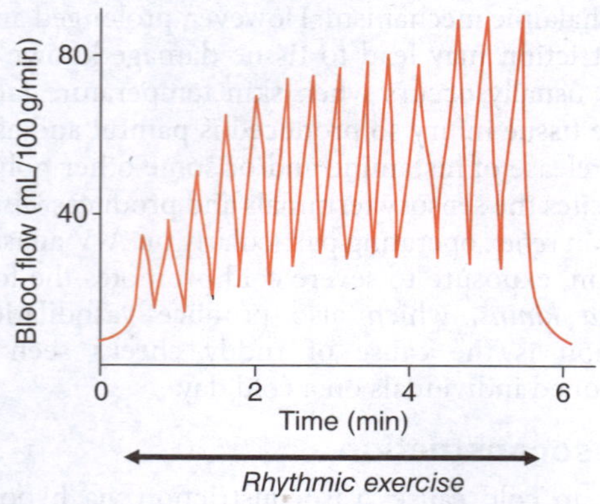

Fig. 4.6.13 Blood flow through skeletal muscles.

- Following heavy phasic exercise, the blood flow does not subside immediately, but falls exponentially from its high level during the exercise to resting values. This is due to the *oxygen debt of exercise* (see page 106).

Reactive hyperaemia When the blood supply to a limb is occluded, the muscular and cutaneous arterioles below the occlusion dilate. When the circulation is re-established, blood flowing into the dilated vessels causes ***muscle hyperaemia*** (muscle blood flow may increase to 35–40 mL/100 g/min). Reactive hyperaemia seems to be mediated by local hypoxia.

White versus red muscle blood flow: White versus red muscles have been described on page 91. Some of the essential differences related to blood flow are enumerated:

- White muscles constitute three-fourth of the total mass and show rapid phasic contractions. In contrast, red muscles constitute one-fourth of total mass and show steady prolonged contraction. These muscles are concerned with maintenance of posture.
- White muscles have a resting blood flow 2–4 mL/min/100 g, which may increase to 50–80 mL/min/100 g, during maximal exercise. In contrast, red muscle fibres employ aerobic metabolism and contract all the times. So, their O_2 demand is much higher (30 mL/min/100 g).
- White muscles are prone to O_2 debt, red muscles are not; because of greater surface area of the capillary bed (three times the size of white muscles) and higher resting blood flow, the red muscles are unlikely to be exposed to O_2 debt.

REGULATION OF MUSCLE BLOOD FLOW

The blood flow to the skeletal muscles is regulated by autoregulation mechanism, metabolic control mechanism and nervous control mechanism. These mechanisms exhibit their role in different situations as described.

1. Autoregulation Mechanism

Autoregulation is the ability of an organ or tissue to adjust its vascular resistance and maintain a relative constant blood flow over a range of arterial pressure. Mechanism of autoregulation is well developed in skeletal muscles like that of kidney, heart and brain. The precapillary resistance vessels in the skeletal muscles have a *high basal myogenic tone.* A rise of the transmural pressure excites a stretch-induced contraction of the sphincter smooth muscles, which by raising the precapillary vessel tone protects the capillaries from an undue rise of pressure (*myogenic theory of autoregulation*) also (see page 307). These responses are particularly important in leg muscles, where they reduce the rate of capillary filtration in erect posture and thus prevent pedal oedema under normal circumstances.

2. Metabolic Control Mechanism

Local metabolic control mechanism is chiefly responsible for the tremendous increase in skeletal muscle blood flow during exercise (exercise hyperaemia). The muscle contraction increases the metabolic rate of tissue, which in turn reduces *oxygen concentration* in the muscle. The decreased tissue pO_2 leads on to vasodilation. In addition, the exercising skeletal muscle, potassium ions, hydrogen ions, lactic acid, carbon dioxide and further rise of *tissue temperature* due to muscular activity may also contribute to the dilation of arterioles and precapillary sphincter. As a result, there is 10- to 100-fold increase in the number of open capillaries in the skeletal muscles.

Metabolic control also explains the *reactive hyperaemia* that occurs following a period of occlusion of arterial blood supply, as discussed above.

3. Nervous Control Mechanisms

Vessels of the skeletal muscles are supplied by both sympathetic vasoconstrictor and sympathetic vasodilator fibres.

Sympathetic vasoconstrictor control Under resting conditions, the noradrenergic sympathetic nerve fibres discharge at a rate of 1 impulse/s in recumbent position and 2–3 impulses/s in the upright position. This sympathetic discharge contributes relatively small part to the high basal tone of the resistance vessels of the muscles. Most of the basal tone of these vessels is myogenic. Because of this relatively low sympathetic contribution to the total basal tone, blockade or the permanent loss (by surgical removal) of sympathetic vasoconstrictor supply to the skeletal muscles only doubles the blood flow.

During muscular exercise: Because of the low sympathetic contribution to total basal tone, it is obvious that *exercise hyperaemia* is independent of sympathetic discharge to muscle vessels and is due to metabolic factors as described above.

Furthermore, skeletal blood vessels contain both α-adrenergic and β-adrenergic receptors. α-Receptors are located in close proximity of the terminals of vasoconstrictor sympathetic nerve fibres, and β-receptors are independent of any innervation. During strenuous exercise, norepinephrine and epinephrine are released into the systemic circulation from adrenal medulla, which tend to produce vasoconstriction and vasodilation by acting on α- and β-receptors, respectively. These two factors tend to counter each other and hence may not contribute significantly to the increased skeletal blood flow during exercise.

During circulatory shock and other type of circulatory stress, the sympathetic vasoconstrictor mechanism assumes a great physiological importance. Sympathetic vasoconstriction reduces muscle blood flow profoundly. Since the muscle capillary bed is very large, these help in diverting substantial amount of blood from the muscles towards the heart and other vital organs.

Sympathetic vasodilator fibres Skeletal blood vessels are also supplied by sympathetic vasodilator fibres. In some animals, these fibres release acetylcholine at their nerve endings, but in primates the vasodilator effect is believed to be caused by epinephrine-exciting β-adrenergic receptors in the skeletal muscle vasculature.

- These fibres are activated by *corticohypothalamic reticulospinal* pathways (see page 328), which are quite separate from the *VMC–thoracolumbar pathways*. Therefore, they are not influenced by the baroreceptor and chemoreceptor afferents and do not participate in changes in peripheral resistance by usual cardiovascular reflexes.
- These fibres probably operate during emergencies, i.e. during mental stress and emotions. Since there is stimulation of different areas in hypothalamus in these situations, due to activation of corticohypothalamic reticular pathway, there occurs vasodilation in muscle blood vessels also.
- Some experiments suggest that the sympathetic vasodilator system might cause initial vasodilation in skeletal muscles to allow anticipatory increase in blood flow, even before the onset of exercise.
- These fibres play an important role in preventing the sudden rise in systemic blood pressure at the beginning of exercise, i.e. these provide a *safety valve mechanism*. Just before the start of exercise, there occurs a considerable increase in the sympathetic activity. This is brought by the mere thought of exercise. As a result, the increase in stroke volume and heart rate should produce a marked increase in the blood pressure to a dangerous level. However, this does not happen so, because the discharge of sympathetic vasodilator fibres reduces the total peripheral resistance and thus lowers the blood pressure to safety level. Since the sympathetic vasodilator fibres dilate only the arterioles and not the precapillary sphincters, they do not increase the blood flow to the muscles. When exercise commences, the precapillary sphincters are dilated by the local metabolites and blood flow to the muscle is increased tremendously.

SPLANCHNIC CIRCULATION

SPLANCHNIC VESSELS

Splanchnic circulation includes the combined vascular beds of the intestines, pancreas, spleen and liver. The main vessels which constitute the splanchnic circulation are as follows:

Arteries supplying the blood to intestines, pancreas, spleen and liver (Fig. 4.6.14) include:

Coeliac trunk: It is approximately 1 cm long and after arising from the abdominal aorta, it divides into three main branches: the *left gastric artery, hepatic artery and splenic artery*.
Superior mesenteric artery.
Inferior mesenteric artery.

Hepatic portal system is formed by the veins draining blood from the abdominal part of the GIT. The veins comprising the hepatic portal system are shown in Fig. 4.6.15. All these veins end in the *portal vein*. The portal vein supplies the blood collected from GIT to the liver by its right and left branches.

Hepatic veins are terminal parts of an elaborate venous tree that permeates the liver. The hepatic veins emerging from the liver tissue end in the inferior vena cava.

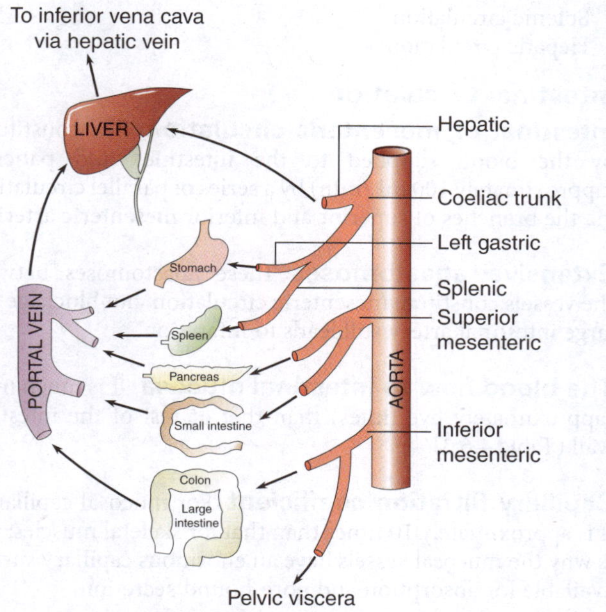

Fig. 4.6.14 Splanchnic circulation.

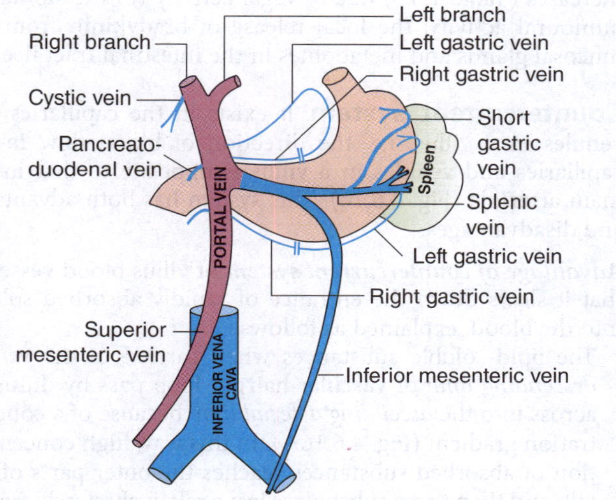

Fig. 4.6.15 Tributaries of portal vein.

SPLANCHNIC CIRCULATION: CHARACTERISTIC FEATURES

- During rest, the abdominal GIT, viscera and liver receive approximately 1500 mL of blood/min (approximately 30% of cardiac output) via coeliac, superior mesenteric and inferior mesenteric arteries (Fig. 4.6.14).
- If the entire GIT becomes simultaneously active, the splanchnic blood flow would have increased to approximately 4.0 L/min. However, since during digestion and absorption, the GIT is sequentially activated, the maximum circulation is approximately 3.0 L/min.
- The unique feature of the splanchnic circulation is that the venous blood from GIT viscera is not directly carried to the heart through systemic veins, but is carried to the liver forming hepatic portal system.

For the purpose of discussion, the splanchnic circulation is considered to consist of three parts:

- Intestinal (mesenteric) circulation

- Splenic circulation
- Hepatic circulation

Intestinal Circulation

Intestinal or mesenteric circulation It is constituted by the blood supplied to the intestines and pancreas (approximately 100 mL/min) by a series of parallel circulations via the branches of superior and inferior mesenteric arteries.

Extensive anastomoses These anastomoses between the vessels constitute mesenteric circulation, but blockage of a large intestinal artery still leads to infarction.

The blood flow to intestinal mucosa It is much more (approximately five times) than that of rest of the intestinal wall (Table 4.6.3).

Capillary filtration coefficient For mucosal capillaries, it is approximately 10 times than that for skeletal muscles; that is why the mucosal vessels have an enormous capillary surface available for absorption and pore-bound secretion.

During metabolic activity The blood flow to GIT increases (Table 4.6.3) due to vagal activity (in the stomach), humoural activity, the local release of bradykinin from the mucosal glands and metabolites in the intestinal tract itself.

Countercurrent system It exists in the capillaries and venules in a villus, i.e. the direction of blood flow in the capillaries and venules in a villus is opposite to that in the main arteriole (Fig. 4.6.16). This system has both advantages and disadvantages.

Advantage of countercurrent system of villus blood vessels is that it slows down the entrance of rapidly absorbed solutes into the blood, explained as follows:

The lipid-soluble substances when carried in the *venous descending limb* of vascular hairpin loop pass by diffusion across into the *ascending arterial limb* because of a concentration gradient (Fig. 4.6.16A). In this way, high concentration of absorbed substances reaches the outer parts of the villi and then these substances leave relatively slowly via the venous blood.

Disadvantage of countercurrent system of villus blood vessels is that it decreases pO_2 at the tip of villi as explained.

This system permits diffusion of O_2 from the ascending arterial limb of villi into the descending venous limb (Fig. 4.6.16B). In this way, at low flow rates, substantial amount of O_2 from the arterioles is shifted to venules near the base of villi resulting in decrease in O_2 supply to the mucosal cells at the tips of villi. When intestinal blood flow is very low, the transfer of O_2 from arterioles to venules is exaggerated and may cause extensive necrosis of intestinal villi.

Table 4.6.3 Blood flow to intestines (in mL/100 g/min)

Structure	At rest	During maximum metabolic activity
• Intestinal mucosa	50–60	300–400
• Rest of the intestinal wall	10	40

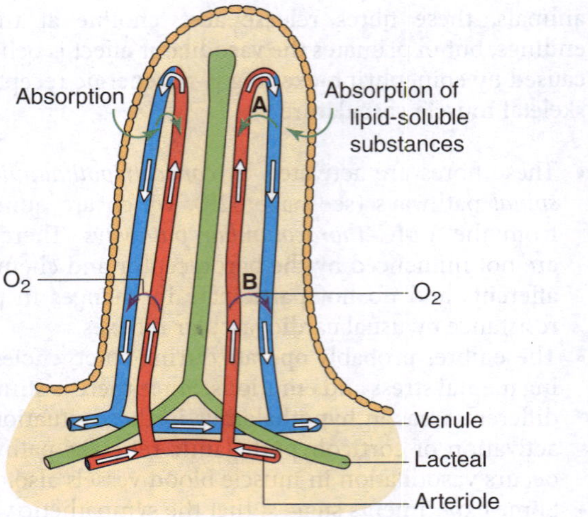

Fig. 4.6.16 Countercurrent system of villus blood vessels depicting transfer of lipid-soluble substances from venous limb to arterial limb **A**, and that of O_2 from arterial to venous limb **B**.

Regulation of Intestinal Circulation

1. Local chemical control (functional hyperaemia): During increased intestinal activity, i.e. after food ingestion, a marked increase occurs in the intestinal blood flow (*functional hyperaemia*). It is proposed that *gastrin, secretin, bradykinin and cholecystokinin*, which are secreted from mucosal glands during food ingestion, cause local vasodilation and augment the blood flow.

The absorption of digested food is also associated with increased intestinal blood flow. The principal mediators of mesenteric hyperaemia present in the digested food are glucose and fatty acids.

- As the digestive and reabsorptive processes proceed in different parts of the alimentary canal in a sequential manner, the blood flow also increases in the same pattern and so the maximum blood flow during these activities is approximately 3 L/min.

2. Neural regulation: The splanchnic vessels are richly innervated by noradrenergic sympathetic nerve fibres. These nerve fibres have mild tonic discharge, which causes a moderate vascular resistance in the splanchnic blood vessels. The direct effect of sympathetic stimulation is intense vasoconstriction of the arterioles leading to decreased blood flow. After few minutes of the vasoconstriction, blood flow returns back to normal by 'autoregulatory escape' phenomenon. Autoregulatory escape is the local metabolic vasodilator mechanism elicited by ischaemia that overrides sympathetic vasoconstriction. Therefore, sympathectomy causes only 25% increase in intestinal blood flow.

The main role of neural regulation of splanchnic vessels is in time of cardiovascular crisis, e.g. sudden hypotension, when more blood is to be transferred from the splanchnic vessels to systemic circulation. Under such situation, the splanchnic vasomotor nerves participate in the baroreceptor-mediated reflexes and their stimulation brings about a rise in systemic blood pressure. The main reason for this rise is not an increase in peripheral resistance but venoconstriction, which squeezes out blood from mesenteric circulation. This role of neural mechanism includes all the splanchnic vessels, i.e. intestinal, splenic and hepatic. The spleen and liver are major reservoirs of the blood. In this way, during hours of crisis, more blood is available to heart muscles and the brain than to the intestine, spleen and liver.

3. Autoregulation, i.e. ability to adjust its vascular resistance and maintenance of relatively constant blood flow over a wide range of arterial blood pressure, is well developed in mesenteric vessels like that in vessels of kidneys, brain, heart and skeletal muscles. The main mechanism responsible for autoregulation in mesenteric vessels is *metabolic*, though the *myogenic* mechanism may also play some role. The principal metabolic mediator here is *adenosine*. However, potassium ions and altered osmolality may also contribute to autoregulation.

Splenic Circulation

Splenic artery It is a branch of coeliac trunk, and supplies approximately 200 mL of blood per minute to the spleen during rest via its splenic branches, which enter the hilum of the spleen.

Spleen serves as reservoir of blood In spleen, two structures are involved in storage of blood, namely splenic venous sinuses and splenic pulp. The small arteries and arterioles open directly into the splenic venous sinuses (Fig. 4.6.17). Due to dilation of venous sinuses, a large amount of blood is stored in spleen and the spleen distends. The capillaries of the splenic pulp are highly permeable. So, lot of blood cells pass through the capillary membrane and are stored in the pulp.

The constriction of splenic venous sinuses It occurs by sympathetic stimulation, and causes release of blood into the circulation.

Regulation of Splenic Blood Flow

It is similar to that of intestinal blood flow. As mentioned earlier, the main role of neural control of splanchnic vessels is to transfer blood to circulation during hours of crisis. The spleen in the dogs and other carnivores contains lot of smooth muscles in its capsule, which contract strongly on sympathetic stimulation and discharge lot of blood into the circulation. This function of spleen is quantitatively not important in humans. However, reservoir function of the whole visceral circulation plays a vital role in this mechanism.

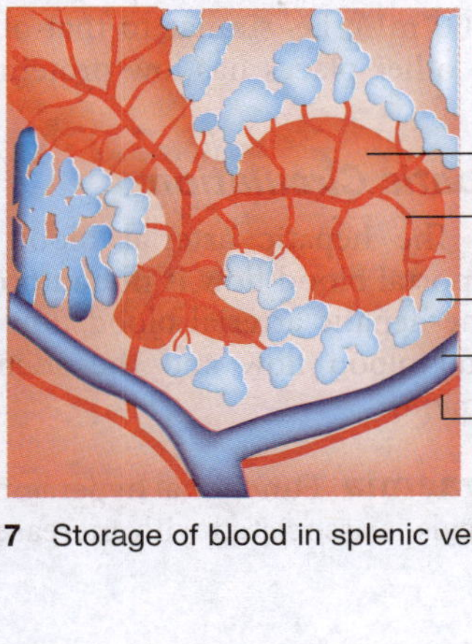

Fig. 4.6.17 Storage of blood in splenic venous sinuses and splenic pulp.

Hepatic Circulation

Characteristic Features of Hepatic Circulation

Source of blood Liver receives approximately 1500 mL of blood per minute from two sources.

Hepatic artery It is a branch of coeliac trunk, and supplies approximately 20%–25% (300–400 mL) of the total blood which caters to the metabolic requirements of the liver tissue.

Portal vein It collects blood from the mesenteric and splenic vascular bed, and supplies approximately 75%–80% (1100–1200 mL/min) of the total blood.

The hepatic and portal bloodstreams meet in the sinusoids.

Functional Unit of Liver

The functional unit of liver is *acinus*. The acini have been likened to grapes or berries, each on a vascular stem. There are approximately 10,000 acini in human liver. Thus, each acinus is at the end of vascular stalk containing terminal branches of portal vein, hepatic arteries and bile ducts (Fig. 4.6.18). Blood flows from these terminal vessels into the sinusoids, which represent the capillary network of the liver. The sinusoids radiate towards the periphery of acinus, where they drain into the terminal branches of hepatic veins. Blood from these terminal hepatic venules drains into progressively larger branches of the hepatic veins, which are tributaries of the inferior vena cava. For details, see page 359.

Zones of acinus Each acinus can be considered to have three zones: 1, 2 and 3 based on the pattern of vessels in the acinus described above (Fig. 4.6.19). The blood supply to different zones of acinus is as follows:

Zone 1 refers to the central portion of acinus immediately surrounding the terminal hepatic arteriole and terminal portal venule. This zone is *well oxygenated*. Enzymes involved in oxidative metabolism and glucogenesis predominate here.

Zone 2, i.e. the intermediate zone which is present in between zones 1 and 3, is *moderately well oxygenated*. It contains a mixed complement of enzymes.

Zone 3 refers to most peripheral part of the acinus. It is least well oxygenated and most susceptible to anoxic injury. It is rich in enzymes involved in glycolysis, lipid and drug metabolism.

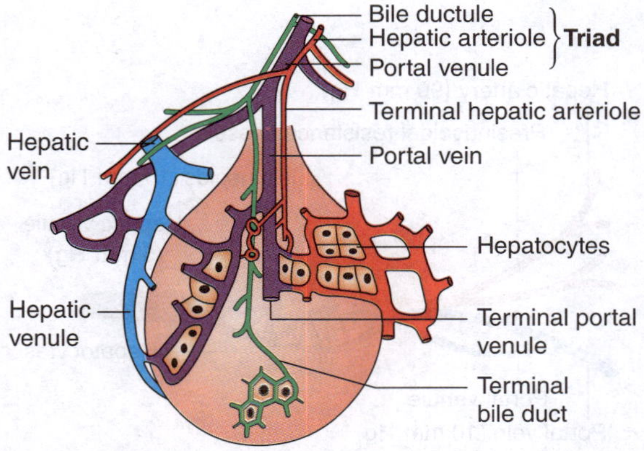

Fig. 4.6.18 Concept of acinus as functional unit of liver.

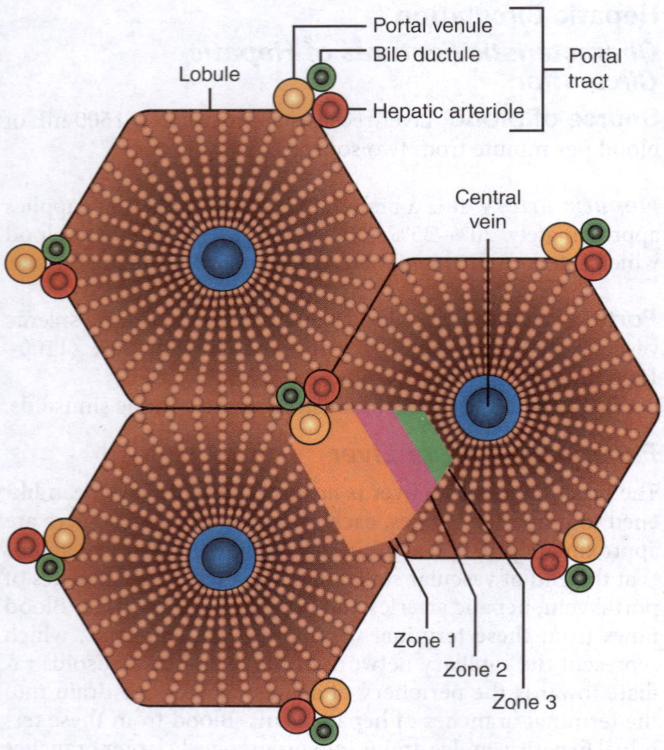

Fig. 4.6.19 Zones of acinus.

Hepatic Artery Versus Portal Vein Blood Flow

Pressure gradients and hepatic arterial and venous blood flow The mean pressure in the hepatic artery branches that converge on the sinusoids is approximately 90 mm Hg and that in the terminal portal venules which converge on the sinusoids is 10 mm Hg. The hepatic venous pressure is approximately 5 mm Hg (Fig. 4.6.20). From the above-mentioned pressures, one would expect sinusoid pressure to be very high. However, the sinusoidal pressure is only 10 mm Hg. This is because of the fact that due to high presinusoidal resistance in hepatic arterial tree, there is a marked pressure drop along the hepatic arterioles. The pressure drop in the hepatic arterial tree is adjusted so that there is an *inverse relationship between hepatic arterial and portal venous blood flow*. That is, when portal venous blood flow is low, the hepatic arterial blood flow increases and when the portal venous blood flow is high, the hepatic arterial blood flow

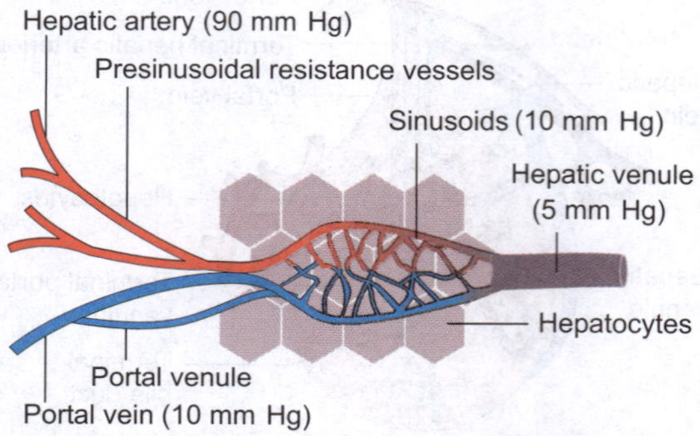

Fig. 4.6.20 Pressure gradient across the blood vessels of an acinus.

decreases. This inverse relationship may be maintained in part by the rate at which adenosine is removed from the region around the arterioles. According to this hypothesis, adenosine is produced by metabolism at a constant rate. When portal flow is reduced, it is washed away more slowly, and local accumulation of adenosine dilates the terminal arterioles increasing the hepatic arterial blood flow and vice versa. Thus, the hepatic arteriolar blood flow has *autoregulation* but the portal vein blood flow system does not have autoregulation.

Applied Aspects

As portal pressures do not increase linearly with portal blood flow, it is important to prevent fluid loss through highly permeable liver sinusoids. *Ascites in cirrhosis of liver* occurs because the parenchymal cells get destroyed and replaced with fibrous tissue that greatly increases resistance to blood flow. High hepatic vascular pressure can cause fluid transudation into the peritoneal cavity from hepatic and portal capillaries (ascites).

Oxygen supply to liver The hepatic arterial flow contributes 30% and rest of the 70% of the O_2 used by the liver is contributed by the portal blood flow. This is because of the fact that approximately 80% of the blood entering the liver is from portal venous system and 20% is from hepatic arterial system. During periods of activity, i.e. ingestion and digestion, there is marked increase of portal blood flow (functional hyperaemia) which compensates for the reduced content of O_2 per 100 mL of blood.

Though the rate of O_2 delivery to the liver is varied, it tends to maintain a constant O_2 consumption. This is made possible because of two reasons: first, the extraction of O_2 from the hepatic blood is very efficient, and second, liver has the capability to compensate by an appropriate change in the fraction of O_2 extracted from the blood. This extraction is facilitated by the distance between the presinusoidal vessels at the centre of acinus and postsinusoidal vessels at the periphery of acinus. In other words, the substantial distance between these types of vessels prevents a countercurrent exchange of O_2 as seen in intestinal villi.

Filtration Across Hepatic Sinusoids

The hepatic sinusoids are perforated and show large fenestrations, and, therefore, allow a free exchange of macromolecules across their wall compared with capillaries elsewhere in the body. Because of this reason, the liver lymph has very high protein content (6 g/100 mL), i.e. similar to that of plasma, while the lymph from other places has low protein content (2 g/100 mL).

Regulation of Hepatic Circulation

1. Autoregulation The hepatic arterial blood flow is autoregulated and the portal blood flow is not autoregulated. As described above, the hepatic arterial blood flow changes reciprocally with portal blood flow and the adenosine is involved in this adjustment.

2. Functional hyperaemia Functional hyperaemia of the intestinal tract after meals is associated with increased portal blood flow to liver.

3. Neural regulation The hepatic vessels are innervated by the noradrenergic sympathetic nerve fibres via T_3 to T_{11} roots and splanchnic nerves and the vasoconstrictor fibres reach the liver from hepatic plexus. There is no known vasodilator innervation to the liver vasculature. The liver serves as a blood reservoir, storing approximately 400 mL of blood in its sinusoids. The sympathetic nerves constrict the presinusoidal resistance vessels in the portal venous system and hepatic arterial system. As described in the neural control of intestinal blood flow (page 360), the neural effects on capacitance vessels are more important. Sympathetic stimulation causes a marked reduction in the capacitance of the portal system and other splanchnic capacitance vessels, and mobilizes approximately 1 L of blood towards the heart in less than a minute. In severe shock, hepatic blood flow gets reduced markedly and may produce patchy necrosis of the liver.

Self-Assessment

1. Discuss the characteristic features and regulation of coronary circulation.
2. Discuss the characteristic features, measurement and regulation of cerebral circulation.
3. Describe briefly about:
   - Hepatic circulation
   - Regulation of muscle blood flow
4. Write notes on:
   - Monro–Kellie doctrine
   - Triple response
   - Cold vasodilation
   - Reactive hypermia

Clinical Cases

Case 1

A 50-year-old male patient brought to the hospital emergency with severe chest pain radiating to inner side of the left arm, sweating, shortness of breath and palpitation. A probable diagnosis of myocardial infarction was made.

Q1. What tests should be performed to confirm the diagnosis and to start immediate treatment?
Q2. What immediate treatment should be started in this case?
Q3. If myocardial infarction (MI) is confirmed, then what further investigations should be carried out for localization of the infarct?

Case 2

A 40-year-old IT sector employee presented with pain in the sternal region radiating to left arm during morning walk. History revealed that the patient is a chronic smoker for more than 20 years. Investigations showed normal ECG and normal X-ray chest.

Q1. What is the probable diagnosis?
Q2. Which drug should be prescribed in this case and what is its mode of action?
Q3. What preventive measures should be followed to avoid further complications?

Case 3

A 60-year-old fatty female patient presented with facial drooping, falling of head on right side, weakness of the right side limbs, blurred vision and slurred speech. There was no history of any type of injury. On examination, the blood pressure was found to be very low.

Q1. What is the probable diagnosis ?
Q2. What is the cause for this condition?
Q3. Name the most important test to confirm the diagnosis.
Q4. Discuss the pathogenesis of this condition.

Case 4

In a class, a classmate had written his name on the friend's forearm with a sharp pencil. Immediately the name letters became red, and a few minutes later, there is diffuse swelling around the letters.

Q1. What is this condition?
Q2. What is the cause of reddening of name letters?
Q3. Why is there diffuse swelling around the letters?

Case 5

A labourer working in the snow for many hours developed pain, tingling sensation and blisters on the fingers.

Q1. What is this condition?
Q2. What is the pathophysiology of this condition?

Case 6

A 45-year-old person employed in a construction company working in a very cold and rainy environment for many hours brought to the emergency with cold red feet, having severe pain and pricking sensation and feeling of heaviness of feet.

Q1. What is the probable diagnosis?
Q2. What is the cause for this condition?
Q3. What is the treatment? What complications can occur if not treated timely?

4.7 Cardiovascular Homeostasis in Health and Disease

CHAPTER OUTLINE

CARDIOVASCULAR HOMEOSTASIS IN HEALTH

Cardiovascular homeostasis in health refers to the compensatory adjustments of the cardiovascular system (CVS) to the challenges faced by the circulation in everyday life. The common situations during which cardiovascular adjustment is required in day-to-day life include:

- Gravitational changes
- Intrathoracic pressure changes
- Exercise

CARDIOVASCULAR ADJUSTMENTS DURING GRAVITATIONAL CHANGES

Gravitational changes occur under the following conditions in life:

- Posture change from lying to standing
- Prolonged quiet standing
- Gravity acceleration (positive *g*), deceleration (negative *g*) and zero gravity (zero *g*)

Adjustments During Posture Change from Lying to Standing

When posture is changed from lying (recumbent) to standing (erect), the haemodynamic changes occur as a result of the effect of gravity on the blood column which tends to reduce the cardiac output and blood pressure. However, in humans, the compensatory mechanisms are so well developed that no effect is felt on posture changes in day-to-day life in normal persons. The sequence of events which occur during change in posture from lying to standing is explained below.

- In standing position, due to *hydrostatic (gravitational) effect of blood column*, for every centimetre below or above the heart level, the pressure increases or decreases, respectively, by 0.77 mm Hg. Therefore, in normal adults, the blood pressure at the level of feet (about 100 cm below heart level) in both arteries and veins is increased approximately by 80 mm Hg. Thus, the mean arterial pressure and venous pressure which are 90 and 10 mm Hg, respectively, in supine position will change to 170 and 90 mm Hg, respectively, on standing.
- Increased intraluminal pressure has no effect on thick-walled arteries, but the thin-walled veins distend and accommodate more blood. If the individual does not move, the *venous pooling* of 300–500 mL of blood occurs in the lower extremities.
- Venous pooling results in decreased venous return and so the cardiac output and thence the blood pressure is also reduced.

A drop in the blood pressure in carotid sinus and aortic arch within seconds triggers the *baroreceptor-mediated compensatory mechanism* which causes the following changes:

Heart rate is increased by 5–10 beats/min.
Force of cardiac contraction is increased leading to increase in stroke volume and cardiac output.
Peripheral resistance is increased due to arteriolar constriction in the cutaneous, renal and splanchnic circulation. Increase in peripheral resistance increases the diastolic pressure.
Venoconstriction in the body transfers blood from the capacitance vessels towards the heart increasing the venous return.

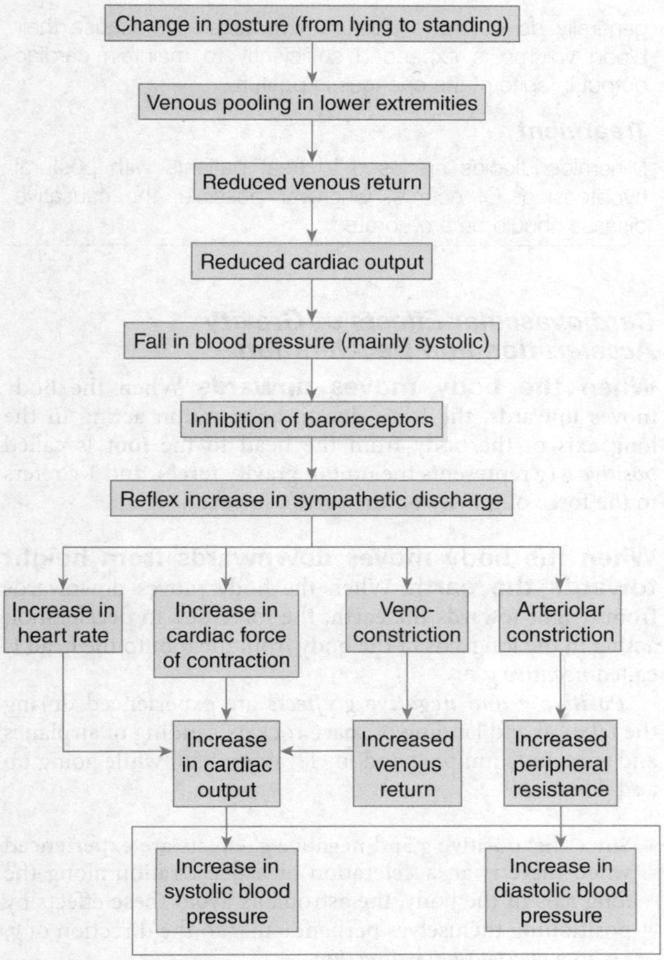

Fig. 4.7.1 Summary of events maintaining normal blood pressure during change of posture from lying to standing.

Increased secretion of renin and aldosterone also helps in normalization of blood pressure.

In spite of the above-mentioned compensatory changes, the stroke volume and cardiac output in standing posture are about 25% less than in supine position. However, due to 25% increase in the total peripheral resistance, the blood pressure becomes almost normal.

The above-mentioned events are summarized in Fig. 4.7.1.

Net Effects on CVS on Rising from the Supine to Upright Position

Average net effects which occur on the CVS on rising from supine to upright position after the compensatory mechanism are as follows:

- *Central venous pressure* is decreased slightly (3 mm Hg).
- *Heart rate* is increased by 25%.
- *Abdominal and limb flow* is decreased by 25%.
- *Stroke volume* is decreased by 40%.
- *Cardiac output* is decreased by 25%.
- *Total peripheral resistance* is increased by 25%.
- *Systolic blood pressure* is slightly reduced due to fall in stroke volume.
- *Diastolic blood pressure* is slightly increased due to increased total peripheral resistance.
- *Pulse pressure* (systolic BP – diastolic BP) is reduced.
- Mean arterial pressure is nearly unchanged.

Maintenance of cerebral blood flow Maintenance of cerebral blood flow in standing position is maintained by certain additional compensatory changes:

Decrease in jugular venous pressure (JVP) to 5 mm Hg due to gravity compensates for the drop in arterial pressure at head level to 20–40 mm Hg by reducing the drop in perfusion pressure (arterial pressure minus venous pressure).

Fall in intracranial pressure due to fall in venous pressure reduces cerebral vascular resistance and thus facilitates cerebral blood flow.

Increased pCO_2 and decreased pO_2 and decreased pH in brain tissues occurring due to decreased cerebral blood flow cause vasodilation, improving the blood flow.

Because of the operation of the above-mentioned *autoregulatory mechanisms*, the cerebral blood flow decreases only 20% on standing. In addition, the amount of O_2 *extracted per unit of blood increases*, and the net effect is that cerebral O_2 consumption is about the same in supine and erect positions.

The above-mentioned events are summarized in Fig. 4.7.2. For details, see page 353.

Changes during Prolonged Quiet Standing

When one changes posture from lying to standing, certain cardiovascular adjustments occur (described above) which maintain the almost normal blood pressure and normal blood flow to various organs of the body.

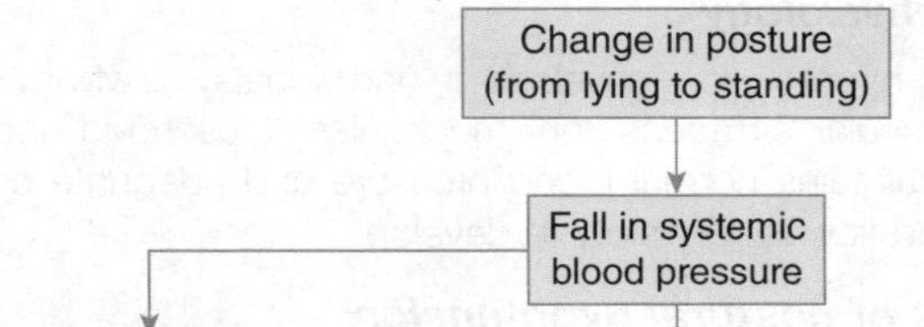

Fig. 4.7.2 Summary of events maintaining normal cerebral O_2 consumption in standing posture.

The prolonged standing presents an additional problem due to increasing interstitial fluid volume in the lower extremities. If the person keeps on moving, the operation of 'muscle pump' (see page 282) keeps the venous pressure below 30 mm Hg at the feet level and maintains adequate venous return. However, on prolonged quiet standing (a situation particularly met with military or police personnel, i.e. standing in attention for long periods), along with the venous pooling, the fluid begins to accumulate in the interstitial spaces because of increased hydrostatic pressure in the capillaries. The cardiac output is decreased due to decreased venous return. A stage may come when cerebral blood flow decreases to less than about 60% and symptoms of cerebral ischaemia develop. The individual may faint and fall down.

The fainting, in a sense, is also a homeostatic mechanism, because falling to horizontal position promptly restores venous return, cardiac output and cerebral blood flow to adequate levels.

Applied Aspects

Postural Hypotension

In postural hypotension or *orthostatic hypotension*, there occurs a sudden fall in blood pressure on changing posture from lying to erect, which causes symptoms of cerebral ischaemia. The individual experiences transient blurring of vision, dizziness or even fainting. It is diagnosed by recording blood pressure in lying and standing postures. A decrease in systolic blood pressure by 30 mm Hg or more on standing from supine position is diagnostic.

Pathophysiology

Postural hypotension develops in individuals in whom the cardiovascular compensatory mechanism (described above) which maintains normal blood pressure and adequate cerebral blood flow is very slow to develop.

Causes of postural hypotension

Causes of postural hypotension include:

1. ***Decreased blood volume:*** The effects of gravity on the circulation in humans depend in part on the blood volume. When the blood volume is low, the compensatory mechanisms are slow to develop and the individual may suffer from postural hypotension.
2. ***Sympatholytic drugs:*** Postural hypotension is common in patients receiving sympatholytic drugs.
3. ***Dysfunctions of sympathetic nervous system*** are obviously associated with postural hypotension. Dysfunction of sympathetic nervous system may be grouped as:
   i. *Surgical sympathectomy*
   ii. *Autonomic neuropathy* occurring in diseases such as diabetes mellitus, syphilis and Parkinson disease
   iii. *Primary autonomic failure* seen in the following conditions:
      - Bradbury–Eggleston syndrome (idiopathic orthostatic hypotension)
      - Shy–Drager syndrome (multiple system atrophy)
      - Riley–Day syndrome (familial dysautonomia)
      - Congenital deficiency of dopamine β-hydroxylase with little or no production of norepinephrine and epinephrine

Note: Patients with *primary hyperaldosteronism* also have abnormal baroreceptor reflexes. However, these patients generally do not have postural hypotension, because their blood volume is expanded sufficiently to maintain cardiac output in spite of the changes in posture.

Treatment

Mineralocorticoids are used to treat patients with postural hypotension. Of course, wherever possible, the causative disease should be ameliorated.

Cardiovascular Effects of Gravity Acceleration and Deceleration

When the body moves upwards When the body moves upwards, the force due to acceleration acting in the long axis of the body from the head to the foot is called *positive g* (*g* represents the unit of gravity force), and 1 *g* refers to the force of gravity on the earth's surface.

When the body moves downwards from height towards the earth When the body moves downwards from height towards the earth, the force due to deceleration acting in the long axis of the body from the foot to the head is called *negative g*.

Positive g and negative g effects are experienced during the take-off and landing of space rockets, landing of airplanes and parachute jumping and in elevators (lifts) while going up and down.

- Since the 'positive *g* and negative *g*' effects are experienced when there is an acceleration or a deceleration along the long axis of the body, the astronauts avoid these effects by positioning themselves perpendicular to the direction of *g*, i.e. in a *chest-to-back direction*.

Effect of positive g The effects of 'positive *g*' on the CVS are due to throwing down of blood in lower part of the body and similar to those occurring from change of posture from lying to standing, but they are multiplied depending on the speed of acceleration.

At acceleration less than 5 g At acceleration less than 5 *g*, the compensatory mechanisms are able to maintain vital cardiovascular status. *Cardiac output* is maintained for a time when blood is drawn from the pulmonary venous reservoir and as the force of cardiac contraction is increased, *cerebral circulation* is protected due to associated fall in the JVP and intracranial pressure.

At acceleration more than 5 g At acceleration more than 5 *g*, with the body in long axis, the pressure in the veins in the lower limbs rises to over 450 mm Hg. The consequent passive dilatation of veins of the lower limbs retains so much blood that the venous return and, therefore, cardiac output is markedly reduced. Under such a situation, vision fails (*blackout*) in about 5 seconds and unconsciousness almost hits immediately thereafter.

Antigravity suit Antigravity suit or the *g*-suit is used by the astronauts to effectively cushion the effects of gravitational force. The '*g*-suit' is a double-walled pressure suit containing water or compressed air. When there is 'positive *g*,' there is a tendency of venous pooling and simultaneously the water in the *g*-suit also rushes to the lower parts. The *g*-suit is regulated in such a way that it compresses the abdomen and legs with a force proportionate to the positive *g*. This decreases venous pooling and helps to maintain venous return.

Effect of negative g The effects of 'negative *g*' on the CVS are due to the rushing up of blood towards the head when the body suddenly moves down. As a result of accumulation of blood in the head and neck, the following changes occur:

Cardiac output is increased due to general increase in venous return. Most of the cardiac output, however, moves towards upper parts of the body.
Cerebral arterial pressure is increased markedly. In spite of the great increase in cerebral arterial pressure, the vessels in the brain do not rupture, because there occurs a corresponding *increase in intracranial pressure and their walls are supported*. In other words, the CSF acts like a *g*-suit.
Blood vessels of the head and neck show intense congestion.
Ecchymosis appears around the eyes.
Severe throbbing headache, pain and, eventually, *mental confusion* (redout) occur.

Effect of zero gravity The 'zero gravity' situation occurs when the astronauts in a spacecraft go out of the earth's gravitational effect, e.g. during orbital flights to other planets. The absence of gravity leads to:

- Weightlessness
- Effortless movements of the body
- Absence of hydrostatic pressure on the blood column

Data of 14-month stay in the zero gravity zone are available, which show the following documental effects:

Effects on the CVS include:

Transient postural hypotension Transient postural hypotension has been present after return to the earth from space flights, and full readaptation to normal gravity has been reported to occur in 4 weeks.
Some atrophy of myocardium Some atrophy of myocardium is reported to occur, because of the fact that the heart did not have to function for increases in cardiac output required in everyday life as on the earth. *More severe disuse atrophy of myocardium* is speculated in prolonged period of weightlessness during future trips to planets.

Other effects of zero gravity are:

Flaccidity and atrophy of skeletal muscles to some extent occurs since, due to zero gravity, the muscular effect is much reduced when objects to be moved are weightless and the normal proprioceptive input is decreased. A programme of regular exercises against resistance, e.g. pushing against a wall of spacecraft or stretching a heavy rubber band, may decrease the muscle atrophy.
Space motion sickness (nausea, vomiting and vertigo) develops in astronauts when they are first exposed to 'zero gravity' and often wears off after a few days of space flight. It can occur with re-entering the gravity. It occurs due to vestibular apparatus dysfunctioning.
Changes in the blood noted are as follows:

- Loss of plasma volume, probably because of headward shift of body fluids, with subsequent diuresis
- Loss of red cell mass
- Alterations in the plasma lymphocytes

Bone mineral is lost steadily with increased Ca^{2+} excretion. A loss of body Ca^{2+} is equivalent to loss of 0.4% of the total body Ca^{2+} per month initially, but later tapers off during prolonged space flight. Furthermore, a high-calcium diet helps to overcome this problem.
Psychological problems associated with isolation and monotony of prolonged space flight are also a matter of concern.

CARDIOVASCULAR ADJUSTMENTS DURING INTRATHORACIC PRESSURE CHANGES

Intrathoracic pressure changes are not uncommon in everyday life. Depending on the mechanism of intrathoracic pressure changes, the activities responsible for these may be grouped into Valsalva manoeuvre and Muller manoeuvre.

Valsalva Manoeuvre

Valsalva manoeuvre refers to a forced expiration against a closed glottis. The common everyday activities in which Valsalva manoeuvre effect is seen on the intrathoracic pressure are straining during defecation, initial phase of coughing and straining during parturition.

Intrathoracic Pressure Changes During Valsalva Manoeuvre and their Effects on CVS

Intrathoracic pressure changes during Valsalva manoeuvre and their effects on CVS are due to a sudden and sharp rise in intrathoracic pressure and can be described in four phases (Fig. 4.7.3):

Phase 1 is characterized by a transient rise in the arterial pressure. It coincides with compression of the aorta due to sudden increase in the intrathoracic pressure.
Phase 2, which follows phase 1, is characterized by:

- A fall in arterial pressure which plateaus after few seconds owing to reflex vasoconstriction.
- Heart rate usually increases slightly.

Mechanism: The phase 2 changes in CVS are initiated by a decrease in venous return which occurs due to increase in intrathoracic pressure changes. The sequence of events which follow decreased cardiac output is depicted in Fig. 4.7.3.

Phase 3 is characterized by a transient fall in blood pressure which follows 1–2 seconds after release of the strain. It coincides with release of pressure compressing the aorta due to decreased intrathoracic pressure. In other words, events in phase 3 are just reverse of the events in phase 1.
Phase 4 is characterized by:

- *Increase in arterial blood pressure* above the resting level within 10 seconds. This overshoot of blood pressure is due to the lingering effect of vasoconstriction induced during phase 2. The blood pressure returns to resting level after about 1.5 minutes of strain release.
- *Slowing of heart rate* occurs due to baroreceptor-mediated vagal stimulation in response to overshoot of blood pressure.

Clinical Application of Valsalva Manoeuvre

In clinical practice, Valsalva manoeuvre is used for testing of baroreceptor reflexes and also as a test for autonomic insufficiency where the vagal response may be impaired.

Procedure: The subject is asked to blow for about 15 seconds into a mouthpiece which is attached to a sphygmomanometer

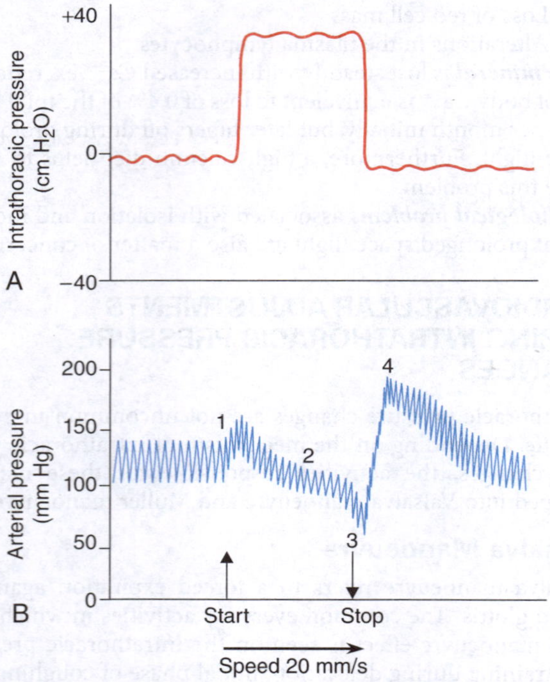

Fig. 4.7.3 Response to Valsalva manoeuvre in a normal person: **A**, intrathoracic pressure changes; **B**, arterial pressure changes in different phases (1, 2, 3, 4).

at a pressure of 40 mm Hg. A continuous recording of electrocardiography (ECG) is made during and after this manoeuvre. ***Interpretation of results:*** Results of this test are interpreted in the form of *Valsalva ratio*. Valsalva ratio is the ratio of the longest RR interval (noted within 20 beats of the end of Valsalva manoeuvre) to the shortest RR interval (noted during the Valsalva manoeuvre). The normal Valsalva ratio is >1.5, but in autonomic insufficiency, the Valsalva ratio is <1.11.

Muller Manoeuvre

Muller manoeuvre refers to forced inspiration against closed glottis. It is just the reverse of the Valsalva manoeuvre, i.e. it reduces the intrathoracic pressure (up to 80 mm Hg). Therefore, the cardiovascular changes occurring during Muller manoeuvre are exactly opposite to those which occur during Valsalva manoeuvre described above.

Cardiovascular Adjustments During Muscular Exercise

Severe muscular exercise is the most stressful physiological condition that the cardiovascular homeostasis mechanisms face in everyday life. In addition to CVS adjustments, respiratory and other adjustments also occur in the body, so they are comprehensively discussed in Chapter 12.1 on 'physiology of exercise' (see page 1169).

CARDIOVASCULAR HOMEOSTASIS IN DISEASES

Cardiovascular homeostasis mechanism operates in almost all cardiorespiratory and many other multiorgan diseases. The most important conditions which need special description are as follows:

- Circulatory shock
- Cardiac failure

CIRCULATORY SHOCK

Circulatory shock or simply called shock is a syndrome (collection of different entities that share certain common features) characterized by *serious reduction of tissue perfusion* with a relatively or absolutely inadequate cardiac output. In other words, the shock is a condition characterized by inadequate delivery of oxygen and nutrients to critical organs such as the heart, brain, liver, kidneys and gastrointestinal tract (GIT).

Types and Causes of Shock

Depending on the cause of inadequacy of cardiac output (relative or absolute), the circulatory shock may be of the following types:

I. Hypovolaemic shock
II. Low-resistance or distributive or vasogenic shock
III. Cardiogenic shock
IV. Obstructive shock

I. Hypovolaemic shock

Hypovolaemic shock, also known as cold shock, is caused by a low blood volume resulting in decreased cardiac output.

Causes Depending on the causes, the hypovolaemic shock may be of the following types:

1. ***Haemorrhagic shock*** occurs as a result of external or internal blood loss caused by ruptured vessels.
2. ***Dehydration shock:*** Fluid loss or insufficient amount of fluid can dehydrate the body and reduce the circulating blood volume. Fluid loss can occur from:
   - *GIT* in diarrhoea or vomiting
   - *Kidney* in diabetes mellitus, diabetes insipidus or excessive use of diuretics
   - *Skin* in burns, exudative lesions and sweating (in burns, large part of the skin gets denuded and large amount of plasma is exuded through the exposed parts; hypovolaemia due to plasma loss is a common complication of severe burns [burn shock])
3. ***Traumatic shock*** is a special type of hypovolaemic shock in which there is associated neurogenic shock caused by severe pain which inhibits the vasomotor centre (VMC).

II. Low-Resistance or Distributive or Vasogenic Shock

Low-resistance or distributive or vasogenic shock occurs when neural reflexes or toxic substances cause excessive vasodilation within the vascular system. Due to vasodilation, the size of capacitance vessels is increased and thus the cardiac output is decreased in spite of normal blood volume. Low-resistance shock is also called *warm shock* because the skin is warm and not cold and moist as it is in hypovolaemic shock.

Depending on the causes, the low-resistance shock is of the following types:

1. Neurogenic shock occurs due to two types of nervous effects:

i. ***Marked reduction in sympathetic vasomotor tone*** is responsible for most cases of neurogenic shock as seen in:
- Deep general anaesthesia
- Spinal anaesthesia
- Brain damage (prolonged ischaemia causes inactivation of VMC [***Note:*** Short periods of medullary ischaemia increase vasomotor activity])
- Effects of antihypertensive drugs
- Postural syncope

ii. ***Pronounced increased in the vagal tone*** of the heart is responsible for neurogenic shock in some cases, as seen in:
- Vasovagal syncope or emotional fainting

2. Anaphylactic shock: Anaphylaxis refers to an acute allergic reaction. Large quantities of histamine and histamine-like substances released in allergic reaction cause widespread and marked *vasodilation* reducing peripheral resistance. Also, there is a marked *increase in capillary permeability* leading to fluid loss and adding hypovolaemic element to the low-resistance shock.

3. Septicaemic shock: Septicaemia is a condition in which bacteria circulate and multiply in the blood and form toxic products and cause high fever. It may occur in conditions like acute peritonitis, perforation of bowel, strangulated bowel and puerperal sepsis. Septicaemic shock develops due to the following effects of bacteria and toxic products:

- Marked vasodilatation due to peripheral arteriolar paralysis
- Sludging of blood, presumably caused by red cell agglutination in response to degenerating tissues
- Disseminated intravascular coagulation (DIC)

4. Endotoxic shock refers to the shock produced by endotoxins released by Gram-negative bacteria. Endotoxins produce shock due to their following effects:

- Marked vasodilation reducing peripheral resistance
- Depressing myocardial contractility reducing cardiac output
- Increasing capillary permeability and causing hypovolaemia

III. Cardiogenic Shock

Cardiogenic shock occurs due to decreased pumping ability of the heart because of some cardiac abnormality. Severe depression of the systolic cardiac performance is the key factor in causing this type of shock. Since the heart is not able to pump out all the venous return, there occurs congestion of the lungs and viscera and that is why it is also called *congested shock.*

Causes Causes of cardiogenic shock are as follows:

1. ***Myocardial*** infarction involving 40% or more of the left ventricular myocardium is the commonest cause.
2. ***Other causes:***
   - Cardiac arrhythmias
   - Congestive heart failure
   - Toxic states of the heart
   - Severe valvular dysfunctions

IV. Obstructive Shock

Obstructive shock or, to be more precise, the extracardiac obstructive shock occurs due to impairment of ventricular filling during diastole due to some external pressure on the heart. Due to decreased ventricular filling, the stroke volume and hence the cardiac output is decreased causing circulatory shock.

Causes Causes of obstructive effusion shock are as follows:

1. Pericardial cardiac tamponade, i.e. bleeding into the pericardium with external pressure on the heart
2. Tension pneumothorax
3. Constrictive pericarditis
4. Pulmonary embolism
5. Post end-expiratory pressure respiration

Stages and Clinical Features of Shock

Stages and clinical features of all types of shock are similar with minor differences. However, since the haemorrhagic shock is more common, the discussion in this section will be centred on it. Depending on the severity, the circulatory shock can be divided into three stages:

- First stage or nonprogressive shock
- Second stage or progressive shock
- Third stage or refractory (irreversible) shock

I. First stage of Shock or Nonprogressive Shock

Nonprogressive shock, also known as *compensated shock* or initial stage of shock, occurs when there is a moderate reduction in cardiac output secondary to fluid loss or venous pooling or negative inotropic effect on the heart depending on the type of shock.

Hypovolaemic shock due to acute blood loss, in other words, the *haemorrhagic shock*, occurs when at least 10%–15% of total blood volume is lost. Thus, about 10% of the total blood volume may be lost without any significant effect.

Compensatory mechanisms of rapid onset (short-term mechanisms) immediately set into motion following the acute loss of blood and try to maintain the blood flow to vital organs in spite of reduced cardiac output. These mechanisms are effective in immediately controlling the blood pressure in nonprogressive shock and are followed by long-term compensatory mechanisms which restore the circulatory plasma proteins and red cell mass in 4–8 weeks. The compensatory mechanisms are described below in detail.

A. Rapid compensatory mechanisms (neural mechanism) Rapid or the so-called short-term control mechanisms primarily include the following three nervous reflexes:

1. Baroreceptor reflex When the blood pressure is decreased, there occurs decrease in the impulse discharge from the arterial baroreceptors (for details, see page 330). Even when the blood pressure has not fallen, the decrease in pulse pressure is sufficient to decrease the impulse discharge from baroreceptors. As a result, there is a generalized increase in the sympathetic vasomotor discharge to the heart, arterioles and veins. There occurs generalized vasoconstriction (sparing vessels of the brain and heart). Vasoconstriction is more marked in the cutaneous, splanchnic, renal and skeletal muscle vessels. This causes shifting of greater amount of blood in circulation. Venoconstriction on account of sympathetic stimulation also causes increased shifting of stored venous blood in circulation leading to increased venous return and cardiac output. In the kidneys, both afferent and efferent blood vessels constrict, but afferent vessels constrict to a greater extent leading to reduction in GFR. All these mechanisms maintain blood pressure at such a level that the blood flow to the vital organs like the heart and brain is not affected. However, blood flow to the vital organs is provided at the cost of other body tissues such as the skin, abdominal viscera, kidney and skeletal muscles.

2. Chemoreceptor reflex Acute haemorrhage causes loss of red blood cells leading to reduced O_2-carrying capacity. The resultant anaemia and stagnant hypoxia as well as acidosis stimulate chemoreceptors which also excite VMC to cause the same effects as those caused by baroreceptor reflex. Fall in blood pressure below 60 mm Hg usually initiates chemoreceptor reflex.

3. CNS ischaemic response When blood pressure falls below 50 mm Hg, this response is initiated (for details, see page 336). It causes more powerful sympathetic stimulation. This effect of central nervous system ischaemic response is called 'last-ditch stand' of sympathetic reflexes.

The rapid compensatory mechanisms discussed above account for the following:

Symptoms and signs Symptoms and signs observed in patients with shock are as follows:

Pale, cold and moist skin occurs due to decreased blood flow to the skin and increased sweating (due to increased sympathetic discharge).

Cyanotic tinge of skin may sometimes occur because of increased O_2 extraction from the blood.

Tachycardia and fall in pulse pressure produce *thin and thready pulse*, the characteristic feature of hypovolaemic shock.

Increased rate and force of respiration is due to greater sino-aortic chemoreceptor discharge.

Oliguria, another important feature of hypovolaemic shock, is due to renal arteriolar constriction.

Restlessness and apprehension may occur due to stimulation of brainstem reticular formation by circulating catecholamines, since haemorrhage is a potent stimulator of secretion of these hormones from the adrenal medulla.

B. Intermediate compensatory mechanisms

1. ***Renin–angiotensin vasoconstrictor mechanism*** (see page 338)
2. ***Reverse stress relaxation*** (see page 320)
3. ***Capillary fluid shift mechanism*** (see page 320)
   - The angiotensin–vasopressin, as well as reverse stress relaxation mechanism, requires 10 minutes to 1 hour to respond completely and help in raising the arterial pressure or circulatory filling pressure, thereby increasing venous return to the heart.
   - Readjustment of blood volume by absorption of fluid from interstitial spaces and intestinal tract, as well as oral ingestion and absorption of additional quantity of water and salt, may require 1–48 hours.

C. Long-term compensatory mechanisms

1. ***Restoration of plasma volume and proteins:*** After a moderate haemorrhage, the plasma volume is restored to normal in 12–72 hours. However, the improvement in blood volume is merely because of the increase in the amount of plasma water along with electrolyte content. The plasma protein concentration and haematocrit value is actually reduced (*haemodilution*). There is rapid entry of preformed albumin from extravascular stores. After this initial influx, albumin and rest of the plasma protein loss are restored by hepatic synthesis over a period of 3–4 days.
2. ***Restoration of red cell mass:*** In the meantime, there is excess release of erythropoietin which increases the rate of cell production in the bone marrow within 10 days. Normal cell mass is restored in 4–8 weeks.

Note: Under normal circumstances, the circulatory compensatory mechanisms described above eventually cause full recovery without help of outside therapy during the stage of nonprogressive shock. However, a timely outside therapy may hasten the recovery.

II. Progressive Shock

Second stage of the circulatory shock is a progressive stage which occurs after a 15%–25% loss of total blood volume. In this stage, the compensatory mechanisms are not able to stop the progression of the shock. In other words, the *intense arteriolar vasoconstriction* seen in this stage is usually not adequate for maintenance of normal blood pressure. In progressive shock, the structures of circulatory system begin to deteriorate and various types of *positive feedback mechanisms* develop. Therefore, timely therapeutic interventions are essential in this stage; otherwise, the vicious cycle of positive feedback mechanisms will cause progressive decrease in the cardiac output and ultimately the patient will go into a stage of refractory shock.

Positive feedback cycles Positive feedback cycles responsible for continuous progression of shock, if not interrupted by therapeutic intervention, leading to refractory stage are as follows (Figs 4.7.4 and 4.7.5):

1. ***Cardiac failure:*** Due to severe decrease in arterial pressure, particularly diastolic pressure, the coronary blood flow also decreases, and coronary ischaemia occurs. This weakens the myocardium and further decreases cardiac output and blood pressure. This positive feedback causes progressive cardiac deterioration and may ultimately cause complete heart failure.
2. ***Vasomotor failure:*** Blood flow to the heart and brain is usually preserved when cardiac output is decreased. However, there occurs very severe fall in blood pressure; there may occur cerebral ischaemia and failure of medullary VMC. Failure of VMC results in marked vascular dilatation causing venous pooling and decreased venous return. The cardiac output and blood pressure are further decreased.
3. ***Peripheral circulatory failure:*** Due to prolonged and intense vasoconstriction, there occurs hypoxia and accumulation of metabolites in the body tissues. The peripheral circulatory failure results from the following changes:
   - Capillaries and venules dilate due to the effect of local metabolites and there occurs peripheral venous pooling.

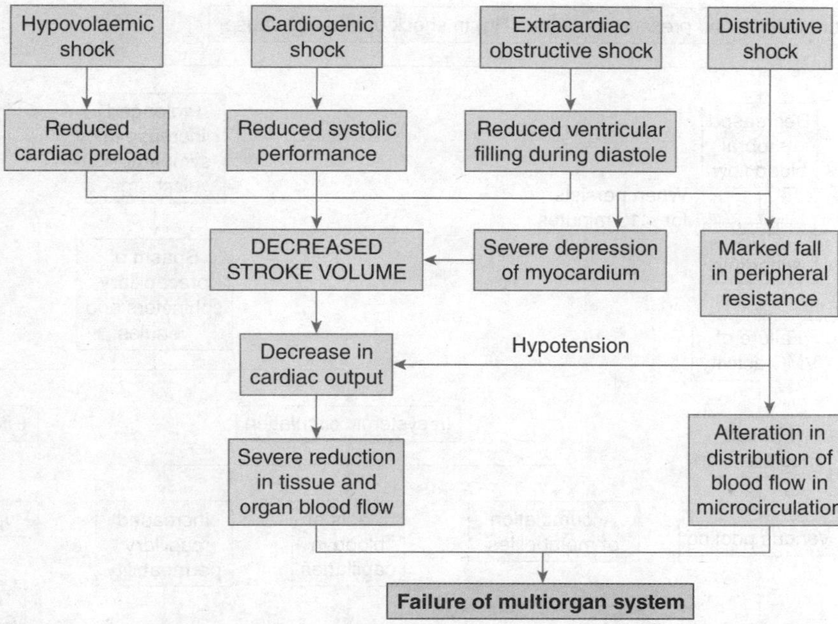

Fig. 4.7.4 Chain of events that ultimately cause failure of multiple organ system and refractive shock in different types of shocks.

- Prolonged capillary hypoxia results in increase in capillary permeability, and large quantity of fluid begins to transudate into the tissues. This decreases the blood volume and increases the shock.
- The pooling and sluggish blood flow in microcirculation leads to *intravascular clotting of blood*. Even if the vessels do not become plugged, the tendency for the cells to stick to each other makes it more difficult for the blood to flow through microvasculature, giving rise to a condition called *sludged blood*.

4. ***Septicaemia and toxaemia:*** Due to prolonged vasoconstriction of splanchnic vessels, there occurs hypoxia of GIT. The hypoxic damage causes a breakdown of normal protective mucosal barrier in the gut leading to the entry of the intestinal bacteria into the portal circulation. Simultaneous deterioration of hepatic functions permits bacteria and bacterial endotoxins to reach the systemic circulation leading to septicaemia and toxaemia. The endotoxins cause widespread failure of arteriolar and precapillary sphincter functions and cardiac depression. There occurs extensive vasodilatation. At this stage, no amount of treatment can restore the circulatory functions to normal.

Effect on body tissues in progressive shock In progressive shock, there occurs *widespread cellular degeneration* in the body tissues. Generalized cellular damage usually occurs first in highly metabolic tissues such as the liver, lung and heart. Liver cells are usually the first to be affected because hepatic cells have very high rate of metabolism and also the liver is the first organ exposed to toxins from the intestine through the portal vein.

The different damaging cellular effects that are known to occur include:

- Great decrease in active transport of sodium and potassium through cell membrane results in the accumulation of sodium in the cells and loss of potassium from the cells. So, the cell begins to swell.
- Mitochondrial activity in liver cells as well as in cells of many other tissues of the body is decreased.
- Lysosomes begin to split in tissues throughout the body, with release of hydrolases that causes widespread intracellular damage.
- Cellular metabolism of nutrients, such as glucose, is eventually greatly depressed in last stages of shock. The activity of some hormones is depressed as well, including a marked suppression of insulin action.
- Poor delivery of oxygen to tissues greatly diminishes oxidative metabolism and the cells switch to anaerobic glycolysis. This leads to the accumulation of lactic acid in the blood. Moreover, the sluggish blood flow through the tissue also results in the accumulation of CO_2 in tissue. The CO_2 dissolves in water to produce H^+ ions causing acidosis. Acidosis causes vasodilation which further aggravates the shock and a vicious cycle starts.

III. Refractory Shock

As mentioned above, when the shock is in the progressive stage and is not treated adequately, a vicious cycle of various positive feedback mechanisms (Fig. 4.7.5) sets in and the patient passes into the third stage of shock, the *refractory shock* (previously known as *irreversible shock*). In this stage, all therapeutic interventions are usually ineffective and eventually the patient dies.

Causes of refractiveness (point of no return) of shock The main factor responsible for irreversibility of shock is the *depletion of high-energy phosphate compounds*. The high-energy phosphate reserves in the cells of the body, especially the liver and heart, are greatly diminished in severe degrees of shock. The adenosine triphosphate is degraded in the cells to adenosine diphosphate and adenosine monophosphate and finally to adenosine. The adenosine diffuses out of the cell and is converted to uric acid, which cannot re-enter the cell. New adenosine is synthesized rather slowly (at a rate of 2% of the total cellular amount per hour); hence, once depleted, the high-energy phosphate stores of the body cells are difficult to replenish during shock and this contributes to the final stage of irreversibility.

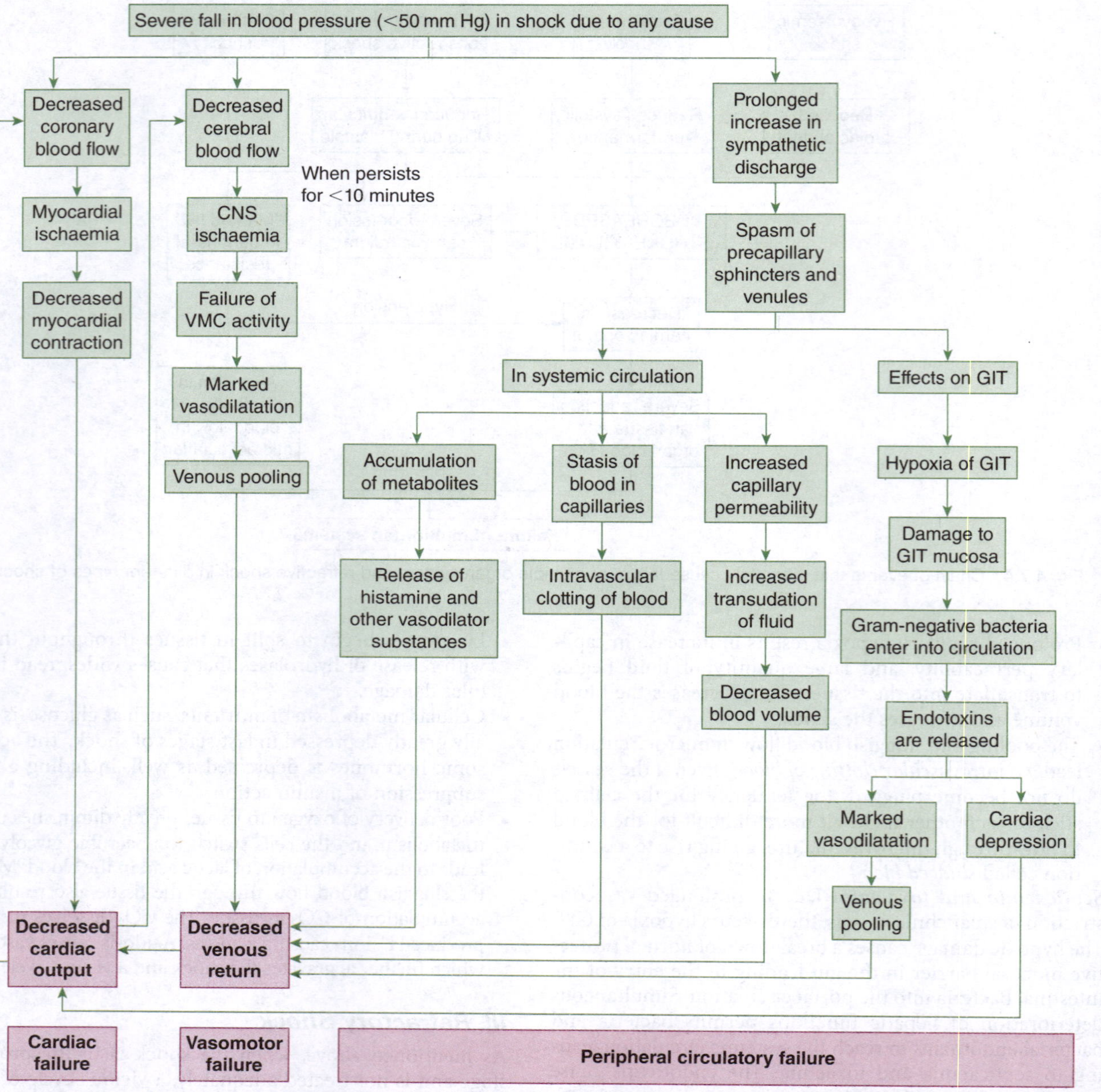

Fig. 4.7.5 Chain of events of various positive feedback cycles which cause progression of shock to refractory stage. ***Note:*** In severe haemorrhage (blood loss >40% of blood volume), the refractory shock develops due to this chain of events.

Tissue damage in refractory shock Slowly, necrosis of some cells of body sets in, especially the cells adjacent to the venous ends of capillaries which receive less nutrition than the cells near the arterial ends of same capillaries. Patchy necrosis first appears in the cells of the liver, kidney tubules, lungs and heart.

- In the kidney, *acute tubular necrosis* may occur, leading to acute renal failure and uraemic death.
- Deterioration of the lungs often leads to respiratory distress, the *shock lung syndrome*.

Treatment of Shock with Physiological Basis

The treatment of shock is aimed at correcting the causes and helping physiological compensatory mechanisms.

1. General measures for shock General measures for shock are as follows:

Room temperature: Where the patients with shock are kept should be cold. If exposed to heat, there will be sweating which will cause further hypovolaemia and aggravate the shock. It is important to note that most patients with shock are cold and therefore reflex warming of the body of a patient with shock with water bottles or providing warm environment, such as covering the patient with blankets, etc., will abolish the sympathetic discharge. So, the compensatory mechanism will be disturbed and shock will be aggravated and the patient may even die.

Raising the foot end of the patient's bed by 6–12 inches (*Trendelenburg position*) helps in promoting the venous return and thereby increasing the cardiac output. It is especially useful in haemorrhagic and neurogenic shock when the blood pressure is too low.

2. Replacement therapy Replacement therapy is very useful in hypovolaemic shock.

In haemorrhagic shock, the best therapy is transfusion of whole *blood*. When whole blood is not available, the *plasma* may be used. Plasma maintains the colloid osmotic pressure of the blood, but the haematocrit decreases with this therapy. If neither whole blood nor plasma is available, a plasma substitute such as *dextran* may be used. Dextran is a large polysaccharide which does not pass through capillary pores. It therefore promotes osmosis of water from the interstitial fluid to the intravascular spaces, thereby increasing the plasma volume.

In hypovolaemic shock with burns or interstitial obstruction, plasma infusion is the appropriate therapy. If plasma is not available, *dextran* can be used.

In hypovolaemic shock due to dehydration, intravenous infusion of *balanced electrolytic solution* (e.g. lactated Ringer's solution) is the appropriate therapy.

3. Sympathomimetic drugs Sympathomimetic drugs are useful as:

- Sympathomimetic drugs are usually not useful in haemorrhagic shock where the sympathetic system is already very active.
- These are especially useful in *neurogenic shock* and *anaphylactic shock* where the cause of shock is marked vasodilation due to lost neurogenic vascular tone.
- *Dopamine* should be the sympathomimetic drug of choice, because it produces renal vasodilation and, at the same time, produces vasoconstriction elsewhere in the body. It also has a positive inotropic effect on the heart.
- Epinephrine or norepinephrine drug may also be used when dopamine is not available.

4. Oxygen therapy Oxygen therapy may have some beneficial effects. In general, it does not have marked effect since the hypoxia of shock is of the anaemic or stagnant type and not of hypoxic type.

5. Glucocorticoids Glucocorticoids are useful in shock because of their below-mentioned effects. They are particularly useful in anaphylactic shock.

- They increase the strength of the heart in the last stages of shock.
- By stabilizing lysosomal membranes, they prevent release of enzymes of cells.
- They help in metabolism of glucose by the severely damaged cells.

HEART FAILURE

Heart failure is a pathophysiological state of the heart when cardiac performance is too low to maintain the cardiac output to meet the demands of the metabolizing tissues.

Pathophysiology

Cardiac failure can occur in the following three situations (Fig. 4.7.6):

1. Increase in Preload

According to *Starling law of the heart*, an increase in preload (end-diastolic volume) augments cardiac function, but when there is too much increase in preload (it operates through descending limb of Starling curve; see page 239), it leads to ventricular dilatation and heart failure.

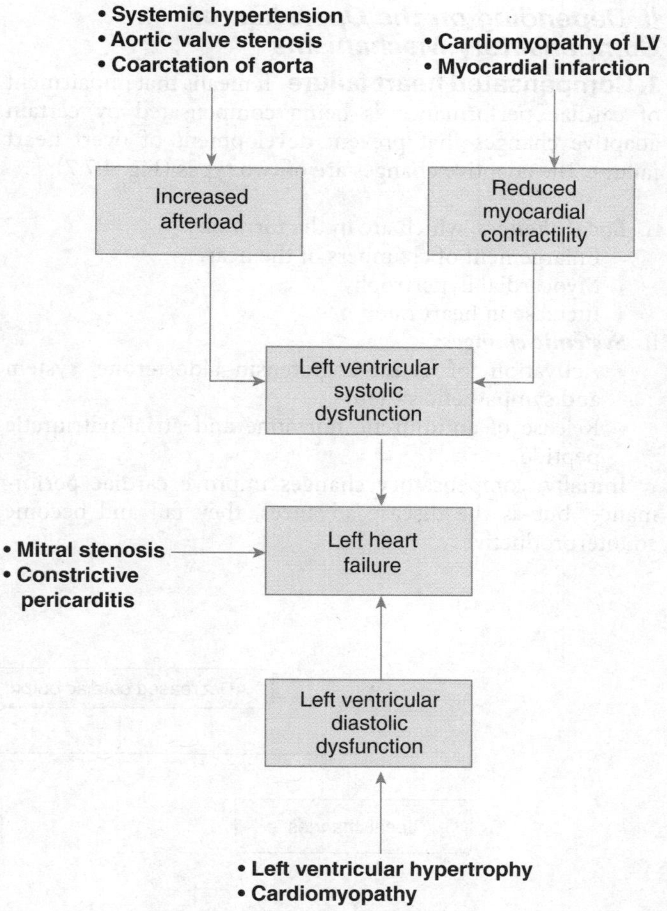

Fig. 4.7.6 Pathophysiology of heart failure.

2. Increase in Afterload

In case of increase in afterload (resistance), e.g. in hypertension, there is resistance to outflow of blood from the heart which causes overstretching leading to ventricular dilatation and heart failure.

3. Reduction in Myocardial Contractility

Reduction in myocardial contractility, i.e. decrease in pumping ability of the heart, decreases the cardiac output.

The interaction of these three variables leads to development of cardiac failure.

Types and Causes of Heart Failure

Heart failures can be classified by the following ways:

I. Depending on the Onset

1. Acute heart failure Acute heart failure develops suddenly as in patients with myocardial infarction.

2. Chronic heart failure Chronic heart failure develops due to gradual deterioration of heart functions, as in patients suffering from valvular diseases.

II. Depending on the Operation of Compensatory Mechanisms

1. Compensated heart failure It means that impairment of cardiac performance is being compensated by certain adaptive changes that prevent development of overt heart failure. The adaptive changes are of two types (Fig. 4.7.7):

i. ***Local changes***, which are in the form of:
- Enlargement of chambers of the heart
- Myocardial hypertrophy
- Increase in heart rate

ii. ***Systemic changes:***
- Activation of renin–angiotensin–aldosterone system and sympathetic system
- Release of antidiuretic hormone and atrial natriuretic peptide

Initially, compensatory changes improve cardiac performance, but as the disease advances, they fail and become counterproductive.

2. Decompensated or overt heart failure In the presence of certain precipitating factors such as infections, anaemia, pregnancy, thyrotoxicosis, arrhythmia and myocardial infarction or due to failure of compensatory mechanisms, compensated heart failure leads to decompensated heart failure.

III. Depending on the Involvement of Side of Heart

1. Left heart failure Anatomically, the left heart comprises left atrium, left ventricle, aortic valve and mitral valve. The left heart failure (LHF), therefore, refers to reduction in left ventricular output leading to elevation of left ventricular volume and pressure and its transmission to left atrium and pulmonary veins. The conditions causing LHF are as follows:

i. ***Left ventricular outflow obstruction*** due to:
- Systemic hypertension
- Aortic valve stenosis
- Coarctation of aorta

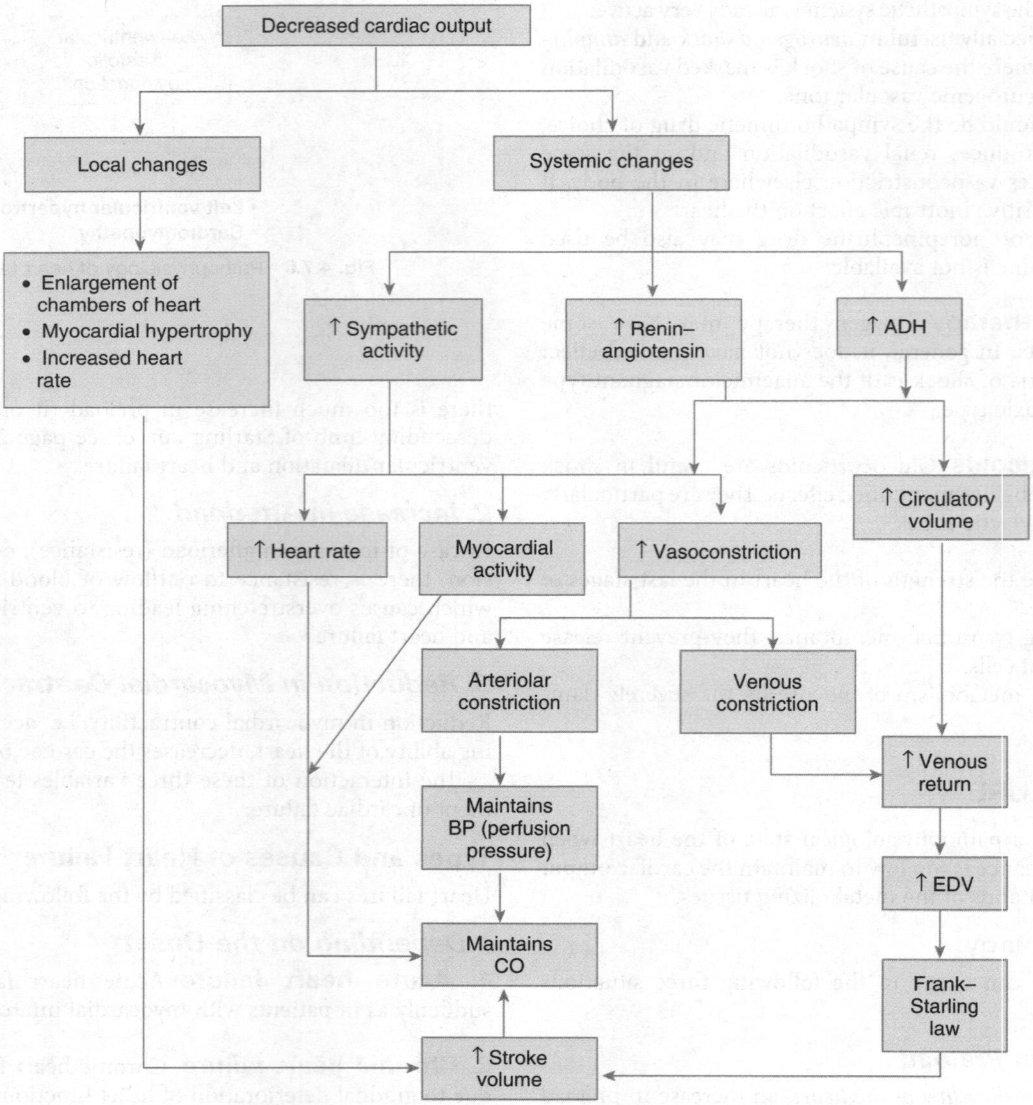

Fig. 4.7.7 Compensatory/adaptive changes in heart failure.

ii. ***Left ventricular inflow obstruction*** due to mitral stenosis
iii. ***Reduced ventricular contractility*** due to:
- Cardiomyopathy particularly involving left ventricle
- Anterior wall myocardial infarction

2. Right heart failure Like the left heart, anatomically, the right heart includes right atrium, right ventricle and tricuspid and pulmonary valves. Right heart failure is a condition in which there is reduction in right ventricular output leading to rise in right ventricular and right atrial pressure, which further causes rise in JVP, oedema, congestive hepatomegaly and congestion of viscera except lungs.

3. Biventricular (congestive) heart failure In this condition, there is simultaneous involvement of the right and left heart due to disease of myocardium, or left ventricular failure, and after sometime involvement of the right heart also.

IV. Depending on Inadequate Cardiac Output

1. Forward heart failure Forward heart failure results due to inadequate cardiac output.

2. Backward heart failure Backward heart failure is the one in which decreased cardiac output results in the elevation of the end-diastolic volume and thus increases the ventricular pressure. The elevation of left and right ventricular pressure results in pulmonary and systemic congestion, respectively.

V. Systolic and Diastolic Heart Failure

1. Systolic heart failure Systolic heart failure occurs due to poor myocardial contractility (systolic dysfunction).

2. Diastolic heart failure Diastolic heart failure results due to poor ventricular filling because of defective relaxation.

Both systolic and diastolic heart failures coexist particularly in myocardial infarction.

VI. High-Output and Low-Output Failure

1. High-output failure High-output failure is a state in which cardiac output remains high, i.e. at the upper limit of normal cardiac output (3.5 L/m^2/min), even though cardiac functions are depressed. Various conditions which result in high output failure are as follows:
- Fever
- Thyrotoxicosis
- Anaemia
- Beriberi

2. Low-output failure In this state, cardiac output remains at its lowest limit (2.5 L/m^2/min) at rest and in stressful conditions becomes further depressed, as in the case of heart failure secondary to ischaemic heart disease, hypertension, and valvular and pericardial diseases.

Clinical Features

Clinical features depend on the underlying disease and type of heart failure and these are as follows (Fig. 4.7.8):

1. *Features due to low cardiac output* are:
- Fatigue
- Hypotension
- Poor tolerance to stress
- Oliguria

2. *Features due to LHF* are:
- Cardiomegaly
- Cardiac arrhythmia
- Dyspnoea and orthopnoea

3. *Features due to right heart failure* are:
- Rise in JVP
- Hepatomegaly
- Peripheral oedema, ascites and hydrothorax

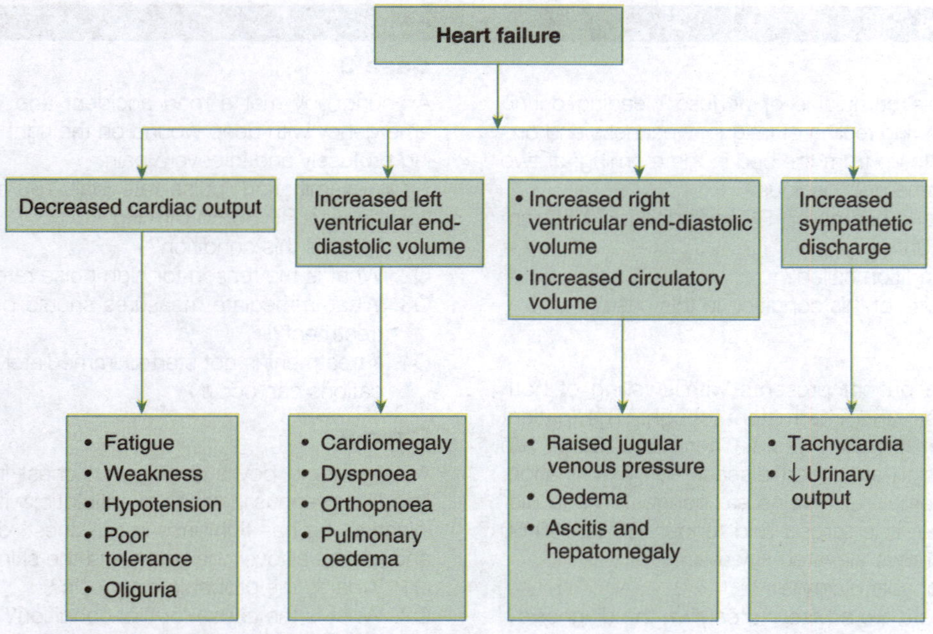

Fig. 4.7.8 Pathophysiological features leading to signs and symptoms in heart failure.

4. Features of chronic heart failure are:

- Raised JVP
- Oedema
- Congestive hepatomegaly

Diagnosis

The diagnosis of heart failure is mainly based on its clinical features and the following investigations are performed to establish the nature, severity and complications which have occurred:

1. Electrocardiography ECG findings may reveal arrhythmia, ventricular hypertrophy and myocardial infarction.

2. Exercise stress test For detail, see page 262.

3. Radiography of chest Radiography of the chest may show enlargement of the heart, congestion of the lungs and certain valvular defects.

4. Biochemical tests Biochemical tests include:

High-sensitivity C-reactive protein (hs-CRP) test helps in determining the risk of heart failure before the symptoms appear. High level of hs-CRP is associated with higher risk of heart stroke and cardiovascular disease.

Cardiac biomarkers are specific enzyme markers. Creatinine phosphokinase (CPK) isoenzyme is found in the heart; the high levels of cardiac enzymes can be the sign of heart attack and other cardiac problems.

Troponin protein is released into the blood when cardiac muscle is damaged. The troponin levels provide quick accurate measure of cardiac myopathy.

Estimation of blood urea and electrolytes for renal failure, hypokalaemia and hyponatraemia.

Echocardiography helps to identify the conditions which cause symptoms of heart failure. *Ultrasound and echocardiography* is used to assess the severity of associated haemodynamic disturbances.

Treatment

The basic principles of treatment of heart failure are aimed to:

- Remove the precipitating factors
- Correct the underlying cause
- Control the congestive heart failure state
- Prevent complications

In general, the following measures are used as a treatment of cardiac failure:

A. To reduce cardiac workload Complete bed rest is advised or the patient is hospitalized for 1–2 weeks.

- Small and light meals are recommended.
- Drugs (like sedatives and antianxiety) are prescribed.

B. To improve myocardial contractility Drugs like cardiac glycosides (digitalis) and sympathomimetic amines (dopamine) are prescribed.

C. To control fluid retention Dietary salt intake is restricted, and diuretics are given.

D. To reduce afterload Use of vasodilator drugs, especially angiotensin-converting enzyme inhibitors (captopril and enalapril), is recommended.

Self-Assessment

1. Discuss the pathophysiology, stages, signs and symptoms, tests for diagnosis and basic principles of treatment of circulatory shock.
2. Discuss in details the effects of gravitational forces on haemodynamics and its clinical implications.
3. Write notes on:
   - Cardiovascular adjustments during changes in intrathoracic pressure
   - Diagnostic tests for heart failure
   - Vasovagal syncope

Clinical Cases

Case 1

A 30-year-old female complains of perfuse bleeding during menstruation and having feeling of fatigue, weakness and dizziness when she gets up from the bed in the morning; at two instances, she became unconscious.

On examination, she has pallor; BP recorded is 80/55 mm Hg and heart rate 100/min.

Q1. What is this condition called?
Q2. What is the cause of this condition in this case?

Case 2

A 60-year-old male patient presents with swelling of both legs, breathlessness and intermittent cough. The patient is a chronic smoker for many years. There is no family h/o diabetes, hypertension and heart disease. On examination, there is pitting oedema, neck veins are congested and distended, and the liver is enlarged and tender. BP is 100/60 mm Hg and ECG shows elevated P wave.

Q1. What is the probable diagnosis?
Q2. What further tests are advised to confirm the diagnosis?
Q3. What is the pathophysiology of this condition?

Case 3

A young boy met a road accident and was brought to the emergency with deep wound on the right leg and arm, bleeding profusely and in severe pain.

On examination, pulse rate was 150/min, feeble and low volume, and BP 80/60 mm Hg.

Q1. What is this condition?
Q2. What is the reason for high pulse rate and low BP?
Q3. What immediate measures should be taken to start the treatment?
Q4. If treatment is not started immediately, then what complications can occur?

Case 4

A 10-year-old boy suffering with chest infection is administered intravenous injection of antibiotic; within 5 minutes of the injection, he has tightness in the chest, difficulty in breathing and rashes all over the body, and the skin becomes red.

Q1. What is the probable diagnosis?
Q2. What is the cause for this condition?
Q3. What is the immediate treatment for this condition?

RESPIRATORY SYSTEM

SECTION 5

SECTION OUTLINE

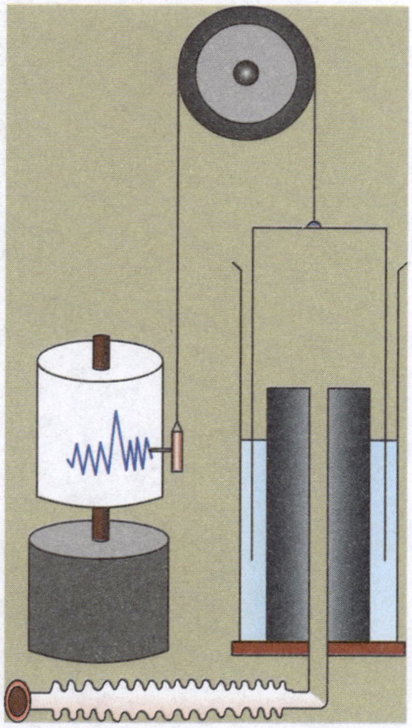

INTRODUCTION

The word respiration has been derived from the Latin word 'respirae' which means to breathe. The primary role of the respiratory system is to provide O_2 to the tissues for metabolic needs and remove the CO_2 formed by them. An adult body consumes about 250 mL of O_2 and produces about 200 mL of CO_2 per minute. Respiration entails two processes – the external respiration and internal respiration.

The *internal respiration* or tissue respiration refers to utilization of O_2 and production of CO_2 by the tissue. It is generally considered the domain of biochemistry.

The *external respiration* includes supply of O_2 to the tissues from the environment and excretion of CO_2 released by the tissues into the atmosphere. The process of external respiration involves three major events:

- *Pulmonary ventilation* refers to exchange of gases between the environment and the lungs. It includes mechanics of respiration.

- *Pulmonary diffusion* refers to transfer of gases from the alveoli to the blood by diffusion across the respiratory membrane. To understand the process of pulmonary diffusion, it is essential to understand facts about *pulmonary circulation* and the *properties of gases* and the laws governing diffusion of gases.
- The process of external respiration also involves transport of gases from the blood to the body cells and back.

The *respiratory adjustments in health and diseases* are essential for life, and to understand these, knowledge about *regulation of respiration* is must.

The study of respiration without the concepts about functional anatomy of the respiratory system will not be easy, and so has been discussed in the very first chapter of this section.

5.1 Respiratory Tract: Structure and Functions

CHAPTER OUTLINE

Functional Anatomy
- Respiratory Passages
- Respiratory Parenchyma
- Respiratory Membrane
- Blood Supply
- Innervation

Functions of the Respiratory System
- Respiratory Functions
- Nonrespiratory Functions

FUNCTIONAL ANATOMY

The chief organs of the respiratory system are right and left *lungs*. The oxygen contained in the atmospheric air reaches the lungs by passing through a series of respiratory passages which also serve for removal of CO_2 from the alveoli to the atmosphere. The respiratory system also includes a pump that ventilates the lung. This pump consists of the chest wall and respiratory muscles. Salient points about functional anatomy of respiratory passages and lungs are discussed here. Functional anatomy of the chest wall and RESPIRATORY muscles is discussed in Chapter 5.2 in 'Pulmonary Ventilation' (page 385) which includes the mechanics of respiration.

RESPIRATORY PASSAGES

Respiratory passages include the following structures (Fig. 5.1.1):

1. Nasal Cavities

The air enters the body through right and left anterior (external) nares which open into the right and left nasal cavities. Through the posterior (internal) nares, the nasal cavities open into the pharynx. The nasal cavities warm up the air to the body temperature, humidify the air to 100% saturation, and clean and filter the air of its particulate content by channelling the air through a tortuous path between the turbinates. The particles are deposited at the bends where they adhere to the mucus layering the nasal cavity.

2. Pharynx

From above downwards, the pharynx is divided into nasopharynx, oropharynx and laryngopharynx. Air from nasal cavities enters the nasopharynx and passes down through the oropharynx and laryngopharynx to the larynx. From the mouth, the air can directly pass to the oropharynx.

3. Larynx

It is continuous above with the laryngopharynx and below with the trachea. The air passes through the glottis (the triangular space between vocal cords) into the trachea. Apart from being a respiratory passage, the larynx also acts as a voice box.

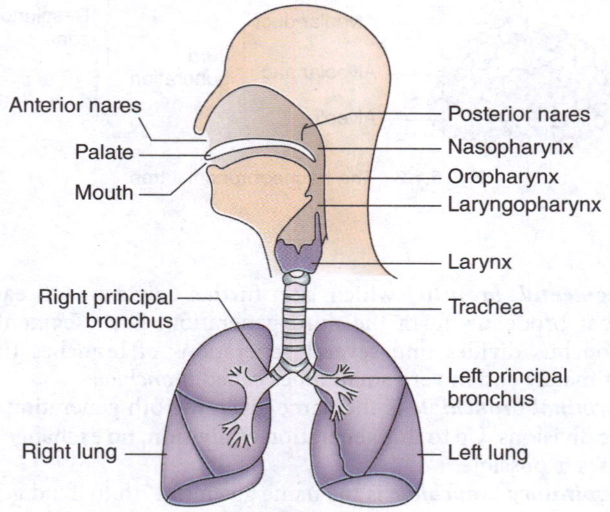

Fig. 5.1.1 The air passages.

4. Tracheobronchial Tree

The air passages between the trachea and the alveoli divide 23 times to form the extensive tracheobronchial tree (Fig. 5.1.2). These multiple divisions greatly increase the total cross-sectional area of the airway from 2.5 cm^2 in the trachea to 11,800 cm^2 in the alveoli. Consequently, the velocity of air flow in the small airway declines to very low values. The 23 generations of divisions of the tracheobronchial tree have been numbered as follows:

The trachea The trachea is designated as generation zero.

The principal bronchi Right and left *bronchi* which are two major divisions of the trachea constitute the first generation.

Lobar bronchi, which are division of the principal bronchus, form the second generation.

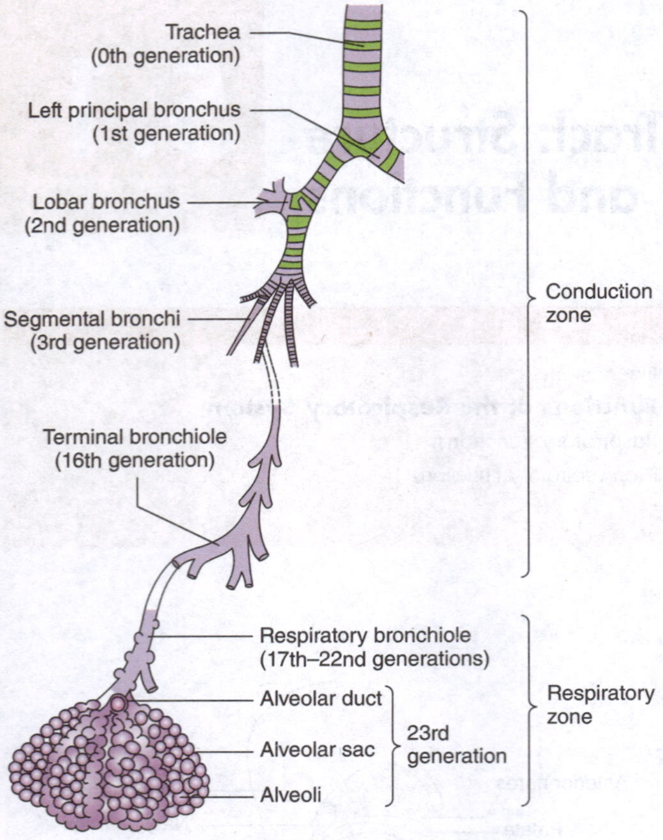

Fig. 5.1.2 The tracheobronchial tree.

Segmental bronchi, which are further division of each lobar bronchus, form the third generation. Each segmental bronchus divides into several generations of branches that ultimately end in very small tubes called *bronchioles*.

Terminal bronchiole is the name given to 16th generation of the divisions. Up to this generation of division, no exchange of gases is possible.

Respiratory bronchiole is the name given to 17th to 22nd generations of divisions. These are labelled as respiratory bronchioles, because some exchange of gases is possible in these tubes.

Alveolar ducts alveoli and alveolar sacs form the 23rd generation of division. It is here that most of the O_2 and CO_2 exchange occurs.

Thus, from the functional point of view, the tracheobronchial tree can be divided into two major zones:

i. Conducting zone Conducting zone of the air passages is formed by the first 16 generations of passages and it only transports gases from and to the exterior. Thus, conducting zone starts from the trachea and extends up to terminal bronchioles. Since no exchange of gases is possible here, starting from the nose to the terminal bronchioles forms the so-called *dead space* which has a total capacity of approximately 150 mL.

ii. Respiratory zone The remaining seven generations of the tracheobronchial tree which include the respiratory bronchioles, alveolar ducts and alveoli form the respiratory zone, where exchange of gases occurs. Its volume is approximately 4 L.

Histological features of the tracheobronchial tree The histological features vary in different generations of the tracheobronchial tree. However, the general characteristics of the wall of the respiratory tract from exterior to interior are as follows (Fig.5.1.3):

1. Cartilaginous rings Cartilaginous rings are present in the trachea and initial bronchi of few generations. These are absent in terminal bronchioles and respiratory bronchioles. The cartilaginous rings of the trachea are incomplete on their posterior aspect. This allows some contraction of the trachea but tracheal lumen cannot be completely obliterated easily.

2. Smooth muscles Ends of cartilaginous rings of the trachea are approximated by transverse smooth muscle fibres. In bronchi, bands of fibres tend to become circular so that in terminal bronchioles they are present in large amount and form a sphincter. Smooth muscles are not present in alveoli.

3. Lamina propria Contains elastic fibres that play a role of elastic recoil of trachea during respiratory movements.

4. Epithelial lining Epithelial lining in the trachea and large bronchi is ciliated pseudostratified columnar and becomes cuboidal in bronchioles and simple squamous in alveoli. The epithelial cells of the tracheobronchial tree are ciliated. Cilia are absent in alveoli.

- Efficiency of ciliated cells of the trachea and bronchi in propelling mucus and waste products is of higher order. Cilia are not influenced by nerve impulses.
- The mucus-secreting goblet cells and deep serous glands are present in the trachea and bronchi but are absent in bronchioles and alveoli (Fig. 5.1.3).

Important Note

- The cartilaginous rings are absent in respiratory bronchioles onwards.
- Mucus-secreting cells are absent in bronchioles and alveoli.

RESPIRATORY PARENCHYMA

Each respiratory unit consists of one respiratory bronchiole which opens into a number of alveolar ducts, and each alveolar duct in turn opens into a number of alveoli. The two lungs contain about 300 million alveoli. Each alveolus has a diameter of about 0.2 μm. The alveoli are surrounded by pulmonary capillaries. The total area of the alveolar walls in contact with capillaries in both the lungs is about 70 m^2.

Microscopic Structure of Alveolus (Fig. 5.1.4)

Each alveolus is lined by two types of epithelial cells.

Type I cells are flat cells with large cytoplasmic extensions and are the primary lining cells that cover around 95% of alveolar epithelial surface. These cells play significant role in alveolar repair.

Type II cells (granular pneumocytes) are thicker and contain numerous lamellar inclusion bodies that cover approximately 5% of alveolar lining. These cells secrete *surfactant*. For detail, see page 394.

The alveolar wall also contains:

Other special types of epithelial cells:

- *Pulmonary alveolar macrophages* (PAMs) which are active phagocytic cells and significant defensive role (for details, see page 382)

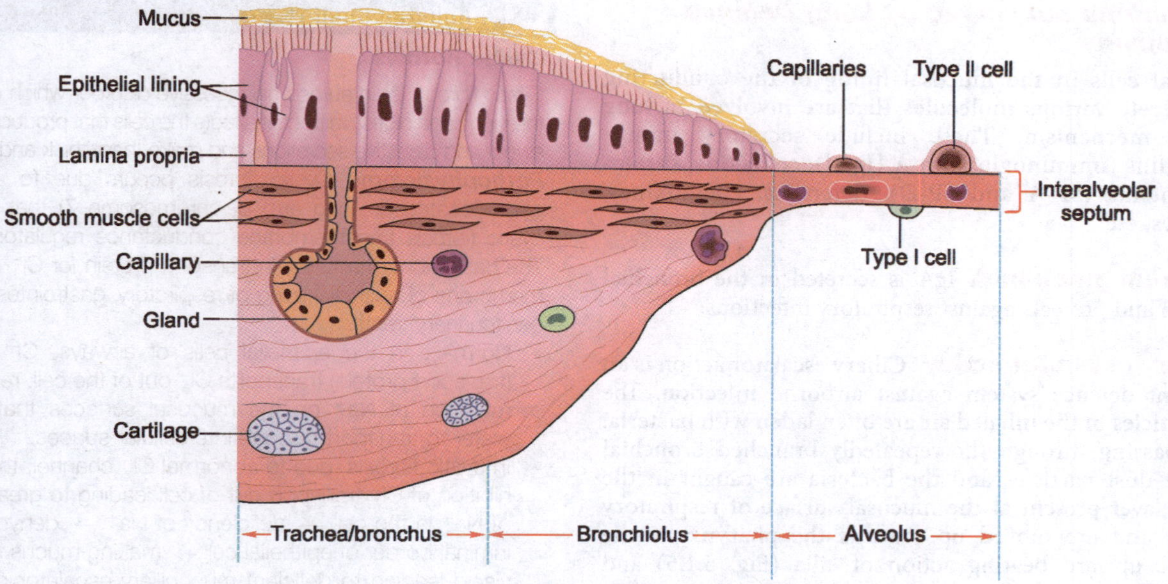

Fig. 5.1.3 Histological features of lining of tracheobronchial tree.

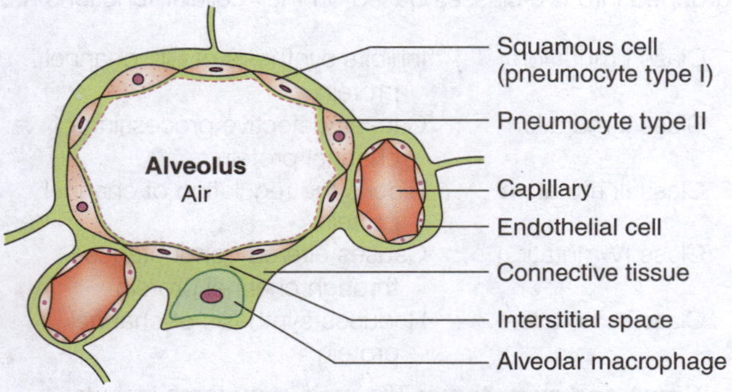

Fig. 5.1.4 Microscopic structure of alveolus.

- *Lymphocytes*
- *Plasma cells* which form and secrete immunoglobulins
- *Amine precursor uptake and decarboxylation* (APUD) *cells* which store and secrete many biologically active peptidases, e.g. vasoactive intestinal peptide (VIP) and substance P
- *Mast cells* which contain heparin, various lipids, histamine and various proteases that participate in allergic reactions

Communication between the two alveoli occurs through small pores, called *pores of Kohn*.

RESPIRATORY MEMBRANE

Respiratory membrane is the name given to the tissues which separate the capillary blood from the alveolar air. It is important to understand the structure of a respiratory membrane for better understanding of diffusion of gases between alveoli and capillary blood, so it is described in detail in Chapter 5.4 (page 414).

BLOOD SUPPLY

Conducting airway is supplied by systemic blood, whereas the respiratory zone of the lung is supplied by deoxygenated (venous) blood coming through pulmonary arteries to lungs. Blood is oxygenated in lungs and is returned to left atrium via pulmonary veins. For details, see Chapter 5.3, page 401.

INNERVATION

The walls of bronchi and bronchioles are innervated by the autonomic nervous system.

Parasympathetic fibres innervate through vagus nerve. Their stimulation causes cholinergic discharge producing bronchoconstriction and increased bronchial secretion via muscarinic receptors.

Sympathetic nerves supplying the lungs when stimulated cause bronchodilation and decreased bronchial secretion via adrenergic receptors, predominantly by β_2-receptors, whereas α_1-adrenergic receptors inhibit bronchial secretions.

Afferents from the lungs pass through vagi nerves.

FUNCTIONS OF THE RESPIRATORY SYSTEM

RESPIRATORY FUNCTIONS

The main function of the respiratory system in general and lung in particular is exchange of gases between atmosphere and body tissue.

It involves:

- Pulmonary ventilation, i.e. exchange of gases between the atmosphere and the lungs. Details are discussed in Chapter 5.2.
- Pulmonary diffusion, i.e. transfer of gases from the lungs to the blood across the respiratory membrane. For details, see Chapter 5.4.
- Transport of gases from blood to tissue and back. Details are discussed in Chapter 5.5.

NONRESPIRATORY FUNCTIONS

Besides the respiratory functions, the respiratory system performs many important nonrespiratory functions which include:

A. Functions Subserved by Lung Defence Mechanisms

Epithelial cells in the mucosal lining of the conducting zone secrete various molecules that are involved in lung defence mechanism. These include secretory immunoglobulins (immunoglobulin A [IgA]), collectins, surfactant proteins (SP-A and SP-D), defensins, chemokines, cytokines, etc.

1. Immunoglobulin A IgA is secreted in the bronchial secretion and protects against respiratory infections.

2. Ciliary escalator action Ciliary escalator action is an important defence system against airborne infection. The dust particles in the inhaled air are often laden with bacteria. While passing through the repeatedly branched bronchial tree, the dust particles and the bacteria are caught in the mucous layer present at the mucosal surface of respiratory passages and are moved up towards the pharynx by the rhythmic upward beating action of cilia (Fig. 5.1.5) and swallowed.

> **Important Note**
>
> Cigarette smoke disturbs the ciliary function. That explains the higher incidence of respiratory infections in smokers than in nonsmokers.

3. Bronchiolar nonciliated epithelial cells are also known as club cells or Clara cells.

- The primary function of these cells is to provide secretory surfactants A, B and D and other specific proteins that contribute airway epithelial lining fluid.
- These cells serve as progenitor cells for ciliated and secretory epithelial cells and thus help during repair.
- These cells metabolize the xenobiotics.

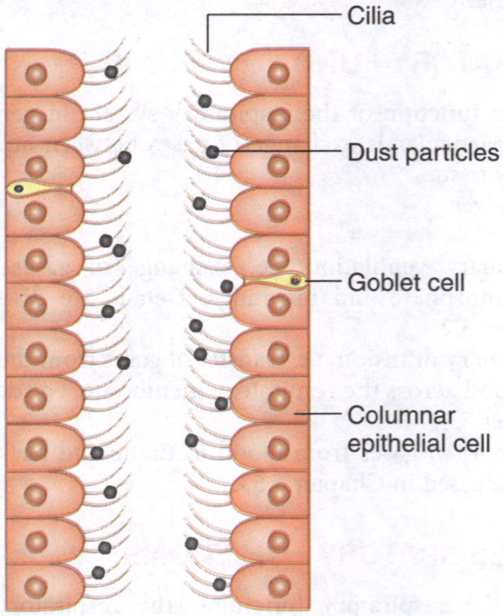

Fig. 5.1.5 Ciliary escalator action of the respiratory mucosa.

> **Applied Aspects**
>
> **Cystic fibrosis**
>
> Cystic fibrosis is an autosomal recessive disorder which damages the lungs and digestive tract. It affects the cells that produce mucus, sweat and digestive secretions and make them thick and sticky
>
> ***Pathophysiology***. Cystic fibrosis occurs due to abnormal gene (located on long arm of chromosome 7) that encodes cystic fibrosis transmembrane conductance regulator (CFTR). The basic abnormality lies in transport protein for Cl^- on apical membrane of epithelial lining of respiratory, gastrointestinal and genitourinary tracts.
>
> - Normally in the epithelial cells of airways, Cl^- channel (transport protein) transports Cl^- out of the cell, resulting in retention of Na^+ on the mucosal surfaces that causes water to transport through intercellular spaces.
> - In cystic fibrosis, due to abnormal Cl^- channel, there is inhibition of Cl^- transport out of cell leading to greater influx of Na^+ in the cell → deficiency of Na^+ → dehydration of luminal border of epithelial cell → making mucus thick and viscid leading to deficient mucociliary escalator clearance → leading to infection.
>
> The mutations in *CFTR* gene that cause cystic fibrosis are grouped into five classes based on their cellular functions as:
>
> | | | |
> |---|---|---|
> | Class I mutation | : | Inhibits synthesis of Cl^- channel protein |
> | Class II mutation | : | Causes defective processing of channel protein |
> | Class III mutation | : | Blocks the regulation of channel protein |
> | Class IV mutation | : | Causes altered conductance through channel protein |
> | Class V mutation | : | Reduces synthesis of channel protein |
>
> ***Signs and symptoms:*** The main symptoms include:
>
> - Recurring lung infections
> - Persistent cough
> - Wheezing and shortness of breath
> - Poor growth
>
> ***Therapeutic measures***. In cystic fibrosis include:
>
> - Chest physiotherapy and mucolytic agents to loosen thick mucus are advised
> - Antibiotics to prevent infection
> - Bronchodilators and anti-inflammatory agents to expand and clear the airways
>
> **Kartagener syndrome**
>
> Kartagener syndrome is also called immotile cilia syndrome, is a rare autosomal recessive genetic disorder characterized by a triad (situs inverts, chronic sinusitis and bronchiectasis). It is also an important cause of male infertility due to lack of sperm motility.

4. Pulmonary alveolar macrophages PAMs play an important role in the defence system by the following mechanisms:

- Being actively phagocytic cells, they ingest the inhaled bacteria and small particles.
- They help in processing inhaled antigens for immunological attack.
- PAMs secrete substances that attract polymorphonuclear cells to the lungs.
- By some secretions, they stimulate granulocyte and monocyte formation in the bone marrow.

Note: The detrimental function of PAM is to digest substances inhaled in cigarette smoke or other irritants. During the digestive process, they release lysosomal products into the extracellular spaces and cause inflammatory reaction.

5. Cough reflex The laryngeal, tracheal and bronchial mucous membranes contain vagal afferent terminals which act as *irritant receptors*. Stimulation of these receptors by chemical or mechanical stimuli (excessive mucus, inadvertently inhaled foodstuff, etc.) produces a bout of coughing which helps in the expulsion of the foreign material. For details of cough reflex, see page 435.

6. The tonsils and adenoids The tonsils and adenoids consist of immunologically active lymphoid tissue. They provide significant defence against inhaled and ingested pathogens.

B. Functions Subserved by Pulmonary Circulation

1. Reservoir for left ventricle When left ventricle output becomes transiently greater than systemic venous return, the blood stored in pulmonary circulation helps in maintaining the left ventricular output for few strokes.

2. Pulmonary circulation acts as a filter Pulmonary circulation acts as a filter and filters out particles from the blood, which may include small fibrin or blood clots, detached cancer cells, fat cells, gas bubbles, agglutinated RBCs, masses of platelets and debris from stored blood.

The filtered particles in the lung are removed by lytic enzyme in capillary endothelium, ingestion by macrophages and penetration into the lymphatic system.

3. Removal of fluid from alveoli Because of low pulmonary hydrostatic pressure, the fluid entering the alveoli is absorbed by the capillaries. This protects the gas exchange function of the lungs and opposes transudation of fluid from the capillaries to the alveoli.

4. Role in absorption of drugs Certain drugs that rapidly pass through the alveolar capillary barrier by diffusion are administered by inhalation, e.g. anaesthetic gases, aerosol and other bronchodilators.

C. Metabolic Functions of Lungs

1. Surfactant Surfactant produced in the lungs plays an important role in respiration (for details, see page 382).

2. Protein synthesis Protein synthesis by lungs helps in maintenance of the structural framework.

3. Conversion of angiotensin I to II Conversion of angiotensin I to II is performed by the enzyme angiotensin-converting enzyme (ACE) present in the pulmonary capillary endothelium.

4. Inactivation partly or completely Inactivation, partly or completely, of many vasoactive substances present in the blood is done by capillary endothelial cells as they pass through pulmonary circulation. These substances include:

- Bradykinin
- Serotonin
- Some prostaglandins
- Norepinephrine
- Acetylcholine

Amount of serotonin and norepinephrine reaching the systemic circulation is decreased by lungs.

Vasoactive substances that pass through the lungs without being metabolized include:

- Epinephrine
- Dopamine
- Oxytocin
- Vasopressin
- Angiotensin I

5. Fibrinolytic mechanism Fibrinolytic mechanism present in the lung lyses clot in the pulmonary vessels.

6. Storage of hormones and certain biologically active peptides Storage of hormones and certain biologically active peptides is done in the APUD cells and nerve fibres present in the alveoli. These substances include VIP, substance P, opioid peptides, cholecystokinin-pancreozymin (CCK-PZ) and somatostatin. These substances are later released into the systemic circulation.

D. Functions Subserved by Respiratory Muscles

Respiratory muscles are also used during pulmonary ventilation laughing and singing and put.

E. Olfaction

Olfactory mucosa having receptors is located in the upper part of the nasal cavity, which helps in sensing the toxic gases and odoriferous substances.

F. Phonation

The vocal cord movement helps in phonation.

G. Water Vaporization

Daily about 400 mL water is being lost through lungs by vaporization.

Applied Aspects

Cold dehydration: In cold environment, during mountaineering, some people develop symptoms such as fatigue, shortness of breath and thirst due to loss of water, because inhaled air gets warm and loaded with water vapours from the respiratory tract, which is exhaled during expiration. Therefore, to prevent dehydration, mountaineers should consciously drink water slowly for several hours.

Panting is rapid shallow breathing commonly seen in dogs during summer leading to loss of water vapours from the upper respiratory tract.

Self-Assessment

1. Discuss the nonrespiratory functions of the respiratory tract.
2. Describe:
   - Significance of respiratory parenchyma
   - Functions of respiratory passages
3. Write notes on:
   - Tracheobronchial tree
   - Lung defence mechanism
   - Cystic fibrosis

Clinical Cases

Case 1

A young boy during hiking developed excessive thirst, fatigue and light-headedness.

Q1. What is this condition known as?
Q2. What is the cause of symptoms in this condition?
Q3. How can the symptoms be prevented during hiking?
Q4. What is the immediate measure in this case?

Case 2

A 36-year-old nonsmoker male presented to the OPD with main complaints of recurrent episodes of common cold, sneezing and cough for the past 10 years; shortness of breath on exertion; and not having any issue despite being married for the last 12 years.

- On examination, vitals were within normal range.
- Physical examination revealed apex beat palpable in the right fifth intercostal space.
- Auscultation of the chest revealed bilateral wheeze (rhonchi) and crackling breath sounds.
- Heart sounds were best heard on the right side.
- History revealed that he was born to nonconsanguineous parents.

Q1. What is the probable diagnosis?
Q2. What further tests are required for confirmation of the diagnosis?

Pulmonary Ventilation 5.2

CHAPTER OUTLINE

INTRODUCTION

As we know, respiration, to be more precise the *external respiration* (supply of O_2 from atmosphere to body tissues and removal of CO_2 from the body to atmosphere), involves three major processes:

- *Pulmonary ventilation* (PV), i.e. exchange of gases between the environment and the lungs
- *Pulmonary diffusion*, i.e. transfer of gases from the alveoli to the capillary blood across the respiratory membrane
- *Transport of gases* from the blood to the tissue cells and back

In this chapter, the following aspects and concepts related to PV are discussed:

- Mechanics of PV
- Lung volumes and capacities
- Pulmonary elastance and compliance
- Work of breathing

MECHANICS OF PULMONARY VENTILATION

MECHANISM OF BREATHING

PV is accomplished by two processes – inspiration and expiration.

Inspiration refers to inflow of atmospheric air into the lungs. This obviously occurs when the intrapulmonary pressure falls below the atmospheric air pressure.

Expiration refers to outflow of air from the lungs into the atmosphere. This obviously occurs when the intrapulmonary pressure rises above the atmospheric air pressure.

Changes in the intrapulmonary pressure which govern the respiratory cycle of inspiration and expiration are related to changes in the intrapleural pressure.

Changes in the intrapleural pressure are brought about by changes in the size of the thoracic cavity. Expansion of the thoracic cage leads to fall in intrapleural pressure and decrease in the size of the thoracic cavity leads to rise in the intrapleural pressure.

Changes in the size of the thoracic cavity are brought about by the actions of respiratory muscles:

Muscles of normal tidal inspiration are diaphragm and external intercostal muscles.

Accessory muscles of inspiration are scaleni, sternomastoid and serratus anterior, and alae nasi.

Muscles of expiration are internal intercostal muscles and abdominal muscles (abdominal recti muscles, transverse abdominis muscles and internal oblique muscles).

Mechanism of Tidal Respiration

Inspiration

Inspiration is an active process, normally produced by contraction of the *inspiratory muscles* (negative-pressure breathing). Use of a respirator to inflate the respiratory system produces positive pressure (*positive-pressure breathing*). During tidal inspiration (quiet breathing), the diaphragm and external intercostal muscles contract and cause an increase in all the three dimensions of the thoracic cavity.

Role of a diaphragm In tidal inspiration (quiet breathing), 70%–75% of the expansion of chest is caused due to the contraction of diaphragm. The diaphragm is a dome-shaped, musculotendinous partition between the thorax and the abdomen. The convexity of this dome is directed towards the thorax. When the diaphragm contracts, the following changes occur:

- The dome becomes flattened, and the level of diaphragm is lowered *increasing the vertical diameter* of the thoracic cavity (Fig. 5.2.1A). During quiet breathing, the descent of diaphragm is about 1.5 cm, and during forced inspiration it increases to 7 cm.
- The descent of diaphragm causes the rise in intra-abdominal pressure which is accommodated by the reciprocal relaxation of the abdominal wall musculature.
- The contraction of diaphragm also lifts the lower ribs causing thoracic expansion laterally and anteriorly (the bucket-handle and pump-handle effect, respectively) (Fig. 5.2.1B and C). The abdominal organs support the diaphragmatic dome and act as a fulcrum, whereas the diaphragmatic contraction raises the lower ribs.

Applied Aspects

Hiccup is a spasmodic contraction of diaphragm and other inspiratory muscles, resulting in inspiration in which there is a sudden closure of glottis, producing sound and a characteristic sensation. Its physiological significance is not yet clear. Usually, hiccup is of short duration, but when it becomes debilitating, use of dopamine antagonist and centrally acting analgesics may help.

In bilateral phrenic nerve palsy, adequate ventilation at rest can be maintained by the external intercostal muscles alone but respiration is somewhat laboured to maintain life.

Spinal cord transaction above the level of the third cervical segment is fatal without artificial respiration, whereas in transaction below the fifth cervical segment, respiration remains normal as the phrenic nerve (C_3, C_4, C_5) that innervates the diaphragm remains intact.

- During swallowing and gagging, the contraction of adductors of larynx closes the glottis, thus preventing aspiration of food, fluid and vomitus into the lungs.

During unconscious state or in deep anaesthesia, incomplete closure of glottis may cause aspiration pneumonitis.

Role of external intercostal muscles The fibres of external intercostal muscles slope downwards and forwards. They are attached close to the vertebral ends of the upper ribs than of the lower ribs (Fig. 5.2.2). From pivot-like joint with the vertebrae, the ribs slope obliquely downwards and forwards. So, when the external intercostal muscles contract (because of the lever effect), the ribs are elevated causing the lateral and anteroposterior enlargement of the thoracic cavity due to the so-called bucket- and pump-handle effects, respectively (Fig. 5.2.1B and C).

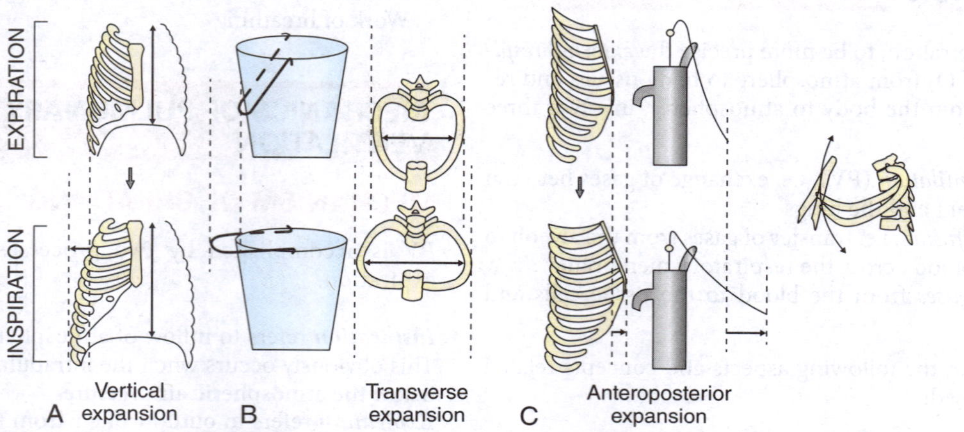

Fig. 5.2.1 Mechanism of increase in diameter of thoracic cavity: **A**, increase in vertical diameter (descent of diaphragm); **B**, increase in transverse diameter (bucket-handle effect); and **C**, increase in anteroposterior diameter (pump-handle effect).

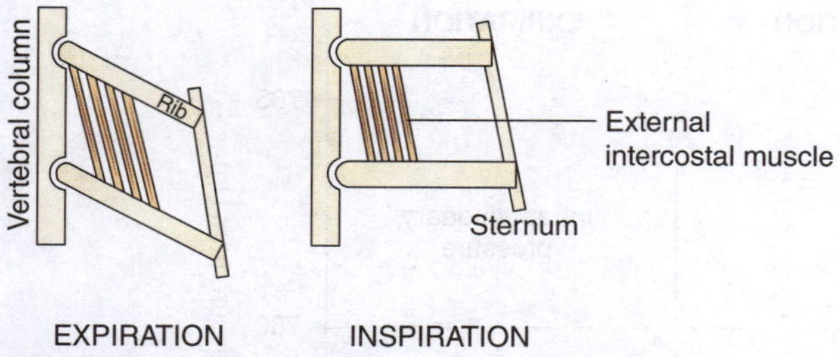

Fig. 5.2.2 Contraction of external intercostal muscle favours elevation of ribs due to mechanical leverage effect of the attachments of its fibres close to the pivot on the upper ribs as compared with that on the lower ribs.

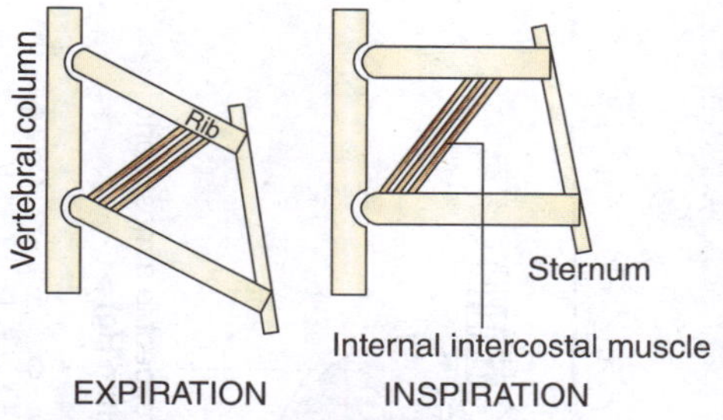

Fig. 5.2.3 Contraction of internal intercostal muscle pulls the ribs down due to mechanical leverage effect of its fibres close to the pivot on the lower ribs as compared with that on the upper ribs.

Role of laryngeal muscles The abductor muscles of the larynx contract during inspiration pulling the vocal cords apart.

Expiration

Expiration in quiet breathing is largely a passive phenomenon and is brought about by the following:

- Elastic recoil of the lungs
- Decrease in the size of the thoracic cavity due to the relaxation of diaphragm and external intercostal muscles
- An increase in the tone of muscle of the anterior abdominal wall which forces the relaxing diaphragm upwards
- The serratus posterior inferior muscles that play a minor role in pulling down the ribs

Mechanism of Forced Respiration

Forced Inspiration

Forced inspiration is characterized by:

1. Forceful contraction of diaphragm Forceful contraction of diaphragm leads to the descent of diaphragm by 7–10 cm as compared with 1–1.5 cm during quiet inspiration.

2. Forceful contraction of external intercostal muscles Forceful contraction of external intercostal muscles causes more elevation of ribs leading to more increase in transverse and anteroposterior diameter of the thoracic cavity.

3. Contraction of accessory muscles of inspiration Contraction of accessory muscles of inspiration causes the following effects:

- *Sternomastoid muscles* contract and lift the sternum upwards.
- *Anterior serrati muscles* contract and lift many of the ribs upwards.
- *Scaleni muscles* contract and lift the first two ribs.

Forced Expiration

Forced expiration is required when respiration is increased during exercise or in the presence of severe respiratory disease. It is an active process that gives rise to the following:

1. Contraction of abdominal muscles

- Compression of the abdominal contents which increases the intra-abdominal pressure and forces the diaphragm upwards, thereby reducing the vertical diameter of the thoracic cavity
- Downward pull on the lower ribs, thus decreasing the anteroposterior diameter of the thoracic cavity
- Fixation of the lower ribs so that internal intercostal muscles act more effectively

2. Contraction of the internal intercostal muscles It causes the effect which is just opposite to that of external intercostal muscles. This is because of the leverage mechanism of the direction of the muscle fibres which slope downwards and backwards, creating a longer force arm for the upper ribs (Fig. 5.2.3). Hence, their contraction tends to pull all the ribs downwards, thereby reducing the anteroposterior diameter (because of the falling of the pump-handle effect) as well as the transverse diameter (because of the action of ribs like the falling of the bucket-handle effect) of the thoracic cavity.

Note: Besides their role in deep breathing, the expiratory muscles are also involved in other forced expiratory efforts, e.g. in coughing, vomiting, defaecation and Valsalva manoeuvre.

PRESSURE AND VOLUME CHANGES DURING THE RESPIRATORY CYCLE

Intrapulmonary Pressure Changes during the Respiratory Cycle (Fig. 5.2.4)

The movement of air in and out of the lungs depends primarily on the pressure gradient between the alveoli and the atmosphere (i.e. *transairway pressure*). The intrapulmonary or alveolar pressure is the air pressure inside the lung alveoli.

At End-Expiration and End-Inspiration

At end-expiration and end-inspiration, i.e. when the glottis is open and there is no movement of air, the pressures in all parts of the respiratory tree are equal to the atmospheric pressure, and the intrapulmonary pressure is considered to be *0* mm Hg (760 mm Hg).

During inspiration During inspiration in quiet breathing, the pressure in the alveoli decreases to about −1 mm Hg (759 mm Hg), which is sufficient to suck in about 500 mL of air into the lungs within 2 seconds of inspiration. At the end-inspiration, the intrapulmonary pressure again becomes zero (760 mm Hg).

During forced inspiration against a closed glottis During forced inspiration against a closed glottis (Muller's manoeuvre), the

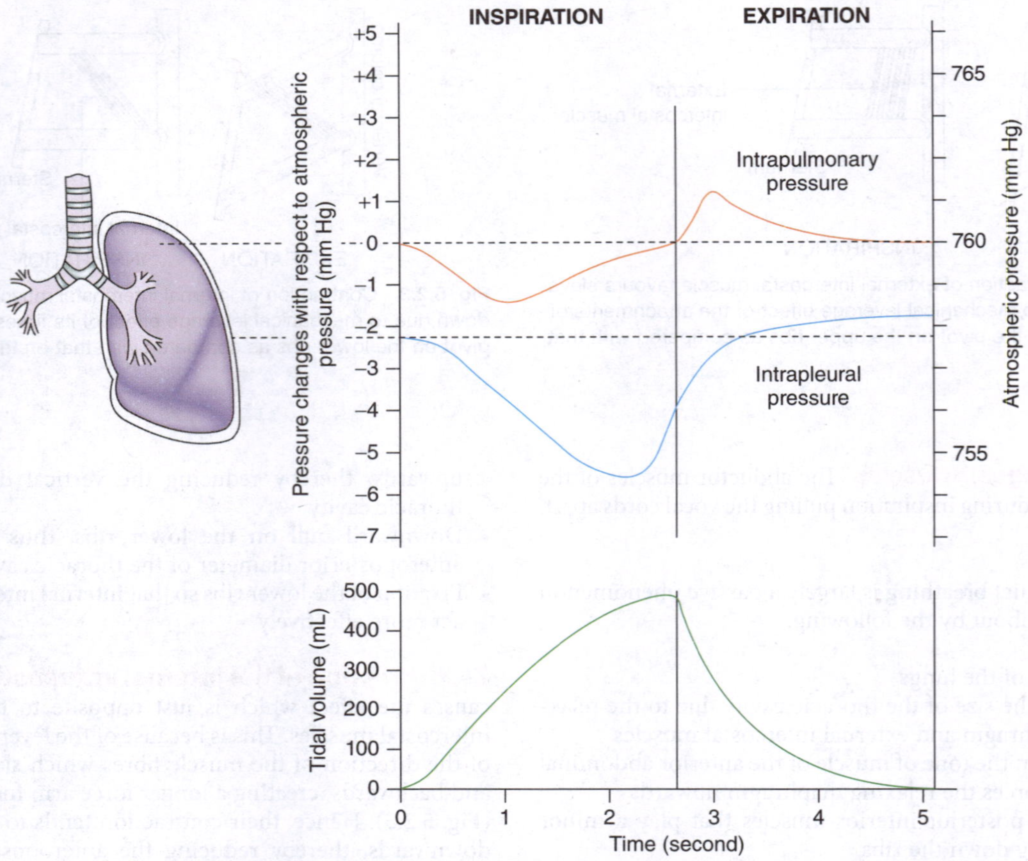

Fig. 5.2.4 Pressure and volume changes during the respiratory cycle.

intrapulmonary pressure may be as low as −80 mm Hg, i.e. below the atmospheric pressure i.e. 680 mm Hg.

During expiration During expiration in quiet breathing, the elastic recoil of the lungs causes the intrapulmonary pressure to swing slightly to the positive side (+1 or 761 mm Hg) which forces 500 mL of inspired air out of the lungs during 2–3 seconds of expiration. At the end-expiration, once again the alveolar pressure regains the atmospheric pressure (0 or 760 mm Hg).

Forceful expiration against closed glottis (Valsalva manoeuvre) may produce the intrapulmonary pressure of as much as 100 mm Hg (860 mm Hg).

Intrapleural (Pleural) Pressure Changes during the Respiratory Cycle (Fig. 5.2.4)

Pleural pressure is the pressure of fluid in the space between the visceral pleura and the parietal pleura.

Normal Pleural Pressure

When the respiratory muscles are completely relaxed and the airways are open, the normal pleural pressure is about −2.5 mm Hg.

- The negative pleural pressure (−2.5 mm Hg) is the amount of suction required to hold the lungs at their equilibrium volume or the functional residual capacity (FRC). FRC is the lung volume at the end of normal (eupnoeic), relaxed expiration and is about 2–2.5 L of gas.
- The negative pleural pressure (−2.5 mm Hg) is the result of balance of two opposite forces – the recoil tendency of the lungs and the recoil tendency of the thoracic cage.
- Recoil tendency of the lungs (continuous tendency to collapse) is caused by:
  - The presence of many elastic fibres in the alveolar walls which are under constant stretch in the inflated lungs
  - Surface tension of the fluid lining the alveoli due to which the alveoli tend to become progressively smaller and collapse
- Recoil tendency of the thoracic cage, i.e. a constant tendency to expand (to pop outwards), is because of the fact that the chest wall is an elastic structure which is normally partially pulled inwards. The elastic property of the thoracic cage is because of the elastic nature of ribs, muscles and tendons.

During inspiration, due to the expansion of the chest wall, the pleural pressure becomes more negative (−6 mm Hg) and pulls the surface of lungs with greater force creating negative intrapulmonary pressure.

During expiration: At the end of inspiration, the inspiratory muscles relax and the recoiling force of lungs begins to pull the chest wall back to expiratory position. At end-expiratory position, where the recoil force of the lungs and the recoil force of thoracic cage balance, the pleural pressure returns back to −2.5 mm Hg.

Factors Affecting Pleural Pressure

1. ***Deep inspirations:*** The pleural pressure may become as low as −30 mm Hg during deep inspiration.

2. During ***Valsalva manoeuvre*** or when expiratory muscles work against closed glottis, there occurs a marked decrease in the thoracic volume causing deflation of lungs. Under such circumstances, the intrapleural pressure can become positive by 60–70 mm Hg (greater than atmospheric pressure), e.g. during defaecation and coughing.
3. ***Gravity:*** The pleural pressure in standing position is more negative (−7 mm Hg) at the apices of the lungs as compared with at the bases (−2 mm Hg). Because of this, lungs are less expanded at the base and even the airway at the base may become closed at the end of expiration. This is why during the first part of inspiration, more of the inspired gas goes to the apices than to the bases of lungs.
4. ***Injury to the chest wall*** causing exposure of the pleural cavity to the exterior causes air to enter the pleural cavity (pneumothorax) and the pleural pressure rises from the subatmospheric level to the atmospheric level. Since there is no opposing force to the elastic recoil of the lung, so in pneumothorax, the lung is collapsed.
5. ***Emphysema*** is a disease of the lungs in which lung elasticity is decreased or lost. Due to the decrease in the recoiling force of lungs, the intrapleural pressure becomes less negative (i.e. increases). Because of this reason, in this disease, the lung alveoli expand and the chest also expands and becomes barrel shaped.

Effects of Pleural Pressure on the Cardiovascular System

1. ***During inspiration***, when the pleural pressure becomes more negative, the mediastinal pressure also becomes more negative, leading to the expansion of the walled structures in the thorax, especially large veins (superior and inferior venae cavae), thereby decreasing pressure on them. This causes blood to be sucked into these veins from extrathoracic regions. Thus, there is *increased venous return* to the heart during inspiration due to suction action of the respiratory pump. The descent of diaphragm during inspiration causes a slight rise in intra-abdominal pressure, thereby increasing the pressure gradient between the abdomen and the thorax further. The increase in the venous return during inspiration *increases the cardiac output*. This respiratory pump action is especially marked during exercise.
2. ***During Valsalva manoeuvre*** or when expiratory muscles are working violently against closed glottis, e.g. during severe bouts of cough, the pleural pressure becomes positive leading to a decrease in the venous return. So the cardiac output is markedly decreased and there may occur cerebral ischaemia, visual blackouts and unconsciousness, especially in old persons.

Important Notes

- In old persons and cardiac patients, a positive intrapleural pressure (e.g. during coughing or straining at stool) causes syncope because of transient cerebral ischaemia.
- High increase in positive intrapleural pressure results in compression of great veins in the thoracic cavity, leading to reduced venous return and thus markedly reduced cardiac output.

MEASUREMENT OF PLEURAL PRESSURE

1. ***Manometric measurement*** can be made by inserting a needle into the intrapleural space whose other end is attached to a water manometer with the help of a rubber tubing.
2. ***Intraoesophageal*** pressure can be recorded with the help of an air-containing rubber balloon sealed over a catheter placed in the lower part of thoracic part of oesophagus. Intraoesophageal pressure in the thoracic part is equivalent to the intrapleural pressure because this part of oesophagus becomes a closed cavity due to the closure of its lower end by the cardiac sphincter and upper end by the closure of glottis.

LUNG VOLUME CHANGES DURING THE RESPIRATORY CYCLE

During tidal inspiration, the volume of air in the lungs increases by 500 mL (tidal volume [TV]).

During tidal expiration, the elastic forces compress the gas in the lungs which starts flowing out and at the end of expiration the volume of air in the lungs decreases by 500 mL (Fig. 5.2.4).

PRESSURE–VOLUME CURVE OF RESPIRATORY SYSTEM

The transrespiratory pressure (TRP) refers to the transmural pressure across the entire respiratory system. It equals alveolar pressure (PA) minus pressure at the body surface (PBs), i.e. TRP = PA − PBs. The pressure at the body surface is usually atmospheric pressure.

Pressure–volume curve of the respiratory system (Fig. 5.2.5) shows that:

- It is a sigmoid-shaped curve which is steepest in the middle and almost flat at both high- and low-lung volumes.
- FRC is determined by the volume at which the TRP is zero.
- Residual volume (RV) and total lung capacity (TLC) are limited by the decreased compliance of the system, as indicated by the reduced slope of the curve at both extremes of volumes.

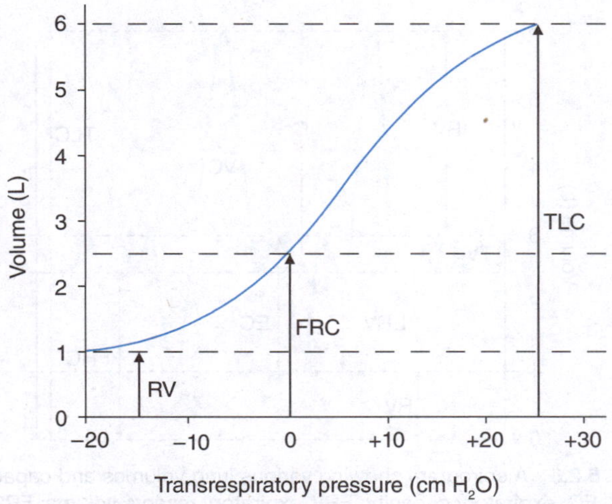

Fig. 5.2.5 Pressure–volume curve of the respiratory system. FRC, functional residual capacity; RV, residual volume; TLC, total lung capacity.

LUNG VOLUMES AND CAPACITIES

STATIC LUNG VOLUMES AND CAPACITIES

Lung Volumes

The maximum volume to which a lung can be expanded has been divided into four nonoverlapping volumes (Fig. 5.2.6).

1. Tidal Volume

It is the volume of air inspired or expired with each breath during normal quiet breathing. It is approximately 500 mL in a normal adult male.

2. Inspiratory Reserve Volume (IRV)

It is the extra volume of air that can be inhaled by a maximum inspiratory effort over and beyond the normal TV. It is about 3000 mL in a normal adult male.

3. Expiratory Reserve Volume (ERV)

It is the extra volume of air that can be exhaled by maximum forceful expiration over and beyond the normal TV, (i.e. after the end of normal passive expiration). It is approximately 1100 mL in a normal adult male.

4. Residual Volume

It is the volume of the air that still remains in the lungs after the most forceful expiration. It is about 1200 mL in a normal adult male.

Lung Capacities

Lung capacities are combination of two or more pulmonary volumes and include (Fig. 5.2.6):

1. Inspiratory Capacity (IC)

This is the maximum volume of the air that can be inspired after normal tidal expiration. Therefore, it equals TV + IRV and is approximately 3500 mL in a normal adult male.

2. Expiratory Capacity (EC)

It is the maximum volume of air that can be expired after normal tidal inspiration. It equals TV + ERV and is approximately about 1600 mL in a normal adult male.

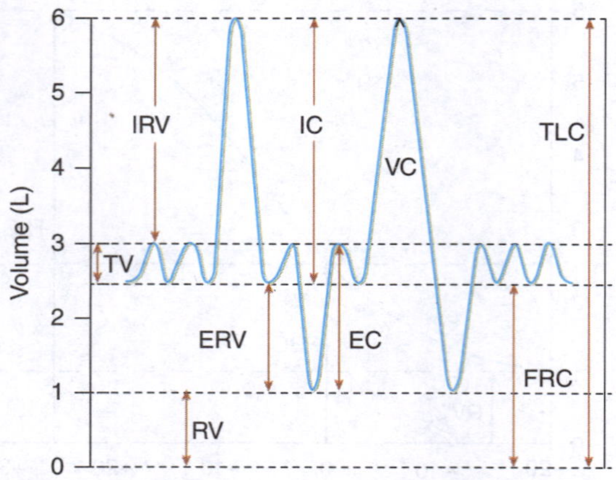

Fig. 5.2.6 A spirogram showing various lung volumes and capacities. EC, expiratory capacity; ERV, expiratory reserve volume; FRC, functional residual capacity; IC, inspiratory capacity; IRV, inspiratory reserve volume; RV, residual volume; TLC, total lung capacity; TV, tidal volume; VC, vitai capacity.

3. Functional Residual Capacity

It is the volume of the air remaining in the lungs after normal tidal expiration. Therefore, it equals ERV + RV and is about 2300 mL in a normal adult male.

Significance of FRC The FRC (RV + ERV) of about 2300 mL represents the air that remains in the lungs most of the times. Even after the most forceful expiration, about 1200 mL (RV) air is always present in the lungs. This has several advantages:

i. ***Continuous exchange of gases*** is possible due to presence of some air always in the lungs, and thereby concentrations of O_2 and CO_2 in blood are maintained constant. Without FRC, pO_2 would have risen to 150 mm Hg during inspiration, and reduced nearly to zero during expiration, which is maintained at about 100 mm Hg due to the FRC.
ii. ***Breath holding*** is made possible due to the FRC.
iii. ***Dilution of toxic inhaled gases*** occurs due to the reserve of 2300 mL of air in the lungs (FRC) most of the times.
iv. ***Load on respiratory mechanism and left ventricle*** would have been much more if there was no FRC, since:
   - Without FRC, lungs would have collapsed at the end of each expiration, and re-expansion would have required tremendous breathing effort.
   - The collapsed lungs would have increased pulmonary vascular resistance and imposed a heavy load on left ventricle.

Factors affecting FRC Hyperinflation of the lungs seen in the following conditions may be associated with increased FRC:

- Old age due to loss of elasticity of lungs
- Emphysema
- Bronchial asthma

Measurement of FRC FRC can be measured by the nitrogen wash-out method or the helium dilution method.

Nitrogen wash-out method This method is based on the assumption that the alveolar air has 80% nitrogen. In this method, the subject is made to wash out nitrogen from the lungs completely by inhaling pure O_2 for 5 minutes and expiring into a large gas bag called the Douglas bag (washed with pure O_2 and, hence, made nitrogen free). The volume of gas collected in the *Douglas bag* and its nitrogen content are measured and the value of FRC is calculated as follows:

- Suppose that the expired gas collected at the end of 5 minutes is 40 L and its nitrogen concentration is 5%.
- Then the volume of nitrogen (V_n) in the expired gas will be

$$\frac{40 \times 5}{100} = 2 \text{ L or } 2000 \text{ mL}$$

- Since the nitrogen content of the expired gas is solely from the subject's lungs where it forms 80% of the gas present in the lungs (FRC), we have

$$\text{FRC} = \frac{2000 \times 100}{80} \text{ mL} = 2500 \text{ mL or } 2.5 \text{ L}$$

Helium dilution method This method is based on the basic principle that the amount (A) of a substance present is

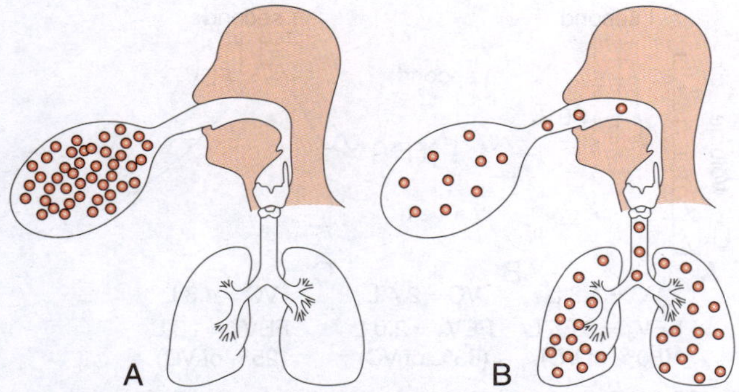

Fig. 5.2.7 Helium dilution method for estimation of functional residual capacity (FRC): **A**, in the beginning, no helium present in the lungs; and **B**, the helium present in closed circuit distributed equally between the bag and the lungs.

equal to its volume (V) multiplied by its concentration (C), i.e.

$$A = V \times C$$

- In this method, a closed circuit system is prepared with a mixture of helium, oxygen and air. The amount of helium is added in the mixture such as to achieve a helium concentration of 10%.
- The subject is then made to breathe in the closed system till the concentration of helium in the lungs and that in the bag become equal. The helium concentration is measured at the end of a normal expiration (because the FRC is the volume of air remaining in the lungs at the end of normal expiration).

Since no helium was present in the lungs to start with, the same amount of helium which was added in the mixture in the closed circuit system gets distributed between the bag and the lungs (Fig. 5.2.7A and B). The FRC can be calculated as follows:

- Suppose that the volume of helium added in the mixture to make its concentration to 10% is 560 mL.
- Volume of the bag is 5000 mL.
- Concentration of helium in the bag and lungs after breathing in the closed circuit system is 8%.

Then,

$$\text{Volume of helium} = \frac{\text{Volume of lungs} + \text{bag}}{\text{Concentration ofh elium}} \times \frac{8}{100}$$

That is,

$$560 = \left(\text{Volume of lungs} + 5000\right) \times \frac{8}{100}$$

or

$$\text{Volume of lungs} + 5000 = \frac{500 \times 100}{8}$$

or

$$\text{Volume of lungs} = 7000 - 5000$$

Hence,

$$\text{FRC} = 2000\ \text{mL}.$$

4. Vital Capacity (VC)

This is the maximum amount of air a person can expel from the lungs after the deepest possible inspiration. Therefore, it equals TV + IRV + ERV and is about 4600 mL in a normal adult male.

Significance of vital capacity Estimation of VC allows the assessment of maximum inspiratory and expiratory efforts and, thus, gives useful information about the strength of respiratory muscles.

- VC also provides useful information about other aspects of pulmonary functions through forced expiratory volume (FEV).

Factors affecting vital capacity Factors affecting VC include:

i. ***Size of the thoracic cavity:*** VC is more in males (2.6 L/m^2 body surface area) because of large chest size and more muscle power than in females.
ii. ***Age:*** In old age, VC decreases due to the decrease in the elasticity of the lungs.
iii. ***Strength of respiratory muscles:*** In swimmers and divers, VC is more because of the increased strength of the respiratory muscles.
iv. ***Gravity:*** In standing position, VC is more than in sitting and lying position because of:
   - Increased size of the thoracic cavity in standing (diaphragm moves down)
   - Reduced pulmonary blood flow due to decreased venous return
v. ***In pregnancy***, VC is reduced due to pushing up of the diaphragm and the reduced capacity of the thoracic cavity.
vi. ***In ascites*** (accumulation of fluid in the abdominal cavity), VC is reduced due to the same reason as in pregnancy.
vii. ***Pulmonary diseases*** such as pulmonary fibrosis, emphysema, respiratory obstruction, pulmonary oedema, pleural effusion and pneumothorax are associated with decreased VC.

5. Total Lung Capacity

It is the volume of air present in the lungs after the maximal inspiration. It equals VC + RV and is about 5800 mL in a normal adult male.

Measurement of Static Lung Volumes and Capacities

All volumes and capacities except RV, FRC and TLC are recorded by a *spirometer.* FRC is determined by the nitrogen wash-out method or the helium dilution method, and then RV and TLC are calculated.

Recording of lung volumes and capacities is an important lung function test (for details, see page 463).

DYNAMIC LUNG VOLUMES AND CAPACITIES

Timed Vital Capacity (TVC) or Forced Vital Capacities (FVC)

Forced VC is the volume of the air that can be expired rapidly with a maximum force following a maximum inspiration. The volume of air expired can be timed by recording the VC on a spirograph moving at the known speed.

Components of TVC or FVC (Fig. 5.2.8)

I. Forced expiratory volume in 1 second (FEV$_1$) It represents the volume expired in the first second of an FVC.

- Estimation of FEV$_1$ is the most commonly used screening test for airway diseases.

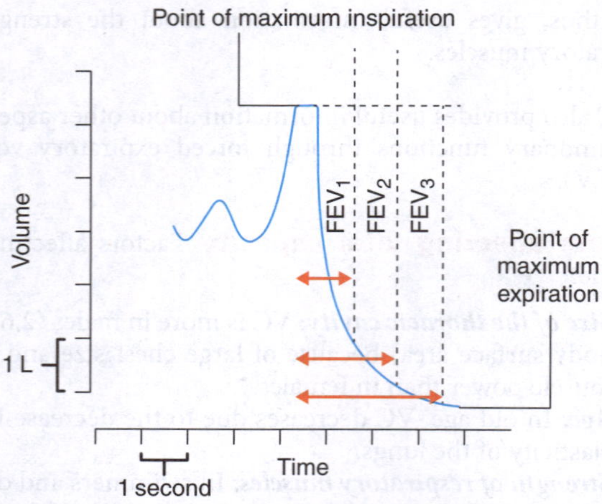

Fig. 5.2.8 Components of timed vital capacity.

- The FEV_1 is actually a flow rate. Its unit is litre per second.
- FEV_1% is the percentage of FVC expired in 1 second (i.e. $FEV_1\% = [FEV_1/FVC] \times 100$); normally, FEV_1% is about 80% of the FVC (Fig. 5.2.9A).

Applied Aspects

FEV is useful in distinguishing between restrictive lung disease (RLD) and obstructive lung disease (OLD) See Table 5.2.1.

- Patients with RLD, e.g. kyphoscoliosis and ankylosing spondylitis, have a reduced FVC, but they are able to achieve relatively high flow rates; therefore, their FEV_1% exceeds 80% (Fig. 5.2.9B).
- Patients with OLD, e.g. bronchial asthma, have low flow rates as a result of high airway resistance; therefore, their FEV_1% is abnormally low (Fig. 5.2.9C).

II. Forced expiratory volume in 2 seconds (FEV_2)

It represents the volume of air expired in the first 2 seconds of FVC; FEV_2% is about 90% of FVC under the normal condition (Fig. 5.2.8).

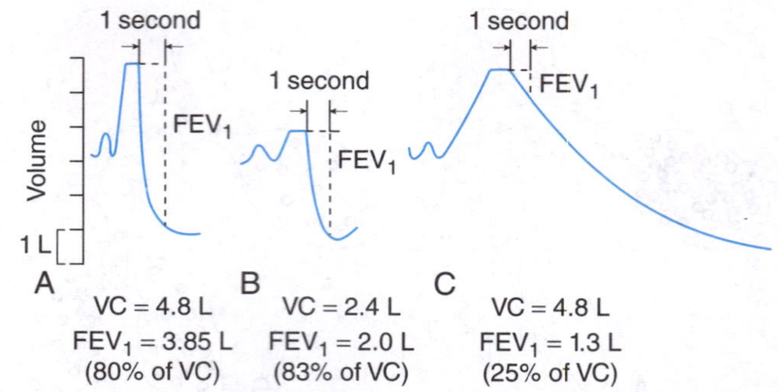

Fig. 5.2.9 Forced expiratory volume in first second (FEV_1) component of timed vital capacity: **A**, in a normal subject; **B**, in a patient with restrictive lung disease (RLD); and **C**, in a patient with obstructive lung disease (OLD).

III. Forced expiratory volume in 3 seconds (FEV_3)

It represents the volume of air expired in the first 3 seconds. Normally FEV_3% is 98%–100% of FVC (Fig. 5.2.8).

Forced expiratory flow during 25%–75% of expiration (FEF 25%–75%)

- It is the mean expiratory flow rate during middle 50% of FVC (Fig. 5.2.10A).
- Normal FEF 25%–75% is 300 L/min.
- Midexpiratory time (MET) refers to the time taken for FEF 25%–75%. Its normal value is 0.5 second which is increased in obstructive lung disorders.

Forced Expiratory Flow during 200–1200 mL of Expiration (FEF 200–1200)

- FEF 200–1200 refers to the mean expiratory flow rate between the 200- and 1200-mL segments of FVC (Fig. 5.2.10B).
- Normal value of FEF 200–1200 is 350 L/min.

Minute Ventilation (MV) or Pulmonary Ventilation

It is the volume of air inspired or expired per minute. It equals the TV multiplied by the respiratory rate. The TV at rest averages 500 mL (0.5 L), and the normal respiratory rate is 12–15 breaths/min; therefore, normal minute volume is 6–7.5 L/min.

Table 5.2.1 Differences between restrictive and obstructive lung diseases

Features	Restrictive lung disease	Obstructive lung disease
Definition	Lung parenchymal damage and restriction in lung expansion with stiff lungs, weak musculature or damage to the nerves	Partial or complete airway obstruction
Examples	Interstitial lung disease, pulmonary fibrosis, sarcoidosis obesity, amyotrophic lateral sclerosis	Bronchial asthma, chronic obstructive pulmonary disease (COPD – emphysema, chronic bronchitis, bronchiectasis), cystic fibrosis
Flow rate	↑	↓
Airway resistance	↓	↑
Total lung capacity	↓	Normal or ↑
FVC	↓↓	↓↓
FEV_1	↓	↓↓
FEV_1/FVC	Normal or ↑	↓↓

↑, increase; ↓, decrease; FEV_1, forced expiratory volume in 1 second.

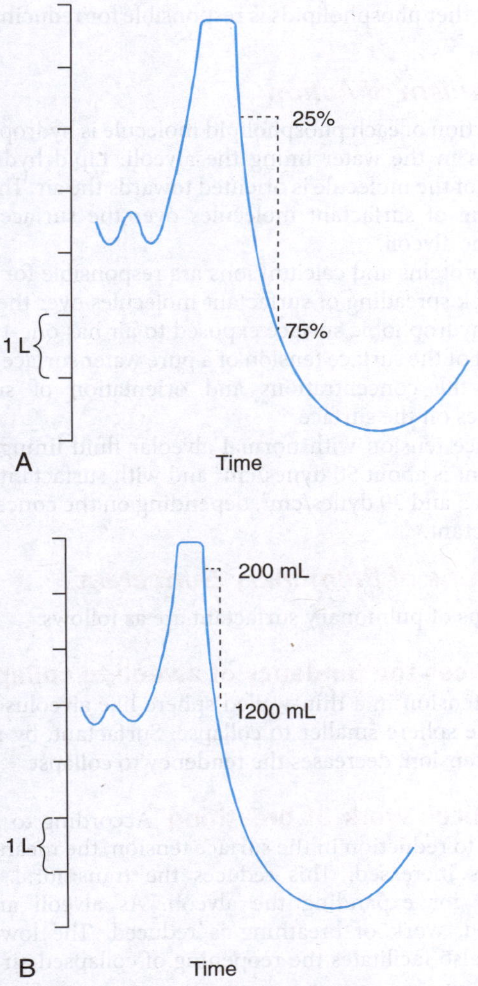

Fig. 5.2.10 Forced expiratory flow: **A**, during 25%–75% of expiration (FEF 25%–75%); and **B**, during 200–1200 mL of expiration (FEF 200–1200 mL).

Maximum Breathing Capacity (MBC) or Maximum Voluntary Ventilation or Maximum Ventilation Volume (MVV)

- It is the maximum volume of air that can be ventilated on command during a given interval.
- This index of ventilatory function depends on the complete cooperation of the subject, who is asked to breathe as rapidly and deeply as he/she can for a 15-second interval. The volume of the air moved is either recorded by a spirometer fitted with a writing point or collected in a Douglas bag; the result is expressed in litre per minute.
- A normal adult male can attain an MVV of 80–170 L/min (average 100 L/min).
- MVV is profoundly reduced in patients with emphysema, airway obstruction and very poor respiratory muscle strength.

> **Important Note**
>
> Hyperventilation causes CO_2 wash-out which leads to respiratory depression. This may result in fainting; therefore, voluntary hyperventilation should be done for brief periods (15 seconds only).

Pulmonary Reserve or Breathing Reserve

- Pulmonary reserve (PR) refers to the maximum amount of the air above the PV that can be inspired or expired in 1 minute.
- It equals the MVV minus PV (MV), i.e.

$$\text{PR} = \text{MVV} - \text{PV/min}$$

- PR is usually expressed as the percentage of MVV and is known as the percentage PR or the dyspnoeic index (DI), i.e.

$$\text{DI} = \frac{\text{MVV} - \text{PV}}{\text{MVV}} \times 100$$

- Normal values of DI or percentage PR range from 60% to 90% with an average of 75%.
- Dyspnoea is usually present when the value of DI becomes less than 60%.

PULMONARY ELASTANCE AND COMPLIANCE

PULMONARY ELASTANCE

Elastance refers to the *recoil* (retractive) tendency of a structure. Both the thoracic cage and the lungs have elastance.

Elastance of Thoracic Cage

Elastance or the recoil tendency of the thoracic cage refers to the constant tendency of the thoracic cage to expand (to pop outward). The elastance of the thoracic cage is because of the fact that the chest wall is an elastic structure which is normally kept partially pulled inward. The elastic property of the thoracic cage is because of the elastic nature of ribs, muscles and tendons.

Elastance of Lungs

Elastance or recoil tendency of the lungs refer to the constant tendency of the lungs to collapse. The recoil forces in the lungs are generated by the following:

1. Tissue forces These are due to the presence of many elastic tissues such as smooth muscle, elastic and collagen in the lung parenchyma which are kept under constant stretch in the inflated lungs. However, the role of these connective tissue fibres in generating elastic (retractile) forces in the lungs is not fully elucidated.

2. Surface forces These are generated at the alveolar surface lined by fluid (*alveolar surface tension*) due to which the alveoli tend to become progressively smaller and tend to collapse. The alveolar surface tension needs further discussion since it is responsible for about two-thirds of total elastic forces in the lungs.

Alveolar Surface Tension

Alveolar surface tension is generated because of the unbalanced attraction of the liquid molecules at the surface of alveolar membrane. A phase change occurs between the alveolar gas and the surface of the alveolar membrane. Alveolar surface tension has a tendency to reduce the size of each alveolus, thus resulting in recoil tendency of the lung, i.e. surface tension increases the tendency of the lungs to deflate.

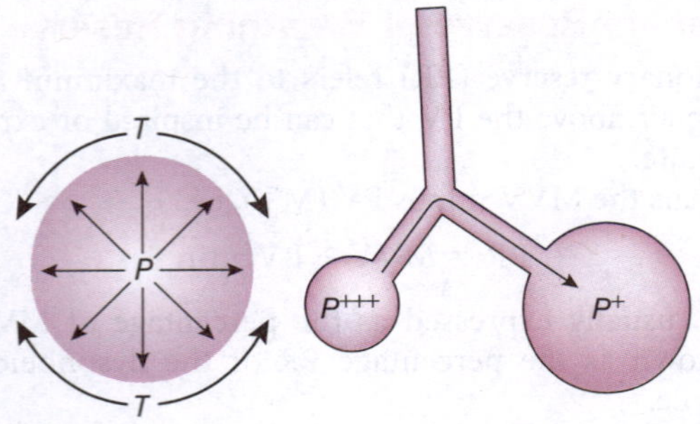

Fig. 5.2.11 Pressure in the alveoli (*P*) is directly proportional to the surface tension (*T*) and inversely proportional to the radii (*r*). Therefore, small alveoli tend to become still smaller and large alveoli tend to become still larger.

An increased transmural pressure is necessary to counteract the effects of surface tension.

- According to the *law of Laplace*, in a spherical structure like alveolus, the transmural pressure generated equals two times the (surface) tension divided by radius, i.e. $P = 2T/r$.
- In other words, the pressure in the alveoli is directly proportional to the surface tension and inversely proportional to the radii.
- Therefore, small alveoli tend to become still smaller, whereas large alveoli tend to become still larger (Fig. 5.2.11). Thus, surface tension tends to produce collapse of the alveoli.

Alveolar surface tension playing a major role in generating elastance forces in the lungs.

Pulmonary Surfactant

The alveolar surface tension opposes the expansion of the lungs during inspiration. The surface tension of pure water and air interface is so high that every inspiration would require an exhausting muscular effort. However, the presence of pulmonary surfactant in the fluid lining the alveoli reduces the surface tension markedly.

Source

Pulmonary surfactant is secreted by type II alveolar epithelial cells (granular pneumocytes). In the cells, it is stored in lamellar bodies. It comes to the surface of alveoli by the process of exocytosis and mixes with the water molecules present there.

Composition

Pulmonary surfactant is a complex mixture of several phospholipids, proteins and ions. It is made up of 70%–80% phospholipids, about 10% proteins and 10% natural fats, mainly cholesterol. Four unique proteins have been identified in surfactant: SP-A, SP-B, SP-C and SP-D. SP-A and SP-D are hydrophilic proteins, and involved in innate immunity of the lungs, whereas SP-B and SP-C are strongly hydrophobic in nature and are main proteins of surfactants.

Synthesis of Surfactant

The substrates (palmate, glucose and choline) for synthesis of surfactant are taken up by the pneumocytes type II and alveolar macrophages. Surfactant is synthesized, assembled, transported and secreted into the alveolus, where it is degraded and recycled. Dipalmitoylphosphatidylcholine (DPPC) along with several other phospholipids is responsible for reducing surface tension.

Mechanism of Action

One portion of each phospholipid molecule is hydrophilic and dissolves in the water lining the alveoli. Lipid hydrophobic portion of the molecule is oriented towards the air. This causes spreading of surfactant molecules over the surface of fluid lining the alveoli.

Apoproteins and calcium ions are responsible for uniform and quick spreading of surfactant molecules over the surface. Such a hydrophobic surface exposed to air has one-twelfth to one-half of the surface tension of a pure water surface depending on the concentrations and orientation of surfactant molecules on the surface.

Surface tension with normal alveolar fluid lining without surfactant is about 50 dynes/cm^2 and with surfactant it varies between 5 and 30 dynes/cm^2, depending on the concentration of surfactant.

Functions of Pulmonary Surfactant

Functions of pulmonary surfactant are as follows:

1. Reduces the tendency of alveoli to collapse The surface tension in a thin-walled sphere like alveolus tends to make the sphere smaller to collapse. Surfactant, by reducing surface tension, decreases the tendency to collapse.

2. Reduces work of breathing According to Laplace's law, due to reduction in the surface tension, the mean alveolar radius is increased. This reduces the transmural pressure required for expanding the alveoli. As alveoli are easily expanded, work of breathing is reduced. The low surface tension also facilitates the reopening of collapsed airway and alveoli.

3. Prevents pulmonary oedema Surface tension is retracting force which not only pulls alveolar wall to the centre of alveolus but also pulls fluid from the capillaries into the interstitial space surrounding the alveoli and into the alveoli leading to pulmonary oedema. Surfactant prevents this phenomenon by lowering the surface tension.

4. Alveolar stabilization Surfactant causes stability of alveoli, i.e. it maintains almost uniform size of alveoli. Due to pulmonary surfactant, pulling pressure in the alveoli is reduced from 18 to 4 cm H_2O. The mechanism of alveolar instability and how the pulmonary surfactant causes alveolar stabilization is explained.

Alveolar instability Alveolar instability due to surface tension effect is produced as follows:

- In the two alveoli (with unequal size) connected to each other, the amount of pressure generated in each according to Laplace's law will be:

$$\text{Pressure} = \frac{2 \times \text{Surface tension}}{\text{Radius}}$$

- Thus, when the surface tension is constant, the pressure developed in the smaller alveolus will be more than in the larger alveolus. This will cause pushing of air from smaller alveolus (with higher pressure) to larger alveolus (with lower pressure). As a result, the smaller alveolar sac will become further smaller and larger alveolar sac will become further larger (Fig. 5.2.11).

- The above-mentioned cycle of pushing air from smaller to larger sac will continue till the smaller sac totally collapses leading to large distension of the other sac, thereby producing instability of the alveoli.

Pulmonary surfactant causes alveolar stabilization

Pulmonary surfactant causes alveolar stabilization by the following mechanisms:

- In the presence of surfactant, the surface tension developed in the alveoli is inversely proportional to the concentration of surfactant per unit area.
- In the smaller alveolus, the surfactant molecules form a thick layer, whereas in a larger alveolus, the surfactant molecules are scattered on the larger surface (as the number of molecules is limited) (Fig. 5.2.12).
- Thus, in a smaller alveolus, the tendency to develop more pressure due to smaller radius will be neutralized by the tendency to develop less pressure due to more concentration of surfactant per unit area, and the reverse will occur in a larger alveolus. In this way, there will not be much pressure gradient between the two alveoli helping to maintain the size of alveolar sac constant. Thus, due to the presence of surfactant, stability of alveoli is maintained.

Other factors which help in alveolar stabilization

Other factors which help in alveolar stabilization along with surfactant are interdependence and fibrous tissue.

Interdependence is a mechanical method of alveolar stabilization. The alveolar septa form a continuous network that is under tension because of lung inflation. Alveoli are tethered together by their adjoining walls and cannot change volume independently of the neighbouring lung tissue.

Fibrous tissue: The lung is constructed of about 50,000 functional units, each of which contains one or a few alveolar ducts and their associated alveoli. All of these are surrounded by fibrous septa that act as additional splints and stabilize the alveoli.

Factors Affecting Pulmonary Surfactant

Factors which decrease the pulmonary surfactant are:

- Long-term inhalation of 100% O_2
- Occlusion of main bronchus
- Occlusion of one pulmonary artery
- Cigarette smoking
- Cutting both the vagi

Factors which increase surfactant production are:

- Thyroid hormones increase the secretion of pulmonary surfactant by increasing the size and number of inclusion bodies in type II alveolar lining epithelial cells.
- Glucocorticoids accelerate the maturation of pulmonary surfactant.

The concentration of glucocorticoids increases in fetal and maternal blood near term; therefore, preterm babies lack surfactant.

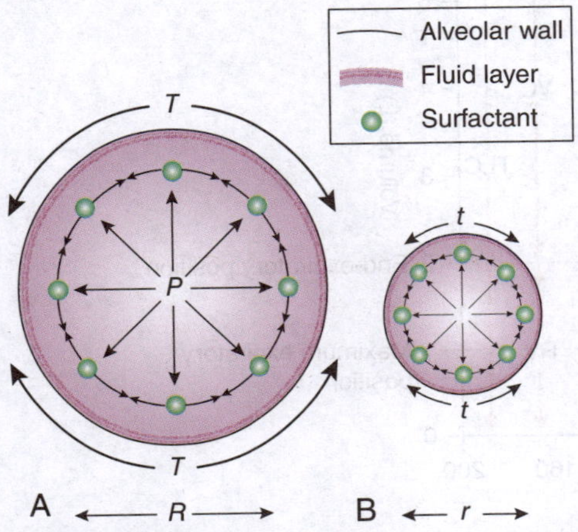

Fig. 5.2.12 Distribution of surfactant in **A,** large and **B,** small alveoli.

Applied Aspects

Clinical significance of pulmonary surfactant is as follows:

1. ***Respiratory distress syndrome (RDS) of newborn*** or the *hyaline membrane disease* occurs in the newborn babies (especially premature) due to inadequate formation of surfactant, resulting in an elevated alveolar surface tension. Retention of fluid in the lung is an additional factor in RDS. During fetal life, pulmonary epithelium secretes Cl^- in the fluid, but at birth, epithelial cells start absorbing Na^+ through epithelial Na^+ channels (ENaCs) and fluid gets absorbed along with Na^+. Immaturity of ENaCs is responsible for pulmonary oedema in RDS. Under this condition, it is extremely difficult to expand the lungs.
   - *Dysfunction/overproduction of surfactant proteins* is the cause of pulmonary alveolar proteinosis and can lead to respiratory distress. Under this condition, it is extremely difficult to expand the lungs.
   - *Signs and symptoms:* Respiratory work is greatly increased and there is inadequate exchange of gases due to alveolar instability, pulmonary oedema and collapse of alveoli (atelectasis) in many areas. This results in severe respiratory insufficiency, and the infant may die.
   - *Diagnosis:* Plasma levels of thyroid hormones and cortisol are low in infants with RDS.
   - *Treatment: Therapy* of RDS includes administration of exogenous surfactant and application of positive end-expiratory pressure (PEEP).
2. ***Adult respiratory distress syndrome*** occurs due to abnormal surfactant function caused by a variety of severe pulmonary injuries. Clinical trials are now underway using exogenous surfactant in an attempt to improve the outcome in adults.
3. ***Patchy atelectasis*** occurs due to surfactant abnormality in patients who have undergone cardiac surgery during which a pump oxygenator is used and the pulmonary circulation is interrupted.

PULMONARY COMPLIANCE

Definition and Normal Value

Compliance refers to the ability of the lungs and thoracic wall to stretch. It can be expressed as change in lung volume (ΔV) per unit change in transpulmonary pressure (ΔP), i.e.

$$C = \frac{\Delta V}{\Delta P}$$

Transpulmonary pressure is the difference in the pressure between alveolar pressure and pleural pressure.

- Compliance expresses the distensibility (expansibility) of the lung and chest wall.
  Normal value of compliance for the lungs and chest wall combined is 0.13 L/cm H_2O and for the lung alone it is 0.22 L/cm H_2O.

Measurement of Total Compliance

Total respiratory compliance (combined compliance of chest wall and lungs) can be measured by the pressure–volume curve of the respiratory system. The pressure–volume curve of the respiratory system can be obtained in living subjects by using a spirometer as follows:

Procedure

The subject is connected to the spirometer and asked to breathe air through the mouth (with nostrils closed). The manometer attached with the spirometer measures airway pressure (transpulmonary pressure). The subject inhales known volume of air from end-expiratory position, and the valve of the spirometer is then shut off to close the airway. The subject holds the breath and then releases the respiratory muscles and change in the airway pressure is measured. The procedure is repeated with actively inhaling or exhaling different air volumes up to the maximum.

The change in the airway pressure is plotted against each air volume and a curve obtained is called the pressure–volume curve of the respiratory system (Fig. 5.2.13).

Observations and Inferences

1. The pressure–volume curve of the respiratory system is a sigmoid-shaped curve which is steepest at the middle and almost flat at both ends (i.e. high and low lung volumes).
2. The volume at which air pressure is 0 mm Hg (atmospheric pressure) is called *relaxation volume* which is equal to FRC. At relaxation volume, the recoil of the chest wall and the recoil of the lung balance each other.
3. Above relaxation volume, on increasing lung volumes, there is increase in the airway pressure, and at maximum inspiration, pressure rises up to 30 mm Hg. On the other hand, decrease in the lung volumes below relaxation volume leads to decrease in airway pressure, and at maximum expiration point, airway pressure decreases up to −30 mm Hg.
4. The RV and TLC are limited by decreased compliance of the system as indicated by the reduced slope at both extremes of volumes.

Factors Affecting Compliance of Lungs and Chest Wall

Downward and right shift of the pressure–volume curve indicates decreased total respiratory compliance. The causes of decreased compliance are as follows:

- Pulmonary congestion
- Interstitial pulmonary fibrosis
- Pulmonary oedema

Upward and left shift of the pressure–volume curve indicates increased total respiratory compliance. The causes of increased compliance are as follows:

- Emphysema
- Old age

Measurement of Pulmonary Compliance

- The compliance of the lung alone can be measured by measuring the intrapleural pressure at different lung volumes.
- The intrapleural pressure (being similar to the intraoesophageal pressure) is measured with the help of an intraoesophageal balloon connected to a manometer.
- The subject is made to inspire air from a spirometer in steps of 100 mL and each time the intrapleural pressure is recorded.
- The relationship of lung volume with intrapleural pressure is plotted on a graph, which gives the *inspiratory compliance curve* (Fig. 5.2.14).
- Similarly expiration is also done in steps and *expiratory compliance* curve is obtained (Fig. 5.2.14).
- The inspiratory and expiratory compliance curves do not coincide but form a loop called *hysteresis loop*.
- So, Fig. 5.2.14 shows that the lung volume at any given pressure is greater during expiration than that during inspiration. This is due to difference in the distensibility (stretchability) of the lungs between inspiratory and expiratory phases. The volume midway between the hysteresis loop (dashed linear line, Fig. 5.2.14) gives the average compliance of the lungs. Had the lungs been a perfectly elastic structure like a spring, the pressure–volume relation line would have been linear (Hook's law).

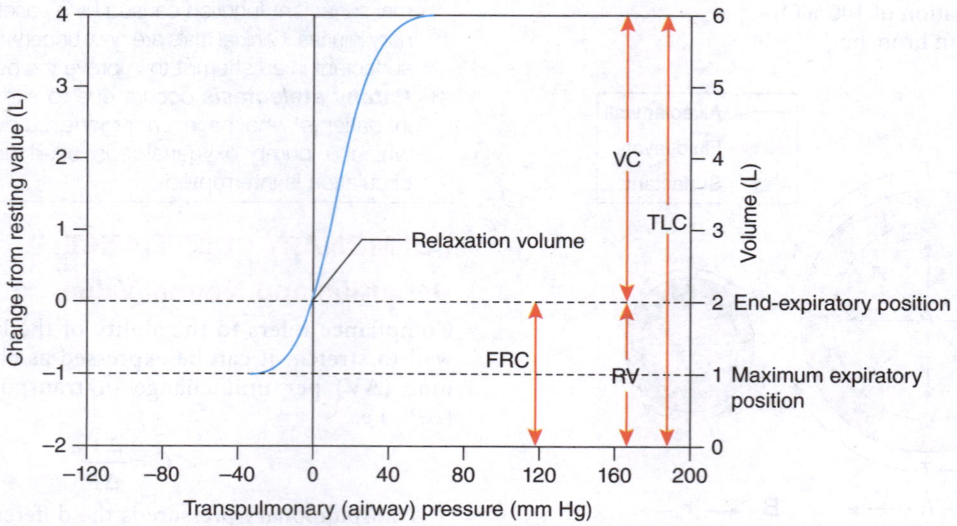

Fig. 5.2.13 Pressure–volume curve of the respiratory system.

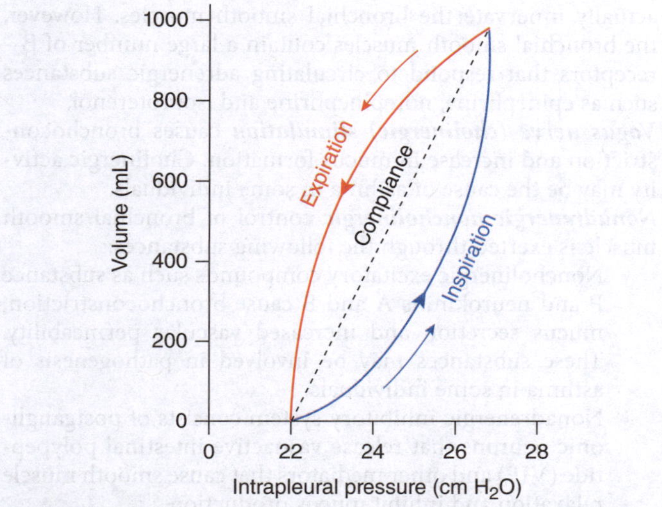

Fig. 5.2.14 Change in volume per unit change in intrapleural pressure during quiet respiration. The dotted line represents the pulmonary compliance.

- The curved lines obtained during inspiration and expiration are because of two resistances:
  Viscous resistance due to nonelastic tissues in the lungs
  Airway resistance
- Therefore, to calculate the compliance of the lung, the point on the graph at the end of inspiration, i.e. when there is no air flow, should be considered. At this point, there is no airway resistance and no viscous resistance. The compliance calculated from pressure and volume changes at this point indicates the compliance of the lung alone due to elastic tissue only.

Static Versus Specific Lung Compliance

Static Compliance

The compliance measured as described above is the *static compliance*. The static compliance of any system is dependent on its size. Thus, the lung compliance depends on the amount of functional lung tissue. Thus, static compliance is not a good measure of absolute distensibility, as is clear from the following example.

For example, if a patient's lung compliance is 0.22 L/cm H_2O, then both lungs together are able to expand 0.22 L for each centimetre of water change in pleural pressure. Assuming equal compliance in both lungs, each lung will take up 0.11 L of gas. If the patient undergoes a pneumonectomy, the compliance measured will be only 0.11 L/cm H_2O, in spite of the fact that distensibility of the remaining lung is normal. Therefore, clinically, term specific compliance is used.

Specific Compliance

Specific compliance is the compliance of the lung at relaxation volume (the point at the end of a tidal expiration), i.e. the FRC. It is expressed per litre of FRC. It is a measure of the absolute distensibility of a structure. For instance, in the above-cited example, if the FRC is 2.2 L, then:

- Specific compliance with both intact lungs will be

$$\frac{0.22}{2.2} = 0.1 \text{ L/cm } H_2O$$

- Specific compliance after pneumonectomy of one lung will be

$$\frac{0.11}{1.1} = 0.1 \text{ L/cm } H_2O$$

Factors Affecting Lung Compliance

Lung compliance is inversely proportional to the lung elastance (elastic recoil force). Therefore, lung compliance is determined on the basis of the following elastic forces:

Elastic forces of the lung: Tissues due to elastic and collagen fibres contribute smaller amount of elasticity.
Elastic forces caused by surface tension within the alveoli account for about two-thirds of total elastic forces in the lungs.
Alveolar surface tension plays a major role in generating elastance forces in the lungs and thus is a very important factor affecting lung compliance. It can be demonstrated experimentally by recording the compliance of an isolated lung of an animal by first distending it with air and then with saline. Filling the lungs with saline theoretically eliminates the force of surface tension so that only the elastic forces of the lung tissue produce recoil. Fig. 5.2.15 shows the results of such an experiment. Compared with air-filled lungs (Fig. 5.2.15A), the saline-filled lungs (Fig. 5.2.15B) markedly reduce recoil forces, leading to the conclusion that the elastic forces caused by alveolar surface tension play a major role in generating elastance forces in the lungs.

Changes in the Lung Compliance

Decreased Compliance

Decreased compliance of the lungs can be caused by lung diseases (e.g. tuberculosis, silicosis) that produce scarring or fibrosis of the lungs, destruction of the functional lung tissue or both. Reduced compliance produces a condition termed restrictive lung disease (RLD). Patients with RLD must generate greater than normal forces to expand the lungs.

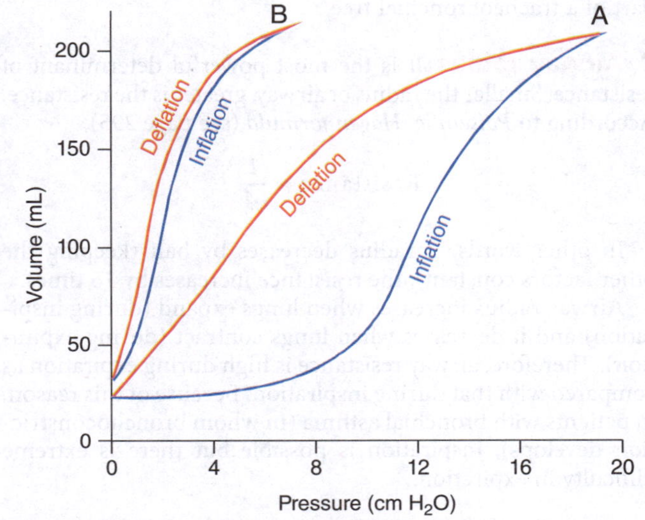

Fig. 5.2.15 Pressure–volume relationship of an isolated lung filled **A,** with air and **B,** with saline. The saline-filled lung has far greater compliance due to absence of surface tension at water–air interface seen with air-filled lung.

Increased Compliance

Increased compliance is produced by the pathological processes that occur in emphysema as well as from the ageing process. Alveolar septa which provide some of the retractive forces in lungs are destroyed under both conditions, but emphysema causes a much more extensive loss of septa than the normal ageing process.

WORK OF BREATHING

The contraction of respiratory muscles causes the expansion of the thoracic cage and thereby causes expansion of lungs and fall in intra-alveolar pressure and allows the atmospheric pressure to push air into the lungs during inspiration. Thus, to move the air into the lungs, the respiratory muscles have to do work to overcome the following *resistances*:

RESISTANCE TO BREATHING

Tissue Resistance

It is the resistance offered by the tissues as they expand or contract. Tissue resistance comprises:

1. Elastic resistance It is the sum of forces of elastic recoil exerted by the lung and the chest wall. The elastic recoil of the lungs is due to the presence of elastic fibres in the lungs and due to the alveolar surface tension.

2. Viscous resistance Viscous resistance is the resistance offered by the nonelastic tissues in the lungs.

Airway Resistance

It is the resistance caused by friction of gas molecules between themselves and the walls of the airways. Factors affecting airway resistance are as follows:

1. Rate of gas flow Greater the rate of gas flow, greater is the resistance. The rate of gas flow is the highest in the intermediate-sized bronchi as they have the highest cross-sectional area; so the highest resistance to flow occurs in this part of a tracheobronchial tree.

2. Airway radius It is the most powerful determinant of resistance. Smaller the radius of airway, greater is the resistance. According to *Poiseuille–Hagen formula* (see page 295),

$$\text{Resistance} \propto \frac{1}{r^4}$$

In other words, if radius decreases by half (keeping the other factors constant), the resistance increases by 16 times.

Airway radius increases when lungs expand (during inspiration) and it decreases when lungs contract (during expiration). Therefore, airway resistance is high during expiration as compared with that during inspiration. Because of this reason, in patients with bronchial asthma (in whom bronchoconstriction develops), inspiration is possible but there is extreme difficulty in expiration.

Control of airway diameter occurs by:

Sympathetic adrenergic stimulation to the airway causes bronchodilation. The sympathetic nerve stimulation causes only slight bronchodilation, because these nerves do not actually innervate the bronchial smooth muscles. However, the bronchial smooth muscles contain a large number of β_2-receptors that respond to circulating adrenergic substances such as epinephrine, norepinephrine and isoproterenol.

Vagus nerve (cholinergic) stimulation causes bronchoconstriction and increase in mucus formation. Cholinergic activity may be the cause of asthma in some individuals.

Nonadrenergic noncholinergic control of bronchial smooth muscle is exerted through the following substances:

- Noncholinergic excitatory compounds such as substance P and neurokinins A and B cause bronchoconstriction, mucus secretion and increased vascular permeability. These substances may be involved in pathogenesis of asthma in some individuals.
- Nonadrenergic inhibitory system consists of postganglionic neurons that release vasoactive intestinal polypeptide (VIP) and other mediators that cause smooth muscle relaxation and inhibit mucus production.

3. Length of airway It does not change much during respiration or in lung diseases and, therefore, is not an important factor.

4. Type of air flow The airway resistance is more in turbulent flow (e.g. during rapid respiration) than in laminar flow or streamline flow in quiet breathing.

COMPONENTS OF WORK OF BREATHING

The total work done by the respiratory muscles during quiet breathing may be divided into the following components:

- Work done to overcome elastic resistance (65%)
- Work done to overcome viscous resistance (7%)
- Work done to overcome airway resistance (28%)

CALCULATION OF WORK OF BREATHING

The work of breathing, i.e. the work of inflating the lungs, can be calculated by plotting the change in lung volume (ΔV) versus the change in intrapleural pressure (ΔP) (Fig. 5.2.16). The total area represented by $\Delta P \times \Delta V$ in Fig. 5.2.16 is proportional to the work that must be performed by the respiratory muscles and to the O_2 utilized by them. The work done by the respiratory muscles can be calculated separately for inspiration and expiration.

Work Done During Inspiration

In Fig. 5.2.16A, the area $A \times BC$ denotes the total work done during normal inspiration. The work of inspiration can be divided into three fractions.

Compliance Work

Compliance work refers to the work done by respiratory muscles to inflate the lungs against the *elastic resistance* of chest wall and lungs. It is represented by the grey triangular area *AYBCA* in Fig. 5.2.16A. Thus, most of the work done (65%) is used to overcome elastic resistance.

Nonelastic Resistance Work

Nonelastic resistance work is done to overcome the nonelastic resistance. It includes the work done to overcome:

- Viscous resistance of lungs (7%)
- Airway resistance (28%)

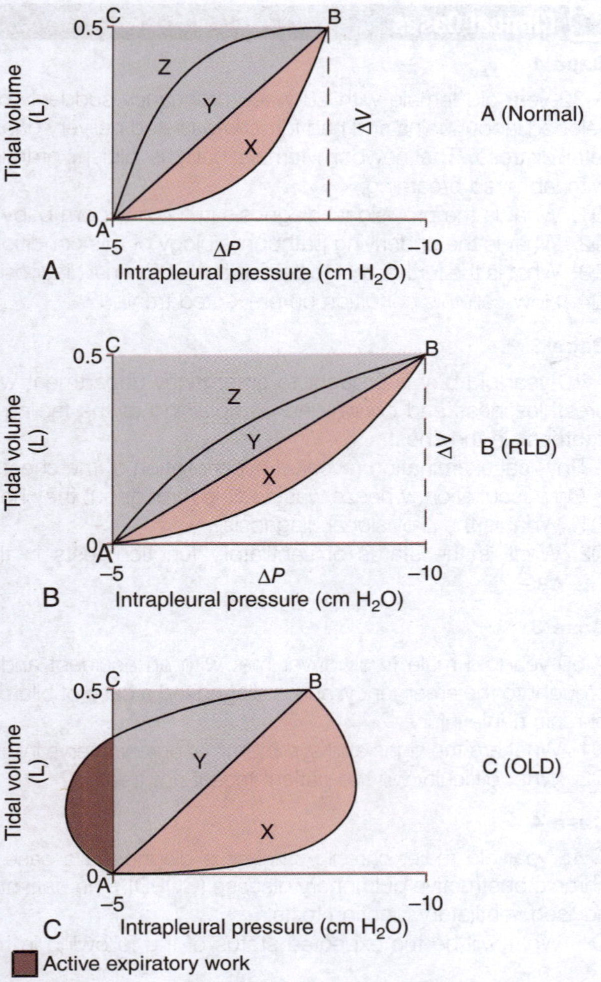

Fig. 5.2.16 Calculation of work done during breathing by plotting the change in volume (ΔV) against change in intrapleural pressure (ΔP): **A**, in normal quiet breathing; **B**, in restrictive lung disease (RLD); and **C**, in obstructive lung disease (OLD).

It is represented by pink area *AXBYA* in Fig. 5.2.16A. Thus, only a small amount (7%) of the work done is used to overcome the viscosity of the lungs and 28% of the work done is utilized to overcome the resistance of air flow through the respiratory passages.

Work Done During Expiration

Since in quiet breathing, expiration is a passive process, no work is done during expiration. The grey triangle *AYBCA* in Fig. 5.2.16A represents the stored elastic energy that is present at the end of inspiration. This stored energy can compress the alveolar gas and create expiratory flow. When the lungs are recoiling back, some energy is required to overcome *nonelastic resistance*, i.e. the airway resistance plus viscous tissue resistance. This is represented by the area which in normal quiet expiration falls within the triangle *AYBZA* (stored energy) and so no extra work is required to overcome this resistance.

Work of Breathing Done in Restrictive Lung Disease

In the presence of RLD, the patient has to overcome significantly higher elastance forces for the normal tidal breathing. So, in RLD, more work has to be performed by the respiratory muscles during inspiration to overcome the decreased compliance (Fig. 5.2.16B).

Minimal Work of Breathing

Minimal work of breathing is a function of airway resistance and respiratory system compliance (Fig. 5.2.17A). All species of animals use the combination of TV and respiratory rate that requires the minimal work of breathing. The increase in the elastance, work done in patients with RLD can be minimized by breathing rapidly and shallow (Fig. 5.2.17B). The TV is decreased but the increased respiratory rate ensures adequate ventilation of lungs.

Work of Breathing Done in Obstructive Lung Diseases

In patients with obstructive lung disease (OLD), the airway resistance is increased due to narrowing of passages. The

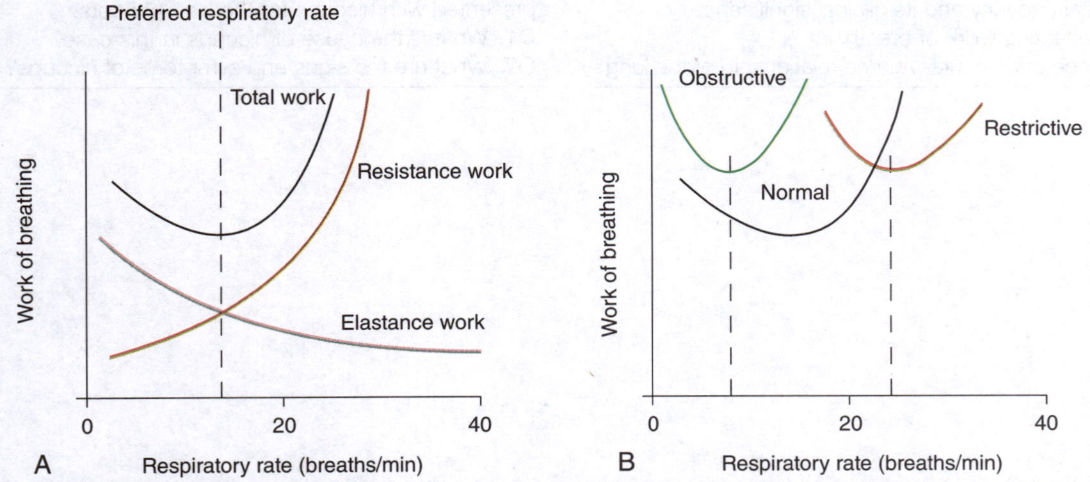

Fig. 5.2.17 Determinants of an optimal breathing to do minimal work of breathing: **A**, variations in different components of work of breathing – the preferred respiratory rate to do minimal work of breathing normally is 12–15 breaths/min, with tidal volume 0.5 L; and **B**, total work of breathing curve reflects that the patients with obstructive lung disease (OLD) minimize their work of breathing by decreasing respiratory rate and increasing tidal volume and those with restrictive lung disease (RLD) do so by decreasing tidal volume and increasing respiratory rate.

patients must generate increased pressure gradients to produce adequate air flow. So, *during inspiration*, more work by respiratory muscles is done to overcome the increased nonelastic resistance; as a result, the work loop broadens significantly as is evident from the pink area *AXBYA* in Fig. 5.2.16C vis-à-vis that in Fig. 5.2.16A. Under such circumstances, when the work loop extends beyond *Y*-axis, active contraction of expiratory muscles is required to accomplish the task of expiration, as the elastic recoil (stored energy represented by grey triangular area) is not sufficient for it. The extra work performed by expiratory muscles is represented by brown area in Fig. 5.2.16C.

Compensatory Mechanism

The resistance work can be minimized by breathing more slowly and deeply (see Fig. 5.2.17B). This prolongs the time of expiration, which reduces the pressure gradient necessary to generate gas flow. The increased TV compensates for the decreased respiratory rate so that normal alveolar ventilation is maintained.

Factors Affecting Total Work of Breathing

Total work of breathing during quiet respiration under normal circumstances ranges from 0.3 to 0.8 kg mt/min. Normally, the work of breathing represents 2%–3% of the resting O_2 consumption.

- If either the respiratory resistance increases or the compliance decreases, the respiratory work will increase and therefore the respiratory muscles will use more O_2 to overcome the added load.
- The work of breathing is also increased markedly during muscular exercise (physiological).

Self-Assessment

1. Discuss the mechanism of respiratory movements.
2. Discuss about elastance and compliance forces in respiratory cycle.
3. Discuss the role of surfactant.
4. Describe briefly:
   - Functional residual capacity
   - Timed vital capacity and its clinical significance
   - Factors affecting work of breathing
   - Significance of pressure–volume relationship of the lung

Clinical Cases

Case 1

A 32-year-old female with 28-week pregnancy suddenly developed labour pains and had forceps-assisted delivery due to fetal distress. The newborn female baby is bluish, grunting with laboured breathing.

Q1. What is the provisional diagnosis in the newborn baby?
Q2. What is the underlying pathophysiology of this condition?
Q3. What is the further test to be carried out for final diagnosis?
Q4. How can this condition be prevented/treated?

Case 2

A 10-year-old boy is brought to emergency department with breathlessness and cough and complaining of the feeling of tightness in the chest.

Physical examination revealed hyperinflation of the chest.

On auscultation, wheeze was audible throughout the chest.

Q1. What is the provisional diagnosis?
Q2. What is the status of ventilatory function tests in this case?

Case 3

A 50-year-old male truck driver met with an accident and is brought to the emergency, and is diagnosed a case of bilateral phrenic nerve injury.

Q1. What are the signs and symptoms of phrenic nerve injury?
Q2. What difficulty will the patient face if not treated?

Case 4

A 45-year-old male, chronic smoker is diagnosed a case of chronic obstructive pulmonary disease (COPD). The patient is advised ventilatory function tests.

Q1. What will be the expected status of the following in this case:
- Vital capacity
- Timed vital capacity
- Total lung capacity
- Functional residual capacity
- Residual volume

Case 5

A 34-year-old male who had spicy food and heavy drinks presented with hiccups for the last 48 hours.

Q1. What is the cause of hiccups in this case?
Q2. What are the signs and symptoms of hiccups?

Pulmonary Circulation 5.3

CHAPTER OUTLINE

FUNCTIONAL ANATOMY

The lungs have three types of circulations – pulmonary, bronchial and lymphatic.

PULMONARY CIRCULATION

The pulmonary trunk arises from the right ventricle and divides into right and left pulmonary arteries which convey deoxygenated blood to the right and left lung, respectively. The blood circulates through a capillary plexus intimately related to the walls of alveoli and receives oxygen from the alveolar air. This blood which is now oxygenated is returned to the heart (left atrium) through the pulmonary veins. There are four pulmonary veins, two each (superior and inferior) on the right and left sides. The pulmonary veins have distensibility characteristics similar to those of veins in the systemic circulation.

BRONCHIAL CIRCULATION

The lungs also receive oxygenated blood like other tissues in the body. This is conveyed through *bronchial arteries* (two left and one right) which are branches of the descending thoracic aorta. Bronchial blood flow amounts to about 1%–2% of total cardiac output. The oxygenated blood in the bronchial arteries supplies the connective tissues, septa and large and small bronchi of the lungs. Because the bronchial blood empties into the pulmonary veins and bypasses the right heart, the bronchial circulation therefore constitutes a *physiological shunt*, i.e. a channel that bypasses oxygenation in the lungs. The other example of physiological shunt is coronary vessels that drain into the left side of the heart. These physiological shunts have two effects:

- They reduce the O_2 saturation of arterial blood slightly.
- They make the left ventricular output greater by about 1%–2% than the right ventricular output.

LYMPHATIC CIRCULATION

Lungs are richly supplied by lymphatics. Lymphatics are present in the walls of the terminal bronchioles and in all the supportive tissues of the lungs. Particulate matter entering the alveoli during inspiration is removed by way of lymphatic channels. Lymphatics also remove the plasma proteins leaking from the lung capillaries and thus help to prevent the pulmonary oedema. The deep lymphatic vessels follow the bronchi and first drain into the *pulmonary nodes* (in the substance of the lungs) and then into *bronchopulmonary nodes*. The superficial lymph vessels lie near the surface of lungs and converge onto bronchopulmonary nodes. From bronchopulmonary node, lymph drains into *tracheobronchial nodes* and from there into the *bronchomediastinal trunk*.

CHARACTERISTIC FEATURES OF PULMONARY CIRCULATION

INTRODUCTION

- The pulmonary arteries and their branches are thin walled and distensible, giving the pulmonary arterial tree a large compliance. The distensibility of pulmonary vessels makes the pulmonary circulation a *low-pressure, low-resistance* and *high-capacitance system*.
- The thickness of the right ventricle and pulmonary artery is approximately one-third of the thickness of the left ventricle and aorta, respectively.
- The pulmonary arterioles have very little smooth muscles in their walls. The pulmonary capillaries are larger in diameter than systemic capillaries and have multiple anastomoses.
- The pulmonary capillaries surround the alveoli and are sandwiched between their walls; as a result, each alveolus seems to be enclosed in a basket of capillaries (Fig. 5.3.1).

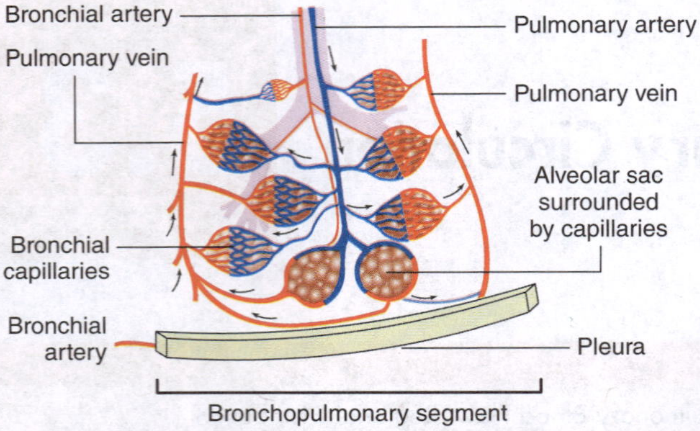

Fig. 5.3.1 Organization of pulmonary circulation.

PRESSURES IN THE PULMONARY SYSTEM (FIG. 5.3.2)

Right Ventricular Pressure

During each cardiac cycle, right ventricular pressure reaches a peak value of 25 mm Hg in systole (if 120 mm Hg in the left ventricle) and falls to 0–1 mm in diastole (if 5 mm Hg in the left ventricle).

Pulmonary Artery Pressures

Pulmonary artery pressures (Pa) vis-à-vis aorta, respectively, are as follows:

- Systolic pressure 25 and 120 mm Hg
- Diastolic pressure 8 and 80 mm Hg
- Mean arterial pressure 15 and 100 mm Hg
- Pulse pressure 17 and 40 mm Hg

Left Atrial Pressure

Left atrial pressure in major pulmonary veins averages about 5 mm Hg in the recumbent human being. Therefore, the pressure gradient in the pulmonary system ([mean Pa] − [mean pulmonary vein pressure]) is 15 − 5 = 10 mm Hg (if 120 mm Hg in the systemic circulation).

Pulmonary Capillary Pressure

The mean value estimated through indirect means is about 10 mm Hg. Since this pressure is far below the colloid osmotic pressure (25 mm Hg), a net suction force of 15 mm Hg tends to draw fluid from alveolar interstitial space into the pulmonary capillaries *which keeps the alveoli dry*. However, if the pulmonary capillary hydrostatic pressure rises above 25 mm Hg, fluid can escape into the interstitial space leading to *pulmonary oedema*. This can happen during exercise, particularly at high altitude, in left heart failure, mitral stenosis and pulmonary fibrosis. It is important to know that even a thin layer of interstitial fluid increases the distance between blood in pulmonary capillaries and gases in alveoli. Since the rate of diffusion is inversely proportional to the diffusion distance, increase in the distance would reduce the rate of gas exchange in the lungs. The resultant hypoxia may be fatal.

Pulmonary Wedge Pressure

Pulmonary wedge pressure is measured to give an estimate of left atrial pressure. Direct measurement of left atrial pressure is difficult because it requires passing a catheter through the left ventricle. Pulmonary wedge pressure is measured by inserting a balloon-tipped catheter through the right side of the heart and pulmonary artery until the catheter wedges tightly in a smaller branch of the artery and stops the blood

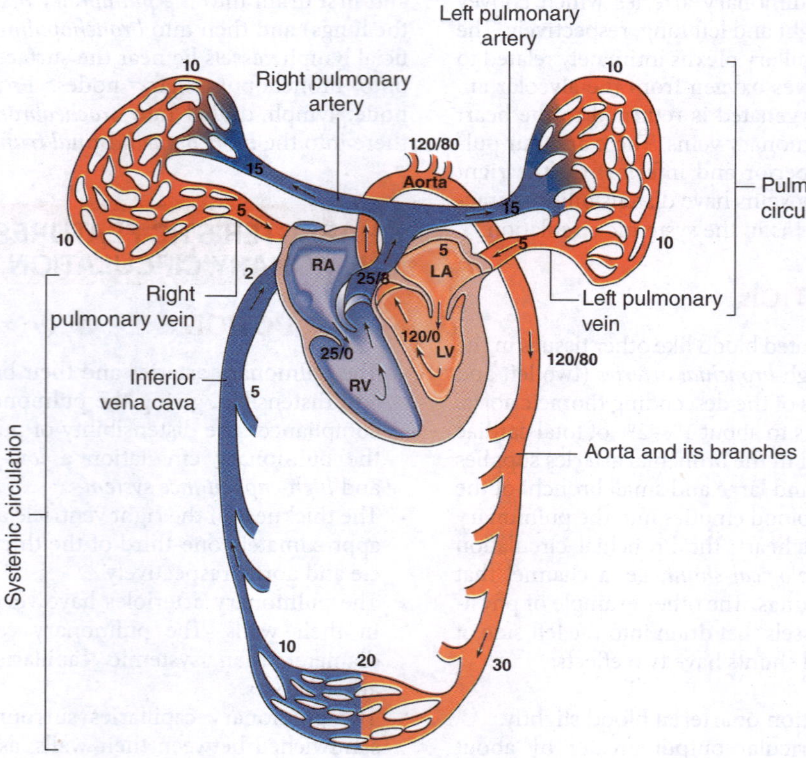

Fig. 5.3.2 Blood pressure (mm Hg) in pulmonary and systemic circulation. LA, left atrium; LV, left ventricle; RA, right atrium; RV, right ventricle.

flowing in it. Under such circumstances, the ballooned tip of the catheter makes an almost direct connection through the pulmonary capillaries with the blood in pulmonary veins which have the pressure similar to that in the left atrium. The wedge pressure so measured is usually only 2–3 mm greater than the left atrial pressure. Clinically, wedge pressure measurements are used frequently for studying changes in left atrial pressure in patients with congestive heart failure.

PULMONARY BLOOD VOLUME

Pulmonary vessels contain about 600 mL of blood at rest. Since the pulmonary vessels act as capacitance vessels, their blood content can vary from 200 to 900 mL.

Pulmonary blood volume decreases under physiological conditions like standing and is shifted to systemic circulation to compensate for the blood pooled in the leg veins due to gravity. Under pathological conditions like haemorrhage, the transfer of blood from pulmonary vessels to systemic circulation can partly compensate for the blood loss. Thus, the pulmonary vessels act as a reservoir of blood.

Pulmonary blood volume increases when changing posture from standing to lying. Pathological conditions in which pulmonary blood volume is increased are mitral stenosis, mitral regurgitation and left heart failure.

PULMONARY BLOOD FLOW: REGIONAL DISTRIBUTION

Pulmonary blood flow is nearly equal to cardiac output, since the right ventricle also pushes the same amount of blood simultaneously into the pulmonary circulation as the left ventricle pushes in the systemic. Blood flow through the lungs depends on the relationship between Pa, pulmonary venous pressure (Pv) and alveolar pressure (PA) as:

- The difference between Pa and Pv is the driving pressure.
- The pulmonary capillary pressure must be above the PA for the blood flow to continue.

Effect of Gravity on Regional Pulmonary Blood Flow

In normal adults in supine position, the mean arterial pressure is same all over the lung and so all regions of the lung are uniformly perfused. However, in erect posture, the gravity affects the regional distribution of blood through the lung by altering the pulmonary vasculature pressure due to hydrostatic pressure effect. The hydrostatic pressure adds or subtracts from the pressure levels in supine position if levels are below or above the zero reference plane, respectively. The zero reference plane is at the level of the right atrium, which is approximately in the middle of the lung in the region of hilum. Therefore, in standing posture, the mean Pa in a 30-cm-long lung will be:

- *In the middle of the lung* (zero reference level), it will be 15 mm Hg.
- *At the apex of the lung*, it will be less by 15 cm H_2O or 11 mm Hg, i.e. about 4 mm Hg.
- *At the base of the lung*, it will be more by 11 mm Hg, i.e. about 26 mm Hg.

Perfusion zones of the lung Depending on the relationship between PA, Pa and Pv, the lung can be divided into three zones in erect posture:

Zone 1 refers to the area of zero flow, i.e. any region of the lung that does not receive blood flow. It *does not exist in normal lungs.* Zone 1 occurs when the regional Pa becomes less than the PA (Pa < PA); under these conditions, the pulmonary capillaries collapse (Fig. 5.3.3) and blood flow becomes zero.

Zone 1 is present under the following abnormal conditions:

- When the Pa is too low as in hypovolaemic shock and pulmonary embolism (PE)
- When the PA is too high to allow flow as in severe obstructive lung disorder

Zone 2 refers to region of the lung that has intermittent blood flow. This occurs during systole when the Pa exceeds the PA which exceeds the Pv (Pa > PA > Pv), but not during diastole when the arterial pressure is less than the PA.

- Zone 2 blood flow is thus determined by the arterial–alveolar pressure gradient, and not the arteriovenous gradient. This condition is known as *waterfall effect*, because changes in the downstream pressure or the venous pressure do not alter blood flow.
- Zone 2 condition normally occurs from the apex to the hilum of the lung. At the middle of the lung, mean Pa is 15 mm Hg, but it varies from 25 mm Hg (in the systole phase) to 8 mm Hg (in the diastole phase).
- These levels of arterial pressure keep on lowering by 1 cm H_2O (0.8 mm Hg) for every 1 cm above the hilum level; therefore, at the apex of the lungs, the mean arterial pressure becomes about 4 mm Hg and varies from 14 mm Hg in systole to −3 mm Hg in diastole. However, the PA remains constant, and thus the blood flow (which depends on arterial–alveolar gradient) increases linearly from the top to the bottom of zone 2 (Fig. 5.3.3).

Zone 3 refers to region of high continuous blood flow where the capillary pressure remains greater than PA during the entire cardiac cycle. So, zone 3 occurs when the Pa exceeds the Pv which exceeds the PA (Pa > Pv > PA). This condition occurs near the bottom of the lung. Since the pulmonary vascular pressure increases as we go down from the middle of the lung to its bottom, the blood flow increases down zone 3 (Fig. 5.3.3).

Effect of exercise on regional pulmonary blood flow

During exercise, the blood flow increases in all the regions of the lungs. During heavy exercise, pulmonary blood flow increases four to seven times. Near the base of the lung, blood flow increases by two to three times, whereas in the upper regions, it can increase to eight times. Thus, the entire lung becomes equivalent to zone 3 during exercise. The marked increase in pulmonary blood flow occurs due to two effects:

- *Recruitment of capillaries*, i.e. increasing the number of open capillaries
- *Distension of the capillaries*, i.e. increasing the rate of flow

Both distension and recruitment of capillaries decrease the resistance to blood flow so much so that even during exercise

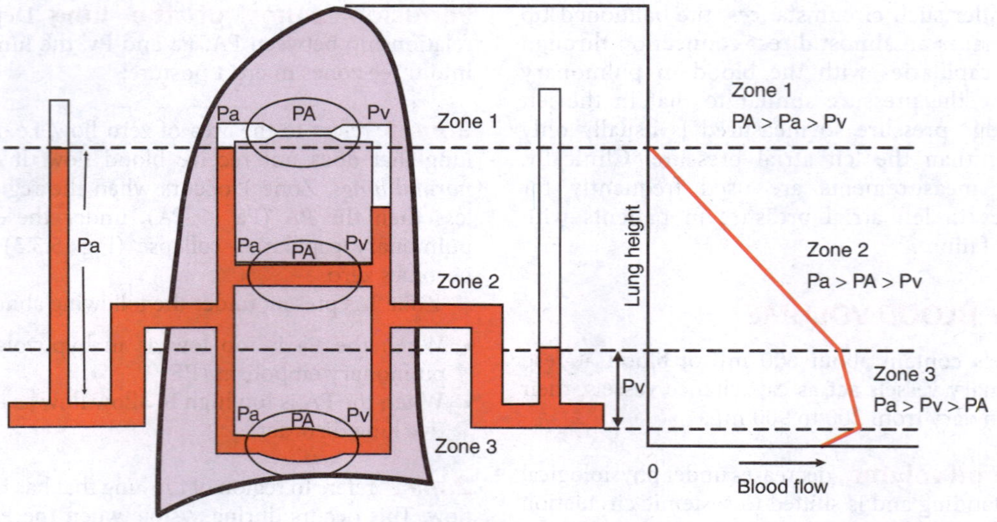

Fig. 5.3.3 Effect of gravity on regional distribution of pulmonary blood flow in standing posture.

the Pa rises very little. This ability of the lungs to accommodate markedly increased flow during exercise has two advantages:

- Conserves the energy of right side of the heart
- Prevents development of pulmonary oedema during the increased cardiac output

PULMONARY CAPILLARY DYNAMICS

Pulmonary Transit Time

The mean transit time in the pulmonary circulation from the pulmonary valves to the left atrium is about 4 seconds. A red cell traverses the pulmonary capillary in approximately 0.8 second at rest (capillary transit time) and 0.3 second during exercise. Even in this brief duration, adequate gaseous exchange between the red cells and the alveolar air can occur.

Capillary Exchange of Fluid in the Lung, and Pulmonary Interstitial Fluid Dynamics

Dynamics of fluid exchange through pulmonary capillaries Dynamics of fluid exchange through pulmonary capillaries are qualitatively the same except for the following quantitative differences from the peripheral tissues in systemic circulation:

- *Pulmonary capillary pressure* is low, about 7 mm Hg (cf. 17 mm Hg in peripheral tissues).
- *Interstitial fluid pressure* is slightly more negative (−5 to −8 mm Hg) than in the peripheral subcutaneous tissue.
- *Capillary permeability* is high, so more proteins leak in the interstitial fluid; consequently, the interstitial oncotic pressure is also high, averaging about 14 mm Hg (cf. 7 mm Hg in peripheral tissues).
- *Alveolar walls are thin* and may rupture when the interstitial pressure becomes greater than atmospheric pressure, which allows dumping of fluid from the interstitial spaces into the alveoli.

Mean filtration pressure at the pulmonary capillaries

Mean filtration pressure at the pulmonary capillaries is +1 mm Hg. This value is derived from the balance of Starling forces at the capillary membrane given as follows:

Outward forces are as follows:

- Interstitial oncotic pressure = 14 mm Hg (pulls fluid out)
- Interstitial hydrostatic pressure = −8 mm Hg (pulls fluid out)
- Capillary hydrostatic pressure = 7 mm Hg (pushes fluid out)
- Total outward force = 29 mm Hg

Inward force

- Plasma oncotic pressure = 28 mm Hg

Net mean filtration pressure = 29 − 28 = 1 mm Hg

Filtration of fluid Filtration of fluid from the pulmonary capillaries into the interstitial space caused by the net filtration pressure of +1 mm Hg is very small in amount. Except for a meagre amount that evaporates in the alveoli, most of this fluid is pumped back to the circulation through the pulmonary lymphatic system. So practically a negligible amount of fluid is present in the interstitial space.

Applied Aspects

Pulmonary oedema

- Theoretically, pulmonary oedema can occur due to change in any of the four Starling forces resulting in increased capillary filtration in the same way as peripheral oedema can occur.
- *Increase in the capillary hydrostatic pressure* is by far the most common factor responsible for pulmonary oedema in conditions leading to left heart failure or mitral valvular disease. The pulmonary capillary pressure normally must rise equal to the plasma colloid osmotic pressure, i.e. above 28 mm Hg. Thus, there is safety factor against pulmonary oedema of about 21 mm Hg.
- *Increase in capillary permeability* due to damage to capillary membrane caused by infections or breathing of irritating gases produces rapid leakage of both plasma proteins and fluid out of the capillaries (exudation).
- *In acute left heart failure*, when capillary pressure rises above the safety level, lethal pulmonary oedema can occur within minutes to hours. When capillary pressure rises

to 50 mm Hg, death frequently ensues within less than 30 minutes from acute pulmonary oedema.

- *In chronic cases of pulmonary oedema*, there occurs a compensatory increase in the lymphatic drainage as much as 10-fold which prevents pulmonary oedema even at higher capillary pressure. In a patient with chronic mitral stenosis, pulmonary capillary pressure of 40–50 mm Hg has been measured without the development of significant pulmonary oedema.

Signs and symptoms of pulmonary oedema are as follows:

- Dyspnoea and orthopnoea occur; sputum becomes pinkish and frothy.
- The patient cannot even speak.

Treatment: Use of diuretics and oxygen therapy may help.

Important Note

Patients with cardiac failure feel more comfortable in sitting position rather than in supine position, because supine posture leads to pulmonary congestion.

Pulmonary hypertension

Pulmonary hypertension (PH) refers to high blood pressure that affects the arteries in the lungs and right side of the heart. It is characterized by raised pulmonary capillary pressure and increased pulmonary vascular resistance, and mainly occurs due to hypoxia.

Signs and symptoms of PH include:

- Shortness of breath while exercising and eventually at rest
- Feeling of chest pressure or pain
- Cyanosis which may occur due to low oxygen level

Treatment: The treatment of PH depends on the severity; the condition worsens over time, but medication in the form of vasodilators and oxygen therapy can help lessen symptoms and improve quality of life.

Complications: If PH is not treated properly, the following complications may occur:

- Right ventricular hypertrophy
- Right ventricular failure
- Pulmonary oedema
- Death may occur

Pulmonary embolism

Pulmonary embolism (PE) is a condition in which one or more arteries in the lungs get blocked by blood clot. Most of the time, blood clot gets dislodged from the legs, travels to lungs and gets lodged in the pulmonary arteries.

Signs and symptoms of PE are as follows:

- Shortness of breath
- Increase in respiratory rate
- Pain in the chest on breathing
- Dry cough
- Tachycardia and palpitation

Treatment: Prompt treatment is essential to prevent serious complications and death.

- Blood thinner and anticoagulants are the most common treatment.
- Analgesics help to relieve pain.
- Oxygen therapy may be required.
- Thrombolysis is required in severe cases.

FUNCTIONS OF PULMONARY CIRCULATION

Respiratory gas exchange is the major function of pulmonary circulation. This function has been discussed in Chapter 5.4 (page 408).

Other functions of pulmonary circulation which have been described on page 383 are as follows:

- Reservoir for the left ventricle
- Filter for removal of emboli and other particles from blood
- Removal of fluid from alveoli
- Role in absorption of drugs
- Synthesis of angiotensin-converting enzyme (ACE)

REGULATION OF PULMONARY BLOOD FLOW

The pulmonary blood flow is affected by autonomic innervation and large number of circulating humoral factors.

NEURAL CONTROL

Efferent Sympathetic Vasoconstrictor Nerves

Efferent sympathetic vasoconstrictor nerves richly innervate the pulmonary blood vessels. But these nerves have *no resting discharge and tone*, which means that they can show only an increase in activity when stimulated. These participate in the vasomotor reflexes, e.g.:

- *Baroreceptor stimulation* produces reflex dilatation of pulmonary vessels.
- *Chemoreceptor stimulation* causes pulmonary vasoconstriction.

However, the effect of vasodilatation and vasoconstriction is more on the capacity rather than on the resistance of pulmonary vessels. The vasoconstriction produced in the lungs due to sympathetic discharge is considerable and results in transfer of pulmonary blood in systemic circulation, e.g. during acute haemorrhage.

Afferent Control

Afferent control through the vagus is mediated through the following receptors:

Pulmonary baroreceptors Pulmonary baroreceptors are present in the tunica adventitia of the pulmonary trunk and its two major branches. These vagal mechanoreceptors detect rise in pressure in the pulmonary artery and produce reflex bradycardia and hypotension.

Pulmonary volume receptors Pulmonary volume receptors are the vagal mechanoreceptors present at the junction of the pulmonary vein with the left atrium. Stimulation of these receptors produces tachycardia and diuresis which help in regulating blood volume. These vagal receptors could be afferent limb of the Bainbridge reflex.

J receptors Juxtapulmonary receptors (J receptors) are present adjacent to pulmonary capillaries in the alveolar interstitial space. These are stimulated by multiple microemboli in the small pulmonary vessels and also by the fluid entrapped in interstitial space, especially after exercise and at high altitude. Stimulation of J receptors leads to *reflex tachypnoea* (increase in rate of breathing) and reduction of skeletal muscle tone. A.S. Paintal, an Indian physiologist who discovered J receptors, postulated that stimulation of these receptors induces dyspnoea, which together with reduction of muscle tone would discourage exercise, thereby taking away the trigger for pulmonary congestion.

Conclusion On the whole, the neural control on the pulmonary circulation is not very strong, since all the cardiac output has to pass through the pulmonary circulation. Mostly pulmonary vessels act as passive distensible tubes that enlarge with increasing luminal pressure and become narrow with the decrease in pressure.

CHEMICAL CONTROL

1. Local Hypoxia

Local hypoxia is responsible for most significant alterations in pulmonary blood flow by producing *vasoconstriction*. This is a local and direct action, since it can be demonstrated in isolated (denervated) perfused lungs. This is exactly opposite to what happens in systemic circulation where low pO_2 produces vasodilatation. Both of these opposite responses are very useful for the body:

Low pO_2 in systemic circulation In systemic circulation, low pO_2 in tissues indicates that oxygen supply is insufficient for the demands of the tissues. Therefore, low pO_2–induced vasodilation increases the blood flow and corrects the deficiency.

Low pO_2 in the lungs In lungs, low pO_2 in the lungs means that the alveoli are not well ventilated. Therefore, blood flow through that region is waste. Since it will not get adequately oxygenated, the local low pO_2–induced vasoconstriction in the lungs is a phenomenon that diverts pulmonary blood flow from the alveoli that are poorly ventilated to better ventilated regions so that blood can be properly oxygenated.

Mechanism: The smooth muscles of pulmonary arteries contain O_2-sensitive K^+ channels, which mediate the vasoconstriction caused by hypoxia. This is in contrast to systemic arteries, which contain adenosine triphosphate (ATP)–dependent K^+ channels that permit more K^+ efflux with hypoxia and cause vasodilation rather than vasoconstriction.

2. Hypercapnia and Acidosis

Hypercapnia and acidosis also produce vasoconstriction. The effects of pCO_2 and acidosis on pulmonary vessels are just opposite to those in the systemic vessels where these stimuli produce vasodilation. The functional significance of this response is same as in the case of local hypoxia.

3. Chronic Hypoxia

Chronic hypoxia, as occurs in high-altitude dwellers, is associated with a marked increase in pulmonary hypertension (PH), which imposes a heavy afterload on the right ventricle that results in right ventricular hypertrophy, right heart failure and pulmonary oedema. This is the reason that:

- Thick pulmonary precapillary vessels develop in high-altitude dwellers.
- Children born and raised at high altitude show PH.

Table 5.3.1 Receptors on smooth muscles of pulmonary vasculature and their effects

Receptor	Subtype	Response
Adrenergic	α_1	Contraction
	α_2	Relaxation
	β_2	Relaxation
Adenosine	A_1	Contraction
	A_2	Relaxation
Angiotensin	A_{T1}	Contraction
ANP	ANP_A	Relaxation
Bradykinin	ANP_B	Relaxation
	B_2	Relaxation
Cholinergic (muscarinic)	M_3	Relaxation
CGRP		Relaxation
Endothelin	ET_A	Contraction
	ET_B	Relaxation
5-HT	$5HT_1$	Contraction
	$5HT_{1C}$	Relaxation
Histamine	H_1	Relaxation
	H_2	Relaxation
Purinergic	P_{2X}	Contraction
	P_{2Y}	Relaxation
Tachykinin	NK_1	Relaxation
	NK_2	Contraction
Thromboxane	T_P	Contraction
Vasopressin	V_1	Relaxation
VIP		Relaxation

HUMORAL CONTROL

The pulmonary vessels respond to circulating agents through their receptors located on smooth muscles of the vasculature (Table 5.3.1).

Self-Assessment

1. Describe the following:
   - Characteristic features of pulmonary circulation
   - Regional distribution of pulmonary blood flow
   - Pulmonary capillary dynamics
2. Discuss the regulation of pulmonary blood flow.
3. Write notes on:
   - Pulmonary oedema
   - Pulmonary hypertension
   - Functions of pulmonary circulation

Clinical Cases

Case 1

A 57-year-old lady presented to the emergency with dyspnoea and episode of dizziness on exertion (during exercise, fast walking and climbing stairs) and twice she had episodes of syncope.

On examination, the respiratory rate was 30 breaths/min, and breathing rapid and shallow; chest auscultation revealed wheeze throughout the chest.

Q1. What is the provisional diagnosis?

Q2. What tests should be carried out to find the cause of this condition?

Case 2

A 24-year-old woman was admitted to the emergency department with shortness of breath, bluish lips and nails, and palpitation.

On examination, pulse rate was 120/min and pulse pressure was normal.

X-ray chest showed bilateral congestion.

Q1. What is the diagnosis?

Q2. What are the causes of this condition?

Q3. What immediate treatment is recommended in this case?

Case 3

A 50-year-old female underwent hip replacement surgery. On the 10th postoperative day, she developed acute chest pain, cough with blood-stained mucus and shortness of breath, and was suspected to be a case of pulmonary embolism.

Q1. What is the main cause of pulmonary embolism?

Q2. What immediate treatment should be given in this condition?

5.4 Pulmonary Diffusion

CHAPTER OUTLINE

INTRODUCTION

As discussed earlier, the external respiration (supply of O_2 from atmosphere to body tissues and removal of CO_2 from the body tissues to atmosphere) is accomplished by three major processes:

- *Pulmonary ventilation* (PV), i.e. exchange of gases between the environment and the lungs
- *Pulmonary diffusion*, i.e. transfer of gases from alveoli to capillary blood across the respiratory membrane
- *Transport of gases* from the blood to the tissue cells and back

To understand the *intricacies* of diffusion of gases across the respiratory membrane, it is essential to have knowledge about the following related aspects and concepts, most of which form the contents of this chapter:

- *Pulmonary perfusion*, i.e. *pulmonary blood flow:* Special problems related to pulmonary haemodynamics have important implications for gas exchange in the lungs. Most of these have been discussed in Chapter 5.3 (page 404).
- *Physics of gas diffusion and gas partial pressures:* The rate at which the respiratory gases diffuse across the respiratory membrane is a much more complicated problem, requiring a deeper understanding of the physics of diffusion and gas exchange.
- *Alveolar ventilation:* It is the rate at which new air reaches the gas exchange area of the lungs. Alveolar ventilation governs the process of pulmonary diffusion in its own way.
- *Alveolar ventilation–perfusion ratio (V/Q):* It is the ratio of alveolar ventilation and pulmonary blood flow. This is a highly quantitative concept which was developed to help in understanding respiratory exchange when there is imbalance between alveolar ventilation and alveolar blood flow.
- *Diffusion of gases through the respiratory membrane:* It is the main process which transfers gases from the alveoli into the capillaries. Various important aspects of this process have also been discussed in this chapter.

PHYSICS OF GAS DIFFUSION AND GAS PARTIAL PRESSURES

It is worthwhile to recapitulate some of the basic principles and laws governing the behaviour of gases, for a better understanding of the process of diffusion between alveolar air and pulmonary capillary blood. Consequently, the present discussion is on some of the important aspects concerning physics of gas diffusion and gas partial pressures.

GAS PRESSURE

The gas molecules have a kinetic energy so they are in a continuous random motion. These molecules bounce against each other and/or against the walls of container and exert a pressure. The gas pressure (P) exerted depends on the following factors:

Concentration of molecules (n) It is obvious that greater the concentration of the molecules of gas, greater would be the force exerted by the molecules against the container walls at any given time. Therefore, the pressure of a gas is directly proportional to its concentration, i.e.

$$P \propto n \qquad \text{(i)}$$

Volume (V) Unlike liquids, gases expand to fill the volume available to them. Therefore, it is obvious that the pressure exerted by a constant number of gas molecules will be more if the volume is less and vice versa. Therefore, at a constant temperature, the pressure (P) of a given mass of gas is inversely proportional to its volume (V), i.e.

$$P \propto \frac{1}{V} \qquad \text{(ii)}$$

This is called *Boyle's law* of gases.

Absolute temperature (T) According to *Charles' law*, at a constant pressure, the volume of gas is directly proportional to its absolute temperature, i.e. $V \propto T$, and, as mentioned above, according to Boyle's law

$$P \propto \frac{1}{V}$$

Therefore, it can be derived that

$$P \propto T \qquad \text{(iii)}$$

From Equations (i)–(iii), it can be derived that

$$P = \frac{nRT}{V}$$

where

P = Pressure of gas
n = Number of molecules of gas
T = Absolute temperature
V = Volume of gas
R = Gas constant

PARTIAL PRESSURE

According to *Dalton's law* of partial pressure, the total pressure exerted by a mixture of gases is equal to the sum of the partial pressure of all gases present in the mixture. Thus, the partial pressure (p) refers to the pressure exerted by any one gas present in a mixture of gases. It is equal to the total pressure exerted by the mixture of gases times the fraction of the total amount of mixture of gases it represents. Hence, the partial pressure (p) of a gas can be calculated by multiplying its fractional concentration by the total pressure. For example, environmental air (which has atmospheric pressure [at sea level] of about 760 mm Hg) is a mixture of 21% oxygen (O_2) and 79% nitrogen (N_2). Therefore, the partial pressure (p) of O_2 and N_2, respectively, will be

$$pO_2 = 760 \frac{21}{100} = 160 \text{ mm Hg, and}$$

$$pN_2 = 760 \frac{79}{100} = 600 \text{ mm Hg.}$$

Partial Pressure of Gases in Water and Tissues

It is important to have knowledge about the partial pressure of gases in water and tissues, because the respiratory gases to cross the respiratory membrane must first dissolve in the tissues and then diffuse into the plasma of pulmonary capillaries. The pressure (p) of a gas in a solution is determined not only by its concentration but also by its solubility coefficient. According to *Henry's law*, when temperature is kept constant, the content of gas (n) dissolved in any solution is directly proportional to the partial pressure of a gas, i.e.

$$n = pc$$

where

n = Concentration (amount) of a gas in a solution
p = Partial pressure of gas
c = Solubility coefficient of the gas

Gas Content, Partial Pressure and Solubility

Gas content, partial pressure and solubility need further clarification. When a gas under pressure comes in contact with a liquid, some of the gas molecules get dissolved in it. As more and more molecules become dissolved, they diffuse all over the liquid medium and some of them start bouncing out of the liquid phase into the gas phase. Ultimately, an *equilibrium* is reached when the number of gas molecules entering the liquid phase equals the number of molecules leaving it.

Gas content Gas content represents the volume of the gas per unit volume of liquid that is present. The units of gas content are volume of gas/volume of solvent (e.g. mL/L, mL, dL).

Partial pressure Partial pressure of a gas in a liquid represents the pressure it would exert in the gas phase. *At equilibrium*, the partial pressure in the liquid phase equals the partial pressure in the gas phase. *In the absence of equilibrium*, the partial pressure of a gas in liquid phase is less than in the gas phase.

Solubility Solubility of a gas is a major determinant of the number of molecules present. A higher solubility increases the rate of diffusion, because this indicates the presence of an increased number of molecules.

Solubility coefficient Solubility coefficient is a constant for each gas that equates gas content and partial pressure. Solubility coefficients of gases (important to respiratory physiology) are given in Table 5.4.1. Increasing the temperature reduces the solubility coefficient of gases (Table 5.4.1).

Important Note

It is important to note that *solubility coefficient of carbon dioxide (CO_2) is about 24 times more and that of nitrogen (N_2) is one-half that of oxygen (O_2).*

Table 5.4.1 Solubility coefficients of important gases in respiratory physiology

	Solubility coefficient (mL gas/mL saline/mm Hg gas tension)			
Temperature (°C)	O_2	N_2	CO_2	CO
0	0.049	0.024	1.71	0.035
20	0.032	0.016	0.90	0.023
37	0.024	0.012	0.58	0.019

WATER VAPOUR PRESSURE

The atmospheric air entering the respiratory passages during inspiration is humidified by the water vapours from the conducting passages. By the time the atmospheric air reaches the alveoli, it is saturated with water vapours. Thus, in the alveolar air, besides O_2 and N_2, water vapour also exerts its partial pressure. Vapour pressure of water is dependent on its temperature. At body temperature (37°C), the vapour pressure of water in alveolar air is 47 mm Hg.

ALVEOLAR VENTILATION

Alveolar ventilation is the volume of the fresh air which reaches the gas exchange area of the lung each minute. During inspiration, some of the air inhaled never reaches the gas exchange areas but instead fills the non–gas exchange areas (conducting zone) of the respiratory tract called the *dead space*, which is equal to about 150 mL. Thus, alveolar ventilation is not equal to PV or the so-called minute respiratory volume (MV), which equals tidal volume (500 mL in quiet respiration) multiplied by the respiratory rate (12 breaths/min), i.e. about 6 L/min.

During expiration, out of 500 mL of tidal volume, 150 mL of the alveolar expired air remains in the conducting passages. Therefore, of 500 mL air entering the lungs, only 350 mL/breath is the fresh air which contributes to alveolar ventilation. Thus, alveolar ventilation can be calculated as:

$$\text{Alveolar ventilation} = \text{Respiratory rate} \times [(\text{tidal volume}) - (\text{dead space volume})]$$

With a normal tidal volume of 500 mL, a normal dead space of 150 mL and a respiratory rate of 12 breaths/min, alveolar ventilation equals 12 × (500 − 150), or 4200 mL/min.

PHYSIOLOGICAL SIGNIFICANCE OF ALVEOLAR VENTILATION

The physiological significance of alveolar ventilation can be understood by comparing the alveolar ventilation of two subjects with the following parameters:

Subject A Subject A having normal breathing with tidal volume of 500 mL and respiratory rate of 12 breaths/min will have:

- PV = 12 × 500 = 6 L/min
- Alveolar ventilation = 12 × (500 − 150) = 4.2 L/min

Subject B Subject B having rapid shallow breathing with tidal volume of 200 mL and respiratory rate 30 breaths/min will have:

- PV = 30 × 200 = 6 L/min
- Alveolar ventilation = 30 × (200 − 150) = 1.5 L/min

On comparison, both the subjects A and B have similar amounts of PV (6 L/min), but the alveolar ventilation of subject B (1.5 L/min) is much less than that of subject A (4.2 L/min). Consequently, subject B is likely to suffer from hypoxia and hypercapnia.

DEAD SPACE AIR

Dead space air is the portion of minute ventilation that does not take part in exchange of gases. There are three types of dead spaces (Fig. 5.4.1).

1. Anatomical Dead Space

Anatomical dead space refers to the volume of air present in the conducting zone of the respiratory passage, i.e. from the nose to the terminal bronchioles. The anatomical dead space ventilation (V_D) is a function of the anatomical dead space and respiratory rate. As mentioned earlier, the anatomical dead space contains approximately 150 mL of air; therefore, at a normal respiratory rate of 12 breaths/min, the anatomical dead space ventilation will be 150 × 12, i.e. 1.8 L/min.

2. Alveolar Dead Space Air

Alveolar dead space air refers to the volume of air present in those alveoli which do not take part in gas exchange. Normally, all the alveoli take part in gas exchange, but in some lung diseases, some alveoli do not take part in gas exchange because of the following reasons:

When alveoli have zero blood flow (Zone 1 condition), the volume of air ventilating such alveoli does not take part in gas exchange.

When alveoli are overventilated, some of the air which is in excess of the volume required to equilibrate with the blood is not able to take part in gas exchange. These alveoli form the alveolar dead space and the air present in them is called the alveolar dead space air.

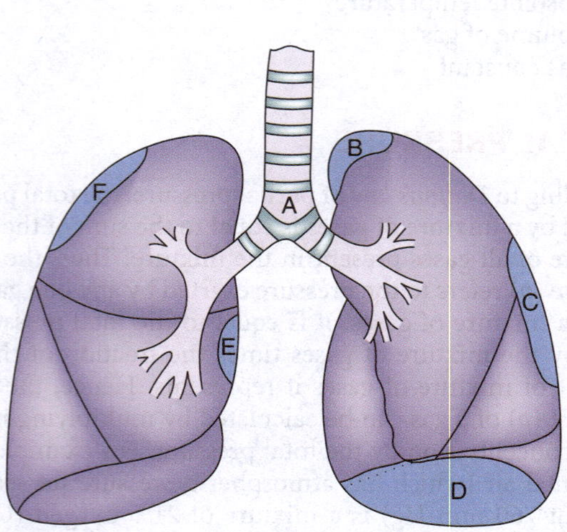

Fig. 5.4.1 Dead space: A, anatomical; B + C + D + E + F, alveolar; A + B + C + D + E + F, physiological.

3. Physiological Dead Space

Physiological dead space refers to the total dead space which includes both the anatomical and alveolar dead spaces. In a normal healthy person, physiological dead space nearly equals the anatomical dead space. However, in certain respiratory disorders with many nonfunctioning alveoli, the physiological dead space may be as much as 10 times the anatomical dead space; obviously, such patients would have very little effective alveolar ventilation which results in respiratory distress. Some of such common respiratory disorders include advanced stages of:

- Emphysema
- Bronchiectasis
- Pulmonary embolism

Measurement of Anatomical Dead Space

Single-Breath Oxygen Technique This technique is also called single-breath nitrogen wash-out test. In this test, nitrogen contents in the expired air are used as an indicator for determining the dead space.

Procedure The subject is asked to take a deep breath of pure oxygen (100% O_2). Then he/she steadily exhales into the nitrometer, which continuously measures N_2 contents in the expired air. The anatomical dead space can be measured by the analysis of single-breath nitrogen curve (Fig. 5.4.2). The curve has four phases labelled by roman letters (I, II, III and IV).

- During inspiration, N_2 contents are nil (0%) as the subject has inspired pure O_2.
- During initial phase of expiration (phase I), N_2 contents are nil (0%) as the expired air is from the dead space (which is filled with pure O_2).
- Subsequently (phase II), there is rise in N_2 contents in the expired air because exhaled air contains mixture of dead space air and alveolar air.
- In phase III, the N_2 contents reach a plateau (60%) and phase III of single-breath nitrogen curve ends at closing volume (CV) and is followed by the phase IV.
  Note: The CV is the lung volume at which the airways in lower (basal) part of the lung begin to close because of lesser transmural pressure in these regions. It is always above residual volume.

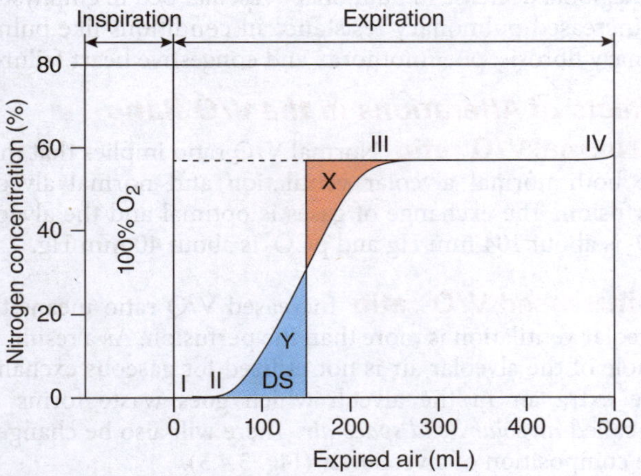

Fig. 5.4.2 Single-breath curve for measuring dead space air. The changes in N_2 concentration of expired air during expiration are indicated by various phases (I–IV). DS, dead space.

- In phase IV, N_2 contents of the expired air are further increased, because the upper parts of the lung are more distended at the beginning of inspiration; therefore, N_2 in these regions gets less diluted with oxygen.
- The volume of the anatomical dead space is measured by placing a vertical line on the record from midportion of phase II of expiration (red area X = blue area Y).

Measurement of Physiological Dead Space

Bohr's Equation is used to measure the physiological (total) dead space by determining CO_2 tensions in the expired and alveolar gases. It is based on the fact that inspired air contains negligible quantity of CO_2 (almost zero). Therefore, all the CO_2 in expired air is derived from the functional alveoli. The equation states that $\boldsymbol{V_D}$ is equal to $\boldsymbol{V_T}$ multiplied by partial pressure of arterial carbon dioxide ($\mathbf{P_ACO_2}$) minus partial pressure of expired air carbon dioxide ($\mathbf{P_ECO_2}$) divided by $\mathbf{P_ACO_2}$.

$$V_D = V_T \times \frac{P_ACO_2 - P_ECO_2}{P_ACO_2}$$

where

V_D = Physiological (total) dead space air
V_T = Tidal volume
P_ECO_2 = Carbon dioxide tension in mixed expired air and is represented by average pCO_2 and of the total expired air
P_ACO_2 = Carbon dioxide tension in alveolar air and is theoretically represented by the pCO_2 of end-tidal samples of expired gases

For example, if

$$P_ECO_2 = 28\text{mm Hg},$$
$$P_ACO_2 = 40\text{ mm Hg},$$
$$V_T = 500\text{mL},$$
$$\text{then } V_D = 150\text{ mL}$$

EFFECT OF GRAVITY ON ALVEOLAR VENTILATION

Alveolar ventilation is more or less evenly distributed in supine position, because hydrostatic effect on intrapleural pressure is reduced. However, in a vertical lung, the alveolar ventilation is unevenly distributed because of variation in compliance in different regions of the lungs as explained (Fig. 5.4.3):

- The alveolar pressure is zero throughout the lung under static conditions.
- The intrapleural pressure shows a gradient of about 8 cm H_2O between apex (−10 cm H_2O) and base (−2 cm H_2O).
- So, transpulmonary pressure ([intrapleural pressure] − [alveolar pressure]) also varies from −10 cm H_2O at the apex to −2 cm H_2O at the base.
- Consequently, the lung compliance (change in lung volume per unit change in transpulmonary pressure) also shows corresponding gradient between apex and base.
- Because of more negative intrapleural pressure at apex (−10 cm H_2O), the apical alveoli are larger but poorly ventilated, whereas the basal alveoli because of less negative (−2 cm H_2O) intrapleural pressure are smaller but better ventilated.

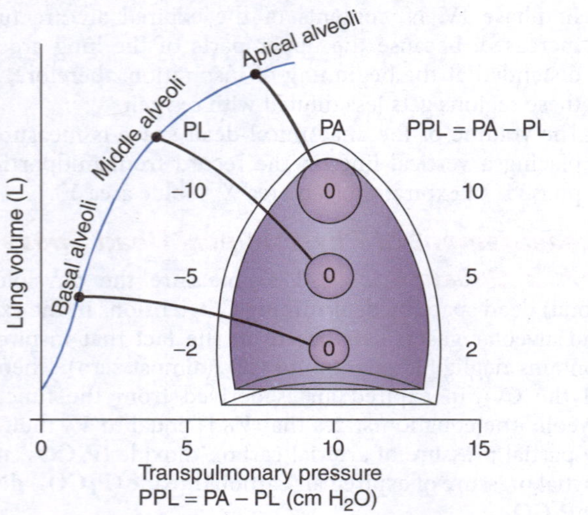

Fig. 5.4.3 Correlation of transpulmonary pressure (PPL = PA – PL) and lung inflation in different regions during erect posture. PA, alveolar pressure; PL, intrapleural pressure; PPL, transpulmonary pressure.

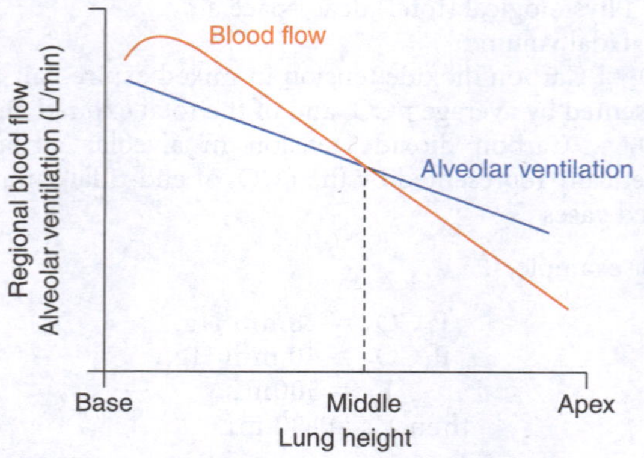

Fig. 5.4.4 Distribution of alveolar ventilation and pulmonary blood flow in different regions of lung during standing.

- There is a linear reduction in regional alveolar ventilation from base to apex in erect position (Fig. 5.4.4).

Clinical Significance of Effect of Gravity on Alveolar Ventilation

Arterial oxygenation can be improved in patients with unilateral lung disease by making them lie on their sides so that the good lung is in the dependent position. Somehow, the situation is opposite in infants, who do better with the diseased lung in dependent position.

ALVEOLAR VENTILATION–PERFUSION RATIO (V/Q)

V/Q is the ratio of alveolar ventilation per minute to quantity of blood flow to alveoli per minute. Normally, alveolar ventilation is 4.2–5.0 L/min, and the pulmonary blood flow (equal to cardiac output) is approximately 5 L/min. So, the normal V/Q is about 0.84–0.9. At this ratio, maximum oxygenation occurs.

Effect of Gravity on V/Q

- Because of the effect of gravity, the basal alveoli are overperfused and apical alveoli are underperfused (see details on page 403). There is almost a linear reduction in the blood flow from base to apex (Fig. 5.4.4).
- The alveolar ventilation also reduces linearly from the base to the apex (Fig. 5.4.4), and thus the basal alveoli are overventilated and the apical alveoli are underventilated (for detailed mechanism, see page 389).
- However, gravity affects perfusion much more than it affects ventilation. Hence, as shown in Fig. 5.4.4, the apical alveoli are more underperfused than underventilated. Because of this relationship, the V/Q is >1. In the middle of the lung, the alveolar ventilation equilibrates the perfusion. As we go up from middle of the lung to apex, the V/Q ratio goes on increasing and is about 3 at the apices. Conversely, at the bases, the alveoli are more overperfused than overventilated; as a result, the V/Q is always less than normal. As we move down from the middle of the lungs to the bases, the V/Q ratio goes on decreasing; at the bases, it is about 0.6.

Applied Aspects

Because of high V/Q ratio, the apical alveolar air has low pCO_2 and high pO_2. Since high alveolar pO_2 provides favourable environment for the growth of *Mycobacterium tuberculosis*, the apices of lungs are more predisposed to tuberculosis.

Causes of Alteration in the V/Q Ratio

Obviously, the factors altering alveolar ventilation or/and pulmonary perfusion will alter the V/Q ratio.

Causes of uneven alveolar ventilation are:

- Bronchial asthma
- Emphysema
- Pulmonary fibrosis
- Pneumothorax
- Congestive heart failure

Causes of uneven pulmonary perfusion are:

- Anatomical shunts, e.g. Fallot's tetralogy
- Pulmonary embolism
- Regional decrease in pulmonary vascular bed in emphysema
- Increased pulmonary resistance in conditions like pulmonary fibrosis, pneumothorax and congestive heart failure

Effects of Alterations in the V/Q Ratio

1. Normal V/Q ratio Normal V/Q ratio implies that there are both normal alveolar ventilation and normal alveolar perfusion. The exchange of gases is optimal and the alveolar pO_2 is about 104 mm Hg and pCO_2 is about 40 mm Hg.

2. Increased V/Q ratio Increased V/Q ratio means that alveolar ventilation is more than the perfusion. As a result, the whole of the alveolar air is not utilized for gaseous exchange. The extra air in the alveoli which goes waste forms the so-called *alveolar dead space air*. There will also be change in the composition of alveolar air (Fig. 5.4.5).

When V/Q ratio increases to infinity, i.e. when alveolar perfusion becomes zero, no exchange of gases can occur. Under such circumstances, the composition of alveolar air becomes

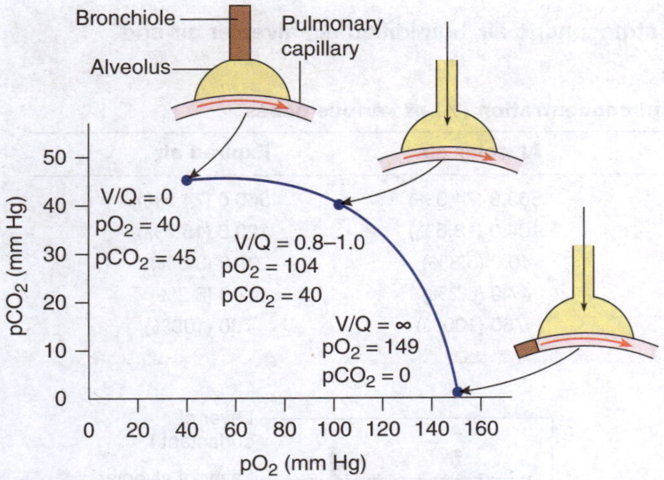

Fig. 5.4.5 Relationship of alveolar ventilation–perfusion ratio (V/Q) with alveolar air pO_2 and pCO_2.

equal to that of the humidified inspired air, which has a pO_2 of 149 mm Hg and a pCO_2 of 0 mm Hg (Fig. 5.4.5).

Thus, the *effects of increased V/Q are as follows*:

- Decreased exchange of gases at the respiratory membrane
- Alveolar dead space formation, leading to increase in physiological (total) dead space
- Change in alveolar air composition

3. Decreased V/Q ratio Decreased V/Q ratio occurs when the rate of blood *flow is more than the rate* of alveolar ventilation. Since the alveolar ventilation is not enough to provide oxygen, a fraction of venous blood passes through the pulmonary capillaries without becoming oxygenated. This fraction is called *shunted blood*. This shunted blood along with additional deoxygenated blood from bronchial veins to pulmonary vein (about 2% of cardiac output) forms the so-called *physiological shunt*. The greater the physiological shunt, the greater is the amount of blood that fails to be oxygenated as it passes through the lungs.

When V/Q becomes zero, there is no alveolar ventilation, so that the air in the alveolus comes to equilibrium with O_2 and CO_2 in the venous blood flowing through the pulmonary capillaries. So, alveolar air will have a pO_2 of 40 mm Hg and a pCO_2 of 45 mm Hg. Thus, the *effects of decreased V/Q ratio are as follows:*

- Decreased exchange of gases at the respiratory membrane
- Shunting of part of venous blood
- Change in alveolar air composition (Fig. 5.4.5)

  Under such circumstances, an *anatomical shunt* is said to exist. The presence of an anatomical shunt means that true venous blood is mixing with oxygenated blood. The anatomical shunt may be intrapulmonary or extrapulmonary. An extrapulmonary anatomical shunt may result from congenital cardiac malformations such as atrial or ventricular septal defect with right-to-left blood flow.

ALVEOLAR AIR

Volume of air which is available for exchange of gases in the alveoli per breath is called alveolar air, which is equivalent to tidal volume minus dead space, i.e. (500 − 150) or 350 mL.

COMPOSITION OF ALVEOLAR AIR

Composition of alveolar air can be studied by *alveolar air sampling* that involves analysis of the last few millilitres of air that issues from the lungs during expiration. Alveolar air composition is considerably different from that of atmospheric air (Table 5.4.2) because of the following reasons:

1. Water Vapours Dilute the other Gases in the Inspired Air

As shown in Table 5.4.2, the atmospheric air is composed mostly of nitrogen (79%) and oxygen (21%). It contains almost no carbon dioxide or water vapour. The dry atmospheric air becomes totally humidified as it passes through the respiratory passages. Water vapour pressure rises to 47 mm Hg at body temperature. As total pressure remains the same, pO_2 decreases from 159 mm Hg in atmospheric air to 149 mm Hg in humidified air and pN_2 decreases from 597 mm Hg in atmospheric air to 563 mm Hg in humidified air.

2. Alveolar Air is Renewed very Slowly by Atmospheric Air

Since with each breath only one-seventh of the alveolar air is replaced by fresh air, the composition of the two is different. This slow replacement of alveolar air prevents sudden changes in gas concentrations in the blood.

3. Oxygen is Constantly Being Absorbed from the Alveolar Air

Oxygen is constantly being absorbed from the alveolar air, so its pO_2 is reduced to 104 mm Hg. The alveolar O_2 concentration is controlled by a dynamic equilibrium between the rate of O_2 absorption into the blood and the rate of entry of new O_2 into the lungs.

4. Carbon Dioxide is Constantly Diffusing from the Pulmonary Blood to Alveoli

Carbon dioxide is constantly diffusing from the pulmonary blood to the alveoli, so the pCO_2 of alveolar air becomes 40 mm Hg which is almost negligible in the atmospheric air.

COMPOSITION OF EXPIRED AIR

As shown in Table 5.4.2, the composition of expired air is different from that of alveolar air. This is because of the fact that the expired air is a combination of dead space air and alveolar air. The expired air can be split into three portions:

First portion of the expired air represents the dead space air and its composition is similar to that of typical humidified air.

Middle portion of the expired air is a mixture of more and more alveolar air with the dead space air until the dead space air is washed out.

Last portion of the expired air represents the alveolar air and so is used to study the alveolar air composition (*alveolar air sampling*).

For alveolar air sampling, last 10 mL of expired air, during quiet breathing, can be collected using modern apparatus with suitable automatic valve.

Alveolar Gas Equation

The alveolar pO_2 and pCO_2 are interrelated to each other, since both are related to alveolar ventilation and alveolar perfusion.

Table 5.4.2 Composition and partial pressure of gases in atmospheric air, humidified air, alveolar air and expired air

	Partial pressure (mm Hg) and concentration (%) of various gases			
Gas	**Atmospheric air**	**Humidified air**	**Alveolar air**	**Expired air**
N_2	597.0 (78.62%)	563.4 (74.09%)	569.0 (74.9%)	566.0 (74.5%)
O_2	159.0 (20.84%)	149.3 (19.67%)	104.0 (13.6%)	120.0 (15.7%)
CO_2	0.3 (0.04%)	0.3 (0.04%)	40.0 (5.3%)	27.0 (3.6%)
H_2O	3.7 (0.5%)	47 (6.20%)	47.0 (6.2%)	47.0 (6.2%)
Total	760.0 (100%)	760 (100%)	760 (100%)	760 (100%)

The alveolar gas equation which gives the relationship between alveolar pO_2 and pCO_2 is as follows:

$$pAO_2 = pIO_2 - p_2 \times \left(FIO_2 + \frac{1 - FIO_2}{RQ} \right)$$

where

pAO_2 = Alveolar air pO_2 (normally 104 mm Hg)
pIO_2 = Inspired air, i.e. atmospheric, pO_2 (normally 159 mm Hg)
$pACO_2$ = Alveolar air pCO_2 (normally 40 mm Hg)
FIO_2 = Fraction of O_2 in dry air (normally 0.2)
RQ = Respiratory quotient, i.e. the ratio of CO_2 output and O_2 intake by tissues per minute (normally 0.8)

The gas analysis for composition of gas mixture or in body fluids is done by the use of O_2 and CO_2 electrodes. These electrodes are small probes which are sensitive to O_2 and CO_2, inserted into the airway, or into blood vessels or tissues, and partial pressure of O_2 and CO_2 (pO_2 and pCO_2) can be recorded continuously.

DIFFUSION OF GASES THROUGH THE RESPIRATORY MEMBRANE

RESPIRATORY UNIT AND RESPIRATORY MEMBRANE

Respiratory Unit

Each respiratory unit is composed of a respiratory bronchiole, alveolar ducts, atria and alveoli. There are about 300 million respiratory units in the 2 lungs. Gas exchange occurs through the membranes of all the structures forming a respiratory unit, not merely in the alveoli themselves.

Respiratory Membrane

Respiratory membrane or pulmonary membrane or the alveolocapillary membrane is the name given to the tissues which separate the capillary blood from the alveolar air. The exchange of gases between the capillary blood and the alveolar air requires diffusion through this membrane.

Structure of respiratory membrane It consists of the following layers (Fig. 5.4.6):

- Layer of pulmonary surfactant and fluid lining the alveolus
- Layer of alveolar epithelial cells
- Basement membrane of the alveolar epithelial cells
- A very thin interstitial space between the epithelial and endothelial cells
- Basement membrane of capillary endothelial cells
- Layer of capillary endothelial cells

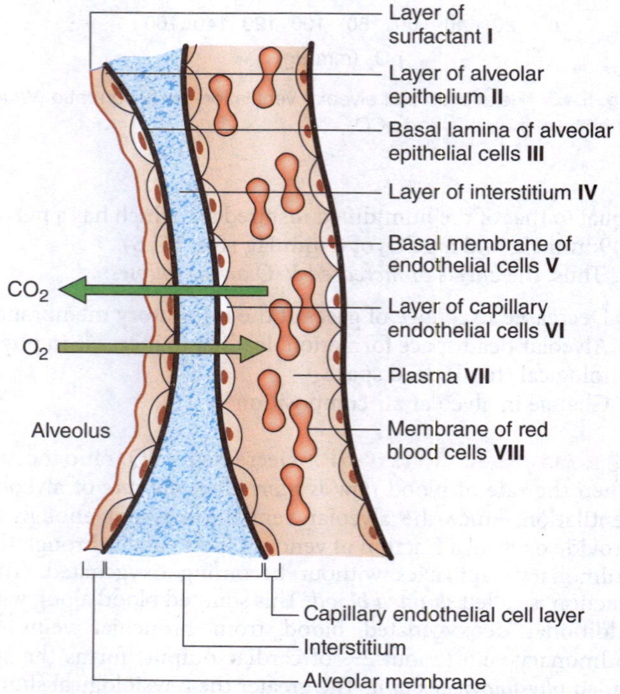

Fig. 5.4.6 Layers of respiratory membrane.

Characteristic features Characteristic features of the respiratory membrane which optimize for the gas exchange are as follows:

Thickness of the respiratory membrane, despite the large number of layers forming it, averages about 0.6 μm.
Surface area of the total respiratory membrane is about 70 m^2 in the normal adult.

Factors Affecting Diffusion Across Respiratory Membrane

The diffusion of gases across the respiratory membrane is affected by the following factors:

1. Thickness of respiratory membrane As mentioned above, the thickness of the respiratory membrane (about 0.6 μm) has been optimized for gas exchange. The rate of diffusion through the membrane is inversely proportional to the membrane thickness (diffusion distance, denoted by *d*), i.e.

$$V_{gas} \text{ (volume of gas diffused)} \propto \frac{1}{d}$$

Any factor which increases thickness will therefore significantly decrease the gaseous exchange. Examples:

- Pulmonary oedema, i.e. collection of fluid in the interstitial space and alveoli
- Pulmonary fibrosis occurring in certain lung diseases which increases the thickness of the respiratory membrane

2. Surface area of respiratory membrane Normally, the total surface area of the respiratory membrane is about 70 m^2. Rate of diffusion is directly proportional to the surface area (*A*), i.e. with the decrease in total surface area, the rate of diffusion of gases decreases, i.e.

$$V_{gas} \propto A$$

Some causes of decrease in surface area are as follows:

- Pulmonectomy, i.e. removal of one complete diseased lung, reduces surface area to half the normal.
- In emphysema, many of the alveoli coalesce, with dissolution of alveolar walls; this often causes the total surface to decrease by as much as fivefold.

3. Diffusion coefficient The rate of diffusion is directly proportional to the diffusion coefficient (*D*) of the gas, i.e.

$$V_{gas} \propto D$$

- The diffusion coefficient of CO_2 is about 20 times that of O_2 through water (and therefore through fluid of the respiratory membrane). Therefore, CO_2 diffuses much more easily through the respiratory membrane.
- The diffusion coefficient of a gas is a function of molecular weight (diffusion is inversely related to the square root of the molecular weight), solubility in a particular solvent and absolute temperature (310 K, normal body temperature), i.e.

$$D = \frac{\text{Solubility of the gas}}{\sqrt{\text{Molecular weight of the gas}}}$$

4. Pressure gradient across respiratory membrane The rate of diffusion across the respiratory membrane is directly proportional to the pressure difference between the partial pressure of a gas in alveoli (pA) and that in pulmonary capillary (pC), i.e.

$$V_{gas} \propto \text{pC} - \text{pA}$$

Further details about pressure gradient during diffusion of gases are discussed later.

From Equations (iv)–(vii), it can be derived that

$$V_{gas} = (\text{pC} - \text{pA})\frac{DA}{d}$$

This is called *Fick's law of diffusion*. Thus, it can be concluded that the rate of pulmonary gas diffusion, i.e. the volume of gas that crosses the respiratory membrane per minute, is determined by several factors as defined by Fick's law of diffusion.

DIFFUSION AND EQUILIBRATION OF GASES ACROSS THE RESPIRATORY MEMBRANE

Diffusion of O_2

- The normal alveolar pO_2 is 104 mm Hg, whereas the blood entering the pulmonary capillary normally has a pO_2 of 40 mm Hg. Pressure gradient therefore is 64 mm Hg in the beginning. After dissolving in the respiratory membrane, the O_2 molecules diffuse into the blood. As O_2 diffuses from alveoli to blood, the pO_2 of blood becomes the same as of alveolar air (104 mm Hg), the gradient becomes zero, and no diffusion occurs (Fig. 5.4.7).
- By the time blood passes to one-third of distance in capillary, the pO_2 of blood equals that of alveoli. This means that the pressure gradient is there only for one-third of blood flow in capillary.
- As stated above, the pressure gradient which is 64 mm Hg in the beginning becomes lesser and lesser with diffusion of O_2 into the blood. Average pressure gradient is therefore calculated considering the pressure gradients at various sites and the time for which particular pressure gradient was present. This time-integrated average pressure gradient is about 11 mm Hg.

Equilibration time The blood remains for about 0.75 second in the capillary (*transit time*). As mentioned above, normally, enough O_2 diffuses across the respiratory membrane so that blood pO_2 and alveolar pO_2 equalize in one-third of the transit time, i.e. about 0.25 second (Fig. 5.4.8); then no further gas transfer normally takes place for the rest 0.50 second of

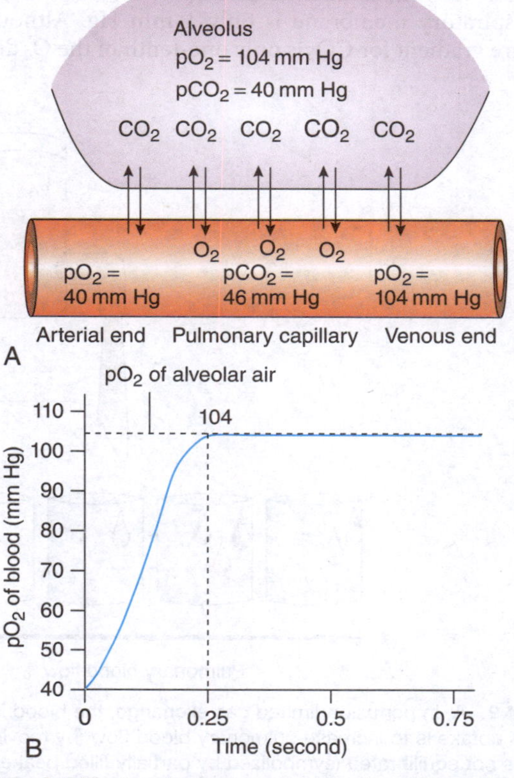

Fig. 5.4.7 **A**, Diffusion of oxygen across respiratory membrane, leading to **B**, progressive increase in capillary blood pO_2.

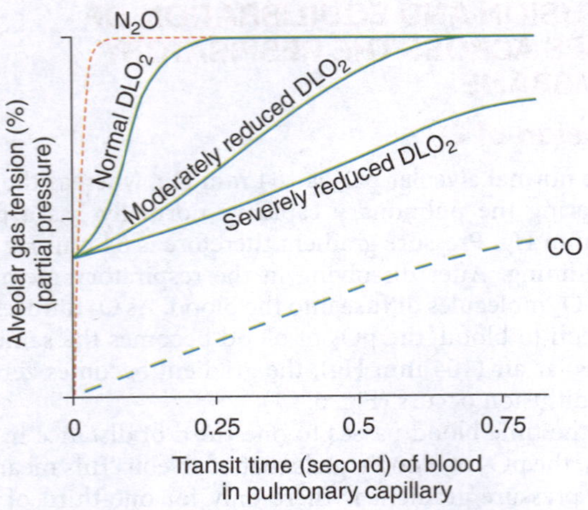

Fig. 5.4.8 Equilibration time of oxygen (in normal DLO_2, moderately decreased DLO_2 and severely reduced DLO_2), nitrous oxide and carbon monoxide. DLO_2, diffusion capacity for O_2.

transit time. This time provides a *safety margin* that ensures adequate O_2 uptake during periods of stress (e.g. exercise, exposure to high altitude) or impaired diffusion. When the normal DL for O_2 is diminished, the equilibrium time is prolonged or never reached.

Diffusion of CO_2

Diffusion of CO_2 occurs from blood to alveoli because pCO_2 is higher in blood than in alveolar air. The average pCO_2 in the pulmonary capillary blood is 46 mm Hg, as opposed to 40 mm Hg in the alveoli. Therefore, pressure gradient in the beginning is 6 mm Hg and time-integrated pressure gradient calculated for CO_2 (in a manner similar to that for O_2) across the respiratory membrane is only 1 mm Hg. Although the pressure gradient for CO_2 is only one-tenth of the O_2 diffusion gradient, CO_2 diffuses almost 20 times more rapidly than O_2 because of higher diffusion coefficient.

Equilibration Time

It is estimated that the time required for the blood pCO_2 and alveolar air pCO_2 to equalize is also approximately 0.25 second.

PERFUSION-LIMITED VERSUS DIFFUSION-LIMITED GAS EXCHANGE

Pulmonary gas exchange is determined by either perfusion or diffusion properties of the system (Fig. 5.4.9).

Perfusion-Limited Gas Exchange

Perfusion-limited gas exchange occurs when equilibration takes place between the alveolar gas and the pulmonary capillary blood. Normally, O_2 and CO_2 are transferred by perfusion-limited gas exchange as they equilibrate in about 0.25 second (whereas transit time is 0.75 second). Therefore, when pulmonary blood flow increases, the diffusion of O_2 and CO_2 across the respiratory membrane also increases.

Nitrous oxide (N_2O), an anaesthetic gas, reaches equilibrium in about 0.1 second; therefore, N_2O taken up is not diffusion limited, but by the amount of blood flowing through pulmonary capillaries (i.e. perfusion limited).

Diffusion-Limited Gas Exchange

Diffusion-limited gas exchange occurs whenever equilibration does not take place between the alveolar and pulmonary gas tensions.

- Carbon monoxide (CO) which does not reach equilibrium in 0.75 second (transit time of blood in pulmonary capillary) has a diffusion-limited transport, i.e. its transport across the respiratory membrane will increase only if the

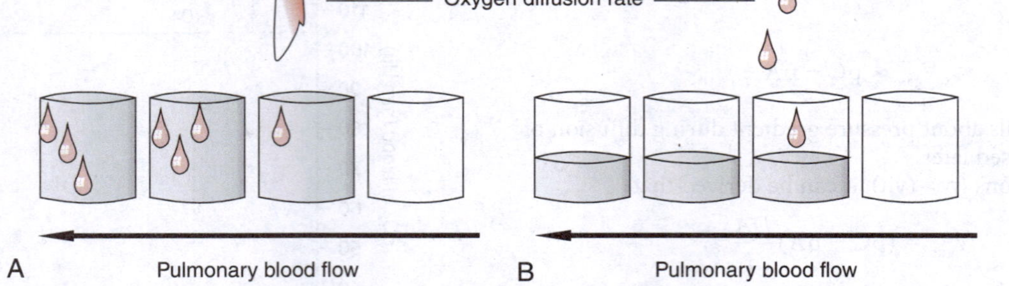

Fig. 5.4.9 **A,** In perfusion-limited gas exchange, the blood is equilibrated (as symbolized by full beakers), so that the only method of increasing gas uptake is to increase pulmonary blood flow (by moving more beakers through the system). **B,** In diffusion-limited gas exchange, the blood is not equilibrated (symbolized by partially filled beakers), so that diffusion rate must be increased to improve the exchange (so that available beaker in the above-mentioned symbolization may become full). The diffusion rate can be increased by raising partial pressure of the alveolar air (pAO_2) and increasing the driving force for diffusion.

rate of diffusion increases. Increase in blood flow will not increase the transport of CO.

- Since CO exchange is diffusion limited, measuring the diffusion capacity of CO is an effective means of evaluating the diffusion properties of the respiratory system.
- In certain systemic diseases and at a significant increase in altitude, pO_2 of alveolar air is reduced, which in turn reduces the diffusion rate. Raising the fraction of inspired O_2 (FIO_2) is one way to treat diffusion-limited gas exchange.

EFFECT OF ALVEOLAR VENTILATION–PERFUSION RATIO ON PULMONARY GAS EXCHANGE

- Optimum gas exchange across the respiratory membrane occurs when the V/Q is normal, i.e. between 0.8 and 1.
- Both a decrease and an increase in V/Q ratio reduce the gas exchange. For details, see page 412.

DIFFUSION CAPACITY OF LUNGS

Diffusion capacity of the lungs (DL) is quantitative expression of the ability of the respiratory membrane to exchange a gas between the alveoli and the pulmonary blood. It is defined as the volume of gas (V_{gas}) that diffuses through the respiratory membrane of the lung each minute for a pressure gradient of 1 mm Hg.

Factors Affecting Diffusion Capacity

All the factors discussed in detail that affect the rate of diffusion through the respiratory membrane (see page 412) will obviously affect the DL. To summarize once again, the DL is:

- Inversely proportional to thickness of the respiratory membrane, i.e. diffusion distance (d)
- Directly proportional to the surface area (A) of the respiratory membrane
- Directly proportional to the diffusion coefficient (D) of the particular gas (diffusion coefficient in turn is directly proportional to the solubility [S] of the gas in the respiratory membrane and inversely proportional to the square root of molecular weight of the gas)
- Directly proportional to the pressure gradient between the partial pressure of gas in alveolar air (pA) and in capillary blood (pC), i.e. pA − pC

Diffusion Capacity of Lungs for Different Gases

Depending on the above-mentioned factors, the diffusion of lungs is bound to be different for different gases. DL for common gases is given below (Table 5.4.3).

Table 5.4.3 Diffusion capacity of lungs for different gases

Gas	Diffusion capacity (mL/min/mm Hg) Rest	Exercise
Oxygen (O_2)	20–25	65
Carbon dioxide (CO_2)	400–500	1200–1300
Carbon monoxide (CO)	17	

Diffusion Capacity of Lungs for O_2

At rest At rest, the DL for O_2 is about 20–25 mL/min/mm Hg. As the mean oxygen pressure gradient across the respiratory membrane is about 11 mm Hg, at rest, about 250 mL of O_2 diffuses through the lungs per minute.

During exercise During exercise, the DL for O_2 is increased. It may reach up to 65 mL/min/mm Hg during strenuous exercise (three times of diffusing capacity for O_2 at rest). It occurs due to:

- *Increase in surface area* of the respiratory membrane caused by opening up of closed pulmonary capillaries and dilation of open capillaries
- *Improvement in V/Q*

Diffusion Capacity of Lungs for CO_2

DL for CO_2 has never been measured because of technical difficulties. Carbon dioxide diffuses across the respiratory membrane so rapidly that the difference between the average pCO_2 of the capillary blood and pCO_2 of the alveolar air is only 1 mm Hg. Such a small difference cannot be detected by any available technique. However, from the available knowledge about diffusion coefficient of CO_2, the DL for CO_2 is estimated.

At rest At rest, the DL for CO_2 is about 20 times that for O_2, i.e. about 400–500 mL/min/mm Hg.

During strenuous exercise During strenuous exercise, the diffusing capacity for CO_2 is increased to 1200–1300 mL/min/mm Hg.

> **Important Note**
>
> ***Clinical significance of higher diffusion capacity of CO_2:*** When diffusing capacity of the respiratory membrane is markedly decreased due to certain diseases, one expects retention of CO_2 and lack of O_2. But due to vast difference in the diffusing capacities for O_2 and CO_2, a serious impairment of diffusion of O_2 causes significant lack of O_2 with little signs of CO_2 retention.

Measurement of Diffusion Capacity of Lungs

DL for different gases can be measured using *Fick's law*, according to which diffusion capacity is given by

$$DL = \frac{V}{pA - pC}$$

where

DL = Diffusion capacity of the lungs for a given gas
V = Volume of the gas uptake in 1 minute (increase in the gas content of blood in 1 minute)
pA - pC = Pressure gradient between alveolar air and pulmonary capillary blood

- Thus, diffusion capacity for O_2 (DLO_2) is

$$DLO_2 = \frac{O_2 \text{ consumption/min}}{pAO_2 - pO_2}$$

- It is easy to measure O_2 consumption per minute and pAO_2, but it is difficult to measure pO_2 in pulmonary capillary blood (because collection of sample is extremely difficult).
- Therefore, DLO_2 is measured from the diffusion capacity for CO (DL CO).

- CO is preferred for measuring the DL because of two reasons:
  - After entering the blood, the CO very rapidly reacts with haemoglobin to form carboxyhaemoglobin and so does not allow the partial pressure of CO to build up in plasma. In this way, pCO in pulmonary capillary blood is almost zero (unless the subject is a smoker or exposed to atmospheric CO levels). Therefore, problem of collecting of CO in the pulmonary capillary blood is avoided.
  - Diffusion of CO across the respiratory membrane is diffusion limited. Therefore, the amount of CO transferred to blood is the correct estimate of the diffusion capacity. Since diffusion of O_2 across the respiratory membrane is flow limited, measuring the amount of O_2 transferred to blood will underestimate the true diffusion capacity.

Procedure of Single-Breath Carbon Monoxide Technique of Measuring Diffusion Capacity of Lungs

- The subject is made to take a single breath of gas mixture containing dilute concentration (0.01%) of CO. He/she is asked to hold the breath for 10 seconds to allow the diffusion.
- The CO uptake per minute is calculated from the difference between the inspired air and expired air CO concentrations, and functional residual capacity (FRC). The pCO of alveolar air is estimated from the end-expiratory sample. The pCO of pulmonary capillary blood is considered zero and so the DL CO is calculated as:

$$\text{DL CO} = \frac{\text{CO uptake/min}}{\text{pCO of alveolar air}}$$

- The diffusion capacity measured for CO at rest is about 17 mL/min/mm Hg.
- DLO_2 is determined by multiplying the DL CO by 1.27, because diffusion coefficient of O_2 is about 1.2 times that of CO: $DLO_2 = 17 \times 1.2$, or about 20 mL/min/mm Hg

Self-Assessment

1. Discuss about alveolar ventilation–perfusion ratio, its significance and effects of its alterations.
2. Discuss the diffusion capacity of lungs for oxygen and carbon dioxide and write brief note on factors affecting diffusion capacity.
3. Write notes on:
   - Physiological significance of alveolar ventilation
   - Bohr's equation
   - Effect of gravity on alveolar ventilation
   - Perfusion-limited gas exchange

Clinical Cases

Case 1

A 6-month-old baby is brought to the paediatric OPD with rapid and heavy breathing, not taking feed and not gaining weight.

On examination, murmur is heard. On the basis of ECG, X-ray chest and MRI findings, the patient is diagnosed to be a case of ventricular septal defect.

Q1. What happens to alveolar ventilation–perfusion ratio (V/Q)?
Q2. What is the effect of altered V/Q?
Q3. What is the normal value of V/Q?

Case 2

A 60-year-old male patient presented with complaints of cough with a lot of mucus, tightness of the chest and breathlessness on exertion.

On examination, the chest is barrel shaped and X-ray chest shows features of chronic obstructive pulmonary disease (COPD); lung function tests are also carried out and the patient is diagnosed to be a case of emphysema.

Q1. What is the status of V/Q in this case?
Q2. What is the status of blood flow to the lungs for exchange?
Q3. What is the status of dead space?

Case 3

A 55-year-old female presented to the emergency department with pain in the chest, shortness of breath and coughing with blood-stained mucus.

Examination and X-ray chest revealed a case of pulmonary oedema.

Q1. What is the main cause of pulmonary oedema?
Q2. What is the status of diffusion capacity of the lungs for O_2 in this case?

Transport of Gases 5.5

CHAPTER OUTLINE

INTRODUCTION

It is being repeated, probably, for the fourth time in this section, but is essential as an introductory remark, that *external respiration* refers to supply of O_2 from atmosphere to tissues and removal of CO_2 from the tissues into the atmosphere. It is accomplished by three major processes:

- *Pulmonary ventilation*, i.e. exchange of gases between the environment and the lungs (discussed in Chapter 5.2)
- *Pulmonary diffusion*, i.e. transfer of gases from alveoli to capillary blood across the respiratory membrane (discussed in Chapter 5.4)
- *Transport of gases* from the blood to the tissue cells and back

TRANSPORT OF OXYGEN

Transport of oxygen from the lungs to the tissues occurs due to constant *circulation of blood*, and *diffusion* of O_2 that occurs at various sites in the direction of concentration gradient which is represented by O_2 tension (pO_2) differences given:

- Alveolar air pO_2: 104 mm Hg
- Arterial blood pO_2: 95 mm Hg
- Venous blood pO_2: 40 mm Hg
- Tissue interstitial fluid pO_2: 40 mm Hg

From the above, it is clear that:

- Oxygen from the alveolar air is taken up by the pulmonary capillary blood along a pressure gradient of 104 − 40 mm Hg, or 64 mm Hg.
- Oxygen from the arterial blood is released into the tissues by a pressure gradient of 95 − 40 mm Hg, or 55 mm Hg.

Transport of oxygen from the lungs to the tissues can be described as follows:

A. Uptake of oxygen in the lungs by pulmonary blood
B. Transport of oxygen in arterial blood
C. Release (diffusion) of oxygen from the blood to the interstitial fluid in tissues

UPTAKE OF OXYGEN BY PULMONARY BLOOD

- As mentioned above, pO_2 of pulmonary arterial blood is about 40 mm Hg and that of alveolar air is 104 mm Hg. Therefore, due to this great concentration gradient, oxygen readily diffuses from the alveoli into the blood.
- The process of diffusion across the respiratory membrane has been described in Chapter 5.4, page 414.

> **Important Note**
>
> It is important to note that this process is very rapid and even if the stay of blood in lungs is reduced (as occurs during strenuous exercise due to increased cardiac output), there occurs complete oxygenation.

TRANSPORT OF OXYGEN IN ARTERIAL BLOOD

pO_2 in pulmonary venous blood is 104 mm Hg; however, by the time blood reaches the aorta, pO_2 falls to about 100 mm

Hg. This happens due to venous admixture, i.e. mixing of venous blood with arterial blood. The venous blood which mixes with arterial blood is:

- Blood present in bronchial veins (which forms about 2% of cardiac output) mixes with the pulmonary capillary blood at the respiratory bronchioles which are supplied by systemic as well as pulmonary capillaries.
- Part of the coronary venous blood flows into the chambers of left side of the heart through Thebesian veins.

Arterial blood contains about 20 mL and venous blood about 15 mL of O_2 per 100 mL. Thus, about 5 mL of O_2 is transported per 100 mL of blood from the lungs to the tissue cells.

Oxygen is transported in the blood in two forms – as dissolved form and in combination with haemoglobin.

Oxygen Transport in Dissolved Form

- The solubility of O_2 in water (plasma) is so little that at pO_2 value of 100 mm Hg, out of the 20 mL of O_2 present in 100 mL of blood, only 0.3 mL is in dissolved form and rest is combined with haemoglobin (as oxyhaemoglobin).
- The dissolved oxygen obeys Henry's law, i.e. amount dissolved is proportional to the pO_2. Thus, there is no limit to the amount of O_2 that can be carried in dissolved form provided the pO_2 is sufficiently high. This is a distinct advantage over O_2 transport as oxyhaemoglobin which cannot exceed a certain limit.

> **Important Note**
>
> It is important to note that dissolved O_2 at high pO_2 (hyperbaric oxygen) is utilized in clinical practice for the oxygenation of tissues when the haemoglobin gets denatured in certain types of poisoning, e.g. carbon monoxide poisoning.

Oxygen Transport in Combination with Haemoglobin

Oxygenation of Haemoglobin

After entering the blood from the alveolar air, most of the oxygen combines with haemoglobin to form a *loose and reversible* combination. The iron present in haem molecule stays in the ferrous form; therefore, this process is called *oxygenation* (not oxidation) and converts deoxyhaemoglobin into oxyhaemoglobin. The reaction is very rapid requiring <0.01 second.

One molecule of oxygen combines with one iron ion of the haem molecule. The O_2 molecule occupies the sixth *coordination* position of the iron atom. Since haemoglobin contains four molecules of haem, each molecule of haemoglobin can combine with as many as *four O_2* molecules. The reaction proceeds in four steps:

$Hb_4 + O_2 \rightarrow Hb_4O_2$
$Hb_4O_2 + O_2 \rightarrow Hb_4O_4$
$Hb_4O_4 + O_2 \rightarrow Hb_4O_6$
$Hb_4O_6 + O_2 \rightarrow Hb_4O_8$

After the first step, affinity of haemoglobin for O_2 increases with each next step because in deoxyhaemoglobin, the globin units are tightly bound (i.e. intense configuration), which reduces affinity for O_2. This happens so, because the insertion of O_2 molecule ruptures all the salt links and changes the quaternary structure of haemoglobin from the tense or *T-configuration* to relaxed or *R-configuration* which exposes more O_2 binding sites, which favours O_2 binding. Subsequent molecules of oxygen, therefore, find it easier to bind to haem moieties and there is 500-fold increase in O_2 affinity. This phenomenon is termed *cooperative binding kinetics.*

Note: The phenomenon of cooperative binding kinetics is the reason for the sigmoid nature of oxygen–haemoglobin association or dissociation curve. In tissues, the reactions are reversed resulting in O_2 release.

Oxygen-Carrying Capacity of Haemoglobin

One gram of haemoglobin can bind with maximum of 1.34 mL of O_2. Thus, 100 mL of blood with haemoglobin level of 15 g% can carry 1.34 × 15 mL, or 20.1 mL of oxygen. However, due to the presence of various physiological shunts (venous admixture), only 97% of the haemoglobin is available for carrying the oxygen. Therefore, practically, 100 mL of the arterial blood carries about 19.8 mL of oxygen, about 19.5 mL as oxyhaemoglobin and 0.3 mL as dissolved form in plasma.

Thus, under normal circumstances, the haemoglobin carries most of the bulk of oxygen present in the blood.

Disadvantage The only disadvantage is that there is a ceiling on the amount of oxygen that can be carried by the haemoglobin (depending on the concentration of haemoglobin in the blood). The limit can never be surpassed.

Haemoglobin saturation is the percentage of haemoglobin that is combined with oxygen. When all the four sites on haemoglobin are occupied by O_2 (1.34 mL), that molecule of haemoglobin is 100% saturated. When 1 g of haemoglobin is combined with 0.67 mL of O_2, it is said to be 50% saturated. The *percentage saturation* is the average saturation of the entire haemoglobin molecules in the blood and is calculated as:

$$\text{Percentage saturation} = \frac{O_2 \text{ content of blood/100 mL}}{O_2\text{-carrying capacity of blood}} \times 100$$

Oxygen–Haemoglobin Dissociation Curve

Oxygen–haemoglobin dissociation curve refers to the curve obtained when the relation between the pO_2 and the percentage of haemoglobin saturation is plotted (Fig. 5.5.1). The O_2–Hb dissociation curve shows that the percentage saturation of haemoglobin increases with the increase in pO_2 of arterial blood. However, the relation is not linear but *sigmoid or*

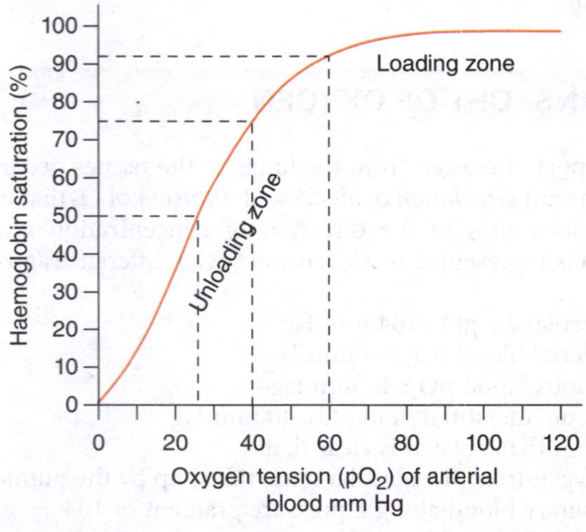

Fig. 5.5.1 Normal oxygen–haemoglobin dissociation curve.

S-shaped (because of the reason explained above), but it has several physiological advantages (vide infra).

Two distinct zones of the O_2–Hb dissociation curve are recognized.

Loading (association) zone Loading (association) zone refers to upper flat part (plateau) of the curve, which is related to the process of O_2 uptake in the lungs. The curve shows that at pO_2 values of 100 mm Hg or above, the haemoglobin is 100% saturated. More important to note is the fact that even if pO_2 falls to 60 mm Hg, the Hb saturation is still 90%. Thus, the loading zone provides a margin of safety, because it ensures fairly high uptake of O_2 by pulmonary blood even when alveolar pO_2 is moderately decreased in situations like:

- Climbing mountains to moderate altitude
- Pulmonary diseases

Unloading (dissociation) zone Unloading (dissociation) zone of the O_2–Hb dissociation curve refers to the *steep portion* of the curve that occurs at pO_2 below 60 mm Hg. The steep part of the curve is concerned with O_2 delivery in the tissues and shows that large amounts of oxygen can be liberated from the blood with relatively minor fall of O_2 tension. This property keeps the O_2 tension in the capillary blood relatively high so that the diffusion gradient for O_2 is maintained. At pO_2 value of 40 mm Hg, Hb is 75% saturated with O_2 (Fig. 5.5.1). Thus, each 100 mL of blood can hold only 15 mL of O_2 as compared with 20 mL at pO_2 of 100 mm Hg (Fig. 5.5.2). Thus, 5 mL of O_2 is extracted by the tissues at rest. At values of pO_2 lower than 40 mm Hg, still larger volume of O_2 would be offloaded and become available to the tissue (e.g. during exercise). The greater release of O_2 with slight decrease in tissue pO_2 (due to increased O_2 consumption) minimizes decrease of tissue pO_2 that would otherwise take place. Thus, it will regulate tissue pO_2 (buffering effect).

Physiological advantages of S-shaped O_2–Hb dissociation curve Physiological advantages of S-shaped O_2–Hb dissociation curve, which can be summarized from the above discussion, are as follows:

- It allows greater uptake of O_2 at lungs despite great variation in alveolar air pO_2.
- Tissues are supplied with O_2 according to their needs.

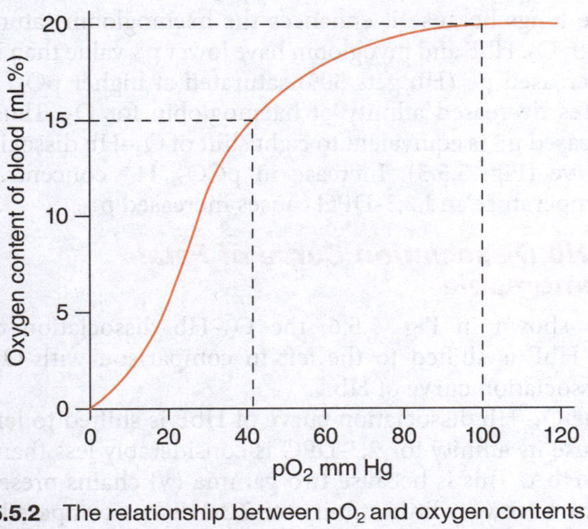

Fig. 5.5.2 The relationship between pO_2 and oxygen contents of the blood.

- Haemoglobin acts as a buffer and maintains tissue pO_2 at about 40 mm Hg.

Shifts in O_2–Hb dissociation curve Several factors affect the affinity of haemoglobin for O_2 and thus shift the O_2–Hb dissociation curve to either right or left.

Shift to right Shift to the right of O_2–Hb dissociation curve signifies decreased affinity of haemoglobin for O_2 (Fig. 5.5.3). Thus, at every level of pO_2, the oxygen saturation of haemoglobin is somewhat lower than the normal curve leading to more offloading of O_2.

Causes The factors causing right shift are as follows:

1. ***Effect of pCO_2 and pH:*** The description of O_2–Hb dissociation curve given above (Fig. 5.5.1) holds true if the blood has pCO_2 value of 40 mm Hg and a pH of 7.4 (pH of normal arterial blood). An increase in pCO_2 shifts the curve to right; this phenomenon is known as *Bohr's effect* (Fig. 5.5.3).
   Bohr's effect
   - When the arterial blood reaches the tissues, it is exposed to not only to low tissue pO_2 (40 mm Hg) but also to higher pCO_2 (45 mm Hg). So, normally in tissues the curve shifts to right and due to Bohr's effect for a given decrease in pO_2 larger volume of O_2 is shed off (about 2% more).
   - A decrease in pH of blood, as occurs in the tissues, also shifts the O_2–Hb dissociation curve to the right.

Important Note

In the fetus, at the level of placenta, both right and left shifts of O_2–Hb dissociation curve occur, which is known as double Bohr's effect (see page 847).

2. ***Effect of temperature:*** An increase in the temperature of blood shifts the curve to right (Fig. 5.5.4).
   During exercise, the demand of O_2 is increased in skeletal muscles. The factors which facilitate the delivery of the required larger amounts of O_2 (by causing right shift in the curve) are as follows:
   - Increased temperature in skeletal muscles due to more heat production

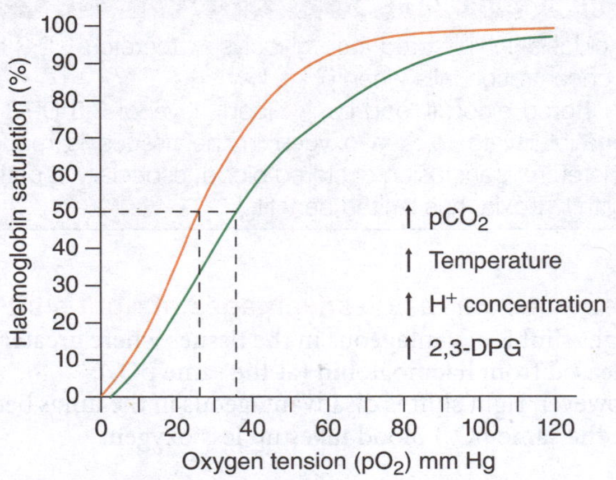

Fig. 5.5.3 Right shift of oxygen–haemoglobin dissociation curve which occurs due to increase in pCO_2, H^+ concentration, temperature or 2,3-DPG. Note: p_{50} value is increased. 2,3-DPG, 2,3-diphosphoglycerate.

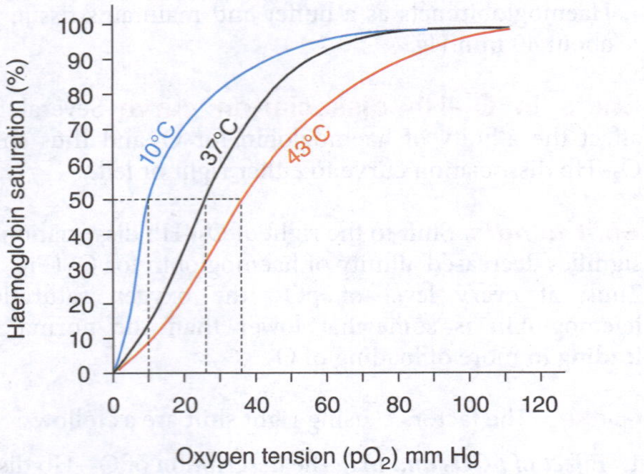

Fig. 5.5.4 Effect of change of temperature of blood on the oxygen–haemoglobin dissociation curve. Note a right shift at increased temperature (43°C) and a left shift at decreased temperature (10°C) as compared with the normal curve (37°C).

- Increased pCO_2 due to accumulation of CO_2 resulting from rapid metabolism
- Decreased pO_2 due to rapid consumption
- Decreased pH due to accumulation of lactic acid produced in muscular exercise

3. ***Effect of diphosphoglycerate or biphosphoglycerate:*** The red blood cells are rich in 2,3-diphosphoglycerate (2,3-DPG) which is formed from 3-phosphoglyceraldehyde produced during glycolysis via *Embden–Meyerhof pathway*. The 2,3-DPG is a highly charged anion that binds to β-chain of deoxygenated adult haemoglobin (HbA).

$$HbO_2 + 2,3\text{-DPG} \rightarrow Hb\text{-}2,3\text{-DPG} + O_2$$

Thus, an increase in the concentration of 2,3-DPG decreases the affinity of Hb for O_2 and shifts the normal O_2–Hb dissociation curve to the right.

Causes of increased levels of 2, 3-DPG are thyroid hormone, growth hormone, androgen, anaemia, exposure to chronic hypoxia at high altitude and certain pulmonary diseases.

Important Note

- Acidosis inhibits red cell glycolysis; therefore, 2,3-DPG concentration falls when pH is low.
- In stored blood (blood bank blood), level of 2,3-DPG falls and ability to release oxygen in the tissues is reduced; therefore, transfusion of stored blood, especially in patients with hypoxia, has limited benefit.

Advantages versus disadvantages of right shift

- Right shift is advantageous in the tissues where greater O_2 is released from haemoglobin (at the same pO_2).
- However, right shift is disadvantageous in the lungs because (at the same pO_2) blood takes up less oxygen.

Shift to left Shift to left of O_2–Hb dissociation curve signifies increased affinity of haemoglobin for O_2 (Fig. 5.5.5). Thus, at every pO_2 level, the oxygen saturation of haemoglobin is somewhat greater than in a normal curve.

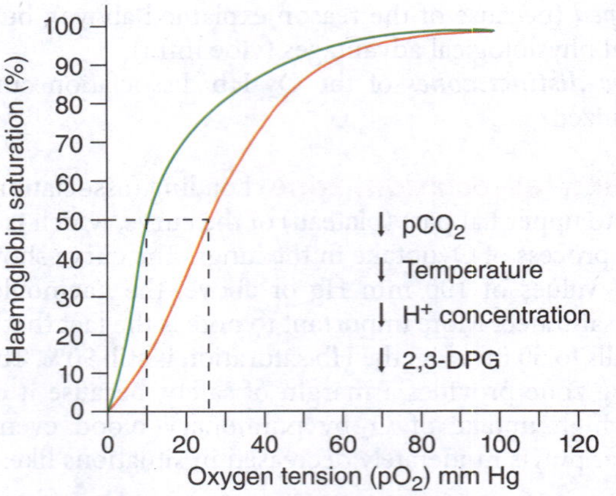

Fig. 5.5.5 Left shift of oxygen–haemoglobin dissociation curve which occurs due to decrease in pCO_2, H^+ concentration, temperature and 2,3-DPG. Note: p_{50} value is decreased. 2,3-DPG, 2,3-diphosphoglycerate.

Causes Causes for left shift of the curve are as follows:

- Decreased pCO_2 of blood
- Increased pH of blood
- Decreased temperature
- Fetal haemoglobin (HbF)

Advantages versus disadvantages of left shift Left shift of the curve has limited advantage because although it allows greater uptake of O_2 at lungs (at same pO_2), it decreases release of O_2 to the tissues (at same pO_2).

Concept of p_{50} and its significance p_{50} refers to the partial pressure of O_2 that produces a 50% saturation of the haemoglobin with O_2. Normal p_{50} for arterial blood in an adult at 37°C body temperature and at pCO_2 of blood 40 mm Hg is 25–27 mm Hg (Fig. 5.5.1). The significance of p_{50} value is related to haemoglobin affinity for oxygen.

Haemoglobin affinity for O_2 is inversely related to the p_{50} value; therefore:

- Decreased p_{50} (Hb gets 50% saturated at lower pO_2) indicates increased affinity of haemoglobin for O_2. Thus, decreased p_{50} is equivalent to shift of Hb–O_2 dissociation curve to left (Fig. 5.5.5). A decreased p_{50} is an obvious benefit in the lungs because it enhances the haemoglobin saturation with O_2. HbF and myoglobin have lower p_{50} value than HbA.
- Increased p_{50} (Hb gets 50% saturated at higher pO_2) indicates decreased affinity of haemoglobin for O_2. Thus, increased p_{50} is equivalent to right shift of O_2–Hb dissociation curve (Fig. 5.5.3). Increase in pCO_2, H^+ concentration, temperature and 2,3-DPG causes increased p_{50}.

O_2–Hb Dissociation Curve of Fetal Haemoglobin

- As shown in Fig. 5.5.6, the O_2–Hb dissociation curve of HbF is shifted to the left in comparison with O_2–Hb dissociation curve of HbA.
- The O_2–Hb dissociation curve of HbF is shifted to left because its affinity for 2,3-DPG is considerably less than that of HbA. This is because two gamma (γ) chains present in HbF have very little affinity for 2,3-DPG as compared with the beta (β) chains of HbA.

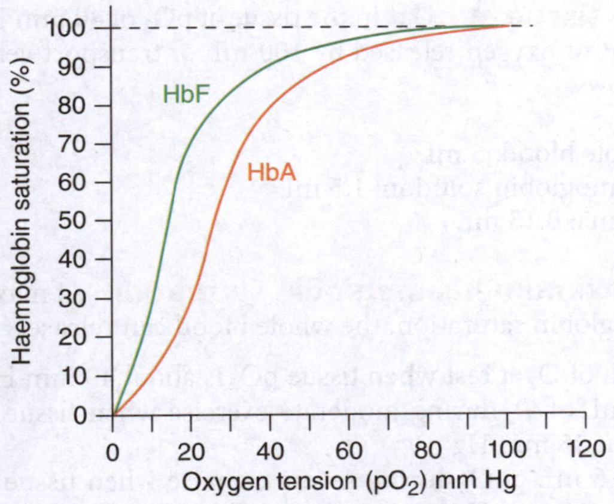

Fig. 5.5.6 Oxygen–haemoglobin dissociation curves of adult haemoglobin (HbA) and fetal haemoglobin (HbF).

- Thus, affinity of HbF to combine with O_2 is more than that of HbA. This property of HbF helps it to take up normal volumes of O_2 in spite of the fact that fetal blood is exposed to rather low pO_2 values of the maternal blood in placenta. As shown in Fig. 5.5.6, at pO_2 20 mm Hg where HbA is only 35% saturated, the HbF is 70% saturated; therefore, HbF can store more O_2.

Effect of Carbon Monoxide on O_2 Transport

- Carbon monoxide (CO) interferes with O_2 transport because it has about 200 times the affinity (of oxygen) for haemoglobin.
- CO combines with Hb at the same site on its molecule as O_2 and forms the carboxyhaemoglobin, and thus decreases the functional haemoglobin concentration.
- Because of the extreme affinity of CO for haemoglobin, the carboxyhaemoglobin curve lies along the *Y*-axis and a CO tension of only 0.5 mm Hg inactivates about 50% of the haemoglobin, i.e. p_{50} for CO is only 0.5 mm Hg (Fig. 5.5.7).
- CO lowers the tissue O_2 tension by decreasing the O_2 content and the p_{50} for O_2.

Oxygen Dissociation Curve for Myoglobin

Myoglobin is present in higher quantities in the muscles specialized for sustained contraction, e.g. muscles of the legs and heart.

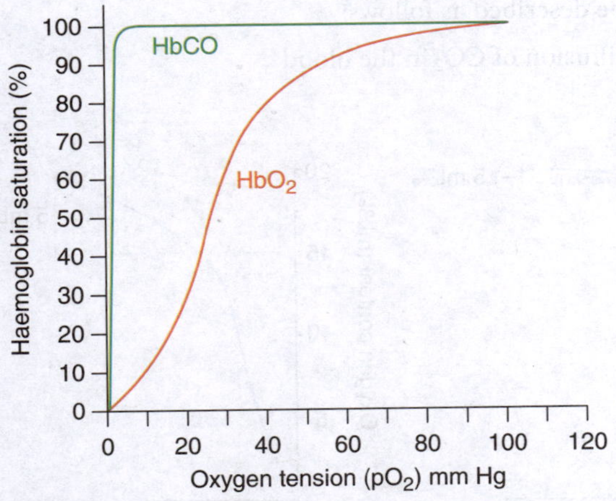

Fig. 5.5.7 Haemoglobin saturation curves for both O_2 (HbO_2) and carbon monoxide (HbCO). Note that HbCO curve lies along the *Y*-axis which indicates extremely high affinity of haemoglobin for carbon monoxide. Note: The p_{50} value for CO is only 0.5 mm Hg.

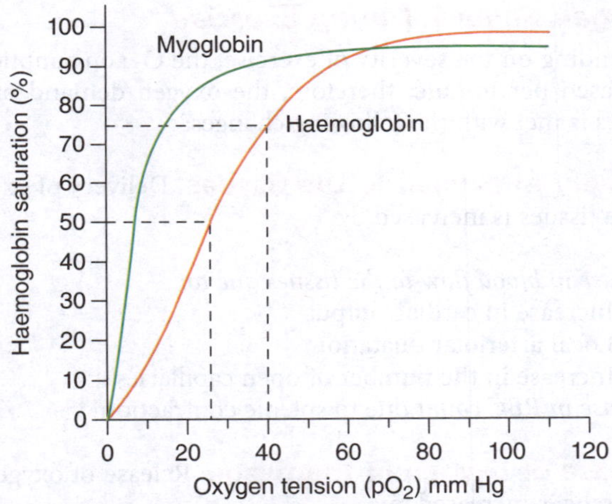

Fig. 5.5.8 Oxygen dissociation curve of myoglobin versus haemoglobin.

The characteristic features of O_2 dissociation curve of myoglobin vis-à-vis haemoglobin are as follows (Fig. 5.5.8):

- Dissociation curve of myoglobin is rectangular hyperbola rather than sigmoid in shape, because it takes up O_2 at low pressure much readily, i.e. rate of association of myoglobin with O_2 is very fast.
- Myoglobin does not show Bohr's effect.
- At pO_2 40 mm Hg, the myoglobin is 95% saturated, whereas haemoglobin is 75% saturated. Even at pO_2 5 mm Hg, myoglobin is saturated by slightly less than 60%. Thus, it acts as a temporary storehouse for O_2 in the muscles.

Release of Oxygen in Tissues

Oxygen Release at Rest

Oxygen delivery Oxygen delivery represents the amount of O_2 that is presented to body cells per minute and is equal to the arterial O_2 content multiplied by cardiac output. Since 100 mL of arterial blood at pO_2 of about 100 mm Hg contains about 20 mL of oxygen, with a cardiac output of about 5 L/min, the normal oxygen delivery to the entire body is about 1 L/min. The oxygen delivery to the tissues decreases with either decrease in arterial O_2 content or decrease in cardiac output.

Oxygen consumption When the arterial blood with approximate pO_2 100 mm Hg reaches the tissues with tissue fluid pO_2 40 mm Hg, because of pressure gradient, about 5 mL of O_2 diffuses from the tissue capillaries to the interstitial fluid out of 100 mL of blood (containing ;19 mL O_2) every minute. Thus, oxygen consumption of the whole body at rest with a cardiac output of 5 L/min is about 250 mL of O_2 per minute.

Utilization coefficient Utilization coefficient refers to the percentage of oxygen consumed out of oxygen delivered to the tissue, i.e.

$$\text{Coefficient of utilization} = \frac{\text{Oxygen consumed/min}}{\text{Oxygen delivered/min}} \times 100$$

$$\text{So, at rest, coefficient of utilization of whole body} = \frac{250 \text{ mL/min}}{1000 \text{ mL/min}} \times 100 = 25\%$$

Oxygen Release During Exercise

Depending on the severity of exercise, the O_2 consumption is increased per minute; therefore, the oxygen demand of the tissues is met with the following changes:

Delivery of oxygen to the tissues Delivery of oxygen to the tissues is increased by:

Increase in blood flow to the tissues due to:
- Increase in cardiac output
- Local arteriolar dilatation
- Increase in the number of open capillaries

Increase in RBC count due to splenic contraction

Release of oxygen in the tissue Release of oxygen in the tissue is increased by:

- Right shift of oxygen dissociation curve occurs due to increase in pCO_2, H^+ concentration, temperature and 2,3-DPG. As a result, more O_2 is released to the tissues at the same pO_2. This can increase the oxygen uptake of tissues to 750 mL/min, i.e. three times the resting level.
- Fall in pO_2 of interstitial fluid: Depending on the degree of activity, the O_2 tension in the interstitial fluid may fall to even zero. This leads to a very steep pressure gradient between blood and tissues increasing release of O_2.

All the above-mentioned factors combined can increase the oxygen released in the tissues by 15 times the resting levels.

Vehicles for Transport of Oxygen: A Comparison of Plasma, Haemoglobin and Whole Blood

The oxygen dissociation curves of plasma, haemoglobin solution and whole blood (Fig. 5.5.9) and the amount of oxygen that can be loaded and unloaded by different transport vehicles reveal the following:

From the lungs at pO_2 From the lungs at pO_2 of about 100 mm Hg, the amount of O_2 loaded by 100 mL of transport vehicle is as follows:

- Whole blood: 19.8 mL
- Haemoglobin solution: 19.5 mL
- Plasma solution: 0.3 mL only

In the tissue at pO_2 In the tissue at pO_2 of 40 mm Hg, the amount of oxygen released by 100 mL of transport vehicle is as follows:

- Whole blood: 5 mL
- Haemoglobin solution: 1.5 mL
- Plasma: 0.18 mL

At maximum haemoglobin saturation At maximum haemoglobin saturation, the whole blood can release:

- 5 mL of O_2 at rest when tissue pO_2 is about 40 mm Hg
- 13 mL of O_2 during moderate exercise when tissue pO_2 is about 25 mm Hg
- 15–16 mL of O_2 during severe exercise when tissue pO_2 is about 15 mm Hg

From the above, it is quite clear that whole blood is an ideal vehicle for transport of O_2, to load itself in lungs with O_2 and to release O_2 in tissues as per requirement.

TRANSPORT OF CARBON DIOXIDE

TRANSPORT OF CARBON DIOXIDE FROM THE TISSUE CELLS TO THE LUNGS

Occurs due to *constant circulation* of blood and diffusion of CO_2 that occurs at various sites in the direction of concentration gradient which is represented by CO_2 tension differences given as follows:

- Intracellular pCO_2: 46 mm Hg
- Interstitial fluid pCO_2: 45 mm Hg
- Arterial blood pCO_2 (in tissue capillaries): 40 mm Hg
- Venous blood pCO_2: 45 mm Hg
- Alveolar air pCO_2: 40 mm Hg

From the above pCO_2 levels, it is clear that:
- CO_2 from the cells diffuses into the interstitial fluid against a tension gradient of 1 mm Hg.
- From the interstitial fluid, the CO_2 diffuses into the capillaries at a tension gradient of 5 mm Hg.
- From the venous blood that is supplied to pulmonary capillaries, the CO_2 diffuses across the respiratory membrane into the alveoli against a tension gradient of 5 mm Hg.

Transport of carbon dioxide from the tissue cells to the lungs can be described as follows:

A. Diffusion of CO_2 in the blood

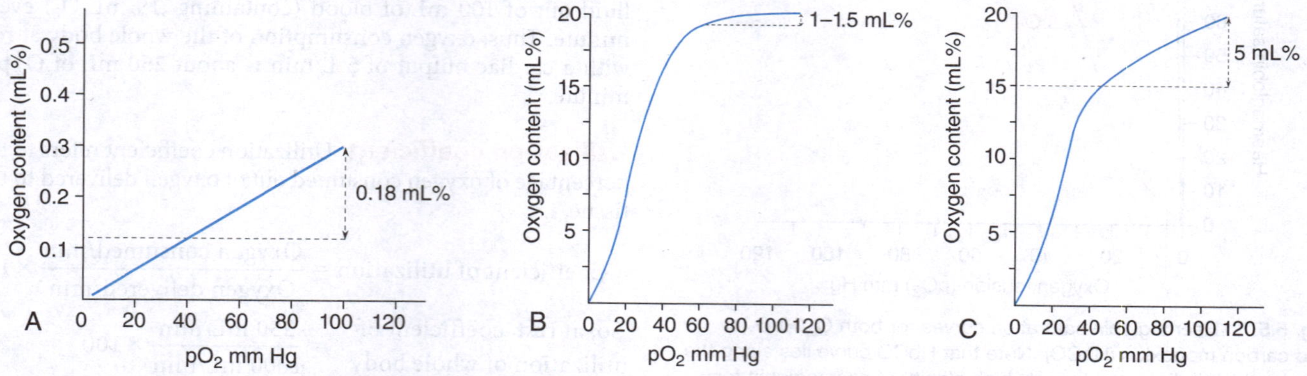

Fig. 5.5.9 Oxygen dissociation curves: **A**, for plasma; **B**, for haemoglobin solution; and **C**, for whole blood.

B. Transport of CO_2 in the blood
C. Release of CO_2 in the lungs

DIFFUSION OF CO_2 IN THE BLOOD

Tissue cells constantly form CO_2 inside the cells due to metabolism. As mentioned above, intracellular pCO_2 is 46 mm Hg and that of interstitial fluid surrounding the cells is 45 mm Hg. Although the cells are continuously forming CO_2, still the CO_2 tension gradient between inside and outside of the cells is only 1 mm Hg. This is owing to the rapid diffusion of CO_2 (20 times that of O_2) out of the cells into the interstitial fluid. Since pCO_2 of the arterial blood flowing in tissue capillaries is lower (40 mm Hg) than that of interstitial fluid, CO_2 diffuses inside the capillary blood which flows in the systemic venous system.

Transport of CO_2 in Blood

Venous blood contains about 52 mL and arterial blood about 48 mL of CO_2 per 100 mL. Thus, 4 mL of CO_2 is transported per 100 mL of blood from the tissue cells to the lungs. Thus, total CO_2 transported from the whole-body tissue cells at rest with a cardiac output of 5 L/min is about $4 \times 5000/100$, or 200 mL/min.

Carbon dioxide is transported in the blood in three forms (Fig. 5.5.10):

- In dissolved state (7%)
- In bicarbonate form (70%)
- In carbamino compound form (23%)

Carbon Dioxide Transport in Dissolved Form

- The venous blood, with pCO_2 45 mm Hg, contains about 2.7 mL/100 mL of CO_2 in the dissolved state.
- The arterial blood with pCO_2 40 mm Hg contains about 2.4 mL/100 mL of CO_2 in the dissolved state.
- Thus, only 0.3 mL of CO_2 is transported in dissolved state per 100 mL of blood from tissues to the lungs. This represents about 7% of all CO_2 that is transported.

Carbon Dioxide Transport in Bicarbonate Form

Approximately 70% of the carbon dioxide is transported in the form of *plasma bicarbonate ions*. However, these bicarbonate ions are formed in the RBCs and then diffuse into plasma, explained as follows:

- After entering the blood, most of the CO_2 enters the RBCs, where it rapidly reacts with water to form carbonic acid (H_2CO_3).
- In the presence of carbonic anhydrase, the carbonic acid (H_2CO_3) dissociates into bicarbonate ions (HCO_3^-) and hydrogen ions (H^+).
- The bicarbonate ions diffuse out of the RBCs into the plasma and are transported as sodium bicarbonate (alkali reserve of blood). Thus, although HCO_3^- is formed within the RBCs, most of the CO_2 is carried in the plasma as HCO_3^- and some in the RBCs as well.
- The H^+ are buffered by deoxygenated haemoglobin, which is a weaker acid than oxyhaemoglobin. This enables the reaction to proceed unabated in the forward direction.
- Chloride shift (*Hamburger phenomenon*): As HCO_3^- diffuses out of the RBCs into the plasma, therefore, the interior of the cells becomes less negatively charged. The RBC membrane is relatively impermeable to cations; in order to neutralize this effect, negatively charged chloride ions (Cl^-) diffuse from the plasma into the RBCs to replace the HCO_3^-. The movement of chloride ions into the RBCs is called chloride shift or Hamburger phenomenon. This process is mediated by band 3, a major ion exchange membrane protein also called anion exchange-I (AE-I). The chloride shift occurs very rapidly and is essentially completed within 1 second.
- As a result of chloride shift, the total number of ions inside the RBCs increases, so the osmotic pressure inside the RBCs becomes higher than that of plasma. This causes

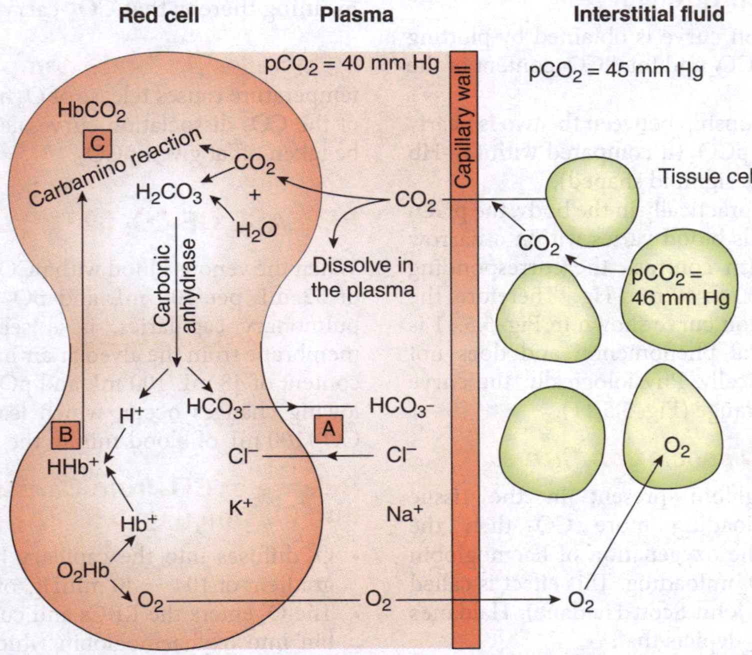

Fig. 5.5.10 **A,** Transport of carbon dioxide (CO_2) in blood demonstrating formation of HCO_3^- and chloride shift phenomenon; **B,** H^+ buffering by haemoglobin; and **C,** formation of carbaminohaemoglobin.

osmotic absorption of fluid into the RBCs. Thus, venous RBCs contain the greater quantity of fluid as compared with the arterial blood RBCs. Because of this:

- Packed cell volume (PCV) of venous blood is slightly higher (~3%) than that of arterial blood.
- Venous RBCs are more fragile than the arterial RBCs.

Transport of Carbon Dioxide in Carbamino Form

Approximately 23% of the total CO_2 is transported in the blood in the form of carbamino compounds. After entering the blood, some of the CO_2 combines with the amino group ($-NH_2$) of proteins to form carbamino compounds.

In the plasma CO_2 combines with amino group of plasma proteins ($PrNH_2$) to form carbamino proteins:

$$CO_2 + PrNH_2 \rightarrow Pr \cdot NH \cdot COOH$$

- This reaction is much less significant because quantity of these proteins is one-fourth that of haemoglobin.

In the RBCs CO_2 combines with amino group of haemoglobin ($HbNH_2$) to form a compound called carbaminohaemoglobin:

$$CO_2 + HbNH_2 \rightarrow Hb \cdot NH \cdot COOH$$

- This combination of CO_2 with haemoglobin is a reversible reaction that occurs with a loose bond, so that the CO_2 is easily released into the alveoli where pCO_2 is lower than that in the tissue capillaries.
- This reaction of CO_2 with Hb is much slower than the reaction of CO_2 with water in RBCs. This is because more CO_2 (70%) is transported as bicarbonates and less as carbamino compounds (23%).
- This reaction of CO_2 with Hb is further decreased to a great extent when 2,3-DPG concentration is more, because both 2,3-DPG and CO_2 compete for the same sites on Hb.

Carbon Dioxide Dissociation Curve

- Carbon dioxide dissociation curve is obtained by plotting the relationship between pCO_2 and total CO_2 content of the blood (Fig. 5.5.11).
- The graph shows that relationship between the two is nearly linear over wider range of pCO_2 (if compared with O_2–Hb dissociation curve, which is sigmoid shaped).
- It is important to note that practically in the body, the pCO_2 value of arterial and venous blood varies within a narrow range of 40–45 mm Hg (in contrast, the corresponding values of pO_2 vary from 100 to 40 mm Hg). Therefore, the full range of CO_2 dissociation curve shown in Fig. 5.5.11 is an experimental theoretical phenomenon and does not operate in the body practically. Physiologically, the curve operates only within A–V range (Fig. 5.5.11).

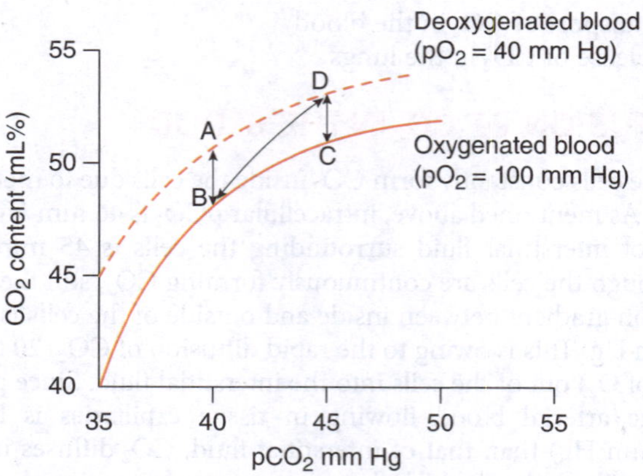

Fig. 5.5.11 Carbon dioxide dissociation curve for oxygenated (solid line) and deoxygenated (dotted line) blood to demonstrate Haldane's effect.

Factors Affecting CO_2 Dissociation Curve

1. Oxygen Deoxyhaemoglobin present in the tissue capillaries is capable of loading more CO_2 than the oxyhaemoglobin. And also the oxygenation of haemoglobin in the lungs increases the CO_2 unloading. This effect is called *Haldane's effect* (named after John Scott Haldane). Haldane's effect on the transport of CO_2 depicts that:

- Blood with pCO_2 40 mm Hg reaching the tissues is capable of drawing CO_2 from the tissues more at pO_2 40 mm Hg (point A) than at pO_2 of 100 mm Hg (point B). Thus, because of Haldane's effect, the CO_2 dissociation curve shifts to the left when blood flows to the tissues.
- Blood with pCO_2 45 mm Hg reaching the lungs is capable of retaining less or in other words releasing more CO_2 in the lungs at pO_2 100 mm Hg (point C) than at pO_2 40 mm Hg (point D). Thus, because of Haldane's effect, the CO_2 dissociation curve shifts to the right when blood flows in the pulmonary capillaries.
- Fig. 5.5.11 also depicts that Haldane's effect is beneficial because it almost doubles the quantity of CO_2 to be carried from the tissues to the lungs and also doubles the amount of CO_2 to be excreted by the lungs.

2. 2,3-DPG 2,3-DPG decreases the formation of carbaminohaemoglobin because it competes with CO_2 for the same sites on Hb especially in case of reduced Hb. Thus, 2,3-DPG shifts the CO_2 dissociation curve to the right, meaning thereby that CO_2-carrying capacity is decreased.

3. Increase in body temperature Increase in body temperature causes release of O_2 from Hb; this causes left shift of the CO_2 dissociation curve, i.e. larger amount of CO_2 can be taken off at given pCO_2.

RELEASE OF CO_2 IN THE LUNGS

When the venous blood with pCO_2 of 45 mm Hg, CO_2 content of 52 mL per 100 mL and pO_2 of 40 mm Hg reaches the pulmonary capillaries, it is separated by the respiratory membrane from the alveolar air having pCO_2 40 mm Hg, CO_2 content of 48 mL/100 mL and pO_2 104 mm Hg. Then the following changes occur, which lead to diffusion of 4 mL of CO_2/100 mL of blood/min in the alveoli (Fig. 5.5.12):

Release of CO_2 from Carbaminohaemoglobin into Plasma (Fig. 5.5.12A)

- O_2 diffuses into the capillary blood with a concentration gradient of 104 − 40 mmHg, or 64 mm Hg.
- The O_2 enters the RBCs and converts the deoxyhaemoglobin into oxyhaemoglobin which has very low affinity for CO_2. In this, CO_2 is released from the carbaminohaemoglobin which diffuses into the plasma.

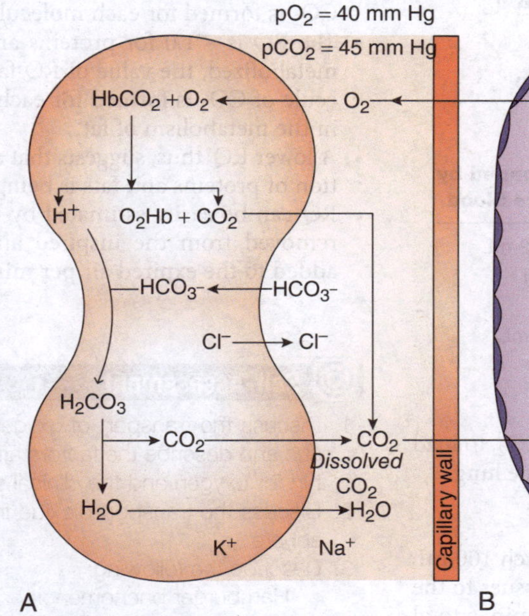

Fig. 5.5.12 **A**, Release of carbon dioxide in the plasma from carbaminohaemoglobin and from bicarbonate ions; and **B**, diffusion of CO_2 from plasma into the alveoli through respiratory membrane.

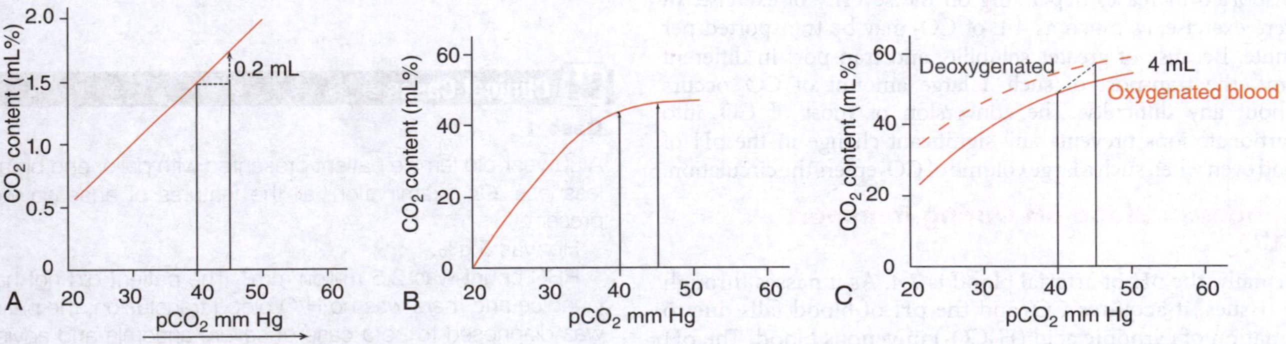

Fig. 5.5.13 Carbon dioxide dissociation curve: **A**, for plasma; **B**, for bicarbonate solution; and **C**, for whole blood.

Release of CO_2 from Carbonate into Plasma (Fig. 5.5.12B)

- The oxyhaemoglobin so formed is a strong acid. Increased acidity of the blood results in increased H^+ concentration. To neutralize it, the bicarbonate (HCO_3^-) ions diffuse into the RBCs where H^+ and HCO_3^- react to form H_2CO_3 (carbonic acid) which dissociates to form H_2O and CO_2. This whole reaction occurs in the presence of enzyme carbonic anhydrase. CO_2 so released diffuses into the plasma.
- With the movement of HCO_3^- inside the RBCs, the inside of the cell becomes more negative. To neutralize it, either the positively charged cations should move in or the negatively charged anions should flow out of the cell. Since RBC membrane is relatively impermeable to cations, the Cl^- anions return in the plasma from the RBC. This whole reaction catalysed by carbonic anhydrase inhibitor is called *reversal of chloride shift*.

Diffusion of CO_2 from plasma to alveoli

The CO_2 dissolved in plasma plus that released from the carbaminohaemoglobin and bicarbonates combinedly exerts pCO_2 of 45 mm Hg. Since the pCO_2 of alveolar air is 40 mm Hg, because of pressure gradient, CO_2 diffuses from blood to alveoli. Due to constant ventilation, CO_2 from alveoli is transported to atmosphere.

OTHER FACTS ABOUT CO_2 TRANSPORT

Comparison of Different Vehicles for CO_2 Transport

The carbon dioxide dissociation curve of plasma, bicarbonate solution and whole blood (Fig. 5.5.13) and the amount of CO_2 that can be loaded and unloaded by different transport vehicles from the tissues at pCO_2 45 mm Hg (Table 5.5.1) reveal that:

- *Plasma* is not a good transport vehicle as very small amount of CO_2 (only 0.2 mL) can be taken from tissues/100 mL of blood/min.
- *Bicarbonate solution* is also not a good transport vehicle because beyond pO_2 40 mm Hg, there is no further transport of CO_2.

Table 5.5.1 Amount of CO_2 that can be loaded and unloaded by different transport vehicles

	Content of CO_2/100 mL/min		
Vehicle	In venous blood at pCO_2 45 mm Hg (mL)	In arterial blood at pCO_2 40 mm Hg (mL)	Loaded by the blood
Plasma	1.8	1.6	0.2 mL
Bicarbonate solution	48	48	Nil
Whole blood	52	48	4 mL

- *Whole blood* is an ideal vehicle for transport of CO_2, to load itself in tissues with CO_2 and to release CO_2 in the lung.

Rate of Total CO_2 Transport

In resting conditions In resting conditions, each 100 mL of blood transports about 4 mL of CO_2 from the tissues to the lungs. Thus, with an average cardiac output of 5 L/min, a total of $(4 \times 5000)/100$ or 200 mL of CO_2 is transported per minute.

During exercise During exercise, the amount of CO_2 transported increases depending on the severity of exercise. In severe exercise, as much as 4 L of CO_2 may be transported per minute. Because of greater solubility and transport in different forms, the transport of such a large amount of CO_2 occurs without any difficulty. The conversion of most of CO_2 into bicarbonate ions prevents any significant change in the pH of blood even when such a large volume of CO_2 enters the circulation.

Changes in Blood pH During Transport of CO_2

Normally, the pH of arterial blood is 7.4. As it passes through the tissues, it acquires CO_2 and the pH of blood falls due to formation of carbonic acid (H_2CO_3) in venous blood. The pH may fall by about 0.4. However, during exercise, the fall in pH may become to the tune of 0.5 and even more. Nevertheless, most of it is neutralized by the blood buffers.

Respiratory Quotient

Definition Respiratory quotient (RQ) refers to the ratio of the rate of CO_2 excretion and rate of O_2 consumption per minute. It is also called the *respiratory exchange ratio*.

Normal value Normally, the rate of CO_2 excretion is 4 mL/100 mL/min, and rate of O_2 consumption is 5 mL/100 mL/min. So, RQ = 4/5, or 0.8.

RQ depends on the type of fuel consumed

- In a person who is utilizing carbohydrates as the entire source of energy for the body metabolism, value of RQ is 1, because in metabolism of carbohydrates, one molecule of CO_2 is formed for each molecule of O_2 consumed.
- The RQ is <1.0 for proteins and fats. When only fats are metabolized, the value of RQ falls to 0.7, because 0.7 molecule of CO_2 is formed for each molecule of O_2 consumed in the metabolism of fat.
- A lower RQ, thus, suggests that a greater than usual proportion of proteins and fats is being catabolized in the body.
- RQ can be easily estimated by knowing the amount of O_2 removed from the inspired air and the amount of CO_2 added to the expired air per minute.

Self-Assessment

1. Discuss the transport of oxygen from the lungs to the tissue and describe the factors affecting affinity of haemoglobin for oxygen and the clinical significance.
2. Discuss the transport dioxide from the tissue to the atmosphere.
3. Describe the following:
   - Hamburger phenomenon
   - Bohr's effect and its significance
   - Haldane's effect
   - Significance of p_{50} in different situations

Clinical Cases

Case 1

A 30-year-old female patient presented with pallor and breathlessness. On examination, all the features of anaemia were present.

Hb was 5 g%.

RBC count was 2.5 million/mm^3. The patient did not have jaundice and there was no H/O blood transfusion; the patient was diagnosed to be a case of severe anaemia and advised blood transfusion.

Two units of compatible stored blood was transfused. On follow-up visit after 10 days, there was no improvement.

Q1. What is the reason for no improvement?

Q2. Explain why stored blood should not transfused in severely hypoxic cases.

Case 2

A 25-year-old farmer developed headache and dizziness while working on a tractor and was brought to the emergency department in an unconscious state. On examination, he was suspected to be a case of carbon monoxide poisoning.

Q1. What is the status of oxygen-carrying capacity of haemoglobin in this case?

Q2. If relationship between pO_2 and haemoglobin saturation is plotted, then what will be the value of p_{50} in this case?

5.6 Regulation of Respiration

CHAPTER OUTLINE

INTRODUCTION

Respiration is regulated by a complex integration of neural control mechanisms which are modified by certain respiratory reflexes and chemical control mechanisms.

Neural control mechanisms include:

- *A system for automatic control* of respiration as an involuntary function. The involuntary control system of respiration is located in the medullary and pontine centres of the brainstem.
- *A system for voluntary control* of respiration is located in the cerebral cortex.

Thus, respiration enjoys the distinction of being an involuntary function which can be influenced voluntarily. This *dual control* has great functional significance, i.e.:

- Involuntary control allows humans to breathe without conscious efforts under all circumstances including sleep and is thus essential for life.
- The voluntary control system facilitates acts like talking, singing, swimming, breath-holding and voluntary hyperventilation.

Respiratory reflexes which modify the effects of neural mechanisms are those initiated by stimulation of stretch receptors, irritant receptors, J-receptors and chest wall receptors.

Chemical control mechanisms are influenced by alterations in arterial pO_2, pCO_2 and H^+ concentration. The chemical control mechanisms are initiated by stimulation of the chemoreceptors (central and peripheral).

Functions of respiratory regulatory mechanisms include:

- *Genesis of normal respiratory spontaneous rhythm:* This is the function of medullary and pontine centres of neural mechanism.
- *Control of rate and depth of respiration*, i.e. adjustment of total ventilation to match metabolic needs of the body so that arterial oxygen tension (pO_2), carbon dioxide tension (pCO_2) and H^+ concentration (pH) are almost maintained constant whether it be during quiet breathing, sleep or muscular exercise: This function is accomplished by all the respiratory control mechanisms acting in unison (Fig. 5.6.1):
  - *Sensors*, i.e. chemoreceptors and other receptors (e.g. stretch, irritant, chest wall and J-receptors), perceive the respiratory needs of the body and convey via afferent nerves to the central controller.
  - *Central controller*, i.e. medullary, pontine and other parts of the brain, adjusts the efferent outputs as per the body needs and conveys to the effectors.

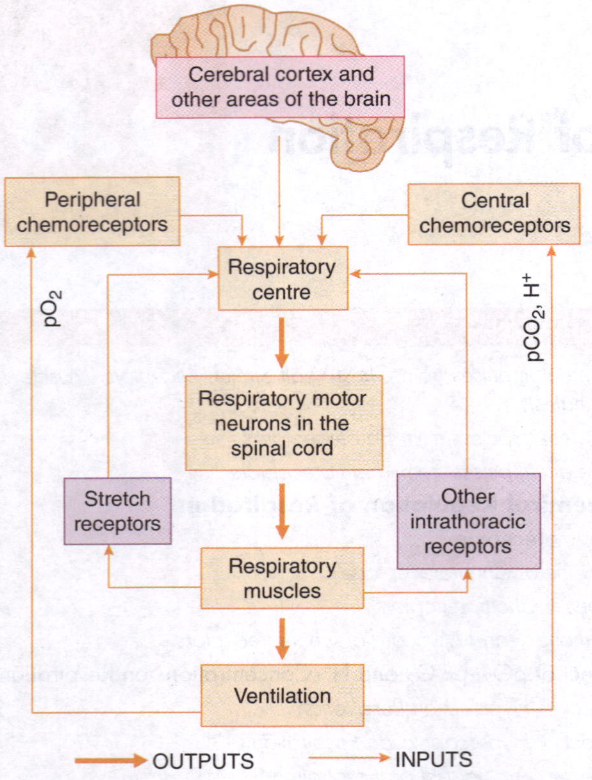

Fig. 5.6.1 Diagrammatic representation of the inputs to respiratory centre that generate the output to the respiratory muscles.

- *Effectors* are the respiratory muscles which perform their activity as per the neural discharges received.

NEURAL REGULATION OF RESPIRATION

The neural mechanisms regulating respiration can be described under two headings:

- Automatic control system
- Afferent impulses to respiratory centres

AUTOMATIC CONTROL SYSTEM

Neural Genesis of Respiratory Rhythm

The involuntary neural control system regulates respiration by several groups of neurons situated bilaterally in medulla and pons which include medullary respiratory centres, pontine respiratory centres and reticular activating system (RAS).

Medullary Respiratory Centres

The medullary respiratory centres include two groups of neurons – the dorsal respiratory group (DRG) and the ventral respiratory group (VRG) – which generate the basic respiratory rhythm.

The respiratory control pattern generator The respiratory control pattern generator, which is responsible for automatic respiration, is located in the medulla. A group of neurons called pacemaker cells form the pre-Bötzinger complex are situated between nucleus ambiguus and lateral reticular nucleus. The rhythmic activity is initiated by these synaptically coupled neurons. These neurons discharge rhythmically and generate rhythmic motor activity in phrenic nerve, hypoglossal nerve and intercostal nerves.

Important Note

On the neurons of pre-Bötzinger complex, the receptors for substance P, tachykinin (NK_1), 5-HT_4 and μ-opioid are present. Opioids are used as analgesic, but at the same time they cause respiratory depression as a side effect. However, it is now known that 5-HT_4 receptor agonists block the inhibitory effect of opioids on respiration without inhibiting analgesic effect.

1. Dorsal Respiratory Group Neurons

Most of the neurons are located within the nucleus of tractus solitarius (NTS) and some in the adjacent reticular substance (Fig. 5.6.2). The neurons of DRG are of three types:

i. Inspiratory neurons The DRG mainly contains inspiratory cells called *I-neurons* that discharge during inspiration only. The axons of I-neurons cross the midline and descend on the contralateral side of spinal cord to make contact with the spinal motor neurons of inspiratory muscles, namely the diaphragm (supplied by the phrenic nerve arising from C_3 to C_5 spinal segments) and the external intercostal muscles (supplied by the intercostal nerves). In other words, the neurons in the DRG are the upper motor neurons of respiratory muscles.

From I-neurons, nerve signals pass to the muscles of inspiration. The signal is not instantaneous but is a ramp signal, i.e. it is weak in the beginning and it steadily increases in a ramp manner for about 2 seconds and is thus called *inspiratory ramp*. This leads to a steady increase in the lung volume during inspiration rather than the respiratory gasps (abrupt distension). Ramp signal then abruptly ceases for approximately next 3 seconds.

ii. Inspiratory off-switch (IOS) neurons IOS neurons refer to a group of neurons that are responsible for terminating the activity of I-neurons and cause turning off of excitation of muscles of inspiration (diaphragm and external intercostal muscles). These muscles, therefore, relax, allowing elastic recoil of the chest wall and the lungs to cause expiration. After expiration, again there is a signal for starting another cycle.

iii. Integrator neurons Integrator neurons are another type of neurons of DRG present near the I-neurons and are stimulated by them. They subserve the following integrating functions:

- The integrator neurons when depolarize to a critical level lead to firing of the so-called IOS neurons which are responsible for terminating the inspiratory ramp. The *I-neurons* trigger the IOS neurons indirectly through integrators and thereby bring about the termination of their own discharge. This forms the basic circuitry of an automatic respiratory rhythm (Fig. 5.6.3). In this way, the cycle of inspiration/expiration goes on continuously to cause tidal respiration.
- The *integrator neurons* receive both excitatory and inhibitory inputs (Fig. 5.6.3) and thus integrate the activity of *I-neurons* and IOS neurons accordingly.

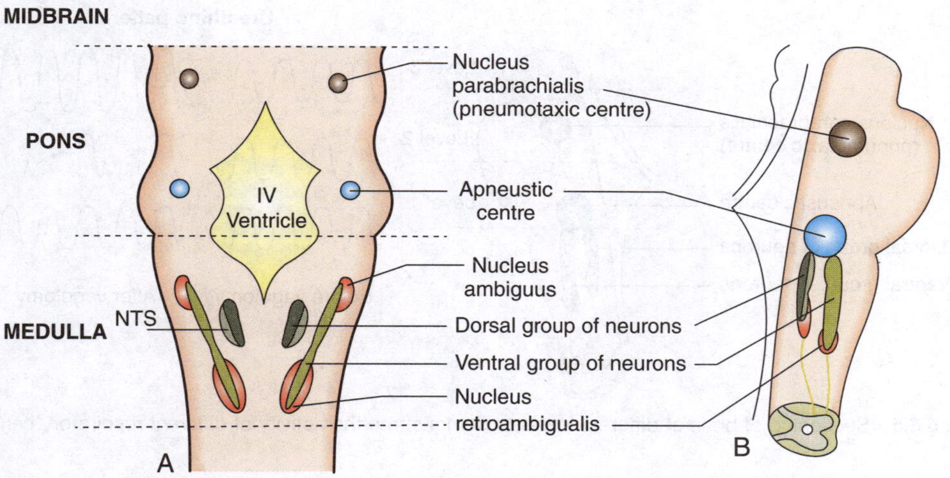

Fig. 5.6.2 Medullary and pontine respiratory centres: **A**, front view; and **B**, lateral view.

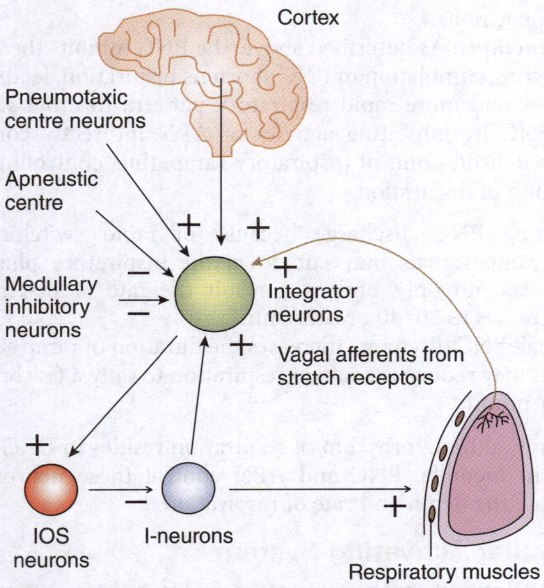

Fig. 5.6.3 Basic circuitry for generation of respiratory rhythm.

- *The excitatory inputs* to integrator neurons come from:
  Cerebral cortex
  Pneumotaxic centre (PNC)
  Vagal afferents from stretch receptors
- *The inhibitory inputs* to integrator neurons come from the *apneustic centre* (APN).

iv. Other neurons Besides the above described, other neurons which form a part of DRG neurons are as follows:

- *P-neurons or pump cells* are the second-order pulmonary stretch receptor sensory neurons. These do not receive other respiratory inputs.
- *Propriobulbar inspiratory ramp interneurons, early inspiratory or early-burst neurons, late-onset inspiratory neurons* and *postinspiration* (PI)-related neurons are other inspiratory neurons of the DRG.

Detailed functioning of these other neurons of the DRG is beyond the scope of this book.

2. Ventral Respiratory Group Neurons

VRG neurons contain both inspiratory cells called I-neurons and expiratory cells called E-neurons (cf. DRG which contain only I-neurons).

Parts of VRG neurons The VRG neurons can be subdivided into three main parts (Fig. 5.6.2):

i. ***Caudal part or nucleus retroambigualis (NRA)*** contains mainly E-neurons which constitute the bulbospinal premotor neurons. Their axons cross the midline and descend on the contralateral side to make contact with the motor neuron pool for the muscles of expiration, i.e. internal intercostal muscles and abdominal muscles. In other words, these neurons in the VRG seem to form the *upper motor neurons of expiratory muscles.*
ii. ***Intermediate part*** of VRG neurons denotes *nucleus parambigualis* because it parallels the ambiguus nucleus. This part mainly contains I-neurons called the bulbospinal inspiratory premotor neurons. These control the activity of inspiratory upper motor neurons.
iii. ***Most rostral part of VRG*** coincides with nucleus retrofacialis (NRF). It contains several types of E-neurons which form a complex called *Bötzinger complex.* Some of these neurons control the pharyngeal and laryngeal musculature which must relax during expiration.

Interaction of I- and E-neurons The I- and E-neurons have inhibitory connections to each other, i.e. there exists *reciprocal innervation* between the two. Therefore, the motor neurons to the expiratory muscles are inhibited when those supplying the inspiratory muscles are active and vice versa. This reciprocal innervation is mediated via collaterals from excitatory pathway that synapse on inhibitory interneurons. Thus, an impulse that stimulates the one will inhibit the other and vice versa (Fig. 5.6.4).

$$\text{I-neurons} \overset{(-)}{\underset{(-)}{\Leftrightarrow}} \text{E-neurons}$$

Fig. 5.6.4 Reciprocal innervation of I- and E-neurons.

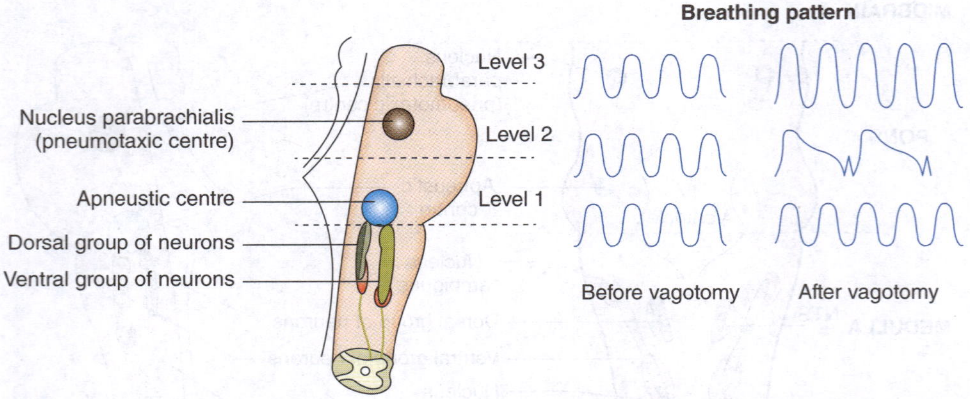

Fig. 5.6.5 Sectioning of brain at different levels to demonstrate the activity of different respiratory centres.

Role of VRG neurons The VRG neurons normally remain totally inactive during quiet breathing. They become active during inspiration (role of I-neurons) as well as expiration (role of E-neurons) during forceful respiration. This area is especially important in providing powerful expiratory signals to expiratory muscles. Thus, VRG operates when high levels of pulmonary ventilation is required, e.g. during exercise.

Pontine Respiratory Centres

The pontine centres include the APN and PNC, both of which modify the activity of medullary respiratory centres.

1. Apneustic Centre

APN refers to a group of inhibitory neurons located bilaterally in the lower part of pons (Fig. 5.6.2). It sends signals to integrator neurons of DRG that affects the IOS neurons and prevents the switch-off of the inspiratory activity (Fig. 5.6.3). This increases the tidal volume and duration of inspiration, resulting in a deeper and more prolonged inspiratory effort termed *apneusis*. However, normally the APN is inhibited by impulses carried by the vagus nerves and also by the activity of PNC. Either of these two influences, PNC or the vagi, seems to be adequate to keep apneusis in check. The above-described facts are based on the experimental observations made in dogs and cats under general anaesthesia. The situation in conscious animals may be different. The existence and functions of APN are based on the following experimental observations (Fig. 5.6.5):

- Sectioning of the brain between the medulla and the pons (level 1 in Fig. 5.6.5) leaves the basic rhythm intact indicating thereby that medullary respiratory centres are working normally.
- Sectioning the brain at midpontine level, i.e. between PNC and APN (i.e. at level 2 in Fig. 5.6.5), along with bilateral vagotomy leads to prolonged periods of inspiration, i.e. apneusis or apneustic breathing. This indicates the removal of two inhibitor influences (PNC and vagi) on the APN and allows APN to exert its influence on medullary centres producing apneusis.
- Sectioning the brain rostral to the pons (level 3 in Fig. 5.6.5) leaves the respiratory rhythm intact even if combined with bilateral vagotomy. This indicates that mere presence of check by PNC is sufficient to control the apneustic effect of APN on medullary centres.

2. Pneumotaxic Centre

The PNCs are located bilaterally in *nucleus parabrachialis* of the upper pons.

Functions: As described above, the PNC inhibits the APN. Therefore, stimulation of PNC shortens inspiration, leading to shallow and more rapid respiratory pattern. In other words, the PNC by inhibiting activity of APN indirectly controls the switch-off point of inspiratory ramp, thus controlling the duration of inspiration.

- Strong PNC discharge because of rapid switching-off of ramp signals may cut down the inspiratory phase to 0.5 second only, and as a result the rate of inspiration increases to 30–40 breaths/min.
- Weak PNC discharge increases the duration of ramp signals and may reduce the rate of respiration to only a few breaths per minute.

Thus, although rhythm of respiration resides in DRG neurons in medulla, PNC and APN control these neurons to regulate the depth and rate of respiration.

Reticular Activating System

The RAS stimulates the respiratory centres to increase respiratory drive. During sleep, RAS activity diminishes, decreasing respiratory drive, which diminishes alveolar ventilation and results in a slight elevation of arterial CO_2 tension.

AFFERENT IMPULSES TO RESPIRATORY CENTRES

The respiratory centres generate the respiratory rhythm and execute their effects through the efferent nerves supplying the respiratory muscles. The activity of respiratory centres in turn is influenced by the afferent impulses from the lungs and various other parts of the body. These afferent impulses guide the respiratory centres to regulate their activity so as to serve a number of purposes in the body such as:

- To cope up with the O_2 demand of the body and get rid of CO_2 from the body
- To help to regulate the H^+ concentration of body
- To maintain the appropriate O_2 tension of blood in certain conditions of anoxia or hypoxia
- To help to maintain the normal body temperature

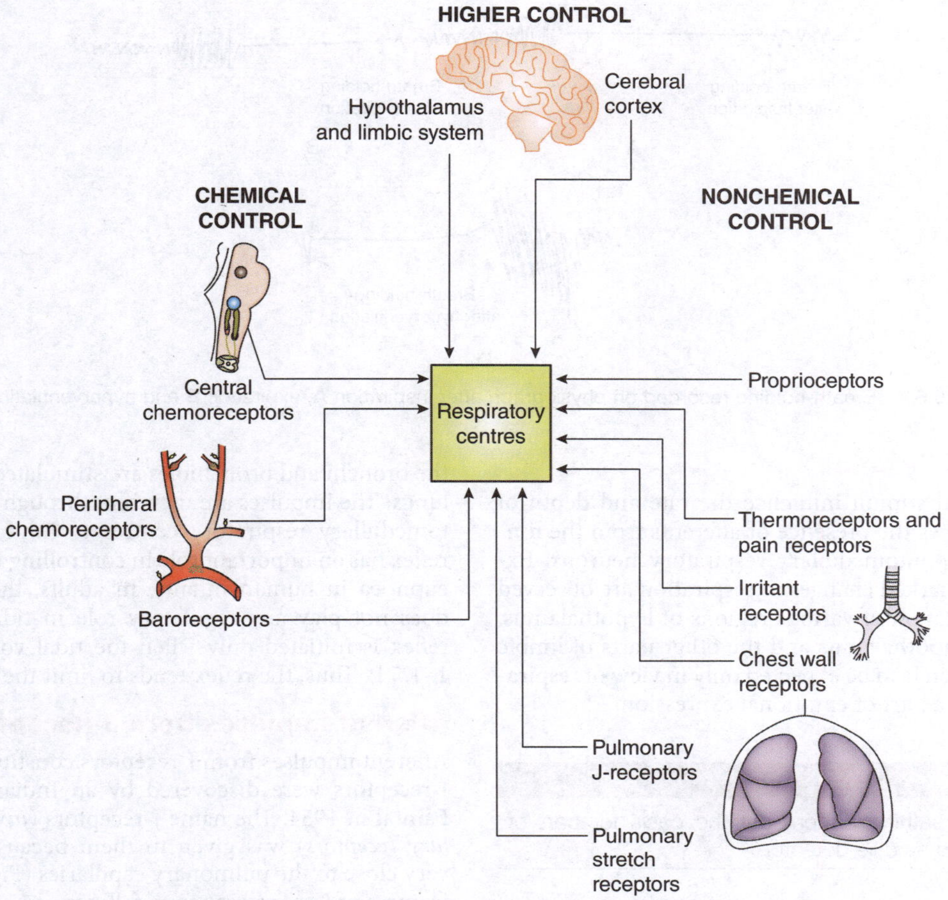

Fig. 5.6.6 Afferent impulses to respiratory centres.

Various afferent impulses to the respiratory centres can be grouped as (Fig. 5.6.6):

- Afferent impulses from higher centres
- Afferent impulses from nonchemical receptors, which may constitute *nonchemical regulation of respiration*
- Afferent impulses from the chemical receptors, which constitute the 'chemical regulation of respiration' and hence have been described separately

AFFERENT IMPULSES FROM HIGHER CENTRES

The afferent impulses from higher centres which influence the involuntary activity of respiratory centres mainly include voluntary control system and limbic control system.

Voluntary control system

As described above, normally, breathing is an involuntary effort and goes on automatically. However, the respiratory muscles are typical skeletal muscle and can also be controlled voluntarily. The voluntary control of respiration is mediated by a pathway which originates from the neocortex and bypasses the medullary respiratory centres to project directly on the spinal respiratory neurons. The voluntary control of breathing is exercised during *activities like* talking, singing and swimming; and breath-holding.

Breath-Holding or Voluntary Apnoea

Breathing can be stopped voluntarily for about 50–60 seconds (breath-holding time). But after this time, the chemical drive overrides the voluntary inhibition and the person has uncontrollable desire to breathe and ultimately breathing is resumed involuntarily. That is why it is impossible to commit suicide by holding the breath voluntarily. The decrease in arterial pO_2 and increase in arterial pCO_2 seem to be the chief causes for the end of breath-holding.

- Breath-holding can be prolonged by 15–20 seconds by an initial hyperventilation which lowers the arterial pCO_2. As a result, it takes longer duration of breath-holding to increase the arterial pCO_2 to the critical level (Fig. 5.6.7).
- Breath-holding may also be increased by prior inhalation of pure O_2. Some mechanical or reflex factors originating from the chest wall also seem to be involved in limiting the duration of breath-holding.
- Breath-holding time is prolonged by doing yogic exercises such as yoga nidra, meditation and motivation. These factors basically induce mental relaxation.

Voluntary Hyperventilation

Voluntary hyperventilation, i.e. voluntary overbreathing, can be done for some time only similar to breath-holding. Effects of hyperventilation are discussed in chemical control of respiration (see page 442).

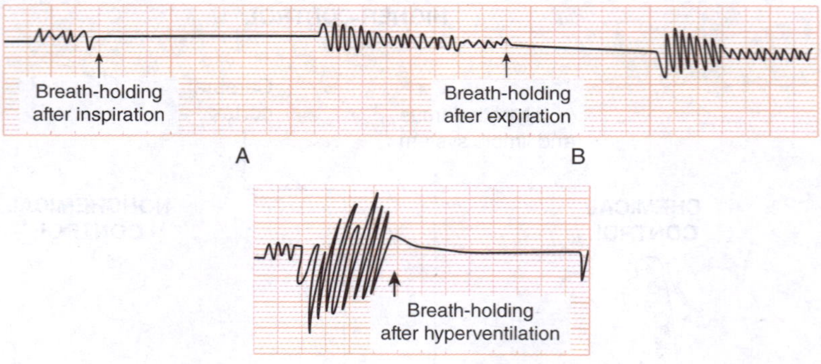

Fig. 5.6.7 Breath-holding recorded on physiograph after inspiration **A**, expiration **B** and hyperventilation **C**.

Limbic Control System

Pain and emotional stimuli influence the rate and depth of breathing. It indicates the presence of afferents from the limbic system to the pontomedullary respiratory neurons. Experimentally also marked changes in respiration are observed on electrical stimulation of various regions of hypothalamus. The influence of hypothalamus and the other parts of limbic system on respiration is to be expected only in view of respiratory changes being a part of emotional expression.

Important Note

Changes in the breathing pattern are the basis for part of polygraph test used as a lie detector.

Applied Aspects

As respiration has two separate controls, voluntary and automatic, sometimes automatic control is disrupted, whereas voluntary control remains intact. Clinically, this condition is known as *Ondine curse*. In this state, a person would stay alive only if he/she is awake and remembers to breathe. Ondine was a water nymph cursed by the king and all his automatic functions were withdrawn. Due to exhaustion, he fell asleep and died because of stoppage of breathing.

Ondine curse is also known as *congenital hypoventilation syndrome* is a rare condition occurs in severe form of sleep apnoea due to decreased sensitivity to hypercapnia and hypoxia and person stops breathing.

This condition usually occurs in the patients suffering from bulbar poliomyelitis or conditions which compress the medulla.

AFFERENT IMPULSES FROM NONCHEMICAL RECEPTORS

Afferent impulses from the receptors other than the chemoreceptors, i.e. from nonchemical receptors, include the following:

Afferent Impulses from Pulmonary Stretch Receptors (Hering–Breuer Reflex)

Hering–Breuer reflex is one of the first examples of negative feedback. In 1868, Hering and Breuer found that lung inflation inhibits output of the phrenic motor neurons, thereby protecting lung from overinflation.

The Hering–Breuer inspiratory inhibitory reflex is initiated when the stretch receptors located in the smooth muscles of the bronchi and bronchioles are stimulated by inflation of the lungs. The impulses are then sent through *vagi nerves* to pontomedullary respiratory centres to inhibit respiration. This reflex has an important role in controlling tidal volume during eupnoea in human infants. In adults, this reflex, therefore, does not play any regulatory role in tidal respiration. This reflex is initiated only when the tidal volume is more than 1–1.5 L. Thus, the reflex tends to limit the tidal volume.

Afferent Impulses from J-Receptors

Afferent impulses from J-receptors constitute the J-reflex. The J-receptors were discovered by an Indian physiologist A.S. Paintal in 1954. The name J-receptors (*juxtapulmonary capillary receptors*) was given to them because of their location very close to the pulmonary capillaries (Fig. 5.6.8). Important features of J-receptors are as follows:

- J-receptors are basically unmyelinated vagal afferent nerve endings (type C fibres).
- These receptors are primarily sensitive to increase in the content of interstitial fluid between the capillary endothelium and the alveolar epithelium; therefore, they are stimulated in conditions like pulmonary congestion, pulmonary

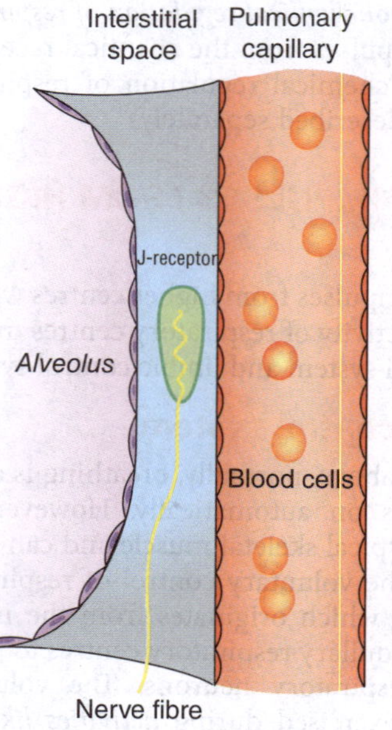

Fig. 5.6.8 Location of J-receptors.

oedema, pneumonia, hyperinflation of lungs and microembolism in pulmonary capillaries.

- J-receptors are also stimulated by some chemical substances like phenyl diguanide, capsaicin, halothane and bradykinin.
- The J-reflex response produced on stimulation of J-receptors is characterized by apnoea followed by hyperventilation, bradycardia, hypotension and weakness of skeletal muscles.

Important Note

Physiological role of J-receptors has been postulated by the discoverer Mr Paintal. He states that after exercise, especially at high altitude, some fluid is entrapped in the alveolar interstitial space which stimulates the J-receptors producing dyspnoea and reduction of skeletal muscle tone. Their combined effect would discourage exercise, thereby taking away the trigger for pulmonary congestion.

Applied Aspects

- J-reflex or pulmonary chemoreflex is a protective reflex during severe exercise and exercise at high altitude.
- Dyspnoea in conditions like pneumonia, pulmonary congestion, pulmonary oedema and hyperinflation of lungs and in left heart failure is attributed to stimulation of J-receptors.

Afferent Impulses from Irritant Receptors in the Respiratory Tract

Irritant receptors are located below the mucosa of the whole respiratory tract. These are stimulated by smoke, noxious gases and particulate matter in the inspired air and in a number of other conditions. These receptors initiate a large number of reflexes some of which are given in the next subsections.

i. Cough Reflex

This is a protective reflex caused by stimulation of irritant receptors in the pharynx, larynx, trachea and bronchi (conducting zone of respiratory tract). Cough begins with a deep inspiration followed by forced expiration with closed glottis. So, intrapleural pressure rises above 100 mm Hg. The glottis is then suddenly opened producing an explosive outflow of air (Fig. 5.6.9). The velocity of the air flow may reach 960 km/h. By this endeavour, the irritants (mucus) may be expelled out of the respiratory tract. The common causes which increase mucus production are infection and allergy.

ii. Sneezing Reflex

Sneezing reflex is also a protective reflex produced on stimulation of irritant receptors of nasal mucosa. The sneezing begins with deep inspiration, followed by forceful expiration with opened glottis (in cough reflex in which glottis is closed) (Fig. 5.6.9).

iii. Hering–Breuer Deflation Reflexs

Hering–Breuer deflation reflex is produced on stimulation of irritant receptors located in bronchial epithelium due to distortion of bronchial epithelium caused by large deflations of the lungs as seen in pneumothorax and lung collapses (atelectasis). This reflex may also be responsible for the *sighs* or *yawning* in response to the increase in compliance that occurs periodically due to the collapse of smaller alveoli. The reflex helps in opening up the collapsed alveoli again.

- Yawning is a peculiar respiratory act. Its physiological basis is uncertain. However, one view suggests that deep inspiration and stretching help in opening up of alveoli and prevent them from collapsing. However, experimentally, atelectasis-preventing effect of yawning could not be demonstrated.
- Yawning increases venous return to the heart.
- In groups of certain animals (monkeys), yawning is used as signal for communication.

iv. Reflex Tachypnoea and Bronchoconstriction

Reflex tachypnoea and bronchoconstriction is produced on stimulation of irritant receptors present in the respiratory zone of the respiratory tract. Rapid shallow breathing results from reflex stimulation of inspiratory motor neurons. Bronchoconstriction is produced by release of histamine and other chemical substances in the lungs, thereby preventing the irritants to reach the gas exchanging surface.

v. Deglutition Reflex

Deglutition reflex refers to temporary apnoea produced during pharyngeal phase of swallowing of food. It is a protective reflex which prevents the entry of food particles into the respiratory tract (Fig. 5.6.10). The afferents travel in the trigeminal, glossopharyngeal and vagus (V, IX and X) nerves and produce *deglutition apnoea* by temporary inhibition of respiratory centres. The receptors for deglutition reflex are present on the pharyngeal mucosa.

Afferent Impulses from Proprioceptors

Proprioceptors are the receptors present in the muscles, tendons and joints and are stimulated during change in the

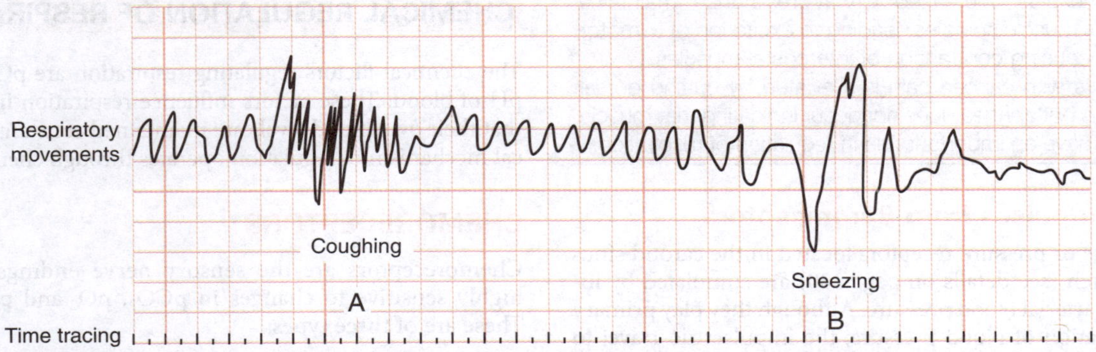

Fig. 5.6.9 Respiration movements, recorded by stethography on physiograph during coughing **A** and sneezing **B**.

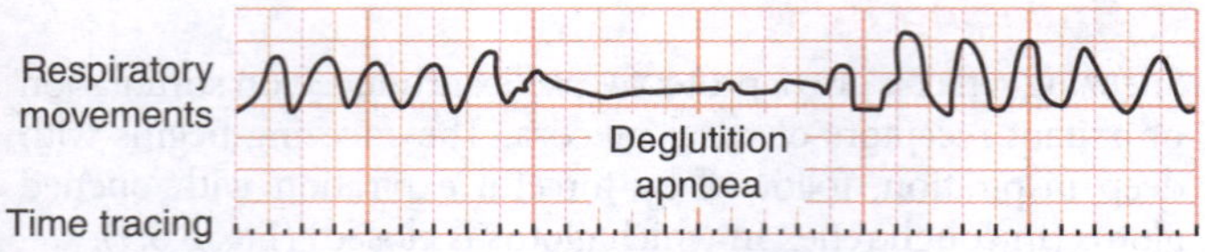

Fig. 5.6.10 Deglutition apnoea recorded on physiograph by stethography.

position of different parts of the body. Afferent impulses from proprioceptors stimulate the inspiratory neurons to increase the rate and depth of respiration.

Important Note

- This reflex helps in increasing ventilation during exercise.
- The paediatricians employ this reflex for initiating first breath in the newborn by slapping it.

Afferent Impulses from Chest Wall Stretch Receptors (Muscle Spindles)

Chest wall stretch receptors are nothing but the *muscle spindles* present in the intercostal muscles. Stretching of the intercostal muscles produces a stretch reflex due to stimulation of muscle spindles that is characterized by contraction of intercostal muscles. The muscle spindles present in respiratory muscles help to coordinate breathing during change in posture or during speech. They play a special role in maintaining normal tidal volume when breathing is impeded by an increase in airway resistance or a decrease in pulmonary compliance.

- When the mechanical load on the respiratory system is increased, intercostal muscles are stretched and their muscle spindles are stimulated leading to increased strength of contraction of intercostal muscles. It has been observed that increase in intercostal nerve afferent activity leads to contraction of neighbouring intercostal muscles. This reflex has been termed the *intercostal-to-intercostal reflex*.
- Although diaphragm contains very few muscle spindles, it also shows reflex contraction. This has been attributed to reflex contraction of diaphragm in response to afferent nerve impulses originating in lower intercostal nerves. This reflex has been termed the *intercostal-to-phrenic reflex*.

Important Notes

- In patients with asthma, tidal volume is maintained due to constant stretching of muscle spindles present in the intercostal muscles. Increased airway resistance maintains stretch of muscle spindles, leading to excitation of α-motor neurons causing contraction of intercostal muscles.
- In patients with cancer, pain is alleviated by cutting dorsal root fibres but apnoea does not occur indicating that muscle spindles have an important role in regulation of respiration.

Afferent Impulses from Baroreceptors

Baroreceptors or pressure receptors located in the carotid sinus and aortic arch (see details on page 330) are stimulated by increase in the arterial blood pressure. Although they play primary role in regulation of blood pressure, the impulses do travel to respiratory centres (via vagus from aortic arch and via

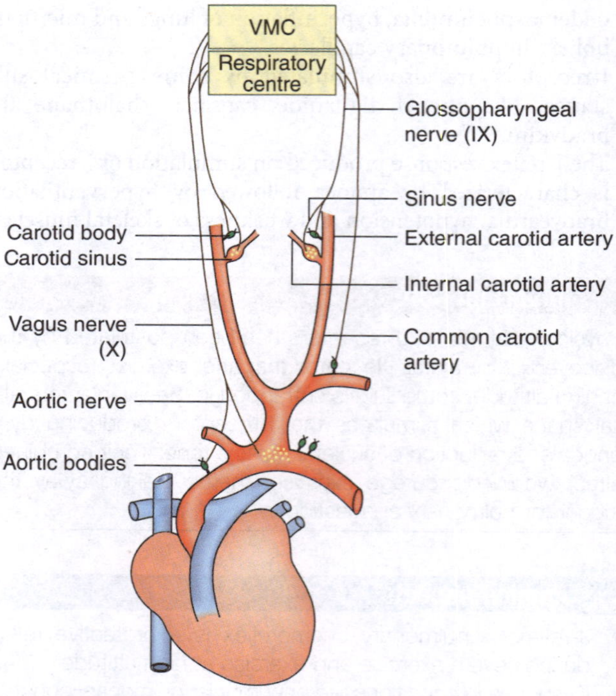

Fig. 5.6.11 Location of carotid and aortic bodies (peripheral chemoreceptors).

glossopharyngeal nerve from carotid sinus) and cause inhibition of respiration; in physiological conditions, the baroreceptors play an insignificant role in regulation of respiration. The *adrenaline apnoea* observed on injection of high doses of adrenaline has been explained due to the fact that the adrenaline causes a large rise in arterial pressure which in turn inhibits respiration by afferent impulses from the baroreceptors to the respiratory centres (Fig. 5.6.11). However, in small doses, adrenaline stimulates respiration by stimulating the peripheral chemoreceptors.

Afferent Impulses from Thermoreceptors

Thermoreceptors are those receptors which are stimulated by a change in the body temperature. They are of two types – the cold receptors and the warm receptors. When warm receptors are stimulated, the impulses are conveyed to cerebral cortex via somatic afferent nerves. Cerebral cortex in turn stimulates the respiratory centres to produce hyperventilation.

Respiration helps to maintain body temperature, as some amount of heat is lost in the expired air. In dogs, panting is one of the major mechanisms of thermoregulation.

CHEMICAL REGULATION OF RESPIRATION

The chemical factors regulating respiration are pCO_2, pO_2 and pH of blood. These factors influence respiration in such a way that their own blood levels are maintained constant. The chemical mechanism of regulation operates through chemoreceptors.

CHEMORECEPTORS

Chemoreceptors are the sensory nerve endings, which are highly sensitive to changes in pCO_2, pO_2 and pH of blood. These are of three types:

- Peripheral chemoreceptors

- Central chemoreceptors
- Pulmonary and myocardial chemoreceptors

Peripheral chemoreceptors

Location

Peripheral chemoreceptors include the carotid and aortic bodies (Fig. 5.6.11).

- *Carotid body* is located on either side near the bifurcation of common carotid artery.
- *Aortic bodies*, two or more in number, are located near the arch of aorta.

Structure

Each carotid and aortic body consists of:

Capsule surrounding each carotid and aortic body is very thin.
Sinusoidal large capillaries present below the capsule surround the main mass of each body.
Epithelial cells: The main mass of the body consists of islands of epithelial cells which are of two types – type I and type II (Fig. 5.6.12).

Type I or glomus cells Type I or glomus cells are similar to chromaffin cells of the adrenal glands. These cells have dense core granules containing catecholamines (dopamine), substance P, met-enkephalin and ACh. Unmyelinated nerve endings are closely applied to these cells; these nerve endings are cup shaped and have dopamine receptors (D_2) on them. When exposed to hypoxia, the type I cells release catecholamine which stimulates the D_2 receptors.

Type II cells Type II cells which are probably glial cells are also closely applied to the type I cells.

Nerve fibres Outside the capsule of each body, the nerve fibres acquire myelin sheath; they are only 2–5 μm in diameter and conduct at relatively low rate of 7–12 m/s.

Afferent Fibres

Afferent fibres from the carotid body join the sinus nerve, a branch of glossopharyngeal (IX) nerve, and ultimately ascend to medulla. Those from the aortic body join the aortic nerve branch of vagus (X cranial) nerve and ascend to medulla.

Blood Flow

Blood flow to each carotid and aortic body is highest in the body (2000 mL/100 g/min). Therefore, the O_2 needs of these cells can be met largely by dissolved O_2 only.

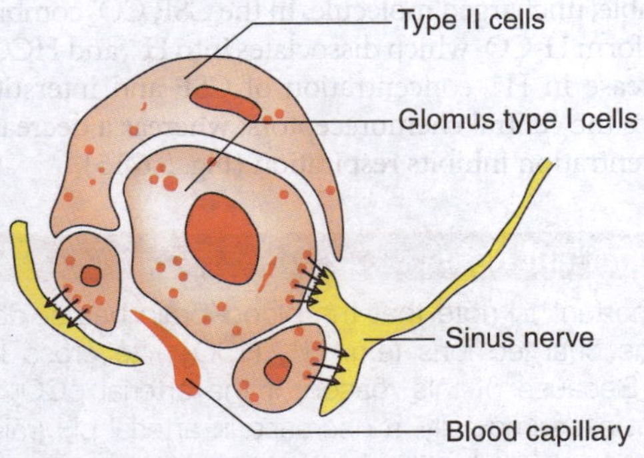

Fig. 5.6.12 Histological structure of carotid body.

Functions

The peripheral chemoreceptors respond to lowered pO_2, increased pCO_2 and increased H^+ concentration in the arterial blood. The afferent impulses from the chemoreceptors stimulate the DRG neurons, which lead to an increased rate and depth of respiration called hyperventilation. Increase in the rate or depth of respiration regardless of patients' subjective sensation is called hyperpnoea. Salient points of their functions are as follows:

- The peripheral chemoreceptors are the only sites that detect changes in pO_2.
- Carotid bodies are seven times more effective than aortic bodies in stimulating respiration.
- Carotid bodies increase both rate and depth of respiration, whereas aortic bodies increase only the frequency of respiration with small increase in ventilation.

Mechanism of Chemoreceptor Stimulation by Hypoxia and Oxygen Transduction in Glomus Cells

The peripheral chemoreceptors are stimulated by the release of neurotransmitter by glomus cells. Oxygen transduction is the process by which changes in the arterial pO_2 result in proportionate changes in the frequency of action potential discharge. The sequence of events is as follows (Fig. 5.6.13):

- Hypoxia leads to decrease in activity of oxygen-sensitive K^+ channels present in the cell membrane of glomus cells leading to decrease in the K^+ efflux depending on the level of pO_2.
- Thus, the glomus cells get depolarized in proportion to the fall in arterial pO_2.
- Depolarization of the glomus cells opens up the L-type Ca^{2+} channels in the glomus cell membrane leading to increase in Ca^{2+} influx.
- The Ca^{2+} influx triggers the release of neurotransmitter which stimulates the afferent nerve endings.

Factors Affecting Peripheral Chemoreceptor Stimulation

i. O_2 Tension Versus O_2 Content The peripheral chemoreceptors monitor the dissolved O_2, i.e. pO_2, rather than its total content. They are stimulated when pO_2 falls below 60 mm Hg. Therefore, they respond to various types of hypoxia differently as:

- *Hypoxic hypoxia* in which arterial pO_2 is reduced stimulates peripheral chemoreceptors.
- *Histotoxic hypoxia* in which there is reduced utilization of O_2 by the tissue cells including glomus cells also stimulates chemoreceptors.
- *Vascular stasis*, in which the amount of O_2 delivered to receptors per unit of time is decreased, leads to chemoreceptor stimulation.
- *Drugs* such as cyanide, nicotine and lobeline prevent O_2 utilization at the tissue level and stimulate peripheral chemoreceptors.
- *Anaemic hypoxia*, methaemoglobinaemia or carbon monoxide poisoning does not stimulate the peripheral chemoreceptors, because under these conditions, although the total content of O_2 may be low, the O_2 tension, which is determined by the amount of dissolved O_2, remains normal.

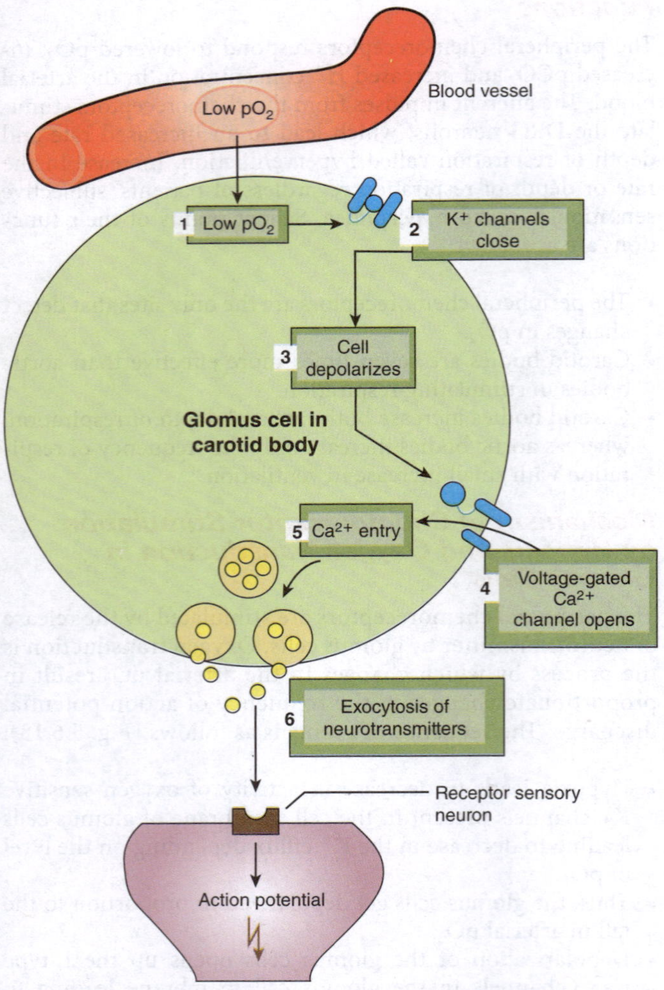

Fig. 5.6.13 Mechanism of stimulation of peripheral chemoreceptors.

ii. Elevated pCO_2 Elevated pCO_2 (by 10 mm Hg) also stimulates the peripheral chemoreceptors, but the major effect of CO_2 is on the central chemoreceptors.

iii. H^+ concentration H^+ concentration when increased in the blood (decreased pH by 0.1 unit) stimulates the peripheral chemoreceptors.

iv. Increase in plasma K^+ levels Increase in plasma K^+ levels may stimulate the peripheral chemoreceptors even in the absence of hypoxia. Increase in plasma K^+ levels during exercise contributes to exercise-induced hyperventilation.

v. Asphyxia Asphyxia, i.e. combination of O_2 lack plus CO_2 excess in blood, stimulates peripheral chemoreceptors.

Effects of Stimulation of Peripheral Chemoreceptors

They regulate the respiration from breath to breath and their stimulation increases the rate and depth of respiration.

- They also cause increase in blood pressure and tachycardia.
- About 15%–20% of resting respiratory drive is due to stimulatory effect of CO_2 on peripheral chemoreceptors.

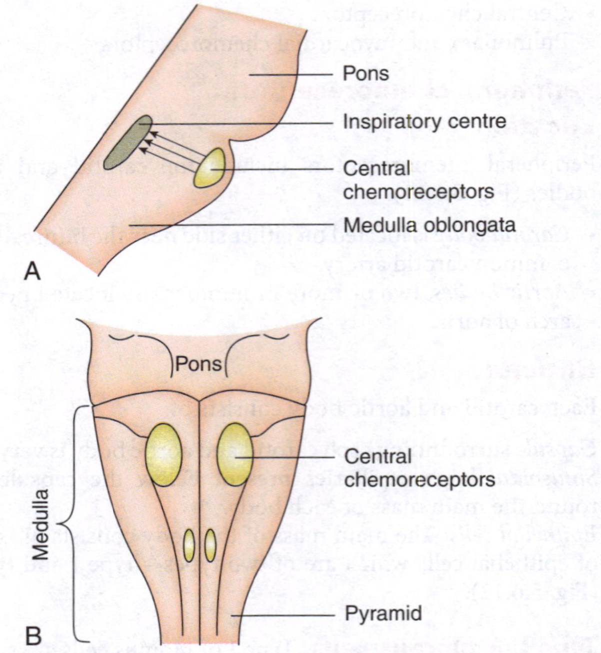

Fig. 5.6.14 Location of central chemoreceptors in medulla: **A**, lateral view; and **B**, front view.

Central Chemoreceptors

Location

Central chemoreceptors are the cells (neurons) that lie just beneath the ventral surface of the medulla oblongata and are therefore also called medullary receptors (Fig. 5.6.14).

Innervation

Nerves from the neurons forming central chemoreceptors project directly over to the respiratory centres which are located slightly deeper to central chemoreceptors.

Stimulation Characteristics

Stimulation characteristics of central chemoreceptors are as follows:

- They respond to H^+ concentration in the surrounding interstitial fluid and cerebrospinal fluid (CSF).
- The magnitude of stimulation is directly proportional to the local H^+ concentration, which in turn parallels arterial pCO_2.

Mechanism by which Increase in CO_2 Concentration Affects Central Chemoreceptors

CO_2 readily crosses the blood–brain barrier, because it is a small, very soluble, uncharged molecule. In the CSF, CO_2 combines with water to form H_2CO_3 which dissociates into H^+ and HCO_3^- ions. The increase in H^+ concentration of CSF and interstitial fluid stimulates the central chemoreceptors, whereas a decrease in the H^+ concentration inhibits respiration (Fig. 5.6.15).

> **Important Note**
>
> It is important to note that the blood–brain barrier does not allow the charged ions (e.g. H^+, HCO_3^-) to cross through readily. Because of this reason, if the arterial pCO_2 is kept constant experimentally, a decrease in arterial pH (raised H^+ concentration) fails to stimulate central chemoreceptors.

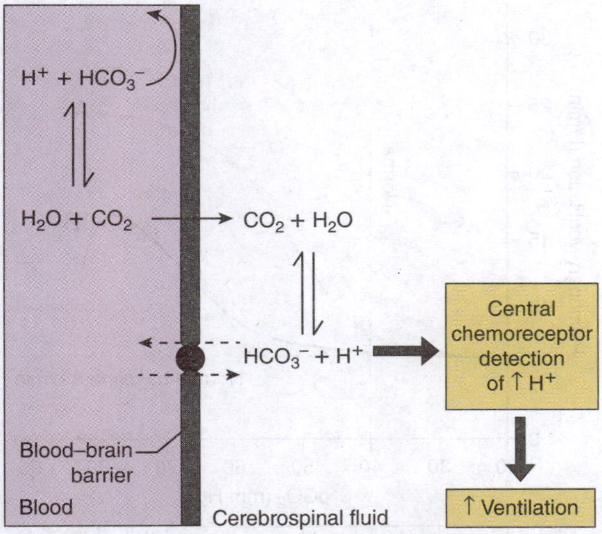

Fig. 5.6.15 Carbon dioxide crosses the blood–brain barrier. The resultant change in the pH of the cerebrospinal fluid is detected by central chemoreceptors. The effect stimulates an increase in alveolar ventilation.

- *Increase in pCO_2* of CSF is more effective in stimulating central chemoreceptors than increased pCO_2 in interstitial fluid of the brain. As mentioned above, actual stimulus for central chemoreceptors is the increased H^+ concentration. In CSF, there are no buffers (proteins) to buffer the H^+ ions formed from H_2CO_3. The interstitial fluid is surrounded by cells having proteins to act as buffers. Therefore, for the same change in CO_2 concentration, H^+ concentration of CSF is more than that of interstitial fluid; thus, increased pCO_2 of CSF is a more important stimulus.
- Central chemoreceptors are not stimulated by hypoxia; rather, like any other cell, they are depressed by hypoxia.
- Central chemoreceptors are also inhibited by anaesthesia and cyanide and during sleep.

Effects of Stimulation

Effects of stimulation of central chemoreceptors are as follows:

- The central chemoreceptors regulate the respiration from minute to minute. Their stimulation leads to increase in the rate and depth of respiration.

> **Important Note**
>
> It is important to note that about 80%–85% of the resting respiratory drive is due to stimulatory effect of CO_2 on the central chemoreceptors. In contrast, peripheral chemoreceptors provide only 15%–20% of initial drive to increase respiration.

Pulmonary and Myocardial Chemoreceptors

Location Pulmonary and myocardial chemoreceptors are located in the pulmonary and coronary blood vessels, respectively.

Innervation These are innervated by the vagus (X cranial) nerve.

Stimulation characteristics and effects Stimulation characteristics and effects of these receptors are as follows:

Pulmonary Chemoreceptors

Pulmonary chemoreceptors are stimulated by injection of veratridine or nicotine into pulmonary circulation and produce the so-called *pulmonary chemoreceptor reflex*, which is characterized by bradycardia, hypotension and apnoea followed by tachypnoea (rapid shallow breathing). Physiological role of this reflex is not established. It occurs in pathological states like pulmonary congestion or embolism.

Myocardial Chemoreceptors

Myocardial chemoreceptors are similarly stimulated when these agents are injected into coronaries supplying the left ventricle and produce the so-called *coronary chemoreflex* or *Bezold–Jarisch reflex* having features similar to those of pulmonary chemoreflex. *Physiological role* of this reflex is not established. It is known to occur after myocardial infarction (see page 335).

EFFECT OF PO_2, PCO_2 AND H^+ CONCENTRATIONS ON RESPIRATION

- The pO_2, pCO_2 and H^+ concentrations influence the respiration by their effects on chemoreceptors.
- The peripheral and central chemoreceptors work in unison to bring about increased ventilation in response to a rise in pCO_2, rise in H^+ concentration or fall in arterial pO_2. Of the three, hypercapnia provides the strongest respiratory drive.
- Chemical regulation of breathing ensures that the arterial pCO_2 is kept constant at normal value of 40 mm Hg, arterial pO_2 is not allowed to fall below 60 mm Hg and changes in blood pH are opposed.
- Denervation or removal of carotid chemoreceptors produces about 40% decrease in response to hypercapnia as well as H^+ concentration and complete abolition of response to drop in pO_2. The predominant effect of hypoxia after denervation of the carotid bodies is a direct depression of the respiratory centre.

With these introductory remarks, effect of each chemical factor on respiration will be discussed followed by the interaction of chemical factors in regulation of respiration.

Effect of Hypoxia on Respiration

Normal arterial pO_2 The normal arterial pO_2 is 100 mm Hg, which may fall in many conditions (see page 450), producing the so-called hypoxic hypoxia.

Decrease in arterial pO_2 A decrease in arterial pO_2 is the most potent stimulus for the peripheral chemoreceptors; consequently, the rate of discharge in the peripheral chemoreceptors begins to increase.

When the arterial pO_2 levels fall between 100 and 60 mm Hg, not much effect is produced on ventilation. However, a marked increase in pulmonary ventilation occurs when the pO_2 falls below 60 mm Hg (Fig. 5.6.16). This can be explained as follows:

- At pO_2 levels from 100 to 60 mm Hg, although there is significant increase in the afferent nerve discharge from the peripheral chemoreceptors, pulmonary ventilation does not increase significantly because of the reasons given in the next subsection.

Breaking effect of CO_2 When decrease in pO_2 of arterial blood stimulates ventilation, increased ventilation causes washing out of CO_2. This leads to decrease in pCO_2 of blood

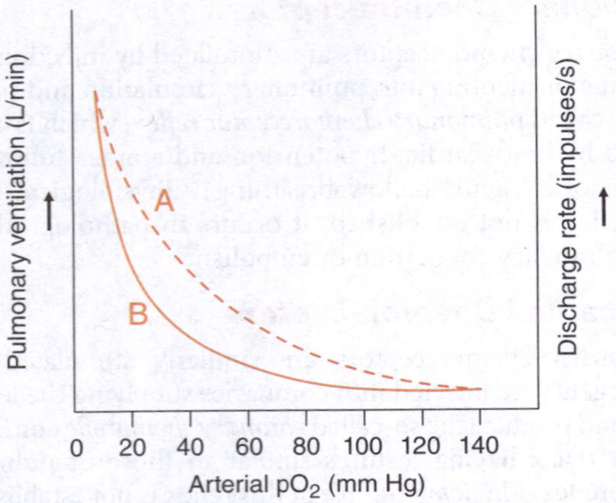

Fig. 5.6.16 Relationship of pO_2 with sinus nerve discharge rate A and pulmonary ventilation B.

which inhibits the respiration through its effect on central chemoreceptors. It opposes and neutralizes the effect of decreased pO_2 and thus there is no marked effect on ventilation. This phenomenon is called breaking effect of CO_2.

This fact can be confirmed experimentally by holding the pCO_2 constant at 40 mm Hg and decreasing arterial pO_2 simultaneously. Under these conditions, hyperventilation is observed even with pO_2 between 100 and 60 mm Hg.

Due to hypoxia the amount of deoxyhaemoglobin is increased which is a weaker acid as compared with oxyhaemoglobin. This results in mild decrease in H^+ concentration of blood which tends to nullify the hypoxic drive on pulmonary ventilation.

At pO_2 levels below 60 mm Hg the stimulation of peripheral chemoreceptors is so strong that it overrides the inhibitory effects of decreased arterial pCO_2 and decreased H^+ concentration and produces a marked increase in pulmonary ventilation.

- Hypoxia stimulating respiration through peripheral chemoreceptors can be proved experimentally by denervating them. Under such circumstances, hypoxia cannot increase pulmonary ventilation; rather it causes direct depression of the respiratory centre.

Effect of Hypercapnia on Respiration

Normal pCO_2 is 40 mm Hg which is kept constant by chemical regulation of respiration.

Hypercapnia i.e. rise in pCO_2, rarely occurs due to an increase in CO_2 production. Clinically, it may occur in restrictive lung disorders (see page 459).

An increase in arterial pCO_2 causes a prompt increase in pulmonary ventilation resulting in CO_2 wash-out and a near restoration of arterial pCO_2 to normal level (40 mm Hg). There exists a linear relation between increase in arterial pCO_2 and increase in pulmonary ventilation. This can be demonstrated experimentally by breathing from a bag of air with different concentrations of CO_2, varying from 4% to 7% (Fig. 5.6.17).

CO_2 increases pulmonary ventilation mainly by stimulating the central chemoreceptors. This can be demonstrated experimentally by removing the peripheral chemoreceptors and then making the person to breathe from a bag of air with different concentrations of CO_2. The same effect is obtained as above (Fig. 5.6.17).

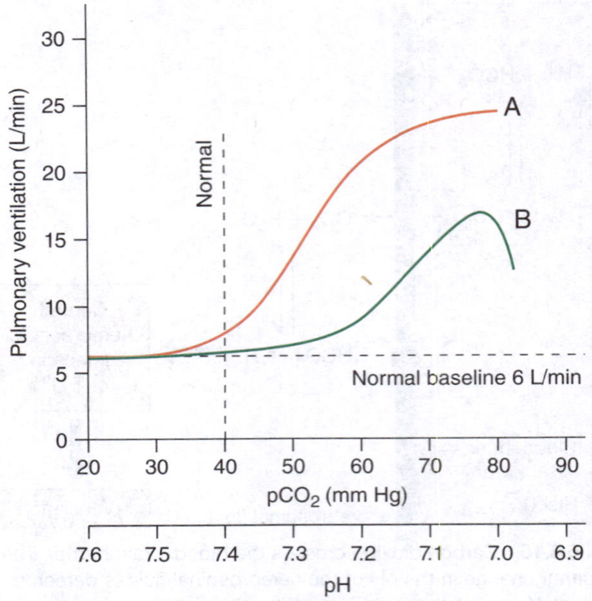

Fig. 5.6.17 Effect of increase in arterial pCO_2 A, and decreased pH on pulmonary ventilation B.

CO_2 is capable of increasing the pulmonary ventilation by stimulating the peripheral chemoreceptors as well When central chemoreceptors are depressed by anaesthesia, CO_2 increases respiration through stimulation of peripheral chemoreceptors.

Important Notes

CO_2 acts as a main regulator of respiration because of the following facts:

- It has a direct effect on respiratory centre through the central chemoreceptors.
- It can cross the blood–brain or blood–CSF barrier easily; therefore, CO_2 concentration in CSF and in interstitial fluid of the brain increases soon after the increase in concentration of CO_2 in the blood.
- CO_2 has a very strong breaking effect on the action of either decreased pO_2 or pH.
- pO_2 or pH does not have a very strong breaking effect on the action of increased CO_2 on ventilation (Fig. 5.6.17).

Applied Aspects

Carbon dioxide narcosis: It develops when arterial pCO_2 increases above 50 mm Hg. Accumulation of such a large amount of CO_2 (hypercapnia) in the body depresses the CNS, including respiratory centres, producing headache, confusion, convulsions and finally coma and death may occur.

Causes: Carbon dioxide narcosis may occur in patients with prolonged severe emphysema or due to accidental inhalation of CO_2 (in breweries, refrigeration plants, etc.). Experimentally, it can be produced by making the person to inhale the air containing more than 7% CO_2. When the inspired air pCO_2 approaches close to the alveolar pCO_2, elimination of CO_2 becomes difficult which causes alveolar and arterial pCO_2 to rise abruptly in spite of the hyperventilation.

Important Note

Clinical significance: Whenever CO_2 is to be used to stimulate respiration in a comatose patient with respiratory depressions, it is always advisable to estimate the CO_2 content of blood, to avoid occurrence of death from carbon dioxide narcosis.

Effect of Arterial pH on Respiration

i. Increased H^+ Concentration

Increased H^+ concentration (metabolic acidosis) produces prolonged respiratory centre stimulation via peripheral chemoreceptors, leading to a decrease in the arterial pCO_2 by elimination of larger amounts of CO_2, producing compensatory fall in blood H^+ concentration (Fig. 5.6.17B). The related aspects of renal correction of acid–base balance are discussed in Chapter 12.3, page 1187.

Applied Aspects

Metabolic Acidosis

Causes of metabolic acidosis, i.e. decrease in HCO_3^- concentration in blood secondary to increase in H^+ concentration of blood, occur in conditions such as:

- Diabetic ketoacidosis (hyperventilation occurring in this condition is called *Kussmaul breathing*)
- Renal failure (when the kidney fails to excrete its normal quota of H^+)
- Due to accumulation of lactic acid in severe muscular exercise
- Ketoacidosis in starvation
- Infantile diarrhoea associated with loss of $NaHCO_3$

ii. Decreased H^+ Concentration

Decreased H^+ concentration (metabolic alkalosis) depresses respiratory centre via peripheral chemoreceptors, leading to retention of CO_2 and an increase in arterial pCO_2. The secondary changes in arterial pCO_2 compensate for the primary metabolic defects and help to restore H^+ concentration of blood.

Applied Aspects

Metabolic Alkalosis

Causes of metabolic alkalosis, i.e. increase in HCO_3^- concentration in blood secondary to decreased H^+ concentration in blood, occur due to excessive vomiting with loss of HCl from the body.

iii. Primary Pulmonary Hypoventilation

Primary pulmonary hypoventilation may lead to elevation of arterial pCO_2 (hypercapnia) producing the so-called *respiratory acidosis*.

Applied Aspects

Respiratory Acidosis

Causes Hypercapnia responsible for respiratory acidosis are:

- Respiratory depression due to narcotic poisoning or cerebral diseases
- Neuromuscular disorders with impaired breathing
- Chronic obstructive pulmonary disease such as emphysema in which effective alveolar ventilation is decreased due to ventilation–perfusion mismatch

Compensatory mechanism through chemoreceptors produces hyperventilation, washes out CO_2 and tries to restore arterial pCO_2.

iv. Primary Pulmonary Hyperventilation

Primary pulmonary hyperventilation may cause a decrease in the arterial pCO_2 producing the so-called *respiratory alkalosis*.

Applied Aspects

Respiratory Alkalosis

Causes of respiratory alkalosis are:

- Voluntary hyperventilation
- Excessive artificial respiration
- Compulsive hyperventilation in patients with hysteria
- Chronic O_2 lack (hypoxia) producing CO_2 wash-out due to hyperventilation, e.g. as seen in high-altitude hypoxia

Signs and symptoms

- *Hypocapnia* produced causes faintness and paraesthesias due to reduction of cerebral blood flow.
- *Respiratory alkalosis* produced causes lowering of ionized Ca^{2+} in plasma and the appearance of symptoms of tetany, e.g. carpopedal spasm.

Compensatory mechanism through chemoreceptors slows down the respiration, leading to retention of CO_2, which in turn restores H^+ concentration of blood towards normal.

Interaction of pO_2, pCO_2 and pH in regulation of respiration

In the above discussion, we have seen that each of hypoxia, increased pCO_2 and acidosis individually causes an increase in the respiration. In many physiological or clinical situations, more than one factor may be present. Their interaction is summarized here.

1. Interaction of pCO_2 and pO_2

Hypoxia sensitizes the respiratory mechanism to excess of CO_2 or H^+ concentration; therefore, increased pCO_2 and H^+ concentration produce a much greater effect (Fig. 5.6.18).

When pCO_2 is held constant at a level 2–3 mm Hg above normal (i.e. in the presence of hypercapnic drive) When pCO_2 is held constant at a level 2–3 mm Hg above normal (i.e. in the presence of hypercapnic drive), there is an inverse relationship between ventilation and alveolar pO_2, even in the 90– to 110–mm Hg range (Fig. 5.6.19A).

When pCO_2 is held constant at a level 2–3 mm Hg below normal When pCO_2 is held constant at a level 2–3 mm Hg below normal (i.e. in the absence of CO_2-related drive), a fall in pO_2 level between 110 and 60 mm Hg does not produce any effect on ventilation. However, a marked increase in pulmonary ventilation occurs when pO_2 falls below 60 mm Hg (Fig. 5.6.19B).

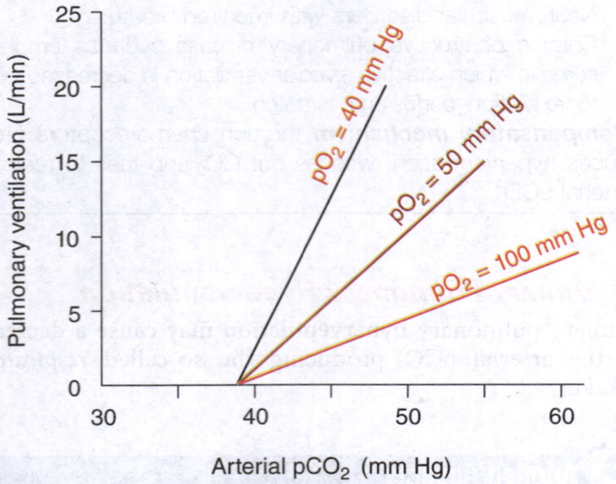

Fig. 5.6.18 Interaction of arterial pO_2 and pCO_2 depicting effect of pCO_2 on pulmonary ventilation at different levels of pO_2.

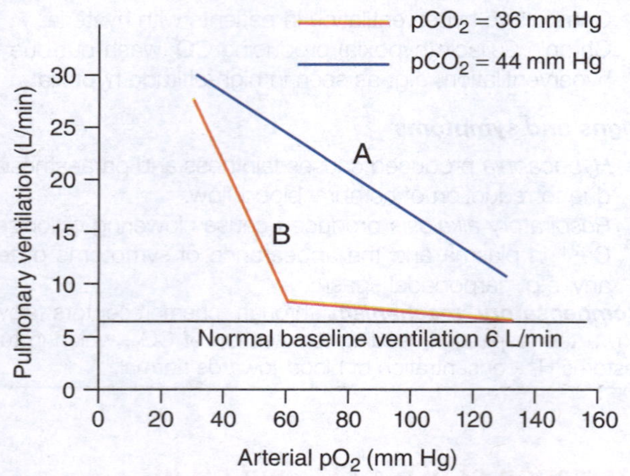

Fig. 5.6.19 Effect of hypoxia (pO_2) on pulmonary ventilation with arterial pCO_2 being kept: A, 2–3 mm Hg above normal; and B, 2–3 mm Hg below normal.

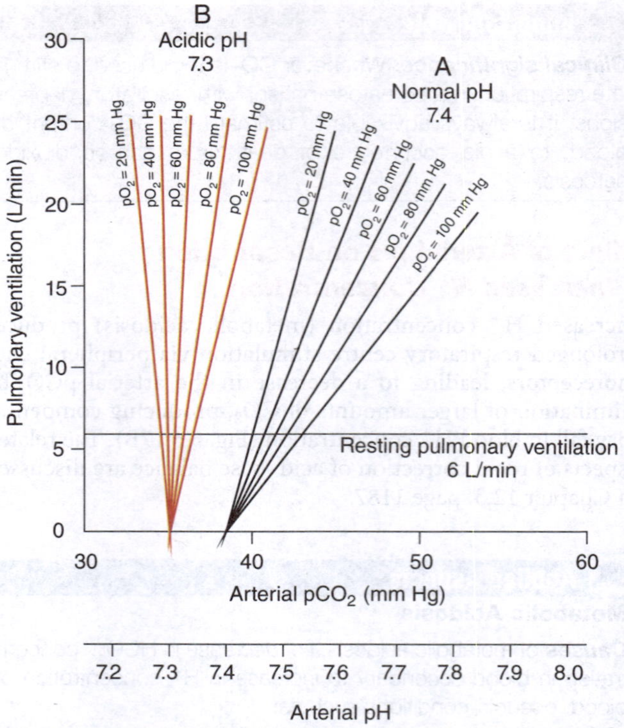

Fig. 5.6.20 Effect on CO_2 response curve of varying amount of hypoxia and pH.

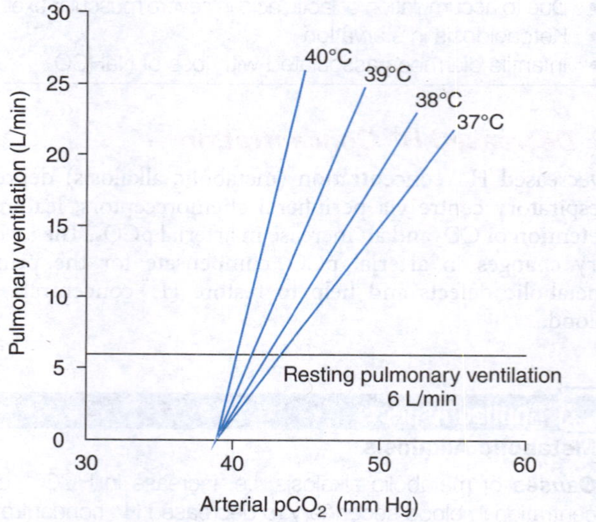

Fig. 5.6.21 Effect of temperature on CO_2 response curve.

2. Interaction of pH and CO_2 Response

The stimulatory effects of H^+ concentration and CO_2 on respiration are additive, i.e. a fall in pH (acidosis) shifts the CO_2 response curve to left without change in slope. In other words, the same amount of respiratory stimulation is produced by lower arterial pCO_2 levels (Fig. 5.6.20).

3. Interaction of CO_2 and Body Temperature

The effect of CO_2 on respiration increases with increase in body temperature (Fig. 5.6.21).

SOME OTHER ASPECTS RELATED TO CHEMICAL REGULATION OF RESPIRATION

Effects of Hyperventilation

Effect of Short-Lasting Severe Hyperventilation

Effects of hyperventilation on respiration can be demonstrated experimentally by making a person to breathe as rapidly and as deeply as possible for him/her for 1–2 minutes and then stopping. The voluntary hyperventilation may show the following effects (Fig. 5.6.22):

i. Effects on respiration After a period of hyperventilation, any of the following patterns of respiration may be seen for a small period before normal respiration is restored:

- *Hypoventilation* for a prolonged period is seen in most of the individuals.
- *Apnoea*, i.e. complete cessation of breathing for 1–2 minutes, may occur in some individuals.

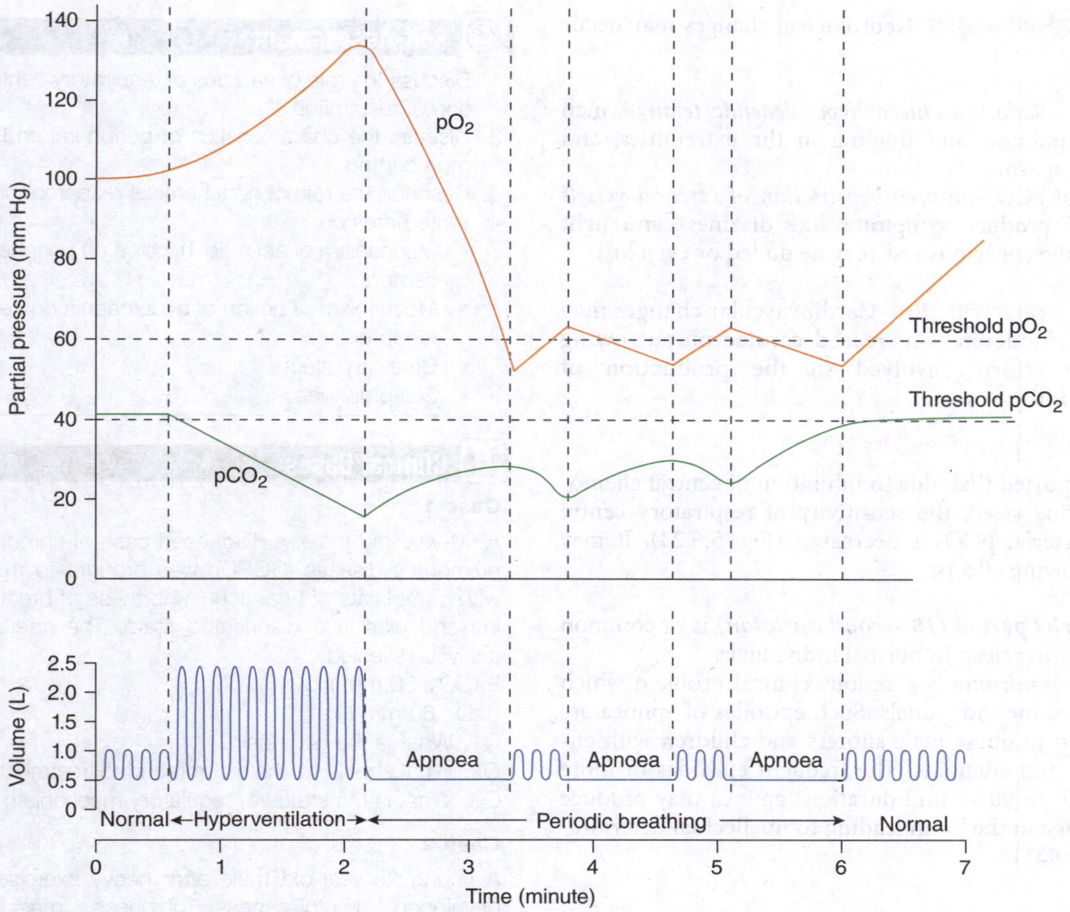

Fig. 5.6.22 Effect of hyperventilation on arterial pO_2, pCO_2 and respiration. Note correlation between pCO_2, pO_2 and periods of hyperventilation, apnoea and periodic breathing and normal breathing.

- *Periodic breathing (Cheyne–Stokes breathing)*, i.e. alternate phases of apnoea and breathing, may occur for some time in a few individuals.

ii. Effects on arterial pCO_2 and pO_2 and their correlation with effect on respiration (Fig. 5.6.22)

- Arterial pO_2 may go as high as 150 mm Hg and pCO_2 as low as 15 mm Hg after a period of voluntary hyperventilation.
- Apnoea occurring in some individuals at the end of hyperventilation seems to be related to lack of CO_2, because it does not occur if the person hyperventilates a gas mixture containing 5% CO_2 and 20% oxygen.
- During phase of apnoea, due to metabolism of body, there occurs a decline in arterial pO_2 and an increase in pCO_2. Depending on the interaction between levels of pO_2 and pCO_2 attained, the following effects can occur on respiration:
  - If the arterial pCO_2 is reached at the threshold level (40 mm Hg), then a normal breathing is resumed.
  - If the hypoxic stimulus (decreased pO_2) becomes strong before the pCO_2 reaches a threshold level, then *periodic breathing* (Cheyne–Stokes breathing) may result, i.e. a few breaths eliminate hypoxic drive, and then breathing stops and restarts when again hypoxic drive stimulates it. Such cycles are repeated till pCO_2 reaches the threshold level to normalize breathing.

Effects of Prolonged Moderate Hyperventilation

Prolonged moderate hyperventilation, i.e. twofold to fivefold increase in pulmonary ventilation, may occur under the following circumstances:

- In residents of high altitude
- In clinically hypoxic patients due to some pulmonary disease
- Voluntarily

The prolonged moderate hyperventilation is associated with decrease in alveolar and arterial pCO_2, since pulmonary ventilation is in excess of the metabolic requirements of the body. The low arterial pCO_2 which lasts for many days may result in the following complications in the body:

Respiratory alkalosis Low levels of pCO_2 reduce the formation of H^+ and HCO_3^- in the blood causing increase in its pH to 7.55 or even 7.6, a condition called respiratory alkalosis.

Renal changes The respiratory alkalosis produced due to decreased arterial pCO_2 interferes with H^+ secretory mechanism in the kidney. There occurs failure of proximal tubular reabsorption of HCO_3^-, which results in excretion of alkaline urine containing HCO_3^-.

Neurological changes Neurological changes may occur due to:

- *Respiratory alkalosis–induced hypocalcaemic tetany* which includes numbness and tingling in the extremities, and carpopedal spasm
- *Low arterial pCO_2–induced constriction of cerebral vessels* which may produce symptoms like dizziness and light headache (the consciousness may be dulled or even lost)

Cardiovascular changes Cardiovascular changes may occur due to moderately increased cardiac output owing to muscular efforts involved in the production of hyperventilation.

Effect of Sleep on Respiration

It has been reported that, due to inhibition of central chemoreceptors during sleep, the sensitivity of respiratory centre neurons to arterial pCO_2 is decreased (Fig. 5.6.23). It may cause the following effects:

Apnoea for brief period (10-second duration) is of common occurrence during sleep in normal individuals.

Sleep apnoea syndrome is a serious clinical problem which may occur in some individuals. Such episodes of apnoea are more common in obese male snorers and children with enlarged tonsils and adenoids. The frequent episodes of more prolonged (30- to 90-second duration) apnoea may produce hypoxic damage to the brain leading to intellectual deterioration (see page 451).

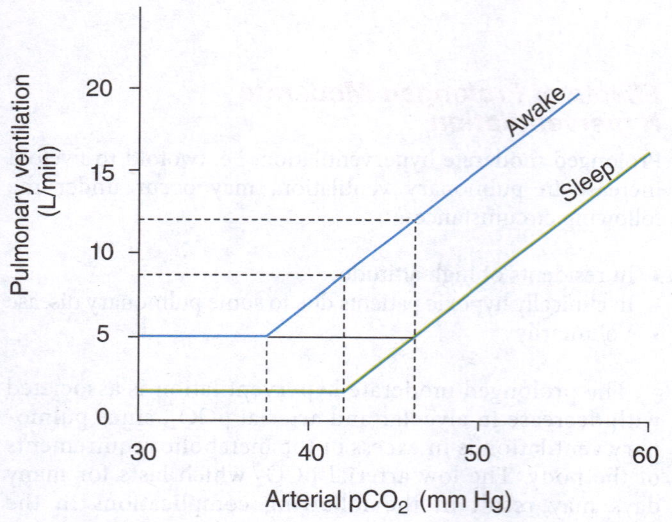

Fig. 5.6.23 Effect of sleep on the sensitivity of respiratory neurons. Note that the amount of pulmonary ventilation of the same level of pCO_2 is less during sleep than during awakening.

Self-Assessment

1. Discuss the role of neurons of respiratory centres in regulation of respiration.
2. Discuss the characteristics of peripheral and central chemoreceptors.
3. Describe the role of nonchemical receptors on respiration.
4. Write notes on:
   - Mechanism of action of hypoxia on peripheral chemoreceptors
   - Mechanism of action of hypercapnia on central chemoreceptors
   - Breaking effect
   - Sleep apnoea

Clinical Cases

Case 1

A 60-year-old male, a diagnosed case of chronic obstructive pulmonary disease (COPD), was brought to the emergency with complaints of headache, shortness of breath and vomiting and was in a disoriented state. The arterial blood gas analysis revealed:

$PaCO_2$: 50 mm Hg
PaO_2: 60 mm Hg

Q1. What is the diagnosis?
Q2. What should be the recommended treatment in this case?
Q3. What is the status of regulatory mechanism in this case?

Case 2

A young 25-year-old male after heavy exercise in the gym developed breathlessness, dizziness, muscle twitching, numbness and tingling sensation in the fingertips and toes and is brought to the emergency.

Q1. What is the probable diagnosis?
Q2. What is the cause of tingling sensation?

Case 3

A 34-year-old male employee of a beverage factory presented with shortness of breath, headache and disoriented state due to leakage of some gas in the factory.

Q1. What is the probable diagnosis?
Q2. What is the status of blood gas analysis in this case?
Q3. What immediate treatment should be given to relieve the symptoms?

Case 4

A 65-year-old male, a diagnosed case of COPD, was admitted due to dyspnoea. The SpO_2 was 85%, and the patient was put on non-breathing mask with oxygen at rate 5 L/min. After half an hour, he developed headache, vomiting and convulsions.

Q1. What is the cause of these symptoms?
Q2. What is the physiological basis?
Q3. During treatment, how can these symptoms be prevented?

5.7 Respiration: Applied Aspects

CHAPTER OUTLINE

INTRODUCTION

Applied respiratory physiology forms a link between the basics of respiration and the clinical manifestations of respiratory diseases. The pulmonary function tests performed to diagnose respiratory disorders require an understanding of basic physiological principles of respiration and gas exchange. In fact, respiratory diseases cannot be managed satisfactorily without a proper understanding of the basic and applied aspects of respiratory physiology. This chapter is concerned with some of the important applied aspects of respiration which include:

- Respiratory adjustments to stresses in health
- Disturbances of respiration
- Artificial respiration (AR)
- Pulmonary function tests

RESPIRATORY ADJUSTMENTS TO STRESSES IN HEALTH

Respiratory adjustments to stresses in health illustrate the integrated operation of the respiratory regulatory mechanisms. The stresses faced by respiration requiring adjustments in day-to-day life include the following:

1. Respiratory Adjustments During Exercise

Exercise is the frequent stress that the body faces in day-to-day life. Since during exercise, many complex adjustments of muscular blood flow, metabolism, respiration, circulation and temperature are required, they have been comprehensively discussed in chapter on 'Physiology of Exercise' (page 1169).

2. Respiratory Adjustments at High Altitude

At high altitude, barometric pressure is low and so the partial pressure of O_2 is also low; however, the amount of O_2 in the atmosphere is same as it is at the sea level. When a person is exposed to high altitude particularly by rapid ascent, the different systems of the body cannot cope with the lowered O_2 tension and the effects of hypoxia start. Respiratory adjustments are thus a part of changes in the body at high attitude, so these have been discussed comprehensively under the title '*Physiology of high altitude*' (see page 1180).

3. Respiratory Adjustments to High Atmospheric Pressure

Respiratory adjustments to high atmospheric pressure form a part of physiological problems faced by the body while going under the sea and have been discussed comprehensively under the title '*Deep sea physiology*' (see page 1183).

4. Respiratory Adjustments on Exposure to Cold and Heat

Respiratory adjustments on exposure to cold and heat have been discussed under the title '*Effects of exposure to heat and cold on the body*' (see page 1204).

5. Respiratory Adjustments at Birth

Birth is the most traumatic event that the respiratory system must withstand during the entire life span of an individual. This forms a part of *fetal physiology* and has been discussed in the concerned chapter on page 1217.

Note: Students are advised to go through the respiratory changes occurring during the above-mentioned situations along with the study of respiratory system for better understanding.

DISTURBANCES OF RESPIRATION

From the physiological viewpoint, disturbances of respiration can be discussed under the following headings:

- Abnormal respiratory patterns
- Disturbances related to respiratory gases
- Pulmonary diseases – pathophysiological aspects

ABNORMAL RESPIRATORY PATTERNS

Eupnoea refers to normal respiratory pattern, which implies a normal rate, rhythm and depth of respiration. Various abnormal respiratory patterns (Fig. 5.7.1) can be produced by changes in the environment or diseases affecting the respiratory system, cardiovascular system or brain. The terms used for the altered pattern of respiration are as follows:

- *Tachypnoea* refers to increase in the rate of respiration.
- *Bradypnoea* means decrease in the rate of respiration.
- *Polypnoea* is used to denote the rapid but shallow breathing resembling panting in dogs. In this, the rate of respiration is increased but the force does not change significantly.
- *Apnoea* refers to temporary cessation of breathing.
- *Hypoventilation* term is used to describe a decrease in rate and force of respiration.
- *Hyperventilation* refers to increase in rate as well as force of respiration.
- *Hyperpnoea* signifies a marked increase in pulmonary ventilation due to increase in rate and/or force of respiration.
- *Dyspnoea:* When hyperpnoea involves fourfold to fivefold increase in pulmonary ventilation, an unpleasant sensation or discomfort is felt. This type of respiration is called dyspnoea.
- *Periodic breathing* refers to a respiratory pattern characterized by alternate periods of respiratory activity and apnoea. Some of the abnormal respiratory patterns are discussed in detail.

Apnoea

Apnoea refers to temporary cessation of breathing. Depending on the cause, apnoea may be of the following types:

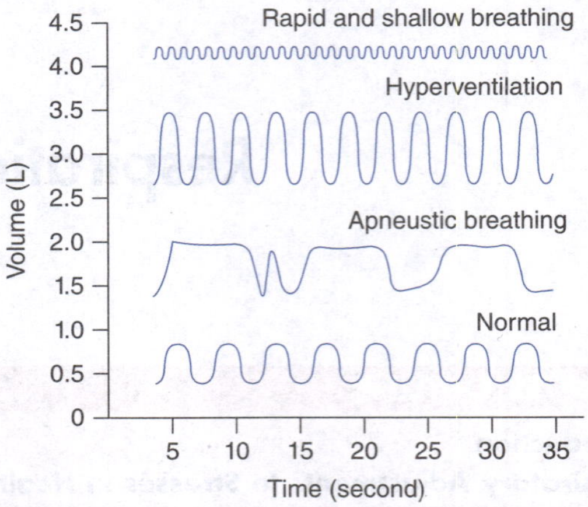

Fig. 5.7.1 Various abnormal respiratory patterns.

1. Voluntary Apnoea

Voluntary apnoea refers to temporary arrest of breathing due to voluntary control of respiration. It is also called breath-holding. The breath-holding time or apnoea time during which breathing can be withheld voluntarily is about 40–60 seconds in a normal person, after a deep inspiration (for details, see page 432).

Breaking point is the point at which breathing can no longer be voluntarily inhibited. At this point, chemical regulation overcomes the neural regulation. The breaking point is due to an increased arterial pCO_2 and a decreased pO_2.

2. Apnoea after Hyperventilation

Apnoea after hyperventilation occurs due to less stimulation of respiratory centre owing to CO_2 wash-out caused by hyperventilation (for details, see page 443; Figs 5.6.22 and 5.7.2).

3. Deglutition Apnoea

Deglutition apnoea occurs reflexly during swallowing (about 0.5 second). During the pharyngeal stage of swallowing, the fluid or food stimulates the sensory nerve endings (V, IX and X cranial nerves) around the pharynx. Nerve impulses from these irritant receptors, via the swallowing centres, specifically inhibit the respiratory centre, stopping the breathing at any point of the cycle (deglutition apnoea). Simultaneously, there is closure of glottis (the opening between vocal cords). Both these effects prevent aspiration of fluid or food into the lungs (also see page 573).

4. Breath-Holding Attacks (Spells)

Breath-holding attacks (spells) are attacks of brief period of apnoea which occur in infants and young children, and are generally precipitated by emotional distress, such as fright, frustration, pain or anxiety. The child starts to cry, and then suddenly holds his/her breath, becomes limp or stiff, and may

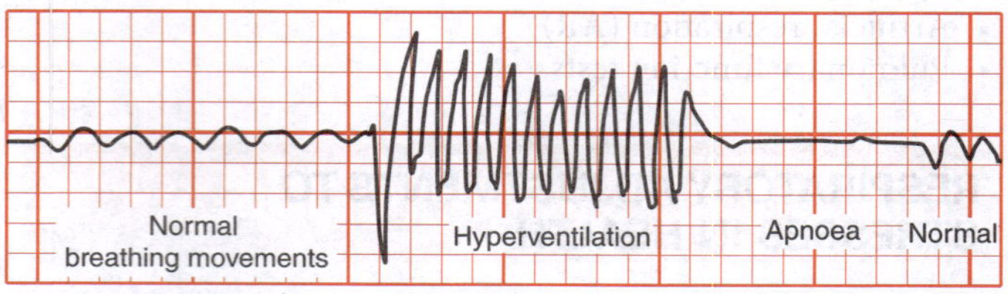

Fig. 5.7.2 Breathing movements recorded by stepthography on physiograph showing apnea after voluantry hyperventilation.

become blue and lose consciousness. The attacks last briefly and recovery is rapid and complete. In some cases, there may be a rigid phase followed by tonic and clonic convulsions. These attacks are harmless and stop by the age of 3 years; they are not considered epileptic in origin.

5. Vagal Apnoea

Vagal apnoea can be produced experimentally in animals by stimulation of vagus nerve. Stimulation of vagus nerve produces apnoea by inhibiting the inspiratory centre.

6. Adrenaline Apnoea

Adrenaline apnoea occurs after injection of high doses of adrenaline (see page 436).

7. Sleep Apnoea

Sleep apnoea refers to cessation of breathing for a brief period (10 seconds) during sleep in normal individuals. It has been related to reduced sensitivity of respiratory centre neurons to arterial pCO_2 owing to inhibition of central chemoreceptors.

Sleep apnoea syndrome Sleep apnoea syndrome has been recognized as a serious clinical problem or disorder of respiratory control that affects middle-aged and elderly men. It may occur in three forms:

Obstructive sleep apnoea (OSA) occurs when inspiration is prevented by transient blockage of the airway due to collapse of hypopharynx as a result of loss of tone of pharyngeal muscles which prevent airflow, although strong contractions of inspiratory muscles occur (Fig. 5.7.3). Partial airway obstruction causes snoring. The association of sleep apnoea with extreme obesity is referred to as the *Pickwickian syndrome*.

Nonobstructive (central) sleep apnoea (CSA) refers to complete stoppage of rhythmic activity from respiratory centres. Obviously, during apnoea, there is no respiratory muscle contraction (Fig. 5.7.3). It is supposed to result from decreased chemoreceptor sensitivity to O_2 and CO_2. CSA has been proposed as one of the many possible causes of *sudden infant death syndrome*.

Mixed sleep apnoea is the combination of OSA and CSA.

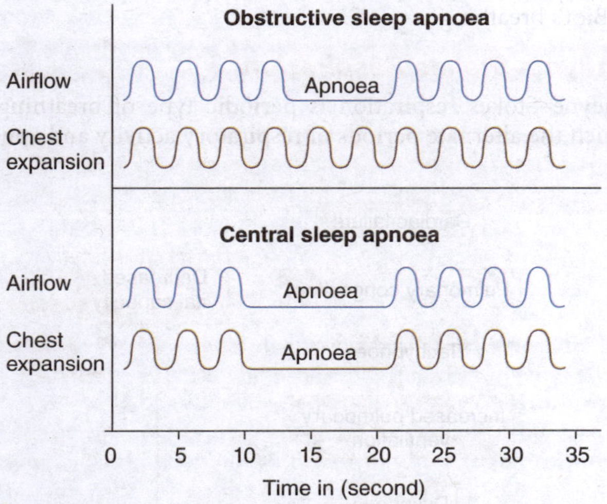

Fig. 5.7.3 Record of airflow and chest movements in patients with obstructive and central sleep apnoea.

In many cases, sleep apnoea is observed by the family members.

Signs and symptoms of sleep apnoea:

Signs observed in sleep apnoea are as follows:

- Breathing pauses during sleep
- Ineffective respiratory movements
- Snoring (high sensitivity and of low pitch)
- Mouth dryness
- Increase in heart rate

Symptoms Symptoms of sleep apnoea include feeling of sleepiness, tiredness in the daytime and frequent feeling of choking.

Diagnosis The sleep apnoea is diagnosed by overnight sleep study in sleep lab. It includes polysomnography (PSG) and in-home tests (IHT).

PSG: During PSG, physiological parameters such as electroencephalogram (EEG), electro-oculogram (EOG), chin electromyogram, airflow, oxygen saturation, breathing movement by electromyography (EMG) and electrocardiogram (ECG) are recorded.

IHT: A portable monitoring device is used that records heart rate, lung and brain activity, breathing pattern, arm and leg movements and blood oxygen level.

A person with sleep apnoea shows breathing interruptions followed by reduction in blood pO_2 and rise in pCO_2 levels. Then scoring of sleep apnoea is evaluated as apnoea–hypoapnoea index (AHI) or respiratory distribution index (RDI).

AHI is the sum of apnoea (pauses of breathing) + number of hypoapnoea (period of shallow breathing) that occurs on an average in each hour:

Minimal: $<5/h$
Mild: >5 but $<15/h$
Moderate: 15–30/h
Severe: $>30/h$

Treatment Treatment may include lifestyle changes, use of breathing devices and surgery.

Lifestyle changes Lifestyle changes may include avoiding alcohol, losing weight, stopping smoking and sleeping on one side.

Breathing devices Breathing devices include the use of continuous positive airway pressure (CPAP) device, bilevel positive airway pressure (BIPAP), automatic servo ventilation (OSV), etc.

- *CPAP* device delivers air pressure through a mask while the person is asleep. The positive air pressure keeps the upper airway patent preventing apnoea and snoring.
- *Auto-CPAP* devices adjust the air pressure automatically when the person is sleeping.
- *Oral appliances* are also available which bring the jaw forward and relieve snoring and mild sleep apnoea.
- *Pacemaker.* Implanting a pacemeker-like device in the neck. This device stimulates phrenic nerve to send signals to the diaphragm, can reduce the frequency and severity of sleep apnoea episodes.

Sleep apnoea surgery Sleep apnoea surgery is performed basically to treat sleep disorders such as: *Snoring, upper airway resistance syndrome, OSA.*

Complications in undiagnosed and untreated sleep apnoea syndrome can lead to serious complications including stroke, hypertension, heart failure, coronary artery disease, occupational accidents and type II diabetes.

Pickwickian syndrome or obesity hypoventilation syndrome In this condition, severely overweight/obese persons have difficulty in breathing rapidly and forcefully, thus resulting in hypoxaemia and hypercapnia.

Hypoventilation

Hypoventilation is used to describe a decrease in rate and force of respiration. Thus, in hypoventilation, the amount of air moving in and out of lungs is reduced.

Causes of hypoventilation are as follows:

- *Depression of respiratory centres by some drugs*
- *Partial paralysis of respiratory muscles*

Effects Hypoventilation leads on to hypoxia and hypercapnia which result in increase in rate and force of respiration and the patient may develop dyspnoea.

Hyperventilation

Hyperventilation refers to increase in rate as well as force of respiration. Thus, in hyperventilation, the amount of air moving in and out of lungs is increased; that is why it is also called increased pulmonary ventilation or overventilation.

Causes of hyperventilation are as follows:

- *During exercise due to stimulation of respiratory centres by increased* pCO_2
- *Voluntary hyperventilation*
- *Secondary to hypoxia*

Effects of hyperventilation on respiration and other systems of the body are described on page 442.

Dyspnoea

Dyspnoea literally means distressed breathing. Increased respiration without discomfort is called *hyperpnoea.* One is not aware of one's respiration till resting pulmonary ventilation becomes more than double. When hyperpnoea involves fourfold to fivefold increase in pulmonary ventilation, an unpleasant sensation or discomfort is felt. This type of respiration is called dyspnoea. The word 'air hunger' is used as a synonym to dyspnoea in general language. Thus, desire for air or mental anguish associated with inability to ventilate enough to satisfy the air demand is the essence of dyspnoea.

Dyspnoea point Dyspnoea point refers to the height of hyperpnoea at which dyspnoea appears.

Predisposing factors for dyspnoea include:

1. *Low vital capacity (VC):* People with low VC are more predisposed to get dyspnoea than those with normal or high VC.
2. *Maximum ventilatory volume (MVV):* Patients with reduced MVV (maximum volume of air that can be taken in or given out per minute; normal value is 120 L/min) are more predisposed to get dyspnoea.
3. *Breathing reserve* (BR) is the difference between MVV and respiratory minute volume (RMV). RMV is the volume of air that is taken in or given out per minute (normal 500 × 12 = 6 L/min). Individuals with RMV increased by four to five times get dyspnoea. Individuals with less BR are more prone to get dyspnoea.

$$BR = MVV - RMV = 114 \text{ L/min}$$

Dyspnoeic index (DI) refers to BR percentage of MVV, i.e.

$$DI = \frac{BR \times 100}{MVV} = \frac{110 \times 100}{120} = 95\%$$

- Normal values of DI range from 70% to 95%.
- Dyspnoea occurs when DI is $<60\%$.

Causes of dyspnoea are as follows:

Physiologically dyspnoea Physiologically, dyspnoea *occurs* in severe muscular exercise.

Pathological causes include:

- *Respiratory disorders* such as bronchial asthma, emphysema, pneumonia, pulmonary oedema and pneumothorax.
- *Cardiac failure:* It causes dyspnoea by the mechanism explained in Fig. 5.7.4.

Important Note

It is important to note that patients with cardiac failure prefer to sit rather than lie down, because in lying position pulmonary congestion is increased which causes dyspnoea. Dyspnoea occurring in lying down position is called *orthopnoea*.

- *Metabolic disorders* causing dyspnoea are diabetic acidosis, uraemia and increased H^+ concentration. Metabolic acidosis causes dyspnoea by increasing pulmonary ventilation.

Periodic Breathing

Periodic breathing is characterized by alternate periods of respiratory activity and apnoea. It is of two types:

- Cheyne–Stokes respiration
- Biot's breathing

Cheyne–Stokes Respiration

Cheyne–Stokes respiration is periodic type of breathing in which the alternate periods of respiratory activity and apnoea

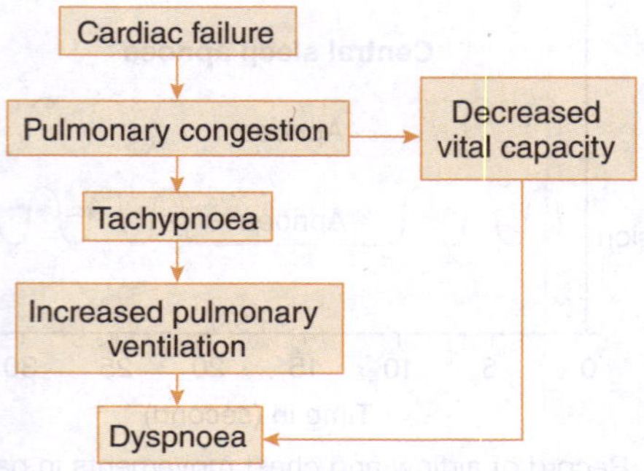

Fig. 5.7.4 Cardiac failure causing dyspnoea: mechanism.

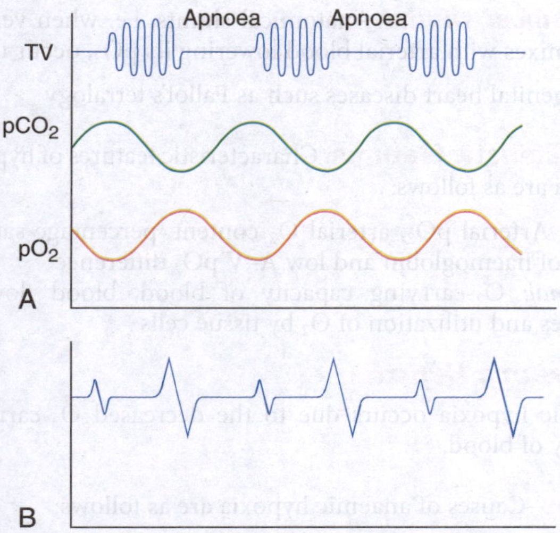

Fig. 5.7.5 Periodic breathing: **A**, Cheyne–Stokes breathing; and **B**, Biot's breathing.

occur at regular intervals, and during the period of respiratory activity there is waxing and waning of tidal volume (TV). The duration of one cycle is about 1 minute. The arterial pO_2 and pCO_2 fluctuate during each cycle. The pO_2 is lowest and the pCO_2 is highest at the end of apnoea (Fig. 5.7.5A).

Causes of Cheyne–Stokes respiration are as follows:

1. ***Physiological causes*** include:
   - Voluntary hyperventilation
   - High altitude
   - During sleep in some normal individuals, especially infants
2. ***Pathological causes*** are as follows:
   - Chronic heart failure, due to increased circulation time from the lungs to the brain
   - Brain damage due to increased negative feedback gain in the respiratory centre
   - Uraemia
   - Poisoning by narcotics

Mechanism of development of Cheyne–Stokes respiration Mechanism of development of Cheyne–Stokes respiration in three most important conditions is described.

Voluntary hyperventilation Mechanism of development of Cheyne–Stokes breathing in hyperventilation has been described on page 442.

Heart failure Mechanism of development of Cheyne–Stokes breathing in heart failure is summarized as:

- Left ventricular failure → pulmonary congestion → hypoxia → stimulation of respiratory centres → increased ventilation → increased alveolar pO_2 and decreased pCO_2 → decreased arterial pCO_2.
- As in heart failure *circulation time* is prolonged, it takes longer than normal time for the blood with low pCO_2 to reach the brain and cause apnoea by inhibiting respiratory centre.
- Since in heart failure the pulmonary congestion is continuously present, hypoxia is maintained and the above-described cycle of apnoea followed by respiratory activity keeps on repeating till the heart failure is treated or alveolar pCO_2 comes back to normal.

Brain damage In brain damage, when supramedullary inhibitory pathway is damaged, the medullary (central) chemoreceptors become more sensitive to the action of CO_2 and produce Cheyne–Stokes breathing as:

- Increased sensitivity of central chemoreceptors to CO_2 → hyperventilation → CO_2 wash-out → apnoea → accumulation of CO_2 → increased pCO_2 → hyperventilation → cycle of respiratory activity and apnoea continues.

Biot's Breathing

Biot's breathing, also known as *ataxic breathing*, is a type of periodic breathing showing alternate periods of respiratory activity and apnoea (Fig. 5.7.5B). It differs from Cheyne–Stokes breathing in the following aspects:

- It occurs at irregular intervals.
- There is no waxing and waning of TV during the period of respiratory activity.
- It can never occur physiologically.

Causes Biot's breathing indicates a disruption of the normal medullary rhythmicity of respiration. It may occur when medulla is involved in disorders such as meningitis, head injury, medullary compressions like pontine haematomas or cerebellopontine herniation. *Central medullary lesions* are the most common cause of Biot's breathing. So, it is rare in cerebral ischaemia, which has to be bilateral to infarct the central medulla.

Apneustic Breathing

Apneustic breathing is an abnormal breathing pattern characterized by long gasping inhalations and irregular exhalations.

Causes: Apneustic breathing occurs due to overstimulation of apneustic centre. This can happen due to stroke or any type of trauma that causes injury to the pons.

Important Note

Apneustic breathing is usually a clear indicator of severe brain injury.

Kussmaul Breathing

Kussmaul breathing is an abnormal breathing pattern characterized by rapid deep breathing at a constant pace. It is sign of an emergency mainly related to diabetic ketoacidosis.

DISTURBANCES RELATED TO RESPIRATORY GASES

Respiratory disturbances related to respiratory gases include:

- Hypoxia
- Hypercapnia
- Hypocapnia
- Asphyxia
- Carbon monoxide (CO) poisoning

Hypoxia

The term hypoxia is used to denote deficiency of oxygen supply at the tissue level. It has almost replaced the term anoxia (complete absence of oxygen), which rarely occurs practically.

Causes and Types

Causes Hypoxia can occur because of any one or more of the following defects:

- Decreased oxygen tension (pO_2) of the arterial blood
- Decreased oxygen-carrying capacity of the blood
- Decreased rate of blood flow to the tissue
- Decreased utilization of oxygen by tissue cells

Types Depending on the mechanism of occurrence, there are four types of hypoxia:

- Hypoxic hypoxia
- Anaemic hypoxia
- Stagnant hypoxia
- Histotoxic hypoxia

1. Hypoxic Hypoxia

Hypoxic hypoxia occurs due to decreased oxygen tension (pO_2) of the arterial blood, hence also called *arterial hypoxia*. Therefore, in this condition, O_2-carrying capacity of blood, rate of blood flow to tissue and utilization of O_2 by tissues are normal.

Causes Causes of hypoxic hypoxia are as follows:

Low oxygen tension (pO_2) in inspired air Examples of low oxygen tension (pO_2) in inspired air include:

- High altitude, where a person is exposed to low atmospheric pO_2
- Breathing artificial gas mixture with low pO_2
- Breathing in a closed space

Hypoventilation Hypoventilation can occur due to any cause, e.g.:

- Obstruction in respiratory passages as in asthma
- Decreased lung compliance as in pneumothorax
- Paresis or paralysis of respiratory muscles, as in poliomyelitis
- Pump failure due to fatigue of respiratory muscles
- Damage to respiratory centres by drugs like morphine (which causes depression of respiratory neurons in the medulla) or brain tumours

Hypoventilation decreases alveolar pO_2 and hence arterial pO_2.

Reduced diffusion of oxygen across respiratory membrane Reduced diffusion of oxygen across respiratory membrane occurs due to:

- Marked reduction in area of respiratory membrane as in emphysema
- Increased thickness of respiratory membrane as in pulmonary oedema
- Nonfunctioning respiratory membrane as in fibrosis

Physiological shunt Physiological shunt formation occurs due to abnormalities of ventilation–perfusion (V/Q) ratio.

Anatomical shunts Anatomical shunts, i.e. when venous blood mixes with arterial blood lowering its pO_2, occur in:

- Congenital heart diseases such as Fallot's tetralogy

Characteristic features Characteristic features of hypoxic hypoxia are as follows:

- *Low:* Arterial pO_2, arterial O_2 content, percentage saturation of haemoglobin and low A–V pO_2 difference
- *Normal:* O_2-carrying capacity of blood, blood flow to tissues and utilization of O_2 by tissue cells

2. Anaemic Hypoxia

Anaemic hypoxia occurs due to the decreased O_2-carrying capacity of blood.

Causes Causes of anaemic hypoxia are as follows:

Decreased RBC count Decreased RBC count occurs in:

- Bone marrow depression
- Haemorrhage

Decreased haemoglobin content Decreased haemoglobin content of blood occurs in:

- Anaemias of all types

Altered haemoglobin Altered haemoglobin is not capable of carrying O_2, e.g.:

- Methaemoglobin, in which iron is present in ferric (Fe^{3+}) form instead of in ferrous (Fe^{2+}) form
- Carboxyhaemoglobin, in which CO combines with haemoglobin due to its 200 times more affinity than O_2

Characteristic features Characteristic features of anaemic hypoxia are as follows:

- Arterial pO_2 is normal (95–100 mm Hg).
- Oxygen-carrying capacity of blood is reduced due to anaemia or altered haemoglobin.
- Percentage saturation of haemoglobin is decreased.
- A–V pO_2 difference is normal ($95 - 40 = 55$ mm Hg).

Pathophysiology of low O_2 supply to tissues in anaemic hypoxia

- Mild to moderate anaemia usually does not produce hypoxia at rest because there is compensatory increase in 2,3-diphosphoglycerate (2,3-DPG) amount in the RBCs which combines with oxyhaemoglobin and results in increased liberation of O_2:

$$HbO_2 + 2,3\text{-DPG} \rightarrow Hb2,3\text{-DPG} + O_2$$

- However, during exercise, the increased demand of O_2 by tissues is not met with and hence symptoms of hypoxia appear.
- Anaemic hypoxia in CO poisoning is severe and needs emergency treatment. CO produces severe hypoxia by:
  - Preventing the Hb to combine with O_2
  - Shifting O_2–Hb dissociation curve to left (Fig. 5.7.6), thereby decreasing the amount of O_2 that can be released

3. Stagnant Hypoxia

Stagnant hypoxia occurs due to decreased blood flow to the tissues so that in spite of normal pO_2 and haemoglobin,

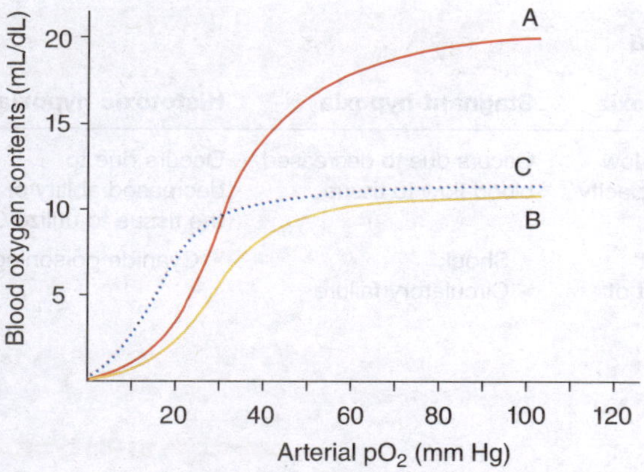

Fig. 5.7.6 Oxygen–haemoglobin dissociation curves: **A**, normal curve (when haemoglobin concentration is 15 g/dL); **B**, anaemic curve (when haemoglobin concentration is 7 g/dL); and **C**, carbon monoxide poisoning curve (when 50% carboxyhaemoglobin) shifted to left of the anaemic curve.

adequate O_2 is not delivered to the tissues. Stagnant or ischaemic hypoxia may be generalized or localized.

Causes Generalized stagnant hypoxia occurs in:

- *Shock* due to circulatory failure and haemorrhage. In this condition, via baroreceptors there occurs reflex vasoconstriction and thus blood flow to the tissues is decreased. Worst affected are the kidneys and heart which have very high O_2 demand.
- *Congestive heart failure* is associated with decreased venous return and hence decreased blood flow to the tissues causing hypoxia. The liver and brain are worst affected by venous congestion. Furthermore, the associated pulmonary congestion produces defect in oxygenation and thus the patients also suffer from hypoxic hypoxia in addition to stagnant hypoxia.

Localized stagnant hypoxia is caused by abnormalities in regional vessels such as:

- Atherosclerosis
- Thrombosis
- Embolism

Characteristic features Characteristic features of stagnant hypoxia are as follows:

- Normal arterial pO_2
- Normal arterial O_2 content
- Normal arterial percentage oxygen saturation of haemoglobin
- A–V pO_2 difference more than normal because resting O_2 uptake of tissues increases from 5% to 10 mL% or the blood stays in the tissue for longer period; thus, in venous blood:
  - pO_2 is reduced from ~40 to ~25 mm Hg.
  - O_2 content is reduced from 14 to 9 mL%.
  - O_2 saturation of Hb is reduced from 75% to 45%.

4. Histotoxic Hypoxia

Histotoxic hypoxia occurs due to decreased ability of the tissues themselves to utilize the oxygen. So, strictly speaking, it is not a true hypoxia, because O_2 supply to the tissues is adequate.

Causes Histotoxic hypoxia is caused by certain poisonous substances which destroy the cellular oxidative enzymes and completely paralyse the cytochrome oxidative system of the cells. These include:

- *Cyanide poisoning*
- *Sulphide poisoning*

Characteristic features Since O_2 supply is adequate and the tissue cells are not able to utilize the O_2, so histotoxic hypoxia is characterized by:

- Normal arterial pO_2
- Normal arterial per cent O_2 saturation of haemoglobin
- No difference in the O_2 content of arterial and venous blood
- Practically nil A–V pO_2 difference

Characteristic Features of Four Types of Hypoxia

Characteristic features of four types of hypoxia are summarized in Table 5.7.1.

Symptoms of Hypoxia

Symptoms of hypoxia depend on:

- Rapidity of development of hypoxia
- Severity of hypoxia
- Effectiveness of the body's compensatory mechanisms

Based on the above, the hypoxia may be fulminant, acute or chronic.

1. Fulminant hypoxia Fulminant hypoxia refers to severe hypoxia developing very fast, i.e. which occurs within seconds after exposure to an arterial O_2 tension of less than 20 mm Hg. Such a situation may occur if an aircraft loses cabin pressure (becomes impressurized) above 20,000 feet and no supplemental O_2 is available. It results in:

Unconsciousness within 15–20 seconds due to lack of O_2 supply to the brain
Brain death which may follow in 4–5 minutes

2. Acute hypoxia Acute hypoxia is produced by exposure to arterial O_2 tensions of 25–40 mm Hg (e.g. as would occur at altitudes of 18,000–25,000 feet). Symptoms of acute hypoxia are very similar to the effects of ethyl alcohol and include:

- Lack of coordination
- Slowed reflexes
- Slurring of speech
- Overconfidence
- Unconsciousness
- Coma and death which can occur in minutes to hours if the compensatory mechanisms of the body are inadequate

3. Chronic hypoxia It occurs due to exposure to low pO_2 (40–60 mm Hg) for long periods (e.g. as would occur after stay for extended period of time at altitudes of approximately 10,000–18,000 feet). Most of the clinical cases of hypoxia are of this category. Patients with chronic hypoxia may be bed-ridden or limited to chair because respiratory and cardiac disease prevents them from increasing O_2 supply to tissues. Symptoms of chronic hypoxia are as follows:

- Severe fatigue
- Dyspnoea

Table 5.7.1 Characteristic features of different types of hypoxia

Features	Hypoxic hypoxia	Anaemic hypoxia	Stagnant hypoxia	Histotoxic hypoxia
Pathophysiology	Occurs due to decreased O_2 tension (decreased arterial pO_2)	Occurs due to low O_2-carrying capacity of blood	Occurs due to decreased blood flow to tissue	Occurs due to decreased ability of the tissue to utilize O_2
Causes	• Low O_2 tension (low pO_2 in inspired air) • Hypoventilation • ↓ Diffusion of O_2 across respiratory membrane • Physiological shunt • Anatomical shunt	• ↓ RBC count • ↓ Hb content of blood • Altered Hb	• Shock • Circulatory failure	• Cyanide poisoning
Arterial pO_2	Decreased	Normal	Normal	Normal
Arterial O_2 contents	Decreased	Markedly decreased	Normal	Normal
Arterial Hb contents	Normal	Reduced	Normal	Normal
Per cent O_2 saturation (in arterial blood)	Decreased	Decreased	Normal	Normal
O_2-carrying capacity of arterial blood	Normal	Decreased	Normal	Normal
Arterial–venous (A–V) pO_2 difference	Decreased	Normal	More than normal	Less than normal (nil)
Cyanosis	Present	Absent	Present	Absent
Peripheral chemoreceptor stimulation	Present (because dissolved oxygen in plasma is reduced)	Absent (because dissolved oxygen in plasma is sufficient)	Present (because arterial pCO_2 increases and pO_2 decreases)	Present (cyanide decreases oxygen utilization at tissue level)
Tachypnoea	Present	Absent	Present	Present

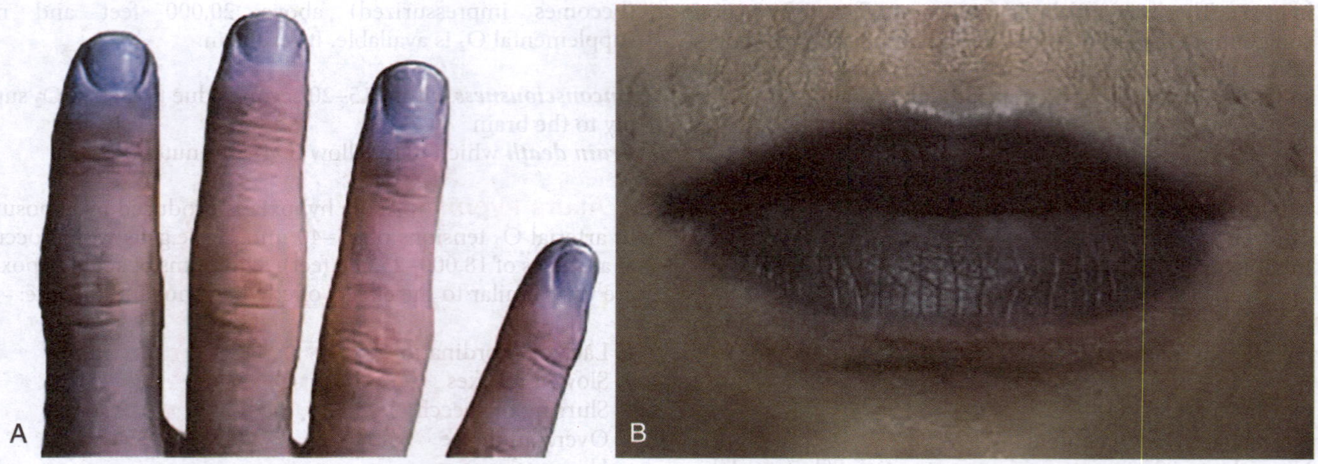

Fig. 5.7.7 Photograph showing: **A**, bluish colour of nails in peripheral cyanosis; and **B**, blue lips in central cyanosis.

- Shortness of breath
- Respiratory arrhythmias (e.g. Cheyne–Stokes breathing) which can occur in patients with chronic hypoxia, especially during sleep, which can contribute to the hypoxic state

Signs of Hypoxia

1. Cyanosis Cyanosis is the bluish discolouration of the skin and mucous membrane caused by presence of more than 5 g of deoxyhaemoglobin/100 mL of the capillary blood. There are two types of cyanosis:

Peripheral cyanosis Peripheral cyanosis is seen in the nail beds and is suggestive of *stagnant hypoxia*. This is because perfusion in these distally located areas is worst affected in hypotensive states. Large amount of O_2 is extracted from haemoglobin and the concentration of deoxyhaemoglobin rises to produce cyanosis (Fig. 5.7.7A).

Causes Peripheral cyanosis may be due to the following causes:

- All common causes of central cyanosis
- Reduced cardiac output (e.g. heart failure or hypovolaemia)

- Cold exposure
- Chronic obstructive pulmonary disease (COPD)
- Arterial obstruction e.g. peripheral vascular disease, (Raynaud phenomenon)

Central cyanosis Central cyanosis is seen in the earlobes where the skin is thin and in the mucous membrane of lips and tongue (Fig. 5.7.7B). These areas receive a good blood supply and become cyanotic only if the O_2 saturation of blood is low, as occurs in *hypoxic hypoxia*.

Causes Central cyanosis is caused by diseases of the lungs or heart or by abnormal haemoglobin like methaemoglobin or sulphaemoglobin.

> **Important Note**
>
> Cyanosis is not a reliable sign of hypoxia because:
> - Patients with anaemia may never develop cyanosis, even though they are extremely hypoxic because of an inadequate haemoglobin concentration.
> - Cyanosis does not occur in histotoxic hypoxia also, because the O_2 saturation of haemoglobin is normal.
> - In contrast, patients with polycythaemia may be cyanotic as a result of high concentration of haemoglobin, even though their tissues are adequately oxygenated.
> - Furthermore, methaemoglobin, with its slate-grey colour, can also impart a bluish colour to tissues.

2. Tachycardia It occurs as a peripheral chemoreceptor reflex response to the low arterial oxygen tension.

3. Tachypnoea Tachypnoea (i.e. rapid breathing) and *hyperpnoea* (i.e. deep breathing) are also reflex responses to hypoxia that are activated by peripheral chemoreceptors. Therefore, tachypnoea and hyperpnoea are as follows:

- Present in hypoxic hypoxia in which arterial pO_2 is low
- Absent in both anaemic hypoxia and stagnant hypoxia in which the arterial pO_2 is normal

Physiological Compensatory Responses to Chronic Hypoxia

Two types of physiological compensatory responses known to occur in hypoxia are *accommodation and acclimatization*.

I. Accommodation Accommodation refers to immediate reflex adjustments of the respiratory and cardiovascular systems to hypoxia. These include:

Hyperventilation As mentioned above, hyperventilation occurs secondary to stimulation of peripheral chemoreceptors by low O_2 tension in the arterial blood. The increased ventilation is compensated by:

- pO_2 is increased and pCO_2 is reduced.
- Reduced pCO_2 causes a respiratory alkalosis, which, in turn, lowers the respiratory drive. The respiratory drive continues to increase during this time as the alkalosis is corrected.

Tachycardia Tachycardia, as mentioned above, also occurs as a peripheral chemoreceptor response to the low arterial oxygen tension. It increases O_2 delivery to the tissues by increasing cardiac output. In the individuals who go to high altitudes, the cardiac output returns to normal after several weeks.

Increase in 2,3-DPG concentration Increase in 2,3-DPG concentration in RBCs occurs in response to hypoxia and alkalosis. The increased 2,3-DPG concentration raises p_{50} of haemoglobin, which helps to maintain the tissue O_2 tension at a slightly higher level than it would be otherwise.

II. Acclimatization Acclimatization refers to the changes in body tissues in response to long-term exposure to hypoxia, such as when a person living at sea level goes and stays at high altitude for a long time. With longer stay, the person gradually gets acclimatized to low pO_2 by the following changes in the body tissues:

i. ***Increase in red blood cell count*** or polycythaemia secondary to tissue hypoxia results from the release of *renal erythropoietic factor*, which acts on plasma globulins to form erythropoietin. Erythropoietin stimulates the production of RBCs by the bone marrow. This leads to:
   - Increase in haemoglobin concentration from 15 g/dL to about 20 g/dL
   - Increase in haematocrit from normal value of 40%–45% to 60% after full acclimatization
   - Increase in blood volume by 20%–30% leading to total increase in circulating haemoglobin by 50%

   These changes allow each unit of blood to carry additional O_2, which compensates for the decreased O_2 tension. Increase in haemoglobin and blood volume starts after 2 weeks, reaches half development in a month and is fully developed only after many months.

ii. ***Increase in pulmonary ventilation:*** When an individual stays at high altitude for many days, there is gradual increase in ventilation to an average of about five times the normal. This is because of loss of breaking effect of CO_2 due to renal correction of alkalosis, leading to decreased HCO_3^- ion concentration in CSF and brain tissues.

iii. ***Cardiovascular changes*** in the form of increased heart rate, force of contraction and increased cardiac output which occur in the initial accommodation period later on decrease back to normal once the O_2 supply to tissues becomes normal due to changes in blood.

iv. ***Pulmonary hypertension*** occurs secondary to the generalized hypoxic pulmonary vasoconstriction. The increased pulmonary artery pressure causes a more even distribution of pulmonary blood flow, which can improve gas exchange. However, the elevated pulmonary artery pressure can induce cor pulmonale if the hypoxia is sufficiently severe.

v. ***Increase in total lung capacity (TLC) and diffusing capacity of the lung*** occurs in high-altitude natives as compared with that in their sea-level counterparts. The increase in TLC is evidenced by the enlarged chest that high-altitude natives develop.

   Diffusing capacity of lungs increases due to increase in surface area of respiratory membrane. The greatly increased pulmonary capillary blood volume expands the capillaries, thereby increasing surface area. Hypoxia increases pulmonary ventilation leading to increase in lung volume which expands surface area of alveolar membrane. Pulmonary hypertension forces blood into a greater number of alveolar capillaries than normally, especially in upper parts of lungs which are poorly perfused.

vi. ***Cellular and tissue acclimatization*** occurs after a long stay at high altitude. This includes:
- *Increase in oxidative enzyme concentrations* within the mitochondria of many tissues, which allows more rapid generation of ATP via oxidative phosphorylation
- *Increase in mitochondrial density* within the cells, which reduces the diffusion distance and provides more sites for O_2 utilization
- *Increase in capillary density* in skeletal and cardiac muscles, which reduces the diffusion distance from the blood into the cells

Important Note

Decreased respiratory drive is caused by lifelong exposure to hypoxia, i.e. for very prolonged periods. The reduced respiratory drive leads to higher CO_2 tension and lower O_2 tension, but it diminishes the work of respiration, which reserves more O_2 for use by other skeletal muscles.

Oxygen Therapy

Physiological Basis of Oxygen Therapy in Hypoxia

Oxygen therapy is of great value in certain types of hypoxia and at the same time of almost no value in other types. With the basic knowledge of physiological principles of different types of hypoxia, one can readily decide when oxygen therapy will be of value and, if so, how valuable.

In general, simple O_2 therapy is not of much help in treatment of hypoxia because diffusion across respiratory membrane depends on partial pressure of gases; therefore, alveolar pO_2 can be increased by:

- Inhalation of 100% pure oxygen, or
- Inhalation of 100% pure oxygen at high barometric pressure, called hyperbaric oxygen therapy

Oxygen therapy with 100% pure oxygen at atmospheric pressure, i.e. at 760 mm Hg

1. Oxygen therapy is useful Oxygen therapy is useful in most types of hypoxic hypoxia. The ways in which the oxygen therapy is useful in different causes of hypoxic hypoxia are highlighted:

In atmospheric hypoxia, oxygen therapy can correct the depressed oxygen level in the inspired gases and therefore provide 100% effective therapy.

In hypoventilation hypoxia, a person breathing 100% oxygen can move five times as much oxygen into the alveoli with each breath as when breathing normal air. Again, here oxygen therapy can be extremely beneficial.

In hypoxia due to impaired respiratory membrane diffusion, oxygen therapy can increase the pO_2 in the lungs from a normal value of about 100 mm Hg to as high as 160 mm Hg, thus raising the oxygen diffusion gradient.

2. Oxygen therapy is of limited value Oxygen therapy is of limited value in anaemic hypoxia, stagnant hypoxia and hypoxic hypoxia caused by physiological or anatomical shunts, because in all these conditions oxygen is already available in the alveoli. However, in these conditions, some extra oxygen can be transported in dissolved state in the blood when alveolar oxygen is increased to the maximum level, and this extra oxygen may sometimes be the difference between life and death.

Therefore, hyperbaric O_2 therapy is more useful in such conditions than O_2 therapy at atmospheric pressure.

3. Oxygen therapy is of no use Oxygen therapy is of no use in histotoxic hypoxia, because in this type of hypoxia, the tissue metabolic enzyme system is simply incapable of utilizing the oxygen that is delivered.

Important Note

Caution is required while giving oxygen therapy to patients with severe pulmonary failure associated with hypercapnia (increased pCO_2), as it may cause death. The central chemoreceptors in these patients are inhibited following excessive overdrive by the pCO_2. In such a situation, whatever respiration is there, it is due to hypoxic stimulation of peripheral chemoreceptors. So, O_2 therapy at such a juncture may produce apnoea by taking away this hypoxic drive and soon death may occur due to direct depression of respiratory centre by severe hypoxia and hypercapnia.

Hyperbaric oxygen therapy (inhalation of 100% pure oxygen at high barometric pressure)

Advantage of hyperbaric O_2 Advantage of hyperbaric O_2 therapy over O_2 therapy at atmospheric pressure is that the former increases the amount of dissolved O_2 in plasma and is therefore unaffected by the haemoglobin concentration.

Amount of O_2 dissolved in plasma Amount of O_2 dissolved in plasma depends on its partial pressures:

- Normally, plasma can have 0.3 mL of dissolved oxygen/100 mL/100 mm Hg pO_2, or 0.003 mL/100 mL/mm Hg pO_2.
- *At atmospheric pressure of 1 (760 mm Hg)*, inhalation of 100% O_2 (in a patient with normal pCO_2 40 mm Hg and pH_2O 47 mm Hg) can raise the arterial pO_2 to a maximum of 760 − (40 + 47), or 673 mm Hg.
- Therefore, the maximum amount of O_2 that can be dissolved in plasma will be:
  At atmospheric pressure of 1: 673×0.003, or 2 mL/100 mL
  At atmospheric pressure of 2: $673 \times 0.003 \times 2$, or 4 mL/100 mL
  At atmospheric pressure of 3: $673 \times 0.003 \times 3$, or 6 mL/100 mL
- The normal demand of the body tissues (5 mL/100 mL/min), thus, can be met only by dissolved O_2 in plasma, if administered at atmospheric pressure of 2.5 or more.

Indications of hyperbaric O_2 therapy Indications of hyperbaric O_2 therapy, thus, include those types of hypoxias in which normal Hb is not available to carry the O_2 to the tissues, and so the main dependence is on dissolved O_2 in plasma. These conditions include:

- CO poisoning
- Anaemic hypoxia (due to severe anaemia)
- Decompression sickness and air embolism
- Wounds with poor blood supply, gas gangrene
- Cerebral palsy
- Skin grafts
- Stagnant hypoxia (very limited value)

Important Note

Caution: For therapeutic use, the pure (100%) hyperbaric O_2 should not be used with pressures beyond two to three times the atmospheric pressure and should not be used more than 5 hours, because of high chances of developing O_2 toxicity.

Side Effects of 100% O_2 (O_2 Toxicity)

Inhalation of 100% O_2 produces side effects (harmful effects) due to conversion of molecular oxygen into active oxygen, i.e. superoxide anion (O_2^-), which is free radical and H_2O. The side effects noted by inhalation of 100% O_2 include:

Irritation of airways Irritation of airways in the form of nasal congestion, sore throat, substernal discomfort, sneezing and coughing and bronchoconstriction may occur after about 8 hours of inhalation.

Bronchopneumonia Bronchopneumonia may be initiated when O_2 therapy is continued for more than 24 hours because of:

- Inhibition of ability of lung macrophages to kill bacteria
- Decreased production of surfactant

Complications in newborn infants Complications in newborn infants are very common, as they are very sensitive to get O_2 toxicity. Therefore, special care is needed while treating newborns in incubators with O_2 therapy. It is cautioned that infants should never be given more than 40% O_2. Special dangers of O_2 therapy in premature infants are occurrence of:

Retinopathy of prematurity (old name, retrolental fibroplasia), which is characterized by retinal neovascularization and proliferation of fibrovascular tissue ultimately forming an opaque retrolental mass, leading to bilateral permanent blindness. Normally, the retinal receptors get matured from central part towards the peripheral part of the retina, and at the same time vascularization also occurs in an orderly manner (centre towards periphery). A large amount of oxygen is being utilized in the process of maturation; therefore, if premature babies are treated with 100% oxygen, the normal pattern of maturation fails and consequently there is proliferation of fibrovascular tissue resulting in formation of opaque retrolental mass.

Bronchopulmonary dysplasia is characterized by formation of lung cysts and opacities.

Nervous system complications Nervous system complications, i.e. derangement of cerebral activity, are especially known to occur with administration of *hyperbaric* O_2 therapy. At high pressures of O_2, dissolved O_2 in plasma is greatly increased, which in turn causes rise in tissue pO_2. As mentioned above, oxygen toxicity is caused by production of free oxygen radicals which oxidize polyunsaturated fatty acids (essential compounds of cells membrane) and also oxidize cellular enzymes (damaging cellular metabolic systems). Nervous tissues are especially susceptible because of their high lipid content. Nervous symptoms include muscular twitching, tinnitus (ringing of bells in ears), convulsions, coma and even death.

Other complications Oxidative damage may occur in any cell in the body. It may cause damage to red blood cells (haemolysis), liver, heart, endocrine glands (adrenal, gonads and thyroid), kidney, ears (tinnitus and loss of equilibrium) and eyes (blurred vision and opacity of vasculature).

Hypercapnia

Hypercapnia refers to increase in arterial pCO_2 (normal value 40 mm Hg). When hypercapnia is the primary problem, it is associated with respiratory acidosis (see page 441) since an increase in CO_2 promptly generates excess H^+ through the following reaction:

$$H_2O + CO_2 \xrightarrow{\text{Carbonic anhydrase}} H_2CO_3 \rightarrow H^+ + HCO_3^-$$

Causes of Hypercapnia

Hypercapnia rarely occurs due to increased production of CO_2: Hypercapnia rarely occurs due to increased production of CO_2, because an increase in arterial pCO_2 causes a prompt increase in pulmonary ventilation through stimulation of central chemoreceptors, resulting in CO_2 wash-out and a near restoration of arterial pCO_2 to normal levels of about 40 mm Hg. There exists a linear relationship between increase in arterial pCO_2 and increase in pulmonary ventilation (see page 440). Increased production of CO_2 without hypercapnia occurs in fever, following excess consumption of carbohydrate, and in metabolic acidosis with respiratory compensation.

Hypercapnia occurs due to

1. ***Defective elimination of CO_2*** as occurs in:
   - Reduced pulmonary ventilation due to restrictive lung disorder, or
   - Reduced effective alveolar ventilation (VA) due to V/Q mismatch as seen in COPD
2. ***Accidental inhalation of CO_2*** in persons working in breweries and refrigeration plants

Signs and Symptoms of Hypercapnia

Signs and symptoms of hypercapnia include:

1. Hyperpnoea Hyperpnoea occurs due to stimulation of respiratory centre through central chemoreceptors. Since, most of the times, clinically hypercapnia occurs due to restrictive lung disorders, hyperpnoea fails to improve pulmonary ventilation.

2. Carbon dioxide narcosis Carbon dioxide narcosis develops when arterial pCO_2 increases above 50 mm Hg. Retention of large amount of CO_2 causes depression of central nervous system leading to confusion, diminution of sensory acuity and eventually coma and death.

These patients present with severe respiratory acidosis; therefore, as a compensation for acidosis, a large amount of HCO_3^- is excreted in urine (for details, see page 440).

Hypocapnia

Hypocapnia, i.e. reduced pCO_2, is usually associated with *respiratory alkalosis*, since decrease in CO_2 promptly drives the following reaction in backward direction, resulting in a decrease in H^+ concentration:

$$H_2O + CO_2 \xleftarrow{\text{Carbonic anhydrase}} H_2CO_3 \leftarrow H^+ + HCO_3^-$$

Causes

Hypocapnia occurs due to hyperventilation (see page 443). The effects of hypocapnia are as follows:

- Vasoconstriction due to direct effect on cerebral blood vessels causes reduction in cerebral blood flow by 30%. The resulting ischaemia causes headache, dizziness and paraesthesia.
- Due to alkalosis, pH increases to 7.5–7.6, and plasma HCO_3^- level becomes low; the renal compensation results in absorption of HCO_3^- due to inhibition of acid secretion.
- Plasma ionic calcium level (Ca^{2+}) falls; therefore, the patient with hypocapnia develops signs of tetany, i.e. *carpopedal spasm* and a *positive Chvostek sign*. For details, see page 719.

Asphyxia

Asphyxia refers to a condition in which hypoxia (decreased pO_2) is associated with hypercapnia (increased pCO_2).

Causes

Asphyxia can be general or local.

Local asphyxia Local asphyxia occurs following complete obstruction or ligation of blood vessel.

General asphyxia General asphyxia can be chronic or acute.

Chronic asphyxia may occur in patients with cor pulmonale, i.e. right ventricular failure due to lung diseases.

Acute asphyxia occurs due to sudden blockage in airways. Common causes are as follows:

- Strangulation
- Drowning
- Acute tracheal obstruction (due to entry of food or due to choking)
- Paralysis of diaphragm, as in acute poliomyelitis

Clinical Stages of Acute Asphyxia

There are three stages of acute asphyxia.

Stage I (stage of hyperpnoea) This stage lasts for 1 minute and is characterized by:

- Increase in rate and depth of respiration, with more pronounced expiratory effort
- Dyspnoea, cyanosis and sudden prominence of eyeballs

This stage occurs due to sudden and powerful stimulation of respiratory centres by acutely occurring rise in pCO_2. (O_2 lack is not yet enough to stimulate ventilation.)

Stage II (stage of central excitation) This stage occurs due to excess CO_2 stimulating the centres directly, and lack of O_2 stimulating the centres reflexly. It lasts for about 1 minute and is characterized by all signs of central excitation, such as:

- Expiration becomes more *violent*.
- Heart rate is increased.
- Systemic blood pressure rises due to widespread vasoconstriction.
- Pupils are constricted.
- All the reflexes are exaggerated.
- Convulsions occur due to excess of pCO_2.
- Consciousness is lost.

Stage III (stage of central depression) This stage occurs due to direct effect of O_2 lack on vital centres causing their inhibition. It lasts for 2–3 minutes and its characteristic features are as follows:

- Convulsions disappear.
- Respiration becomes slow and finally it becomes gasping (shallow and with low frequency).
- Heart rate is decreased.
- Blood pressure falls.
- Pupils are dilated.
- All the reflexes are abolished.
- The whole body lies still.
- Duration between the gasps is gradually increased.
- Finally death occurs.

Drowning

Drowning is defined as respiratory impairment as a result of being in or under liquid.

There are two main mechanisms by which drowning ultimately causes death which are as follows:

1. Asphyxia is the cause of death in only 10% of cases of drowning. It occurs initially due to *breath-holding*, and after the breaking-in effect due to the severe *laryngospasm* induced by the first gasp of water. The laryngospasm prevents entry of water into the lungs, but soon produces death due to asphyxia. Thus, the lungs remain dry in asphyxial deaths due to drowning.

2. Flooding of Lungs with Water occurs in 90% of cases of drowning. The muscles of glottis relax and allow entry of water into the lungs. Further events depend on the type of water:

Fresh water drowning is associated with rapid absorption of water (since it is hypotonic) into the circulation, which causes plasma dilution and intravascular haemolysis.

Sea water drowning is associated with hypovolaemia due to draining of water from the circulation into the lungs (since the sea water is hypertonic).

Management Management in drowning cases includes check on circulation, airway and breathing (CAB). When the patients with drowning are timely rescued and resuscitated with AR, the above-described circulatory effects must be taken care of depending on the type of water.

- Treat hypothermia.
- Manage hypovolaemia by infusion therapy.

Carbon Monoxide Poisoning

CO is a dangerous gas present in exhaust of gasoline engines, coal mines, gases from deep wells and underground drainage systems.

Toxic Effects

CO produces anaemic hypoxia and derangement of cellular metabolic system.

1. Anaemic hypoxia When CO is inhaled accidently from the above-mentioned sources, CO having 200 times more affinity than O_2 for haemoglobin combines with it to form *carboxyhaemoglobin*. The carboxyhaemoglobin produces severe anaemic hypoxia by the following mechanisms:

- It does not allow the haemoglobin to take up oxygen from alveolar air.

- The presence of carboxyhaemoglobin decreases the release of oxygen from haemoglobin, i.e. the oxygen–haemoglobin dissociation curve shifts to the left (Fig. 5.5.7); see page 423.

2. Derangement of cellular metabolic system CO causes toxic effects on cytochrome system of the cells causing derangement of the cellular metabolic system but the amount of CO required for producing cytochrome toxic effects is 1000 times (the lethal dose).

Signs and Symptoms of CO Poisoning

Signs and symptoms of CO poisoning depending on its concentration in the inspired air are as follows:

- *When the inspired air contains 1% CO*, saturation of haemoglobin with CO becomes 15%–20%. Patients get headache and nausea within 1 hour of inhalation.
- *When the inspired air contains more than 1% CO*, the haemoglobin saturation becomes 30%–40%. This causes loss of consciousness.
- *When haemoglobin saturation with CO* becomes 50%, death occurs.
- The symptoms of CO poisoning are of hypoxia, but there is no stimulation of respiration because arterial blood pO_2 remains normal.
- The cherry red colour of COHb is visible on the skin, nail bed and mucous membrane.

Diagnosis

Diagnosis is mainly based on the signs and symptoms, but for management, amount of carboxyhaemoglobin present in the blood must be quantitated using various techniques, like spectrophotometric method or by chromatographic method, the CO oximeter and breath CO monitoring.

Treatment of CO Poisoning

When diagnosed timely, the following measures should be taken promptly:

- Immediate termination of exposure to CO:
  Hyperbaric 100% O_2 therapy: Hyperbaric oxygen helps in dissociation of Hb from carboxyhaemoglobin.
- Administration of air with few per cent of CO_2 to stimulate respiratory centres

PULMONARY DISEASES: PHYSIOLOGICAL PECULIARITIES

Physiological peculiarities of some of the common pulmonary diseases are described to understand the pathophysiology of respiratory insufficiency occurring in these diseases.

From the physiological point of view, the pulmonary diseases can be divided into two groups:

- Obstructive lung diseases
- Restrictive lung diseases

Obstructive Lung Diseases

The chronic obstructive lung diseases include asthma, chronic bronchitis and emphysema. The obstructive lung diseases are characterized by increased resistance to airflow.

The airway resistance mainly depends on the radius of the airway and on the type of airflow. Resistance is low when airflow is laminar and high when airflow is turbulent. Upper airway resistance usually does not increase, except in conditions like nasal congestion, deviated nasal septum or enlarged adenoids. Mouth breathing is common in these conditions.

Lower Airway Resistance

Lower airway resistance chiefly lies in the medium-sized bronchi (2–4 mm diameter). Smooth muscle contraction mainly increases airway resistance by reducing airway's radius. The diameter of these bronchi is altered by the following factors:

Bronchomotor tone is chiefly regulated by autonomic neural discharge (see page 381) and also by local chemical mediators like prostaglandins, leukotrienes and kinins.

Radial traction by lung parenchyma: Bronchi and bronchioles are surrounded by lung parenchyma. The constant pull of lung parenchyma helps in maintaining patency of the airway. This supportive action is known as radial traction. During expiration, small airways (bronchioles) collapse.

Transmural pressure: In quiet breathing, during inspiration, pressure is negative (because of negative intrapleural pressure with respect to intrapulmonary pressure). Therefore, the airways remain patent. Same situation prevails during tidal expiration; however, in forced expiration, transmural pressure becomes positive, which tends to collapse the small airways. The condition is worsened in emphysema due to loss of radial traction.

Mucus secretion: Presence of mucus or any other material in airways also increases airway resistance.

Mechanisms of Airway Obstruction

Mechanisms of airway obstruction in the obstructive lung diseases include:

The airway lumen may be partially obstructed by excessive secretions (chronic bronchitis), oedema fluid or aspiration of food or fluids.

The airway wall smooth muscles may be contracted (asthma) or thickened because of inflammation and oedema (asthma, bronchitis), or mucous glands may be hypertrophied (chronic bronchitis).

Outside the airway, the destruction of lung parenchyma may decrease radial traction, causing the airways to be narrowed (emphysema).

1. Asthma

Asthma is considered an inflammatory disease of the bronchioles caused by the hypersensitivity of the bronchioles to foreign substances in the air. It is a chronic lifelong disease with periods of *remissions* and *exacerbation*.

Aetiopathogenesis Functional abnormality in asthma is airway narrowing produced by the following effects of allergic reactions:

Spasm of bronchial smooth muscle, which is triggered by exposure to provoking agents such as allergen or exercise

Inflammation of bronchial wall (predominantly eosinophilic/ producing mucosal oedema)

Secretion of thick mucus into the lumen of bronchioles

Symptoms The above-mentioned changes increase the airway resistance; thus, asthma is an obstructive lung disease. The person with asthma can usually inspire adequately but has great difficulty during expiration. During attack of asthma, the patient may have:

- Dyspnoea, or air hunger may occur.
- Cough may be present.
- With repeated acute attacks, the patient may get progressive fatigue and even eventual respiratory arrest.
- Pulmonary function abnormalities may occur in patients over the years. During asthmatic attack, because of difficulty in expiring air, there occurs:
  - *Reduced maximum* expiratory rate
  - Increase in functional residual capacity (FRC) and in residual volume (RV)
  - Reduction in TV, VC and forced expiratory volume in the 1st second (FEV_1)

Important Note

Gas exchange abnormalities

There is no decrease in diffusion capacity in asthma. VA is uneven and decreased causing *mild hypoxia*. However, with increasing severity of attack, pO_2 decreases in direct proportion to the drop in FEV_1. Hyperventilation in response to hypoxia leads to decreased pCO_2. When the attack is prolonged, the patient may get acidosis, dyspnoea and cyanosis. A normal or increased pCO_2 in asthma along with increasing hypoxaemia is an ominous sign of impending respiratory arrest.

Treatment Therapeutically the drugs used are as follows:

- β-Adrenergic agonists are used to treat mild to moderate asthmatic attack.
- Steroids both as inhaler and systemically may be used to reduce inflammation.
- Agents that block synthesis of leukotrienes or their receptors are also useful in certain cases.

2. Chronic Bronchitis and Emphysema

Chronic bronchitis Chronic bronchitis, i.e. inflammation of the bronchial tree, occurs due to cigarette smoking and exposure to oxidant gases, dust and irritants. Mucosal inflammation is exacerbated by superadded infection. It is characterized by an increase in volume of submucosal glands and increase in the number of goblet cells in the surface epithelium.

- Chronic cough and hypersecretion of mucus are the hallmark of chronic bronchitis.
- Increased airflow resistance occurs due to chronic inflammation of the small airways and the condition is termed *small airway disease.*

Pulmonary emphysema Pulmonary emphysema literally means excess air in the lung. Chronic pulmonary emphysema, however, signifies a complex obstructive and destructive process of the lungs and is usually a consequence of long-term smoking. Development of emphysema involves two main events:

Airway obstruction Airway obstruction is caused by changes of chronic bronchitis (as described above) which include chronic infection, excess mucus and inflammatory oedema of the bronchial epithelium. Furthermore, the smaller peripheral bronchi are thickened and distorted by the scar tissue and at the segmental level there may be loss of bronchial cartilage. All these changes are termed *small airway disease.*

Destruction of alveolar walls The obstruction of the airway makes it especially difficult to expire, causing entrapment of air in the alveoli and overstretching of the alveoli. This combined with lung infection causes marked destruction of alveolar cells. Usually there is loss of some elastic tissues because of the proteolytic enzyme called elastase.

Consequences or sequelae of emphysema include:

- Increase in physiological dead space
- Altered V/Q ratio
- Decrease in diffusion capacity
- Decreased arterial pO_2 and rise in pCO_2
- Hypoxia, polycythaemia and hypercapnia
- Increase in work of breathing due to decreased recoil of the lungs leading to barrel-shaped chest

3. Chronic Obstructive Pulmonary Disease

COPD is the term used to denote the clinical entity having combined effects of chronic bronchitis and chronic pulmonary emphysema. Genetic factors also predispose to COPD by producing deficiency of antitrypsin activity. In the lungs, normally action of elastase and other proteolytic enzymes (produced by leucocytes) is antagonized by antitrypsin activity. It is characterized by the following respiratory physiological changes:

Increased airway resistance Increased airway resistance occurs due to chronic bronchial obstruction. So, the movement of air through the respiratory passages becomes difficult. Expiration is especially difficult because the force on the outside of the lung compresses the bronchioles, which further increases their resistance.

Decreased diffusing capacity Decreased diffusing capacity of the lungs results from destruction of alveolar membrane. So, ability of the lungs to oxygenate the blood and to remove the carbon dioxide is reduced.

Abnormal ventilation–perfusion ratio Abnormal V/Q ratio occurs as:

Very low V/Q ratio Very low V/Q ratio occurs in the areas of lungs with bronchiolar obstruction. In these areas, VA is much less than the blood supply (perfusion), resulting in poor aeration of blood (*physiological shunt formation*).

Very high V/Q ratio Very high V/Q ratio occurs in the areas of lungs having marked loss of alveolar walls. In such areas, VA is much more as compared with perfusion, resulting in wasted ventilation (*physiological dead space formation*).

Increased pulmonary resistance Increased pulmonary resistance may occur due to decrease in the number of capillaries owing to the destruction of lung parenchyma. It may in turn cause pulmonary hypertension.

Pulmonary function tests Pulmonary function tests in patients with moderate to severe COPD may reveal the following abnormalities:

- *Decreased forced expiratory flow* occurs due to loss of lung elasticity, increase in airway resistance upstream from equal pressure point and an increase in compliance of the airway downstream from equal pressure points.

- *Forced vital capacity (FVC)* may be normal or decreased (reflecting increased RV).
- FEV_1 is reduced as is the ratio of FEV_1/FVC.
- RV and FRC are increased. TLC may also be increased in some cases.

Restrictive Lung Diseases

The restrictive lung diseases include pulmonary fibrosis, silicosis, asbestosis, tuberculosis, pneumothorax, pleural effusion and paresis of respiratory muscles (e.g. in poliomyelitis and myasthenia gravis).

Characteristic features Restrictive lung diseases are characterized by low lung volumes. Patients with restrictive lung disease find it easier to breathe at low lung volumes because it is difficult to expand the lungs.

Mechanisms of restriction of lung expansion Mechanisms of restriction of lung expansion include:

- *Abnormalities of lung parenchyma* – diseases in which excessive pulmonary fibrosis decreases lung elasticity as occurs in pulmonary fibrosis, pneumonia, silicosis, asbestosis and tuberculosis
- *Abnormalities of pleura* as occur in pneumothorax and pleural effusion
- *Paresis of respiratory muscles* as occurs in poliomyelitis and myasthenia gravis

i. Lung Parenchymal Diseases

1. Pneumonia The term pneumonia includes an inflammatory condition of the lung in which alveoli are filled with fluid and inflammatory cells. It is characterized by clinical and radiological consolidation of the involved parts of lung parenchyma.

Causes The pneumonia is usually an infective process caused by bacteria (commonly pneumococci) and viruses, but can also result from noninfective causes such as chemical or radiation injury to the lungs.

Functional abnormalities Functional abnormalities which occur in patients with pneumonia are as follows:

- *Restrictive pulmonary function defect* occurs due to total replacement of alveolar gases by the inflammatory exudates in the involved part of the lung.
- *V/Q* is decreased because in the involved areas of the lung, perfusion is normal but VA is markedly decreased, resulting in *physiological shunt formation.*
- *Hypoxia* may develop depending on the extent of involvement of lung parenchyma.

Clinically Clinically, the patient may develop:

- *Fever* occurs in response to infection.
- *Compression of the chest* and feeling of chest pain may occur.
- *Respiratory efforts may be increased* due to stimulation by hypoxia and associated fever, leading to hypocapnia and respiratory alkalosis.
- *Heart rate* may be increased in response to hypoxia.
- *Retention of CO_2* occurs only in later stages in severe disease when the patient gets exhausted and respiratory effort is failing.
- *Cerebral hypoxia* may develop in severe cases causing delirium which is characterized by confused mental state, illusion, hallucination, disorientation, hyperexcitability and loss of memory.

ii. Pulmonary Tuberculosis

Pulmonary tuberculosis is a chronic infection of the lung parenchyma caused by the acid-fast bacteria called *Mycobacterium tuberculosis* or tubercle bacilli.

- The invasion of lung parenchyma by tubercle bacilli causes infiltration of the infected area by macrophages and walling off of the lesion by fibrous tissue to form the so-called tubercle.
- Tuberculosis in its late stages causes many areas of fibrosis and reduces the total amount of lung tissue.
- Initially, the alveoli in the affected part become nonfunctioning due to thickness of respiratory membrane. When a large part of the lung is involved, the diffusing capacity is very much reduced.

iii. Atelectasis

Atelectasis refers to the collapse of alveoli with absence of air in the involved parts.

Causes Atelectasis may develop due to:

- *Obstruction of bronchus or a bronchiole:* Air trapped distal to the bronchial obstruction is absorbed causing collapse of the alveoli attached to the bronchus or bronchiole.
- *Lack of surfactant* increases the surface tension of alveolar fluid and causes collapse of the alveoli. Marked lack of surfactant is seen in a disease called hyaline membrane disease or the so-called respiratory distress syndrome.
- *Pressure from the pleural cavity* caused by presence of air (pneumothorax), fluid (hydrothorax) or blood (haemothorax) in the pleural cavity may cause collapse of the lung, depending on their amount present.

Functional abnormality When a large portion of the lung is collapsed, the partial pressure of oxygen is reduced in blood leading to respiratory disturbances. Marked collapse is a common cause of dyspnoea.

iv. Pulmonary Oedema

Pulmonary oedema refers to collection of serous fluid in the alveoli and the interstitial spaces of the lung tissue.

Causes Causes of pulmonary oedema are as follows:

- *Increased pulmonary capillary pressure* as occurs in left ventricular failure or mitral valve disease
- *Pneumonia*
- Effect of harmful chemicals like chlorine or sulphur dioxide

Functional abnormalities Functional abnormalities produced by pulmonary oedema are as follows:

- *Diffusion capacity of the lung* is decreased due to increased thickness of respiratory membrane. So, the ability of the lungs to oxygenate the blood and to remove the carbon dioxide is reduced.
- *Marked alveolar oedema* is fatal and causes sudden death due to suffocation.

II. Diseases of Pleura

The diseases of pleura include the following:

i. Pleural effusion Pleural effusion refers to accumulation of a large amount of fluid in the pleural cavity. Normally, there is very little pleural fluid because the fluid which is produced by a pressure gradient pushing fluid from parietal capillaries to pleural space is promptly absorbed by a net force driving pleural fluid from pleural space to visceral capillaries and lymphatics.

Causes Causes of pleural effusion include:

Excessive transudation of fluid from the pulmonary capillaries due to:

- Increased hydrostatic pressure as occurs in left ventricular failure
- Decreased oncotic pressure as occurs in hypoproteinaemia

Exudation in inflammatory conditions of pleura (pleuritis or pleurisy) results due to damage of capillary membranes, allowing leakage of fluid and plasma proteins into the pleural cavity. The high-protein content of pleural fluid increases its osmotic pressure which pulls more fluid.

Obstruction to lymphatics in inflammatory and neoplastic conditions also leads to collection of fluid in the pleural cavity.

Functional abnormalities Functional abnormalities produced in pleural effusion depend on the size of effusion and the rate at which fluid accumulates.

- Pleural effusion essentially produces a *restrictive abnormality* with decrease in FVC, FRC, TLC and RV.
- When large pleural effusion develops quickly, it causes atelectasis which is associated with dyspnoea and *hypoxia* producing hyperventilation and hypocapnia.
- Moderate to massive effusion causes shift of the mediastinal structures to the opposite side. When this occurs rapidly, this may compromise cardiac output and hypotension.

ii. Pneumothorax Pneumothorax refers to presence of air in the pleural cavity. Normally, there is a negative pressure in the pleural space (about −0.66 kPa), which becomes positive in pneumothorax.

Causes Pneumothorax occurs due to entry of air into the pleural cavity due to either a hole in the chest wall and parietal pleura or a hole in the lung parenchyma and visceral pleura as may occur in accidents, bullet injuries or stab injuries.

Types of pneumothorax and functional abnormalities Types of pneumothorax and functional abnormalities produced in them are as follows:

i. ***Open pneumothorax*** refers to the condition in which an open communication is developed between the pleural cavity and the atmosphere. So the air is present in the pleural cavity at atmospheric pressure which reduces all lung volumes. Thus, there occurs a restrictive ventilatory impairment leading to reduction in FVC, FRC and TLC in proportion to the volume of pneumothorax. Depending on the degree of lung collapse produced, there occurs proportionate hypoxia, hypocapnia, dyspnoea and cyanosis.

ii. ***Closed pneumothorax*** develops when the hole in the pleura is sealed after the entry of air into the pleural cavity. As normally, the partial pressure of gases in the capillaries in the pleura is about 5.3–6 kPa less than the atmospheric pressure, there is a significant gradient for absorption of gases from pleural space to capillaries. Thus, the air entrapped in the pleural cavity is slowly absorbed, and so not much functional abnormalities are produced.

iii. ***Tension pneumothorax*** occurs when the hole produced in pleura is valvular which allows entry of air into the pleural cavity during inspiration but prevents the exit of air during expiration. As a result, the intrapleural pressure keeps on rising progressively leading to collapse of the ipsilateral lung and pushing the mediastinum and contralateral lung.
   - Squeezing of both lungs leads to marked hypoxaemia.
   - Displacement of mediastinal structures leads to progressive fall in cardiac output.
   - Decreased cardiac output and hypoxia combined produces loss of consciousness and hypotension, and ultimately may prove fatal soon.

Tension pneumothorax requires treatment as a medical emergency.

Treatment of pneumothorax consists of supportive care and procedures

Supportive care Supportive care includes oxygen therapy and monitoring for changes/improvement.

Medical procedure When pneumothorax is large, a needle or tube is used to remove excess air.

Surgery (thoracotomy) is usually performed when there are two or more episodes of pneumothorax and partially collapsed lung.

> **Important Note**
>
> ***Treatment of tension pneumothorax*** requires decompressive needle thoracostomy.

III. Pulmonary Vascular Disorders

Pulmonary vascular disorders include pulmonary hypertension and pulmonary embolism.

i. Pulmonary hypertension The mechanisms responsible for genesis of pulmonary hypertension are as follows:

Increased pulmonary resistance: The most common cause of pulmonary hypertension occurs due to:

- Pulmonary vasoconstriction because of alveolar hypoxia (see page 406)
- Obstruction of pulmonary vessels, e.g. thromboembolism
- Pulmonary capillaries obliteration, e.g. in emphysema

Increase in left atrial pressure: For details, see page 374.

Increased pulmonary blood flow due to congenital heart diseases like atrial septal defect (ASD), ventricular septal defect (VSD) or patent ductus arteriosus; the high blood flow is accommodated by recruitment and distension of pulmonary blood vessels. However, sustained high blood flow results in structural changes in smaller vessels leading to rise in pulmonary arterial pressure and ultimately shunt in the heart is reversed (i.e. instead of left to right, becomes right to left).

Treatment Pulmonary hypertension is treated by use of:

Vasodilators such as prostacyclin (PGI_2) and its analogues

Endothelin antagonists (ETA)

Complications Pulmonary hypertension, when not treated properly, may result in complications such as right ventricular hypertrophy, right ventricular failure and pulmonary oedema, and death may occur.

ii. Pulmonary embolism Occlusion of pulmonary vessels by an embolus results in the following effects:

A. ***When a large embolus gets lodged in a major branch of the pulmonary artery***, it results in reduction in cardiac output and cor pulmonale. In contrast, when small segmental arteries get blocked by medium-sized emboli, pulmonary infarction, cyanosis, tachypnoea and pleural pain occur. In a nutshell, there is high V/Q ratio due to increase in physiological dead space and hypoxia, and pulmonary hypertension occurs.
B. ***The substances released from the thromboemboli*** (e.g. histamine, serotonin and prostaglandins) cause constriction in pulmonary vasculature and bronchoconstriction.
C. ***Surfactant synthesis*** also gets reduced due to compromised blood flow, and results in collapse of alveoli and exudation of fluid (pulmonary oedema).

The above-mentioned effects ultimately lead to the following:

Clinical features include:
- Tachypnoea and dyspnoea
- Pleuritic chest pain
- Haemoptysis
- Coughing

In severe cases In severe cases, due to reduced blood flow to the lungs, the patient becomes cyanosed and may collapse; left heart failure results in circulatory shock.

Treatment of pulmonary embolism includes: Anticoagulant therapy and analgesics to reduce pain, and may require thrombolysis in severe cases

ARTIFICIAL RESPIRATION AND CARDIOPULMONARY RESUSCITATION

ARTIFICIAL RESPIRATION (AR)

AR or artificial ventilation (AV) is any means of assisting or stimulating respiration when natural respiration has ceased. AR is required as an emergency life-saving procedure:

I. ***When there is sudden stoppage of breathing*** as seen in:
   - Drowning
   - Electrocution
   - Anaesthetic accidents
   - CO poisoning
   - Strangulation
   - Accidents

II. ***AR may also be needed when breathing is expected to stop gradually*** as in paralysis of muscles in:
   - Poliomyelitis
   - Diphtheria
   - Ascending paralysis

> **Important Note**
>
> *It is important to note* that the tissues of the brain, particularly cerebral cortex, develop irreversible damage if oxygen supply is stopped for 5 minutes. So, the resuscitation must be started quickly without any delay, before the development of cardiac failure.

METHODS OF ARTIFICIAL RESPIRATION

Presently, AR can be given by two types of methods:
- Manual methods, e.g. mouth-to-mouth breathing method
- Mechanical methods

Mouth-to-Mouth Breathing Method

Various manual methods of AR have been described in the past and discarded. Presently, the only manual method used is mouth-to-mouth breathing (exhaled air ventilation) because:

- It can be applied quickly without waiting for the availability of any aid.
- It is a simple and effective measure of resuscitation.
- It can be applied in all age groups.
- It is the only technique capable of producing adequate ventilation.
- It also works by expanding the lungs.

Procedure

The procedure should be performed swiftly and alertly.

- The procedure is performed after placing the patient in supine position.
- It is essential to provide and maintain a clear airway for the procedure to be effective. Therefore, any foreign material present in the mouth cavity must be removed with fingers, e.g. grass and straw (in case of drowning patients), and artificial denture if any – mucus, saliva and blood clot. The tongue must be drawn forward and it must be prevented from falling posteriorly causing airway obstruction. The clothes around the neck and chest region must be loosened. If the mouth is full of blood, mouth-to-nose respiration should be given.
- To begin with, the patient's neck is extended by placing one hand under the neck and lifting it and pressing the forehead with the other hand (Fig. 5.7.8A). This prevents the flaccid tongue from falling back into the pharynx.
- Then the patient's nostrils are closed by the thumb and index finger of the hand (Fig. 5.7.8B).
- The resuscitator then takes a deep breath and exhales air into the patient's airway after tightly placing his/her mouth over the patient's mouth and noting the expansion of the chest at the same time. The volume of the air exhaled must be twice the normal TV. This expands the patient's lungs.
- Then, the resuscitator removes his/her mouth from that of the patient, allowing expiration to occur passively due to the elastic recoil of the lungs and chest (Fig. 5.7.8C).
- Some of the air is likely to enter the stomach through the oesophagus. It can be easily expelled by pressure on the epigastrium.
- The above procedure is repeated 12–16 times per minute till spontaneous breathing returns, or till the patient is shifted to a hospital.

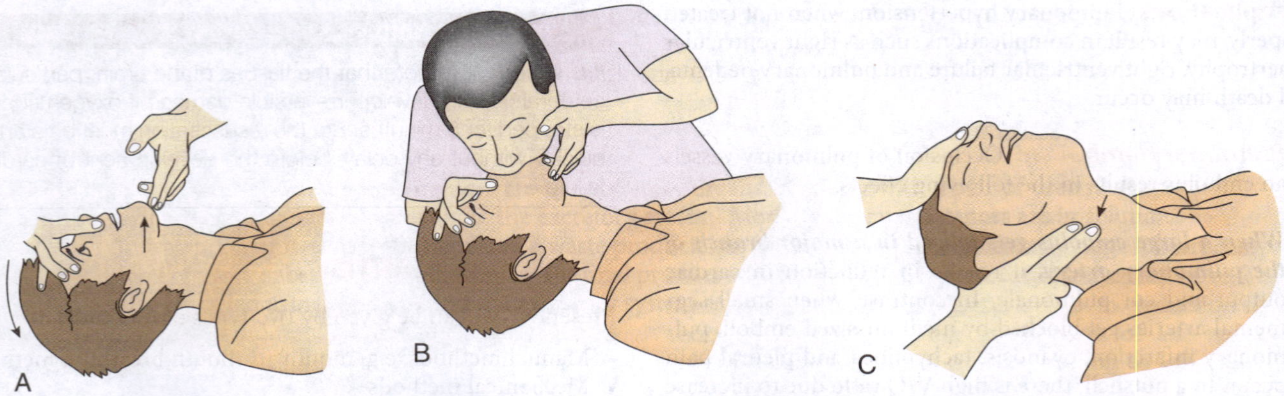

Fig. 5.7.8 Mouth-to-mouth breathing: **A**, the neck is extended by placing one hand under the neck and pressing the forehead with other hand; **B**, nostrils are closed with thumb and index finger and resuscitator exhales into the patient's airway by tightly placing his/her mouth over the patient's mouth; and **C**, the resuscitator allows the patient to exhale passively by unsealing nose and mouth.

Important Notes

It is important to remember that:

- Mouth-to-mouth method is the most effective manual method, because the CO_2 present in the expired air by the resuscitator can also directly stimulate the respiratory centres and facilitate the onset of respiration.
- The expired air by the resuscitator contains 16% oxygen which is sufficient to revive the patient.

Mechanical Methods of AR

The mechanical respirators are used when AR has to be continued for long periods. The mechanical respirators are of two types:

- Tank respirators
- Ventilators

1. Tank Respirators

Tank respirators or the so-called iron lung chambers as the name indicates consist of an airtight chamber made of iron or steel. There are various types of mechanical respirators. A commonly used respirator is the Drinker respirator. In this respirator, the patient is kept inside the tank by placing the head outside the chamber. In the Drinker method, alternate positive and negative pressure breathing machines produce periodic inflation and deflation of the lungs.

2. Ventilators

Ventilators are the AR machines by which air or oxygen is pumped into the lungs with pressure intermittently through a rubber tube introduced into the patient's trachea. Inflation occurs when air is pumped and expiration occurs by elastic recoil of the chest and lungs when it is stopped. Therefore, based on mode of ventilation, presently two types of ventilators are available:

Manual ventilator Manual ventilators include bag, valve masks and anaesthesia bags.

For operation of these bags, an operator is required to hold the ventilator onto an artificial airway and maintain breathing with his/her hands.

Mechanical ventilators Mechanical ventilators do not require operator efforts. These are either computer controlled or pneumonic controlled. Different types of mechanical ventilators are as follows:

- Transport ventilators
- Intensive care ventilators
- Neonatal ventilators
- Positive airway pressure ventilators

Mechanical mode of ventilation is of two types – positive-pressure ventilation and negative-pressure ventilation.

- *In positive-pressure ventilation*, air or gas mixture is pushed into the lungs through the trachea.
- *In negative-pressure ventilation*, air is sucked into the lungs.

Volume ventilator Volume ventilator pumps a constant volume of air into the patient's lungs intermittently with minimum pressure.

Pressure ventilator Pressure ventilator pumps the air with a constant high pressure into the patient's lungs.

CARDIOPULMONARY RESUSCITATION

Cardiopulmonary resuscitation (CPR) is an emergency procedure that combines chest compression with AV to preserve intact brain functions until further measures are taken to restore spontaneous blood circulation and breathing. It is required in some patients when both the heart and the respiration stop. Breathing usually stops before the heart stops, so AR should be started immediately. The CPR may be required in patients with:

- Ventricular fibrillation following a heart attack
- Victim of electrocution
- Drowning

Emergency plan of CPR

The following plan called ABC of CPR has proved useful in reviving such patients:

A. Airway Care

Airway care is required in unconscious patients. Immediately, tilt the head back with a hand under the neck to maintain an open airway (Fig. 5.7.8A).

B. Breathing

Breathing by the AR method is required when the patient is not breathing. Mouth-to-mouth respiration should be immediately started (see page 461). Feel carotid pulse; if present, continue AR only (Fig. 5.7.8B).

C. Cardiac Massage

Cardiac massage is required when carotid pulse cannot be felt. During external cardiac massage (procedure described below), the sternum should be depressed by 4–5 cm at a rate of 80–90 times per minute. The cardiac compression should be alternated with mouth-to-mouth respiration at a rate of one ventilation to five chest compressions (1:5).

Procedure Effective cardiac massage can be carried out without opening the chest. The person conducting external cardiac massage places the heel of one hand on the lower sternum above the xiphoid process and the heel of the other hand on top of the first (Fig. 5.7.9). Pressure is applied straight down, depressing the sternum 4 or 5 cm towards the spine. This procedure is repeated 100–110 times per minute. Manually squeezing the ventricles is also effective, if the chest is already open, but emergency thoracotomies should not be performed.

Compression/ventilation (C/V) ratio: To be followed:

In adults: C/V ratio is 30:2 when one or two rescuers are available.

In children: C/V ratio is 15:2 when only one rescuer is available.

In infants: C/V ratio should be 3:1.

Advanced Life Support

Advanced life support (ALS) includes:

Oxygen administration

ECG recording (to know the status of the heart)

Tracheostomy to maintain airway

Precautions Precautions to be taken during CPR are as follows:

- CPR must be started at the earliest, because a delay of more than 4–5 minutes may cause irreversible damage to the brain.
- The patient should not be made to sit or stand. No pillow should be put under his/her head, because it will bend the head and occlude the trachea.
- Nothing orally should be given to an unconscious person.
- The feet and legs should be raised with a pillow under the hip to improve cerebral blood flow.
- While giving cardiac massage, the pressure should not be applied over the ribs as they are likely to fracture.

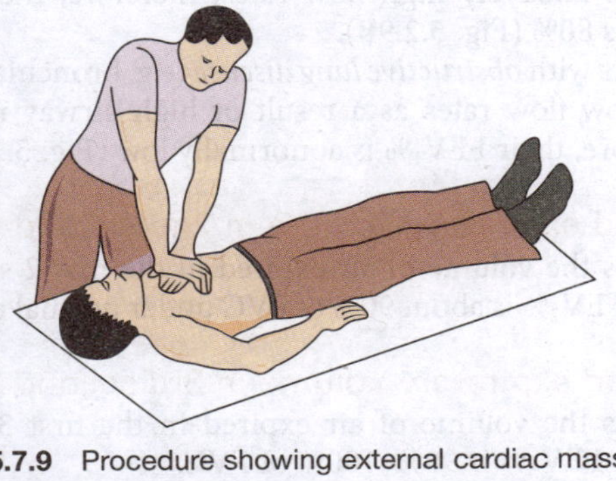

Fig. 5.7.9 Procedure showing external cardiac massage.

PULMONARY FUNCTION TESTS

ROLE OF PULMONARY FUNCTION TESTS IN CLINICAL PRACTICE

The evaluation of pulmonary function begins with a careful history taking, meticulous clinical examination and radiographs of the chest. In addition, various pulmonary function tests are used to help the clinician to make a physiological assessment of lung function rather than to make a pathological diagnosis. The roles of pulmonary function tests in clinical practice are as follows:

1. In diagnosis of pulmonary diseases, pulmonary function tests may be used:
   - For early diagnosis of a disease, e.g. decreased diffusing capacity is the earliest change seen in interstitial lung disease
   - For confirmation of clinical diagnosis
   - For exclusion of a diagnosis
2. To follow the progress of disease and its response to treatment
3. To objectively assess the severity of disease
4. To assess respiratory status before anaesthesia and also to assess the capacity of the individual to tolerate the risk of surgery, especially cardiothoracic surgery involving removal of a lung or its part
5. To assess physical fitness for certain jobs such as those involving strenuous physical exercise and flying at high altitude
6. To obtain medicolegal information in certain situations

Classification Pulmonary function tests can be classified into the following groups:

A. Ventilatory function tests
B. Tests of diffusion
C. Tests of ultimate purpose of respiration
D. Tests during exercise

VENTILATORY FUNCTION TESTS

Ventilatory function tests are meant for the assessment of the expansion of the lungs and chest wall, and for the assessment of restrictive and obstructive ventilatory defects. The assessment of ventilatory functions can be accomplished by:

I. Measurement of various lung volume and capacities
II. Measurement of dead space
III. Measurement of compliance
IV. Measurement of airway resistance

Measurement of Various Lung Volumes and Capacities

Various lung volumes and capacities have been described on page 390. Most of the lung volumes and capacities except RV, FRC and TLC can be measured by spirometry. FRC is determined by nitrogen wash-out method or helium dilution method, and then RV and TLC are calculated.

Spirometry Spirometry refers to recording of volume changes during various clearly defined breathing manoeuvres. It can be performed using a simple spirometer, a modified spirometer called respirometer or computerized spirometer.

Simple spirometer Simple spirometer (Fig. 5.7.10) is made of metal. It consists of the following parts:

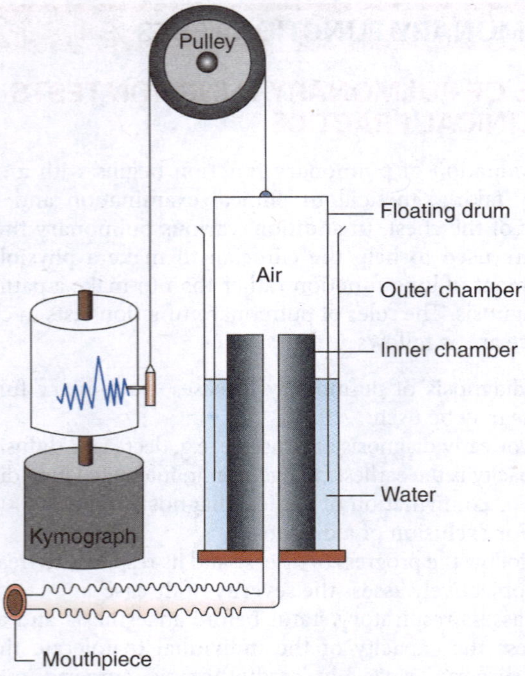

Fig. 5.7.10 Simple spirometer.

Outer chamber or container is filled with water.
Floating drum or a gas bell with 6-L capacity floats in the water in an inverted manner. It is attached to a chain which passes over a pulley bearing a balancing weight and a writing needle (pen). The needle (pen) moves with the movement of the floating drum. The floating drum is thus counterpoised and has very little inertia and friction.
Inner chamber is open at the top end which lies above the water level in outer chamber and is connected to a tube at the bottom end. At the end of the tube, a mouthpiece is attached through which the subject is made to respire.
Kymograph is a recording drum on which the movements of the needle are recorded.

Procedure The whole procedure is explained to the subject thoroughly and then he/she is made to breathe through the mouthpiece of the spirometer. As explained above and shown in Fig. 5.7.10, the arrangement in spirometer is such that when the subject expires, the floating drum (gas bell) moves up and the counterweight along with writing needle (pen) moves down, and thus the expiration is recorded as downward deflection on the kymograph. Conversely, when the subject inspires, the floating drum moves down and the counterweight with writing pen moves up, and thus the inspiration is recorded as an upward deflection on the kymograph. The record of various lung volumes and capacities so obtained on the kymograph is called spirogram.

To measure the various lung volumes and capacities, the subject is instructed to expire or inspire as described:

- First, he/she is asked to breathe normally (tidal respiration) for a few times.
- Then he/she is asked to inspire as deeply and fully as possible.
- Thus, while keeping the nostrils closed with his/her thumb and index finger, he/she is asked to expire with a maximum effort. It is preferable to take three recordings, at intervals of 5 minutes, for each determination. The maximum volume of the three readings should be considered the reporting value. The various lung volumes and capacities are then calculated from the record (spirogram so obtained) (see page 390; Fig. 5.2.6) which in general give information about the ventilatory functions.

The various static and dynamic lung volumes and capacities which serve as more useful pulmonary function tests are as follows:

1. Vital Capacity

Measurement of VC under different conditions is the most commonly performed pulmonary function test.

Slow vital capacity Slow VC is the volume of air expired (after maximum inspiration) during a slowly performed maximum expiratory effort. It is used to evaluate the size of the lungs (see Fig. 5.2.6). The VC can be decreased either by decrease in TLC as seen in restrictive lung disease or by increase in reserve volume as seen in obstructive lung disease.

Forced vital capacity FVC (or TVC) is the volume of air that can be expired rapidly with a maximal expiratory effort after a maximal inspiration.
FVC is reduced in:

- *Conditions producing restrictive defect*, such as kyphoscoliosis, pleural effusion and pneumonia
- *Conditions producing trapping of air* due to collapse of distal air during a forced expiratory manoeuvre

Components of FVC The volume of air expired can be timed by recording the FVC on a spirograph moving at the known speed. From the graph so obtained (Fig. 5.2.8), the FVC can be divided into the following components:

I. Forced expiratory volume in 1st second (FEV_1)

- FEV_1 is the volume of air expired during the 1st second of FVC.
- It is the most commonly used screening test for airway diseases.
- The FEV_1 is actually a flow rate; its unit is litre per second.
- FEV_1% is the percentage of VC expired in 1 second, i.e. $FEV_1\% = FEV_1/(FVC \times 100)$, normally FEV_1% or about 80% of the FVC (Fig. 5.2.9A).

Clinical application: useful in distinguishing between restrictive and obstructive lung diseases

- Patients with *restrictive lung disease* (e.g. kyphoscoliosis and ankylosing spondylitis) have a reduced FVC but are able to achieve relatively high flow rates; therefore, their FEV_1% exceeds 80% (Fig. 5.2.9B).
- Patients with *obstructive lung disease* (e.g. bronchial asthma) have low flow rates as a result of high airway resistance; therefore, their FEV_1% is abnormally low (Fig. 5.2.9C).

II. Forced expiratory volume in 2nd second (FEV_2) It represents the volume of air expired in the first 2 seconds of an FVC; FEV_2% is about 90% of FVC under normal condition.

III. Forced expiratory volume in 3rd second (FEV_3) It represents the volume of air expired in the first 3 seconds. Normally FEV_3% is 98%–100% of FVC.

Flow–volume curve The rate of airflow noted during maximum expiration can be plotted versus volume change to give a flow–volume curve (Fig. 5.7.11). This curve may be altered dramatically in obstructive and restrictive diseases. However, due to technical problems, flow–volume curve is not routinely plotted in clinical respiratory laboratories.

Flow–volume loop Flow–volume loop is a relationship between volume and flow during maximum inspiratory and expiratory efforts, which can be recorded with recent computerized recorders for ventilatory function. The normal pattern of pressure–volume loop is a 'triangle sitting on a semicircle' (Fig. 5.7.12).

Clinical significance of flow–volume loop During expiration, depending on the mechanical properties of the lung and resistance to airflow, the flow is effort dependent in early part but, in later part, it is effort independent. Therefore:

- In case of airflow obstruction, the flow rate at any given volume is decreased, particularly in later part of expiration, and the expiratory curve has a scooped-out appearance (Fig. 5.7.13). Therefore, in obstructive lung disease, an abnormal flow–volume loop may appear before any abnormality is appreciated in FEV_1/FEV or forced expiratory flow rate during 25%–75% of expiration ($FEF_{25\%–75\%}$).

2. Forced Expiratory Flow Rate During 25%–75% of Expiration

- It is the mean expiratory flow rate during middle 50% of FVC (Fig. 5.2.10A), and so is also called the mid-expiratory flow rate.
- This measurement can be done from the same record as FEV_1. The total expired volume is divided into four equal parts. The flow rate is calculated for the middle two parts (25%–75%), i.e. the middle half.
- Mid-expiratory time (MET) refers to the time taken for $FEF_{25\%–75\%}$. Its normal value is 0.5 second which is increased in obstructive lung disorders. It may be the only abnormality indicating early disease in smokers with COPD.

3. Peak Expiratory Flow Rate

Park expiratory flow rate (PEFR) refers to the maximum rate of airflow observed during a sudden forced expiration, from the position of full inspiration. It can be measured by a simple device known as peak flow meter (Fig. 5.7.14) which can be used by the patients even at home. The best of three efforts should be noted as the value of PEFR. It is a good and reproducible measure of degree of airflow obstruction.

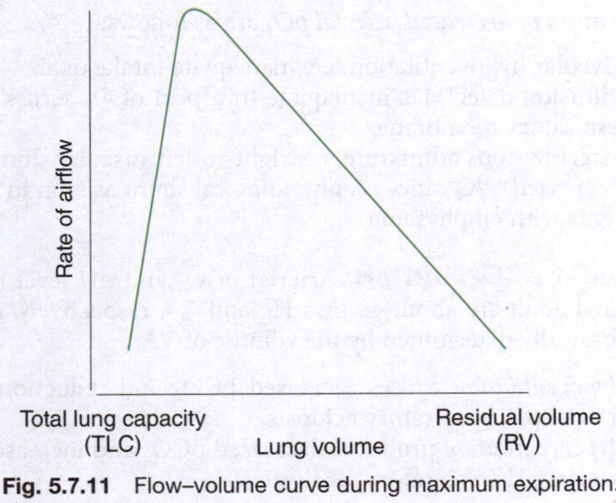

Fig. 5.7.11 Flow–volume curve during maximum expiration.

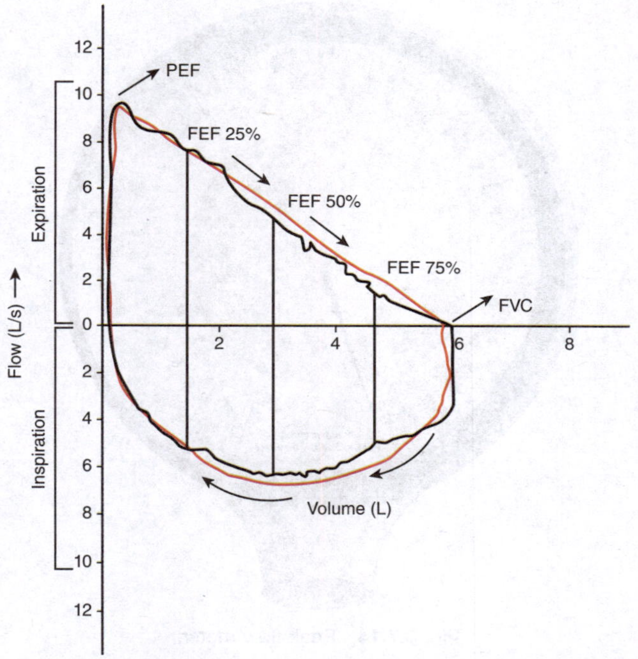

Fig. 5.7.12 Computerised recording of flow–volume curve during inspiration and expiration.

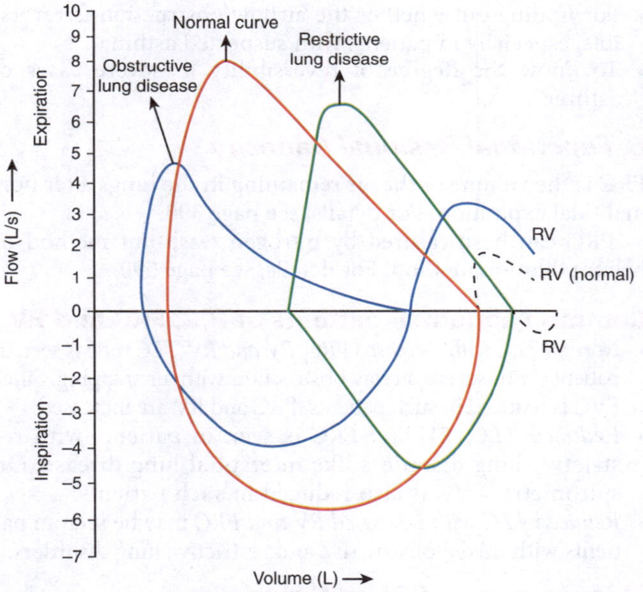

Fig. 5.7.13 Computerised recording of flow–volume loop in restrictive and obstructive lung diseases in comparison to normal.

4. Maximum Breathing Capacity (MBC) or Maximum Voluntary Ventilation (MVV)

For details, see page 393.

5. Spirometric Response to Inhaled Bronchodilators

In this test, forced expirogram is recorded before and 10–20 minutes after inhalation of two puffs of salbutamol

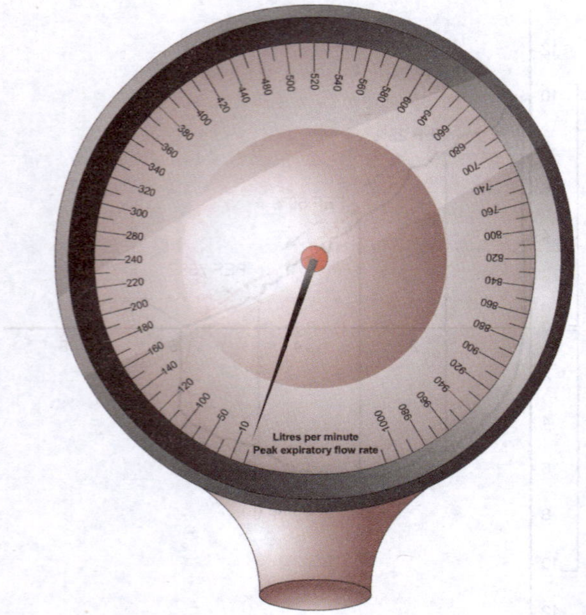

Fig. 5.7.14 Peak flow meter.

inhaler (separated by 30- to 60-second interval). Each puff delivers 100 µg of bronchodilator. Test is used:

- For finding out whether the airflow obstruction is reversible, especially in patients with suspected asthma
- To know the degree of reversibility in severe cases of asthma

6. Functional Residual Capacity

FRC is the volume of the air remaining in the lungs after normal tidal expiration. For details, see page 390.

FRC can be measured by nitrogen wash-out method or helium dilution method. For details, see page 390.

Common abnormal patterns of TLC, FRC and RV

- *Normal TLC with increased FRC, RV and RV/TLC ratio* is seen in patients with severe airway obstruction with air trapping. Since FVC is reduced in such patients, FRC and RV are increased.
- *Reduced TLC, RV and FRC* is seen in patients with restrictive lung disorders like interstitial lung disease. On spirometry, FVC is also reduced in such patients.
- *Reduced TLC with increased RV and FRC* may be seen in patients with mixed obstructive and restrictive lung disorders.

Measurement of Dead Space

Dead space air is the portion of minute ventilation that does not take part in exchange of gases. Normally, it is constituted by the air present in the conducting zone of respiratory passages (*anatomical dead space*), but in some diseases may additionally include also poorly perfused alveoli (physiological dead space). For details, see page 410.

Measurement of Compliance

Compliance (*C*) expresses the distensibility (expansibility) of the lungs and chest wall. Reduced compliance produces a condition called restrictive lung disease. In clinical testing, the restrictive lung diseases are evaluated indirectly by measurement of various lung volumes and capacities as described above. Thus, direct measurement of compliance in the respiratory system is rarely done for clinical use; however, it may be required for research purposes. For details, see page 396.

Measurement of Airway Resistance

Airway resistance is the resistance caused by friction of gas molecules between themselves and the walls of the airways. It is increased in many obstructive lung diseases. Like compliance, airway resistance is also seldom measured directly for clinical use. However, it may be required for research purposes (for details, see page 398).

TESTS OF DIFFUSION

Pulmonary diffusion refers to transfer of gases from alveoli to capillary blood across the respiratory membrane. The exchange of gases in the lungs was earlier believed to be dependent merely on the ability of the gases to diffuse across the respiratory membrane. This term led to the use of the term *diffusion capacity*. However, later it was realized that many other factors like V/Q balance, pulmonary capillary blood volume, Hb concentration of the blood and rate of reaction of gases with Hb are also involved in the exchange of gases. Therefore, nowadays, the term *transfer factor*, rather than diffusion capacity, is used.

For estimation of transfer factor (diffusion capacity) of O_2, see page 417.

TESTS OF ULTIMATE PURPOSE OF RESPIRATION

Since the ultimate purpose of respiration is to supply O_2 from the atmosphere to the tissues and removal of CO_2 from the tissues into the atmosphere, the estimation of arterial blood pO_2, pCO_2 and pH (blood gas analysis) is most fundamental of all the pulmonary function tests.

Estimation of Arterial pO_2, pCO_2 and pH

For blood gas analysis, arterial blood sample is usually taken from the radial artery or femoral artery. The estimation of pO_2, pCO_2 and pH can be done within a minute or so using a very small sample of blood with the help of miniaturized glass electrodes.

Arterial pO_2 Arterial pO_2 levels in a young healthy adult vary from 85 to 105 mm Hg with a mean of 95 mm Hg. The value may drop by up to 15% in healthy elderly subjects due to an increase in V/Q inequality.

Causes of decreased arterial pO_2 are as follows:

- Alveolar hypoventilation, i.e. inadequate intake of air
- Diffusion defect, i.e. inadequate transport of O_2 across the respiratory membrane
- Arteriovenous admixture, i.e. right-to-left vascular shunt
- Decreased V/Q ratio, i.e. physiological shunt as seen in patients with emphysema

Arterial pCO_2 and pH Arterial pCO_2 and pH level in a normal adult are about 40 mm Hg and 7.4, respectively, and are basically determined by the volume of VA:

- *Hypoventilation* causes increased pCO_2 and reduction in arterial pH (respiratory acidosis).
- *Hyperventilation* produces decreased pCO_2 and increase in arterial pH (respiratory alkalosis).

TESTS DURING EXERCISE

Because of enormous physiological reserves, both the cardiac and pulmonary functions may be normal at rest in early stages of the disease. Exercise testing provides information about the total cardiopulmonary performance of the individual and unmasks the abnormality not detected by the function tests performed at rest. The exercise may be performed on a treadmill or a cycle ergometer. Measurement of pulse rate, minute ventilation, O_2 uptake and arterial blood gas tension during graded exercise is extremely useful especially when the cause of dyspnoea is obscure.

Self-Assessment

1. Discuss the causes, types and characteristics of different types of hypoxia.
2. Discuss the physiological compensatory responses to chronic hypoxia.
3. Discuss the physiological basis of oxygen therapy in hypoxia.
4. Discuss the pathophysiology of chronic obstructive lung disease.
5. Describe the causes and clinical stages of asphyxia.
6. Discuss the clinical significance of ventilatory function tests.
7. Describe the following:
   - Sleep apnoea syndrome
   - Periodic breathing
   - Oxygen toxicity
   - Carbon monoxide poisoning
   - Cardiopulmonary resuscitation
8. Write notes on:
   - Drowning
   - Pneumothorax
   - Pulmonary embolism
   - Pulmonary hypertension

Clinical Cases

Case 1

A 25-year-old female presented with breathlessness, palpitation and tightness in the chest.

Examination and laboratory tests revealed cyanosed lips and tongue, heart rate 120/min, respiratory rate 30/min, BP 84/50 mm Hg, Hb 8 g% and RBC count 2.8 million/mm^3.

Q1. What is the probable cause for cyanosis?
Q2. What other tests should be advised in this case to reach the final diagnosis?
Q3. What is the physiological basis for cyanosis?
Q4. What immediate measures should be taken to relieve breathlessness?
Q5. Oxygen therapy should be helpful in this case. Explain.

Case 2

An 18-year-old female was transferred from a local hospital to a tertiary care centre for treatment of shortness of breath and dyspnoea.

On examination, the heart rate was 110 beats/min, BP 98/60 mm Hg and respiratory rate 26/min.

Auscultation of the chest revealed heavy second heart sound and bilateral basilar crackling.

Ankle oedema and hepatomegaly were present.

Q1. The patient is suffering from which type of hypoxia?
Q2. Oxygen therapy will be useful in this case. Yes/no?
Q3. If yes, which type of oxygen therapy should be given and why? Explain.

Case 3

A 27-year-old obese man was referred to a sleep clinic due to loud snoring, daytime sleepiness and spells of apnoea, and was diagnosed a case of sleep apnoea syndrome.

Q1. What tests should be done for clinical diagnosis of sleep apnoea syndrome?
Q2. Which clinical condition can cause sleep apnoea?
Q3. What are the risks of sleep apnoea?
Q4. How can sleep apnoea be treated?

Case 4

A 60-year-old patient with diabetes presented with gasping breath, loss of appetite, excessive thirst and fruity smelling breath.

Q1. What is the cause of these signs and symptoms in this case?
Q2. What treatment should be given?
Q3. If not treated timely, what complications can occur?

Case 5

A 56-year-old male working in a plastic factory entrapped in factory building fire was brought to the emergency with difficulty in breathing, vomiting, severe headache and flushing of the face and in a confused state, and provisionally diagnosed a case of cyanide poisoning.

Q1. What will be the expected results of arterial blood gas analysis in this case?
Q2. The patient is suffering with which type of hypoxia?
Q3. Will oxygen therapy be helpful or not? Give explanation for both the situations.

Case 6

A 35-year-old traffic policeman presented with sudden attack of difficulty in breathing and tightness in the chest. There was a history of smoking for more than 10 years and the patient usually had difficulty in breathing, particularly in cold and dusty weather.

On chest auscultation, rhonchi were heard all over the chest.

Spirometry revealed normal vital capacity and reduced FEV_1 (<60%).

Q1. What is the probable diagnosis?
Q2. Why is FEV_1 reduced in this condition?
Q3. What is the pathophysiology of the condition?

Case 7

A 50-year-old man while walking on river bank in winter slipped into the river and was rescued and brought to emergency department. The presenting signs and symptoms were hypothermia, dyspnoea, respiratory rate 25 breaths/min, heart rate 60/min and BP 90/64 mm Hg. Chest auscultation showed wheezing all over the chest.

Q1. What first aid treatment should be given to a patient of drowning?
Q2. What is the common cause of death in drowning?
Q3. What is the difference between fresh water drowning and sea water drowning?

EXCRETORY SYSTEM

SECTION 6

SECTION OUTLINE

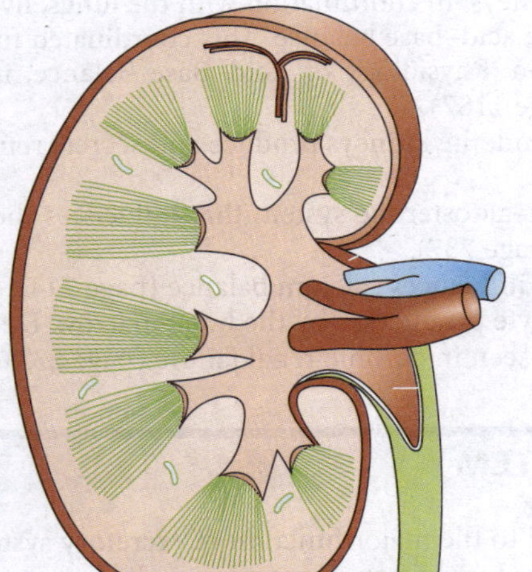

INTRODUCTION

CONCEPT OF EXCRETORY SYSTEM

Excretion

Literally, the word excretion means elimination of any matter from the body of an organism. The organs that are involved in the process of excretion include:

- *Kidneys*, which excrete water and water-soluble waste products
- *Lungs*, which excrete carbon dioxide, water vapour and other volatile substances such as acetone
- *Skin*, which excretes water and salts mainly in the form of sweat
- *Gastrointestinal tract*, which excretes faeces (excreta)

However, *sensu stricto*, the term excretion refers to elimination of principal products of metabolism except carbon dioxide. The principal products of metabolism, other than carbon dioxide, are ammonia, urea, uric acid, creatinine, various pigments and inorganic salts. Of these, carbon dioxide is a universal metabolic waste which is discharged by the respiratory organs. The remaining excretory substances, in bulk, are excreted by the kidneys. Small quantities of some of the excretory substances are also eliminated by the skin.

Excretory Organs

Thus, in the strictest sense, kidneys are the excretory organs. Together with a pair of ureters and a urinary bladder, kidneys constitute the excretory system. Most excretory substances are in solution in water. Water itself is not considered a waste product, but any excess of it is eliminated along with the excretory substances dissolved in it. The final product is called urine. Therefore, the kidneys may also be called urinary organs and the excretory system as urinary system.

FUNCTIONS OF EXCRETORY ORGANS

Excretory organs, i.e. the kidneys, serve several major functions:

1. *Excretory function:* As mentioned above, the kidneys excrete a number of end products of metabolism in urine. Thus, formation of urine is the major function of the kidneys. The kidneys eliminate these substances from the body at a rate that matches their production. Thus, they regulate their concentration within the body fluids. In addition to the metabolic wastes, they also excrete foreign substances from the body, such as drugs, pesticides and other chemicals ingested in food.
2. *Regulation of water and inorganic ion balance:* Control of volume of body fluids and their inorganic ion balance is an important homeostatic role of the kidneys. The kidneys accomplish this task by working in concert with components of cardiovascular system, endocrine system and central nervous system. Therefore, it has been discussed in the chapter on 'Regulation of Body Fluid, Osmolality, Composition and Volume' on page 519.
3. *Regulation of acid–base balance:* The kidneys, in coordination with the lungs, liver and buffers in the body, play a role in regulation of the acid–base balance. This coordinated function has been discussed in a separate Chapter 12.3 on 'Physiology of Acid–Base Balance', in Section 12 on 'Specialized Integrative Physiology' (page 1187).
4. *Hormonal function:* As an endocrine gland, the kidneys produce and secrete renin, calcitriol and erythropoietin.
   - *Renin* activates the renin–angiotensin–aldosterone system that influences the blood pressure and sodium and potassium balance (page 737).
   - *Calcitriol* (1,25-dihydroxyvitamin D_3) influences calcium balance (page 714).
   - *Erythropoietin* stimulates the erythrocyte production by the bone marrow. Decreased erythrocyte production is a cause of anaemia seen in chronic renal failure (page 533).

OVERVIEW OF EXCRETORY SYSTEM

This section on excretory system is devoted to the major function of excretory system – the formation of urine and physiology of micturition. In addition, important applied aspects have also been included. This section begins with a chapter on 'functional anatomy of kidneys and renal blood flow', which is mandatory to understand renal physiology.

Kidneys: Functional Anatomy and Blood Flow

6.1

CHAPTER OUTLINE

FUNCTIONAL ANATOMY OF KIDNEYS

GROSS ANATOMY

External Features

Gross anatomical features of a human kidney, illustrated in Fig. 6.1.1A, are as follows.

Location The kidneys are bean-shaped organs that lie retroperitoneally on the posterior abdominal wall, one on each side of the vertebral column at the level of T_{12} to L_1 vertebrae. The right kidney lies slightly inferior to the left kidney.

Size and shape During life, the kidneys are reddish-brown in colour. Each kidney in an adult human weighs about 150 g and measures approximately 10 cm in length, 5 cm in width and 2.5 cm in thickness.

Surface, borders and poles Each kidney has anterior and posterior surfaces, medial and lateral margins, and superior and inferior poles. The lateral margin is convex and the medial margin is concave, where the renal sinus and renal pelvis are located.

Renal hilum and sinus The renal hilum is a vertical cleft present on the concave medial margin. It is the entrance to space within the kidney – the renal sinus. Through the renal hilum, the renal artery enters and the renal vein and renal pelvis leave the renal sinus. The *renal sinus* is thus occupied by the renal pelvis, calyces, vessels, nerves and a variable amount of fat.

Renal pelvis and calyces The renal pelvis is the flattened, funnel-shaped expansion of the superior end of the ureter. Within the renal sinus, the pelvis divides into two (or three) parts called *major calyces.* Each major calyx divides into a number of *minor calyces.* The end of each minor calyx is shaped like a cup into which fits a projection of kidney tissue called renal papilla (the apex of renal pyramid).

Gross Internal Structure

Gross internal structure of the kidney, as seen in coronal section through the organ, exhibits that kidney tissue consists of an outer region called the cortex and an inner region called the medulla (Fig. 6.1.1B).

Medulla It is made up of triangular areas of renal tissue that are called the renal pyramids. Pyramids are 4–14 in number and separated from each other by cortical columns of Bertin. Each pyramid has a base directed towards the cortex, and an apex (or renal papilla) which is directed towards the renal pelvis and fits into the minor calyx. Pyramids show striations that pass radially towards the apex. These striations are due to straight portion of the nephron and extend some distance

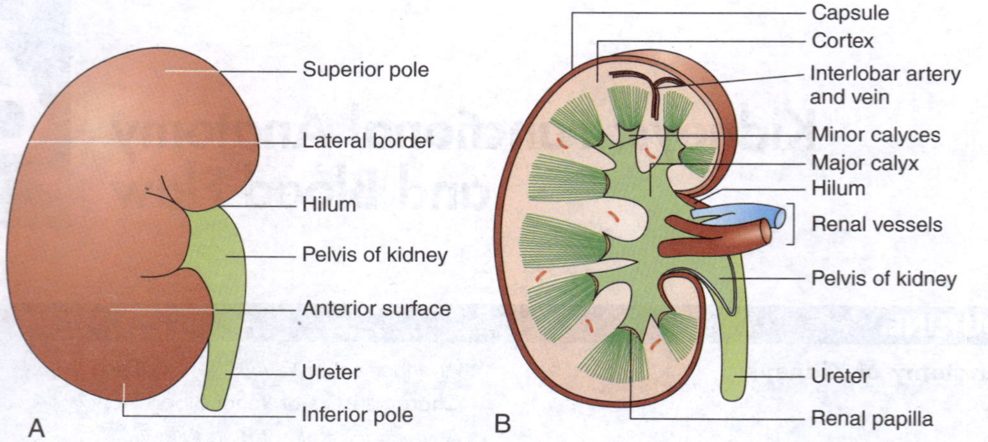

Fig. 6.1.1 **A**, Gross anatomical features; and **B**, coronal section through human kidney.

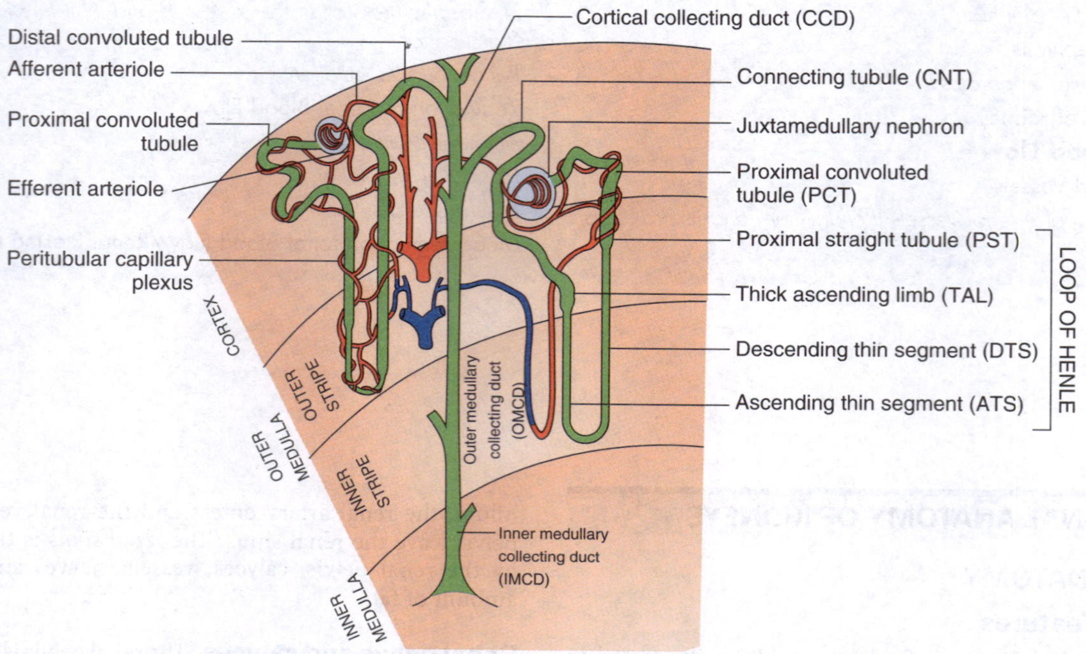

Fig. 6.1.2 Part of a typical nephron. Organization of cortical and juxtamedullary nephrons showing different parts. Note the differences between two types of nephrons.

upwards into the cortex where they are called medullary rays. The medulla can be subdivided into two parts:

Outer medulla is further subdivided into the outer stripe and the inner stripe.

Inner medulla is also called papillary zone.

Cortex The renal cortex can be divided into two parts which are continuous with each other:

Cortical arches or cortical lobules refer to the tissue lying between the bases of pyramids and the surface of the kidney.

Renal columns *refer* to the cortical tissue that lies in between the pyramids.

Lobe of kidney: Each pyramid, surrounded by a shell of cortex, constitutes a lobe of the kidney. This lobulation is obvious in the fetal kidney.

MICROSCOPIC STRUCTURE OF KIDNEY

Microscopically, the cortex and medulla of the kidney are composed of nephrons, blood vessels, lymphatics and nerves.

Nephron is a structural and functional unit of the kidney. Each kidney contains approximately 1.2 million nephrons. Each nephron is capable of forming urine.

Structure of the Nephron

A nephron consists of two major parts (Fig. 6.1.2):

- Renal corpuscle
- Renal tubule

Renal Corpuscle

Renal corpuscle or Malpighian corpuscle is a rounded structure comprising glomerulus surrounded by glomerular capsule (Fig. 6.1.3A).

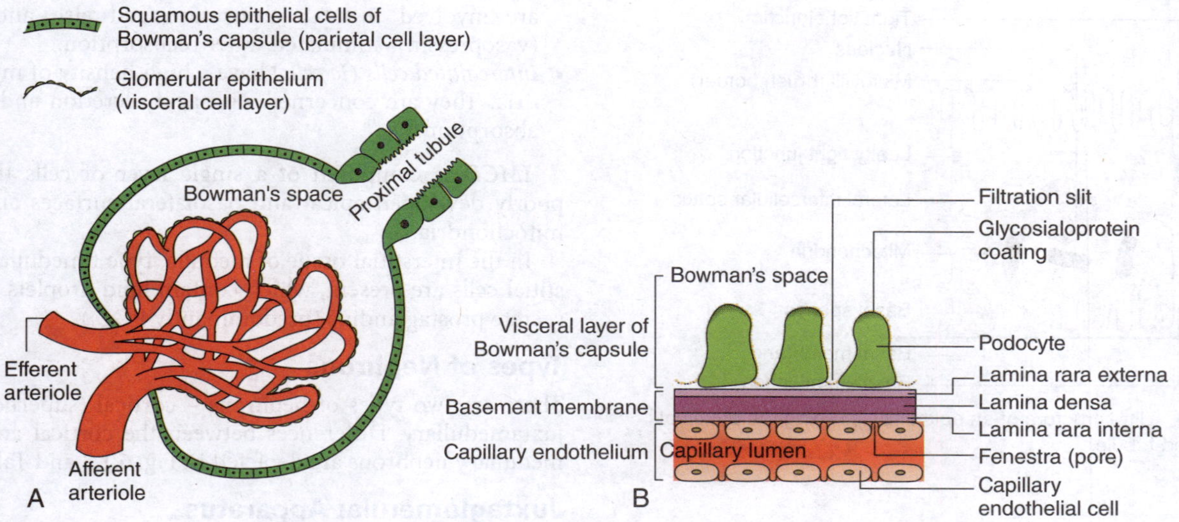

Fig. 6.1.3 **A**, Structure of a glomerulus; and **B**, glomerular membrane.

Glomerulus refers to a rounded tuft of anastomosing capillaries about 200 μm in diameter. Blood enters the glomerulus through an *afferent arteriole* and leaves it through an *efferent arteriole* (note that the efferent vessel is an arteriole and not a venule). The afferent and efferent arterioles lie close together at a point that is referred to as the *vascular* pole of the renal corpuscle.

Glomerular capsule also known as Bowman's capsule, encloses the glomerulus and is formed of two layers – the inner layer covering the glomerular capillaries is called *visceral layer*, and the outer layer is called *parietal layer*. In fact, the Bowman's capsule represents the cup-shaped blind beginning of the renal tubule. The space between the visceral and parietal layers of the capsule (called Bowman's space or urinary space) is continuous with the lumen of the renal tubule.

Ultrastructure of glomerular membrane refers to the membrane that separates blood of glomerular capillaries from the fluid present in the Bowman's space. It is also called *filtration barrier* and consists of three major layers (Fig. 6.1.3B):

1. ***Capillary endothelium*** is fenestrated (i.e. it contains pores with diameter 70–90 nm) and is freely permeable to water, small solutes and even small proteins.
2. ***Basement membrane*** consists of a matrix of glycoproteins and mucopolysaccharides. Compared with typical membranes, the glomerular basement membrane is very thick. It comprises three layers:
   - *Lamina rara externa or outer cement layer*
   - *Lamina densa*
   - *Lamina rara interna*

   No pores have been demonstrated in the basement membrane; however, its permeability corresponds to pore size (of about 8 nm).
3. ***Bowman's visceral epithelium*** or the inner layer of Bowman's capsule, which forms the third layer of glomerular membrane, is formed by special cells called *podocytes*.

Podocytes have finger-like processes that encircle the outer surface of capillaries. The processes of podocytes interdigitate to cover the basement membrane and are separated by gaps called the *filtration slits* (~25 nm diameter). Each filtration slit is covered by a layer of fine filaments that constitute the diaphragm.

Mesangium is an important component of renal corpuscle; it consists of mesangium cells that are present between the capillary endothelial cells and the basement membrane, especially where the basement membrane encloses more than one capillary. These cells provide structural support for the glomerular capillaries, secrete the extracellular matrix and exhibit phagocytic activity.

Renal Tubule

Renal tubule is a long complicated tubule, which is divisible into the following main parts (Fig. 6.1.2), and is about 15 mm long and 55 μm in diameter:

1. ***Proximal tubule*** initially forms several coils, *proximal convoluted tubule (PCT)*, followed by a straight segment, *proximal straight tubule (PST)* or *pars recta* that descends towards the medulla.
2. ***Intermediate tubule or loop of Henle*** consists of:
   - *Descending thin segment (DTS)*
   - *Ascending thin segment (ATS)*
   - *Thick ascending limb (TAL)*

   In juxtamedullary nephrons, the DTS joins ATS to form the hairpin band (loop). The ATS reaches up to the junction of outer and inner medulla. In *cortical nephrons*, there is no ATS; the DTS is continuous at the bend of loop with the TAL. Near the end of TAL, the nephron passes between its afferent and efferent arterioles. This short segment of the TAL is called the *macula densa*.
3. ***Distal convoluted tubule (DCT)*** is about 5 mm long. It begins a short distance beyond the macula densa and extends to a point in the cortex where the connecting tubules (CNT) of two or more nephrons join to form the cortical collecting ducts (CCDs).
4. ***Collecting duct*** is about 20 mm long which passes through the renal cortex and medulla. The collecting duct, strictly

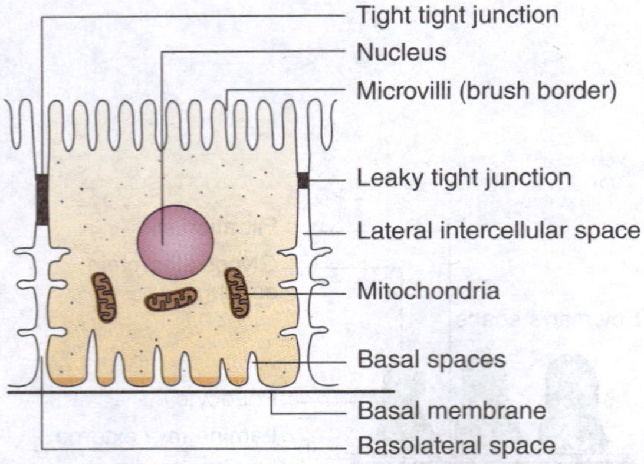

Fig. 6.1.4 Ultrastructure of an epithelial cell lining the proximal convoluted tubule.

speaking, is not a part of the nephron, since embryologically it is derived from the ureteric buds. It is divisible into three parts:

- *CCD*, i.e. the portion present in the cortex
- *Outer medullary collecting duct* (*OMCD*), i.e. the portion present in the outer medulla
- *Inner medullary collecting duct (IMCD)*, i.e. the portion present in the inner medulla (several IMCDs coalesce together before finally opening at the tip of the renal papilla)

Characteristics of epithelium lining the renal tubule The epithelium lining the different segments of renal tubule has some special characteristic features which are suited to perform specific transport functions (Figs 6.1.2 and 6.1.4).

Type of cells The cells lining the renal tubule are mostly cuboidal, except in the thin segment where these are flat or squamous type.

Apical surface Apical surface of cuboidal cells bears a few microvilli in general, which are numerous, dense and amplified in proximal tubule cells to form the so-called brush border.

Basolateral membrane Basolateral membrane of the PCT cells, thick ascending segment cells and DCT cells is highly invaginated and contains many mitochondria. These infoldings create basal spaces. In contrast, the cells of descending thin limb and ascending thin limb of loop of Henle have poorly developed basolateral surfaces and contain a few mitochondria.

Lateral surfaces Lateral surfaces of the cells of renal tubules bear the lateral cell process which interdigitate with lateral processes of the adjacent cells. *Lateral intercellular* spaces are present in between the interdigitations. They do not communicate with the basal spaces. The lateral surfaces of cells form two types of tight junctions:

Leaky tight junctions permit water and solutes to diffuse across them. These are present in the *proximal tubule*.
Tight tight junctions do not permit water and solutes to diffuse across them easily. They are present in the *distal tubule*.

CCD is composed of two cell types:

- *Principal cells (P cells)* have a moderately invaginated basolateral membrane and contain few mitochondria. They are involved in Na^+ absorption and also antidiuretic (vasopressin)–stimulated water reabsorption.
- *Intercalated cells (Ic cells)* have a high density of mitochondria. They are concerned with acid secretion and HCO_3^- absorption.

IMCD is composed of a single layer of cells that have poorly developed apical and basolateral surfaces and a few mitochondria.

In the interstitial tissue of medulla, type I medullary interstitial cells are present, which contain lipid droplets and also secrete prostaglandins (predominantly PGE_2).

Types of Nephrons

There are two types of nephrons – cortical (superficial) and juxtamedullary. Differences between the cortical and juxtamedullary nephrons are depicted in Fig. 6.1.2 and Table 6.1.1.

Juxtaglomerular Apparatus

Juxtaglomerular (JG) apparatus, as the name indicates (juxta – near), refers to collection of specialized cells located very near to the glomerulus. It forms the major component of renin–angiotensin–aldosterone system The JG apparatus comprises three types of cells (Fig. 6.1.5):

- JG cells
- Macula densa cells
- Mesangial cells

1. Juxtaglomerular cells JG cells are specialized *myoepithelial* (modified vascular smooth muscle) cells located in the media of the *afferent arteriole* in the region of JG apparatus.

Table 6.1.1 Differences between cortical and juxtamedullary nephrons

Features	Cortical nephron	Juxtamedullary nephron
• Location of glomerulus	Upper region of cortex	Near junction of cortex and medulla
• Percentage of total nephron	85	15
• Size of glomeruli	Small	Larger
• Size of loop of Henle	Small, extends up to outer layer of medulla	Large, extends deep into the medulla
• Descending limb of loop of Henle comprises	Thin segment	Thin segment
• Ascending limb of loop of Henle comprises	Thick segment	Thin segment
• Efferent arterioles	Have large diameter, and break up into peritubular capillaries	Have small diameter and continue as vasa recta
• Rate of filtration	Slow	High
• Major function	Excretion of waste products in urine	Concentration of urine by counter-current system

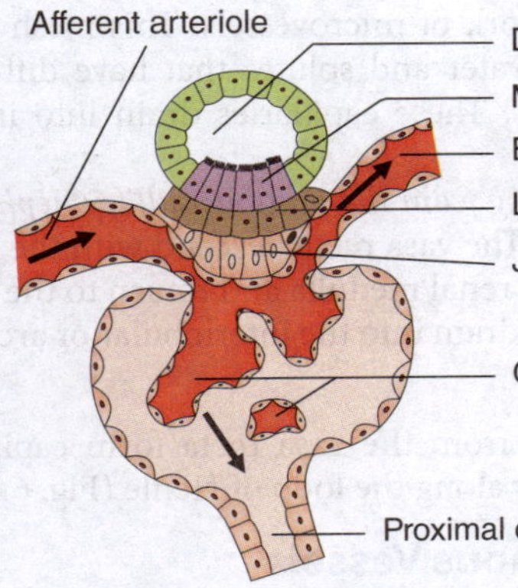

Fig. 6.1.5 Juxtaglomerular apparatus.

Characteristic features Characteristic features of JG cells are as follows:

- They have well-developed Golgi apparatus and endoplasmic reticulum, abundant mitochondria and ribosomes.
- They synthesize, store and release an enzyme called *renin*. Renin is stored in the secretory granules of JG cells and, therefore, these are also called *granular cells*.
- They act as *baroreceptors* (tension receptors) and respond to changes in the transmural pressure gradient between the afferent arterioles and the interstitium.
- They are densely innervated by *sympathetic nerve* fibres and release their renin content in response to sympathetic discharge.
- As these cells act as vascular volume receptors, they monitor renal perfusion pressure and are stimulated by hypovolaemia or decreased renal perfusion pressure. The granulation of these cells increases when there is sustained hypotension in afferent arteriole, in sodium deficiency.

2. Macula densa cells Macula densa cells refer to the specialized renal tubular epithelial cells of a short segment of the TAL of loop of Henle which passes between the afferent and efferent arterioles supplying its glomerulus of origin.

Characteristic features Characteristic features of macula densa cells are as follows:

- They are not well adapted for reabsorption.
- They are not innervated.
- They have prominent nuclei, and their Golgi complex is usually located between the nucleus and the cell base (i.e. towards the afferent arteriole), whereas in other tubular cells, the Golgi complex is located near the apical membrane. These characteristics suggest that these cells may be secreting a substance towards the arteriole.
- These cells are in direct contact with the mesangial cells and in close contact with the JG cells.
- They act as chemoreceptors, are stimulated by decreased NaCl concentration and cause increased renin release.

3. Mesangial cells Mesangial cells or *lacis* cells are the interstitial cells of the JG apparatus.

Characteristic features Characteristic features of these cells are as follows:

- They are in contact with both the macula densa cells (on one side) and the JG cells (on the other side).
- Structurally, these cells act as supporting cells and plugging device at the glomerular entrance.
- Functionally, these cells possibly relay the signals from macula densa to granular cells after modulating the signals. In this way, a decreased intraluminal Na^+ load, Cl^- load or both in the region of macula densa stimulates the JG cells to secrete renin.
- They also show granulation to secrete renin in conditions of extreme hyperactivity.
- They also secrete various substances and take up immune complexes.

INNERVATION OF KIDNEY

Renal vessels are innervated by sympathetic and parasympathetic fibres.

Parasympathetic innervation Parasympathetic innervation is by vagus nerve, but its function is uncertain.

Sympathetic innervation Preganglionic sympathetic fibres arise from the neurons of lower thoracic and upper lumbar (T_{10}–L_2) intermediolateral segments of the spinal cord. The cell bodies of the postganglionic neurons are located in the ganglia of sympathetic chain and superior mesenteric ganglion. The fibres from these neurons are carried by the renal nerves, which travel along the renal blood vessels as they enter the kidney. The efferent fibres are mainly distributed to afferent and efferent arterioles, to cells of renal tubule and also to JG cells.

Afferents from the kidney Afferents from the kidney (afferents of renorenal reflex and pain fibres) run along with the efferent fibres and enter the spinal cord through the thoracic and upper lumbar dorsal roots.

Important Note

Renorenal reflex: An increase in ureteral pressure of one kidney reflexly reduces efferent nerve activity of contralateral kidney and causes increased excretion of sodium and water, known as renorenal reflex.

Applied Aspects

Polycystic kidney disease (PKD) is an autosomal dominant disorder that runs in the families. In PKD, clusters of cysts develop in the kidneys, which contain fluid and can grow very large.

Signs and symptoms include high blood pressure, pain in the back and sides, and fullness of the abdomen, ultimately affecting kidney functions and leading to kidney failure.

Diagnosis is based on ultrasound and CT scan/MRI.

Treatment includes medications to slow down the growth of cysts (tolvaptan therapy is recommended) and to keep the blood pressure within the normal range, low-salt diet and physical exercise.

Prevention: Genetic counselling is very important as the disease runs in the family, and children of the parents suffering from this disease can develop it.

RENAL BLOOD FLOW

RENAL BLOOD VESSELS

Arrangement of Arterial Vessels (Renal Artery and its Branches) in the Kidney (Fig. 6.1.6)

Renal artery (one for each kidney), a major branch from the aorta, divides into a number of lobular arteries at the hilum of the kidney.

Lobular artery (one for each pyramid) divides into two or more interlobar arteries.

Interlobar arteries enter the tissue of the renal columns and run towards the surface of the kidney. Reaching the level of the bases of the pyramids, the interlobar arteries divide into arcuate arteries.

Arcuate arteries run at right angles to the parent interlobar arteries. They lie parallel to the renal surface at the junction of pyramid and cortex. They give a series of interlobular arteries.

Interlobular arteries run through the cortex at right angles to the renal surface to end in a subcapsular plexus. It has been held that interlobular arteries divide the renal cortex into small lobules. Each interlobular artery gives off a series of afferent arterioles.

Afferent arterioles: Each afferent arteriole enters the Bowman's capsule and divides into a rounded tuft of anastomosing capillaries called *glomerulus*. As mentioned earlier, this capillary network has special features owing to which it works as a sieve allowing plasma filtration with retention of plasma proteins and blood cells. The glomerular capillaries join to form the efferent arteriole.

Efferent arterioles leaving the glomeruli of two types of nephrons exhibit different behaviour:

- *Efferent arterioles arising from the cortical nephrons* divide into *peritubular capillaries* that surround the PCT and DCT forming a rich meshwork of microvessels. This meshwork functions to remove water and solutes that have diffused from the renal tubules. These capillaries drain into interlobular veins.
- *Efferent arterioles arising from the juxtamedullary nephrons* give rise to vasa recta. The vasa recta descend with the long loops of Henle into the renal medulla and return to the area of the glomerulus, and drain into the interlobular or arcuate vein.

Side branches arising from the vasa recta form capillary network at different levels along the loop of Henle (Fig. 6.1.7).

Arrangement of Venous Vessels (Renal Veins)

The pattern of the renal venous system is similar to that found in the end arterial system, except for the presence of multiple anastomoses between veins at all levels of the venous circulation. The corresponding veins which run parallel to the arterial vessels are the interlobular veins, the arcuate veins, the interlobar veins and the renal veins which exit the kidney at the hilus.

CHARACTERISTICS OF RENAL BLOOD FLOW

Amount and Rate of Blood Flow

Rate of renal blood flow (RBF) under basal conditions, approximately 1200 mL/min (400 mL/100 g tissue/min), is very high compared with other tissues, e.g.:

- Coronary blood flow: 80 mL/100 g/min
- Brain blood flow: 55 mL/100 g/min
- Skeletal muscle blood flow: 4 mL/100 g/min

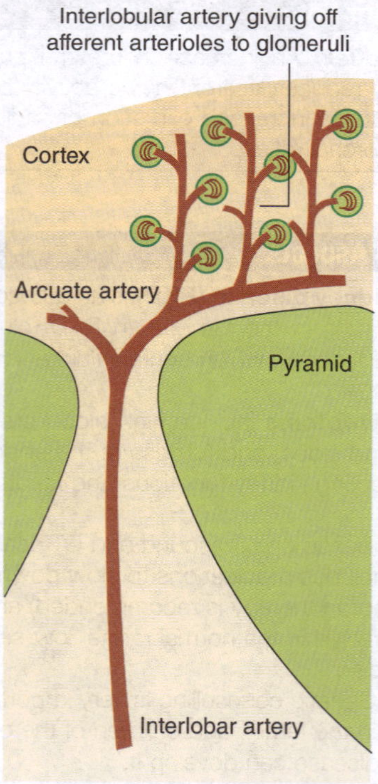

Fig. 6.1.6 Scheme to show arrangement of arteries within the kidney.

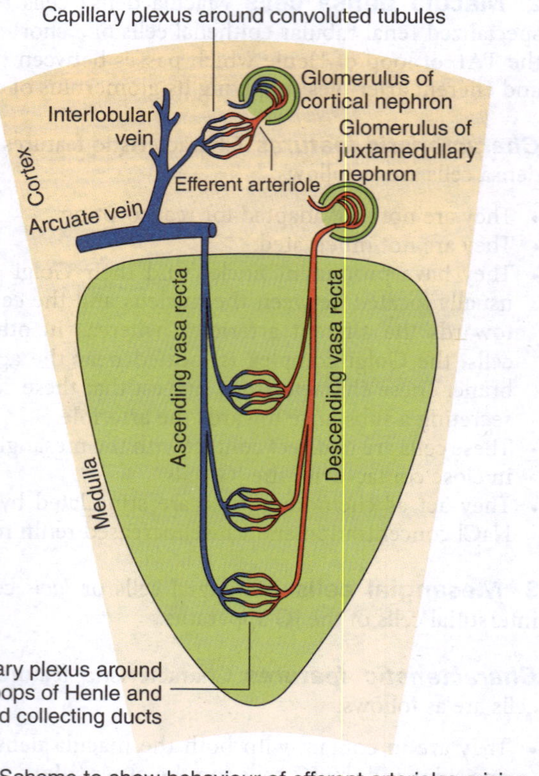

Fig. 6.1.7 Scheme to show behaviour of efferent arterioles arising from the glomeruli of cortical and juxtamedullary nephrons.

Total RBF is approximately 20% of resting cardiac output, whereas the two kidneys make <0.5% of total body weight.

Range of blood flow to the kidney is rather narrow. It allows only a 25% increase (300 mL) over the basal RBF of 1200 mL/min. This reserve is much higher in other organs.

Higher blood flow to the kidney is related to its excretory function rather than to its metabolic requirement.

Blood flow to the kidneys is directly proportional to the pressure difference between the renal artery and the renal vein, and is inversely proportional to the resistance of the renal vasculature. Because the afferent arteriole, the efferent arteriole and the intralobular artery are the major resistance vessels in the kidneys, they determine renal vascular resistance.

In face of blood pressure changes, the RBF shows remarkable constancy due to autoregulation.

During exercise, sympathetic tone to renal vessels increases and shunts RBF to the skeletal muscles.

Renal Blood Flow and Oxygen Consumption

- *Renal O_2 consumption* (approximately 6 mL/100 g tissue/min) is very high, being only second to the heart (i.e. 8 mL/100 g tissue/min) in the body.
- *Arteriovenous O_2* difference (approximately 1.5 mL/dL) of blood is the smallest of the major organ systems (Table 6.1.2).
- *Oxygen consumption* (VO_2) in the kidneys is directly proportional to the RBF, and arteriovenous O_2 difference does not change in spite of massive alteration in blood flow. This is a unique feature of the kidneys, because in most body organs, the (A–V) O_2 difference is inversely proportional to their blood flow. Thus, unlike other organs, where the blood flow is related to O_2 requirements of the organ, in the kidneys, the O_2 consumption is a function of blood flow.
- *Renal oxygen consumption correlates* best with the active reabsorption of Na^+, but a significant fraction is also required for H^+ secretion via the H^+-ATPase pumps.
- Some basic differences in the determinants of blood flow in the kidney vis-à-vis other organs, notably the muscular vascular bed, are summarized in Table 6.1.3.

Applied Aspects

- Hypoxic medullary interstitial cells produce prostaglandins (PGs), which cause vasodilation of local arterioles and wash out hypertonic environments which is necessary for concentration of urine. This fact impairs urine concentration ability.
- Prostaglandins also reduce Na^+–K^+-ATPase activity and limit oxygen consumption.
- Nonsteroidal anti-inflammatory drugs (NSAIDs) block the prostaglandin production, thus interfere with delicate balance and lead to papillary necrosis.

Table 6.1.2 Arteriovenous O_2 difference in major organ systems of the body

Organ	Arterial O_2 content (mL%)	Venous O_2 content (mL%)	A–V O_2 difference (mL%)
Kidneys	19	17.5	1.5
Heart	19	8	11
Brain	19	12	7
Whole body	19	14	5

Table 6.1.3 Basic differences in the determinants of renal blood flow vis-à-vis muscle blood flow

Muscle blood flow (MBF)	Renal blood flow (RBF)
MBF increases or decreases to maintain a constant O_2; MBF changes according to O_2 demands	RBF is regulated to maintain a constant GFR; O_2 consumption changes with GFR, which in turn changes with RBF
When O_2 consumption increases, the blood flow increases in excess of the requirement; hence, the (A–V) O_2 difference falls	O_2 consumption parallels the change in RBF; hence, (A–V) O_2 difference remains constant despite marked changes in RBF

GFR, glomerular filtration rate.

Intrarenal Distribution of Renal Blood Flow

Of the total RBF, approximately 90% perfuses the cortex, whereas only 10% perfuses the medulla (9% outer medulla and 1% inner medulla). As the main function of the renal cortex is filtration, renal cortical blood flow is relatively greater. Low blood flow to the medulla is due to relatively high vascular resistance in vasa recta because of the following three reasons:

Long length (40 mm) of vasa recta (vascular resistance is proportional to the length of the vessel)

Increased viscosity of blood near the hairpin bend of loop of Henle (resistance is proportional to the viscosity of blood) (sudden increase in the viscosity of blood in the region of inner medulla occurs due to loss of large amounts of water, as the osmotic pressure of interstitium in this region is very high [(2000 mOsm/L])

Low hydrostatic pressure head, because the diameter of efferent arterioles arising from the juxtamedullary nephrons is small

Important Note

Physiological significance of low perfusion of medulla: Low medullary blood flow plays an important role in the urinary concentration mechanism (page 570).

Applied Aspects

Acute kidney injury (AKI) or acute renal failure is most commonly caused by renal hypoperfusion due to hypotension (occurs due to heart failure, haemorrhage or dehydration). AKI progresses to acute tubular necrosis.

Hydrostatic Pressure in Renal Vessels and Their Physiological Significance

Glomerular capillaries have relatively high hydrostatic pressure (45 mm Hg), which is an important factor in the formation of glomerular filtrate.

Peritubular capillaries have very low hydrostatic pressure (8 mm Hg only) due to drop in the pressure in efferent arterioles. This low hydrostatic pressure in peritubular capillaries facilitates the reabsorptive function of PCT and DCT.

Renal veins have hydrostatic pressure of only 4 mm Hg.

Renal Portal Circulation

It has been mentioned above that the afferent arterioles arise from the interlobular arteries and each breaks up into a bunch of capillaries, called the glomerulus. The glomerular capillaries drain into efferent arterioles which again break up into peritubular capillary network which ultimately drains into an interlobular vein. In this way, two sets of capillaries are formed and thus renal circulation becomes a sort of portal circulation.

REGULATION OF RENAL BLOOD FLOW

The regulatory mechanisms affect the RBF and glomerular filtration rate (GFR) by changing the arteriolar resistance. Therefore, before discussing the various regulatory mechanisms, it will be worthwhile to understand the relationship between selective changes in the resistance of afferent and/or efferent arterioles and RBF and GFR (Fig. 6.1.8):

- *Constriction of afferent arteriole* decreases both RBF and GFR, without change in filtration fraction (FF) (Fig. 6.1.8A).
- *Dilatation of the afferent arteriole* increases both RBF and GFR, without change in FF (Fig. 6.1.8B).
- *Constriction of the efferent arteriole* decreases the RBF and increases GFR and FF (Fig. 6.1.8C).
- *Dilatation of the efferent arteriole* increases the RBF and decreases the GFR and FF (Fig. 6.1.8D).

Regulatory mechanisms of RBF include:

Autoregulation
Hormonal regulation
Nervous regulation

Autoregulation of Renal Blood Flow

RBF and thus the GFR remains constant over a wide range of renal arterial pressures (80–200 mm Hg) (Fig. 6.1.9). This occurs due to an intrarenal mechanism known as autoregulation (also see page 478). Autoregulation of RBF is accomplished by changing renal vascular resistance. When arterial pressure changes (between 80 and 200 mm Hg), a proportionate change occurs in the renal vascular resistance which maintains a constant RBF.

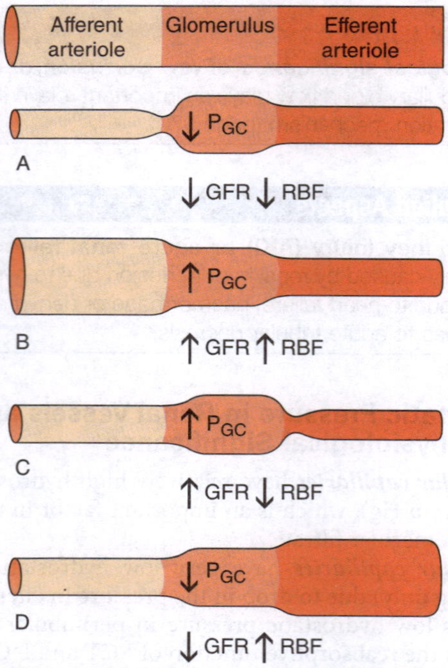

Fig. 6.1.8 Relationship between selective changes in arteriolar resistance and of either afferent or efferent arteriole and renal blood flow (RBF) and glomerular filtration rate (GFR). P_{GC}, hydrostatic pressure in glomerular capillaries.

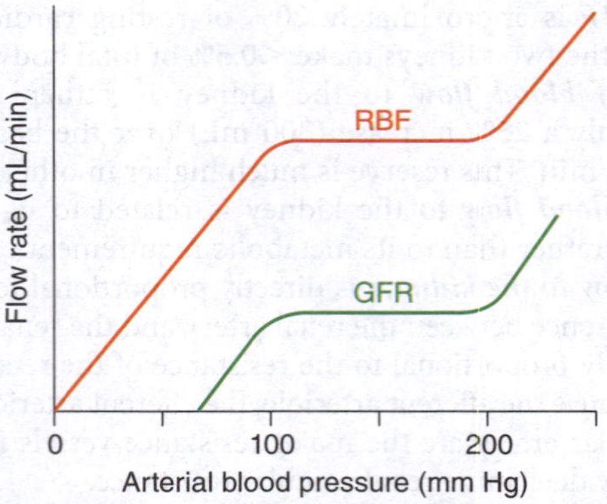

Fig. 6.1.9 Autoregulation maintains renal blood flow (RBF) and glomerular filtration rate (GFR) constant over a wide range of arterial pressure (80–200 mm Hg).

Mechanisms of Autoregulation

Autoregulation has been observed to persist after renal denervation, in the isolated perfused kidney, in the transplanted kidney, after adrenal demedullation, and even in the absence of erythrocytes, thus ruling out the role of all these factors.

Two mechanisms are considered responsible for autoregulation of RBF and GFR – one mechanism that responds to changes in arterial pressure, and another that responds to changes in NaCl concentration of tubular fluid.

1. Myogenic mechanism It is related to an intrinsic property of vascular smooth muscle – the tendency to contract when it is stretched. Thus, when renal arterial pressure is raised, the afferent arterioles are stretched, which contract and increase the vascular resistance. The increased vascular resistance offsets the effect of increased arterial pressure and thereby maintains a constant RBF and GFR (Fig. 6.1.9).

2. Tubuloglomerular feedback (TGF) mechanism It is based on the NaCl concentration of tubular fluid. It involves a feedback loop which operates as (Fig. 6.1.10):

- Changes in the GFR cause changes in NaCl concentration of fluid in the loop of Henle.
- Changes in the NaCl concentration are sensed by the macula densa cells and converted into a signal.
- The signal from the macula densa cells changes the vascular resistance in afferent arterioles.
- Signals obtained due to increased concentration of NaCl produce vasoconstriction; conversely, signals obtained due to decreased NaCl cause vasodilatation of afferent arterioles.
- Mechanism responsible for vasoconstriction and vasodilatation is not exactly known. Perhaps, it involves the concept of purinergic signalling, in which an increased sodium chloride concentration in distal convoluted tubular fluid causes basolateral release of adenosine from the macula densa cells. Adenosine triphosphate (ATP), which selectively constricts the afferent arterioles and metabolites of arachidonic acid, may contribute to TGF mechanism. The

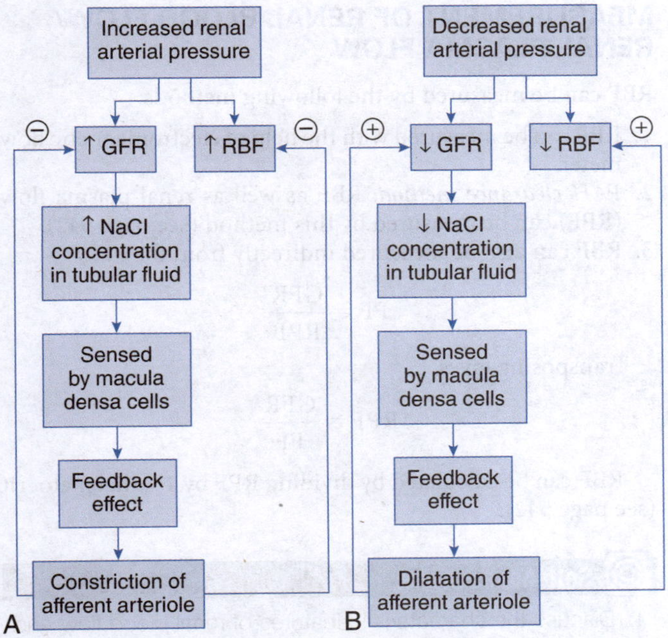

Fig. 6.1.10 Tubuloglomerular feedback mechanism which maintains a constant renal blood flow (RBF) and glomerular filtration rate (GFR) when renal arterial pressure increases **A,** or decreases **B.**

following cascade of events that ultimately bring GFR to appropriate level are depicted in Fig. 6.1.11:

Physiological Significance and Certain Important Facts About Autoregulation

A small change in GFR has a great effect on urinary output and therefore on loss of solutes and water. If RBF and GFR were to change suddenly in proportion to change in blood pressure, urinary excretion of fluid and solute would also change suddenly. Such changes in water and solute excretion, without comparable alterations in intake, would prove disastrous due to alterations in fluid and electrolyte balance. Thus, autoregulation of RBF and GFR is an effective mechanism for uncoupling renal function from fluctuations in arterial pressure and maintaining fluid and electrolyte balance.

Certain important facts about autoregulations to be noted are as follows:

- Autoregulation of RBF and GFR is virtually absent at the mean arterial blood pressure below 80 mm Hg.
- Autoregulation is not a perfect mechanism, i.e. RBF and GFR do change slightly with variation in arterial blood pressure.
- Several hormones and other factors can change RBF and GFR, despite autoregulation mechanisms.

Hormonal Regulation

As mentioned above, despite autoregulation, several hormones and other factors have a major effect on RBF and GFR by affecting afferent and/or efferent arteriolar resistance (Table 6.1.4).

1. Hormones that Cause Vasoconstriction

Hormones that cause vasoconstriction and thereby decrease RBF and GFR include:

Norepinephrine causes an intense vasoconstriction of both afferent and efferent arterioles.

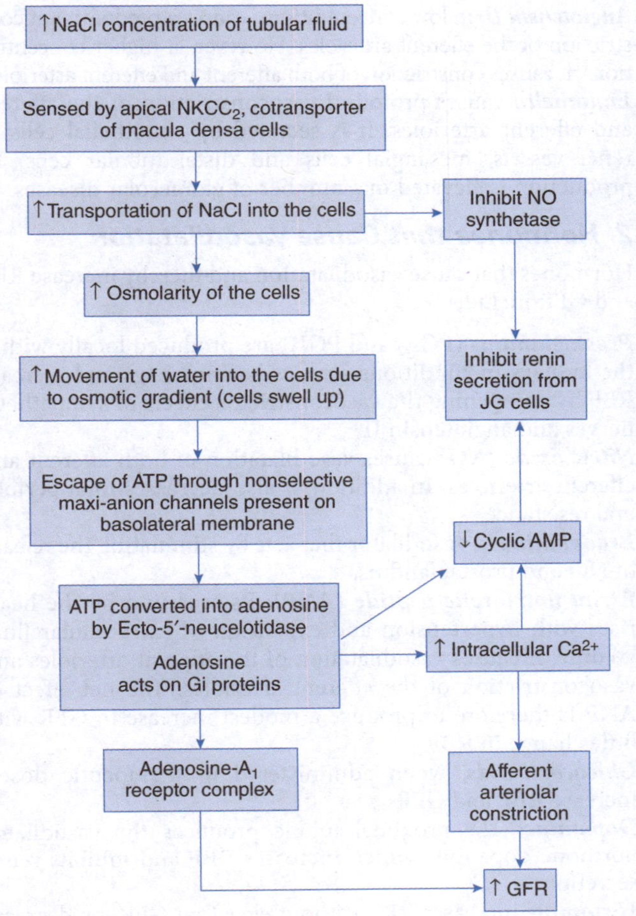

Fig. 6.1.11 Cascade of events maintaining glomerular filtration rate (GFR).

Table 6.1.4 Hormones influencing RBF and GFR

Hormone	Stimulus	Effect on GFR	Effect on RBF
Vasoconstrictors			
• Norepinephrine	↓ ECV	↓	↓
• Angiotensin II	↓ ECV	↓	↓
• Endothelin	↑ Stretch, ↓ ECV, angiotensin II, bradykinin, epinephrine	↓	↓
Vasodilators			
• Prostaglandins (PGI_2 and PGE_2)	↓ ECV, stretch, angiotensin II	NC	↑
• Nitric oxide (NO)	↑ Stretch, ACh, histamine, bradykinin, ATP	↑	↑
• Bradykinin	Prostaglandin, ↓ ACE	↑	↑
• ANP	↑ ECV	↑	↑
• Glucocorticoids	Administration in therapeutic dose	↑	↑
• Dopamine	–	NC	↑
• Histamine	Inflammation, injury	NC	↑

ACE, angiotensin-converting enzyme; ANP, atrial natriuretic peptide; ATP, adenosine triphosphate; ECV, effective circulatory volume; GFR, glomerular filtration rate; NC, no change; RBF, renal blood flow.

Angiotensin II, in low concentrations, causes a predominant constriction of the efferent arterioles. However, at higher concentrations, it causes constriction of both afferent and efferent arterioles.
Endothelin causes profound vasoconstriction of the afferent and efferent arterioles. It is secreted by endothelial cells of renal vessels, mesangial cells and distal tubular cells. Its production is elevated in a number of glomerular diseases.

2. Hormones that Cause Vasodilatation

Hormones that cause vasodilatation and thereby increase RBF and GFR include:

Prostaglandins (PGE_2 and PGI_2) are produced locally within the kidneys in conditions such as haemorrhage and increase RBF by dampening the vasoconstrictor effects of sympathetic nerves and angiotensin II.
Nitric oxide (NO) causes vasodilatation of both afferent and efferent arterioles. In addition, it also decreases total peripheral resistance.
Bradykinin is a vasodilator that acts by stimulating the release of NO and prostaglandins.
Atrial natriuretic peptide (ANP): Its secretion by the heart rises with hypertension and expansion of extracellular fluid volume. It causes vasodilatation of the afferent arterioles and vasoconstriction of the efferent arterioles. The net effect of ANP is therefore to produce a modest increase in GFR with little change in RBF.
Glucocorticoids, when administered in therapeutic doses, increase RBF and GFR.
Dopamine: The proximal tubule produces the vasodilator hormone dopamine which increases RBF and inhibits renin secretion.
Histamine increases RBF without elevating GFR, by decreasing the resistance of afferent and efferent arterioles.

Nervous Regulation

The afferent and efferent arterioles are innervated by sympathetic nerve fibres from T_{10} to L_2 intermediolateral grey segments of the spinal cord through the splanchnic nerves. The sympathetic cell bodies are located in the superior mesenteric ganglion.

Under normal circulatory conditions, sympathetic tone is minimum.
Mild to moderate stimulation of sympathetic nerves usually has mild effects on RBF because of autoregulation mechanism.
Strong acute stimulation of sympathetic nerves may produce marked fall in RBF (even to 10%–30% of normal) temporarily due to constriction of both afferent and efferent arterioles. This effect is mediated mainly by α_1-adrenergic receptors and to a lesser extent by postsynaptic α_2-adrenergic receptors.

Important Note

This system works to preserve arterial pressure at the expense of maintaining normal RBF in conditions of acute hypotension due to severe haemorrhage. Furthermore, an increase in sympathetic activity also increases the release of epinephrine and angiotensin II, enhancing vasoconstriction (vide infra).

MEASUREMENT OF RENAL BLOOD FLOW/ RENAL PLASMA FLOW

RBF can be measured by the following methods:

1. RBF can be measured with the help of electromagnetic flow meter.
2. *PAH clearance method:* RBF as well as renal plasma flow (RPF) can be measured by this method (see page 542).
3. RBF can also be measured indirectly from the FFs:

$$FF = \frac{GFR}{RPF}$$

Transposing gives

$$RPF = \frac{GFR}{FF}$$

RBF can be calculated by dividing RPF by 1 − haematocrit (see page 542).

Self-Assessment

1. Discuss the characteristic features of renal blood flow and its regulation.
2. Describe briefly:
   - Juxtaglomerular apparatus and its functions
   - Tubuloglomerular feedback mechanism
   - Autoregulation of renal blood flow and glomerular filtration

Clinical Cases

Case 1

A 45-year-old female, a known case of hypertension, presented in a hypertension clinic with pain in the abdomen and back, and feeling of fullness of the abdomen.

On examination, BP was 150/94 mm Hg, pulse rate 74/min and CVS normal.

Kidney function tests were normal.

Ultrasound, CT scan and MRI showed cysts of variable size in both kidneys. The case is diagnosed as polycystic kidney disease.

Q1. What is the type of disease?
Q2. What is the treatment?

Case 2

A 60-year-old woman presented with symptoms of pain in the back and sides, increase in frequency and urgency in urination, and feeling of fatigue. The patient also revealed a history of taking drug diclofenac (ibuprofen) for the last 1 year for treatment of joint pain.

On examination, she has shortness of breath, ankle oedema, BP 90/54 mm Hg and heart rate 82/min.

Laboratory tests revealed haematuria and the patient was diagnosed a case of analgesic nephropathy.

Q1. What is the mechanism of action of the drug on the kidney in this condition?
Q2. What is the pathophysiology of analgesic nephropathy?

6.2

Mechanism of Urine Formation: Glomerular Filtration and Tubular Transport

CHAPTER OUTLINE

INTRODUCTION

The main function of the kidneys is to clear waste products from blood and excrete them in the urine. In addition to the metabolic wastes, the kidneys also excrete foreign substances from the body such as drugs, pesticides and other chemicals ingested in food. The kidneys accomplish their excretory function by formation of urine.

Processes concerned with urine formation Three processes are involved in urine formation (Fig. 6.2.1):

- *Glomerular filtration*, i.e. filtration of plasma from the glomerular capillaries into the renal tubules, is the first step in the formation of urine.
- *Tubular reabsorption*, i.e. the return of needed solutes and water from the tubules into the blood, is the second step in the process of urine formation. It changes the composition of glomerular filtrate and reduces its volume markedly.
- *Tubular secretion* involves net movement of water and unwanted solutes (which could not be filtered) from the blood into the tubules.

Thus, the excretion of each substance in the urine involves a specific combination of filtration, reabsorption and secretion as expressed by the following relationship: urinary excretion = filtration − reabsorption + secretion (Fig. 6.2.1).

GLOMERULAR FILTRATION

Glomerular filtration refers to the process of ultrafiltration of plasma from the glomerular capillaries into the Bowman's capsule. The understanding of the process of glomerular filtration involves a review of:

- Characteristics of filtration membrane
- Composition of glomerular filtrate
- Dynamics of glomerular filtration
- Glomerular filtration rate (GFR)
- Filtration fraction (FF)
- Factors affecting glomerular filtration
- Regulation of glomerular filtration
- Measurement of glomerular filtration

CHARACTERISTICS OF FILTRATION MEMBRANE

As described on page 473 (Fig. 6.1.3B), the filtration membrane consists of three layers: capillary endothelium, glomerular

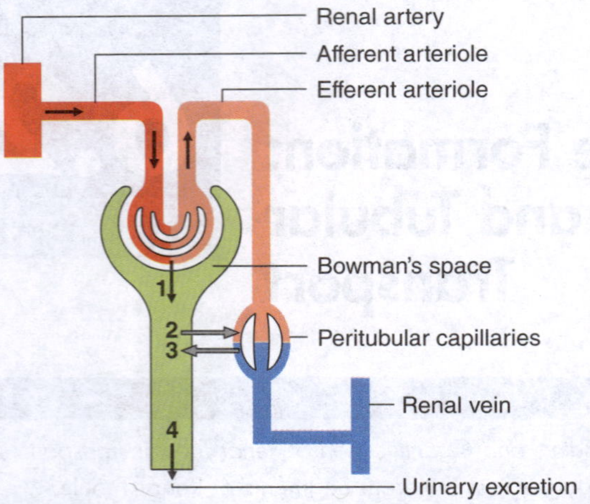

Fig. 6.2.1 Steps involved in the formation of urine: 1, filtration; 2, reabsorption; 3, secretion; and 4, excretion.

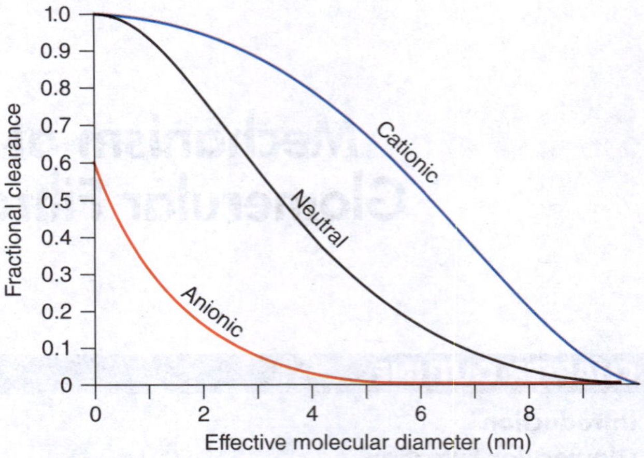

Fig. 6.2.2 Effect of electrical charge and effective molecular diameter on filterability of dextran molecule through glomerular filtration membrane. A value of 1 indicates that it is filtered freely, whereas a value of zero indicates that it is not filtered.

basement membrane (GBM) and Bowman's visceral epithelium (podocytes). Glomerular filtration occurs across this membrane.

Characteristic features of the filtration membrane are as follows:

High permeability The glomerular membrane is highly permeable to water and 100% dissolved substances because of its porous nature.

Permeability selectivity The filtration membrane exhibits a high degree of permeability selectivity based on two factors:

Pore size The capillary endothelial cells have pores that are 70–90 nm in diameter, the GBM has no pores but its permeability corresponds to pore size of 8 nm, and the podocytes form filtration slits which are approximately 25 nm wide. From this, it is clear that the glomerular filtration barrier for solutes resides at the level of GBM. The permeability of the membrane to various neutral solutes depending on their effective molecular diameter is as follows (Fig. 6.2.2):

- Molecules less than 4 nm in size are freely filtered.
- Molecules with diameter more than 8 nm are not filtered at all (i.e. zero permeability).
- Filtration of molecules having diameter between 4 and 8 nm is inversely proportional to their diameter.

Electrical charge It may, however, be realized that permeability of the filtration membrane is not simply related to molecular size but also to its shape and electrical charge. The pores in the filtration membrane are negatively charged due to the presence of glycoproteins rich in sialic acid. Thus, with the same molecular size, compared with anionic particles, there is, in order, increasing permeability for neutral and cationic particles (Fig. 6.2.2). This explains why albumin (with a molecular diameter of 7 nm but a negative charge) is not filtered.

COMPOSITION OF GLOMERULAR FILTRATE

The unique characteristic features of the glomerular filtration membrane determine the composition of glomerular filtrate; it is like that of plasma except for the absence of proteins (colloids) and cells. Capillary permeability alterations in disease do not alter rate of filtration of diffusible molecules. Thus, transfer of such substances into glomerular filtrate depends only on GFR. Filtration membrane permeability alteration in diseases, however, may alter diffusibility of colloids and cells. For example, in a number of glomerular diseases, the negative charge on the filtration membrane is reduced because of immunological damage and inflammation. As a result, filtration of proteins is increased, and albumin appears in the urine in significant amounts (albuminuria or proteinuria). It is important to note that normally the amount of proteins in the urine is less than 100 mg/dL, and most of this is not filtered but comes from the shedded tubular cells.

DYNAMICS OF GLOMERULAR FILTRATION

The forces which determine the bulk flow or ultrafiltration of protein-free plasma across the glomerular membrane are the same which determine formation of tissue fluid, i.e. fluid exchange across capillaries in the rest of the body. Thus, the driving force for glomerular filtration is the net ultrafiltration pressure across the glomerular capillaries. Filtration is always favoured in the glomerular capillaries because the net ultrafiltration pressure always favours the movement of fluid out of the capillaries.

The GFR will depend on the balance of Starling forces (Fig. 6.2.3). For detailed information about Starling forces, see page 309. According to Starling hypothesis, the GFR can be expressed as:

$$\text{GFR} = \text{Kf}\left[\left(P_{\text{GC}} - P_{\text{BS}}\right) - \left(\pi_{\text{GC}} - \pi_{\text{BS}}\right)\right]$$

where:

GFR is the filtration across the glomerular membrane.
***Kf** or the filtration coefficient of the glomerular membrane*:
- It is the product of glomerular membrane hydraulic permeability and the effective filtration surface area.
- The filtration coefficient (Kf) normally equals 12.5 m^2/min/mm Hg.

P_{GC} is the glomerular capillary hydrostatic pressure.
- It tends to force the fluid out through the glomerular membrane.

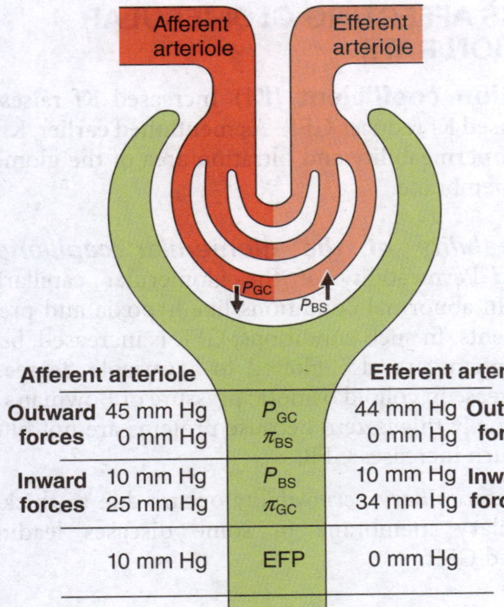

Fig. 6.2.3 Depiction of Starling forces across the glomerular filtration membrane. π_{BS}, Bowman's space oncotic pressure; π_{GC}, glomerular capillary oncotic pressure; P_{BS}, Bowman's space hydrostatic pressure; P_{GC}, glomerular capillary hydrostatic pressure.

- It depends on the arterial blood pressure, and preglomerular and postglomerular capillary resistance.
- It is the major determinant of GFR.
- Its normal value is about 45 mm Hg.

P_{BS} *or Bowman's space hydrostatic pressure*:

- It is analogous to P_i (hydrostatic interstitial pressure) in systemic circulation.
- It tends to force fluid inwards through the glomerular membrane.
- Its normal value is about 10 mm Hg.

π_{GC} *or glomerular capillary oncotic pressure:*

- It results from the osmotic pressure of plasma proteins.
- It tends to pull fluid inward through the glomerular membrane.
- Its normal value is 25 mm Hg.
- At the efferent arteriolar end, the concentration of plasma proteins increases by 20% as the glomerular fluid gets filtered into the Bowman's space.

π_{BS} *or Bowman's space oncotic pressure:*

- It is the oncotic pressure of the fluid in Bowman's space.
- Its normal value is zero, because glomerular filtrate contains no proteins.

Effective filtration pressure (EFP) is the net outward force and is calculated as the difference between the outwardly (i.e. P_{GC} and π_{BS}) and inwardly (P_{BS} and π_{GC}) directed forces (Fig. 6.2.3).

Thus, under normal circumstances:

$$GFR = 12.5[(45 - 10) - (25 - 0)] = 125 \text{ mL/min}$$

NORMAL GLOMERULAR FILTRATION RATE

As calculated above, the normal GFR in an average-sized man is about 125 mL/min (range 90–140 mL/min). Its magnitude correlates fairly well with surface area, but values in women are 10% lower than those in men even after correction for surface area. Thus, in a 24-hour period, as much as 180 L/day of plasma is filtered at the glomerulus. In other words, in 1 day, kidneys filter an amount of fluid equal to 4 times the total body water, 15 times the extracellular fluid (ECF) and 60 times the plasma volume. Of the 180 L/day of glomerular filtrate which passes through the remaining part of the nephron, 99% or more is reabsorbed and only 1% or less is excreted as urine.

After age of 30 years, GFR declines with age. However, this decline in GFR usually does not adversely affect the kidneys' excretory function, or their ability to maintain fluid, electrolyte and acid–base balance.

FILTRATION FRACTION (FF)

The FF is the ratio of GFR to the renal plasma flow (RPF).

At normal values of GFR 125 mL/min and RPF 650 mL/min, the FF is approximately 0.2% (125/650). In other words, normally only about 20% of the RPF is actually filtered per minute.

Glomerular Versus Systemic Filtration

Total Filtration

Approximately 180 L of fluid is filtered from the glomerular capillaries; in contrast, only 20 L of fluid is filtered out per day in the rest of the systemic capillaries of the body. These figures demonstrate the massive scale at which glomerular filtration occurs.

Filtration coefficient (Kf) The considerable greater rate of filtration in glomerular capillaries than in systemic capillaries is mainly because the Kf is approximately 100 times higher in glomerular capillaries.

Hydrostatic pressure Hydrostatic pressure within the glomerular capillaries is approximately twice as high in systemic capillaries. It also contributes to greater glomerular filtration.

Important Note

The reasons for higher hydrostatic pressure in glomerular capillaries are as follows:

- The afferent arteriole has little resistance being short and wide; therefore, drop in pressure is smaller as compared with that in capillaries of other tissues.
- The glomerular capillaries do not cloacae into venule, rather into an efferent arteriole, which is a high-pressure vessel with muscular wall.
- The diameter of the efferent arteriole is smaller than that of the afferent arteriole.

Total capillary exchange area The total glomerular capillary exchange area is estimated to be 1.6 m^2, of which 2%–3% is available for filtration. Thus, the glomerular filtration surface area measures between 500 and 810 cm^2. In contrast, the total exchange area of the systemic capillary bed is estimated to be 1000 m^2, of which only 25% is open at any time at rest. Thus, the systemic filtration area at rest measures about 250 m^2.

Balance of starling forces In the systemic capillary, the oncotic pressure does not vary over the length of capillary, as

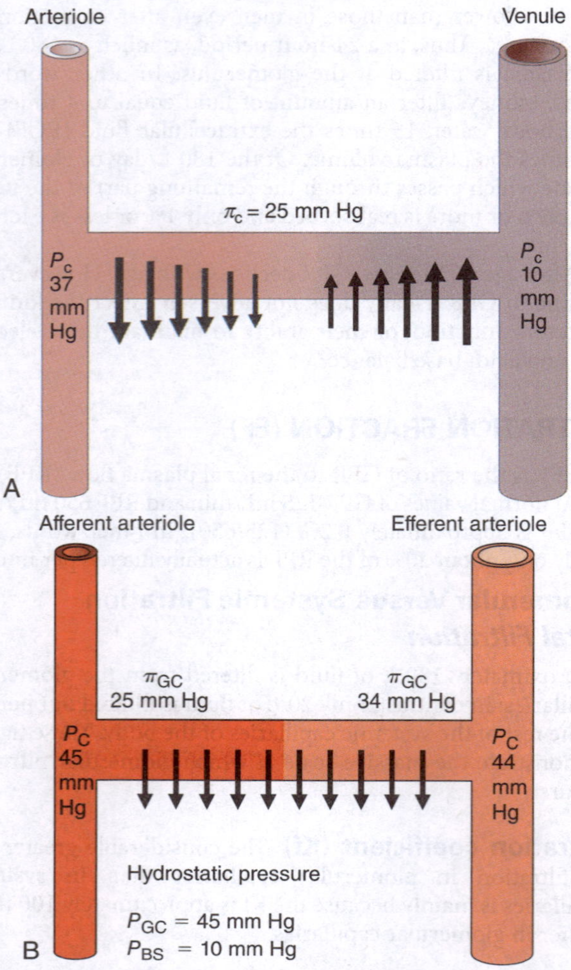

Fig. 6.2.4 Balance of Starling forces: systemic capillary (**A**) versus glomerular capillary (**B**).

the filtration of fluid is small. The hydrostatic pressure at the arteriolar end exceeds the oncotic pressure of plasma proteins and favours filtration. However, over the length of the capillary, the hydrostatic pressure gradually declines and the net filtration pressure (NFP) becomes zero near the middle of the capillary. From here, the inward forces become dominant and the reabsorption process starts to reach its maximum at the venular end (Fig. 6.2.4A).

IN THE GLOMERULAR CAPILLARY

In the glomerular capillary, the hydrostatic pressure does not decline over the length, because of the efferent arteriolar resistance. But, because of massive filtration of fluid, the oncotic pressure in the glomerular capillary increases over the length and becomes equal to hydrostatic pressure at the efferent end. Thus, there is no filtration of fluid in distal 25% of glomerular capillary (Fig. 6.2.4B).

However, if the rate of renal blood flow is increased, the equilibrium between the hydrostatic pressure (P_{GC}) and the oncotic pressure (π_{GC}) would be reached more slowly, i.e. filtration would continue over a larger length of the glomerular capillary. From this, it can be concluded that besides Starling forces, the rate of renal blood flow is also an important factor determining the GFR.

FACTORS AFFECTING GLOMERULAR FILTRATION RATE

1. Filtration coefficient (Kf) Increased Kf raises GFR and decreased Kf reduces GFR. As mentioned earlier, Kf is the product of permeability and filtration area of the glomerular capillary membrane.

i. Permeability of the glomerular capillaries is increased Permeability of the glomerular capillaries is increased in abnormal conditions like hypoxia and presence of toxic agents. In such conditions, GFR is increased, because plasma proteins are also filtered to a variable degree. This causes increase in colloid osmotic pressure of Bowman's space fluid (normally this is zero because proteins are not filtered), which in turn increases GFR.

- *Decreased capillary permeability* occurs due to thickening of capillary membrane in some diseases leading to decreased GFR.

ii. Alteration in GFR filtration area of glomerular capillaries Alteration in GFR filtration area of glomerular capillaries can alter the Kf. *Mesangial* cell contraction or relaxation is associated with alteration in coefficient of filtration.

- *Contraction of mesangial cells* leading to decreased Kf is caused by vasoconstrictors like angiotensin II, endothelin, norepinephrine, thromboxane A_2, leukotrienes C_4 and D_4, and histamine.
- *Relaxation of mesangial cells* leading to increased Kf is caused by vasodilators like dopamine, cyclic adenosine monophosphate (cAMP), atrial natriuretic peptide (ANP), nitric oxide (NO) and prostaglandins (PGE).

2. Hydrostatic pressure in Bowman's space fluid (P_{BS}) Hydrostatic pressure in Bowman's space fluid (P_{BS}) opposes filtration, and therefore GFR is inversely related to it. It is increased in acute obstruction of the urinary tract (e.g. a ureteric obstruction by stone).

3. Glomerular capillary hydrostatic pressure (P_{GC}) GFR is directly related to P_{GC}. Changes in P_{GC} serve as a primary means for physiological regulation of GFR. P_{GC} is mainly dependent on arterial pressure, renal blood flow, afferent arteriolar resistance and efferent arteriolar resistance.

i. Arterial pressure GFR is autoregulated between arterial pressure of 80 and 200 mm Hg. Increased arterial pressure above 200 mm Hg may raise GFR and decreased arterial pressure below 70 mm Hg may lower GFR.

ii. Renal blood flow GFR is directly proportional to the renal blood flow. However, renal blood flow is controlled by autoregulatory mechanisms.

iii. Afferent and efferent arteriolar resistances Relation of afferent and efferent arteriolar resistances with GFR is described on page 479.

Note: In *acute renal failure*, GFR declines because of fall in P_{GC}.

4. Glomerular capillary oncotic pressure (π_{GC}) GFR is inversely proportional to π_{GC}. In hyperproteinaemia and in haemoconcentration ratio, the π_{GC} is raised leading to decrease in GFR. Conversely, in hypoproteinaemia and haemodilution, the π_{GC} is reduced leading to increased GFR.

5. Sympathetic stimulation See page 480.

REGULATION OF GFR

Regulation of GFR, like that of renal blood flow, includes:

- Autoregulation
- Nervous regulation
- Hormonal regulation
  For details, see page 479.

MEASUREMENT OF GFR

GFR can be measured by renal clearance of inulin, urea and creatinine. For details, see page 504.

TUBULAR REABSORPTION AND SECRETION

Of the 180 L glomerular filtrate formed per day, about 1.5 L (i.e. <1%) per day is excreted as urine. The different segments of the renal tubule, i.e. proximal tubule, loop of Henle, distal tubule (DT) and collecting duct (CD), determine the composition and volume of the urine by the process of *selective reabsorption* of solutes and water and *selective secretion* of solutes. Consequently, the tubules precisely control the volume, osmolality, composition and pH of intracellular fluid and ECF compartments. For conceptual understanding, this section on renal tubular reabsorption and secretion can be considered in the following subsections:

General principles of renal tubular transport:

- Transport mechanisms across cell membranes
- Transepithelial transport pathways
- Tubular mechanisms and patterns of renal handling of a substance and concept of renal clearance
- Parameters of renal active transport

Transport across different segments of renal tubule:

- Transport across proximal tubule
- Transport across loop of Henle
- Transport across DT
- Transport across CD

Tubular transport of common solutes and water:

- Tubular transport of Na^+
- Tubular transport of Cl^-
- Tubular transport of K^+
- Tubular transport of glucose
- Tubular transport of water

GENERAL PRINCIPLES OF RENAL TUBULAR TRANSPORT

Transport Mechanisms Across Cell Membrane

The water moves across the cell membrane of renal tubular cells passively, whereas the solute movement occurs by both passive and active mechanisms.

Passive transport does not need energy and occurs spontaneously, down an electrochemical gradient, by the following mechanisms:

- Diffusion
- Facilitated diffusion (channels, uniport, coupled transport, uniport or symport)
- Solvent drag

Active transport requires direct input of energy and is abolished if cell metabolism is inhibited. It can occur against an electrochemical gradient, but it does not mean that it occurs only against such gradients in the body. Most of the active transports are carrier mediated. Endocytosis is also a type of active transport and it will prove prudent to revise the various transport mechanisms described in Chapter 1.3, page 25, before proceeding further.

Transepithelial Transport Pathways

In the renal tubule, a substance can be reabsorbed or secreted by two pathways:

Paracellular pathway refers to transport between the cells (Fig. 6.2.5A). Examples of paracellular pathway include:

- Reabsorption of Ca^{2+} and K^+ occurs across the proximal tubule.
- Some of the water reabsorbed across the proximal tubule crosses the paracellular pathway.
- Some solutes dissolved in this water (in particular, Ca^{2+} and K^+) are carried along with the reabsorbed fluid across the paracellular pathway by the process of solvent drag.

Transcellular pathway refers to transport through the cells. Its example includes transcellular Na^+ reabsorption by the proximal tubule, which is a two-step process (Fig. 6.2.5B):

- *Movement of Na^+ into the cell* across the apical membrane occurs down an electrochemical gradient established by Na^+–K^+-ATPase.
- *Movement of Na^+ into the ECF* across the basolateral membrane occurs against an electrochemical gradient via Na^+–K^+-ATPase.

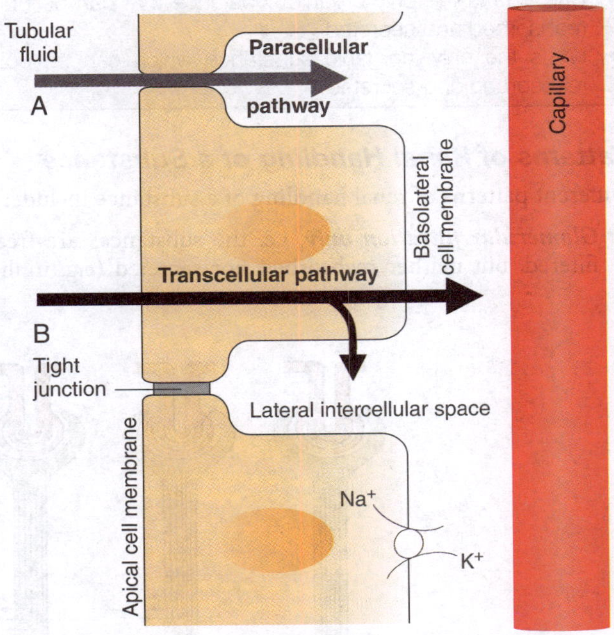

Fig. 6.2.5 Pathways of transepithelial transport: **A**, paracellular pathway; and **B**, transcellular pathway.

Tubular Mechanisms, Patterns of Renal Handling of Substances and Concept of Renal Clearance

Tubular mechanisms As mentioned earlier, the two main tubular mechanisms involved in renal handling of a substance are tubular reabsorption and tubular secretion.

Tubular reabsorption Tubular reabsorption denotes the active transport of solutes and passive movement of water from the tubular lumen into the peritubular capillaries. In other words, reabsorption is the removal of substances of nutritive value such as glucose, amino acids, electrolytes (Na^+, K^+, Cl^-, HCO_3^-) and vitamins from the glomerular filtrate. Small proteins and peptide hormones are reabsorbed in the proximal tubules by endocytosis.

Tubular secretion Tubular secretion refers to the transport of solutes from the peritubular capillaries into the tubular lumen, i.e. it is the addition of a substance to the glomerular filtrate.

Active secretion of substances occurs into the tubular fluid (TF) with the help of certain nonselective carriers. The carrier which secretes *para*-aminohippuric acid (PAH) can also secrete uric acid, bile acids, oxalic acid, penicillin, probenecid, cephalothin and furosemide. It is because of the common carrier that probenecid can block secretion of penicillin and maintain its plasma concentration for a longer time. For bases, there is another carrier, which is also nonselectively involved in secretion of substances like acetylcholine, creatinine, dopamine, histamine, 5-HT, thiamine, quinine, procaine, morphine and other bases.

Important Notes

The ensuing discussion includes the list and mechanism of the substances reabsorbed and/or secreted in different segments of renal tubule (page 487).

- Only two natural constituents of plasma (K^+ and H^+) are secreted by the distal tubules.
- Proximal tubular cells may secrete uric acid and many drugs.
- Uric acid is the only organic substance that can be both reabsorbed and secreted.
- K^+ is the only inorganic substance which can be both reabsorbed and secreted.

Patterns of Renal Handling of a Substance

Different patterns of renal handling of a substance include:

1. ***Glomerular filtration only***, i.e. the substances are freely filtered, but neither reabsorbed nor secreted (e.g. inulin) (Fig. 6.2.6A). Such substances are called glomerular markers and are said to have renal clearance equal to GFR.
2. ***Glomerular filtration followed by partial reabsorption*** (Fig. 6.2.6B): Such substances have renal clearance less than GFR.
3. ***Glomerular filtration followed by complete tubular reabsorption*** (Fig. 6.2.6C): Such substances have the lowest renal clearance, e.g. Na^+, glucose, amino acids, HCO_3^- and Cl^-. The substances that are not filtered at all (e.g. protein) also have the lowest renal clearance.
4. ***Glomerular filtration followed by tubular secretion*** (Fig. 6.2.6D): Such substances that are both filtered across the glomerular capillaries and secreted from the peritubular capillaries into urine have the highest renal clearances (e.g. PAH).
5. ***Glomerular filtration followed by partial reabsorption and secretion*** (Fig. 6.2.6E): In such circumstances, depending on which of the two processes is dominant, there may be net reabsorption or net secretion of the substance. Net absorption is said to occur if the amount of substance excreted in urine is less than GFR in the same time. Similarly, net secretion is said to occur when the amount excreted is more than GFR in the same time.
6. ***No glomerular filtration, no absorption, only secretion*** (Fig. 6.2.6F): Many organic compounds are bound to plasma proteins and are therefore unavailable for ultrafiltration. Secretion is thus their major route of excretion in urine.

Concept of Renal Clearance

From the above, the renal clearance can be defined as the volume of plasma that is cleared of a substance in 1 minute by excretion of the substance in the urine. Furthermore, from the above description and examples, the relative clearances of the common substances are as follows:

$$\text{PAH} > K^+(\text{high-}K^+\text{diet}) > \text{inulin} > \text{urea} > Na^+ > \text{glucose, amino acids and } HCO_3^-$$

Parameters and Quantification of Renal Tubular Transport

The parameters used for quantitative analysis of renal tubular transport include:

- Filtered load (F^o)
- Excretion rate (E^o)
- Reabsorption rate (R^o)
- Secretion rate (S^o)
- Renal tubular transport maximum (T_m)
- TF concentration and plasma concentration (P) ratio

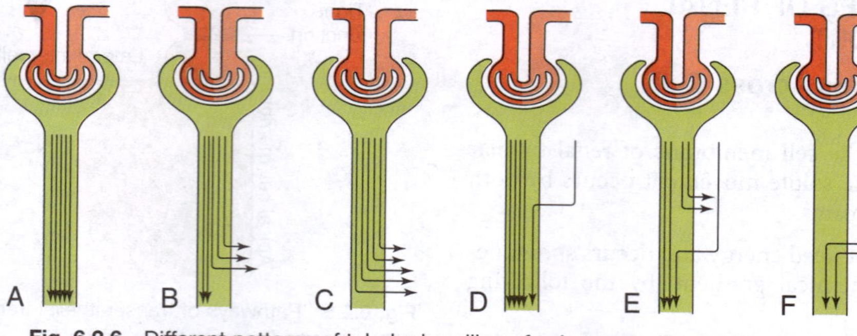

Fig. 6.2.6 Different patterns of tubular handling of substances (for details, see text).

Filtered load It is the amount of a substance entering the renal tubule by glomerular filtration per unit time.

- Filtered load (F^o) is calculated by multiplying the GFR with the plasma concentration of the substance (P_x), i.e. F^o = GFR × P_x mg/min. As described on page 540, the GFR is equal to the clearance of inulin (C_{in}); therefore, $F^o = C_{in} \times P_x$.

Excretion rate It is the amount of substance that appears in the urine per unit time. The excretion rate (E^o) can be calculated by multiplying the urine flow rate (V) *and the urinary concentration of the substance* (U_x), i.e.

$$E^o = V \times U_x \text{ mg/min}$$

Reabsorption rate (R^o) Reabsorption of a substance is said to occur when the filtered load exceeds the excretion rate. The reabsorption rate of a substance is calculated by subtracting the excretion rate from the filtered load, i.e.

$$R^o = F^o - E^o$$

Secretion rate (S^o) The net secretion of a substance is said to occur when the excretion rate is more than the filtered load. Under such circumstances, the secretion rate is calculated by subtracting the filtered load from the excretion rate, i.e.

$$S^o = E^o - F^o$$

Renal tubular transport maximum (T_m) Renal tubular transport maximum (T_m) refers to the maximal amount of a solute that can be actively transported (reabsorbed or secreted) per minute by the renal tubules. In other words, the point at which carriers are saturated is the T_m.

> **Important Note**
>
> - It is important to note that T_m pertains to solutes that are actively transported only.
> - The substances that are passively transported (e.g. urea) do not exhibit T_m.

Maximum tubular secretory capacity (T_s) is the highest attainable rate of secretion. All substances secreted by the kidney do not have T_m.

- Secreted substances that have T_m include PAH, penicillin, certain diuretics, salicylate and thiamine (vitamin B_1).
- Secreted substance that does not have T_m is K^+ which is secreted by the DTs.

Maximal tubular reabsorptive capacity (T_r) is the highest attainable rate of reabsorption. All substances reabsorbed by an active carrier-mediated mechanism do not have T_m.

- Substances that have T_m are phosphate ion, sulphate, glucose, many amino acids, uric acid and albumin, acetoacetate, β-hydroxybutyrate and α-ketoglutarate (αKG).
- Substances that do not have T_m include reabsorption of Na^+ along the nephron and HCO_3^-.

Threshold concentration is defined as the plasma concentration at which a substance first appears in the urine.

Tubular fluid concentration/plasma concentration ratio TF/P_x The TF/P_x ratio compares the concentration of a substance in TF at any point along the nephron with its concentration in plasma.

> **Important Note**
>
> The TF, for such studies, is collected by micropuncture technique. A micropipette is inserted into the Bowman's space and different portions of the tubules of the living kidney in experimental animals and the composition of aspirated TF is determined by the use of microchemical techniques.

Significance of TF/P_x Ratio The TF/P_x ratio may be 1, <1 or >1.

TF/P_x ratio of 1.0 signifies that either there has been no reabsorption or reabsorption of the substance has been exactly proportional to the reabsorption of water.

For example, a TF/P_x of 1.0 indicates that concentration of Na^+ in TF and plasma is identical. For any freely filterable substance, TF/P_x ratio is 1.0 in Bowman's space (before any reabsorption or secretion has taken place to modify the TF).

TF/P_x ratio of <1.0 signifies that reabsorption of a substance has been greater than the reabsorption of water and its concentration in TF is less than that of plasma.

For example, a TF/P_{Na^+} of 0.8 indicates that the concentration of Na^+ in TF is 80% of Na^+ concentration in plasma.

TF/P_x ratio of >1.0 signifies that either the reabsorption of a substance has been less than the reabsorption of water or there has been secretion of the substance.

Tubular fluid concentration/plasma concentration of inulin (P_{inulin}) The substance inulin is freely filtered by glomerular capillaries but is neither reabsorbed nor secreted into the tubules. Thus, its concentration in TF is determined solely by how much water remains in the TF. So, TF/P_{inulin} is used as a marker for water reabsorption along the nephron. Its value increases as water is reabsorbed. From the value of TF/P_{inulin}, the *fraction of the filtered water that has been reabsorbed* can be calculated by the following equation:

- Fraction of filtered H_2O reabsorbed = 1 − 1/TF/P_{inulin}.
- When TF/P_{inulin} is 2, FF of H_2O reabsorbed is 1 − 1/2 = 0.5 = 5%.
- Similarly, when TF/P_{inulin} is 3, FF of H_2O reabsorbed is 1 − 1/3 = 0.67 = 67%.

[TF/P_x]/[TF/P_{inulin}] ratio The double ratio corrects the TF/P_x ratio for water reabsorption and gives the fraction of the filtered load remaining at any point along the nephron.

For example, a [TF/P_K]/[TF/P_{inulin}] ratio of 0.3 at the end of proximal tubule indicates that 30% of filtered K^+ remains in the TF and 70% has been reabsorbed into the blood.

TRANSPORT ACROSS DIFFERENT SEGMENTS OF RENAL TUBULE

The substances transported across the different segments of renal tubules are described below and enlisted in Table 6.2.1.

Transport Across Proximal Tubule

The proximal tubule reabsorbs:

- Approximately 67% of the filtered water, Na^+, Cl^-, K^+ and other solutes

Table 6.2.1 Transport of substances across different segments of renal tubule

Reabsorption			
Active	**Passive**	**Non-reabsorption**	**Secretion**
Proximal tubule			
Na^+	Cl^-	Inulin	H^+
K^+	HCO_3^-	Creatinine	Water
Ca^{2+}	HPO_4^-	Sucrose	Penicillin
Mg^{2+}	Water	Mannitol	Sulphonamide
HPO_4^{2-}	Urea	Creatinine	
SO_4^{2-}			
NO_3^-			
Glucose			
Amino acids			
Protein			
Urate			
Vitamins			
Acetoacetate			
β-Hydroxybutyrate			
Loop of Henle			
Na^+	Cl^-		
K^+	HCO_3^-		
Ca^{2+}	Water		
Distal tubule and collecting duct			
Na^+	Cl^-		K^+
Ca^{2+}	HCO_3^-		H^+
Mg^{2+}	Water		
Water			

- Almost all the glucose and amino acids filtered by the glomerulus

The proximal tubule does not reabsorb inulin, creatinine, sucrose and mannitol.

The proximal tubule secretes H^+, PAH, urate, penicillin, sulphonamides and creatinine.

Reabsorption

Characteristics of proximal tubule cells As shown in Fig. 6.1.3, the proximal tubular cells are characterized by the presence of brush border on their luminal surfaces. The brush is composed of thousands of villi which increase the absorptive surface area of each cell 20-fold. The substances absorbed are transferred to the peritubular capillaries from the basolateral membrane of the cells.

Note: Key element in the proximal tubular reabsorption is Na^+–K^+-ATPase in the basolateral membrane. The reabsorption of every substance including water is linked in some way to the operation of Na^+–K^+-ATPase.

Sodium reabsorption The process of sodium reabsorption in proximal tubule is *isosmotic*, i.e. the reabsorptions of sodium and water are exactly proportional. Therefore, both TF/ and TF/P_{osm} are 1.0.

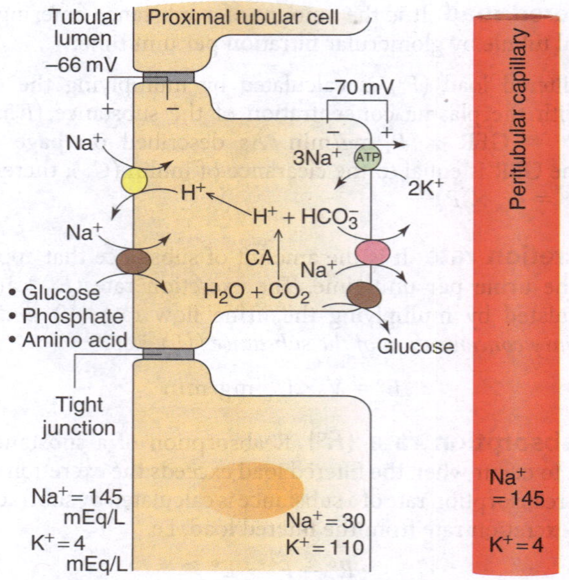

Fig. 6.2.7 Mechanism of reabsorption of sodium and other solutes across early proximal tubule.

Mechanisms of Na^+ reabsorption Mechanism of Na^+ reabsorption in the early proximal tubule and late proximal tubule is different.

In early proximal tubule, Na^+ is reabsorbed by *cotransport with* H^+ or organic solutes (glucose, amino acids, phosphate and lactate). The Na^+ absorption is a two-step process (Fig. 6.2.7):

Across the basolateral membrane, Na^+ moves against an electrochemical gradient via Na^+–K^+-ATPase pump, which pumps Na^+ into the paracellular spaces and lowers the intracellular Na^+ concentration.

Across the apical membrane, the sodium moves down an electrochemical gradient as above. The entry of Na^+ is mediated by specific antiporter and symporter proteins, and not by diffusion through channels:

- *Na^+–H^+-antiporter* is the main determinant of Na^+ and H_2O reabsorption in the proximal tubule. Na^+–H^+ exchange is linked directly to the reabsorption of HCO_3^-.

Important Note

Carbonic anhydrase inhibitors (e.g. acetazolamide) are diuretics that act in the early proximal tubule by inhibiting the reabsorption of filtered HCO_3^-.

Na^+–glucose (and other organic solutes) symporter mechanisms are also involved in the entry of Na^+ in the proximal cells. The glucose, amino acids, phosphate and lactate are almost completely absorbed along with Na^+ (Fig. 6.2.8) by the symporter (carrier) proteins which are different for different molecules. The carrier for glucose in proximal tubule is called sodium-dependent glucose transporter-1 (SGLT-1). The glucose and other organic solutes that enter the cell with Na^+ leave the cell across the basolateral membrane by passive transport mechanism.

Note: The reabsorption of Na^+–HCO_3^- and Na^+–organic solutes across the proximal tubule establishes a transtubular osmotic gradient that provides the driving force for the passive absorption of water by osmosis. Because more water than Cl^- is reabsorbed in the early segment of proximal tubule, the

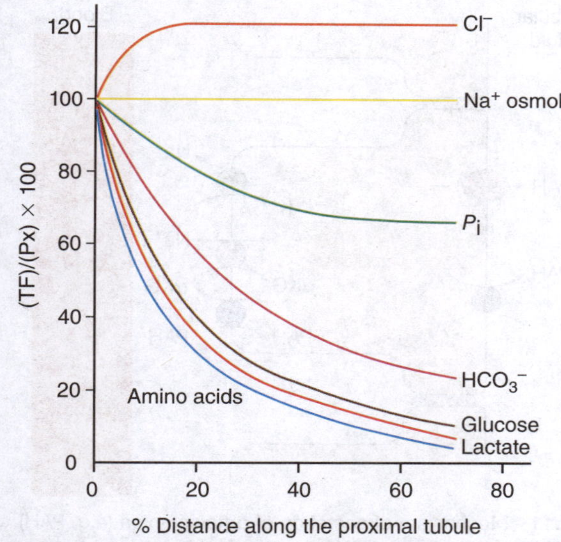

Fig. 6.2.8 Concentration of solutes in tubular fluid as a function of length along the proximal tubule. TF is the concentration of substance in the tubular fluid, and P_x is the concentration of substance in the plasma. Values above 100 indicate that relatively less of substance than water was absorbed, and values below 100 indicate that relatively more of substance than water was reabsorbed.

Cl^- concentration in TF rises along the length of the early proximal tubule (Fig. 6.2.8).

In the late proximal tubule In the late proximal tubule, the Na^+ is reabsorbed primarily by *chloride-driven sodium transport mechanism* across both the transcellular and paracellular pathways.

Reabsorption via paracellular pathway: The filtered glucose, amino acids and HCO_3^- have already been almost completely removed from the TF by reabsorption in the early proximal tubule. So the fluid entering the late proximal tubule contains very little of these substances but contains a high concentration of Cl^- (140 mEq/L) compared with that in the early proximal tubule (105 mEq/L). This high Cl^- (140 mEq/L) concentration in the lumen of late proximal tubule and comparatively low concentration (105 mEq/L) in the interstitium creates a concentration gradient which favours the diffusion of Cl^- from the tubular lumen across the tight junctions into lateral intercellular space. Movement of negatively charged Cl^- causes the TF to become positively charged relative to the blood. This causes the diffusion of Na^+ across the tight junctions into the blood. ***Transcellular Na^+*** reabsorption across the luminal membrane of late proximal tubule cells occurs due to parallel operation of Na^+–H^+ and one or more Cl^- anion (formate) antiporters (Fig. 6.2.9). ***Across the basolateral membrane***, the Na^+ leaves the cell by the action of Na^+–K^+-ATPase pump, and Cl^- leaves by K^+–Cl^- cotransporter (Fig. 6.2.9).

Water reabsorption Approximately 67% of the filtered water is absorbed in the proximal tubule by osmosis in response to a transtubular osmotic gradient established by the solute reabsorption (i.e. Na^+–Cl^-, Na^+–glucose and so forth).

- Two-thirds of H_2O reabsorption occurs through the transcellular pathway and one-third through the tight junction's paracellular pathway (Fig. 6.2.10).

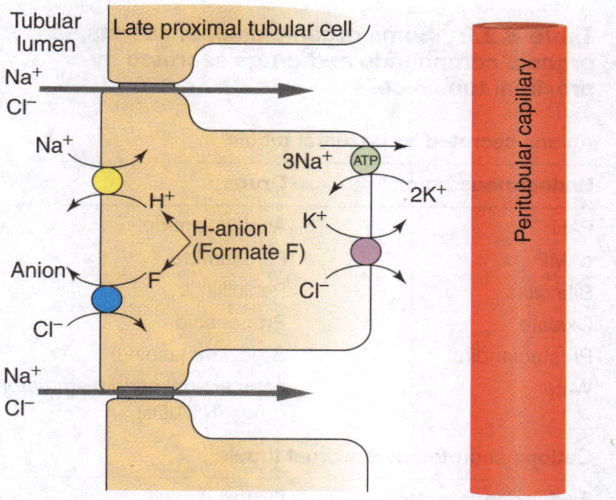

Fig. 6.2.9 Mechanism of reabsorption of sodium and other solutes across late proximal tubule (for understanding, see text).

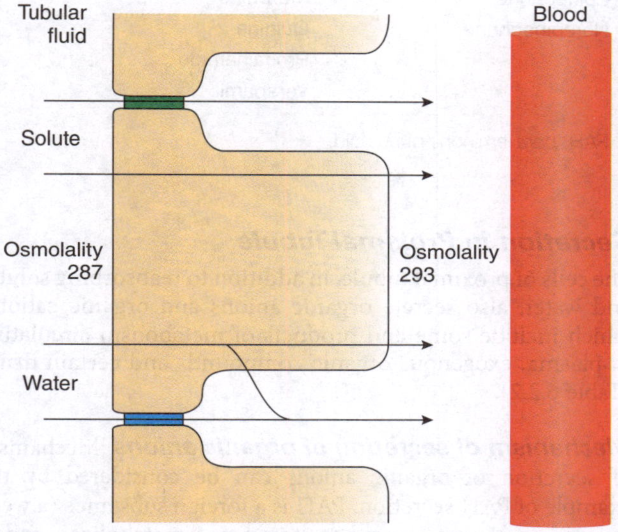

Fig. 6.2.10 Routes of water and solute reabsorption across the proximal tubule (for understanding, see text).

- The osmotic water flowing across the proximal tubule also causes some reabsorption of K^+ and Ca^{2+} by the process of *solvent drag*.
- The osmotic water absorption is termed *obligatory water absorption* as it cannot be changed according to the needs of the body.

Protein reabsorption Normally, only a small amount of proteins is filtered by the glomerulus (40 mg/L). However, because of high GFR (180 L/day), the total amount of protein filtered per day is significant (180 L/day × 40 mg/L = 7.2 g/day). Normally, the proteins are completely taken into the cells of proximal tubules by the process of endocytosis. Once inside the cells, enzymes digest the proteins and peptides into their constituent amino acids which exit across the basolateral membrane and return to the blood in the peritubular capillaries.

When the amount of filtered proteins increases (due to disruption of glomerular filtration barrier in kidney diseases), the reabsorbing mechanisms saturate and the proteins may appear in the urine (*proteinuria*).

Table 6.2.2 Some organic anions, cations, organic compounds and drugs secreted by proximal tubule cells

Anions secreted by proximal tubule	
Endogenous anion	**Drugs**
PAH	Acetazolamide
cAMP	Furosemide
Bile salts	Penicillin
Oxalate	Probenecid
Prostaglandins	Salicylate (aspirin)
Water	nonsteroidal anti-inflammatory drugs (NSAIDs)
Cations secreted by proximal tubule	
Endogenous cation	**Drugs**
Creatinine	Atropine
Dopamine	Cimetidine
Epinephrine	Morphine
Norepinephrine	Quinine
	Procainamide
	Verapamil

PAH, *para*-aminohippuric acid.

Secretion in Proximal Tubule

The cells of proximal tubule, in addition to reabsorbing solutes and water, also secrete organic anions and organic cations, which include some end products of metabolism circulating in plasma, exogenous organic compounds and certain drugs (Table 6.2.2).

Mechanism of secretion of organic anions Mechanism of secretion of organic anions can be considered by the example of PAH secretion. PAH is a foreign substance (a weak organic acid) that is neither stored nor metabolized and is excreted virtually unchanged in the urine. Because 10% of PAH is bound to plasma proteins, it is cleared from the plasma, by both glomerular filtration and tubular secretion through the kidney. As with glucose, the filtered load of PAH increases in direct proportion to the plasma PAH concentration.

Secretion of PAH occurs from the peritubular capillary blood into TF via carriers in the proximal tubule by a transport maximum T_m-limited process.

- The carrier which secretes PAH is nonselective, i.e. it can transport most of the organic anions listed in Table 6.2.2.
- At low plasma concentration of PAH, the secretion rate increases as the plasma concentration increases. But, once the carriers are saturated, further increase in plasma PAH concentration does not cause further increase in secretion rate T_m (Fig. 6.2.11).
- The PAH is taken into the cell across the basolateral membrane against its chemical gradient, in exchange for αKG via a PAH–αKG *antiport mechanism*. The resultant high intracellular concentration of PAH provides the driving force for PAH exit across the luminal membrane into the TF via a PAH–anion (A^-) antiporter and possibly a voltage-driven PAH transporter (Fig. 6.2.11).

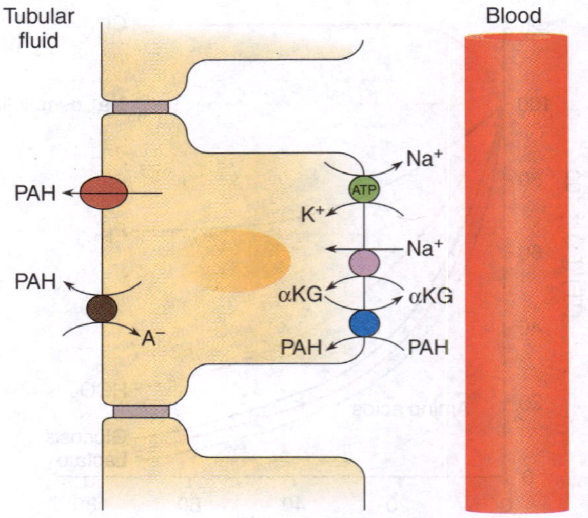

Fig. 6.2.11 Mechanism of secretion of organic anion (e.g. PAH) across the proximal tubule. PAH, *para*-aminohippuric acid.

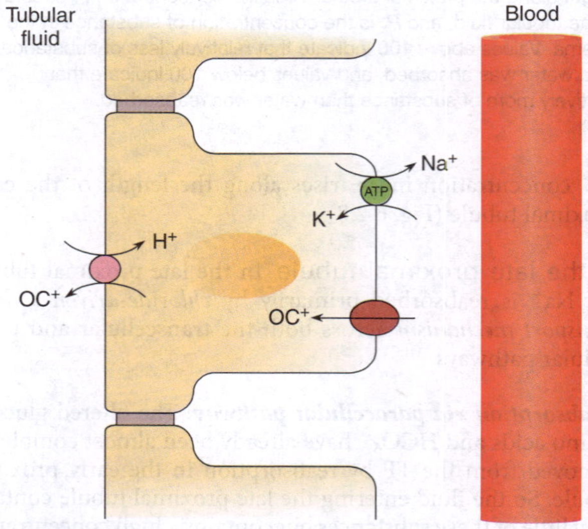

Fig. 6.2.12 Mechanism of secretion of organic cations (OC^+) across the proximal tubule (for understanding, see text).

Note: PAH clearance can be used to measure RPF (see page 542).

Mechanism of secretion of organic cations Mechanism of secretion of organic cations in proximal tubule occurs as follows:

Across the basolateral membrane, the organic cations enter the cell by facilitated diffusion. This mechanism is driven by the magnitude of the voltage difference (negative potential) across the basolateral membrane.

Across the luminal membrane, the organic cations enter the TF by an OC^+–H^+ antiport (Fig. 6.2.12).

- The carrier which secretes organic cation into the TF is nonselective, i.e. it can transport most of the organic cations listed in Table 6.2.2.

Transport Across Loop of Henle

About 20% of filtered Na^+ and Cl^-, 15% of filtered water and cations such as K^+, Ca^{2+} and Mg^{2+} are reabsorbed in the loop of Henle. Reabsorption occurring in different parts of the loop of Henle is as follows:

Thin descending limb of loop of Henle Water absorption occurs passively (because of hypertonic interstitial fluid) exclusively in this part of loop of Henle. It is accompanied by diffusion of sodium ions from interstitial fluid into tubular lumen.

Thin ascending limb of loop of Henle Limited passive reabsorption of Na^+ and Cl^- occurs in this water-impermeable limb. Because of impermeability to water, the fluid leaving this limb is hypotonic relative to plasma.

Thick ascending limb of loop of Henle Thick ascending limb (TAL) of loop of Henle is impermeable to water but is involved in the reabsorption of 20% of the filtered Na^+, Cl^- and other cations. About half of the Na^+ is reabsorbed actively and transcellularly, whereas the other half of the Na^+ is reabsorbed passively by paracellular pathway along with other cations, as described:

Na^+, K^+–$2Cl^-$ symporter-mediated active transport of sodium: Salient points are as follows (Fig. 6.2.13):

- The key element involved is Na^+–K^+-ATPase located in the basolateral membrane which extrudes Na^+, leading to low intracellular Na^+ concentration.
- Due to low intracellular Na^+, a chemical gradient is created which favours movement of Na^+ from the lumen into the cell.
- The movement of Na^+ across the apical membrane is mediated by Na^+–K^+–$2Cl^-$ symporter.
- This symporter, with downhill movement of Na^+ and Cl^-, drives the uphill movement of K^+ influx.

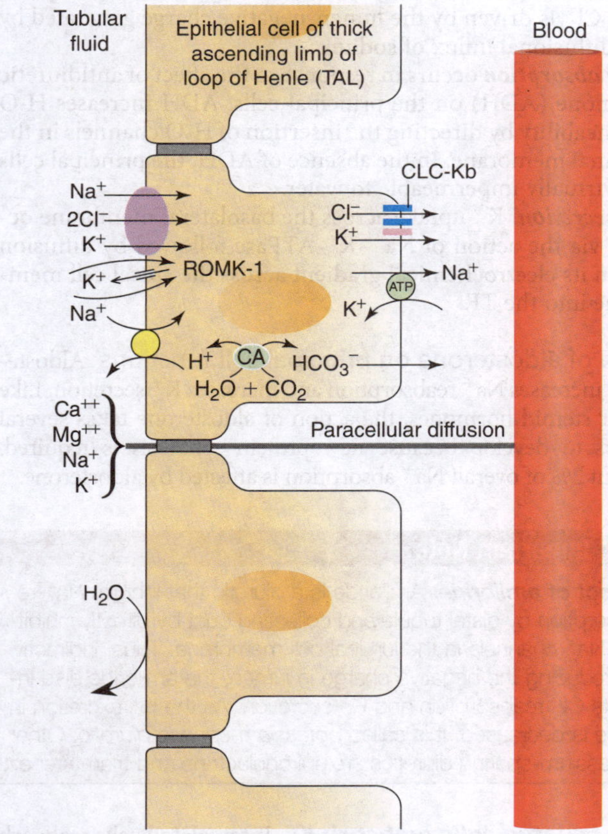

Fig. 6.2.13 The active (transcellular) and passive (paracellular) transport mechanisms operating across the tubular cells in thick ascending limb (TAL) of loop of Henle.

- Cl^- delivery is rate-limiting, as NaCl transport increases directly with the TF Cl^- concentration.
- Na^+ leaves the cell across the basolateral membrane by the action of Na^+–K^+-ATPase.
- Cl^- exits into interstitium via Clc–kbCL$^-$ channels. Barttin (an integral membrane protein) present in the cell membrane is necessary for normal functioning of Clc–kbcl$^-$ channel.
- Due to the presence of 'tight' tight junctions, Na^+ is unable to leak back into the tubule to produce a luminal potential; however, some of the K^+ which enters the cell leaks back across the apical membrane into the tubular lumen, by ROMK and other K^+ channels, generating a lumen-positive transepithelial potential difference (TEPD) of +6 to +10 mV.

Important Note

TAL is the site of action of the loop diuretics (e.g. furosemide, ethacrynic acid), which inhibit Na^+–K^+–$2Cl^-$ transporter.

Applied Aspects

Dent disease: Some of Cl^- absorption in thick ascending loop of Henle occurs with Na^+, K^+ and Ca^{2+}. In kidneys, a type of Cl^- channel has been identified which is linked with Ca^{2+}. Gene mutation of this channel is associated with Ca^{2+}-containing renal stones and hypercalciuria, and is known as Dent disease.

Na^+–H^+ antiporter-mediated active reabsorption of sodium also occurs transcellularly leading to H^+ secretion (HCO_3^- reabsorption) (Fig. 6.2.13).

Paracellular passive reabsorption of Na^+, K^+, Ca^{2+} and Mg^{2+} is the function of voltage across the TAL. Because of the unique location of transport proteins in the apical and basolateral membranes, the TF is positively charged relative to the blood. The increased salt reabsorption by the TAL increases the magnitude of positive charge in the lumen which plays a major role in driving the passive paracellular reabsorption of cations (Fig. 6.2.13).

Important Note

TAL is *impermeable* to water. Thus, NaCl and other solutes are reabsorbed without water. As a result, TF Na^+ and TF osmolarity decrease to less than their concentration in plasma (i.e. $TF/P_{osm} < 1.0$). This segment is therefore called the *diluting segment*. Furthermore, Na^+ reabsorbed from this segment is the main driving force behind the countercurrent multiplier system which concentrates Na^+ and urea in medullary interstitium. (For details, see page 507.)

Applied Aspects

Bartter syndrome: Bartter syndrome is a rare disease that most often presents in neonatal period or early childhood. It may result due to mutation affecting any of the ion transport proteins in TAL: Na^+–K^+–$2Cl^-$ symporter, the ROMK K^+ channel, Clc–kbcl channel or barttin. The TAL transporters function in an integrated manner to maintain electrical potential difference and Na^+ gradient between the tubular lumen and the cell.

- Loss of lumen-positive electric transport potential (which normally derives paracellular absorption of Na^+, Ca^{2+}

and Mg^{2+}) causes NaCl wasting, hypercalciuria and hypomagnesemia.
- Bartter syndrome due to mutation of barttin is also associated with deafness, because stria vascularis in the inner ear is responsible for maintaining high K^+ concentration in scala media.

Signs and symptoms vary with severity of the disease. In children, the typical signs of Bartter syndrome are excessive urination and thirst, chronic dehydration, growth failure, muscle weakness and cramps.

Transport Across Distal Tubules and Collecting Duct

Approximately 7% of the filtered NaCl and about 8%–17% of water are reabsorbed and K^+ and H^+ are secreted in these segments.

Early DT Early DT (initial segment of DT) reabsorbs Na^+, Cl^- and Ca^{2+}, and is impermeable to water.

- *Na^+–Cl^- symporter* mechanism is involved in the transport of Na^+–Cl^- across the apical membrane. Across the basolateral membrane, Na^+ leaves the cell via the action of Na^+–K^+-ATPase, and Cl^- leaves the cell by diffusion via channels (Fig. 6.2.14).
- Because of *impermeability to water*, the reabsorption of NaCl in this segment occurs without water leading to dilution of TF. This is why it is also called cortical diluting segment.

Important Note

Thiazide diuretics reduce NaCl reabsorption by inhibiting Na^+–Cl^- cotransport.

Late DT and CD Late DT and CD have two cell types (principal cells and intercalated cells) which perform both reabsorption and secretory functions:

Principal cells Principal cells reabsorb Na^+, Cl^- and H_2O and secrete K^+ (Fig. 6.2.15):

Na^+ reabsorption: Na^+ is actively transported using Na^+–K^+-ATPase across the basolateral membrane. Across the apical membrane, Na^+ diffuses passively due to chemical gradient.

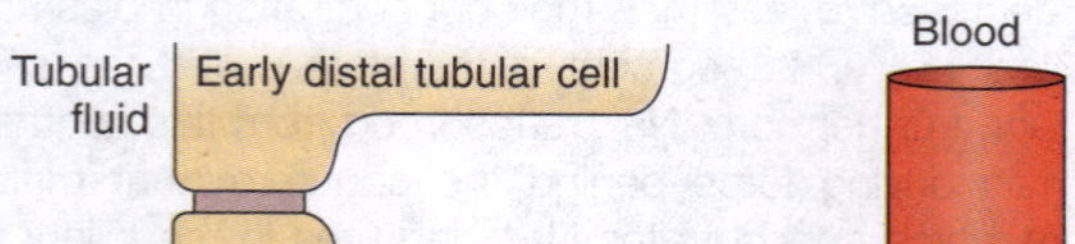

Fig. 6.2.14 Mechanism of reabsorption of Na^+ and Cl^- in the early distal tubule. This segment is impermeable to water (see text for details).

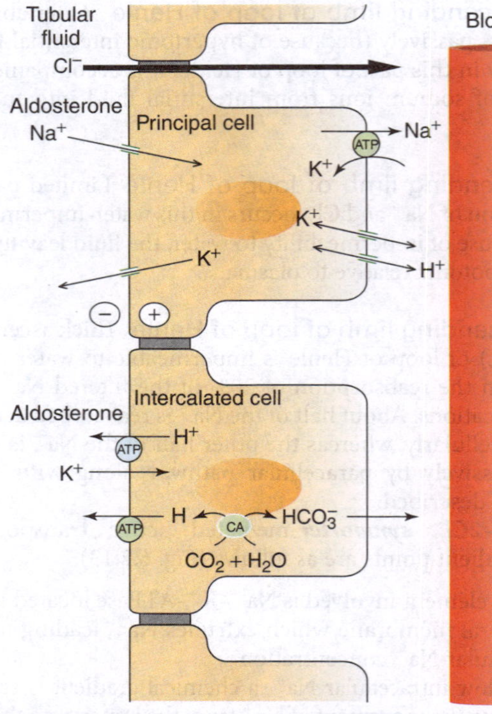

Fig. 6.2.15 Mechanism of transport in principal cells and intercalated cells of the late distal tubule and collecting duct (see text for details). CA, carbonic anhydrase.

Cl^- reabsorption occurs passively through paracellular pathway. Cl^- is driven by the lumen-negative charge generated by the diffusional influx of sodium.

H_2O absorption occurs in response to the effect of antidiuretic hormone (ADH) on the principal cells. ADH increases H_2O permeability by directing the insertion of H_2O channels in the luminal membrane. In the absence of ADH, the principal cells are virtually impermeable to water.

K^+ secretion: K^+ uptake across the basolateral membrane occurs via the action of Na^+–K^+-ATPase followed by diffusion down its electrochemical gradient across the apical cell membrane into the TF.

Role of aldosterone on principal cell functions Aldosterone increases Na^+ reabsorption and increases K^+ secretion. Like other steroid hormones, the action of aldosterone takes several hours to develop because new protein synthesis is required. About 2% of overall Na^+ absorption is affected by aldosterone.

Important Note

Effect of amiloride: Amiloride is a diuretic that inhibits Na^+ reabsorption by distal tubule and collecting duct by directly inhibiting Na^+ channels in the luminal cell membrane. Thus, indirectly, by reducing the negative charge in lumen, the amiloride also inhibits Cl^- reabsorption and K^+ secretion. As the K^+ excretion in urine is decreased, it is called *potassium-sparing diuretic*. Other potassium-sparing diuretics are spironolactone and triamterene.

Intercalated cells reabsorb K^+ Intercalated cells reabsorb K^+ and secrete H^+:

K^+ reabsorption occurs probably by an H^+–K^+-ATPase located in the apical cell membrane.

***H^+* secretion** (HCO_3^- reabsorption) or HCO_3^- secretion (H^+ reabsorption) can occur by H^+-ATPase. This function is important for acid–base balance (see page 514).
Aldosterone increases H^+ secretion by intercalated cells by stimulating the H^+-ATPase (in addition to its actions on the principal cells).

RENAL HANDLING OF COMMON SOLUTES AND WATER

After discussing the transport across different segments of renal tubule, it will be worthwhile to discuss briefly the renal handling of common solutes and water, which include:

- Renal handling of sodium and water
- Renal handling of potassium
- Renal handling of glucose
- Renal handling of urea
- Renal handling of uric acid
- Renal handling of PAH
- Renal handling of acid–base balance (see page 1187)

Renal Handling of Sodium and Water

Site and mechanisms of reabsorption of sodium

Reabsorption of the filtered sodium in different segments of the renal tubule is as follows:

- Proximal tubule: 60%
- Loop of Henle (mainly TAL): 30%
- DT: 7%
- Cortical CD: 3%

Mechanisms of reabsorption Mechanisms of reabsorption, as described in detail in the section 'Transport across Proximal Tubule,' are summarized in Table 6.2.3.

Sodium recycling: The sodium which is actively pumped out from the TAL into the outer medullary interstitium mostly enters the outer medullary descending thin segment (DTS). This results in recycling of Na^+ in the long loops of the juxtamedullary nephrons. The recycling causes accumulation of Na^+ in the interstitium of the renal medulla.

Table 6.2.3 Summary of mechanism of Na^+ absorption across different segments of renal tubule

Segment of the tubule	Absorption (active/passive/ impermeable)	Mediated by
Proximal tubule		
• Early proximal tubule	Active	• Na^+–K^+ antiporter • Na^+–H^+ antiporter • Na^+ glucose (and other organic solutes) symport
• Late proximal tubule	Active	• Cl^--driven Na^+ transport
Loop of Henle		
• Descending thin segment (DTS)	Passively secreted in interstitium	
• Ascending thin segment (ATS)	Passive	
• Thick ascending limb (TAL)	Active (transcellular)	• Na^+–K^+–Cl^- symporter • Na^+–H^+ antiporter
Distal tubule and collecting duct		
• Early distal tubule	Active	• Na^+–Cl^- symporter
• Late distal tubule and collecting duct (principal cell)	Active	• Na^+ channels (ENa) • Regulated by aldosterone

Reabsorption of Water

Site and mechanism of reabsorption Water is absorbed passively by osmosis in response to a transtubular osmotic gradient. Rapid diffusion of water across the cell membrane occurs through water channels made up of proteins called *aquaporins*. Different types of aquaporins are aquaporin-1, -2, -5 and -9. Mostly, these aquaporins are present in the kidney. The other sites included are leucocytes, liver, lung and lacrimal gland. In the CDs, reabsorption of water is controlled by ADH. Renal handling of water by different segments of renal tubule is as follows:

Proximal tubule. Passively reabsorbed (67%)

Loop of Henle (15%):

- DTS: Passively reabsorbed (15%)
- Ascending thin segment (ATS): Impermeable
- TAL: Impermeable

DT and CD (8%–17%):

- Distal convoluted tubule (DCT): Impermeable
- Connecting tubule (CNT): Impermeable
- Cortical collecting duct (CCD): Reabsorbed (ADH)
- Outer medullary collecting duct (OMCD): Reabsorbed (ADH)
- Inner medullary collecting duct (IMCD): Reabsorbed (ADH)

Obligatory and facultative reabsorption of water

Obligatory reabsorption About 85% of the filtered water is always reabsorbed, irrespective of the body water balance. This reabsorption occurs by osmosis in response to a transtubular osmotic gradient and is called obligatory (must occur) reabsorption.

- About 67% of obligatory reabsorption occurs in the proximal tubules.
- About 15%–18% of obligatory reabsorption occurs in the DTS of loop of Henle.

Facultative reabsorption The remaining 15%–18% of the water may or may not be absorbed depending on the body water balance. It is called facultative (optional) reabsorption.

Facultative reabsorption of water occurs from the collecting tubule and is under the control of ADH.

Regulation of NaCl and Water Absorption

1. Hormonal regulation Various hormones including angiotensin II, aldosterone, ADH, ANP, urodilatin, epinephrine and norepinephrine (released from sympathetic nerves) and dopamine regulate NaCl reabsorption. ADH is the only major hormone that directly regulates the amount of water excreted by the kidney. Table 6.2.4 summarizes for each hormone the major stimulus for secretion, the nephron site of action and the effect on transport.

Table 6.2.4 Hormonal regulation of NaCl and water reabsorption

Hormone	Major stimulus for secretion	Nephron (site of action)	Effect on transport
Angiotensin II	↑ Renin	PT	↑ Na^+, Cl^- and H_2O reabsorption
Aldosterone	↑ Angiotensin and ↑ $[K^+]_P$	TAL, DT/CD	↑ NaCl and H_2O reabsorption
Atria natriuretic peptide	↑ ECV	CD	↓ NaCl and H_2O reabsorption
Urodilatin	↑ ECV	CD	↓ NaCl and H_2O reabsorption
Sympathetic nerves	↓ ECV	PT, TAL, DT/CD	↑ NaCl and H_2O reabsorption
Dopamine	↑ ECV	PT	↓ NaCl and H_2O reabsorption
ADH	↑ P_{osm}	DT/CD	↑ H_2O reabsorption

ADH, antidiuretic hormone; DT/CD, distal tubule and collecting duct; ECV, effective circulatory volume; $[K^+]_P$, plasma K^+ concentration; P_{osm}, plasma osmolarity; PT, proximal tubule; TAL, thick ascending limb.

2. Role of Starling forces Although Na^+ reabsorption is an active process, it is affected by the passive Starling forces operating between the intercellular spaces and the peritubular capillaries in the proximal tubule.

Starling forces that favour the movement of reabsorbed substances into the capillaries are capillary oncotic pressure (π_C) and the hydrostatic pressure in the intercellular spaces (P_i).
Opposing Starling forces are the interstitial oncotic pressure (π_i) and the capillary hydrostatic pressure (P_C).

- Starling forces do not affect transport by the loop of Henle, DT and CD because these segments are less permeable to water than the proximal tubule.
- Starling forces across the peritubular capillaries around the proximal tubule are changed by:
  - Dilatation of efferent arteriole (↑ P_C)
  - Constriction of efferent arteriole (↓ P_C)

3. Role of glomerulotubular balance (GTB) in the proximal tubule GTB in the proximal tubule maintains reabsorption at a constant fraction (two-thirds or 67% of the filtered Na^+ and H_2O). For example, if GFR spontaneously increases, the filtered load of Na^+ also increases. Without a change in reabsorption, this situation would lead to increased Na^+ excretion. However, GTB functions such as Na^+ reabsorption will also increase, ensuring that a constant fraction is reabsorbed.

Mechanism of GTB Mechanism of GTB is based on Starling forces in the peritubular capillaries, which alter the reabsorption of Na^+ and H_2O in the proximal tubule (Fig. 6.2.16):

- *Route of isosmotic fluid reabsorption* is from the lumen to the proximal tubule cell, to the lateral intercellular space and then to the peritubular capillary blood.

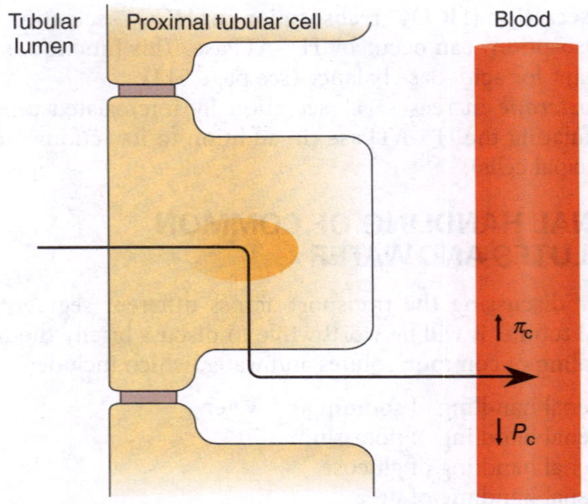

Fig. 6.2.16 Mechanism of glomerulotubular balance (isosmotic reabsorption).

- *Starling forces in the peritubular capillary blood* govern how much of this isosmotic fluid will be reabsorbed.
- *Fluid reabsorption* is increased by increase in oncotic pressure of the peritubular capillary blood (π_C) and decreased by decrease in π_C.
- *Increase in GFR and FF* causes the protein concentration and π_C of peritubular capillary blood to increase. This increase, in turn, produces an increase in fluid reabsorption. Thus, there is matching of filtration and reabsorption, i.e. GTB.

4. Effects of ECF volume on proximal tubular reabsorption

ECF volume contraction increases reabsorption. ECF volume contraction increases peritubular capillary protein concentration and oncotic pressure (π_C) and decreases peritubular capillary hydrostatic pressure (P_C). Together, these changes in Starling forces in peritubular capillary blood cause an increase in proximal tubular reabsorption.
ECF volume expansion decreases reabsorption. ECF volume expansion decreases peritubular capillary protein concentration and oncotic pressure (π_C) and increases peritubular capillary hydrostatic pressure (P_C). Together, these changes in Starling forces in peritubular capillary blood cause a decrease in proximal tubular reabsorption.

Renal Handling of Potassium and Potassium Homeostasis

General Considerations

Functions of K^+ Potassium (K^+) is one of the most abundant cations in the body. It is the *principal intracellular cation*, and is equally important in the ECF for specific functions. Potassium is required for the following biochemical functions:

- Maintenance of intracellular osmotic pressure
- Optimal activity of enzyme pyruvate kinase (of glycolysis)
- Proper synthesis of DNA and proteins by ribosomes
- Optimal cell growth
- Transmission of nerve impulse
- Generation of cell membrane potential and muscle contraction
- Influencing cardiac muscle activity by extracellular K^+
- Regulation of acid–base balance and water balance in the cells

Daily Requirement and Sources

Daily requirement of K^+ is about 3–4 g/day.
Sources of K^+ are bananas, oranges, pineapples, potatoes, beans, chicken, liver and tender coconut water.

Potassium Homeostasis

Distribution of K^+

Total body K^+ constitutes about 50 mEq/kg of body weight, or 3500 mEq, for a 70-kg individual.

Intracellular K^+: K^+ is predominantly an intracellular cation. Ninety-eight per cent of the K^+ in the body is located within cells, where its average concentration is 150 mEq/L.
ECF contains only 2% of the total body K^+, where its normal concentration is approximately 4 mEq/L.

Shifts of K^+ between ICF and ECF

occurs:
Hyperkalaemia, i.e. ECF K^+ concentration >5.0 mEq/L, occurs when K^+ is shifted out of cells in the following conditions:

- Insulin deficiency
- β-Adrenergic antagonists
- Acidosis (exchange of extracellular H^+ for intracellular K^+)
- Hyperosmolarity (H_2O flows out of the cells, K^+ diffuses out with H_2O)
- Inhibition of Na^+–K^+ pump (e.g. digitalis), as when pump is blocked, K^+ is not taken up into cells
- Exercise
- Cell lysis (therefore, care should be taken to avoid haemolysis of RBCs for the estimation of serum K^+)

Hypokalaemia, i.e. ECF K^+ concentration <3.5 mEq/L, occurs when K^+ is shifted into the cells, as is caused by:

- Insulin
- β-Adrenergic agonists
- Alkalosis (exchange of intracellular H^+ for extracellular K^+)
- Hypo-osmolarity (H_2O flows into the cell, K^+ diffuses in with H_2O)

External Versus Internal K^+ Balance

Despite wide fluctuations in dietary K^+ intake, its concentration in ICF and ECF remains constant. Two sets of regulatory mechanisms safeguard K^+ homeostasis – one type of mechanism maintains external K^+ balance and the second set of mechanism maintains the internal K^+ balance.

External K^+ balance

External K^+ balance refers to maintenance of constant amount of K^+ in the body. It is accomplished by adjusting renal K^+ excretion to match the dietary K^+ intake. Normally, all the K^+ absorbed by GIT is excreted by the kidneys. However, it is a slow process and at least takes 6 hours. This arrangement ensures a long-term, chronic constancy of K^+ content. However, rapid losses of large amount of K^+ can cause serious hypokalaemia. Conversely, hyperkalaemia can occur when K^+ is absorbed from GIT or infused intravenously much faster than the kidney can excrete it.

Internal K^+ balance

Internal K^+ balance refers to the constancy of K^+ distribution in ICF and ECF. Rapid changes in ECF are not uncommon. After a meal, the K^+ absorbed by the GIT enters the ECF within minutes and, as mentioned above, the kidney takes at least 6 hours to excrete it. Therefore, certain mechanisms are required to keep a balance between ECF and ICF; otherwise, even after normal meals, the plasma K^+ levels will rise to fatal levels. The internal K^+ balance is maintained by various hormones which allow a rapid to-and-fro shift between ECF and ICF (Fig. 6.2.17).

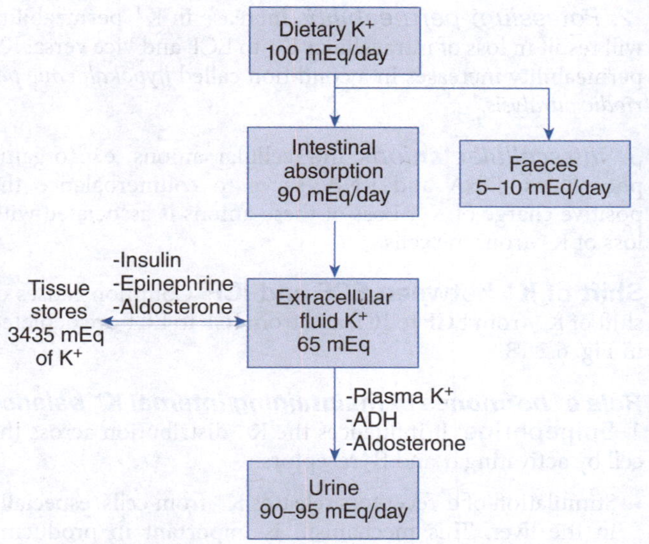

Fig. 6.2.17 An overview of potassium homeostasis (for explanation, see text).

Maintenance of internal K^+ balance

The internal K^+ balance is maintained by rapid redistribution of K^+ between ICF and ECF. Factors involved in it are summarized in Fig. 6.2.17. Before discussing the role played by each factor, it will be worthwhile to understand the mechanism involved in the regulatory process.

Mechanism of control of K^+ entry into the cells

The primary mechanisms which affect the movement of K^+ into and out of the cells are as follows:

1. Na^+–K^+-ATPase activity Na^+–K^+-ATPase activity is the main factor controlling entry of K^+ into the cells. All the major hormones involved in maintaining internal K^+ balance (i.e. epinephrine, insulin and aldosterone) increase K^+ uptake of cells (particularly of skeletal muscle, liver, bone and red blood cells) by stimulating activity of the Na^+–K^+-ATPase pump. The activity of Na^+–K^+-ATPase is increased:

- *Rapidly* (within minutes) by increased turnover rate of existing Na^+–K-ATPase to handle the acute changes in plasma K^+ levels
- *Slowly* (within hour to day) by an increase in the number of Na^+–K^+-ATPase units in the membrane (the slow increase in Na^+–K^+-ATPase activity is required to produce a chronic increase in K^+ uptake by the cells)
  For example, an increase in plasma K^+ levels that follows K^+ absorption by GIT stimulates insulin secretion from the pancreas, aldosterone release from the adrenal cortex and epinephrine secretion from the adrenal medulla to stimulate Na^+–K^+-ATPase activity for handling the raised K^+ plasma levels. In contrast, a decrease in plasma K^+ levels inhibits the release of these hormones.

Important Note

It is important to note that insulin and epinephrine act within a few minutes, whereas aldosterone requires about 1 hour to stimulate K^+ uptake into the cells.

2. Potassium permeability Increase in K^+ permeability will result in loss of intracellular K^+ to ECF and vice versa. K^+ permeability increases in a condition called *hypokalaemic periodic paralysis*.

3. Intracellular anions Intracellular anions, e.g. organic phosphates, DNA and RNA, serve to counterbalance the positive charge of K^+. Loss of these anions is associated with loss of K^+ from the cells.

Shift of K^+ between ECF and ICF Common causes of shift of K^+ from ECF to ICF and from ICF to ECF are depicted in Fig. 6.2.18.

Role of hormones in maintaining internal K^+ balance

1. Epinephrine It influences the K^+ distribution across the cell by activating α and β_2 receptors.

- Stimulation of α receptors releases K^+ from cells, especially in the liver. This mechanism is important in producing local hyperkalaemia in the muscle, which subserves two beneficial functions – vasodilatation and activation of glycogenolysis. Both activities support vigorous exercise.
- Stimulation of β_2 receptors causes K^+ uptake by cells. This mechanism lowers plasma K^+ during acute stress, e.g. myocardial ischaemia.

2. Insulin It is the most important hormone that shifts K^+ into cells after ingestion of K^+ in a meal by stimulating Na^+–K^+-ATPase. The role of insulin explains:

- Greater rise in plasma K^+ after a K^+-rich meal in an individual with diabetes mellitus (insulin deficiency) as compared with in a normal person
- Role of insulin infusion (with glucose to prevent insulin-induced hypoglycaemia) in correcting hyperkalaemia

3. Aldosterone It promotes K^+ uptake into the cells by activating Na^+–K^+-ATPase; therefore:

- *Hypokalaemia* occurs when aldosterone levels are increased (e.g. in primary aldosteronism).
- *Hyperkalaemia* occurs when aldosterone level falls (e.g. in Addison disease).

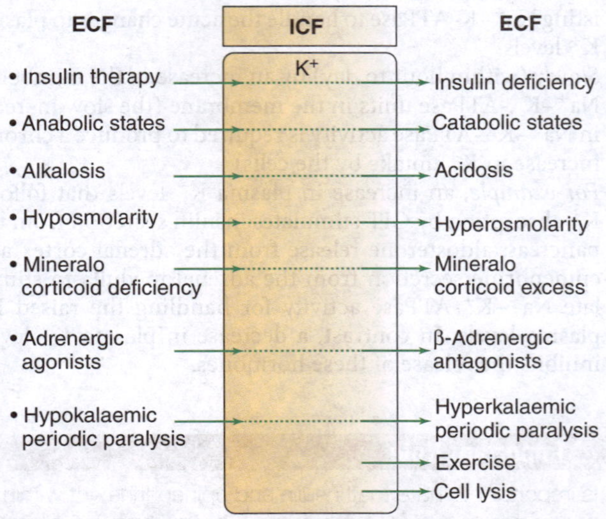

Fig. 6.2.18 Causes of shift of K^+ between ECF and ICF. ECF, extracellular fluid.

The aldosterone also stimulates urinary K^+ excretion (discussed later in this chapter).

Effect of other factors on internal K^+ balance Certain factors which do not contribute to K^+ homeostasis, but do affect the internal K^+ balance are described below. The extent to which these factors are able to alter plasma K^+ depends on the integrity of homeostatic mechanisms that regulate plasma K^+ (e.g. secretion of epinephrine, insulin and aldosterone).

1. Acid–base balance influences the internal K^+ balance in the following ways:

Metabolic acidosis produced by inorganic acids (e.g. HCl and H_2SO_4) is associated with entry of H^+ into the cells and movement of K^+ into the ECF, producing hyperkalaemia.

Metabolic acidosis produced by organic acids (e.g. lactic acid, acetic acid and keto acids) usually does not produce hyperkalaemia. It is because in such circumstances, the anions enter the cell along with H^+, and thereby eliminate the need for K^+/H^+ exchange across the cell membrane. Furthermore, organic anions may stimulate insulin secretion which moves K^+ into the cells. This movement may counteract the direct effect of acidosis, which moves K^+ out of the cell.

Respiratory acidosis has very little effect on plasma K^+ levels, because the resting membrane potential does not change when CO_2 enters the cells, or when it reacts with water to form H^+ and HCO_3^-.

Metabolic alkalosis decreases plasma K^+ because K^+ enters the cells in exchange of H^+.

2. Plasma osmolarity influences the internal K^+ balance as:

Hyperosmolarity: In this condition, water moves out of the cells because of the osmotic gradient across the cell membrane until the intracellular osmolarity equals that of ECF. The loss of water shrinks cells and causes K^+ to rise. The rise in intracellular K^+ leads to diffusion of K^+ into the ECF, producing hyperkalaemia.

Hypo-osmolarity results in hypokalaemia because of movement of K^+ into the cells by the effect just opposite to that seen in hyperosmolarity.

3. Exercise During exercise, more K^+ is released from the skeletal muscle cells than during rest. This is because during the depolarization that accompanies muscle contraction, K^+ exits from the muscle cells. However, most of the K^+ released enters the T tubules, from which K^+ is rapidly taken back into the cell on repolarization, but a little K^+ does enter the interstitial fluid and plasma. Therefore, the ensuing hyperkalaemia depends on the degree of exercise. After slow walking, plasma K^+ level increases by 0.3 mEq/L, but with more vigorous exercise the K^+ levels may increase up to 2.0 mEq/L above normal. However, exercise-induced hyperkalaemia usually does not produce symptoms and is reversed after several minutes of rest.

Applied Aspects

Exercise-induced hyperkalaemia is unusual under the following circumstances:

- *Patients with disturbed T tubule architecture of muscles* may develop hyperkalaemia with minimal exercise. For example, even fist clenching may be associated with significant hyperkalaemia.

- *Patients with certain endocrine disorders* that affect release of insulin, epinephrine or aldosterone may develop potentially life-threatening hyperkalaemia.
- *Patients with impaired K^+ excretion* (e.g. renal failure) may also develop significant hyperkalaemia after exercise.
- *Individuals taking β-blockers*, e.g. propranolol, for treatment of hypertension may get significant hyperkalaemia after exercise.

4. Drug-induced hyperkalaemia for one-third of total cases of clinically significant hyperkalaemia. Drugs that induce hyperkalaemia include:

- Potassium supplements
- Angiotensin-converting enzyme (ACE) inhibitors
- K^+-sparing diuretics
- Heparin
- PGE-suppressing drugs

Applied Aspects

Risk for drug-induced hyperkalaemia is increased in:

- Elderly individuals
- Patients with diabetes mellitus
- Patients with renal insufficiency

Signs and symptoms of hyperkalaemia include chest and abdominal pain, irregular heartbeat and palpitation, muscle weakness and numbness in the limbs. Sometimes nausea and vomiting may occur.

Treatment: Hyperkalaemia is a common disorder that can be fatal if untreated. The immediate treatment of hyperkalaemia includes intravenous administration of calcium gluconate and insulin with glucose.

Maintenance of external potassium balance As mentioned earlier, external potassium balance refers to maintenance of constant body potassium, i.e. renal excretion matches dietary intake.

Intestinal absorption versus renal excretion

Absorption: The average diet contains approximately 100 mEq/day (~5 g/day) of potassium. Normally, 90% of the dietary K^+ is absorbed and about 10% is lost through faeces and sweats (Fig. 6.2.17). This amount (90%) of absorption is essentially constant, and not physiologically regulated, and, therefore, plays little role in maintenance of the external potassium balance.

Excretion: Normally, kidneys excrete 90%–95% of K^+ ingested in the diet (Fig. 6.2.17) and thus play a major role in maintaining external potassium balance. Excretion equals intake, even when intake increases by as much as 10-fold. Therefore, the K^+ excretion can vary widely from 1% to 110% of the filtered load, depending on the dietary intake, aldosterone levels and acid–base balance. The transport pattern of K^+ by the major nephron, i.e. renal handling of the K^+, is described. It will be noted that the *main event that regulates external potassium balance is K^+ secretion* from the blood into the TF by the cells of the DT and CD system, and not the reabsorption in the proximal tubule which is load dependent.

Transport of Potassium Across Major Nephron

Glomerular filtration Filtration occurs freely across the glomerular capillaries and potassium is not bound to plasma proteins. Therefore, TF/PK^+ in Bowman's space is 1.00.

Tubular reabsorption and secretion As shown in Fig. 6.2.19, 67% of the filtered K^+ is reabsorbed in the proximal tubule, 20% in the loop of Henle and approximately 10% is delivered to the early DT. In contrast to proximal tubule and loop of Henle, which are capable of only reabsorbing K^+, the DT and CD are able to either reabsorb or secrete K^+. The role of reabsorption or secretion by DT and CD depends on a variety of hormones and factors.

Reabsorption of K^+ by proximal tubule In proximal tubule, potassium reabsorption is load dependent like that of Na^+. Two mechanisms involved in K^+ reabsorption are as follows:

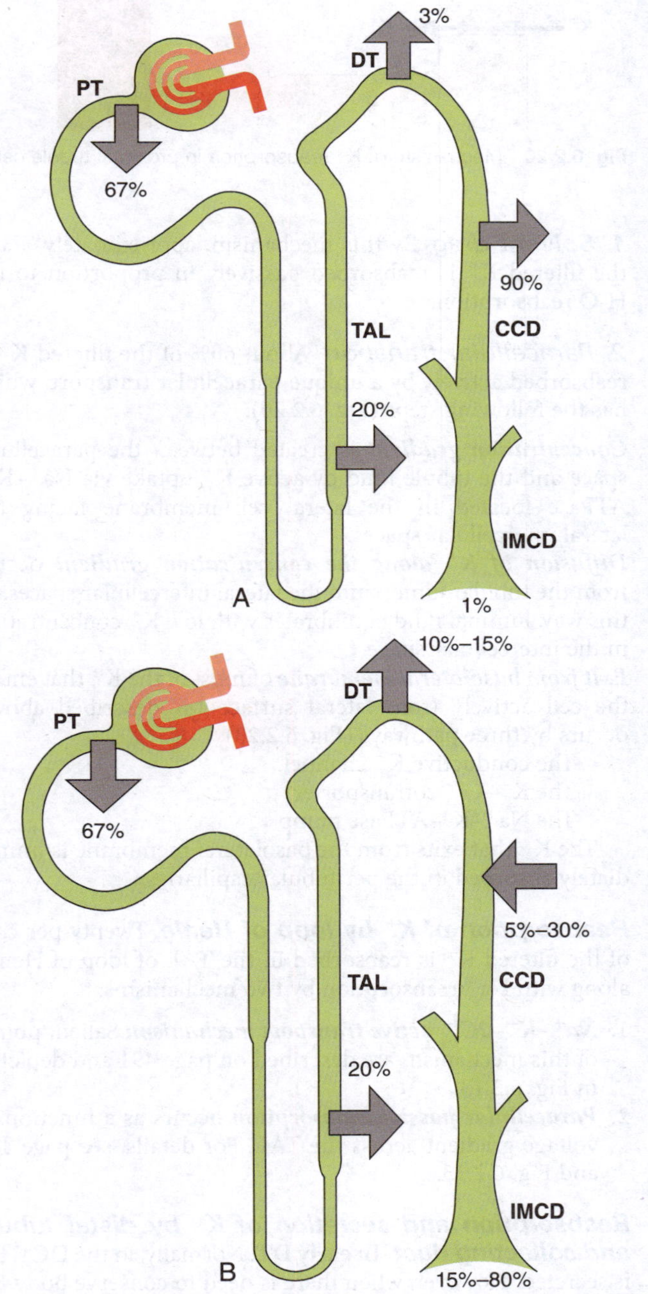

Fig. 6.2.19 Potassium transport along the nephron: **A**, during dietary potassium depletion; and **B**, during normal and increased dietary intake.

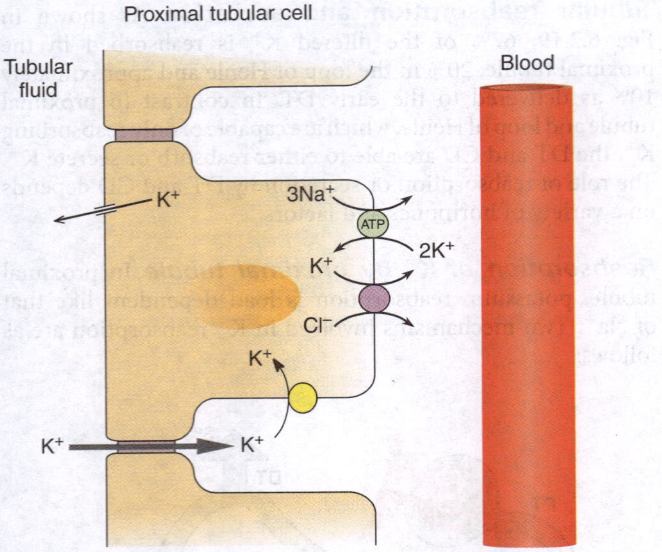

Fig. 6.2.20 Mechanism of K^+ reabsorption in proximal tubule cells.

1. Solvent drag By this mechanism, approximately 7% of the filtered K^+ is reabsorbed passively in proportion to the H_2O reabsorption.

2. Paracellular transport About 60% of the filtered K^+ is reabsorbed actively by a unique paracellular transport, which has the following steps (Fig. 6.2.20):

Concentration gradient is created between the paracellular space and the tubule fluid by active K^+ uptake via Na^+–K^+-ATPase located in the lateral cell membrane facing the lateral intercellular spaces.

Diffusion of K^+ along the concentration gradient occurs from the tubular lumen into the lateral intercellular spaces. In this way, luminal fluid equilibrates with low K^+ concentration in the intercellular space.

Exit from basolateral membrane of most of the K^+ that enters the cell actively from lateral surface (as described above) occurs by three pathways (Fig. 6.2.20):

- The conductive K^+ channel
- The K^+–Cl^- cotransporter
- The Na^+–K^+-ATPase pump

The K^+ that exits from the basolateral membrane is immediately absorbed in the peritubular capillaries.

Reabsorption of K^+ by loop of Henle Twenty per cent of the filtered K^+ is reabsorbed in the TAL of loop of Henle, along with Na^+ reabsorption by two mechanisms:

1. ***Na^+–K^+–$2Cl^-$ active transport mechanism:*** Salient points of this mechanism are described on page 491 and depicted in Fig. 6.2.13.
2. ***Paracellular passive reabsorption*** occurs as a function of voltage gradient across the TAL. For details, see page 491 and Fig. 6.2.13.

Reabsorption and secretion of K^+ by distal tubule and collecting duct **In early DT:** Normally, in the DCT, K^+ is secreted. However, when there is need to conserve body K^+ (e.g. during K^+ depletion), K^+ is reabsorbed. Both secretion and reabsorption occur in the same cell, i.e. distal tubular cell, depending on the status of K^+ balance in the body.

Late DT and CD either reabsorb or secrete K^+, depending on the dietary intake.

- ***Reabsorption of K^+*** occurs only when the dietary intake is very low (i.e. during K^+ depletion). Under these circumstances, K^+ excretion can be as low as 1% of the filtered load (Fig. 6.2.19A), because the kidneys conserve as much K^+ as possible.
- ***Intercalated cells*** are involved in the reabsorption of K^+. Exact mechanism and cellular pathway of reabsorption is still not known. Probably, H^+–K-ATPase located in the apical cell membrane plays a role.
- ***Secretion of K^+*** is variable and accounts for the wide range of urinary K^+ excretion, depending on the dietary K^+ intake, aldosterone levels, acid–base status and urine rate of flow. *Principal cells* are involved in the K^+ secretion.

Mechanism of K^+ secretion is as follows (Fig. 6.2.15):

- At the basolateral membrane, K^+ is actively transported into the cell by Na^+–K^+-ATPase. As in all cells, this mechanism maintains a high intracellular K^+ concentration.
- At the apical membrane, K^+ is passively secreted into the lumen through K^+ channels, down its electrical and chemical gradient.
- *Regulation of K^+ secretions.* See 'Hormones and Factors that Regulate Urinary K^+ Excretion.'

Hormones and Factors that Regulate Urinary K^+ Excretion

As mentioned earlier, regulation of urinary K^+ excretion is achieved mainly by alterations in K^+ secretion by principal cells of the DT and CDs. In a nutshell, K^+ secretion by the principal cells is increased when the electrochemical driving force for K^+ across the apical membrane is increased and vice versa. Hormones and other factors involved in regulation of K^+ tubular secretion and thus of urinary K^+ excretion include:

- Plasma K^+ level
- Aldosterone
- Glucocorticoids
- ADH
- Acid–base balance
- Flow of TF
- Luminal anions

1. Plasma K^+ level mainly depends on:

Dietary intake of K^+ is an important determinant of K^+ secretion by principal cells (Fig. 6.2.21). Hyperkalaemia, resulting from a high-K^+ diet or any other factor (e.g. rhabdomyolysis), stimulates K^+ secretion within minutes.

Mechanisms involved in high secretion of K^+ in hyperkalaemia are as follows:

Stimulation of Na^+–K^+-ATPase, caused by hyperkalaemia, increases K^+ uptake across the basolateral membrane. Increased levels of intracellular K^+ increase the electrochemical gradient across the apical membrane.

Permeability of apical membrane to K^+ is increased by hyperkalaemia.

Aldosterone secretion is increased by hyperkalaemia, which (as discussed below) acts synergistically with plasma K^+ levels to stimulate K^+ secretion.

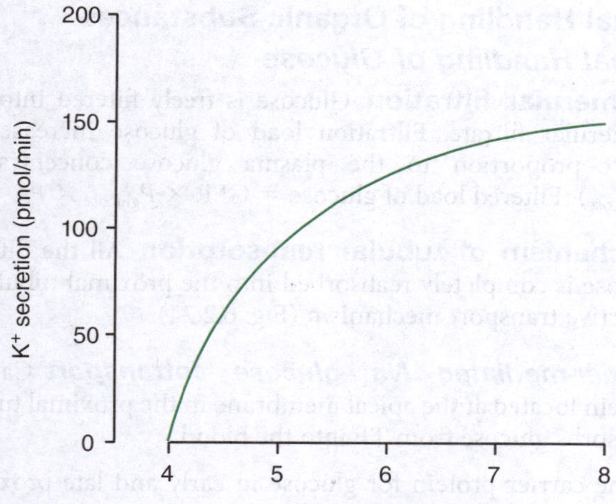

Fig. 6.2.21 Relationship between plasma K^+ level and K^+ secretion by principal cells.

Flow rate of TF is increased by hyperkalaemia, which (as discussed below) stimulates K^+ secretion by principal cells.

Hypokalaemia, resulting from a low K^+ diet or other factors (e.g. diarrhoea), decreases K^+ secretion by mechanisms opposite to those described for hyperkalaemia. In addition, hypokalaemia also *stimulates* α-intercalated cells to reabsorb K^+ by the H^+–K^+-ATPase.

2. Aldosterone Salient points on the role of aldosterone in regulating K^+ secretion by principal cells are as follows:

- *Aldosterone secretion is increased* by hyperkalaemia and angiotensin II (after activation of renin–angiotensin system).
- *Aldosterone secretion is decreased by* hypokalaemia and ANP.

Acute increase in aldosterone does not increase K^+ secretion This is because of the fact that due to acute increase in Na^+ and water reabsorption caused by aldosterone, the tubular flow is decreased, which in turn decreases K^+ secretion (as discussed below in detail).

Chronic rise in aldosterone level increases K^+ Chronic rise in aldosterone level increases K^+ secretion by the principal cells via the following mechanisms:

i. ***By increasing Na^+–K^+-ATPase activity:*** Aldosterone increases the amount of Na^+–K^+-ATPase in principal cells. This leads to increased pumping of Na^+ out of the cell in the basolateral membrane and increased Na^+ entry into the cells across the luminal membrane. Stimulation of Na^+–K^+-ATPase simultaneously increases K^+ uptake into the principal cells, increasing the intracellular K^+ concentration and the driving force for K^+ secretion.

> **Important Note**
>
> It is important to note that chronic stimulation of Na^+ reabsorption results in volume expansion and thereby returns tubular flow to normal and thus does not affect the K^+-secreting action of aldosterone. Furthermore, like other steroid hormones, the action of aldosterone takes hours to develop because new protein synthesis is required.

ii. ***By making the TEPD more lumen negative:*** By increasing the Na^+ reabsorption from lumen, the aldosterone makes the TEPD more lumen negative which in turn favours K^+ secretion.

iii. ***By increasing the permeability*** of apical membrane to K^+, aldosterone increases K^+ secretion.

3. Glucocorticoids Glucocorticoids indirectly increase K^+ excretion by increasing GFR, which increases tubular flow. Increased tubular flow increases K^+ secretion (as discussed below).

4. ADH ADH increases Na^+ and water reabsorption and decreases the tubular flow, which in turn decreases K^+ secretion (as discussed below). However, the ADH-induced increased Na^+ uptake across the luminal membrane of the principal cells creates an electrochemical gradient which increases K^+ secretion into the lumen. In this way, the inhibitory effect (through decreasing tubular flow) and stimulatory effect (through increasing electrochemical driving force for K^+) of ADH on K^+ secretion enable urinary K^+ excretion to be maintained constant, despite wide fluctuations in water excretion.

5. Flow of TF Salient points of effect of flow of TF on K^+ secretion are as follows:

Tubular flow rate is increased by ECF volume expansion and with diuretic therapy, whereas it is decreased in volume contraction caused by severe haemorrhage, or vomiting or diarrhoea.

Increase in TF flow increases K^+ secretion rapidly, whereas decrease in TF flow decreases the secretion of K^+ by DT and CDs by the following two mechanisms:

- *Change in the electrochemical driving force for K^+ across the apical membrane:* K^+ secretion in the TF leads to increased K^+ levels in the fluid and thus reduces the electrochemical driving force for K^+ exit across the apical membrane. The increased TF flow rate prevents the rise in K^+ concentration as the secreted K^+ is immediately washed down the stream.
- *Stimulation of K^+ uptake across basolateral membrane:* Increased tubular flow rate increases the amount of Na^+ reabsorbed across the apical membrane of principal cells. The increased Na^+ reabsorption in turn increases the K^+ uptake across the basolateral membrane by increasing the Na^+–K^+-ATPase activity.

Note: The increase in K^+ secretion with the increase in TF flow rate is directly proportional to the dietary intake of K^+ (Fig. 6.2.22).

> **Important Note**
>
> Thiazide and loop diuretic increase the K^+ secretion by increasing the TF flow through the DT and CDs.

6. Acid–base balance Acid–base balance affects the K^+ secretion by DT and CDs in the following manner:

Acute acidosis reduces K^+ secretion by two mechanisms:

By decreasing Na^+–K^+-ATPase activity across the basolateral membrane, it reduces the intracellular K^+ concentration and thus reduces the electrochemical driving force for K^+ exit across the apical membrane.

- *By reducing the permeability of apical membrane K^+*, it decreases K^+ secretion and also tends to increase intracellular K^+ concentration.

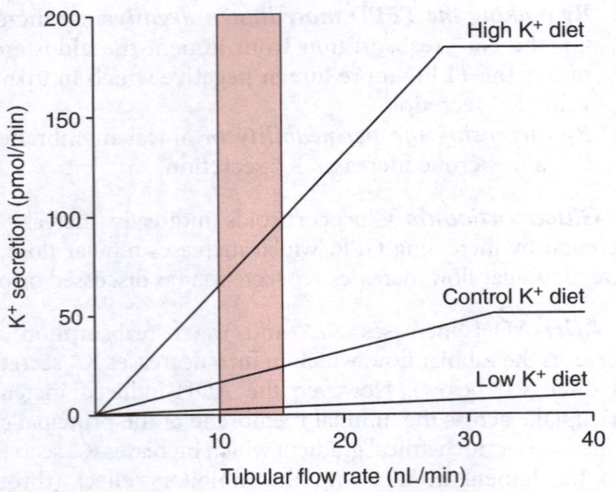

Fig. 6.2.22 Effect of dietary intake of K^+ on the relationship between tubular flow rate and K^+ secretion by the distal tubule and collecting duct.

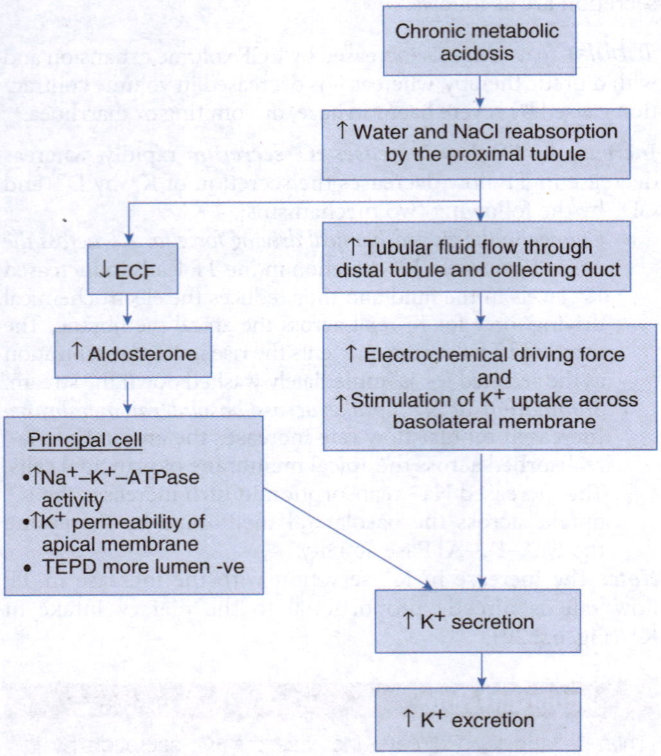

Fig. 6.2.23 Mechanism of increase in K^+ secretion in patients with chronic metabolic acidosis.

So, as a net result of the above-mentioned two mechanisms, K^+ secretion by the principal cells is decreased, whereas their K^+ content remained unchanged.

Acute alkalosis has exactly the opposite effect to acute acidosis and thus as a net result increases K^+ secretion by the principal cells.

Chronic acidosis, i.e. when metabolic acidosis lasts for several days, there occurs an increase in K^+ secretion by the mechanisms depicted in Fig. 6.2.23.

Renal Handling of Organic Substances

Renal Handling of Glucose

Glomerular filtration Glucose is freely filtered into the glomerular filtrate. Filtration load of glucose increases in direct proportion to the plasma glucose concentration ($P_{glucose}$). Filtered load of glucose = GFR × $P_{glucose}$ × P_G.

Mechanism of tubular reabsorption All the filtered glucose is completely reabsorbed into the proximal tubule by an active transport mechanism (Fig. 6.2.24):

Carrier-mediated Na^+–glucose cotransport Carrier protein located at the apical membrane in the proximal tubule reabsorbs glucose from TF into the blood.

- The carrier protein for glucose in early and late proximal tubule is called SGLT-2 and SGLT-1, respectively.
- The carrier is driven by the Na^+ concentration gradient which exists between the high tubular (Na^+) concentration and the low intracellular (Na^+) gradient produced by the pumping out of Na^+ through the basolateral surface.

Important Note

Phlorizin (a plant glucoside) inhibits glucose transport in the kidney by binding with carrier protein SGLT-2.

Facilitated diffusion moves the glucose out of the cell through the basolateral membrane. The carrier for facilitated diffusion across the basolateral membrane in early and late proximal tubule is called GLUT-2 and GLUT-1, respectively (glucose transporter).

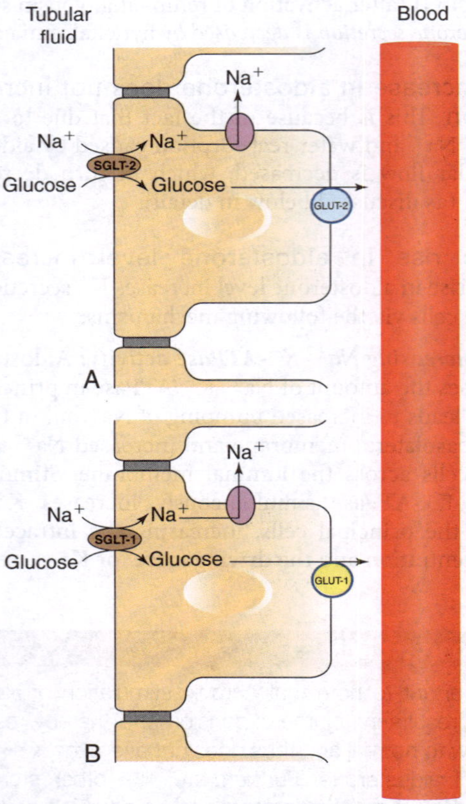

Fig. 6.2.24 Mechanism of glucose reabsorption in: **A**, early proximal tubule; and **B**, late proximal tubule.

Characteristics of glucose transport and glucose excretion Glucose is reabsorbed by a transport maximum process, i.e. there is a limited number of Na^+–glucose carriers. The characteristics of glucose transport and glucose excretion can be elicited from the glucose titration curve which is constructed by plotting the following pairs of variables:

- The filtered load against plasma glucose concentration
- The excretion rate against plasma glucose concentration
- The difference between the filtered load and the excretion rate (i.e. maximum tubular reabsorption capacity, T_r) against plasma concentration

Glucose titration curve Glucose titration curve (Fig. 6.2.25) depicts that:

Filtered load increases with the plasma glucose concentration (P_G).

Renal threshold, i.e. the plasma glucose concentration at which glucose first appears in the urine (glycosuria), is about 180–200 mg%. At plasma levels below the renal threshold, the reabsorption of glucose is complete (100%), i.e. all of the filtered glucose can be reabsorbed because plenty of carriers are available and hence no glucose is excreted in urine. In this region, the line of reabsorption is the same as that of filtration.

Transport maximum (T_m) refers to the plasma concentration at which carriers are fully saturated. As shown in Fig. 6.2.25, beyond plasma glucose concentration of 350 mg% (T_{mG}), the reabsorption rate does not increase, i.e. becomes constant and is independent of P_G. Thus, beyond T_{mG} levels, all the additional filtered glucose is excreted in the urine. Therefore, as the T_{mG} is reached, the urinary excretion rate increases linearly with increase in plasma glucose concentration (Fig. 6.2.25).

Splay refers to the region of the glucose curve between threshold and T_{mG}, i.e. between P_G 180 and 350 mg%. It represents the excretion of glucose in urine before the T_{mG} is fully achieved.

Important Note

It is important that in the region of splay, the reabsorption curve is rounded, indicating that although the reabsorption rate is increasing with increase in P_G, the reabsorption is less than filtration. Similarly, the excretion curve is also rounded in the region of splay, indicating that although the urinary excretion is increasing with increase in P_G, there is no linear relation.

Causes of splay are as follows:

- *Heterogenicity in glomerular size*, proximal tubular length and number of carrier proteins for glucose reabsorption: For example, a nephron with a large glomerulus (i.e. a high filtered load) or a short proximal tubule (i.e. low reabsorptive capacity) will spill glucose into the urine at a lower P_G than predicted from the T_{mG} for the whole kidney.
- *Variability in T_{mG}* of the nephron: For example, there is variability in the number of glucose carriers, the transport rate of the carriers and the binding affinity of the Na^+–glucose carriers.

Renal Handling of Proteins, Peptides and Amino Acids

Normally, a small amount of protein is filtered by the glomerulus and almost all is absorbed in the proximal tubule (see page 489). Normally, up to 150 mg of proteins is excreted daily in urine and of this only 15 mg is albumin and the rest are low-molecular-weight proteins (LMWP). About 25 mg of

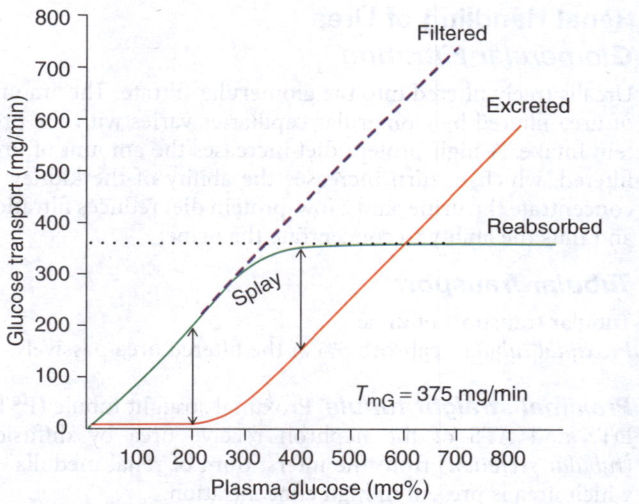

Fig. 6.2.25 Glucose titration curve (for details, see text).

LMWP are the *Tamm–Horsfall* proteins or uromodulin, which are glycoproteins derived from the cells of TAL and are normal constituents of urinary casts. The rest are derived from plasma proteins and include microproteins, lysozymes and light chains of immunoglobulins.

Important Note

Tamm–Horsfall proteins are basically crystallization of tubular fluid. These proteins play a significant role by providing defence against urinary tract infection caused by uropathogenic bacteria.

Applied Aspects

Proteinuria

Proteinuria is labelled when excretion of proteins in urine is more than 150 mg/day. It may be of the following types:

1. ***Glomerular proteinuria*** occurs when the glomerular permeability increases and allows albumin and other large proteins to be filtered.
2. ***Tubular proteinuria:*** Normally, LMWP enter the glomerular filtrate in fairly large amounts. When tubular reabsorption for these proteins is impaired, e.g. in *tubulointerstitial disorders and Fanconi syndrome*, large amounts of LMWP are excreted in urine.
3. ***Overflow proteinuria*** occurs when the amount of LMWP filtered exceeds the reabsorptive capacity of the tubules. Such a situation may arise when plasma levels of LMWP are increased, e.g. in multiple myeloma, in which large amounts of an abnormal protein called *Bence–Jones* proteins appear in the plasma.
4. ***Nephrogenic proteinuria*** occurs when tubular enzymes such as *N*-acetyl-β-glucosaminidase (NAG) and γ-glutamyltransferase (γ-GT) are released following damage to the proximal tubular cells.

Cause The most common cause of nephrogenic proteinuria is glomerulonephritis due to infection (leading to excessive filtration of proteins) and tubular damage leading to reduced reabsorption of proteins.

Signs and symptoms mainly occur due to hypoproteinaemia leading to swelling around the eyes and swelling of the body mainly in the dependent parts (legs and ankle).

Renal Handling of Urea

Glomerular Filtration

Urea is freely filtered into the glomerular filtrate. The amount of urea filtered by glomerular capillaries varies with the protein intake. A high-protein diet increases the amount of urea filtered, which in turn increases the ability of the kidney to concentrate the urine, and a low-protein diet reduces filtration and thus the ability to concentrate the urine.

Tubular Transport

Tubular transport of urea:
Proximal tubules reabsorb 5% of the filtered urea passively.

Proximal straight tubule Proximal straight tubule (PST), DTS and ATS of the nephron receive urea by diffusion (*tubular secretion*) from the interstitium of renal medulla, in which urea is present in high concentration.

TAL, DCT, CNT, CCD and OMCD are all impermeable to urea.

Inner medullary collecting duct IMCD reabsorbs large amounts of urea using a specialized *urea transport protein* (UT-A). There are four isoforms of UT-A in the kidneys (UTA_1 to UTA_4). This protein is stimulated by ADH which consequently increases urea permeability of the IMCD; UT-B is found in erythrocytes.

Urea Recycling

Urea recycling involves the following steps (Fig. 6.2.26):

1. ***Concentration of urea in CD*** (CCD and OMCD): As mentioned above, the nephron segments distal to ATS (i.e. TAL, DCT, CNT, CCD and OMCD) are all impermeable to urea. Therefore, as water is reabsorbed from the CCD, OMCD and the initial part of IMCD, urea gets more and more concentrated within the CD.
2. ***Rapid and massive reabsorption of urea by IMCD***, as described above, increases the concentration of urea in medullary interstitium. Urea transport in CD is mediated by $UT\text{-}A_1$.

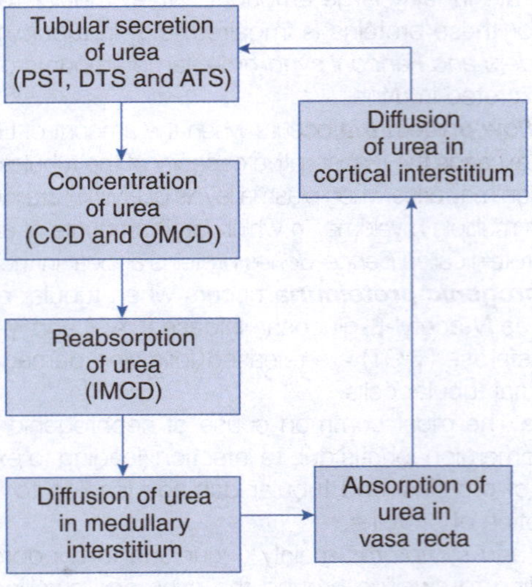

Fig. 6.2.26 Steps involved in urea recycling.

3. ***Carriage of urea by vasa recta to renal cortex interstitium:*** From the medullary interstitium, most of the urea enters the vasa recta and is carried upwards towards the renal cortex by the ascending vasa recta.
4. ***Tubular secretion of urea*** from the renal cortical interstitium occurs into the PST of cortical nephrons. Some of the urea also enters the thin segment of the long loops of the juxtamedullary nephrons. In this way, the urea is again carried back to the IMCD from where it diffuses out again resulting in a constant recycling.

Urea recycling plays an important role in the countercurrent system (see page 507).

Renal Handling of Uric Acid

Glomerular Filtration

Urate is freely filtered by the glomerular capillaries.

Tubular Transport

Tubular transport of uric acid is limited almost exclusively to the proximal tubule (Fig. 6.2.27):

- Early proximal tubule (S1 segment) reabsorbs 90% of the filtered uric acid.
- Mid-proximal tubule (S2 segment) secretes a moderate amount of uric acid equivalent to 50% of glomerular filtrate.
- Late proximal tubule (S3 segment) reabsorbs a moderate amount of uric acid (equivalent to 40% of glomerular filtrate). This is called postsecretory reabsorption.

Mechanism of uric acid reabsorption The uric acid is reabsorbed by two mechanisms:

Passive reabsorption occurs through *paracellular* pathway.

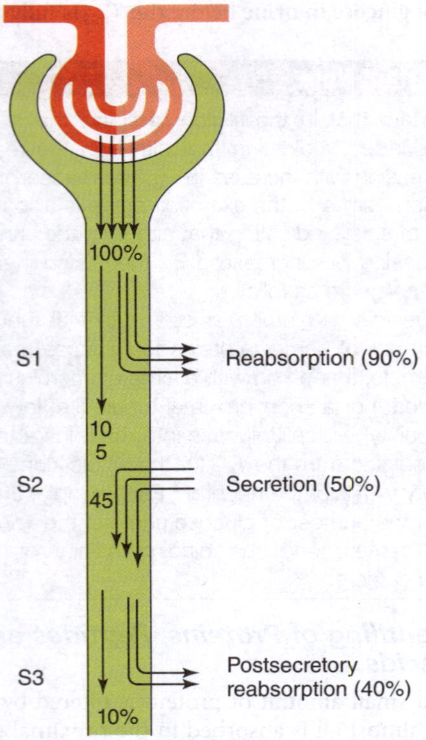

Fig. 6.2.27 Tubular transport of uric acid – reabsorption, secretion and postsecretory reabsorption.

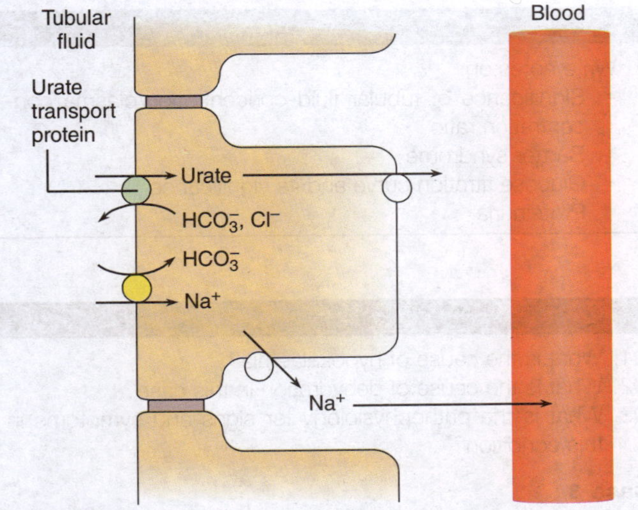

Fig. 6.2.28 Mechanism of urate reabsorption in proximal tubule cell.

Secondary active transport, which occurs through transcellular pathways, involves the following steps (Fig. 6.2.28):

- Across apical membrane, the uric acid enters the cell by countertransport with intracellular anions like Cl^-, HCO_3^- and also organic anions like lactate. The carrier protein involved is called *urate transport protein*.
- Across the basolateral membrane, the urate moves out using another anion exchanger. The same anion exchangers are used for urate secretion also.

Renal Handling of Para-Aminohippuric Acid (PAH)

The cells of proximal tubule, in addition to reabsorbing solutes and water, also secrete organic anions and organic cations, which include some end products of metabolism circulating in plasma, exogenous organic compounds and certain drugs (see Table 6.2.2).

Mechanism of secretion of organic anions

Mechanism of secretion of organic anions can be considered by the example of PAH secretion. PAH is an exogenous weak organic acid that is neither stored nor metabolized and is excreted virtually unchanged in the urine. Because 10% of PAH is bound to plasma proteins, it is cleared from the plasma both by glomerular filtration and by tubular secretion through the kidney. As with glucose, the filtered load of PAH increases in direct proportion to the plasma PAH concentration.

Secretion of PAH occurs from the peritubular capillary blood into the TF via carriers in the proximal tubule by a transport maximum T_m-limited process.

- The carrier which secretes PAH is nonselective, i.e. it can transport most of the organic anions.
- At low plasma concentration of PAH, the secretion rate increases as the plasma concentration increases. But, once the carriers are saturated, further increase in the plasma PAH concentration does not cause further increase in the secretion rate T_m.
- The PAH is taken into the cell across the basolateral membrane against its chemical gradient, in exchange for αKG via a PAH–αKG *antiport mechanism*. The resultant high intracellular concentration of PAH provides the driving force for PAH exit across the luminal membrane into the TF via a PAH–anion (A^-) antiporter and possibly a voltage-driven PAH transporter.

Note: PAH clearance can be used to measure RPF (see page 542).

SUMMARY OF EFFECTS OF RENAL HANDLING OF COMMON SOLUTES AND WATER

Effects of renal handling (glomerular filtration and tubular transport) of common solutes and water are summarized in Table 6.2.5.

Table 6.2.5 Effects of glomerular and tubular function on water, electrolytes and solutes in a normal human adult on an average diet

Substance	Measure	Filtered	Reabsorbed	Secreted	Excreted	Percentage reabsorption	Location
Na^+	mEq	26,000	25,850	–	150	99.4	P, L, D, C
K^+	mEq	720	620		100	86.1	P, L, D, C
Cl^-	mEq	18,000	17,850	–	150	99.2	P, L, D, C
HCO_3^-	mEq	4900	4900	–	–	100	P, D
Ca^{2+}	mEq	540	530	–	10	98.2	P, L, D, C
Glucose	mmol	800	800	–	0	100	P
Urea	mmol	870	435	–	435	50	P, L, D, C
Creatinine	mmol	12	1	1	12	–	–
Uric acid	mmol	50	49	4	5	98	P
Total solutes	mOsm	54,000	53,400	100	700	98.9	P, L, D, C
Water	L	180	178.5	–	1.5	99.2	P, L, D, C

C, collecting duct; D, distal tubule; L, loop of Henle; P, proximal tubule.

Self-Assessment

1. Discuss the mechanism of glomerular filtration, factors affecting it and filtration rate.
2. Describe the tubular mechanisms, pattern of renal handling of substances and concept of renal clearance.
3. Describe the renal handling of sodium and water.
4. Describe potassium metabolism and its renal handling.
5. Write notes on:
   - Significance of tubular fluid concentration/plasma concentration ratio
   - Bartter syndrome
   - Glucose titration curve and its significance
   - Proteinuria

Clinical Cases

Case 1

A 2-year-old male child presented with inability to walk for 1 year. History revealed that the child was born to nonconsanguineous parents and had birth weight 2.8 kg. He was able to stand and walk properly at 11 months, but within few weeks he was not able to walk properly, and was not able to even stand properly without support and was not gaining weight.

Physical examination and laboratory tests revealed frontal bossing; the child was irritable; BP was 90/56 mm Hg; hypoproteinaemia, hypocalcaemia and renal stones were present; and the child was diagnosed a case of Dent disease.

Q1. What is cause of this disease?
Q2. What is the pathophysiology of this disease?
Q3. What are the complications?

Case 2

A 5-year-old male child was brought to the paediatric OPD with complaints of excessive urination and thirst, not gaining weight and growing as per age, and frequent muscle cramps in the legs.

Examination and tests revealed:

- The child was dehydrated.
- Electrolyte measurement showed K^+ 1.24 mmol/L, Na^+ 110 mmol/L, Mg^{2+} 0.72 mmol/L, Ca^{2+} 1.17 mmol/L, Cl^- 60.5 mmol/L and HCO_3^- 36.1 mmol/L.
- Kidney function tests showed normal blood urea and creatinine.
- Urine analysis revealed increased level of calcium and potassium (>20 mmol/L).
- Arterial blood gas analysis revealed pH 7.60, pO_2 763 mm Hg and pCO_2 37.2 mm Hg.

The patient was treated with IV high concentration of potassium, but hypokalaemia was not corrected and the patient was suspected to be a case of Bartter syndrome.

Q1. What is the cause of hypokalaemia?
Q2. What is the cause of dehydration in this case?
Q3. What is the pathophysiology for signs and symptoms in this condition?

Case 3

A 50-year-old male was admitted to the hospital with complaints of pain in the abdomen, diarrhoea, nausea, numbness in the legs and arms, muscle weakness and fatigue. History revealed that the patient was on drug (ACE inhibitor) for treatment of hypertension for 1 year.

Examination and tests showed irregular heartbeat, hyperkalaemia and deranged renal function tests.

Q1. What is the cause of hyperkalaemia?
Q2. What is the mechanism of action of ACE inhibitor on potassium metabolism?
Q3. What immediate measures should be adopted to treat hyperkalaemia?

Case 4

A 2-year-old female child presented with swelling around the eyes and both legs; the child had a history of fever, chest infection and reduced urinary output.

Examination revealed bilateral pedal oedema (pitting) and weight gain.

Laboratory investigations showed proteins in the urine, serum albumin 2.1 g/dL and increased levels of serum lipids.

Based on examination and laboratory investigations, the child was diagnosed a case of paediatric nephrotic syndrome.

Q1. What are the causes?
Q2. What is the pathophysiology of signs and symptoms of the disease?

6.3 Concentration, Dilution and Acidification of Urine

CHAPTER OUTLINE

CONCENTRATION AND DILUTION OF URINE: A MECHANISM TO REGULATE URINE VOLUME AND OSMOLALITY

INTRODUCTION

The kidneys possess a unique property of regulating the volume and osmolality of the urine formed by the mechanism of concentrating and diluting the urine as per the need of the body.

Purpose of concentration and dilution of urine: The main purpose is to maintain the osmolality and volume of the body fluids within a narrow range, which is accomplished by the kidneys in concert with other systems by regulating the excretion of water and NaCl, respectively. The present discussion pertains to urine concentration and dilution, the mechanism which controls the amount of water excreted relative to the amount of solute excreted and thus regulates the plasma osmolality by varying urine osmolality.

The kidney can produce urine with osmolality as low as 30 mOsm/kg H_2O to as high as 1400 mOsm/kg H_2O by changing the water excretion as high as 23.3 L/day to as low as 0.5 L/day, respectively (Table 6.3.1). From the figures shown in Table 6.3.1, the following two important facts need to be noted:

- First, at least 87% of the filtered water is reabsorbed even when urine volume is 23.3 L/day.
- Second, the reabsorption of the remainder of the filtered water should be varied without affecting the total solute excretion, i.e. when the urine is concentrated, water is retained in excess of solutes, and when it is dilute, water is lost from the body in excess of solutes.

Principal Factors

Principal factors responsible for the mechanism of concentration and dilution of urine are as follows:

- Antidiuretic hormone (ADH)
- Hyperosmolality and osmolality gradient in medullary interstitium of the kidneys

The details about ADH are described on page 677. It will be useful to go through these pages before proceeding further. After an overview of hyperosmolality and osmolality gradient of medullary interstitium, the role of these two principal factors is concentration and dilution of the urine, which is discussed separately.

MEDULLARY HYPEROSMOLALITY AND MEDULLARY GRADIENT

Interstitial fluid of the medulla is critically important in concentrating the urine, because the osmotic pressure of this fluid provides the driving force for reabsorbing water from both the descending thin segment (DTS) and the collecting duct.

Normal osmolality of plasma and other body fluids is about 300 mOsm/kg H_2O. The interstitial fluid of the renal cortex has the same osmolality as that of plasma, i.e. 300 mOsm/kg H_2O with virtually all osmoles attributable to NaCl. The osmolality of the renal medulla is higher than that of the plasma (i.e. *hyperosmolar*) and it goes on increasing progressively from about 300 mOsm/kg H_2O at corticomedullary junction to about 1200 mOsm/kg H_2O at papilla (medullary gradient) where a maximally concentrated urine is excreted (Fig. 6.3.1). This hyperosmolality and medullary

Table 6.3.1 Effects of concentration and dilution mechanism on volume and osmolality of urine

Character of urine formed	GFR (mL/min)	Percentage of filtered water reabsorbed	Urine volume (L/day)	Urine concentration (mOsm/kg H_2O)	Gain or loss of urine formed of water in excess of solute (L/day)
Urine isotonic to plasma	125	98.7	2.4	290	–
Concentrated urine (vasopressin: maximal antidiuresis)	125	99.7	0.5	1400	1.9, gain
Diluted urine (no vasopressin or diabetes insipidus)	125	87.1	23.3	30	20.9, loss

Note: In each case, the osmotic load excreted is same (700 mOsm/day). GFR, glomerular filtration rate.

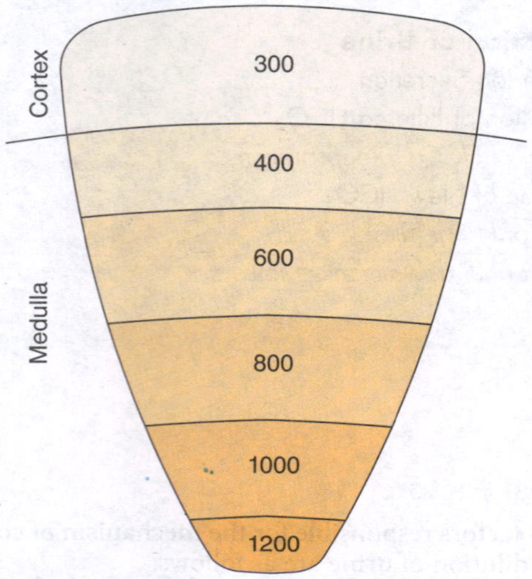

Fig. 6.3.1 Osmolality gradient of renal medullary interstitium (values are in mOsm/kg H_2O).

gradient is generated and maintained by the so-called countercurrent system.

Countercurrent System

A countercurrent system refers to a system in which the inflow runs parallel to, counter to and in close proximity to the outflow for some distance. The countercurrent flow system is formed by U-shaped tubules. The effect of countercurrent system can be best understood by studying the effect of a heater on a straight water pipe and a pipe bent in U shape (Fig. 6.3.2). Let us suppose that the heater raises the temperature of flowing fluid through the straight tube at a constant flow rate by 10°C from 30°C to 40°C (Fig. 6.3.2A). Now, if the pipe is bent in a U shape and the two limbs are brought in close proximity, the temperature at the outlet is again 40°C, but a gradient of temperature is set up along the pipe in such a way that at the bend of the pipe the temperature is not raised from 30°C to 40°C but from 30°C to 100°C (Fig. 6.3.2B). This is because the outgoing fluid warms the incoming fluid and sets up the countercurrent system.

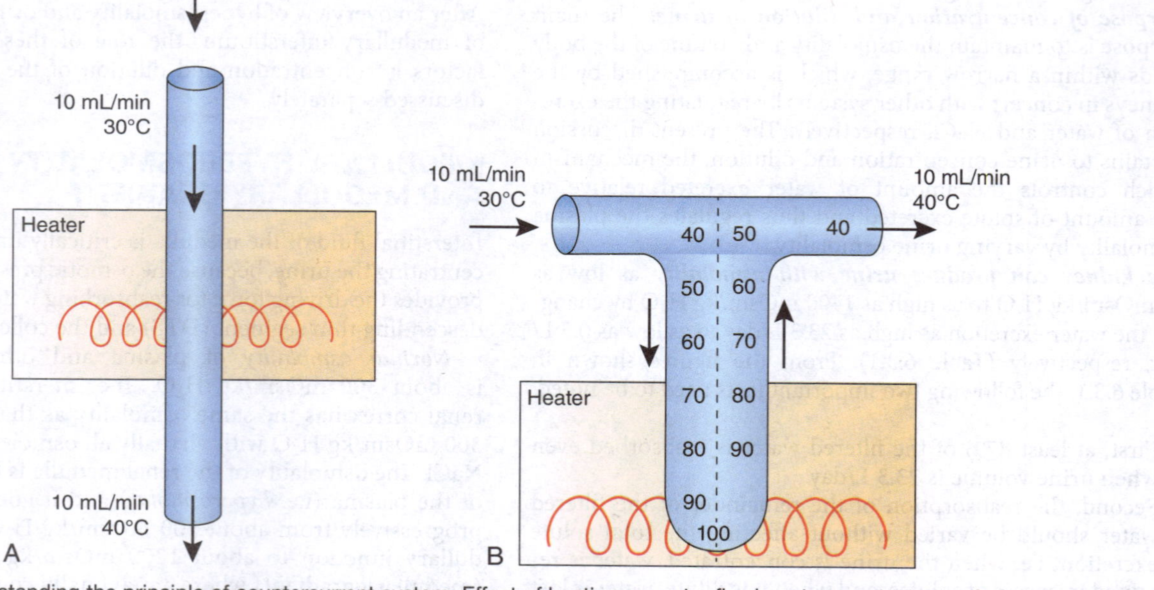

Fig. 6.3.2 Understanding the principle of countercurrent system. Effect of heating on water flowing at a constant rate: **A**, from a straight pipe; and **B**, from a U-shaped bent pipe (countercurrent effect).

In the kidney, the structures which form the countercurrent system are the loop of Henle and the vasa recta. In both, the direction of flow of fluid in the descending limb is just the opposite to that in the ascending limb. Thus, the countercurrent system of the kidney consists of two components:

Countercurrent multiplier, which is formed by the operation of loop of Henle and is responsible for the production of hyperosmolality and a gradient in renal medulla
Countercurrent exchanger, which is formed by the operation of vasa recta and is responsible for maintenance of the medullary gradient and hyperosmolality

Countercurrent Multipliers

The working of countercurrent multiplier, which operates in the loop of Henle and generates hyperosmolarity and medullary gradient, can be best understood by describing it as two processes:

- Origin of single effect
- Multiplication of the single effect

Origin of single effect The single effect is the main driving force behind the countercurrent multiplier. It is the name given to the osmotic gradient of approximately 200 mOsm that exists between the ascending limb of loop of Henle and the surrounding interstitial fluid. These are the juxtamedullary nephrons which are more important for the production of medullary hyperosmolarity. The cortical nephrons contribute to production of hyperosmolarity in the outer medulla mainly. The mechanism of origin of single effect in the outer medulla is different from that in the inner medulla.

Mechanism of origin of single effect in outer medulla
As shown in Fig. 6.3.3, the thick ascending limb (TAL) of loop of Henle is located in the outer medulla, and not in the inner medulla. TAL is impermeable to water. So NaCl and other solutes are actively absorbed in this segment without water; as a result, the tubular fluid osmolality decreases to less than that of plasma. Therefore, this segment is called the diluting segment. The NaCl reabsorbed in this segment raises the osmolality of outer medullary interstitium by about 200 mOsm. This separation of solute and water by the TAL leading to osmolality difference between that tubular fluid and interstitial fluid is called single effect and is the main driving force behind the countercurrent multiplier.

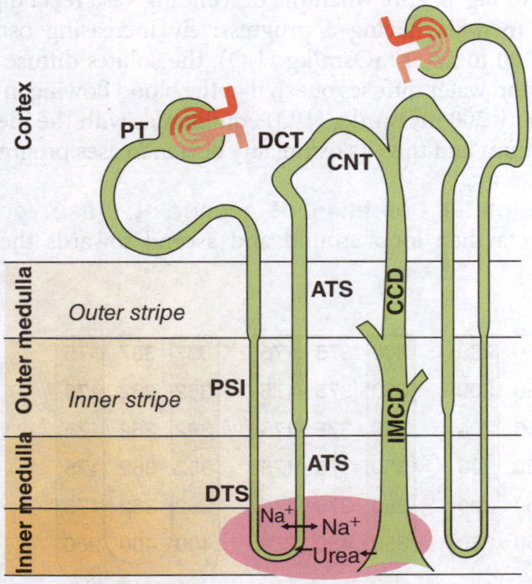

Fig. 6.3.3 Location of different components of cortical nephron and juxtacortical nephron with particular reference to origin of single effect in outer versus inner medulla.

Origin of single effect in inner medulla Three different mechanisms contribute to the origin of single effect (and, thus, ultimately to the development of medullary gradient and hyperosmolality after multiplication) in the inner medullary interstitium. These include:

- Passive transport of sodium ions from ascending thin segment (ATS) into the interstitium
- Active transport of sodium from the inner medullary collecting duct (IMCD)
- Diffusion of urea from the collecting duct into the medullary interstitium (when ADH concentration is high in blood)

1. Passive transport of sodium ions from ATS As shown in Fig. 6.1.2, the inner medulla contains ATS of loop of Henle of juxtamedullary nephrons, which is impermeable to water and does not have the property to actively absorb solutes (cf. TAL). The single effect is, therefore, produced by the passive diffusion of solutes, which occurs because of difference in the composition of tubular fluid and that of interstitium. The tubular fluid in the ATS is relatively rich in NaCl and but has less urea in it compared with the interstitium. Consequently, NaCl moves out from the ATS into the interstitium and urea moves into the ATS from the interstitium. However, the rate at which NaCl diffuses out far exceeds the rate at which urea diffuses into the lumen of ATS. Thus, as a net result, more solute diffuses out in the interstitium, raising the inner medullary osmolality (single effect).

2. Reabsorption of sodium ions from medullary part of collecting duct In addition to the passive diffusion of Na^+ from ATS, smaller quantities of ions are also transported from medullary part of the collecting duct into the medullary interstitium, particularly in the inner part of medulla near renal sinus. As described on page 492, Na^+ is actively transported by the principal cells of the collecting duct, which is followed by electrogenic passive absorption of chloride ions.

3. Role of urea Urea plays an important role in the development of medullary osmotic gradient, especially when concentration of ADH is high in the blood. Under such circumstances, IMCD absorbs large amount of urea using a specialized urea transport protein (UT-A) (see page 502). Furthermore, there occurs urea recycling (see page 502), which plays an important role in the countercurrent system.

Multiplication of the single effect The hyperosmolality and medullary gradient is in fact generated by the multiplication of the single effect by the countercurrent multiplier. The main characteristics of the components of countercurrent multiplier which play a role in multiplication of single effect are as follows (Table 6.3.2):

- High permeability of a DTS to water is present.
- They are impermeable to water but highly permeable to NaCl.
- They are impermeable to water and have the ability to actively absorb solutes by TAL.

Table 6.3.2 Permeability and transport in various segments of the nephron

Segment of nephron	Permeability and transport of H_2O	Urea	NaCl	Na^+
Loop of Henle	4+	+	±	0
• Thin descending limb	0	+	4+	0
• Thin ascending limb	0	±	±	4+
• Thick ascending limb	±	±	±	3+
Distal convoluted tubule	±	±	±	3+
Collecting duct				
• Cortical collecting duct (CCD)	3+[a]	0	±	2+
• Outer medullary collecting duct (OMCD)	3+[a]	0	±	1+
• Inner medullary collecting duct (IMCD)	3+[a]	3+	±	1+

[a]These values are in the presence of ADH. In the absence of ADH, these values are positive. ADH, antidiuretic hormone.

- In renal medulla, all other tubular structures (except ascending limb) are in osmotic equilibrium. The descending limb, therefore, acquires the increased osmolality of the surrounding fluid. The effect is multiplied as new iso-osmolar filtrate arrives at the descending limb and forces the concentrated tubular contents towards the tip of loop of Henle (hairpin band).

The process of multiplication of single effect can be best understood by dividing the whole process in hypothetical steps, leading to normal equilibrium condition. These steps are summarized as follows (Fig. 6.3.4):

- *Initially*, let us assume that the osmolality of fluid in the descending limb and the ascending limb of loop of Henle and medullary interstitium is 300 mOsm/kg H_2O (Fig. 6.3.4A).
- Furthermore, let us assume that the TAL actively pumps out 100 mOsm/kg H_2O of NaCl into the medullary interstitium. Since the TAL is impermeable to water, this effect will lower the osmolality of fluid in TAL to 200 mOsm/kg H_2O and raise the osmolality of the adjacent interstitium to 400 mOsm/kg H_2O (Fig. 6.3.4B). Establishment of this osmotic gradient of 200 mOsm/kg H_2O, as described earlier, is called single effect.
- The portion of DTS which is located in the outer medulla is moderately permeable to Na^+ and highly permeable to water.
- Due to osmotic gradient created, the water moves out and Na^+ from the interstitium (osmolality 400 mOsm/kg H_2O) moves into the DTS (osmolality 300 mOsm/kg H_2O) till equilibrium is reached with osmolality of 350 mOsm/kg H_2O (Fig. 6.3.4C).
- The fresh iso-osmolar filtrate at 300 mOsm/kg H_2O trickles down into the descending loop and pushes some of the hyperosmolar fluid (350 mOsm/kg H_2O) into the ascending limb (Fig. 6.3.4D).
- In the meanwhile, hypotonic fluid flows into the distal tubule, and isotonic and subsequently hypertonic fluid (Fig. 6.3.4E and F) flows into the ascending thick limb.
- As the process with above-mentioned steps keeps repeating, the final result is a gradient of osmolality from top to bottom of the loop and surrounding interstitium.

Countercurrent Exchanger

Vasa recta (the countercurrent exchanger) If the vasa recta would have been a straight blood vessel, the osmotic gradient in the medullary pyramid would not last long, as the Na^+ and urea in the interstitial spaces would have been removed by the circulation (Fig. 6.3.5A). However, because of the hairpin (U-shaped) anatomical arrangement, the vasa recta operate as countercurrent exchanger and retain these solutes in the medullary interstitium (Fig. 6.3.5B). Thus, the countercurrent exchanger formed by the vasa recta is responsible for the maintenance of the hyperosmolality medullary gradient generated by the countercurrent multiplier.

Operation of countercurrent exchanger The vasa recta, the capillary network supplying blood to the medulla, are highly permeable to the solute and water. So, in addition to bringing nutrients and oxygen to tubules within the medulla, these capillaries more importantly remove excess water and solutes, which are continuously added to the medullary interstitium by the nephron segments in this region.

Operation at the level of descending vasa recta As shown in Fig. 6.3.5B, when the descending vasa recta dip down in the medulla having a progressively increasing osmolality (from 300 to 1200 mOsm/kg H_2O), the solutes diffuse into its lumen and water diffuses out so that the blood flowing in it (with osmolality 300 mOsm/kg H_2O) equilibrates with the medullary interstitium and thus its osmolality also increases progressively.

Operation at the level of ascending vasa recta The vasa recta then loop around and ascend towards the cortex

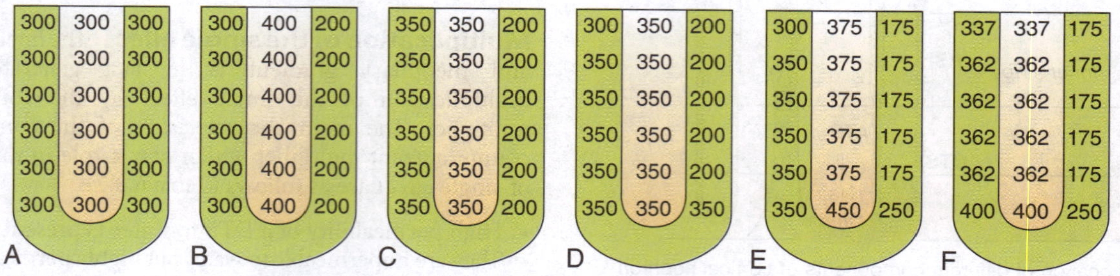

Fig. 6.3.4 Operation of loop of Henle as countercurrent multiplier producing a gradient of hyperosmolality in the medullary interstitium: **A–F**, hypothetical steps involved in the process of generation of the gradient (see text for details).

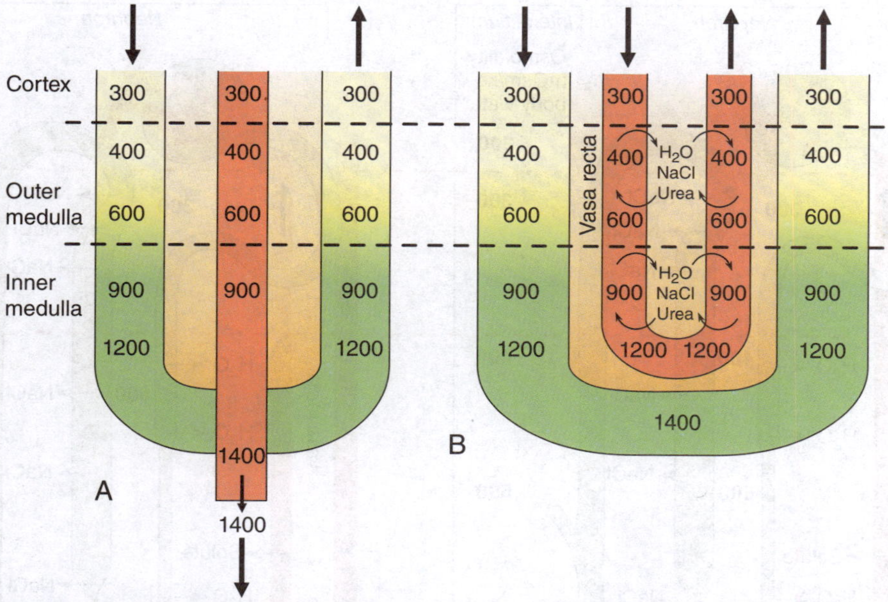

Fig. 6.3.5 Operation of vasa recta as countercurrent exchangers in the kidney: **A**, effect on medullary osmolality if vasa recta would be straight vessels without hairpin arrangement; and **B**, as they are U-shaped vessels.

(Fig. 6.3.5B). As at the beginning of the ascending vasa recta, their blood has attained an osmolality of 1200 mOsm/kg H_2O and when they pass through an interstitium, the osmolality is progressively decreasing from 1200 to 300 mOsm/kg H_2O, the solutes move out and water diffuses in, and thus the blood in them once again equilibrates with the interstitium around them.

Effect of operation of countercurrent exchanger on the medullary interstitium By the above-described operations, the solutes tend to recirculate in the medulla and water tends to bypass it, so that hypertonicity of the medulla is maintained. Since solutes (sodium and urea) are exchanged for water between the ascending and descending limbs of vasa recta, this system has been named countercurrent exchanger.

Another factor which ensures retention of sodium in the medullary interstitium is very slow rate of blood flow through the medullary parenchyma. Some important facts about working of countercurrent exchanger which need elaboration are as follows:

Important Notes

- *The ability of the vasa recta to maintain the medullary interstitial gradient is flow dependent.* A substantial increase in blood flow through the vasa recta will ultimately dissipate the medullary gradient, i.e. wash out the medullary gradient. Alternatively, if blood flow is reduced, the nephron segments within the medulla will receive inadequate oxygen. Under such conditions, the tubular transport, especially by the thick ascending limb (TAL), is impaired. As a result, the medullary interstitial osmotic gradient cannot be maintained.
- Countercurrent exchanger is a passive process, as it depends on the diffusion of water and solutes in both directions across the permeable walls of the vasa recta. Therefore, it could not maintain the osmotic gradient along the medullary pyramids if the process of countercurrent multiplier were to cease.

MECHANISM OF URINE DILUTION AND CONCENTRATION

Production of Diluted Urine

Conditions in Which Dilute Urine is Formed

Dilute urine is called hypo-osmotic urine, in which urine osmolality is less than blood osmolality. It is produced under the following circumstances:

- When the circulating levels of ADH are low (e.g. after water drinking), central diabetes insipidus (see page 681)
- When ADH is ineffective (e.g. nephrogenic diabetes insipidus) (see page 681)

Principal Factors Governing Formation of Dilute Urine

As mentioned earlier, the principal factors governing formation of dilute and concentrated urine are hyperosmolality medullary gradient and the presence or absence of ADH. The renal medullary osmotic gradient is smaller in the absence of ADH. This is because ADH stimulates both countercurrent multiplication and urea cycling.

Segmental changes in Tubular Fluid During Formation of Dilute Urine

Segmental changes occurring in tubular fluid during the formation of dilute urine are summarized (Fig. 6.3.6A) as follows:

Proximal tubule The osmolality of glomerular filtrate entering the proximal tubule is identical to that of plasma (300 mOsm/L). About 60%–70% of the H_2O is reabsorbed isosmotically (with Na^+, Cl^-, HCO_3^-, glucose, amino acids and so forth). As H_2O is reabsorbed isosmotically, the TF/Posm = 1.0 throughout the proximal tubule.

DTS of loop of Henle DTS of loop of Henle receives isosmotic fluid (i.e. osmolarity 300 mOsm/L) from the

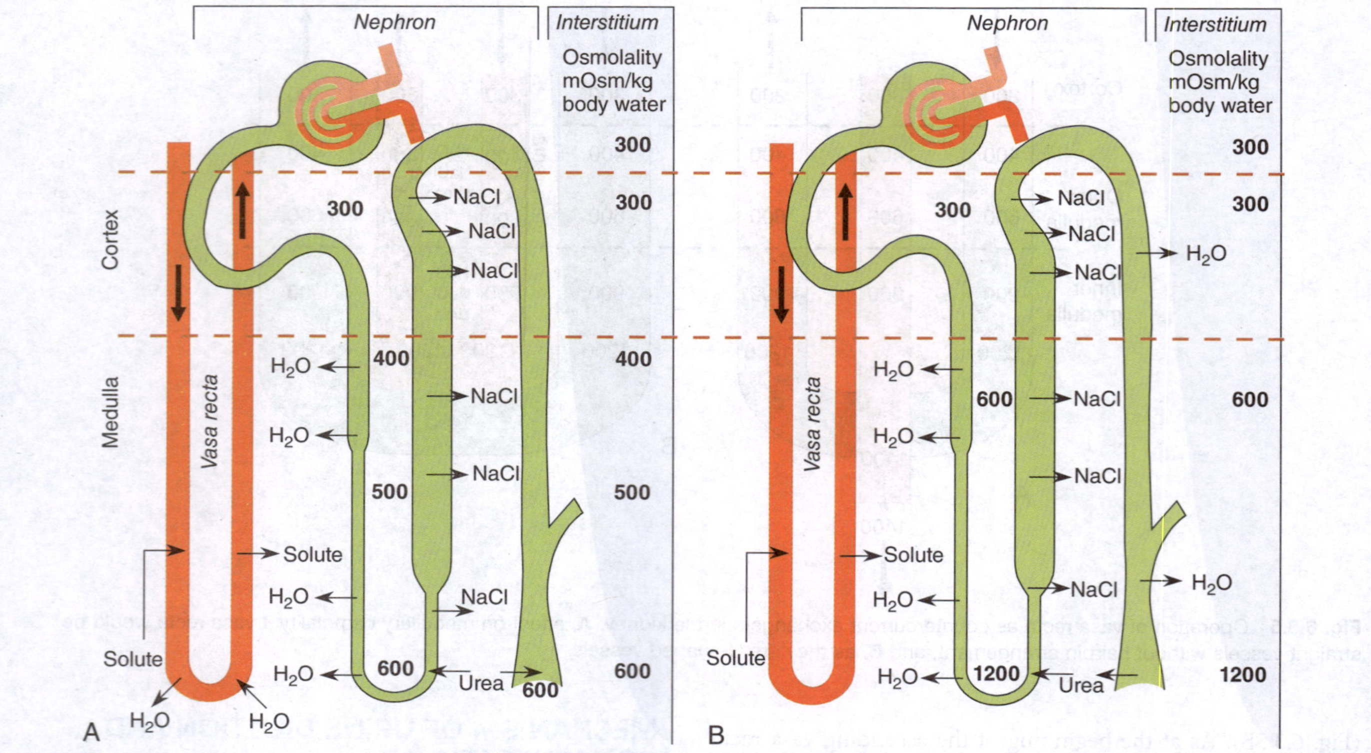

Fig. 6.3.6 Mechanism of producing: **A**, dilute urine in the absence of ADH; and **B**, concentrated urine in the presence of ADH. ADH, antidiuretic hormone.

proximal tubule, because this segment is highly permeable to water but much less to solutes (Table 6.3.2). As thin segment descends deeper in the renal medulla, water is reabsorbed owing to the osmotic gradient set up by the progressive increasing hyperosmolality of the medulla. At the bend of loop of Henle, although the osmolalities of tubular fluid and interstitium are equal, their composition differs. The NaCl concentration is higher and that of urea is lower in the tubular fluid than in the interstitial fluid.

ATS of loop of Henle ATS of loop of Henle is impermeable to water but permeable to NaCl and urea (Table 6.3.2). As the tubular fluid moves up in this segment, NaCl moves out and urea moves in. As a net result, the volume remains the same, osmolarity decreases and the concentration of NaCl decreases, but that of urea increases in the tubular fluid.

TAL TAL of loop of Henle is impermeable to water and urea. Because of active absorption of NaCl without water, the tubular fluid becomes dilute (although not quite as dilute as in the presence of ADH). In this diluting segment, urine becomes hypo-osmolar for the first time, and the only time. The minimum possible osmolarity of the tubular fluid is 100 mOsm/L (i.e. 200 mOsm less than the surrounding interstitium).

Early distal tubule Early distal tubule behaves like TAL and the tubular fluid is further diluted.

Late distal tubule and cortical collecting ducts Cells of these segments actively reabsorb NaCl but are impermeable to urea. In the absence of ADH, the cells of these segments are impermeable to water. So, due to reabsorption of NaCl without the water, the osmolality of the tubular fluid is further reduced.

Medullary collecting duct Medullary collecting duct actively reabsorbs NaCl. Even in the absence of ADH, this segment is slightly permeable to H_2O and urea. So, some urea enters the collecting duct from the interstitium and about 2% of H_2O is reabsorbed. So, in the absence of ADH, the urine will have an osmolality between 30 and 50 mOsm/L and will contain low NaCl and urea ($TF/P_{osm} < 1.0$). The volume of urine excreted can be about 18 L/day or approximately 10% of glomerular filtrate: however, in extreme conditions, it may reach 23–32 L/day (Table 6.3.2).

Production of Concentrated Urine

Conditions in which Concentrated Urine is Formed

Concentrated urine is also called *hyperosmotic urine*, in which urine osmolality is more than that of blood. It is produced when circulating ADH levels are high, e.g.:

- Water deprivation
- Haemorrhage
- Syndrome of inappropriate antidiuretic hormone (SIADH) (see page 681)

Principal Factors Governing Formation of Concentrated Urine

The high level of ADH is the main factor governing the formation of concentrated urine, because it:

- Increases the size of hyperosmolality medullary gradient

- Augments the urea cycling from the IMCDs into the medullary interstitial fluid

Segmental Changes in the Tubular Fluid During Formation of Concentrated Urine

Segmental changes occurring in the tubular fluid during the formation of concentrated urine are summarized as follows (Fig. 6.3.6B):

From proximal tubule to ascending thick limb and even early distal tubule From proximal tubule to ascending thick limb and even early distal tubule, the changes occurring in the tubular fluid are the same as during the formation of dilute urine. Only point to be noted here is that the ADH stimulates NaCl reabsorption in the TAL and therefore increases the size of medullary gradient by *countercurrent multiplier*, which is important for formation of concentrated urine.

Late distal tubule The tubular fluid entering the late distal tubule is *hypo-osmolar* (osmolality about 150 mOsm/L). In the presence of ADH, H_2O permeability of the principal cells is increased and consequently H_2O is reabsorbed until the osmolality of distal tubular fluid equals that of the surrounding cortical interstitium (300 mOsm/L) (Fig. 6.3.6B). So, at the end of the distal tubule, TF/Posm = 1.0, because osmotic equilibrium occurs in the presence of ADH. It is important to note that although the osmolality of the fluid in this segment is similar to that of the fluid, which entered the DTS from the proximal tubule, its composition has altered dramatically. Because of NaCl reabsorption by the preceding nephron segments (NaCl accounts for a much smaller portion of the total tubular fluid osmolality), urea, filtered and that added in descending thin and ascending thin limb of loop of Henle, mainly accounts for the osmolality at this juncture.

Note: ADH increases the H_2O permeability of the principal cells of late distal tubule and collecting duct through aquaporin-2 (for details about mechanism of action, see page 678).

Collecting ducts ADH markedly increases the permeability of the principal cells (see page 492). As the tubular fluid flows through the collecting ducts, it passes through the corticopapillary gradient (regions of increasingly higher osmolality, from 300 to 1200 mOsm/L), which was previously established by countercurrent multiplication (see page 507) and urea cycling (see page 502). Consequently, H_2O is reabsorbed from the collecting ducts until the osmolality of tubular fluid equals that of the surrounding interstitial fluid. Because initial portion of the collecting duct is impermeable to urea, it remains in the tubular fluid, and its concentration in the tubular fluid increases. In the presence of ADH, the urea permeability of the last portion of the medullary collecting duct is increased, and so some urea diffuses out into the medullary interstitium.

The final osmolality of urine is about 1200 mOsm/L, and it contains high concentration of urea and other non-reabsorbed solutes. TF/Posm >1.0, because osmotic equilibrium occurs with the medullary gradient in the presence of ADH. In humans, the osmolality of urine may reach even 1400 mOsm/L, almost five times the osmolality of plasma, with a total of 95.7% or more of the filtered water being reabsorbed, and urine under this condition can be as low as 0.5 L/day (Table 6.3.1).

Note: In other species, the ability to concentrate urine is even greater. Maximal urine osmolality is about 2500 mOsm/kg H_2O in dogs, about 3200 mOsm/kg H_2O in laboratory rats and as high as 5000 mOsm/kg in certain desert rodents. In fact, the ability to concentrate urine depends on the number of long-looped juxtamedullary nephrons, which form about 15% of total nephrons in humans.

> **Important Note**
>
> It is important to note that the tubular response to ADH is not an all-or-none phenomenon, but a graded response. Therefore, varying grades of plasma ADH concentrations can produce proportionate increase in permeability of collecting ducts to H_2O. Consequently, depending on the status of body water and plasma osmolality, considerable variations in the rate of urine flow and urinary osmolality normally occur in different parts of the day. After an overnight fast, the morning urine samples tend to be relatively more concentrated.

Urine Volume and Osmolality Changes in Response to Water Intake and Water Deprivation

Water Diuresis Versus Osmotic Diuresis

Water diuresis Water diuresis refers to increased urinary output following excessive intake of water or hypotonic solution.

Pathophysiology It occurs due to the absence of ADH in the plasma. Steps involved in its occurrence are summarized in Fig. 6.3.7. Due to the absence of ADH, the distal tubule and collecting ducts become impermeable to water leading to marked decrease in reabsorption. However, water reabsorption in the proximal tubule and loop of Henle is not affected.

Characteristic features Characteristic features are as follows:

- Water diuresis begins about 15 minutes after ingestion of water and reaches its maximum in 40 minutes.

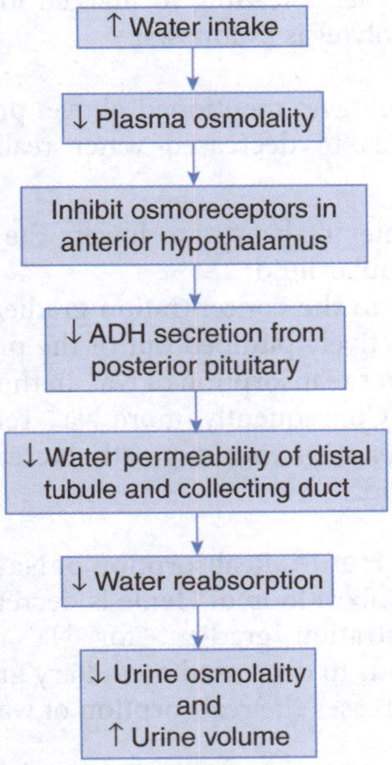

Fig. 6.3.7 Steps involved in urine osmolality changes in response to increased water intake.

- Urine output may be increased to 20 L/day.
- Urine formed is diluted; osmolality is low (50 mOsm/kg H_2O).
- Specific gravity of urine is always below 1.010.

Applied Aspects

Water intoxication

Water intoxication occurs when water is being consumed in high quantity without adequate electrolyte intake. When water ingestion exceeds this limit of water excretion, there occurs water stasis, leading to a marked increase in extracellular fluid (ECF). Similar situation may also occur when water intake is not reduced after administration of exogenous vasopressin or secretion of endogenous vasopressin in response to nonosmotic stimuli such as surgical trauma. It is common among people with psychosis (schizophrenia) and personality disorders.

Consequently, the body cells are swollen because of uptake of water by the cells from increased hypotonic ECF. Symptoms of water intoxication occur rarely when swelling of the brain cells may cause altered mental status, disorientation, confusion, nausea and vomiting, convulsions, coma and eventually death.

Osmotic diuresis Osmotic diuresis refers to increased urine output because of an osmotic effect.

Pathophysiology Presence of large quantities of nonabsorbable solutes in the proximal tubules exerts an appreciable osmotic effect. Osmotic diuresis may occur under the following circumstances:

- When the filtered load of naturally occurring substances such as Na^+, glucose (e.g. in diabetes mellitus) and urea exceeds the maximum capacity of the tubules to reabsorb (T_m)
- Following administration of compounds such as mannitol and related polysaccharides that are filtered but not reabsorbed
- Following infusion of large amounts of sodium chloride and urea

Sequence of events leading to marked loss of Na^+, water and other electrolytes is as follows:

Proximal tubule As mentioned above, presence of excessive solutes leads to decreased water reabsorption in the proximal tubule.

- Decreased water reabsorption lowers the Na^+ concentration in the tubular fluid.
- When a limit to the concentration gradient against which Na^+ can be actively pumped out of the proximal tubule is reached, further reabsorption of Na^+ in the proximal tubule is prevented. Consequently, more Na^+ remains in the tubule, and water stays with it, greatly increasing the volume of isotonic fluid.

In the loop of Henle Reabsorption of Na^+, K^+ and Cl^- in the ascending limb of loop of Henle is decreased because the limiting concentration gradient for Na^+ reabsorption is reached. This leads to decreased medullary gradient, which in turn further decreases the reabsorption of water and Na^+.

Collecting ducts Collecting ducts thus receive a large volume of fluid but can reabsorb very less amount of water because of decreased medullary gradient. Consequently, the urine output and excretion of Na^+ and other electrolytes increase.

Characteristic features

- Urine output may be >20 L/day, in spite of maximal ADH secretion.
- Urine osmolality is higher than 300 mOsm/kg H_2O.
- Urine specific gravity is over 1.010.

Water Deprivation

Water deprivation is followed by a sequence of changes which consume water for the body needs. As a consequence, urine volume is decreased but urine osmolality is increased (Fig. 6.3.8).

Factors Affecting Urinary Concentration and Dilution Mechanisms

1. Functioning of thick ascending limb of loop of Henle The active reabsorption of NaCl in TAL is the most important event for the generation of medullary hyperosmolality by the countercurrent system. If this event is blocked (e.g. by loop diuretics), the entire medullary gradient of hyperosmolality disappears within minutes. As a result, urine can be neither concentrated nor diluted.

2. Length of loop of Henle In the human kidney, long-looped juxtamedullary nephrons, which are mainly responsible for the development of hyperosmolality gradient, constitute 15% of the total nephrons. Consequently, the human kidney can produce urine with a maximum osmolality of 1400 mOsm/kg H_2O. Animals with a large number of long-looped nephrons (e.g. cat, dog) can produce more concentrated urine (with osmolality of 2500 mOsm/kg H_2O).

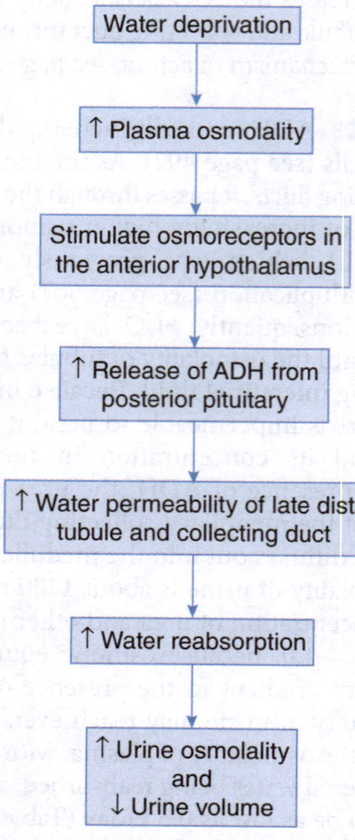

Fig. 6.3.8 Steps involved in urine osmolality changes in response to water deprivation.

3. Availability of urea Development of single effect in the inner medulla (and subsequently development of hyperosmolality) requires the presence of high concentration of urea in the medullary interstitium (see page 507). Therefore, factors which affect the availability of urea will affect urine-concentrating mechanism. For example:

- Individuals who genetically lack the urea transport protein (UT) have lesser urine-concentrating ability.
- Low-protein diet makes lesser quantity of urea available and thus decreases urine-concentrating ability. The reverse occurs in high-protein diet.

4. Effect of tubular fluid flow rate Increased tubular fluid flow is associated with reduced medullary hyperosmolality because of the following reasons:

- Greater reabsorption of water from the thin descending limb dilutes the solutes in the medullary interstitium.
- Active transport of Na^+ is not able to dilute the tubular fluid in TAL, and the single effect is reduced in magnitude.
- The reabsorption of water from the collecting tubule is not able to sufficiently concentrate urea in the IMCD.

Causes of increased tubular flow rate

- Increased glomerular filtration rate (GFR) leads to increased tubular flow rate.
- Osmotic diuretics (like mannitol or excessive glucose) when present in the proximal convoluted tubules interfere with reabsorption of NaCl and water. Therefore, intratubular flow rate is increased throughout the nephron leading to impairment of urinary concentration ability.
  Conversely, a decrease in tubular flow rate (e.g. due to decreased GFR) tends to cause increased urinary concentration even in the absence of ADH.

5. Blood flow through vasa recta It affects the ability of countercurrent exchanger to maintain medullary gradient (see page 508).

6. Effect of prostaglandins Certain prostaglandins impair the urinary concentration ability by:

- Increasing blood flow through vasa recta
- Inhibiting active transport of NaCl in the TAL of loop of Henle
- Inhibiting the enzyme adenylyl cyclase which is involved in the genesis of cAMP (required for ADH action)

Assessment of Renal Diluting and Concentrating Ability

Assessment of renal dilution and concentration process can be made by performing the following tests:

- Measurement of urine osmolality
- Measurement of urine specific gravity
- The urine concentration test
- The urine dilution test
- Estimation of free water clearance (CH_2O)

All these tests are described in detail in the subsection 'Kidney Function Tests' (see page 542).

Applied Aspects

Clinical Disorders Related to the Concentration and Dilution of Urine

Common clinical disorders related to the concentration and dilution of urine include:

- Primary psychogenic polydipsia (compulsive water drinking)
- Diabetes insipidus, which may be:
  Central diabetes insipidus
  Nephrogenic diabetes insipidus
- Water deprivation
- (SIADH

Most of these have been described in detail on page 527, and for a ready reference are summarized in Table 6.3.3.

ACIDIFICATION OF URINE

The pH of urine is variable depending on the concentration of H^+ ions. Under normal circumstances, the pH of urine is acidic (~6.0). This clearly indicates that the kidneys have contributed to the *acidification of urine*, when it is formed from the plasma (pH 7.4). In other words, H^+ ions generated in the body in the normal circumstances are eliminated by acidified urine. Thus, the role of the kidneys in the maintenance of

Table 6.3.3 Summary of clinical disorders related to the concentration and dilution of urine

Clinical disorder	Serum ADH	Serum osmolality/ serum Na^+	Urine osmolality	Urine flow rate	Free water clearance (CH_2O)
Primary polydipsia	Decreased	Decreased	Hypo-osmotic	High	Positive
Central diabetes insipidus	Decreased	Increased (because of excretion of too much water)	Hypo-osmotic	High	Positive
Nephrogenic diabetes insipidus	Increased (because of increased plasma osmolality)	Increased (because of excretion of too much water)	Hypo-osmotic	High	Positive
Water deprivation	Increased	High/normal	Hyperosmotic	Low	Negative
SIADH	Markedly increased	Decreased (because of reabsorption of water)	Hyperosmotic	Low	Negative

ADH, antidiuretic hormone; SIADH, syndrome of inappropriate antidiuretic hormone.

acid–base balance of the body (blood pH) is highly significant, as the renal mechanism tries to provide a permanent solution to the acid–base disturbances. This is in contrast to the temporary buffering systems of the blood and short-term respiratory mechanisms described in the chapter 'Physiology of Acid–Base Balance' (see page 1187).

The kidneys regulate the blood pH by three main mechanisms:

- Reabsorption of the filtered HCO_3^-
- Generation of $NaHCO_3^-$ of the alkali reserve of the body
- Excretion of acid in the form of titrable acid and ammonium ions

All these mechanisms are accomplished through the process of H^+ secretion by the nephron.

HYDROGEN ION SECRETION

The tubular cells of proximal tubule, distal tubule and collecting ducts are capable of secreting H^+. The kidney is the only organ which can eliminate the fixed acids by active secretion of H^+.

Mechanism of H^+ secretion by proximal tubule

Steps involved are as follows (Fig. 6.3.9):

Formation of carbonic acid: Carbonic acid (H_2CO_3) is first formed in the cells of proximal tubules from CO_2 and H_2O by a reaction that is catalysed by the intracellular *carbonic anhydrase*. Therefore, the carbonic anhydrase inhibitors depress the secretion of acid by proximal tubule.
Dissociation of carbonic acid (H_2CO_3) then occurs in H^+ and HCO_3^-.
Secretion of H^+ into the lumen occurs via Na^+–H^+ exchange mechanism in the luminal membrane. This is an example of secondary active transport, in which first Na^+ is extruded actively from the cell into the interstitium by Na^+–K^+-ATPase, and intracellular Na^+ is lowered. This is followed by the entry of Na^+ into the cell from the lumen coupled with H^+ secretion into the lumen by Na^+–H^+ antiporter (Fig. 6.3.9).

- The secreted H^+, in the lumen, combines with the filtered HCO_3^- and helps its reabsorption (as described below). Therefore, this process does not result in net secretion of H^+.
- *HCO_3^- formed in the cell* (from the dissociation of H_2CO_3) diffuses into the interstitial fluid. Thus, for each H^+ secreted, one Na^+ ion and one HCO_3^- ion enter the interstitial fluid. The latter adds up to the alkali reserve of the body.

Mechanism of H^+ secretion by distal tubules and collecting ducts

In the distal tubule and collecting ducts, H^+ secretion occurs independent of Na^+. Two mechanisms involved in secretion of H^+ by the intercalated cells in these parts of tubules are the following (Fig. 6.3.10):

- ATP-driven proton pump is mainly responsible for the secretion of H^+ in the distal tubules and collecting ducts. It can increase the H^+ concentration of the luminal fluid 1000 times the plasma concentration. Aldosterone acts on this pump to increase distal H^+ secretion.
- H^+, K^+–ATPase is also responsible for secretion of some of the H^+ coupled with reabsorption of K^+ in these parts of renal tubules.

Fate of H^+ secreted in the renal tubule

The secretion of H^+ in the renal tubule can continue only if the H^+ is immediately buffered in the luminal fluid. The tubular cells can secrete H^+, up to a luminal fluid pH of about 4.5, i.e. an H^+ concentration in the urine that is 1000 times the concentration in plasma. In the absence of buffering of H^+ in the lumen, this pH would be reached rapidly, stopping further H^+ secretion.

- The pH 4.5 is thus the *limiting pH*. However, the free H^+ secreted in the renal tubules is immediately buffered (permitting more acid to be secreted):
  In proximal tubule, the secreted H^+ ions are buffered by the filtered HCO_3^- (i.e. consumed in reabsorption of filtered HCO_3^-, vide infra).
  In distal tubule and connecting ducts, the secreted H^+ ions are buffered by Na_2HPO_4 and NH_3 and are excreted as titrable acid and ammonium ion (NH_4^+) (vide infra).

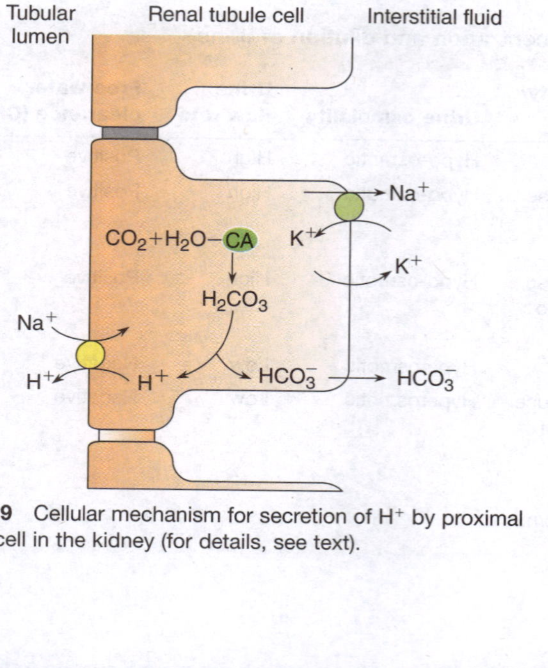

Fig. 6.3.9 Cellular mechanism for secretion of H^+ by proximal tubular cell in the kidney (for details, see text).

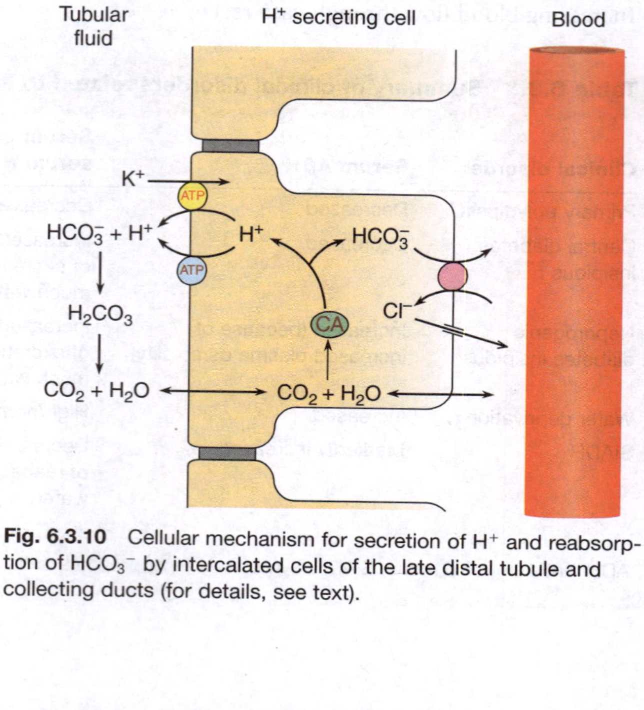

Fig. 6.3.10 Cellular mechanism for secretion of H^+ and reabsorption of HCO_3^- by intercalated cells of the late distal tubule and collecting ducts (for details, see text).

REABSORPTION OF FILTERED HCO_3^-

The concentration of HCO_3^- in plasma, and consequently in the glomerular filtrate, is about 24 mEq/L. Thus, glomerular filtration delivers about 4320 mEq of HCO_3^- (180 L × 24 mEq/L) per day to the nephron. The reabsorption of the filtered HCO_3^- is critically important for the prevention of its loss in the urine and thus for the maintenance of acid–base balance in the body. Under normal circumstances, virtually all the filtered HCO_3^- is reabsorbed by different segments of nephron (Fig. 6.3.11) and none appears in the urine. The mechanisms involved in reabsorption of filtered HCO_3^- in different segments are summarized.

Proximal tubule Proximal tubule reabsorbs approximately 80% of the filtered HCO_3^-. Steps of cellular mechanism involved are as follows:

- H^+ secreted in the lumen of proximal tubule (as described above [Fig. 6.3.9]) combines with the filtered HCO_3^- to form carbonic acid (H_2CO_3) (Fig. 6.3.12).
- The H_2CO_3 is rapidly converted to CO_2 and H_2O. This reaction is catalysed by the brush border carbonic anhydrase.
- The CO_2 diffuses into the tubular cell along the concentration gradient. In the tubular cell, the CO_2 again combines with H_2O to form H_2CO_3, which then dissociates into H^+ and HCO_3^-, followed by secretion of H^+ in tubule and diffusion of HCO_3^- in the interstitial fluid as described above (Figs 6.3.9 and 6.3.12). Thus, for each mole of HCO_3^- reabsorbed from the lumen, 1 mole of HCO_3^- diffuses from the tubular cell into the blood, even though it is not the same mole that disappeared from the tubular fluid.

Important Note

Furthermore, it is important to note that, although there occurs net reabsorption of filtered HCO_3^-, the process neutralizes the H^+ secreted into lumen, meaning thereby that there is no net secretion of H^+ in the lumen, and consequently pH of fluid in proximal tubule is changed very little.

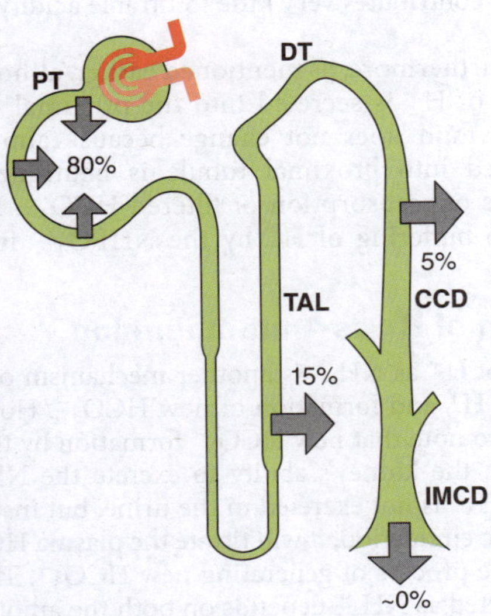

Fig. 6.3.11 Reabsorption of filtered HCO_3^- load along various segments of nephron.

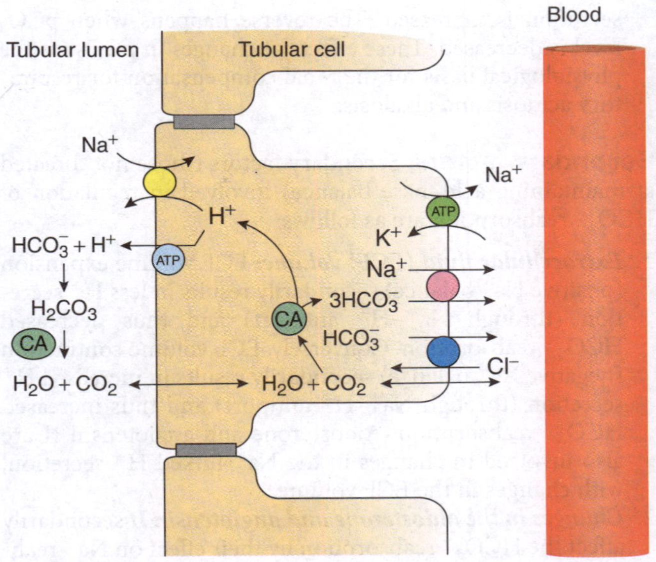

Fig. 6.3.12 Cellular mechanism involved in reabsorption of filtered HCO_3^- in proximal tubular cell.

Loop of Henle Loop of Henle reabsorbs 15% of the filtered HCO_3^-, mainly in the region of TAL. The mechanism involved is exactly the same as described for proximal tubule, except that brush border carbonic anhydrase is not present in the apical membrane of TAL cells.

Distal tubules and convoluted tubules Distal tubules and convoluted tubules reabsorb only 5% of the filtered HCO_3^- which escapes absorption in the proximal tubule and TAL. So, some of the H^+ secreted by intercalated cells of these parts of tubule is utilized in reabsorption of HCO_3^- (Fig. 6.3.10), whereas most of the H^+ secreted in these segments is excreted with non-HCO_3^- urinary buffers (described in later discussion).

Regulation of HCO_3^- Reabsorption

Various factors that regulate HCO_3^- reabsorption (i.e. H^+ secretion) can be divided into two groups of primary and secondary factors.

Primary factors Primary factors (those directed at maintaining acid–base balance) involved in regulation of HCO_3^- reabsorption include:

1. ***Plasma HCO_3^- level:*** An increase in the plasma HCO_3^- increases the filtered load of HCO_3^-, resulting in increased HCO_3^- reabsorption. However, if the plasma concentration becomes very high (above 28 mEq/L, e.g. metabolic alkalosis), the filtered load will exceed the reabsorptive capacity (the renal threshold for HCO_3^-), the HCO_3^- appears in the urine and the urine becomes alkaline. Conversely, with the decrease in plasma HCO_3^-, the filtered load is decreased and this results in decreased HCO_3^- secretion. Under such circumstances, more H^+ becomes available to combine with other buffer anions. Therefore, lower the plasma HCO_3^- concentration drops, the more acidic the urine becomes and the greater is the NH_4^+ content.
2. ***pCO_2 level*** when increased results in increased rates of HCO_3^- reabsorption, as the supply of intracellular H^+ for

secretion is increased. The reverse happens when pCO_2 level is decreased. These effects of changes in pCO_2 are the physiological basis for the renal compensation for respiratory acidosis and alkalosis.

Secondary factors Secondary factors (those not directed at maintaining acid–base balance) involved in regulation of HCO_3^- reabsorption are as follows:

1. ***Extracellular fluid (ECF) volume:*** ECF volume expansion (positive Na^+ balance) secondarily results in less H^+ secretion (through Na^+–H^+ antiport) and thus decreased HCO_3^- reabsorption. Conversely, ECF volume contraction (negative Na^+ balance) secondarily results in increased H^+ secretion (through Na^+–H^+ antiport) and thus increased HCO_3^- reabsorption. Aldosterone and angiotensin II are also involved in changes in the Na^+-linked H^+ secretion, with changes in the ECF volume.
2. ***Changes in the aldosterone and angiotensin II*** secondarily affect the HCO_3^- reabsorption by their effect on Na^+ reabsorption and associated H^+ secretion through Na^+–H^+ antiporter.
3. ***Parathyroid hormone (PTH)*** also inhibits HCO_3^- reabsorption by proximal tubules. It is mainly involved in the maintenance of Ca^{2+} and phosphate balance (see page 672). However, PTH also inhibits the Na^+–H^+ antiporter in the apical membrane of proximal tubule cells.
4. ***Plasma K^+*** levels also influence the secretion of H^+ by the proximal tubules, with hypokalaemia stimulating and hyperkalaemia inhibiting secretion.

GENERATION OF NEW HCO_3^-

As discussed above, the kidneys play an important role in the maintenance of acid–base balance of the body by completely reabsorbing the filtered HCO_3^-. However, in reality, HCO_3^- reabsorption alone does not replenish the HCO_3^- lost during the titration of nonvolatile acids which are daily added to the plasma, from the diet and produced by metabolism. Therefore, to maintain acid–base balance, the kidneys replace this lost HCO_3^- with new HCO_3^- by the following processes:

- Excretion of H^+ as titrable acid
- Excretion of H^+ as NH_4

As discussed below, by these processes, the kidneys not only synthesize new HCO_3^- but also result in net secretion of H^+.

Excretion of H^+ as Titrable Acid

Excretion of H^+ as titrable acid (as explained below) refers to the excretion of secreted H^+ along with the primary urinary buffer, the dibasic phosphate (HPO_4^{2-}). This reaction occurs in the distal tubules and collecting ducts, because it is here that the phosphate which escapes proximal reabsorption is greatly concentrated by the reabsorption of water. The cellular mechanisms involved in the synthesis of new HCO_3^- and net excretion of H^+ with dibasic phosphate urinary buffer are as follows (Fig. 6.3.13):

- H^+ and HCO_3^- are produced in the cell from CO_2 and H_2O.
- The new HCO_3^- is reabsorbed into the blood.
- H^+ secreted into the lumen (mainly by H^+-ATPase) combines with filtered HPO_4^{2-} to form $H_2PO_4^-$, which is excreted as titrable acid. The amount of H^+ excreted as titrable acid is determined by the amount of urinary buffer and the p*K* of the buffer.

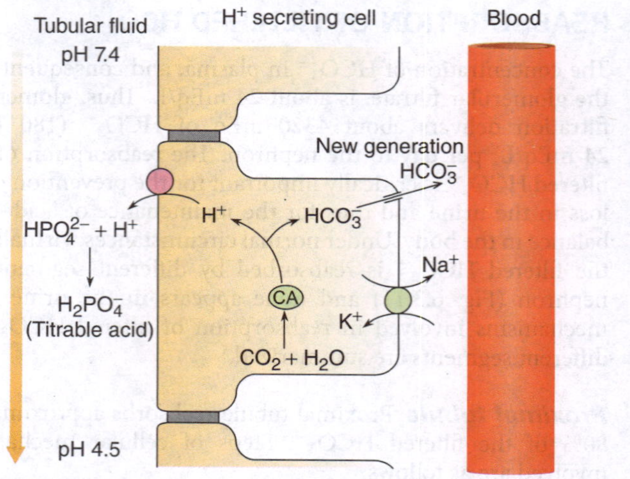

Fig. 6.3.13 Mechanism for excretion of H^+ as titrable acid and synthesis of new HCO_3^-.

As a result of H^+ excretion in the form of titrable acid, the pH of urine is progressively decreased (from 7.4, that of blood). The *acidification of the urine* may lower its pH to a minimum of 4.5, i.e. H^+ concentration of urine is approximately 1000 times the concentration of H^+ in the plasma. Thus, titrable acidity is a measure of acid excreted in the urine by the kidney. This can be estimated by titrating urine back to normal pH of blood (7.4).

- In quantitative terms, titrable acidity refers to the number of millilitres of N/10 NaOH required to titrate 1 L of urine to pH 7.4. However, the titrable acidity obviously measures only a fraction of the acid secreted, since it does not account for the H_2CO_3 that has been converted to H_2O and CO_2.
- In addition, the p*K* of ammonia system is 9.0, and the ammonia system is titrable only from the pH of urine to pH 7.4, so it contributes very little to titrable acidity.

Note: Furthermore, as mentioned earlier, although nearly 4000 mEq of H^+ is secreted into the proximal tubule, the pH of the fluid does not change because almost all the H^+ secreted into proximal tubule is neutralized during the process of reabsorption of filtered HCO_3^-. Practically, there is no buffering of H^+ by the $NHPO_4^{2-}$ in proximal tubules.

Excretion of H^+ as Ammonium Ion

Excretion of H^+ as NH_4^+ is another mechanism of excretion of secreted H^+ and formation of new HCO_3^-. However, it is important to note that new HCO_3^- formation by this process depends on the kidney's ability to excrete the NH_4^+ in the urine. If NH_4^+ is not excreted in the urine, but instead enters the systemic circulation, it will titrate the plasma HCO_3^-, thus negating the process of generating new HCO_3^-. The amount of H^+ excreted as NH_4^+ depends on both the amount of NH_3 synthesized by renal cells and the urine pH. The process by which the kidneys excrete NH_4^+ is complex and can be

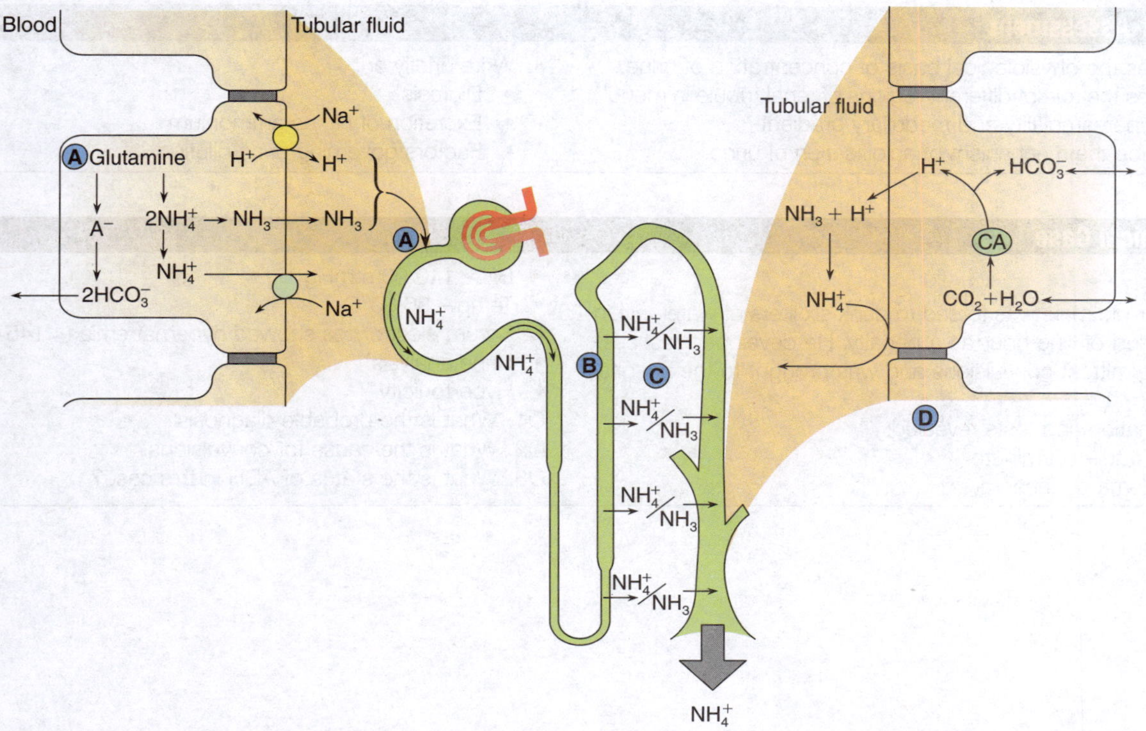

Fig. 6.3.14 Excretion of H^+ as NH_4^+ and generation of new HCO_3^- can be considered in four stages: **A**, synthesis of NH_4^+ and HCO_3^- from glutamine in proximal tubule; **B**, reabsorption of NH_4^+ across thick ascending limb; **C**, accumulation of NH_4^+ in medullary interstitium in equilibrium with NH_3^+; and **D**, anionic diffusion and diffusion trapping in collecting ducts.

described to have four stages (for the purpose of understanding only) (Fig. 6.3.14):

A. Synthesis of NH_4^+ and new HCO_3^- in proximal tubule Ammonium ions (NH_4^+) are produced in the cells of proximal tubules from the metabolism of *glutamine.* Each molecule of glutamine is metabolized into two molecules each of NH_4^+ and HCO_3^-.

- HCO_3^- diffuses across the basolateral membrane into the peritubular blood as new HCO_3^-.
- NH_4^+ is secreted into the lumen via Na^+–H^+ antiporter, with NH_4^+ substituting for H^+. Some NH_4^+ is converted into NH_3^+ and H^+. NH_3^+ diffuses into the lumen where it combines with the secreted H^+ to form NH_4^+.

B. Reabsorption of NH_4^+ across thick ascending limb NH_4^+ then moves along the tubular fluid. In the TAL of loop of Henle, a significant amount of NH_4^+ is reabsorbed via two mechanisms:

- *Transcellularly*, via $1Na^+$–$1K^+$–$2Cl^-$ symporter with NH_4^+ substituting for K^+
- *Paracellularly* driven by the lumen-positive transepithelial voltage in this segment

C. Accumulation of NH_4^+ in medullary interstitium The NH_4 reabsorbed across the TAL accumulates in the medullary interstitium, where it exists in chemical equilibrium with NH_3^+.

D. Anionic diffusion and diffusion trapping in collecting ducts The cells of collecting duct are not permeable to NH_4^+, but permeable to NH_3^+. From the medullary interstitium, NH_3^+ diffuses into the lumen of collecting ducts by a process called nonionic diffusion and is protonated to NH_4^+ by combining with H^+ secreted by the cells of collecting duct. Since the cells of collecting ducts are impermeable to NH_4^+, NH_4^+ is trapped in the lumen of collecting duct (*diffusion trapping*) and is excreted in the urine. Thus, for every NH_4^+ excreted in the urine, a new HCO_3^- is returned to the systemic circulation. Therefore, excretion of NH_4^+ can be used as a marker of proximal tubule glutamine metabolism, which in turn determines new HCO_3^- formation.

Important Note

Certain important points to note about NH_4^+ are as follows:

- *NH_4^+* is a major urine acid. It is estimated that about half to two-thirds of body acid load is eliminated in the form of NH_4^+ ions. For this reason, renal regulation via NH_4^+ excretion is very effective to eliminate large quantities of acids produced in the body.
- The ammonium content of urine is negligible until the urinary pH falls below 6. Below this urinary pH, the ammonium secretion increases linearly with the fall in pH.
- Unlike phosphate buffer, the capacity of ammonia buffer is not limited by the amount filtered in the glomerular filtrate. In states of chronic acidosis (e.g. diabetic ketoacidosis, respiratory acidosis), the amount of H^+ excreted as NH_4^+ may increase to 10-fold, due to an *adaptative increase in NH_3 synthesis.*
- Since the p*K* value of this buffer system is 9, H^+ excreted as NH_4^+ does not contribute to titrable acidity of the urine.

Self-Assessment

1. Discuss the physiological basis of concentration of urine.
2. Discuss the role of different regions of renal tubule in medullary hyperosmolality and medullary gradient.
3. Describe the mechanism of acidification of urine.
4. Write briefly on:
   - Diuresis
   - Excretion of H^+ as ammonium
   - Factors governing urine dilution

Clinical Case

Case 1

A 22-year-old male was forced to drink six liters of water within short period of one hour as a penalty. He developed restlessness, intermittent convulsions and was brought to the hospital emergency.

Examination and tests revealed:

- Pulse rate – 60/minute
- No edema on face
- BP – 140/90 mmHg
- Temp – 36.80°C
- Serum electrolytes showed hypernatremia (<145 mmol/L)
- Urine analysis
- Hypertonicity

Q1. What is the probable diagnosis?

Q2. What is the cause for convulsions?

Q3. What is the status of ADH in this case?

6.4

Regulation of Body Fluid Osmolality, Composition and Volume

CHAPTER OUTLINE

INTRODUCTION

The control of body fluid osmolality, composition and volume, and thus the water and electrolyte balance in the body, is concerted function of the kidneys, blood, skin, lungs, digestive system, certain hormones and neural mechanisms. However, the kidneys play a major role in these homeostatic mechanisms. For the ease of understanding, this chapter has been divided into the following sections:

- The body fluid compartments
- Control of body fluid osmolality
- Regulation of extracellular fluid (ECF) volume and composition
- Defence of specific ion composition
- Water and electrolyte disturbances

BODY FLUID COMPARTMENTS

VOLUMES AND COMPOSITION OF BODY FLUID COMPARTMENTS

The total body water (TBW) and the body fluid compartments have been described in Chapter 1.1 (see page 6). The salient features are summarized here:

- TBW, intracellular fluid (ICF) and ECF form 60%, 40% and 20% of the total body weight, respectively (60–40–20 rule).
- Percentage of TBW is the highest in newborns and adult males, and the lowest in adult females and in adults with a large amount of adipose tissue.
- The major cation of ECF is Na^+, whereas that of ICF is K^+.
- The major anions of ECF are Cl^- and HCO_3^-, whereas those of ICF are protein and organic phosphates (adenosine

triphosphate [ATP], adenosine diphosphate [ADP] and adenosine monophosphate [AMP]).

FLUID EXCHANGE BETWEEN BODY FLUID COMPARTMENTS

Basic Principles

Basic principles of fluid exchange which are also useful for analysis of fluid shifts between ICF and ECF are as follows:

Osmolalities of ECF and ICF are equal at steady state. Because the plasma membranes of cells are highly permeable to water, a change in the osmolality of either ECF or ICF results in the rapid movement of water between these compartments to achieve the equality in osmolality.

Movement of water across plasma membrane between ECF and ICF is determined mainly by the osmotic difference between the two compartments, whereas fluid exchange between plasma and interstitial fluid across the capillary wall is determined by Starling forces (see page 309).

Movement of ions across the cell membrane is variable and depends on the presence of specific membrane transporters. However, for the sake of simplification in analysing fluid shifts between compartments, it can be assumed that equilibration between ECF and ICF occurs only by the movement of water and that solutes like NaCl and mannitol do not cross cell membranes and are confined to the ECF.

Exchanges of solutes and water with external environment occur through the ECF (e.g. intravenous administration, oral intake or loss via GIT and urinary tract). Changes in ICF are secondary to changes in ECF, and occur only if perturbation of the ECF alters its osmolality.

Gross estimation of volume of various fluid compartments in the normal adult can be made from their standard ratio:

- TBW = 0.6 × body weight
- ICF = 0.4 × body weight
- ECF = 0.2 × body weight
- Interstitial fluid = 0.75 × ECF
- Plasma volume = 0.25 × ECF

CONTROL OF BODY FLUID OSMOLALITY

At steady state, the major fluid compartments of the body, i.e. ECF and ICF, are in osmotic equilibrium and thus have the same osmolality. This equilibrium is maintained by free water shifts between the ECF and ICF compartments. Therefore, a measurement of plasma osmolality provides a measure of both ECF and ICF osmolality. It is important to note that although the osmolalities of ECF and ICF are similar, there is marked difference in the concentration of electrolytes (cations and anions) between the ECF and the ICF. As described in body electrolytes (Chapter 1.1, page 8), Na^+ is the principal cation of ECF, whereas in the ICF, the principal cation is K^+. This difference in the concentration is essential for the cell survival, and is maintained by Na^+–K^+ pump.

Normal plasma osmolality ranges from approximately 280 to 295 mOsm/kg H_2O. Table 6.4.1 shows the distribution of constituents in plasma osmolality. Sodium and its associated anions make the largest contribution (~90%) to plasma osmolality.

Computation of plasma osmolality, for practical purposes, can be done from the concentration (mmol/L) of Na^+, K^+, urea and glucose:

$$\text{Plasma osmolality} = 2(Na^+) + 2(K^+) + \text{urea} + \text{glucose}$$

Table 6.4.1 Distribution of constituents in plasma osmolality

Constituent (solute)	Osmolality (mOsm/kg H_2O)
Sodium	135
Associated anions	135
Potassium	3.5
Associated anions	3.5
Calcium	1.5
Associated anions	1.5
Magnesium	1.0
Associated anions	1.0
Urea	5.0
Glucose	5.0
Protein	1.0
Total	293

The factor of 2 is used for Na^+ and K^+ ions to account for the associated anion concentration. Since plasma Na^+ is the most predominant contributor to osmolality, the above-given calculation can be simplified (provided plasma glucose and urea are in the normal range) as follows:

$$\text{Plasma osmolality (mmol/kg)} = 2 \times \text{plasma } Na^+ \text{ (mmol/L)}$$

Plasma (Na^+) and ECF: It is important to realize that Na^+ and its associated anions (mainly Cl^-) are mainly confined to ECF. Therefore, the retention of water in the ECF is directly related to the osmotic effect of these ions. Thus, the amount of Na^+ in the ECF ultimately determines its volume.

Note: When evaluating abnormal plasma (Na^+) in an individual, it is tempting to suspect a problem in Na^+ balance. The problem most often relates to water balance, and not with Na^+ balance, alterations in the volume of ECF and its osmolality.

Determinants of body fluid osmolality: The total body osmolality is directly proportional to the total body sodium plus the total body potassium divided by the TBW. Therefore, changes in the body fluid occur when there is disproportion between the amounts of these electrolytes and the amount of water ingested or lost from the body. In other words, water balance in the body is the most important determinant of the body fluid osmolality.

REGULATION OF WATER BALANCE

The kidneys possess tremendous capacity to regulate the body water balance. In a healthy individual, this is achieved by balancing the daily water input and output.

Water Input

Water is added to the body fluids by:

1. ***Ingestion of water*** in the form of fluid and as constituent of foodstuffs (Table 6.4.2). The water intake is highly variable, which may range from 0.5 to 20 L/day depending on the social and personal habits and environmental conditions. In general, people living in hot climate drink more water. Ingestion of water is mainly controlled by the thirst centre. Increase in the plasma osmolality stimulates the thirst centre and promotes water ingestion.

Table 6.4.2 Water balance in the body represented by daily water input and output in adults at room temperature (23°C)

Water intake (mL/day)		Water output (mL/day)	
Source	**Volume**	**Route**	**Volume**
Ingested water	1200[a]	Insensible	700
In food	1000	Sweat	100
Metabolic water	300	Faeces	200
		Urine	1500[b]
Total	2500		2500

[a]Fluid ingestion varies from 1000 to 2000 mL/day; obligatory water ingestion is 400 mL/day.
[b]Urine flow varies depending on the water ingested; obligatory urine volume is 500 mL/day.

2. ***Endogenous production of water*** during oxidation of foodstuffs adds about 300 mL of water to the body fluids per day (Table 6.4.2).

Water Output

A variable amount of water is lost from the body in urine, faeces and sweat and as insensible loss (Table 6.4.2).

1. Insensible loss of water Insensible loss of water (about which the individual is unaware) occurs by evaporation from the cells of the skin and respiratory passages.

2. Water loss in sweat Water loss by the production of sweat from the skin can vary from 100 mL/day in routine at room temperature of 23°C to 1400 mL in hot weather, to 5000 mL following prolonged exercise (Table 6.4.3).

3. Water loss in faeces Most of the water entering the GIT is reabsorbed by the intestine. About 200 mL/day is lost through faeces in a healthy individual (Table 6.4.2). Faecal loss of water is tremendously increased in diarrhoea. GIT water losses can also occur with vomiting.

Table 6.4.3 Effect of environmental temperature and exercise on water loss and intake in adults

	Volume (mL/day)		
Route of water loss	**Normal temperature**	**Hot weather**	**Prolonged heavy exercise**
• Insensible loss			
Skin	350	350	350
Lungs	350	250	650
• Sweat	100	1400	5000
• Faeces	200	200	200
• Urine	1500	1200	500
• Total loss	2500	3400	6700
• Water intake to maintain balance	2500	3400	6700

4. Water loss in urine About 1500 mL of water is eliminated from the body in urine. Water losses through the kidney are highly variable.

It is important to note that water loss in sweat, faeces and evaporation from the lungs and skin is *not regulated*. However, the renal loss, though variable, is well regulated to maintain the water balance. For water balance, the water output is precisely matched with water intake by the kidneys:

- The kidneys produce a small amount of concentrated urine (hyperosmotic with respect to plasma) when the intake is low or losses are more.
- Conversely, the kidneys produce a large amount of dilute urine (hypo-osmotic with respect to plasma) when the water intake is high.

Thus, in a normal individual, depending primarily on the antidiuretic hormone (ADH) concentration, the urine osmolality may vary from 500 to 800 mOsm/kg H_2O with a corresponding urine volume of 800–2000 mL/day.

Applied Aspects

Disorders of water balance alter body fluid osmolality. Changes in body fluid osmolality are manifested by a change in plasma (Na^+):

Positive water balance (intake > excretion) results in decrease in body fluid osmolality and hyponatraemia.

Negative water balance (intake < excretion) results in an increase in body fluid osmolality and hypernatraemia.

Factors Controlling Water Balance

Both the input of water (i.e. thirst) and the output of water (i.e. urinary excretion) are controlled by plasma osmolality and blood volume.

1. ***Plasma osmolality*** controls water balance by stimulating the thirst centre and ADH secretion through the osmoreceptors as mentioned in the subsequent text. Significant changes in ADH secretion occur by a small (2%) change in the plasma osmolality.
2. ***Blood volume:*** Under normal circumstances, the water balance of the body is mainly regulated through osmoreceptors. However, a significant (more than 10%) decrease in blood volume also stimulates thirst and ADH secretion from the posterior pituitary. If blood volume is markedly decreased, ADH release is stimulated even if plasma osmolality is low. Whenever there is conflict between plasma osmolality and blood volume, the latter is maintained at the cost of plasma osmolality. Decreased blood volume is sensed by low-pressure receptors in the atria and pulmonary vessels.

For further details, see page 334.

MECHANISMS CONTROLLING BODY FLUID OSMOLALITY

The control of body fluid osmolality, i.e. defence of the tonicity of the ECF, is primarily the function of the vasopressin secretion and thirst mechanisms:

When the effective osmotic pressure of plasma rises When the effective osmotic pressure of plasma rises,

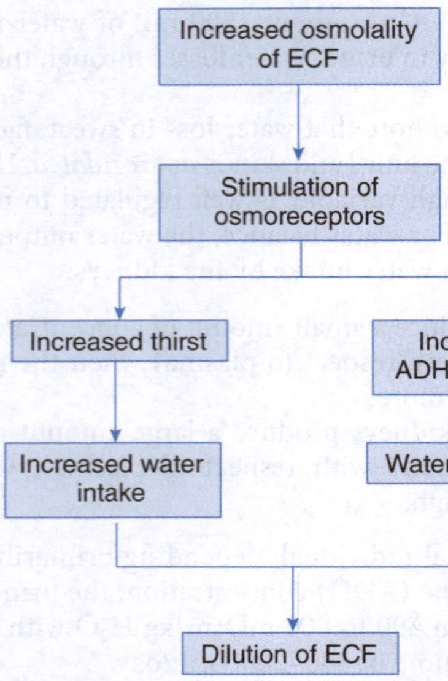

Fig. 6.4.1 Mechanisms regulating body fluid osmolality.

the *osmoreceptors* located in the anterior hypothalamus are stimulated. The stimulation of receptors results from their shrinkage caused by cellular dehydration. Cellular dehydration may occur because of:

- Deficiency of TBW
- Excessive intake of NaCl, which causes the water to shift from ICF to ECF

The *stimulated osmoreceptors* in turn cause (Fig. 6.4.1):

- Increase in thirst, which regulates water intake
- Increase in vasopressin release, which regulates water excretion by the kidneys

When the effective osmotic pressure of plasma decreases When the effective osmotic pressure of plasma decreases, i.e. when plasma becomes hypotonic, the vasopressin secretion is decreased (increasing water excretion in excess of solute) and thirst is decreased (decreasing water intake).

Thus, the main mechanisms which are related with regulation of body fluid osmolality are as follows:

- Role of ADH (see page 338)
- Role of thirst mechanism
- Renal mechanisms for dilution and concentration of urine (see page 509)

REGULATION OF EXTRACELLULAR FLUID VOLUME AND COMPOSITION

The regulation of ECF volume is primarily mediated through the regulation of the amount of osmotically active solute in it. The major solutes of the ECF are the salts of Na^+; of these, NaCl is the most abundant. Since the kidneys are the major route of NaCl excretion from the body, they play an important role in the regulation of ECF. The kidneys get signals from the volume-sensing system to make appropriate adjustment in NaCl excretion. The volume sensors generate signals in response to changes in the effective circulatory volume (ECV). The volume sensor signals then control the volume of ECF by controlling the renal excretion of NaCl and water. Therefore, the process of regulation of ECF volume can be described in the following subsections:

- Concept of effective circulating volume and volume-sensing system
- Neural and hormonal control of NaCl excretion
- Sodium balance

EFFECTIVE CIRCULATORY VOLUME AND VOLUME SENSORS

Concept of Effective Circulating Volume

Effective circulatory volume ECV is not a measurable and distinct body fluid compartment. In physiologically conceptual term, the ECV refers to the portion of ECF volume that is present in the arterial system under particular pressure and is effectively perfusing the tissues. Thus, ECV cannot be simply regulated with the volume of fluid in the vascular tree. In a 70-kg man with 42 L of TBW (60% of body weight), the ECF volume is about 14 L (20% of body weight), out of which interstitial fluid volume is 10.5 L (75% of ECF) and plasma volume (vascular volume) is 3.5 L (25% of ECF). Only about 0.7 L of vascular volume (i.e. 20% of plasma, or 5% of ECF or 1.7% of TBW or 1% of the body weight) forms the ECV. The ECV is regulated by the volume sensors which are located entirely within the vascular tree. Sensation of ECV is related to 'fullness', i.e. 'volume and pressure' in the vascular tree.

In the normal state In the normal state, variations in ECV are reflected as parallel variations in ECF volume and also in vascular volume, arterial blood pressure and cardiac output. In other words, a decrease in ECF, vascular volume, arterial pressure or cardiac output will be sensed in the body as decrease in ECV.

Maintenance of ECV Maintenance of ECV and regulation of Na^+ balance are closely related. Therefore, Na^+ loading produces expansion of ECV and Na^+ loss leads to depletion of ECV. In other words, when ECV is decreased, the renal NaCl excretion is reduced. This adaptive response restores the ECV to normal and thereby maintains adequate tissue perfusion. Conversely, an increase in ECV results in an enhanced renal NaCl excretion termed the *natriuresis*. Again, this is an adaptive response to restore the ECV to its normal point.

Applied Aspects

In pathological conditions such as congestive heart failure and hepatic cirrhosis, the ECV may be independent of ECF volume, i.e. ECV is reduced, although ECF volume is markedly increased. Since the kidneys regulate the excretion of NaCl in response to changes in ECV rather than in ECF volume, there occurs renal retention of Na^+ and H_2O, despite the increased content of total body Na^+ and H_2O, which is a paradoxical renal response. The increase in ECF and retention of Na^+ in such patients manifests as accumulation of fluid in the lungs (*pulmonary oedema*) and peripheral tissues (*generalized oedema*).

ECV Sensors (Volume-Sensing System)

The ECV sensors, commonly known as volume sensors or volume receptors, refer to the receptors which are located in the vascular system and respond to the degree of stretch of the vessel wall and not to the volume of the vessel (hence, also called baroreceptors). Various volume sensors known are as follows:

I. ***Vascular volume receptors***
  a. *Low-pressure volume receptors* are located in:
    - Cardiac atria
    - Pulmonary vasculature
  b. *High-pressure volume receptors* include:
    - Carotid sinus
    - Aortic arch
    - Juxtaglomerular apparatus of the kidney

II. ***Hepatic volume receptors (sensors)***

III. ***Central nervous system (CNS) Na^+ sensors***

The sensors within the liver and CNS are less well understood, and do not seem to be as important as the vascular sensors in monitoring the effective circulating volume. The vascular receptors are described in detail in Chapter 4.5 (see page 334); only salient points are mentioned here.

Vascular low-pressure volume sensors (receptors)

Located within the walls of cardiac atria and large pulmonary vessels, these sensors respond to fullness of vascular tree. *Afferents from these receptors* travel to the solitary tract nucleus of the medulla oblongata via vagus nerve and reflexly modulate:

- Sympathetic discharge
- ADH secretion
- Atrial natriuretic peptide (ANP) secretion (only by cardiac atrial receptors)

Vascular high-pressure volume sensors (receptors)

These are located in carotid sinus and aortic arch.

The sinoaortic baroreceptors respond primarily to the arterial blood pressure. Afferents from these receptors travel to the solitary tract nucleus of the medulla via glossopharyngeal and vagus nerves and reflexly regulate:

- Sympathetic discharge to the heart and resistance vessels including the renal arterioles
- ADH secretion

Juxtaglomerular apparatus of the kidneys (see page 474), particularly the afferent arterioles, responds directly to change in the pressure and modulates the renin–angiotensin mechanism.

Hepatic volume sensors Hepatic volume sensors, though not as important as vascular volume receptors, do play a role in regulating renal NaCl excretion by reflexly regulating renal sympathetic discharge. The hepatic sensors also appear to be involved in the regulation of gastrointestinal Na^+ absorption. For example, when the Na^+ concentration of the portal vein blood is increased, there is reflex reduction in jejunal NaCl absorption.

CNS Na^+ sensors (receptors) CNS Na^+ sensors (receptors), like the hepatic sensors, play only a little role in regulating renal NaCl excretion. Probably, these are located in the hypothalamus and respond to Na^+ concentration in carotid blood or cerebrospinal fluid (CSF), and regulate renal sympathetic nerve activity.

NEURAL AND HORMONAL REGULATION OF RENAL SODIUM CHLORIDE EXCRETION

Both neural and hormonal volume sensor signals arise in response to afferents from the above-described volume sensors and regulate the renal excretion of NaCl (Table 6.4.4).

Neural Regulation

As described in Chapter 6.1 (page 480), the sympathetic nerve fibres innervate the afferent and efferent arterioles of the glomerulus as well as nephron cells.

Renal sympathetic stimulation Renal sympathetic stimulation, which is induced by vascular low- and high-volume sensors, in conditions of negative Na^+ balance (i.e. decreased ECV), leads to decrease in NaCl excretion by the following mechanisms:

1. ***Reduction in glomerular filtration rate (GFR)*** occurs due to vasoconstriction of afferent arterioles induced by sympathetic stimulation. Reduced GFR leads to a decrease in the filtered load (filtered load = GFR × plasma Na^+ concentration). Reduction in filtered load does help in Na^+ conservation; however, changes in filtered load of Na^+ are not reflected in parallel changes in the urinary Na^+ excretion because of the following effects:
   - Glomerular tubular balance (see page 494)
   - Tubuloglomerular feedback (see page 478)
2. ***Increased Na^+ reabsorption*** along the nephron is directly produced by stimulation of α-adrenergic receptors. Proximal tubule is the most important segment influenced by sympathetic nerve stimulation.
3. ***Stimulation of renin secretion*** from the cells of afferent arterioles is produced by the activation of β-adrenergic receptors. As described below, it results in increased plasma concentration of angiotensin II and aldosterone.

Renal sympathetic inhibition Renal sympathetic inhibition, which is induced by vascular low- and high-pressure volume receptors in conditions of positive Na^+ balance (i.e. increased ECV), leads to increased NaCl excretion by the reverse effect of the above-described mechanisms.

Hormonal Regulation

1. Renin–angiotensin–aldosterone system Renin–angiotensin–aldosterone system when stimulated with volume depletion results in decreased NaCl excretion; conversely, when suppressed with volume expansion, it enhances NaCl excretion.

Renin is secreted by smooth muscles of afferent arterioles of the kidney in response to:

- Reduced perfusion pressure
- Increased renal sympathetic discharge (as mentioned above)
- Decreased delivery of NaCl to the macula densa cells (tubuloglomerular feedback mechanism) (see page 478)

Renin converts angiotensinogen (produced by the liver) into angiotensin I, which is converted to angiotensin II by angiotensin-converting enzyme (ACE) (Fig. 6.4.2).

Angiotensinogen II subserves the following physiological functions:

- Stimulates aldosterone secretion by the adrenal cortex
- Increases blood pressure by arteriolar vasoconstriction
- Stimulates ADH secretion and thirst
- Enhances NaCl reabsorption by proximal tubules

Table 6.4.4 Summary of neural and hormonal control of renal NaCl and water excretion

Neural control
↑ Sympathetic activity decreases NaCl excretion by:
• ↓ Glomerular filtration rate
• ↑ Renin secretion
• ↑ Tubular NaCl reabsorption
Hormonal control
↑ Renin–angiotensin–aldosterone secretion decreases NaCl excretion by:
• ↑ Proximal tubule absorption
• ↑ ADH secretion by angiotensinogen II
• ↑ Tubular reabsorption by aldosterone
↑ ANP secretion increases NaCl excretion by:
• ↑ Glomerular filtration rate
• ↓ Renin secretion
• ↓ Aldosterone secretion
• ↓ NaCl and water reabsorption by the collecting duct
• ↓ ADH secretion and action of ADH on the collecting duct
↑ ADH secretion decreases H_2O excretion by:
• ↑ H_2O absorption by the collecting duct
ADH, antidiuretic hormone; ANP, atrial natriuretic peptide.

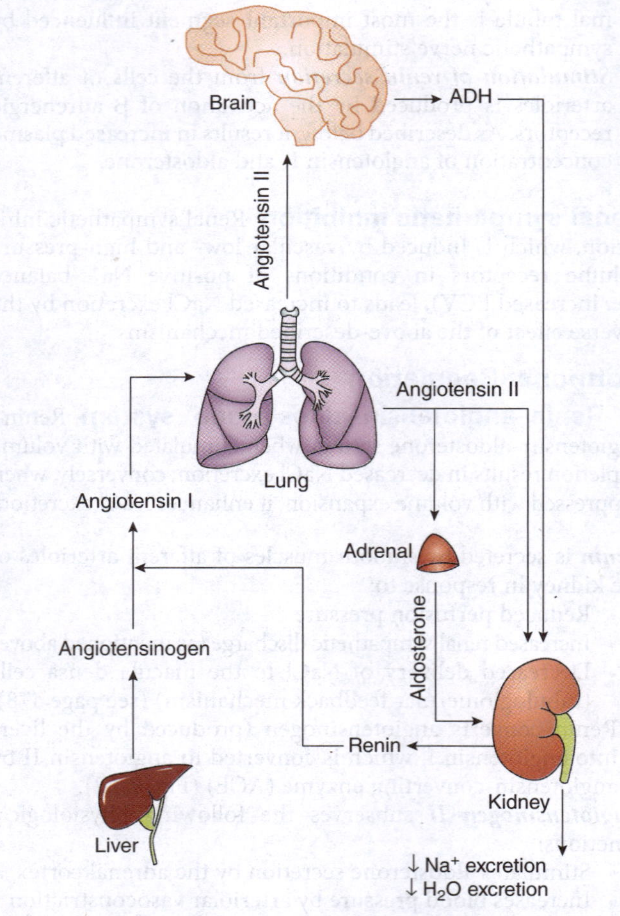

Fig. 6.4.2 Mechanism of decreased Na^+ excretion by the renin–angiotensin–aldosterone system (for explanation, see text).

Aldosterone enhances NaCl reabsorption from the thick ascending limb (TAL) of loop of Henle by stimulating Na^+–K^+–$2Cl^-$ symporter at the apical membrane and Na^+–K^+-ATPase at the basolateral membrane.

2. ANP ANP is released from the atrial myocytes by the atrial stretch caused by volume expansion (increased ECV). Its actions are opposite to those of renin–angiotensin–aldosterone system and result in increased urinary excretion of NaCl by the following mechanisms:

- *Increased GFR* by vasodilation of afferent and vasoconstriction of efferent arterioles
- *Inhibition of renin secretion* by the afferent arterioles
- *Inhibition of aldosterone secretion* by inhibiting renin secretion and also by its direct effect on the adrenal cortex cells
- *Inhibition of ADH secretion* by posterior pituitary and inhibition of ADH action on the collecting duct
- *Inhibition of NaCl reabsorption* by the collecting duct by inhibiting aldosterone secretion, by inhibiting ADH secretion and also by its direct effect on the collecting duct cells

3. ADH ADH secretion by the posterior pituitary is increased with volume depletion (decreased ECV) leading to retention of water by the kidneys and thus re-establishing euvolaemia. Reverse occurs in volume expansion (see page 678).

SODIUM BALANCE

Sodium is actively pumped out of the cells by Na^+–K^+-ATPase pump. As a result, 85%–90% of all Na^+ is extracellular, and the ECF volume is reflection of total body Na^+ content. Normal volume regulatory mechanisms ensure that Na^+ loss balances Na^+ gain. If this does not occur, conditions of Na^+ excess or deficit ensure and manifest as oedematous or hypovolaemic states, respectively.

Sodium Intake

An individual consumes about 150 mmol of NaCl daily. This normally exceeds basal requirements. Since Na^+ is the principal extracellular cation, the dietary intake of Na^+ results in ECF volume expansion. This, in turn, promotes enhanced renal Na^+ excretion to maintain steady-state Na^+ balance.

Sodium Excretion

The neural and hormonal regulation of the Na^+ excretion, as described above, is multifactorial and is the major determinant of Na^+ balance. Therefore, further discussion is devoted to:

- Characteristics and mechanisms of responses to varying salt intake
- Regulation of Na^+ excretion during euvolaemia
- Regulation of Na^+ excretion with volume expansion
- Regulation of Na^+ excretion with volume contraction

Characteristics and Mechanisms of Responses to Varying Salt Intake

Wide range of Na^+ excretion The kidneys can maintain normal ECF volume and normal ECV by varying the amount of NaCl excretion over a wide range depending on the circumstances. Consequently, under conditions of salt restriction (e.g. low-NaCl diet), the kidneys conserve all the Na^+, and virtually no Na^+ appears in the urine. Conversely, with large quantities of intake, renal excretion can exceed 1000 mEqL/day.

Response to variation in salt intake takes a few days and during the transition period, excretion does not match intake, explained as follows:

1. ***When NaCl intake is suddenly increased***, the individual remains in a positive balance (intake > excretion) for 2–3 days. With positive balance, water retention occurs, which manifests as an increase in the body weight. After a period of adaptation (which depends on the magnitude of change in NaCl intake), the daily urinary excretion of NaCl matches the amount ingested (Fig. 6.4.3).

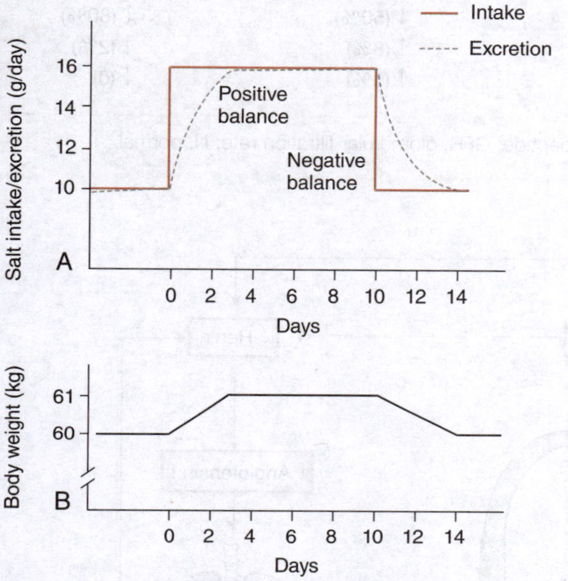

Fig. 6.4.3 Effect of sudden increase and decrease in dietary salt intake on sodium and water balance: **A**, the positive and negative balance during adaptive period; and **B**, corresponding increase and decrease in body weight.

2. ***When the salt intake is abruptly decreased***, the individual remains in a negative balance (intake < excretion) for 2–3 days. With negative balance, there occurs loss of water, which manifests as decrease in the body weight. After a period of adaptation, the daily urinary excretion of NaCl matches the amount ingested (Fig. 6.4.3).

Mechanism The role of different regulatory mechanisms (described above) in controlling Na^+ excretion in different situations is described.

Regulation of Na^+ excretion during euvolaemia During euvolaemia, the kidneys match Na^+ excretion with intake simply by adjusting the reabsorption in the collecting duct. A change of about 2% in fractional excretion of Na^+ can produce more than 3 L of change in the volume of ECF.

Aldosterone is the primary regulator of collecting duct Na^+ reabsorption.

As long as variations in dietary intake of NaCl are minor, this mechanism can regulate renal Na^+ excretion appropriately, and thereby maintain euvolaemia (Fig. 6.4.4A; Table 6.4.5).

Regulation of Na^+ excretion with volume expansion Volume expansion, i.e. a large increase in ECF volume and ECV, may occur following excessive salt intake or excessive administration of intravenous saline.

An increase in ECV (volume expansion), as detected by the vascular volume receptors, initiates a response that ultimately leads to increased sodium excretion by the following mechanisms (Fig. 6.4.5):

- Decreased renal sympathetic discharge
- Suppression of the renin–angiotensin–aldosterone system
- Increased ANP secretion from the atrial myocytes
- Suppression of ADH release

Renal response to the above-mentioned signals, which results in increased Na^+ excretion, consists of (Fig. 6.4.4B; Table 6.4.5):

- Increased GFR

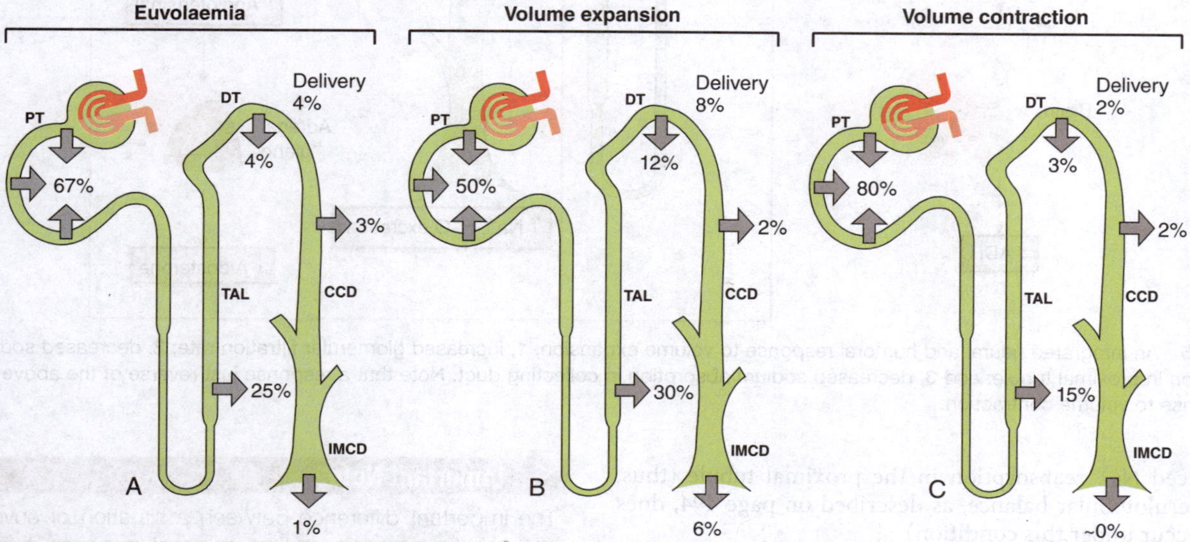

Fig. 6.4.4 Segmental Na^+ reabsorption during: **A**, euvolaemia; **B**, volume expansion; and **C**, volume contraction. Note that the delivery of Na^+ to collecting duct in euvolaemia, volume expansion and volume contraction is 4%, 8% and 2%, respectively, and Na^+ excretion is 1%, 6% and 0%, respectively.

Table 6.4.5 Neural and hormonal signals producing different renal response in euvolaemia, volume expansion and volume contraction

Signals	Euvolaemia	Volume expansion	Volume contraction
Neural signal			
• Renal sympathetic activity	N	↓	↑
Hormonal signal			
• Renin–angiotensin–aldosterone system activity	↑	↓	↑
• ANP secretion	N	↑	↓
• ADH secretion	N	↑	↓
Renal response			
• GFR	N		
• Na^+ reabsorption in proximal tubule	N (67%)	↓ (50%)	↑ (80%)
• Delivery of Na^+ to collecting duct	(4%)	↑ (8%)	↓ (2%)
• Na^+ excretion	(1%)	↑ (6%)	↓ (0)

↑, increased; ↓, decreased; ADH, antidiuretic hormone; ANP, atrial natriuretic peptide; GFR, glomerular filtration rate; N, normal.

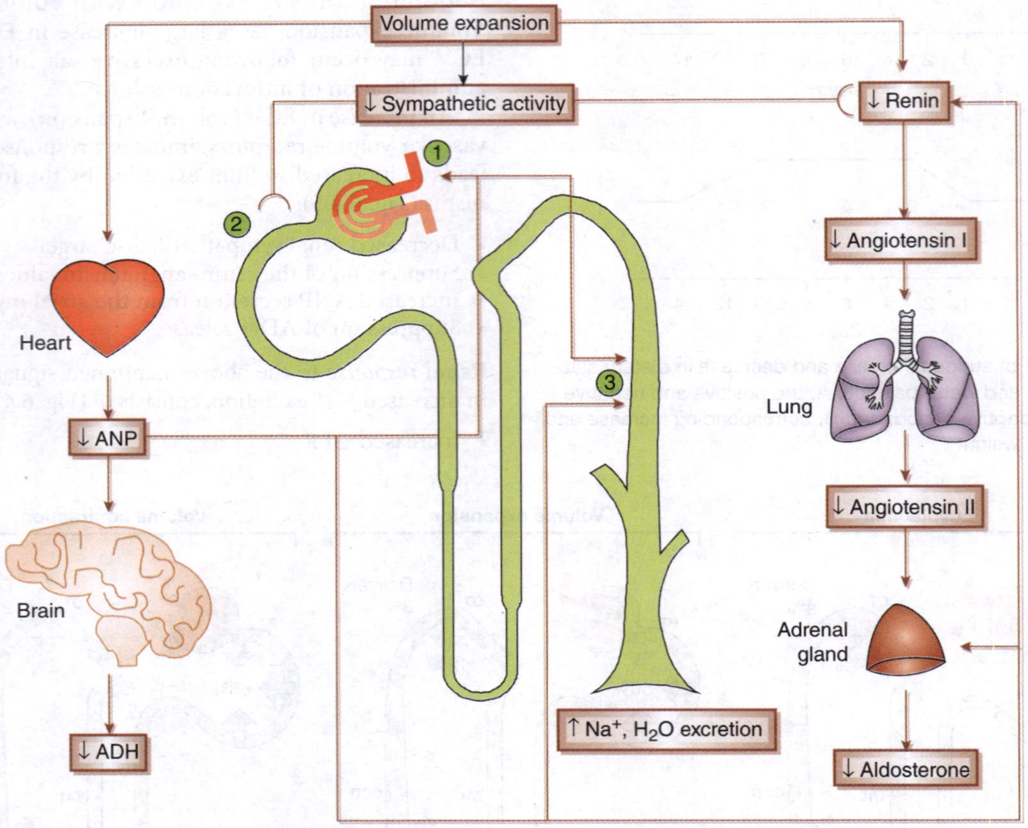

Fig. 6.4.5 An integrated neural and humoral response to volume expansion: **1**, increased glomerular filtration rate; **2**, decreased sodium reabsorption in proximal tubule; and **3**, decreased sodium absorption in collecting duct. Note that a response just reverse of the above occurs in response to volume contraction.

- Reduced Na^+ reabsorption in the proximal tubule (thus, glomerulotubular balance, as described on page 494, does not occur under this condition)
- Increased delivery of NaCl to the beginning of the collecting duct (i.e. about 8%)
- Decreased Na^+ reabsorption in the collecting duct

Important Note

The important difference between a situation of euvolaemia and volume expansion is that the renal response in the latter involves the entire nephron and is not limited to the collecting duct as in the former.

Regulation of Na^+ excretion with volume contraction Volume contraction, i.e. a large decrease in ECF and ECV, may occur due to severe extrarenal loss of NaCl, e.g. due to heavy sweating or diarrhoea. A decrease in ECV as detected by vascular volume sensors initiates a response that ultimately leads to decreased excretion by the following mechanisms, and the reverse effects to these are shown in Fig. 6.4.5:

- Increased renal sympathetic discharge
- Stimulation of renin–angiotensin–aldosterone mechanism
- Decreased ANP secretion from the atrial myocytes
- Stimulation of ADH release

Renal response to the above-mentioned signals, which results in decreased Na^+ excretion, consists of (Fig. 6.4.4C; Table 6.4.5):

- Decreased GFR
- Increased Na^+ reabsorption in the proximal tubule (thus, G–T balance, as described on page 494, does not occur under this condition)
- Decreased delivery of NaCl to the beginning of the collecting duct (i.e. about 2%), and increased Na^+ reabsorption in the collecting duct

Important Note

The important difference between a situation of euvolaemia and volume contraction is that the renal response in the latter involves the entire nephron and is not limited to the collecting duct as in the former.

DEFENCE OF SPECIFIC ION COMPOSITION

The regulation of ion composition of ECF is the function of special regulatory mechanisms that maintain the level of these ions as follows:

- *Maintenance of ionized Ca^{2+} level* is governed by the feedback of Ca^{2+} on the parathyroids and the calcitonin secretory cells (see page 711).
- *Maintenance of Mg^+ level:* The magnesium concentration of ECF is closely regulated, but the mechanisms controlling Mg^+ metabolism are incompletely understood (see page 704).
- *Maintenance of Na^+ level* is primarily the function of the kidneys. It has been described above as part of the regulation of ECF volume.
- *Maintenance of K^+ level* is discussed on page 495.
- *Maintenance of H^+ concentration* is the function of buffer system, respiratory mechanisms and renal mechanisms (see page 514).

DISTURBANCES OF VOLUME AND CONCENTRATION OF BODY FLUID

Broadly, disturbances of fluid volume include:

Dehydration (i.e. fluid loss) and overhydration (i.e. fluid gain) Depending on the osmolality relative to plasma, a fluid may be:

Isotonic fluid, i.e. the fluid having the same osmolality as the plasma, e.g. 0.9% NaCl solution, 5% glucose, 10% mannitol and 20% urea. These solutions do not change the volume of the body cells.

Hypotonic fluid, i.e. the fluid having osmolality less than plasma. Such solutions cause the cells to swell and, if sufficiently dilute, to burst (lyse).

Hypertonic fluid, i.e. the fluid having osmolality more than plasma. Such solutions cause cells to shrink (i.e. to undergo crenation).

Disturbances of fluid volume and concentration can be classified as follows:

- Iso-osmotic volume expansion
- Iso-osmotic volume contraction
- Hyperosmotic volume expansion
- Hyperosmotic volume contraction
- Hypo-osmotic volume expansion
- Hypo-osmotic volume contraction

The causes, consequences and corrective responses of disturbances of volume and concentration in dehydration and overhydration are summarized in Table 6.4.6.

ISO-OSMOTIC VOLUME EXPANSION

Cause Cause of iso-osmotic volume expansion includes:

Infusion of isotonic fluids, e.g. 0.9% NaCl solution

Consequences Consequences of iso-osmotic volume expansion are as follows (Fig. 6.4.6A):

- *ECF volume* increases.
- *ECF osmolality* does not change. So water does not shift between the ECF and ICF compartments.
- *Plasma protein* concentration decreases because of dilution effect of additional fluid, resulting in decreased plasma colloid osmotic pressure. Due to decreased colloid osmotic pressure, water moves out of blood vessels and gets distributed in the interstitial compartment.
- *Haematocrit* decreases because the addition of fluid to ECF dilutes the RBCs. Because ECF osmolality is unchanged, the RBCs will neither shrink nor swell.
- *Arterial blood pressure* increases because ECF volume increases.

Corrective response Change in plasma volume is sensed by vascular volume receptors and brings about excretion of large volumes of hypotonic urine (water diuresis), which gradually restores the plasma volume and osmolality to normal.

ISO-OSMOTIC VOLUME CONTRACTION

Causes Iso-osmotic volume contraction occurs because of loss of isotonic fluid in the following conditions:

- Diarrhoea, vomiting
- Haemorrhage
- Ascites and burns

Consequences Consequences of iso-osmotic volume contraction are as follows (Fig. 6.4.6B):

- *ECF volume* is decreased.
- *ECF osmolality* does not change. So, water does not shift between the ECF and ICF compartments.
- *Plasma protein* concentration is increased because loss of ECF concentrates the protein. Due to presence of plasma protein (which hold fluids), the plasma volume is less reduced compared with interstitial fluid.

Table 6.4.6 Summary of disturbances of volume and concentration of body fluids

Type of disturbance	Volume (L) ICF	Volume (L) ECF	Osmolality (mOsm/L) ICF	Osmolality (mOsm/L) ECF	Causes	Consequences	Corrective response
Dehydration							
Iso-osmotic contraction	—	↓	— (Fig. 6.4.6B)	—	• Water loss due to: • Diarrhoea • Vomiting • Haemorrhage • Burns • Ascites	• Plasma protein concentration *increases* • Haematocrit increases • Arterial BP falls	Decrease plasma volume → inhibition of volume sensors → reflexly **restoration of plasma volume** due to decreased excretion of Na^+ and water ***Note:*** Thirst sensation is quenched by drinking isotonic salt solution
Hyperosmotic contraction	↓	↓	↑ (Fig. 6.4.6D)	↑	• Water loss due to: • Decreased water intake • Excessive sweating • Diabetes (mellitus and insipidus) • Alcoholism • Patients with tracheostomy (if loss >500 mL)	• Increased plasma protein concentration due to decreased ECF volume • Haematocrit increases	↑ ECF osmolality → stimulate osmoreceptors and decrease plasma volume → inhibit volume receptors → **restoration of plasma volume and osmolality**
Hypo-osmotic contraction	↑	↓	↓ (Fig. 6.4.6F)	↓	• Loss of NaCl or hypertonic fluid from body, e.g. vomiting • Adrenocortical insufficiency (Addison disease)	• Increased plasma protein concentration causes increased oncotic pressure, therefore shift of fluid from plasma to interstitial fluid • However, in grave salt depletion, plasma volume decreases • Thirst is inhibited because thirst cells swell up • Haematocrit increases due to decreased ECF • Arterial BP decreases	• The ECF volume is decreased but thirst is absent • Salt craving or salt appetite stimulates person to consume more NaCl → ECF osmolality restoration → shift of water from ICF to ECF → shrinkage of thirst centre cells → thirst stimulation → drinking of water → **normalization of plasma volume and osmolality**
Overhydration							
Iso-osmotic expansion	—	↑	— (Fig. 6.4.6A)	—	• Infusion of isotonic fluids (0.9% NaCl)	• Plasma protein concentration decreases • Haematocrit decreases • Arterial pressure increases (due to increase in ECF volume)	• Change in plasma volume sensed by volume receptors → excretion of large volume of hypotonic urine (water diuresis) → **normalization of ECF volume**

Hyperosmotic expansion	↓ (due to fluid shift from ICF to ECF)	↑	↑ (equalization with ECF) (Fig. 6.4.6C)	↑	• Administration of excessive amount of hypertonic saline	• Plasma protein concentration decreases • Haematocrit decreases • Arterial pressure increases (due to increase in ECF volume)	• Increased plasma osmolality promotes water retention • Increase in plasma volume • Thirst and ADH secretion are suppressed (increased *plasma volume oversides osmolality*) → excretion of excessive hypotonic urine → **plasma volume normalized** • ANP secretion increases → promotes Na excretion → **osmolality normalized**
Hypo-osmotic expansion	↑ (shift of water from ECF to ICF)	↑ due to water retention)	↓ (Fig. 6.4.6E)	↓	• Syndrome of inappropriate ADH (SIADH) secretion • Ingestion of large volume of water	• Water shifts from ECF to ICF → decreased ICF osmolality • Plasma protein concentration decreases • Haematocrit remains unchanged (because water shifts from plasma into RBCs)	Vascular volume receptors and osmoreceptors sense volume changes → excretion of large amount of hypotonic urine → **volume and osmolality normalized**

↑, increased; ↓, decreased; —, no change; ADH, antidiuretic hormone; ANP, atrial natriuretic peptide; ECF, extracellular fluid; ICF, intracellular fluid.

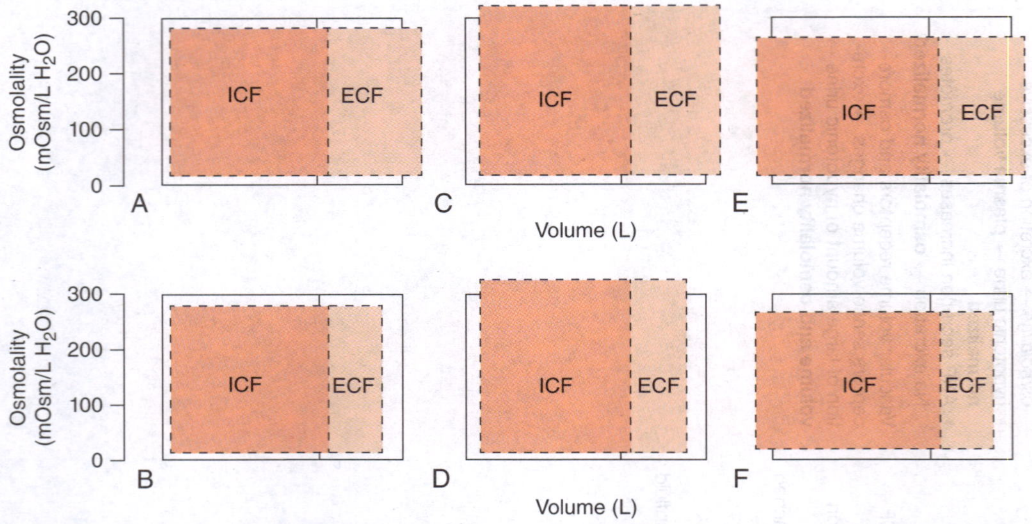

Fig. 6.4.6 Volume and osmolality of ECF and ICF and shift of water between two compartments during disturbances of fluid volume: **A**, iso-osmotic volume expansion; **B**, iso-osmotic volume contraction; **C**, hyperosmotic volume expansion; **D**, hyperosmotic volume contraction; **E**, hypo-osmotic volume expansion; and **F**, hypo-osmotic volume contraction. Volume and osmolality of normal ECF and ICF are indicated by solid lines. Changes in volume and osmolality as consequences of various situations are indicated by dashed lines. ECF, extracellular fluid; ICF, intracellular fluid.

- *Haematocrit* is increased because loss of ECF concentrates the RBCs. Because ECF osmolality is unchanged, the RBCs will neither shrink nor swell.
- *Arterial blood pressure* is decreased because of decrease in ECF volume.

Corrective response Decreased plasma volume inhibits the vascular volume sensors and reflexly restores the plasma volume by decreasing Na^+ and water excretion.

> **Important Note**
>
> It is important to note that the thirst produced by volume receptors is quenched with isotonic salt solution, instead of with plain water.

HYPEROSMOTIC VOLUME EXPANSION

Causes Hyperosmotic volume expansion results when excessive amount of hypertonic saline is administered.

Consequences Consequences of hyperosmotic volume expansion are as follows (Fig. 6.4.6C):

- ECF osmolality is increased, because osmoles (NaCl) have been added to ECF.
- *Water shifts from ICF to ECF.* As a result of this shift, ICF osmolality increases until it equals that of ECF.
- *ECF volume* increases because of addition of fluid as well as shift of fluid from ICF to ECF (volume expansion).
- *ICF volume* is decreased due to fluid shift.
- *Plasma protein* concentration decreases because of the increase in ECF volume.
- *Haematocrit* decreases because of increase in ECF volume. RBCs shrink and ECF osmolality is increased.
- *Arterial blood pressure* is increased because of increase in ECF volume.

Corrective response Increased plasma osmolality promotes water retention, whereas an increase in plasma volume inhibits the same. Under such circumstances, volume overrides tonicity. Therefore, the increased plasma volume would suppress thirst and ADH, leading to excretion of large volume of hypotonic urine, which brings down the plasma volume. The natriuretic hormones, which are secreted only in response to osmolality and not to volume changes, promote Na^+ excretion and correct osmolality.

HYPEROSMOTIC VOLUME CONTRACTION

Causes Hyperosmotic volume contraction occurs due to loss of water in the following conditions:

- Decreased water intake
- Diabetes mellitus
- Diabetes insipidus
- Excessive sweating in a desert
- Alcoholism
- In patients with tracheostomy (insensible loss of water up to 500 mL occurs from the lungs)

Consequences Consequences of hyperosmotic volume contraction (Fig. 6.4.6D) are as follows:

- *ECF volume* is reduced because of loss of water.
- *ECF osmolality* increases because more water is lost.
- *Water shifts from ICF to ECF.* As a result of this shift, ICF osmolality increases until it equals that of ECF.
- *ICF volume* decreases because of shift of water.
- *Plasma protein concentration* increases because of the decrease in ECF volume.

Haematocrit is also expected to increase, but it remains unchanged because water shifts out of RBCs decreasing their volume and offsetting the concentrating effect of the decreased ECF volume.

Corrective response Increased ECF osmolality stimulates the osmoreceptors, whereas reduced plasma volume inhibits the volume receptors. Either of them would reflexly restore the plasma volume and plasma osmolality to the normal level.

HYPO-OSMOTIC VOLUME EXPANSION

Causes Hypo-osmotic volume expansion occurs due to gain of water in the following conditions:

- Syndrome of inappropriate ADH (SIADH) secretion
- Ingestion of large volume of water
- Rectocolonic wash-outs with plain water

Consequences (Fig. 6.4.6E)

- *ECF osmolality* decreases because of excess water retention.
- *ECF volume* increases because of excess water retention.
- *Water shifts from ECF to ICF* increasing the volume of ICF.
- *ICF osmolality* decreases until it equals ECF osmolality.
- *Plasma protein concentration* decreases because of the increase in the ECF volume.
- *Haematocrit* might be expected to decrease, but actually it remains unchanged because water shifts into the RBCs, increasing their volume and thus offsetting the diluting effect in the gains of ECF volume.

Corrective response The vascular volume receptors and osmoreceptors sense the changes in plasma volume and osmolality, respectively. The signals from either of them lead to excretion of large amount of hypotonic urine (*water diuresis*) which gradually restores the plasma volume and osmolality to normal.

HYPO-OSMOTIC VOLUME CONTRACTION

Causes Hypo-osmotic volume contraction results from loss of NaCl or hypotonic fluid from the body in the following conditions:

- Adrenocortical insufficiency is associated with renal loss of NaCl.
- Vomiting or aspiration of gastric secretions is associated with hypertonic fluid loss from the body.

Consequences Consequences of hypo-osmotic volume contraction (Fig. 6.4.6F) are as follows:

- *ECF osmolality* is decreased because of loss of NaCl or other solutes.
- *Water shifts from ECF to ICF*, increasing the volume of ICF and decreasing the ECF volume.
- *ICF osmolality* decreases until it equals ECF osmolality.
- *Plasma volume* and osmolality changes tend to parallel those of ECF. However, a decrease in plasma volume raises *plasma protein* concentration. Due to the raised colloid oncotic pressure, the shift of fluid from the plasma to the interstitial fluid is decreased. Because of this, plasma volume is better preserved than the volume of interstitial fluid. However, in severe cases (*grave salt deficiency syndrome*), the plasma volume reduces sufficiently to produce a shock-like state with signs of renal failure. But, unlike in shock, there is no sensation of thirst, as explained:
  Cells of the thirst centre swell up due to shift of water from ECF to ICF. The thirst centre interprets this as the presence of excess water in the body. Consequently, thirst is inhibited.
- *Haematocrit* increases because of the decrease in ECF volume and because the RBCs swell as a result of water entry.
- *Arterial blood pressure* decreases because of the decrease in ECF volume.

Corrective response The ECF volume is decreased but thirst is absent; this seems to be nature's defence mechanism, since any water ingested would promptly leave the ECF and expand the ICF further. Therefore, salt craving or salt appetite which stimulates the individual to consume a large amount of NaCl is useful in restoring ECF osmolality. Normalization of ECF osmolality shifts water from ICF to ECF, leading to partial restoration of ECF volume shift of fluid from ICF to ECF which shrinks the cells of the thirst centre and restores the thirst. Consequently, drinking of water restores the remaining deficit in ECF volume.

Self-Assessment

1. Discuss the water balance of the body and its maintenance.
2. Describe the mechanism of control of plasma osmolality.
3. Describe the role of various hormones in regulation of sodium and water balance.
4. Describe in short the following:
   - Volume-sensing system
   - Significance of renin–angiotensin system
   - Effective circulatory volume
   - Hyperosmotic and hypo-osmotic contractions and their consequences

Clinical Cases

Case 1

A 54-year-old male was brought to the emergency department in the state of confusion, with blurred vision and increased frequency of urination. The patient was suffering from type 2 diabetes for which he was not taking the prescribed drug for the last 20 days. The examination and laboratory tests showed:
The patient was severely dehydrated, with blood sugar level 655 mg/dL.

Q1. Which type of disturbance of volume and concentration of body fluid has occurred in this case?
Q2. What should be the state of ECF and ICF in this condition?
Q3. What will be the expected status of plasma proteins and haematocrit in this case?
Q4. What complications can occur if not treated timely?

Case 2

A 40-year-old labourer working in desert area in scorching heat was brought to the emergency in a state of dizziness, with blurred vision and muscular cramps. Examination and laboratory tests revealed BP 86/59 mm Hg, pulse110 beats/min and low volume. Tendon reflexes slowed and the patient was diagnosed a case of hypotonic contraction.

Q1. What will be the osmolality of ECF and ICF?
Q2. What happens to plasma volume and why?
Q3. What is cause of this condition in this case?

6.5 Applied Renal Physiology Including Renal Function Tests

CHAPTER OUTLINE

PATHOPHYSIOLOGY OF COMMON RENAL DISORDERS

The applied aspects of common renal disorders which need some elaboration are as follows:

- Common urinary symptoms
- Renal failure
- Nephrotic syndrome

COMMON URINARY SYMPTOMS

Polyuria, Nocturia and Urinary Frequency

Polyuria Normal urine output per day is 800–2500 mL. Therefore, a reasonable criterion to satisfy the definition of polyuria is excretion of 3.0 L of urine daily provided the patient is not on high-fluid diet.

Nocturia Nocturia means excessive amount of urine passed at night.

Urinary frequency Urinary frequency means the increase in the number of times the patient goes for urination. Polyuria is differentiated from increased frequency by measuring the 24-hour urine output.

Common causes of polyuria are:

I. ***Physiological*** (primary polydipsia or excessive water drinking), which can be:
   - Psychogenic
   - Drug-induced (chlorpromazine, anticholinergics)

II. ***Pathological*** (defective water conservation by the kidney):
   - Diabetes insipidus
   - Solute diuresis, as in chronic renal failure (CRF), diabetes mellitus and mannitol infusion
   - Natriuresis as occurs in salt-losing nephropathy and effects of diuretics

Dysuria and Urgency of Micturition

Dysuria Dysuria refers to pain or burning during micturition.

Urgency of micturition Urgency of micturition is the exaggerated sense or urge to micturate. It is due to either irritative or inflammatory disorders of the urinary bladder. This is often associated with increased frequency of urination.

Incontinence

Incontinence refers to inability to retain urine in the bladder. It results from neurological or mechanical disorders of the complicated system that controls normal micturition.

Common causes of incontinence are:

- Neurogenic incontinence due to disturbances of neural control of micturition
- Stress incontinence, e.g. in postmenopausal parous women
- Mechanical incontinence, e.g. damage to urethral sphincters following transurethral resection of prostate (TURP)
- Overflow incontinence, e.g. in obstruction due to benign prostatic enlargement
- Psychogenic incontinence, as in anxious children
- Functional incontinence seen in very old persons who have mental derangement

Enuresis

Enuresis refers to the involuntary passage of urine at night or during sleep. It is also called night bedwetting or nocturnal enuresis. It is normal in children up to 2–3 years of age. In some children, it continues for long.

Oliguria

Oliguria refers to urine output less than 500 mL/day in an average adult. It invariably occurs in acute-on-chronic renal failure or acute renal failure (ARF).

Anuria

Anuria is said to occur when the patient does not pass any urine or passes less than 50 mL of urine/day. In a physiological sense, the term anuria means less formation or absence of formation of urine by the kidney.

Causes: Common causes of anuria are as follows:

- Complete urinary tract obstruction
- Total bilateral renal arterial or venous occlusion
- Bilateral renal cortical necrosis
- Rapidly progressive acute glomerulonephritis

RENAL FAILURE

Renal failure refers to the deterioration of renal functions resulting in a decline in glomerular filtration rate (GFR) and rise in urea and non-nitrogenous substances in the blood. It is of two types:

- Acute renal failure (ARF)
- Chronic renal failure (CRF)

Acute Renal Failure

ARF refers to the sudden decline in GFR over a period of days or weeks associated with a rapid rise in blood urea.

Pathophysiology of acute renal failure Common causes of ARF can be grouped as follows:

1. Prerenal causes Prerenal causes include:

Reduced blood supply to the kidneys: Normally, the kidneys receive about 20%–25% of the cardiac output (1100 mL/min). Decreased renal blood flow (RBF) is usually accompanied by decreased GFR and reduced urinary output. When blood flow is reduced below the basal requirements (i.e. 20%–25% less than normal RBF), renal ischaemia occurs causing damage to renal cells, particularly tubular epithelial cells. The common causes of reduced blood flow to the kidney are severe haemorrhage, shock, severe burns, hypovolaemia, septicaemia, cardiac failure and so on.

2. Intrarenal causes Intrarenal causes include acute glomerulonephritis and acute tubular necrosis (ATN).

Acute glomerulonephritis is usually caused by an abnormal immune reaction, which causes damage to the glomeruli. In more than 90% of cases of glomerulonephritis, streptococcal infection involving other parts of the body (tonsillitis or skin infection) and the antibodies develop against the streptococcal antigen (within few weeks), which react and form insoluble antigen–antibody complexes, which get deposited in the glomeruli and evoke an inflammatory reaction. The glomeruli get blocked and the permeability of those which are not blocked increases which allows leak of proteins and red cells from the glomerular capillaries into the glomerular filtrate. In severe cases, there is renal shutdown and this results in ARF.

ATN means destruction of tubular epithelial cells. Tubular necrosis occurs due to diminution of oxygen and nutrition to epithelial cells. Toxins, poisons and certain drugs also damage the tubular epithelium resulting in ARF due to toxins or ischaemia.

3. Obstructive causes Obstructive causes include urinary tract obstruction at any site.

Postrenal or obstructive renal failure occurs due to abnormalities of the lower urinary tract which partially or completely blocks urinary flow (although RBF is normal). If the urine output of only one kidney is blocked, no major changes occur in body fluid composition because the contralateral kidney undergoes compensation. The causes of postrenal ARF include:

- *Bilateral obstruction of ureters*, or of renal pelvis, by large stones or blood clots
- *Bladder or urethral obstruction*

Physiological effects of ARF are:

i. ***Retention of salt and water***, waste metabolites and electrolytes (rise in creatinine and urea) in blood and extracellular fluid can lead to oedema and hypertension.
ii. ***Excessive retention of potassium*** (hyperkalaemia) is a serious threat to a patient with ARF.
iii. ***Kidneys are unable to excrete hydrogen ions*** resulting in metabolic acidosis and that itself is a fatal condition and also aggravates hyperkalaemia.
iv. **In *severe cases of ARF***, oliguria or complete anuria occurs and the patient may die unless kidney functions are restored.

Characteristic features of ARF include:

- No history of pre-existing renal disease
- Presence of oliguria or anuria
- Rapid rise in blood urea and creatinine levels
- High urine osmolality (>400 mOsm/kg H_2O)

Management during the oliguria phase is directed with the sole aim of keeping the patient alive with appropriate measures till diuretic phase sets in:

1. ***Medical management*** consists of:
   - Maintenance of adequate water and electrolyte balance
   - Control of infection
   - Control of blood pressure
   - Control of metabolic acidosis by i.v. use of sodium bicarbonate, so that the bicarbonate levels are maintained around 18 mmol/dL
   - Control of diet – protein, Na^+, K^+, Mg^+ and water (about 20–40 g of protein should be given per day to prevent endogenous breakdown of proteins)
2. ***Dialysis*** is frequently needed in cases with oliguria, hyperkalaemia, or acidosis or fluid overload (for details, see page 545).

Chronic Renal Failure

CRF refers to a slow, insidious, irreversible deterioration of renal functions resulting in the development of clinical syndrome of *uraemia*, manifested by excretory, metabolic, neurological, haematological and endocrinal abnormalities.

Common causes which lead to slow, progressive nephron loss and ultimately CRF can be grouped as follows:

1. ***Congenital disorders***, e.g. polycystic kidney, can lead to slow, progressive nephron loss.
2. ***Vascular diseases of the kidney e.g. renal hypertension:*** Injury to renal vasculature can lead to renal ischaemia. The most common cause of renal vascular injury is atherosclerosis. Atherosclerosis of the larger renal arteries leads to hypertension and involvement of smaller arteries (interlobular arteries and efferent arterioles) results in thickening of vessel walls due to deposits of fibrinoid tissue (nephrosclerosis), eventually leading to constriction (ischaemic injury).
3. ***Glomerular diseases, e.g. proliferative glomerulonephritis and diabetic nephropathy:*** In chronic glomerulonephritis, injury to glomeruli can be caused by several diseases. In most cases, it begins with accumulation of antigen-antibody complexes in the glomerular membrane and ultimately glomeruli are replaced by fibrous tissue, therefore unable to filter the fluid. Therefore, glomerular capillary filtration coefficient gets markedly reduced.
4. ***Tubulointerstitial disease, e.g. chronic pyelonephritis and analgesic nephropathy:*** These diseases are referred to as interstitial nephritis. Injury to renal interstitium can be caused by bacterial infection (called pyelonephritis) or as a result of vascular, glomerular and tubular damage by poison and toxic drugs.
5. ***Obstructive renal diseases***, e.g. benign enlargement of prostate, renal calculi and ureteral constriction, can also lead to slow, progressive nephron loss.

Pathophysiology of chronic renal failure CRF, like ARF, also occurs in a wide variety of diseases, but the end result is reduction of functional nephrons and deterioration of the kidney function to the point where the patient must be placed on dialysis treatment or transplanted with a functional kidney for survival. This condition is referred to as *end-stage renal disease (ESRD)*.

The exact mechanism of this stage is not well understood, but a slowly progressing vicious cycle due to renal adaptive changes may be responsible (Fig. 6.5.1).

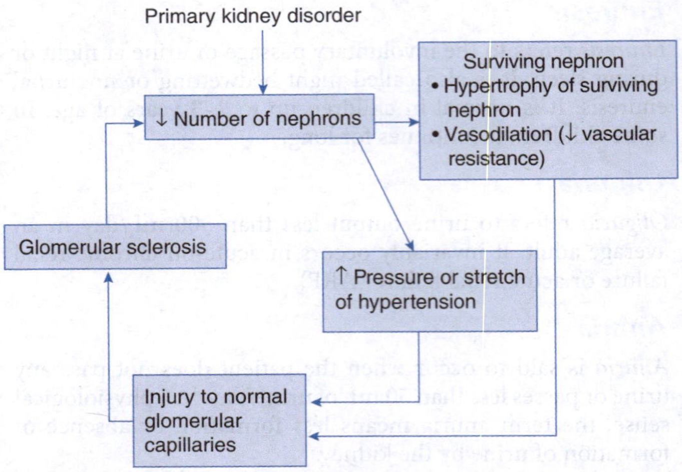

Fig. 6.5.1 Flow diagram depicting sequence of events in pathophysiology of chronic renal failure.

Acute versus chronic renal failure Differentiating features of ARF and CRF are summarized in Table 6.5.1.

Treatment of chronic renal failure

I. ***Medical management*** consists of:
   a. Treat, if the cause is reversible, e.g. hypertension and urinary tract obstruction.
   b. Nephrotoxic drugs should be avoided.
   c. Measures to limit the adverse effects of uraemia and to prevent further progression include:
      - Control of infection
      - Control of hypertension
      - Control of diet as regards proteins, Na^+, K^+, water and Mg^+ content
      - Control of anaemia
      - Control of metabolic acidosis
      - Maintenance of electrolyte and water balance

II. ***Dialysis and renal transplantation*** is frequently needed (see page 545).

Table 6.5.1 Distinguishing features of acute and chronic renal failure

Features	Acute renal failure	Chronic renal failure
Onset	Sudden, over days or weeks	Gradual, over months or years
Reversibility	Invariably reversible	Usually irreversible
Causes	May be prerenal	Mostly renal or postrenal but may be extrarenal
Urinary volume	Oliguria and anuria	Polyuria and nocturia
Signs and symptoms of uraemia	Of recent onset	Of duration more than 3 months
Characteristic features	Of acute reduction in GFR, e.g. oedema, hypertension, salt and water retention	Of chronicity, i.e. uraemic symptoms of long duration, small-sized kidneys, anaemia, hypertension and so on
Renal failure casts (broad casts) in urine	Absent	Present
Specific gravity of urine	High	Low and fixed
Past history of renal disease	Absent	Present
Dialysis	Required for short period	Repeated chronic maintenance dialysis required
Renal transplantation	Usually not required	Usually is the final answer

GFR, glomerular filtration rate.

NEPHROTIC SYNDROME

Nephrotic syndrome refers to massive proteinuria (more than 3.5 g/day), mainly albuminuria and its associated consequences which include:

- Hypoalbuminaemia
- Oedema
- Hyperlipidaemia
- Lipiduria
- Hypercoagulability

Pathophysiology A wide variety of disease processes including immunological disorders, toxic injuries, metabolic abnormalities, biochemical defects and vascular disorders involving glomeruli contribute to development of the nephrotic syndrome. The sequence of events involved in pathophysiology of the nephrotic syndrome is summarized in Fig. 6.5.2.

Minimal change nephrotic syndrome Minimal change nephrotic syndrome is a condition in which there is no abnormality of the glomerular capillary membrane. Minimal change nephropathy is associated with loss of normal negative charges from the basement of the glomerular membrane resulting in easy passage of albumin. Normally, negative charges in the basement membrane repel negatively charged plasma protein molecules. Incidence of minimal change nephropathy in children between ages 2 and 6 years is more. Plasma protein concentration usually falls below 2 g/L, leading to a decrease in colloidal osmotic pressure (<10 mm Hg). Therefore, a large amount of fluid leaks out from the capillaries all over the body into the tissue, causing oedema.

Recently it has been reported that podocytes play a key role in proteinuria.

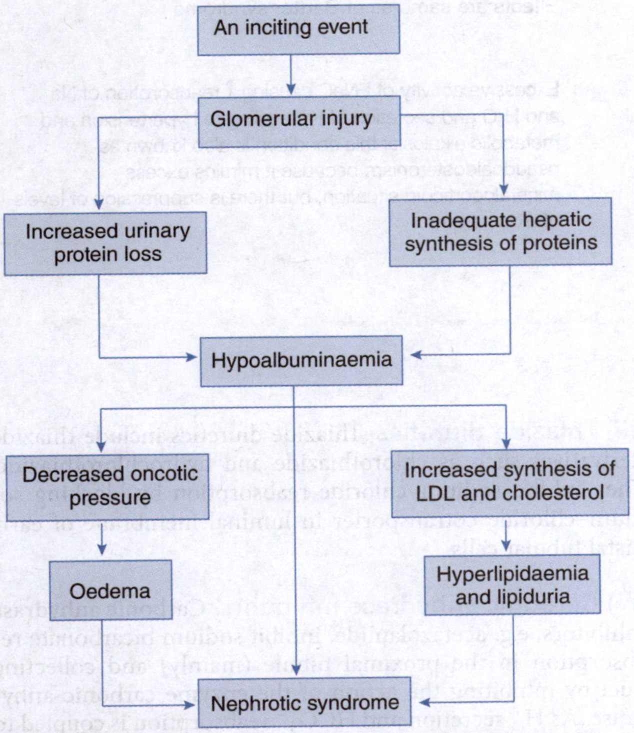

Fig. 6.5.2 Flow diagram showing sequence of events of pathophysiology of nephrotic syndrome.

SPECIFIC TUBULAR DISORDERS

There are many tubular disorders due to abnormal transport of individual or groups of substances through the tubular epithelial membrane. These disorders mainly occur due to an absence of enzyme, deficiency or mutations of genes encoding carrier proteins required for transport. The specific tubular disorders are summarized in Table 6.5.2.

DIURETICS

The diuretics are the drugs which primarily cause a net loss of Na^+ (*natriuresis*) associated with water loss (secondary to natriuresis) and thus increase the rate of urine flow.

CLASSIFICATION

Depending on their efficacy, the diuretic drugs can be classified as follows:

1. ***High-efficacy diuretics*** (inhibitors of Na^+–K^+–$2Cl^-$ transport), also called loop diuretics, e.g.:
   - Furosemide
   - Bumetanide
   - Ethacrynic acid
2. ***Medium-efficacy diuretics*** (inhibitors of Na^+–Cl^- symport):
   - Thiazide diuretics, e.g. chlorothiazide, hydrochlorothiazide and benzthiazide
   - Thiazide-like, e.g. metolazone
3. ***Weak or adjunctive diuretics:***
   - Carbonic anhydrase inhibitors, e.g. acetazolamide
   - Potassium-sparing diuretics, e.g. spironolactone, triamterene and amiloride
   - Osmotic diuretics, e.g. mannitol, isosorbide and glycerol
   - Xanthines, e.g. theophylline

SITE OF ACTION, MECHANISM OF ACTION AND MAJOR EFFECTS

Site of action The different sites of a nephron where the diuretics act are as follows (Table 6.5.3):

1. Proximal tubule Diuretics acting on proximal tubules have limited efficacy since the thick ascending loop (TAL), which has a great reabsorptive property, compensates for any decrease in Na^+ and H_2O reabsorption that might occur in proximal tubule.

2. TAL Diuretics acting on TAL are called loop diuretics. They abolish the urine concentrating ability of the nephron and, therefore, are also classified as high-efficacy diuretics.

3. Early distal convoluted tubule Thiazide diuretics act on this cortical diluting segment and have medium efficacy, because only a small part of the filtered solute load reaches this part of the tubule.

4. Late distal convoluted tubule and collecting duct Various K^+-sparing diuretics act on this site. These diuretics have weak efficacy.

Mechanism of action and major effects Mechanism of action and major effects of the diuretics are summarized in Table 6.5.3.

Table 6.5.2 Specific tubular disorders, their causes and effects

Tubular disorder	Cause	Effect
1. Renal glycosuria	Tubular transport mechanism of glucose is limited or absent	• Blood–glucose level: Normal • Renal excretion of glucose: Greatly increases
2. Aminoaciduria	Rare condition, occurs due to deficiency of specific carrier proteins for cystine, glycine and β-aminoisobutyric acid	• Essential cystinuria → cystine stone (renal stone) due to crystallization • β-Aminoisobutyric aciduria • Glycinuria
3. Renal phosphataemia	Failure to absorb phosphate	• Long-standing low level of phosphate leads to reduced calcification of bones resulting in rickets • Rickets is refractory to vitamin D therapy
4. Renal tubular acidosis	Hereditary disorder, failure to secrete H^+	• Loss of $NaHCO_3^-$ in the urine leading to continued state of metabolic acidosis
5. Nephrogenic diabetes insipidus	Deficiency of vasopressin receptors or renal tubules does not respond to ADH	• Water diuresis leading to dehydration
6. Fanconi syndrome	A generalized reabsorptive defect.	Children with Fanconi syndrome are usually short statured, have low muscle mass, frontal bossing, signs of rickets and hyperpigmentation of skin • In severe cases: • ↓ Excretion of all amino acids • ↓ Absorption of HCO_3^- leading to metabolic acidosis • ↑ Excretion of potassium and calcium • Nephrogenic diabetes insipidus • ↑ Urinary excretion of Na^+ and water ↑ Water depletion leads to activation of renin–angiotensin–aldosterone system ↑
7. Bartter syndrome	Autosomal recessive disorder, occurs due to defect in: • Na^+–K^+–$2Cl^-$ cotransporter Or • K^+ channels on luminal surface Or • Cl^- channels on basolateral membrane of thick ascending loop of Henle (for details, see page 491)	Stimulates K^+ and H^+ secretion in collecting duct ↑ Hypokalaemia and metabolic alkalosis
8. Gitelman syndrome	An autosomal recessive disorder due to thiazide-sensitive sodium chloride cotransporter	• Effects are same as of Bartter syndrome
9. Liddle syndrome	An autosomal dominant disorder due to mutations in amiloride-sensitive epithelial sodium channel (ENaC) in distal and collecting tubules	• Excessive activity of ENaC causing ↑ reabsorption of Na^+ and H_2O and secretion of K^+ leading to hypertension and metabolic alkalosis; this condition is also known as pseudoaldosteronism because it mimics excess mineralocorticoid situation, but there is suppression of levels of aldosterone

ADH, antidiuretic hormone.

(i) Osmotic diuretics Osmotic diuretics such as urea, mannitol and sucrose are not easily absorbed by the renal tubules. The increased concentration of osmotically active molecules causes an increase in osmotic pressure resulting in reduced water reabsorption. Therefore, a large amount of tubular fluid is excreted. In diabetes mellitus, polyuria is an example of osmotic diuresis (see page 512).

(ii) Loop diuretics Loop diuretics (such as furosemide, ethacrynic acid and bumetanide) decrease the active transport of sodium–chloride–potassium reabsorption by blocking Na^+–K^+–$2Cl^-$ cotransporter at luminal surface of epithelial cells of thick ascending limb (TAL) of loop of Henle.

(iii) Thiazide diuretics Thiazide diuretics include thiazide derivatives such as chlorothiazide and hydrochlorothiazide. They inhibit sodium–chloride reabsorption by blocking sodium–chloride cotransporter in luminal membrane of early distal tubular cells.

(iv) Carbonic anhydrase inhibitors Carbonic anhydrase inhibitors, e.g. acetazolamide, inhibit sodium bicarbonate reabsorption in the proximal tubule (mainly) and collecting duct by inhibiting the action of the enzyme carbonic anhydrase. As H^+ secretion and HCO_3^- reabsorption is coupled to sodium reabsorption through sodium–hydrogen ion countertransport (see page 515). Increased concentration of sodium and bicarbonate in tubular fluids acts as osmotic diuresis. The

Table 6.5.3 Site of action, mechanism of action and major effects of various classes of diuretics

Class of diuretic	Site of action	Mechanism of action	Major effects	Other effects	K^+ depletion	Acidosis/ alkalosis
High-efficacy diuretics Loop diuretics, e.g.: • Furosemide • Bumetanide • Ethacrynic acid	TAL	Inhibition of $Na^+–K^+–2Cl^-$	• ↑ NaCl excretion • ↑ K^+ excretion • ↑ Ca^{2+} excretion • ↓ Ability to concentrate urine • ↓ Ability to dilute urine	↑ Venous capacitance by venodilatation	Yes	Alkalosis
Medium-efficacy diuretics Thiazide diuretics, e.g.: • Chlorothiazide • Hydrochlorothiazide	Early distal tubule	Inhibition of $Na^+–Cl^-$ symport	• ↑ NaCl excretion • ↑ K^+ excretion • ↓ Ca^{2+} excretion • ↓ Ability to dilute urine	Antihypertensive	Yes	Alkalosis
Weak or adjunctive diuretics						
i. Carbonic anhydrase inhibitor, e.g.: • Acetazolamide	Proximal tubule	Inhibition of carbonic anhydrase	↑ HCO_3^- excretion	↓ Formation of aqueous humour (antiglaucoma drug)	Yes	Acidosis
ii. Potassium-sparing diuretics, e.g.: • Spironolactone • Triamterene • Amiloride	Late distal tubule and collecting duct	Inhibition of Na^+ reabsorption, inhibition of K^+ secretion	• ↑ Na^+ excretion • ↓ K^+ excretion • ↓ H^+ excretion	–	No	Acidosis
iii. Osmotic diuretics, e.g.: • Mannitol • Isosorbide	Proximal tubule	Retain water iso-osmotically and inhibit NaCl reabsorption	• ↑ Na^+ excretion • ↑ K^+ excretion • ↑ Cl^- excretion		Yes	Acidosis

TAL, thick ascending loop.

carbonic anhydrase inhibitors cause some degree of acidosis due to loss of HCO_3^- in the urine.

(v) Potassium-sparing diuretics Potassium-sparing diuretics, e.g. spironolactone and eplerenone, are mineralocorticoid receptor antagonists, which act as competitive inhibitors of aldosterone for receptors present on the epithelial cells in cortical collecting ducts. Mineralocorticoids (aldosterone) normally act through their receptors. The aldosterone–receptor complex in the principal cells of the collecting tubule increases mRNA synthesis which induces the formation of aldosterone-induced protein (AIP). The AIP leads to:

a. Translocation of $Na^+–K^+$-ATPase towards basolateral membrane
b. Translocation of amiloride-sensitive Na^+ channels towards luminal membrane which can decrease reabsorption of sodium and secretion of potassium (therefore, sodium remains in tubules causing osmotic diuresis; spironolactone inhibits formation of AIPs by combining with mineralocorticoid receptors)

(vi) Sodium channel blockers Sodium channel blockers like amiloride and triamterene inhibit sodium reabsorption and potassium secretion by blocking sodium channels present on the luminal membrane of epithelial cells of the collecting duct.

Other substances which act as diuretics In addition to the above-described drugs, the following other substances also act as diuretics, e.g.:

- *Water* acts by inhibiting antidiuretic hormone (ADH) secretion.
- *Alcohol* also acts by inhibiting ADH secretion.
- *Glucose* (e.g. in diabetes mellitus) acts as osmotic diuretic.
- *Caffeine* increases GFR and probably decreases renal tubular Na^+ reabsorption.
- *V_2 receptor antagonists* like tolvaptan inhibit the action of vasopressin on collecting duct.

RENAL FUNCTION TESTS

Renal function tests are carried out to assess the functional capacity of the kidneys. The main aim of these tests in clinical medicine is the detection of renal impairment as early as possible in its course and the quantitative measure of change in function with time. However, it must be remembered that about two-thirds of renal tissue must be functionally damaged to show any abnormality by these tests. Renal function tests can be divided into the following groups:

- Analysis of urine
- Analysis of blood
- Renal clearance tests
- Radiology and renal imaging
- Renal biopsy

ANALYSIS OF URINE

Analysis of urine helps, of course, to a limited degree, to assess kidney functioning. In patients with suspected renal disorder, the urine analysis should be performed for volume, specific gravity, osmolality, pH, abnormal constituents, microscopic examination and bacteriological finding.

1. Volume Normal urine output per day is 800–2000 mL. Abnormalities of urine volume include polyuria (>3000 mL/day), oliguria (<500 mL/day) and anuria (<50 mL/day) (see page 533).

2. Physical appearance Normally the appearance of the urine is clear, but becomes turbid when it is alkaline (in bacterial infection) and due to pus in the urine.

3. Colour The normal light yellow colour of the urine is due to the presence of urochrome pigment (a compound of urobilin and urobilinogen with peptide). On standing, the colour deepens due to oxidation of urobilinogen into urobilin. Abnormalities of urine colour include:

- *Brownish-yellow* colour is due to the presence of conjugated bilirubin in patients with hepatic and posthepatic jaundice.
- *Cloudy appearance* is seen in strongly alkaline urine due to precipitation of calcium phosphate and due to precipitation of urates.
- *Frothy appearance* is indicative of proteinuria.
- *Red-dark brown* tinge of urine is seen in porphyria.

4. Osmolality and specific gravity Normal urinary osmolality varies from 500 to 2000 mOsm/kg H_2O and specific gravity from 1.003 to 1.030, depending on the state of hydration of the body. If the early morning urine sample after an overnight fast has an osmolality of >600 mOsm/kg H_2O (and specific gravity >1.018), then the patient has a normal urine concentrating ability. Certain abnormalities are as follows:

- Fixed urinary osmolality of 300 mOsm/kg H_2O (specific gravity 1.010) is an evidence of fairly advanced urinary failure.
- Persistently low urinary osmolality (<100 mOsm/kg H_2O) even after 8 hours of fluid deprivation is diagnostic of diabetes insipidus.

5. Urine pH Normal pH of urine varies from 4.5 to 8.0. Urine is normally slightly acidic, except for a short postprandial alkaline tide. Intake of high-protein nonvegetarian diet shifts the urinary pH towards the acidic side, whereas vegetarian diet shifts it towards the alkaline side.

Causes of abnormal pH include:

- Infection with urea-splitting organisms which raises the pH
- Impairment of tubular acidification

6. Odour Normal odour of urine is aromatic.

In certain conditions, there is change in the odour:

- Fruity odour in diabetes mellitus
- Musty odour in liver diseases
- Foul smell in infection of the urinary bladder
- Ammonium odour in severe dehydration

7. Chemical analysis for abnormal urinary constituents Chemical analysis for abnormal urinary constituents may reveal:

i. Proteinuria Normally, up to 150 mg of proteins is excreted daily in urine (see page 501). Excretion of >150 mg/day of proteins is called proteinuria. Depending on the cause, proteinuria may be of the following types:

- *Mild transient proteinuria* occurs in congestive heart failure, high fever and severe anaemia.
- *Orthostatic proteinuria* occurs after prolonged walking or standing, in some otherwise healthy individuals.
- *Glomerular proteinuria* occurs in diseases in which permeability of glomerular membrane is increased. Massive glomerular proteinuria is seen in nephrotic syndrome. Other causes of glomerular proteinuria are acute glomerulonephritis, pyelonephritis and toxaemia of pregnancy.
- *Tubular proteinuria* occurs in conditions in which tubular reabsorption of low-molecular-weight proteins (which are normally filtered by glomeruli) is impaired, e.g. tubulointerstitial disorders and Fanconi syndrome.

Important Note

Tamm-Horsfall proteins (uromodulin) are glycol-proteins produced by epithelial cells of ascending limb of loop of Henle. These proteins are the main constituent of urinary casts.

Functions

Prevent Ca^{2+}-induced crystallization

Prevent formation of renal stones

Provide defence against bacterial infection by entrapping pathogenic bacteria

ii. Glycosuria Glycosuria refers to the presence of glucose in the urine. It may be due to diabetes mellitus, renal disorders (renal glycosuria) or GIT disorder (alimentary glycosuria). Other sugars like galactose and fructose may also be present in urine in certain inborn errors of metabolism.

iii. Ketonuria Ketonuria refers to the presence of ketone bodies (acetoacetic acid, β-hydroxybutyric acid and acetone) in the urine. It occurs in patients suffering from ketosis due to severe diabetes mellitus or prolonged starvation.

iv. Bilirubinuria Bilirubinuria refers to the appearance of bilirubin in the urine in patients with elevated conjugated bilirubin levels, in hepatic or posthepatic jaundice. Normally, 1–3.5 mg of urobilinogen is excreted daily in the urine. Its excessive excretion in the urine is one of the characteristic features of haemolytic jaundice.

v. Haemoglobinuria Haemoglobinuria, i.e. presence of haemoglobin in the urine, indicates intravascular haemolysis, as seen in blackwater fever, due to *falciparum* malarial infection.

vi. Porphobilinogen Porphobilinogen appears in urine in acute intermittent porphyria. This is not detected in fresh voided urine but gives a red-brown colour (Burgundy wine) to urine on standing for some time.

vii. Haematuria Haematuria, i.e. presence of blood in the urine, is seen in acute glomerulonephritis, renal stone disease and malignancy of the urinary tract. Urine becomes reddish in colour in gross haematuria.

viii. Aminoaciduria Aminoaciduria occurs in a variety of congenital tubular disorders.

Dipstick test: Dipstick test is the quickest way of urine analysis. It consists of a thin plastic dipstick with stripes of chemicals (Fig. 6.5.3). When dipstick is placed in the urine, the change in the colour of the chemical stripes occurs.

Certain substances present in the urine are detected by this test and values above or below the normal range are recorded. The parameters of urine which can be detected by dipstick test

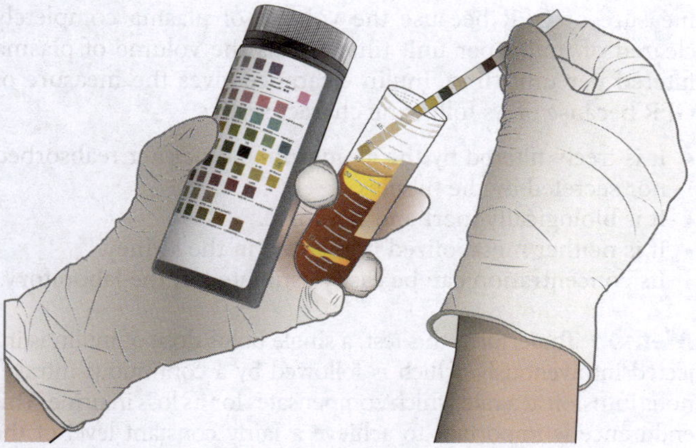

Fig. 6.5.3 Dipstick test for urine analysis.

are leucocytes, blood urobilinogen bilirubin, nitrite, pH, specific gravity, ketone bodies and glucose.

8. Microscopic examination Examination of centrifuged sediment of urine may show casts, cells and crystals.

i. Casts Casts are proteinaceous plugs formed by coagulation of Tamm–Horsfall protein within the renal tubules and washed out by the flow of tubular fluid. They have cylindrical shapes, broken ends and various shapes corresponding to the tubule in which the formed casts may be cellular or noncellular.

In cellular casts, certain cells are coagulated with the protein material. Cellular casts include:

Red cell casts are typically seen in acute glomerulonephritis.
Leucocytic casts are a feature of acute bacterial pyelonephritis.
Epithelial casts made of tubular epithelial cells are present in ATN.
Fatty casts containing epithelial cells laden with fat drops are seen in nephrotic syndrome.
Noncellular casts are hyaline and granular casts.

ii. Crystals Crystals are usually present in normal urine and thus have no pathological significance. Commonly seen are crystals of calcium oxalate, calcium phosphate, calcium ammonium–magnesium phosphate (triple phosphate) or uric acid. Uric acid crystals and cysteine crystals, when present in large amounts, have some diagnostic significance.

iii. Cells Cells found on microscopic examination may be RBCs, leucocytes, tubular epithelial cells and squamous epithelial cells.

9. Bacteriological examination of urine The midstream sample of urine is examined for pus cells and bacteria. Bacteriuria and pyuria indicate urinary tract infection.

ANALYSIS OF BLOOD

Estimation of blood levels of the substances that are excreted by the kidneys throws some light on the functional status of the kidney, although these tests are less sensitive than clearance tests.

1. Blood urea Blood urea level (normal 20–40 mg%) is an index of glomerular function. The blood urea levels begin to rise after about 50% glomerular damage has occurred.

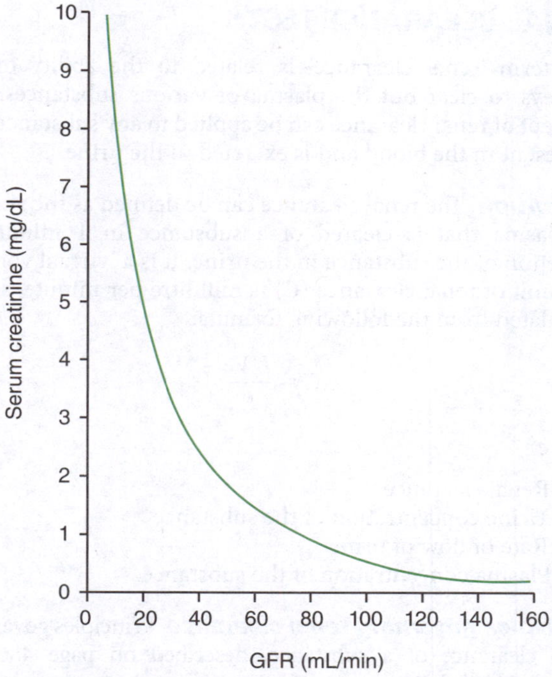

Fig. 6.5.4 Relationship between plasma creatinine concentration and glomerular filtration rate.

2. Plasma creatinine concentration Plasma creatinine concentration (normal 0.6–1.5 mg%) is more reliable than blood urea, as the latter is subjected to variations by dietary proteins, hydration and tissue breakdown. The relationship between GFR and serum creatinine levels depicts that GFR must fall to about 50% of its normal value before a significant increase in serum creatinine occurs (Fig. 6.5.4). Therefore, a normal serum creatinine level does not necessarily mean that all is well with the kidney.

> **Important Note**
>
> Cystatin C, a member of the superfamily of cysteine protease inhibitors, is produced by nucleated cells. The production of cystatin C is not affected by diet or nutrition status. Hence, it is a more sensitive marker of renal function than creatinine. Even minor changes in GFR in the early stages of chronic renal diseases are associated with increased cystatin C (normal range is 0.8–1.2 µg/dL).

3. Serum protein levels Serum protein levels (normal: total protein, 6.7–8 g%; albumin, 3–5 g%; globulins, 2–3 g%; and A/G ratio, 1.7:1) are reduced if there is significant proteinuria with renal failure. In nephrotic syndrome, the albumin levels decrease and globulin levels increase, leading to reversal of A/G ratio.

4. Serum cholesterol levels Serum cholesterol levels (normal 150–200 mg%) are increased in nephrotic syndrome.

5. Serum electrolytes Serum electrolyte levels (normal: Na^+, 152 mEq/L; K^+, 5 mEq/L; Ca^{2+}, 9–11 mg%; PO_4^{3-}, 3–4.5 mg%; SO_4^{2-}, 0.5–1.5 mEq/L; and Mg^{2+}, 1.5–2.5 mEq/L) are of value in a variety of renal disorders. For example, CRF is mostly accompanied by high potassium and phosphate but low sodium and calcium levels in blood.

RENAL CLEARANCE TESTS

The term 'renal clearance' is related to the ability of the kidneys to clear out the plasma of various substances. The concept of renal clearance can be applied to any substance that is present in the blood and is excreted in the urine.

Definition The renal clearance can be defined as the volume of plasma that is cleared of a substance in 1 minute by excretion of the substance in the urine. It is a 'virtual volume'. The unit of renal clearance (*C*) is millilitre per minute, and is calculated from the following formula:

$$C = \frac{UV}{P}$$

where

C = Renal clearance
U = Urine concentration of the substance
V = Rate of flow of urine
P = Plasma concentration of the substance

Principles governing renal clearance Principles governing renal clearance of a substance, described on page 486, are summarized briefly:

- Substances that are freely filtered but neither reabsorbed nor secreted (e.g. *inulin*) have renal clearance rate equal to GFR, and hence are called glomerular markers.
- Substances that are freely filtered but are partially reabsorbed in the tubules have renal clearance rate less than GFR.
- Substances that are freely filtered but are completely reabsorbed (e.g. Na^+, glucose, amino acids, Cl^- and HCO_3^-) have the lowest renal clearance rate.
- Substances that are filtered and also secreted by the tubules but not reabsorbed (e.g. para-aminohippuric acid [*PAH*] and diodrast) have the highest renal clearance rate. Such substances are thus entirely excreted by a single passage of blood through the kidneys. Clearance of such substances represents the range of blood flow.

Renal clearance as kidney function test Renal clearance of a substance is correlated more directly with the status of kidney function. It shows a deviation from normal (earlier) in the course of renal damage.

Renal clearance tests, therefore, can be used to assess the different functions of a nephron, e.g.:

- To assess glomerular filtration
- To assess tubular secretory capacity
- To assess renal plasma flow (RPF) and RBF
- To assess 'osmotic' and 'free water' clearance ability

Renal Clearance Tests to Measure GFR

GFR can be accurately measured by renal clearance of inulin, urea and creatinine. In practice, however, measurement of clearance for the substances already present in the blood is preferred. Furthermore, the renal clearance tests are not commonly used in the clinical practice. The plasma levels of urea and creatinine are used as indicators of glomerular function.

1. Inulin Clearance Test

Inulin is a dye (chemically a fructopolysaccharide) with molecular weight 5200 that does not exist naturally in the body. It is found in roots of certain plants. Inulin clearance (C_{in}) is a measure of GFR because the volume of plasma completely cleared of inulin per unit time equals the volume of plasma filtered per unit time. Inulin clearance gives the measure of GFR because of its following characteristics:

- It is freely filtered by the glomeruli and neither reabsorbed nor secreted by the tubules.
- It is biologically inert and nontoxic.
- It is neither metabolized nor stored in the kidney.
- Its concentration can be easily estimated in the laboratory.

Method To perform this test, a single bolus dose of inulin is injected intravenously, which is followed by a continuous intravenous infusion at a rate which compensates for its loss in urine. This endurance is important to achieve a fairly constant level of the plasma concentration of inulin. The inulin clearance (C_{in}) and, thus, the GFR is then calculated from the values of urine concentration of inulin (U_{in}; 35 mg/mL), urine flow rate (V; 0.9 mL/min) and plasma concentration of inulin (P_{in}; 0.25 mg/mL), as follows:

$$C_{\text{inulin}}(\text{or GFR}) = \frac{U_{\text{in}}V}{P_{\text{in}}}$$

$$\text{GFR} = \frac{35 \times 0.9}{0.25} = 126\ \text{mL/min}$$

Clinical applications (significance) of inulin clearance In addition to its use as a measure of GFR, the inulin clearance rate is also used as an indicator of plasma clearance mechanisms. A comparison of the clearance of a given substance (*Cx*) with the clearance of inulin (C_{in}) provides information about the renal transport processes used to remove the substance from the plasma (Fig. 6.5.5):

i. When *Cx* equals C_{in} When *Cx* equals C_{in}, i.e. when clearance ratio is 1 (ratio of clearance of given substance [*Cx*] and clearance of inulin [C_{in}]), such a substance has characteristics similar to those of the inulin, i.e. it is filtered only by glomeruli and neither reabsorbed nor secreted by the tubules. Furthermore, the mass of such a substance excreted in the urine per unit time (U_xV) equals the mass of the substance filtered during the same time (GFR*Px*), i.e.:

$$U_x V = C_{\text{in}} P_x \text{ or GFR } P_x = C_{\text{in}}$$

Examples of substances with clearance ratio close to 1 are mannitol, sorbitol, ferricyanide, vitamin B_{12} and sucrose. Although inulin is used most commonly, these substances can also be used to measure GFR.

ii. When *Cx* is less than C_{in} When *Cx* is less than C_{in}, i.e. clearance ratio (*Cx*/C_{in}) is less than 1. Such substances with clearance below that for inulin (Fig. 6.5.5) are filtered and reabsorbed, i.e. excretion is by filtration and reabsorption. *Examples* of substances with clearance ratio <1 are glucose, xylose and fructose.

iii. When *Cx* is greater than C_{in} When *Cx* is greater than C_{in}, i.e. when clearance ratio (*Cx*/C_{in}) is more than 1. Such substances with clearance above that of inulin (Fig. 6.5.5) are filtered and secreted, i.e. excretion is by filtration and secretion. Examples of substances with clearance ratio more than 1 are PAH and phenol red.

2. Creatinine Clearance Test

Although the creatinine clearance test is less accurate than the inulin clearance test for measurement of GFR, in clinical

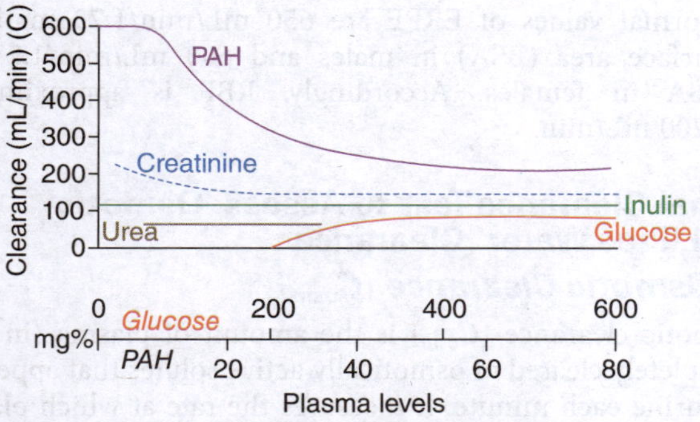

Fig. 6.5.5 Clearance of various substances plotted against their plasma concentration.

practice, the former is preferred over the latter because the latter is more cumbersome as it requires a continuous intravenous infusion. Creatinine is an endogenous substance (a by-product of muscle metabolism) having a fairly constant plasma value (*P*) of about 0.6–1.5 mg/dL. It is filtered by the glomeruli and only marginally secreted by the tubules. The value of creatinine clearance is close to GFR; hence, its measurement is a fairly good method of measuring GFR.

Method In the traditional method, creatinine content of 24-hour urine collection and the plasma concentration in a sample collected at midpoint of the urinary collection period are estimated. The creatinine clearance (*C*) is then calculated by the usual formula:

$$C_{cr} = \frac{U_{cr}V}{P_{cr}}$$

Normal value of creatinine clearance ranges from 80 to 110 mL/min in an adult and declines with age in healthy individuals. Because creatinine clearance is an index of GFR, it reflects the normal decline in GFR with age, although plasma creatinine concentration remains constant because of decreased muscle mass.

Sometimes, it is difficult to collect urine for measuring creatinine clearance. In such cases, the approximate GFR changes can be obtained by plasma concentration of creatinine, which is inversely proportional to GFR:

$$\text{GFR} = C_{cr} = \frac{U_{cr} \times V}{P_{cr}}$$

where
C_{cr} = Creatinine clearance
U_{cr} = Urine concentration of creatinine
P_{cr} = Plasma concentration of creatinine

Creatinine Clearance as Kidney Function Test in Disease

As shown in Fig. 6.5.4, the plasma creatinine concentration varies inversely with GFR and the product of GFR and plasma creatinine concentration is constant. Thus, a fall in GFR may be the earliest clinical sign of renal disease (i.e. a decline in functional renal mass).

3. Urea Clearance Test

Urea is the end product of protein metabolism. After being filtered by the glomeruli, it is partly reabsorbed by the renal tubules. Hence, urea clearance is less than the GFR, and, furthermore, it is influenced by the protein content of the diet. For these reasons, urea clearance is not as sensitive as creatinine clearance for assessing renal function. Despite this fact, several laboratories traditionally use this test.

Method At the beginning of the test, the patient is asked to completely empty the bladder by voiding the urine and the exact time is recorded. Exactly after 1 hour, the patient is asked to void again and the quantity of urine is exactly measured. The levels of urea are estimated in the urine and the blood sample collected at the midpoint of the test. Since the urea clearance drastically changes when the volume of urine is less than 2 mL/min, two empirical indices have been developed to calculate the urea clearance, which are called the maximal urea clearance and standard urea clearance.

i. ***Maximal urea clearance [$C_{urea(m)}$]*** is calculated from the usual formula. This is applicable when the urine output is more than 2 mL/min.

$$\text{Maximum urea clearance} = \frac{U \times V}{P}$$

where
U = Urea concentration in urine (mg/mL)
V = Volume of urine excreted (mL/min)
P = Urea concentration in plasma (mg/mL)

ii. ***Standard urea clearance [$C_{urea(s)}$]:*** When the volume of urine is less than 2 mL/min, $C_{urea(s)}$ is calculated by a modified formula:

$$C_{urea(s)} = \frac{U \times \sqrt{V}}{P}$$

Normal value of maximal urea clearance is 75 mL/min, whereas that of standard urea clearance is 54 mL/min.

Diagnostic importance A urea clearance value below 75% of the normal is viewed seriously. Since it is an indicator of renal damage, blood urea level as such is found to increase only when the clearance falls below 50% normal.

Calculation of GFR from urea clearance Since the proportion of urea reabsorbed by the renal tubules remains relatively constant at about 40% of the filtered, the urea clearance test can serve as a measure of GFR. The urea clearance expressed as a percentage of normal multiplied by 1.2 is a rough clinical estimation of GFR. As already mentioned, creatinine clearance test is a better indicator of GFR compared with urea clearance.

Renal Clearance Tests to Assess Tubular Secretory Capacity

The tubular secretory capacity can be assessed by the renal clearance of substances that are actively secreted by the tubular cells. As described on page 490, secretion of PAH occurs into the tubular fluid via carriers in the proximal tubule by a transport maximum (T_m)–limited process. Once T_m of PAH is reached, the clearance of PAH (C_{PAH}) becomes progressively more a function of glomerular filtration and hence the C_{PAH} approaches C_{in}, and the constant amount of PAH secreted becomes a smaller fraction of the total amount excreted. Because the T_m (PAH) is nearly constant, it is used clinically to estimate tubular secretory capacity (T_s).

Renal Clearance Test to Assess Renal Plasma Flow

The RPF can be calculated by applying *Fick's principle* to the kidneys. According to this principle, the amount of a substance excreted by the kidney per unit time (*UV*) is equal to the RPF multiplied by the arteriovenous difference in its plasma concentration:

$$UV = \text{RPF}(P_a - P_v)$$

$$\text{RPF} = \frac{UV}{P_a - P_v}$$

where

P_a = Concentration of the substance in renal arterial plasma (mg/mL)
P_v = Concentration of the substance in renal venous plasma (mg/mL)
U = Concentration of the substance in urine (mg/mL)
V = Volume of urine excreted (mL/min)

PAH Clearance is used to Measure RPF

Method PAH is continuously infused at low doses, so as to keep its plasma concentration constant. The RPF is calculated as follows:

$$\frac{U_{PAH}V}{P_{a(PAH)} - P_{v(PAH)}}$$

- At low plasma concentration of PAH, all the PAH is excreted into the urine and none is returned to the circulation via the renal vein. As a result, the PAH concentration in the renal vein is zero and can be eliminated. The equation now becomes

$$\text{RPF} = \frac{U_{PAH}V}{P_{a(PAH)}}$$

- Since $\frac{U_{PAH}V}{P_{PAH}}$ is equal to clearance of PAH (C_{PAH}), so the equation can be written as follows:

$$\text{RPF} = C_{PAH}$$

- About 10% of total RPF perfuses the nonexcretory portions of the kidney. Therefore, RPF calculated from the clearance of PAH is referred to as the effective RPF (ERPF) because only 90% of the plasma PAH is excreted. Therefore, the equation can be written as follows:

$$\text{ERPF} = C_{PAH}$$

Normally:
- Concentration of PAH in urine (U_{PAH}): 14 mg/mL
- Urine flow (V): 0.9 mL/min
- Concentration of PAH in plasma (P_{PAH}): 0–02 mg/mL

Therefore, ERPF = 14 × 0.9/0.02 = 630 mL/min.

- To obtain true RPF, it is necessary to divide C_{PAH} by 0.9:

$$\text{True RPF} = \frac{C_{PAH}}{0.9}$$

Therefore, actual RPF = 630/0.9 = 700 mL/min.

- From the value of true RPF, the value of RBF can be easily determined, if haematocrit value (Hct) is known as follows:

$$\text{RBF} = \text{RPF} \times \frac{1}{1 - \text{Hct}}$$

Normally, Hct is 45%; therefore:

$$\text{RBF} = \frac{700 \times 1}{1 - 0.45} = \frac{700 \times 1}{0.55} = 1273 \text{ mL/min}$$

- Normal values of ERPF are 650 mL/min/1.73 m^2 body surface area (BSA) in males and 600 mL/min/1.73 m^2 BSA in females. Accordingly, RBF is approximately 1200 mL/min.

Renal Clearance Test to Assess 'Osmotic' and 'Free Water' Clearance

1. Osmotic Clearance (C_{osm})

Osmotic clearance (C_{osm}) is the amount of plasma (in mL) completely cleared of osmotically active solutes that appear in the urine each minute. It measures the rate at which plasma is cleared of osmotic particles and is calculated by the usual renal clearance formula:

$$C = \frac{U \times VV}{P}$$

which can be written as follows:

$$C_{osm} = \frac{U_{osm} \cdot V}{P_{osm}}$$

where

U_{osm} = Urinary osmolality
V = Rate of urine flow (mL/min)
P_{osm} = Plasma osmolality

Normal value of C_{osm} is about 3 mL/min. It is increased in osmotic diuresis and decreased in fasting or diet deficient in proteins.

2. Free Water Clearance (C_{H_2O})

The quantitative measure of the kidney's ability to excrete water is termed *free water clearance* (C_{H_2O}). Free water clearance (C_{H_2O}) denotes the volume of pure (i.e. solute-free) water that must be removed from, or added to, the flow of urine (in mL/min) to make it iso-osmotic with plasma. In other words, it is a measure of the ability of the kidneys to generate solute-free water. It is not a true clearance, because no osmotically free water exists in plasma.

Free water, or solute-free water, is generated in the diluting segments of the kidney (i.e. TAL and early distal tubule), where NaCl is reabsorbed and free water is left in the tubular fluid.

In the absence of ADH, this solute-free water is excreted and is positive.

In the presence of ADH, this solute-free water is not excreted but is reabsorbed by the late distal tubule and collecting ducts and C_{H_2O} is negative.

Calculation of C_{H_2O}

$$C_{H_2O} = V - C_{osm}$$

where

C_{H_2O} = Free water clearance (mL/min)
V = Urine flow rate (mL/min)
C_{osm} = Osmolal clearance

$$\frac{U_{osm}V}{P_{osm}} \text{ mL/min}$$

Example: If the urine flow rate (V) is 10 mL/min, urine osmolality (U_{osm}) is 100 mOsm/kg H_2O and when plasma osmolality is 300 mOsm/kg H_2O, the C_{H_2O} can be calculated as follows:

$$C_{H_2O} = V - C_{osm}$$
$$= 10\ \text{mL/min} - \frac{100\ \text{mOsm/kg H}_2\text{O} \times 10\ \text{mL/min}}{300\ \text{mOsm/kg H}_2\text{O}}$$
$$= 10 - 3.33\ \text{mL/min} = 6.7\ \text{mL/min}$$

Relationship Between Free Water Clearance, Urine Volume and Osmolal Clearance

1. With ISO-Osmotic Urine (Fig. 6.5.6A)

With iso-osmotic urine (Fig. 6.5.6A), neither excretion nor reabsorption of solute-free water occurs, i.e.:

- Solute-free water clearance (C_{H_2O}) = 0
- Urine flow (V) = osmolal clearance (C_{osm})
  Clinical situation when C_{H_2O} ***is zero*** can occur in treatment with a loop diuretic. Treatment with loop diuretic inhibits NaCl reabsorption in the TAL, inhibiting both dilution in TAL and production of the corticopapillary osmotic gradient. Therefore, the urine cannot be diluted during water drinking (because a diluting segment is inhibited) or concentrated during water deprivation (because the corticopapillary gradient has been abolished).

2. With Hypo-Osmotic Urine (Fig. 6.5.6B)

With hypo-osmotic urine (Fig. 6.5.6B), the urine is divided into two virtual volumes – one that contains solutes that is iso-osmotic to plasma (C_{osm}) and a volume that is solute-free water (C_{H_2O}). Thus:

- Osmolal clearance (C_{osm}) is equal to solute-free water clearance (C_{H_2O}), i.e. $C_{osm} = C_{H_2O}$.
- Urine flow rate (V) is equal to the sum of osmolal clearance (C_{osm}) and free water clearance, i.e. $V = C_{osm} + C_{H_2O}$. C_{H_2O} is positive.
  Clinical situations in which a positive C_{H_2O} occurs include:
- Excessive water intake (in which ADH release from the posterior pituitary is suppressed)
- Central diabetes insipidus (in which pituitary ADH is insufficient)
- Nephrogenic diabetes insipidus (in which the collecting ducts are unresponsive to ADH)

3. With Hyperosmotic Urine

With hyperosmotic urine, TC_{H_2O} ($-C_{H_2O}$) represents the volume of free water that would have to be added to the urine to make it iso-osmotic to plasma (Fig. 6.5.6C), i.e.:

- Urine volume (V) is equal to the difference between osmolal clearance (C_{osm}) and free water reabsorption.

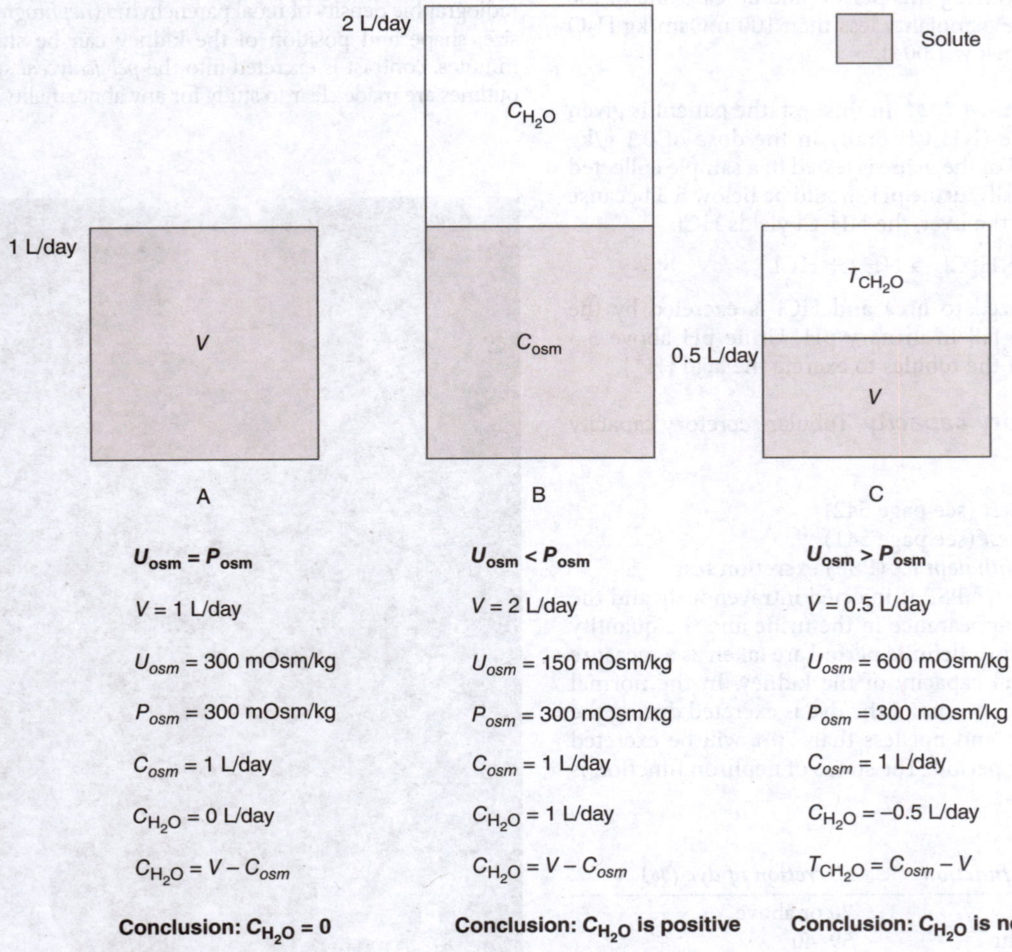

Fig. 6.5.6 Relationship between free water clearance (C_{H_2O}), urine volume (V) and osmolal clearance (C_{osm}): **A**, with iso-osmotic urine; **B**, with hypo-osmotic urine; and **C**, with hyperosmotic urine.

- The osmolal clearance (C_{osm}) is equal to the sum of urine volume (V) and free water reabsorption (TC_{H_2O}).
- C_{H_2O} is thus negative.

Clinical situations in which negative C_{H_2O} or positive free water reabsorption, i.e. tubular conservation of water (TC_{H_2O}), occurs include:

- Water deprivation (ADH release from the pituitary is stimulated)
- Syndrome of inappropriate ADH (SIADH)

TESTS FOR TUBULAR FUNCTIONS

The reabsorptive and secretory functions of renal tubules can be tested by the following tests:

1. Urine concentration test The ability of tubules to concentrate the urine is assessed by measuring the specific gravity of urine either after 12 hours of water deprivation or 12 hours after injection of vasopressin (ADH). In either case, if the specific gravity of urine is above 1.020, the tubular function is considered to be normal.

2. Urine dilution test In this test, the patient is asked to drink 1 L of water and the urine sample is collected every hour for the next 4 hours. Normally, at least 750 mL (75%) of urine should be excreted during this period and at least one of the samples should have osmolality less than 100 mOsm/kg H_2O (or specific gravity below 1.004).

3. Urine acidification test In this test, the patient is given ammonium chloride (NH_4Cl) orally in the dose of 0.1 g/kg body weight and pH of the urine is tested in a sample collected after 6 hours. Normally, urine pH should be below 5.3 because after metabolism in the liver, the NH_4Cl yields HCl:

$$NH_4Cl \rightarrow NH_3 + HCl$$

NH_3 is metabolized to urea and HCl is excreted by the kidney leading to a fall in urinary pH. Urine pH above 5.3 indicates inability of the tubules to excrete the acid (H^+).

4. Tubular secretory capacity Tubular secretory capacity is also tested by:

i. *PAH clearance test* (see page 542)
ii. *Urea clearance test* (see page 541)
iii. *Phenolsulphonphthalein Px* (PSP) excretion test
In this test, the dye PSP is injected intravenously and the time of its first appearance in the urine and the quantity eliminated within a definite period are taken as a measure of the functional capacity of the kidney. In the normal individual, 25% or more of the dye is excreted during the first 15 minutes and not less than 70% will be excreted during a 2-hour period. The status of nephron function is graded as follows:

Status of nephron function	*Excretion of dye (%)*
• Normal	70 or above
• Slight impairment	59–40
• Moderate impairment	39–25
• Marked impairment	24–11

5. Other methods of study of the tubular function Other methods of study of the tubular function usually used in research laboratory include:

i. *Micropuncture technique* to analyse the tubular fluid at various levels
ii. *Microcryoscopic studies* of renal tissue slices at different depths
iii. *Microelectrode studies* to measure the membrane potential of the tubular cells

RADIOLOGY AND RENAL IMAGING

Although not strictly speaking, kidney function tests are quite useful investigations in present-day clinical practice to assess anatomical and physiological abnormalities of the kidneys.

1. Plain radiograph of abdomen Plain radiograph of the abdomen is useful in detecting calcium-containing (radiopaque) renal stones. However, a radiograph from a well-prepared patient gives enough of an idea of the size, shape and position of the kidneys.

2. Intravenous pyelography Intravenous pyelography (IVP) is performed by injecting a radiopaque dye like urografin intravenously and taking radiographs of the abdomen at short intervals (1, 5, 10 and 30 minutes). The dye is filtered by the glomeruli and concentrated in the renal tubules increasing the radiographic density of renal parenchyma (*nephrogram*), by which size, shape and position of the kidney can be studied. Within minutes, contrast is excreted into the *pelvicalyceal system* and the outlines are made clear to study for any abnormality (Fig. 6.5.7).

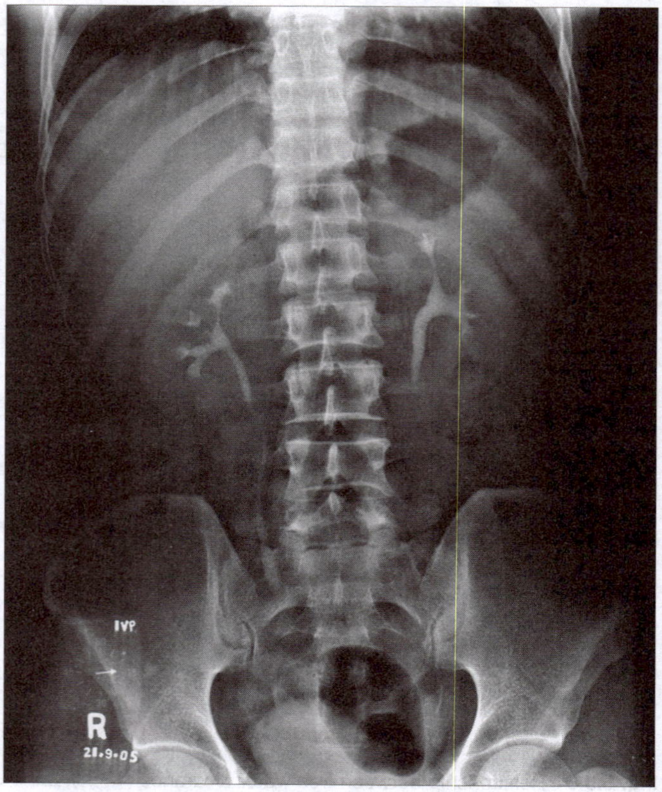

Fig. 6.5.7 Intravenous pyelogram.

3. Ultrasonography Ultrasonography is a quick, noninvasive, inexpensive and harmless method to evaluate size, shape and position of the kidney and to detect tumour, stones, cysts, etc., of the kidneys, ureter, prostate and urinary bladder.

4. Computed tomography The kidney is a retroperitoneal structure. To visualize the details of renal structure, computed tomography (CT) is performed to detect abnormalities in and around the kidneys as mentioned above in 'Ultrasonography'.

5. Radionuclide studies Radionuclide studies are carried out by injecting radioactive compounds which are concentrated and excreted by the kidneys. Radioactivity of the kidneys is recorded by a gamma camera.

RENAL BIOPSY

Renal biopsy is performed percutaneously with the help of *Vim–Silverman* needle. This is useful in diagnosis of patients with proteinuria of unknown origin, an unexplained renal failure with normal-sized kidneys or systemic diseases associated with abnormal urinary constituents. The biopsy specimen is subjected to light, electron and immunofluorescence microscopic studies. This technique has increased knowledge and a better understanding of glomerular and tubular diseases.

DIALYSIS AND RENAL TRANSPLANTATION

DIALYSIS

The term dialysis in physiological sense refers to the diffusion of solutes from an area of higher concentration to an area of lower concentration through a semipermeable membrane.

Indications This principle has been used to dialyse the blood of patients with renal failure, especially those developing uraemia.

Uraemia Uraemia develops when more than 75% of nephrons are damaged and is characterized by:

- Accumulation of nitrogenous waste products in the blood
- Metabolic acidosis
- Hyperkalaemia

Uraemic coma Uraemic coma is the terminal event in CRF. It has been attributed chiefly to acidosis and hyperkalaemia. Accumulation of nitrogenous waste products contributes relatively less to the loss of consciousness in uraemic coma.

Types of dialysis By dialysis, the dissolved crystalloids of the plasma pass through a semipermeable membrane so that their levels are brought down to lower levels. Two types of dialysis procedures are available:

- Haemodialysis or artificial kidney
- Peritoneal dialysis

Haemodialysis or Artificial Kidney

Haemodialysis can save a life in many types of *ARF* produced by reversible pathological processes, especially circulatory shock or mercury poisoning. The intermittent haemodialysis may prolong the life of many patients with CRF, which may lead to an active life for many years.

The dialysis can partially replace the excretory function of the kidneys but does not replace endocrine and metabolic functions.

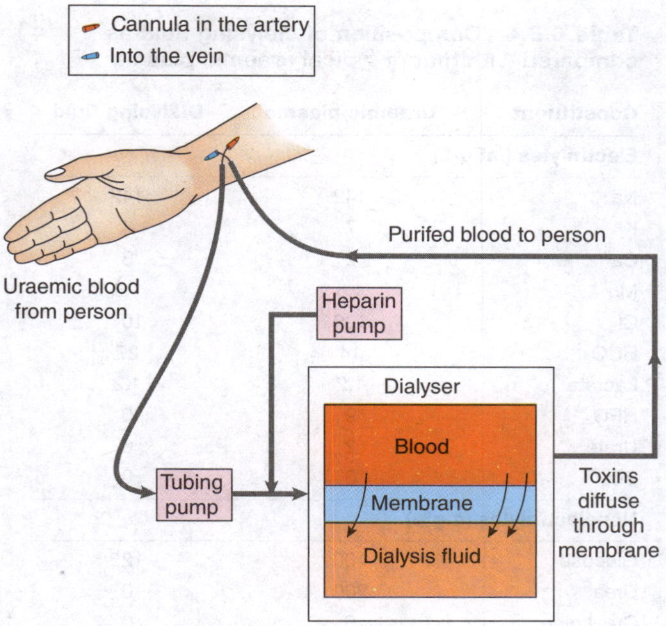

Fig. 6.5.8 Basic principle of haemodialysis.

Procedure The haemodialysis machine is also called artificial kidney. Haemodialysis is done in a hospitalized patient through an intravenous line for 3–5 hours. During haemodialysis, the patient's radial artery is connected to the haemodialysis machine. Inside the haemodialysis machine, the blood is passed through a long and coiled cellophane tube immersed in a dialysis fluid (Fig. 6.5.8). Heparin is used as an anticoagulant while passing the blood through the machine.

Dialysing fluid The composition of dialysing fluid is similar to that of plasma, except it is free of waste products like urea and uric acid. The fluid contains less amounts of sodium, potassium and chloride ions than uraemic blood. But the quantity of glucose, bicarbonate and calcium ions is more in the dialysing fluid than in the uraemic blood (Table 6.5.4).

During haemolysis the semipermeable cellophane membrane permits the free diffusion of the constituents of plasma, except proteins. In this way, the dialysis of the patient's blood removes the toxic waste products and restores normal electrolyte concentration in the plasma. The dialysed blood is returned back to the patient's body through a peripheral vein (Fig. 6.5.8). At a time, about 500 mL is passed through the artificial kidney. Haemodialysis is done usually thrice a week in severe uraemia.

Important Note

The rate of diffusion or movement of solutes depends on concentration gradient, permeability of the cellophane membrane, size (length), surface area and time of contact between blood and fluid.

Table 6.5.4 Composition of dialysing fluid as compared with that of typical uraemic plasma

Constituent	Uraemic plasma	Dialysing fluid
Electrolytes (mEq/L)		
Na^+	142	142
K^+	7	4
Ca^{2+}	2	3
Mg^{2+}	1.5	1.5
Cl^-	103	107
HCO_3^-	14	27
Lactate	1.2	1.2
HPO_4	9	0
Urate	2	0
SO_4^{2-}	3	0
Nonelectrolytes (mg%)		
Glucose	100	125
Urea	200	0
Creatinine	6	0

Table 6.5.5 Peritoneal dialysis versus haemodialysis

Peritoneal dialysis	Haemodialysis
Costly machine not required	Costly machine required
Less effective	More effective
Takes nearly 24 h to bring down urea level from 200 to 100 mg/dL	Takes 6 h to bring down urea level from 200 to 150 mg/dL
May be uncomfortable	Usually not uncomfortable
Haemodynamic disturbances are less	Haemodynamic disturbances are more
Suitable to patients with coagulopathy	May have haemorrhagic problems following heparinization
May be done in patients with low blood pressure	Difficult in patients with hypotension
Not very suitable for drug poisoning cases	Very helpful in drug poisoning with toxic kidney
Not very effective in patients with gross fluid overload	Very effective in patients with gross fluid overload and water can be filtered out very fast by haemofiltration

Peritoneal Dialysis

In peritoneal dialysis, the peritoneum is used as a semipermeable membrane. Continuous ambulatory peritoneal dialysis is a form of long-term dialysis done by the patients at home or at work.

Procedure Two litres of dialysing fluid is introduced through a permanent intraperitoneal catheter. It is then kept in the peritoneal cavity for exchange to take place for a period of 15–20 minutes, called dwell time. Fluid is then drained out and measured. A strict input and output chart is maintained. The whole procedure constitutes one cycle. It is done at 6-hour intervals (four cycles per day), even when the patient is ambulatory or mobile. There is no need for hospitalization and it is useful for young children and old patients with cardiovascular disorders. It prolongs survival in patients with CRF for many years.

Peritoneal Dialysis Versus Haemodialysis

Table 6.5.5 compares and contrasts peritoneal dialysis with haemodialysis.

RENAL TRANSPLANTATION

The haemodialysis is an expensive procedure and needs to be repeated almost every week. Therefore, it cannot be regarded as a remedy in individuals with irreversible terminal renal failure (*ESRD*). Renal transplantation is the final answer to all the problems in cases with CRF. It reverses metabolic and excretory abnormalities. The graft is taken from a cadaver donor or from a sibling or a parent. Usually the left kidney of the donor is transplanted to the right iliac fossa of the recipient. Long-term immune suppression with prednisolone and cyclosporine is needed. It offers complete rehabilitation and is the most cost-effective option.

Self-Assessment

1. Discuss the concept of renal clearance test and its significance.
2. Describe the pathophysiology of renal failure.
3. Describe the classification of diuretics, mechanism of action and site of action.
4. Describe briefly about the following renal function tests:
   - Analysis of urine
   - Analysis of blood
   - Dipstick test
5. Describe the principle, indications and types of dialysis.
6. Write notes on:
   - Glycosuria
   - Renal transplantation
   - Renal imaging
   - Liddle syndrome

Clinical Cases

Case 1

A 35-year-old male patient suffering from fever for the last 3–4 days was brought to the hospital with complaints of sudden weakness in the muscle, frequent cramps and swelling in the legs, nausea, vomiting and also difficulty in breathing.

Examination and laboratory tests revealed:

- Temperature 38°C
- BP 100/60 mm Hg
- Pulse 120/min
- Oedema in the ankle and legs
- Dry skin
- Reduced urinary output
- Raised blood urea and creatinine levels

Urine analysis showed proteinuria, serum electrolytes and hyperkalaemia.

Q1. What is the probable diagnosis?

Q2. What are the causes for this condition?

Q3. What immediate measures should be taken in this case to prevent complications.

Case 2

A 9-year-old male child was brought to the paediatric OPD with complaints of generalized hyperpigmentation on the trunk and neck region. Some drug (antibiotic) had been given to the child for infection. The examination and laboratory tests showed that the child was short statured for his age, with malformed thumbs of both hands, broad nasal base and diminished vision. Urine analysis revealed glycosuria and proteinuria

Q1. What is the diagnosis?

Q2. What is the cause of this condition?

Q3. Which part of the nephron is damaged to cause glycosuria in this condition?

6.6 Physiology of Micturition

CHAPTER OUTLINE

URINARY BLADDER AND URETHRA

GROSS ANATOMY

External features The urinary bladder, a hollow muscular viscus, is a temporary reservoir for urine. The main body of an empty bladder is pyramidal, having an apex, a base, and a superior and two inferolateral surfaces. The lowest part of the bladder is called neck, which is the most fixed part of the bladder. The neck continues as posterior urethra.

Interior of the bladder In an empty bladder, the greater part of the mucosa shows irregular folds due to its loose attachments to the muscular coat. The interior of the base (posterior surface) of the bladder presents a triangular area, the trigone where the mucosa is smooth due to its firm attachment.

Internal urethral orifice The internal urethral orifice is located at the apex (inferior angle) of the trigone. The ureters open into the bladder at superior angles of the trigone (Fig. 6.6.1). The ureters pierce the bladder wall obliquely, and this provides a valve-like action, which prevents a reverse flow of urine towards the kidneys as the bladder fills.

STRUCTURE OF THE BLADDER

The wall of the urinary bladder consists of three layers – an outer serous layer, a thick coat of smooth muscle and the inner mucous membrane.

Mucous membrane The mucous membrane is lined by transitional epithelium. Its characteristic features are as follows:

- It stretches when the bladder distends.
- It forms a complete barrier to the passage of fluid and electrolytes. Therefore, urine stored in the bladder remains unchanged in chemical composition.
- It secretes a glycosaminoglycan barrier that prevents bacterial adherence.

Muscular layer The muscular layer is formed by smooth muscle fibres which constitute the detrusor muscle. The detrusor muscle is arranged in interlacing longitudinal, circular and spiral bundles. Contraction of this muscle coat is responsible for emptying of the bladder.

URETHRA AND ITS SPHINCTERS

Male urethra The male urethra, about 20 cm in length, is divided into three parts – prostatic urethra (3 cm), membranous urethra (1.25 cm) and penile urethra (15.75 cm). The membranous urethra is surrounded by the external sphincter.

Female urethra The female urethra is about 3.8 cm long. It extends from the neck of the bladder to the external meatus. It traverses the external sphincter and lies immediately in front of the vagina.

Sphincters of the Urethra

1. Internal Sphincter

The circular smooth muscle fibres in the area of the neck of the bladder are thickened to form the internal sphincter (sphincter vesicae). The natural tone of the internal sphincter prevents emptying of the bladder until the pressure in the body of the bladder rises above a threshold level.

2. External Sphincter

Beyond the bladder neck, as the urethra passes through the urogenital diaphragm, it is encircled by a ring of voluntary

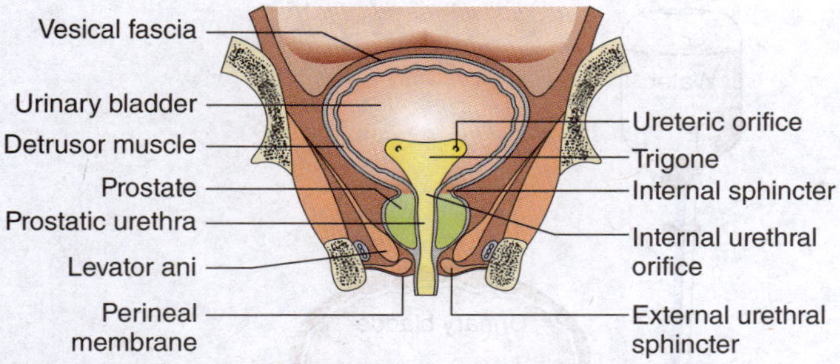

Fig. 6.6.1 Coronal section through the bladder and prostate to show the interior of the bladder, internal urethral sphincter and external urethral sphincter.

(skeletal type) muscle known as external sphincter of the bladder. The external sphincter provides voluntary control over micturition. In males, its stronger action can stop micturition midstream even after it has been reflexly initiated.

INNERVATION OF THE URINARY BLADDER (FIG. 6.6.2)

Motor Innervation

Parasympathetic innervation The parasympathetic efferent fibres (nervi erigentes) are derived from the second, third and fourth sacral segments (mainly S_2 and S_3). These fibres carry motor impulses to the urinary bladder causing contraction of detrusor muscle and emptying of the bladder. These fibres are inhibitory to the internal sphincter. If these fibres are destroyed, normal micturition is not possible.

Sympathetic innervation These nerves arise in the 11th thoracic to the 2nd lumbar segments (T_{11}–L_2). These fibres are said to be inhibitory to detrusor muscle and motor to the

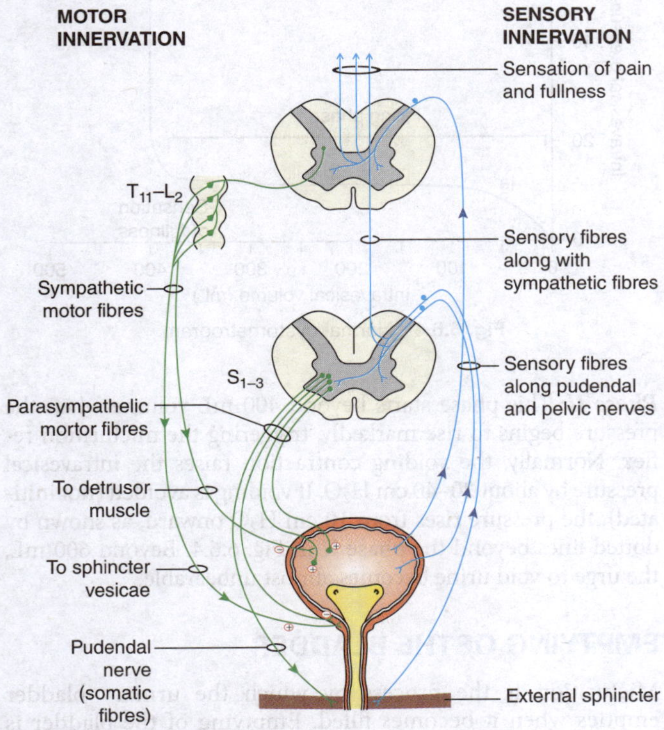

Fig. 6.6.2 Innervation of urinary bladder.

sphincter vesicae. Many workers regard them to be chiefly vasomotor.

Sympathetic activity is not involved in micturition. Increased sympathetic discharge to the bladder occurs during ejaculation and helps to prevent the reflux of sperms from the prostatic urethra into the bladder.

Somatic motor innervation The somatic pudendal nerve (S_2, S_3 and S_4) supplies the external sphincter which is voluntary.

Sensory Innervation

Sensation of bladder distension Afferents from the detrusor stretch receptors travel to the spinal cord via the pelvic splanchnic nerve (nervi erigentes). From the region of the bladder neck and trigone, the afferents travel via the hypogastric plexus to spinal cord segments T_{11}–L_2.

In the spinal cord In the spinal cord, the fibres of awareness of bladder distension run in the posterior column (fasciculus gracilis) to reach the spinal micturition centre, pontine micturition centre (PMC) and suprapontine micturition centres.

Sensation of bladder pain The pain fibres are stimulated by excessive distension or spasm of the bladder wall, or by stone, inflammation or malignant disease irritating the bladder. The pain fibres run predominantly in the hypogastric plexus but are also present in the nervi erigentes.

In the spinal cord In the spinal cord, the fibres carrying pain sensation run in the lateral spinothalamic tract.

> **Important Note**
>
> Bilateral anterolateral cordotomy, therefore, selectively abolishes pain without affecting the awareness of bladder distension and the desire to micturate (which runs in the posterior column).

Urethral sensations Urethral sensations, including sensation of imminent voiding associated with maximal bladder filling, reach the spinal cord via the pudendal nerve.

In the spinal cord In the spinal cord, fibres carrying urethral sensations travel in the dorsal column.

PHYSIOLOGY OF MICTURITION

Micturition is the process by which the urinary bladder empties when filled. It begins in the fifth month of intrauterine life with the onset of urinary secretion. It remains purely a reflex act until approximately 2–2.5 years of age, at which time it begins to come under voluntary control. The main physiological events in the process of micturition are as follows:

- Filling of the urinary bladder
- Emptying of the urinary bladder

FILLING OF URINARY BLADDER

Transport of Urine into Urinary Bladder Through Ureters

As urine collects in the renal pelvis, the pressure in the pelvis increases and initiates a peristaltic contraction beginning in the pelvis and spreading along the ureter to force urine towards the bladder. This peristaltic wave, travelling at a velocity of about 3 cm/s, occurs from once every second to once every 2–3 minutes. The peristaltic wave can move urine against an obstruction with a pressure as high as 25–50 mm Hg.

Capacity of the Bladder

Physiological capacity Physiological capacity of the bladder varies with age, being 20–50 mL at birth, about 200 mL at 1 year and can be as high as 600 mL in young adult males. In all cases, the physiological capacity is about twice that at which the first desire to void is felt.

Anatomical capacity Anatomical capacity refers to the capacity of the bladder beyond which rupture occurs. It is about 1 L or more, and is never approached under physiological conditions.

Volume and Pressure Changes in Bladder During Filling

The normal bladder is completely empty at the end of micturition and the intravesical pressure is equal to the intra-abdominal pressure. As the bladder is filled up, it adjusts its tone and a fairly large volume of urine can be accommodated with minimal alterations in the intravesical pressure. This is possible because of the phenomenon of adaptation. The *adaptation* occurs because of the inherent property of *plasticity*, the smooth muscles of detrusor and *law of Laplace*. According to Laplace's law, pressure in a hollow organ is inversely proportional to its radius, the tone remaining constant. That is, if tone remains constant, an increase in radius decreases the pressure and vice versa:

$$P = \frac{T}{R}$$

where P = pressure, T = tension and R = radius.

In the bladder, as volume of fluid rises, the radius increases due to relaxation of detrusor and therefore the pressure rise is almost nil. It is important to note that adaptation is independent of nervous mechanism and it, therefore, presents in the denervated bladder, but not after birth.

Cystometry This refers to the process of studying the relationship between the intravesical volume and the pressure; the cystometrogram refers to graphical record of this relationship.

Method of recording cystometrogram A double-lumen catheter is introduced into the bladder. The fluid is introduced through one lumen and pressure changes are recorded by connecting the other lumen to the pressure transducer of a polygraph (Fig. 6.6.3). The bladder is filled with 50-mL increments of water and at each volume, the intravesical pressure is recorded.

Normal cystometrogram Normal cystometrogram shows three phases of filling (Fig. 6.6.4):

Phase Ia: It is the initial phase of filling in which pressure rises from 0 to 10 cm H_2O, when about 50 mL of fluid is collected in the bladder.

Phase Ib: It is the phase of plateau which lasts till the bladder volume is 400 mL. During this phase, the pressure in the bladder does not change much and remains approximately at 10 cm H_2O. This is because of adaptation of the urinary bladder by relaxation, as described above.

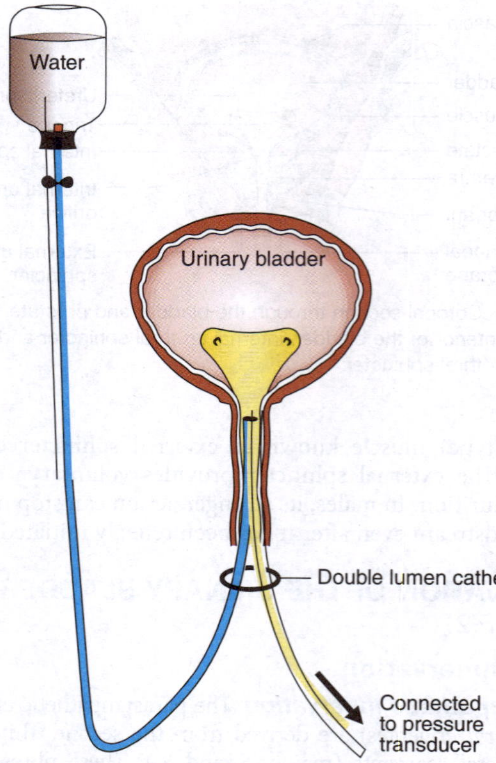

Fig. 6.6.3 Procedure of cystometry to demonstrate pressure–volume relationship in urinary bladder.

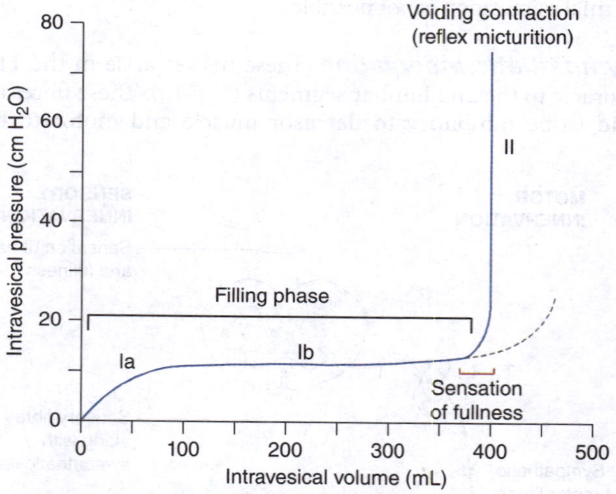

Fig. 6.6.4 Normal cystometrogram.

Phase II: This phase starts beyond 400 mL volume when the pressure begins to rise markedly, triggering the micturition reflex. Normally, the voiding contraction raises the intravesical pressure by about 20–40 cm H_2O. If voiding is avoided (not initiated), the pressure rises from 10 cm H_2O onward, as shown by dotted lines beyond the phase II in Fig. 6.6.4. Beyond 600 mL, the urge to void urine becomes almost unbearable.

EMPTYING OF THE BLADDER

Micturition is the process by which the urinary bladder empties when it becomes filled. Emptying of the bladder is basically a reflex action called the micturition reflex, which is controlled by supraspinal centres and is assisted by contraction of perineal and abdominal muscles. Therefore, discussion on emptying of the urinary bladder focuses on:

- Micturition reflex
- Voluntary control of micturition
- Role of perineal and abdominal muscles in micturition

Micturition Reflex

Initiation Micturition reflex is initiated by stimulation of the stretch receptors located in the wall of the urinary bladder.

Stimulus Filling of the bladder by 300–400 mL of urine in adults constitutes the adequate stimulus for the micturition reflex to occur. Although, under natural circumstances, the first urge to empty the bladder occurs at approximately 150 mL of urinary volume, it can be easily suppressed.

Afferents Micturition reflex is a spinal reflex. The afferents from the stretch receptors in the detrusor muscle and urethra travel along the pelvic splanchnic nerves and enter the spinal cord through dorsal roots to S_2, S_3 and S_4 segments to reach the sacral micturition centre (SMC) (Fig. 6.6.5).

SMC SMC is formed by the sacral detrusor nucleus and sacral pudendal nucleus.

Sacral detrusor nucleus Sacral detrusor nucleus is a cluster of preganglionic parasympathetic neurons located in the intermediolateral grey matter of S_2, S_3 and S_4 segments. Afferents of micturition reflex excite the neurons of this nucleus.

Sacral pudendal nucleus Sacral pudendal nucleus refers to a cluster of neurons found in the ventral horn primarily of the S_2 and to a lesser degree of S_3 and S_4 segments. The afferents from the stretch receptors in the bladder wall inhibit this nucleus, thereby exciting the external sphincter of the urethra.

Efferents Efferents arising from the sacral detrusor nucleus are the preganglionic parasympathetic fibres which relay in the ganglia near or within the bladder and urethra (Fig. 6.6.5). The postganglionic parasympathetic fibres are excitatory to the detrusor muscle and inhibitory to the internal sphincter.

Response Once micturition reflex is initiated, it is self-regenerative, i.e. initial contraction of the bladder wall further activates the receptors to increase sensory impulses (afferents) from the bladder and urethra which cause further increase in reflex contraction of detrusor muscle of the bladder. The cycle thus keeps on repeating itself again and again until the bladder has reached a strong degree of contraction. After a few seconds, reflex fatigues and regenerative cycle ceases. Once a micturition reflex has occurred but not succeeded in emptying the bladder, the nervous elements of the reflex usually remain in an inhibited state for at least a few minutes to an hour before another micturition reflex occurs.

Once the micturition reflex becomes powerful enough, this causes another reflex which passes through pudendal nerves to

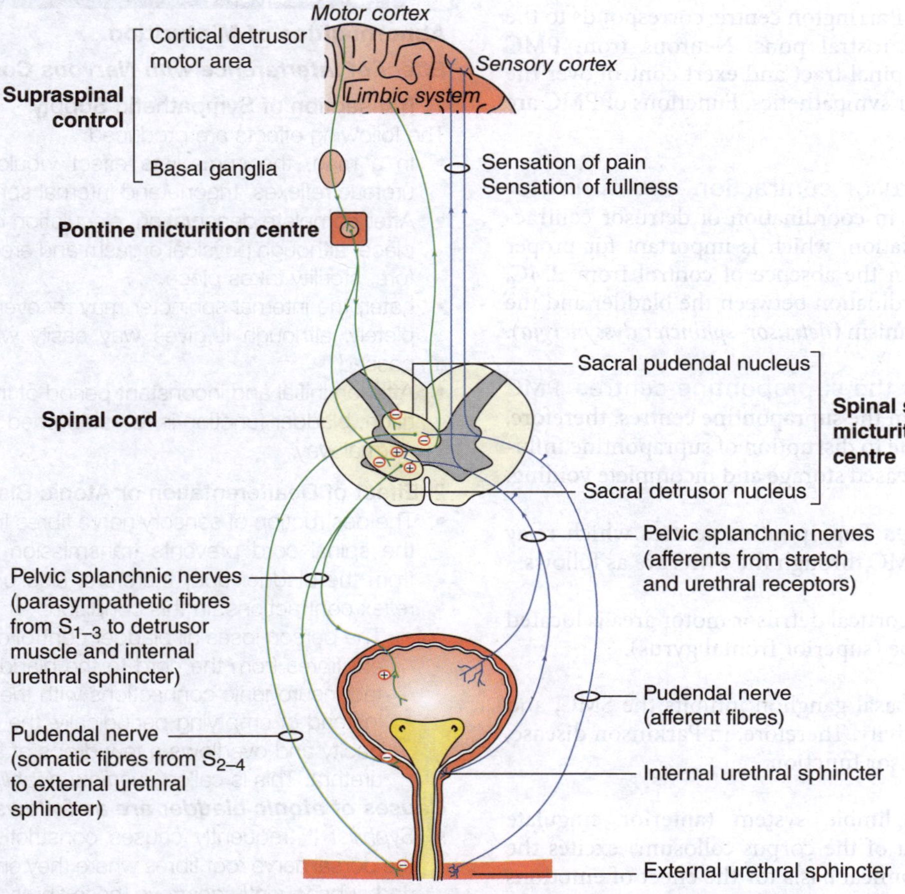

Fig. 6.6.5 Pathway and supraspinal control of micturition reflex.

the external sphincter to cause its inhibition. If this inhibition is more potent than the voluntary constrictor signals from the brain, then urination will not occur. If not so, urination will not occur unless the bladder fills still more and micturition reflex becomes more powerful.

Voluntary Control of Micturition

Role of Supraspinal Centres

The micturition reflex is fundamentally a *spinal reflex* facilitated and inhibited by higher brain centres (*supraspinal centres*) and, like defaecation, is subjected to voluntary facilitation and inhibition. In infants and young children, micturition is purely a reflex action. *Voluntary control* is gradually acquired as a learned ability of the toilet training. Once voluntary control is acquired, the supraspinal control centres exert final control of micturition by the following means:

- The higher centres keep the micturition reflex partially inhibited all the time except when it is desired to micturate.
- Even if the micturition reflex occurs, the higher centres can prevent micturition by continual tonic contraction of external urinary sphincter until a convenient time presents.
- When the convenient time to urinate presents, the higher centres facilitate the SMC to initiate a micturition reflex and inhibit the external urinary sphincter so that urination can occur.

Supraspinal control centres which control the micturition reflex (a completely automatic cord reflex) include the PMC and suprapontine centres.

PMC PMC, also called Barrington centre, corresponds to the locus coeruleus of the rostral pons. Neurons from PMC descend in the reticulospinal tract and exert control over the SMC and thoracolumbar sympathetics. Functions of PMC are as follows:

Coordination of detrusor contraction and sphincter relaxation PMC helps in coordination of detrusor contraction and sphincter relaxation, which is important for proper micturition. Therefore, in the absence of control from PMC, there occurs loss of coordination between the bladder and the external sphincter mechanism (*detrusor–sphincter dyssynergia*).

To relay inputs from the suprapontine centres PMC helps to relay inputs from the suprapontine centres; therefore, in the lesions of PMC due to disruption of suprapontine influences, there occurs decreased storage and incomplete voiding.

Suprapontine centres Suprapontine centres which relay their influence on the SMC through the PMC are as follows:

Cerebral cortex The cortical detrusor motor area is located in the medial frontal lobe (superior frontal gyrus).

Basal ganglion The basal ganglion inhibits the SMC, and thereby the detrusor activity. Therefore, in Parkinson disease, there may be poor detrusor function.

Limbic system The limbic system (anterior cingulate gyrus and anterior genu of the corpus callosum) excites the SMC. It forms the anatomical basis for the effect of emotions on voiding.

Role of Perineal and Abdominal Muscles in Micturition

Certain muscular movements which aid the emptying of the bladder, but are not the essential component of micturition process, are as follows:

- At the onset of micturition, the levator ani and perineal muscles are relaxed, thereby shortening the posturethra and decreasing the urethral resistance.
- The diaphragm descends.
- The abdominal muscles contract, accelerating the flow of urine by raising intra-abdominal pressure which in turn secondarily increases the intravesical pressure, thereby increasing the flow of urine.

Important Note

Certain important facts about micturition are as follows:

- A voiding contraction, once initiated, is normally maintained until all the urine has been discharged from the urinary bladder. This is a function of facilitating impulses from the higher centres. However, if required so, the micturition can be voluntarily stopped in between by inhibitory impulses from the higher centres.
- The bladder contracts in all directions like a toy balloon deflating from its neck.
- After urination, the female urethra empties by gravity, whereas the urine remaining in the urethra of a male is expelled by several contractions of bulbospongiosus muscle.

Applied Aspects

Abnormalities of Micturition

Effect of Interference with Nervous Control of Bladder

1. Transection of Sympathetic Supply

The following effects are produced:

- In a man, the immediate effect would be relaxation of ureteric reflexes, trigone and internal sphincter.
- After complete denervation, ejaculation no longer can take place, although physical orgasm and erection occur; therefore, sterility takes place.
- Later, the internal sphincter may recover and closes completely, although it gives way easily when a catheter is passed.
- After an initial and inconstant period of frequency of micturition, bladder function is re-established in a comparatively normal way.

2. Effect of Deafferentation or Atonic Bladder

- The destruction of sensory nerve fibres from the bladder to the spinal cord prevents transmission of stretch signals from the bladder and, therefore, also prevents micturition reflex contractions. In this condition:
  - The person loses all bladder control despite intact efferent fibres from the cord to the bladder and despite intact neurogenic connections with the brain.
  - Instead of emptying periodically, the bladder fills to capacity and overflows a few drops at a time through the urethra. This is called *overflow dribbling*.

Causes of atonic bladder are as follows:

- *Syphilis:* It frequently causes constrictive fibrosis around the dorsal nerve root fibres where they enter the spinal cord and subsequently destroys these fibres.

- *Crushing injuries to spinal cord:* They damage the sensory roots.

3. Effect of Denervation.

When there is interruption with both afferent and efferent nerves of the bladder, the following consequences are observed:

- The bladder is flaccid and distended for a while.
- Gradually, however, the muscle of the *decentralized bladder* becomes active, with many contraction waves that expel dribbles of urine out of the urethra.
- The bladder becomes shrunken and the bladder wall hypertrophies.

The reason for the difference between the *small, hypertrophic bladder* seen in this condition and the *distended, hypotonic bladder* seen only when afferent nerves are interrupted is not known. The hyperactive stage in the former condition suggests the development of denervation hypersensitization even though the neurons interrupted are preganglionic rather than postganglionic.

Conditions: e.g. tumours of the cauda equina

4. Effect of Spinal Cord Transection.

During spinal shock Voluntary micturition is completely abolished. The activity of detrusor muscle remains in abeyance for a long period, but the activity of the sphincter now returns very soon. At this stage, the bladder responds to filling in the same manner as the dead organ or an elastic bag. Retention of urine is therefore complete from an early stage. If no catheter is passed, the bladder becomes increasingly overstretched. The sphincter is finally forced open by a high intravesical pressure and small quantities of urine escape at frequent intervals – a condition of *retention with overflow*.

- The capacity is reduced and its walls become hypertrophied. This type of bladder is sometimes called *spastic neurogenic bladder*.
- Owing to excessive stretching of bladder wall, its nutrition suffers and it becomes very prone to infection. *Cystitis* may occur, and death results from the usual complications of *ascending urinary infection*.

After spinal shock has passed After spinal shock has passed, the voiding reflex returns, although there is no voluntary control. Some paraplegic patients train themselves to initiate voiding by pinching or stroking their thighs, provoking a mild mass reflex.

Conditions causing obstruction to the outflow of urine from the bladder may be:

- *Anatomical obstacles*, e.g. enlarged prostatic or urethral stricture
- *Functional derangements*, e.g. atonic sphincter with a relatively weak detrusor

5. Effects of Obstruction

- Retention of urine consequently tends to occur, and the intravesical pressure rises till it causes expulsion of urine.
- When the obstruction is mechanical, the stretching of bladder wall acts at first as a growth stimulus resulting in hypertrophy of its fibres and increase in their expulsive power which for a time enables the obstacle to overcome. But when, finally, the bladder wall is overstretched, it becomes paralysed and normal evacuation no longer takes place.

Self-Assessment

1. Discuss the physiology of micturition.
2. Describe the micturition reflex and its control.
3. Write briefly about:
   - Atonic bladder
   - Cystometry and its significance
   - Effects of spinal cord transaction on urination

Clinical Cases

Case 1

A 50-year-old patient had a fall from a building under construction and is on the bed for the last 1 month; he is unable to control urination and every time only a small volume of urine is voided; urinary frequency and urgency has increased and dribbling of urine is present.

Q1. What is this condition called?

Q2. What is the most common cause of this condition?

Case 2

A 60-year-old female presented with urinary urgency and reported urinary loss on coughing or lifting heavy weight.

Q1. What is this condition known as?

GASTROINTESTINAL SYSTEM

SECTION 7

SECTION OUTLINE

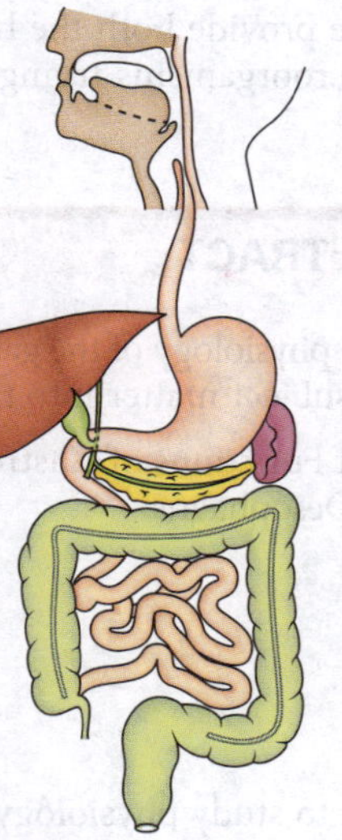

INTRODUCTION

To sustain life, the body needs a continual supply of water, electrolytes and nutrients. This function is served by the gastrointestinal or the so-called digestive system.

The gastrointestinal system comprises the alimentary canal and other associated organs such as the liver, gall bladder and pancreas. The alimentary canal is a long tube starting at the mouth; passing through the pharynx, oesophagus, stomach, small intestine, large intestine and rectum; and ending at the anus.

FUNCTIONS OF GASTROINTESTINAL SYSTEM

I. Digestive functions The major function of the gastrointestinal system is to transfer nutrients, minerals and water from the external environment to the circulating body fluids for distribution to all the body tissues. This function is accomplished by the following processes:

1. ***Ingestion of food:*** It involves:
   - Placing the food into the mouth. Most of the foodstuffs are taken into the mouth as large particles, mainly made of carbohydrates, proteins and fats.

- Chewing the food into smaller pieces is carried out with the help of teeth and jaw muscles. This process is called mastication.
- Lubrication and moistening of the food is done by the saliva.
- Swallowing the food (deglutition). It refers to pushing the bolus of food from the mouth into the stomach. It is accomplished in three phases – oral phase, pharyngeal phase and oesophageal phase.

2. ***Digestion of food:*** It refers to conversion of complex, insoluble, large organic molecules (food) into simpler, soluble, smaller molecules which can be easily absorbed. Digestion of food is accomplished with the help of hydrochloric acid and digestive juices containing various enzymes.
3. ***Absorption of digested food:*** Absorption of food refers to movement of digested molecules from the lumen of the alimentary canal across its epithelial lining to the blood or lymph. The absorbed water, electrolytes and nutrients are carried away to the various tissues by the circulating blood.
4. ***Egestion:*** Excretion of unwanted undigested food by the alimentary canal in the form of faeces is called defaecation.

To understand the digestive function of the gastrointestinal system, it is imperative to have knowledge about:

- Functional anatomy and organization of the gastrointestinal system
- Gastrointestinal motility
- Gastrointestinal blood flow
- Role of salivary glands, liver, gall bladder and pancreas
- Neural and hormonal control of gastrointestinal functions

II. Nondigestive functions The main nondigestive function of the gastrointestinal system is its role as immune system. The lymphoid tissue in the tonsils, adenoids and Peyer's patches constitute an important part of the body's immune system. These provide both the humoral and the cellular immunity which is especially effective against the microorganisms trying to enter the body from the alimentary canal.

PHYSIOLOGY OF GASTROINTESTINAL TRACT

Two different approaches can be adopted to study the physiology of the gastrointestinal tract (GIT).

The approach adopted in this book divides the subject matter into the following chapters:

7.1 Functional Anatomy and General Principles of Functions of Gastrointestinal System
7.2 Physiological Activities in Mouth, Pharynx and Oesophagus
7.3 Physiological Activities in Stomach
7.4 Pancreas, Liver and Gall Bladder
7.5 Physiological Activities in Small Intestine
7.6 Physiological Activities in Large Intestine
7.7 Digestion and Absorption

The alternative approach which can be adopted to study physiology of GIT is summarized with reference page numbers given in parentheses:

1. Functional anatomy of GIT (page 559)
2. Motility of GIT:
   - Chewing (page 567)
   - Deglutition (page 572)
   - Gastric motility (page 586)
   - Motility of the small intestine (page 618)
   - Motility of the large intestine (page 626)
   - Defaecation (page 628)
3. Gastrointestinal secretions:
   - Salivary secretion (page 569)
   - Gastric secretion (page 579)
   - Pancreatic secretion (page 596)
   - Bile secretion (page 606)
   - Secretions of the small intestine (page 617)
   - Secretion of the large intestine (page 624)

4. Gastrointestinal hormones:
   Gastrin family of hormones:
   - Gastrin (page 581)
   - Cholecystokinin (page 600)

   Secretin family of hormones:
   - Secretin (page 659)
   - Gastric inhibitory polypeptide (GIP) (page 589)
   - Vasoactive intestinal peptide (VIP) (page 617)
   - Glucagon (page 764)

   Glucagon-like immunoreactivity (GLI) (page 565)
   Other GIT hormones:
   - Motilin (page 565)
   - Neurotensin (page 565)
   - Substance P (page 565)
   - Gastrin-releasing peptide (GRP) (page 582)
   - Somatostatin (page 583)
5. Digestion and absorption in GIT (page 632)
6. Gastrointestinal function tests:
   - Gastric function tests (page 593)
   - Pancreatic function tests (page 601)
   - Liver function tests (page 511)
   - Tests of intestinal absorption (page 646)
7. Physiology of gastrointestinal disorders:
   - Disorders of swallowing (page 574)
   - Disorders of the stomach (page 590)
   - Disorders of the pancreas (page 600)
   - Disorders of the small intestine (page 621)
   - Disorders of the liver and gall bladder (page 610)
   - Disorders of the large intestine (page 630)
   - Disorders of absorption (page 644).

7.1

Functional Anatomy and General Principles of Functions of Gastrointestinal System

CHAPTER OUTLINE

FUNCTIONAL ANATOMY

FUNCTIONAL ORGANIZATION

The digestive system comprises the gastrointestinal tract (GIT) and accessory organs of digestion like teeth, tongue, salivary glands, liver and exocrine part of the pancreas.

GIT, also known as alimentary canal, is basically a muscular tube extending from the mouth to the anus (Fig. 7.1.1). At either end, the lumen is continuous with external environment. It measures about 10 m (30 feet) and comprises the following parts:

Mouth Mouth is a loosely used term to denote the external opening and for the cavity it leads to. Strictly speaking, the term mouth should be applied only for the external opening which is also called oral fissure. The cavity containing anterior two-thirds of the tongue and teeth is the *mouth cavity* or *oral cavity* or *buccal cavity* (Fig. 7.1.2). The oral cavity extends from the lips to the oropharyngeal isthmus, i.e. junction of the mouth with the pharynx. The oral cavity is subdivided into two parts – the vestibule and oral cavity proper (Fig. 7.1.2).

Vestibule lies between the lips and the cheeks externally, and the gums and the teeth internally.
Oral cavity proper lies within the alveolar arches, gums and teeth.

Tongue Tongue, in the digestive system, plays two important roles:

- Tells the taste of food
- Helps in chewing and swallowing of the food

Teeth Teeth are accessory organs of digestion which help in chewing of food. They are present in the sockets of alveolar processes of upper and lower jaws. There are two sets of teeth:

- *Deciduous set* (primary or milk teeth) comprises 20 teeth (10 in each jaw). The eruption of milk teeth starts in the sixth month after the birth and is completed by the second year. These teeth shed off by the sixth to seventh years of age and are replaced by permanent teeth.
- *Permanent set* comprises 32 teeth (8 in each quadrant of upper and lower jaws): 2 incisors, 1 canine, 2 premolar and 3 molars.

Structure of tooth: Each tooth consists of three parts:
Root is made of three or four anchoring branches by which the tooth is attached in the alveolar sockets.
Crown is that part of the tooth which projects above the level of gums.
Neck is the constricted part that lies between the root and the crown.

Functions of different types of teeth in chewing:

- *Incisors* provide strong cutting action.
- *Canines* are responsible for tearing action.
- *Premolars and molars* have grinding action.

Pharynx. The pharynx is a median passage that is common to the gastrointestinal and respiratory systems. It is divisible, from above downwards, into three parts:

Nasal part or nasopharynx into which nasal cavities open
Oral part or oropharynx which is continuous with the posterior end of the oral cavity
Laryngeal part or laryngopharynx which is continuous in front with the larynx, and below with the oesophagus

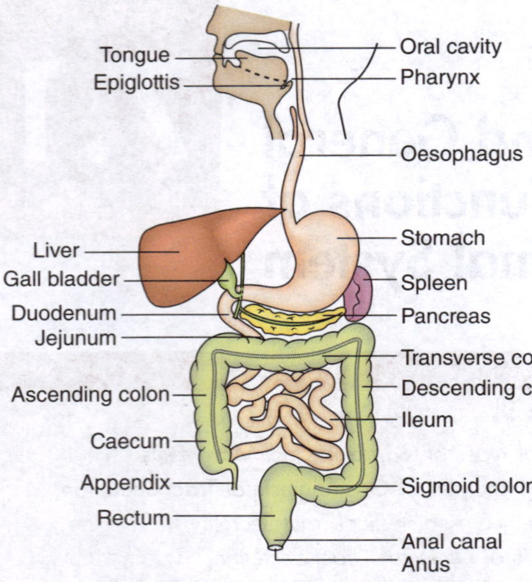

Fig. 7.1.1 The gastrointestinal system.

Oesophagus It is a fibromuscular tube about 25 cm long. At its junction with the pharynx, upper oesophageal sphincter is present and at its junction with the stomach, lower oesophageal sphincter is present. During swallowing, the upper oesophageal sphincter opens and food passes into the oesophagus. The peristaltic movements of the oesophagus propel the food into the stomach.

Stomach It is a hollow muscular bag connected to the oesophagus at its upper end and to the duodenum at its lower end. It serves the following motor functions:

- Storage of food till it can be accommodated in the duodenum
- Mixing of food with gastric secretions to form a semiliquid mixture called chyme
- Slow emptying of food into the small intestine

Small intestine It is a long tubular structure which can be divided into three parts:

Duodenum is the first part of the small intestine. It is C shaped and measures about 25 cm in length.
Jejunum, the middle part of the small intestine, is about 25 m long.
Ileum, the last part of the small intestine, is about 3.5 m long.

Gastric chyme enters the duodenum where it meets with pancreatic juice, bile and secretions of the small intestine (succus entericus). The partially digested foodstuffs in the gastric chyme are digested further and the final products of digestion are absorbed by the villi of the small intestine. The movements of the small intestine help in mixing, digestion and absorption of the food. The peristaltic activity of the small intestine also helps in moving the undigested and unabsorbed food material to the large intestine.

Large intestine It arches around and encloses the coils of the small intestine and tends to be more fixed than the small intestine. It is divided into the following parts (Fig. 7.1.1):

Caecum is a blind-ended sac into which opens the lower end of ileum. The ileocaecal junction is guarded by the ileocaecal valve which allows onflow but prevents backflow of intestinal contents.
Appendix is a worm-shaped tube that arises from the medial side of caecum which in humans is a vestigial organ.
Ascending colon extends upward from the caecum along the right side of the abdomen up to the liver. On reaching the liver, it bends to the left, forming the *right hepatic flexure*.
Transverse colon extends from the right hepatic flexure to the *left splenic flexure*. It forms a wide U-shaped curve.
Descending colon extends from the left splenic flexure to the pelvic inlet below.
Sigmoid colon begins at the pelvic inlet as continuation down of the descending colon and joins the rectum in front of the sacrum.
Rectum descends in front of the sacrum to leave the pelvis by piercing the pelvic floor. Here it becomes continuous with the anal canal in the perineum.
Anal canal opens to the exterior through the anus, the opening which is guarded by two sphincters.

In the large intestine, there occurs absorption of water and electrolytes from the intestinal contents. The remaining material is called *faecal matter*. The mucus secreted from the wall of the large intestine lubricates the faecal matter. The faecal matter is stored in the sigmoid colon (pelvic colon) till expelled by the process of defaecation which is assisted by the movements of the large intestine, activity of the anal canal and anal sphincters.

STRUCTURAL CHARACTERISTICS OF GIT WALL

Different parts of GIT are specialized for carrying out different functions, particularly digestion and absorption, but the

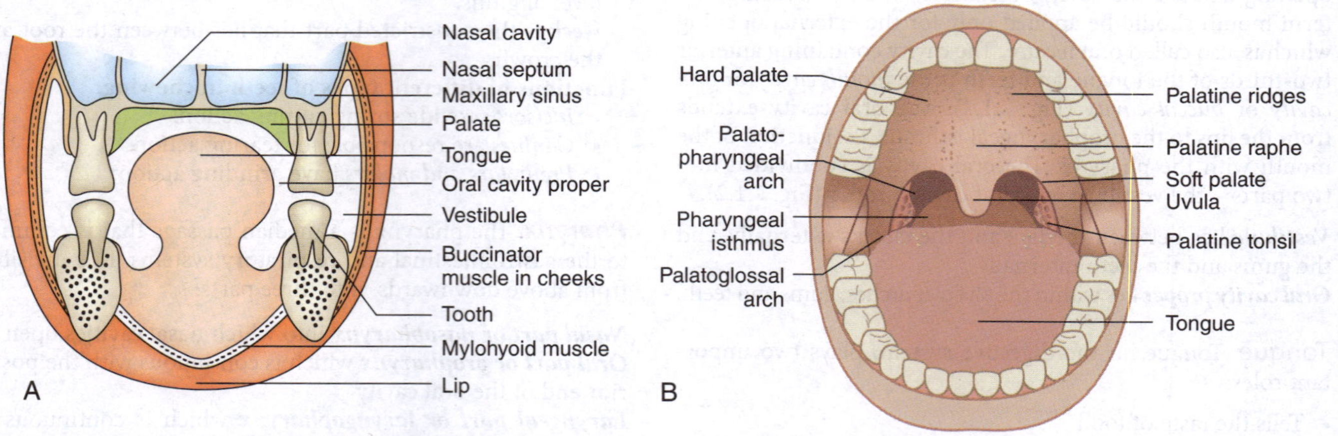

Fig. 7.1.2 **A**, schematic of coronal section through oral cavity; and **B**, structure of oral cavity shown in open mouth.

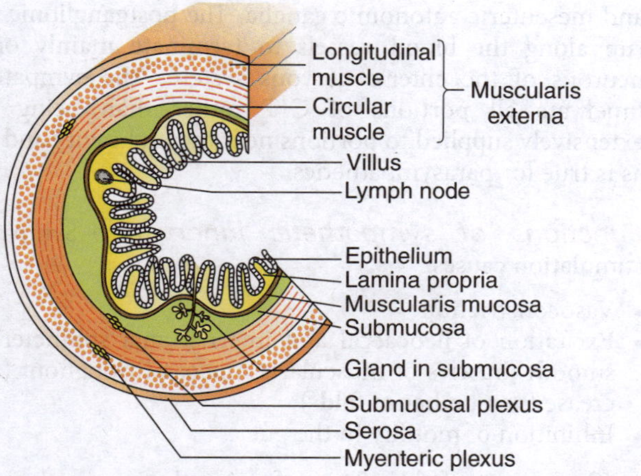

Fig. 7.1.3 Cross-section of the alimentary canal depicting structural characteristics of its wall.

basic structural characteristics of the wall of the whole GIT are similar. The intestinal wall from inside to outwards consists of the following layers (Fig. 7.1.3):

1. Mucosa (mucous layer) It is the innermost coat consisting of three layers:

Surface epithelium lining the luminal surface consists of epithelial cells which vary in type from simple squamous to tall columnar depending on the function of the part of GIT.
Lamina propria is composed of loose connective tissue which contains numerous glands, small blood vessels, lymphatics and nerve fibres.
Muscularis mucosa is composed of two thin layers of smooth muscle fibres which help in localized movements of the mucosa.

2. Submucosa This refers to the layer of connective tissue present outside the mucosa. It contains blood vessels, lymphatics and a network of nerve fibres and nerve cells called submucosal nerve plexus (Meissner's plexus).

3. Muscle coat It is formed by a thick layer of smooth muscle fibres surrounding the submucosa. The smooth muscle fibres are arranged in two layers:

Circular muscle fibres form the inner layer.
Longitudinal muscle fibres form the outer layer.

In between the circular and longitudinal muscle fibres is present an extensive network of nerve cells and fibres named *Auerbach's plexus* (myenteric plexus).

4. Serosa (serous layer) This is the outermost layer consisting of a layer of connective tissue. This layer helps in the attachment of the gut to the surrounding structures.

INNERVATION OF GIT

The innervation of GIT includes intrinsic and extrinsic systems (Fig. 7.1.4).

1. Intrinsic Innervation

The intrinsic nervous system, also called *enteric nervous system*, consists of nerve cells and fibres which originate and are located in the intestinal wall itself. This system supplies the smooth muscles of GIT (i.e. musculature of GIT except upper oesophagus and external anal sphincter which contain striated muscle). This system controls most of the gastrointestinal functions like secretion and motility. The enteric nervous system is composed mainly of two plexuses:

Myenteric plexus Myenteric plexus or Auerbach's plexus is present in between the circular and longitudinal muscle fibres of muscular coat of GIT. Stimulation of myenteric plexus

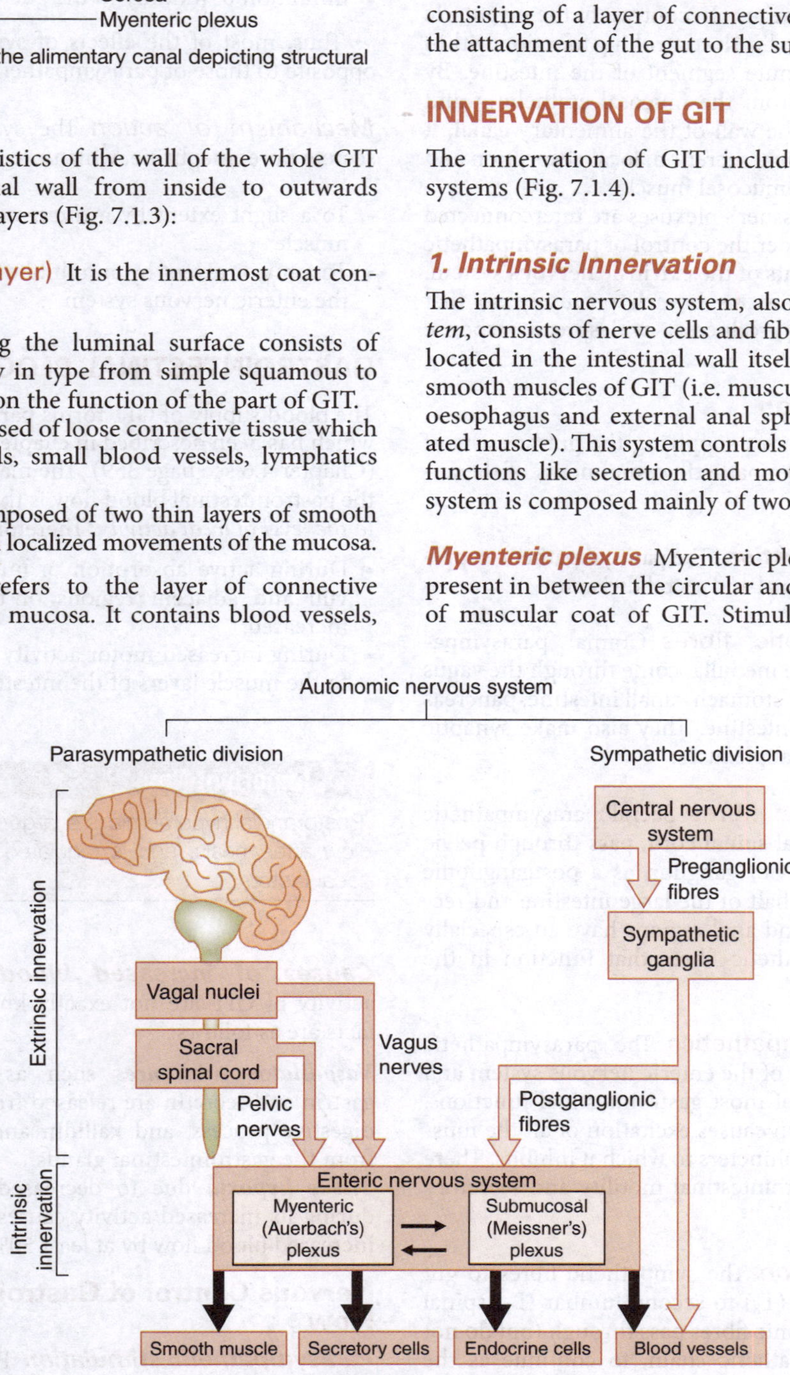

Fig. 7.1.4 Schematic illustration of the innervation of gut.

causes increase in tone of the gut wall, intensity of rhythmical contractions of the gut wall, rate of contraction and velocity of contraction.

Functions of myenteric plexus include:

- *Control of motility of gut*, which is the main function of this plexus
- *Inhibition of pyloric sphincter*, which controls the emptying of the stomach
- *Inhibition of the ileocaecal valve*, which controls the emptying of the small intestine into the caecum

Meissner's plexus Meissner's plexus or submucosal plexus is present in the submucosal layer. It *controls the secretory activity* and blood flow to the gut. In contrast to the myenteric plexus, it is mainly concerned with controlling function within the inner wall of each minute segment of the intestine. By receiving sensory signals from the mucosal epithelium and from stretch receptors in the wall of the alimentary canal, it helps to control local intestinal secretion, local absorption and local contraction of the submucosal muscle.

The Auerbach's and Meissner's plexuses are interconnected with each other and are under the control of parasympathetic and sympathetic components of the extrinsic nervous system. In both the plexuses, the axons branch profusely, so that stimulation of one region produces a widespread response in GIT.

2. Extrinsic Innervation

The extrinsic system of nerves supplying the gut consists of the parasympathetic and sympathetic components of the autonomic nervous system.

Parasympathetic innervation The parasympathetic supply to the gut is made up of cranial and sacral divisions:

Cranial parasympathetic fibres Cranial parasympathetic fibres originate in the medulla, come through the vagus and supply the oesophagus, stomach, small intestine, pancreas and first half of the large intestine. They also make synaptic connections with intramural plexuses.

Sacral parasympathetic fibres Sacral parasympathetic fibres originate in the sacral spinal cord, pass through pelvic nerves to hypogastric (pelvic) ganglion as a postganglionic fibre and supply the distal half of the large intestine and rectum. The sigmoid, rectal and anal regions have an especially rich supply of parasympathetic fibres that function in the defaecation reflex.

Functions of parasympathetics The parasympathetic nerves increase the activity of the enteric nervous system and thus enhance the activity of most gastrointestinal functions. Parasympathetic stimulation causes excitation of all the musculature of gut except the sphincters to which it inhibits. There occurs an increase in gastrointestinal motility and secretory activity.

Sympathetic innervation The sympathetic fibres to gut arise from eighth thoracic (T_8) to second lumbar (L_2) spinal segments. These preganglionic fibres pass through (but do not relay in) the lateral sympathetic chain, to continue as the *splanchnic nerves*. The preganglionic fibres relay in the coeliac and mesenteric autonomic ganglia. The postganglionic fibres run along the blood vessels to terminate mainly on the neurons of the enteric nervous system. The sympathetics innervate all portions of GIT rather than being more extensively supplied to portions near the oral cavity and anus, as is true for parasympathetics.

Functions of sympathetic innervation Sympathetic stimulation causes:

- Vasoconstriction
- Excitation of ileocaecal and internal anal sphincters and smooth muscles of muscularis mucosa throughout (to increase the number of folds)
- Inhibition of motility in the gut

Thus, most of the effects of sympathetic stimulation are opposite to those of parasympathetic stimulation.

Mechanism of action The sympathetic nerve endings secrete norepinephrine, which exerts its effects in two ways:

- To a slight extent by a *direct action* that inhibits smooth muscle
- To a major extent by an inhibitory effect on the neurons of the enteric nervous system

GASTROINTESTINAL BLOOD FLOW

The blood supply of GIT forms part of splanchnic circulation which has been described in chapter on 'Regional Circulation' (Chapter 4.6 see page 359). The main characteristic feature of the gastrointestinal blood flow is that it is *usually proportional to the level of local activity*. Therefore:

- During active absorption of nutrients, blood flow in the villi and adjacent regions of the submucosa is greatly increased.
- During increased motor activity of the gut, the blood flow to the muscle layers of the intestinal wall is increased.

Important Note

Postprandial hyperaemia is a large increase in intestinal blood flow after meals, and is regulated by neural, hormonal and local factors.

Causes of increased blood flow during increased activity of GIT are not exactly known; some of the known facts are as follows:

Vasodilator substances such as cholecystokinin (CCK), gastrin and secretin are released from the mucosa during the digestive process, and kallidin and bradykinin are released from the gastrointestinal glands.

Tissue hypoxia due to decreased oxygenation of the gut during its increased activity causes marked vasodilation and increased blood flow by at least 50%.

Nervous Control of Gastrointestinal Blood Flow

Parasympathetic stimulation Parasympathetic stimulation increases glandular secretion and local blood flow in the gut.

Sympathetic stimulation Sympathetic stimulation causes vasoconstriction and decrease in blood flow. This phenomenon is especially useful when blood is to be shifted from the splanchnic circulation to the heart in conditions like heavy exercise and circulatory shock.

GENERAL PRINCIPLES OF GASTROINTESTINAL FUNCTIONS

The main activities involved in the functioning of GIT are GIT motility and GIT secretion. The general principles governing these activities are discussed here.

GENERAL PRINCIPLES OF GASTROINTESTINAL MOTILITY

Characteristics of Gastrointestinal Smooth Muscle Functioning

The motor functions of the gut are performed by different layers of smooth muscles in its wall. The *gastrointestinal smooth muscle functions as a syncytium*, i.e. when an action potential is elicited within the muscle mass, it travels in all directions in the muscle and it contracts as a whole mass. The distances that it travels depend on the excitability of the muscle. This occurs because of the fact that the smooth muscle fibres in the longitudinal and circular muscle layers are electrically connected through the gap junctions that allow the ions to move from one cell to the next.

Electrical Activity of Gastrointestinal Smooth Muscle

Resting Membrane Potential

Resting membrane potential (RMP) of gut smooth muscle fluctuates between −50 and −60 mV and thus shows undulating changes in the form of slow waves. The cause of these waves is not exactly known; it probably might be due to slow undulation of the activity of sodium–potassium pump. These waves determine the rhythm of most gastrointestinal contractions.

Factors affecting RMP of gastrointestinal smooth muscles The basic level of RMP of gastrointestinal smooth muscle can be increased or decreased.

Factors that depolarize the membrane Factors that depolarize the membrane include:

- Stretching of the muscle
- Stimulation by acetylcholine
- Stimulation by parasympathetic nerves that secrete acetylcholine at their endings
- Stimulation by gastrointestinal hormones

Factors that hyperpolarize the membrane

- Effect of norepinephrine or epinephrine on the muscle membrane
- Stimulation by sympathetic nerves that secrete norepinephrine at their endings

Action Potentials

Action potentials that cause muscle contraction occur in the form of spike potentials. They occur when the RMP becomes more positive than about −40 mV. The channels responsible for the action potentials are called *calcium–sodium channels*. These channels allow a particularly large number of calcium ions to enter along with a smaller number of sodium ions. For details, see page 111.

Functional Types of Gastrointestinal Movements

Peristalsis refers to the movement of gut. Functionally, two types of peristalsis are recognized – propulsive movements and mixing movements.

1. Propulsive Movements

The propulsion of food in the gut towards the anus is accomplished by peristalsis:

Contraction ring Contraction ring around a segment of the intestine appears when it is distended, which moves forward propelling the food a few centimetres before ending.

Receptive relaxation Receptive relaxation of the gut several centimetres towards the anus occurs along with appearance of contraction ring. This allows the food to be propelled more easily towards the anus.

The propulsive movements comprising appearance of contraction rings and receptive relaxation do not occur in the absence of myenteric plexus; therefore, it is also called *myenteric reflex* or *peristaltic reflex*. The peristaltic reflex plus the direction of movement towards the anus is called *law of the gut*.

2. Mixing Movements

The mixing of food in the gut is accomplished by peristalsis and local constrictive contractions:

Peristaltic contractions cause most of the mixing of food. The churning is made possible more effectively when forward propulsion of intestinal contents is blocked by a sphincter.
Local constrictive contractions which occur every few centimetres in the gut cause mixing of intestinal contents by their chopping action.

GENERAL PRINCIPLES OF GASTROINTESTINAL TRACT SECRETION

Functions of Gastrointestinal Tract Secretions

The secretions of GIT subserve three primary functions.

1. Lubrication of food Lubrication of food is carried out by the mucus present in the secretion. Lubrication helps in propulsion of the intestinal contents.

2. Protection of mucosa Protection of mucosa of the alimentary tract is also done by the mucus present in the secretion.

3. Digestion of food Digestive enzymes present in the secretions degrade the food into usable nutrients. For example:

- *Starches* are degraded by amylases into monosaccharides.
- *Proteins* are degraded by a variety of enzymes (e.g. pepsin and trypsin) into dipeptides and amino acids.
- *Fats* are digested by lipases and esterases into monoglycerides and free fatty acids.

Stimulation of Alimentary Tract Secretion

The alimentary tract secretion is initiated by direct mechanical stimulation of glandular cells by food. The stimulated local glands secrete digestive juices.

REGULATION OF GASTROINTESTINAL MOTILITY AND SECRETION

Regulation of gastrointestinal motility and secretion provides optimal conditions for digestion and absorption of the foodstuffs. The regulation reflexes are initiated by stimulation of receptors located in the walls of the intestinal tract, especially in the mucosa. ***Receptors*** located in the gut wall include:

- Mechanoreceptors
- Chemoreceptors
- Osmoreceptors

Stimulation of above-mentioned receptors activates the enteric nervous system of the gut wall. The types of stimuli that do this are as follows:

- Distension of the gut wall by luminal contents
- Tactile stimulation by the foodstuff
- Chemical stimulation by acidity of the chyme
- Stimulation of osmoreceptors by the osmolality of the chyme
- Chemical stimulation by products of protein, fat and carbohydrate digestion, e.g. peptides and fatty acids

The regulation of gastrointestinal motility and secretion is mediated through neural and hormonal mechanisms.

Neural Regulation

Neural Innervation

Neural innervation involved in the regulation of gastrointestinal function is described on page 561.

Characteristics of neural regulation Characteristics of neural regulation are as follows:

- *Enteric nervous system* is responsible for basic gut motility and secretions.
- *Stimulation of receptors* present in the gut mucosa modifies the activity of the enteric nervous system.
- *Sensory signals* arising from one part of the gut may modify the secretory activity of another part of the gut, e.g. low pH of chyme in the duodenum decreases the acid secretion in the stomach.
- *Extrinsic nervous system* is involved in the regulation of gut motility and secretion in response to changes in the environment, e.g. effect of emotions, smell or taste on the gastric secretion and motility. This system is also involved in the long-loop reflexes in the gut, e.g. gastrointestinal reflex.

Gastrointestinal reflexes Gastrointestinal reflexes that essentially control the gut motility and secretion can be grouped as follows:

Reflexes that occur entirely within the enteric nervous system of gut These reflexes control the gastrointestinal secretion, peristalsis, mixing contractions and local inhibitory effects.

Reflexes involving sympathetic innervation Such reflexes transmit signals for long distances (long-loop reflexes). These include:

Gastrocolic *reflex* involves the signals from the stomach to cause evacuation of the colon.
Enterogastric *reflex* involves the signals from the small and large intestines that inhibit gastric motility and secretion.
Coloileal *reflex* involves the signals from the colon which inhibit emptying of ileal contents into the colon.

Reflexes involving central nervous system, spinal cord or brainstem These include:

- *Reflexes* that control motor and secretory activity of the stomach through the vagus nerve
- *Pain reflexes* that cause general inhibition of the entire GIT
- *Defaecation reflexes* that travel to the spinal cord and back again to produce the powerful colonic, rectal and abdominal contraction required for defaecation

Autonomic control of gastrointestinal tract Autonomic control of the GIT can be summarized as follows:

Motility of the gut Motility of the gut exhibits the following effects:

Parasympathetic stimulation produces increase in motility and tone of the gut wall but causes relaxation of sphincters.
Sympathetic stimulation produces decrease in motility and tone of the gut wall but causes contraction of sphincters.

Secretions of the gut Secretions of the gut exhibit the following effects:

Parasympathetic stimulation Parasympathetic stimulation increases the secretions. This is especially true of salivary glands, oesophageal glands, gastric glands, the pancreas, Brunner's glands in the duodenum and the glands of distal portion of the large intestine. Secretions in the remaining part of the small intestine and in the first two-thirds of the large intestine occur mainly in response to local neural and hormonal stimuli.

Sympathetic stimulation Sympathetic stimulation can have a dual effect on glandular secretion, i.e. may increase or decrease, depending on the existing secretory activity of the gland. This dual effect is highlighted:

- *Sympathetic stimulation alone* usually slightly increases secretions.
- *When secretion is already increased*, superimposed sympathetic stimulation usually inhibits the secretion by reducing blood flow to the gland.

Hormonal Regulation

Gastrointestinal Hormones: An Overview

- Gastrointestinal hormones regulate the secretions and even to some extent the motility of GIT.
- The *glandular cells* secreting gastrointestinal hormones are individually scattered in the epithelium of the stomach and small intestine and not in the form of clusters of cells as in the endocrine glands.
- The luminal surface of glandular cells when stimulated by various chemicals present in the chyme releases hormone from the opposite surface into blood capillaries of portal circulation.

- Through portal circulation, the released hormone reaches the target tissue situated in the nearby region of GIT and exhibits physiological actions on the target cells with specific receptors for the hormone. For example, the hormone gastrin released by G cells present in mucosa of pyloric part of the stomach in response to presence of peptides in chyme reaches the body of the stomach via portal circulation and increases the acid secretion as well as motility of the stomach.
- The effects of gastrointestinal hormones persist even after nervous connections between the site of release and the site of action have been severed.
- Gastrointestinal hormones are characterized by two specific features:
  - Each hormone (even at physiological concentration) may affect more than one target tissue. For instance, the secretin increases the secretion of not only pancreatic juice but also bile.
  - Each target tissue usually responds to more than one gastrointestinal hormone. For example, acid-secreting cells of gastric glands are stimulated by gastrin but inhibited by secretin.

Classification of Gastrointestinal Hormones

The gastrointestinal hormones, based on their physioanatomical similarities, can be broadly classified into three types:

1. ***Gastrin family of hormones*** includes:
   - Gastrin (for details, see page 581)
   - CCK-PZ
2. ***Secretin family of hormones*** includes:
   - Secretin (for details, see page 659)
   - Gastric inhibitory polypeptide (GIP) (for details, see page 589)
   - Vasoactive intestinal peptide (VIP) (for details, see page 617)
   - Glucagon (for details, see page 764)
   - Glucagon-like immune reactivity (GLI) or glicentin
3. ***Other gastrointestinal hormones*** include:
   - Motilin
   - Neurotensin
   - Substance P
   - Gastrin-releasing peptide (GRP) (see page 582)
   - Somatostatin (see page 583)

Actions of Gastrointestinal Hormones

The details about the action of various gastrointestinal hormones are described somewhere else (see pages given in parentheses above). However, the outlines of the action of each gastrointestinal hormone as well as the stimulus for secretion and site of secretion are depicted in Table 7.1.1.

IMMUNOLOGY OF THE GASTROINTESTINAL TRACT

GIT helps in replenishment of nutrient supply that comes from the external environment, and also is equipped with defence mechanisms against harmful microbes that enter

Table 7.1.1 Stimuli for secretion, site of action and actions of gastrointestinal hormones

			Actions						
Hormone	**Stimuli for secretion**	**Site of secretion**	**Gastric secretion**	**Gastric motility**	**Pancreatic secretion**	**Bile secretion**	**Gall bladder contraction**	**Small intestine secretion**	**Small intestine motility**
• Gastrin	Small peptides, amino acids, gastric distension, vagal stimulation	G cells of gastric antrum	+	+	+	0	0	0	0
• Cholecystokinin (CCK)	Small peptides, amino acids, fatty acids	Type I cells of duodenum and jejunum	0	–	+	0	+	0	+
• Secretin	Acid low pH (<3.5) of chyme due to gastric HCl	S cells of duodenum	–	0	+	+	0	0	0
• Gastric inhibitory polypeptide (GIP)	Fatty acids, amino acids and oral glucose	Duodenum and jejunum	–	–	0	0	0	+	–
• Vasoactive intestinal polypeptide (VIP)	Fatty acids	Jejunum	–	–	0	0	0	0	0
• Somatostatin	Acid in stomach	D cells of islets of Langerhans	–	–	–	0	–	0	0

0, no effect; +, stimulatory effect; –, inhibitory effect.

along with food and other foreign invaders. The gut immunity protects and acts as barrier in different ways:

Saliva: Salivary secretion contains lysozyme (bactericidal) and lactoferrin (bacteriostatic). It also dilutes the irritant food and prevents the injury of buccal mucosa.

HCl of gastric secretion kills most of the pathogen due to highly acidic pH.

Architecture

The human intestinal tract is the largest immune organ of the body. The gut and immune system are very closely linked; about 70%–80% of the immune tissue is located in the gut. Indeed gut-associated lymphoid tissue (GALT) is the prominent part of mucosal-associated lymphoid tissue (MALT). About 80% of plasma cells, and immunoglobulin A (IgA)–bearing cells, reside in GALT.

The immunological architecture of gut comprises cells from nonhaematopoietic (epithelia, Paneth cells, goblet cells) and haemopoietic (macrophages, dendritic cells, T cells) tissues and also microbiota i.e. microbes of gut.

Epithelium: The mucosal epithelium overlying the Peyer's patches in the small intestine has specialized microfold cells (M cells) for absorption of antigenic substances.

Peyer's patches are dense aggregates of lymphoid tissue having a collection of T and B lymphocytes.

Paneth cells: These are large columnar cells named after Joseph Paneth, located at the base of crypts of Lieberkühn. These cells have prominent defensin-secreting granules, which are secreted in response to stimuli such as bacterial products.

Lamina propria: In the lamina propria of the small intestine, a large number of lymphocytes and plasma cells are scattered. The antigens absorbed by M cells get processed in these lymphocytes and get converted into lymphoblasts that ultimately form plasma cells.

Plasma cells are responsible for secretion of IgA antibodies which provide secretory immunity against ingested antigens.

Intestinal microbiota: The intestinal microflora has protective, metabolic, trophic and immunological functions and establishes with the intestinal innate and adaptive immune system and plays a pivotal role in maintenance of gut ecosystem.

Peritoneal lymphoid tissue: A large number of lymph nodes present in the greater omentum of the peritoneum also play an important role in gastrointestinal immunity.

Physiological Role of Immune Mechanism of GIT

- It prevents the absorption of intestinal-derived antigens such as food antigens and microorganism-origin antigens (bacteria and viruses). IgA antibodies present in the intestinal lumen prevent their access to the epithelial lining. The mechanism is known as *immune exclusion*.
- Luminal IgAs check bacterial colonization in the gut by preventing adherence of bacteria to the mucous membrane.
- IgAs play some role in bacteriolysis in the presence of complement system.
- IgAs neutralize the adverse effect of viral toxins by inactivation of viruses.

The lymphocytes interspread in the epithelial lining mount an antigen-specific cell-mediated immune response that is especially useful in viral infection and tumour surveillance.

Important Notes

Probiotics and prebiotics

Probiotics are foods or supplements that contain useful live microorganisms like yeast, fermented foodstuffs and beverages which maintain and improve the useful bacterial flora of the gut.

Prebiotics are the group of nutrients that are degraded by gut microbiota. Many vegetables and fruits like whole grain, banana, green vegetables, onion and garlic are useful prebiotics which provide beneficial effects on human health. Fructo-oligosaccharides and galacto-oligosaccharides are two important groups of prebiotics.

Benefits of probiotics for gut health are as follows:

- Improve gut functions by balancing the normal bacteria of the gut
- Reduce the symptoms of gut disorders such as infective diarrhoea and ulcerative colitis
- Reduce gas and bloating
- Reduce the stress and improve the mood
- Improve body resistance against allergies
- Reduce the serum cholesterol level

Probiotics can be used as an ecological therapy in the treatment of immune diseases.

Self-Assessment

1. Discuss the structural characteristics of the gastrointestinal tract and its functions.
2. Discuss the general principles of gastrointestinal functions.
3. Write briefly about:
   - Innervation of gut
   - General overview of gastrointestinal hormones
   - Immunology of GIT and its significance

Clinical Case

Case 1

A 10-year-old male child was brought to the emergency department with fever, pain in the abdomen, cramps, loose watery stools and blood in the stools.

Examination and laboratory tests showed that the patient was dehydrated. Blood and stool analysis revealed acute infective diarrhoea.

Q1. What are the immediate measures to treat the condition?

Q2. What is the benefit of the use of probiotics and prebiotics?

7.2 Physiological Activities in Mouth, Pharynx and Oesophagus

CHAPTER OUTLINE

INTRODUCTION

The digestive system is responsible for breaking down food and supplying the body with water, nutrients and electrolytes needed to sustain life. The functioning of the digestive system starts from the mouth (oral cavity) and ends at the anus.

Ingestion of food involves the following processes:

- Placing of food into the mouth
- Mastication, i.e. chewing the food into smaller pieces
- Lubrication of the food with saliva
- Swallowing, i.e. deglutition

The aforementioned physiological activities which take place in the mouth, pharynx and oesophagus are discussed in this chapter.

MASTICATION

Mastication or chewing refers to the process by which the food placed in the mouth is cut and ground into smaller pieces. It involves:

- Movements of the jaws
- Action of teeth (the incisors provide a strong cutting action, whereas the molars have a grinding action)
- Coordinated movements of the tongue and muscles of the oral cavity

CHEWING REFLEX

Mastication or chewing, though a voluntary act, is coordinated by a chewing reflex that facilitates the opening and closing of the jaw. The chewing reflex operates as follows:

- When the mouth is opened to place the food inside it, the muscles of the jaw are stretched which leads to their contraction due to stretch reflex, thereby raising the jaw to cause closure of the mouth.
- When the mouth is closed, the food comes into contact with buccal receptors which cause reflex inhibition of the muscles of mastication and also initiate a reflex contraction of the digastric and lateral pterygoid muscles, causing the mouth to open.
- When the jaw drops, again there occurs contraction of jaw muscles due to stretch reflex and causes the entire cycle to be repeated. Again and again repetition of the cycle of opening and closing the jaw leads to mastication. The tongue contributes to the grinding process by positioning the food between the upper and lower teeth.
- Jaw muscles working together are capable of exerting a force of about 11–25 kg for incisors and about 29–30 kg for molars. As the force is exerted over a small area, the pressure exerted is hundreds of kilograms per square centimetre.

MUSCLES OF MASTICATION

Masseter raises the mandible, *clenches* the teeth and helps to protract the mandible.

Temporalis raises the mandible and helps to retract the mandible after protraction.

Internal and external pterygoids protrude the mandible, depress the chin and, therefore, help in opening the mouth. Grinding movements are produced by these when right and left muscles are acting alternatively.

Buccinator is an accessory muscle of mastication which prevents accumulation of food between the cheek and the teeth.

FUNCTIONS OF MASTICATION

1. Breaking of food into smaller pieces increases the total surface area. As the digestive enzymes act mainly on the surface of food particles, the digestion rate is increased.
2. Undigestive cellulose membrane present around the nutrition portion of most fruits and raw vegetable is broken, making it easier for them to be digested.
3. Mixing of food with saliva initiates the process of starch digestion by salivary amylase, and lipid digestion by lingual lipase.
4. Swallowing becomes easy because of breaking of food into smaller pieces, and lubrication and softening of the food bolus by saliva.
5. Chewing brings food into contact with taste receptors and releases odour that stimulates the olfactory receptors. Stimulation of taste receptors and olfactory receptors increases the pleasure of eating and stimulates gastric secretions.

Net Effect of Mastication

The bolus of food becomes a homogenized mixture of small food particles, saliva and mucus, which is easy to swallow and digest.

LUBRICATION OF FOOD BY SALIVA

SALIVARY GLANDS

In addition to the chewing, another important physiological activity which takes place in the mouth is lubrication of food by saliva. Saliva is secreted by three pairs of major salivary glands (Fig. 7.2.1).

1. Parotid Glands

Location

Parotid glands are the largest salivary glands (each weighing 20–30 g), located near the angles of the jaw.

Acini

The parotid glands are purely serous glands (Fig. 7.2.2) which secrete watery saliva containing more than 90% water. They secrete 25% of the total salivary secretion (which is about 1500 mL/day).

Ducts

Ducts of the parotid glands open on the inner side of the right and left cheeks and pour their secretions in the vestibule.

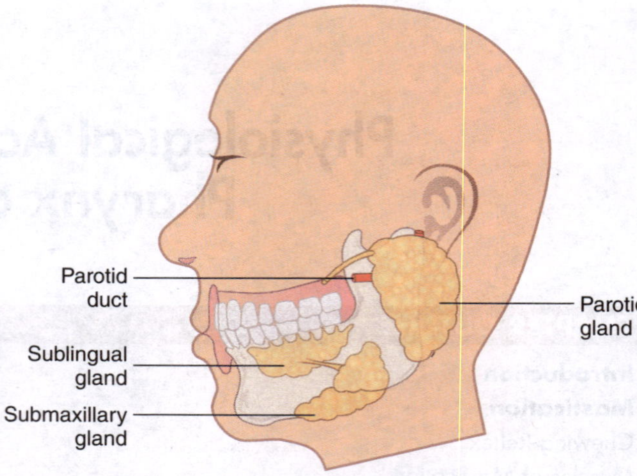

Fig. 7.2.1 Salivary glands and their ducts.

2. Sublingual Glands

Location

The sublingual gland is the smallest of the three main salivary glands. It lies just below the mucosa on the floor of the mouth. Each gland raises a ridge of mucosa which starts at the sublingual papilla and runs laterally and backwards. The ridge is called the sublingual fold.

Acini

The sublingual gland contains both serous and mucous acini (Fig. 7.2.2), the latter predominating.

Ducts

Ducts of the sublingual gland are 8–20 in number. Most open into the mouth on the summit of sublingual fold but a few may open into the submandibular duct.

3. Submandibular Glands

Location

The submandibular glands are large salivary glands which lie (one on each side) partly under cover of the body of the mandible. Each gland is made up of a large superficial part and a small deep part.

Acini

The submandibular gland is composed of a mixture of serous and mucous acini, the former predominating (Fig. 7.2.2).

Ducts

S-shaped duct of each submandibular gland opens on the sublingual papilla located just lateral to the frenulum lingua.

Note: The sublingual and submandibular glands secrete a fluid that contains a higher concentration of proteins and so is

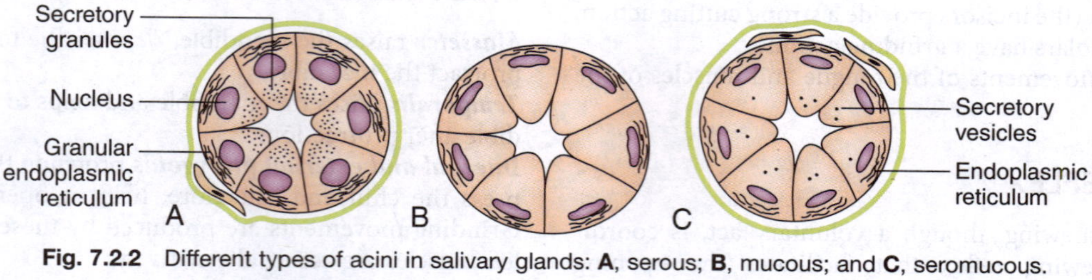

Fig. 7.2.2 Different types of acini in salivary glands: **A**, serous; **B**, mucous; and **C**, seromucous.

more viscous compared with the watery secretion of parotid glands.

Smaller Salivary Glands

In addition to the three pairs of salivary glands described above, several smaller glands are located throughout the oral cavity. Those in the tongue secrete lingual lipase.

SALIVA

Secretion and Composition

The composition of salivary secretion depends on its source and rate of secretion. Serous secretion is watery and mainly contains electrolytes and amylase, whereas mucus secretion is viscous in nature, and it contains electrolytes and mucin.

Amount

Under normal circumstances, the salivary glands secrete about 500–1500 mL of saliva every day. pH of saliva varies from 6 to 7.4.

Composition

Saliva is composed of:

Water: 99%
Solids: 1%, which include:

- *Organic* substances are L-amylase (ptyalin), lingual lipase, kallikrein, lysozyme, small amounts of urea, uric acid, cholesterol and mucin.
- *Inorganic* substances are Na^+, Cl^-, K^+ and HCO_3^-.

Note: Composition of saliva varies with the salivary flow rate.

Mechanism of Formation of Saliva

Mechanism of formation of saliva involves two processes.

1. Primary secretion of saliva The acinar cells of salivary glands secrete the initial saliva into the salivary ducts. The initial saliva is formed by transudation (pressure filtration) of plasma and therefore is isotonic, i.e. has the same Na^+, Cl^-, K^+ and HCO_3^- concentrations as plasma (Fig. 7.2.3).

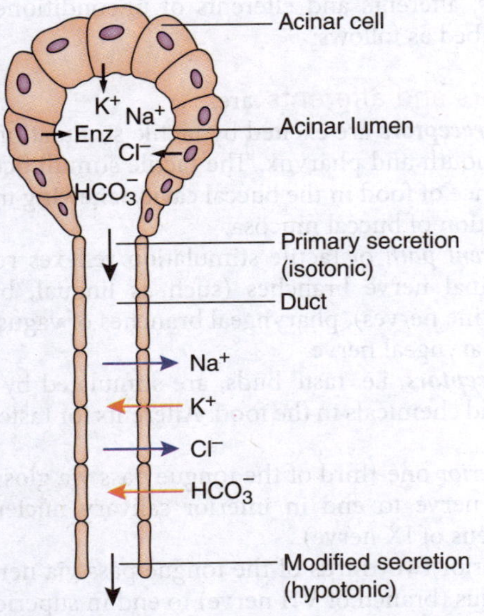

Fig. 7.2.3 Mechanism of formation of saliva.

However, the initial saliva is soon modified by the salivary ducts.

2. Modification of saliva The ductal cells that line the tubular portions of the salivary ducts change the composition of initial saliva by the following processes (Fig. 7.2.3):

Reabsorption of Na^+ and Cl^- occurs in the ductal cells; therefore, the concentration of these ions is lower than their plasma concentration.

Secretion of K^+ and HCO_3^- is caused by the ductal cells; therefore, the concentration of these ions is higher than their plasma concentrations.

Modified saliva becomes hypotonic in the ducts because the ducts are relatively impermeable to water. Because more solutes than water are reabsorbed by the ducts, the saliva becomes dilute relative to plasma.

Note: Aldosterone acts on the ductal cells to increase the reabsorption of Na^+ and Cl^- from salivary ducts (analogous to its actions on renal tubule). Thus, a high Na^+/Cl^- ratio is seen when aldosterone is deficient in Addison disease (see page 736). Conversely, in the presence of excess aldosterone, the greatly increased sodium chloride concentration of saliva falls almost to zero and increases K^+ concentration equal to or higher than that of plasma.

Effects of Flow Rate on the Composition of Saliva

Effects of flow rate on the composition of saliva occur due to changes in the contact time available for reabsorption and secretion processes to occur in the ducts.

1. At high flow rates At high flow rates, there is less time for reabsorption and secretion, and therefore the saliva is most likely the initial secretion by the acinar cells. Thus, with the increase in flow rate, the concentration of ions changes (Fig. 7.2.4):

- *Sodium ion (Na^+)* concentration increases progressively to a plateau value of 80–90 mEq/L.
- *Chloride ion (Cl^-)* concentration increases to about 50 mEq/L.

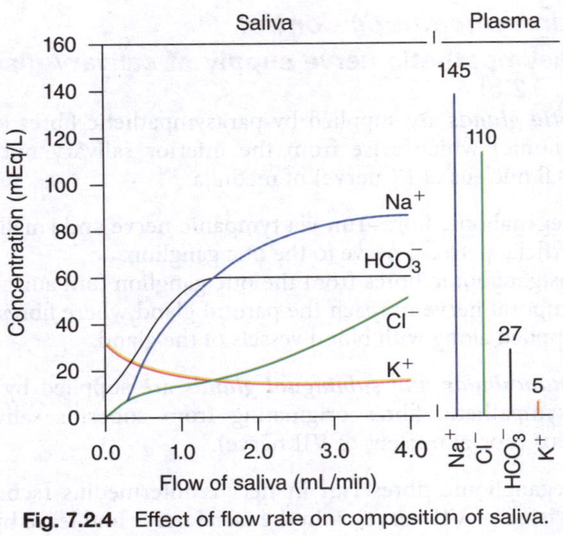

Fig. 7.2.4 Effect of flow rate on composition of saliva.

Note: Na^+ and Cl^- concentrations of saliva are always lower than those in the plasma.

- Potassium ion (K^+) concentration decreases to 15–20 mEq/L.
- Bicarbonate ion (HCO_3^-) concentration increases when salivary flow rate increases, because HCO_3^- secretion is increased when salivary glands are stimulated by the parasympathetic nervous system. HCO_3^- concentration then increases in saliva than that in plasma at high flow rates (up to 50–70 mEq/L).

2. At low flow rates At low flow rates, there is more time for reabsorption and secretion; therefore, the modified saliva under resting conditions contains:

- Low concentration of Na^+ (about 15–20 mEq/L)
- Low concentration of Cl^- (15–20 mEq/L)
- Low concentration of HCO_3^- (10–15 mEq/L)
- High concentration of K^+ (25–30 mEq/L)

Phases of Salivary Secretion

1. ***Cephalic phase*** refers to secretion of saliva before entering of food into the mouth. It is caused by a conditioned reflex initiated by the mere sight or smell of food.
2. ***Buccal phase*** refers to secretion of saliva caused by stimulation of buccal receptors by the presence of food in the mouth. It is an unconditioned reflex, partially regulated by the appetite area of the brain.
3. ***Oesophageal phase*** occurs due to stimulation of salivary glands to a slight degree by the food passing through the oesophagus.
4. ***Gastric phase*** refers to secretion of saliva by the presence of food in the stomach. It especially occurs when irritant food is present in the stomach (e.g. increased salivation before vomiting).
5. ***Intestinal phase*** refers to salivary secretion caused by presence of irritant food in the upper intestine.

Control of Salivary Secretion

- Salivary secretion is controlled entirely by autonomic nervous system (ANS) reflexes.
- Unlike other gastrointestinal glands, there is no hormonal regulation of salivary secretion.
- Salivary secretion production is unique in that it is increased by both parasympathetic and sympathetic activities; however, the activity of former is more important.

I. Parasympathetic Control

Parasympathetic nerve supply of salivary glands (Fig. 7.2.5)

Parotid glands are supplied by parasympathetic fibres (preganglionic) which arise from the inferior salivary nucleus (dorsal nucleus of IX nerve) of medulla.

- Preganglionic fibres run via tympanic nerve and small superficial petrosal nerve to the otic ganglion.
- Postganglionic fibres from the otic ganglion join auriculotemporal nerve to reach the parotid gland where fibres are supplied along with blood vessels of the gland.

Submandibular and sublingual glands are supplied by the parasympathetic fibres originating from superior salivary nucleus (dorsal nucleus of VII nerve).

- Preganglionic fibres run in nervus intermedius (sensory division of VII nerve), join the facial nerve and leave by its chorda tympani branch to join the lingual nerve. They synapse in the ganglia present near the glands.
- Postganglionic fibres arising from the ganglia present near the glands are supplied to the glands along with the blood vessels.

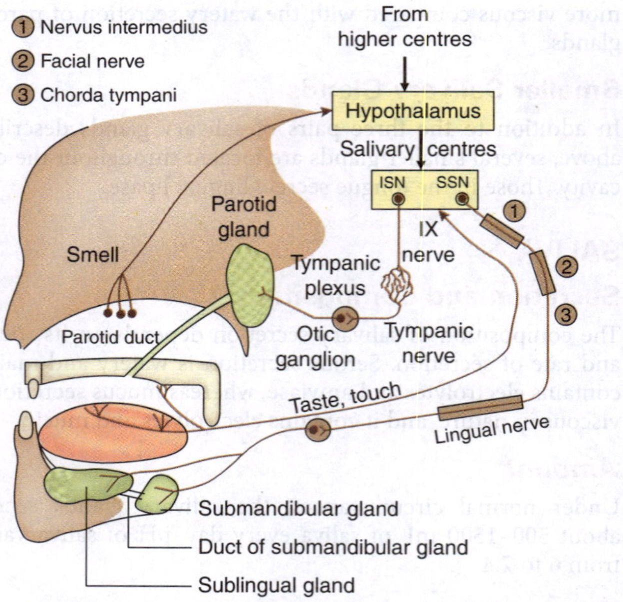

Fig. 7.2.5 Parasympathetic nerve supply to salivary glands.

Parasympathetic reflexes Parasympathetic nerves are secretomotor to the salivary glands and control their secretion via the following reflexes:

1. Conditioned reflexes Sight, smell or even thought of palatable food increases the salivary secretion by conditioned reflexes. In conditioned reflexes, the parasympathetics supplying the salivary glands are stimulated by impulses coming from higher centres of the brain.

2. Unconditioned reflexes Unconditioned reflexes are initiated by stimulation of receptors in the buccal cavity. Receptors, afferents and efferents of unconditioned reflexes are described as follows:

Receptors and afferents are:

Mechanoreceptors are excited by tactile stimulation from the tongue, mouth and pharynx. The tactile stimuli occur due to the presence of food in the buccal cavity, chewing movements and irritation of buccal mucosa.

- *Afferent path* of tactile stimulation reflexes runs in trigeminal nerve branches (such as lingual, buccal and palatine nerves), pharyngeal branches of vagus and glossopharyngeal nerve.

Chemoreceptors, i.e. taste buds, are stimulated by sensation of taste and chemicals in the food. Afferents for taste sensation from:

- *Posterior* one-third of the tongue pass via glossopharyngeal nerve to end in inferior salivary nucleus (dorsal nucleus of IX nerve).
- Anterior two-thirds of the tongue pass via nervus intermedius (branch of VII nerve) to end in superior salivary nucleus (dorsal nucleus of VII nerve).

Salivary centre is thus constituted by superior and inferior salivary nuclei.

Efferents from the superior salivary nucleus stimulate the submandibular and sublingual salivary glands, whereas those from the inferior salivary nucleus stimulate the parotid glands.

Effects of parasympathetic stimulation Parasympathetic nerve stimulation causes the salivary gland cells to secrete a large volume of watery fluid that is high in electrolytes but low in proteins. Parasympathetic stimulation (cranial nerves VII and IX) increases saliva production by the mechanisms given next (Fig. 7.2.5).

Stimulation of parasympathetic nerves liberates a proteolytic enzyme kallikrein from the gland cells which acts on α_2-globulin in interstitial fluid to form bradykinin. It also causes local release of vasoactive intestinal peptide (VIP). These increase the saliva production by:

- Increasing transport processes in the acinar and ductal cells
- Causing vasodilatation of blood vessels of the salivary gland

Important Notes

It is important to note that:

- Cholinergic receptors on acinar and ductal cells are muscarinic.
- The second messenger is inositol 1,4,5-triphosphate (IP_3) and increased in transcellular calcium (Ca^{2+}) (Fig. 7.2.6).
- Anticholinergic drugs (e.g. atropine) inhibit the production of saliva and cause dry mouth.

II. Sympathetic Control

Sympathetic nerve supply to salivary glands

Preganglionic fibres originate from the lateral horn cells of T_1 and T_2 segments of the spinal cord and enter paravertebral sympathetic chain via ventral roots to synapse with the cells in *superior cervical ganglion*.

Postganglionic fibres run along the carotid artery branches and are supplied to the three pairs of salivary glands along with their blood supply.

Effects of sympathetic stimulation Stimulation of sympathetic fibres causes vasoconstriction in the salivary glands, and transient secretion of a very small amount of thick viscid saliva rich in mucus and other organic constituents. Sympathetic stimulation causes salivary secretion if the gland is already activated by parasympathetic activity. However, in humans, the role of sympathetic nerves in physiological stimulation of salivary secretion is doubtful.

Receptors on acinar and ductal cells are β-adrenergic and the second messenger is cyclic adenosine monophosphate (cAMP) (Fig. 7.2.6).

Applied Aspects

Salivary Gland Disorders

Hypersalivation (sialorrhea) refers to excessive salivation, and is a common clinical feature of various neurological disorders (neurological impairment in children and Parkinson disease and stroke in adults).

Hyposalivation/xerostomia: The most common cause of hyposalivation is dehydration and certain medical conditions like depression and anxiety. The effects of xerostomia include:

- Impairment of speech occurs.
- Chewing and swallowing become difficult.
- Ulcerations occur in the mouth.
- The person becomes predisposed to infection.

Paralytic secretion: *Claude Bernard* observed that cutting the chorda tympani nerve (parasympathetic) in a dog or cat produces scanty secretion of thin turbid saliva, which increases to peak on the 7th day and diminishes in 3 weeks. He called it paralytic secretion because it was caused by cutting the nerve supply. However, later on, it was shown that the increased secretion is due to increased sensitivity of the gland to adrenaline after cutting the chorda tympani nerve.

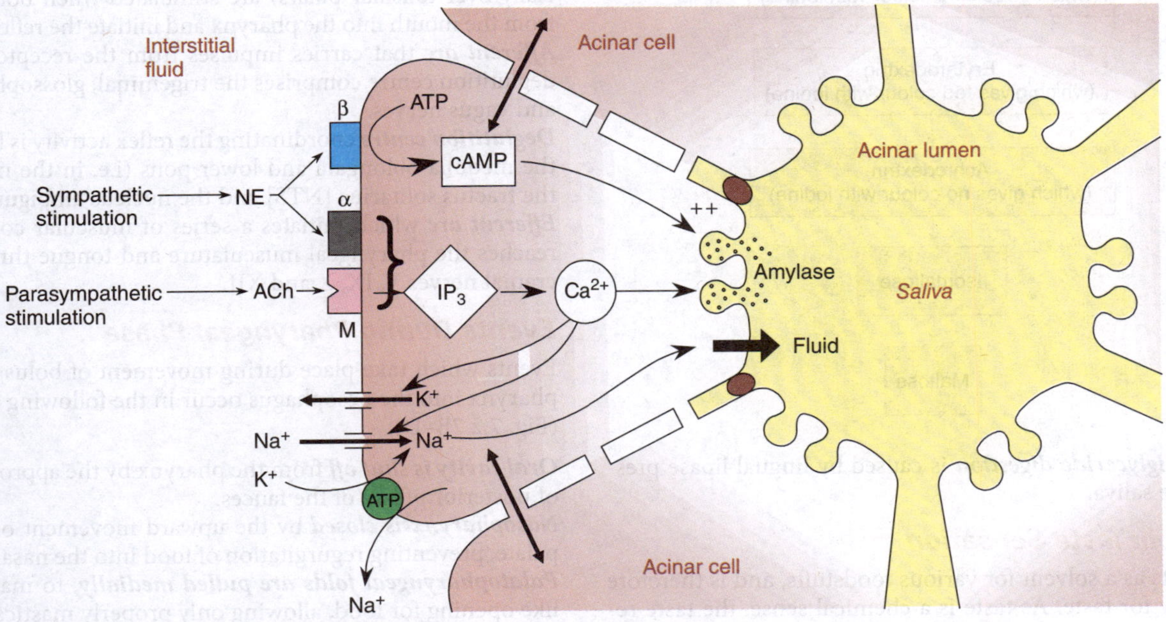

Fig. 7.2.6 Mechanism of salivary regulation by parasympathetic and sympathetic nerves.

Functions of Saliva

1. Protective Function

Dilutes hot and irritant food substances, thus preventing injury to the buccal mucosa.

Washes away food particles that remain in the oral cavity at the end of meal and thus cleans the oral cavity, i.e. helps in maintaining oral hygiene. In this way, growth of several harmful bacteria in the oral cavity is prevented.

Destroys harmful bacteria in the mouth and thus minimizes risk of buccal infection and dental caries because of its following constituents:

- *Lysozymes* which have bactericidal action
- *IgA* which provides immunological defence against bacteria and viruses
- *Lactoferrin* which has bacteriostatic action, i.e. prevents multiplication of bacteria

Thiocyanate: Saliva also contains thiocyanate ions (which are bactericidal) and an enzyme that facilitates the entry of thiocyanate ions into the bacteria.

Dilutes any hydrochloric acid (HCl) and bile which regurgitate into the oesophagus and mouth.

2. Role in Mastication and Deglutition

- Salivary mucus lubricates the food and buccal mucosa and thus aids in mastication and swallowing.
- It helps bolus formation by acting as a glue.

3. Digestive Functions

Initial starch digestion starts by α-amylase (ptyalin) present in the saliva. However, the role of salivary amylase in the digestion of polysaccharides is limited by the short duration of salivary action. When the bolus of food reaches the stomach and mixes with the gastric juice, the gastric acidity (pH 1) stops the action of salivary amylase (which acts at an optimum pH of 6.5–7). Salivary amylase is an alpha-amylase, therefore acts on alpha 1–4 linkage (but not on alpha 1–6 linkage) and digests starch to maltose in the following way:

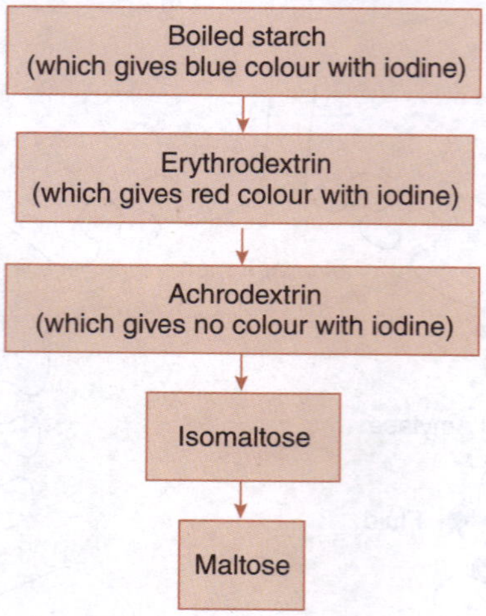

Initial triglyceride digestion is caused by lingual lipase present in the saliva.

4. Role in Taste Sensation

Saliva acts as a solvent for various foodstuffs, and is therefore necessary for taste. As taste is a chemical sense, the taste receptors respond only to dissolved substances.

5. Role in Speech

Salivary mucus lubricates the oral mucosa and thus aids speech by facilitating movements of the lips and tongue.

6. Excretory Function

Saliva acts as a vehicle for excretion of certain heavy metals, thiocyanate ions, alcohol and morphine.

7. Role in Temperature Regulation

- *During state of dehydration,* the salivary secretion is reduced which induces thirst.
- *Panting mechanism:* In dogs, saliva is evaporated from the surface of the tongue to cause evaporative heat loss.

DEGLUTITION (SWALLOWING)

PHASES OF SWALLOWING

Deglutition or swallowing refers to passage of food from the oral cavity into the stomach. It comprises three phases:

- Oral phase (voluntary)
- Pharyngeal phase (reflex or involuntary)
- Oesophageal phase (reflex or involuntary)

Oral Phase

Oral phase or the first stage of swallowing is a voluntary phase.

- During this phase, the bolus of food formed after mastication is put over the dorsum of the tongue. The tongue forces the bolus into the oropharynx by pushing up and back against the hard palate (Fig. 7.2.7A).

Pharyngeal phase

Pharyngeal phase or second stage of swallowing is an involuntary phase (swallowing reflex).

Components of Swallowing Reflex (Fig. 7.2.8)

Receptors present around the opening of the pharynx (especially over tonsillar pillars) are stimulated when bolus moves from the mouth into the pharynx and initiate the reflex activity.

Afferent arc that carries impulses from the receptors to the deglutition centre comprises the trigeminal, glossopharyngeal and vagus nerves.

Deglutition centre coordinating the reflex activity is located in the medulla oblongata and lower pons (i.e. in the nucleus of the tractus solitarius [NTS] and the nucleus ambiguus).

Efferent arc which initiates a series of muscular contraction reaches the pharyngeal musculature and tongue through the cranial nerves V, IX, X and XII.

Events During Pharyngeal Phase

Events which take place during movement of bolus from the pharynx into the oesophagus occur in the following sequence (Fig. 7.2.7B–D):

Oral cavity is shut off from the pharynx by the approximation of posterior pillars of the fauces.

Nasopharynx is closed by the upward movement of the soft palate, preventing regurgitation of food into the nasal cavities.

Palatopharyngeal folds are pulled medially, to make a slit-like opening for food, allowing only properly masticated food to pass through (selective action).

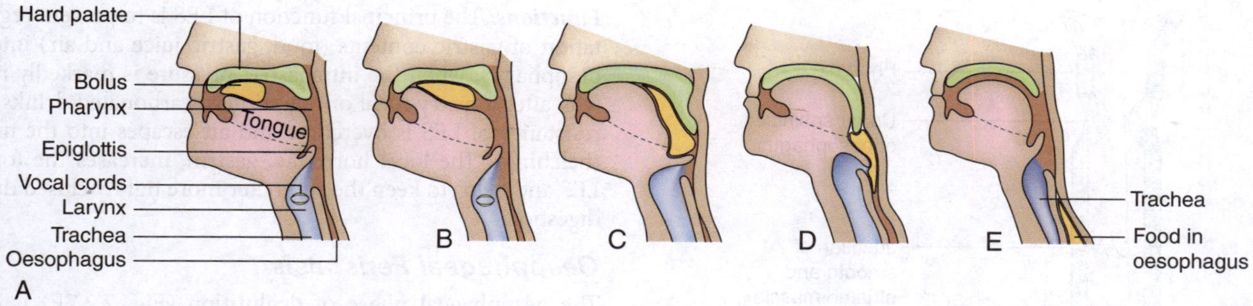

Fig. 7.2.7 Phases of swallowing: **A**, oral phase; **B–D**, early, middle and late pharyngeal phases; and **E**, oesophageal phase.

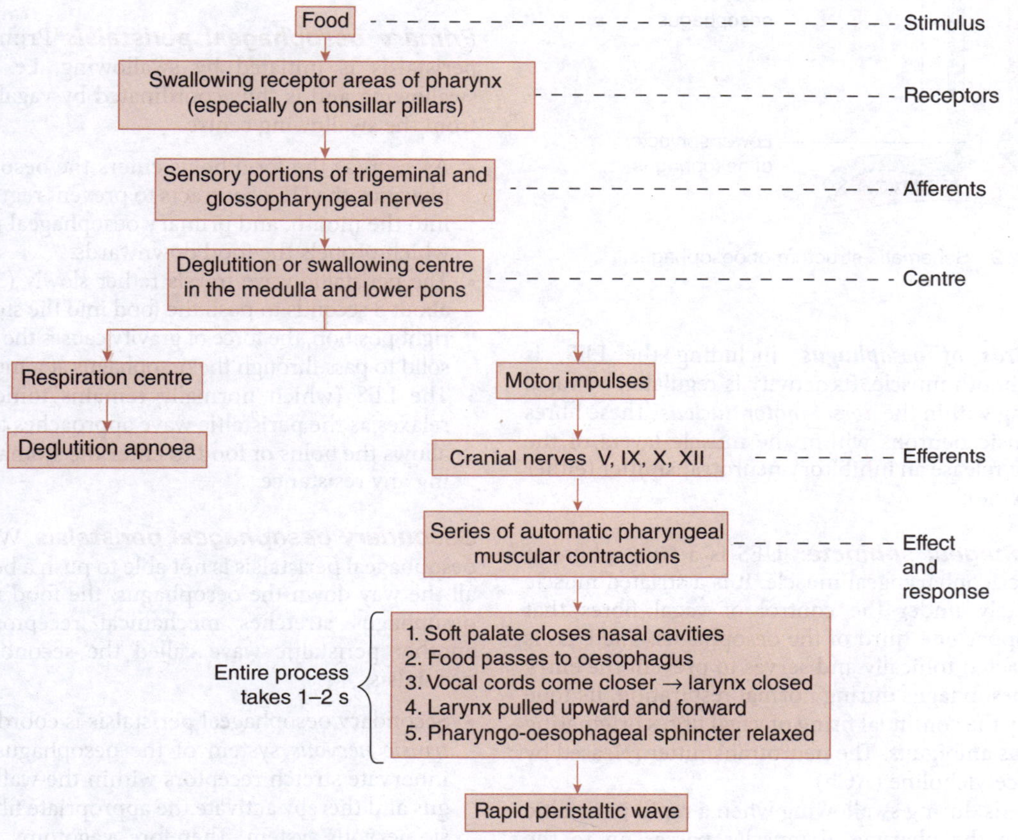

Fig. 7.2.8 Summary of swallowing reflex.

Vocal cords strongly approximate stopping the breathing temporarily (*deglutition apnoea*), the *larynx* is pulled upward and anteriorly by neck muscles enlarging the opening of the oesophagus which is normally a slit and the *epiglottis* swings backwards to close the laryngeal opening. All this guides the food towards the oesophagus and prevents its entry into the trachea.

Upper oesophageal sphincter (UES) which normally remains contracted tonically opens up and allows the bolus of food to be pushed into the upper part of the oesophagus by the rapid peristaltic contraction wave of the pharynx which also continues in the oesophagus.

Once the bolus of food has passed into the oesophagus, the cricopharyngeus contracts, vocal cords open up allowing normal breathing to be resumed and the UES once again goes into tonic contraction.

The entire process of pharyngeal phase is completed in 1–2 seconds.

Oesophageal Phase

During oesophageal phase, the food bolus is propelled from the upper part of the oesophagus to the stomach by the oesophageal peristalsis and aided by gravity. Before describing the features of oesophageal peristalsis, it will be worthwhile to discuss briefly the applied anatomy of the oesophagus (Fig. 7.2.9).

Applied Anatomy of Oesophagus

Oesophagus is a fibromuscular tube about 25 cm long. It is separated from the pharynx by the UES and from the stomach by the lower oesophageal sphincter (LES).

Musculature of oesophagus consists of:

Upper one-third of oesophagus, including the UES, like the pharynx is made up of striated muscle that is under the control of vagal fibres emerging from the nucleus ambiguus.

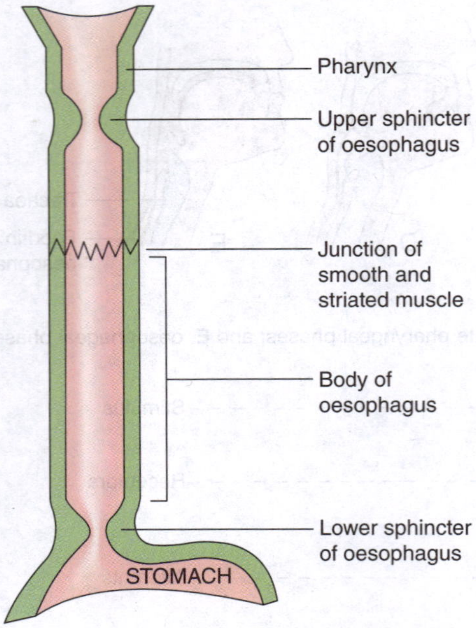

Fig. 7.2.9 Schematic structure of oesophagus.

Lower two-thirds of oesophagus, including the LES, is composed of smooth muscle. Its activity is regulated by vagal fibres originating within the *dorsal motor nucleus*. These fibres innervate intrinsic neurons within the muscle layers of the oesophagus that release an inhibitory neurotransmitter (either VIP or nitric oxide).

Upper oesophageal sphincter UES is a true sphincter formed by the cricopharyngeal muscle. It is a striated muscle and is completely under the control of vagal fibres that innervate the upper one-third of the oesophagus. The UES is normally contracted tonically and serves to prevent the entry of air into the oesophagus during normal respiration. Its tone is maintained by the continual firing of vagal fibres originating from the nucleus ambiguus. The neurotransmitter released by these fibres is acetylcholine (ACh).

The UES opens during swallowing when a rapid peristaltic wave starting in the pharyngeal muscles passes on to the oesophagus.

Lower oesophageal sphincter LES, also known as cardiac sphincter, refers to distal 2 cm of the oesophagus. Although LES is not separately identifiable histologically, its contractile characteristics are quite different from those of the rest of oesophageal smooth muscle (that is why it is called physiological sphincter).

The components of LES are as follows:

- The oesophageal smooth muscle is more prominent at the junction of the oesophagus and the stomach.
- The skeletal muscle fibres of the crura of the diaphragm surround at this point and act as pinchcock.
- The oblique sling fibres of the gastric wall act as flap valve at this junction and prevent regurgitation of gastric contents when there is increase in intragastric pressure.

During quiescent (nonperistaltic) periods, the LES is tonically contracted, whereas the remainder of smooth muscle within the oesophagus is relaxed.

Functions: The principal function of LES is to prevent regurgitation of gastric contents (food, gastric juice and air) into the oesophagus; when the intragastric pressure is markedly raised (e.g. after a heavy meal or ingestion of carbonated drinks), the resistance of LES is overcome and air escapes into the mouth (belching). The local hormone, gastrin, increases the tone of LES and helps to keep the sphincter more tightly closed during digestion.

Oesophageal Peristalsis

The oesophageal phase of deglutition (Fig. 7.2.7E) is completed by two types of oesophageal peristalsis – primary and secondary.

Primary oesophageal peristalsis Primary oesophageal peristalsis is initiated by swallowing, i.e. it is a part of swallowing and is thus coordinated by vagal fibres emerging from the swallowing centre.

- As soon as the food bolus enters the oesophagus from the pharynx, the UES contracts to prevent regurgitation of food into the mouth, and primary oesophageal peristalsis begins which propels the food downwards.
- The peristaltic wave travels rather slowly (3–4 cm/s), taking about 8 seconds to push the food into the stomach. In the upright position, the force of gravity causes the liquids and semisolid to pass through the oesophagus at a much faster rate.
- The LES (which normally remains tonically contracted) relaxes as the peristaltic wave approaches the sphincter and allows the bolus of food to enter the stomach without causing any resistance.

Secondary oesophageal peristalsis When the primary oesophageal peristalsis is not able to push a bolus of solid food all the way down the oesophagus, the food remaining in the oesophagus stretches mechanical receptors and initiates another peristaltic wave called the secondary oesophageal peristalsis.

- Secondary oesophageal peristalsis is coordinated by the *intrinsic nervous* system of the oesophagus. Afferent fibres innervate stretch receptors within the wall of the oesophagus and thereby activate the appropriate fibres in the intrinsic nervous system. Therefore, vagotomy would have little or no effect on secondary oesophageal peristalsis.
- Thus, the secondary oesophageal peristalsis is initiated by the presence of food within the oesophagus and the waves continue until all the swallowed food is removed from the oesophagus.

Note: After the food enters the stomach, the LES contracts to prevent regurgitation of food into the oesophagus. With this, the oesophageal phase of deglutition is completed.

Applied Aspects

Disorders of Swallowing

1. Abolition of Deglutition Reflex

Abolition of deglutition reflex causes regurgitation of food into the nose or aspiration into the larynx and trachea. It may occur:

- When IX or X nerve is paralysed in lesions of the medulla
- When the pharynx is anaesthetized with cocaine (deglutition reflex is abolished temporarily)

2. Aerophagia

Aerophagia refers to unavoidable swallowing of air along with the swallowing of food bolus and liquids.

- It usually occurs in nervous individuals having low tone of the UES.
- Some of the gases present in the air swallowed are absorbed; partly the air is regurgitated into the oral cavity and out in the atmosphere (belching), and majority of it passes on the colon and is then expelled as flatus through the anus.

3. Cardiac Achalasia

Cardiac achalasia is a neuromuscular disorder of the lower two-thirds of the oesophagus, characterized by absence of oesophageal peristalsis and failure of the LES to relax during swallowing.

- Because of this, food transmission to the stomach is impeded. In severe cases, the oesophagus fails to empty the swallowed food into the stomach for several hours.
- Over months and years, the oesophagus becomes enlarged and infected due to long-standing stasis of food.

Causes: The myenteric plexus of the oesophagus is usually deficient in the region of LES, due to destruction of ganglion cells of Auerbach's plexus by *Trypanosoma cruzi*, stress and emotions. Therefore, the release of VIP and NO is also defective leading to increased resting tone of LES and incomplete relaxation during swallowing.

Diagnosis is based on the following tests:

- Endoscopy
- Barium meal swallow
- Oesophageal manometry

Treatment: Cardiac achalasia can be treated by the following procedures:

- Pneumatic dilatation of the LES
- Incision of oesophageal smooth muscle (myotomy)
- Injection of botulinum toxin into LES to prevent release of ACh (this treatment is effective for about several months)

4. Gastro-Oesophageal Reflux Disease

Gastro-oesophageal reflux disease (GERD) refers to a condition in which incompetence of LES causes reflux of acidic gastric contents into the oesophagus. Reflux of stomach acid causes oesophageal pain (heartburn) and may lead to irritation of the oesophagus or bronchioles (due to aspiration).

Conditions associated with GERD include:

- *Zollinger–Ellison syndrome* (in this condition, there is increased release of gastrin causing increase in acidic gastric secretion)
- Conditions in which emptying of the stomach is not normal (e.g. as in pyloric sphincter disease)
- When the gastric contents are pushed up against the oesophagus (e.g. when the patient is lying down)
- When the LES is forced through the diaphragm into the thoracic cavity (e.g. hiatal hernia)
- When, during pregnancy, the growing fetus may push the top of the stomach into the thorax (the low intrathoracic pressure [compared with the higher intra-abdominal pressure] causes the LES to expand, allowing reflux to occur)
- Conditions in which LES fails to contract between swallows
- Obesity

Diagnosis is mainly based on the signs and symptoms; however, to confirm the diagnosis, the following tests are done:

- *Endoscopy with biopsy* may detect inflammation of the oesophagus and other complications.
- *pH impedance test* is carried out by a flexible catheter which is inserted through the nose and stays in the oesophagus for 24 hours. The data of the amount of acid and non-acid reflux material collected from the stomach into the oesophagus are analysed.

Treatment of GERD includes:

a. *Lifestyle* alteration is done and measures are taken for weight control.
b. *Drugs like* proton pump inhibitors and antacid are used to decrease gastric HCl secretion.
c. *Fundoplication:* In severe cases of GERD, to reduce regurgitation, fundoplication is used. Fundoplication is a procedure in which LES is strengthened by wrapping the upper part of the stomach around the lower part of the oesophagus.

Complications: In severe and long-standing cases, oesophageal stricture and oesophagus adenocarcinoma (Barrel's adenoma) may occur.

5. Dysphagia

Dysphagia is a term used to denote difficulty in swallowing due to sialolithiasis.

Sialolithiasis refers to the formation of stones in the ducts of salivary glands/salivary glands. They block the drainage of saliva, thus causing swelling and pain and dryness of the mouth. The salivary gland stones are usually made of precipitates of calcium and phosphates.

Treatment: The treatment of sialolithiasis mainly consists of:

- *Supportive measures* in the form of:
  - Hydration by drinking plenty of water
  - Gland message (i.e. milking of gland towards duct)
  - Warm compresses (by placing heated damp towels on the swollen area)
  - Sialogogues (in the form of chewing gums)
  - Maintenance of proper oral hygiene
- *Medication* includes nonsteroidal anti-inflammatory drugs and antibiotics.
- *Probing* into the duct through the mouth with a thin blunt instrument can free the stone, which falls into the mouth.
- *Sialendoscopy:* Small and some medium-sized salivary gland stones are primarily treated with sialendoscopy, which is a minimally invasive procedure to extract the stones.

Self-Assessment

1. Discuss the composition, functions, mechanism and regulation of salivary secretion.
2. Discuss about phases and events related to deglutition.
3. Describe briefly:
   - Cardiac achalasia
   - Pathophysiology of gastro-oesophageal reflux disease
4. Write notes on:
   - Dysphasia
   - Oesophageal motility
   - Significance of pH impedance test

Clinical Cases

Case 1

A 67-year-old woman presented with difficulty in swallowing, pain in the chest, regurgitation of food, mouth ulcers and weight loss. On the bases of symptoms and physical findings, the patient was provisionally diagnosed a case of cardiac achalasia.

Q1. What further tests should be carried out to confirm the diagnosis?

Q2. What is the cause of cardiac achalasia?

Q3. What is the treatment to be advised?

Case 2

A 56-year-old male presented to the hospital with symptoms of heartburns, regurgitation and chronic cough, and also a history of asthma.

From symptoms and history, the patient was diagnosed a case of gastro-oesophageal reflux disease (GERD).

Q1. What is the main cause of GERD?

Q2. What further tests should be done to confirm the diagnosis and to find the cause?

Q3. What treatment should be prescribed in this condition?

7.3 Physiological Activities in Stomach

CHAPTER OUTLINE

FUNCTIONAL ANATOMY

GROSS ANATOMY

General Features

- Stomach is a J-shaped hollow muscular bag connected to the oesophagus at its upper end and to the duodenum at its lower end.
- Gastric contents are isolated from the rest of the gastrointestinal tract proximally by the lower oesophageal sphincter (LES) and distally by the pyloric sphincter.
- The *volume* of the stomach is 1200–1500 mL, but its *capacity* is greater than 3000 mL.
- The stomach has two curvatures. The concavity of the right inner curve is called *lesser curvature* and the convexity of the left outer curve is the *greater curvature*. An angle along the lesser curvature, the *incisura angularis*, marks the approximate point at which the stomach narrows before its junction with the duodenum.

Parts of Stomach

The stomach can be divided into five anatomic regions (Fig. 7.3.1):

Cardia is the narrow conical portion of the stomach immediately distal to the gastroesophageal junction.

Fundus is the dome-shaped proximal portion of the stomach.

Body or corpus is the main part of the stomach that extends up to the incisura angularis.

Pyloric antrum extends from the incisura angularis to the pyloric canal.

Pyloric canal or pylorus is the distal-most 1-inch-long tubular part of the stomach.

> **Important Note**
>
> Anatomically, the antrum and pylorus are continuous and respond to the nervous control as a unit. Functionally, the first part of the duodenum is associated with the pyloric part of the stomach.

STRUCTURAL CHARACTERISTICS

The gastric wall consists of mucosa, submucosa, muscular coat and serosa (serous layer). The mucosa and muscular coats of the stomach need to be described in detail to understand the physiology of the stomach.

Gastric Mucosa

- The inner surface of the stomach exhibits coarse *rugae*. These infoldings of mucosa and submucosa extend longitudinally and are most prominent in the proximal stomach.

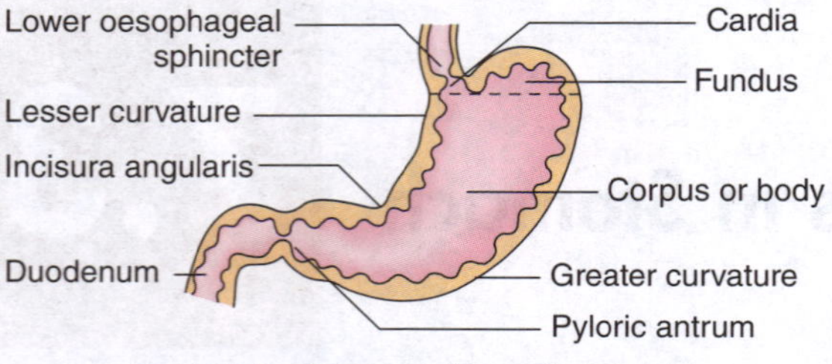

Fig. 7.3.1 Gross anatomy of stomach.

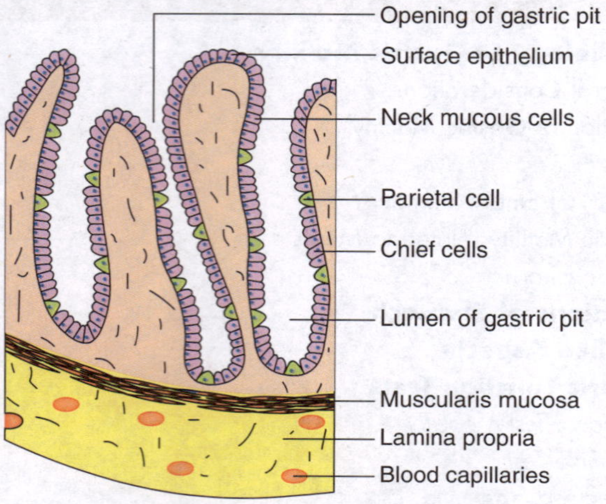

Fig. 7.3.2 Histological features of gastric mucosa.

- A finger mosaic-like pattern is delineated by small furrows in the mucosa.
- The delicate texture of the mucosa is punctured by millions of gastric *foveolae* or pits, leading to the mucosal glands.

Histological features Gastric mucosa comprises (Fig. 7.3.2):

Surface foveolar cells Surface foveolar cells are tall columnar mucin-secreting cells which line the entire gastric mucosa, as well as the gastric pits. These cells have basal nuclei and mucin-containing granules in the supranuclear region.

Mucous neck cells Mucous neck cells are present deeper in the gastric pits. These cells have a lower content of mucin granules and are thought to be the progenitors of both the surface epithelium and the cells of gastric glands.

Glandular cells Glandular cells form the gastric glands. There are three types of gastric glands – main gastric glands, cardiac tubular glands and pyloric (antral) glands.

1. Main gastric glands Main gastric glands, found in the body and fundus of the stomach, are much more in number than in the other gastric glands. These are simple tubular glands (Fig. 7.3.2). The alveoli of main gastric glands contain two types of cells:

Chief cells, also known as peptic or zymogen cells, are basophilic. These cells are concentrated at the base of the main gastric glands. These cells secrete proteolytic proenzymes and pepsinogen I and II.
Parietal cells, also known as oxyntic cells, are acidophilic. These cells predominantly line the upper half of the glands and have an extensive intracellular canalicular system. These secrete *hydrochloric acid* (HCl) and the *intrinsic factor* (IF).

2. Cardiac tubular glands Cardiac tubular glands are found in the mucosa of cardia (a small conical part of the stomach), just around the distal end of the oesophagus. These secrete *soluble mucus*.

3. Pyloric (antral) glands Pyloric (antral) glands are found in the antrum and pylorus region of the stomach. These glands contain two types of cells:

Mucous cells, which secrete *soluble mucus*
G-cells, which are responsible for release of the hormone gastrin

Other cells include:

- Amine precursor uptake decarboxylate (APUD) cells secrete somatostatin are distributed throughout the stomach.
- Enterochromaffin-like (ECL) cells (ECC) are present mainly in the corpus and fundus region near the parietal cells. These cells secrete histamine to stimulate parietal cells.

MUSCULATURE OF STOMACH

Characteristic Features of Gastric Musculature

- The muscle coat of the stomach has three layers – an outer longitudinal, a middle circular and an inner oblique (Fig. 7.3.3).
- As elsewhere in the gut, each muscle layer in the stomach forms a *functional syncytium* and, therefore, acts as a unit. In the fundus, where the layers are relatively thin, the strength of contraction is weak; in the antrum, where the muscle layers are thick, the strength of contraction is greater.
- The stomach and duodenum are divided by a thickened, circular smooth muscle layer called the *pyloric sphincter*.

INNERVATION OF STOMACH

Innervation of the stomach, as elsewhere in the gut (page 561), includes an intrinsic and an extrinsic system.

1. Intrinsic innervation Intrinsic innervation comprises two interconnected plexuses:

Myenteric (Auerbach's) plexus, located between the layers of circular and longitudinal muscles of the stomach
Submucosal (Meissner's) plexus, located in the submucosal layer

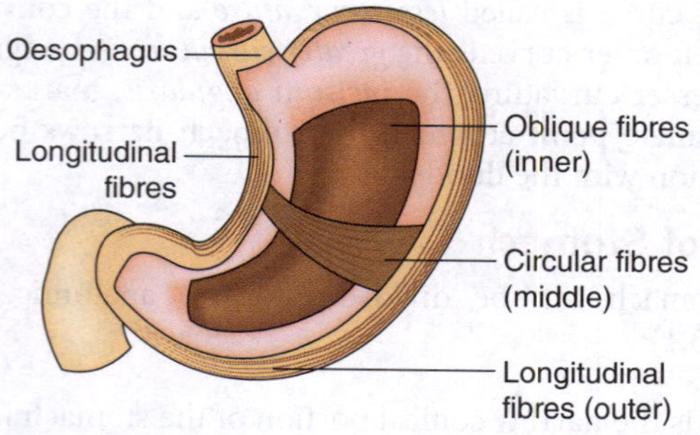

Fig. 7.3.3 Three layers of gastric mucosa.

The intrinsic innervation is directly responsible for peristalsis and other contractions. Because this system is continuous between the stomach and the duodenum, peristalsis in the antrum influences the duodenal bulb.

2. Extrinsic innervation Extrinsic innervation modifies the coordinated motor activity that arises independently in the intrinsic nervous system. It consists of the two components of the autonomic nervous system:

Sympathetic innervation comes via the coeliac plexus and inhibits motility.

Parasympathetic innervation comes via the vagus nerve and stimulates motility

PHYSIOLOGY OF GASTRIC SECRETION

The gastric secretions include:

- *Exocrine secretions*, i.e. gastric juice
- *Endocrine secretions*, i.e. gastrin hormone (see regulation of gastric secretion, page 581)

GASTRIC JUICE

Composition

Gastric glands secrete about 2–2.5 L of gastric juice in the lumen of the stomach per day. It is acidic with a pH varying from 1 to 2. Important constituents of gastric juice are as follows:

Water: 99.45%

Solids: 0.55%, which include:

Electrolytes such as Na^+, K^+, Mg^{2+}, Cl^-, HCO_3^-, HPO_4^{2-} and SO_4^{2-}. The electrolyte content of gastric juice varies with the rate of secretions. At low secretory rates, Na^+ concentration is high and H^+ concentration is low, but as acid secretion increases, Na^+ concentration falls.

Enzymes present in the gastric juice are as follows:

- *Pepsin* is a proteolytic enzyme which is secreted by chief cells of gastric glands in an inactive form pepsinogen. Pepsinogen is activated to pepsin in the presence of HCl at an optimal pH of about 2.
- *Gastric lipase* is a weak fat-splitting enzyme. It is of little importance in fat digestion except in pancreatic insufficiency.
- *Gastric gelatinase* liquefies gelatin, a protein contained in connective tissue.
- *Gastric amylase* is present in small amounts.
- *Lysozyme* is bactericidal.
- *Carbonic anhydrase* is present in small amounts.

Mucin or mucus is of two types:

- ***Soluble mucus*** secreted by mucous cells of pyloric and cardiac glands
- ***Insoluble mucus*** secreted by surface foveolar cells (tall columnar mucin-secreting cells) lining the entire gastric mucosa

Intrinsic factor (IF) is secreted by parietal cells of gastric glands.

Secretion of Gastric Juice

Secretion of HCl

General consideration HCl is secreted by the *parietal cells* (also called oxyntic cells). These cells show under electron microscope as a complex network of *intracellular canaliculi* (Fig. 7.3.4) into which HCl is secreted.

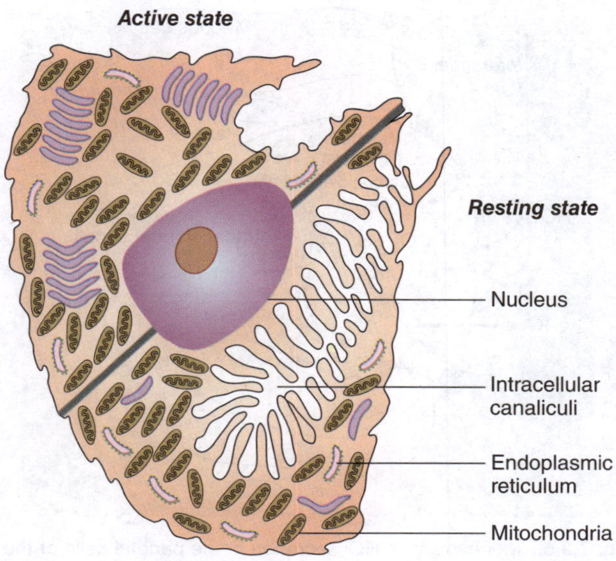

Fig. 7.3.4 Parietal cell showing secretion of H^+ and Cl^- in the intracellular canaliculi which pour HCl into the stomach. Note the presence of numerous mitochondria which provide energy for the active transport process. HCl, hydrochloric acid.

- Gastric glands secrete about 2.5 L of HCl in a day. The HCl secreted by gastric glands is concentrated having a pH of approximately 1.0.
- The gastric HCl dissociates completely into H^+ and Cl^-. The concentration of H^+ in the gastric juice increases with the increase in the rate of its secretion. At high rates of secretion, H^+ concentration may be as high as 155 mEq/L, i.e. about 3 million times greater than its concentration in the blood.

Mechanism of HCl secretion Various theories have been put forward to explain the origin of H^+ of HCl (e.g. Davenport and Fisher theory, Davies theory and Hollander hypothesis). However, it is still not known exactly. The hypothesis more widely accepted is shown in Fig. 7.3.5. HCl is made up of hydrogen (H^+) and chloride (Cl^-) ions and, therefore, its secretion can be described in two steps, i.e. secretion of H^+ and secretion of Cl^-.

Secretion of H^+ ions The H^+ ions are believed to be generated inside the parietal cell from metabolic CO_2 and H_2O present in the cell.

- The enzyme carbonic anhydrase present in abundance in the parietal cells is essential for the secretion. It accelerates the formation of H_2CO_3 which dissociates to release H^+ and HCO_3^- as follows:

$$CO_2 + H_2O \xrightarrow{\text{Carbonic anhydrase}} H_2CO_3 \rightarrow H^+ + HCO_3^-$$

- The H^+ ions generated by the above reaction are then secreted into the lumen of the canaliculi in exchange for K^+ by a primary active transport mediated by H^+–K^+-ATPase pump or proton pump (Fig. 7.3.5). This H^+–K^+ exchange is obviously electroneutral.

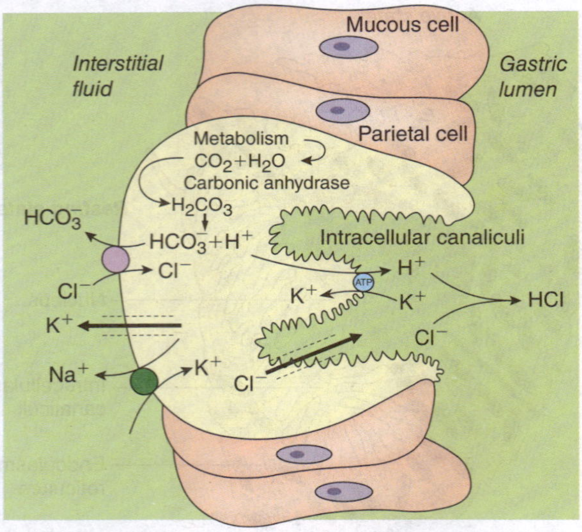

Fig. 7.3.5 Mechanism of HCl secretion in the parietal cells of the stomach. HCl, hydrochloric acid.

> **Important Note**
>
> The drug omeprazole, used to decrease HCl formation, inhibits the H^+–K^+-ATPase and blocks H^+ secretion.

- In resting condition, the proton pumps are sequestered as tubulovesicles within the parietal cell membrane. In active stage, these proton pumps get fused with the canaliculi present on the apical membrane; thus, positioning of proton pumps on the membrane helps in acid secretion.
- The K^+ channels present on the apical membrane supply K^+ for exchange of H^+ secretion.
- The HCO_3^- ions produced in the parietal cell are transported by an antiport in the serosal (basolateral) membrane into the blood in exchange of Cl^- by an active transport via Cl^-/HCO_3^- exchange. The HCO_3^-/Cl^- exchange is again electroneutral.

> **Important Note**
>
> The HCO_3^- released into the blood is responsible for the postprandial alkaline tide associated with increased gastric acid secretion after meals, which is characterized by alkaline urine, slightly depressed breathing and raised alveolar pCO_2.

Note: Eventually, this HCO_3^- from the blood will be secreted in pancreatic secretion to neutralize H^+ in the small intestine. If vomiting occurs, gastric H^+ never arrives in the small intestine, there is no stimulus for pancreatic HCO_3^- secretion and the arterial blood becomes alkaline (metabolic alkalosis).

Secretion of Cl^- Because of the high intracellular negativity, the Cl^- present in the parietal cell is forced out into the lumen of gland through the Cl^- channels located on the apical membrane of the cell. These Cl^- channels are activated by cAMP. The high intracellular negativity is the result of the following (Fig. 7.3.5):

- The Na^+–K^+ pump located on the basolateral membrane of parietal cells pumps out three Na^+ for every two K^+ pumped in, thereby creating intracellular negativity.
- The K^+ pumped in diffuses out through the K^+ channels present on the basolateral as well as apical membranes. This diffusion further increases intracellular negativity of parietal cells.

> **Important Note**
>
> It is important to note that the active transport processes involved in the generation of HCl require a large amount of adenosine triphosphate (ATP). The ATP generated by mitochondria is found in very high concentration (40% of cell volume) within the parietal cell (Fig. 7.3.4).

Factors affecting HCl secretion include:

Factors stimulating HCl secretion:

- Vagal stimulation
- Gastrin
- Histamine

Factors that inhibit HCl secretion:

- Low pH in the stomach (<3) by negative feedback mechanism
- Intestinal influences
- Somatostatin
- Prostaglandins (PGE_2 and PGI_2), epidermal growth factor (EGF) and transforming growth factor (TGF)

Functions of HCl are:

- HCl participates in the breakdown of protein.
- It provides an optimal pH for the action of pepsin.
- It hinders the growth of pathogenic bacteria.

Pepsinogen Secretion

Pepsinogen is an inactive precursor (proenzyme) of pepsin. It is mainly secreted by *chief cells* of the main gastric glands. A small amount of pepsinogen is also secreted by pyloric glands. The pepsinogen secreted by chief cells is called *pepsinogen I* and that secreted by pyloric glands is called *pepsinogen II*. Pepsinogen I and II can be differentiated by the immunological method but their physiological significance is not known.

Pepsinogen is synthesized and stored as zymogen granules in the apical region of chief cells.

Pepsinogen secretion is stimulated by vagal stimulation, gastrin and histamine.

Pepsinogen is converted to pepsin (the active form) by the action of HCl or preformed pepsin.

$$\text{Pepsinogen} \xrightarrow{\text{HCl}} \text{Pepsin}$$
$$\text{Pepsinogen} \xrightarrow{\text{Pepsin}} \text{Pepsin}$$

Function of pepsinogen Pepsin, the active form of pepsinogen, is a proteolytic enzyme that begins the process of protein digestion. It splits protein into proteoses, peptones and polypeptides; for details, see page 636. It is important to note that the optimum pH for the action of pepsin is 2.0; therefore, acid secretion by the stomach is as essential as pepsinogen secretion for the digestion of proteins.

Secretion of Mucus

Mucus is of two types – insoluble and soluble.

Insoluble mucus is secreted by the mucus-secreting cells lining the entire gastric mucosa. The insoluble mucus is such a viscid that it forms a gel-like coat over the mucosa. These cells also secrete bicarbonate ions which make the mucus with alkaline pH of 7 that forms an extremely important protective layer saving the stomach from the destruction of HCl and substances known as trefoil peptides that stabilize the mucus bicarbonate layer.

Soluble mucus is secreted by mucous cells of pylorus and cardiac glands.

Mucus secretion is increased by direct stimulation of mucosa by the rough food. Neural or hormonal control over secretion of mucus, if any, is not known.

Secretion of Intrinsic Factor (IF)

Secretion IF, a glycoprotein, is secreted by the parietal cells of gastric mucosa, chiefly by those in the fundus. The secretion of IF by the parietal cells is linked to the action of histamine through cAMP mechanism.

Functions The IF is essential for the absorption of vitamin B_{12}. It forms a complex with vitamin B_{12}, which is carried to the terminal ileum where the vitamin is absorbed.

Applied Aspects

Deficiency of IF in some patients with idiopathic atrophy of gastric mucosa may cause a serious disorder called pernicious anaemia (see page 155).

REGULATION OF GASTRIC SECRETION

Regulation of gastric secretion can be discussed under three subheads:

- Regulatory mechanisms
- Phases of gastric secretion and their regulation
- Experimental demonstration of the role of regulatory mechanisms

Regulatory Mechanisms

Mechanisms regulating the gastric secretion include neural control and chemical control.

Neural Control

Neural control over the gastric glands is exerted by local enteric plexus involving cholinergic neurons and impulses from the CNS via vagal (extrinsic) innervation.

Vagal stimulation increases the secretion of HCl by parietal cells and pepsin by chief cells. It increases H^+ secretion by a direct path and an indirect path (Fig. 7.3.6):

In the direct path, the vagus nerve fibres innervating parietal cells stimulate H^+ secretion by releasing neurotransmitter acetylcholine (ACh), originating from the dorsal vagus complex, which acts on the muscarinic receptors on parietal cells. The second messengers involved in it are IP_3 and increased intracellular Ca^{2+}. In addition, ACh also potentiates the effects of histamine on H_2 receptors of parietal cells.

In the indirect path, the vagus nerve innervates G-cells and stimulates the release of gastrin into circulation through gastrin-releasing peptide (GRP). GRP is a neurotransmitter released from enteric plexus nerve endings. The gastrin, in turn, stimulates H^+ secretion by the mechanism, described a bit later.

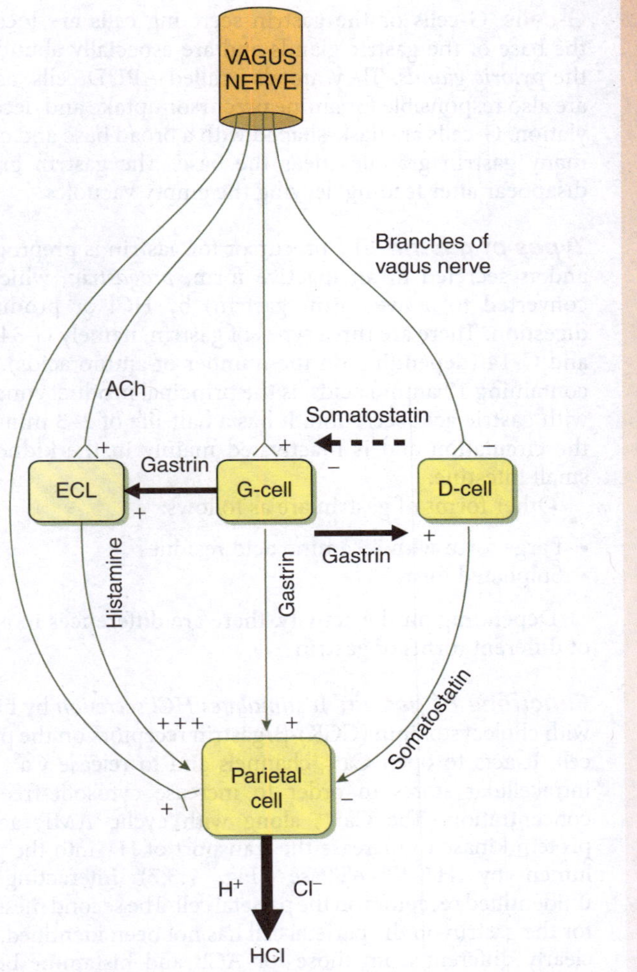

Fig. 7.3.6 Mechanisms by which vagal stimulation increase H^+ secretion in parietal cells.

Furthermore, vagal stimulation also inhibits the release of *somatostatin* and thus indirectly stimulates H^+ secretion by removing the inhibitory effect of somatostatin on the parietal cells.

- ACh released on vagal stimulation also acts on the ECC, which release histamine. Histamine increases H^+ secretion by acting on H_2 receptors on the parietal cells.

Chemical Control

Chemical control on gastric glands is exerted mainly through:

- *Gastrin*, a hormone secreted by G-cells
- *Histamine*, a paracrine agent released from the mast cells of gastric mucosa
- *Somatostatin*, secreted by D-cells
- *Low pH* (<3.0) in the stomach which acts in a negative feedback mechanism
- *Local hormones* released in the duodenum which inhibit the gastric secretion, in addition to promoting the secretion of pancreatic juice and bile

1. Role of gastrin Gastrin, a hormone, is secreted by the G-cells into the blood circulation (and not into gastric juice). It reaches the stomach through the arterial circulation and stimulates secretory activity of the parietal cells and chief cells.

G-cells G-cells or the gastrin-secreting cells are located at the base of the gastric glands and are especially abundant in the *pyloric glands.* They are also called APUD cells, as these are also responsible for amine precursor uptake and decarboxylation. G-cells are flask-shaped with a broad base and contain many gastrin granules near the base. The gastrin granules disappear after feeding, leaving the empty vacuoles.

Types of gastrin The precursor for gastrin is preprogastrin and is secreted in an inactive form, *progastrin,* which gets converted to active form (gastrin) by HCl or products of digestion. There are three types of gastrin, namely G-34, G-17 and G-14 (depending on the number of amino acids). G-17, containing 17 amino acids, is the principal product concerned with gastric acid secretion. It has a half-life of 2–3 minutes in the circulation and is inactivated mainly in the kidney and small intestine.

Other forms of gastrin are as follows:

- Large form with 45 amino acid residues
- Sulphated form

Depending on the activity, there are differences in activity of different forms of gastrin.

Functions of gastrin It *stimulates HCl secretion* by binding with cholecystokinin (CCK)-β/gastrin receptors on the parietal cell. It acts to open Ca^{2+} channels and to release Ca^{2+} from intracellular stores in order to increase cytosolic-free Ca^{2+} concentration. The Ca^{2+}, along with cyclic AMP, acts via protein kinase to increase the transport of H^+ into the gastric lumen by H^+–K^+-ATPase (Fig. 7.3.7) interacting with unidentified receptors on the parietal cell. The second messenger for the gastrin on the parietal cell has not been identified, but is clearly different from those for ACh and histamine because their actions are additive with those of gastrin.

Gastrin also increases the HCl secretion by stimulating secretion of histamine from the *ECC* present in the body of the stomach.

- *Increases gastric and intestinal motility* (it also causes contraction of LES and it has a feeble influence on gall bladder contraction)
- *Increases pancreatic secretion* of insulin and glucagon, but only after a protein meal
- *Trophic action,* i.e. it is necessary for the proper growth of gastrointestinal mucosa

Factors stimulating gastrin secretion are:

Vagal stimulation: Vagal stimulation increases gastrin release through GRP and not through release of neurotransmitter ACh. Because of this, atropine (which blocks muscarinic receptors) does not affect release of gastrin from G-cells.

Distension of the pyloric antrum increases gastrin secretion through the intrinsic innervation. This fact can be proved experimentally by Heidenhain's pouch (see page 585).

Products of protein digestion (e.g. peptides and amino acids), alcohol and coffee also increase gastrin secretion.

Calcium and epinephrine are also reported to increase gastrin secretion.

Factors inhibiting gastrin secretion are:

Low pH of gastric juice (<3) inhibits gastrin secretion and forms the basis of negative feedback mechanism controlling HCl release.

Somatostatin, released by D-cells (located adjacent to G-cells or parietal cells in gastric mucosa), inhibits gastrin secretion by G-cells.

Other substances that inhibit gastrin secretion are secretin, gastric inhibitory peptide (GIP), vasoactive intestinal peptide (VIP), glucagon and calcitonin.

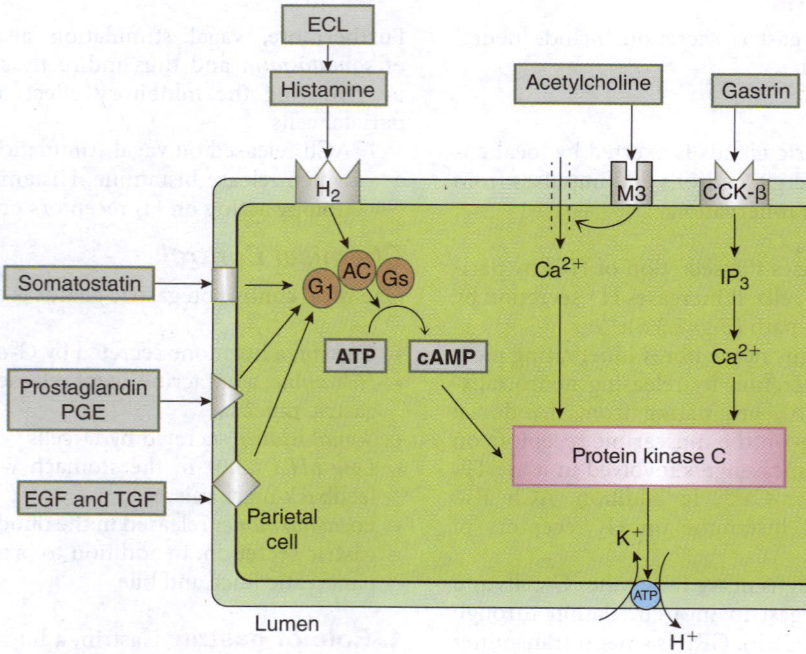

Fig. 7.3.7 Control of HCl secretion at the parietal cell level. Acetylcholine (ACh), histamine and gastrin act as agonists of HCl secretion by distinct mechanism (for details, see text). Somatostatin, prostaglandins (PGE), epidermal growth factor (EGF) and transforming growth factor (TGF) act as endogenous antagonists of HCl secretion by inhibiting adenylyl cyclase. HCl, hydrochloric acid.

2. Role of histamine Histamine is released from the ECC found in the oxyntic region of the stomach in the base of the gastric gland. ECC bear both gastrin receptors and ACh receptors.

- They release histamine in response to both circulating gastrin and ACh released by vagal fibres. The histamine released stimulates *HCl secretion* from parietal cells by acting on H_2 receptors.
- The H_2 receptors increase intracellular cAMP via Gs. The cAMP acts as a second messenger to activate cAMP-dependent protein kinase.
- These events stimulate HCl secretion by activating basolateral K^+ channels, and also cause H^+–K^+-ATPase molecules and Cl^- channel to be inserted into apical plasma membrane (Fig. 7.3.7). The second messenger for histamine is cyclic AMP.

Important Note

Histamine is classified as a paracrine agent because it diffuses from its release site to the parietal cells (rather than travelling within the circulation, as does a hormone).

Applied Aspects

H_2 receptor–blocking drugs, such as cimetidine and ranitidine, inhibit H^+ secretion by blocking the stimulatory effect of histamine.

3. Role of somatostatin Somatostatin, a growth-inhibiting hormone, is released from D-cells in gastrointestinal mucosa and of pancreatic islets. There are two types of somatostatins, i.e. somatostatin 14 and 28.

- Somatostatin is secreted by D-cells located adjacent to G-cells or the parietal cells in the gastric glands.
- Somatostatin secretion by D-cells is stimulated by secretin, enteroglucagon, GIP and VIP.
- Somatostatin inhibits HCl secretion in two ways:
  - *Directly* by its action on parietal cells
  - *Indirectly* by inhibiting gastrin secretion by G-cells
- Somatostatin, prostaglandins, EGF and TGF act on parietal cells to inhibit HCl secretion by inhibiting adenylyl cyclase (Fig. 7.3.7).

4. Role of low pH (<3) in stomach Low pH (<3) in the stomach inhibits the secretion of H^+ by parietal cells by a negative feedback mechanism:

- After a meal is ingested, H^+ secretion is stimulated by cephalic and gastric influences.
- After the meal is digested and the stomach emptied, further H^+ secretion decreases the pH of stomach contents.
- When the pH of stomach contents is <3.0, *gastrin secretion is inhibited*, which in turn inhibits H^+ secretion. This forms the so-called *negative feedback mechanism*.
- On the other hand, if the pH of gastric contents rises above 3.5 (due to buffering action of food), the release of gastrin is stimulated. In this way, the negative feedback control over gastrin release maintains the pH of gastric contents near 3.

5. Intestinal influences When chyme containing acid, fats and products of protein digestion reaches the duodenum, it causes the release of several intestinal hormones like secretin, CCK and GIP.

Interaction of Neural and Chemical Regulatory Mechanisms

The neural and hormonal mechanisms *potentiate* each other's effect. Potentiation is said to occur when the response to simultaneous administration of two stimulants is greater than the sum of responses to either agent given alone.

Potentiation of gastric H^+ secretion can be explained in part, because each agent has a different mechanism of action on the parietal cell. Fig. 7.3.6 demonstrates that:

- Histamine potentiates the actions of ACh and gastrin.
- ACh potentiates the actions of histamine and gastrin.

Phases of Gastric Secretion and their Regulation

Meal-related gastric secretion can be divided into three phases:

- Cephalic phase
- Gastric phase
- Intestinal phase

1. Cephalic phase Cephalic phase of gastric secretion occurs before the entry of food into the stomach.

- Rate of gastric juice secretion during this phase is high, about 500 mL/h, but this phase lasts for a short time and accounts for about 45% of total gastric juice secretion during a meal.
- Cephalic phase of gastric secretion is *initiated* by the thought, sight, smell or taste of food. Neurogenic signals originate in the cerebral cortex and appetite centres of the amygdala or hypothalamus. The impulses are transmitted to dorsal vagal nuclei and from there through the vagi to the stomach (Fig. 7.3.8). The vagal efferent fibres stimulate secretion of HCl from parietal cells, gastrin from G-cells and pepsinogen from peptic (chief) cells.
- Emotions also influence this vagally mediated gastric secretion. *Anger and hostility* are associated with increased gastric secretion and motility. *Fear and depression* decrease the gastric secretion and motility. In high-strung and aggressive individuals, increased vagal discharge produces gastric secretion even during nondigestive periods, leading to hyperacidity or even peptic ulceration.

2. Gastric phase Gastric phase of gastric secretion occurs when food enters the stomach.

- Rate of gastric juice secretion during this phase is less (200 mL/h) as compared with that in the cephalic phase. But this phase lasts for a long time (as long as food remains in the stomach) and so accounts for about 50% the total gastric secretion.
- The presence of food in the stomach induces gastric secretion by the following *mechanisms*:
  Distension of the body of the stomach acting through local myenteric and vagovagal reflexes results in increase in HCl secretion.
  Distension of the antrum initiates vagally mediated and local reflexes that result in gastrin release from the antral G-cells. Gastrin release is inhibited when pH becomes low (<3).
  Products of partial protein digestion also stimulate gastrin secretion and this increases secretion mainly of gastric acid.
  Low pH causes increased pepsinogen secretion through local reflexes.

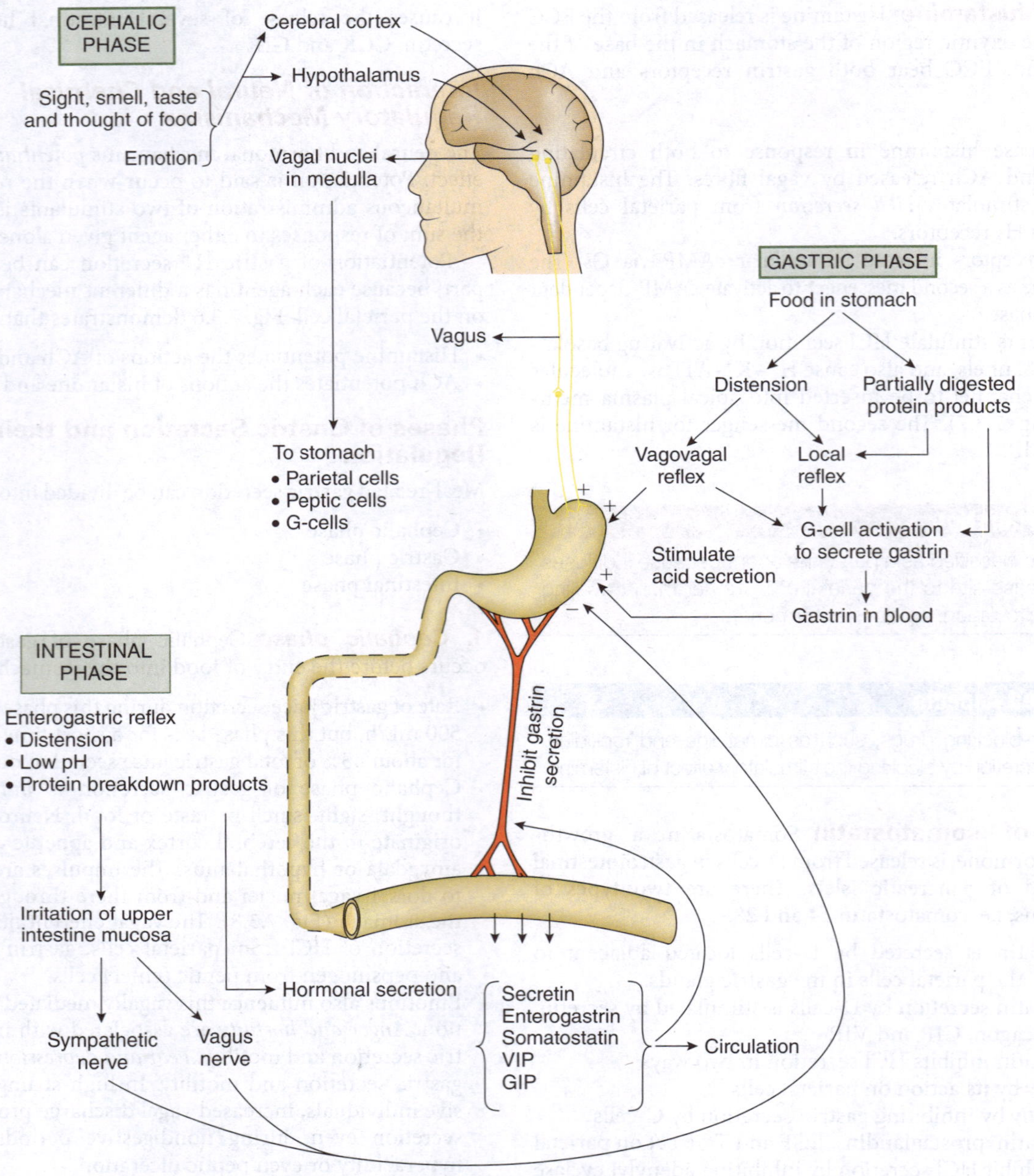

Fig. 7.3.8 Phases and regulation of gastric secretion.

3. *Intestinal phase* Intestinal phase of gastric secretion begins as the chyme begins to empty from the stomach into the duodenum.

- In contrast to the excitatory cephalic and gastric influences, the intestinal influence on the gastric secretion is chiefly inhibitory in nature. Intestinal factor inhibits gastric secretion by the following mechanisms:
  Enterogastric reflex is initiated by the distension of the small intestine, presence of acid or protein breakdown products in the upper intestine and irritation of mucosa. The reflex activity involves intrinsic as well as extrinsic sympathetic and vagus nerves and inhibits gastric secretion.
  Hormonal mechanism: Presence of acid, fat, hypertonic or hypotonic solution and irritating factors in the upper small intestine releases several hormones such as secretin, CCK, GIP, VIP and somatostatin which inhibit gastric secretion.
- The inhibitory influences discussed above help to terminate the gastric secretion when all the food has left the stomach.
- Products of protein digestion, however, have a slight stimulatory effect on gastric acid secretion.

Experimental Demonstration of Regulation of Gastric Secretion

Phases and regulation of gastric secretion have been studied by certain experiments which are described briefly.

1. Sham feeding: an experiment to demonstrate cephalic phase of gastric secretion Cephalic phase of gastric secretion, i.e. secretion of gastric juice before the entry of food, can be demonstrated by sham feeding experiment. For this, the oesophagus of a dog is exposed and divided in the middle of the neck and the two cut ends are brought to the

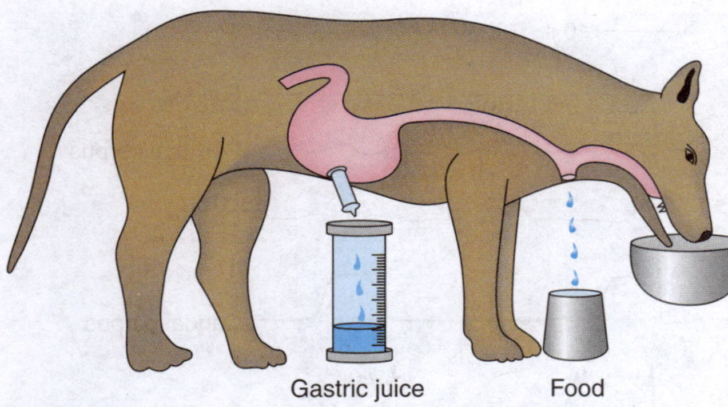

Fig. 7.3.9 Sham feeding experiment to demonstrate initiation of cephalic phase of gastric secretion.

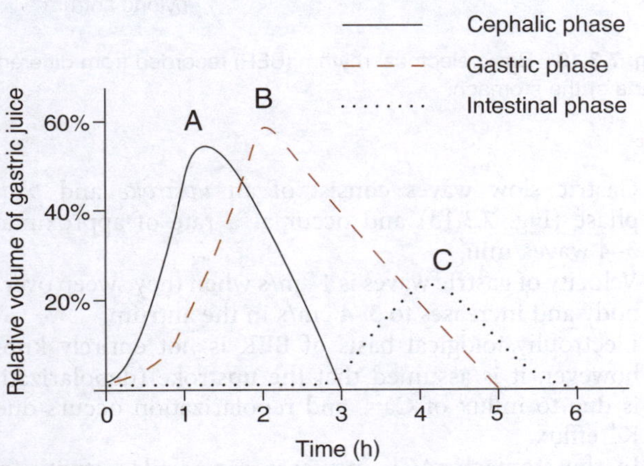

Fig. 7.3.10 Volume and time curve of different phases of gastric secretion: **A**, cephalic phase; **B**, gastric phase; and **C**, intestinal phase.

surface (Fig. 7.3.9). When a dog swallows, the food comes out through the upper cut end of the oesophagus and does not enter the stomach. Gastric secretion, which occurs before the entry of food into the stomach (caused by sight, smell and taste of food), represents the *cephalic phase* and is collected for study by passing a tube in the stomach through the lower cut end of the oesophagus.

Study of gastric juice so collected shows that (Fig. 7.3.10):

- Cephalic phase of the so-called appetite juice begins after a latency of 5–7 minutes.
- The volume reaches the peak within an hour.
- Gastric secretion continues for 3 hours.
- Gastric juice so collected is highly acidic and rich in pepsin.

2. Pavlov's pouch experiment to demonstrate that vagus is secretomotor nerve to stomach For this, under general anaesthesia, a pouch of the stomach with intact nerve and blood supply is separated from the body of the stomach by incising the mucosa and keeping the muscle layer intact. The intactness of a larger, main part of the stomach is restored by applying sutures. An outlet is made in the smaller part (pouch) so separated and is brought out through the abdominal wall to provide drainage for the pouch secretion (Fig. 7.3.11). The vagus nerve is exposed and divided in the neck and the animal is allowed to recover.

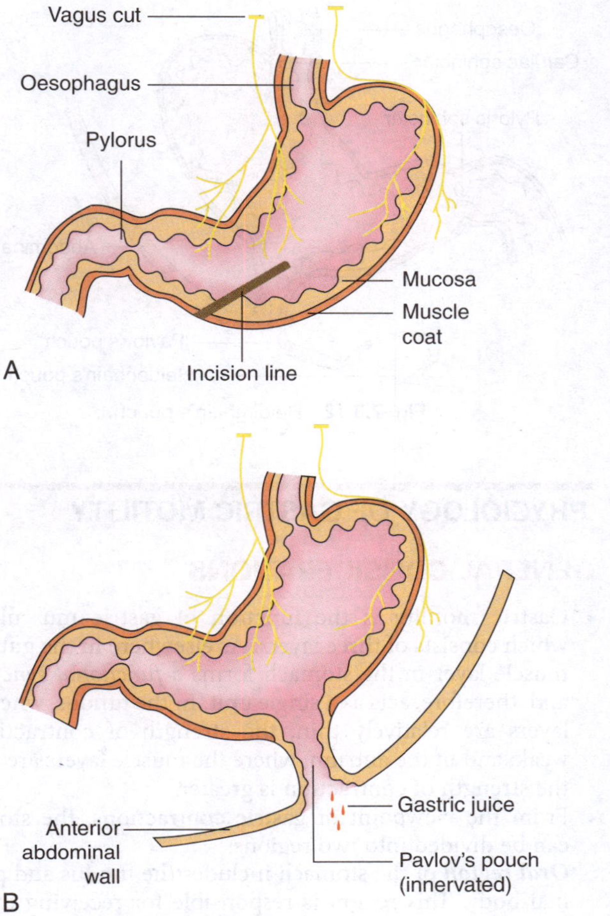

Fig. 7.3.11 Preparation of Pavlov's pouch: **A**, site of incision; and **B**, Pavlov's pouch opening outside through anterior abdominal wall.

After some days, the peripheral cut end of the vagus is stimulated in the unanaesthetized dog. Flow of gastric juice rich in HCl and pepsin after a short latent period demonstrates that the vagus nerve is the secretomotor to the stomach.

3. Heidenhain's pouch experiment to demonstrate existence of some blood-borne mechanism regulating gastric secretion

- Heidenhain's pouch is a modified Pavlov's pouch, which is separated in such a way from the antral part of the stomach that it is denervated but with intact blood supply (Fig. 7.3.12).
- Distension of the denervated pouch (with intact blood supply) induces gastric secretion. Occurrence of gastric secretion in a denervated pouch of the stomach demonstrates that there exists some blood-borne mechanism which also regulates gastric secretion.
- Intravenous injection of gastrin is followed after 5 minutes by secretion of gastric juice from the denervated Heidenhain's pouch. This demonstrates that the blood-borne mechanism is mediated by the gastrin hormone released from the antral mucosa.

Note: Bickel's, Farrell's and Ivy's pouches are other examples of completely denervated pouches, which have been used to study the gastric secretion.

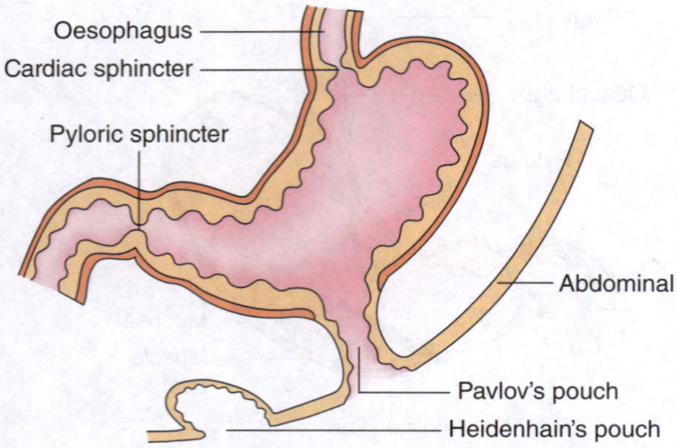

Fig. 7.3.12 Heidenhain's pouch.

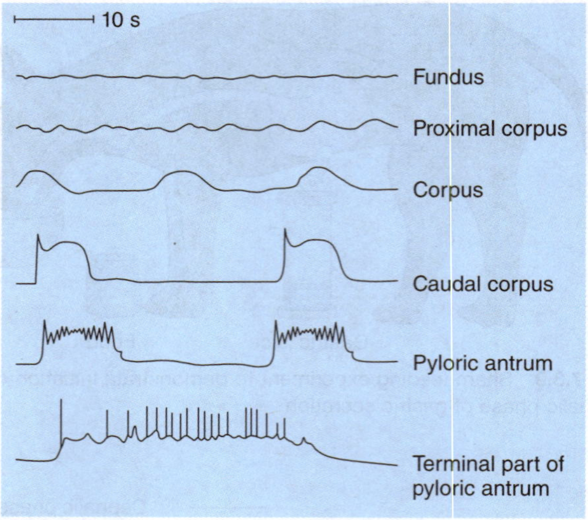

Fig. 7.3.13 Basic electrical rhythm (BER) recorded from different parts of the stomach.

PHYSIOLOGY OF GASTRIC MOTILITY

GENERAL CONSIDERATIONS

- Gastric motility is the function of gastric musculature, which consists of three layers. As elsewhere in the gut, each muscle layer in the stomach forms a *functional syncytium* and, therefore, acts as a single unit. In the fundus, where the layers are relatively thin, the strength of contraction is weak; and in the antrum, where the muscle layers are thick, the strength of contraction is greater.
- From the viewpoint of gastric contractions, the stomach can be divided into two regions:
  Oral region of the stomach includes the fundus and proximal body. This region is responsible for receiving the ingested food.
  Caudal region of the stomach includes the antrum and the distal part of the body of the stomach. This region is responsible for the contractions that mix food and propel it into the duodenum.

Motor functions of stomach Motor functions of the stomach observed by gastric motility are as follows:

Storage of food is accomplished by a special gesture of gastric musculature of the oral region called the receptive relaxation.
Mixing of food with gastric juice to form semisolid paste (chyme) is accomplished by enhanced contractile activity (combination of peristalsis and retropulsion) in the caudal region.
Slow emptying of food into the small intestine is carried out by contractions in the caudal region of the stomach.

INITIATION OF GASTRIC MOTILITY

Basic Electrical Rhythm

- The musculature of the stomach, being a single-unit smooth muscle, has its only rhythmic contractile myogenic tone called the *basic electrical rhythm* (BER) or *gastric slow waves*. Thus, the BER represents a wave of depolarization of smooth muscle cells proceeding from the circular muscles of the fundus of the stomach to the pyloric sphincter.
- The gastric slow waves are initiated by *pacemaker cells* (interstitial cells of Cajal) located in the outer circular muscle layer and near the myenteric plexus near the fundus on the greater curvature of the stomach.
- Gastric slow waves consist of an *upstroke* and *plateau* phase (Fig. 7.3.13) and occur at a rate of approximately 3–4 waves/min.
- Velocity of gastric waves is 1 cm/s when they sweep over the body and increases to 3–4 cm/s in the antrum.
- Electrophysiological basis of BER is not entirely known; however, it is assumed that the upstroke (depolarization) is due to influx of Ca^{2+} and repolarization occurs due to K^+ efflux.
- In the stomach, ACh increases contractile activity (produces peristalsis) by increasing the amplitude and duration of plateau phase of slow gastric waves. Other agents that initiate contraction of smooth muscles of the stomach are gastrin, histamine, nicotine, barium and K^+. Agents that inhibit the activity are enterogastrone, epinephrine, norepinephrine, atropine and Ca^{2+}.

Types of gastric motility *The peristaltic activity of the gastric musculature has been given various names depending on its features and motor function subserved by it. Gastric motility can be described as follows:*

Motility of the empty stomach, which includes:
- Migrating motor complex (MMC)
- Hunger contractions

Gastric motility related to meal includes:
- Receptive relaxation
- Mixing peristaltic waves
- Gastric emptying

MOTILITY OF EMPTY STOMACH

Migrating motor complexes MMC is the name given to the peristaltic wave that begins in the oesophagus and travels through the entire gastrointestinal tract (migratory motor activity) during interdigestive period.

- The MMCs remove any food remaining in the stomach during interdigestive period.
- The MMC wave travels at a regular rate (5 cm/min) and occurs every 60–90 minutes during the interdigestive period.

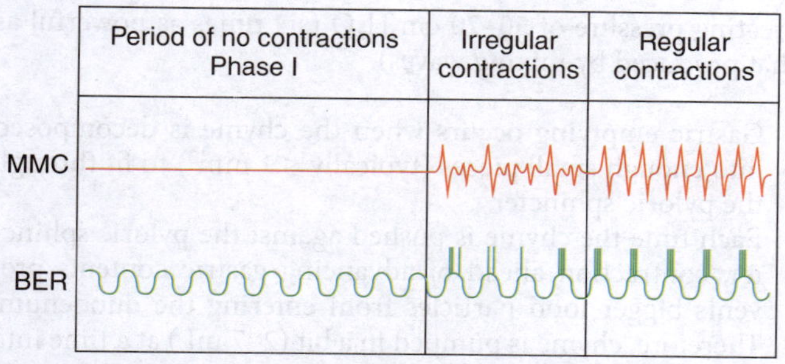

Fig. 7.3.14 Relation of basic electrical rhythm (BER) with migratory motor complexes (MMCs).

- Each cycle of MMC has three phases – each MMC begins with a quiescent period (phase I), continues to a period of irregular electrical and mechanical activity (phase II) and ends with a burst of regular activity (phase III).
- There is a close correlation of the basic electrical rhythm (BER) and migratory motor complexes (MMCs). When there are no MMCs, the BER consists of rhythmic oscillation of the resting membrane potential (RMP) between about −65 and −45 mV. During the MMC, the electrical oscillations are superimposed with spikes (Fig. 7.3.14).
- Each MMC is associated with increase in gastric secretion, bile flow and pancreatic secretion.
- As the MMCs clear the stomach and small intestine of luminal contents in preparation for the next meal, they have been called the *interdigestive housekeepers*.
- The hormone motilin, which is released from the endocrine cells within the epithelium of the small intestine, increases the strength of MMC.
- The MMCs are abolished immediately after the entry of food in the stomach.

Hunger contractions Mild peristaltic contractions occur in the empty stomach, which over a period of hours increase in intensity and are called hunger contractions. MMCs are probably responsible for hunger contractions. When they become extremely strong, they fuse to cause *tetanic* contraction lasting for 2–3 minutes which can be felt and may even be painful. These are associated with the sensation of hunger.

GASTRIC MOTILITY RELATED TO MEALS

Receptive relaxation and accommodation Storage function of the stomach is accomplished by receptive relaxation and accommodation.

- The empty stomach has a volume of about 50 mL only and the diameter of its lumen is only slightly more than that of the small intestine.
- As stated earlier, as soon as the food enters the stomach, the MMCs are abolished and the fundus and upper part of the body of the stomach, i.e. the *oral region*, relaxes to accommodate the ingested food without any increase in intramural pressure. This phenomenon is called *receptive relaxation* (Fig. 7.3.15).
- The passage of each bolus of food stimulates the stretch *receptors of oral region* and produces further relaxation. By the end of the meal, the smooth muscles of the oral region of the stomach relax to such an extent that 1–2 L of food can be accommodated.

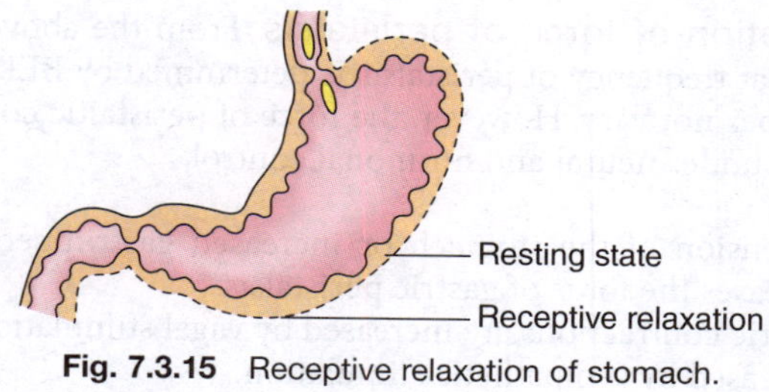

Fig. 7.3.15 Receptive relaxation of stomach.

- Receptive relaxation is a *vagovagal reflex* initiated by distension of the stomach and is synchronized with the primary peristaltic waves in the oesophagus.
- CCK participates in receptive relaxation by increasing the distensibility of the oral stomach.
- The inhibitory neurotransmitter responsible for receptive relaxation and accommodation is either VIP or NO.
- Vagotomy abolishes receptive relaxation.

Mixing peristaltic waves The presence of food in the caudal region (distal body and antral part) of the stomach increases the contractile activity of this part of the stomach. This enhanced contractile activity (a combination of peristalsis and retropulsion) is called mixing waves which mix the food with stomach acid and enzymes and break it into smaller and smaller pieces. When the food is mixed into a pasty consistency, it is called *chyme*.

Initiation and production of peristalsis Peristalsis is the coordinated pattern of smooth muscle contraction and relaxation in which a wave of relaxation precedes the wave of contraction. Peristaltic contractions are produced by periodic changes in membrane potential (BER, described earlier). The rhythmicity of gastric peristalsis is determined by the BER which has a frequency of 3–4/min (slow waves). Certain neurotransmitters like ACh or hormone gastrin cause generation of depolarizing spikes at the peak of BER cycles resulting in mechanical contraction (peristalsis). The number of spikes fired in a slow wave determines the force of each peristaltic contraction (Fig. 7.3.16).

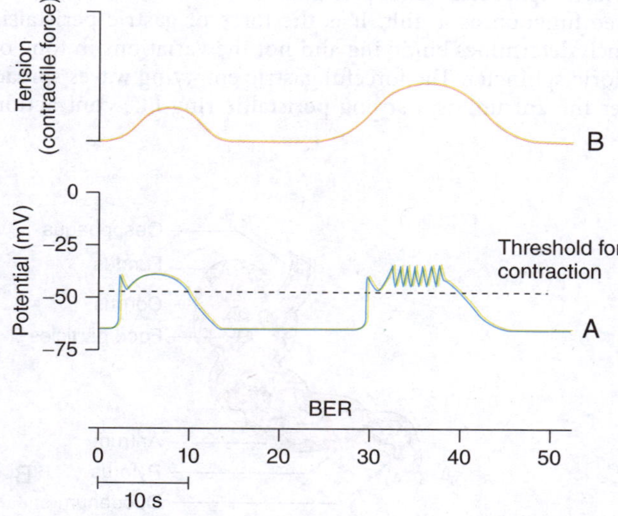

Fig. 7.3.16 **A**, membrane potentials of smooth muscle of stomach; and **B**, and their relation with mechanical response.

Regulation of force of peristalsis From the above, it is clear that frequency of peristalsis is determined by BER, and, thus, does not vary. However, the force of peristaltic contractions is under neural and hormonal control.

- Distension of the stomach or increased gastrin secretion increases the force of gastric peristalsis.
- Gastric contractions are increased by vagal stimulation and decreased by sympathetic stimulation.
- ACh and gastrin increase the size of slow-wave plateau potential, which increases the amount of Ca^{2+} entering the cell from the extracellular fluid (ECF), and activate second messengers that release Ca^{2+} from the sarcoplasmic reticulum. The amount of Ca^{2+} present in the smooth muscle cell determines the force of contraction.

Mixing mechanism of peristalsis and retropulsion

Peristaltic contractions begin in the mid-stomach (Fig. 7.3.17A) and proceed caudally. As the wave proceeds towards the pylorus, it deepens. Thus, the peristaltic waves are most marked in the distal half of the stomach (called antral systole).

- The food particles also move towards the pylorus (Fig. 7.3.17B), along with the deep wave of contraction, but the wave of contraction reaches pyloric sphincter and causes its contraction before the food reaches there.
- When the food reaches the pylorus, it strikes against the closed pyloric sphincter with a force. As a result, most of the antral contents are forced back into the body of the stomach and only a small amount of chyme passes into the duodenum (Fig. 7.3.17C). The backward movement of the food is called *retropulsion*.
- The forward and backward movements (caused by forceful propulsion and retropulsion) of the gastric contents help to break the food particles into smaller pieces and mix them with gastric secretion, converting them into a semiliquid paste called chyme.

Gastric Emptying

Gastric emptying results from a progressive wave of forceful contraction, which sequentially involves the antrum, pylorus (pyloric sphincter) and proximal duodenum; thus, all the three function as a unit. It is the force of gastric peristalsis which determines emptying and not the variations in tone of pyloric sphincter. The forceful gastric emptying waves spread over the antrum as a strong peristaltic ring-like contraction creating pressure of 50–70 cm H_2O (six times as powerful as that produced by mixing waves).

- Gastric emptying occurs when the chyme is decomposed into enough small pieces (typically <1 mm^3) to fit through the pyloric sphincter.
- Each time the chyme is pushed against the pyloric sphincter, contraction ahead of advancing gastric contents prevents bigger food particles from entering the duodenum. Therefore, chyme is pumped in a bit (2–7 mL) at a time into the small intestine.
- The peristaltic waves which provide this pumping action are known as *pyloric pump*.
- Regurgitation from the duodenum, normally, does not occur, because the contraction of the pyloric segment tends to persist slightly longer than that of the duodenum. The prevention of regurgitation may also be due to the stimulating action of CCK and secretin on the pyloric sphincter.

Factors Regulating the Gastric Emptying

After a normal meal, the emptying time is 2–3 hours. The gastric emptying is regulated by various factors:

1. Fluidity of the chyme The rate of gastric emptying of solids depends on the rate at which the chyme is broken down into smaller particles. Liquids empty much faster than solids. The rate at which liquids empty is proportional to the pressure within the oral stomach, which increases slowly during the digestive period.

2. Gastric factors Gastric factors which affect emptying are as follows:

Volume of food in the stomach: Greater the volume of food in the stomach, greater is the stretching of the stomach wall. Distension of the stomach triggers long (vagally mediated) and short (intrinsic neural plexus mediated) reflexes leading to strong peristalsis waves and increased rate of gastric emptying.
Gastrin hormone: Presence of certain types of food (e.g. meat) causes release of gastrin from antral mucosa. Gastrin enhances the activity of pyloric pump and therefore promotes gastric emptying.
Type of food ingested (present in the stomach) affects the gastric emptying as follows:

- Carbohydrate-rich food causes rapid gastric emptying.
- Protein-rich food causes slow gastric emptying.
- Fat-rich food causes the slowest gastric emptying.

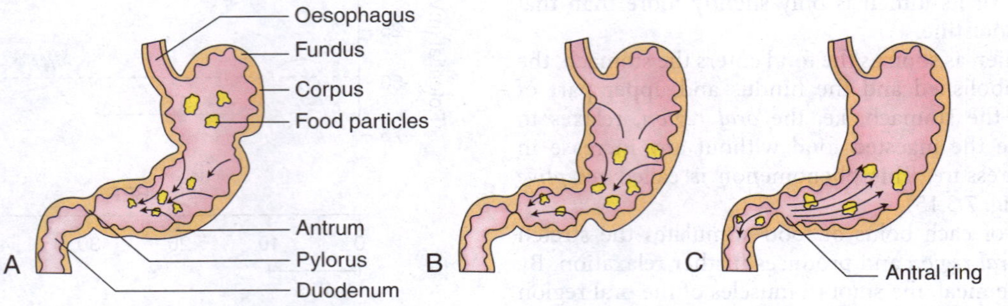

Fig. 7.3.17 Mixing peristaltic waves of stomach: **A**, peristaltic contractions begin in the mid-stomach and push the food towards pylorus; **B**, when food reaches the pylorus, it strikes against closed pyloric sphincter; and **C**, antral contents forced back (retropulsion).

Important Note

Some people consume fats before a cocktail party. The fat keeps the alcohol in the stomach longer, slowing the absorption and reducing the chances of intoxication.

3. Duodenal factors Duodenal factors which inhibit gastric emptying are as follows:

Enterogastric reflex: It is a neural-mediated reflex. It is initiated by stimulation of receptors in the duodenal mucosa. The important stimuli are distension of the duodenum, acidity of the contents (pH < 4), high or low osmolarity of chyme, and presence of fat and protein digestion products in the chyme.

The enterogastric reflex is initiated in the duodenum and passes to the stomach through the myenteric plexus and also extrinsic nerves to inhibit or even stop emptying by inhibiting antral propulsive contractions and increasing slightly the tone of the pyloric sphincter.

Enterogastric hormones: A variety of intestinal hormones, collectively called enterogastrones, inhibit gastric contractions. Some of the hormones which have been identified are as follows:

- *CCK:* It is released from the duodenum in response to fat or protein digestion product. CCK probably acts by blocking the excitatory effects of gastrin on gastric smooth muscles.
- *Secretin:* It is released from the duodenum in response to presence of acid. Secretin most likely has a direct inhibitory effect on smooth muscle.
- *GIP:* It is released from the upper small intestine in response to fat in chyme and reduces gastric motility under some conditions.

Important Note

Purpose of Duodenal Inhibitory Effect on Gastric Emptying

The duodenal inhibitory effects (exerted through enterogastric reflex and enterogastrones) prevent the flow of chyme from exceeding the ability of intestine to handle it (especially longer time is required for fat digestion). It does not allow disturbance in electrolyte balance even if hypotonic or hypertonic solutions are drunk.

Size of osmoreceptors: The rate of gastric emptying is also controlled by the size of osmoreceptors present in the duodenum; these receptors respond to the osmolarity of the chyme that enters the duodenum. Thus, hypo-osmolar chyme causes distension (increase in the size) of the osmoreceptors and thereby inhibits gastric emptying, whereas hyperosmolar chyme causes shrinkage of the osmoreceptors, and markedly inhibits the gastric emptying. As osmolarity of the food profoundly affects gastric emptying, both hypertonic and hypotonic solutions (pure water) are emptied slowly as compared with isotonic solutions.

4. Other factors affecting gastric emptying

- *Emotions* have a strong effect on gastric motility. Anger and aggression increase gastric motility, whereas depression and fear decrease it.
- *Vagotomy* decreases the magnitude and coordination of stomach contractions and thus slows emptying.

FUNCTIONS OF STOMACH

After studying the physiological activities of the stomach, its functions can be summarized as follows.

1. Mechanical or motor functions include:

Storage of food: The stomach serves as a reservoir for the food ingested. It can store about 1 L of food. Food remains in the stomach for several hours.

Mixing of food with gastric juice is performed by gastric motility until it forms a semisolid paste known as chyme.

Slow emptying of food into the duodenum occurs to provide proper time for digestion and absorption by the small intestine.

2. Digestive functions Only small amounts of foods are digested in the stomach as follows:

Carbohydrate digestion in the stomach depends on the action of salivary amylase, which remains active until halted by the low pH of the stomach.

Protein digestion: About 10% of ingested protein is broken down completely in the stomach. *Gastric pepsin* facilitates later digestion of protein by breaking protein into peptone.

Fat digestion in the stomach is minimal due to the restriction of gastric lipase activity to triglycerides containing short-chain ($<$10 carbon) fatty acids. Acid and pepsin break emulsions so that fats coalesce into droplets, which float and empty last.

3. Absorptive function The stomach contributes little in the absorption function.

Absorption of nutrients: Very little absorption of nutrients takes place in the stomach. The only substances absorbed to any appreciable extent are highly lipid-soluble substances (e.g. the nonionized triglycerides of acetic, propionic and butyric acids). *Aspirin* at gastric pH is nonionized and fat soluble and after absorption it ionizes intracellularly, damaging mucosal cells and ultimately producing bleeding.

Ethanol is absorbed rapidly in proportion to its concentration.

Water absorption: Water moves in both directions across the gastric mucosa. It does not, however, follow osmotic gradients. Water-soluble substances, including Na^+, K^+, glucose and amino acids, are absorbed in insignificant amounts.

IF released from gastric glands helps in absorption of vitamin B_{12} from the small intestine.

4. Excretory function The stomach excretes the following substances:

- Certain toxins, as in case of uraemia
- Certain alkaloids, such as morphine

5. Stimulating functions The stomach performs stimulatory function for release of:

- Gastrin
- Enterogastrin
- IF of Castle

6. Reflex functions Various reflexes initiated from the stomach are as follows:

- Gastrosalivary reflex
- Gastroileal reflex
- Gastrocolic reflex

- Secretion of pancreatic juice and expulsion of bile because of presence of food in the stomach

7. Antiseptic action HCl present in the gastric juice kills the bacteria and other harmful substances.

Applied Aspects

Important applied aspects of the stomach which need special attention are as follows:

- Gastric mucosal barrier and pathophysiology of peptic ulcer
- Physiology of vomiting
- Gastrectomy
- Gastric function tests

I. Gastric Mucosal Barrier and Pathophysiology of Peptic Ulcer

Gastric Mucosal Barrier

The gastric mucosal barrier protects the gastric mucosa from damage by intraluminal HCl, i.e. autodigestion. Indeed, it is a physiological marvel, or gastric walls would suffer the same fate as a piece of swallowed meat. It is created by the following:

Mucin secretion: The thin layer of surface mucus in the stomach and duodenum exhibits a diffusion coefficient for H^+ that is one-fourth that of water. Acid- and pepsin-containing fluid exits the gastric glands as jets passing through the surface mucus layer, entering the lumen directly without contacting surface epithelial cells.

Bicarbonate secretion: Surface epithelial cells, in both the stomach and the duodenum, secrete bicarbonate into the boundary zone of adherent mucus, creating an essentially pH neutral microenvironment immediately adjacent to the cell surface.

Epithelial barrier: Intercellular tight junctions provide a barrier to the back-diffusion of H^+. Any damaged cells are quickly replaced, as the turnover rate of gastric mucosa is very high. Approximately, 5×10^5 mucosal cells are shed each minute, replacing the entire mucosa in 1–3 days.

High mucosal blood flow: It rapidly carries away any acid that penetrates the cellular lining. The rich mucosal blood supply also provides oxygen, bicarbonate and nutrients to epithelial cells.

Chemical factors include gastrin and EGF.

Prostaglandins are responsible for maintaining the gastric mucosal barrier.

Role of diet: The diet also contains polyamines that are required for growth. The trophic agents like gastrin stimulate polyamine synthesis in the proliferative cells, and also increase release of luminal polyamines from diet. Thus, diet also plays an important role in mucosal growth.

Pathophysiology of Peptic Ulcer

Peptic ulcer refers to excavation of mucosa of the duodenum or pyloric part of the stomach caused by the digestive action of gastric juice. It can be caused by either of the following two ways:

1. ***Diminished ability of the gastroduodenal mucosal barrier*** to protect against the digestive properties of the acid–pepsin complex. Factors that disturb the mucosal barrier include:

   Bacterial infection by Helicobacter pylori breaks down the gastroduodenal mucosal barrier. At least 75% of patients with peptic ulcer have recently been found to have chronic infection by *H. pylori*. The sequence of events in the pathology of the peptic ulcer by *H. pylori* infection is as follows:

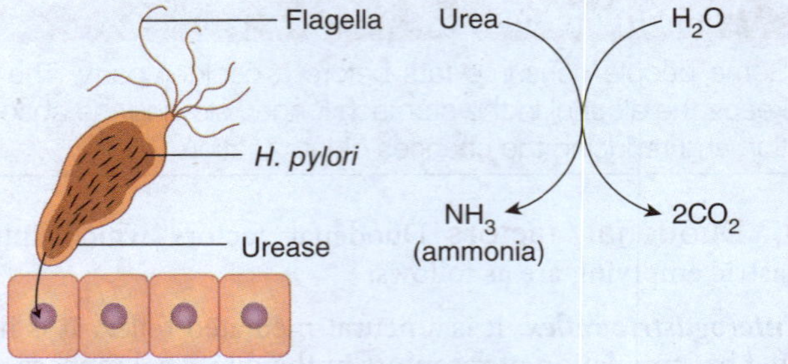

Fig. 7.3.18 Buffer action of *H. pylori* by production of urease enzyme.

   - *H. pylori* is a Gram-negative bacterium, with multiple flagella at one end which makes it highly motile. The bacterium burrows into the mucus layer and lives deeply adherent to the epithelial surface.
   - *H. pylori* uses an adhesion molecule (Bab A) to bind itself to the antigen called *Lewis b* antigen present on the epithelial cells. The surface pH nearly remains neutral because if there occurs any acidity, it gets buffered by production of urease (an enzyme produced by the bacteria), which produces ammonia from urea that raises the pH (Fig. 7.3.18). The bacterium stimulates gastritis by local inflammatory reaction in the underlying epithelium that depends on expression of gene, i.e.:
     - Cytotoxin-associated gene A (Cag A), which interacts with various cell signalling pathways involved in cell replication
     - Vacuolating cytotoxin gene A (Vac A), which is a pore-forming adhesin (Bab A)
     - Cytokine interleukin-1β (IL-1β) associated with gastric atrophy
   - *H. pylori* causes gastritis due to depletion of somatostatin from D-cells and increased gastrin release from G-cells (Fig. 7.3.19).

     The bacterium releases digestive enzymes that liquefy the barrier, which allows gastric secretion to digest the epithelial cells leading to peptic ulceration.

   Nonsteroidal anti-inflammatory drugs (NSAIDs), such as aspirin, ibuprofen and diclofenac sodium:

   - NSAIDs act through inhibition of prostaglandin H synthase and cyclooxygenase (COX) enzyme. They damage the gastric mucosal barrier by reducing prostaglandin synthesis.

   Other factors which can disrupt the mucosal barrier are ethyl alcohol, vinegar, bile salts and cigarette smoking.

2. ***Excessive secretion of gastric acid.*** Hyperacidity leads to ulcer formation in the duodenum and pyloric part of the stomach. Hyperacidity may occur due to:

   Increased parietal cell mass

   Increased sensitivity for secretory stimuli (it has been observed that in most of the patients with gastric and duodenal ulcer, the resting gastrin levels are normal, but response of parietal cells to gastrin after feeding is greater than normal)

   Increased basal acid secretory drive and conditions, such as pernicious anaemia in which there is damage to the parietal cells (as a result, the basal secretion of gastrin is chronically elevated)

H. pylori
↓
Depletion of antral D-cell somatostatin
↓
Increased gastrin release from G-cells
↓
Increased HCl secretion
↓
Increased acid load on duodenum leads to gastric metaplasia
↓
Further inflammation results in ulceration (due to reduced gastric mucosal resistance)

Fig. 7.3.19 Sequence of events of pathophysiology of peptic ulcer by *H. pylori*.

Important Notes

- The incidence of duodenal and prepyloric ulcer is more in patients with pernicious anaemia.
- Excess gastric secretion is seen in Zollinger–Ellison syndrome, in which patients have *gastrinomas* (tumours that secrete gastrin).[a]
- Pepsinogen-I: The acid-secreting activity is related to pepsinogen-I level. It has been observed that the patients congenitally having high levels of pepsinogen-I have a greater incidence of peptic ulcer as compared with those with normal levels.

[a]*Zollinger–Ellison syndrome* is a rare condition in which tumours called gastrinomas grow in the pancreas/small intestine. These tumours produce a large amount of gastrin, which increases HCL level of gastric secretion (>100 pg/mL).

Investigations

1. **Endoscopy** is the procedure by which microscopic details can be observed with the help of an endoscope. It is used for both diagnostic and therapeutic purposes.
2. ***Tests for diagnosis of H. pylori infection*** include both noninvasive and invasive tests.
   Noninvasive tests are serology, C urea breath test for higher sensitivity and faecal antigen test (a specific test).
   Invasive tests include biopsy for histology, microbiological culture and rapid urease test.
   - Rapid urease test or *Campylobacter*-like organism (CLO) test: This test is used to detect the presence of urease that converts urea to carbon dioxide and ammonia. Ammonia causes change in the colour of phenol red due to rise in pH. This test is performed during gastroscopy.
   - Urea breath test: In this test, C-13- or C-14-labelled urea is ingested with liquid meal and the labelled CO_2 will split off and is expired if urease is present in the stomach.

Clinical Features of Peptic Ulcer

The signs and symptoms of peptic ulcer include:

- Burning
- Nausea
- Haematemesis
- Weight loss

Physiological Basis of Management of Peptic Ulcer

The aims of peptic ulcer management are to:

- Reduce symptoms
- Induce healing
- Prevent recurrence

Commonly used measures for treatment of peptic ulcer, along with their physiological bases, are as follows:

Antacids: These form a gel that coats the mucosa and neutralizes the acid. Most of the antacids contain aluminium hydroxide, magnesium hydroxide or calcium bicarbonate.

H_2 receptor–blocking drugs such as cimetidine, ranitidine and nizatidine decrease HCl secretion by blocking the effect of histamine on H_2 receptors of parietal cells.

M_1 muscarinic receptor–blocking drugs such as atropine and pirenzepine decrease H^+ secretion by blocking the effect of ACh on M_1 muscarinic receptors of parietal cells.

Gastric H^+–K^+-ATPase–inhibiting drugs such as omeprazole obviously decrease H^+ secretion by blocking the action of gastric H^+–K^+-ATPase in the parietal cell.

H. pylori eradication: All proven cases of acute or chronic gastric ulcer with *H. pylori* should be given eradication as primary therapy.

Bilateral vagotomy combined with resection of gastrin-producing pyloric part of the stomach is performed in very severe cases of duodenal and pyloric ulcers. This surgical treatment abolishes the effects of both ACh and gastrin, and thus markedly reduces HCl production.

Pyeloplasty: In this procedure, vagotomy is combined with distension of pylorus. Pyeloplasty is done to prevent retention of gastric contents due to increased pyloric sphincter tone because of simple vagotomy.

Complications

Peptic ulcer if not treated properly, then complications can occur, such as bleeding, perforation, gastric carcinoma and duodenal ulcer.

Haematemesis refers to presence of blood in the vomit, and can be due to bleeding in the stomach, duodenum and oesophagus.

Causes

The causes of haematemesis are as follows:

- Gastritis due to bacterial infection, heavy use of alcohol, and routine use of painkillers (NSAIDs)
- Ulcers in the stomach, oesophagus or intestines
- Acid reflux which occurs mainly when the oesophagus does not close properly, e.g. gastroesophageal reflux disease (GERD)
- Bleeding veins in the oesophagus and stomach
- Liver damage which can cause swollen veins that can bleed with vomiting

Symptoms

The vomit contains dark/bright red or dark brown blood with or without food contents.

Management

Depending on the severity and physical condition of the patient, the treatment includes fluids, blood transfusion, oxygen therapy and medication to reduce acid production in the stomach and to treat underlying cause.

II. Vomiting

Vomiting refers to forceful expulsion of contents from the stomach and intestine. It is a complex reflex involving both autonomic and somatic pathways.

Initiation of Vomiting

Vomiting may be initiated either by activation of the vomiting centre or by activation of the chemoreceptor trigger zone.

1. Activation of vomiting centre. Vomiting centre is situated in the reticular formation of medulla oblongata near the vagal nucleus. It may be activated directly or through afferents:

i. ***Direct activation of the vomiting centre*** occurs due to initiation caused by injury to the area or by raised intracranial pressure, and causes projectile vomiting – a rapid, forceful emesis not accompanied by nausea.

ii. ***Afferent impulses*** activating vomiting centre include (Fig. 7.3.20):
Visceral afferent pathway in the sympathetic and vagus nerves relays impulses arising due to irritation of mucosa of upper GIT. There are 5-HT receptors in the stomach and small intestine, and 5-HT (serotonin) released from the enterochromaffin cells appears to initiate impulses in afferents that trigger nausea and vomiting. These receptors are stimulated by local irritants such as drugs, viruses, radiations, bacteria, $CuSO_4$ and cytotoxic agents.
Afferent impulses from the vestibular nuclei mediate nausea and vomiting of motion sickness.

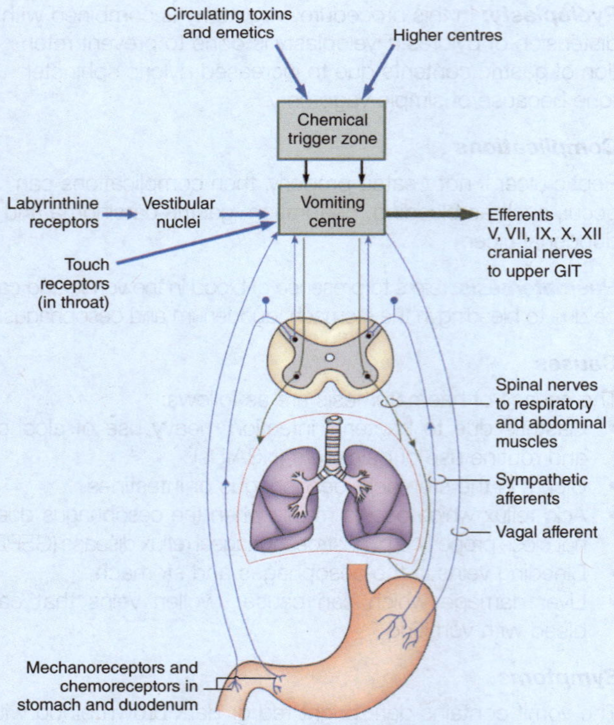

Fig. 7.3.20 Pathway for vomiting reflex.

Afferents from higher centres (diencephalon and limbic system) mediate emetic response to emotionally charged stimuli such as nauseating smell, sickening sights and memory, fear, dread and anticipation of vomiting.

2. Activation of chemoreceptor trigger zone. Chemoreceptor trigger zone (CTZ) is located in the area *postrema* (a V-shaped band of tissue on the lateral walls of the fourth ventricle near the obex), which is outside the blood–brain barrier and is thus more permeable to many substances than the underlying medulla (Fig. 7.3.20). Chemoreceptor cells present in CTZ contain dopamine (D_2) receptors and $5HT_3$ receptors and initiate vomiting when they are stimulated by:

- Circulating emetic substances in patients with uraemia and radiation sickness
- Drugs such as NSAIDs, opioids, glycoside (digoxin) antibiotics and cytokines
- Infections – viral and bacterial infections, hepatitis, gastroenteritis and urinary tract infection
- Emetic agents such as apomorphine and emetin, digitalis and glucosides

Note: $5\text{-}HT_3$ antagonists such as ondansetron and D_2 antagonists such as chlorpromazine and haloperidol, cannabinoids, corticosteroids and benzodiazepines are effective antiemetic agents.

Efferent Impulses from Vomiting Centre and CTZ. Efferent impulses from the vomiting centre and CTZ, which give effect to the act of vomiting, are transmitted via V, VII, IX, X and XII cranial nerves to the upper GIT and through spinal nerves to the muscles of respiration.

Sequence of mechanical events of vomiting. Vomiting is a complex process and consists of the following phases:

1. ***Pre-ejection phase:*** During this phase, there occurs gastric relaxation and retroperistalsis. It is characterized by a feeling of nausea, excessive salivation, and deep, rapid and irregular breathing.
2. ***Retching phase*** may precede in many cases. It is characterized by:
   Closure of glottis, which remains so till the end of the act of vomiting. It increases intrapulmonary pressure causing compression of the oesophagus. It also prevents aspiration of vomitus in the trachea.
   Rhythmic action of respiratory muscles precedes vomiting and consists of contraction of abdominal, intercostal and diaphragmatic muscles against a closed glottis.
3. ***Ejection phase***, during which the GIT contents are actually expelled out, consists of events which occur in the following sequence:
   - Closure of the glottis is continued.
   - Pyloric part of the stomach contracts firmly and its contents are transferred to flaccid body of the stomach.
   - Simultaneous intense contraction of abdominal muscles and the descent of the diaphragm raise the intra-abdominal pressure to such an extent that all the contents are squeezed out of the stomach into the oesophagus as a reflex relaxation of its cardiac sphincter, which also occurs at this moment.
   - From the oesophagus, the contents are expelled into the mouth due to the effect of positive intrapulmonary pressure and antiperistaltic waves in the oesophagus.

At this juncture, a soft palate is raised and it shuts off the nasal cavity from the throat.

- Towards the end of the act of vomiting, the diaphragm relaxes (i.e. ascends) and the expiratory muscles and abdominal wall contract.

III. Total Gastrectomy

In the patients who undergo a surgical removal of the stomach or gastric bypass surgery (in which the stomach is stapled), the loss of reservoir function of the stomach may produce the following effects:

Nutritional Disturbances After Gastrectomy

1. Effect on Carbohydrate Metabolism. The carbohydrates directly enter the duodenum and are digested and absorbed rapidly resulting in *hyperglycaemia*. As a result of *hyperglycaemia*, there occurs an abrupt rise in insulin secretion, which leads to hypoglycaemia after about 2 hours of meals. Thus, there occur sharp oscillations between hypoglycaemia and hyperglycaemia.

2. Effect on Protein Metabolism. The stomach plays an important role in the digestion of protein, but the near-normal digestion of protein can occur in the absence of pepsin and nutrition can be maintained.

3. Effect on Fat Digestion. Almost no effect on fat digestion is seen except on butter fat, for which gastric juice has an enzyme tributarase.

4. Effect on Absorption of Vitamin B_{12}. Due to deficiency of IF, absorption of vitamin B_{12} is affected markedly and there may occur *pernicious anaemia*.

5. Effect on Iron Absorption. Conversion of iron from ferric (Fe^{3+}) to ferrous (Fe^{2+}) form requires HCl. Therefore, iron absorption, which occurs in ferrous form, is affected, predisposing the individual to iron-deficiency anaemia. However, only traces of iron are absorbed in the stomach.

IV. Dumping Syndrome

Dumping syndrome refers to a condition characterized by development of weakness, dizziness and sweating after meals. This is seen in the cases of partial or total gastrectomy, where the oesophagus is directly anastomosed with duodenum.

Causes of symptoms of dumping syndrome

1. Main cause of symptoms in dumping syndrome is sharp oscillations between hyperglycaemia and hypoglycaemia, as described above.
2. Another cause of symptoms is the rapid entry of hypertonic meals into the intestine. It provokes the movement of so much water into the gut that the resultant reduction of plasma volume is great enough leading to a significant decrease in cardiac output.

Treatment. The following are recommended in case of dumping syndrome:

- Avoid a large meal.
- Meals should be small in bulk and dry.
- Milk and carbohydrate meals should be avoided and meals should have some dietary fibres.
- Daily and regular supplement of iron and vitamin B complex is necessary to prevent development of anaemia.

GASTRIC FUNCTION TESTS

Gastric function tests are used to establish the presence of *hyperchlorhydria* (associated with peptic ulcer) or achlorhydria (complete absence of acid secretion) associated with pernicious anaemia. Gastric function tests include the following:

Fractional Test Meal Test

Fractional test meal (FTM) test was previously used commonly for analysis of gastric juice. Presently, it is no more used because of its relative insensitivity and inconvenience.

Procedure, in brief, is described as follows:

- After an overnight fast, the gastric fluid present in the stomach is aspirated with the help of Ryle's tube passed into the stomach through the nose or throat.
- A test meal is then given to stimulate the gastric juice. Any one of the standard test meals can be given – 300 mL of oatmeal gruel or dry toast and cup of tea or wheat biscuits and 300 mL of water.
- After 15 minutes of giving test meal, a sample of gastric content (10 mL of fluid) is aspirated. The procedure is repeated every 15 minutes for 3 hours. Thus, including the fasting sample, a total of 13 samples are collected in separate containers.
- Each sample is analysed for free acidity, combined acidity (Fig. 7.3.21), starch and sugar, bile, total chlorides, blood lactic acid and mucus.

Histamine Test

Histamine test is a comparatively more sensitive test than the FTM test for studying the gastric acid secretion. It is because:

- First, the histamine is a powerful stimulator of acid secretion.
- Second, due to histamine injection, acid level increases very rapidly and therefore there is no time for neutralization of acid.

Procedure: After overnight fast, in the morning, the stomach is aspirated and washed with distilled water. Then, 0.5 mg

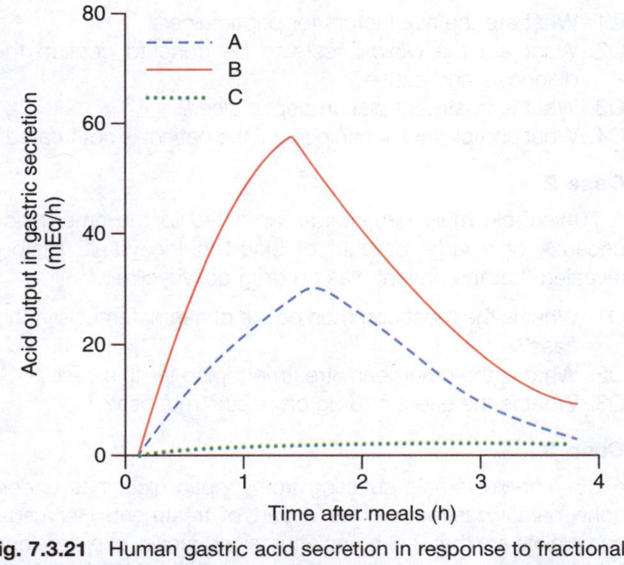

Fig. 7.3.21 Human gastric acid secretion in response to fractional test meal: **A**, normal response; **B**, hyperchlorhydria in duodenal ulcer; and **C**, hyposecretion or achlorhydria.

histamine is injected subcutaneously and the gastric samples are aspirated and analysed as described in FTM test.

If there is no free acid present in any of the samples, then it is called true achlorhydria or histamine-fast achlorhydria.

Augmented Histamine Test

- This test is performed with progressively increasing doses of histamine in a stepwise manner till a maximal secretory response is obtained.
- The maximal secretory response correlates well with the total number of parietal cells in the gastric mucosa.

Pentagastrin Test

This test is also performed to assess the gastric acid status. It is performed similar to the histamine test except that in this, instead of histamine, 6 mg of pentagastrin (a synthetic gastrin) is given as subcutaneous injection.

Insulin Test

- This test is based on the fact that hypoglycaemia (blood sugar below 45 mg%) produces vagal stimulation through the hypothalamus and that vagal stimulation causes secretion of acid from the stomach.
- In this test, 7 units of insulin is given intravenously and the gastric samples are tested for the presence of free acid, as done in histamine test.
- Acid secretion occurs after insulin injection (positive test) only if vagus is intact. Therefore, insulin test is performed after vagotomy operation (for gastric ulcer) to know whether all the fibres of nerves supplying the stomach are cut or not. If vagotomy is done properly, insulin test is negative.

Barium Meal Study

Barium meal study is a radiographic evaluation of the status of mucosa and lumen of the upper intestinal tract. In this test, the patient swallows a suspension of radiopaque barium sulphate, while its passage through the GIT is observed by radiograph on a fluorescent screen and films are taken to provide a permanent record. Diagnosis of gastric ulcer, duodenal ulcer or other abnormalities in the lumen of GIT is made from the typical finding.

Endoscopic Examination and Biopsy

Nowadays, the condition of the oesophagus and gastric and duodenal mucosa can be directly visualized by endoscopic examination. This is a more reliable method than the conventional barium meal studies. The endoscopes carry a channel through which biopsy forceps or a brush can be introduced to obtain specimens for histological and cytological examination.

Self-Assessment

1. Discuss about composition. mechanism, phases and regulation of gastric secretion.
2. Describe:
   - Gastric emptying and factors affecting it
   - Gastric mucosal barrier
   - Physiology of vomiting
   - Migrating motor complexes
3. Write notes on:
   - Achlorhydria
   - Peptic ulcer
   - Gastric function tests

Clinical Cases

Case 1

A 36-year-old male was admitted to the hospital with complaints of blood in the vomit, epigastric pain and heartburns. Physical examination revealed rapid and low-volume pulse and low BP. On the basis of history and signs and symptoms, the patient was provisionally diagnosed a case of peptic ulcer.

Q1. What are the risk factors for peptic ulcer?
Q2. What are the clinical tests to be done to confirm the diagnosis and cause?
Q3. What is treatment plan in peptic ulcer?
Q4. What complications can occur if the patient is not treated?

Case 2

A 70-year-old male patient was admitted to the emergency because of a large amount of blood in the vomit. History revealed that the patient was on drug doxycycline.

Q1. What is the most common cause of haematemesis in this case?
Q2. What is the emergency treatment plan for this case?
Q3. What is the effect of drug on gastric mucosa?

Case 3

A 55-year-old female suffering from peptic ulcer has undergone partial gastrectomy as a part of treatment. Her usual complaints are that 2–3 hours after taking meals, she develops light-headedness, sweating, dizziness and flushing of the face.

Q1. What is the probable diagnosis?
Q2. What is the main cause for the symptoms?
Q3. What is the pathophysiology of peptic ulcer?
Q4. What is the treatment basis for this condition?

Case 4

A 30-year-old woman was admitted with complaints of abdominal pain, diarrhoea, weight loss and feeling of abdominal bloating after taking meals for 2–3 months.

The patient was examined and investigated.

- The physical findings revealed glossitis, pallor, koilonychia, breathlessness and decreased vibratory sensation.
- Haemogram showed decreased Hb, RBC count, increased MCV and decreased MCHC.
- Biochemical findings indicated raised bilirubin level and reduced levels of iron and vitamin B_{12}.

The case was provisionally diagnosed pernicious anaemia and treated by oral haematinics and vitamin B_{12}, but no improvement was observed after 1 month, and the patient was suspected a case of achlorhydria/hypochlorhydria.

Q1. What is the most common cause of pernicious anaemia?
Q2. What further investigations should be done for the final diagnosis of achlorhydria?
Q3. What special investigation should be advised to find the cause of pernicious anaemia?
Q4. What should be the treatment of pernicious anaemia in this case?

Pancreas, Liver and Gall Bladder

7.4

CHAPTER OUTLINE

INTRODUCTION

Pancreas, liver and gall bladder are accessory organs of the digestive system. After studying the physiological events occurring in the stomach and before considering the physiological activities of the small intestine, it will be worthwhile to know about the physiological role of the pancreas, liver and gall bladder in the digestive system, because secretions of these organs affect the activities of the small intestine.

PANCREAS

FUNCTIONAL ANATOMY

General Considerations

The pancreas is an elongated, accessory digestive gland that lies retroperitoneally and transversely across the posterior abdominal wall, posterior to the stomach between the duodenum on the right and the spleen on the left (Fig. 7.4.1).

Anatomically, for the purpose of description, the pancreas is divided into four parts – head, neck, body and tail.

Physiologically, on the basis of functions performed, the pancreas consists of two parts:

Exocrine part produces a secretion called pancreatic juice that contains enzymes capable of hydrolysing proteins, fats and carbohydrates.

Endocrine part of the pancreas, the islets of Langerhans, produces the hormones insulin and glucagon, which play a key role in the carbohydrate metabolism. The endocrine part is discussed in Section 8 (page 753).

Structural Characteristics of Exocrine Part of Pancreas

The exocrine part of the pancreas is in the form of a serous compound, tubuloalveolar gland, very similar to the parotid gland in the general structure (Fig. 7.4.2).

Acinar cells lining the alveoli appear triangular in section. Numerous secretory (or zymogen) granules can be demonstrated in the cytoplasm, especially in the apical part of the cells. These granules are eosinophilic and decrease considerably after the cells have poured out their secretions.

The acinar cells produce a thick secretion containing numerous enzymes (listed in composition of pancreatic juice).

Centroacinar cells: In addition to the secretory acinar cells, the alveoli of the exocrine pancreas contain centroacinar cells that are so called because they appear to be located near the centre of the acinus (alveolus). These cells really belong to the intercalated ducts which are invaginated into the acinus (Fig. 7.4.2).

Ductal cells lining the ductal system of the pancreas produce a watery secretion rich in bicarbonate ions (HCO_3^-), which mixes with the thick secretion produced by acinar cells to constitute the pancreatic juice.

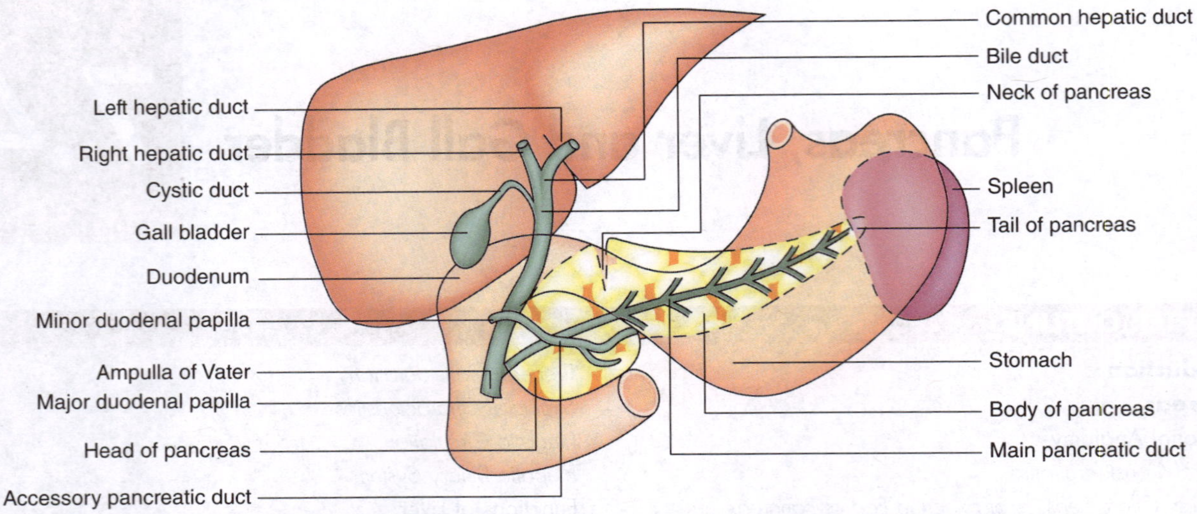

Fig. 7.4.1 Anatomical relations of pancreas, pancreatic duct and extrahepatic biliary system.

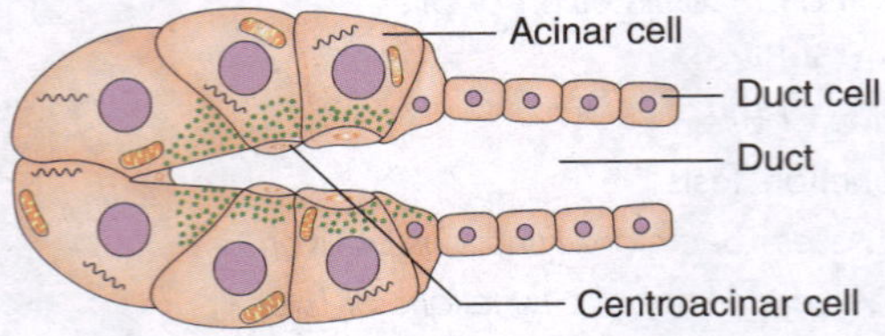

Fig. 7.4.2 Histology of functional unit of pancreas.

Pancreatic Ducts

The intercalated ducts, which receive secretions produced by acini, pass them on to interlobular ducts. Ultimately, the pancreatic secretion passes into the duodenum through the main pancreatic duct and the accessory pancreatic duct.

Main pancreatic duct, also known as *duct of Wirsung*, begins in the tail and runs the length of the gland, receiving numerous tributaries on the way. It joins the common bile duct (CBD) to form the ampulla of Vater, which opens into the second part of the duodenum at about its middle on the major duodenal papilla (Fig. 7.4.1). The ampulla of Vater is guarded by the sphincter of Oddi.

Accessory pancreatic duct, also called the *duct of Santorini*, when present, drains the upper part of the head and then opens into the duodenum about 2 mm above the main duct on the minor duodenal papilla. The accessory duct frequently communicates with the main duct.

Vessels and Nerves of Pancreas

Arterial supply to the pancreas comes from the splenic and superior as well as inferior pancreaticoduodenal arteries.

Veins, corresponding to arteries, drain into the portal system.

Lymphatics drain into the lymph nodes situated along the arteries that supply the gland. The efferent vessels ultimately drain into the coeliac and superior mesenteric lymph nodes.

Nerve supply comes from both sympathetic and parasympathetic (vagi) nerves. Preganglionic vagal fibres synapse with ganglionic cells embedded in the pancreatic tissue; the postganglionic fibres innervate both the acinar cells and the smooth muscles of the ducts. Vagal stimulation increases pancreatic juice secretion.

PANCREATIC SECRETION

Properties and Composition

- Pancreatic juice is a transparent, colourless fluid isotonic with plasma.
- About 1200–1500 mL of pancreatic juice is secreted per day.
- Its specific gravity varies from 1.010 to 1.018.
- Pancreatic juice is markedly alkaline (pH 7.8–8.4), due to very high concentration of HCO_3^- (113 mEq/L, about four to five times that of plasma).

Composition

Pancreatic juice is composed of 99.5% water and 0.5% solids, which include organic and inorganic substances.

Organic constituents of pancreatic juice are certain enzymes and other substances.

- ***Enzymes:*** The pancreas secretes four major types of enzymes – amylase, lipase, protease and trypsin inhibitor.
- ***Other organic substances*** present in traces are albumin and globulin.

Inorganic substances present in the pancreatic juice are cations like Na^+, K^+, Ca^{2+}, Mg^{2+} and Zn^{2+}, and anions such as HCO_3^-, Cl^- and traces of SO_4^{2-} and HPO_4^{2-}. Electrolyte composition varies with rate of secretion (see page 598).

Pancreatic enzymes Pancreatic acini secrete four major types of enzymes – amylase, lipase, protease and trypsin inhibitor.

1. ***Pancreatic amylase:*** It is secreted in its active form. It is the only amylolytic enzyme present with pancreatic juice. Its action on the carbohydrates is like that of salivary amylase. It hydrolyses glycogen, starch and most other complex carbohydrates, except cellulose, to form disaccharides.
2. ***Pancreatic lipases*** or lipolytic enzymes include pancreatic lipase, cholesterol ester hydrolase and phospholipase A_2.
   - *Pancreatic lipase* is a powerful lipolytic enzyme. It hydrolyses neutral fats to glycerol esters and fatty acids. Its activity is accelerated in the presence of bile salts.
   - *Cholesterol ester hydrolase* converts cholesterol esters to cholesterol.
   - *Phospholipase A_2* is secreted in an inactive form prophospholipase A_2 and gets converted to active form

phospholipase A_2 by the action of trypsin. Phospholipase A_2 splits fatty acid phosphatidylcholine (PC) forming lyso-PC. Lyso-PC damages the cell membrane.

Important Note

It is *important to note* that in acute pancreatitis, phospholipase A_2 gets activated in the pancreatic ducts causing disruption of pancreatic tissue and necrosis of surrounding fat, which may be fatal. Acute pancreatitis is invariably associated with high serum amylase level.

3. ***Pancreatic proteases*** or proteolytic enzymes include three endopeptidases (trypsin, chymotrypsin and elastase) and two exopeptidases (carboxypeptidase A and B). Endopeptidases break the peptides somewhere in the middle. Exopeptidases break the peptide chain near its end, releasing single amino acid.
   - *Trypsin:* It is the most powerful proteolytic enzyme of the pancreatic juice. It is secreted in an inactive form of trypsinogen, which is activated by the enzyme enterokinase (enteropeptidase) secreted by the duodenal mucosa. Once formed, trypsin also activates trypsinogen – an autocatalytic reaction.

$$\text{Trypsinogen} \xrightarrow{\text{Enterokinase}} \text{Trypsin}$$
$$\text{Trypsinogen} \xrightarrow{\text{Trypsin}} \text{Trypsin}$$

     - Trypsin hydrolyses proteins into proteoses and to polypeptides.
     - It activates trypsinogen and other pancreatic enzymes.
   - *Chymotrypsin:* It is also secreted in an inactive form chymotrypsinogen and is activated by trypsin. It hydrolyses the proteins into small polypeptides.
   - *Elastase:* It is secreted as proelastase, which is activated by trypsin. It digests elastin.

   Carboxypeptidase A and B: These are secreted as procarboxypeptidase A and B and are activated by enterokinase and trypsin.
     - Carboxypeptidase A cleaves the carboxyl-terminal amino acid that has aromatic or branched aliphatic side chains.
     - Carboxypeptidase B cleaves the carboxyl-terminal amino acids that have basic side chains.
   - *Nucleases* (ribonuclease and deoxyribonuclease): They split nucleic acids of ribose and deoxyribose type into nucleotides.
   - *Collagenase:* It is also activated by trypsin and digests collagen.
4. ***Trypsin inhibitor:*** If even a small amount of trypsin is released into the pancreas, the resulting chain reaction would produce active enzymes that could digest the pancreas. It is, therefore, not surprising that the pancreas normally contains a trypsin inhibitor, which is secreted by the same cells and at the same time as the pancreatic proenzymes. The trypsin inhibitor protects the pancreas from autodigestion.

Functions of Pancreatic Juice

1. Digestive functions The pancreatic juice is the major source of digestive enzymes that digest all components of the food – proteins, carbohydrates, fats and nucleic acid. For details, see page 633.

2. Neutralizing function Pancreatic juice is highly alkaline due to high concentration of HCO_3^- and neutralizes the gastric HCl in the chyme that enters the duodenum.

Mechanism of Pancreatic Secretion

Secretion of Pancreatic Enzymes

- The acinar cells of the exocrine part of the pancreas produce the pancreatic enzymes which are synthesized in the ribosomes of the rough endoplasmic reticulum. The raw material for the synthesis of enzymes is amino acids derived from the blood.
- After synthesis in the rough endoplasmic reticulum, the enzymes pass to the Golgi complex where they are surrounded by membranes and then released into the cytoplasm as *secretory (zymogen) granules.*
- The zymogen granules move to the luminal surface of the cells. When stimulated, the acinar cells pour the enzymes in the lumen of acini by *exocytosis.* After passing through the intercalated and interlobar ducts, ultimately the pancreatic juice containing these enzymes is poured into the duodenum through the main and accessory pancreatic ducts.
- Within the cells, these enzymes are stored in inactive form (proenzymes). They become active only after mixing with duodenal contents. Activation is initiated by the brush border enzyme enteropeptidase (enterokinase) present in the epithelial cells lining the duodenum.

Formation of Aqueous Component of Pancreatic Secretion

The aqueous component of the pancreatic juice is produced principally by the columnar epithelial cells which line the pancreatic ducts. However, acinar cells, which are primarily responsible for secreting pancreatic enzymes, also have some contribution towards aqueous component. The characteristics of the aqueous component of pancreatic juice secreted by acinar cells, intralobular ductal cells and extralobular ductal cells (Fig. 7.4.3) are as follows:

Secretion by acinar cells The acinar fluid is isotonic and resembles plasma in its concentrations of Na^+, K^+, Cl^- and HCO_3^-. Cl^- is secreted across the apical membrane down its concentration gradient through cystic fibrosis transmembrane conductance regulator (CFTR) channels. The concentration gradient is established by basolateral uptake through Na^+/

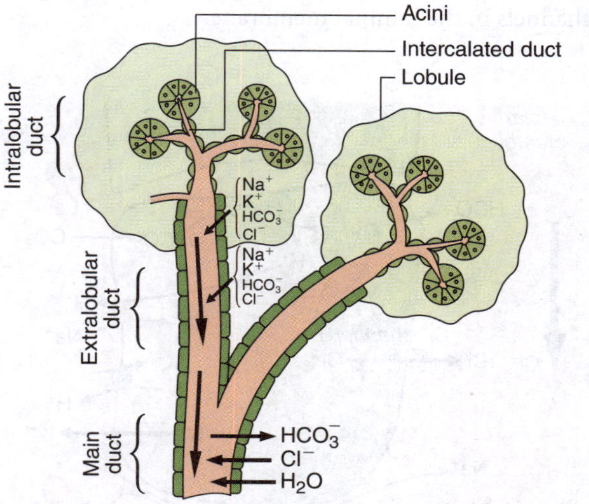

Fig. 7.4.3 Formation of the aqueous component of pancreatic juice at the level of acinar cells, intralobular ductal cells and extralobular ductal cells, and modification at the level of the main collecting duct.

$K^+/2Cl^-$ cotransporter. Water and Na^+ follow Cl^- movement through paracellular transport.

The secretion of acinar fluid and the proteins it contains is stimulated by cholecystokinin (CCK) and acetylcholine.

Applied Aspects

In the absence of cystic fibrosis (CFTR), the pancreatic secretions become thick and viscus (due to inadequate Cl^- and water), which block the pancreatic ducts causing chronic pancreatitis.

Secretion by intralobular ductal cells The spontaneous secretion that is produced by intralobular ductal cell has a higher concentration of K^+ and HCO_3^- than plasma.

Secretion by extralobular ductal cells Secretion by extralobular ductal cells is stimulated by the hormone secretin. The secretin-stimulated secretion by the extralobular ductal cells is still richer in HCO_3^- than the spontaneous secretion.

Cellular mechanism for secretion of HCO_3^--rich fluid by the ductal epithelial cells Bicarbonate in the blood, perfusing the pancreatic duct, rather than HCO_3^- that is produced by the ductal epithelial cells, is the major source of the HCO_3^- that is secreted into the lumen of the extralobular duct. The steps involved in the secretion of HCO_3^- are as follows (Fig. 7.4.4):

- Blood perfusing the ducts is acidified by Na^+–H^+ exchangers and H^+–K^+-ATPase in the basolateral membrane resulting in the formation of CO_2 from blood HCO_3^-.
- CO_2 diffuses into the ductal cells, where it combines with water (H_2O) to form carbonic acid (H_2CO_3) in the presence of enzyme carbonic anhydrase (CA).
- Dissociation of H_2CO_3 to H^+ and HCO_3^-, together with extrusion of H^+ across the basolateral membrane, produces a high intracellular HCO_3^-.
- HCO_3^- flows down its electrochemical potential gradient across the luminal membrane via the Cl^-, HCO_3^- exchanger.
- Cl^- is recycled back into the lumen by the electrogenic Cl^- channels in the luminal membrane.

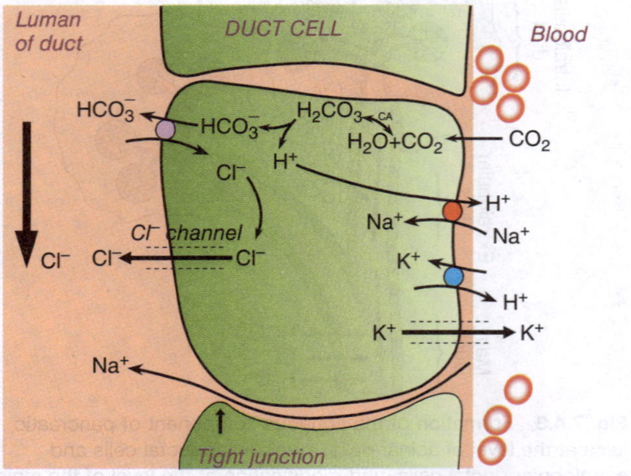

Fig. 7.4.4 Mechanism of secretion of HCO_3^- by the ductal epithelial cells.

- Na^+ enters the luminal fluid by flowing through the tight junctions in response to the negative electrical potential in the lumen that is produced by electrogenic Cl^- transport.
- Efflux of K^+ through basolateral K^+ channels maintains the intracellular electronegativity that is part of the driving force for the transport of Cl^- and HCO_3^- across the luminal membrane.

Modification in the main collecting ducts As the secretion flows through the main ducts, water moves into the duct across the epithelium (because the pancreatic duct cells are permeable to water), and makes the pancreatic juice isotonic to plasma. In addition, some HCO_3^- moves out of the ducts in exchange for Cl^- (Fig. 7.4.3).

Effect of flow rate on composition of aqueous component of pancreatic juice The electrolyte composition of pancreatic juice varies with the secretion rate (Fig. 7.4.5).

Bicarbonate ion (HCO_3^-) Bicarbonate ion (HCO_3^-) concentration of pancreatic juice at low secretory rate is as high as 80 mEq/L (much more that of plasma, 26 mEq/L) and increases up to 120 mEq/L at high flow rates.

Chloride ion (Cl^-) Chloride ion (Cl^-) concentration decreases as the flow rate of pancreatic juice increases; in other words, the HCO_3^- concentration rises. Thus, the total concentration of HCO_3^- and Cl^- remains constant and there exists a reciprocal relationship between their concentrations (Fig. 7.4.5).

Sodium (Na^+) and potassium (K^+) Sodium (Na^+) and potassium (K^+) concentrations in the pancreatic juice, unlike the saliva, are similar to those in the plasma and do not vary with the rate of secretion.

Tonicity of pancreatic juice From the above, it is clear that regardless of the flow rate, pancreatic secretions are *isotonic*. ***At low flow rates***, the pancreas secretes an isotonic fluid that is composed mainly of Na^+ and Cl^-, as at low flow rates, equal volume of pancreatic juice comes from acinar and ductal cells. At high flow rates, the pancreas secretes an isotonic fluid that is composed mainly of Na^+ and HCO_3^-, as at high flow rates, the proportion of the pancreatic juice secreted by

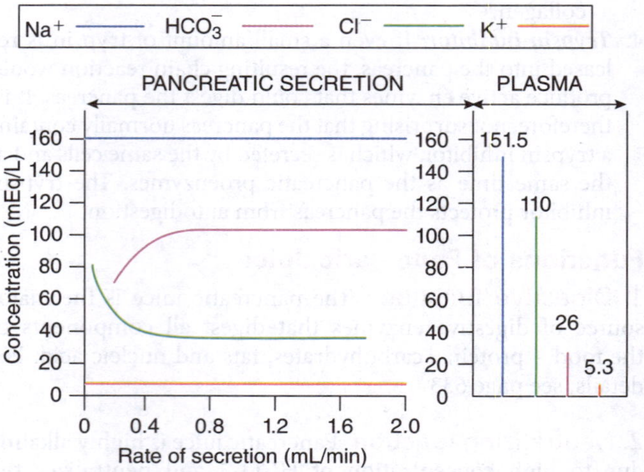

Fig. 7.4.5 Effect of rate of secretion of pancreatic juice on its electrolyte composition.

the ductal cells, which have a high concentration of HCO_3^-, increases.

Regulation of Pancreatic Secretion

Both neural and hormonal mechanisms are involved in the regulation of pancreatic secretion, with the latter playing the predominant role.

Neural regulation is through vagal efferents supplying the exocrine gland of the pancreas and hormonal regulation is through secretin, CCK, gastrin and somatostatin. The exact role of these regulatory mechanisms in regulating the different phases of pancreatic secretion, viz. cephalic phase, gastric phase and intestinal phase, is summarized in Table 7.4.1.

1. Regulation of cephalic phase

Cephalic phase of pancreatic secretion like that of gastric secretion occurs before the entry of food into the stomach. This phase is characterized by very little flow of secretions from pancreatic ducts into the juice.

Regulation of this phase is mainly through the reflex vagal stimulation, which occurs by:

Conditioned reflexes, initiated by sight, smell and thought of food.

Unconditioned reflexes are initiated by stimulation of taste buds by the food in the mouth cavity, the act of chewing and swallowing.

Afferent impulses, from the cerebral cortex (during conditioned reflexes) and from the mouth (during unconditioned reflexes), reach the dorsal nucleus of vagus.

Efferents in vagus nerve supplying the exocrine part of the pancreas enhance secretion from both acinar and ductal cells:

- *Enzyme secretion* from acinar cells is enhanced due to stimulation of enteric neurons, which release acetylcholine. Acetylcholine exerts its effect on the acinar cells by activating *phospholipase*.
- *Bicarbonate secretion* from the ductal cells is enhanced by stimulation of enteric neurons which release noradrenergic transmitters.

2. Regulation of gastric phase

Gastric phase of pancreatic secretion occurs when the stomach is distended by the food. This phase is regulated by *neural control* exerted through the vagus and *hormonal control* executed through the hormone gastrin:

Vagus stimulation (vagovagal reflex), which occurs due to distension of the body of the stomach by the food, results in secretion of low volumes of pancreatic juice containing HCO_3^- and enzymes. Acetylcholine is the transmitter.

Gastrin hormone is released from antral G-cells by the food breakdown products (primarily amino acids and peptides). Gastrin released into the blood, while reaching the pancreas, stimulates the acinar cells and produces a low-volume, high-enzyme pancreatic secretion.

3. Regulation of intestinal phase

The intestinal phase of pancreatic secretion begins when the chyme enters the duodenum and jejunum. It is characterized by a marked increase in the secretion of both enzymes and aqueous component of pancreatic juice. This phase is regulated by the hormones secretin and CCK.

i. Role of secretin

Secretin was the first hormone ever discovered by Bayliss and Starling in 1902. It is a polypeptide with 27 amino acids.

Source Source of secretin is endocrinal S-cells located among the epithelial cells of the mucous membrane of the duodenum and jejunum.

Stimulant Stimulant for release of secretin is *low pH* (<4.5) of chyme caused by the presence of gastric HCl.

Actions Secretin is released in an inactive form – *prosecretin*, which is converted into secretin by the gastric HCl and salts of fatty acids present in the chyme. Secretin enters the blood circulation and after reaching the pancreas it *acts on the duct* cells via cyclic AMP (second messenger) and produces large amounts of watery juice with a high concentration of HCO_3^-. The alkaline pancreatic juice with high concentration of HCO_3^- subserves the following functions:

- *Neutralizes the HCl* present in the chyme and thus protects the intestinal mucosa from the acid
- *Provides a required pH* (7–9) for the activation of pancreatic enzymes

Table 7.4.1 Summary of regulation of cephalic, gastric and intestinal phases of pancreatic secretion

Phase	Stimulus	Mediator	Pancreatic response
Cephalic	Conditioned reflex initiated by: • Taste • Smell • Thought of food Unconditioned reflex initiated by taste of food in mouth	Vagus	Little secretion of pancreatic enzymes and HCO_3^-
Gastric	• Distension of stomach by food	Vagus	Low volume of pancreatic HCO_3^- and enzymes
	• Amino acids and peptides	Gastrin	Low-volume, high-enzyme secretion
Intestinal	• Low pH of chyme in duodenum	Secretin	Large amount of aqueous secretion with high HCO_3^- concentration
	• Amino acids and peptides in chyme in duodenum	CCK	Pancreatic juice rich in enzymes
	• Food in small intestine	Vagus through: • Secretin • CCK	Pancreatic juice rich in enzymes and HCO_3^-

CCK, cholecystokinin.

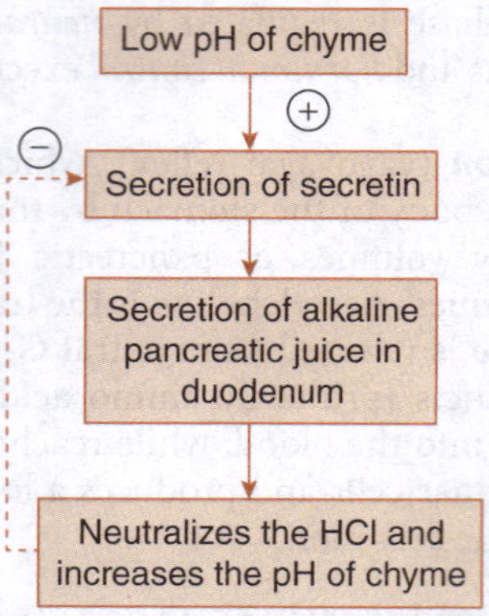

Fig. 7.4.6 Regulation of secretin secretion.

Other actions of secretin are as follows:

- Also stimulates bile secretion
- Potentiates the effect of CCK on the pancreas
- Along with CCK causes contraction of the pyloric sphincter delaying gastric emptying and thus preventing the reflux of duodenal contents into the stomach

Regulation of secretin Regulation of secretin occurs through a negative feedback mechanism shown in Fig. 7.4.6.

ii. Role of cholecystokinin CCK is a polypeptide containing 33 amino acids. Previously it was thought that two separate hormones – CCK (which causes contraction of the gall bladder) and pancreozymin (PZ, which stimulates the pancreas) – are released from the duodenal mucosa. However, now it has been proved that both the actions (on the gall bladder and pancreas) are brought about by a single hormone which is called CCK-PZ or simply CCK.

Source of secretion of CCK Source of secretion of CCK is the *endocrinal I-cells* located among the epithelial cells of the mucosa of the duodenum and jejunum. CCK, produced from the precursor prepro-CCK, contains 58 amino acid residues (CCK-58) processed into many fragments. Different forms of CCK are CCK-39, CCK-12, CCK-8 and CCK-4. Like gastrin, all these forms of CCK have five amino acids same at the carboxyl terminal. The half-life of CCK is 5 minutes; very little is known about its metabolism.

Stimulants Stimulants for release of CCK are amino acids (primarily phenylalanine), fatty acids and monoglycerides present in the chyme.

Actions CCK passes via blood to the pancreas and causes *secretion of pancreatic juice rich in enzymes* by causing discharge of zymogen granules from the pancreatic acinar cells via second messenger inosine triphosphate (IP_3) and increased intracellular Ca^{2+}.

Other actions Other actions of CCK are as follows:

- Contraction of the gall bladder to release bile
- Potentiates the effect of secretin to produce more alkaline pancreatic juice
- Increases the secretion of enterokinase (enteropeptidase) from the duodenum
- Inhibits the gastric motility and gastric emptying
- Increases the motility of small and large gut
- Increases the pancreatic growth (trophic effect)
- Is also found in neurons in the brain (especially in the cerebral cortex) where it is involved in the regulation of food intake and is related to the production of anxiety and analgesia

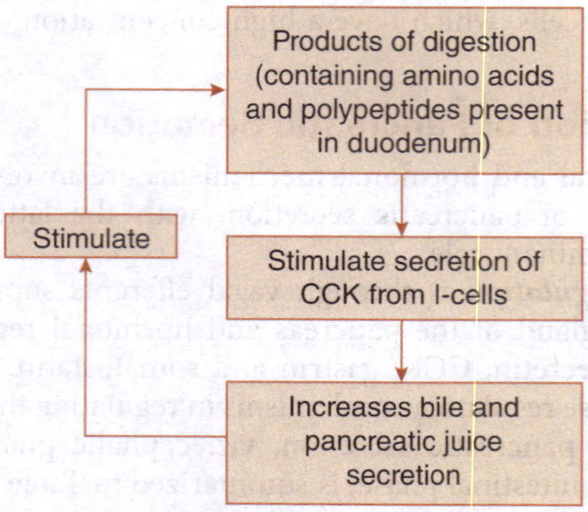

Fig. 7.4.7 Regulation of cholecystokinin secretion.

Mechanism of action CCK acts through its receptors. Two types of CCK receptors have been identified. CCK-A receptors are located primarily in the periphery, whereas both CCK-A and CCK-B receptors are found in the brain. Both types of receptors cause activation of phospholipase-C, causing increased production of IP_3 and diacylglycerol (DAG).

Regulation of CCK secretion Regulation of CCK secretion occurs through a positive feedback mechanism (Fig. 7.4.7).

The secretion of CCK is increased by contact of intestinal mucosa with product of digestion (particularly peptides of amino acid and fatty acid containing more than 10 carbon atoms). Two releasing factors that activate CCK secretion have been identified, which are CCK-releasing peptide (from intestinal mucosa) and monitor peptide (from the pancreas).

Potentiation of effect of secretin and CCK

- Secretin potentiates the effect of CCK. By itself, secretin has no effect on enzyme secretion.
- CCK potentiates the effect of secretin. By itself, CCK has no effect on HCO_3^- secretion.
- Because they are potentiators of each other's action, small concentrations of CCK and secretin together can produce significant amounts of pancreatic HCO_3^- and enzyme secretions.

Interaction of nervous and humoral regulation A vagovagal reflex is initiated during intestinal phase of digestion, which greatly potentiates the effects of secretin and CCK through the acetylcholine. Thus, vagus stimulation is much more potent in stimulating pancreatic secretions when CCK and secretin are present in the plasma.

Applied Aspects

Disorders of Pancreas

Common disorders of the pancreas are as follows:

1. Acute Pancreatitis

It is an acute inflammatory disease of the pancreas, thought to result from autodigestion of pancreatic tissue by the proteolytic enzymes which leak out of the acini and are activated within the pancreas. Recently, it has been hypothesized that the proteolytic enzymes become activated by lysosomal hydrolases within the pancreatic acini itself. The patient usually presents with acute pain in the upper abdomen, nausea and vomiting. Acute pancreatitis is a serious disease and may be fatal sometimes. Marked elevation of serum amylase (threefold rise) usually *clinches* the diagnosis.

Pathophysiology of Acute Pancreatitis. Acute pancreatitis occurs as a consequence of premature activation of zymogen granules, releasing proteases which digest the pancreatic epithelium and surrounding tissue. The severity of the condition depends on the balance between the activity of released proteolytic enzymes and antiproteolytic factors such as intracellular pancreatic trypsin inhibitor protein, circulating β_2-macroglobulin, α_1-antitrypsin and Cl-esterase inhibitor. The conditions that can cause acute pancreatitis have been given in Fig. 7.4.8.

Clinical Presentation of Acute Pancreatitis:

- Abdominal pain, vomiting, fever and anorexia are the main symptoms.
- Multisystem failure may occur due to hypoxia and hypotension.
- In severe cases, widespread intravascular bleeding may occur.

Diagnosis. Diagnosis of acute pancreatitis is made by signs, symptoms and investigations.

- *Blood tests* show elevated levels of pancreatic enzymes (amylase and lipase).
- *Inflammatory markers* such as C-reactive proteins are raised.
- *Abdominal ultrasonography*, computed tomography (CT) and MRI indicate enlarged pancreas.

Management. Acute pancreatitis is often self-limiting. The management comprises several steps:

- Proper diagnosis and its severity to be established

Early treatment depending on the severity of the disease, i.e. management of analgesia by:

- Analgesics such as pethidine are given.
- Hypovolaemia is corrected using normal saline/colloids.

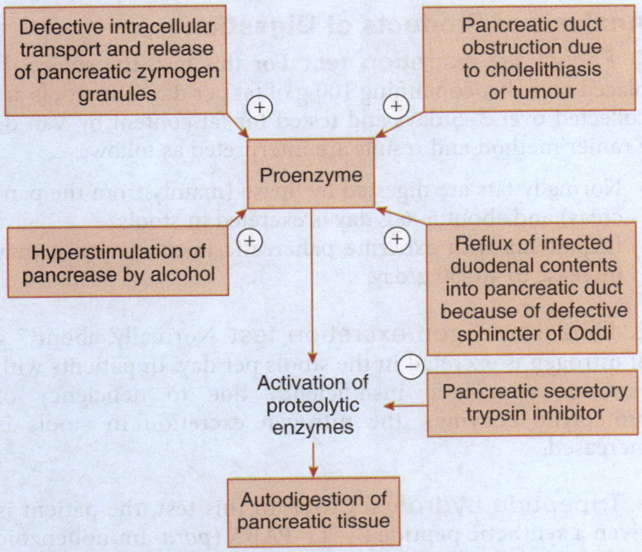

Fig. 7.4.8 Pathophysiology of acute pancreatitis.

- To minimize pancreatic enzyme production, the patient should be kept on nil orally and the stomach is emptied by nasogastric suction.
- Antibiotics are recommended to control infection.

Detection and treatment of complications

Treatment of underlying cause, especially gallstones

Complications include diabetes mellitus, kidney failure and bleeding.

2. Chronic Pancreatitis

Chronic pancreatitis is a chronic inflammation of the pancreas which results in slow destruction of the tissue resulting in the deficiency of pancreatic secretions.

Causative Factors include:

- *Toxic* metabolic factors which include alcohol, smoking and hypercalcaemia
- *Chronic* renal failure
- *Genetic factors* (hereditary pancreatitis occurs due to trypsinogen mutation, SPINK-1 mutation and cystic fibrosis)
- *Autoimmunity* (it may be isolated or involve multiple organs)
- *Recurrence* of acute pancreatitis
- *Obstructive cause due to stenosis of the sphincter of Oddi or tumours*

Patients with Extensive Destruction of Pancreas

Patients with extensive destruction of the pancreas may develop:

- *Digestive disturbances* due to deficiency of pancreatic enzymes mainly affect the fat metabolism resulting in *steatorrhoea* which is characterized by bulky, foul-smelling, pale and greasy stools (due to increase in faecal fat content). The condition resembles *intestinal malabsorption*, from which it can be differentiated by the secretin CCK test (see page 602).
- *Diabetes mellitus* occurs due to pancreatic endocrine deficiency of insulin (see page 769).
- Damage to sensory nerves, scarring and obstruction of pancreatic duct causes abdominal pain.

Treatment. Treatment involves:

- Replacement of pancreatic enzymes with oral supplements
- Treating diabetes mellitus with insulin therapy
- Relief of abdominal pain

3. Cystic Fibrosis

Cystic fibrosis is a disorder of pancreatic secretion. It results from a defect in the Cl^- channel that is caused by a mutation in the cystic fibrosis transmembrane conductance regulator (CFTR) gene. It is associated with a deficiency of pancreatic enzymes resulting in steatorrhoea (features described above).

4. Pancreatectomy

Pancreatectomy, i.e. surgical removal of the pancreas, is usually performed in carcinoma of the pancreas. It results in deficiency of pancreatic enzymes characterized by the same features as described in 'Chronic Pancreatitis'.

PANCREATIC FUNCTION TESTS

Pancreatic function tests are performed to evaluate the normal functioning of the pancreas and to detect abnormality, if

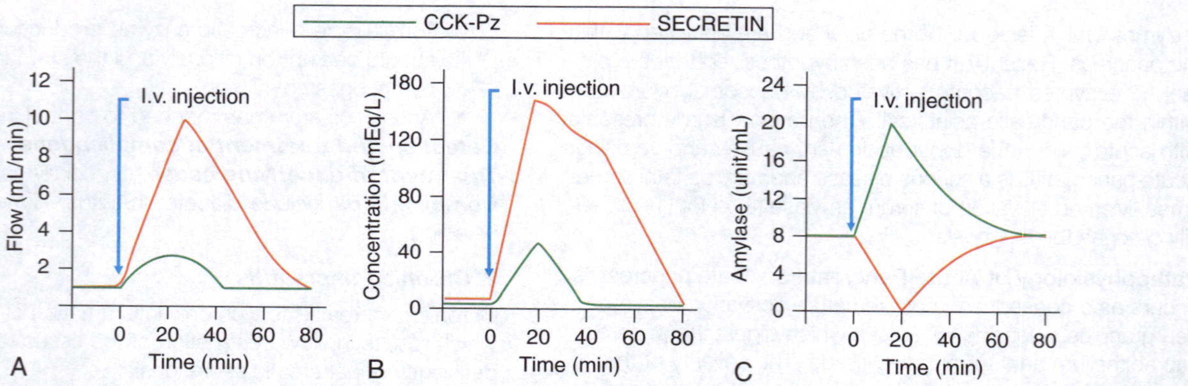

Fig. 7.4.9 Normal curves for combined secretin–cholecystokinin test: **A**, volume of pancreatic juice; **B**, HCO_3^- concentration of pancreatic juice; and **C**, enzyme (amylase) level of pancreatic juice.

any. The function tests to evaluate the functioning of the exocrine part of the pancreas can be divided as follows:

- Analysis of pancreatic juice
- Analysis of products of digestion
- Estimation of serum amylase levels

Analysis of Pancreatic Juice

Collection of pancreatic juice *A double-lumen radiopaque* tube (D veiling tube) is inserted through the nose or mouth, till the tip of the tube reaches the duodenum near the ampulla of Vater. The tube has a weighted bulbous end and contains two sets of holes, one for duodenal and the other for gastric aspiration. In this way, uncontaminated pancreatic juice can be collected from the duodenum.

The recent, advanced method of collecting pure pancreatic juice involves use of a *fibreoptic catheter* introduced under direct vision into the pancreatic duct.

Analysis of pancreatic juice collected after direct stimulation Analysis of pancreatic juice collected after direct stimulation of the pancreas is done by:

1. Secretin test Secretin, which stimulates ductal cells, is used to measure the secretory capacity of these cells:

- After overnight fasting, duodenal and gastric contents are aspirated in the morning.
- Intravenous infusion of secretin (12.5 units/kg body weight) is given, and duodenal aspirate is collected at 10-minute intervals over the next 80 minutes.
- Aspirated contents are examined for volume, pH, HCO_3^- concentration and HCO_3^- output.
- Normal values are as follows:
  - *Volume output:* 2.0 mL/kg in 80 minutes
  - *HCO_3^- concentration:* 80 mEq/L
  - *HCO_3^- output:* 10 mEq/L in 30 minutes
  - *Secretory activity of ductal cells:* Decreased in chronic pancreatitis

2. Combined secretin and CCK test Combined secretin and CCK test is used to evaluate the secretory capacity of both ductal cells and acinar cells. The test is performed as follows:

- First, secretin test is performed as described above.
- Then, CCK is given intravenously and the whole process is repeated.
- Curves for normal values of volume of pancreatic juice, HCO_3^- concentration and enzyme levels obtained by this test are shown in Fig. 7.4.9.
- Abnormalities can be detected from the results. With mild pancreatic damage, there is dissociation between the bicarbonate and enzyme output, i.e. only the former is affected, although with advanced damage, both are affected.
- This test helps to differentiate patients with steatorrhoea due to intestinal malabsorption (in which the test will be normal) from that due to chronic pancreatitis (in which there will be decreased secretion of enzymes).

Analysis of pancreatic juice collected after indirect stimulation Analysis of pancreatic juice collected after indirect stimulation of the pancreas is done by:

1. Lundh test In this test, the pancreas is stimulated indirectly, by ingestion of a test meal (containing fats, proteins and carbohydrates), and assessment of trypsin activity is made from the pancreatic juice collected. The mean trypsin activity of <6 IU/L indicates presence of pancreatic exocrine insufficiency.

Analysis of Products of Digestion

1. Faecal fat excretion test For this test, the subject is placed on a diet containing 100 g of fat per day. The stools are collected over 3–5 days and tested for fat content by Van de Kramer method and results are interpreted as follows:

- Normally fats are digested by lipase (mainly from the pancreas) and about 5–6 g/day is excreted in stools.
- In patients with exocrine pancreatic insufficiency, it may increase to 40–50 g/day.

2. Faecal nitrogen excretion test Normally, about 7 g of nitrogen is excreted in the stools per day. In patients with exocrine pancreatic insufficiency due to deficiency of proteolytic enzymes, the nitrogen excretion in stools is increased.

3. Tripeptide hydrolysis test In this test, the patient is given a synthetic peptide B_2–T_4–PABA (*para*-aminobenzoic acid). Normally, B_2–T_4–PABA is cleaved by the chymotrypsin into B_2–T_4 and PABA. PABA is rapidly absorbed and excreted in urine. In exocrine pancreatic insufficiency, cleavage of B_2–T_4–PABA is decreased leading to decreased excretion of PABA in the urine. Thus, from the values of PABA in urine, activity of pancreatic chymotrypsin can be studied.

4. Dual-label Schilling test In this test, ability of the gut to absorb vitamin B_{12} is studied. It is based on the fact that pancreatic proteases (trypsin) play an important role in the absorption mechanism of vitamin B_{12} and that in pancreatic insufficiency the absorption of vitamin B_{12} is abnormal.

Estimation of Serum Amylase Levels

This test is particularly useful in ruling out acute pancreatitis in patients presenting with acute pain in the upper abdomen. Normal values of serum amylase are 50–120 units/L. The levels of serum amylase are markedly raised in patients with acute pancreatitis.

LIVER AND GALL BLADDER

LIVER: PHYSIOLOGICAL ANATOMY

General Considerations

- Liver, the largest gland in the body, weighs approximately 1500 g and accounts for approximately 1/40th of adult body weight.
- Traditionally, the liver has been divided into *right and left lobes*. The right lobe is much larger and includes the caudate and quadrate lobes. The left lobe is much smaller and consists of one-sixth of total weight of the liver.
- In current terminology, the liver consists of right and left functionally independent parts called the *portal lobes* that are approximately equal in size. Thus, functionally the left part of the liver includes the caudate lobe and most of the quadrate lobe (Fig. 7.4.10).
- The right and left functional parts of the liver have their own blood supply from the hepatic artery and portal vein and their own venous and biliary drainage.
- The liver has got considerable physiological reserve. Even after removal of 80% of liver tissues, all *physiological* functions of the liver can be accomplished normally. Furthermore, even if 90% of bile ducts are ligated, the volume of bile secreted remains normal.
- The liver possesses considerable *regeneration power*. Original liver mass is restored within 6–8 weeks of removal of up to three-fourths of the liver. This occurs due to active mitotic division of the cells.

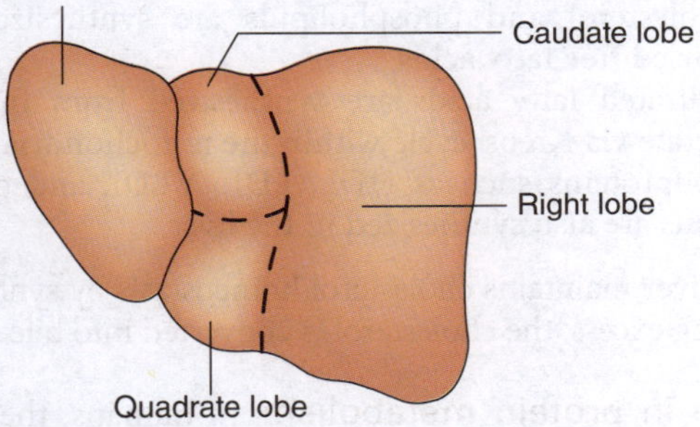

Fig. 7.4.10 Gross anatomy of the liver (viewed from the back).

Structural Characteristics

- The liver tissue comprises about 1 lakh hexagonal areas that constitute the *hepatic lobules* (Fig. 7.4.11A).
- Each hepatic lobule is made up of ramifying columns of hepatic cells (*hepatocytes*) that are arranged in the form of one-cell-thick plates. In between the cells are present bile canaliculi. These hepatic cell plates are tunnelled by a communicating system of lacunae called *blood sinusoids*. The sinusoids open into a central vein present in the centre of each lobule (Fig. 7.4.11B).
- Blood sinusoids are lined by endothelial cells. Few tissue macrophages called *Kupffer* cells are found at regular intervals in between the endothelial cells. The endothelial cells have large fenestrations, thereby forming an intimate contact between the blood and hepatic cells. This helps the liver to transform or modify many of the constituents of blood.
- Along the periphery of each lobule are present *portal triads* consisting of a branch of portal vein, a branch of hepatic artery and an interlobular bile duct. Blood from the branch of the portal vein and hepatic artery enters the sinusoids which drain into the central vein.
- Concept of portal lobule has been suggested by some workers. It has been described to consist of adjoining parts of three hepatic lobules centred on a portal triad.
- Presently, acinus is considered the functional unit of the liver. Each acinus is considered to have three zones – 1, 2 and 3. ***Zone 1*** refers to the central portion of the acinus immediately surrounding the terminal hepatic arteriole and terminal portal venule. This zone is well oxygenated. Enzymes involved in oxidative metabolism and glucogenesis predominate here.

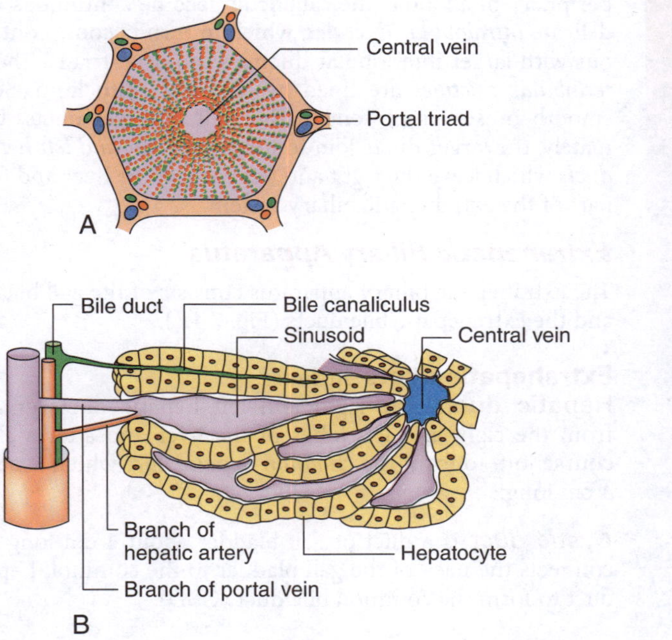

Fig. 7.4.11 Histological characteristics of the liver: **A**, hexagonal lobule with portal triad; and **B**, hepatocyte, sinusoid and biliary canaliculi seen under high magnification.

Zone 3 refers to the most peripheral part of the acinus. It is the least oxygenated and most susceptible to anoxic injury. It is rich in enzymes involved in glycolysis, lipid and drug metabolism.

Zone 2, i.e. the intermediate zone, which is present in between zones 1 and 3, is moderately well oxygenated. It contains a mixed complement of enzymes.

For details, see page 361 and Fig. 4.6.19.

Hepatic Circulation

The liver receives about 1500 mL blood/min from two sources:

Hepatic artery, which is a branch of the coeliac trunk, supplies about 20%–25% (300–400 mL/min) of total blood which caters to the metabolic requirement of the liver tissue.

Portal vein, which collects blood from the mesenteric and splenic vascular bed, supplies about 75%–80% (1100–1200 mL/min) of the total blood.

Hepatic vein: The hepatic and portal streams of blood meet in the sinusoids. The various substances produced by liver cells, the waste products and CO_2 are discharged into the sinusoids. The sinusoids drain into the central vein of the lobule. The central veins from different lobules unite to form bigger veins. These veins ultimately form the right and left hepatic veins which open into the inferior vena cava.

For details about the hepatic circulation and oxygen consumption, see page 362.

Hepatic Biliary System

Intrahepatic Biliary System

The bile is secreted by liver cells into bile canaliculi. These canaliculi have no walls of their own. In fact, the bile canaliculi are the spaces bounded by canalicular surfaces of adjacent hepatic cells. On either side of the canaliculus, the two cell membranes are united by junctional complexes. These canaliculi form a hexagonal network around the liver cells. At the periphery of a lobule, the canaliculi become continuous with delicate *intralobular ductules*, which in turn become continuous with larger interlobular ductules of portal triads. The *interlobular ductules* are lined by cuboidal epithelium. Some smooth muscle is present in the wall of larger ducts. Ultimately, the larger ducts join to form the *right and left hepatic ducts* which leave the right and left parts of the liver and form part of the extrahepatic biliary system.

Extrahepatic Biliary Apparatus

The extrahepatic biliary apparatus consists of the gall bladder and the extrahepatic bile ducts (Fig. 7.4.1).

Extrahepatic ducts includes:

Hepatic ducts The right and left hepatic ducts emerge from the right and left lobes of the liver and after a short course join to form the *common hepatic duct* which is about 4 cm long.

Cystic duct is a duct of gall bladder about 4 cm long and connects the neck of the gall bladder to the common hepatic duct to form the common bile duct (CBD).

CBD is about 8 cm long. It joins the pancreatic duct to form the common hepatopancreatic duct which is otherwise called the ampulla of Vater. Ampulla of Vater opens into the duodenum at major duodenal papilla. The terminal parts of bile ducts and ampulla of Vater are surrounded by circular muscle fibres known as sphincter of Oddi, which play an important role in the storage and release of bile from the gall bladder.

FUNCTIONS OF LIVER

The fact that mitochondria are maximally present in the liver emphasizes that the liver is involved in many biochemical functions. Although details of the various functions performed by the liver are discussed under their respective places, they are summarized here briefly.

I. Secretory functions Liver cells act as exocrine glands and continuously secrete bile which is important for digestion and absorption of fats. Various aspects of the bile juice are discussed in this chapter.

II. Metabolic functions The liver is the key organ and the principal site where the metabolism of carbohydrates, lipids and proteins takes place. It is also involved in the metabolism of vitamins and minerals to a certain extent.

1. Role in carbohydrate metabolism The liver acts as a glucostat in three ways:

Glycogenesis, i.e. formation of glycogen from glucose and storage in the liver

Glycogenolysis, i.e. breaking down of liver glycogen to glucose

Glucogenesis, i.e. formation of glucose from noncarbohydrate sources such as non-nitrogenous residues of amino acids

The liver plays an important role in maintaining blood glucose level. In the postprandial period, the liver removes excess of glucose from blood and returns it back when needed. Therefore, this action is called *glucose buffer function*.

- The liver is the main site of alcohol metabolism for which liver cells contain the enzyme *alcohol dehydrogenase*.
- The interconversion of three monosaccharides, as glucose, galactose and fructose, also occurs in the liver.

2. Role in fat metabolism Both degradation and synthesis of fats take place in liver.

Degradation of fat: The liver contains the enzyme lipoprotein lipase which hydrolyses triglycerides, cholesterol and phospholipids into fatty acids.

- β-Oxidation, i.e. a process which oxidizes the fatty acids into acetoacetic acid, occurs within the mitochondria.

Synthesis of fat also takes place in the liver.

- The liver synthesizes triglycerides from carbohydrates.
- Cholesterol and phospholipids are synthesized from unused free fatty acids.
- Saturated fatty acids are synthesized from the active acetate via Krebs' cycle within the mitochondria.
- Lipoproteins such as HDL, LDL, VLDL and chylomicrons are also synthesized in the liver.

The liver maintains cholesterol homeostasis by synthesizing it. During excess, the cholesterol is converted into bile acids.

3. Role in protein metabolism In humans, the protein turnover involves breakdown and resynthesis of 80–100 g of tissue protein per day, and its 50% part (i.e. 40–50 g) occurs in the liver. Important activities are as follows:

- The liver brings about *deamination* of amino acids and this is essential for energy production, and their conversion into carbohydrates or fats.
- The liver is the main site of *urea formation*.
- The liver is the main site for formation of all nonessential amino acids by transamination of ketoacids.
- Albumin is solely resynthesized in the liver and also to some extent α- and β-globulins.

III. Detoxicating and protective functions

- Kupffer cells efficiently remove bacteria and other foreign bodies from portal circulation. This is the blood cleansing action of the liver.
- The biochemical detoxifying action of the liver is brought about by a large number of cytochrome P_{450} enzymes from hepatocytes. These enzymes convert xenobiotics and other toxins into their inactive form. The detoxification reactions can be divided into two phases:
  Phase I reactions, e.g. oxidation and hydroxylation, are mediated by P_{450} enzymes.
  Phase II reactions include esterification.
- The liver detoxifies certain drugs by oxidation, hydrolysis, reduction or conjugation and excretes out through bile.

IV. Storage functions The liver stores glucose (in the form of glycogen), vitamin B_{12} and vitamin A.

- The liver acts as a blood iron buffer and iron storage medium. It stores 60% of excess of iron mainly in the form of ferritin and partly as haemosiderin.

V. Excretory functions

Ammonium excretion The liver is the only site where circulating ammonia is converted into urea and then excreted by the kidney into the urine.

- In the circulating blood, ammonium is derived from the colon, kidney, breakdown of red blood cells and metabolism in the muscles.
- In the liver, ammonium is taken up by the hepatocytes. In the mitochondria of the hepatocyte, it is converted into carbonyl phosphate, which reacts with ornithine to generate citrullin, and by series of cytoplasmic reactions produces arginine, which can be dehydrated to form urea and ornithine (Fig. 7.4.12A).

The ornithine taken back into the mitochondria begins another urea cycle, whereas urea diffuses back into sinusoidal circulation and gets excreted by the kidney into the urine (Fig. 7.4.12B). Ammonia is critically handled by the liver, as it is freely permeable across the blood–brain barrier; therefore, it is toxic to CNS tissue.

(i) Certain exogenous dyes like bromsulphthalein (BSP) and rose Bengal dye are exclusively excreted through liver cells.
(ii) Cholesterol, alkaline phosphate and bilirubin are excreted in the bile.
(iii) A number of drugs and adrenocortical and other steroid hormones are excreted in the bile.

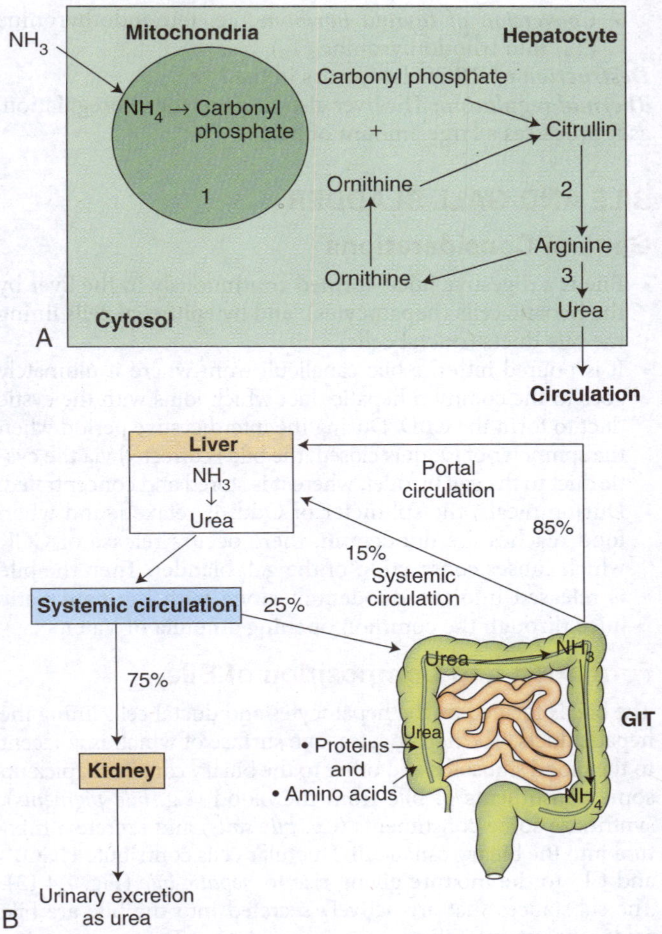

Fig. 7.4.12 **A**, urea cycle; and **B**, ammonia excretion as urea by the kidney.

VI. Synthesis function Liver is the site for synthesis of:

Plasma proteins, especially albumin and to some extent α- and β-globulins

Some blood coagulation factors (liver cells are responsible for conversion of preprothrombin [inactive] to active prothrombin in the presence of vitamin K; they also produce other clotting factors such as fibrinogen factor [I] and factors V, VII, IX and X)

Enzymes, such as alkaline phosphatase, serum glutamic oxaloacetic transaminase (SGOT), serum glutamic pyruvic transaminase (SGPT) and serum isocitrate dehydrogenase (SICD)

Urea (the liver removes ammonia from the body to synthesize urea)

Cholesterol (it is synthesized from the active acetate)

VII. Miscellaneous functions

Reservoir of blood: The liver acts as a reservoir of blood and it stores about 650 mL of blood. It also helps in regulation of blood volume.

Erythropoiesis: The liver is an important site of erythropoiesis in fetal life.

Hormone metabolism: The liver causes:

- *Inactivation* of some hormones such as insulin, glucagon and vasopressin
- *Reduction and conjugation* of adrenal and gonadal steroid hormones such as cortisol, aldosterone, oestrogen and testosterone

- *Conversion of thyroid hormone*, i.e. tetraiodothyronine (T_4) into triiodothyronine (T_3)

Destruction of RBCs also occurs in the liver.

Thermal regulation: The liver also helps in thermoregulation, as it produces a large amount of heat.

BILE AND GALL BLADDER

General Considerations

- Bile is a digestive juice, formed continuously in the liver by the hepatic cells (hepatocytes), and by epithelial cells lining the bile ducts (ductal cells).
- It is poured into the bile canaliculi from where it ultimately goes to the common hepatic duct which joins with the cystic duct to form the CBD. During the interdigestive period when the sphincter of Oddi is closed, the bile is directed via the cystic duct to the gall bladder, where it is stored and concentrated.
- During meals, the sphincter of Oddi is relaxed, and when food reaches the duodenum, there occurs release of CCK which causes contraction of the gall bladder. Then the bile is released into the duodenum along with the pancreatic juice through the common opening ampulla of Vater.

Formation and Composition of Bile

The bile is formed by the hepatocytes and ductal cells lining the hepatic ducts. The hepatocytes, one surface of which is adjacent to the blood sinusoids and other to the biliary canaliculi, pick up some constituents of bile from the blood (e.g. *bile pigments*), synthesize some constituents (e.g. *bile salts*) and secrete a mixture into the biliary canaliculi. Ductular cells contribute HCO_3^- and Cl^- to the mixture giving rise to *hepatic bile* (Fig. 7.4.13). The substances that are actively secreted into the bile are bile acids, cholesterol, bilirubin and xenobiotics. There are specific canalicular transporters for their excretion. The canalicular bile is transiently hypertonic, because a number of substances such as glucose, glutathione, water, calcium and urea passively diffuse from plasma through tight junctions. In the bile ductules and ducts, it undergoes modifications. The tight junctions of epithelial cells of ductules (cholangiocytes) are less permeable than those of hepatocytes, but freely permeable to water, making the bile isotonic. The bile so formed is an alkaline juice comprising:

Water

Solids include organic and inorganic substances:

- *Organic substances* are bile salts, bile pigments, cholesterol, lecithin, fatty acids, lipid-soluble end products of fat metabolism and xenobiotics, PC, glucose, glutathione, amino acid, urea and enzyme alkaline phosphatase.
- *Inorganic substances* are Na^+, K^+, Ca^{2+}, HCO_3^- and Cl^-.

Since the bile is concentrated in the gall bladder, the concentrations of its ingredients in the liver bile and gall bladder bile are bound to differ as shown in Table 7.4.2.

Salient features of the some of the ingredients of bile are described here.

1. Bile salts

Formation of bile salts Bile salts are sodium and potassium salts of bile acids conjugated with either taurine or glycine. They are of two types – primary and secondary. Steps in the formation of bile salts are as follows (Fig. 7.4.14):

Primary bile acids are cholic acid and chenodeoxycholic acid. These are synthesized by hepatocytes from cholesterol.

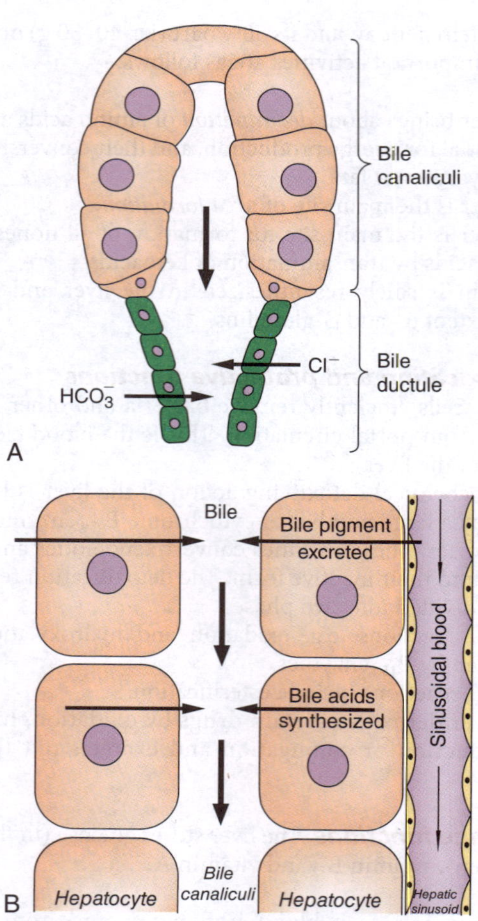

Fig. 7.4.13 Mechanism of bile formation: **A**, secretion by hepatocytes and ductal cells; and **B**, bile pigments picked up from blood sinusoids are excreted, whereas bile salts are synthesized and secreted by hepatocytes.

Table 7.4.2 Liver bile versus gall bladder bile

Properties and composition	Liver bile	Gall bladder bile
• pH	8–8.6	7–7.6
• Specific gravity	1010–1011	1026–1032
• Water	97.5%	87.5%
• Solids	2.5%	12.5%
Organic substances		
• Bile salts	1.10 g%	8.0 g%
• Bile pigments	0.20 g%	1.0 g%
• Cholesterol	0.10 g%	0.5 g%
• Fatty acid	0.15 g%	0.5 g%
• Fat	0.10 g%	0 g%
• Lecithin	0.1 g%	0.8 g%
• Mucin	Absent	Present
Inorganic substances	0.75 g%	8.7 g%

Secondary bile acids are deoxycholic acid and lithocholic acid. These are formed from the primary bile acids in the colon by the action of intestinal bacteria and a small quantity of ursodeoxycholic acid is formed from chenodeoxycholic acid.

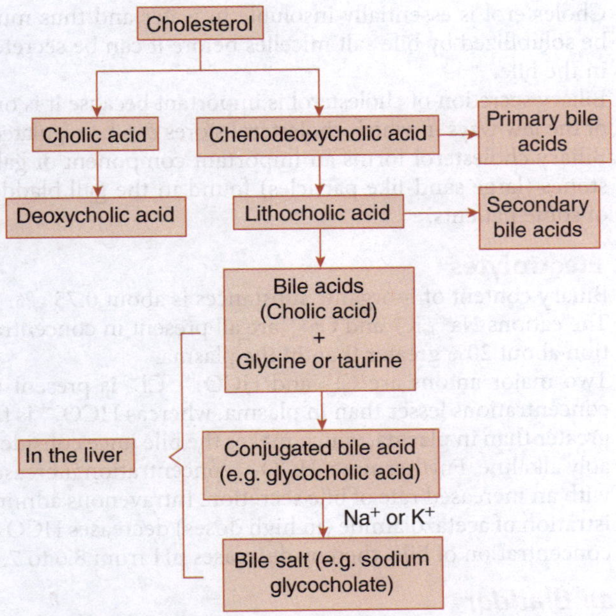

Fig. 7.4.14 Formation of bile salts from the bile acids.

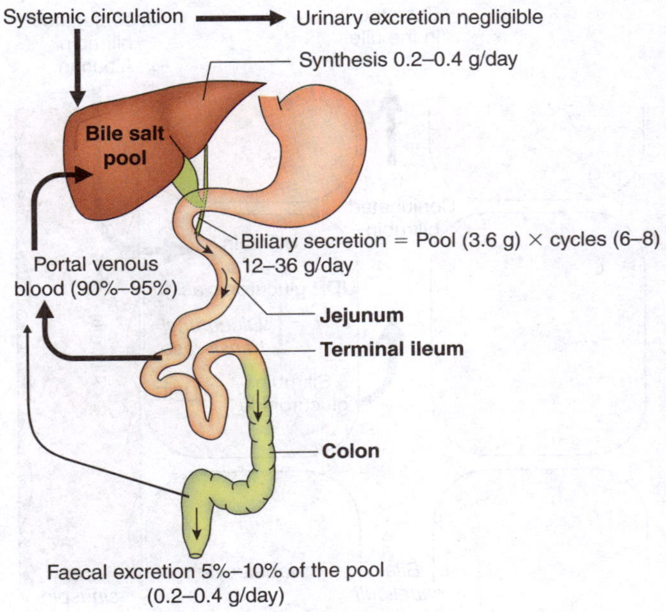

Fig. 7.4.15 Enterohepatic circulation of bile salts.

The conjugation of bile acids: In the liver, the bile acids are conjugated with either glycine (an amino acid) or taurine (an amino acid derivative) forming the conjugated bile acids.

The conjugated bile acids, namely glycocholic acid and taurocholic acid, form bile salts in combination with sodium or potassium.

Functions of bile salts Bile salts help in digestion as well as absorption of fat by their following actions:

Emulsification of fat, i.e. breaking of large fat droplets into smaller droplets, and their stabilization is caused by the bile salts because of their power of lowering surface tension. The emulsification is a prerequisite for action of pancreatic lipase, which is water soluble and acts only on the surface of a lipid droplet.

Acceleration of action of pancreatic lipase occurs in the presence of bile salts due to binding of colipase for the lipase.

Micelle formation: The bile salts combine with the products of hydrolysis of triglycerides to form *small water*-soluble cylindrical disc-shaped particles called micelles, which are transported to the brush border of the epithelial cells for absorption.

Absorption of fat-soluble vitamins (A, D, E and K) is aided by the bile salts by forming complexes more soluble in water (hydrotropic action).

Choleretic action, i.e. they stimulate the liver to secrete bile (as long as bile salts are absorbed) and then make more bile salts available for fat digestion.

Cholesterol is kept in soluble form in the gall bladder bile by the bile salts. This property of bile salts prevents formation of gallstone.

Intestinal motility is stimulated by bile salts. This action of bile salts helps in defaecation (laxative action).

Enterohepatic circulation of bile salts Enterohepatic circulation is the recirculation of bile salts from the liver to the small intestine and back again. This circulation is necessary because of the *limited pool of bile salts available* to help break down and to absorb fat.

Path of circulation Bile salts travel from the liver to the duodenum via the CBD (Fig. 7.4.15).

- When the bile salts reach *terminal ileum*, 90%–95% of bile salts is reabsorbed into the portal circulation. It is important to note that no absorption of bile salts occurs in the duodenum and jejunum. The liver then extracts the bile salts from the portal blood and secretes them once again into the bile.
- The remaining 5%–10% of bile salts is excreted into the faeces.

Circulating pool: The total circulating pool of bile salts (consisting of salts of primary and secondary bile acids) is approximately 3.6 g. About 4–8 g of bile salts is required (more if the meal is high in fat) for digestion of fats during each meal; thus, of the total content of bile salts in the body (3.6 g), most circulate twice during the digestion of each meal. Consequently, the bile salts usually circulate six to eight times daily.

Bile salt synthesis and replacement: The rate of bile salt synthesis is determined by the rate of return to the liver by enterohepatic circulation. Usually only 0.2–0.4 g (5%–10% of 3.6 g) of bile salts is lost in the faeces, which is replaced by synthesis. The maximal synthesis rate can go up to 3–6 g/day. If faecal losses exceed this rate, the total pool size decreases.

Clinical implications of enterohepatic circulation: As bile salts are required for proper digestion and absorption of fats, any condition that disrupts enterohepatic circulation (e.g. ileal resection or small intestinal diseases such as sprue or Crohn disease) leads to decreased bile salt pool and malabsorption of fat and fat-soluble vitamins. The clinical manifestations of such conditions are as follows:

- Steatorrhoea, i.e. increased fat content in the stools
- Nutritional deficiency due to malabsorption
- Watery diarrhoea because the bile salts which inhibit water and sodium absorption from the colon are decreased due to excessive loss in stools

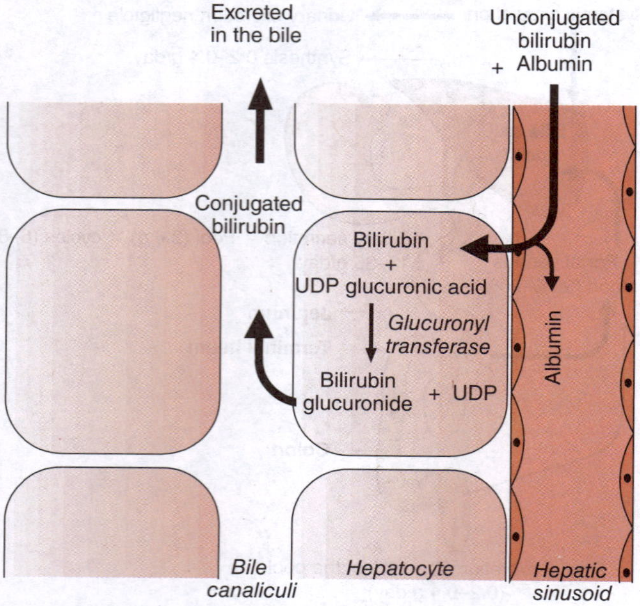

Fig. 7.4.16 Bile pigment metabolism in the hepatocyte.

2. Bile pigments

- The two principal bile pigments, *bilirubin* and *biliverdin*, are the other major constituents of bile which have no digestive function.
- Bile pigments are metabolites of haemoglobin formed in the liver.
- The hepatic cells extract bilirubin and biliverdin from the blood, conjugate them with glucuronic acid and transfer them into the bile canaliculi by an active transport mechanism (Fig. 7.4.16). They are responsible for the golden yellow colour of bile.
- Intestinal bacteria metabolize bilirubin further to urobilinogen, which is responsible for the brown colour of stools.

Applied Aspects

Hepatocellular dysfunction leading to failure of bilirubin passages causes accumulation of bile pigments in the blood producing hepatic or posthepatic jaundice, respectively.

Formation and circulation of bile pigments and jaundice are described on page 416.

3. Phospholipids

- The phospholipids (primarily lecithins) are, after bile salts, the most abundant organic compound in the bile.
- Phospholipids, which are normally insoluble in water, are solubilized by the bile salt micelles.
- Micelles are able to solubilize other lipids more effectively when they are composed of bile salts and phospholipids than when they are composed of bile salts alone.

4. Cholesterol

- Cholesterol is another important constituent of bile that does not have a digestive function. Its presence in the bile seems to be a by-product of bile salt synthesis in the hepatic cells. Normal biliary content of cholesterol is about 100 mg% (60–170 mg%) as compared with 150–240 mg% in blood.
- Cholesterol is essentially insoluble in water and thus must be solubilized by bile salt micelles before it can be secreted in the bile.
- Biliary secretion of cholesterol is important because it is one of the few ways in which cholesterol stores can be regulated.
- Biliary cholesterol forms an important component of gallstones (large sand-like particles) found in the gall bladder of some patients.

5. Electrolytes

- Biliary content of inorganic substances is about 0.75 g%.
- The cations Na^+, K^+ and Ca^{2+} are all present in concentration about 20% greater than in the plasma.
- Two major anions are Cl^- and HCO_3^-. Cl^- is present in concentrations lesser than in plasma, whereas HCO_3^- is far greater than in plasma, which makes the bile juice considerably alkaline. Furthermore, HCO_3^- concentration increases with an increased rate of bile secretion. Intravenous administration of acetazolamide (in high doses) decreases HCO_3^- concentration of bile, thereby decreases pH from 8.6 to 7.4.

Gall Bladder

The gall bladder is a pear-shaped sac lying on the undersurface of the liver. It has a capacity of about 30–50 mL and stores bile and concentrates by absorbing water. For descriptive purposes, the gall bladder is divided into fundus, body and neck. The neck becomes continuous with the *cystic duct*. It is not essential for life. Removal of the gall bladder (cholecystectomy) in patients suffering from dysfunction of the gall bladder does not result in any major disadvantages. Functions of the gall bladder are:

1. Storage of bile The bile secreted during the interdigestive period is stored in the gall bladder. The gall bladder typically stores 30–50 mL of bile. During meals, the gall bladder contracts and releases its contents into the duodenum.

2. Concentration of bile The mucosa of the gall bladder is extensively folded and can actively absorb fluid and electrolytes. In this way, the following are noted in the gall bladder bile, in comparison to that in liver bile (also see page 606):

- It becomes thicker, viscous and darker in colour.
- Water content is decreased (from 97% to 87.5%).
- All organic constituents which are not absorbed become five to six times concentrated.
- Cl^- and HCO_3^- ions decrease by five to six times (due to active absorption).
- Ca^{2+} and K^+ which are not absorbed increase by two times.

3. Effect on the pH of bile In the gall bladder, alkalinity of the stored bile is reduced due to rapid absorption of HCO_3^- (mainly), Na^+ and Cl^-. The pH of bile is decreased from 8–8.6 to 7–7.6.

4. Secretion of mucus The gall bladder secretes mucin which is added to the bile stored in it. The mucin acts as a lubricant in the intestine for the chyme.

5. Regulates equalization of pressure in biliary system Due to continuous absorption of water from the stored bile, the gall bladder regulates equalization of pressure in the biliary system. This fact can be understood by the following observations:

- When both the bile duct and the cystic duct are clamped, the pressure in the biliary system rises to above 30 cm of bile in 30 minutes, and bile secretion is stopped.

- When the bile duct is clamped alone, water is continuously reabsorbed in the gall bladder, and the pressure in the biliary system rises to only 10 cm of bile in several hours. Thus, the gall bladder prevents the rise of pressure in the biliary system.

Applied Aspects

Effects of Cholecystectomy

As mentioned earlier, bile, and not the gall bladder, is essential for digestion and absorption of fats. After removal of the gall bladder (cholecystectomy), the bile empties slowly but continuously into the intestine, allowing digestion of fats sufficient to maintain good health and nutrition. Only high-fat meals need to be avoided.

- Bile ducts become dilated to accommodate some of the bile which is continuously secreted by the liver.

Functions of Bile

Functions subserved by the bile poured into the duodenum are because of its constituents (mainly bile salts), which have already been discussed. However, they are compiled and summarized once again:

1. ***Digestive function:*** Bile salts help in digestion of fats by *emulsifying fat drops* (see page 638).
2. ***Absorptive functions:*** Bile salts help in absorption of fats (by micelle formation) and fat-soluble vitamins (see page 639).
3. ***Excretory function:*** Bile pigments are the major excretory products of the bile. The other substances excreted in bile are heavy metals (e.g. copper and iron), some toxins, some bacteria (e.g. typhoid bacteria), cholesterol, lecithin and alkaline phosphatase.
4. ***Laxative action:*** Bile salts increase the gastrointestinal motility and act as a laxative.
5. ***Protective action:*** Bile is a natural detergent. So, it inhibits the growth of certain bacteria in the lumen of the intestine.
6. ***Choleretic action***, i.e. bile salts stimulate the liver to secrete bile.
7. ***Maintenance of pH of GIT:*** Being highly alkaline, the bile juice neutralizes the gastric HCl present in the chyme entering the small intestine. Thus, an optimum pH is maintained for the action of digestive enzymes.
8. ***Prevention of gallstone formation:*** Bile salts keep the cholesterol and lecithin in solution and thus prevent the formation of gallstones. In the absence of bile salts, the cholesterol precipitates along with lecithin and may form gallstones.
9. ***Lubricating function:*** The mucin secreted by gall bladder mucosa into the bile lubricates the chyme in the intestine.
10. ***Cholagogue function:*** Cholagogue is an agent which increases the release of bile from the gall bladder into the intestine. The bile salts perform this function indirectly. The bile salts stimulate the secretion of hormone CCK, which has got the cholagogue action.

Regulation of Bile

The regulation of bile juice released into the duodenum after the meals is performed at two levels:

- Regulation of biliary secretion
- Regulation of release of bile from the gall bladder

A. Regulation of Biliary Secretion

The secretion of aqueous component (water and electrolytes) and that of the bile (containing bile salts and other organic substances), though occurring together, are controlled separately by the following mechanisms (Fig. 7.4.17A):

- Regulation of bile-independent fraction of biliary secretion
- Regulation of bile-dependent fraction of biliary secretion

1. Regulation of bile-independent fraction of biliary secretion The bile-independent fraction of biliary secretion refers to the amount of *fluid containing water and electrolytes.* Secretion of this fraction of the bile juice is (similar to the fluid secreted by ductal cells of the pancreas) controlled by secretin and vagal stimulation.

Secretin is a hormone secreted by S-cells of the duodenum and jejunum in response to stimulation of acidic chyme (for details, see page 659). It acts on the ductal cells of hepatic ducts (Fig. 7.4.17A) via cyclic AMP, second messenger, and produces large amounts of watery fluid with high concentration of HCO_3^-.

Vagovagal reflex initiated during intestinal phase of digestion also affects the ductal secretion by potentiating the effects of secretion through the acetylcholine.

Important Note

The agents (e.g. secretin and acetylcholine) which cause secretion of bile from the liver with more amount of water and less amount of solids are called hydrocholeretics.

2. Regulation of bile-dependent fraction of biliary secretion The bile-dependent fraction of biliary secretion refers to the quantity of bile salts secreted by the liver. It depends on the following factors (Fig. 7.4.17):

- The amount of bile salts secreted by the hepatocytes is directly proportional to the *amount of bile salts reabsorbed* by them from portal circulation. As the bile salts are recycled in the enterohepatic circulation, they maintain a high level of bile secretion during the digestive period. The secretion

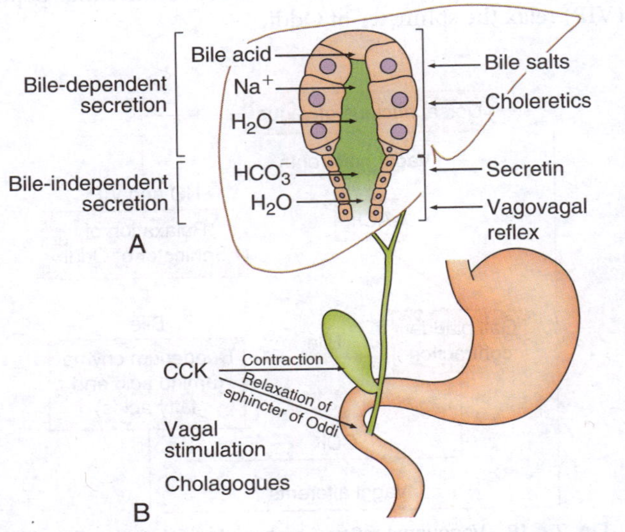

Fig. 7.4.17 A, regulation of bile secretion; and B, release from gall bladder.

of bile increases about 1 hour after a meal (when the gastric emptying starts). The maximum rate of bile secretion is achieved 3–5 hours after intake of food.

- Synthesis of bile salts in hepatocytes occurs to a limited amount. Bile salts and bile acids are the major agents which enhance synthesis of bile salts. Substances that enhance the secretion of bile salts by the hepatocytes are called choleretics.

Note: Synthesis of bile salts by the liver is not controlled by any hormonal or nervous factor.

B. Regulation of Release of Bile from Gall Bladder

Filling of gall bladder by the bile is simply controlled by a pressure gradient. During the interdigestive period, the sphincter of Oddi remains closed. As bile is secreted continuously, it gets accumulated in the CBD. When pressure of bile in the CBD rises, it forces its way through the cystic duct into the gall bladder. During the interdigestive period, the pressure in the CBD and gall bladder reaches 7 cm H_2O.

Emptying of gall bladder: When the chyme enters the duodenum, the gall bladder is contracted along with relaxation of the sphincter of Oddi, raising the pressure to about 20 cm H_2O. Because of the increase in pressure, the bile from the gall bladder enters the duodenum. The contraction of the gall bladder and relaxation of the sphincter of Oddi are regulated by the following factors (Fig. 7.4.17B):

1. Hormonal control The hormone *CCK* is the major stimulus for gall bladder contraction and sphincter of Oddi relaxation. When chyme enters the small intestine, *fat and protein digestion products* directly stimulate the secretion of CCK (for details about CCK, see page 600).

2. Neural control Vagal stimulation also causes contraction of the gall bladder and relaxation of the sphincter of Oddi. It occurs directly during the cephalic phase of digestion and indirectly via a vagovagal reflex during the gastric phase of digestion (Fig. 7.4.18).

Note: Substances that cause contraction of the gall bladder are called cholagogues. Thus, CCK is a well-known cholagogue and acetylcholine released on vagal stimulation also acts as a cholagogue. NO and vasoactive intestinal peptide (VIP) relax the sphincter of Oddi.

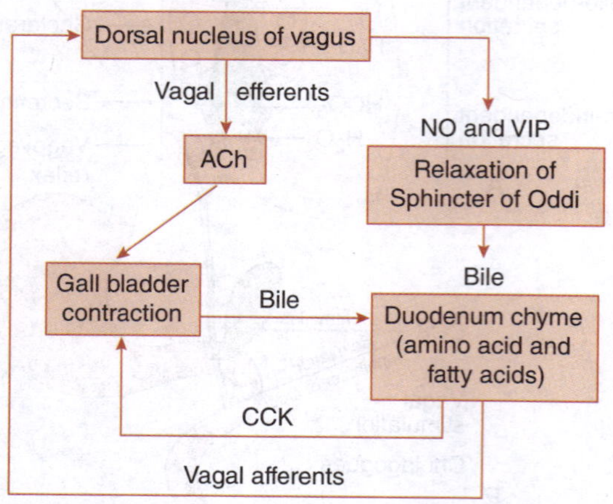

Fig. 7.4.18 Vagovagal reflex – a physiological choleretic reflex.

Applied Aspects

Disorders of Liver and Gall Bladder

Some of the important disorders of the gall bladder and liver which need emphasis are mentioned here.

I. Jaundice or Icterus

Jaundice or icterus refers to yellow discolouration of the skin and mucous membrane due to raised levels of bilirubin in the blood.

- *Normal values* of serum bilirubin range between 0.3 and 1 mg%.
- *Latent jaundice*, which cannot be detected clinically, occurs when serum bilirubin level is between 1 and 2 mg%.
- *Jaundice* manifests when serum bilirubin becomes more than 2 mg%.

Types of Jaundice. Jaundice is of three types:

Haemolytic jaundice, also called prehepatic jaundice, occurs due to overproduction of unconjugated bilirubin due to excessive destruction of RBCs owing to any reason.

Hepatocellular jaundice occurs due to damage to hepatocytes, as seen in viral hepatitis, cirrhosis and drug-induced hepatitis. In this condition, bilirubin is conjugated but cannot be excreted into the bile by the hepatocytes. So, the conjugated bilirubin returns to the blood, producing jaundice.

Obstructive jaundice, also called posthepatic jaundice, occurs due to blockage in bile duct due to either a stone or any growth (e.g. in carcinoma of the head of pancreas). The bile cannot be poured into the intestine, so due to back pressure, the biliary ducts and canaliculi are dilated and the bile salts and bile pigment enter the blood producing jaundice.

For further details and differences in the three types of jaundice, see page 148.

II. Cirrhosis of Liver

Cirrhosis of the liver refers to an irreversible chronic damage to the liver with extensive fibrosis and regenerative nodule formation.

Causes. Depending on the cause, the cirrhosis of the liver may be alcoholic, postviral (hepatitis B and hepatitis D), postnecrotic, biliary, cardiac, metabolic and drug induced (acetaminophen, antidepressants and some antibiotics), and may occur due to miscellaneous causes.

Clinical features cirrhosis liver are: Loss of functioning of liver tissue may lead to jaundice, oedema, a variety of metabolic disorders and portal hypertension (due to fibrosis and disordered vasculature). Ascites and hepatic encephalopathy result from both hepatocellular insufficiency and portal hypertension.

Diagnosis is based on the following tests:

- Liver function tests (LFTs; see page 611)
- Ultrasonography and MRI of the liver
- Liver biopsy

III. Viral Hepatitis

Aetiology. Viral hepatitis (inflammation of the liver) is caused by hepatitis virus A, B, C, D or E.

Hepatitis A is caused by the hepatitis A virus and spread by faecal–oral route. The infected individual excretes the virus in faecal matter for about 2–3 weeks.

Hepatitis B is more common, and is caused by hepatitis B virus. The sources of hepatitis B infection are by horizontal (blood) transmission, i.e.:

- Injection of unscreened blood products
- Tattoo/acupuncture needle
- Sexual

Clinical Features. Patients usually present with a history of anorexia, fever and malaise, followed by yellow discolouration of urine, eyes and skin. The liver may be enlarged, and the patient may have some discomfort in the upper abdomen.

Investigations to diagnose hepatitis A and B are:

- In *hepatitis A*, presence of antibodies against hepatitis A virus (anti-HAV) is of IgM type. Detection of anti-HAV can be used as a marker for previous HAV infection.
- In *hepatitis B*, presence of hepatitis B surface antigen (HBsAg) is detected on serology. Vertical transmission occurs in 90% of cases, i.e. from HBsAg-positive mother to child.

Treatment. Treatment is usually strict bed rest and ingestion of high-carbohydrate diet.

Medication include antiviral drugs such as interferon; bepirovirsen is the drug of choice.

Hepatitis B vaccine prevents occurrence of hepatitis B.

IV. Liver Failure

Any cause of liver damage can produce liver failure. Liver failure, though uncommon, is a serious syndrome. Hepatic encephalopathy is the cardinal presentation of acute liver failure. The mental changes start as confusion, but extend to stupor and coma.

Hepatic encephalopathy in liver failure occurs due to an increased ammonia level due to defective hepatic ammonia metabolism.

Treatment: The treatment of liver failure is primarily to reduce the ammonia load on the liver:

- Amounts of nonabsorbable carbohydrates such as lactulose, which is converted into short-chain fatty acids in the colon, which can trap ammonia in its ionized form, are increased.
- In severe disease, the only effective treatment is liver transplantation.

V. Cholecystitis

Cholecystitis refers to the inflammation of the gall bladder. It is not uncommon, although it is more common in fatty, fertile females in their forties (4Fs). It is of two types:

Acute cholecystitis: The patient usually presents with acute pain in the upper abdomen (biliary colic). The triad of symptoms – sudden onset of tenderness in right upper quadrant of the abdomen, fever and leucocytosis – is highly suggestive of acute cholecystitis.

Chronic cholecystitis is almost always associated with gallstones. The patient gets repeated attacks of pain in the abdomen and vomiting.

Cholecystectomy, i.e. surgical removal of the gall bladder, is indicated in patients with continued and recurrent discomfort.

VI. Gallstones (cholelithiasis)

Gallstone formation is not an uncommon problem. Two types of gallstones are known:

Cholesterol stones account for 80%–85% of the cases. These are formed due to precipitation of cholesterol. Normally, cholesterol is present in soluble form due to a proper ratio of cholesterol and bile salts (1:20 to 1:30). When this ratio falls below 1:13, the cholesterol is precipitated forming many small crystals. This stimulates further formation of crystals, so that the crystals grow larger and larger. In these crystals, bile pigments and calcium also get inspirated forming gallstones. These stones are *radiolucent*, i.e. cannot be visualized on radiograph.

Pigment stones, also called *calcium bilirubinate stones*, account for 15%–20% of cases of gallstones. These stones are formed when the conjugated bilirubin in the bile is disconjugated by the action of β-glucuronidase found in certain bacteria. The free bilirubin combines with calcium to form calcium bilirubinate, which is highly insoluble in bile. These stones are radiopaque.

- *Symptoms:* Gallstones may be asymptomatic or may produce symptoms due to either inflammation (biliary colic) or obstruction (obstructive jaundice) following their migration into the cystic duct or CBD. The most specific and characteristic symptom of gallstones is biliary colic.
- *Treatment* of gallstones, when required, is surgical removal of the gall bladder (cholecystectomy).

LIVER FUNCTION TESTS

The liver function tests (LFTs) are the investigations to assess the capacity of the liver to carry out any of the functions it performs. Thus, LFTs help in:

- Assessing the extent of functional damage to the liver
- Diagnosing the cause of hepatic insufficiency
- Assessing the progress/regress of the disease

The major LFTs may be classified as follows:

I. Tests to assess secretory functions
II. Tests to assess metabolic functions
III. Tests to assess synthesis functions
IV. Tests to assess detoxicating functions
V. Tests to assess hepatic cellular integrity
VI. Miscellaneous tests

Tests to Assess Secretory Functions of Liver

1. Serum Bilirubin The normal values are as follows:

- Total serum bilirubin: 0.3–1.0 mg%
- Conjugated bilirubin: 0.1–0.3 mg%
- Unconjugated bilirubin: 0.2–0.7 mg%

Van den Bergh test is specific to identifying the increase in serum bilirubin (above reference level). For procedure, see page 147. The results of the test are interpreted as follows:

- *Normal serum:* Negative reaction
- *Haemolytic jaundice:* Indirect positive reaction
- *Obstructive jaundice:* Direct positive reaction
- *Hepatic jaundice:* Biphasic reaction

2. Urine bilirubin and bile salts Normally, urine does not contain bilirubin and bile salts. In liver insufficiency, when the serum bilirubin levels increase above 2 mg%, the bilirubin is excreted in the urine (*bilirubinuria*).

3. Urine urobilinogen In normal individuals with urine flow of about 1 mL/min, less than 4 mg of urobilinogen is excreted in the urine. In liver insufficiency, initially there occurs a mild increase in the daily excretion of urine urobilinogen. However, in the later stages, urobilinogen is absent in the urine. This occurs because of the fact that the swollen liver cells block the bile canaliculi and prevent excretion of conjugated bilirubin in the bile.

4. Faecal stercobilinogen The normal levels are 20–25 mg%.

- Increased initially in liver insufficiency producing dark brown stools
- Decreased in later stages of liver insufficiency producing pale-coloured stools

5. Faecal fat levels Normally, 5%–6% of total fat intake per day is excreted in the faeces.

- In liver insufficiency, fat excretion in faeces increases up to 40%–50% of total intake (steatorrhoea). This is because of the fact that due to deficiency of bile salts, emulsification and absorption of fat is inadequate in the intestine.

Tests to Assess Metabolic Functions of Liver

1. Galactose tolerance test This test is based on the principle that galactose after absorption from the gut gets converted into glycogen in the liver. Therefore, in liver insufficiency, its level in the blood rises.

Procedure: In a fasting individual, 40 g galactose is administered orally and blood samples are collected at 30-minute intervals for 2 hours. From the blood galactose levels in these samples, the galactose index (GI) is calculated. GI is the sum of the four values of blood galactose levels in milligram per cent. Its normal value is 68–160 mg%. In hepatic insufficiency, GI value is markedly increased.

2. Blood glucose level The normal fasting blood glucose level is 70–90 mg%. In hepatic insufficiency, its level decreases.

3. Blood and urine amino acid levels Blood and urine amino acid levels are estimated to assess protein metabolism. In liver damage, blood amino acid levels (normal 30–65 mg%) and urine amino acid levels are increased.

4. Lipid profile In hepatic insufficiency, lipid profile is affected as follows:

- Plasma NEFA and FFA: Increase (normal 10–30 mg%)
- Serum cholesterol: Decreases (normal 150–240 mg%)
- Serum triglycerides: Decrease (normal 30–150 mg%)
- Serum phospholipids: Decrease (normal 150–300 mg%)
- Total lipids: Decrease (normal 350–800 mg%)
- Ketone bodies: Increase (normal 7–15 mg%)

Abnormalities of serum lipid levels are sensitive but nonspecific indicators.

Tests to Assess Synthesis Functions of Liver

1. Estimation of plasma proteins

Albumin: Liver cell damage causes hypoalbuminaemia (normal 6.4–8.3 g%).

Globulins: Hyperglobulinaemia is usually associated with hypoalbuminaemia.

A:G ratio: In liver disorder, there occurs reversal of A:G ratio (normal 1.7:1).

2. Serum levels of liver enzymes

Transaminases: The activity of transaminases like SGPT and SGOT increases in hepatic insufficiency. Serum SGPT levels are increased by 10–1000 times in acute phase (normal value <40 IU%). Raised levels of SGPT are more specific as it is primarily present in the liver, whereas SGOT is also present in other cells like red blood cells, skeletal muscle, GIT, brain and kidney.

Alkaline phosphatase: Alkaline phosphatase is not a liver-specific enzyme because it arises from bone, intestine and also liver and is secreted into the bile. In obstructive jaundice, its level is markedly increased (>30 KA units).

Gamma-glutamyl transferase is a microsomal enzyme. Raised level of GT is a sensitive index of liver damage.

3. Blood urea The liver is the main site for urea formation from ammonia. Decreased levels of blood urea (normal 20–40 mg%) and raised blood ammonia level (normal 20–80 mg%) occur in liver insufficiency.

4. Blood ammonia Raised blood ammonia level indicates severe liver disease (hepatic encephalopathy).

5. Urine ammonia Urine ammonia level also increases (normal 350–1200 mg/day).

6. Coagulation factors Factors II, V, VII, IX and X and vitamin K needed to activate these factors are synthesized by the liver. The integrity and activity of these factors is determined by prothrombin time test (PTT) (for prothrombin test, see page 216). Prolonged prothrombin time (PT) (normal 10–16 seconds) indicates severe liver disease.

- *Prothrombin time index (PTI):* It is calculated as follows:

$$\text{PTI} = \frac{\text{Normal PT}}{\text{PT of patient}} \times 100$$

Normal PTI is 100%. Its value less than 70% is indicative of severe liver damage.

Tests to Assess Detoxification Functions of Liver

1. Bromsulphthalein excretion test BSP is taken up by the liver cells from the blood and detoxified and excreted in the bile. The rate of removal of BSP from the blood depends on the functional efficiency of the liver and rate of hepatic blood flow.

Procedure: BSP is injected intravenously (dose 5 mg/kg body weight) and its concentration in blood samples (collected at an interval of 5 and 45 minutes) is measured.

Assuming BSP concentration as 100% at the beginning, normally its concentration should fall to 85% in the blood sample collected after 5 minutes and 5% only in the blood sample collected after 45 minutes. A concentration of >10% indicates liver insufficiency. Nowadays, this test is used only for diagnosis of Dubin–Johnson syndrome (congenital hyperbilirubinaemia).

2. Hippuric acid excretion test Sodium benzoate when ingested orally gets conjugated with glycine in the liver and excreted as hippuric acid in the urine.

Normally, when 6 mg of sodium benzoate is ingested orally, about 2.7–3.5 g is excreted in the urine as hippuric acid within 4 hours, provided the kidneys are functioning normally. Decreased excretion of hippuric acid occurs in liver damage.

Tests to Assess Hepatic Cellular Integrity

1. Ultrasonography Ultrasonography is done to detect diffuse disease of parenchyma of the liver (cirrhosis of the liver, fatty liver), abscess, cysts, tumours, gallstones and dilatation of biliary system proximal to site of obstruction.

2. Computed tomography CT scan has the same diagnostic significance as ultrasonography except that it can also detect even smaller lesions.

3. Radionucleotide imaging Technetium (^{99m}Tc) is a sulphur colloid, which is easily taken up by the liver cells, monocyte macrophage system (Kupffer cells), and emits gamma (γ)-rays. Gamma camera picks up these rays and is used to find out the size of the liver and the lesions of the liver (such as filling defect, diffuse liver disease and portal hypertension).

4. Liver biopsy This is performed by a special needle passed through intercostal space under local anaesthesia to obtain tissue for histopathological examination.

5. Fine needle aspiration (FNA) A very fine needle is usually guided by ultrasound and material is aspirated for cytological, histopathological and bacteriological examination.

6. Cholecystography Cholecystography is done to assess the functions and diseases of the gall bladder. Iodinated compounds given orally are concentrated in the gall bladder and excreted in bile. The gall bladder gets opacified on cholecystography. Therefore, conditions like gallstones and nonfunctioning gall bladder fail to produce opacification. Nowadays, this test is less commonly performed than ultrasonography.

7. Other elaborate tests Other elaborate tests include:

- Percutaneous cholangiography (PTC)
- Portal venography
- Endoscopic retrograde cholangiography (ERCP)

Miscellaneous Tests

Serological tests to detect hepatitis viruses, antigens and antibodies

Self-Assessment

1. Describe the composition, mechanism of secretion and regulation of pancreatic secretion.
2. Discuss the composition, functions of the constituents, mechanism of secretion and regulation of bile.
3. Discuss briefly:
   - Significance of pancreatic function tests.
   - Enterohepatic circulation of bile salts and its significance
   - Role of cholecystokinin
4. Write notes on:
   - Cholelithiasis
   - Liver failure and its effects
   - Pancreatitis

Clinical Cases

Case 1

A 30-year-old male patient was admitted with complaints of severe abdominal pain, vomiting and fever. Physical examination revealed temperature 38.2°C, tachycardia and low BP. Abdominal examination revealed tenderness on palpation and guarding. Blood and biochemical tests showed increased levels of amylase and lipase enzymes. From above observations, the patient was diagnosed a case of acute pancreatitis.

Q1. What is the pathophysiology of acute pancreatitis?
Q2. What are the basis of management of acute pancreatitis?
Q3. If not treated, what complications can occur?

Case 2

A 42-year-old male was admitted with haematemesis. History revealed that the patient was a chronic alcoholic, and had loss of appetite and weight loss.

Examination showed tenderness and pain around the liver area, tiny red lines on the skin of upper part of the abdomen and jaundice.

From history and signs and symptoms, the patient was provisionally diagnosed a case of liver cirrhosis.

Q1. What further tests should be carried out for final diagnosis?
Q2. What is the cause of haematemesis in this case?
Q3. What is the cause for jaundice in this case?

Case 3

A 45-year-old male patient presented with loss of appetite, weight loss, weakness and fatigue, abdominal discomfort and fever. Examination revealed jaundice and hepatomegaly; history revealed that he had blood transfusion at the age of 25 years when he met a road accident. From signs and symptoms and history, the patient was provisionally diagnosed a case of hepatitis B.

Q1. To confirm the diagnosis, what are the tests to be carried out?
Q2. What is the causative organism?
Q3. What are the treatment measures?
Q4. What are the preventive measures?

Case 4

A 40-year-old obese woman was admitted with right upper abdominal pain, vomiting and fever. History revealed recurrent attacks of same type of pain and vomiting. On examination, there was no jaundice, temperature was 37.8°C, and the patient was found to have low BP and bradycardia.

Lab investigations showed the following: TLC, DLC and absolute count were normal, and total bilirubin was within normal range. From signs and symptoms, the case was diagnosed biliary colic.

Q1. What is the cause of biliary colic?
Q2. What further investigations are required to know the exact cause?
Q3. What immediate treatment should be given?

Case 5

A 42-year-old fatty female presented with severe pain in the upper abdomen and vomiting. History revealed that the pain was radiating to the right shoulder and towards the back between the shoulder blades. Laboratory tests showed bilirubin, TLC, DLC and absolute count to be within normal range.

On ultrasonography of the abdomen, stones were seen in the gall bladder.

Q1. What is the main cause of cholelithiasis?
Q2. What is the pathophysiology of formation of gallstones?
Q3. What are the types of gallstones?
Q4. What is the treatment basis of cholelithiasis?
Q5. What are the complications of cholelithiasis?

7.5 Physiological Activities in Small Intestine

CHAPTER OUTLINE

FUNCTIONAL ANATOMY

GROSS ANATOMICAL CONSIDERATIONS

The small intestine is a convoluted tube that extends from the pylorus to the ileocaecal valve, where it joins with caecum, the first part of the large intestine. It is about 6–7 m in length, and its diameter gradually diminishes from its commencement to its termination. It is divided into three parts – the duodenum, the jejunum and the ileum (see Fig. 7.1.1).

Duodenum The first and *shortest* part (25 cm long) of the small intestine is also the *widest* and most fixed part. It is C shaped, and for descriptive purposes is divided into four parts – superior (first) part, descending (second) part, horizontal (third) part and ascending (fourth part). Superior part of duodenum is also called *duodenal cap* or bulb. It is the region which is struck by acidic gastric contents when they pass through pylorus and is a *common site for the peptic ulcer*. The bile and pancreatic ducts open by a common hepatopancreatic ampulla of Vater on the posteromedial wall of descending (second) part of duodenum. Ligament of Treitz demarcates the continuation of duodenum with jejunum.

Jejunum and ileum Jejunum and ileum form the proximal two-fifths and distal three-fifths, respectively, of the remaining part of the small intestine. There is no sharp demarcation between jejunum and ileum. The inner mucosal surfaces of jejunum and ileum, however, can be differentiated from each other.

STRUCTURAL CHARACTERISTICS OF SMALL INTESTINE

Histologically, the wall of the small intestine is made up of four layers, which from within to outwards consist of mucosa, submucosa, muscle coat and serosa (for details, see page 561).

Characteristic Features of Mucous Membrane of Small Intestine

Characteristic features of mucous membrane of the small intestine need special emphasis.

Although the small intestine is about 6 m long, it has an absorptive area of over 250 m^2. This larger surface is created by:

- Numerous folds of the intestinal mucosa *plicae circulares* (Fig. 7.5.1)
- Densely packed villi, which line the entire mucosal surface
- *Microvilli*, which protrude from the surface of intestinal cells
- The presence of numerous depressions (crypts of Lieberkuhn) that invade the lamina propria

Plicae circulares The mucosal surface shows numerous circular folds (*plicae circulares* or valvulae conniventes), which are absent in the first 2 inches of duodenum but are larger, more numerous and closely set in rest of the duodenum and jejunum, whereas in the upper part of ileum, they are smaller and more widely separated and in the lower part they are absent (Fig. 7.5.1). Unlike the folds in the stomach, the plicae circulares are permanent and do not obliterate when the intestine is distended. Each fold is made up of all layers of the

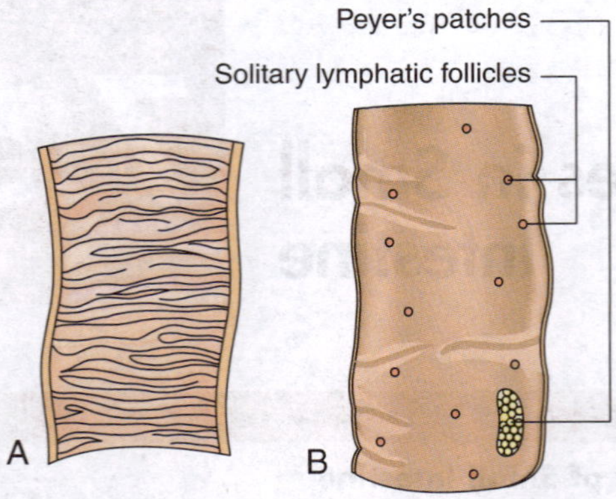

Fig. 7.5.1 The mucosal surface of jejunum **A** and ileum **B**.

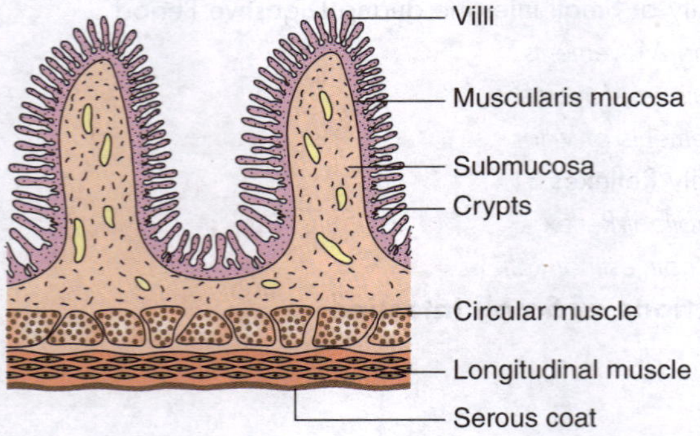

Fig. 7.5.2 Longitudinal section of small intestine showing plicae circulares and villi.

mucosa (lining epithelium, lamina propria and muscularis mucosa). The submucosa also extends into the fold. The circular folds serve the following functions:

- They increase the surface area for absorption, and also slow down the passage of contents through the small intestine, which facilitate absorption.

Villi Villi are finger-like projections of mucous membrane seen throughout the length of the small intestine (Fig. 7.5.2).

Total number of villi The total number of villi is about 5 million and they are distributed about 20–40 villi/mm^2. Each villus is about 0.5–1 mm long.

Structure Each villus is covered by a single layer of columnar epithelial cells called enterocytes. The core of each villus contains (Fig. 7.5.3):

- An arteriole and a venule with their communicating capillary plexus; the venules of the villi, which carry absorbed nutrients that ultimately drain into the portal vein; blind-ended lymphatic vessels called lacteals which carry the absorbed fats to the thoracic duct; and few smooth muscle fibres extending from the muscularis mucosa
- A fine network of nerves, which has connections with submucosal and myenteric plexus

Activity During digestion and absorption, the villi contract quickly with an irregular rhythm and relax slowly. Their muscular fibres serve to pump the lymph from core of villi towards the submucosal lacteals.

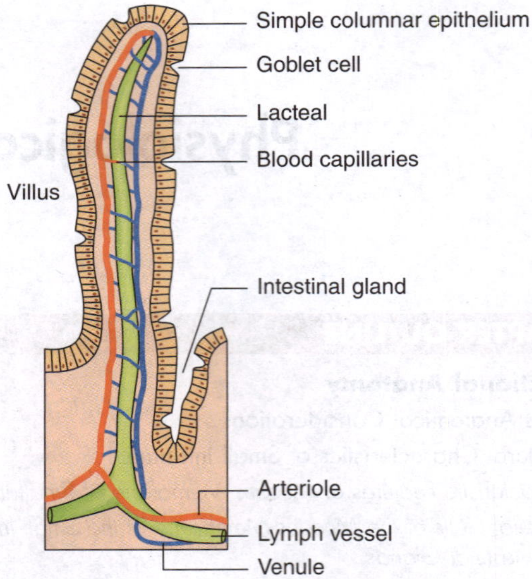

Fig. 7.5.3 Structure of an intestinal villus, an enterocyte and crypts of Lieberkuhn.

Crypts of Lieberkuhn The crypts of Lieberkuhn are single tubular intestinal glands that invaginate deep into the lamina propria and are present between the villi throughout the length of the small intestine (Fig. 7.5.3). These glands are lined by undifferentiated columnar cells, and also contain goblet cells, argentaffin cells and Paneth cells.

Epithelial Cells of the Mucous Membrane of the Small Intestine and Intestinal Glands

The mucous membrane of the small intestine is made up of the following types of epithelial cells:

1. Absorptive columnar cells Absorptive columnar cells or the so-called enterocytes are the cells of epithelium which cover the villi, and the areas of the mucosal surface intervening between them. These cells are specialized for absorptive function. The luminal surface of each enterocyte shows small multiple projections of the cell membrane called the *microvilli* or the *brush border* (Fig. 7.5.3), which increase the surface area to about 30-fold. Each enterocyte has about 1000 microvilli. Whole of the system of folds, villi and microvilli combinedly increases the surface area about 600 times as follows: folds (3 times) × villi (10 times) × microvilli (20 times) = 600 times. The surface of each microvillus is covered by a layer of fine fibrils and mucus (glycocalyx).

The lateral surfaces of adjacent enterocytes are joined by *tight junctions*. Enzymes *capable of breaking down* small peptides and disaccharides are associated with microvilli of the absorptive columnar epithelial cells.

2. Undifferentiated columnar cells Undifferentiated columnar cells line the crypts of Lieberkuhn. They are similar to absorptive cells, but their microvilli are not as developed and their cytoplasm contains secretory granules. The cells of the lower parts of the crypts *proliferate actively* by mitosis. The newly formed cells migrate upwards from the crypt to reach the walls of villi. Here they differentiate into typical absorptive cells, or into goblet cells. These cells migrate towards the tips of villi, from where they are *shed off in the lumen* of the intestine. Thus, the epithelial lining of the small intestine is being replaced constantly. The *total cycle* of *cell migration*, from the bases of crypts to the tips of villi and then shedding off, takes about up to 5 days only. In this way, about 17 billion cells containing nearly 3 g of proteins are shed into the intestine per day.

3. Goblet cells Fairly large number of mucus-secreting goblet cells can be seen among the epithelial cells of the mucous membrane. They increase in number, as we pass down the small intestine, being few in the duodenum and most numerous in the terminal ileum.

4. Argentaffin or enterochromaffin cells Argentaffin or enterochromaffin cells are also present in the intestinal mucous membrane, being most numerous near the *lower ends of crypts*. These cells secrete 5-hydroxytryptamine (5-HT or serotonin).

5. Zymogen cells or Paneth cells Zymogen cells or Paneth cells are found only in the deeper parts of intestinal crypts. They are large acidophilic cells containing secretory granules. They are known to produce lysozyme, which destroys bacteria. They may also produce other enzymes.

6. Duodenal glands of Brunner Duodenal glands of Brunner are limited only to the duodenum. These are compound tubuloalveolar glands present in submucosa of duodenum. Their ducts pass through the muscularis mucosa to open into the crypts of Lieberkuhn. They are situated mostly near the pylorus; beyond pylorus, their number greatly diminishes and they disappear at the junction of duodenum and jejunum. Secretions of these glands contain *mucus and* HCO_3^-, which neutralizes gastric acid entering the duodenum and thus protects its mucosa.

SMALL INTESTINAL SECRETIONS

COMPOSITION AND FORMATION

The intestinal juice, also called succus entericus, comprises the intestinal secretions which include:

- Aqueous component (water and electrolytes)
- Intestinal enzymes
- Mucus

Aqueous Component of Intestinal Juice

Aqueous component of intestinal juice primarily refers to water and electrolytes secreted by the epithelial cells of the small intestine, especially those present in the crypts of Lieberkuhn. About 2 L of secretion is produced per day by these cells, whose chemical composition is almost similar to that of the extracellular fluid, except that it is slightly more alkaline (pH 7.5–8.6). This fluid is colourless; however, it becomes slightly cloudy due to admixture of mucus, shed epithelial cells and cholesterol.

Mechanism of formation There is an active secretion of chloride and bicarbonate ions into the crypts, which causes electrical force leading to diffusion of sodium ions. All these ions cause osmotic movement of water. Thus, there is marked secretion of watery fluid without enzymes.

Functions The watery secretion provides a solvent into which the products of digestion are dissolved. This fluid is rapidly reabsorbed by the intestinal villi. Thus, circulation of this fluid from the crypts to the villi supplies a watery vehicle for absorption of foodstuffs from the small intestine. For details, see page 621.

Intestinal Enzymes

Brush border of epithelial cells covering the villi contains a large number of intracellular digestive enzymes. It is believed that these brush border enzymes produce final hydrolysis of the food particles on the surface of the epithelial cells prior to the absorption of end products of digestion like amino acids, monosaccharides and fatty acids into the cell. When the epithelial cells at tip of villi, the various enzymes along with the cells, enter the intestinal secretion, this mode of secretion of enzymes is known as *holocrine mode of secretion*. The enzymes which have been identified in the brush border are as follows:

1. ***Peptidases*** (proteolytic enzymes) which digest peptides into amino acid, e.g. aminopeptidases, dipeptidases, nuclease and related enzymes
2. ***Disaccharidases*** such as sucrase, maltase and lactase which split the respective disaccharidases into the monosaccharides
3. ***Intestinal lipases*** that split triglycerides present in small amount
4. ***Enterokinase*** or enteropeptidase which activates trypsinogen to trypsin

Mucus

Mucus in the small intestine is secreted by:

1. ***Brunner's glands***, which are located in the duodenum, secrete thick, alkaline mucoid secretion that serves a protective role, preventing HCl and chyme from damaging the duodenal mucosa.
2. ***Goblet cells***, located along the length of the intestinal epithelium and in the intestinal crypts of Lieberkuhn, secrete lot of mucus which protects the intestinal mucosa and lubricates the chyme.

REGULATION OF SMALL INTESTINAL SECRETIONS

1. ***Local stimuli:*** Local mechanical and chemical stimuli to the intestinal mucosa form the most important means of regulation of intestinal secretions. Mechanical distension of intestinal mucosa by the food or irritation by chemicals, via local myenteric reflexes, increases the volume and total enzyme output of the small intestine; that is why, the greater is the chyme, greater is the secretion of intestinal secretion.
2. ***Role of vasoactive intestinal polypeptide (VIP):*** Although the secretion of the crypts of Lieberkuhn is mainly regulated by the local stimuli, the local hormone VIP is also reported to increase its secretion.
3. ***Secretion of Brunner's gland*** is increased by:
   - Vagus stimulation
   - Direct tactile stimulation or irritation of the duodenal mucosa
   - Secretin

FUNCTIONS OF INTESTINAL SECRETION

See 'Functions of Small Intestine' (page 621).

MOTILITY OF SMALL INTESTINE

Motility of the small intestine can be described as follows:

A. ***Motility of the small intestine during interdigestive period,*** which includes:
  - Migrating motor complexes (MMCs)

B. ***Motility of the small intestine during digestive period*** (related to meals), which includes:
  - Mixing movements such as segmentation contractions and pendular movements
  - Propulsive movements such as peristaltic contractions and peristaltic rush
  - Movements of villi

C. ***Motility reflexes,*** which include:
  - Peristaltic reflex
  - Gastroileal reflex
  - Intestinointestinal reflex

MOTILITY OF SMALL INTESTINE DURING INTERDIGESTIVE PERIOD

Migrating Motor Complexes

- MMC is the name given to the peristaltic wave that begins in the oesophagus and travels through the entire gastrointestinal tract during the interdigestive period.
- The MMCs sweep out the chyme remaining in the small intestine.
- The MMCs occur every 60–90 minutes and last for about 10 minutes.
- For further details about MMCs, see page 586.

MOTILITY OF SMALL INTESTINE DURING DIGESTIVE PERIOD

Mixing Movements

The mixing movements of the small intestine are responsible for proper mixing of chyme with digestive juices like pancreatic juice, bile juice and intestinal juice. These include:

- Segmentation contractions
- Pendular movements

i. Segmentation Contractions

Features Segmentation is the most common type of intestinal contractions, which occurs throughout the digestive period in a rhythmic fashion, and hence is also called *rhythmic segmentation contractions.*

- During segmentation contraction, a section of the small intestine (about 2–5 cm) contracts, sending the intestinal contents (chyme) in both oral and caudal directions. That section of the small intestine then relaxes, and the contents move back into the segment. At the same time, the adjoining segment which was relaxed now contracts (Fig. 7.5.4A).
- The alternate contracted and relaxed segments give a ring-like appearance resembling the chain of sausages (Fig. 7.5.4B).

Functions These back-and-forth movements of chyme, produced by segmentation contractions, cause thorough mixing without any net forward movement of chyme (Fig. 7.5.4A).

- The segmentation contractions slow down the transit time in the small intestine and thus increase the contact time with the absorption surfaces of the intestinal mucosa.
- The higher frequency of segmentation in the proximal intestine (duodenum) than in the distal intestine (ileum) also propels the chyme slowly towards the colon.

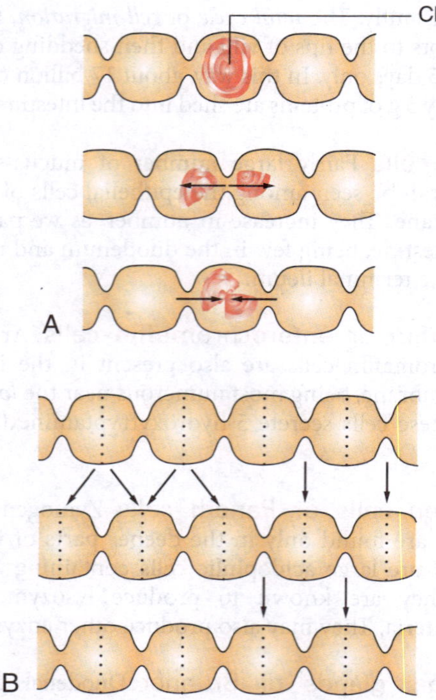

Fig. 7.5.4 Segmentation contraction of small intestine: **A**, steps of segmentation are shown to reveal back-and-forth movements of chyme; and **B**, the alternate contracted and relaxed segments give a ring-like appearance resembling the chain of sausages.

Rate and duration Segmentation contractions occur about 12 times/min in the duodenum and 8 times/min in the ileum. The contractions last for 5–6 seconds.

Types Two types of segmentation contractions have been described:

Eccentric contractions: They consist of contractions located in a localized segment less than 2 cm in length, and are eccentric in appearance. They are mainly due to contraction of outer longitudinal smooth muscle layer.

Concentric contractions: The segments are usually longer than 2 cm and are of relatively uniform circumference. They are mainly due to contraction of inner circular smooth muscle layer.

Tonic contractions are variants of segmentation contractions, which last somewhat longer, isolating one segment of the intestine from another for quite some time.

Control of segmental contractions

Initiation: Segmentation contractions can occur only if the slow waves (basal electrical rhythm [BER]) produce spikes, or action potentials. Spikes appear on the slow waves when the membrane potential is sufficiently depolarized. The slow waves (BER) are initiated by the pacemaker cells (interstitial cells of Cajal) which are stellate mesenchymal cells having long branched processes reaching up to intestinal smooth muscles located in second part of duodenum near the entry of common bile duct. The BER is conducted caudally by the longitudinal muscle fibre layer and is coordinated by the myenteric plexus.

Frequency of segmentation contractions is directly related to the frequency of slow waves and is thus controlled by pacemaker cells within the walls of the small intestine and is not influenced by the neural activity or circulating hormones.

Strength of segmentation contractions is proportional to the frequency of spikes generated by slow waves which in turn is controlled by the amplitude of slow waves. Therefore, the greater the slow-wave amplitude, the greater is the frequency of spikes generated, and the greater is the strength of the contraction. The slow-wave amplitude and thus the strength of segmentation contraction is controlled by the hormones released during digestion:

- Slow-wave amplitude is increased by gastrin, cholecystokinin (CCK), motilin and insulin.
- Slow-wave amplitude is decreased by secretin and glucagon.

ii. Pendular Movements

These are small constrictive waves which sweep forward and backward or upward and downward in pendular fashion. These mixing movements can be noticed only by close observation.

Propulsive Movements

The propulsive movements of the small intestine are involved in pushing the chyme towards the aboral end of the intestine. These include:

- Peristaltic contractions
- Peristaltic rush

i. Peristaltic Contractions

Characteristic features Peristalsis refers to a wave of contraction preceded by a wave of relaxation. Ideally, in the small intestine, peristalsis is superimposed over the segmentation contractions after digestion and absorption have taken place.

- The peristaltic contractions are highly coordinated, and, typically, a peristaltic contraction involves contraction of a segment behind the bolus, and simultaneous relaxation of the segment in front of the bolus, causing the chyme to be propelled caudally (Fig. 7.5.5).
- A peristaltic contraction consists of deep circular ring of contraction, which passes down the intestine at a rate of 0.5–2 cm/s. Each contraction travels for a variable but short distance and then dies out. A new contraction is then initiated from a site little distal to the site of origin of the previous contraction. In this way, a continuous peristaltic wave is set up in the intestine. Several of these wave-like contractions occur simultaneously along the length of the intestine, resulting in vermiform movements (worm-like movements). That is why they are called vermicular or peristaltic movements.
- Along with the peristaltic movements, the chyme moves at a rate of about 1 cm/min. Thus, the net movement of chyme in anal direction is very slow and it takes about 3–5 hours for the chyme to move from the pylorus to the ileocaecal valve.

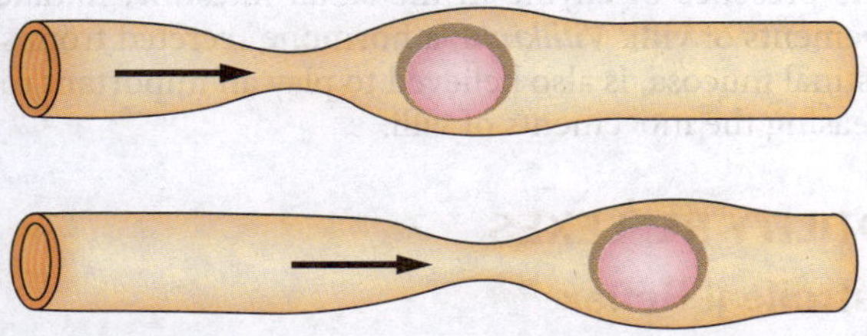

Fig. 7.5.5 Peristaltic contraction moves the food through intestine by pushing bolus ahead of muscle contraction.

Law of intestine As a matter of fact, the peristaltic contraction travels from the point of stimulation in both directions. But under normal conditions, the progress of contraction in an oral direction is inhibited quickly and the contraction disappears. Only the contraction that travels in the aboral direction persists. In this way, the peristaltic waves always travel from the oral end towards the aboral end of the intestine. This phenomenon has been labelled as the *law of the intestine*, by Starling in 1901. The other names which have been given to this phenomenon are 'polarity of intestine', 'polar conduction of intestine', 'electrical activity of intestine', 'law of gut' and 'theory of receptive relaxation'.

Proof: The law of the intestine can be proved experimentally. When a piece of gut is resected, and the resected segments are resutured in the same position, the peristaltic wave passes easily over the resected segment (Fig. 7.5.6B). But if the resected segment is resutured in the reverse position, the peristalsis stops at the beginning of the reversely sutured segment, proving the law of the intestine.

Explanation: The law of the intestine has been attributed to the *descending* rate of rhythmicity of BER from duodenum (12/min) towards ileum (9/min).

Functions Functions subserved by peristaltic waves are as follows:

- Help to propel the intestinal contents aborally
- Also help in digestion and absorption of the food particles, because different types of nutrients are digested and absorbed in different segments of the small intestine

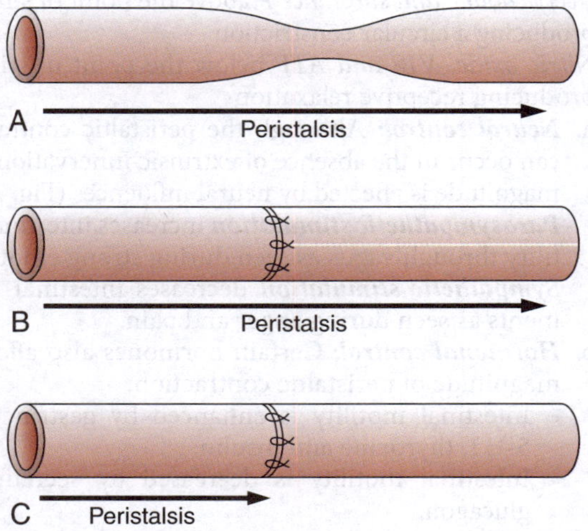

Fig. 7.5.6 Experiment to prove 'law of intestine': **A**, normal peristaltic movements of a segment of small intestine; **B**, normal peristalsis continues when a part of small intestine is cut and sutured in the same position; and **C**, when the resected segment is sutured in reverse position, the peristalsis stops at proximal sutured end.

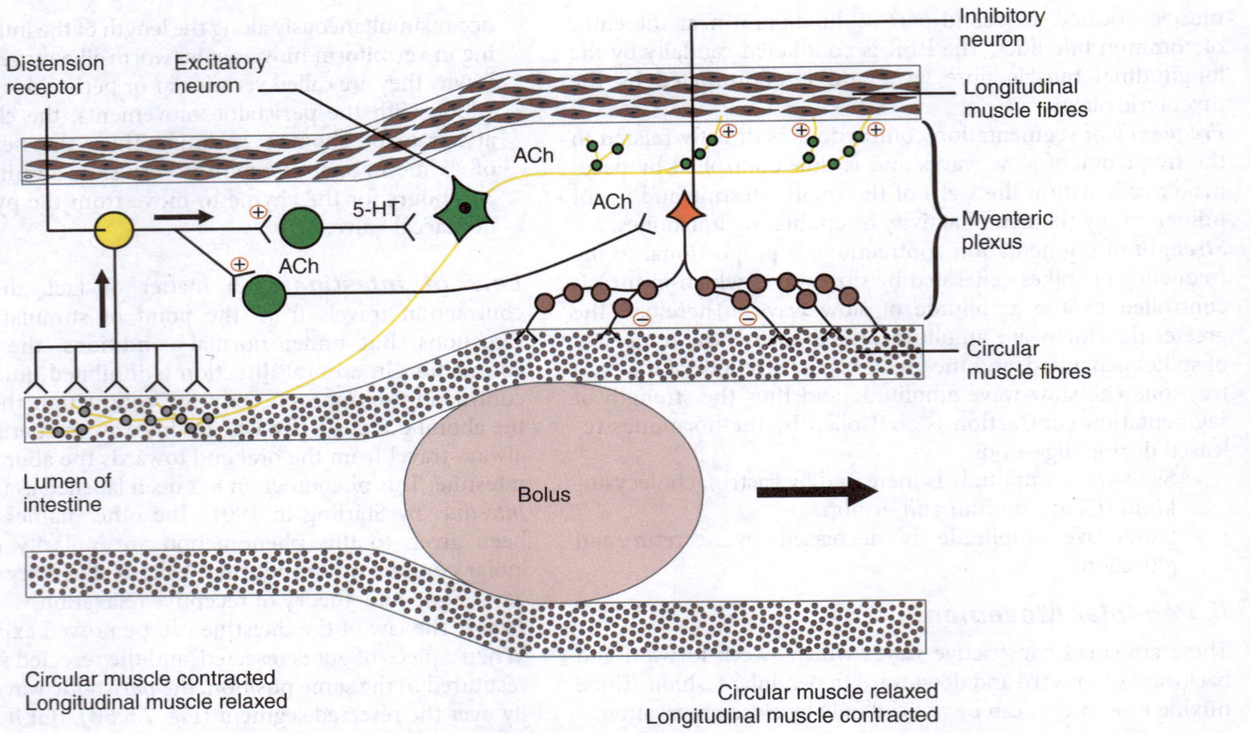

Fig. 7.5.7 The postulated connection in the myenteric plexus to coordinate the peristaltic contraction. +, excitatory synapse; –, inhibitory synapse; ACh, acetylcholine; 5-HT, 5-hydroxytryptamine.

Control of peristaltic contractions ***Initiation:*** The coordinated peristaltic activity is dependent on the integrity of enteric nerve plexus.

- The usual stimulus for peristalsis is distension. When the wall of the intestine is stretched, the wave of peristalsis is initiated which passes along the intestine towards the rectum at a rate of 2–2.5 cm/s. This response to stretch is called *myenteric reflex*.
- The local stretch releases serotonin, which activates sensory neurons that stimulate the myenteric plexus. Activity of the myenteric plexus from a stimulus point travels in either direction to activate neurons that release (Fig. 7.5.7):
  - *Acetylcholine and substance P* above the point of stimulus, producing a circular constriction
  - *Nitric oxide, VIP and ATP* below the point of stimulus producing receptive relaxation
    a. ***Neural control:*** Although the peristaltic contractions can occur in the absence of extrinsic innervation, their magnitude is affected by neural influences (Fig. 7.5.8). ***Parasympathetic stimulation*** increases intestinal motility through vagus as seen during strong emotions. ***Sympathetic stimulation*** decreases intestinal movements as seen during anger and pain.
    b. ***Hormonal control:*** Certain hormones also affect the magnitude of peristaltic contraction:
       - Intestinal motility is enhanced by gastrin, CCK, 5-HT, thyroxine and insulin.
       - Intestinal motility is decreased by secretin and glucagon.

ii. Peristaltic Rush

- Peristaltic rush refers to a very powerful peristaltic contraction which occurs when intestinal mucosa is irritated intensely as in some infectious processes.
- It is partly initiated by extrinsic nervous reflex and partly by myenteric reflex.
- This type of powerful contraction begins in duodenum and passes through the entire length of the small intestine, and finally reaches the ileocaecal valve within few minutes. Thus, it sweeps the contents of the intestine into the colon, thereby relieving the small intestine of irritant or excessive distension, as occurs in cases of diarrhoea.

Movements of Villi

As the smooth muscle fibres of the intestinal wall extend into the villi, movements of villi also occur during the movements of the small intestine.

Features Movements of villi consist of alternate shortening and elongation of the villi caused by contraction and relaxation of the muscle.

Functions Movements of villi help in emptying lymph from the central lacteal into the lymphatic system. The surface area of villi is increased during elongation. This helps in the absorption of digested foodstuffs from the lumen of the intestine.

Initiation Local nervous reflexes, which occur in response to the presence of chyme in the small intestine, initiate the movements of villi. *Villikinin*, a hormone secreted from small intestinal mucosa, is also believed to play an important role in increasing the movements of villi.

MOTILITY REFLEXES

Gastroileal Reflex

- Gastroileal reflex refers to marked increase in peristaltic contractions of ileum associated with relaxation of ileocaecal

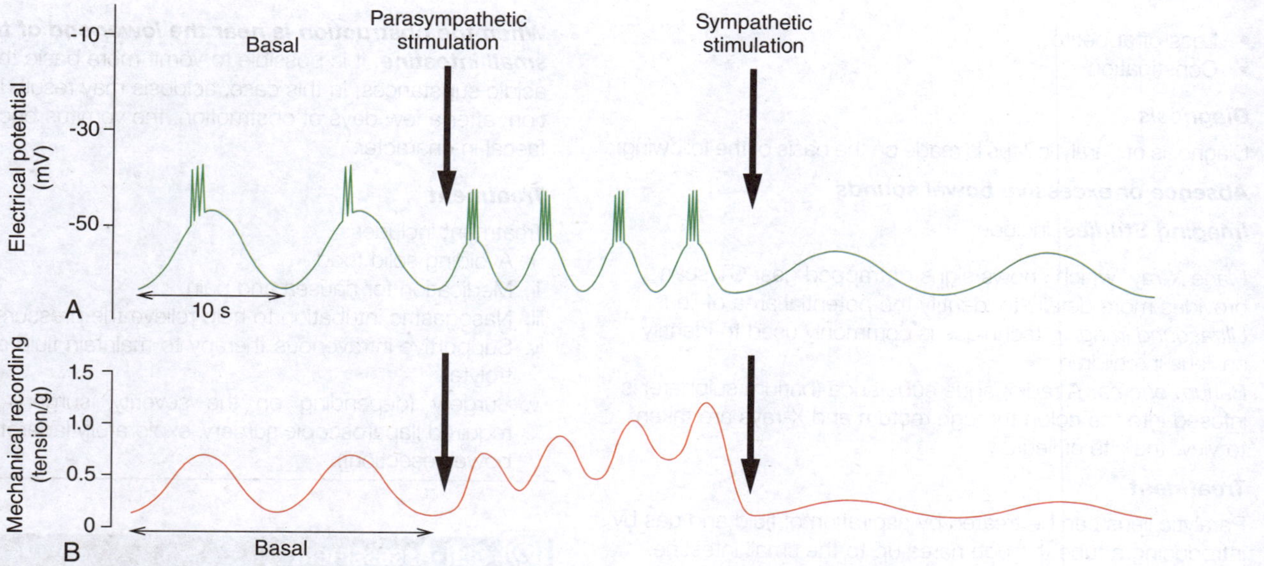

Fig. 7.5.8 Effect of parasympathetic stimulation and sympathetic stimulation on membrane potential **A**, and mechanical activity **B**, of small intestine.

sphincter which occur immediately after the meals. As a result, the intestinal contents are delivered to the large intestine.

- This reflex is initiated by the distension of the stomach by the food.
- The peristaltic contractions are caused by reflex stimulation of vagus and the relaxation of ileocaecal sphincter seems to be produced by the hormone gastrin.

Intestinointestinal Reflex

Intestinointestinal reflex refers to relaxation of smooth muscles of rest of the small intestine in response to overdistension of one segment of the intestine.

FUNCTIONS OF SMALL INTESTINE

After going through the physiology of intestinal secretion and intestinal motility, the functions of the small intestine can be summarized as follows:

1. Mechanical functions The mixing and propulsive movements of the small intestine help in thorough mixing of chyme with the digestive juices (pancreatic juice, bile juice and succus entericus), and propel it towards the large intestine.

2. Digestive functions Digestive functions of the small intestine are carried out by the digestive enzymes present in the succus entericus (see page 617), pancreatic enzymes (see page 596) and bile (see page 606).

3. Absorptive function Absorptive function is accomplished by the huge surface area created by the presence of plicae circulares, villi and microvilli. The end products of digestion of carbohydrates, proteins and fats are absorbed through portal system or through the lymph. For details of absorption, see page 632.

4. Hormonal functions The small intestine secretes certain hormones that exert their effect on the secretions and motility of the gastrointestinal tract. These hormones include *enterogastrone, secretin* (page 599) and *CCK* (page 600).

5. Activator function The enzyme enterokinase secreted by the small intestine activates trypsinogen into trypsin, which in turn activates other enzymes.

6. Protective function The mucus secreted into the succus entericus protects the intestinal wall from the gastric acid chyme.

7. Hydrolytic function The aqueous component of the succus entericus provides water, and thus helps in all the hydrolytic processes of enzymatic reactions of digestion of various food particles.

Applied Aspects

I. Paralytic Ileus

Paralytic ileus or the adynamic ileus refers to a condition in which the intestinal motility is markedly decreased leading to retention of its contents (because the contents cannot be propelled into the colon). This produces irregular distension of the small intestine by pockets of gas and fluid.

Causes

Paralytic ileus may occur due to:

1. ***Direct inhibition of smooth muscles of the small intestine*** due to handling of the intestine:
   - During intra-abdominal operations
   - During trauma
2. ***Reflex inhibition of smooth muscles of the small intestine*** due to increased discharge of noradrenergic fibres in splanchnic nerves, as seen in irritation of peritoneum (in patients with peritonitis and injury to peritoneum)

Signs and Symptoms

An ileus can lead to intestinal obstruction causing:

- Crampy abdominal pain

- Loss of appetite
- Constipation

Diagnosis

Diagnosis of paralytic ileus is made on the basis of the following:

Absence or excessive bowel sounds

Imaging Studies include:

Plane X-ray, which shows signs of trapped gas; CT scan provides more details to identify the potential area of ileus.
Ultrasound imaging technique is commonly used to identify an ileus in children.
Barium enema: A radiopaque substance (barium sulphate) is infused into the colon through rectum and X-rays are taken to view the site of ileus.

Treatment

Paralytic ileus can be treated by aspiration of fluid and gas by introducing a tube through nares up to the small intestine.

- The occurrence of paralytic ileus can be reduced by using laparoscopic surgery.
- Postsurgical, early ambulation also enhances intestinal motility.
- Use of specific opioid antagonists is also helpful in relieving this condition.
- Supportive care is provided by intravenous fluid and electrolytes.

Intestinal Obstruction

Causes

Obstruction of the lumen of the small intestine may occur due to many causes, such as tumours, strictures and fibrotic bands in the abdomen.

Features

The intestinal obstruction is characterized by:

Intestinal colic, i.e. severe abdominal pain. Pain is caused by peristaltic rush (intense peristaltic wave initiated due to irritation of intestinal mucosa at the site of obstruction).
Distension of the small intestine with pockets of fluid and gas occurs proximal to the site of obstruction.
Local ischaemia of intestinal wall may occur due to increased intraluminal pressure.
Stimulation of visceral afferent nerves by the increased intraluminal pressure may cause sweating, hypotension and severe vomiting.
When the obstruction is in the upper half of the small intestine, the antiperistaltic reflux causes intestinal juices to flow into the stomach, and these juices are vomited along with the secretions of the stomach. The person becomes severely dehydrated, but the loss of acids and bases may be approximately equal, so that little change occurs in acid–base balance.
When the obstruction is near the lower end of the small intestine, it is possible to vomit more basic than acidic substances; in this case, acidosis may result. In addition, after a few days of obstruction, the vomitus becomes faecal in character.

Treatment

Treatment includes:

i. Avoiding solid food
ii. Medication for nausea and pain
iii. Nasogastric intubation to help relieve the pressure
iv. Supportive intravenous therapy to maintain fluid and electrolyte
v. Surgery (depending on the severity, surgery may be required [laparoscopic surgery, exploratory laparotomy and bowel resection]).

Self-Assessment

1. Discuss the composition, mechanism of secretion and regulation of succus entericus.
2. Discuss the various types of intestinal movements.
3. Describe briefly:
   - Characteristics and significance of small intestinal mucosa
   - Adynamic ileus
   - Gastroileal reflex
   - Peristaltic rush

Clinical Cases

Case 1

A 40-year-old male patient had abdominal surgery and postoperatively developed vomiting and abdominal discomfort. On examination, abdominal sounds were not heard and the patient did not pass flatus.

Q1. What is this condition called?
Q2. Why are bowel sounds absent?
Q3. Which tests should be carried out to find the cause?
Q4. What is the most common cause of this condition?

Case 2

A 92-year-old male patient was admitted with complaints of severe abdominal pain, swelling of the abdomen, cramping sensations and loud gargling sound. History revealed that the patient suffered with this type of episode 2 months back also but that was not so severe. On the basis of signs and symptoms, this case was diagnosed a case of intestinal obstruction.

Q1. What are the causes of intestinal obstruction?
Q2. What further tests should be carried out to find the cause?
Q3. What are the immediate treatment measures?
Q4. What are the types of intestinal obstructions?

7.6 Physiological Activities in Large Intestine

CHAPTER OUTLINE

FUNCTIONAL ANATOMY

GROSS ANATOMICAL CONSIDERATIONS

Functional Organization

The large intestine is a tube about 6 cm in diameter and 100 cm in length. It normally arches around and encloses the coils of the small intestine and tends to be more fixed than the small intestine. It is divided into the following parts (Fig. 7.6.1):

Caecum is a blind-ended sac into which opens the lower end of ileum. The ileocaecal junction is guarded by the ileocaecal valve which allows inflow but prevents backflow of intestinal contents.
Appendix is worm-shaped tube that arises from the medial side of caecum which in humans is a vestigial organ.
Ascending colon extends upward from the caecum along the right side of the abdomen up to the liver. On reaching the liver, it bends to the left, forming the right hepatic flexure.
Transverse colon extends from the right hepatic flexure to the left splenic flexure. It forms a wide U-shaped curve.
Descending colon extends from the left splenic flexure to the pelvic inlet below.
Sigmoid colon begins at the pelvic inlet as continuation of the descending colon and joins the rectum in front of the sacrum.
Rectum descends in front of the sacrum to leave the pelvis by piercing the pelvic floor. Here, it becomes continuous with the anal canal in the perineum.
Anal canal opens to the exterior through the anus, the opening of which is guarded by two sphincters.

Ileocaecal Valve

Structure Ileocaecal valve functioning occurs due to invagination of the ileum into the caecum at the ileocaecal junction and a very small ileal opening (only 2–3 mm in diameter) (Fig. 7.6.1).

Functions The principal function of the ileocaecal valve is to prevent backflow of the faecal matter from the caecum into the ileum. The valvular mechanism works in such a way that when the caecal pressure is increased, the ileocaecal opening is closed.

Role of ileocaecal sphincter Ileocaecal sphincter refers to thickened band of circular muscle coat of the terminal part of ileum just above the ileocaecal junction. The rhythmic contractions of ileocaecal sphincter leading to rhythmic opening and closing occur after every 30 seconds after a meal. During every rhythmic opening, a small jet of ileal fluid (approximately 15 mL) escapes into the caecum. The ileocaecal sphincter slows down the emptying of ileal contents into the caecum and thus helps in completion of the absorption of nutrients in the ileum.

Control Gastrin produces relaxation and secretin causes contraction of ileocaecal sphincter. It is important to note that these hormones show opposite effects on cardiac sphincter.

STRUCTURAL CHARACTERISTICS

Histological structure of the large intestine is similar to that described in general (see page 561) with the following special characteristics.

Mucosa of the large intestine is characterized by:

- Plicae circulares and villi are absent (seen in the small intestine).
- It is thrown into folds opposite to the contractions seen in the wall of the large intestine which produce sacculations.
- A large number of simple tubular glands (crypts of Lieberkuhn) lined by simple columnar epithelial cells with a large number of goblet cells which secrete mucus are the histological characteristics of mucosa of the large intestine (Fig. 7.6.2). Epithelial cells contain no enzyme.

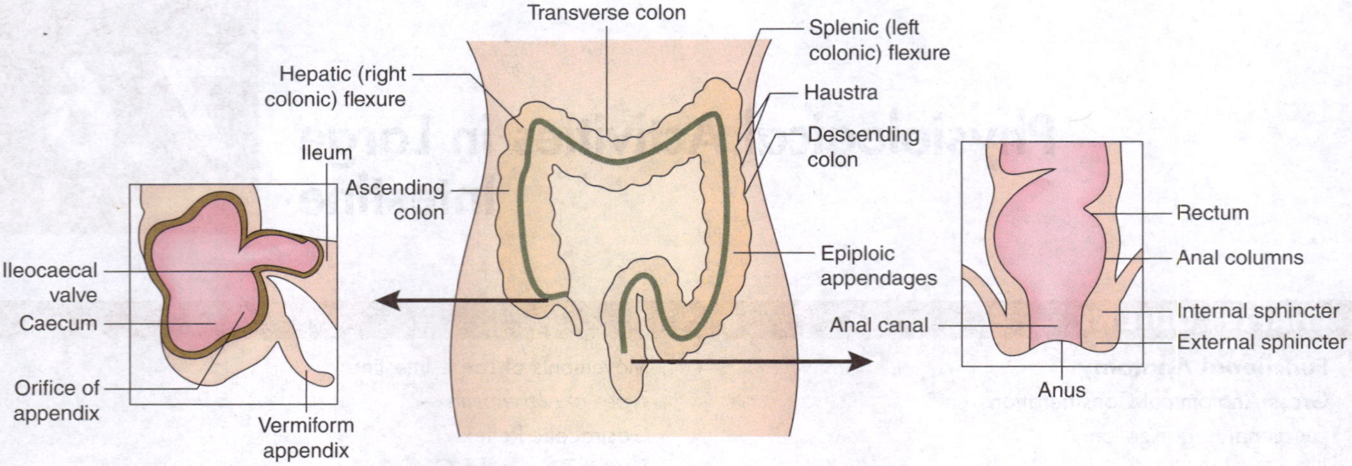

Fig. 7.6.1 Functional organization of the large intestine.

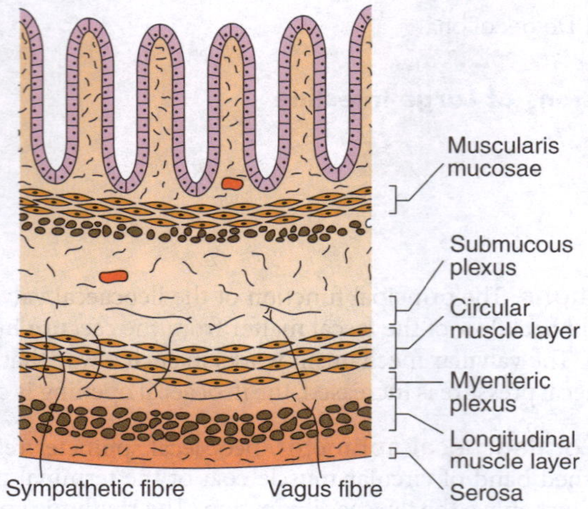

Fig. 7.6.2 Histological structure of the colon.

- The epithelium overlying solitary lymphatic follicles (in the ascending colon, caecum and appendix) contains M-cells similar to those seen in the small intestine.

Longitudinal layer of muscle coat of colon is unusual

- Most of the fibres in it are collected to form three thick bands, the *taenia coli*, which can be seen through the serous layer (Fig. 7.6.1). A thin layer of longitudinal fibres is present in the intestines between the taenia.
- The taenia coli are shorter in length than other layers of the wall of the colon. This results in the production of *sacculations* (also called *haustrations*) on the wall of the colon.

Serous layer is missing over the posterior aspect of the ascending and descending colon. At places, small peritoneal bags of fat, called *appendices epiploicae*, project from the colonic serosa.

LARGE INTESTINAL SECRETIONS AND BACTERIAL ACTIVITY

LARGE INTESTINAL SECRETIONS

- The large intestinal secretions mainly comprise mucus secreted by the goblet cells which are in abundance among the epithelial cells of mucosa and some water, and lot of HCO_3^- is secreted by glands of Lieberkuhn.
- The mucus lubricates the faecal matter and also protects the mucous membrane of the large intestine by preventing the damage caused by mechanical injury or chemical substances.
- The alkaline nature (pH 8.0) of the mucoid secretions of the large intestine is due to the presence of HCO_3^-. It serves to neutralize the acids formed by bacterial action on the faecal matter.
- Large quantities of water and electrolytes are secreted by mucosa of the large intestine only when it is intensely irritated.

INTESTINAL BACTERIAL ACTIVITY

Bacterial flora At birth, the colon is sterile, but the colonic bacterial flora becomes established early in life and includes:

- *Harmless bacteria* such as *Escherichia coli* and *Enterobacter aerogenes*
- *Potentially dangerous bacteria* such as *Bacteroides fragilis*, various types of cocci and gas gangrene bacilli (these bacteria can cause serious disease in tissues outside the colon)

Intestinal bacterial activities Intestinal bacterial activities can be grouped as follows:

- Beneficial bacterial activities
- Indifferent bacterial activities
- Detrimental bacterial activities

Beneficial bacterial activities Beneficial bacterial activities include:

Synthesis of vitamins: Vitamins such as vitamin C, a number of B-complex vitamins, folic acid and vitamin K are synthesized.

Recycling of bile salts: Bile salts needed for transport and absorption of lipids are recycled.

Trophic effects on colonic mucosa: Unabsorbed carbohydrates are converted to short-chain fatty acids (SCFAs) by colonic bacteria. Some of the SCFAs produced have a trophic effect on colonic mucosa.

Role in cholesterol metabolism: Bacterial activities play a role in cholesterol metabolism by decreasing plasma cholesterol and low density lipids (LDL) levels.

Indifferent bacterial activities Indifferent bacterial activities include:

Production of intestinal gases: The colonic bacteria produce gas in large volumes up to 7–10 L/day, which contribute towards flatus. The gas is produced chiefly through breakdown of undigested nutrients that reach the colon. The gases produced by colonic bacteria include carbon dioxide (CO_2), hydrogen sulphide (H_2S), hydrogen (H_2) and methane (CH_4) which contribute to flatus. Nitrogen gas (N_2) derived from the swallowed air accounts for most of the flatus passed through the rectum, or other gases diffuse readily through the intestinal mucosa. Therefore, the volume of flatus expelled is reduced to about 600 mL/day.

Organic acids formed by the colonic bacteria from the carbohydrates are responsible for the slight acidic reaction of the stools (pH 5–7).

Substances responsible for odour of the faeces such as indole, skatole and mercaptans are synthesized by colonic bacteria.

Potentially toxic amines like histamine and tyramine are synthesized by some colonic bacteria. These substances were earlier thought to produce 'autointoxication' in patients with constipation, but are now known to be harmless.

Pigments formed by the colonic bacteria from the bile pigments are responsible for the known colour of stools.

Detrimental bacterial activities Detrimental bacterial activities include:

Consumption of nutrients like vitamin C, vitamin B_{12} and choline by some bacteria may lead to deficiency symptoms, unless these are supplemented in adequate amounts in the diet.

Production of ammonia: Colonic bacteria also produce ammonia, which is absorbed by blood and is normally detoxified quickly by the liver. However, in liver dysfunction, hyperammonaemia results, producing neurological symptoms (hepatic encephalopathy); osmotic cathartic such as lactulose is useful in the treatment of such a condition, by its following actions:

- Reduces the colonic load of ammonia-forming proteins
- Acidifies the colonic contents and promotes the growth of bacteria that form ammonia
- Ferments dietary starches to form SCFAs, which are two- to five-carbon weak acids, such as acetate, propionate and butyrate (these fatty acids are the main source of nutrition for epithelial cells; the SCFAs also help in sodium absorption)
- Mutually dependent relationship with immune system (the colonic bacterial flora represents a potentially vast array of foreign antigen that must be tolerated by the immune system; this relationship between gut microbes and development of GIT and systemic immune system is involved in immune regulation; for example, they influence the systemic immune tolerance to antigens that would otherwise provoke a strong immune response in the form of autoimmune disease or allergy)

Important Notes

The small intestine is relatively sterile as compared with the colon, but bacterial growth can occur if there is any structural change (e.g. due to surgery or radiotherapy) or metabolic change (e.g. in diabetes mellitus).

Probiotics such as *Lactobacillus* and *Bifidobacterium* are now widely used as dietary supplements. These contain live cultures of bacteria and yeast that are beneficial to colonic host function.

Probiotics are quite useful as treatment of *Clostridium difficile*–associated diarrhoea.

Prebiotics are nondigestible oligosaccharides that are helpful in stimulating the growth of certain species of beneficial bacteria in the host. Inulin is the best example of probiotics. For details, see page 566.

MOTILITY OF LARGE INTESTINE

SLOW-WAVE ACTIVITY

Like other parts of the gastrointestinal tract, the motility of the large intestine is also coordinated by the 'basic electrical rhythm (BER)' or the so-called slow-wave activity (SWA). However, the frequency of SWA gradually increases down the large intestine (from 9/min at the ileocaecal valve to 16/min at the sigmoid colon), in contrast to gradually decreasing frequency of SWA in the small intestine (from about 12/min in the duodenum to about 9/min in the lower ileum).

MOVEMENTS OF LARGE INTESTINE

Functions The principal functions of the colon are absorption of water and electrolytes from the chyme and storage of faecal matter until it can be expelled. The proximal half of the colon is concerned principally with absorption, and the distal half is concerned with storage. The contractile activity of the large intestine serves two main functions:

- It increases the efficiency of the colon for water and electrolyte absorption.
- It promotes the excretion of the faecal matter remaining in the colon.

Types of Movements

The movements of the colon have been studied by different methods and have been differently classified. The different types of movements (most accepted nomenclature) of the colon are as follows:

1. Haustral Shuttling

The haustral shuttling or haustral contractions are similar to the segmentation contractions of the small intestine, which vigorously mix the contents of the colon by exposing more of the contents to mucosa (facilitate absorption). During haustral contractions, the pressure rises to about 10–16 mm Hg in the distal colon, and their frequency is 2–3 contractions/min. Contraction of circular and longitudinal muscles in the large intestine causes haustrations to develop as follows:

- Contraction of circular muscle produces constriction rings at regular intervals.
- Contraction of longitudinal muscle (taenia coli) causes the unstimulated portion of the large intestine in between the constriction rings to bulge in bag-like sacs called haustration.
- Contraction disappears within 60 seconds. After a few minutes, haustral contractions are initiated in a nearby area. The dynamic formation and disappearance of haustrations squeeze the chyme, moving it back and forth in a manner

similar to that described for the segmentation contractions in the small intestine.

Functions The haustral contractions perform two main functions:

Mixing: Haustral contractions dig into and roll over the faecal material in the large intestine. In this way, all the faecal material is gradually exposed to the surface of the large intestine, and fluid and dissolved substances are progressively absorbed.
Propulsion: Haustral contractions at times move slowly towards the anus during the period of contraction and thereby provide forward propulsion of the colonic contents.

2. Peristalsis

Peristalsis is a progressive contractile wave preceded by a wave of relaxation. In the colon, the peristaltic waves are very small pressure waves of prolonged duration.

Function They propel the contents towards the rectum very slowly (5 cm/h). It can take up to 48 hours for the chyme to traverse the colon.

3. Mass Movements

The mass movements are special type of peristaltic contractions which are observed in the colon only.

- These occur three to four times a day, generally after meals, and each contraction lasts for about 3 minutes.
- A mass movement is characterized by appearance of a constriction ring at a distended or irritated point in the colon followed by a simultaneous contraction of the smooth muscle as a unit over large confluent areas distal to the constriction.
- The mass movements force the faecal material rapidly in mass down the colon. These powerful peristaltic movements empty about <20 cm segment of the colon. They also move material into the rectum, and rectal distension initiates the defaecation reflex.
- A mass movement can be initiated by:
  - Gastrocolic or duodenocolic reflexes
  - Intense stimulation of the parasympathetic nerves
  - Overdistension of a segment of the colon

GASTROCOLIC REFLEX

Gastrocolic reflex refers to contraction of the colon induced by entry of food into the stomach. This reflex results in an urge to defaecate after a meal. Because of this, defaecation after meals is a rule in children. However, in adults, the bowel training suppresses this reflex.

Initiation It has been reported that perhaps this reflex consists of two phases:

Early or rapid phase The early or rapid phase (which occurs within 10 minutes of meals) is initiated by distension of the stomach and is conducted through the extrinsic nerves of the autonomic nervous system. It can be abolished by anticholinergic drugs.

Late or slow phase The late or slow phase is considered to be mediated by gastrointestinal hormones like gastrin and cholecystokinin (CCK) which are secreted into the bloodstream in significant amounts shortly after a meal.

TRANSIT TIME IN THE GUT

The transit time in various parts of the gut studied after a test meal is as follows:

Up to *caecum*: 4 hours
Up to *hepatic flexure*: 6 hours
Up to *splenic flexure*: 8 or 9 hours
Up to *pelvic colon*: 12 hours

- From *the pelvic colon to the anus*, transport is made slower, and as much as one-quarter (25%) of the residue of a test meal may still be in the rectum for up to 3 days.
- Complete expulsion of the meal in stool takes more than a week. It has been observed that when beads of three different colours are consumed on 3 consecutive days (e.g. red on first day, green on second day and blue on third day), beads of all the three colours are found in the stool from the fourth day onward and complete expulsion occurs after a week of the consumption. It indicates that there is a pool probably in the caecum and sigmoid colon where residues get mixed.
- It has been observed that a high-residue diet passes more rapidly through the entire gut. This is mainly because of its effect on the colonic movements, as addition of fibres to the diet is actually reported to decrease the rate of flow through the jejunum.

Note: Recent advances have made it possible to study the transit time, pressure fluctuations and changes in pH in the gastrointestinal tract by monitoring the progress of a small pill that contains sensors and a miniature radio transmitter.

DEFAECATION

FUNCTIONAL ANATOMY

A brief description of functional anatomy of the anal sphincters which play the most important role in the process of defaecation needs special emphasis.

1. Internal or involuntary anal sphincter Internal or involuntary anal sphincter consists of thickened circular smooth muscles at the pelvic–rectal flexure. This sphincter relaxes reflexly in response to stimulation of stretch receptors when the rectum is distended.

Innervation Innervation of internal anal sphincter is by:

- *Parasympathetic* pelvic splanchnic nerves which are inhibitory
- *Sympathetic nerves* which are excitatory

2. External or voluntary anal sphincter External or voluntary anal sphincter consists of somatic skeletal muscle fibres innervated by the pudendal nerves.
Characteristic features are as follows:

- It is maintained in a state of tonic contraction.
- Mild to moderate distension of the rectum increases its force of contraction.
- Moderately severe distension of the rectum initiates a reflex which inhibits the discharge of somatic pudendal nerves (which cause tonic contraction) and thus relaxes the internal anal sphincter.
- The external anal sphincter can be voluntarily relaxed, the action which aids the reflex emptying of the distended rectum.

ACT OF DEFAECATION

Defaecation, the process of excretion of faecal material, involves both voluntary and reflex activities:

- Reflex contraction of smooth muscles of the distal colon and rectum which propel the faecal matter in the anal canal
- Reflex relaxation of internal anal sphincter
- Reflex relaxation with voluntary control of external anal sphincter and voluntary contraction of abdominal muscles

The events associated with the process of defaecation proceed as follows:

Distension of rectum Usually the rectum is empty. This is because the frequency of contractions is greater in the rectum than in the sigmoid colon, which causes retrograde movement of faecal material (because of this movement, material placed into the rectum, such as suppository, is pushed up into the colon).

Usually, once or twice a day, the gastrocolic reflex drives the faeces into the rectum which increases the intrarectal pressure passively (Fig. 7.6.3A, I and II).

Defaecation reflexes As the rectum starts filling, the resultant rise in the intrarectal pressure stimulates the stretch receptors, sets up defaecation reflexes and produces an urge to defaecate (when intrarectal pressure increases to about 18 mm Hg). The voluntary external anal sphincter which normally remains tonically contracted further contracts when there is moderate rise in the rectal pressure (Fig. 7.6.3C, I–III).

Intrinsic reflex It is mediated by intrinsic nerve plexus. Distension of the rectum with faeces initiates afferent signals that spread through the myenteric plexus:

- Initiates peristaltic waves in the descending colon, sigmoid colon and rectum causing the active contraction of smooth muscles and further raising intrarectal pressure, thus forcing the faeces towards the anus (Fig. 7.6.3A, III and IV)
- Relaxation of internal anal sphincter by inhibitory signals from the myenteric plexus, when the peristaltic wave approaches the anus (Fig. 7.6.3B)

The intrinsic defaecation reflex functioning by itself is relatively weak. To be effective in causing defaecation, this reflex usually must be fortified by a spinal cord reflex.

Spinal cord reflex Distension of the rectum by faeces causes transmission of afferent impulses through the pelvic nerves to sacral segments of the spinal cord. This induces reflex parasympathetic discharge in nervi erigentes (mainly from S_2–S_4) and the pelvic splanchnic nerves (Fig. 7.6.4) to cause:

- Intensification of colonic peristaltic contraction occurs, further raising the intrarectal pressure (Fig. 7.6.3A, V).
- When the rectal pressure reaches about 55 mm Hg, there occurs further relaxation of internal anal sphincter (Fig. 7.6.3B, V) and external sphincter as well (Fig. 7.6.3C, V).

Role of voluntary control on defaecation Once the above-described reflex effects are obtained, the voluntary control mechanism depending on the convenience may or may not allow the act of defaecation to occur.

When defaecation is not allowed When defaecation is not allowed, the voluntary control mechanism maintains the contraction of external anal sphincter, which is composed of skeletal muscle innervated by the pudendal nerves (also see page 626). Soon, the internal anal sphincter also closes, and the rectum relaxes to accommodate the faecal matter within it. Once the defaecation reflex dies out, it recurs after some hours.

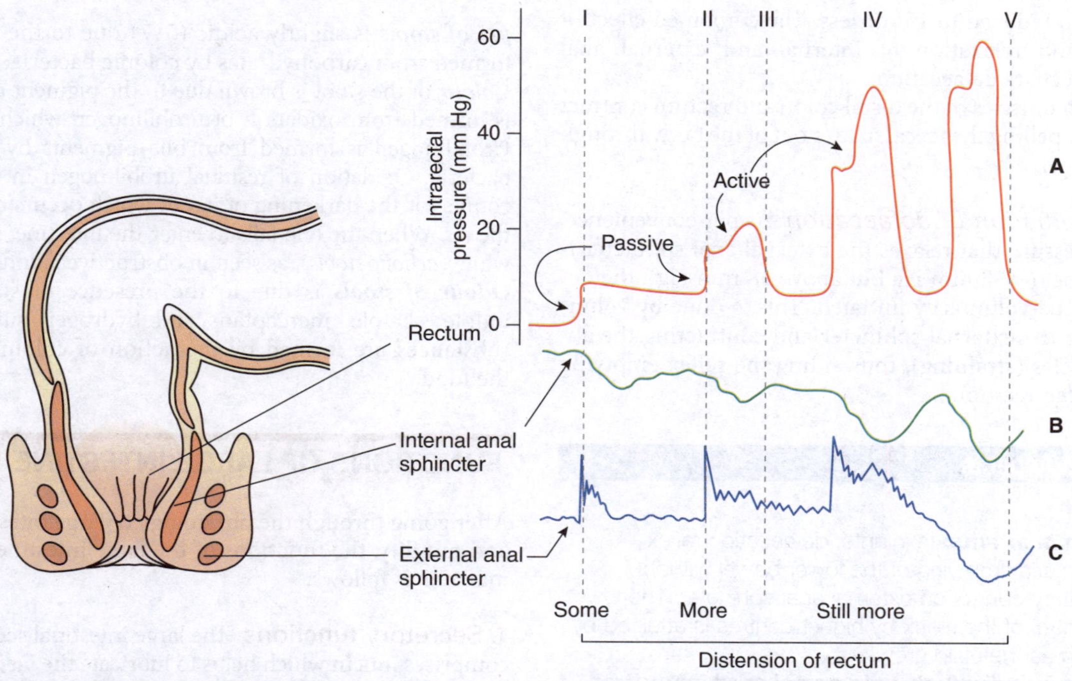

Fig. 7.6.3 Changes in **A**, intrarectal pressure, **B**, tone of internal anal sphincter and **C**, tone of external anal sphincter during distension of rectum by the faeces.

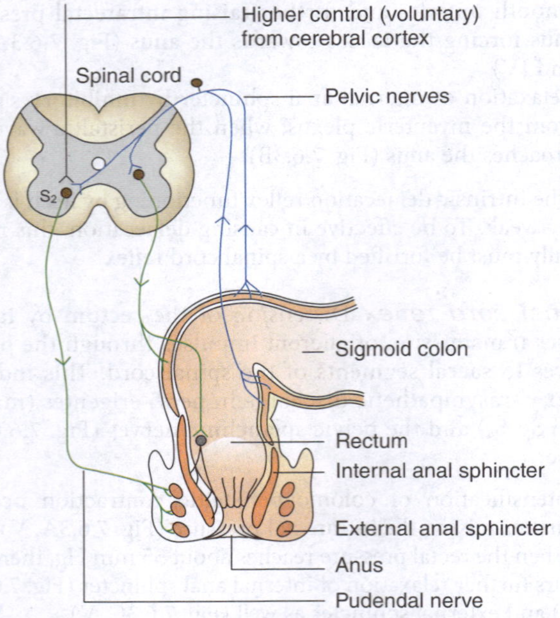

Fig. 7.6.4 Pathway of spinal defaecation reflex and its voluntary control.

When it is convenient to defaecate When it is convenient to defaecate, the external anal sphincter is relaxed voluntarily. Thus, both internal and external sphincters are relaxed.

- The intra-abdominal pressure is increased by contraction of abdominal and diaphragmatic muscles (a process of expiring against closed glottis, i.e. Valsalva manoeuvre).
- Normally, the defaecation is inhibited because of a 90° angle between the rectum and the anus (anorectal angle) and contraction of puborectalis muscle. Straining causes contraction of abdominal muscles and lowers the pelvic floor by 1–3 cm, and relaxation of puborectalis. The anorectal angle is also reduced to 15° or less. The combined effect of straining and relaxation of internal and external anal sphincters causes defaecation.
- The smooth muscles of the distal colon and rectum contract forcibly, propelling the faecal matter out of the body through the anal canal.

Voluntary initiation of defaecation As per convenience, before the pressure that relaxes the external anal sphincter is reached (i.e. below 55 mm Hg but above 18 mm Hg), the defaecation can be voluntarily initiated. This is done by voluntarily relaxing the external sphincter and contracting the abdominal muscles (straining), thus aiding the reflex emptying of the distended rectum.

Applied Aspects

Defaecation

Defaecation in infants: In infants, defaecation reflex causes automatic emptying of the lower bowel without normal voluntary control on external anal sphincter. The voluntary control of the reflex by higher centres is attained by social training as the child grows.

Defaecation in individuals with spinal cord injury/transection: In individuals with spinal cord transection, initially there occurs retention of faeces. But defaecation reflex returns quickly. However, reflex evacuation occurs automatically, without voluntary control, when the rectal pressure increases to about 55 mm Hg.

- When spinal cord injury occurs between the conus medullaris and the brain (lower spinal cord injury), the defaecation reflex remains intact, but voluntary control is blocked. In these patients, enema is usually given in the morning shortly after meals to excite defaecation reflex.

Role of dietary fibres: Dietary fibres increase bulk of faeces; this plays a role in defaecation reflex by distending the rectum (for details, see page 629).

FAECES

Composition Faeces or the faecal matter is derived mainly from the intestinal secretion and partly from the undigested material. If vegetables and coarsely ground cereals are excluded from the diet, faeces have a fairly uniform composition. The faecal matter consists of 75% *water*, which forms the main bulk of faeces, and 25% *solids*. These include inorganic material, mostly calcium and phosphate, undigested plant fibres, epithelial cells, dead bacteria, constituents of intestinal secretions including bile pigments, fats and proteins. It is important to note that:

- *Proteins* in the stools are not of dietary origin but come from bacteria and cellular debris.
- Some of the *fats* in the stools come from the dietary intake but most of them are also derived from desquamated epithelial cells and from bacterial synthesis. On an average, for a fat intake of 100 g/day, 5–6 g/day is normally lost in faeces. Stool fat content is increased in steatorrhoea.
- Since a large fraction of the faecal matter is of nondietary origin, faeces during starvation, though decreased in bulk, differ little in composition from those of normally fed persons.

pH of stools is slightly acidic (5–7) due to the organic acids formed from carbohydrates by colonic bacteria.
Colour of the stool is brown due to the pigment *urobilin* which is formed from oxidation of urobilinogen which is colourless. Urobilinogen is formed from bile pigments by the intestinal bacteria. Oxidation of residual urobilinogen in the stools accounts for the darkening of faeces which occurs on standing in the air. When the bile fails to enter the intestine, stools become white (*acholic stools*), as seen in obstructive jaundice.
Odour of stools is due to the presence of substances like indole, skatole, mercaptans and hydrogen sulphide. These substances are formed by the action of colonic bacteria on the food.

FUNCTIONS OF LARGE INTESTINE

After going through the physiology of large intestine secretion and motility, the functions of the large intestine can be summarized as follows:

1. Secretory functions The large intestinal secretion mainly comprises mucin which helps to lubricate the faecal matter. The alkaline nature (pH 8) of the secretion serves to neutralize the acids formed by bacterial action on the faecal matter.

2. Synthesis functions The bacterial flora of the large intestine synthesizes folic acid, vitamin B_{12} and vitamin K.

3. Absorptive functions Absorption of water and electrolytes is the chief function of proximal part of the colon. Organic substances like glucose, alcohol and some drugs like anaesthetic agents, sedatives and steroids can also be absorbed in the large intestine. Vitamin K and a number of B-complex vitamins which are synthesized in the colon by bacterial flora are also absorbed in the large intestine.

4. Excretory functions Heavy metals like mercury, lead, bismuth and arsenic are excreted by the large intestine through the faeces.

5. Storage function After the absorption of nutrients, water and other substances, the unwanted substances form faeces. The faeces are stored in the pelvic colon until they can be expelled by the process of defaecation.

Applied Aspects

Role of Dietary Fibres

Dietary fibres are mainly plant material of diet which is resistant to enzymatic digestion. They are also called roughage. The main sources of dietary fibres are cereal grains, fruits and vegetables.

Dietary fibres are basically classified into two types:

Water-insoluble (less fermented) dietary fibres include cellulose, hemicellulose and lignin.

Water-soluble (fermented) dietary fibres include pectin, gums and mucilages.

Physiological Role of Dietary Fibres on Intestinal Food Transit

In humans, there is no appreciable digestion of the dietary fibres at all.

- The ingested dietary fibres reach the large intestine in an essentially unchanged state and thus add bulk to the faeces and play a role in defaecation reflex by distending the rectum.
- If the amount of dietary fibres is small, the diet is said to lack bulk. Since the material in the colon is small, the colon is inactive and colon movements are infrequent.
- The bulk laxatives such as pectin work by providing a larger volume of indigestible material to the colon.

Role of Dietary Fibres in Prevention of Diseases. In addition to their role in activating the colon movements, epidemiological evidences indicate that groups of people who consume a diet which contains large amounts of vegetable fibres have a low incidence of diverticulitis, cancer of the colon, diabetes mellitus and coronary artery disease. However, the definitive researches on relationship between dietary fibres and the incidence of such diseases are needed to establish the epidemiological observations. Probably, the dietary fibres might be playing role by their following effects:

Reduction in absorption of digested foodstuffs is caused by dietary fibres by forming a mechanical barrier between the nutrients and the absorptive surface. Due to this effect, the dietary fibres reduce chances of postprandial hyperglycaemia and are thus especially useful in patients with diabetes.

Reduction in blood cholesterol level by dietary fibres is caused by increasing excretion of bile salts in faeces, summarized as follows:

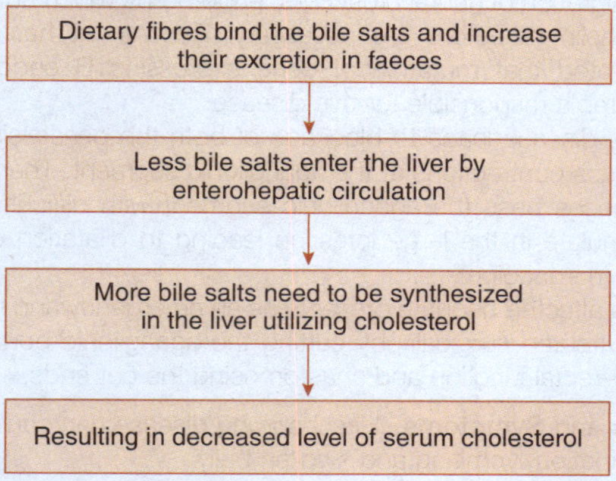

Therefore, dietary fibres are especially useful in patients with atherosclerosis, obesity, hypercholesterolaemia and diabetes mellitus.

Prevention of colonic cancers by dietary fibres is caused by their following effects:

- Dilution of carcinogens by the water held in them
- Reduction of duration of contact between carcinogens and mucous membrane of the colon, as they decrease the intestinal transit time
- Excretion of carcinogens which get bound to dietary fibres

Therapeutic Role of Dietary Fibres

The daily recommended intake of dietary fibres is about 25–35 g/day. High-fibre supplements have therapeutic role in the following conditions:

In constipation, the dietary fibres work as bulk laxatives by providing a larger volume of indigestible material to the colon. *Plantago lanata* or isabgol rich in hemicellulose is being used since ages as ancient Indian medicine for constipation.

In spastic colon and diverticular disease, the dietary fibres are useful by making the stools softer and thus lowering the intraluminal pressure.

In diabetes and high cholesterol levels, the role of dietary fibres has already been discussed.

In diarrhoea, complete avoidance of dietary fibres is useful by increasing the transit time, and decreasing the frequency and volume of stools.

Precautions for Consuming Fibre Supplements

Should be taken at least 2 hours before meals, to avoid impairment in absorption of iron and calcium from the diet

Should not be taken at bedtime, to avoid the risk of reflux and aspiration

Should be avoided in disorder of oesophageal motility as the smaller dietary fibres can make a solid mass inside the oesophagus called bezoar

Disorders of Large Intestine Motility

1. Hirschsprung Disease

Hirschsprung disease, or the aganglionic megacolon, occurs due to congenital absence of the ganglion cells in the myenteric as well as submucous plexus (as a result of failure of migration of neural crest cells during development). For normal migration of neural crest cells, endothelins which act on B endothelin receptors are necessary. Recently, it has been postulated that mutation of gene expressing B endothelin receptor is responsible for this disease.

This disease leads to blockage of both the peristalsis and the mass contractions at the aganglionic segment. Therefore, the faeces pass the aganglionic segment with difficulty and accumulate in the large intestine leading to dilatation of the colon (megacolon).

The affected neonate presents as an emergency and needs to be treated surgically by cutting the aganglionic portion of pelvic–rectal junction and anastomosing the cut ends.

Signs and Symptoms. Hirschsprung disease can cause constipation, vomiting and swollen belly.

2. Constipation

Constipation refers to failure of voiding of faeces which produces discomfort. It results from infrequent mass movement in the colon. As a result, the faecal matter remains in the colon for a longer time, so a large amount of fluid is absorbed and the faeces become hard and dry.

Aetiopathogenesis. Constipation, most of the time, results from irregular bowel habit. If the sensation of fullness of the rectum (i.e. urge to defaecate) is repeatedly ignored voluntarily, over the time there occurs adaptation. Progressively, increasing weakness of the defaecation reflex results in problematic constipation, which is a fairly common problem.

Constipation also occurs due to imbalance between secretion and absorption in the colon.

Symptoms. Persons suffering from constipation may develop anorexia, nausea and abdominal distension and discomfort. Patients may have headache, restlessness and irritability. Symptoms of constipation are not due to absorption of any toxic substances from the colon, as they are quickly relieved with evacuation of the rectum.

Treatment. Addition of dietary fibres (which are neither digested nor absorbed) in the meals adds to the bulk of faeces which helps in initiating the colonic peristalsis by distending the colon. Bulk laxatives may be used. In severe cases, even finger evacuation of the rectum may be needed.

Lubiprostone is used to relieve constipation. It acts by enhancing chloride secretion and water into the colon, resulting in increased fluidity of colonic contents.

3. Diarrhoea

Diarrhoea is a condition which is characterized by increased frequency of defaecation with increased water content of the faeces. It may develop in a number of bacterial, protozoal and viral infections of the intestinal tract, food poisoning, ulcerative colitis, etc.

Enteritis. Enteritis (inflammation of the intestinal tract) is usually caused by viral or bacterial infection. The mucosa gets irritated resulting in increased rate of secretions. At the same time, there is several-fold increase in motility of the gut.

Cholera. Cholera is a severe secretory diarrhoea caused by cholera bacillus which usually occurs in epidemics.

Pathogenesis. Cholera bacillus stays in the gut lumen but produces a toxin that binds to receptors (GM-1 ganglioside receptors) present on the apical membrane of enterocytes, leading to entry of toxins into the enterocytes. The cholera toxin increases cyclic AMP concentration by activation of adenyl cyclase which stimulates excessive secretion of electrolytes and reduces NaCl absorption by reducing mucosal transport for Na^+.

Thus, increase in intestinal water and electrolyte contents causes diarrhoea leading to about 20 L stool volume/day.

Treatment. The main physiological basis is replacement therapy to prevent dehydration by infusing fluid intravenously.

- In cholera, however, Na^+–K^+-ATPase and Na^+–glucose transporter are unaffected; therefore, oral administration of solution containing NaCl and glucose is useful in diarrhoea.
- Oral rehydration solution (prepacked mixture of sugar, salt) dissolved in water is effective to reduce mortality in epidemic of cholera.

Ulcerative colitis. In this condition, there is inflammation of the large intestine leading to ulcerations. The exact cause of ulcerative colitis is not known, but may be allergic or immune response. The irritation occurring in ulcerative colitis causes increased motility which is so great that mass movements occur and colon secretions are greatly increased.

Psychogenic diarrhoea. Psychogenic diarrhoea accompanies nervous tension and anxiety (such as during examination). This type of diarrhoea, also called psychogenic diarrhoea, occurs due to excessive stimulation of the parasympathetic system causing increased motility and mucous secretion in the distal colon.

Complications: Severe diarrhoea may cause dehydration, hypovolaemia and electrolyte imbalance due to marked loss of water, Na^+, K^+ and HCO_3^- in the stools. There may occur shock, cardiovascular collapse and even death (especially in infants).

Treatment: Treatment consists of maintenance of water and electrolyte balance by oral rehydration therapy (ORT), which is life-saving. In very serious cases, intravenous administration of fluids is required.

Self-Assessment

1. Discuss the role of colonic bacterial activity.
2. Describe the following:
   - Role of dietary fibres
   - Defaecation and its control
   - Types of large intestinal movements
   - Hirschsprung disease
3. Write notes on:
   - Significance of anal sphincters
   - Gastrocolic reflex

Clinical Cases

Case 1

A newborn baby developed swollen belly, vomiting having greenish brown–coloured vomitus and constipation.

Q1. What is the probable diagnosis?
Q2. What is the most common cause of this condition?
Q3. What is the best treatment for this condition?
Q4. What complications can occur if this condition is not treated timely?

Case 2

An 18-year-old male student was admitted to the emergency with watery diarrhoea, sunken eyes, dry mouth and extreme thirst. History revealed that the student was staying in the hostel and eating food from the street vendor to avoid ragging.

Examination revealed low BP and rapid and low-volume pulse indicating hypovolaemia due to dehydration. From history, signs and symptoms and examination, the probable diagnosis made was cholera.

Q1. What is the pathophysiology of cholera?
Q2. What is the cause of watery diarrhoea?
Q3. What are the risk factors of this condition?
Q4. What is the causative organism of cholera?
Q5. Which blood test detects cholera?

7.7 Digestion and Absorption

CHAPTER OUTLINE

DIGESTION AND ABSORPTION OF CARBOHYDRATES

DIETARY CARBOHYDRATES

Dietary intake of carbohydrates is 250–850 g/day, which represents 50%–60% of the diet. Major carbohydrates in the human diet are present in the following forms:

1. Polysaccharides Polysaccharides are made up of many monosaccharides, may be up to 1 million. These may be present in the following forms:

Starch Starch is the carbohydrate reserve of plants. It consists of two polysaccharide components:

- *Amylose* (15%–20%): It is a water-soluble straight-chain polysaccharide.
- *Amylopectin* (80%–85%): It is a water-insoluble branched-chain polysaccharide.

Glycogen It is available in nonvegetarian diet and so often referred to as animal starch. In it, glucose molecules are mostly long chains (1:4 α glycoside linkages and 1:6 glycoside linkages) at branching points.

Cellulose Cellulose is another plant polysaccharide, which is present in diet in large amounts. But there is no enzyme in the human GIT to digest it, so it is excreted.

2. Oligosaccharides Undigested oligosaccharide contains 2–10 monosaccharide molecules which are liberated on hydrolysis. Based on the number of monosaccharide units present, oligosaccharides are further subdivided into disaccharide, trisaccharide, tetrasaccharide and pentasaccharide.

Disaccharides Disaccharides include:

- Sucrose (glucose + fructose) is also known as table sugar (cane or beet sugar).
- Lactose (glucose + galactose) is also called milk sugar.

- Maltose (glucose + glucose) is a product of starch hydrolysis. It is present in germinating seeds.

3. Monosaccharides Monosaccharides consumed mostly in human diet are *hexoses* such as:

- Glucose (in fruits, vegetables and honey)
- Fructose in fruits

Pentoses do not occur in free form, but are found in nucleic acid and in certain polysaccharides such as pentosans of fruits and gums.

Other carbohydrates Other carbohydrates that may be present in the human diet are alcohol, lactic acid, pyruvic acid, pectin, dextrin and minor quantities of carbohydrate derivatives in the meat.

DIGESTION OF CARBOHYDRATES (FIG. 7.7.1)

The digestion of carbohydrates begins in mouth and continues in the stomach but occurs mainly (almost all) in the small intestine.

Digestion of Carbohydrates in the Mouth

Initial starch digestion starts in the mouth by the enzyme α-amylase (ptyalin) present in the saliva. However, the role of salivary amylase in the digestion of carbohydrates is limited by the short duration of stay of the food in the mouth.

α-Amylase present in the saliva acts on the 1–4 linkages (but not on 1–6 linkages). It digests cooked starch to maltose (see page 596).

Digestion of Carbohydrates in the Stomach

In the stomach, there occurs minimal carbohydrate digestive activity:

α-Amylase (which enters the stomach with food) activity continues in the stomach for 20–30 minutes till the highly acidic gastric juice mixes with the food and makes it inactive. The optimum pH for the action of salivary amylase is 6–7, and its activity in the stomach completely stops when pH falls below 4. ***The HCl*** of the gastric juice may hydrolyse some sucrose.

Digestion of Carbohydrates in the Small Intestine

In the small intestine, the carbohydrates are digested by the amylolytic enzymes present in the pancreatic juice and brush border enzymes of the small intestine (Table 7.7.1).

Pancreatic α-amylase Pancreatic α-amylase is present in the pancreatic juice which is poured into the duodenum. Its actions on the carbohydrates are similar to those of salivary amylase, but it is much powerful and so it acts on boiled as well as unboiled starch and a variety of other carbohydrates except cellulose. It hydrolyses almost all the starch within 15–30 minutes of the entry of chyme into the duodenum. Its action occurs before the chyme passes beyond the duodenum or upper jejunum.

Pancreatic amylase acts in an alkaline medium and its digestive activity is increased by the presence of bile salts. It converts the starch (polysaccharides) into oligosaccharides such as maltose, maltotriose and dextrin (Fig. 7.7.1).

Brush border enzymes of small intestine The carbohydrate-splitting brush border enzymes of the small intestine include *dextrinase, maltase, sucrase* and *lactase*. It is believed that these brush border enzymes digest the oligosaccharides into monosaccharides on the surface of epithelial cells of villi as follows:

α-Limiting dextrinase: It is the only enzyme in GIT which attacks 1,6 α-glycoside linkage, at the branching points of α-limit dextrins. It also attacks 1,4 α-glycoside linkages, resulting in sequential removal of glucose monomers from the dextrins (the breakdown products of starch by the enzyme amylase).

Maltase, sucrase and lactase hydrolyse the corresponding disaccharides into monosaccharides as follows:

End Products of Carbohydrate Digestion

The carbohydrate digestion is completed in the small intestine (mainly in the jejunum and proximal ileum).

- The end products of carbohydrates are monosaccharides such as glucose, fructose and galactose. Glucose represents

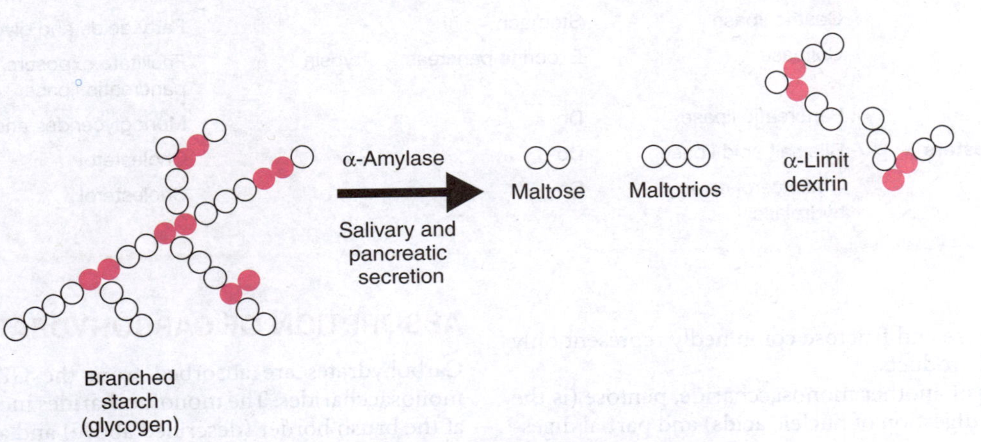

Fig. 7.7.1 Digestion of carbohydrates.

Table 7.7.1 Principal digestive enzymes

Substrate	Enzyme	Source	Activator	Function and product
A. Carbohydrate Starch (polysaccharide)	• Salivary α-amylase • Pancreatic amylase	Salivary gland Exocrine pancreas	Cl^- Cl^-	Hydrolyses 1:4 α-linkages, producing α-limit dextrin, maltotriose and maltose Same as above
Disaccharides				
Maltose	• Maltriose • Maltase • α-Dextrins	Intestinal mucosa	–	Glucose
Lactose	• Lactase	Do-	–	Galactose and glucose
Sucrose	• Sucrase	Do-	–	Fructose and glucose
α-Dextrins, maltriose and maltose	• α-Dextrinase	Do-	–	Glucose
Trehalose	• Trehalase	Do-	–	Glucose
B. Nucleic acid	• Nuclease and related enzymes	Do-	–	Pentoses, purines and pyrimidines
RNA	• Ribonuclease	Exocrine pancreas		Nucleotides
DNA	• Deoxyribonuclease	Do-		Nucleotides
C. Proteins and polypeptides	• Pepsinogen (pepsin)	Gastric glands	HCl	Cleave peptide bonds adjacent to aromatic amino acids
	• Trypsinogen (trypsin)	Exocrine pancreas	Enteropeptidase	Cleave peptide bonds on carboxyl side of basic amino acids (arginine and lysine)
	• Chymotrypsin	Do-	Trypsin	Cleave peptide bonds on carboxyl side of aromatic amino acids
Elastin and some other proteins	Proelastase (elastase)	Do-	Trypsin	Cleave peptide bonds on carboxyl side of aliphatic amino acids
	Exopeptidase, procarboxypeptidase A (carboxypeptidase)	Do-	Do-	Cleave carboxyl terminal aromatic amino acids having branched aliphatic side chains
	Carboxypeptidase B	Do-	Do-	Cleave carboxyl terminal amino acid having basic amino acid side chains
Polypeptides	Endopeptidase	Brush border of intestinal mucosa	–	Cleave amino terminal amino acid from peptide
	Carboxypeptidase	Do-	–	Cleave carboxyl terminal amino acid from peptide
	Endopeptidase	Do-	–	Cleave between residue of midportion of peptide
Dipeptides	Dipeptidase	Do-	–	Two amino acids
Dipeptides, tripeptides and tetrapeptides	Various peptidases	Cytoplasm of mucosal cells	–	Amino acids
D. Fats (lipids), triglycerides	Lingual lipase	Lingual gland	–	1,2-Diacylglycerol and fatty acids
	Gastric lipase	Stomach	–	Fatty acids and glycerol
	Colipase	Exocrine pancreas	Trypsin	Facilitate exposure of active site of pancreatic lipase
	Pancreatic lipase	Do-	–	Monoglycerides and fatty acids
Cholesterol esters	Bile salt acid lipase	Do-	–	Cholesterol
	Cholesterol ester hydrolase	Do-	–	Cholesterol

80% and galactose and fructose combinedly represent only 20% of the end products.

- A little amount of another monosaccharide, pentose (is the end product of digestion of nucleic acids) and partial digestion of pentosans.

ABSORPTION OF CARBOHYDRATES

Carbohydrates are absorbed from the GIT in the form of monosaccharides. The monosaccharides include those formed at the brush border (described above) and also those ingested as such (e.g. glucose and fructose in fruits).

Site of absorption Most of the monosaccharides are absorbed from the mucosal surface of the jejunum and upper ileum. The absorption is almost completed before the remains of a meal reach the terminal ileum. Negligible absorption also occurs in the stomach and colon.

Mechanism of absorption Various monosaccharides are absorbed by the following mechanisms:

- *Glucose* and *galactose* are absorbed by a common *Na^+-dependent* active transport system.
- *Fructose* is absorbed by *facilitated diffusion*. Fructose absorption occurs readily, because most of the fructose is rapidly converted into glucose and lactic acid within the epithelial cells, thus maintaining a high concentration gradient for diffusion.
- *Pentoses* are absorbed by simple diffusion.

Absorption of glucose and galactose Glucose and galactose are absorbed into the epithelial cells (enterocytes) lining the mucous membrane of the small intestine from their brush border surface (luminal surface) by an *active transport mechanism* – the *sodium cotransport* mechanism. *Salient points of glucose absorption are* as follows (Fig. 7.7.2):

Binding of glucose and Na^+ to carrier protein The carrier protein (present in the cell membrane) has two binding sites, one for sodium and another for glucose. It is called *sodium-dependent glucose transporter-1 (SGLT-1)*. The conformational change in the carrier protein occurs only when the binding sites are occupied by the sodium and glucose present in the gut lumen forming the sodium–glucose–carrier complex.

Creation of electrochemical gradient across the epithelial cell The active transport of sodium by Na^+–K^+-ATPase pump through the basolateral membrane into the paracellular spaces lowers the intracellular Na^+ concentration. This creates an electrochemical gradient.

Movement of sodium and glucose inside the cell Because of the electrochemical gradient created, sodium moves into the cell (downhill transport). The flow of sodium ions down the gradient is so forceful that the glucose (or galactose) molecule attached to the carrier protein also enters the cell, even against concentration gradient for glucose (uphill movement). Because two Na^+ are transported down their electrochemical gradient, a large amount of energy is available for transport. Thus, almost all of the glucose and galactose present in the intestine can be absorbed (against the concentration gradient). The energy so released is required for Na^+–K^+ pump activity to maintain the sodium gradient.

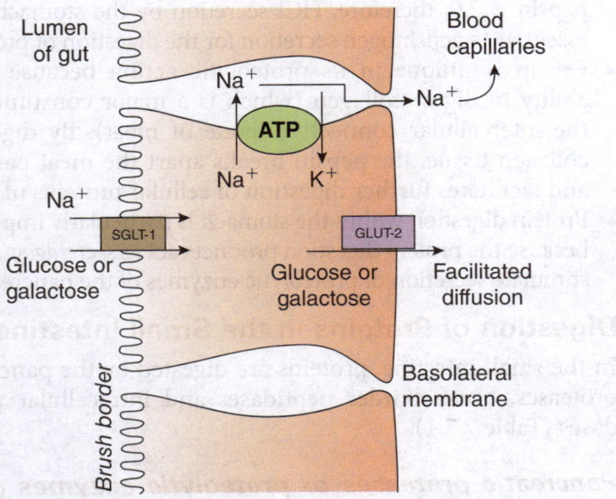

Fig. 7.7.2 Mechanism of glucose absorption across intestinal epithelial cell.

Transport of glucose into blood capillaries From the epithelial cell, the glucose is transported into the interstitial space and thence to blood capillaries of the portal system, through *facilitated diffusion* by *glucose transporter-2 (GLUT-2)*.

Note: Fructose absorption is independent of Na^+ transport. It is absorbed from intestinal lumen into the enterocyte by GLUT-5, and from enterocyte to interstitium by GLUT-2.

Factors affecting glucose absorption Factors affecting glucose absorption are as follows:

1. ***Presence of Na^+ in the intestinal lumen:*** Due to common carrier protein, the entry of glucose/galactose into the epithelial cells is favoured by the presence of Na^+ in the intestinal lumen (similarly, the presence of glucose and galactose in the lumen favours the absorption of Na^+).
2. ***State of mucous membrane:*** Absorption of glucose is decreased in abnormal states of mucous membrane such as in enteritis and coeliac disease.
3. ***Duration of time during which the carbohydrate remains in contact with mucous membrane:*** Absorption of glucose is decreased because of intestinal hurry in conditions like diarrhoea, excision of the small intestine and gastrocolic fistula.
4. ***Role of endocrines*** in glucose absorption is as follows:
   Thyroid: Thyroxine increases the glucose absorption by directly acting on the mucosa. Therefore, in thyrotoxicosis, glucose absorption is increased and in myxoedema it is decreased.
   Anterior pituitary affects the glucose absorption by its effects on the thyroid gland. Hyperpituitarism causes hyperthyroidism and thus increases the glucose absorption and vice versa.
   Adrenal cortex deficiency decreases glucose absorption by decreasing the Na^+ concentration.

Important Notes

Regulation of absorption of monosaccharides does not exist, i.e. absorption of monosaccharides is *not regulated*. The intestines can absorb over 5 kg of sucrose per day. Therefore, after ingestion of a high-carbohydrate diet, glycosuria can occur, i.e. glucose appears in the urine. This condition is called *alimentary glycosuria*.

Rate of absorption of monosaccharides is variable, being:

- Fastest with glucose and galactose
- Intermediate with fructose
- Slowest with mannose or pentoses

FATE OF GLUCOSE IN THE BODY

1. Storage as glycogen About 5% of the total glucose absorbed is stored as glycogen in the liver and muscles.

2. Catabolism to produce energy About 50%–60% of the glucose absorbed is catabolized in the body tissues to produce energy. A total of 1 g of glucose produces about 4 kcal of energy, when it is completely oxidized to CO_2 and H_2O. Amino acids are formed on transamination of some intermediary products of glucose breakdown.

3. Conversion into fat About 30%–40% of glucose is converted into fat and is stored in the fat depot.

Applied Aspects

Abnormalities of Carbohydrate Digestion and Absorption

Lactose intolerance is the inability to digest lactose, the main carbohydrate of dairy products. It is caused by reduced production of the enzyme lactase in the gut. Lactose intolerance is mainly of three types which have different causes:

Congenital lactose intolerance refers to a condition in which lactose (milk sugar) cannot be digested due to congenital deficiency of enzyme lactase.
Primary lactose intolerance is the most common. It is caused by a decreased production of lactase with advancing age.
Secondary lactose intolerance is rare. It is caused by inflammation in the gut secondary to infection or diseases such as stomach bug and coeliac disease.

Signs and Symptoms

Lactose intolerance can cause severe digestive problems. The most common symptoms are bloating, abdominal cramps, diarrhoea, nausea and vomiting.

- The undigested lactose acts as osmotic particles and draws excessive fluids into the intestine resulting in *diarrhoea*.

In the colon, the undigested lactose is metabolized by bacteria producing a variety of gases (e.g. hydrogen, methane and CO_2) and a variety of intestinal irritants, which increase the colonic motility.

The diarrhoea so produced can lead to life-threatening dehydration and electrolyte imbalance.

Treatment

Treatment for lactose intolerance includes:

- Avoidance of milk and milk products which prevents the symptoms from developing if the infant can be fed synthetic milk containing sucrose instead of lactose
- Use of enzyme supplements
- Use of probiotics

DIGESTION AND ABSORPTION OF PROTEINS

SOURCES OF PROTEINS

The proteins that are digested and absorbed in the GIT come from two sources – exogenous and endogenous.

1. Exogenous (Dietary) Proteins

Daily requirement of dietary proteins for adults is 0.5–0.7 g/kg body weight and for children (1–3 years), it is 4 g/kg.

Quantity of dietary proteins Quantity of dietary proteins varies with the socioeconomic status of the individuals; a balanced diet contains about 95–100 g/day.

Sources of dietary proteins Sources of dietary proteins with high biological value are meat, fish, eggs, cheese and other milk products. Soya beans, wheat and various types of pulses are also a rich source of proteins.

Proteins of important dietary items are the following:

- Wheat: Glutenin, glycinin and gliadin
- Milk: Casein, lactalbumin, albumin and myosin
- Egg: Albumin and vitelline
- Meat: Collagen, albumin and myosin

Structure of dietary proteins: Dietary proteins are made of long chains of amino acids bound together by peptide linkages.

2. Endogenous Proteins

Endogenous proteins, totalling 30–50 g/day, are the proteins which reach the intestine through various gastrointestinal secretions and those which are present in the desquamated epithelial cells of the gut.

DIGESTION OF PROTEINS

Proteins are digested by the proteolytic enzymes to amino acids and small polypeptides, before they are absorbed. Digestion of proteins does not occur in the mouth, as there are no proteolytic enzymes in the saliva. It thus begins in the stomach and is completed in the small intestine.

Digestion of Proteins in the Stomach

Pepsin, secreted by chief cells of the main gastric glands in an inactive form (pepsinogen), is responsible for digesting about 10%–15% of proteins entering the gastrointestinal tract.

- Pepsinogen is converted into pepsin (active form) by the action of HCl or preformed pepsin (see page 580).
- Pepsin hydrolyses the bond between aromatic amino acid (phenylalanine or tyrosine) and a second amino acid. Therefore, pepsin splits proteins into proteoses, peptones and polypeptides (Fig. 7.7.3).
- It is important to note that the optimum pH for the action of pepsin is 2.0; therefore, HCl secretion by the stomach is as essential as pepsinogen secretion for the digestion of proteins.
- Pepsin is unique in its proteolytic action because of its ability to digest collagen (which is a major constituent of the intercellular connective tissue of meat). By digesting collagen tissue, the pepsin breaks apart the meat particles and facilitates further digestion of cellular proteins of meat.
- Protein digestion within the stomach is particularly important because the protein digestion products act as *secretagogues*, i.e. stimulate secretion of proteolytic enzymes of the pancreas.

Digestion of Proteins in the Small Intestine

In the small intestine, proteins are digested by the pancreatic proteases, brush border peptidases and intracellular peptidases (Table 7.7.1).

Pancreatic proteases or proteolytic enzymes of the pancreas play a major role in protein digestion. These can digest all the proteins, even if gastric pepsin is absent.

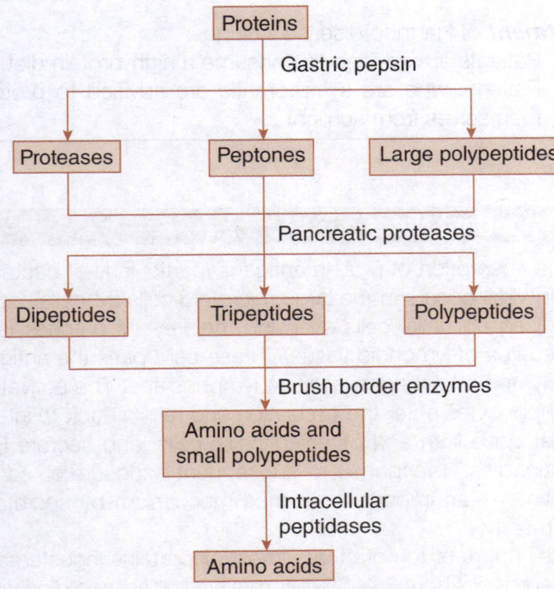

Fig. 7.7.3 Digestion of proteins.

Various types of proteases along with their functions are described on page 597.

Pancreatic proteases digest the proteins and split them into dipeptides, tripeptides and small polypeptides, which are further digested by brush border peptidases (Fig. 7.7.3).

- Some of the dipeptides and tripeptides are absorbed directly into the epithelial cells of mucosa of the small intestine, and are further digested by intracellular enzymes into amino acids.

Brush border peptidases are the proteolytic enzymes which form an integral constituent of the epithelial cell membrane with active sites projecting into the lumen.

- Brush border peptidases include aminopeptidases, dipeptidases, tripeptidases, nuclease and related enzymes.
- These enzymes continue the digestive process initiated by the pancreatic proteases, eventually converting the proteins to small polypeptides and amino acids (Fig. 7.7.3).

Intracellular peptidases are the proteolytic enzymes present in the cytosol of epithelial cells of the small intestine. The multiple peptidases present in the enterocytes are specific for linkages between the various amino acids. Within minutes, these digest the last dipeptides and tripeptides into amino acids which then enter the blood.

Digestion of Nucleic Acid and Nucleoproteins

Nucleic acid and nucleoproteins are found in abundance in the foodstuffs which are rich in nuclei such as the liver, kidney, pancreas and yeast.

In the stomach In the stomach, HCl hydrolyses the nucleoproteins, removing proteins which are digested together with other proteins as described above.

In the small intestine In the small intestine, the free nucleic acids are digested by the pancreatic enzymes and brush border enzymes.

Pancreatic enzymes, such as ribonuclease and deoxyribonuclease in the duodenum, digest free nucleic acids into nucleotides and nucleosides.

Brush border enzymes, such as nucleases, nucleotidases and nucleosidases, convert nucleotides and nucleosides into pentoses (purine and pyrimidine).

End Products of Protein Digestion

Protein digestion, which starts in the stomach, is completed in the enterocyte of the small intestine. The end products of protein digestion are amino acids.

ABSORPTION OF PROTEINS

Mechanisms of Absorption into the Intestinal Epithelial Cells

The end products of protein digestion (amino acids, dipeptides and tripeptides) are absorbed through the luminal membrane of the epithelial cells of the small intestine. Absorption of amino acids is faster in the duodenum and jejunum and slower in the ileum. The following mechanisms of absorption are known:

1. Transport systems There are seven different transport systems existing for amino acid transport from the intestinal lumen into the enterocytes. Five of them require Na^+ (Na^+-dependent cotransport), and out of these, two also require Cl^-, whereas the other two are Na^+-independent transporters.

(i) Na^+-dependent active transport mechanism The laevo-amino acids, dipeptides and tripeptides are absorbed by a Na^+-dependent active transport mechanism.

- Separate transporters (carriers) are present for the absorption of basic, acidic and neutral amino acids. At least two different polypeptide transporters exist.
- Steps of active transport mechanism are similar to those described for glucose absorption (see page 635). These include (Fig. 7.7.4):
  - Binding of amino acid and Na^+ to carrier protein
  - Creation of electrochemical gradient across the epithelial cells
- Movement of Na^+ and amino acids inside the cell

(ii) Na^+-independent active transport mechanism The carrier is known as $PepT_1$ (peptide transporter-1) that

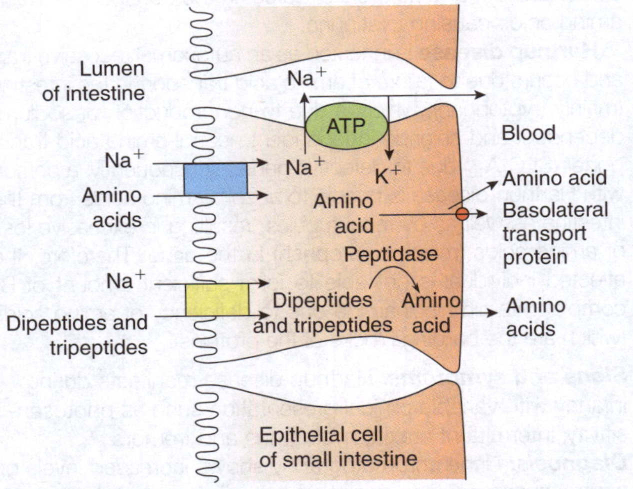

Fig. 7.7.4 Mechanism of absorption of amino acids, dipeptides and tripeptides by intestinal epithelial cells.

requires H^+ instead of Na^+ for transport of dipeptides and tripeptides.

2. Simple diffusion The dextro-amino acids are absorbed solely by passive diffusion.

3. Endocytosis Larger polypeptides cannot be absorbed into the epithelial cells. Occasionally, small amounts of larger polypeptides are absorbed by endocytosis. Proteins absorbed by endocytosis usually excite immunological/allergic reaction. In newborn infants, immunoglobulins present in the colostrum are absorbed in the intestinal mucosa by endocytosis and impart passive immunity to the child.

Further Digestion in the Epithelial Cells

Once amino acids and polypeptides are absorbed into the intestinal epithelial cells, the intracellular peptidases break the remaining linkages of tripeptides and dipeptides causing release of amino acids.

Transport of Amino Acids into Blood Capillaries

From inside the epithelial cells, the amino acids are transported into the interstitial space across the basolateral membrane of the cells by a series of basolateral transport proteins. From the interstitium, the amino acids enter the capillaries of villus by simple diffusion, and then via the portal vein, they reach the liver and general circulation. Therefore, after ingestion of a high-protein meal, there occurs a sharp transient rise in the free amino acid content of the portal blood, which provides the whole body requirements of proteins.

Applied Aspects

Abnormalities of Protein Digestion and Absorption

1. Inadequate Absorption of Proteins

Inadequate absorption of proteins due to lack of trypsin is a common consequence of pancreatic diseases.

2. Malabsorption of Amino Acids

Malabsorption of amino acids due to lack of transporters is relatively rare. For example, in *Hartnup disease*, there occurs malabsorption of neutral amino acids due to lack of specific carrier protein, and congenital defect in the transport for basic amino acids causing cystinuria.

Hartnup disease is inherited as an autosomal recessive trait, and occurs due to failure of amino acid transport in the intestine (mainly tryptophan), which is due to nonproduction of sodium-dependent and chloride-independent neutral amino acid transporter (SLC_6A_{19}) due to defective gene. Consequently, a person with Hartnup disease is unable to absorb amino acids from the intestine as well as by renal tubules, resulting in excessive loss of amino acids (mainly tryptophan) in the urine. Therefore, the affected individual is not able to form sufficient amount of B-complex vitamin niacinamide due to deficiency of amino acids (which are the building blocks of the proteins).

Signs and symptoms: Hartnup disease manifests during infancy with variable clinical presentation such as photosensitivity, intermittent ataxia, nystagmus and tremors.

Diagnosis: Urine chromatography shows increased levels of neutral amino acids (e.g. glutamine, valine, phenylalanine and tryptophan).

Treatment of Hartnup disease includes:

- Patients are advised to consume a high-protein diet.
- Patients who are symptomatic are advised to protect themselves from sunlight.

Important Notes

- The absorption of protein antigens (particularly of bacterial and viral) occurs in the large microfold cells (M-cells), specialized epithelial cells overlying the Peyer's patches (aggregates of lymphoid tissue). These cells pass the antigen to lymphoid cells and activate lymphocytes. The activated lymphocytes enter the circulation and return back to intestinal epithelium and other epithelial cells, and secrete IgA antibodies in response to subsequent exposure to same antigen – an important defence mechanism by secretory immunity.
- It is important to note that almost all proteins ingested are absorbed. About 2%–5% of proteins that escape digestion and absorption in the small intestine enter the colon and are finally digested by bacterial digestion. Therefore, the proteins that appear in the stool are not of dietary origin, but are derived from the bacterial and cellular debris.

DIGESTION AND ABSORPTION OF FATS

DIETARY FATS

Types of fats Fats are of three types:

- Simple fats or neutral fats, e.g. triglycerides and cholesterol
- Compound fats, e.g. phospholipids
- Associated fats, e.g. steroids and fat-soluble vitamins

Dietary fat is of both vegetable and animal origin. Mostly, it is in the form of neutral fat (triglycerides). It also includes small amounts of phospholipids, cholesterol, some free fatty acids, lecithin and cholesterol esters.

Daily intake of fats in the diet varies widely, from about 25 to 160 g.

DIGESTION OF FATS

Site of Digestion

Although lipolytic enzymes are secreted in the mouth (*lingual lipase*) and stomach (*gastric lipase*), their action is so insignificant that practically digestion of all the dietary fats occurs in the small intestine. Gastric lipase which initiates fat digestion acts only on butter. Under normal conditions, gastric lipase is soon inactivated by gastric juice (pH 1–2), as it is inactivated at pH 2.5 and acts at an optimum pH of 4.5. Some fat digestion in the stomach may occur under the following exceptional circumstances:

Achlorhydria (i.e. gastric juice cannot inactivate gastric lipase)
Regurgitation of pancreatic lipase from the duodenum into the stomach
In young suckling animals which ingest large quantities of milk (in such animals, the fat of milk is present in an emulsified form and digested, and this inhibits the secretion of gastric juice)

Mechanism of Digestion of Fats

The digestion of fat includes three steps:

Emulsification of fat by bile salts
Hydrolysis of fat by pancreatic and intestinal lipolytic enzymes
Acceleration of fat digestion by micelle formation

1. Emulsification of fat by bile salts Emulsification, i.e. breaking of large fat drops into smaller droplets, is a prerequisite for action of pancreatic lipase. It is so because the pancreatic lipase being water soluble acts only on the oil–water interface of fat. The surface area available for the action of lipase is increased many thousand times by the emulsification of fats.

- Emulsification of fat is caused by bile salts because of their property of lowering the surface tension (detergent-like action). With the lowered surface tension of the fats, the segmentation movements of the small intestine break up large fat globules into fine droplets (1 μm in diameter).
- Lecithin (a component of bile), which has a stabilization action on the emulsions, greatly enhances the emulsifying action of bile salts. The bile salts surround the fine fat droplets in such a way that their lipophilic nonpolar ends are towards the fat and their hydrophilic polar ends separate the fat droplets from the aqueous phase (Fig. 7.7.5).

2. Hydrolysis of fat droplets by pancreatic and intestinal lipolytic enzymes Pancreatic juice is markedly alkaline (pH 7.8–8.4). When it mixes with the acidic chyme (pH 6.0) coming from the stomach into the duodenum, the pH of chyme is adjusted to about 7 (which is optimal pH for the action of pancreatic lipases).

Pancreatic lipolytic enzymes Pancreatic juice contains three types of lipolytic enzymes. Their hydrolysing effects on fats are given as follows (Table 7.7.1):

i. ***Pancreatic lipase:*** Pancreatic lipase is a very powerful lipolytic enzyme. Fat digestion by it occurs very rapidly after emulsification because of the large surface-to-volume ratio of the small globules. Colipase, a protein present in the pancreatic juice, displaces the bile salts from the fat droplet and allows the action of lipase. Pancreatic lipase hydrolyses almost all the triglycerides (neutral fat) of the food to produce two fatty acids and a 2-monoglyceride.
Note: Colipase is secreted in an inactive form and is activated by trypsin in the intestinal lumen. When activated, colipase binds to –COOH terminal domain of pancreatic lipase; the activity of this enzyme is facilitated by opening of lid (helix-like structure) that covers its active site.

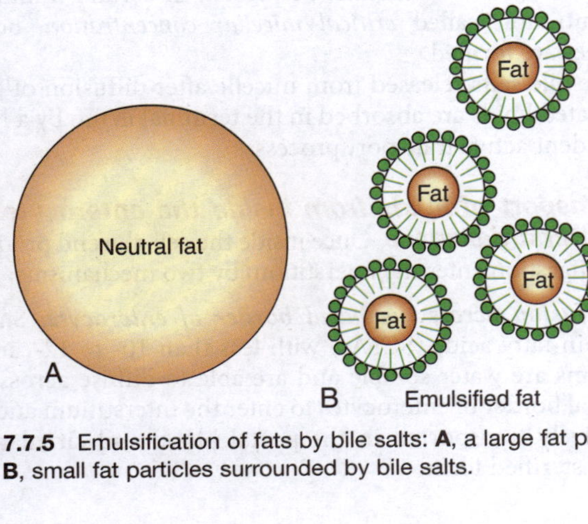

Fig. 7.7.5 Emulsification of fats by bile salts: **A**, a large fat particle; and **B**, small fat particles surrounded by bile salts.

ii. ***Cholesterol ester hydrolase:*** Most of the dietary cholesterol is in the form of cholesterol esters, which are hydrolysed to cholesterol and fatty acid by the cholesterol ester hydrolase. The cholesterol esterase is activated by the bile salts. It represents about 4% of the total protein contents of pancreatic juice. The bile salt–activated pancreatic lipase hydrolyses cholesterol esters, esters of fat-soluble vitamins, phospholipids and triglycerides. A similar type of lipase is also present in the human milk.
iii. ***Phospholipase A_2:*** It is secreted in an inactive form prophospholipase A_2, and gets converted to active form. It hydrolyses phospholipids and separates fatty acid from them.

Intestinal lipolytic enzymes
Brush border of epithelial cells covering the intestinal villi contains small amount of lipase and cholesterol esterase. Their effects, though minor, are similar to those of pancreatic lipase.

3. Acceleration of fat digestion by micelle formation
The hydrolysis of triglycerides is highly reversible; therefore, accumulation of monoglycerides and free fatty acids in the vicinity of digesting fats quickly blocks further digestion. This problem is solved by the property of bile salts to form micelle. ***Micelle formation*** depends on critical micelle concentration of bile salts in the aqueous solution. At a critical micelle concentration, all the bile salts in a solution form micelles. The lipids get collected in the centre of micelle.

Structure Micelles are small, water-soluble, cylindrical disc-shaped particles. Each micelle is composed of a central fat globule surrounded by about 30 molecules of bile salts in such a way that their lipid-soluble nonpolar ends are in the central fat globule and water-soluble polar ends fan out to form the outer covering of micelle. Monoglycerides and free fatty acids released from the digestion of fat are quickly incorporated into the central fatty portion of the micelles forming, what are known as, the *mixed micelles* (Fig. 7.7.6). In this way, bile salts accelerate the fat digestion by allowing the lipolytic action to continue.

ABSORPTION OF FATS

Most of the fat absorption occurs in the duodenum; almost all the digested lipids are totally absorbed by the time the chyme reaches the mid-jejunum. Absorption of fats is accomplished by the following steps (Fig. 7.7.7):

1. Transportation as micelles to the brush border membrane The micelles so formed (as described above) not only accelerate the fat digestion but are also essential for the fat absorption as explained.

The insolubility of fat globules prevents their diffusion through the aqueous medium of the intestinal lumen to reach the brush border. This problem is solved by the bile salts by forming the micelle. As described above (Fig. 7.7.6), the outer surface of micelle is formed by water-soluble polar ends of bile salts, which help the micelle to diffuse through the aqueous medium to reach the brush border membrane. Thus, the bile salt micelle acts as a transport vehicle for the products of fat digestion.

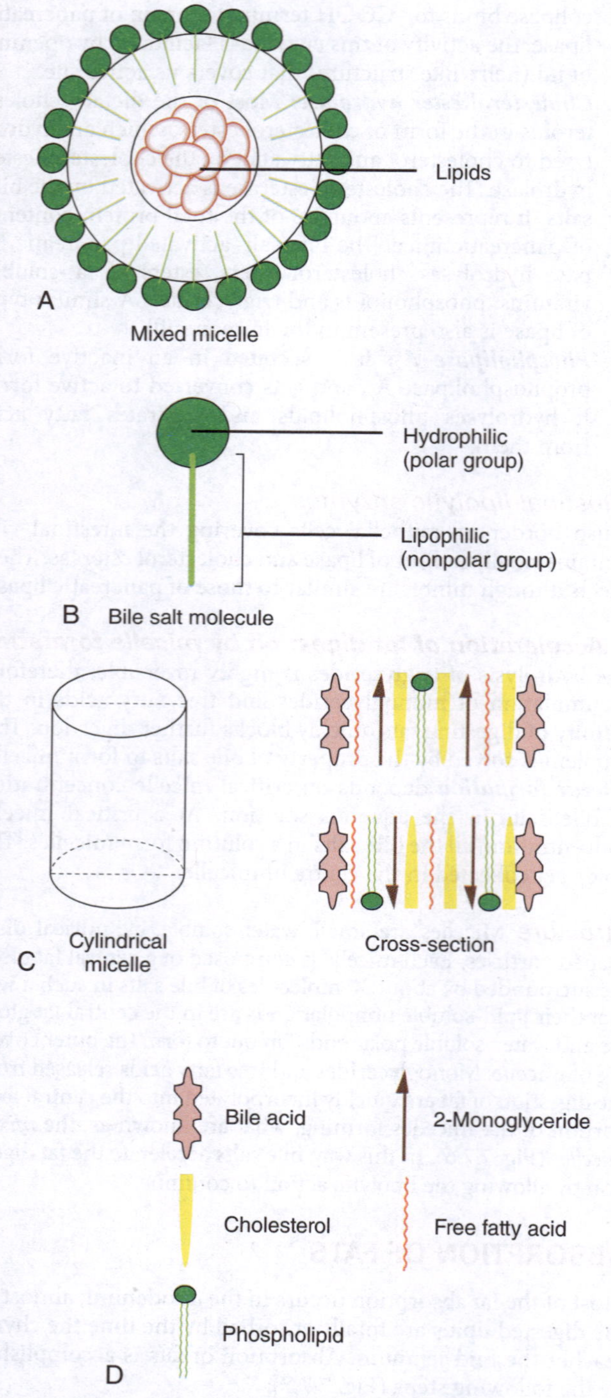

Fig. 7.7.6 Structure of micelle: **A**, a mixed micelle composed of lipids (monoglycerides, fatty acids and cholesterol) in the centre surrounded by bile salts; **B**, bile salt molecule showing globular (hydrophilic or polar) end and lipophilic (nonpolar) end; **C**, a model of the structure of mixed (bile salt and lipid) micelle and its cross-section showing arrangement of various lipid molecules; and **D**, diagrammatic structure of different lipid molecules.

2. Diffusion of lipids across the enterocyte cell membrane Once the micelle comes in contact with the cell membrane, the monoglycerides, free fatty acids, cholesterol and fat-soluble vitamins (being soluble in the cell membrane) *diffuse passively* at a rapid speed through the enterocyte cell

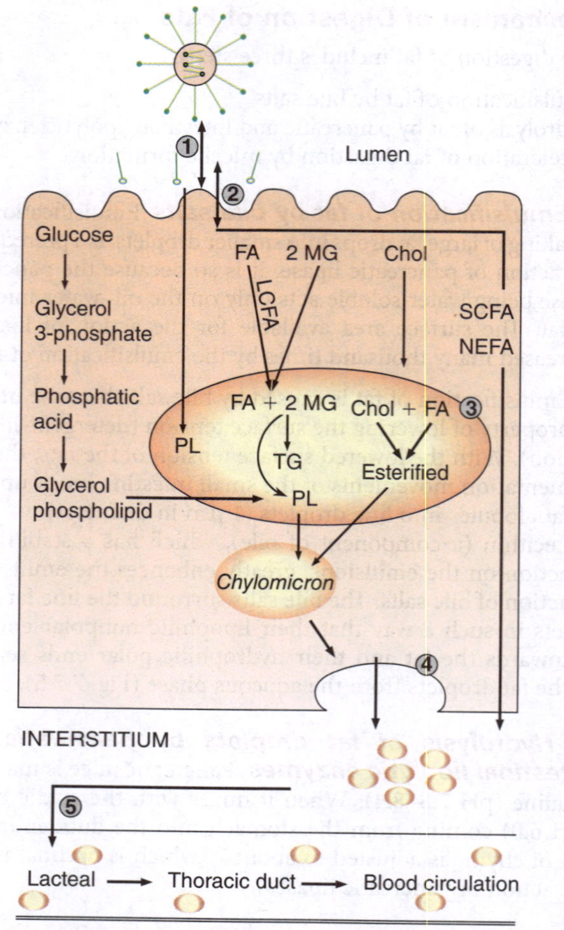

Fig. 7.7.7 Steps of fat absorption: 1, transportation of micelle to enterocyte brush border; 2, diffusion of lipids across the enterocyte membrane leaving bile salt in the lumen; 3, formation of chylomicron in the endoplasmic reticulum; 4, release of lipids into interstitium by exocytosis; and 5, diffusion of lipids from interstitium into lacteal (from where lipids enter lymphatic circulation) and through thoracic duct into circulation. chol, cholesterol; FA, fatty acid; LCFA, long-chain fatty acid; MG, monoglyceride; NEFA, nonesterified fatty acid; PL, phospholipid; SCFA, short-chain fatty acid; TG, triglyceride.

membrane to the interior of the cell, leaving bile salts in the intestinal lumen. Thus, the *rate-limiting* step in lipid absorption is the formation and migration of the micelles from the intestinal chyme to the microvilli surface. It is important to note that the bile salts must be present in certain minimum concentration called *critical micellar concentration*, before micelles are formed.

The bile salts released from micelle after diffusion of their associated lipids are absorbed in the terminal ileum by a Na^+-dependent active transport process.

3. Transport of lipids from inside the enterocytes to the interstitial space Once inside the cell, the end products of fat digestion enter the interstitium by two mechanisms:

i. ***Diffusion across the basal border of enterocyte:*** Small-chain fatty acids (SCFAs) with less than 10- to 12-carbon atoms are water soluble and are able to diffuse across the basal border of enterocytes to enter the interstitium and are actively transported in the portal blood and circulate in unesterified form.

ii. ***Formation and excretion of chylomicrons from enterocytes by exocytosis:*** Large-chain fatty acids, which are more than 12-carbon atoms, cholesterol and lysophosphatides enter the smooth endoplasmic reticulum, where they are reconstituted:
- 2-Monoglycerides are combined with fatty acids to produce triglycerides. Some of the triglycerides are also formed from glycerophosphate (a product of glucose catabolism). Glycerophosphate is also converted into glycerophospholipids and participates in chylomicron formation.
- Lysophosphatides are combined with fatty acids to form phospholipids.
- Cholesterol is re-esterified.

The reformed lipids coalesce to form small lipid droplets (about 1 nm in diameter) called chylomicrons, which are lined by the synthesized β-lipoproteins. The chylomicrons are then excreted into the interstitium by exocytosis from the basolateral membrane of enterocyte. Covering of β-lipoproteins is essential for the exocytosis to occur. Therefore, in the absence of β-lipoprotein, exocytosis will not occur, and the enterocytes become engorged with lipids.

4. Transport of lipids into circulation After exiting the enterocytes (i.e. in the interstitium), the chylomicrons merge into larger droplets that vary in size from 50 to 500 nm, depending on the amount of lipid being absorbed. From the interstitium, the lipids diffuse into the *lacteals*, from where they enter the lymphatic circulation, and via the thoracic duct gain access into the blood circulation. In an adult, more than 95% of the fat gets absorbed on moderate intake.

Note: The process involved in fat absorption at birth is not fully matured; thus, infants are more susceptible to ill effects of disease that reduces fat absorption.

Fate of SCFAs in the colon is as follows:

The SCFAs (two- to five-carbon atoms) are weak acids produced by the action of colonic bacteria on unabsorbed complex carbohydrates, resistant starches and components of dietary fibres. They are absorbed from the colon by specific transporter.

Functions of SCFAs are as follows:
- SCFAs provide significant calories.
- They have trophic effect on colonic epithelium and play an important role during inflammation.
- They help in maintaining acid–base balance.

The principal digestive enzymes, their source and functions are summarized in Table 7.7.1.

Applied Aspects

Lipid Malabsorption

Lipid malabsorption is much more common than carbohydrate and protein malabsorption.

Causes of lipid malabsorption include:
- Deficiency of pancreatic lipase in certain pancreatic diseases
- Bile deficiency in disorders of the liver and gall bladder

Steatorrhoea, i.e. increased amount of fat in the stools, is a common manifestation of fat malabsorption. For details, see page 644.

Serum Lipid Profile

Lipids are present as lipoprotein complexes. Depending on the density, the lipoproteins are of the following types:

i. Very low-density lipoproteins (VLDL; density is <1.060)
ii. Low-density lipoproteins (LDL)
iii. High-density lipoproteins (HDL; density is 1.060–1.200)

Normal Values
- Serum triglycerides: 30–150 mg%
- Serum cholesterol: 150–240 mg%
- Serum phospholipids: 150–300 mg%
- Serum free fatty acids (FFA or nonesterified fatty acid [NEFA]): 10–30 mg%

ABSORPTION OF WATER, ELECTROLYTES, MINERALS AND VITAMINS

WATER ABSORPTION

Water Balance in the GIT

The gastrointestinal tract receives about 9 L of water per day, which includes about 2 L of ingested water and about 7 L contained in salivary, gastric, biliary, pancreatic and intestinal secretions (Table 7.7.2).

The gastrointestinal tract absorbs about 8.8 L of water (about 95% of total water received) per day. About 60% of absorption occurs in the jejunum, 20%–25% in the ileum and 10%–15% in the colon (Table 7.7.2).

The gastrointestinal tract excretes about 0.2 L of water in the faeces per day.

Mechanism of water absorption In general, water is absorbed passively and iso-osmotically across the gastrointestinal mucosa, following the osmotic gradient created by the active absorption of electrolytes and nutrients.
- Because osmotic equilibrium is rapidly achieved, the fluid in the intestine is always isotonic to plasma.

Table 7.7.2 Daily water balance in GIT

Input (L)		Absorption (L)		Faecal excretion (L)
Water ingested	2	Jejunum (60%)	5.5	0.2
Water in GIT	7	Ileum (25%)	2.0	
		Colon (10%–15%)	1.3	
Secretions				
• Saliva	• 1.5			
• Gastric juice	• 2.5			
• Bile	• 0.75			
• Pancreatic juice	• 0.75			
• Intestinal juice	• 1.5			
Total	**9.0**		**8.8**	**0.2**

- Only a small amount of water moves across the gastric mucosa, but water moves in both directions across the mucosa of the small intestine and colon in response to the osmotic gradient.
- In the duodenum, the osmotic pressure created by the entering chyme causes water to flow into it.
- In the jejunum and ileum, reabsorption of sodium chloride (NaCl) creates an osmotic gradient favouring the reabsorption of water.

ABSORPTION OF SODIUM

Sodium Balance in GIT

The gastrointestinal tract receives about 40 g of sodium per day, out of which about 10 g is ingested with food and about 30 g is contained in the gastrointestinal secretions. All of it is reabsorbed.

Site of absorption Although sodium can be reabsorbed in the entire length of the intestine, maximum absorption occurs in the jejunum.

Mechanisms of absorption Absorption of sodium is a two-step process:

1. Transport of sodium from the lumen into the enterocyte Transport of sodium from the lumen into the enterocyte occurs by the following mechanisms (Fig. 7.7.8):

- Na^+–glucose, Na^+–amino acids and Na^+–dipeptide or Na^+–tripeptide cotransport system account for 30% of Na^+ transport into the cell.
- Neutral Na^+–Cl^- cotransport system also transports about 30% of Na^+.
- Na^+–H^+ exchange also helps in transport of sodium.
- Passive diffusion (through Na^+ channels) down an electrochemical gradient is responsible for transport of remainder 40% of Na^+.

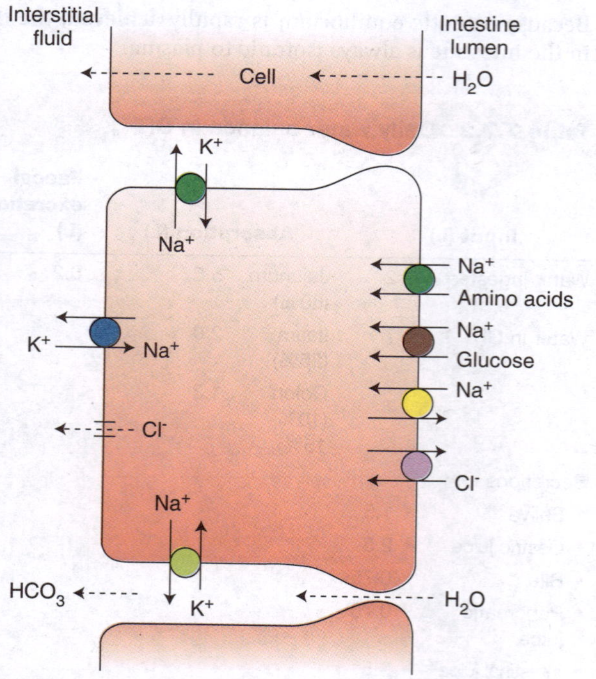

Fig. 7.7.8 Absorption of sodium, chloride, glucose and amino acids through the intestinal epithelium. The absorption of water 'follows' sodium through the epithelial membrane.

In the small intestine In the small intestine, Na^+–glucose cotransport, Na^+–amino acid cotransport and Na^+–H^+ exchange mechanisms are the most important (these cotransport and exchange mechanisms are similar to those in renal proximal tubule) (see page 488). Thus, the presence of glucose in the intestinal lumen facilitates the reabsorption for Na^+. Because of this reason, in the treatment of Na^+ and water loss in diarrhoea, glucose is added to the orally administered NaCl solution. Cereals containing carbohydrates are also useful in the treatment of diarrhoea.

In the colon In the colon, passive diffusion via Na^+ channels is the most important. These channels of the colon are similar to those in the renal distal tubules, and are stimulated by aldosterone (which greatly enhances sodium absorption). This mechanism is especially useful in dehydration, which leads to aldosterone secretion by the adrenal medulla.

2. Transport of Na^+ out of the enterocytes into the interstitium Transport of Na^+ out of the enterocytes into the interstitium occurs against its electrochemical gradient across the basolateral membrane by Na^+–K^+-ATPase active transport system.

ABSORPTION OF CHLORIDE

In the jejunum and proximal ileum, most of the Cl^- is absorbed passively through the enterocytes down the electrochemical gradient established by the active transport of Na^+. The mechanisms involved in the transport of Cl^- are the following:

- Passive diffusion by a paracellular route through the leaky (permeable) junction between the enterocytes
- Neutral Na^+–Cl^- cotransport system

In the distal ileum and large intestine, the Cl^- is absorbed by an active Cl^-–HCO_3^- exchange mechanism. In this mechanism, Cl^- is absorbed from the lumen in exchange of HCO_3^-, which is secreted into the lumen. Bicarbonate (HCO_3^-) secreted into the lumen helps to neutralize the acidity produced by the action of colonic bacteria on the food.

ABSORPTION OF BICARBONATE

To neutralize acidic chyme in the duodenum and acidic pH in the colon (due to bacterial activity), a large amount of bicarbonate ions is secreted into pancreatic secretion and bile is poured into the duodenum. At the same time, epithelial cells on the surface of villi in the ileum and large intestine also secrete bicarbonate ions in exchange for chloride ion absorption. The bicarbonate ion is absorbed indirectly as follows:

- During sodium ion absorption, moderate amount of hydrogen ions gets secreted into the lumen of the gut in exchange of Na^+. These H^+ combine with bicarbonate to form carbonic acid (H_2CO_3), which then dissociates to form water and carbon dioxide.
- The water remains in the intestine; however, CO_2 is readily absorbed into the blood and ultimately eliminated during expiration through the lungs.

ABSORPTION OF POTASSIUM

Passive diffusion via paracellular route down its electrochemical gradient is the mechanism involved in the absorption of dietary K^+ from the small intestine.

Net movement of K^+ across the intestinal mucosa is directly proportional to the potential difference between the blood and the intestinal lumen, with the magnitude as follows:

- Jejunum: 5 mV
- Ileum: 25 mV
- Colon: 50 mV

Therefore, the concentration of K^+ is approximately 6 mEq/L in the jejunum, 13 mEq/L in the ileum and 30 mEq/L in the colon. This accounts for hypokalaemia occurring due to ileal and colonic fluid loss in chronic diarrhoea.

ABSORPTION OF CALCIUM

Body Calcium

Calcium is the most abundant among the minerals in the body. The total content of calcium in an adult man is about 1–1.5 kg of which about 99% is present in the bones and teeth. A small amount (10%) found outside the skeletal tissue performs a wide variety of functions.

Dietary Calcium

Best sources of dietary calcium are milk and milk products. Good sources of calcium are beans, leafy vegetables, fish, cabbage and egg yolk.

Dietary requirements Dietary requirements of calcium are as follows:

- Infants (younger than 1 year) : 300–500 mg/day
- Children (1–18 years) : 800–1200 mg/day
- Adult men and women : 800 mg/day
- Women during pregnancy, lactation and postmenopause : 1500 mg/day

Site of absorption Most of the ingested calcium is absorbed in the upper small intestine (duodenum and jejunum).

Mechanism of absorption Normally, about 75%–80% of the daily intake (about 1000 mg) of calcium is absorbed from the upper small intestine. Most of the calcium is absorbed by an active transport mechanism in the following two steps:

Entry of calcium inside the enterocyte across its luminal border occurs by the active transport mechanism involving a membrane-bound carrier that is activated by vitamin D.

Transport of calcium out of the cell into the interstitium, from where it is absorbed into the blood capillaries, occurs by a Ca^{2+}-ATPase active transport system and by a Na^+–Ca^{2+} exchange system.

Regulation of Calcium Absorption

Calcium absorption from the small intestine is well regulated to maintain the plasma calcium (*homeostasis of calcium*) levels within a narrow range (9–11 mg%). Vitamin D and parathyroid hormone (PTH) play main role in the regulation of calcium absorption as follows:

Vitamin D_3 is converted to 25-hydroxyvitamin D_3 by the liver.

- *25-Hydroxyvitamin D_3* is converted to 1,25-dihydroxyvitamin D_3 (also known as 1,25-dihydroxycholecalciferol [1,25-DHCC] or calciferol) in the kidneys by a process that is regulated by the PTH.

1,25-Dihydroxyvitamin D_3 (which is the physiologically active form of vitamin D, acting as hormone) enters the enterocyte and activates the formation of 'calcium-carrier protein' that inserts in the luminal surface of the enterocyte.

- *Calcium-carrier protein* is responsible for carrier-bound transport of calcium inside the cell.

Factors promoting calcium absorption include:

- *Vitamin D* (through its active form calciferol) promotes calcium absorption by inducing synthesis of calcium-binding protein (as described above).
- *PTH* enhances Ca^{2+} absorption by influencing synthesis of calciferol (as described above).
- *Low pH* is more favourable for Ca^{2+} absorption.
- *Lactose promotes* Ca^{2+} intake by the intestinal cells.
- *Amino acids* (lysine and arginine) facilitate Ca^{2+} absorption.

Factors inhibiting calcium absorption include:

- *Phytates and oxalates* inhibit Ca^{2+} absorption by forming insoluble salts with Ca^{2+} in the intestine.
- *High content of dietary phosphate* also prevents Ca^{2+} absorption by forming insoluble calcium phosphate. The dietary ratio of Ca^{2+} and P between 1:2 and 2:1 is ideal for optimum Ca^{2+} absorption.
- *Free fatty acids* inhibit Ca^{2+} absorption by forming insoluble calcium soaps. It occurs particularly when the fat absorption is impaired.
- *High pH* (alkaline conditions) is unfavourable for Ca^{2+} absorption.
- *Dietary fibres* in high content interfere with calcium absorption.

Importance of Ca:P ratio: The ratio of Ca:P is important for calcification of bones. The product of Ca × P (in mg/dL) in children is about 50 and in adults it is around 40. This product is less than 30 in rickets.

Excretion of calcium Excretion of calcium occurs mainly in faeces and partly in urine.

Excretion of Ca^{2+} into the faeces is a continuous process and this is increased in vitamin D deficiency.

Excretion of Ca^{2+} into the urine occurs when the serum Ca^{2+} goes beyond 10 mg/dL. Ingestion of excess proteins causes increased Ca^{2+} excretion in the urine. This is mainly due to an increase in the acidity of urine.

For details of calcium balance, see page 700.

ABSORPTION OF IRON

Absorption of iron is discussed in Chapter 3.2, on page 515.

ABSORPTION OF VITAMINS

Absorption of Fat-Soluble Vitamins

Fat-soluble vitamins (A, D, E and K) become part of micelle formed by bile salts, and are absorbed along with other lipids in the upper part of the small intestine (for details, see page 639).

The absorption of fat-soluble vitamins is deficient if fat absorption is depressed because of lack of pancreatic enzymes or if bile is excluded from the intestine by the obstruction of bile duct.

Absorption of Water-Soluble Vitamins

Absorption of water-soluble vitamins is rapid as compared with that of fat-soluble vitamins.

Most vitamins are absorbed in the upper part of the small intestine (jejunum) except vitamin B_{12}, which is absorbed in the ileum.

Most water-soluble vitamins, e.g. vitamin C and the vitamins B (biotin; folic acid; nicotinic acid; B_8, i.e. pyridoxine; B_2, i.e. riboflavin; and B_1, i.e. thiamine), are absorbed by facilitated transport or by Na^+-dependent active transport system in the proximal small intestine.

Vitamin B_{12} absorption is most complex than that of other water-soluble vitamins and needs separate description.

Absorption of vitamin B_{12} Absorption of vitamin B_{12} involves the following steps:

In the stomach In the stomach, vitamin B_{12} is exposed to specific binding protein R and vitamin B_{12}–binding protein called intrinsic factor (IF). As the affinity of R proteins for vitamin B_{12} is much more than that of IF, most of the vitamin B_{12} gets bound to R protein in the stomach.

In the lumen of intestine In the lumen of the intestine, the pancreatic proteases cleave vitamin B_{12} from the R protein. Then, vitamin B_{12} binds to IF to form a complex.

On the brush border of enterocyte On the brush border of enterocyte, IF–B_{12} complex becomes bound to the specific receptors. Following this, the vitamin B_{12} is transported into the cytosol of enterocyte by endocytosis, leaving behind IF at the brush border. It is important to note that absorption of vitamin B_{12} from the IF–B_{12} complex can occur only after the complex binds to the receptors. In the absence of IF, vitamin B_{12} absorption is markedly decreased and the patient may develop pernicious anaemia (see page 155).

From the basolateral border of enterocyte Vitamin B_{12} enters the portal circulation after binding with plasma globulin called transcobalamin-11.

In the liver In the liver, vitamin B_{12} is stored in large amounts after binding with another globulin called *transcobalamin-1*. The storage of water-soluble vitamin is unique to vitamin B_{12}. The liver may store up to 3 years of supply. Vitamin B_{12} is also stored in the muscles for some extent. Whenever required, it is transported from the liver to the bone marrow.

Applied Aspects

Malabsorption Syndrome

Malabsorption syndrome is not a simple disease but a group of disorders in which multiple nutritional deficiency states are produced.

Pathophysiology

Malabsorption occurs due to abnormalities of three processes, which are important for normal digestion and absorption.

i. ***Intraluminal maldigestion:*** When there is deficiency of pancreatic enzymes and bile, there occurs inadequate solubilization and hydrolyses of nutrients leading to fat and protein malabsorption.
ii. ***Mucosal malabsorption*** results when there is damage of small intestinal epithelium, thereby diminishing the surface area for absorption and depleting brush border enzyme activity.
iii. ***Postmucosal lymphatic obstruction*** prevents the uptake and transport of absorbed lipids into lymphatic vessels. Increased pressure in these vessels results in leakage into intestinal lumen leading to protein-losing enteropathy (PLE).

General Features of Malabsorption

Deficient absorption of amino acids, fats and carbohydrates results in general weakness.

- Malabsorption of vitamins may produce anaemia and signs of hypovitaminosis.
- Malabsorption of iron results in iron-deficiency anaemia.
- Malabsorption of fats produces steatorrhoea (see page 641).
- Water and electrolyte depletion may result in dehydration.

Common conditions which can produce malabsorption are the following:

- Coeliac disease
- Sprue
- Lactose intolerance (see page 636)
- Crohn disease
- Resection of the small intestine
- Malabsorption after gastric surgery (see page 593)
- Gastrocolic fistula
- Blind loop syndrome
- Chronic pancreatitis (see page 601)
- Obstruction of common bile duct (see page 148)

Coeliac Disease

Aetiopathogenesis

Aetiopathogenesis is an autoimmune disorder that is caused by a reaction to gluten, which primarily affects the small intestine.

It occurs due to deficiency of the enzyme gluten hydrolase. As a result, gluten, the principal protein of wheat, rye, barley and oats, is not properly hydrolysed. Consequently, gliadin, a toxic polypeptide, is formed, which produces an inflammatory response in the intestinal mucosa leading to destruction of microvilli.

Clinical Features

Clinical features of gluten-induced enteropathy are those of generalized malabsorption. It may occur as follows:

- *Congenital disease* manifesting usually within first 3 years of life
- *Acquired disease* in adults due to unknown aetiology

The coeliac disease symptoms may include diarrhoea, excessive wind and/or constipation, persistent nausea and vomiting, stomach cramps, mouth ulcers, fatigue and anaemia.

Diagnosis

There are specific blood tests to diagnose coeliac disease:

- Detection of tissue transglutaminase antibodies (tTG test) is the most commonly used test.

Treatment

Treatment consists of withdrawal of wheat and other sources of gluten in the diet.

Sprue

Sprue or the tropical sprue is a disorder of malabsorption, an acquired malabsorption condition commonly found in tropical regions that causes progressive atrophy of the small intestine villi.

Causes

Tropical sprue is associated with infection of the small intestine with aerobic bacteria.

Clinical features

Clinical features are particularly characterized by acute or chronic diarrhoea, weight loss and malabsorption of nutrients and vitamin B_{12}. So, general features of malabsorption with megaloblastic anaemia, which is conspicuous, occur.

Treatment

Tropical sprue is treated with antibiotics; tetracycline is the most commonly used antibiotic along with folic acid.

Crohn Disease

Aetiopathogenesis

It is an inflammatory bowel disease (IBD) characterized by idiopathic, nonspecific granulomatous inflammation of the bowel. Scientists believe that Crohn disease is caused by a combination of factors such as immune system problem, genetics and environmental factors.

Clinical Features

Clinical features vary depending on the part and extent of the bowel involved. Common clinical features are off and on fever, chronic diarrhoea, abdominal discomfort and pain, and weight loss, which is frequent; many patients have moderate anaemia and other features of malabsorption. Ultimately, the patient may develop narrowing and obstruction of intestinal lumen, fistula formation or intestinal perforation.

Radiological Examination

Radiological examination (barium meal study) shows pathognomonic features in the form of *string sign* due to marked narrowing of the lumen and *skip lesions* due to patchy involvement.

Treatment

It is a chronic disease with remissions and relapses over many years. Although there is no specific cure, *corticosteroids* may induce remission in patients with active disease.

Resection of Small Intestine

Removal of Short Segment

Removal of short segment from the jejunum or ileum generally does not produce any severe symptoms. Because there occurs compensatory hypertrophy and hyperplasia of remaining mucosa (*intestinal adaptation*), the capacity of the jejunum to adapt is less than that of the ileum.

Removal of Ileum

Removal of ileum produces a greater degree of malabsorption compared with removal of the jejunum. Because ileal resection prevents absorption of bile salts causing decreased fat absorption, the entry of unabsorbed bile salts in the colon inhibits Na^+ and water reabsorption producing diarrhoea.

Removal of Large Segment of Ileum

Removal of large segment of ileum leaving behind duodenum, jejunum and a very small length of ileum produces malabsorption which is characterized by:

- *Normal carbohydrate absorption* (99% of ingested carbohydrates are absorbed)
- *Adequate protein absorption* (70% of ingested proteins are absorbed)
- *Markedly decreased fat absorption* which may produce:
  - Steatorrhoea, i.e. increase in faecal fat (see page 148)
  - Deficiency symptoms of fat-soluble vitamins (A, D, E and K)
  - Fatty infiltration of liver and cirrhosis
- *Markedly decreased calcium absorption* due to the formation of insoluble calcium salts (decreased serum calcium [hypocalcaemia] may produce tetany)

Gastrocolic fistula. In this condition, chyme enters the transverse colon directly from the stomach. It is characterized by the following additional features, over and above the features of large segment resection of ileum described above:

- *Pernicious anaemia*, due to the failure of absorption of vitamin B_{12}
- *Hypovitaminosis* due to both water-soluble and fat-soluble vitamins
- *Amino acid malabsorption*, which produces hypoproteinaemia (causing generalized oedema) and marked muscular weakness with wasting

Blind loop syndrome. Blind loop syndrome is characterized by formation of the areas of the intestine where bacteria can proliferate without being subjected to movement down the intestine.

Causes

Causes of blind loop formation are multiple diverticula in the small intestine, afferent loop after partial gastrectomy, areas of disordered peristalsis in the small intestine and fistula from the upper small intestine to the colon.

Features

Colonization of small bowel by bacteria in blind loop syndrome may produce:

- *Malabsorption of fat* (steatorrhoea) (it occurs due to deconjugation of bile salts by bacteria)
- *Megaloblastic anaemia*, due to vitamin B_{12} deficiency (which is taken up by bacteria)
- *Amino acid deficiency* (due to consumption by the bacteria) resulting in weakness and hypoproteinaemia
- *Diarrhoea* and other nutritional deficiencies

Diagnosis

Diagnosis is confirmed by radiological demonstration of blind loop areas.

Treatment

Treatment consists of broad-spectrum antibiotics and dietary and vitamin supplements. Occasionally, it may be necessary to correct a structural abnormality by surgical means.

Investigations to Confirm the Malabsorption and its Cause

These include:

i. ***Routine blood tests:*** If steatorrhoea is suspected, these include urea, electrolyte, immunoglobulins, Ca^{2+}, Mg^{2+}, blood counts, clotting tests, albumin, folate and coeliac antibodies.
ii. ***To investigate the small intestine***, the tests include duodenal biopsy, barium studies and sugar absorption test.
iii. ***To investigate the pancreas***, the tests include pancreatic function test, ultrasonography/CT scan.
iv. ***To investigate bile salt malabsorption (BMA)***, the tests include:
    SeHCAT scan is a diagnostic procedure to determine the efficiency of the gut to absorb bile acids.
    Procedure: On the first day, the person is asked to swallow a capsule having radionucleotide tracer

(75-seleno-homotaurocholic acid) with a glass of water. Then after 3 hours, a scan will be taken. Then on the seventh day, only scan using a standard gamma camera will be taken. The amount of bile acids (percentage) remaining in the bowel is calculated. Retention value of 7-day SeHCAT more than 15% is normal and less than 15% signifies excessive bile acid loss.

Serum 7α-hydroxycholestenon: Serum 7α-hydroxy-4-cholesten-3-one is an intermediate in the biochemical synthesis pathway of bile acid. Measurement of 7α-hydroxy-4-cholesten-3-one is an effective test in diagnosis of BMA diarrhoea.

Tests of Intestinal Absorption

General Principle. General principle of the commonly performed tests of intestinal absorption is to give a fixed quantity of nutrient, and measure its blood level, urinary excretion or faecal excretion (Fig. 7.7.9). The nutrient used for the test will depend on the region to be tested (Fig. 7.7.10).

Carbohydrate Absorption Tests. Carbohydrate absorption tests include:

1. ***D-Xylose test:*** D-Xylose is a pentose sugar that is completely absorbed from the small intestine as such but is neither metabolized nor stored in the body. The test is conducted in the fasting state, by giving 25 g D-xylose orally with three to four glasses of water and measuring its urinary excretion over the next 5 hours.
   - Absorption is considered normal if more than 4 g of xylose appears in the urine over the 5-hour period.
   - Lesser excretion in urine indicates malabsorption.
   - The diagnostic value of this test is compromised if the patient's kidney function is subnormal.
2. ***Lactose tolerance test:*** After overnight fasting, blood glucose level and hydrogen concentration in the end-expiratory air is estimated. The subject is made to ingest 50 g of lactose. Results are interpreted as follows:
   - Absorption is considered normal if the rise in blood glucose is more than 50 mg/100 mL.
   - Lack of diarrhoea, abdominal discomfort and flatulence also point to adequate absorption.
   - Hydrogen concentration in the end-expiratory air, 90 minutes after ingestion of lactose, is a fairly reliable indicator of lactose tolerance. Normally, H_2 concentration is less than 15 ppm; a concentration greater than 20 ppm indicates lactose intolerance (in lactose intolerance, the unabsorbed lactose enters the colon, where it generates H_2 after fermentation; the H_2 is absorbed in bloodstream and eliminated by the lungs).

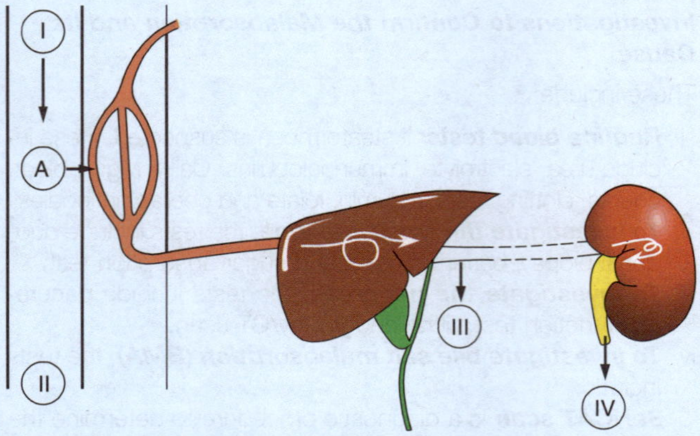

Fig. 7.7.9 General principle of commonly performed tests of intestinal absorption. The intake is known (I); the quantity absorbed (A) may be estimated from the values of faecal loss (II) and/or blood levels (III) and urinary excretion (IV) of the substance.

Tests for Absorption of Fats and Related Substances

Tests for absorption of fats and related substances are as follows:

1. ***Faecal fat:*** See page 602.
2. ***^{131}I-triolein test:*** A measured quantity of radioactive triolein (a triglyceride) is given orally. The fraction excreted in the stool is assessed by radioactivity.
3. ***Absorption of fat-soluble vitamins*** can also be used as an index of fat absorption.
4. ***^{14}C-glycine–bile acid test*** is performed to test the absorption of bile acids.

Protein Absorption Tests

Protein absorption tests include:

1. ***Faecal nitrogen excretion test:*** See page 602.
2. ***Serum protein estimation:*** Serum protein concentration is a fair indicator of protein absorption provided:
   - Protein intake is normal.
   - The liver is manufacturing adequate albumin.
   - There is no loss of proteins in urine.
   - There is no PLE.
3. ***Tests for PLE:*** In PLE, the absorption of proteins is normal but loss from the bowels is abnormally fast, leading to high protein content in stools. It can be tested by tagging the albumin with ^{51}Cr and then radioactive chromium is followed in the blood and stool.

Tests for absorption of water-soluble vitamins

Tests for absorption of water-soluble vitamins include:

Schilling test (see page 603)

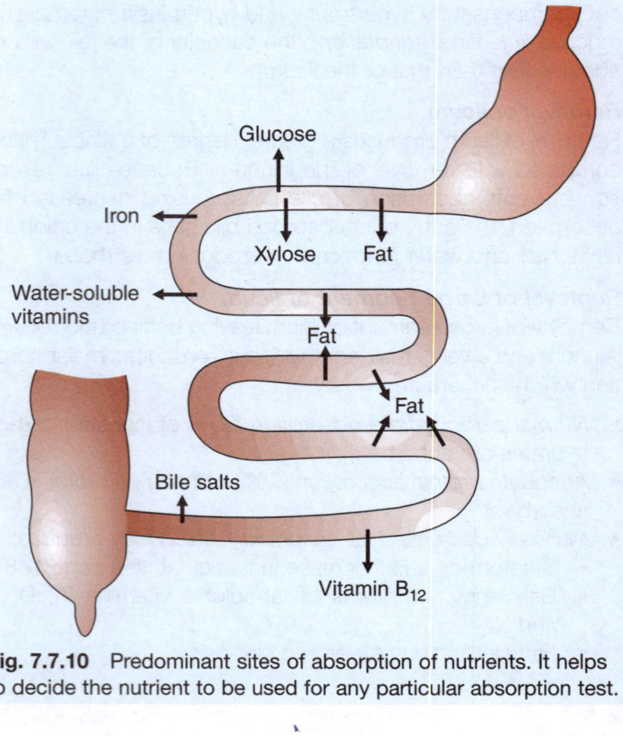

Fig. 7.7.10 Predominant sites of absorption of nutrients. It helps to decide the nutrient to be used for any particular absorption test.

Table 7.7.3 Common causes of malabsorption and tests for differential diagnosis

Test	Coeliac disease	Crohn disease	Pancreatic insufficiency
1. Faecal fat contents	Increased	Increased	Increased
2. D-Xylose absorption test	Impaired	Normal	Normal
3. Schilling test	Normal	Abnormal	Normal
4. Radiological examination of intestines	Abnormal	Abnormal	Normal

In practice, usually few screening procedures are sufficient to differentiate between the common causes of malabsorption (Table 7.7.3). Coeliac disease is an example of generalized malabsorption, Crohn disease is a localized disease of distal ileum and colon, and chronic pancreatitis is an example of exocrine pancreatic insufficiency.

Self-Assessment

1. Discuss the mechanism and absorption of carbohydrates.
2. Discuss the mechanism and absorption of proteins.
3. Discuss the mechanism and absorption of fats.
4. Describe the following:
   - Proteolytic enzymes of the gut
   - Mechanism and regulation of calcium absorption in the gut
   - Lactose intolerance
   - Malabsorption
5. Write notes on:
   - Crohn disease
   - Bile salt malabsorption tests
   - D-Xylose test

Clinical Cases

Case 1

A 6-year-old boy started having diarrhoea, abdominal pain, vomiting and bloating sensation 1–2 hours after drinking milk.

Q1. What is the probable diagnosis?
Q2. What is the pathophysiology of this condition?
Q3. What further tests should be carried out for confirmation of the diagnosis?
Q4. What are the precautions and treatment measures for this condition?

Case 2

An 8-year-old child presented with frequent diarrhoea for the last 2 years, passing four to five loose motions per day. History revealed that the patient had weight loss and growth failure, and the stools were bulky and foul smelling. The probable diagnosis made was a case of malabsorption syndrome.

The blood tests carried out showed low RBC count, picture of macrocytic hypochromic anaemia, raised levels of CRP protein and IgA test for coeliac disease.

Q1. On the basis of history, signs and symptoms, what is the cause of malabsorption?
Q2. What is the pathophysiology of the causative disease?
Q3. How can the disease be treated?

Case 3

A 17-year-old girl was admitted with complaints of recurrent blood-stained diarrhoea, abdominal pain, mouth ulcers, weight loss and scanty periods.

Physical examination revealed cachexia appearance, abdominal tenderness, muscle wasting and features of malnutrition.

Laboratory findings showed microcytic hypochromic anaemia, hypoalbuminaemia and positive faecal fat test; CT scan showed an inflammatory picture.

The provisional diagnosis made was Crohn disease.

Q1. What is the cause of this disease?
Q2. What is the aetiology?
Q3. What are the radiological findings?
Q4. How can the condition be managed?

ENDOCRINAL SYSTEM

SECTION 8

SECTION OUTLINE

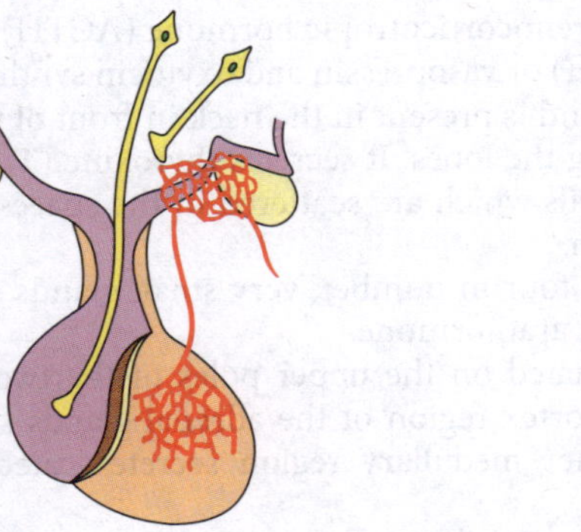

INTRODUCTION

The biological functions of the multicellular living organisms are very well coordinated. This coordination is achieved by two main control systems, nervous system and the endocrinal system.

Nervous system is principally related to functions of the body in an external and internal environment. The nervous system coordinates the body functions through transmission of electrochemical impulses via nerve fibres.

Endocrinal system is mainly concerned with different metabolic functions of the body, especially the chemical reactions and transport of various substances. The endocrinal functions are accomplished through a wide range of chemical messengers, the hormones.

RELATIONSHIP BETWEEN ENDOCRINE AND NEURAL PHYSIOLOGY

In a conceptual sense, the nervous system and the endocrine system have important functional similarities. Each is basically a system for signalling. In fact, the nervous system and the endocrine system often respond together to incoming stimuli so as to integrate the organism's response to changes in its external and internal environment. The coordinated function of these systems is well illustrated by the following example.

A significant decrease in the circulating blood volume is sensed by baroreceptors, the cardiac atria, the kidney and the brain. The sympathetic nervous system, a neurohormone from the posterior pituitary gland and hormones from the cardiac atria and ventricles, the adrenal medulla, the adrenal cortex and the kidneys act on target cells in blood vessels and kidneys to restore blood volume. Further, this *close relationship between the nervous and endocrine systems is illustrated by the following common characteristics*:

- Both nervous and endocrine cells can secrete substances into the bloodstream.
- Some endocrine cells and neurons generate electrical potentials and can be depolarized.
- Peptides originally discovered as products of endocrine cells have neurotransmitter function as well. Likewise, molecules normally considered to be neurotransmitters can act as hormones.
- Both biogenic amine neurotransmitters and peptide hormone molecules can be produced by a single cell.
- Certain factors such as neurogenin and nerve growth factor play a role in the development of both endocrine cells and nervous system.
- Structural similarities exist between the receptors for hormones and neurotransmitters.

ORGANIZATION OF ENDOCRINE SYSTEM

The endocrinal system consists of various endocrine glands and neurosecretory cells located in the hypothalamus. The neurosecretory cells of hypothalamus secrete certain neurohormones called releasing and inhibitory factors which influence the secretion of hormones from other endocrine glands. Certain other substances act as neurotransmitters in the brain and influence the secretion of neurosecretory cells of hypothalamus. The environmental factors through these neurotransmitters influence the whole endocrine system. The various endocrine glands present in the body are as follows:

1. ***Pituitary gland (hypophysis):*** Pituitary gland is also known as hypophysis, which in Greek means undergrowth of the brain. It has two main parts: adenohypophysis and neurohypophysis. *Adenohypophysis* secretes growth hormone (GH) or somatotropins, follicle-stimulating hormone (FSH), luteinizing hormone (LH), prolactin, thyrotropin or thyroid-stimulating hormone (TSH) and corticotropin or adrenocorticotropic hormone (ACTH). The *neurohypophysis* stores the antidiuretic hormone (ADH) or vasopressin and oxytocin synthesized by the hypothalamus.
2. ***Thyroid gland:*** The thyroid gland is present in the neck in front of trachea. It has two lobes and an isthmus (bridge) connecting the lobes. It secretes thyroxine ($\mathbf{T_4}$) and triiodothyronine ($\mathbf{T_3}$). The C cells or parafollicular cells which are scattered in the spaces between the follicles of the thyroid gland secrete calcitonin.
3. ***Parathyroid glands:*** These are four in number, very small glands situated behind the lobes of the thyroid gland, and secrete parathormone.
4. ***Adrenal glands:*** These are situated on the upper poles of the two kidneys, hence also called suprarenal glands. The outer cortex region of the adrenal glands secretes cortisol, aldosterone and sex steroids, and the inner medullary region secretes catecholamines (adrenaline and noradrenaline).
5. ***Pancreatic islets (islets of Langerhans):*** These are small groups of cells which secrete insulin, glucagon and somatostatin.
6. ***Gonads:*** These include ovaries in females and testes in males. The ovaries secrete oestrogens and progesterone (female sex steroids), and testes secrete male sex hormone (testosterone).
7. ***Pineal gland:*** It is a small gland present in the roof of third ventricle in the brain. It secretes melatonin and other biogenic amines.
8. ***Placenta:*** During pregnancy, the placenta secretes various hormones like human chorionic gonadotropin (hCG), oestrogen, progesterone, somatotropins and relaxin.
9. ***Gastrointestinal mucosa:*** It also secretes various hormones collectively known as gastrointestinal (GIT) hormones, e.g. gastrin, secretin and cholecystokinin-pancreozymin (CCK-PZ).
10. ***Kidneys:*** In addition to their renal functions, the kidneys secrete erythropoietin, prostaglandins and 1,25-dihydroxycholecalciferol, and also help in activation of angiotensin production.
11. ***Atrial muscle cells:*** These secrete atrial natriuretic peptides (ANPs) and many other peptides.
12. ***Skin:*** This is also considered to act as an endocrine structure by producing vitamin D, which is now considered to be a hormone.

General Principles of Endocrinal System

8.1

CHAPTER OUTLINE

HORMONES: DEFINITION AND CLASSIFICATION

DEFINITION

The word hormone is derived from the Greek word *hormaein*, which means to execute or to arouse (to set in motion). In the classic definition, hormones are secretory products of the ductless glands which are released in catalytic amounts into bloodstream and transported to specific target cells (or organs), where they elicit physiological, morphological and biochemical responses. In reality, the requirement that hormones be secreted into the bloodstream is too restrictive, because they can also act locally. Therefore, the chemical messengers that perform hormonal functions are defined as follows (Fig. 8.1.1).

1. Endocrine hormones These include the chemical messengers whose function is the transmission of a molecular signal from a classic endocrinal cell through the bloodstream to a distant target cell (Fig. 8.1.1A).

2. Neurocrine hormones Nervous communication involves the release of chemical messengers from nerve terminals, which may reach their target cells via one of three routes:

Neurotransmitters can be released directly into the intercellular space, cross the synaptic junction and inhibit or activate the postsynaptic cell, e.g. acetylcholine (ACh) and norepinephrine.

Neural signals can be transferred via gap junction, which is a membrane stabilization between the nerve cells, between nerve terminals and endocrine cells and between endocrine cells.

Neurohormones or peptides are released from a neurosecretory neuron into the bloodstream and then carried to distant target cells (Fig. 8.1.1B). Examples of such neurocrine substances are oxytocin and antidiuretic hormone (ADH). The effector sites of neurohormones are not always endocrine cells.

3. Paracrine hormones These chemical messengers, which, after getting secreted by a cell, are carried over short

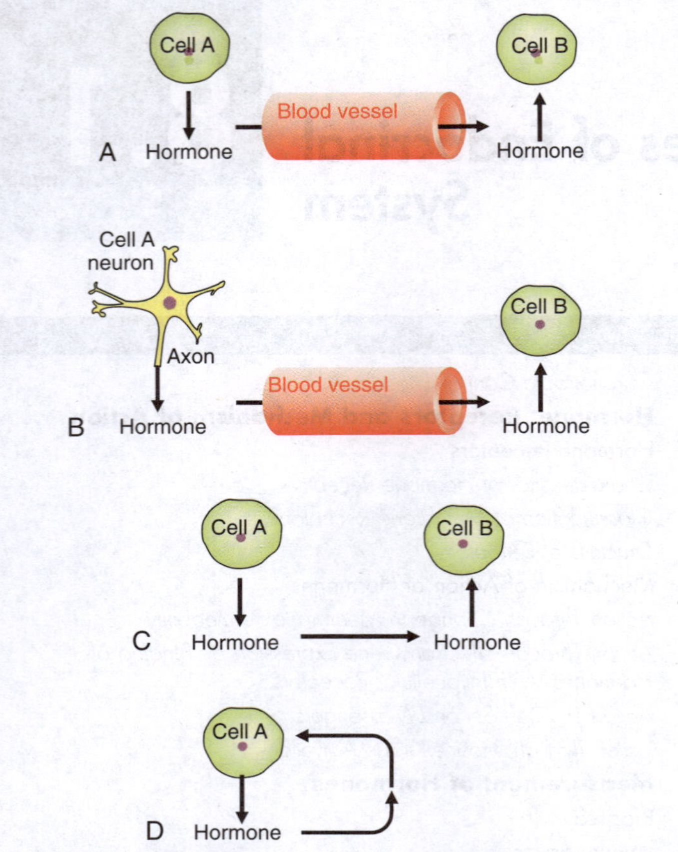

Fig. 8.1.1 Different types of hormones (by their mechanism of action): **A**, endocrine hormone; **B**, neurocrine hormone; **C**, paracrine hormone; **D**, autocrine hormone.

distance by diffusion through the interstitial spaces (extracellular fluid) to act on the neighbouring different cell types as or a regulatory substance (Fig. 8.1.1C). For example, in islets of Langerhans, somatostatin secreted by the delta cells acts on the alpha and beta cells.

4. Autocrine hormones These refer to those chemical messengers which regulate the activity of neighbouring similar type of cells (Fig. 8.1.1D). Examples of autocrine hormones are prostaglandins.

Important Note

It is important to note that according to the route by which it is transmitted, the same chemical messenger may act as endocrinal hormone (bloodstream conveyance), or as a paracrine or as an autocrine hormone (local conveyance), e.g. insulin secreted by beta cells in the pancreatic islets may act as:

- *Endocrine hormone:* When released into bloodstream, insulin acts on the adipose tissue, muscle, liver and brain to regulate energy stores and carbohydrate, fat and protein metabolism.
- *Paracrine hormone:* Insulin, when released into the islets interstitial fluid, inhibits the neighbouring alpha cells of the islets.
- *Autocrine hormone:* The insulin released in the islets interstitial fluid can regulate growth and function of beta cells themselves, as they possess insulin receptors.

CLASSIFICATION OF HORMONES

Depending on the Chemical Nature

1. ***Amines or amino acid derivatives***, e.g.:
   - Catecholamines (epinephrine and norepinephrine)
   - Thyroxine (T_4) and triiodothyronine (T_3)
2. ***Proteins and polypeptides***:
   i. ***Short-chain polypeptides include:***
      - Posterior pituitary hormones
      - ADH
      - Oxytocin

   ii. ***Long-chain polypeptides include:***
      - Insulin
      - Glucagon
      - Parathormone
      - Other anterior pituitary hormones
3. ***Steroid hormones include:***
   - Glucocorticoids
   - Mineralocorticoids
   - Sex steroids
   - Vitamin derivatives

Depending on the Mechanism of Action

Group I hormones: These act by binding to intracellular receptor and mediate their actions via formation of a hormone–receptor complex. These include steroid, retinoid and thyroid hormones.

Group II hormones: These involve second messenger to mediate their effect. Depending on the chemical nature of the second messengers, group II hormones are further divided into four subgroups A, B, C and D (Table 8.1.1).

HORMONES: GENERAL CONSIDERATIONS

HORMONE CHEMISTRY, SYNTHESIS, STORAGE AND RELEASE

Amines or Amino Acid Derivatives

Synthesis

These hormones include catecholamines, thyroid hormone and calciferol, which are derived from the amino acid tyrosine. Thyroid hormones are derived from two iodinated tyrosine residues. Thyroid hormones are the only substances in the body that contain iodine. These are synthesized in the cell cytoplasm.

Storage and release

Catecholamines are stored in secretory granules inside the cytoplasm of chromaffin cells. Secretion occurs when the membrane of granule fuses with the plasma membrane, causing the granular contents to be extruded into the circulation.

Thyroid hormones are stored outside the follicular cells in the form of thyroglobulin. Following endocytosis and proteolysis of thyroglobulin, thyroid hormones are secreted into the bloodstream by simple diffusion.

Calciferol (1,25-dihydroxyvitamin D_3) is stored as a precursor in the form of 7-dehydrocholesterol or cholecalciferol (vitamin D_3) in the skin.

Table 8.1.1 Types of group II hormones based on the chemical nature of second messenger involved in their mechanism of action

Group	Second messenger	Hormones
Group II-A	Cyclic AMP (cAMP)	Adrenocorticotropic hormone (ACTH) Antidiuretic hormone (ADH) Angiotensin II Calcitonin Corticotropic hormones (CRH) Catecholamine (α_2-adrenergic) Follicle-stimulating hormone (FSH) Glucagon Luteinizing hormone (LH) Parathormone (PTH) Somatostatin Thyroid-stimulating hormone (TSH)
Group II-B	Cyclic GMP (cGMP)	Atrial natriuretic factor (ANF) and nitric oxide
Group II-C	Calcium or phosphatidylinositol or both	Acetylcholine (ACh), catecholamines (α_1-adrenergic), gastrin, oxytocin, thyrotropin-releasing hormone (TRH), gonadotropin-releasing hormone (GnRH), platelet-derived growth factor (PDGF) and substances
Group II-D	Kinase or phosphatase cascade	Human chorionic somatotropin (hCS), erythropoietin, growth hormone, insulin and insulin-like growth factors (IGF-I and IGF-II), nerve growth factor (NGF), prolactin and other growth factors

Protein and Polypeptide Hormones

Synthesis

The peptide and protein hormones are composed of chains of amino acids linked by peptide bonds. These are synthesized in the granular endoplasmic reticulum of glandular cells in the same manner as other proteins:

- The amino acid sequence is determined by specific deoxyribonucleic acid (DNA) molecules through the messenger ribonucleic acid (mRNA).
- First, the precursor hormone (prohormone, or preprohormone) is synthesized in the rough endoplasmic reticulum.
- Then the precursor hormone is converted into proper hormone within the Golgi complex by post-translational cleavage.

Storage and release

Protein and polypeptide hormones are stored exclusively in subcellular membrane-bound secretory granules within the cytoplasm of endocrine cell until a release signal is received. On receiving the release signal, these hormones are released into the blood by exocytosis.

Steroid Hormones

Synthesis

Steroids are hydrophobic lipid-soluble substances. These are synthesized from cholesterol.

Storage and release

There is little storage of steroids. Instead, different precursors of cholesterol and intermediate compounds are present in the cells. These serve as precursors and when the necessity of hormone arises, the enzymatic action converts them into steroids which are released in the circulation by simple diffusion.

Vitamin Derivatives

Two important vitamins, i.e. vitamin A and vitamin D, act as hormones.

HORMONE TRANSPORT, PLASMA CONCENTRATION AND HALF-LIFE

Hormone Transport

After secretion into bloodstream, the hormones may circulate in two forms.

Unbound form Some hormones circulate as free molecule, e.g. catecholamines and most peptide and protein hormones circulate unbound.

Bound form Some hormones, such as steroids, thyroid hormones and vitamin D, circulate bound to specific globulins that are synthesized in the liver. The binding of hormones to proteins is advantageous as it:

- Protects the hormone against clearance by the kidney
- Slows down the rate of degradation by the liver
- Provides circulating reserve of the hormone

Some hormones are carried in the blood as inactive forms with proteins. They become active at the target site only. Only unbound hormones pass through capillaries to produce their effects or to degrade.

Plasma Concentration

Hormones are usually secreted into the circulation in extremely low concentrations:

- *Peptide hormone concentration is between* 10^{-12} and 10^{-10} mol/L.
- *Epinephrine and norepinephrine concentrations are* 2×10^{-10} and 13×10^{-10} mol/L, respectively.
- *Steroid and thyroid hormone concentrations are* 10^{-9} *and* 10^{-6} *mol/L, respectively.*

Table 8.1.2 Half-life of some of the important hormones

Class of hormone	Hormone	Half-life
Protein and peptide hormones	ADH	<1 min
	Oxytocin	<1 min
	Insulin	5 min
	Prolactin	12 s
	Growth hormone	<30 min
	ACTH	15–25 s
	LH	15–45 min
	FSH	180 min
Amines	Epinephrine	10 s
	Norepinephrine	15 s
	Thyroxine (T_4)	5–7 days
	Triiodothyronine (T_3)	1–3 days
Steroid hormones	Aldosterone	30 min
	Cortisol	90–100 min
	1,25-Dihydroxycholecalciferol	15 h
	25-Hydroxycholecalciferol	15 days

Half-life

Most hormones are metabolized rapidly after secretion. In general:

- Peptide hormones have short half-life.
- Steroids and thyroid hormones have significantly longer half-life because they are bound to plasma proteins. Table 8.1.2 depicts half-life of some of the hormones.

FUNCTIONS OF HORMONES

Hormones regulate existing fundamental processes but do not initiate reactions de novo.

1. Regulation of biochemical reactions Hormones regulate the metabolic functions in a variety of ways:

- They stimulate or inhibit the rate and magnitude of biochemical reactions by controlling enzymes and thereby cause morphological, biochemical and functional changes in target tissues.
- They modulate energy-producing processes and regulate the circulating levels of energy-yielding substances (e.g. glucose, fatty acids). However, they are not used as energy sources in biochemical reactions.

2. Regulation of bodily processes Hormones regulate different bodily processes such as growth, maturation, differentiation, regeneration, reproduction and behaviour. Thus, the main function of endocrine glands is to maintain homeostasis in an internal environment. For these functions, the hormones do not act directly on the intracellular machinery.

HORMONE DISPOSAL

Mechanisms of Hormone Disposal

The circulating hormones are disposed of by the following mechanisms:

- Target cell uptake and intracellular degradation
- Metabolic degradation/inactivation
- Urinary or biliary secretion

1. Target cell uptake and intracellular degradation The interaction of hormones with their target cells is followed by intracellular degradation.

Degradation of protein and amine hormones occurs after binding to membrane receptors, and then internalization of hormone–receptor complex.

Degradation of thyroid and steroid hormones occurs after binding the hormone–receptor complex to the chromatin.

2. Metabolic degradation/inactivation Only a small fraction of the circulating hormone is removed by target tissue cells; most of the hormone extraction and degradation occurs in the liver and kidneys. Metabolic degradation occurs by enzymatic processes that include proteolysis, oxidation, reduction, hydroxylation, decarboxylation and methylation. Virtually all the hormones are extracted from the plasma and degraded to some extent by the liver. In addition, glucuronidation and secretion of hormones or their metabolites may be carried out, and the conjugates are subsequently excreted in the bile or urine.

Metabolic clearance rate Metabolic clearance rate (MCR) refers to the sum of all the removal processes, i.e. target cell uptake and degradation, metabolic degradation and urinary or biliary excretion. In a steady rate, MCR is defined as the volume of plasma cleared/unit time, which equals mass removed/unit time divided by circulating mass/unit volume, that is,

$$\text{MCR} = \frac{\text{mg/min removed}}{\text{mg/mL of plasma}} = \frac{\text{mL cleared}}{\text{minute}}$$

MCR is inversely correlated with plasma half-life.

Functional turnover rate (k) Functional turnover rate (k) refers to the ratio of MCR to the volume of distribution of a hormone. The plasma half-life, which is inversely related to k, is a *wider* but more conveniently determined index of hormone disappearance.

3. Urinary and biliary excretion Renal clearance of hormones is reduced greatly by protein binding in the plasma, e.g. less than 10% of secreted cortisol appears unchanged in the urine, because only the small, free fraction of plasma cortisol is filtered by the glomerulus. On the other hand, approximately 30% of cortisol metabolites are excreted in urine, because they are generally unbound or only loosely bound to protein. Peptide and smaller protein hormones are filtered to some degree by the glomerulus. However, they may subsequently undergo tubular reabsorption and degradation within the kidney, so that only a small fraction appears in the final urine. Further, as mentioned above, the conjugated hormones are excreted in the bile or urine.

REGULATION OF HORMONE SECRETION

The quantity of hormones secreted is regulated in accordance with their requirement. General mechanisms that govern the secretion of hormone include:

- Feedback control
- Neural control
- Chronotropic control

Feedback Control

Regulation of a hormone in terms of requirement is best accomplished through feedback from the blood concentration

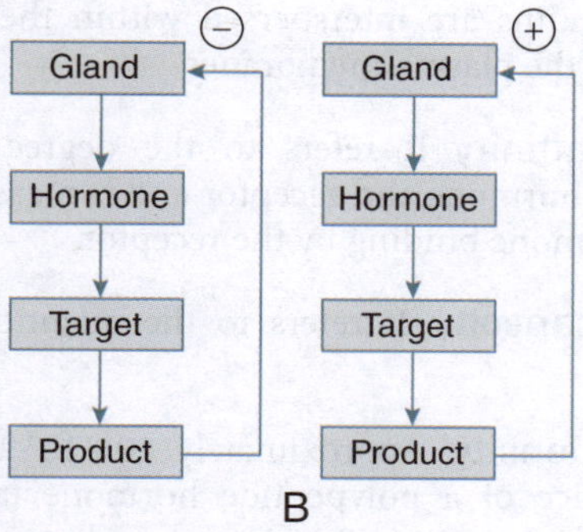

Fig. 8.1.2 Hormonal regulation by feedback control mechanism: **A**, negative feedback; **B**, positive feedback.

of the hormone concerned (hormone–hormone) or some result of action of the hormone (substrate–hormone). Feedback control is of two types:

- Negative feedback control
- Positive feedback control

Negative feedback control Generally, the influence of blood concentration of the hormone concerned or its effect is to inhibit further secretion of the hormone and is called negative feedback control (Fig. 8.1.2A).

Positive feedback control This is less common and acts to amplify the initial biological effects of the hormone (Fig. 8.1.2B).

Depending on the product involved, the feedback mechanism may be:

- Hormone–hormone feedback
- Substrate–hormone feedback
- Mineral–hormone feedback

i. Hormone–hormone feedback control The best example of hormone–hormone negative feedback control is regulation of hormone secretions by hypothalamus and pituitary, which involves three loops (Fig. 8.1.3):

Long-loop feedback (Fig. 8.1.3A): The peripheral gland hormone (e.g. thyroid, adrenocortical and gonads) can exert long-loop negative feedback control on both the hypothalamus and the anterior lobe of pituitary.
Short-loop feedback (Fig. 8.1.3B): The pituitary tropic hormones decrease the secretion of hypophysiotropic hormone (e.g. GHRH, GHIH, TRH, GnRH) by short-loop feedback.
Ultrashort-loop feedback (Fig. 8.1.3C): The hypophysiotropic hormones may inhibit their own synthesis and secretion via an ultrashort-loop feedback mechanism.

ii. Substrate–hormone feedback control The best example of substrate–hormone feedback control is regulation of insulin secretion from pancreatic beta cells of islets of Langerhans and glucagon secretion from alpha cells by blood glucose levels. A rise in blood glucose level promotes the secretion of insulin, while a fall in blood glucose promotes secretion of glucagon. These responses keep the blood glucose level within narrow limits in spite of variation in carbohydrate intake in diet.

iii. Mineral–hormone feedback The best example of mineral hormonal feedback is regulation of blood calcium level. The parathyroid glands secrete parathyroid hormone

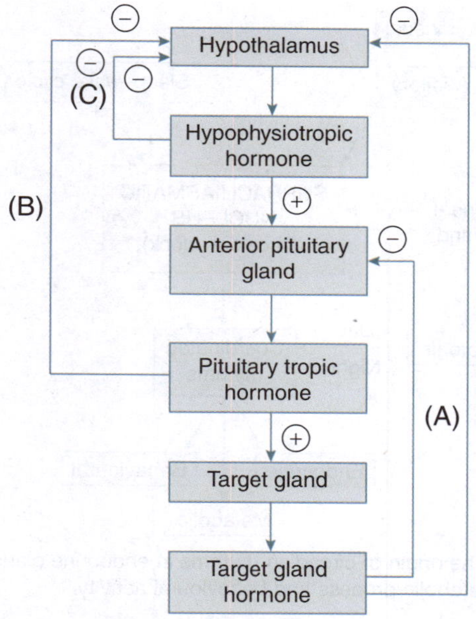

Fig. 8.1.3 Hormone–hormone negative feedback control by hypothalamus and pituitary: **A**, long-loop feedback; **B**, short-loop feedback; and **C**, ultrashort-loop feedback.

(PTH), which regulates the level of calcium in the blood. If calcium level decreases, parathyroid glands sense the decrease and secrete more PTH.

Neural Control

Neural control acts to evoke or suppress hormone secretion in response to both external and internal stimuli.

External stimuli which can modulate hormone release through neural mechanisms may be visual, auditory, olfactory, gustatory and tactile.
Internal stimuli which influence hormonal release through neural mechanism include pain, emotion, sexual excitement, fright, stress and changes in blood volume.
Neural control depending on the type of nerve fibres involved may be:

- Adrenergic
- Cholinergic
- Dopaminergic
- Serotoninergic
- GABAergic

Examples of neural control of hormones:

- *Release of oxytocin*, which fills the milk ducts in response to the stimulus of suckling
- *Release of aldosterone*, which augments the circulatory volume in response to upright posture
- *Release of melatonin* in response to darkness

Chronotropic Control

Chronotropic control of hormone secretion accounts for:

- Oscillating and pulsatile release of certain hormones
- Diurnal variation in hormonal levels
- Menstrual rhythm
- Seasonal rhythm
- Developmental rhythm

The source of regular oscillatory cycles is a pulse generator(s) located in the suprachiasmatic nucleus (SCN) of the hypothalamus (Fig. 8.1.4).

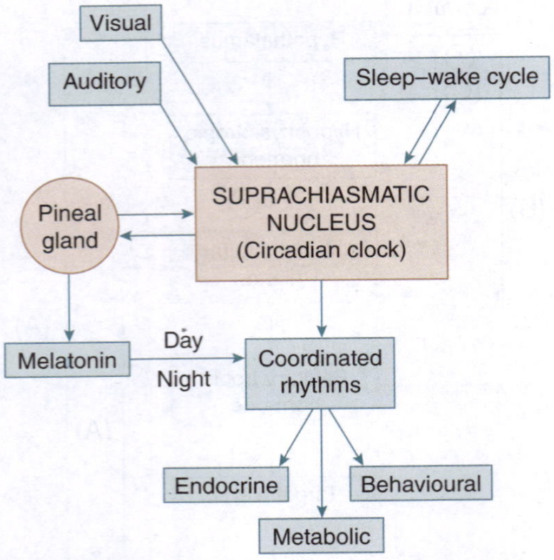

Fig. 8.1.4 The origin of circadian rhythms in endocrine gland secretion, metabolic process and behavioural activity.

The intrinsic circadian clock is also located in the SCN, which is responsible for endocrinal, metabolic and behavioural coordinated rhythms. For details, see page 931.

HORMONE: RECEPTORS AND MECHANISM OF ACTION

HORMONE RECEPTORS

All hormones act through specific receptors. Almost all hormone receptors are large proteins present in hormone-sensitive target cells.

Characteristics of Hormone Receptors

Receptor specificity There are specific receptors for each hormone. This is the reason that all hormones circulate to all parts of the body, yet each hormone has a specific target tissue for its action (Fig. 8.1.5).

Receptor location Depending on the location, receptors are of two types:

i. ***Internal receptors*** are located inside the cells, e.g. receptors for steroid hormones and thyroid hormones are localized within the nucleus of target cells.
ii. ***External receptors*** are located on the plasma membrane of target cells, e.g. peptide and protein hormones, amines and prostaglandins are interspersed within the phospholipid bilayer of the plasma membranes.

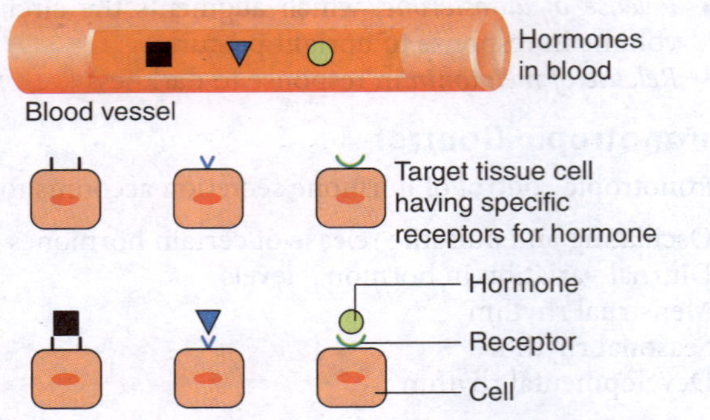

Fig. 8.1.5 Specificity of hormone action is because of specific receptors.

Receptor affinity It refers to the degree of attraction between the hormone and receptor and is measured from the speed of hormone binding by the receptor.

Receptor capacity It refers to the quantity of hormone binding.

Receptor density Approximately 10^4–10^5 receptors exist on the surface of a polypeptide hormone target cell, and approximately 3×10^3 to 3×10^4 intracellular receptors exist per steroid target cell.

Change in receptor number The number of receptors of a cell varies depending on the situation. It is regulated by two mechanisms: downregulation and upregulation.

i. ***Downregulation*** refers to decrease in the number of active receptors. It occurs to regulate the hormone sensitivity when it is present in excess. For example, elevated ambient insulin concentration causes a loss or inactivation of insulin receptors in liver cells, fat cells and white blood cells (WBCs).
ii. ***Upregulation*** refers to increase in the number of active receptors on a cell. It occurs to regulate the hormone action when its concentration is less. This phenomenon tends to reduce the effect of hormone deficiency.

Spare receptors A maximum physiological response of a target cell is observed even when the concentration of a hormone is lower than required to occupy all of the receptors on that cell. Therefore, most of the receptors (~97%) are referred to as spare (reserve) receptors.

Classification of Membrane Receptors

Cell membrane receptors have been classified into four classes (Fig. 8.1.6).

1. Receptor kinases These include membrane receptors that contain enzyme activity. For example, receptors for insulin hormone contain tyrosine or serine kinase as an intrinsic part of structure.

2. Receptor-linked kinases These have no intrinsic enzyme activity, e.g. receptors for growth hormone, prolactin and cytokines.

3. G-protein–coupled receptors Examples: receptors for pituitary tropic hormones, glucagon, epinephrine, norepinephrine, PTH and prostaglandins.

4. Ligand-gated ion channels These act as receptors for neurotransmitters such as ACh, γ-aminobutyric acid (GABA) and glycine.

Structure of Receptor

The receptors in general have two parts or domains: a recognition domain (R) and a coupling domain (C) (Fig. 8.1.7).

Recognition domain (R): It is that part of the receptor where the hormone binds. It is formed by extracellular N-terminus portion of the receptor (extracellularly projected NH_2 group).
Coupling domain (C): It is that part of receptor which initiates signals for intracellular activities after the recognition. It

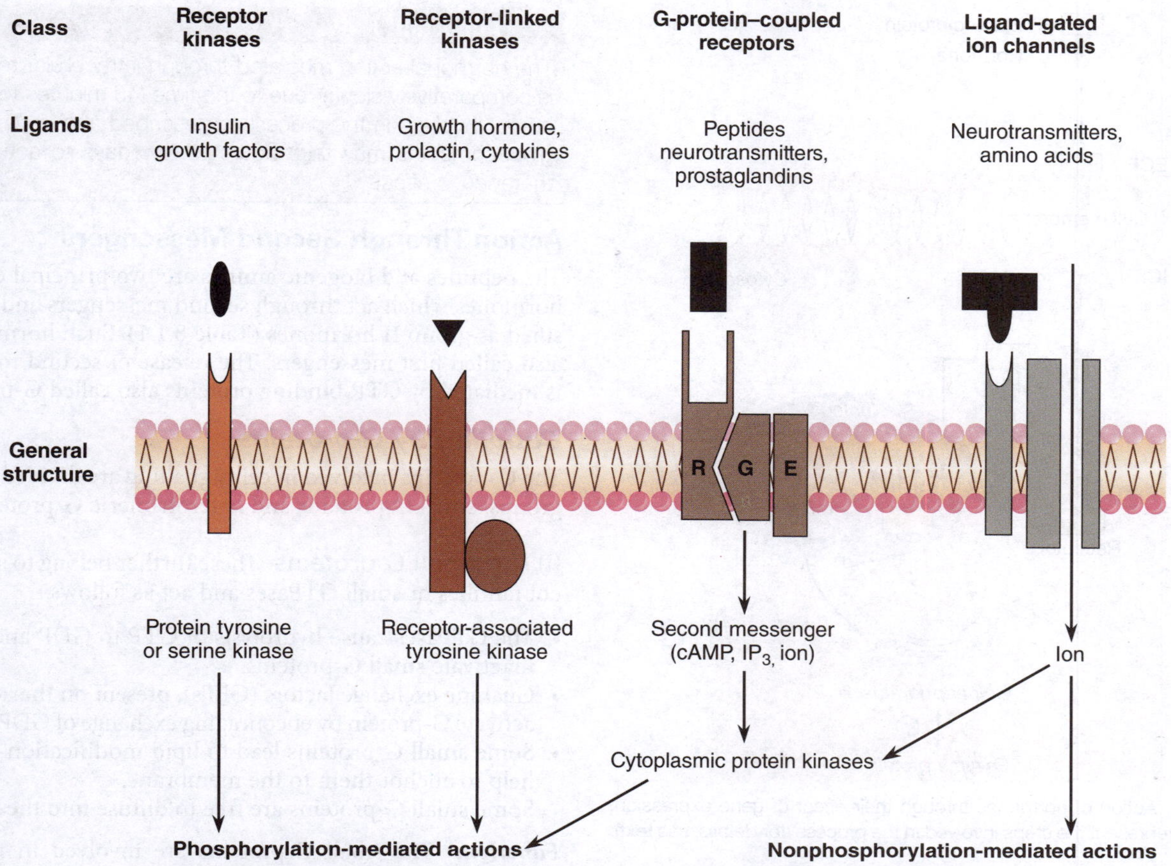

Fig. 8.1.6 Schematic general structure of four major classes of membrane receptors.

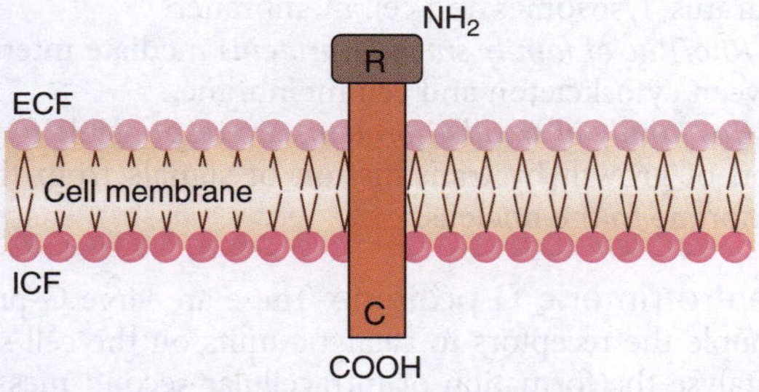

Fig. 8.1.7 General structure of a hormonal receptor.

is formed by the intracellular C-terminus tail of the receptor (intracellularly projected carboxyl, i.e. COOH). The membrane receptors wind in and out of the plasma membrane by means of seven transmembrane segments.

MECHANISM OF ACTION OF HORMONES

As mentioned previously, all hormones act through specific receptors, and depending on the mechanism of action hormones, they have been divided into group I and group II (Table 8.1.1).

Group I hormones act by affecting gene expression at cellular level.

Group II hormones act through intermediary molecules called second messenger, and depending on the chemical nature of second messenger, the group II hormones have been further divided into subgroups A, B, C and D (Table 8.1.1).

The main mechanisms of hormone actions:

- Action through change in membrane permeability
- Action through effect on gene expression by binding of hormones with intracellular receptors
- Action through secondary messengers which activate intracellular enzymes when hormones combine with membrane receptors
- Action through tyrosine kinase activation

Action Through Change in Membrane Permeability

Certain hormones bind with the receptors present in the cell membrane (external receptors) and cause conformational change in the protein of the receptors; this results in either opening or closing of the ion channels (such as Na^+ channels, K^+ channels and Ca^{2+} channels). The movement of ions through Ca^{2+} channels causes the subsequent effect, e.g. adrenaline and noradrenaline act by this mechanism.

Action Through Effect on Gene Expression by Binding of Hormones With Intracellular Receptors

Group I hormones act by their effect on gene expression which include steroid hormones, retinoids and thyroid hormones. These hormones are lipophilic in nature and can easily pass across the cell membrane. They act through intracellular receptors located either in the cytosol or in

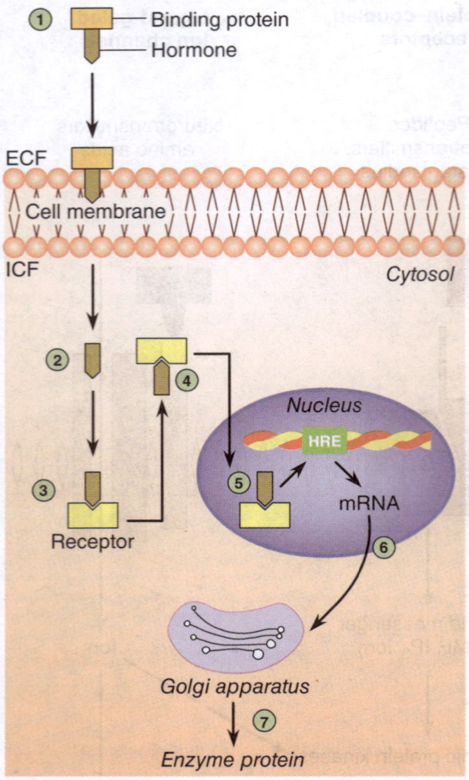

Fig. 8.1.8 Action of hormones through their effect of gene expression. Note: 1–7 represent the steps involved in the process (for details, see text).

the nucleus. The sequence of events involved is as follows (Fig. 8.1.9):

1. ***Transport:*** After secretion, the hormone is carried to the target tissue on serum-binding protein.
2. ***Internalization:*** Being lipophilic, the hormone easily diffuses through the plasma membrane.
3. ***Receptor–hormone complex:*** It is formed by binding of hormone to the specific receptor inside the cell. There are three distinct pathways by which primary messenger alter transcription and gene expression as follows:
   - Primary messenger (in case of steroid and thyroid hormone) directly binds to nuclear receptor and directly interacts with DNA to alter gene expression.
   - By activation of cytoplasmic receptor protein (kinase) that moves into the nucleus and activates latent transcription factor causing phosphorylation, e.g. *mitogen-activated protein kinase (MAP)*.
   - The third pathway is the activation of latent transcription factor present in the cytosol. This pathway is shared by nuclear factor kappa B (NF-κB) and signal transducers and activators of transcription (STATs).
4. ***Conformational change:*** This occurs in receptor proteins leading to activation of receptors.
5. ***That the activated receptor–hormone complex then diffuses*** into the nucleus and binds on the specific region on the DNA known as hormone response element (HRE), which initiates gene transcription.
6. ***Binding of the receptor–hormone complex to DNA:*** This alters the rate of transcription of mRNA.
   - The mRNA diffuses in the cytoplasm, where it promotes the translation process at the ribosomes. In this way, new proteins are formed which result in specific responses. Some of the new proteins synthesized are enzymes.

> **Important Note**
>
> The hormonal action mediated through intracellular receptors is comparatively slower due to the time (45 minutes to several hours) involved in the processes described above. Therefore, glucocorticoids may take hours to few days to achieve the therapeutic effect.

Action Through Second Messengers

The peptides and biogenic amines are two principal classes of hormones which act through second messengers and are classified as group II hormones (Table 8.1.1). Such hormones are also called first messengers. The release of second messenger is mediated by GTP-binding proteins also called G-proteins.

Coupling by G-proteins

The G-proteins involved in cell signalling are divided into two groups: small G-proteins and heterotrimeric G-proteins.

(i) The small G-proteins These further belong to six different families or small GTPases and act as follows:

- The GTPases cause hydrolysis of GTP to GDP and tend to inactivate small G-proteins.
- Guanine exchange factors (GEFs), present on the active site, activate G-protein by encouraging exchange of GDP for GTP.
- Some small G-proteins lead to lipid modification and thus help to anchor them to the membrane.
- Some small G-proteins are free to diffuse into the cytosol.

Functions: The small G-proteins are involved in following functions:

- *The Rab family members of small G-proteins* regulate vesicular movement between endoplasmic reticulum, the Golgi apparatus, lysosomes and cell membrane.
- *The Rho/Rac of family small G-proteins* mediate interaction between cytoskeleton and cell membrane.
- *The Ras family of small G-proteins* are responsible for regulation of growth by transmission of signals from the cell membrane to the nucleus.

(ii) Heterotrimeric G-proteins These are large G-proteins that couple the receptors to catalytic units on the cell surface and catalyse the formation of intracellular second messenger. The heterotrimeric G-proteins are made up of three subunits (α, β and γ). The α- and γ-subunits help in anchoring of G-protein to the cell surface (Fig. 8.1.8). The α-subunit is bound to GDP. When hormone or ligand binds to G-protein–coupled receptor (GPCR), the GDP is exchanged with GTP and α-subunit separates from the β- and γ-subunits and is responsible for various biological activities. The intrinsic GTPase activity of separated α-subunit converts GTP into GDP and leads to reassociation of α-subunit with β- and γ-subunits.

- The regulators of G-protein signalling (RGS) accelerate α-subunit GTPase activity.
- The heterotrimeric G-protein is involved in relaying signals for more than 1000 G-protein receptors (GPCRs). ***GPCRs*** structurally are barrel like.

Mechanism of action

When a ligand binds the GPCR, a conformational change occurs, which activates heterotrimeric G-protein–associated cytoplasm, i.e. leaf of plasma membrane which in turn activates many G-proteins, thus leading to amplification of the

Table 8.1.3 The ligands act via G-protein–coupled receptors

Type of ligands	Examples
Neurotransmitters	Epinephrine, norepinephrine, dopamine, 5-HT, acetylcholine, opioids and adenosine
Tachykinins	Substance P, neuropeptide K and neurokinin
Hormones	Vasopressin, angiotensin II, oxytocin, VIP, GRP, parathyroid, TRH, TSH, FSH, LH, hCG
Arachidonic acid derivatives	Thromboxane A_2
Other	Endothelins, odorants and tastants, platelet-activating factor, cannabinoid and light

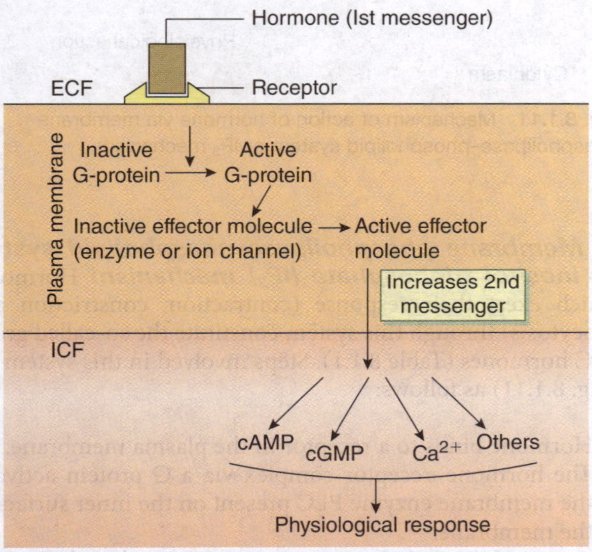

Fig. 8.1.9 Schematic mechanism of coupling by G-protein leading to increase in second messenger which mediates hormone's physiological response.

effect. A large number of ligands act through G-protein–coupled proteins (Table 8.1.3).

Events involved in coupling by G-protein which lead to changes in the cellular concentration of the second messengers are summarized (Fig. 8.1.9):

- Group II hormones are water soluble and bind to the plasma membrane of the target cell via cell surface receptors.
- The hormone-bearing receptor then interacts with a G-protein and activates it by binding GTP. There are two classes of G-proteins: stimulatory G-protein (Gs) and inhibitory G-protein (Gi).
- In its activated ('on') state, the G-protein interacts with one or more of the effector proteins (most of which are enzymes or ion channels such as adenylyl cyclase, Ca^{2+} or K^+ channels or phospholipase C [PLC], A_2 or D) to activate or inhibit them.
- The changed effector molecules in turn generate second messenger that mediates the hormone's intracellular action.

Second Messenger Systems

The second messenger systems that are activated through coupling of hormone–receptor complexes by G-protein include:

- Adenylyl cyclase–cAMP system
- Guanylyl cyclase–cGMP system
- Membrane phospholipase–phospholipid system
- Calcium–calmodulin system

1. Adenylyl cyclase–cAMP system The adenylyl cyclase–cAMP system was the first to be described by Sutherland in 1961 that initiated the concept of second messenger. The hormones which act through this system constitute the group IIA hormones (Table 8.1.1). The steps involved in the hormone action via adenylyl cyclase–cAMP system are summarized as follows (Fig. 8.1.10):

i. ***Binding of hormone*** *(Step 1)* to a specific receptor in the cell membrane.
ii. ***Activation of G-protein*** *(Step 2):* After formation of hormone–receptor complex, the GDP is released from the G-protein and is replaced by GTP, i.e. G-protein is activated.
iii. ***Activation of enzyme adenylyl cyclase*** *(Step 3):* The hormone–receptor complex via activated G-protein (stimulatory or inhibitory) either stimulates or inhibits the enzyme adenylyl cyclase which is also located in the plasma membrane.
iv. ***Formation of cAMP*** *(Step 4):* A part of the enzyme adenylyl cyclase protrudes through the inner surface of the cell membrane and when activated it catalyses the formation of cAMP from cytoplasmic ATP with Mg^{2+} as cofactor.

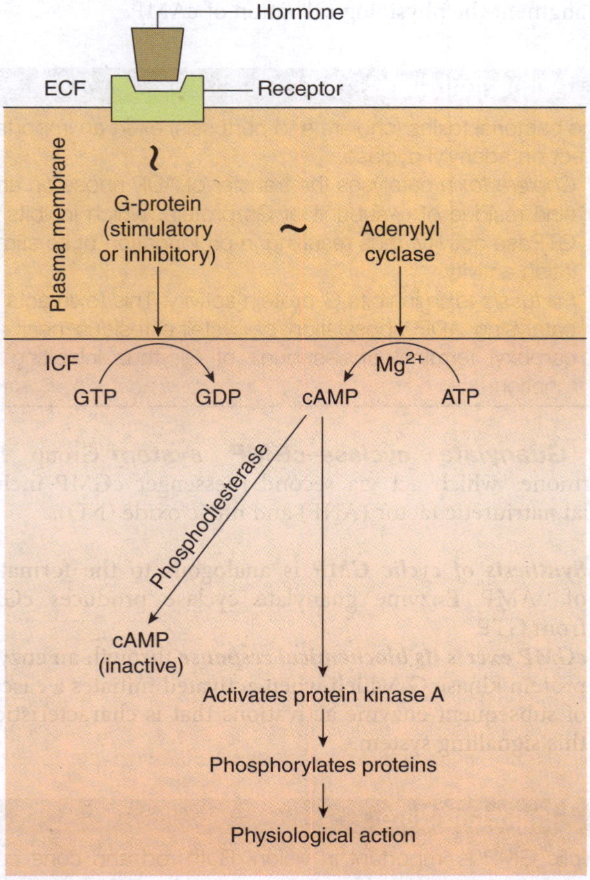

Fig. 8.1.10 Mechanism of action of hormone through adenylyl cyclase (cAMP) system as second messenger.

A stimulatory G-protein (Gs) therefore increases intracellular cAMP levels, whereas an inhibitory G-protein (Gi) decreases cAMP levels.

v. ***Action of cAMP:*** The cAMP once formed stimulates a cascade of enzyme activation. One molecule of cAMP may stimulate many enzymes. Therefore, even the slightest amount of hormone acting on the cell surface can initiate a very powerful response. The cyclic AMP so formed initiates response by different mechanisms in eukaryotic and prokaryotic cells.
   - *In eukaryotic cells,* the cAMP activates protein kinase A *(Step 5)* which phosphorylates the specific proteins, producing highly specific physiological actions *(Step 6)*:
     - Increase in cell permeability (e.g. ion transport and secretion)
     - Increase in synthesis of enzyme system (enzyme induction)
     - Activation of enzymes present in the cell
     - Release of hormones from storage pack cells and steroidogenesis
     - Gene regulation and so on
   - *In prokaryotic cells,* in contrast to eukaryotic cells, the cAMP acts directly at the gene level. It binds to a specific protein called *catabolic regulatory protein (CRP).* In association with CRP, it binds to DNA and influences gene expression or transcription. Therefore, cAMP in prokaryotic cells acts just like steroid hormones.

vi. ***Inactivation of cAMP:*** The cAMP is degraded to 5′-AMP (inactive form) by enzyme phosphodiesterase. Hence, the effect of cAMP is short lived if the hormone stimulating adenylyl cyclase is removed. Phosphodiesterase inhibitors such as caffeine and theophylline would be expected to augment the physiological action of cAMP.

Important Notes

The bacterial toxins (cholera and pertussis) exert an important effect on adenylyl cyclase.

- *Cholera toxin* catalyses the transfer of ADP ribose on arginine residue of α-subunit of Gs protein, which inhibits its GTPase activity, thus resulting in prolongation of its stimulation activity.
- *Pertussis toxin* inhibits G-protein activity. This toxin acts by catalysing ADP ribosylation of cysteine residue near the carboxyl terminal of α-subunit of Gi, thus inhibiting its function.

2. Guanylate cyclase–cGMP system Group II-B hormones which act via second messenger cGMP include atrial natriuretic factor (ANF) and nitric oxide (NO).

i. ***Synthesis of cyclic GMP*** is analogous to the formation of cAMP. Enzyme guanylate cyclase produces cGMP from GTP.

ii. ***cGMP exerts its biochemical response*** through an enzyme protein kinase G, which when activated initiates a cascade of subsequent enzyme activations that is characteristic of this signalling system.

Important Note

Cyclic GMP is important in vision. Both rod and cone cells contain ion channels which are regulated by cGMP.

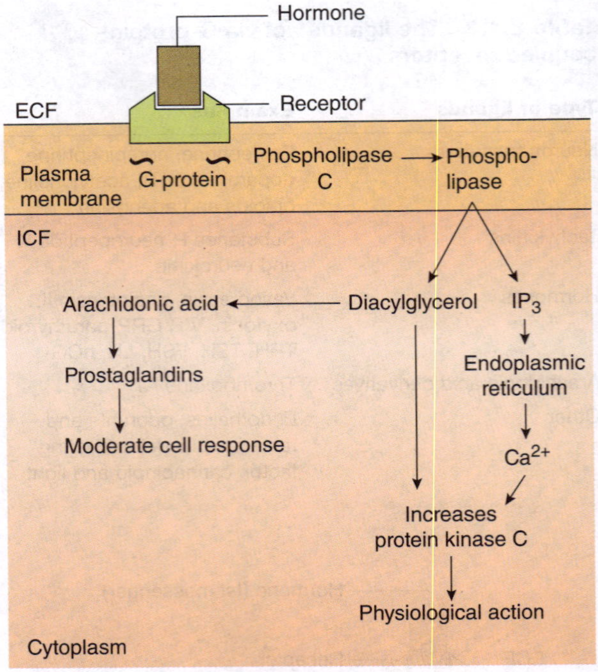

Fig. 8.1.11 Mechanism of action of hormone via membrane phospholipase–phospholipid system or IP_3 mechanism.

3. Membrane phospholipase–phospholipid system or inositol triphosphate (IP_3) mechanism Hormones which exert their response (contraction, constriction and exocytosis) through this system constitute the so-called group II-C hormones (Table 8.1.1). Steps involved in this system are (Fig. 8.1.11) as follows:

- Hormone binds to a receptor in the plasma membrane.
- The hormone–receptor complex via a G-protein activates the membrane enzyme PLC present on the inner surface of the membrane.
- Activated PLC then releases diacylglycerol and IP_3 from membrane phospholipid.
- IP_3 (1,4,5-triphosphate) then mobilizes Ca^{2+} from the endoplasmic reticulum.
- Calcium ions (Ca^{2+}) and diacylglycerol together activate protein kinase C.
- Activated protein kinase C phosphorylates proteins and causes specific physiological action.
- Diacylglycerol also yields arachidonic acid which serves as a substrate for rapid synthesis of prostaglandins that modulate cell response.

4. Calcium–calmodulin system Hormones that act through this system as second messenger are also included in the so-called group II-C hormones (Table 8.1.1). Steps involved in this system (Fig. 8.1.12):

- Hormone binds to a specific receptor in the plasma membrane.
- Then the hormone–receptor complex, via G-protein, opens the Ca^{2+} channels on the cell membrane and also activates mobilization of Ca^{2+} bound to the endoplasmic reticulum.
- Ca^{2+} binds to a specific binding protein, calmodulin, in various proportions.

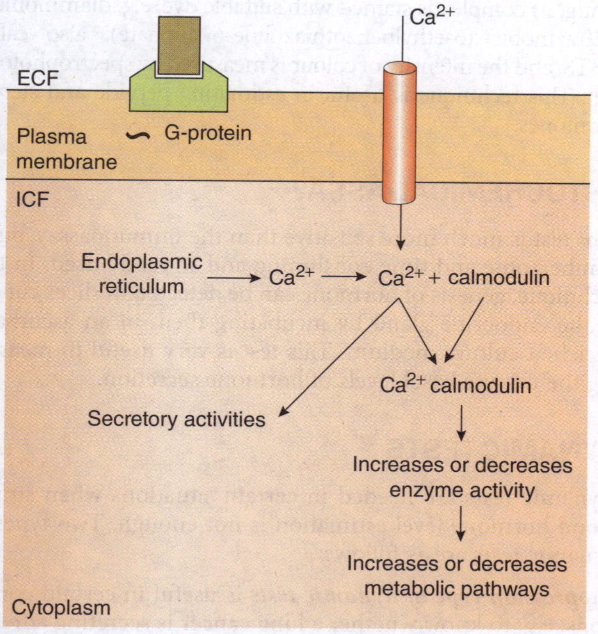

Fig. 8.1.12 Mechanism of action of hormone via calcium–calmodulin system.

- The different calcium–calmodulin complexes activate or deactivate various calcium-dependent enzymes producing different physiological actions.

Action Through Tyrosine Kinase Activation

Certain hormones act by activating tyrosine kinase system and have been classified as group II-D hormones (Table 8.1.1). This mechanism of signal generation from plasma membrane receptors does not require G-protein intermediaries. These receptors have an extracellular hormone-binding portion, a single transmembrane portion and an intracytoplasmic C-terminal portion.

The activation of tyrosine kinase occurs by two mechanisms:

1. ***Hormone receptors possessing intrinsic tyrosine activity,*** e.g. those for insulin and epidermal growth factor (EGF), involve the following steps (Fig. 8.1.13A):
   - Binding of hormone to the receptor changes its conformation and exposes sites on its intracellular portion that are capable of receptor autophosphorylation at specific tyrosine sites.
   - As a result, the receptor itself becomes a tyrosine kinase that phosphorylates tyrosine residue on intracellular protein substrates.
   - The latter activity sets into motion a cascade of events leading to enzyme activation and gene transcription.
   - The most important function of tyrosine kinase is to control cell growth and differentiation.
   - Tyrosine kinase receptors serve as receptor for insulin, insulin-like growth factor-I (IGF-I), EGF, nerve growth factor (NGF), platelet-derived growth factor (PDGF) and fibroblast growth factor (FGF).
2. ***Hormone receptors that do not possess intrinsic tyrosine activity***, e.g. those for growth hormone, prolactin-releasing hormones, cytokines erythropoietin and leptin, act by activation of JAK_2–STAT pathway. JAK_2 belongs to Janus family of tyrosine kinases. The phosphorylation of tyrosine kinases

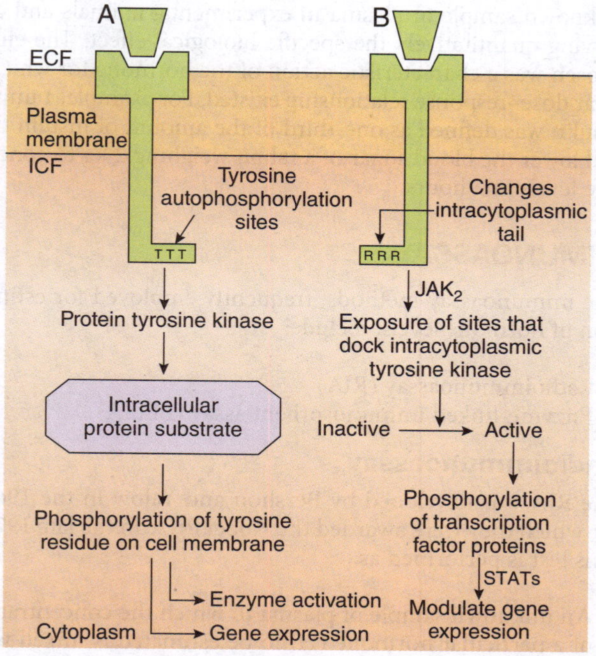

Fig. 8.1.13 Mechanism of action of hormone via tyrosine kinase activity: **A**, by receptors that possess intrinsic tyrosine activity; **B**, by receptors that act by activation of JAK_2–STAT pathway.

causes activation of signal transducer and activators of transcription (STATs) which are cytoplasmic transcription factors. On activation, STATs migrate into the nucleus and causes transcription of various genes as follows (Fig. 8.1.13B):
   - Hormone binding to extracellular portion of the receptor changes its intracytoplasmic tail.
   - The changes produced in intracytoplasmic tail of receptor expose sites which attract and dock the intracytoplasmic tyrosine kinases (such as JAK kinases and STAT kinases) and then activate them.
   - The activated intracytoplasmic tyrosine kinases phosphorylate cytoplasmic substrates such as transcription factor proteins and ultimately modulate gene expression.

MEASUREMENT OF HORMONES

Measurement of blood level of hormones is essential to confirm the endocrinal disorders associated with either deficiency or excess of a hormone. Since hormones exist in the blood at very low concentrations, the conventional methods of estimation, such as colorimetry, are not of much use. Therefore, they are measured by hormone assays and some special techniques which include:

- Bioassay
- Immunoassay
- Cytochemical assay
- Dynamic tests

BIOASSAY

Biological assay that was frequently used earlier to measure the level of a hormone in the plasma is now an obsolete technique. In this method, hormone levels were assessed by injecting the unknown sample of plasma in experimental animals and observing quantitatively the specific biological effect. The effect chosen was a characteristic action of the hormone for which a clear dose–response relationship existed. For example, 1 unit of insulin was defined as one-third of the amount of insulin that will lower the blood sugar of a rabbit weighing 2 kg to conclusive levels in 3 hours.

IMMUNOASSAY

The immunoassay methods, frequently employed for estimation of hormone levels, include:

- Radioimmunoassay (RIA)
- Enzyme-linked immunosorbent assay (ELISA)

Radioimmunoassay

The RIA was developed by Bershon and Yalow in the 1960s, for which they were awarded the Nobel Prize in the late 1970s. This test is performed as:

- An unknown sample of plasma in which the concentration of a particular hormone (H) to be estimated is mixed with commercially available purified specific antibody (anti-H) and an appropriate amount of the purified hormone tagged with radioactive isotope (H^+). The mixture is incubated in cold.
- The antibodies have high affinity for the hormone. There occurs a competition between the free hormone (H) present in the unknown sample of plasma and the tagged hormone (H^+) for binding to the specific antibody (anti-H).

Enzyme-Linked Immunosorbent Method

ELISA method is principally similar to RIA, i.e. it is also based on the principle of antigen–antibody reaction. Any antigen that is protein can be measured by this technique. In this method, radioactivity is not measured; instead, specific antibody–hormone (antigen) complex is stained with suitable dye, e.g. diammonium 2,2′-azinobis (3-ethylbenzothiazoline-6-sulphate), also called ABTS, and the intensity of colour is measured by spectrophotometer. This technique is useful in estimating peptide and steroid hormones.

CYTOCHEMICAL ASSAY

This test is much more sensitive than the immunoassay, but is cumbersome and time consuming and so rarely used. In this technique, genesis of hormone can be detected in slices cut out of the endocrine gland by incubating them in an ascorbate-enriched culture medium. This test is very useful in measuring the minute basal levels of hormone secretion.

DYNAMIC TESTS

Dynamic tests are needed in certain situations when simple blood hormone level estimation is not enough. Two types of dynamic tests are as follows:

Suppression type of dynamic tests is useful in certain conditions, e.g. to know whether a lung cancer is secreting adrenocorticotropic hormone (ACTH).

Stimulation type of dynamic tests is useful in certain other conditions, e.g. metyrapone test is performed to know whether the corticotrophs of the pituitary (which secrete ACTH) are normally functioning or not. For details, see page 741.

Self-Assessment

1. Discuss the mechanism of action of hormones.
2. Discuss the regulation of secretion of hormones.
3. Describe:
   - Methods of measurement of hormones
   - JAK–STAT pathway
   - Characteristics of hormonal receptors

8.2

Endocrinal Functions of Hypothalamus and Pituitary Gland

CHAPTER OUTLINE

INTRODUCTION AND FUNCTIONAL ANATOMY

The hypothalamic–pituitary unit forms a unique component of the entire endocrine system that regulates growth, lactation, fluid homeostasis and the functions of the thyroid gland, adrenal glands and gonads.

To appreciate the functional relationship between the hypothalamus and pituitary gland, it is necessary to have knowledge of the functional anatomy and embryological development of the pituitary gland.

GROSS ANATOMY AND DEVELOPMENT OF PITUITARY GLAND

Gross Anatomy

Pituitary gland, also called *hypophysis cerebri*, is a small gland, weighs approximately 0.5 g and is approximately 1 cm in diameter. It is situated in the hypophyseal fossa (sella turcica) of the sphenoid bone. A reflection of the dura mater, called the *diaphragma sellae*, extends across the top of sella and separates the pituitary gland from the brain. The diaphragma sellae is perforated in the middle through which the *pituitary stalk* passes that connects the pituitary gland with the hypothalamus.

Physiologically, the pituitary gland consists of three distinct parts or lobes (Fig. 8.2.1):

- Anterior lobe or adenohypophysis
- Posterior lobe or neurohypophysis
- Intermediate lobe or pars intermedia

Development of Pituitary Gland

Anterior pituitary is ectodermal in origin. It develops from *Rathke's pouch*, which is an embryonic upward outpouching from the roof of the primitive oral cavity. This pouch eventually gets separated from the oral cavity by the sphenoid bone of the skull and its lumen is reduced to a small cleft (residual cleft).

Posterior pituitary or neurohypophysis develops from a lowered outpouching of neuroectodermal tissue from the central areas of the hypothalamus (tuber cinereum and median eminence). The lumen of this pouch is obliterated inferiorly and the median eminence continues as infundibular stem and ends as infundibular processes of the posterior pituitary. Superiorly, the lumen remains contiguous with and forms a recess in the adult third ventricle.

From the above, it is quite clear that the anterior and posterior pituitaries develop independently from widely different origins and it is only a coincidence that when fully formed, they happen to lie so close together that they are considered parts of the same organ.

Parts of Pituitary Gland

Adenohypophysis

The glandular anterior lobe of the pituitary gland is called adenohypophysis. It constitutes approximately 80% of the pituitary gland. It can be further divided into three parts (Fig. 8.2.1):

Pars distalis: It forms the main bulk of the anterior lobe and is a highly vascular area.

Pars intermedia: It is an avascular zone that lies between pars distalis and neurohypophysis. In humans, this area is rudimentary, but in lower animals it forms the intermediate lobe of the pituitary.

Pars tuberalis: It is the most vascular zone and contains many secretory cells. Superficially, it is surrounded by the pituitary stalk.

Neurohypophysis

The posterior lobe of the pituitary is a neural structure and hence called neurohypophysis. It consists of three parts (Fig. 8.2.1):

Pars posterior: It is also called pars nervosa or neural lobe or infundibular process and forms the main bulk of neurohypophysis.

Infundibular stem: It is the funnel-shaped extension arising from the median eminence at the floor of the third ventricle.

Median eminence: It is a small protrusion from the base of the hypothalamus (tuber cinereum). It is situated just beneath the third ventricle and is highly vascular.

Pituitary Stalk

The median eminence and infundibulum constitute the neural stalk. The posterior pituitary maintains its neural connection with the hypothalamus by this neural stalk. The neural stalk surrounded by pars tuberalis of adenohypophysis constitutes the pituitary stalk.

Intermediate lobe of pituitary gland is rudimentary in humans as well as in a few other mammalian species and thus does not secrete melanocyte-stimulating hormone (MSH). In certain lower animals, this lobe secretes MSH in response to changes in exposure to light and other environmental factors. This hormone, in fish, reptiles and amphibians, controls the change of the colour of their skin (during thermoregulation, camouflage and behavioural display) by controlling the dispersal and aggregation of pigment granules in the melanophores.

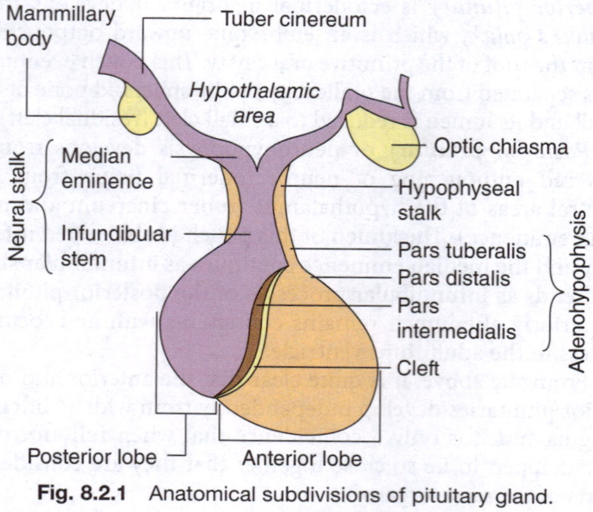

Fig. 8.2.1 Anatomical subdivisions of pituitary gland.

> **Important Notes**
>
> In humans, there are no melanophore-containing pigment granules that disperse and aggregate, but there are *melanocytes*, which have multiple processes containing melanin granules. The adrenocorticotropic hormone (ACTH; having sequence of first 13 of the amino acids same as that of MSH) has a weak MSH-like activity. It binds to melanotropin-1 receptors present on the melanocytes. This may probably be the reason why patients with hypersecretion of ACTH develop hyperpigmentation of the skin (e.g. in Addison disease), and those with hypopituitarism develop abnormal pallor.

HISTOLOGICAL STRUCTURE OF PITUITARY GLAND

Adenohypophysis

Pars distalis It consists of cords of cells separated by fenestrated sinusoids. The cells can be divided into two main types: the chromophobes and chromophils. In addition, folliculostellate cells are also present.

1. Chromophobes These are agranular cells and contain very few granules in their cytoplasm. It is considered that the chromophils are derived from the chromophobes.

2. Chromophils These are granular cells, which constitute 50% of the cells of anterior pituitary. Chromophils are further classified as: acidophils (35%) and basophils (15%).

Acidophilic cells (α-cells) The granules of acidophilic cells stain with acidic dyes (like eosin or orange G). The size of granules varies from 200 to 700 nm. Depending on the size and nature of granules, the acidophils are further divided into the following subtypes:

Somatotrophs: These cells are located mainly in the lateral part of the anterior lobe and constitute 20%–40% of acidophilic series of cells and secrete growth hormone (GH) or somatotropin (STH).

Mammotrophs or lactotrophs: These are scattered throughout the anterior lobe and produce mammotropic hormones, prolactin (PRL) or lactogenic hormone (LTH).

Basophilic cells (β-cells) The granules of basophilic cells are stained with basic dyes (like haematoxylin) and contain abundant dense core vesicles. The basophils are also further divided into functional subtypes:

Corticotrophs: The staining characteristics of these cells are intermediate between those of acidophilic and basophilic cells. The granules in these cells contain complex molecules of pro-opiomelanocortin. These secrete ACTH and β-lipotropins.

Thyrotrophs: These cells produce thyrotropic hormone (thyrotropin or thyroid-stimulating hormone [TSH]), which stimulates the activity of the thyroid gland.

Gonadotrophs (delta [δ] cells): These basophilic cells are present all along the anterior lobe. They produce two types of hormones: follicular-stimulating hormone (FSH) and luteinizing hormone (LH). Gonadotrophs subserve different actions in males and females.

3. Folliculostellate cells These cells send processes between established secretory cells. Recently, it has been demonstrated

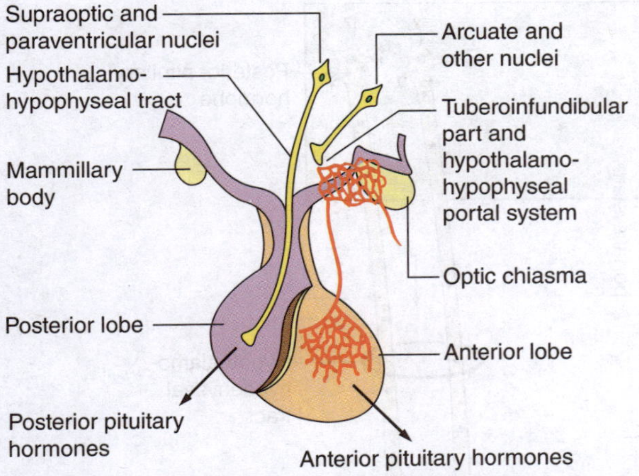

Fig. 8.2.2 Anatomical and functional relationship between hypothalamus and pituitary gland through hypothalamo-hypophyseal tract and hypothalamo-hypophyseal portal system.

that these contain and secrete the cytokine IL-6. Though their physiological role is still not clear, they may act paracrineally to regulate growth and functions of secretory cells.

Capillary network In addition to the above-mentioned cells, the anterior pituitary also contains an extensive network of capillaries. The endothelium of the capillaries is fenestrated like that in other endocrine organs. The secretory cells outpour secretory granules by exocytosis. These granules presumably break down in the pericapillary space and the hormones released enter the capillaries.

Pars tuberalis It mainly consists of undifferentiated cells with few acidophils and basophils.

Pars intermedia It contains β-cells, few secretory cells and chromophobe cells.

Neurohypophysis

Histologically, posterior pituitary contains the following structures:

1. ***Unmyelinated nerve fibres:*** These are the axons of the neurons located in the supraoptic and paraventricular nuclei of hypothalamus. These carry precursor of posterior pituitary hormones and end as closed terminals near the blood capillaries (Fig. 8.2.2).
2. ***Pituicytes:*** These are the special type of supporting cells, having long dendritic processes. These are present in between the axons.
3. ***Glial cells*** like astrocytes and oligodendrocytes are also seen.

BLOOD SUPPLY OF PITUITARY GLAND

Arterial Supply

The arterial blood to the pituitary gland is supplied by the branches of internal carotid artery and circle of Willis:

- Internal carotid arteries (superior and inferior hypophyseal branches)
- Anterior cerebral artery
- Posterior cerebral artery

HYPOTVHALAMO-HYPOPHYSEAL PORTAL SYSTEM (FIGS 8.2.2 AND 8.2.3)

- The branches from the superior hypophyseal artery form a ring around the upper part of the pituitary stalk and further branch to form a *capillary network* called primary plexus on the ventral surface of the hypothalamus.
- The blood from this capillary network is drained by *long portal veins* in the infundibulum.
- Then, in the anterior lobe, these long portal veins break up into another set of capillary network and are represented as *sinusoids of pars anterior*. This arrangement is called *hypothalamo-hypophyseal portal system*.
- The inferior hypophyseal (branch of internal carotid artery) branches to form a capillary network at the lower end of infundibulum stem called secondary capillary plexus.
- The short portal vessels arise from this capillary network and supply blood mainly to the posterior pituitary and some parts of the anterior pituitary.
- The short portal vessels provide a link between the anterior and posterior pituitary.

VENOUS DRAINAGE

The blood from anterior pituitary is drained to cavernous sinus and then into the jugular vein.

Important Notes

Important Points Regarding Circulation of Hypophysis

- The whole of neurohypophysis (median eminence to pars posterior) is permeated by a continuous network of capillaries, in which blood flows in either direction.
- The anterior pituitary lies outside the blood–brain barrier; hence, it is accessible to influences from general circulation (hormones and neurotransmitter by the brain and hormones secreted in general circulation).

HYPOTHALAMIC–PITUITARY RELATIONSHIP

The influences from the hypothalamus are conveyed to the pituitary gland by two different tracts.

1. Hypothalamo-hypophyseal tract It is composed of axons of the large neurosecretory cells of the supraoptic and paraventricular nuclei of the hypothalamus. These fibres pass to neurohypophysis through the infundibular stem and form a series of dilated terminals known as *Herring bodies* (Fig. 8.2.2).

- The neurosecretory cells of supraoptic and paraventricular nuclei secrete peptide hormones (vasopressin and oxytocin [OTC]), which travel down their axons in neurosecretory granules to be stored in the nerve terminals lying in the neurohypophysis.
- Upon stimulation of the cell bodies, the granules are released from the axonal terminals by exocytosis. The peptide hormones then enter the peripheral circulation via the capillary plexuses of inferior hypophyseal artery (Fig. 8.2.3). Thus, a single neural cell performs the entire process of hormone synthesis, storage and release.

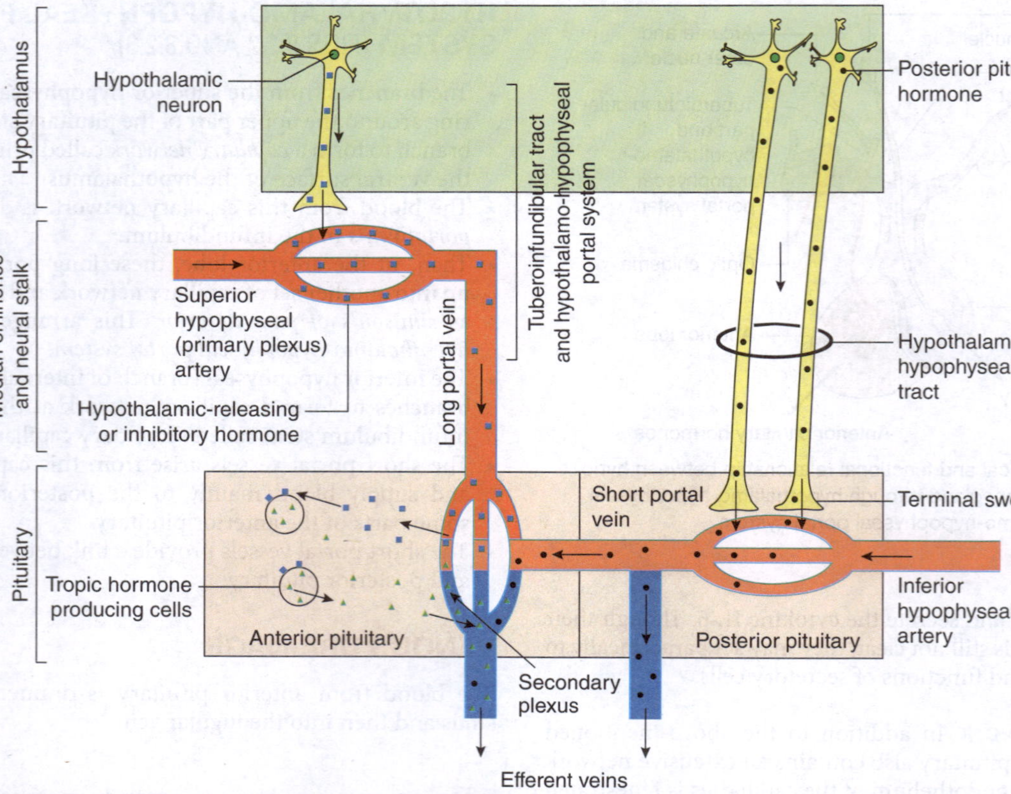

Fig. 8.2.3 Schematic diagram to explain anatomical and functional relationship between hypothalamus and pituitary gland.

2. Tuberoinfundibular tract and hypothalamo-hypophyseal portal system It consists of fibres arising from the arcuate nuclei of the tuberal region of the hypothalamus and extends to the median eminence (Fig. 8.2.2). The cell bodies of these hypothalamic neurons synthesize certain releasing and inhibiting hormones which are conveyed as membrane-bound vesicles by the tuberoinfundibular tract to the median eminence region where they are stored in the nerve terminals. After these hypothalamic neurons are stimulated by nerve impulses, the releasing or inhibiting hormones are discharged into the median eminence and enter the capillary plexus of the superior hypophyseal artery. From here, they are transported down the portal vessels (long portal veins) and then exit from the secondary capillary plexus to reach the specific endocrine target cells in the adenohypophysis where they regulate the secretion of tropic hormones of anterior pituitary (Fig. 8.2.3). The tropic hormones released from the secretory cells of adenohypophysis enter the same secondary capillary plexus through which they ultimately reach the peripheral circulation (Fig. 8.2.3).

ENDOCRINAL ASPECTS OF HYPOTHALAMUS

FUNCTIONAL ANATOMY

Hypothalamus is a specialized centre in the brain that functions as a master coordinator of hormonal action. It is a part of the brain situated below the thalamus and is very closely connected to the pituitary gland, as described above. Thus, the hypothalamus provides an important link between the endocrine system and the nervous system. Before proceeding further, see details of functional anatomy of hypothalamus on page 928.

ENDOCRINAL FUNCTIONS OF HYPOTHALAMUS

The functions of hypothalamus, in general, are described on page 931. The hypothalamus serves its endocrinal functions through the neurosecretory cells which are arranged in different nuclei of hypothalamus (see page 928 before proceeding further).

The main endocrinal functions of hypothalamus:

- Control of anterior pituitary function
- Control of posterior pituitary function

Control of Anterior Pituitary Function

Hypothalamus controls the functioning of the anterior pituitary through various hypothalamic–hypophysiotropic hormones, i.e. various hypothalamic-releasing and hypothalamic-inhibiting hormones. These hormones are synthesized by neurosecretory cells forming the arcuate nucleus and the periventricular nucleus of the medial basal hypothalamus. Some of these neurons are also located in the paraventricular nucleus. These are small (parvicellular) neurons and their axons project to the median eminence in close proximity to capillary loops.

Release of Hypothalamic–Hypophysiotropic Hormones

The hypothalamic-releasing and hypothalamic-inhibiting hormones are released in response to neural stimuli. The

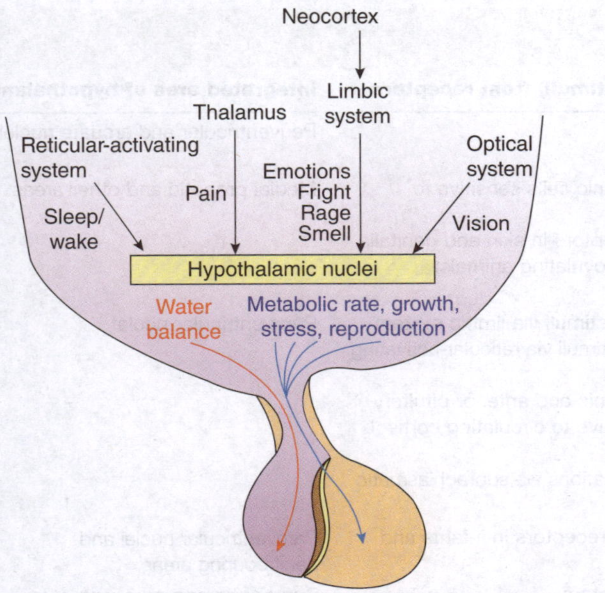

Fig. 8.2.4 Afferent impulses to different hypothalamic nuclei leading to release of hypothalamic-releasing or hypothalamic-inhibiting hormones controlling pituitary gland.

lateral hypothalamus receives afferent impulses and it relays them to neurosecretory nuclei of the anterior and medial basal portions of the hypothalamus. The hypothalamus receives afferent nerve tracts from the thalamus, the reticular-activating system, the limbic system, the eyes and remotely the neocortex (Fig. 8.2.4). In response to these afferent stimuli, the hypothalamic–hypophysiotropic hormones are released in the regions of median eminence and reach the anterior pituitary (to control its function) through the hypothalamic–hypophyseal portal vessels as described above and shown in Figs 8.2.2 and 8.2.3. Through these inputs (Fig. 8.2.4), the pituitary functions can be influenced by pain, sleep, wakefulness, emotion, fright, rage, olfactory sensations, light and possibly even thought (Table 8.2.1).

Various hypothalamic-releasing and hypothalamic-Inhibiting Hormones These include (Fig. 8.2.5):

- Growth hormone–releasing hormone (GHRH)
- Growth hormone–inhibiting hormone (GRIH), also called somatostatin
- Corticotropin-releasing hormone (CRH)
- Thyrotropin-releasing hormone (TRH)
- Gonadotropin-releasing hormone (GnRH)
- Prolactin-releasing hormone (PRH)
- Prolactin-inhibiting hormone (PIH)

Functions of hypothalamic-releasing and hypothalamic-Inhibiting Hormones These have been described at different places in the context (e.g. TRH has been discussed along with TSH and thyroid hormones in Chapter 8.3 on Thyroid Gland, see page 688). In general, they control the release of various tropic hormones from the anterior pituitary. Initially, it was thought that each tropic hormone was controlled by a unique hypothalamic-releasing and hypothalamic-inhibiting hormone. Also, each hypothalamic hormone was presumed to have only one target anterior pituitary cell. However, now it is known that besides regulating the secretion of specific tropic hormone, a hypothalamic hormone may also influence the secretion of another anterior pituitary hormone. For example:

- TRH, besides promoting secretion of TSH, also stimulates the secretion of PRL.
- Somatostatin, discovered as a growth hormone–inhibiting hormone (GRIH), also inhibits the secretion of TSH.
- GHRH also stimulates the secretion of ACTH and PRL.
- GnRH promotes the release of both LH and FSH.

Mechanism of action of hypothalamic–hypophysiotropic hormones The hypothalamic-releasing and hypothalamic-inhibiting peptides are secreted in pulses, and they induce effects via cAMP, Ca^{2+} and phosphatidylinositol products as second messengers. They stimulate or inhibit transcription, modulate translation and stimulate or inhibit secretion of the target anterior pituitary hormones.

Control of Posterior Pituitary Function

The large (magnocellular) neurosecretory cells forming the supraoptic and paraventricular nuclei of hypothalamus are responsible for synthesis of the two posterior pituitary peptide hormones (OTC and antidiuretic hormone [ADH]). These hormones reach the posterior pituitary through the hypothalamic–hypophyseal tract described above (Figs 8.2.2 and 8.2.3).

ANTERIOR PITUITARY HORMONES

Anterior pituitary is truly the master endocrine organ. It secretes various hormones that influence, either directly or indirectly, many biochemical processes in the body. The hormones of adenohypophysis are broadly classified into three categories:

- GH (PRL group)
- Glycoprotein hormones
- Pro-opiomelanocortin (POMC) peptides

I. ***Hormones of GH family:*** GH, PRL and human chorionic somatomammotropin (hCS) belong to this family and have been thought to have arisen from the same ancestral gene. There is 85% homology between GH and hCS. These hormones have primary regulatory actions of their own.

II. ***Glycoprotein hormone family:*** The hormones of glycoprotein family secreted by anterior pituitary include:
   - TSH
   - LH
   - FSH

   These hormones contain an α- and a β-subunit. The α-subunits of all the hormones are identical. The β-subunit of each hormone is different and is responsible for the unique biological activity of each hormone. Each subunit is a product of a separate gene. Hence, synthesis of the whole hormone requires the coordinated expression of the α- and β-subunit genes. The α- and β-subunits are noncovalently linked and the three-dimensional structures are determined by intramolecular S–S bonds.

III. ***POMC peptides:*** The hormones of this group are derived from a single precursor, the POMC, consisting of 241 amino acids.

   The gene for POMC is expressed in anterior pituitary cells, the intermediate lobe (absent in humans) and cells of other tissues like brain, placenta, gastrointestinal tract,

Table 8.2.1 Neuroendocrinal control by hypothalamus

Hormone	Factor	Afferents (stimuli) from receptors	Integrated area of hypothalamus
Growth hormone	Somatostatin and growth hormone–releasing hormone		Periventricular and arcuate nuclei
Gonadotropins: • Follicular-stimulating hormone (FSH) • Luteinizing hormone (LH)	Gonadotropin-releasing hormone (GnRH)	• Hypothalamic cells sensitive to oestrogen • Touch receptors in skin and genitalia (in reflexly ovulating animals) • Eyes	Medial preoptic and other areas
Adrenocorticotropic hormone (ACTH) and β-lipotropin	Corticotropic-releasing hormone (CRH)	• Emotional stimuli via limbic system • Systemic stimuli via reticular-activating system • Hypothalamic and anterior pituitary cells sensitive to circulating cortisol level • Diurnal variations via suprachiasmatic nuclei	Paraventricular nuclei
Thyroid-stimulating hormone (TSH)	Thyrotropin hormone (TRH)	Temperature receptors in infants and others	Paraventricular nuclei and neighbouring areas
Antidiuretic hormone (ADH) or vasopressin		• Osmoreceptors • Volume receptors • Others	Supraoptic and paraventricular nuclei
Oxytocin	–	Touch receptors present in breast, uterus and genitalia	Supraoptic and paraventricular nuclei
Catecholamines	–	Limbic area related to emotions	Dorsal and posterior hypothalamus

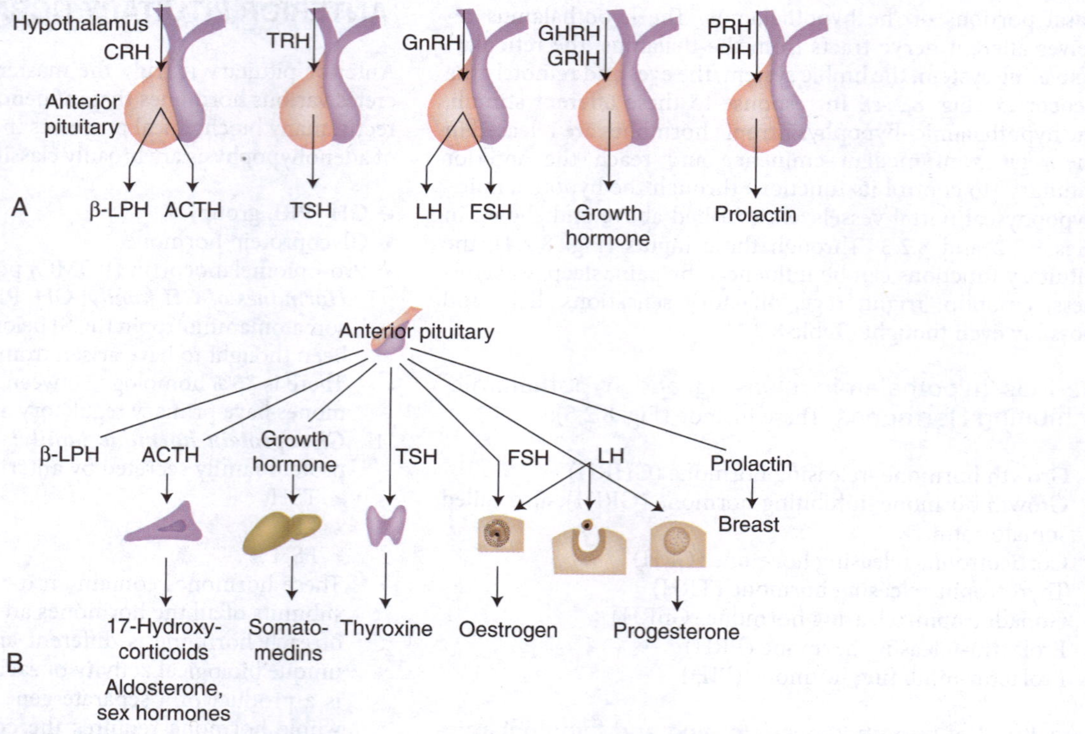

Fig. 8.2.5 Effect of hypophysiotropic hormones on anterior pituitary **A**, and their effects **B**.

lungs and platelets. The precursor molecule (POMC) is first glycosylated and phosphorylated at certain sites and then cleaved into fragments (Fig. 8.2.6), which include:

- ACTH
- MSH, α-MSH and β-MSH are produced in the intermediary lobe (which is rudimentary in humans)
- β-Lipotropin (β-LPH)
- β-Endorphin

Physiological aspects of the GH are discussed in detail in this chapter. Other hormones are discussed in different chapters (e.g. TSH with thyroid hormone and ACTH with adrenal gland).

GROWTH HORMONE

GH, also called somatotropic hormone (*STH*), is the most important hormone for postnatal growth and development to

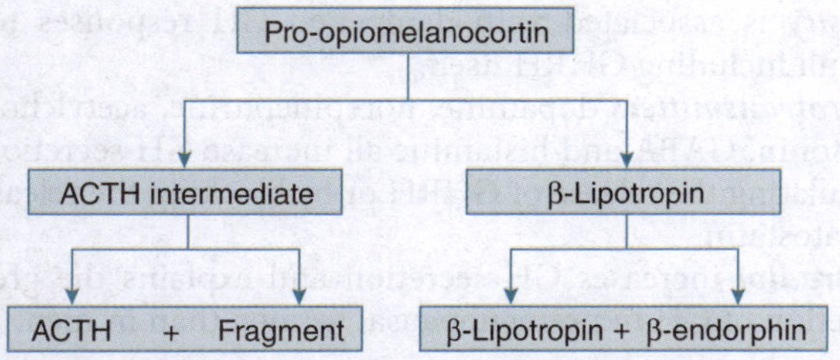

Fig. 8.2.6 Pro-opiomelanocortin is the precursor of ACTH, β-lipotropin and β-endorphin.

adult size. It also helps to maintain lean body mass and bone mass in adults.

Structure, Synthesis and Secretion

Structure GH consists of a single unbranched chain containing 191 amino acids and 2 disulphate bondages. Its molecular weight is 2000. It is a member of the large family of 'helix bundle proteins'.

The genes that code human GH (hGH) are present on the long arm of the chromosome 17 and are in cluster form. There are five genes for GH.

First two genes encode GH:

- hGH-N – normal hGH
- hGH-V – variant form of GH

Two other genes encode hCS and fifth gene is hCS pseudogene.

The transcription factors during development for GH are prop-1 and pit-1.

Species specificity GHs obtained from different species show chemical and immunological variations, i.e. exhibit species specificity. Because of species specificity, the bovine and porcine GHs do not even have a significant transient effect on growth in humans and monkeys. However, in humans, the hGH and monkey GH have similar biological activity. Therefore, GH preparation from monkey origin is therapeutically effective.

- Bovine GH is effectively used for increasing milk production in dairy animals and also used as a GH supplement by body builders.
- Recombinant hGH is therapeutically used for increasing the height of those who have short stature, but otherwise there is no deficiency of GH.

Synthesis GH is synthesized by acidophilic cells called *somatotrophs*, which are approximately 40% of the total cell population of the anterior pituitary. The GH gene transcribes a messenger RNA that directs synthesis of a prehormone. Subsequently, a single peptide is removed and the final form of the hormone is stored in granules.

Secretion GH is released in *pulsatile* fashion. Binding of GHRH to its plasma membrane receptor stimulates the release of GH. Primary mediators of GH release are cAMP and Ca^{2+} and phosphatidylinositol products are secondary mediators of GHRH action.

Secretion is increased by the stimuli, which are categorized into three parts:

(i) The conditions which decrease the substrate for energy production in the cell, such as: hypoglycaemia, fasting and exercise
(ii) The conditions in which the amount of certain amino acids is increased in the plasma, e.g. protein meal, infusion of arginine and other amino acids
(iii) Stressful stimuli, such as fever, psychological stress-sleep, hormones related to puberty, starvation, exercise and hypoglycaemia

Secretion of GH is decreased by somatostatin, somatomedins, obesity, hyperglycaemia, cortisol, free fatty acids and pregnancy.

Regulation of Growth Hormone Secretion

1. Hypothalamic Control

Hypothalamus controls GH secretion by releasing two hormones, growth hormone–releasing hormone (GHRH) and growth hormone release–inhibiting hormone (GRIH) (Fig. 8.2.7).

Growth hormone–releasing hormone It is a polypeptide with 44 amino acids that stimulates the secretion of GH from the anterior pituitary.

Mechanism of action GHRH acts through guanylate cyclase, which releases cyclic GMP, which, in turn, stimulates the release of GH from the anterior pituitary. Influx of Ca^{2+} into pituitary cells is an essential event associated with the GHRH-stimulated release of GH.

Factors stimulating GHRH secretion Factors stimulating GHRH secretion and thus increasing GH release:

Hypoglycaemia increases GHRH secretion through glucoreceptor cells in the ventromedial nucleus of the hypothalamus. Neurotransmitter involved is epinephrine.

Emotions, exercise and physical stress (pain, trauma, cold, surgery, inflammation, etc.) stimulate GHRH release through

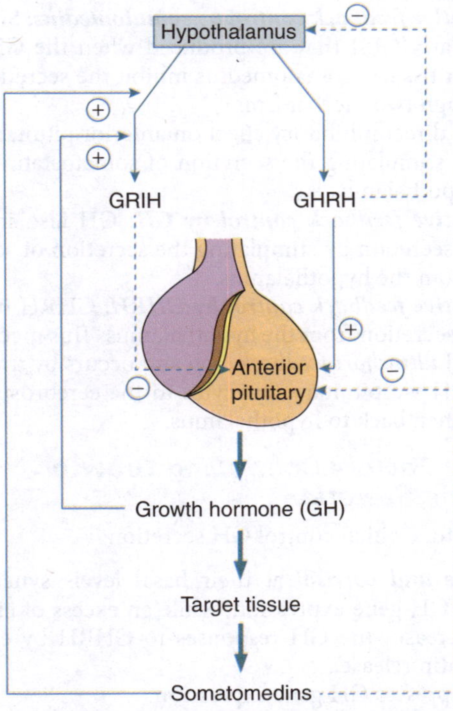

Fig. 8.2.7 Control of growth hormone secretion. GHRH, growth hormone–releasing hormone; GRIH, growth hormone release–inhibiting hormone.

nervous pathways (therefore, the effect is seen within a couple of minutes).

Slow-wave phase of sleep (NERM stages 3 and 4) is associated with increase in GHRH. The neurotransmitter involved is serotonin.

Increase in plasma levels of certain amino acids such as arginine (after protein meal or infusion of amino acids) increases GHRH secretion by α-adrenergic stimulation of the receptors in neurons that release GHRH.

Growth hormone–releasing peptide (GHRP), also called 'ghrelin', increases GHRH secretion. GHRP is synthesized by the oxyntic glands of the stomach. It increases GH release by its direct action on the anterior pituitary.

Growth hormone release–inhibiting hormone

It is also called somatostatin, and is a polypeptide with 14 amino acids. It inhibits the release of GH from the anterior pituitary.

Mechanism of action GRIH blocks GHRH stimulation in a noncompetitive manner. It acts through its own plasma membrane receptor in part, by decreasing intracellular cAMP and calcium levels.

Factors stimulating GRIH secretion Factors stimulating GRIH secretion and thus decreasing GH secretion:

- Hyperglycaemia
- High plasma FFA concentration
- Insulin-like growth factor-I (IGF-I)
- Cortisol
- During REM sleep

2. Negative Feedback Control of Growth Hormone Secretion

The negative feedback control mechanism for GH involves the role of somatomedins, GH and GHRH (Fig. 8.2.7).

i. ***Negative feedback control by somatomedins:*** Somatomedins are IGF-I that are produced when the GH acts on target tissues. Somatomedins inhibit the secretion of GH through two mechanisms:
   - By direct inhibitory effect on anterior pituitary
   - By stimulating the secretion of somatostatin from the hypothalamus

ii. ***Negative feedback control by GH:*** GH also inhibits its own secretion by stimulating the secretion of somatostatin from the hypothalamus.

iii. ***Negative feedback control by GHRH:*** GHRH inhibits its own secretion from the hypothalamus. This mechanism is called *ultrashort feedback loop* and occurs by transport of GHRH via pituitary tanycytes to the cerebrospinal fluid and then back to hypothalamus.

3. Other Factors Controlling Growth Hormone Secretion

Other factors which control GH secretion:

Thyroxine and cortisol at their basal levels synergistically stimulate GH gene expression, while an excess of either hormone decreases the GH responses to GHRH by enhancing somatostatin release.

Insulin represses GH gene expression.

Placental GH and placental lactogen are responsible for decreased GH secretion noted during later part of pregnancy.

Obesity is associated with dampened GH responses to all stimuli including GHRH itself.

Neurotransmitters dopamine, norepinephrine, acetylcholine, serotonin, GABA and histamine all increase GH secretion by stimulating the release of GHRH or by blocking the release of somatostatin.

Oestradiol increases GH secretion and explains the greater secretion of GH in premenopausal women than in men.

Plasma Levels

Basal plasma GH level It varies from 2 to 4 ng/mL. Its concentration graph shows fluctuations, i.e. after every 1- to 2-hour interval, there is a rise in plasma GH level, i.e. GH is released in 10–20 pulses per day. This pulsatility arises from some combination of the pulsatile release of GHRH and of GRIH into the portal blood.

Diurnal variation in plasma levels of GH Diurnal variation in plasma levels of GH is noted. The nocturnal peak occurs 1–2 hours after deep sleep (which corresponds to stage three or stage four of slow-wave sleep). This supports the adage, 'If you don't sleep, you won't grow'.

The nocturnal sleep bursts account for nearly 70% of the daily GH secretion. These secretory bursts are greater in children and decrease with age.

Variation in plasma GH levels with age (Fig. 8.2.8):

From birth to early childhood, plasma GH levels increase progressively.

Children versus adults: In general, children have only slightly higher plasma GH levels than adults. So, it should not be assumed that plasma GH levels would be very high during childhood and low in adults.

Puberty is associated with peak period of plasma GH levels (Fig. 8.2.8).

Senescence is associated with a reduction in GH secretion in response to GHRH and other stimuli. This decline in GH secretion is partly responsible for the decline in lean body mass, physical fitness, protein synthesis and metabolic rate, as well as the increase in adipose mass that characterizes elderly humans.

Circulation, Half-life and Metabolism

Circulation Circulating GH is bound to a plasma protein that is a large fragment of the extracellular domain of the GH receptor. This GH-binding protein (GHBP) appears to arise by cleavage of the receptor at the cell's surface. One molecule of GH binds two of the circulating binding protein molecules.

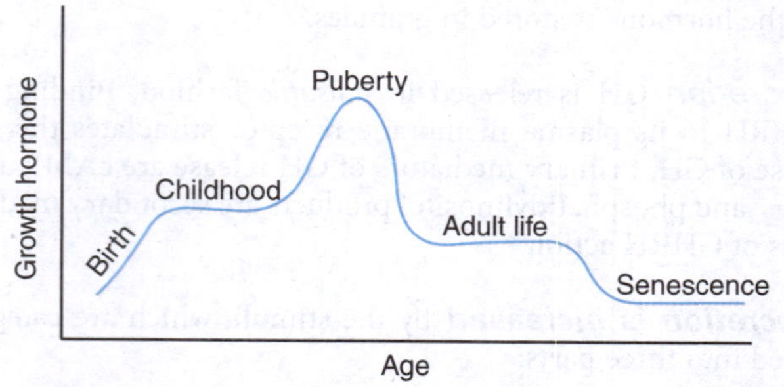

Fig. 8.2.8 Variations in plasma growth hormone levels with age.

Half-life of circulating GH in humans is 6–20 minutes and the daily GH output has been calculated to be 0.2–1.0 mg/day in adults.

Metabolism GH is rapidly metabolized, probably at least in part in the liver. Metabolic clearance rate (MCR) is 350 L/day. Although only a trivial portion of secreted GH is excreted unchanged by the kidneys, daily urinary GH excretion correlates well with the integrated 24-hour plasma GH profile.

Growth Hormone Receptors and Mechanism of Action of Growth Hormone

Growth Hormone Receptors

GH receptors of various sizes are present on the cell membrane in target tissues, including the liver and adipose tissue. The GH receptor belongs to the cytokine family of receptors and is a 620–amino acid protein. It comprises a large extracellular portion, a transmembrane domain and a large intracellular cytoplasmic portion.

Mechanism of Action of Growth Hormone

Originally, it was thought that GH promotes growth by its direct action on the target tissues, but later it was proposed that it acts solely by indirect action through the somatomedins, also known as insulin growth factor (IGF). However, the current view is that it acts by a combination of both direct and indirect effects. By indirect effect, GH increases the circulating IGF-I. By direct effect on the cartilages, GH produces IGF-I locally and also converts stem cells into the cells that respond to IGF-I. Then the locally produced and circulating IGF-I makes the cartilage grow.

Insulin-like growth factors As mentioned above, IGF ultimately exerts its growth-promoting effect via peptide mediators (IGFs or somatomedins) that are produced in the liver and many GH target cells.

Steps involved in the production of IGFs The steps are summarized as follows (Fig. 8.2.9):

- GH has two binding sites for receptors. Binding of two GH receptor molecules at different sites on one molecule of GH produces a homodimer (Fig. 8.2.9, step 1). This process of dimerization activates the receptors.
- The activated receptor dimer then initiates GH actions. The intracytoplasmic portions of the receptors attract, dock and activate *Janus kinases* (JAK-1) (Fig. 8.2.9, step 2). These phosphorylate the signal transducer and activator of transcription factors (STAT) (Fig. 8.2.9, step 3) and induce or repress expression of GH target genes such as IGF genes (Fig. 8.2.9, step 4).
- GH-stimulated expression of IGF genes leads to production of IGFs, primarily, but not solely, in the liver. IGFs circulate, bound to at least six carrier proteins known as insulin growth factor–binding proteins (IGFBP 1–6). Approximately 95% of IGF binding is related to IGF-binding protein-3 (IGFBP-3). The characteristic features of IGF-I and IGF-II are depicted in Table 8.2.2.

Structure, types and properties of somatomedins

Structure IGFs are closely related to insulin except that their C chains are not separated and they have an extension of A chain called D domain.

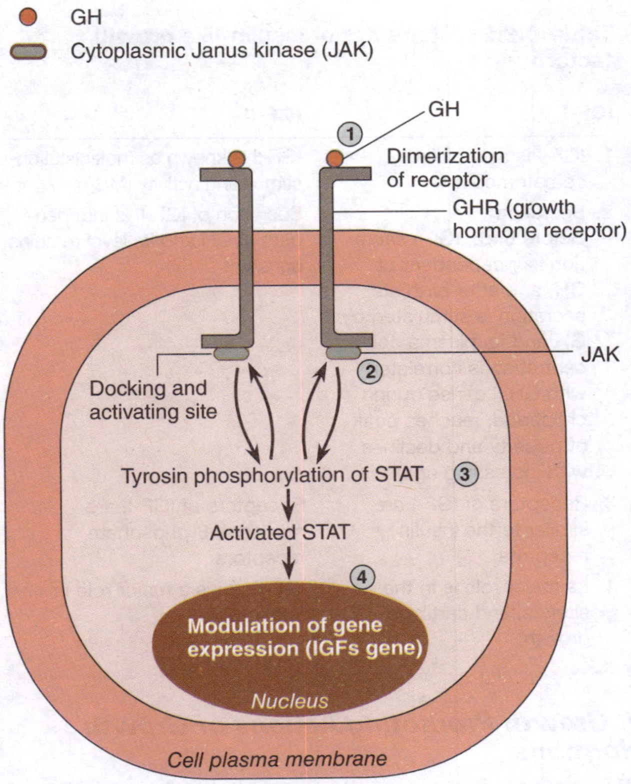

Fig. 8.2.9 Steps involved in the GH-stimulated expression of the IGF genes. For description of steps 1–4, see text.

Types In humans, two types of IGF are known, IGF-I and IGF-II. Variants of IGF-I and IGF-II are also known. The mRNAs for IGF-I and IGF-II are found in the liver, in cartilage and in many other tissues, indicating that they are synthesized in these tissues.

IGF-I, also known as somatomedin-C, is primarily involved in skeletal and cartilage growth. Secretion of IGF-I before birth is independent of GH, but after birth it is stimulated by GH and its plasma concentration like that of GH (Fig. 8.2.8) rises during childhood, peaks at the time of puberty and then declines to low levels in old age. The IGF-I receptor is very similar to the insulin receptor and probably uses much of the same intracellular machinery.

IGF-II, also known as multiplication-stimulating activity (MSA), is independent of GH. It plays a role in growth during fetal development. Its overexpression in the fetus leads to disproportionate growth of organs, especially the tongue, other muscles, kidneys, heart and liver. The *IGF-II receptor* is mannose-6-phosphate receptor, which is involved in the intracellular targeting of acid hydrolases and other proteins to intracellular organelles.

The characteristic features of IGF-I and IGF-II are depicted in Table 8.2.2.

Actions of Growth Hormone

GH promotes growth and also influences the normal metabolism; therefore, besides acting on one specific organ, its actions are generalized (Fig. 8.2.10).

Table 8.2.2 Character of insulin-like growth factors

IGF-I	IGF-II
1. IGF-I is also called somatomedin-C	IGF-II is known as multiplication-stimulating activity (MSA)
2. Secretion Before birth, IGF-I secretion is independent of GH, and after birth, its secretion is stimulated by GH and its plasma concentration is correlated with GH (i.e. rise during childhood, reaches peak at puberty and declines with increasing age)	Secretion of IGF-II is independent of GH and its level remains constant
3. Receptors of IGF-I are similar to the insulin receptors	Receptors of IGF-II are mannose-6-phosphate receptors
4. Its major role is in the skeletal and cartilage growth	IGF-II plays a major role in fetal growth

1. Growth-Promoting Actions of Growth Hormone

GH promotes linear growth of an individual by its effects on the bone, cartilage and other connective tissues.

Effects on cartilage GH stimulates the proliferation of chondrocytes (cartilage cells) present in the epiphyseal end plates of long bones and thus increases the thickness of the epiphyseal cartilage by depositing new cartilage.

Effects on bone GH stimulates osteoblastic activity which converts cartilage into bone. This process continues up to adolescence till there is fusion of epiphyseal end plate with shaft of the bone. The bone mass also increases during this period.

Mode of action As described above, the effects of GH on growth are mediated by somatomedins, also called IGFs.

This action of GH is independent of adrenal glands; probably these electrolytes are diverted from kidney to the growing tissue.

Excretion of amino acid 4-hydroxyproline increases during growth and reflects the stimulation of synthesis of collagen by the GH.

2. Metabolic Actions of Growth Hormone

The actions of GH on protein metabolism resemble those of insulin, while actions on fat and carbohydrate metabolism are antagonistic to those of insulin and synergistic with those of cortisol. It appears that influence of GH on carbohydrate and fat metabolism is produced directly and is not mediated through IGF-I.

i. Effects on protein metabolism GH has an anabolic effect on protein metabolism. It promotes the protein deposition in the tissues by the following effects:

- Increases the rate of amino acid uptake into the cells
- Increases protein synthesis in ribosomes
- Stimulates transcription (RNA synthesis from DNA)

The overall effect of GH on protein metabolism is positive nitrogen balance that leads to increase in body weight. In addition, GH also decreases protein breakdown, as well as the rate of amino acid degradation for energy purposes.

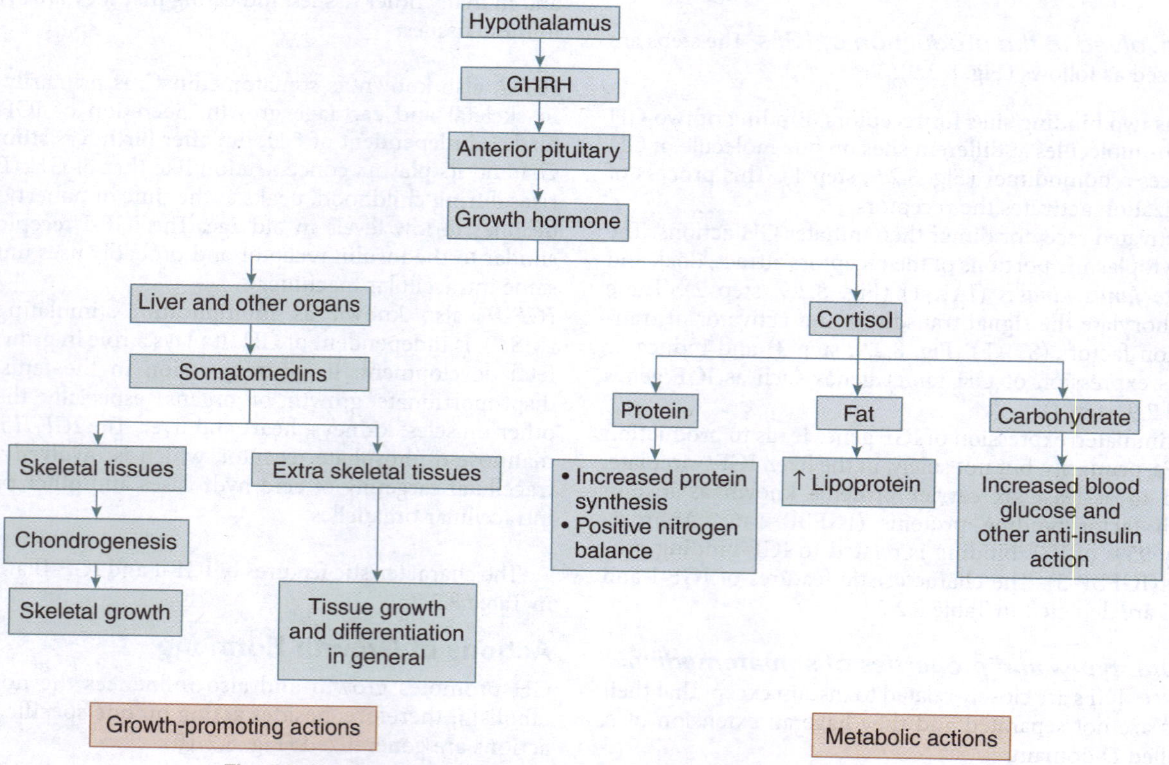

Fig. 8.2.10 Growth-promoting and metabolic actions of growth hormone.

ii. Effects on fat metabolism GH promotes lipolysis in adipose tissue (catabolic effect) and then increases fat utilization for energy. Administration of GH is associated with:

- Increased levels of circulating FFA. The plasma FFAs provide a ready source of energy for the tissues during hypoglycaemia, fasting and stressful stimuli.
- Increased hepatic oxidation of FFA produces ketone bodies (ketogenic effect).

iii. Effects on carbohydrate metabolism GH is antagonistic to insulin and produces hyperglycaemia by the following effects on carbohydrate metabolism:

- Increases gluconeogenesis, i.e. increases hepatic glucose output.
- Decreases the uptake as well as utilization of glucose by the tissues for energy production.
- Inhibits glycolysis, and thus glycogen stores tend to increase. This occurs as a consequence of increased mobilization and use of FFA for energy production.

As a consequence of hyperglycaemia (produced by above-mentioned effects), insulin secretion increases. This is an additional way GH promotes growth, since insulin has a protein anabolic effect.

iv. Effects on mineral metabolism GH promotes bone mineralization in growing children. This effect of GH is probably mediated through IGF-I, which causes positive balance of calcium, phosphate and magnesium. It promotes renal absorption of Ca^{2+}, phosphate and Na^{+}. It also promotes the retention of Na^{+}, K^{+} and Cl^{-} in the body.

3. Effect on Lactation

GH enhances milk production in lactating animals. It acts like PRL; therefore, this action is referred to as PRL-like effect of GH.

Applied Aspects

Abnormalities of Anterior Pituitary Hormones

The abnormalities related to pituitary hormones occur due to either excess or deficiency of the hormones secreted. The most common causes of pituitary hormone disturbances are pituitary tumours which may cause symptoms of excess of one or more hormones and simultaneous deficiency of other hormones; hence, a mixed picture may evolve. The various hormones of pituitary, their site of action and disease produced by them are given in Table 8.2.3.

Pituitary disorders seen in clinical practice:

- Hypopituitarism
- Abnormalities of GH
- PRL deficiency (see page 861)
- Cushing syndrome (see page 739)

I. Hypopituitarism

Hypopituitarism is a clinical condition of hyposecretion of one or more pituitary hormones.

Causes Hypopituitarism can be due to hypothalamic causes or pituitary causes.

A. ***Hypothalamic causes of hypopituitarism:***

1. Congenital conditions:
- GnRH deficiency, i.e. Kallmann syndrome
- Isolated GH deficiency

2. Acquired conditions involving hypothalamus include:
- Tumours such as craniopharyngioma
- Radiation
- Head injury
- Tuberculosis
- Sarcoidosis
- Histiocytosis 'X'

B. ***Pituitary causes of hypopituitarism:***
- Tumours of anterior pituitary
- Supracellar cysts
- Remnants of Rathke's pouch that enlarge and compress the pituitary
- Surgery
- Radiotherapy
- Head injury
- Postpartum necrosis in females (Sheehan syndrome)
- Autoimmune
- Pituitary infarction as occurs in haemorrhagic fever

Effects of Hypopituitarism Since anterior pituitary has a large reserve, the endocrine abnormalities are produced only when the large part of pituitary is destroyed. The effects of hypopituitarism are as follows:

1. GH deficiency This appears, first of all, with progressive loss of pituitary tissue. Effects of hyposecretion of GH are described on page 676.

Table 8.2.3 Pituitary hormones: site of action and diseases associated with their deficiency and excess

		Diseases	
Hormone	**Site of action**	**Excess**	**Deficiency**
Anterior pituitary			
Growth hormone (GH)	All somatic cells	Gigantism in adolescents	Dwarfism
Adrenocorticotropic hormone (ACTH)	Adrenal cortex	ACTH-dependent Cushing syndrome	Hypoadrenalism (rare)
Thyroid-stimulating hormone (TSH)	Thyroid	Hyperthyroidism	Hypothyroidism
Prolactin	Breast	Hyperprolactinaemia	–
Gonadotropins	Gonads	Hypergonadism	Hypogonadism
Melanocyte-stimulating hormone (MSH)	Skin	Hyperpigmentation	–
Posterior pituitary			
Antidiuretic hormone	Kidneys	–	Diabetes insipidus

2. *Gonadotropin secretion* The secretion is decreased when 70%–90% of anterior pituitary is destroyed. It leads to gonadal atrophy, thus decreasing sex hormone levels, which causes:

- *In males,* loss of spermatogenesis, loss of libido, impotency and gynaecomastia.
- *In females,* abolition of ovulation and stoppage of menstrual cycle results in sterility.
- Some of the secondary sex characteristics disappear (especially loss of axillary and pubic hair in both the sexes).
- Urinary gonadotropin excretion stops within 2 weeks to 2 months.

3. *Thyrotropic hormone (TSH) secretion* The secretion is decreased leading to impairment of thyroid function when 90%–95% of anterior pituitary is destroyed. Clinical features of hypothyroidism due to hypopituitarism are less marked. Tolerance to cold *is rare*. Frank's myxoedema is not seen.

4. *Adrenocorticotropic hormone deficiency* It leads to atrophy of adrenal cortex and adrenal insufficiency occurs when almost the whole of the anterior pituitary is destroyed. ACTH-dependent Addison disease is produced. For details, see page 741. In brief, there occurs:

- Pallor of the skin due to decreased ACTH.
- Sensitivity to stress is increased due to decreased glucocorticoids.
- Mineralocorticoid deficiency does not occur, as secretion of aldosterone is controlled by renin secreted from juxtaglomerular apparatus (JGA). Hence, salt loss and hypovolaemic shock do not occur.

5. *Effect on water metabolism* Though deficiency of ADH, the posterior pituitary hormone, produces diabetes insipidus (DI), removal of both anterior and posterior pituitary usually causes no more than a transient polyuria. This occurs because of the following effects:

- Fewer osmotically active products of catabolism are filtered (because ACTH deficiency decreases rate of protein catabolism and TSH deficiency decreases metabolic rate).
- GH deficiency also contributes to the depression of the glomerular filtration rate.

As a consequence of the above, the urine volume decreases even in the absence of ADH. The diuretic activity of anterior pituitary thus can be explained in terms of effects of decreased ACTH, TSH and GH levels.

6. *Effect on insulin sensitivity* Sensitivity to insulin is markedly increased in hypophysectomized animals. It occurs because of two reasons:

- Due to deficiency of adrenocortical hormones
- Due to lack of anti-insulin effect of GH

II. Abnormalities of Growth Hormone Secretion

The abnormalities of GH secretion include:

- Hypersecretion of GH
- Hyposecretion of GH

Hypersecretion of Growth Hormone

Hypersecretion of GH occurs in tumours of acidophilic cells (particularly of somatotrophs) of anterior pituitary. Hypersecretion of GH is also associated with hypersecretion of PRL. Depending on the age of an individual, excess of GH may cause:

- Gigantism
- Acromegaly
- Acromegalic gigantism (mixed disorder)

1. Gigantism It is a clinical condition resulting from hypersecretion of GH in growing children before the closure of epiphysis of long bones.

Clinical features Clinical features of gigantism include those caused by excess of GH and those produced by compressive and other effects of pituitary tumours.

Features due to excess of GH These include gigantism and acromegaly (Figs 8.2.11 and 8.2.12).

Features due to tumour mass These include:

- Headache
- Visual field defects

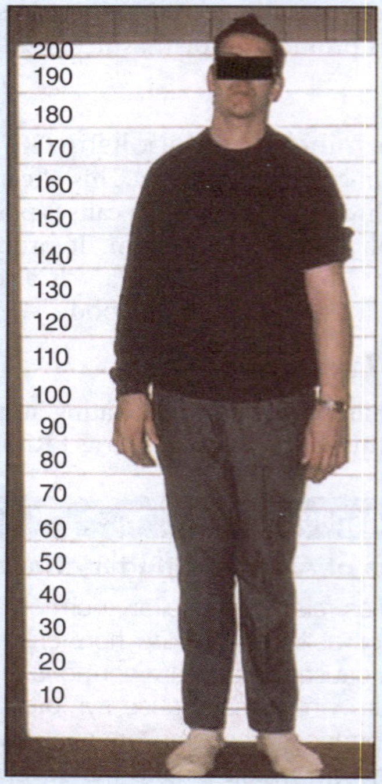

Fig. 8.2.11 Photograph showing tall stature in a patient with gigantism.

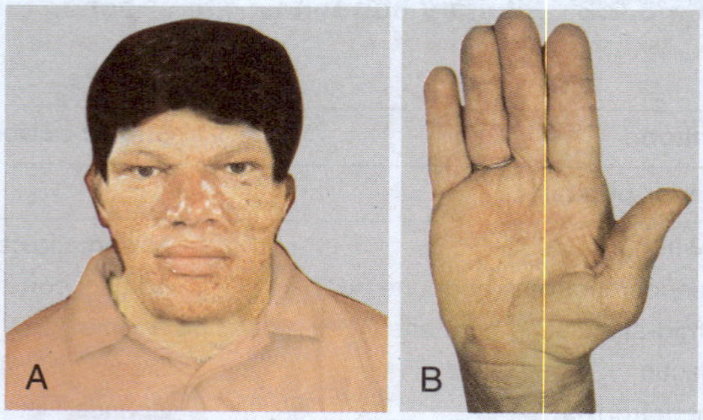

Fig. 8.2.12 Clinical features of acromegaly: **A,** Note coarse facial features, broad and thick nose, prognathism, prominent eyebrows and thickened skin; **B,** large spade-like hand with short, thick, wide fingers.

- Cranial nerve palsies
- Enlargement of pituitary fossa with destruction of clinoid processes may be detected on radiograph of skull
- Hypopituitarism may ultimately result due to compression of other cells of pituitary gland by the tumour

2. Acromegaly It is a clinical condition that occurs due to excess of GH in adults (after epiphyseal closure of long bones has occurred) and causes excessive growth in those areas where cartilage persists.

Causes GH hypersecretion occurs mainly due to GH-secreting somatroph adenoma of anterior pituitary.

- It also occurs in paraneoplastic syndrome in cancers of pancreas, ovaries, lung and blood.
- Hypersecretion of GH can be due to high level of GHRH; therefore, acromegaly is also associated with hypothalamic choristoma and carcinoid tumours.
- Acromegaly occurs as part of Carney syndrome due to mutation of protein kinase-A.

Clinical features Clinical features of acromegaly include those caused by excess of GH and those produced by compressive and other effects of tumour mass.

Features due to excessive GH These include (Fig. 8.2.12):

Acromegalic face, which is characterized by thick lips, macroglossia, broad and thick nose, prominent eyebrows, thickened skin and coarse facial features.

Prognathism, i.e. protrusion of the lower jaw due to elongation and widening of mandible associated with increased spacing of the teeth.

Acral part abnormalities include large spade-like hands, thick and wide fingers, increase in heel pad thickness and large feet with increase in size of the shoes. Height is normal; build is stout and stocky.

Kyphosis may occur due to improper vertebral growth.

Excessive growth of internal organs, i.e. cardiomegaly, hepatomegaly, splenomegaly and renomegaly, may be associated.

Increased sympathetic activity may cause increased sweating and hypertension.

Poor gonadal functions due to hyperprolactinaemia or due to lactogenic effects of GH (galactorrhoea).

Cardiomyopathy, hypertension and coronary heart disease.

These patients also have sleep apnoea (due to upper airway obstruction).

Biochemical features include:

- Poor glucose tolerance and even occurrence of diabetes in 15% of cases
- Hypertriglyceridaemia
- Reduced hepatic and lipoprotein lipase activities
- Hypercalcaemia and hyperphosphataemia due to their increased intestinal absorption

Features due to tumour mass These are similar to those seen in gigantism as described above.

3. Acromegalic gigantism Acromegalic gigantism, i.e. a mixed picture of acromegaly and gigantism, is evolved when the excess of GH occurring in adolescence continues during adult life.

Diagnosis In patients with acromegaly and gigantism, the following tests are performed to confirm the diagnosis:

1. ***Basal plasma GH:*** Level is high.
2. ***Plasma PRL level:*** It is high in 30% of cases.
3. ***Glucose tolerance suppression test:*** In the fasting patient, blood is withdrawn to measure baseline hGH, then a drink containing 75 g of glucose is given orally and GH and blood glucose levels are estimated every 30 minutes for 2 hours.
   Interpretation For adult male, the normal range of GH is <0.5 μg/L.
   - In normal persons, hyperglycaemia suppresses GH secretion.
   - In acromegaly or gigantism, there is either no suppression or paradoxical rise in GH (Fig. 8.2.13).
4. ***Radiography of skull for pituitary fossa*** may show enlargement of pituitary fossa with destruction of clinoid processes.
5. ***Visual fields*** may be normal or bitemporal; hemianopia or scotoma may be seen due to pressure of pituitary adenoma on the optic chiasma.
6. ***CT scan of skull*** may show a small or large hypodense microadenoma.

Treatment It may be surgical or medical.

Surgical treatment It consists of transsphenoidal resection of pituitary tumour (adenoma) without damaging other functions.

Radiotherapy: If acromegaly persists even after surgery, then radiotherapy is second line of treatment to stop tumour growth.

Medical treatment It includes employing medical therapy usually to lower GH level to <1.5 μg/L and to normalize IGF-I concentration by use of somatostatin analogues:

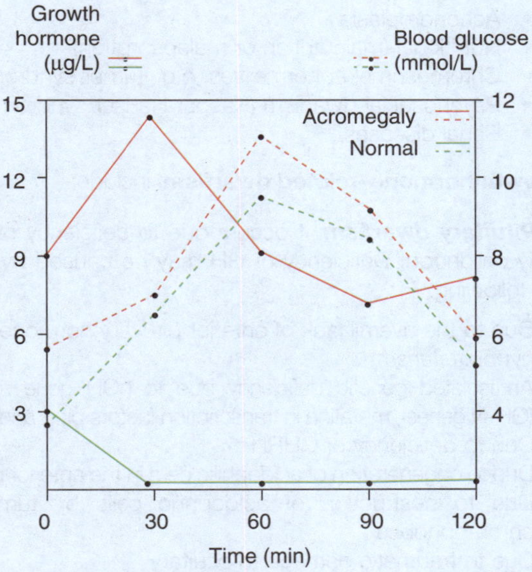

Fig. 8.2.13 Oral glucose tolerance tests in a normal subject and a patient with acromegaly with measurement of blood glucose and plasma growth hormone. Note the suppression of growth hormone secretion to <0.5 μg/L in the normal subject, and failure to suppress (sometimes accompanied by paradoxical elevation) in acromegaly. Glucose tolerance may also be impaired in acromegaly. (To convert GH in μg/L to μU/L multiply by 3; to convert glucose in mmol/L to mg/dL multiply by 18.)

Octreotide and lanreotide (somatostatin analogues) are effective in the treatment of long-term acromegaly, but their use is associated with increased chances of gallstone formation.

Sandostatin – LAR is a long-acting somatostatin analogue which is used for long-term treatment.

Bromocriptine, which is a stimulator of GH secretion in normal individuals, is effective in suppressing GH levels in most acromegalic patients.

Dopamine agonists (cabergoline) may be helpful if GH hypersecretion is also associated with PRL excess.

Pegvisomant as GH-receptor antagonist may be indicated, when GH and IGF-I concentration fails to lower with somatostatin analogue therapy.

Hyposecretion of Growth Hormone

Deficiency of GH in childhood: It leads to stunted growth or *dwarfism*.

Deficiency of GH in adulthood: Growth is not impaired; GH deficiency communally occurs as part of hypopituitarism; the affected individuals are characterized by:

- *Mild anaemia* which is refractory to usual treatment with haematinics like iron.
- Reduction in muscle mass.
- Hypoglycaemia may also occur.

Dwarfism

Causes Short stature or dwarfism may be due to endocrinal or nonendocrinal causes.

Endocrinal causes of dwarfism:

- GH deficiency (pituitary dwarf)
- Panhypopituitarism
- Hypothyroid dwarf (see page 695)
- Cushing syndrome (see page 739)

Nonendocrinal causes of dwarfism include:

- Familial dwarfism
- Achondroplasia
- Nutritional (malnutrition or malabsorption)
- Chromosomal abnormalities, e.g. Turner syndrome
- Psychosocial dwarfism (Kaspar Hauser syndrome)
- Renal diseases

Growth hormone–related dwarfism include:

1. Pituitary dwarfism It occurs due to deficiency of GH in early childhood. Deficiency of GH may be caused by any of the following:

- Due to the overall lack of anterior pituitary hormones (*panhypopituitarism*)
- An isolated genetic deficiency due to hGH gene mutation (GH-N genes), mutation in transcription factors pit-1 and prop-1
- Due to deficiency of GHRH
- Due to degeneration of acidophilic cells in the anterior pituitary
- Due to destruction of acidophilic cells by tumour of chromophobes
- Due to traumatic damage to pituitary

Characteristic features Deficiency of GH causes retardation of growth in all parts of the body proportionately. Consequently, a pituitary dwarf with a chronological age of 20 years has the body structure like that of a normal child of 7–10 years of age. Thus, a pituitary dwarf has the following features (Fig. 8.2.14):

- Shortness of stature.

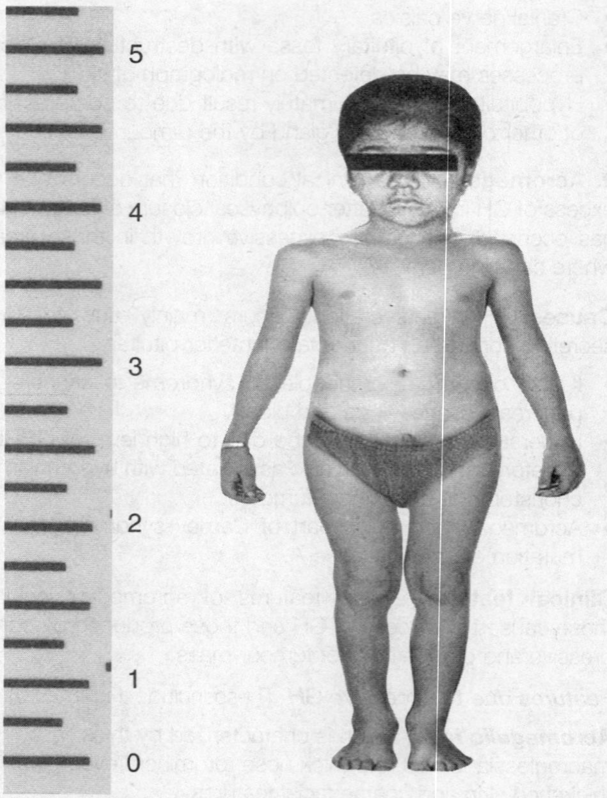

Fig. 8.2.14 Clinical features of pituitary dwarf.

- Normal mental activity.
- Plumpness (fatness).
- Immature face and high-pitched voice.
- Delicate extremities.
- Sexual maturity does not occur when associated with gonadotropin deficiency. In one-third of the pituitary dwarfs, there is deficiency of GH only. Such individuals do mature occasionally but do not reproduce.
- More prone for hypoglycaemia.

Functional tests These include:

i. ***Plasma levels of GH*** are low. Since GH levels are undetectable normally in any sample taken during daytime, sample for GH should be taken any of the following:
   - Postexercise
   - One to 2 hours after going to sleep (at this time, there is physiological increase in GH)
   - Frequent samples at night

ii. ***Stimulation test:*** Stimulation of GH secretion by insulin-induced hypoglycaemia is a golden standard to confirm or exclude the diagnosis. This test is performed by giving 0.15 U/kg of soluble insulin intravenously to produce hypoglycaemia (blood sugar <40 mg%). The samples are collected at 0, 30, 60, 90 and 120 minutes for blood glucose and GH. In normal individuals, hypoglycaemia raises GH levels above 20 ng/mL. But in patients with deficiency of GH, the hormone level remains below 7 ng/mL.

Treatment In children with documented GH deficiency, replacement therapy with recombinant hGH is useful.

2. African pygmies In this condition, short stature is due to lack of GH receptors in the tissues, though both GH and somatomedin levels are normal. In addition, their plasma IGF-I levels fail to increase at the time of puberty.

3. Laron dwarfism In this condition, there is congenital abnormality of the GH receptors, so it is also called *GH insensitivity syndrome*. The plasma concentration of GH-binding protein decreases and IGF-I is not secreted in sufficient amount. The level of GH is either normal or elevated.

Treatment Drugs used are as follows:

- Mecasermin is recombinant human IGF-I.
- Recombinant human insulin-like growth factor binding proteins (rhIGFBP-3).
- The drug mecasermin rinfabate is a combination of mecasermin and its binding protein.

POSTERIOR PITUITARY HORMONES

The two important hormones released from posterior pituitary:

- ADH
- Oxytocin (OTC) (see page 857)

ANTIDIURETIC HORMONE

ADH, as the name indicates, prevents diuresis and is chiefly concerned with conservation of body water. Since it also causes vasoconstriction, it is also called vasopressin or more precisely arginine vasopressin (AVP).

Structure, Synthesis, Storage, Release, Transport and Metabolism

Structure, synthesis, storage and release of ADH and OTC being similar are discussed together.

Structure Both ADH and OTC are homologous neurohormones, polypeptide in nature, containing nine amino acids each, but the amino acids in positions 3 and 8 differ in the two hormones.

Synthesis ADH, as well as OTC, is nonapeptide synthesized in the cell bodies of magnocellular neurons of both paraventricular and supraoptic nuclei of hypothalamus. However, supraoptic nucleus predominately contains ADH-forming neurons while paraventricular nucleus contains mainly the OTC-synthesizing neurons.

- Like all other peptides, they are formed on rough endoplasmic reticulum.
- The ADH and OTC are synthesized as large molecules, the prohormones known as *prepropressophysin* and *preprooxyphysin*, respectively.
- In prepropressophysin, the ADH molecule is associated with neurophysin II and in preprooxyphysin, the OTC molecule is associated with neurophysin I. The neurophysins were originally thought to be binding polypeptides, but it now appears that they are simply parts of the precursor molecules.
- The precursor molecules have their leader molecules removed in the endoplasmic reticulum and are packaged into secretory granules in the Golgi apparatus.

Storage The axons of ADH- and OTC-synthesizing neurons end in the posterior pituitary gland as terminal swelling. The secretory granules containing hormone precursors, known as Herring bodies, are transported down the axons by axoplasmic flow to the nerve endings in the posterior pituitary. Cleavage of the precursor molecules occurs as they are being transported, and thus the storage granules in the endings contain free ADH or OTC and the corresponding neurophysin. In the case of ADH, a glycopeptide is also present.

Secretion ADH and OTC are released when a nerve impulse is transmitted from the cell body in the hypothalamus down the axon, where it depolarizes the neurosecretory vesicles. An influx of calcium into the neurosecretory granule then by exocytosis results in secretion of hormones, neurophysins and glycopeptides. Thus, the factors which increase the discharge activity of these neurons cause increased release of hormones and vice versa. All these products are secreted but the functions of the components other than ADH and OTC are not known.

Transport The hormone and other secreted products separately enter the closely adjacent capillary. Subsequent transport of the hormone into the bloodstream is accomplished by endocytosis into the endothelial cells and then by diffusion through pores in the fenestrated capillary endothelium. The hormone then reaches the target cells and, by circulatory interconnections, also to the anterior pituitary.

Evidence to support that ADH and OTC are synthesized in hypothalamus and only stored in posterior pituitary It includes:

- Herring bodies (coarse large granules) containing ADH and OTC can be visualized in hypothalamus and posterior pituitary by special staining techniques.
- After sectioning of the hypothalamo-hypophyseal tract, Herring bodies disappear below the section and fill up proximal to the point of section, suggesting that the granules are coming from the hypothalamus.
- Destruction of supraoptic nucleus causes disappearance of Herring bodies with symptoms of ADH deficiency, confirming that the neurons of supraoptic nucleus synthesize ADH.
- Newly synthesized hormone can be released into the circulation from the hypothalamus even in the absence of posterior pituitary depicting that this is not the site of hormone synthesis.

Other sources of ADH and OTC In addition to the above-described magnocellular neurons of hypothalamus, the ADH and OTC are also present in the:

- Endings of neurons which project onto brainstem and spinal cord
- Gonads
- Adrenal cortex
- Thymus

Biological half-life of ADH is 16–20 minutes after its release into the circulation.

Metabolism The circulating vasopressin is rapidly inactivated in the liver and kidney.

Vasopressin Receptors

The action of vasopressin is mediated by stimulation of G-protein–coupled receptors, called vasopressin receptors, which are classified into three subtypes:

V_{1A} receptors: These act through phosphatidylinositol hydrolysis to increase the intracellular Ca^{2+} concentration. These are involved in the vasoconstrictor effect of ADH.
V_{1B} receptors: These also act by a mechanism similar to that of V_{1A} and are involved in the action of ADH on anterior pituitary.
V2 receptors: These act through Gs to increase cAMP levels and are involved in the action of ADH on the kidney.

Actions of Antidiuretic Hormone

1. Action on kidney The main role of ADH is regulation of water balance in the body by acting on the kidney, where it decreases the excretion of free water (i.e. antidiuretic and concentrating effect on kidney).

Site of action ADH acts on the basolateral membrane of the renal cells that are responsible for reabsorbing free (i.e. osmotically unencumbered) water from the glomerular filtrate. These ADH responsive cells line the distal convoluted tubules and collecting ducts of the renal nephron. ADH increases the permeability of these cells to water. ADH also acts on the ascending limb of the loop of Henle to enhance sodium transport into the medullary interstitium. The resultant increase in the osmolality of the interstitium helps to create the osmotic gradient for water reabsorption. In this way, ADH increases the osmolality of urine to a maximum that is fourfold greater than that of glomerular filtrate. For details, see page 511.

Mechanism of action The ADH exerts its antidiuretic effect by binding to a specific plasma membrane receptor (known as V_2 receptor) on the capillary (basal) side of the cell, where it activates adenylyl cyclase. The increase in intracellular cAMP activates a protein (kinase) on the opposite (luminal apical) side of the cell. The activated protein kinase leads to rapid insertion of protein water channels (known as aquaporins) in the plasma membranes of the principal cells of the collecting ducts. Through these protein water channels (i.e. aquaporin), water rapidly moves from the tubular lumen into the collecting duct cells.

Aquaporins are of different types: aquaporin 1, 2 and 3 are found in the kidneys; aquaporin 4 is found in the brain and aquaporin 5 is found in the salivary and lacrimal glands and in respiratory tract.

- ADH responsive aquaporin 2 is stored in the endosomes inside the cells and is translocated by the ADH into the luminal membrane of the principal cells of collecting ducts. Through these protein water channels (i.e. aquaporin 2), water rapidly moves from the tubular lumen into the cells of collecting ducts.
- From inside the cells, the water moves into extracellular fluid (ECF) through aquaporin 3 and 4, which are inserted into the basolateral membrane of the cells.

2. Vasoconstrictor effect ADH in large doses, referred to as supraphysiological or pharmacological doses, causes vasoconstriction and leads to rise in blood pressure. Haemorrhage is a potent stimulus to ADH secretion, and it has been reported that ADH plays an important role in blood pressure homeostasis by causing constriction of splanchnic vascular bed. This effect has been exploited therapeutically in controlling serious gastrointestinal bleeding.

Mechanism of action The ADH exerts its vasoconstrictor effect by binding to the V_{1A} receptors on the arterial smooth muscles and causes them to constrict. This action is mediated by Ca^{2+} and phospholipase C–generated second messengers.

- Vasopressin also acts as a neurotransmitter on the brain through the V_{1A} receptor to decrease cardiac output. The site for this action is area postrema (also known as circumventricular organs) having fenestrated capillaries (out of blood–brain barrier). Therefore, vasopressin plays an important role in blood pressure homeostasis.

3. Action on anterior pituitary ADH travels to the anterior pituitary via the portal veins and combines with the V_{1B} receptors (also called V_3 receptors) which appear to be unique to the anterior pituitary. The binding of ADH to V_{1B} receptor generates phospholipase C–released second messengers, which cause increased ACTH secretion from the corticotrophs.

4. Action on the liver In the liver, ADH causes *glycogenolysis* by combining with the V_{1A} receptor.

5. Action on the brain V_{1A} receptors are also found in brain, where ADH acts as neurotransmitter and is involved in memory, regulation of temperature, regulation of blood pressure, circadian rhythms and brain development.

Synthetic agonists and antagonists of ADH are:
Synthetic agonists of ADH that have selective actions and are more active than naturally occurring ADH have been produced by altering the amino acid residues. For example, 1-deamino-8-D-arginine vasopressin (DDAVP), also called *desmopressin*, has very high antidiuretic activity with little pressure activity, making it valuable in the treatment of ADH deficiency.
Synthetic antagonists that selectively block the pressure or antidiuretic activity of ADH have also been synthesized.

Regulation of Antidiuretic Hormone Secretion

The main factors which regulate the ADH secretion are effective osmotic pressure of the plasma and changes in blood volume. In addition, some other factors also effect ADH secretion.

1. Effective Osmotic Pressure of Plasma or Plasma Osmolality

Plasma osmolality in normal individuals is maintained very close to 285 mOsm/L by ADH. In other words, change in plasma osmolality is a very potent regulator of ADH secretion. A significant change in ADH secretion occurs when plasma osmolality is changed as little as 1%. Thus, water deprivation (which increases plasma osmolality) stimulates ADH secretion, and it thereby decreases free water clearance and enhances water conservation. On the other hand, a water load (which decreases plasma osmolality) decreases ADH secretion, and thus increases free water clearance and the efficiency of water excretion.

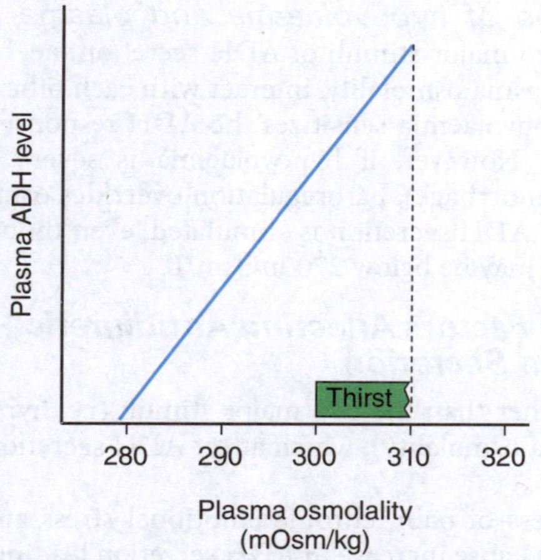

Fig. 8.2.15 Correlation between plasma osmolality, ADH secretion and onset of thirst in healthy human in whom the plasma osmolality was increased by infusing hypertonic sodium chloride.

Thus, ADH and water form a negative feedback loop. When plasma osmolality is increased by infusing hypertonic sodium chloride, ADH secretion is stimulated, and plasma ADH rises over a linear concentration range (Fig. 8.2.15). It is important to note that this response of ADH to hyperosmolality just precedes the response of thirst (Fig. 8.2.15). Both ADH release and thirst lead to increase in body water that limits further increments in the osmolality of plasma.

Mechanism of action Changes in plasma osmolality affect the osmoreceptors.

Osmoreceptors These refer to the group of neurons located in the anterior hypothalamus in the region of circumventricular organs and organum vasculosum of lamina terminalis (this region is outside the blood–brain barrier). These cells are distinct from the cells which produce ADH.

Osmoreceptors are very sensitive to osmolality of the plasma As mentioned earlier, the normal plasma osmolality is 285 mOsm/L. The rise in plasma osmolality even by 1%–2% results in shrinkage of osmoreceptors causing increased rate of discharge and reflexly increased ADH secretion and thus maintained plasma osmolality (Fig. 8.2.16).

Solutes which stimulate osmoreceptors: The osmoreceptors are stimulated by those solutes to which the cells are relatively impermeable and cross the blood–brain barrier slowly. Therefore, substances like Na^+, mannitol and sucrose are potent stimulators for ADH secretion.

- *Na^+*: It is a very important stimulator of ADH because 95% of effective plasma osmotic pressure is due to plasma Na^+ only.
- *Glucose and urea:* The hyperglycaemia and uraemia are comparatively less potent stimulators for ADH releases, but in uncontrolled diabetes mellitus (hyperglycaemia associated with insulin deficiency), glucose acts as an effective stimulus for ADH release.

2. Changes in Blood Volume

Changes in circulating blood volume, central blood volume, cardiac output and blood pressure (Fig. 8.2.17) affect the secretion of

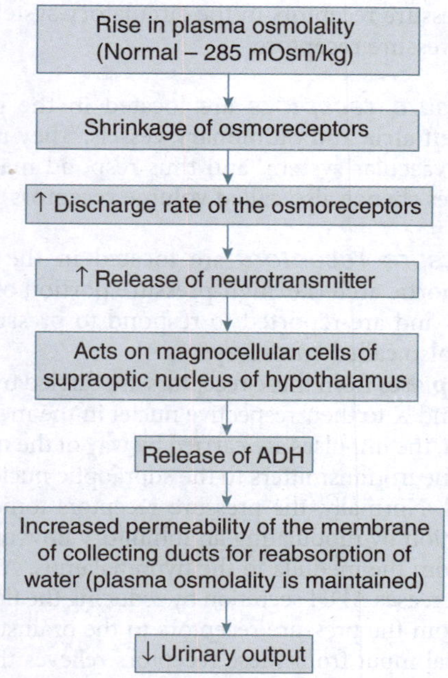

Fig. 8.2.16 Mechanism of regulation of ADH by plasma osmolality.

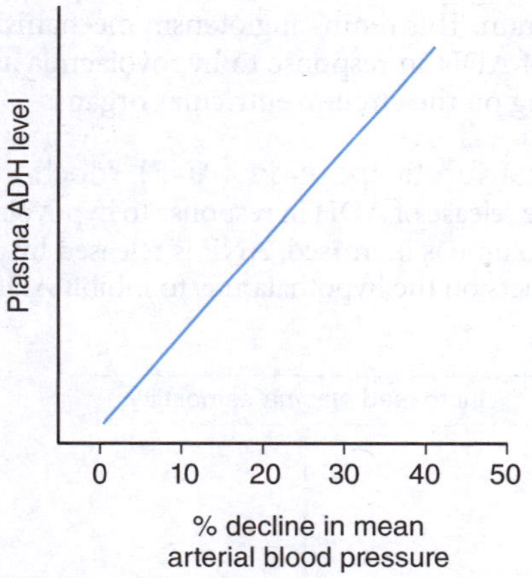

Fig. 8.2.17 Correlation between declining blood pressure and plasma ADH levels in healthy adult human in whom a progressive decline in blood pressure was induced by infusing trimethaphan (a sympathetic blocking agent).

ADH. ADH secretion is increased when ECF volume is low and decreased when ECF volume is high. Quiet standing, tilting or positive-pressure breathing also reduces central blood volume, and, therefore, increases ADH secretion, particularly when blood pressure falls. On the other hand, administration of blood or isotonic saline solution increases total circulating blood volume, or immersion of body up to the neck in water increases central blood volume and decreases ADH release.

Mechanism of action The changes in blood volume regulate ADH secretion by the following mechanisms:

i. Pressure receptor mechanism Variations in the discharge from pressure receptors in the circulatory system are inversely related to the rate of ADH secretion. There are two types of pressure receptors in the circulatory system: the low- and high-pressure receptors.

Low-pressure receptors are located in the great veins, right and left atria and pulmonary vessels. They monitor the fullness of vascular system, and thus respond mainly to volume changes (hence also called volume receptors).

High-pressure receptors are located in the carotid sinuses and aortic arch (i.e. high-pressure portion of the vascular system) and are reported to respond to pressure changes and so are also called baroreceptors.

Afferent impulses from these receptors are carried by the cranial nerves IX and X to their respective nuclei in the medulla. From the medulla, the impulses are carried by way of the midbrain via adrenergic neurotransmitters to the supraoptic nuclei of the hypothalamus. Normally, the pressure receptors tonically inhibit ADH secretion by modulating an inhibitory flow of adrenergic impulses from the medulla to the hypothalamus. A decrease in pressure increases ADH secretion by reducing the flow of neural impulses from the pressure receptors to the brainstem. The reduced neural input from these receptors relieves the source of tonic inhibition on the hypothalamic cells that secrete ADH.

ii. Renin–angiotensin mechanism Hypovolaemia also stimulates the generation of renin and angiotensin directly within the brain. This renin–angiotensin mechanism reinforces the release of ADH in response to hypovolaemia and hypotension by acting on the circumventricular organs.

iii. Atrial natriuretic peptide (ANP) mechanism *It* also reinforces the release of ADH in response to hypovolaemia. When circulating volume is increased, ANP is released by cardiac myocytes which acts on the hypothalamus to inhibit ADH release.

Interaction of hypovolaemia and plasma osmolality The two major stimuli of ADH secretion, i.e. hypovolaemia and plasma osmolality, interact with each other.

The hypovolaemia sensitizes the ADH response to hyperosmolality. However, if hypovolaemia is severe (e.g. after severe haemorrhage), baroregulation overrides osmotic regulation, and ADH secretion is stimulated, even though plasma osmolality may be below 270 mOsm/L.

3. Other Factors Affecting Antidiuretic Hormone Secretion

Factors, other than the two major stimuli (i.e. hypovolaemia and plasma osmolality), which affect ADH secretions:

Stress: Stress of pain, chronic emotional stress and surgical procedures cause increase in ADH secretion leading to reduction in urine formation under these conditions.
Adrenaline: It decreases the ADH. Hence, one experiences increased frequency of micturition during such acute emotional stresses, such as during interviews or examinations.
Alcohol: It reduces ADH secretion and thus leads to diuresis.
Sex: The size of ADH neurons, the rate of ADH secretion and the plasma level of ADH are all greater in men than in women.
Age: Elderly individuals secrete more ADH than younger individuals, probably in compensation for a diminished ability of their kidneys to concentrate urine.
Cortisol and thyroid hormones: These restrain ADH release. Therefore, in their absence, ADH may be secreted, even though plasma osmolality is low.
Some other factors: Other factors that increase ADH secretion include nausea, vomiting, standing posture and drugs like clofibrate, carbamazepine and cytokines.

Summary of factors regulating ADH secretion is given in Fig. 8.2.18.

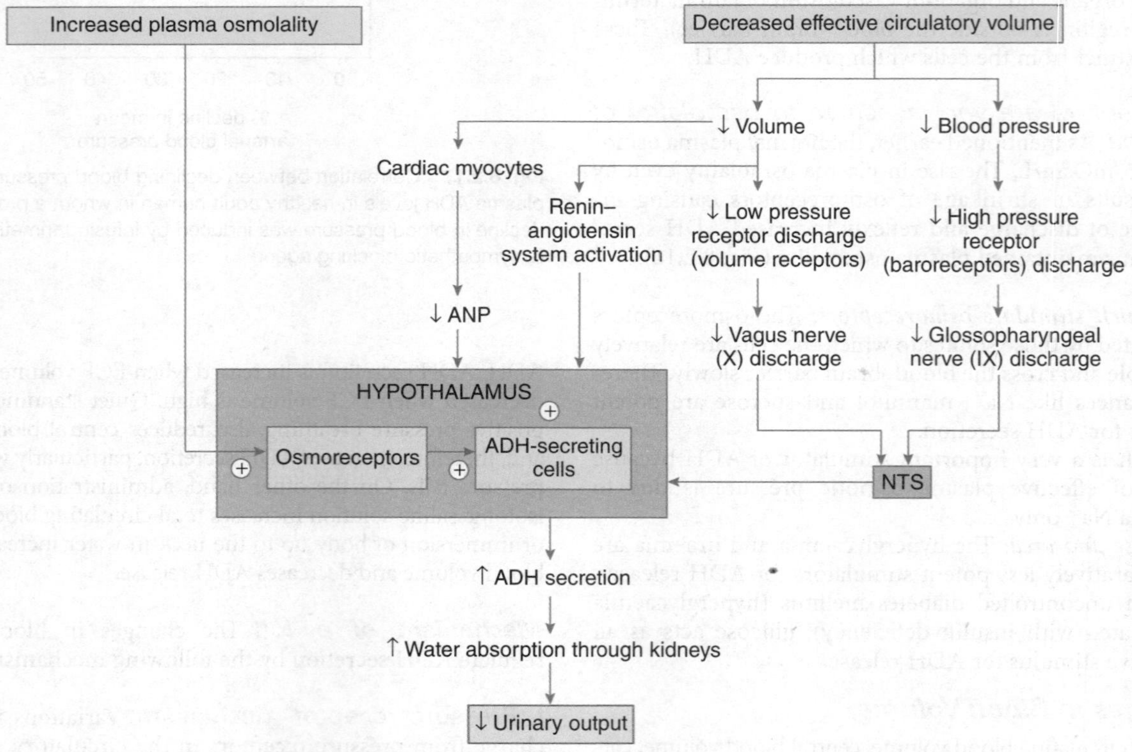

Fig. 8.2.18 Summary of factors regulating ADH secretion.

Applied Aspects

Abnormalities of ADH Secretion

Abnormalities of ADH secretion include:

- Syndrome of inappropriate hypersecretion of ADH (SIADH)
- Diabetes insipidus (DI)

I. Syndrome of Inappropriate Hypersecretion of ADH

SIADH refers to a condition in which ADH secretion is increased despite the presence of hypo-osmolality. Excessive ADH secretion leads to water intoxication, i.e. overhydration, and because of this SIADH is also called *dilution syndrome*.

Causes. The causes are as follows:

I. ***Excessive secretion of ADH from posterior pituitary*** may occur during surgical stress, because of pain and hypovolaemia.

II. ***Excessive secretion of ADH from some ectopic sources***, e.g.:
   - In cerebral disease (cerebral salt wasting)
   - In pulmonary diseases (pulmonary salt wasting) such as bronchogenic carcinoma

III. ***Excess of ADH due to its decreased metabolic degradation*** may occur in patients with liver cirrhosis and cardiac failure. In such cases, half-life of ADH is prolonged.

Characteristic features. Characteristic features of SIADH are as follows:

1. ***Water retention:*** Excessive ADH leads to water retention causing expansion of blood volume and ECF volume.
2. ***Hypernatriuria:*** The expansion in ECF volume reduces aldosterone secretion causing hypernatriuria, i.e. excessive urinary excretion of Na^+.
3. ***Hyponatraemia***, i.e. decrease in plasma Na^+ level (<135 mmol/L): It is caused by ADH by its dilatational effect (water retention) as well as by causing hypernatriuria.
4. ***Oedema:*** Water retention and excessive urinary excretion of Na^+ cause hypo-osmolality of blood (since ADH secretion is increased despite hypo-osmolality of blood, which is why the condition is called SIADH). The low plasma osmolality causes shift of water from plasma into the interstitial spaces producing the so-called oedema. The decreased osmolality of fluid in interstitial spaces, i.e. ECF, causes shift of water from ECF into the cells.
5. ***Increased urinary osmolality:*** It occurs due to decreased urinary excretion of water and continued excretion of Na^+. The urinary osmolality exceeds plasma osmolality and urinary Na^+ excretion may be more than 20 mEq/L.

Important Note

In this situation, if water intake is restricted, then water retention does not occur and ADH secretion has no effect on plasma Na^+ and oedema does not occur. This is because reduced water intake does not cause an increase in ECF volume, and thus aldosterone secretion is not suppressed and hence there is no excessive urinary excretion of Na^+.

- In animals (rats), studies have demonstrated that a prolonged exposure to high vasopressin levels can lead to:
  - Decreased production of aquaporin 2 channels resulting in sudden increase in urinary output
  - Fall in plasma osmolality

Treatment. The treatment of SIADH depends on the symptoms and its severity of hyponatraemia and its duration. The management of SIADH includes:

- Removal of underlying cause
- Adequate solute intake including salt and protein and fluid restriction
- Use of frusemide along with replacement of sodium and potassium loss with 0.9% saline
- SIADH with severe neurological symptoms – hypertonic saline (3%) 1–2 mL/kg intravenously in 3–4 hours
- Drugs include:
  Urea – oral daily ingestion of urea has shown favourable long-term result.
  Antagonists of vasopressin receptors – conivaptan (an antagonist of both V_{1A} and V_2 vasopressin receptors) and *tolvaptan (an* antagonist V_2 receptor).

II. Diabetes insipidus (DI)

DI refers to a clinical condition of polyuria that occurs due to either deficiency of ADH (vasopressin) release or failure of renal response to ADH.

Causes. Depending on the cause, DI is of two types:

A. ***Central (cranial) or neurogenic DI*** results from failure of ADH secretion. Causes of failure of ADH secretion can be:

I. Congenital, e.g. DIDMOAD (diabetes insipidus, diabetes mellitus, optic atrophy and deafness) syndrome

II. Acquired causes include:

- *Neoplasia* of hypothalamus or pituitary, such as:
  - Craniopharyngioma
  - Chromophobe adenoma
  - Pinealoma
  - Metastatic tumour
  - Sarcoidosis
  - Histiocytosis
- *Surgery of pituitary or hypothalamus*
- *Post-traumatic, i.e. following head injury*
- *Vascular lesions such as intracranial blood and subarachnoid haemorrhage*
- *Intracranial infections*
- *Systemic diseases*
- *Mutation of gene for prepropressophysin*

B. ***Nephrogenic DI*** occurs due to failure of renal response to ADH.

Congenital defect in vasopressin receptor (V_2) due to mutation of gene is the main cause of nephrogenic DI. It is an X chromosome–linked disorder or defect in gene aquaporin 2.

Other causes of nephrogenic DI are hypokalaemia and hyperkaliuria.

Characteristic features. DI is characterized by decreased renal absorption of water leading to the following features:

- Polyuria
- Polydipsia
- Dehydration

1. ***Polyuria***, i.e. passage of large amounts of urine: It is the most important single feature of DI. Patient passes up to 3–20 L of urine of pale colour and of low specific gravity per day. Patient goes for urination after every 0.5–l hour. In nephrogenic DI, urine output is directly related to the volume of water delivered to collecting ducts.

2. ***Polydipsia:*** Polyuria is followed by obligatory polydipsia (drinking of large amount of water). It occurs due to stimulation of thirst mechanism. In fact, polydipsia is an important mechanism which helps to maintain water balance with near-normal plasma Na^+ level in patients with DI.
3. ***Dehydration:*** **It** may occur in severe cases. Its signs and symptoms include dry tongue and dry mouth. Fall of blood pressure and loss of consciousness may be seen in acute severe cases.

Tests for diagnosis. These are as follows:

1. ***Water deprivation test:*** This test is performed to differentiate DI from primary psychogenic polydipsia (compulsive water drinking).
   - Normally, after 8 hours of (overnight) water deprivation, plasma osmolality rises and it also raises the urine osmolality, which may reach even up to 800 mOsm/kg.
   - In DI, initially, plasma osmolality is high and urine osmolality rises due to ADH deficiency. After water deprivation test, blood osmolality rises further but there is negligible rise in urine osmolality, which is usually less than 300 mOsm/kg.
   - In primary psychogenic polydipsia, initial plasma osmolality and urine osmolality are low, which rise significantly after water deprivation test. Thus, significant rise of urine osmolality after water deprivation differentiates primary psychogenic polydipsia from DI.
2. ***Vasopressin test:*** This test is performed immediately after deprivation test and may even form the second part of the test. It helps to differentiate central DI. A total of 5 IU of vasopressin is injected subcutaneously and the response is observed.
   - A positive response, i.e. rise in urine osmolality, is diagnostic of central DI.
   - A negative response, i.e. no rise in urine osmolality even after administration of vasopressin, is diagnostic of nephrogenic DI.
3. ***Other tests*** to find out the cause of DI:

   For central DI:
   - Radiograph of skull may show pituitary fossa enlargement.
   - Visual field test may be defective.
   - CT scan and MRI may reveal tumours or other lesions of pituitary or hypothalamus.

   For nephrogenic DI:
   - Serum sodium
   - Serum potassium
   - Serum calcium
   - Radiology of urinary tract
   - Renal function tests

Treatment for two types of DI is as follows:

1. ***Central or neurogenic DI*** can be treated by:
   Hormonal therapy, i.e. ADH or desmopressin administration
   Nonhormonal therapy, i.e. via drugs which increase ADH secretion, such as:
   - Chlorpropamide (an oral hypoglycaemic agent), thiazides (diuretics), clofibrate and carbamazepine
2. ***Nephrogenic DI*** is treated by diuretics, e.g. hydrochlorothiazide. These inhibit Na^+ reabsorption in thick segment of loop of Henle and so urine osmolality does not fall below 300 mOsm/kg.

Complications. DI if not treated can lead to the following complications in a child: brain damage, impaired mental function, poor growth, irritability and restlessness.

Self-Assessment

1. Discuss the endocrinal aspects of hypothalamo-hypophyseal relationship.
2. Discuss the mechanism of action and functions of growth hormone.
3. Describe the mechanism of action, functions and regulation of antidiuretic hormone.
4. Write notes on:
   - Panhypopituitarism
   - Features of hypersecretion of growth hormone
   - Diabetes insipidus
   - SIADH

Clinical Cases

Case 1

A 76-year-old woman presented to emergency department with abdominal pain, constipation and decreased urinary output. History and examination revealed that the patient is on drug duloxtine for a few months as a part of treatment for depression. There was swelling on the face and hands, and the patient was feeling tired.

Laboratory tests showed the following:

- Plasma osmolality – 254 mmol/L; Na^+ – 118 mmol/L
- Urine osmolality – 400 mmol/L; Na^+ – 150 mmol/L
- TSH, cortisol, T_4 and T_3 – within normal range

Depending on history, examination and laboratory tests, answer the following:

Q1. What is the probable diagnosis?

Q2. What are the side effects of the drug prescribed?

Q3. What further tests should be advised to confirm the diagnosis?

Q4. What are the common causes of this condition?

Case 2

A 25-year-old woman was suffering from increased body growth and enlargement of body parts since the age of 14. History revealed that her menstruation has not started yet and for the last 3–4 months she was having low back pain and light headache. Physical examination revealed that her height was 220 cm and weight 140 kg; facial features were coarse; the hands were larger; voice was deep and husky; and axillary and pubic hair were scanty. A probable diagnosis of acromegaly gigantism was made.

Q1. What is the probable cause of these signs?

Q2. To reach the final diagnosis, what further tests should be done?

Q3. Explain the pathophysiology of this condition.

Q4. What is the physiological basis for treating this case?

Case 3

A 24-year-old diabetic female after giving birth to a baby girl by vaginal delivery, on 10th day developed severe headache associated with nausea and vomiting, generalized weakness and dizziness.

On examination, the BP, temperature and heart rate were found to be normal. To find out the cause of headache, a few tests were done, which showed hypernatremia, raised urinary osmolality, and a provisional diagnosis of panhypopituitarism was made.

Q1. What further tests should be done to find the cause?

Q2. What are the causes of this condition?

8.3 Thyroid Gland

CHAPTER OUTLINE

FUNCTIONAL ANATOMY

GROSS ANATOMY

The thyroid gland has two distinctions: (i) it was the first endocrine gland to be recognized as such on the basis of symptoms associated with excess or deficient functions, and (ii) it is the largest endocrine gland in the body (weighing approximately 15–25 g in adults). It consists of two lobes joined together by a narrow isthmus and is located on either side of the trachea, just below the larynx. It receives high blood supply with its rate of blood flow, 400–600 mL/100 g/min, which is higher than even the myocardium or kidneys.

HISTOLOGICAL STRUCTURE (FIG. 8.3.1)

Histologically, each *lobe* of the thyroid gland is divided into various *lobules* by fibrous tissue septa. Each lobule is made up of an aggregation of several *follicles*. Follicle (acinus) is the functional unit of the thyroid gland. Each follicle is lined by *follicular cells* that rest on a basement membrane. The reabsorption lacunae are the areas where the colloid is being actively absorbed into the thyrocytes by endocytosis. The follicle is surrounded by a rich capillary plexus.

Follicular cells These vary in shape with the degree of glandular activity. Normally (at an average level of activity), the cells are *cuboidal* and the colloid in the follicles is moderate in amount. During high degree of activity, the cells become columnar and flat when inactive (Fig. 8.3.1B). These cells secrete thyroid hormones.

Parafollicular cells In addition to follicular cells, the thyroid gland contains parafollicular cells or *C cells*. These do not border on the follicular lumen but are scattered between the follicular cells and basement membrane (Fig. 8.3.1A). They may also lie in the intervals between the follicle cells. These cells secrete calcitonin, which is described in Chapter 8.4, page 715.

Colloid This is a homogeneous material that fills the cavity of each follicle. When stimulated, the follicles are depleted of colloid, and when unstimulated, the follicles accumulate colloid. The major constituent of the colloid is thyroglobulin (TG), a glycoprotein with a molecular weight of 660,000.

THYROID HORMONES

INTRODUCTION

The two principal thyroid hormones include thyroxine (T_4) and triiodothyronine (T_3). Both T_4 and T_3 consist of iodine-containing amino acids.

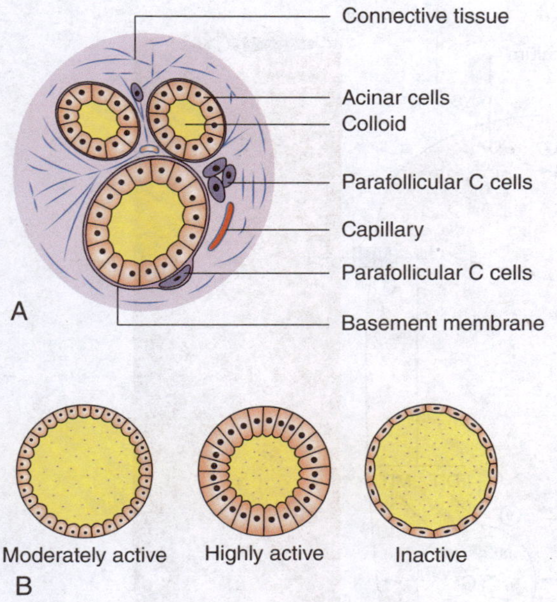

Fig. 8.3.1 **A**, Histological structure of thyroid gland. **B**, variations in follicular cell size with activity.

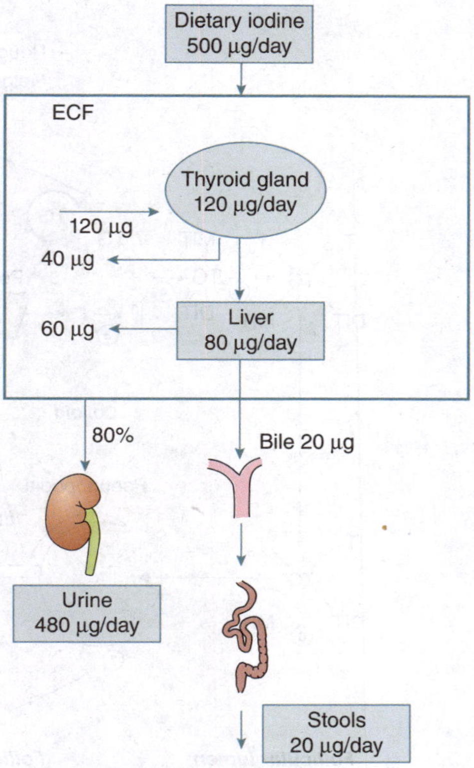

Fig. 8.3.2 Iodine metabolism.

- *Thyroxine* or T_4 (3,5,3′,5′-tetraiodothyronine) constitutes 90% of thyroid output.
- *Triiodothyronine* or T_3 (3,5,3′-triiodothyronine) constitutes 10% of thyroid output; however, it is responsible for most of the tissue actions of thyroid hormone.
- *Reverse triiodothyronine* (3,3′,5′-triiodothyronine) or reverse T_3 or RT_3, is a biologically inactive thyronine, which forms less than 1% of thyroid output.
- *Calcitonin* is a hormone secreted by the parafollicular cells of the thyroid gland. It is concerned with calcium homeostasis and is discussed in Chapter 8.4.

Thyroid hormones: For all practical purposes, refer thyroxine (T_4) and triiodothyronine (T_3).

- *Molar activity ratio* of T_3 to T_4 is 10:1 in most systems.
- *Storage ratio* of T_4 to T_3 bound to TG is 10:1.
- *Secretory ratio of* T_4 to T_3 is 10:1.
- *Plasma concentration ratio* of free T_4 to free T_3 is 2:1.

Iodine Metabolism

Dietary intake Iodine is essential for the synthesis of thyroid hormones. It is ingested in the form of iodides. ***Sources*** of iodine are sea fish (richest), bread, milk and vegetables. Iodine is added to table salt to prevent iodine deficiency.

- Daily average intake of iodine is 500 µg.
- Daily requirement of iodine is 100–200 µg.
- Minimum intake required to prevent goitre is 75 µg/day.
- Neonatal iodine requirement is 40 µg/day.
- During pregnancy, iodine requirement is 200 µg/day.

Fate of dietary iodide Most of (i.e. 500 µg/day) the iodides absorbed from the gastrointestinal tract (GIT) are rapidly excreted through kidneys, but 120 µg/day is selectively removed from circulation by cells of the thyroid gland. Thyroid uses it for synthesis of the thyroid hormone. Thyroid secretes approximately 80 µg/day in the form of T_4 and T_3, whereas 40 µg/day diffuses back into the ECF. The circulating T_4 and T_3 are metabolized in the liver and other tissues, with release of 60 µg/day iodine into the ECF and some derivatives excreted into the bile. Some of the iodine is then absorbed by enterohepatic circulation, while approximately 20 µg/day iodine is lost in the stools (Fig. 8.3.2).

Plasma iodide Its level is 0.15–0.3 µg%.

Thyroid iodide Thyroid gland contains 5–8 mg of iodide, i.e. approximately 95% of total iodine content of the body. Thus, the thyroid serves as a store for iodine which is sufficient to maintain a euthyroid state for 3 months without hormone synthesis. Of the total thyroid iodide, only 5% is present within the cells of the follicular epithelium. The remaining 95% is present in the follicular lumen, and stored in the colloid as TG. In the colloid, two-thirds of the total iodine is present in the form of biologically inactive iodotyrosines and one-third is in the form of biologically active thyronine (T_4 and T_3).

BIOSYNTHESIS AND STORAGE OF THYROID HORMONES

Thyroxine (T_4) and triiodothyronine (T_3) are synthesized from tyrosine and iodide by the enzyme complex, peroxidase. The steps involved in the synthesis of thyroid hormones are given next (Fig. 8.3.3).

1. Iodine trapping The first step in the synthesis of thyroid hormones is *uptake of iodide* by the thyroid gland which occurs against the chemical (approximately 30:1) and electrical gradients by a Na^+–I^- cotransport/symport (NIS) system that is located in the basal membrane of the thyroid epithelial

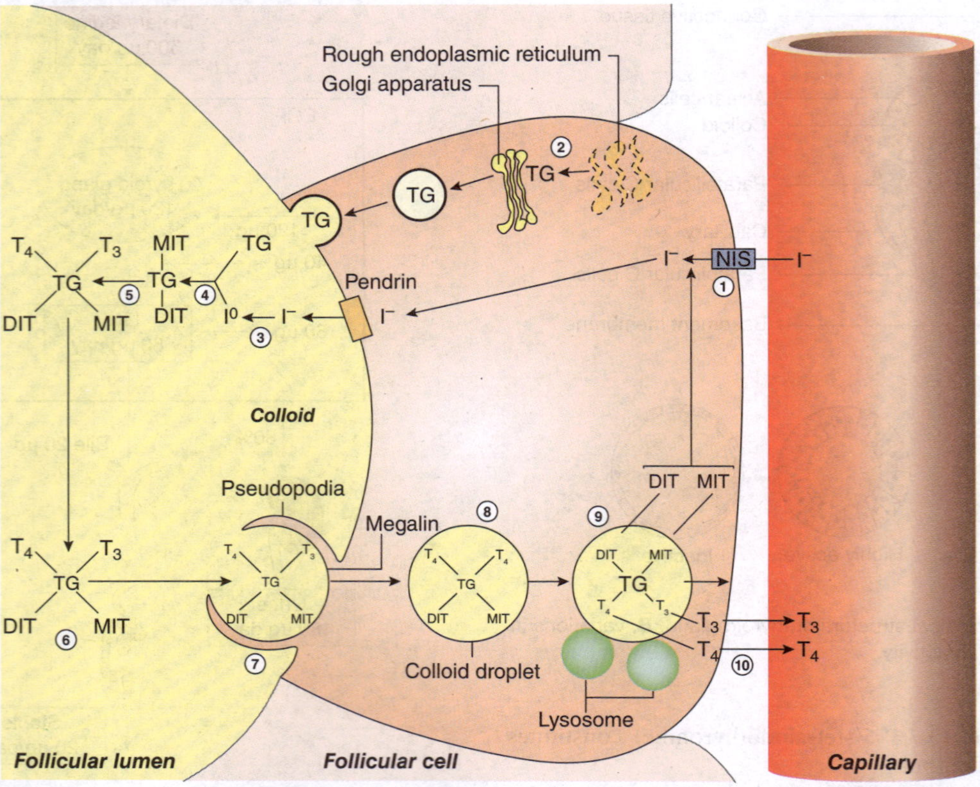

Fig. 8.3.3 Steps in the synthesis and release of thyroid hormones: 1, iodine trapping; 2, synthesis of thyroglobulin; 3, oxidation of iodine; 4, organification of thyroglobulin; 5, coupling reaction; 6, storage of thyroid hormone in colloid; 7, take-up of colloid by epithelial cell by endocytosis; 8, colloid vesicle; 9, release of T_3 and T_4 after proteolysis; and 10, diffusion of T_3 and T_4 into the capillary.

cells. It is an energy-requiring process and is linked to the ATPase-dependent Na^+–K^+ pump.

- *Thyroid-stimulating hormone (TSH) controls* the iodide uptake. The thyroid and plasma-free iodide ratio, which is normally maintained at 30, may exceed 100 when the gland is maximally activated by TSH.
- *Antithyroid agents* such as thiocyanate and perchlorate inhibit iodide transport.

2. Synthesis and secretion of thyroglobulin TG is a large glycoprotein that is synthesized on the rough endoplasmic reticulum of thyroid epithelial cells as peptide units of molecular weight 330,000 (the primary translation product of its messenger RNA). These units combine into a dimer, after which carbohydrate moieties are added as the molecule moves to the Golgi apparatus. The completed glycoprotein is contained in small vesicles, which move to the apical plasma membrane and release into the lumen of the follicle (Fig. 8.3.3).

- Each molecule of TG contains approximately 140 tyrosine residues which can serve as substrate for iodine for the formation of thyroid hormones. It is also the storage site of the two hormones within the thyroid gland.

3. Oxidation of iodide Once within the gland, iodide rapidly moves to the apical surface of the epithelial cells. From there, it is transported into the lumen of the follicles by a sodium-independent iodide/chloride transporter called *pendrin*. The iodide (1) is then immediately oxidized to iodine (1°) by the enzyme *peroxidase* present near the apical border of the epithelial cells. The immediate oxidant (electron acceptor) for this reaction is H_2O_2, which is supplied by an NADPH-dependent system (Fig. 8.3.4).

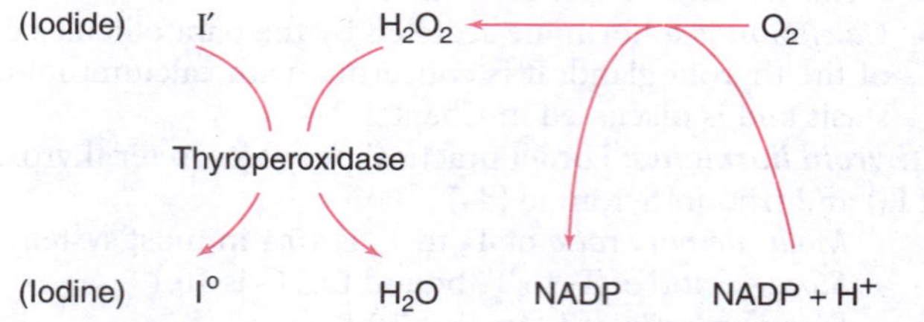

Fig. 8.3.4 Oxidation of iodide by the enzyme thyroperoxidase.

Thyroid is the only tissue that can oxidize iodide to iodine. TSH promotes this reaction while antithyroid drugs (thiourea, thiouracil, methimazole) inhibit.

Note. Pendrin is an ion exchanger protein in nature, first identified in patients suffering with Pendred syndrome with thyroid dysfunction.

4. Organification of thyroglobulin It refers to iodination of tyrosine residues present in the TG molecule. This reaction occurs at the apical membrane of the cell as soon as TG molecule is released by the secretory granules by exocytosis and requires thyroid peroxidase (TPO). Tyrosine (of TG) is first iodinated at position 3 to form monoiodotyrosine (MIT) and then at position 5 to form diiodotyrosine (DIT).

5. Coupling reaction The process of iodination of tyrosine residues is followed by a coupling reaction, which lasts for the next

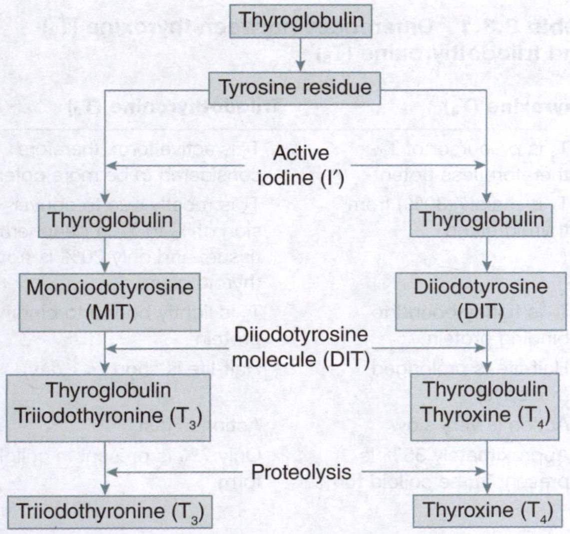

Fig. 8.3.5 Coupling reaction to form T_3 and T_4.

few minutes to an hour. Two molecules of DIT couple to form thyroxine (T_4). Triiodothyronine (T_3) is produced when one molecule of MIT is coupled with one molecule of DIT (Fig. 8.3.5). The mechanism of coupling is not well understood. The enzyme peroxidase is required during coupling as well as for iodination. There are two theories regarding the coupling reaction.

As the process of iodination and coupling is completed, each molecule of TG contains approximately 7 molecules of MIT, 6 molecules of DIT, 2 molecules of T_4 and 0.2 molecule of T_3. Thus, the ratio of T_4 to T_3 in a molecule of TG is 10:1.

6. Storage Once TG has been iodinated, it is stored in the lumen of the follicle as colloid for several months. It is estimated that the stored thyroid hormones can meet the body requirement for 1–3 months.

SECRETION, TRANSPORT AND METABOLISM OF THYROID HORMONES

Hormone Secretion

Secretion of the thyroid hormone from the colloid stored in the lumen of follicle involves the following steps (Fig. 8.3.3).

Endocytosis The colloid containing iodinated TG is retrieved from the lumen of the follicle by the epithelial cells through endocytosis. This process is facilitated by the TG receptor *megalin* located on the apical membrane. By this process, the colloid enters the cytoplasm in the form of *colloid droplets*, which move through the cytoplasm towards the basal membrane probably as a result of microtubule and microfilament functions (Fig. 8.3.2).

Proteolysis The colloid droplets fuse with the lysosome vesicles containing proteolytic enzymes. The proteases digest the TG molecule releasing T_4, T_3, DIT, MIT and other amino acid constituents into the cytoplasm of the epithelial cells.

- T_4 and T_3 diffuse through the basal border of epithelial cells into the bloodstream via adjacent rich capillary plexus.
- MIT and DIT are rapidly deiodinated within the follicular cells by the enzyme iodotyrosine *deiodinase*. In this way, iodide is retrieved for recycling along with the tyrosine into T_4 and T_3 synthesis (Fig. 8.3.3).

> **Important Note**
>
> In patients with congenital absence of iodotyrosine deiodinase, MIT and DIT get excreted into the urine and symptoms of iodine deficiency appear.

Transport of T_4 and T_3

Secreted T_4 and T_3 circulate in the bloodstream in two forms: bound and free.

1. Bound form Most of the circulating T_4 (99.95%) and T_3 (99.5%) are bound to specific binding proteins.

Thyroxine-binding globulin (TBG) is the major binding protein which binds approximately 70% of T_4 and T_3.
Thyroxine-binding prealbumin (TBPA) or transthyretin (TTR) binds approximately 15%–20% of T_4.
Thyroxine-binding albumin (TBA) binds approximately 10% of the T_4.
Binding of the hormone with plasma protein serves the following functions:

- It constitutes a reservoir for the supply of free hormones which buffers any acute changes in thyroid gland function.
- It prevents renal loss of hormone in urine, and thereby helps conserve iodide.

T_4 is more tightly bound to plasma protein than T_3. The tight binding of T_4 with plasma proteins is shown by its prolonged half-life (approximately 7 days). The half-life of T_3 is approximately 1 day only, due to its lesser affinity for the plasma proteins.

2. Free form Only approximately 0.05% of T_4 and 0.5% of T_3 circulate unbound (free form) in the plasma. These free, unbound hormones represent the biologically active hormone. The lower affinity of T_3 for the plasma binding proteins (and thus the higher concentration of unbound T_3) contributes to the greater biological activity of T_3.

> **Important Note**
>
> It is important to note that most of the circulating T_3 is not of thyroid origin but diffuses from the tissues, which convert T_4 into T_3 as described below.

Metabolism and Excretion of Thyroid Hormones

The major pathways of peripheral metabolism of the circulating thyroid hormone include deiodination, deamination (decarboxylation) and conjugation with glucuronic acid.

1. Deiodination In the peripheral tissues, T_4 is deiodinated as:

- Approximately one-third of T_4 is deiodinated into T_3 (3,5,3′-triiodothyronine) by the enzyme 5′-deiodinase. T_3 so formed remains within the cells to produce metabolic effects but some of it diffuses into circulation to act in other tissues. In this way, 80% of the T_3 present in plasma is formed in the liver, kidney and pituitary.

- Remaining T_4 is deiodinated to reverse T_3, i.e. RT_3 (3,3′,5′-triiodothyronine), by 5-deiodinase. RT_3 is physiologically inert. During fetal life, prolonged fasting and prolonged illness or even after administration of glucocorticoids, a still greater percentage of T_4 is converted into RT_3. On the other hand, in obesity, T_3 production is more than the RT_3.

Important Note

Since T_4 is deiodinated to T_3, which produces physiological effects, T_4 itself may be metabiologically inert and hence called a *prohormone*. Therefore, only 13% of circulating T_3 is secreted by thyroid, whereas 87% is formed by deiodination of T_4. Similarly, only 5% of circulating RT_3 is secreted by the thyroid and 95% is formed by deiodination of T_4.

- T_3 and RT_3 are deiodinated to DIT (T_2) and MIT (T_1). DIT (T_2) is further deiodinated to MIT (T_1) (Fig. 8.3.6).

Note. Deiodinases that act on thyroid hormones are mainly of three types: D_1, D_2 and D_3.

- D_1, primarily responsible for conversion of T_4 into T_3, is present in high concentration in the liver, kidney, thyroid, pituitary and brown fat.
- D_2 is present in brain (astroglia) and responsible for supply of T_3 to neurons.
- D_3 is present in reproductive tissues and also in brain.

2. Decarboxylation Very small amounts of T_4 and T_3 are metabolized by decarboxylation to form tetraiodothyroacetic acid (TETRAC) and triiodothyroacetic acid (TRIAC).

3. Conjugation Approximately 15% of thyroid hormones (T_4 and T_3) are conjugated in the liver to form glucuronides and sulphates. The conjugate then is secreted via the bile duct into the intestine. In normal individuals, metabolites of T_4 and T_3 are excreted mainly in the faeces with a small amount appearing in the urine.

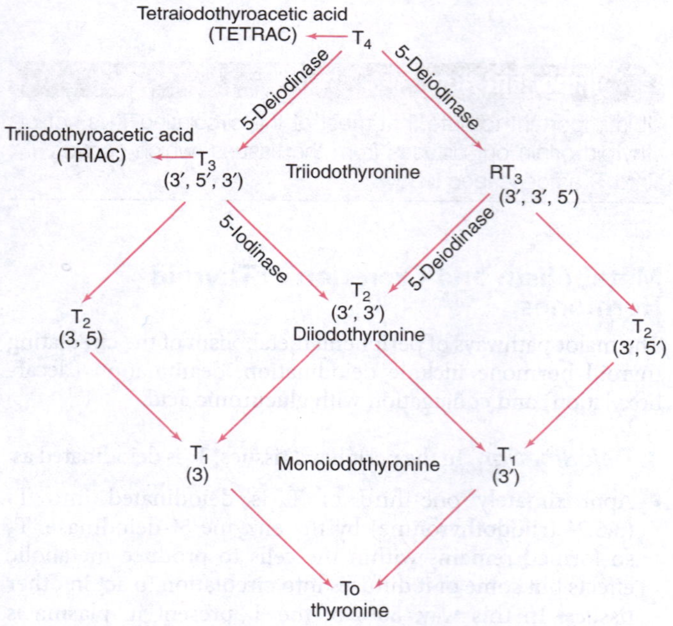

Fig. 8.3.6 Deiodination of T_4 and T_3 in peripheral tissues.

Table 8.3.1 Differences between thyroxine (T_4) and triiodothyronine (T_3)

Thyroxine (T_4)	Triiodothyronine (T_3)
• T_4 is precursor of T_3, therefore less potent	• T_3 is active form, therefore considered to be more potent
• T_4 is mainly (80%) from thyroid gland	• T_3 is mostly due to conversion of T_4 to T_3 in peripheral tissue, and only 20% is from thyroid gland
• T_4 is tightly bound to binding protein	• T_3 is lightly bound to binding protein
• Half-life is prolonged (>7 days)	• Half-life is short (<1 day)
• Action is very slow	• Action is fast
• Approximately 35% is present in the colloid form	• Only 7% is present in colloid form

The differences between thyroid hormones, thyroxine (T_4) and triiodothyronine (T_3), are depicted in Table 8.3.1.

REGULATION OF THYROID HORMONE SECRETION

The secretion of thyroid hormones is regulated by:

- Negative feedback mechanism through hypothalamus–anterior pituitary–thyroid gland axis
- Autoregulation of thyroid gland

Regulation Through Negative Feedback Mechanism Operating Through Hypothalamus–Anterior Pituitary–Thyroid Gland Axis

The negative feedback mechanism operating through hypothalamus–anterior pituitary–thyroid gland axis (Fig. 8.3.7) plays the essential role in controlling secretion of thyroid hormones.

- T_3 appears to be more actively involved than T_4 in the regulation process.
- The production of TSH by pituitary and thyrotropin-releasing hormone (TRH) by hypothalamus is inhibited by T_3 and to a lesser degree by T_4.
- The increased synthesis of TSH and TRH occurs in response to decreased circulatory levels of T_3 and T_4.

Thyroid-Stimulating Hormone

TSH is a dimer (αβ) glycoprotein. The α-subunit is identical to the α-subunit of FSH, LH and hCG, whereas functional specificity of TSH is conferred by β-subunit and its:

- Molecular weight — 30,000
- Biological half-life — 60 min
- Normal secretion rate — 110 μg/day
- Average plasma level — 2.3 μIU/mL (range 0.2–0.5 μIU/mL)

TSH secretion is pulsatile; its output starts rising at approximately 9 p.m., peak reaches at midnight, and then starts declining during the day.

Mechanism of action: TSH binds with plasma membrane receptors of thyroid cells and stimulates adenylyl cyclase with

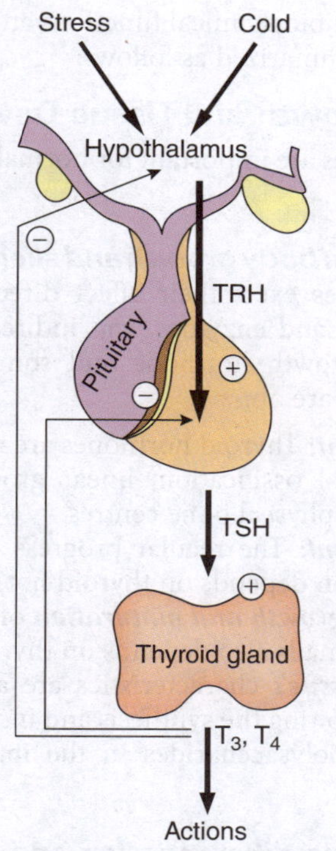

Fig. 8.3.7 Regulation of thyroid hormone secretion by negative feedback control mechanism through hypothalamus–anterior pituitary–thyroid gland axis.

a consequent increase in intracellular cAMP (second messenger), which initiates cascade of reactions to produce biochemical effects (also see page 659).

Action of TSH: TSH, through the mediation of cAMP, exerts the following effects on thyroid gland:

1. ***Increases the secretion of thyroid hormones*** by accelerating all the steps in biosynthesis, which include:
   - Iodide trapping
   - Conversion of iodide to active iodine
   - Synthesis of TG
   - Iodination of TG
   - Coupling reaction
   - Proteolysis of TG leading to increased secretion of T_3 and T_4
2. **Increases the number (hyperplasia) and size** (hypertrophy) *of the follicular epithelial cells*
3. ***Increases the vascularity of thyroid gland***

Important Notes

- Removal of pituitary gland is associated with depressed thyroid functions and ultimately results in atrophy.
- Administration of TSH (chronic TSH treatment): The thyroid gland increases in weight and size due to hypertrophy of the cells (goitre).

Regulation of TSH Production

1. ***Feedback control by plasma T_4 and T_3:*** Day-to-day secretion of TSH depends on the negative feedback control exerted by plasma levels of free T_4 and T_3 (Fig. 8.3.6):
   - A fall in T_4 and T_3 levels stimulates TSH secretion from anterior pituitary.
   - A rise in T_4 and T_3 levels inhibits TSH secretion.

Important Note

Since there exists an established inverse relationship between the plasma levels of thyroid hormones and TSH, measurement of the plasma TSH levels is a reliable test for assessing the status of thyroid hormones.

2. ***Hypothalamic control of TSH:*** Hypothalamus adjusts TSH secretion under certain special circumstances, such as exposure to cold, warmth, stress, anxiety and excitement. It exerts its effect by secreting TRH.

Thyrotropin-Releasing Hormone

TRH is a tripeptide secreted by arcuate nucleus of hypothalamus and stored in median eminence from where it is released into the hypothalamo-hypophyseal portal vessels to reach the anterior pituitary.

Mechanism of action TRH acts on the basophils (thyrotrophs) in the anterior pituitary via the adenylyl cyclase AMP system, and controls the release of TSH.

Important Note

It is important to note that TRH, and T_3 and T_4 act competitively on pituitary thyrotrophs to control TSH secretion.

Control of TRH Secretion of TRH by hypothalamus is controlled by:

- *Nervous stimuli* like emotion, stress and exposure to cold
- *Negative feedback control* exerted by plasma T_3 and T_4 levels on the hypothalamus (Fig. 8.3.6)

Autoregulation of Thyroid Gland

The secretions of thyroid gland are regulated by dietary iodine contents. It has been observed that if there is deficiency of iodine content in the diet, then the *iodine trapping* mechanism of the follicular cells becomes superefficient and vice versa is also true, i.e. when there is an excess of iodine content in the food, iodine trapping becomes less efficient and organification of the excess amount of iodine does not occur. In this way, iodine availability for thyroxine synthesis remains constant and this phenomenon is called autoregulation of thyroid gland.

MECHANISM OF ACTION OF THYROID HORMONES

The thyroid hormones do not have any discrete target organs. They affect cellular activity of almost all the tissues of the body. The multitude of thyroid hormone action cannot be explained by a single common mechanism. Basically, they act through genes (transcription and translation effect). Overall scheme of thyroid hormone effects is described (Fig. 8.3.8).

Entry of thyroid hormone in the tissue cells: Both free T_4 and T_3 enter the cells by a carrier-mediated energy-dependent process. The transport of T_4 is rate limiting for intracellular production of T_3. The different specific types of transporters are as follows:

- Monocarboxylate 8 transporter (MCT8)
- Monocarboxylate 10 transporter (MCT10)
- Organic-anion-transporting polypeptide (OATP)

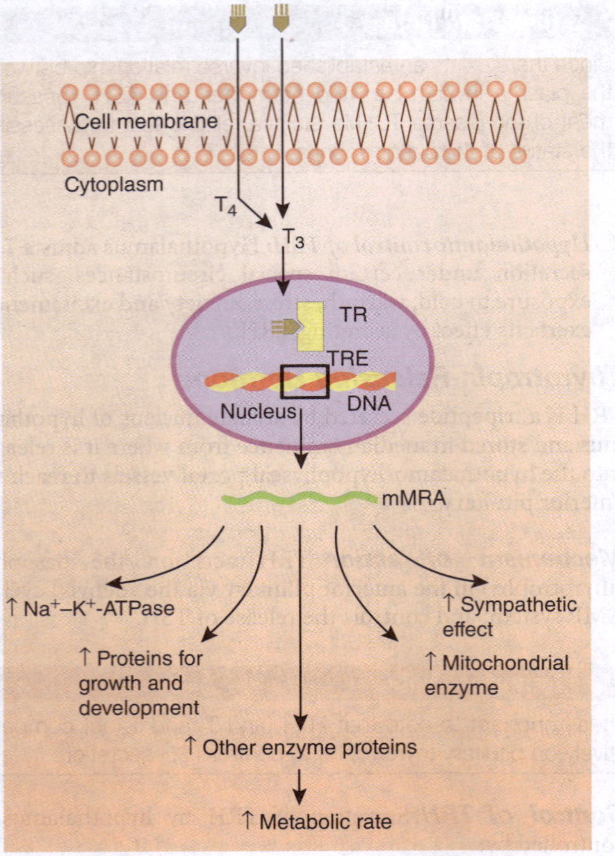

Fig. 8.3.8 Mechanism of intracellular actions of thyroid hormone.

Intracellular production of T_3: Within the cell, most, if not all, of the T_4 is converted into T_3 or RT_3 (Fig. 8.3.8).

Effects of T_3 on gene expression: T_3 (and to a much lesser extent T_4) diffuses into the nucleus and binds to three thyroid receptor (TR) subtypes that exist linked to thyroid regulatory elements (TREs) in target DNA molecules, particularly the retinoid X receptor (RXR). This causes activation and inhibition of transcription process resulting in increased synthesis of mRNA. This ultimately results in (Fig. 8.3.8):

- *Increased synthesis of enzymes and specific structural or functional proteins:* This mechanism can explain the anabolic action and other metabolic actions of thyroxine.
- *Increased synthesis of Na^+–K^+-ATPase:* It explains the calorigenic action of thyroxine. Increased metabolic rate has been attributed to increased energy consumption associated with increased Na^+ transport.
- *Increase in the number and activity of mitochondria* in the cells of the body: These increase the rate of ATP synthesis. Extremely high concentrations of thyroid hormones cause uncoupling of oxidative phosphorylation process. As a result, a large amount of heat is produced, but little ATP.

ACTIONS OF THYROID HORMONES

As explained above, thyroid hormones bind to the specific TRs on the target cell nuclei and bring about the biochemical action. T_3 is nearly 10 times more potent than T_4 in binding to the receptors. The biochemical functions attributed to thyroid hormones are summarized as follows:

Effects on Growth and Tissue Development

Thyroid hormones are important for normal body growth and development.

i. Role in normal body growth and skeletal maturation

Thyroid hormones exert their effect directly by increasing protein synthesis and enzymes, and indirectly by increasing production of growth hormone and somatomedins. Some important effects are on:

Bone development: Thyroid hormones are reported to stimulate endochondral ossification, linear growth of bone and maturation of epiphyseal bone centres.

Teeth development: The regular progress of tooth development and eruption depends on thyroid hormone.

Normal cycle of growth and maturation of the epidermis, its hair follicles and nails also depends on thyroid hormone.

Subcutaneous tissue's characteristics are altered by thyroid hormone by inhibiting the synthesis and increasing the degradation of mucopolysaccharides in the intercellular ground substance.

ii. Role in tissue differentiation and maturation The role of thyroid hormones is evidenced by the absence of metamorphosis of tadpoles into baby frogs after experimental removal of thyroid gland in the former. Conversely, administration of T_4 in tadpoles causes early metamorphosis of tadpole into adult dwarf frog, which is not more than the size of the housefly, confirming thereby the role of T_4 in tissue differentiation.

iii. Role in development of nervous tissue T_3 seems to be necessary for proper axonal and dendritic development as well as normal myelination in the nervous system. The parts of the central nervous system affected are cerebral cortex, basal ganglia and internal ear (cochlea). This is the reason for mental retardation being a striking feature in a child with congenital hypothyroidism. In such children, the disorder must be detected at the earliest and replacement hormonal therapy should be started; otherwise, the mental retardation becomes irreversible.

Effect on the Metabolic Rate in General

Thyroid hormone in general stimulates the metabolic activities and increases the basal rate of oxygen consumption and heat production in most tissues of the body except the brain, retina, gonads, lungs and spleen.

Resting oxygen use in humans ranges from approximately 150 mL/min in hypothyroid state to approximately 400 mL/min in the hyperthyroid state (normal 225–250 mL/min).

The magnitude of calorigenic action of thyroxine partly depends on the level of circulating catecholamines.

Increased metabolic rate is associated with increased utilization of many hormones, vitamins and certain drugs. Therefore, patients with hyperthyroidism require a larger vitamin intake. On the other hand, patients with hypothyroidism may show toxic effects at usual doses of certain drugs.

Effects on Metabolism

The increased O_2 consumption and metabolic rate ultimately depends on an increased supply of necessary substrate for oxidation. Thyroid hormones stimulate the provision of these substrates by their effect on carbohydrate, fat and protein metabolism.

i. Effect on carbohydrate metabolism T_4 and T_3 lead on to overall increase in enzymes, causing:

- Increased glucose absorption from GIT
- Acceleration in almost all aspects of glucose metabolism, i.e. rapid uptake of glucose by the cells, enhanced glycolysis, enhanced gluconeogenesis and increased insulin secretion and its effects on carbohydrate metabolism

ii. Effect on fat metabolism Thyroid hormones cause:

- Mobilization of fat from adipose tissue
- Increase in the levels of fatty acids and enhanced oxidation of free fatty acids by cells
- Decrease in the quantity of cholesterol, phospholipids and triglycerides in plasma and plasma cholesterol level is lowered due to increased excretion in bile

Important Note

Hypothyroidism is associated with elevated plasma cholesterol levels, which can be reversed by thyroid hormone administration.

iii. Effect on protein metabolism *In physiological amounts, the thyroid hormones* function as anabolic hormones. That is, they cause an increase in RNA and protein synthesis leading to positive nitrogen balance.

Important Note

In high concentrations, thyroid hormones have a catabolic effect leading to negative nitrogen balance. Therefore, muscle weakness and creatinuria are characteristic features of a hyperthyroid patient.

iv. Metabolic effects through other hormones T_4 and T_3 potentiate the respective stimulatory effects of epinephrine, norepinephrine, glucagon, cortisol and growth hormone on gluconeogenesis, lipolysis, ketogenesis and proteolysis of the labile protein pool.

v. Effect on vitamin metabolism Thyroid hormones increase the quantity of enzymes. Vitamins are the essential parts of some of the enzymes and coenzymes. Therefore, thyroid hormones cause increased need for vitamins leading to relative vitamin deficiency in hyperthyroidism.

T_4 is essential for conversion of carotene to vitamin A. In hypothyroidism, this reaction is very slow and carotene accumulation in the blood and tissues (carotenaemia) gives a yellow colour to the skin.

Important Note

Carotenaemia can be clinically differentiated from jaundice by the fact that sclerae of the eyeballs are not affected in the former condition.

vi. Effect on water and electrolyte balance Thyroid hormones play a role in regulation of water and electrolyte balance. This fact is clear from the observation that impairment of the thyroid function is associated with retention of water and electrolytes, which can be reversed by hormonal administration.

Note. The overall metabolic effect of thyroid has been aptly described as accelerating the response to starvation.

Respiratory Effects

Thyroid hormones cannot stimulate O_2 utilization for long without also enhancing oxygen supply, which is accomplished by the following effects of T_4 and T_3:

i. ***Increase in the resting respiratory rate, minute ventilation and ventilatory responses*** to hypercapnia and hypoxia: These actions maintain a normal pO_2 when O_2 utilization is increased and a normal pCO_2 when CO_2 production is increased.

ii. ***Increase in oxygen-carrying capacity of blood*** by slightly increasing the red blood cell mass: This increase in red blood cell mass results from stimulation of erythropoietin production, which arises directly by alteration of its gene expression and indirectly by way of the renal tissue hypoxia that results from increased O_2 use.

Cardiovascular Effects

Thyroid hormone increases cardiac output, ensuring sufficient oxygen delivery in the tissues. This is accomplished by direct and indirect mechanisms, the latter being probably quantitatively more important (Fig. 8.3.9). In general, the thyroid hormones have the following effects on cardiovascular system:

i. Vasodilatation and increased blood flow to tissues occur by two mechanisms:

Indirect mechanism: Thyroid hormones cause rapid utilization of O_2 and increased production of heat and CO_2. These

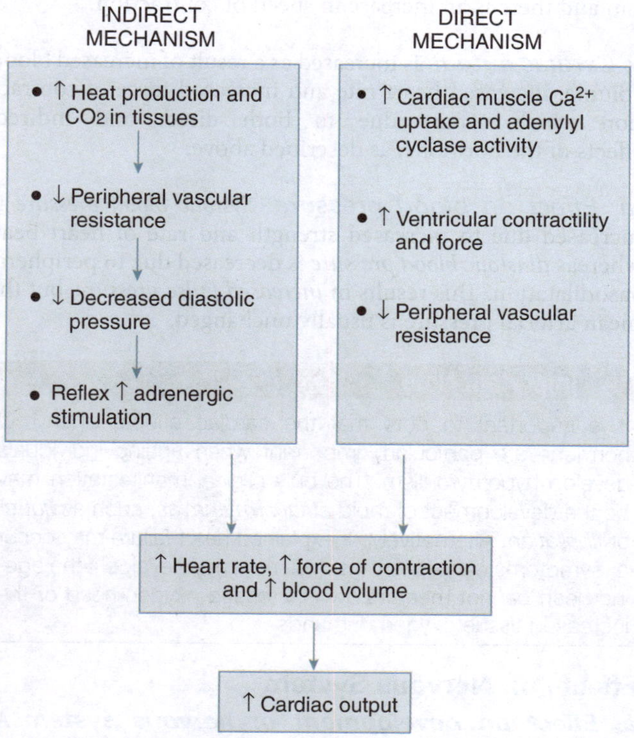

Fig. 8.3.9 Direct and indirect mechanisms by which thyroid hormones increase cardiac output. The indirect mechanisms are probably quantitatively more important.

effects cause vasodilatation and increase in blood flow in most of the tissues, especially skin, muscle and heart. Cutaneous vasodilatation is particularly a prominent feature, which helps in dissipation of excessive heat produced.

Direct mechanism: Thyroid hormones directly decrease systemic vascular resistance by dilating arterioles in the peripheral circulation.

ii. Blood volume in circulation is increased because of:

- The effect of vasodilatation produced, as described above
- Activation of the renin–angiotensin–aldosterone axis, thereby increasing renal tubular sodium reabsorption

iii. Tachycardia, i.e. increased heart rate (at rest, even during sleep), is an important physical sign which is used by clinicians in assessing the function of the thyroid gland. Thyroid hormone produces tachycardia by directly increasing the excitability of the heart and indirectly via adrenergic stimulation.

iv. Force of cardiac contraction is increased by moderate increase in thyroid hormone. The cardiac inotropic effects are partly indirect, via adrenergic stimulation and partly by direct effect of hormones on cardiac muscle. Myocardial calcium uptake and adenylyl cyclase activity are increased and enhance contractile force.

Mechanism: In the cardiac myocytes, T_3 is not formed from T_4. When circulatory T_4 enters the cardiac myocytes, it enhances genes for α-myosin heavy chain (α-MHC), sarcoplasmic reticulum Ca^{2+}, ATPase and certain K^+ channels. At the same time, thyroid hormone depresses the gene expression for β-myosin heavy chain (β-MHC). The myosin containing β-MHC has less ATPase activity as compared to that containing α-MHC. Therefore, α-MHC is predominant in hyperthyroidism and there is an increase in speed of contraction.

v. Cardiac output is increased as a result of increased blood volume, increased heart rate and increased force of contraction which occurs due to both direct and indirect effects of the hormone, as described above.

vi. Effect on blood pressure: *Systolic blood pressure* is increased due to increased strength and rate of heart beat, whereas *diastolic blood pressure* is decreased due to peripheral vasodilatation. This results in *increased pulse pressure*, but the mean arterial pressure is usually unchanged.

Important Note

It is important to note that the cardiac effects of thyroid hormone are particularly important when ageing individuals develop hypothyroidism. The only clinical manifestation may be the development of rapid *atrial arrhythmias*, such as *flutter* or *fibrillation*. Alternatively, unexplained heart failure may occur or symptoms of coronary insufficiency may develop if the ageing heart cannot meet its own increased oxygen need or the increased tissue oxygen demands.

Effects on Nervous System

a. Effect on development of nervous system As described above, thyroid hormones play an essential role in the development of the nervous system. Critical period for development of nervous system is up to 1 year of life.

b. Effect on functioning of nervous tissue in adults

i. On central nervous system: Besides its role during neonatal development of the nervous system, the thyroid hormone seems to be required for normal functioning of the brain.

T_4 enhances wakefulness, alertness, responsiveness to various stimuli, auditory sense, awareness of hunger, memory and learning capacity. Normal emotional tone also depends on proper thyroid hormone availability.

Hypothyroid adults, therefore, develop:

- Loss of intellectual functions
- Impairment of memory
- Somnolence
- Slowness of sleep
- Mental and physical lethargy
- Eventually psychosis (myxoedema madness)

Hyperthyroid adults: Excess of T_4 in adults increases the number of beta-adrenergic receptors and hence potentiates the biological activity of circulating catecholamines. Catecholamines stimulate the reticular activating system (RAS) producing:

- Emotional instability, anxiety, nervousness
- Overexcitability and nervousness
- Irritability
- Insomnia
- Fatigue with fine rhythmic tremors in hands, tongue and eyeballs

ii. Effects of thyroid hormones on peripheral nervous system: Thyroid hormone increases the speed and amplitude of peripheral nerve reflexes.

In hypothyroid adults, therefore, knee-jerk reaction time increases (normal 20 milliseconds) and in thyrotoxicosis decreases.

Thyroid Hormone Versus Sympathetic Nervous System or Catecholamines

- Certain effects of thyroid hormone, such as the increase in metabolic rate, heat production, heart rate, motor activity and central nervous system excitation, are also produced by the adrenergic catecholamines, epinephrine and norepinephrine.
- The exact relationship between thyroid hormone and catecholamines is not known. Most studies show that the thyroid hormone does not increase the level of catecholamines or their metabolites in blood, urine or tissues. In fact, norepinephrine levels (marker of sympathetic activity) are reduced by thyroid hormone.
- Probably, the thyroid hormones produce catecholamine-like effects by increasing levels of cAMP (a beta-adrenergic second messenger), as increased levels of cAMP are found in plasma, urine and muscle after T_4 administration. At least one mechanism for this important effect is that T_3 increases the number of beta-adrenergic receptors in the heart muscle.
- The catecholamines and T_4 potentiate the actions of each other. Further synergism between catecholamines and thyroid hormones is also required for maximal thermogenesis, lipolysis, glycogenolysis and gluconeogenesis to occur.

Important Note

A useful *adjunct therapy* in hyperthyroidism is treatment with a beta-adrenergic blocking agent, such as propranolol, which is extensively used in severe exacerbation of hyperthyroidism called thyroid storms.

Effects on Gastrointestinal Tract

Effects of thyroid hormones on GIT include:

- Increase in appetite and therefore increase in food intake.
- Increase in rate of secretion of digestive juices.
- Increase in motility of GIT; excess of thyroid hormone often causes diarrhoea.

Effects on Skeletal Muscles

Slight increase in thyroid hormones makes the muscle react with vigour.

Excessive quantities of thyroid hormones weaken the muscles because of increased protein catabolism (thyrotoxic myopathy). Muscle tremors occurring very rapidly at the rate of 10–15 times per second in hyperthyroidism are due to increased reactivity of neuronal synapses in the areas of the spinal cord that control muscle tone.

Lack of thyroid hormones causes weakness, cramps, stiffness and sluggishness in muscles.

Effects on Reproductive System

In both women and men, the thyroid hormone plays an important permissive role in the regulation of reproductive functions. The normal ovarian cycle of follicular development, maturation and ovulation; the homologous testicular process of spermatogenesis; and the maintenance of the healthy pregnant state are all disrupted by significant deviations of thyroid hormone levels from the normal range:

In males, lack of thyroid hormones causes complete loss of libido and excess of hormones causes impotence.

In females, lack of thyroid has varying effects:

- Menorrhagia and polymenorrhagia.
- Irregular periods or even amenorrhoea occurs in some women.

In hyperthyroid women, there is oligomenorrhoea (reduced bleeding). The effects of thyroid hormones on gonads are due to direct metabolic effects on the gonads as well as indirectly through alterations in the anterior pituitary hormones.

Effects on Other Endocrine Glands

Thyroid hormones also have significant effects on other parts of the endocrine system.

Pituitary production of growth hormone is increased, whereas that of prolactin is decreased.

Adrenocortical secretion of cortisol, as well as metabolic clearance of this hormone, is stimulated, but plasma-free cortisol levels remain normal.

Oestrogen and androgen ratio, in males, is increased. It accounts for occurrence of breast engorgement in males in hyperthyroidism.

Parathyroid hormone and 1,25-(OH)2 vitamin D are decreased as a compensatory consequence of the effects of thyroid hormone on bone resorption. Bone resorption is possibly stimulated by the T_3-induced release of interleukin-6 and interleukin-8 from osteoblasts.

Effects on Kidney

Kidney size, renal tubular epithelium, renal plasma flow, glomerular filtration rate and tubular transport maximum for a number of substances are also increased by thyroid hormone.

Applied Aspects of Thyroid Hormones

Abnormalities of Thyroid Gland

- Hyperthyroidism
- Hypothyroidism

Hyperthyroidism

Hyperthyroidism refers to increased secretion of thyroid hormones. Its common causes are as follows:

Graves disease (described below).

Toxic nodular goitre (multinodular or solitary nodule): Nodule of thyroid tissue causes large amounts of thyroid hormone secretion. There is no evidence of autoimmune disease.

Other causes of hyperthyroidism:

- Thyroiditis (inflammation of thyroid gland)
- Excessive pituitary secretion of TSH
- Ingestion of exogenous T_4 and T_3
- Activating mutations of TRs
- Too much consumption of iodine (in either food or supplement or medication)

Graves Disease. Graves disease or toxic goitre or thyrotoxicosis is the most common cause of hyperthyroidism.

It was first described by Sir Robert Grove in the 19th century.

Aetiology It is an autoimmune disease characterized by development of thyroid-stimulating antibodies (TSAb) against the TSH receptors, also called long-acting thyroid stimulator (LATS). These antibodies bind to TSH receptors and mimic TSH action on thyroid growth and hormone synthesis. The entire thyroid gland undergoes hyperplasia as a result of autoimmune stimulation.

Symptoms and signs of Graves disease include:

1. ***General features of Graves disease are:***
   - Marked increase in basal metabolic rate (BMR).
   - Weight loss, despite an increased intake of food.
   - Increased heat production causes discomfort in warm environments, excessive sweating and a greater intake of water.
2. ***Goitre:*** Goitre refers to swelling of thyroid gland. Graves disease is characterized by diffuse goitre, while a single or more nodules indicate toxic nodular goitre.
3. ***Cardiovascular features include:***
   - Increased pulse rate or sinus tachycardia.
   - Wide pulse pressure (difference between systolic and diastolic pressure) is more than 60 mm Hg.
   - Exertional dyspnoea.
   - Arrhythmias (atrial fibrillation is commonest).
   - Precipitation of angina in patients with ischaemic heart disease.
4. ***Neuromuscular features include:***
   - Nervousness, irritability
   - Restlessness, psychosis
   - Tremors of hand
   - Muscular weakness
   - Exaggerated tendon reflexes
5. ***Gastrointestinal features include:***
   - Diarrhoea or steatorrhoea
   - Vomiting
6. ***Dermatological features are:***
   - Perspiration (increased sweating or hyperhidrosis)
   - Loss of hair

- Redness of palm
- Pretibial myxoedema

7. ***Reproductive features include:***
   - Impotence in males
   - Oligomenorrhoea or amenorrhoea, abortions and infertility in females
8. ***Ophthalmological signs of Graves disease are:***
   - Lid retraction producing staring look (*Dalrymple's sign*).
   - Lid lag (von Graefe's sign).
   - Wide palpebral fissure.
   - Exophthalmos, i.e. bulging out of eyeballs: Exophthalmos occurs due to cytokine-mediated proliferation of fibroblasts which secrete hydrophilic glycosaminoglycans, leading to increase in interstitial fluid contents combined with chronic inflammatory cells, resulting in marked swelling and ultimately fibrosis of extraocular muscles and rise in retrobulbar pressure. The eyes displace forward (proptosis and exophthalmos) (Fig. 8.3.10).
   - Diplopia with ocular motility defect because of extraocular muscle involvement.

Diagnosis For diagnosis, the investigations are as follows:

Investigations show:

- Both T_3 and T_4 plasma levels are elevated.
- TSH is low or may become undetectable.
- ^{131}I uptake is increased, i.e. >35% at 5 hours.
- TR antibodies may be increased >7 units/L (*N* ≤7 units/L).
- Serum cholesterol is less.
- ECG shows tachycardia and arrhythmia.
- Ultrasonography of thyroid gland shows diffuse goitre.

Treatment include:

1. Drug therapy consists of antithyroid drugs and beta-blockers.

Antithyroid drugs: These drugs block the iodination of tyrosine and hence reduce the synthesis of thyroid hormones. Common antithyroid drugs include carbimazole, propylthiouracil and methimazole.

- *Methimazole* is the first choice of drug but prolonged use of this drug has side effects.

Note: In pregnant women, methimazole is not used especially during first trimester because of risk of birth defects.

- *Carbimazole* also has an immunosuppressive action, leading to reduction of serum TR_{Ab} concentration.
- *Beta-blockers:* A nonselective beta-blocker is useful for symptomatic relief but it does not abolish thyrotoxicosis. Propranolol and metoprolol are preferred drugs.

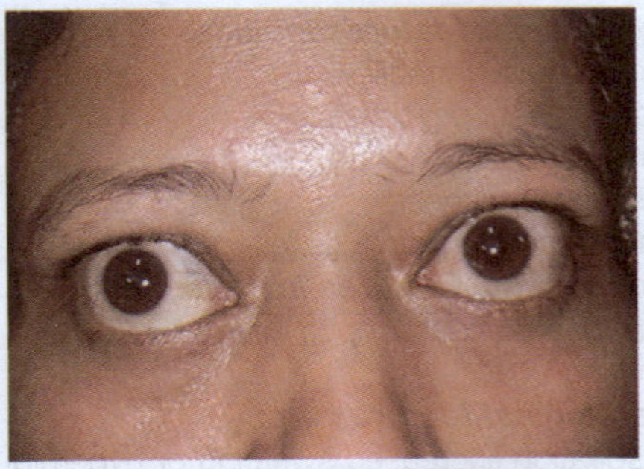

Fig. 8.3.10 Patient with Graves disease having exophthalmos.

Note: Beta-blockers are not often prescribed for asthmatic patients, because these drugs may trigger asthma attack.

- Beta-blockers may also affect diabetic management.

2. Surgical subtotal thyroidectomy is indicated in large goitre with frequent relapses on drug treatment.

3. Radioactive ablation of thyroid by ^{131}I is indicated in cases with recurrence following surgery. ^{131}I has long-lasting inhibitory effect on survival and replication of follicular cells.

4. For Graves ophthalmopathy, depending on the severity of symptoms, the following management is prescribed:

Artificial tears during daytime and lubricating gel at night.
Corticosteroids (prednisone) – to diminish swelling of the eyeballs.

- Use of prisms in glasses may help in correction of double vision (diplopia).
- *Orbital compression surgery* is recommended when pressure on the optic nerve threatens loss of vision.

5. For Graves dermopathy, use of creams/ointments containing hydrocortisone to relieve swelling and redness.

Note: During pregnancy, some women tend to develop inflamed thyroid known as postpartum thyroiditis.

Hypothyroidism

Hypothyroidism is a clinical syndrome caused by low levels of circulating thyroid hormones.

Aetiology. Depending on the aetiology, hypothyroidism can be primary or secondary.

Primary hypothyroidism is caused by the disorder of thyroid gland. Causes include:

1. ***Idiopathic or spontaneous or atrophic hypothyroidism***
2. ***Goitrous hypothyroidism occurs in:***
   - Hashimoto thyroiditis
   - Deficiency of iodine:
     - Drug-induced, e.g. *para*-aminosalicylic acid and lithium are the most common medications that cause hypothyroidism
     - Dyshormonogenesis
3. ***Postablative hypothyroidism,*** i.e.:
   - Following surgery
   - Following ^{131}I administration
4. ***Transient due to thyroiditis*** (self-limiting)
5. ***Maternally transmitted*** (iodide, antithyroid drugs)

Secondary hypothyroidism is caused by diseases of anterior pituitary and hypothalamus.

Thyroid hormone resistance usually inherited as autosomal dominant disorder, occurs due to mutation in TRβ gene that codes TSH receptor β (TRβ), associated with resistance to the effects of T_3 and T_4.

Attention-deficit hyperactivity disorder is a condition associated with thyroid hormone resistance, usually common in hyperactive and impulsive children.

Clinical Features. Clinical features depend on the age at which deficiency manifests, duration and severity of the disease. Three different clinical entities are as follows:

- Infantile hypothyroidism (cretinism)
- Juvenile hypothyroidism
- Adult hypothyroidism (myxoedema)

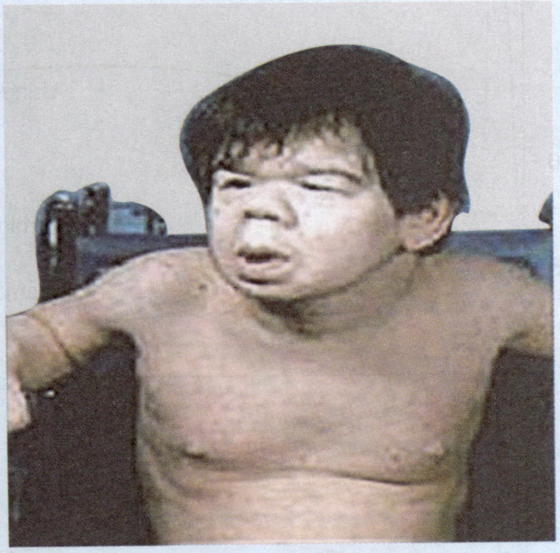

Fig. 8.3.11 Clinical features of cretinism. Note short stature, pot belly and idiotic look.

1. ***Infantile hypothyroidism (cretinism):*** It occurs when thyroid deficiency occurs during the first year of life and is characterized by (Fig. 8.3.11) mental retardation, marked retardation of growth, delayed milestones of development, potbelly, protruding tongue, flat nose, dry skin and sparse hair.

   Radiograph of bone shows delayed bone age.

   Treatment should be prompt; otherwise, mental deficiency will persist.
2. ***Juvenile hypothyroidism (dwarf)*** manifests at adolescence and is characterized by short stature, poor performance at school, and delayed puberty and sexual maturation. Other features of adult hypothyroidism are present in variable degrees.
3. ***Adult hypothyroidism*** is also called myxoedema because of the characteristic infiltration of skin by myxoedematous tissue (Fig. 8.3.12). Paradoxically, iodide itself inhibits thyroid functions. In normal individuals, a high dose of iodide acts directly on the thyroid gland and inhibits organification and decreases hormone synthesis. The effect is known as *Wolff–Chaikoff effect*. In hypothyroidism, there is infiltration of body tissues by polymucopolysaccharides, hyaluronic acid and chondroitin sulphate. Infiltration of the dermis causes nonpitting oedema (myxoedema) which is most marked on the skin of the hands, feet and eyelids (periorbital puffiness). Symptoms and signs include:

   General features: Tiredness and weight gain without an appreciable increase in caloric intake (due to lower than normal metabolic rate). Decreased heat production, lower body temperature, intolerance to cold and decreased sweating.

   Cardiovascular features: Adrenergic activity is decreased causing bradycardia. Other features include hypertension, pericardial effusion and precipitation of angina.

   Neuromuscular features: Movement, speech and thought are all slowed, and lethargy, sleepiness, delayed relaxation of ankle jerks (termed Woltman sign or hung-up deep tendon reflex), aches and pain are common and pressure palsy of peripheral nerves (e.g. carpal tunnel syndrome) due to entrapment in excess ground substance.

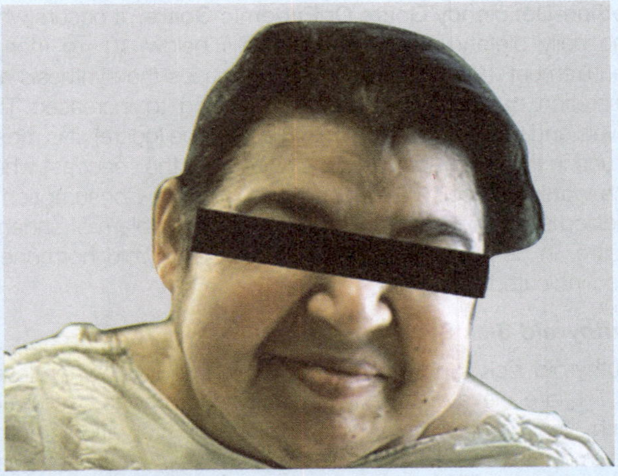

Fig. 8.3.12 Photograph of a patient with myxoedema showing puffy face, thick lips and periorbital oedema.

Reduced levels of thyroid hormones lead to mental retardation, forgetfulness, hearing loss, hypotonia, ataxia and psychosis termed myxoedema madness.

Dermatological features: Dry, thick skin (toad skin), sparse hair, nonpitting oedema due to infiltration by myxoedematous tissue (myxoedema). Lemon yellow tint of the skin occurs due to carotenaemia.

Reproductive features: Menorrhagia and infertility (common), galactorrhoea and impotence (less common).

Gastrointestinal features: Constipation (common) and adynamic ileus (less common).

Haematological feature: It includes anaemia.

Investigations of hypothyroidism are:

- Serum T_3 and T_4 levels low.
- Serum TSH levels high in primary hypothyroidism, low in secondary hypothyroidism.
- Serum cholesterol high.
- Peripheral blood film shows macrocytic anaemia.
- ECG classically demonstrates sinus bradycardia, low-voltage complexes, and ST-segment and T-wave abnormalities.
- Photomotogram – delayed ankle jerk.

Treatment. Treatment of hypothyroidism is lifelong replacement of thyroid hormones by l-thyroxine.

Goitre

Goitre refers to any abnormal increase in the size of the thyroid gland. The term goitre does not denote the functional status of thyroid gland, because it may be associated with:

- *Euthyroid*, i.e. normal thyroid hormone level
- *Hypothyroidism*, i.e. low thyroid hormone level
- *Hyperthyroidism*, i.e. high thyroid hormone levels, as seen in Graves disease and toxic nodular goitre

Goitrogenic Substances (goitrogens). These are the substances that interfere with the production of thyroid hormone and cause thyroid enlargement, i.e. goitre. These include thiocyanates, nitrates and perchlorates and drugs such as thiourea, thiouracil and thiocarbamide. Certain plant foods such as cabbage, cauliflower and turnip contain goitrogenic factors, mostly thiocyanates.

If the goitrogen reduces thyroid hormone synthesis to subnormal levels, TSH secretion is increased, chronically producing hypertrophy of thyroid gland (goitre).

Iodine-Deficiency Goitre Or Endemic Goitre. It occurs when the daily dietary intake of iodine falls below 10 µg (normal requirement 100–200 µg/day). It decreases the synthesis and secretion of the thyroid hormone leading to increased TSH levels and proliferation of thyroid gland tissue (goitre). It is mostly found in the geographic regions away from the seacoast where the water and soil are low in iodine content. Consumption of iodized salt is advocated to overcome the problem of endemic goitre. In certain cases, administration of thyroid hormone is also indicated.

Euthyroid Sick Syndrome

Euthyroid sick syndrome refers to the condition when levels of RT_3 are elevated. Euthyroid sick syndrome is associated with various conditions like prolonged starvation, burns, trauma, cirrhosis and chronic kidney diseases. It is basically an adaptive response to conserve calories and proteins. This condition is characterized by low levels of T_3 and T_4 and high levels of RT_3.

THYROID FUNCTION TESTS

1. Measurement of basal metabolic rate Theoretically, it is the physiological test of thyroid functions, since it measures the tissue response (O_2 consumption). However, because of poor sensitivity and specificity, BMR is now seldom used as a thyroid function test.

- Normal values of BMR: ±20%.
- In hyperthyroidism, BMR may increase to 100%.
- In hypothyroidism, it may decrease to −30% to −40%.

2. Estimation of protein-bound iodine (PBI) It reflects the level of circulating T_3 and T_4 bound to plasma protein. However, because of poor sensitivity and specificity, estimation of PBI is no longer considered as a thyroid function test.

- Normal values – 6 g/100 mL.
- Decreased levels of PBI are seen in hypothyroidism, pregnancy and acute thyroiditis.
- Increased levels of PBI occur in hyperthyroidism and patients on oral contraceptives.

3. Radioactive iodine uptake (RAIU) This test, being a cumbersome and time-consuming procedure, is no longer used nowadays as a routine thyroid function test. To perform this test, 25 Ci of radioactive iodine (^{131}I) is given orally in 100 mL water and thyroid uptake is determined by placing an X-ray counter over the neck. An area over the thigh is also counted and count in this region is subtracted from the neck count to correct for nonthyroidal radioactivity in the neck.

- Normal value of RAIU by thyroid (at 24 hours) is 20%–40%.
- In hyperthyroidism, this value may be 60%.
- In hypothyroidism, this value may be <20%.

The analysis of RAIU is helpful in understanding the physiology of the thyroid gland. The RAIU in a normal person is plotted in Fig. 8.3.13A.

- In hyperthyroidism, the amount of radioactivity in the thyroid gland rises sharply because iodide is rapidly incorporated into T_4 and T_3 and then starts declining within 24 hours (Fig. 8.3.13B).
- In hypothyroidism, the uptake is low (Fig. 8.3.13C).

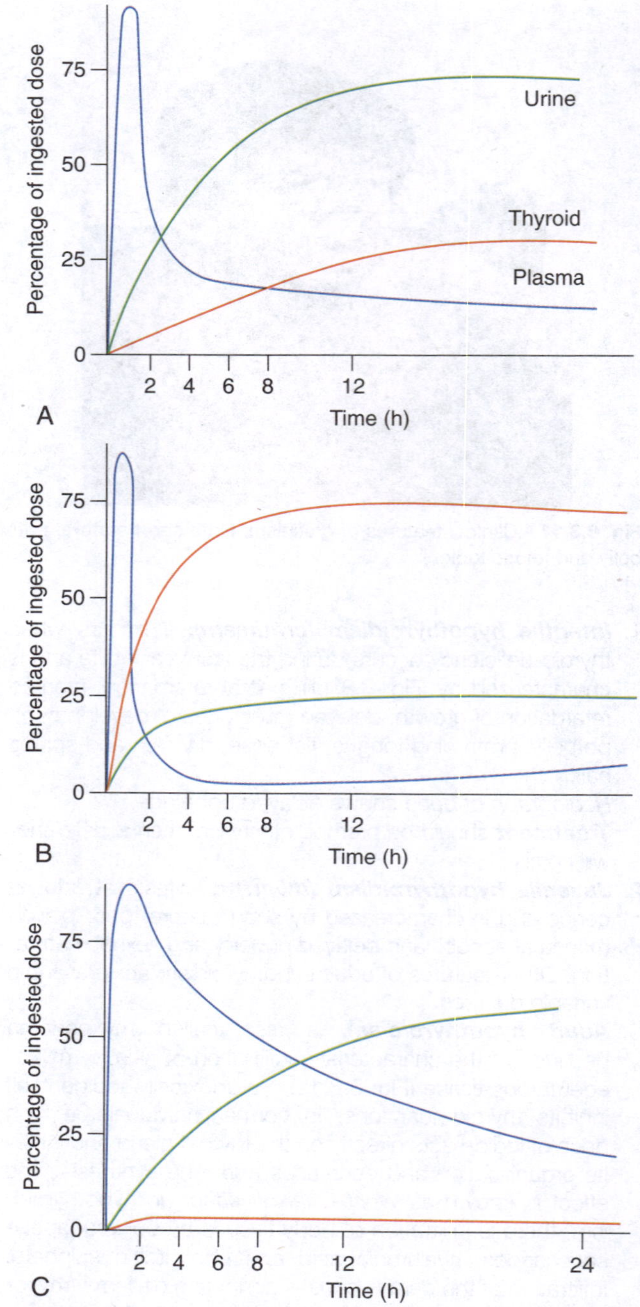

Fig. 8.3.13 Distribution of radioactive iodine (^{123}I) uptake: **A**, in normal (euthyroid); **B**, hyperthyroid; and **C**, hypothyroid individuals.

> **Important Note**
>
> A large amount of radioactive iodine destroys thyroid tissue; therefore, radioactive iodine therapy is useful in some cases of Graves disease and thyroid carcinomas.

4. Measurement of total and free T_3 and T_4 and TSH levels in blood These tests are considered best and are widely used for the diagnosis of various thyroid disorders. An accurate estimation of thyroid hormones can be done by

Table 8.3.2 Normal values of T_3, T_4, TSH and changes in hyperthyroidism and hypothyroidism

	Normal values	Hyperthyroidism	Hypothyroidism
• Total serum T	0.12 μg/dL	↑	↓
• Total serum T_4	8 μg/dL	↑	↓
• Free serum T_3	0.28 ng/dL	↑	↓
• Free serum T_4	2 ng/dL	↑	↓
• Serum TSH	0.2–5 μIU/mL	↑	↓

radioimmunoassay (RIA) or by the ELISA method. Their normal values and changes in hyperthyroidism and hypothyroidism are shown in Table 8.3.2.

Note. *Total T_3 and T_4* estimation has the following drawbacks:

- It measures the total amount of the hormone, the major portion of which is bound and does not take part in metabolism.
- The values are liable to be altered with the fluctuations in the levels of thyroid-binding proteins (TBG), such as during pregnancy and other related conditions.
- *Free T_3 and T_4 estimation* truly represents thyroid activity, hence are preferred to total T_3 and T_4.
- *TSH levels* are an important parameter of thyroid disorder which tests the integrity of hypothalamus–pituitary–thyroid axis.

5. Ultrasonography of thyroid gland Ultrasonography (B-scan) allows evaluation of an enlarged thyroid gland. It elucidates shape and dimension of nodules in the thyroid gland.

6. Thyroid scan A radionucleotide scan of thyroid by either ^{131}I or ^{99m}Tc is useful in demonstrating functioning thyroid tissue. It detects hot (functioning) and cold (nonfunctioning) nodule/nodules in the thyroid, in cases with single or multinodular goitre.

7. Antithyroid antibodies Detection of antithyroid antibodies is useful in diagnosing autoimmune thyroid disorder, such as Hashimoto thyroiditis.

8. Fine-needle aspiration biopsy (FNAB) It is carried out in patients with nodular goitre to detect any malignant process.

ANTITHYROID DRUGS

Secretions of the thyroid gland can be reduced by antithyroid drugs. These drugs act by different ways; therefore, depending on the mechanism of action, these drugs are of the following types:

A. ***Drugs inhibiting iodide trapping by thyroid:*** These drugs act by two ways:
   - *Competitive inhibition* (monovalent ions, such as chlorate, perchlorate, thiocyanate compete with I_2 for active transport into the thyroid gland)
   - *Metabolic poisons* such as dinitrate and cyanide

B. ***Drugs inhibiting oxidation of iodide and coupling:*** Thioureylenes (e.g. thiouracil and carbimazole) inhibit iodination of MIT and block the coupling reaction to form T_3 and T_4.

C. ***Drugs inhibiting release of thyroxine (T_4 and T_3):*** A large dose decreases release of thyroid hormones, thus decreases serum concentration of T_4 and T_3.
   This effect is called *Wolff–Chaikoff effect.*

Important Note

Patients with hyperthyroidism are more responsive to *iodide* as compared with normal individuals because the Wolff–Chaikoff effect is greater and more prolonged as a result of increased iodine transport.

Excess amount of iodine can cause both hypothyroidism and hyperthyroidism.

Jod-Basedow effect: This effect is just opposite to the Wolff–Chaikoff effect, i.e. excess iodine induces hyperthyroidism.

Self-Assessment

1. Discuss the biosynthesis of thyroid hormone and its mechanism of action.
2. Describe the following:
   - Regulation of secretion of thyroid hormone
   - Functions of thyroid hormone
3. Write notes on:
   - Graves disease
   - Wolff–Chaikoff effect
   - Hypothyroidism
   - Thyroid function tests
   - Antithyroid drugs

Clinical Cases

Case 1

A 56-year-old woman presented in the ENT department with loss of appetite, difficulty in swallowing and weight loss since last 3 months. Examination revealed swelling in the neck, so she was referred to the endocrinology department.

Thyroid function tests revealed the following: Total thyroxin level within normal range, TSH level low, clinically absence of goitre and labelled as euthyroid. After few weeks, thyroid function tests were repeated that showed raised level of thyroxine and suppressed TSH.

Q1. What is the probable diagnosis?
Q2. What is the aetiology of this condition?
Q3. What are the typical signs and symptoms?
Q4. What are the changes expected in the ECG?
Q5. What is the treatment basis in this condition?

Case 2

A 40-year-old female presented with complaints of weight gain, puffiness of face, weakness and slowness. History revealed that she is having cold intolerance, constipation and depression.

Examination observations showed hypothermia, dry skin, scanty hair and non-pitting oedema.

Q1. What is this condition called as?
Q2. What is the cause for non-pitting oedema in this condition?
Q3. What biochemical tests to be done to reach the final diagnosis?
Q4. What should be the treatment plan for this case?

Case 3

A 9-year-old female child was admitted with the following symptoms:

- Short strature by her age.
- Reduced muscle power and incoordination.

Family history revealed that mother is a case of hypothyroidism. The probable diagnosis made was a case of cretinism.

Q1. What is the main cause of this condition?
Q2. How this condition can be treated?
Q3. What are the consequences is not treated properly and timely?

8.4

Endocrinal Control of Calcium Metabolism and Bone Physiology

INTRODUCTION

Calcium, phosphorus and magnesium belong to a group of seven principal elements which constitute 60%–80% of the body's inorganic material. Calcium and phosphorus form important structural components of bones and teeth, and are important determinants of neuromuscular excitability. Various hormones involved in the regulation of metabolism of these minerals include:

Calcitropic hormones refer to three hormones, namely parathyroid hormone (PTH), calcitonin and cholecalciferol (vitamin D_3), which are primarily concerned with the regulation of calcium, phosphate and magnesium metabolism in the body. These hormones act on three organ systems, bones, kidneys and intestinal tract, to maintain calcium and phosphate levels in the face of environmental changes.

Parathyroid hormone–related protein (PTHrP) is the fourth local hormone that acts on the PTH receptor and is important for skeletal development in utero.

Other hormones which also have some effect on calcium metabolism include glucocorticoids, growth hormone, oestrogens and various growth factors.

Discussion in this chapter is limited to regulatory role of PTH, calcitonin and cholecalciferol (vitamin D_3) only. An overview is presented of calcium and phosphate metabolism, as well as of the related structural and functional aspects of bone physiology.

CALCIUM, PHOSPHORUS AND MAGNESIUM METABOLISM

CALCIUM METABOLISM

Physiological and Biochemical Functions

Calcium ions regulate a number of important physiological and biochemical processes. To ensure that these processes operate normally, the plasma concentration is maintained within a very narrow limit (9–11 mg%). Free, ionized calcium is the biologically active form of calcium.

Important physiological and biochemical functions subserved by calcium are as follows:

1. ***Development of bone and teeth:*** Calcium along with phosphorus is essential for the formation (of hydroxyapatite) and physical strength of skeletal tissue. Bones which are in dynamic state serve as reservoir of calcium.
2. ***Neuromuscular excitation:*** Calcium is essential for the transmission of nerve impulse. It interacts with troponin C to trigger muscle contraction. Calcium also activates ATPases and increases the interaction between actin and myosin.
3. ***Blood coagulation:*** Calcium (factor IV) is involved in several reactions in the cascade of blood clotting mechanism.
4. ***Membrane integrity and plasma membrane transport:*** Permeability and transport of water and several ions across the cell membrane are influenced by calcium.
5. ***Mediation of intracellular action of hormones:*** Calcium mediates the intracellular actions of certain hormones by acting as a second messenger (e.g. epinephrine in liver glycogenolysis) and third messenger (e.g. antidiuretic hormone acts through cAMP, and then Ca^{2+}).
6. ***Activation of enzymes:*** Calcium is needed for direct activation of enzymes, such as lipase (pancreatic), ATPase and succinate dehydrogenase.
7. ***Release of hormones and neurotransmitters:*** Calcium facilitates the release of certain hormones and neurotransmitters, e.g. insulin, PTH and calcitonin.
8. ***Calmodulin-mediated action of calcium:*** Calmodulin is a calcium-binding protein. Calcium–calmodulin complex activates certain enzymes, e.g. adenylyl cyclase and calcium-dependent protein kinases.
9. ***Regulation of secretory processes:*** The microfilament- and microtubule-mediated processes such as endocytosis, exocytosis and cell motility are regulated by calcium.
10. ***Contact inhibition:*** Calcium is believed to be involved in cell-to-cell contact and adhesion of cells in tissues. It may also be required for cell-to-cell communication.
11. ***Action on heart:*** By acting on myocardium, calcium prolongs the systole.

Calcium Distribution in the Body

Calcium is the most abundant mineral in the body. The total content of calcium in an adult man is approximately 1100 g (27.5 mol). As much as 99% of it is present in the bones and teeth as hydroxyapatite. A small fraction (1%) of the calcium found outside the skeletal tissues performs a wide variety of functions.

Calcium in bones Calcium in bones is present in two pools:

1. ***Pool of stable calcium*** is much larger (99% of total bone calcium) and is formed by the calcium present in stable mature bones. It represents the calcium pool that is not readily exchangeable, but can be mobilized only through the action of PTH.
2. ***Pool (reservoir) of readily exchangeable calcium*** is much smaller (only 1% of the total bony content) and consists of labile (young) newly formed bone.

Calcium in plasma Most of the blood calcium is present in the plasma, since blood cells contain very little of it. In the plasma, calcium is present in nondiffusible (40% of total plasma calcium) and diffusible forms. The diffusible form includes further two forms: the ionized calcium (50% of total plasma calcium) and that complexed to HCO_3^-, citrate, etc. (10% of total plasma calcium). The diffusible form of calcium, as the name indicates, is diffusible from blood to the tissues, while the nondiffusible form is not. The nondiffusible form refers to the calcium which is bound to plasma proteins, mostly albumin and to a lesser extent globulin.

Normal values of different forms of plasma calcium are as follows:

Total plasma calcium

	10 mg% (2.5 mmol/L) (range 9–11 mg%)
Diffusible calcium	6 mg% (1.5 mmol/L)
• *Ionized calcium*	5 mg% (1.25 mmol/L) (50% of total plasma calcium)
• **Complexed** to HCO_3^-, citrate, etc.	1 mg% (0.25 mmol/L) (10% of total plasma calcium)
Nondiffusible calcium	4 mg% (1 mmol/L)
• Bound to albumin	That is, 40% of total plasma calcium

Dietary Requirement and Sources of Calcium

Dietary requirements of calcium per day are as follows:

• Adult man and woman	800 mg/day
• Women during pregnancy, lactation and postmenopause	1500 mg/day
• Children (1–18 years)	800–1200 mg/day
• Infants (<1 year)	300–500 mg/day

Dietary sources of calcium:

- *Best sources* are milk and milk products.
- *Good sources* include beans, leafy vegetables, fish, cabbage, egg yolk and cereals (ragi).
- Drinking water provides approximately 200 mg/day.

Calcium Balance

The calcium ion is fundamentally important to all biological systems. Therefore, the concentration of calcium must be maintained within specific limits of physiological tolerance in several compartments. The overall calcium homeostasis (calcium balance) or the normal daily calcium turnover is maintained by an interplay of the following processes (Fig. 8.4.1):

- Absorption of ingested calcium
- Exchange of calcium between bone and extracellular fluid (ECF)
- Secretion of calcium from ECF
- Excretion of calcium in the faecal matter and urine

Absorption of Calcium

The daily dietary intake of calcium, depending on the amount of milk and milk products consumed, may vary from 200 to 2000 mg. Unfortunately, in many adults, the daily intake of calcium is below the recommended minimum of 800 mg.

Process of absorption The absorption of calcium mainly occurs in the duodenum by an energy-dependent active process. This process involves the activity of calcium-dependent

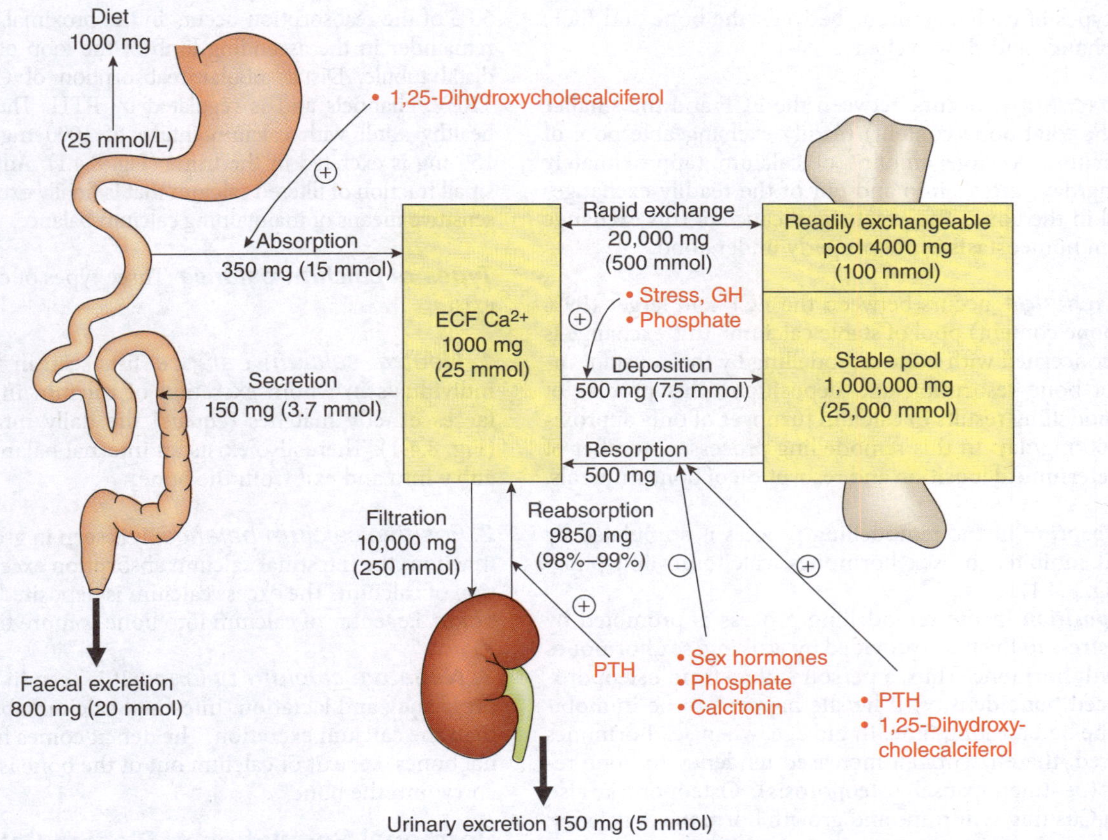

Fig. 8.4.1 Hormonal maintenance of calcium balance in an adult human ingesting 1000 mg (25 mmol) of calcium per day.

ATPase at brush border of epithelial cells and is regulated by 1,25-dihydroxycholecalciferol.

Across the brush border, Ca^{2+} is transported via channels known as transient receptor potential vanilloid type-6 (TRPV-6) and binds to an intracellular protein (calbindin-D_{qK}).

From the basolateral border of intestinal epithelial cells, absorbed Ca^{2+} is transported into the blood by either Na^+/Ca^{2+} exchanger (NCX_1) or Ca^{2+}-dependent ATPase.

Factors promoting absorption

1,25-Dihydroxycholecalciferol directly affects the absorption by its regulatory role.

PTH indirectly promotes the intestinal absorption of calcium by increasing the renal synthesis of 1,25-dihydroxycholecalciferol.

Dietary lactose promotes calcium intake by intestinal cells by some unknown mechanism.

Amino acids lysine and arginine facilitate calcium absorption.

Low pH is more favourable for calcium absorption.

Factors inhibiting calcium absorption

Phytates and oxalates present in the diet form insoluble salts with calcium and thereby decrease its absorption.

Phosphates present in high amount in diet result in the formation of insoluble calcium phosphate and prevent calcium uptake. The dietary ratio of calcium:phosphate between 1:2 and 2:1 is ideal for optimum calcium absorption.

Free fatty acids react with calcium to form insoluble calcium soaps. This is particularly observed when fat absorption is impaired.

High pH is unfavourable for calcium absorption.

Dietary fibre in high content interferes with calcium absorption.

Adaptive mechanism for absorption The percentage of dietary calcium absorbed from the intestine is inversely related to intake.

Adaptive increase in fractional absorption is one mechanism for maintaining normal body calcium start when the dietary intake of calcium is chronically low. The adaptation seems to be produced through greater synthesis of 1,25-dihydroxycholecalciferol.

Adaptive decrease in calcium absorption occurs when the diet supplies too much calcium. This adaptation prevents overload and seems to be produced through lesser synthesis of 1,25-dihydroxycholecalciferol.

Normal absorption: Normally, at a daily intake of 1000 mg of calcium, approximately 35% (i.e. 350 mg) is absorbed (Fig. 8.4.1), approximately half passively and half stimulated by vitamin D.

Important Note

In elderly individuals, both the dietary calcium intake and the absorption of calcium from the intestine are diminished. This decreased calcium input contributes to a declining bone mass and the increased risk of fracture in the aged due to osteoporosis.

Exchange of Calcium Between Bone and Extracellular Fluid

The ECF contains approximately 1000 mg of calcium, which is in dynamic equilibrium with the calcium present in the bones.

Two types of exchange occur between the bone and ECF: rapid exchange and slow exchange.

Rapid exchange occurs between the ECF and the smaller (1% of the total bony content) readily exchangeable pool of bone calcium. A large amount of calcium (approximately 20,000 mg/day) moves into and out of the readily exchangeable pool in the bone. The exact significance of this exchange in calcium homeostasis is not properly understood.

Slow exchange occurs between the ECF and larger (99% of total bone content) pool of stable calcium. This exchange is the one concerned with bone remodelling by the constant interplay of bone resorption and deposition. This process of bone remodelling results in calcium turnover of only approximately 500 mg/day. In this remodelling process, a number of factors determine deposition and resorption of bone minerals.

Bone resorption in the remodelling process is stimulated by PTH and inhibited by sex hormones, calcitonin and phosphate (Fig. 8.4.1).
Bone deposition in the remodelling process is promoted by physical stress to the bone provided by walking, sex hormones and growth hormone. Thus, a person suffers from osteoporosis (reduced bone density) if he/she happens to be immobilized in the bed for long time. In old age, when sex hormones are reduced, there occurs an increased tendency to bone resorption (postmenopausal osteoporosis). Osteoporosis also occurs in Cushing syndrome and growth hormone deficiency.

Excretion of Calcium

The same amount of calcium as absorbed from the gut, i.e. approximately 350 mg, must ultimately be excreted to maintain balance. Excretion of calcium occurs in the faecal matter as well as urine.

Faecal excretion of calcium Approximately 150 mg calcium is secreted into the intestine through bile, pancreatic juice and intestinal secretions, and excreted in the stools along with the unabsorbed fraction (650 mg) from the diet. In this way, approximately 800 mg of calcium is excreted in the faecal matter (Fig. 8.4.1).

Urinary excretion of calcium A large amount (approximately 10,000 mg) of calcium is filtered in the kidneys per day, but 98%–99% of the filtered calcium is reabsorbed. Approximately 60% of the reabsorption occurs in the proximal tubules and the remainder in the ascending limb of the loop of Henle and the distal tubule. Distal tubular reabsorption of Ca^{2+} occurs via $TRPV_5$ channels and is regulated by PTH. Thus, in a normal healthy adult with calcium intake of 1000 mg, approximately 150 mg is excreted in the urine (Fig. 8.4.1). Adjustment of this small fraction of filtered calcium that is finally excreted provides a sensitive means of maintaining calcium balance.

Types of calcium balance Three types of calcium balance exist.

1. Neutral calcium balance It is seen in normal healthy individuals in whom excretion of calcium in the urine and faeces exactly matches (equals) the daily intake of calcium (Fig. 8.4.1). There also exists an internal balance between the entry into and exit from the bone.

2. Positive calcium balance It is seen in growing children, in whom the intestinal calcium absorption exceeds total excretion of calcium. The excess calcium is deposited in the growing bones, i.e. entry of calcium into bone is more than the exit.

3. Negative calcium balance It is seen in women during pregnancy and lactation. Intestinal calcium absorption is less than the calcium excretion. The deficit comes from the maternal bones, i.e. exit of calcium out of the bone is more than the entry into the bone.

Hormonal Regulation of Plasma Calcium Level

As mentioned earlier, maintenance of plasma calcium level within narrow range (9–11 mg/dL) is essential as it is involved in a number of important physiological and biochemical processes. Deviations of the ionized calcium from the normal range cause many disorders and can be life-threatening. The hormones regulating plasma calcium levels include the following.

A. Calcitropic hormones The three primarily involved in the calcium homeostasis are as follows:

- PTH
- Active form of vitamin D (1,25-dihydroxycholecalciferol)
- Calcitonin

Main role of these hormones in calcium metabolism is summarized in Table 8.4.1 and Fig. 8.4.1.

Table 8.4.1 Summary of calcitropic hormones that regulate calcium balance

	PTH	1,25-Dihydroxycholecalciferol	Calcitonin
Stimulus for secretion	↓ Serum Ca^{2+}	↓ Serum Ca^{2+} ↑ PTH ↓ Serum phosphate	↑ Serum Ca^{2+}
Actions on			
• Bone	↑ Resorption	↑ Resorption	↓ Resorption
• Kidney	↓ P reabsorption ↑ Ca^{2+} reabsorption	↑ P reabsorption ↑ Ca^{2+} reabsorption	– –
• Intestine	↑ Ca^{2+} absorption	↑ Ca^{2+} absorption	–
Overall effect on			
• Serum Ca^{2+}	↑	↑	↓
• Serum phosphate	↓	↑	–

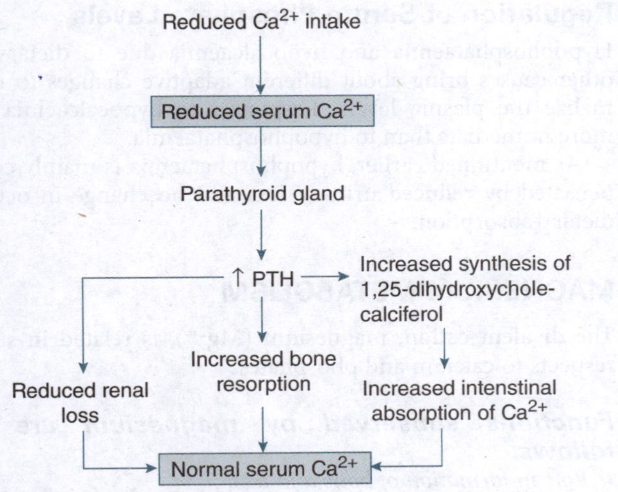

Fig. 8.4.2 Mechanism of regulation of serum calcium levels in hypocalcaemia.

B. Parathyroid hormone–related protein It is a local hormone that acts on the PTH receptors and is important for skeletal development in utero (for details, see page 717).

C. Other hormones Other hormones which have some effect on calcium metabolism include:

- *Growth hormone* has stimulatory effect on bone deposition.
- *Sex hormones* have inhibitory effect on bone resorption.
- *Glucocorticoids* have stimulatory effect on bone resorption.
- *Growth factors* have stimulatory effect on bone deposition.

Important Note

Hypocalcaemia is compensated by (Fig. 8.4.2):

- Release of calcium from the bones
- Increased fractional reabsorption in the kidney
- Increased absorption from the intestine

PHOSPHORUS METABOLISM

Physiological and Biochemical Functions

The phosphate ion is also critically important to all biological systems. Important functions subserved by phosphate are as follows:

1. ***Development of bone and teeth.***
2. ***Structural part of:***
   - *High-energy* transfer and storage compounds such as ATP, GTP, creatine phosphate
   - *Cofactors* such as NAD, NADP and thiamine pyrophosphate
   - Second messengers, e.g. cAMP, inositol triphosphate
   - Nucleic acids (DNA, RNA), phospholipids and phosphoproteins
3. ***Activation of enzymes*** by phosphorylation.
4. ***Role in carbohydrate*** metabolism.
5. ***Phosphate buffer system*** is important for the maintenance of pH in the blood as well as in the cells.
6. ***Important intracellular anion*** that balances certain cations (K^+ and Mg^{2+}) inside the cells.

Distribution of Phosphate in the Body

An adult body contains approximately 1 kg phosphate (P) which is distributed as:

- *Bones and teeth* — 80% (in combination with Ca^{2+})
- *Muscles and blood* — 10% (in association with proteins, carbohydrates and lipids)
- *Chemical compounds* — 10% widely distributed in body

Blood phosphate

- *Plasma levels* (P_I) — 3–5 mg%
- *Whole blood* — 40 mg% (because RBCs and WBCs have very high content of phosphate)
- *Plasma phosphate exists in* three forms:
  - Protein bound — 10%
  - Free ions — 40%
  - Complexed with cations — 50% (Ca^{2+}, Mg^{2+}, Na^+, K^+)

Important Note

Fasting plasma phosphate levels are higher than the postprandial levels. It is because of the reason that after ingestion of carbohydrates, the phosphate from the plasma is drawn by the cells for metabolism (phosphorylation reaction).

Phosphorus Balance (Fig. 8.4.3)

1. Intake and absorption Recommended intake is approximately 800 mg/day. The recommended ratio of Ca^{2+}: P in adults is 1:1 and in infants 2:1. Sources of phosphorus are milk, cereals, leafy vegetables, meat and eggs. Ca^{2+} and phosphorus are distributed in the majority of natural foods in a 1:1 ratio. Therefore, it is generally held that one should take

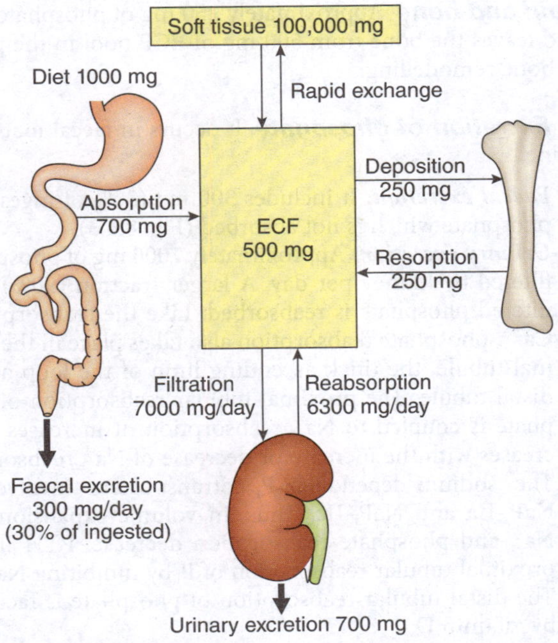

Fig. 8.4.3 Maintenance of phosphorus balance in an adult human ingesting 1000 mg of phosphorus.

care of one's protein intake and calcium intake, and this will automatically take care of requirement of phosphorus.

- On an average, dietary intake of phosphorus in adults is approximately 1000 mg/day. Phosphorus is absorbed actively and maximally in duodenum. Approximately 70%–80% of phosphorus, compared with 30%–40% of Ca^{2+}, is absorbed from the gut.
- The total plasma phosphorus is approximately 12 mg/dL, approximately two-third in inorganic compound form and remaining one-third is present as inorganic phosphorus (P_i). The uptake of P_i occurs by two related sodium-dependent P_i cotransporters (i.e. NaP_i-IIa and NaP_i-IIc).
- The low concentration of Na^+ in the enterocyte is established by Na^+–K^+-ATPase on the basolateral membrane.

Factors affecting phosphorus absorption are as follows:

- Vitamin D, PTH and GH promote absorption. 1,25-Cholecalciferol increases P_i absorption via increasing expression of NaP_i-IIa transporter and their insertion onto apical membrane of the enterocytes.
- Cortisol and heavy metal ions inhibit absorption.

Important Note

The fraction of dietary phosphate (unlike calcium) absorbed does not change with the change in amount of dietary intake. Therefore, urinary excretion provides the major mechanism for maintaining phosphorus balance.

2. Exchange of phosphate between extracellular fluid and soft tissues The soft-tissue stores of phosphate, such as those in the muscle mass, undergo rapid exchange with the ECF pool of phosphate (Fig. 8.4.3). This process plays an important role in the minute-to-minute regulation of plasma phosphate concentration.

3. Exchange of phosphate between extracellular fluid and bone Approximately 250 mg of phosphate enters and leaves the bone from 500 mg of ECF pool in the process of bone remodelling.

4. Excretion of phosphate It occurs in faecal matter and urine.

i. ***Faecal excretion:*** It includes 300 mg (30% of ingested) of phosphate which is not absorbed (Fig. 8.4.3).
ii. ***Urinary excretion:*** Approximately 7000 mg of phosphate is filtered by kidney per day. A larger fraction (90%) of the filtered phosphate is reabsorbed. Like the reabsorption of Ca^{2+}, phosphate reabsorption also takes place in the proximal tubule, the thick ascending limb of the loop and the distal tubule. The proximal tubular reabsorption of phosphate is coupled to Na^+ reabsorption. It increases or decreases with the increase or decrease of Na^+ reabsorption. The sodium-dependent P_i cotransporters involved are NaP_i-IIa and NaP_i-IIc. Thus, in volume expansion, both Na^+ and phosphate reabsorption decrease. PTH inhibits proximal tubular reabsorption of P_i by inhibiting NaP_i-IIc. The distal tubular reabsorption of phosphate is facilitated by vitamin D.

Thus, in a healthy adult, approximately 700 mg (10% of total filtered load) is excreted in urine (Fig. 8.4.3).

Regulation of Serum Phosphate Levels

Hypophosphataemia and hypocalcaemia due to dietary or other causes bring about different adaptive changes to normalize the plasma levels. Responses to hypocalcaemia are more immediate than to hypophosphataemia.

As mentioned earlier, hypophosphataemia is mainly compensated by reduced urinary loss and no change in occurs dietary absorption.

MAGNESIUM METABOLISM

The divalent cation, magnesium (Mg^{2+}), is related in some respects to calcium and phosphates.

Functions subserved by magnesium are as follows:

- *Role in formation of bone and teeth.*
- *Serves as a cofactor for several enzymes* requiring ATP, e.g. hexokinase, glucokinase, phosphofructokinase and adenylyl cyclase.
- *Required for proper neuromuscular function:* Low levels of Mg^{2+} lead to neuromuscular irritability.
- *Required for release of PTH* in response to hypocalcaemia and also for the actions of the hormone on its various target tissues.

Distribution of Mg^{2+} in the body The body contains a total of 25 g of Mg^{2+}, which is distributed as:

- Ten per cent in bones, in combination with calcium and phosphate
- Fifty per cent in soft tissues and body fluids

Plasma levels These range from 1.8 to 2.4 mg%. Approximately 60% is present in ionized form, 10% in combination with other ions and 30% bound to proteins.

Magnesium balance Daily requirement of magnesium is 300–500 mg. Leafy vegetables, nuts and soya bean are rich sources of magnesium. Magnesium is mainly absorbed in the distal part of small intestine (while more Ca^{2+} absorption occurs in proximal parts). No active transport has been demonstrated; only passive and facilitated transport occur. Consumption of large amounts of calcium, phosphate and alcohol diminishes Mg^{2+} absorption. PTH increases Mg^{2+} absorption. On an average, 40% (i.e. 120–200 mg) of intake is absorbed daily. In a steady state, the same amount is excreted in the urine. Magnesium deficiency is compensated by decreased urinary excretion. Adaptative responses to reduced dietary intake of Mg^{2+} are poorly developed as compared to similar responses for hypocalcaemia.

Applied Aspects

Magnesium deficiency causes muscular irritation, weakness and convulsions. These symptoms are similar to those observed in tetany (Ca^{2+} deficiency), which are relieved only by magnesium.

Causes of magnesium deficiency:

- Malnutrition, alcoholism and liver cirrhosis.
- Mg deficiency may be observed in uraemia and rickets.

BONE PHYSIOLOGY

FUNCTIONS AND COMPOSITION OF BONE

Functions of Bone

Bone is a specialized tough connective tissue that forms the skeleton of the body. It subserves the following functions:

1. ***Protective function:*** The framework formed by the bones protects the vital organs and soft tissues of the body, e.g. thoracic cage protects lungs and heart, and skull protects brain.
2. ***Mechanical functions:*** These functions served by the bones include:
   - *Support* to body.
   - *Attachment* to muscles and tendons.
   - *Movements* are performed at the joints by leverage effects of bones.
3. ***Metabolic functions:*** These functions of bone include their important role in homeostasis of calcium and phosphate metabolism.
4. ***Haemopoietic function:*** It includes the formation of blood cells in the red bone marrow.

Types and Parts of a Bone

Types

Bones, depending on the size and shape, have been classified as:

- *Long bones*, e.g. limb bones
- *Short bones*, e.g. wrist and ankle bones
- *Flat bones*, e.g. scapula, skull bones and mandible
- *Irregular bones*, e.g. vertebrae
- *Sesamoid bones*, e.g. patella

Parts of a typical long bone (Fig. 8.4.4)

- Diaphysis (shaft) is the mid-portion of the long bone.
- Epiphysis is the widened part on either end of the bone.
- Metaphysis is the portion between the diaphysis and epiphysis.
- Epiphyseal cartilage or growth plate refers to a layer of cartilage that is present between the epiphysis and metaphysis during growing age. The growth of the bone stops when epiphysis fuses with shaft of the bone.

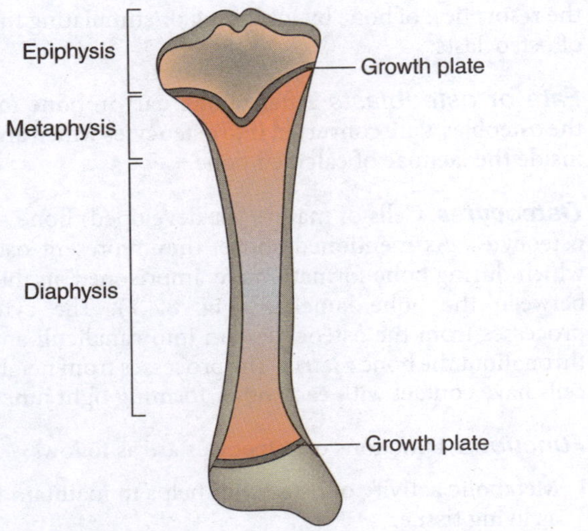

Fig. 8.4.4 Parts and gross structure of long bones as seen in longitudinal cut section.

Composition of Bone

Bone, a special form of connective tissue, is composed of a collagenous framework (matrix) impregnated with bone salts. The dry, fat-free bone consists of one-third organic bone matrix, and two-thirds minerals (inorganic).

Bone matrix Bone matrix, also called osteoid, consists of collagen fibres embedded in the gelatinous ground substance.

Collagen fibres These are arranged in lamellae. The fibres of one lamellus run parallel to each other, but those of adjoining lamellae run at varying angles to each other. Over 90% of the organic matrix is type I collagen.

Ground substance Ground substance of a lamellus is continuous with that of adjoining lamellae. It is formed by the ECF and proteoglycans (which include chondroitin sulphate and hyaluronic acid). These substances are concerned with the regulation and deposition of bone salts.

Bone salts The bone salts constitute the inorganic component of bone which primarily comprises calcium and phosphate in the form of hydroxyapatite crystals ($Ca_{10}(PO_4)_6(OH)_2$). Each crystal measures approximately 400 Å units in length, 100 Å units in breadth and 10–30 Å units in thickness. Adsorbed on the surface of hydroxyapatite crystals are present small amounts of other salts such as sodium, potassium, magnesium and carbonate. The bone salts strengthen the bone matrix.

STRUCTURAL CONSIDERATIONS

Structure of Bone

Structurally, two types of bones are known: compact or cortical bone, and trabecular or spongy or cancellous bone. In most of the bones, both compact and cancellous forms are present, but thickness of each type varies in different regions of the bone. For example, in long bones, the *epiphyseal region* contains large amount of cancellous bone and outer thin compact bone. While in *diaphyseal regions*, the amount of compact bone is more and cancellous (spongy) bone is very thin (Fig. 8.4.4).

Structure of compact bone The compact bone makes the outer layer of most bones and accounts for 80% of the bone in the body. Histologically, the compact bony tissue is made up of several minute cylindrical structures called *osteons* or *Haversian system* (Fig. 8.4.5). Each osteon is formed by several layers of collagen lamellae (Haversian lamellae) arranged concentrically around a centrally placed canal called the

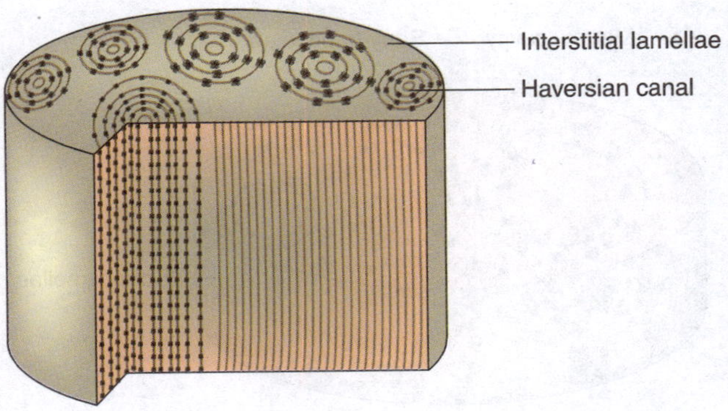

Fig. 8.4.5 Structure of compact bone.

Haversian canal which contains the blood vessels, lymph vessels and nerve fibres. Many *lacunae* (small cavities) which contain *osteocytes* are present in between the concentric layers of collagen tissue. The osteocytes send long processes called canaliculi all around. The canaliculi from neighbouring osteocytes unite to form tight junctions.

The Haversian canals (and therefore the osteons) run along the longitudinal axis of long bones and branch and anastomose with each other. They also communicate with the external surface of the bone through channels that are called *canals of Volkmann*. Blood vessels and nerves pass through all these channels, so that compact bone is permeated by a network of blood vessels that provide nutrition to it. The compact bone is lined externally by periosteum and internally by endosteum. Both periosteum and endosteum of the long bones contain osteoprogenitor cells which can differentiate into osteoblasts or osteoclasts.

Structure of trabecular or spongy bone The trabecular or spongy or cancellous bone is present inside the compact bone and makes up 20% of bone in the body. It is made up of spicules or plates or trabeculae which are separated by wide spaces that are filled in by bone marrow. Nutrients diffuse from the bone ECF to trabeculae. The surface to volume ratio is much higher in trabecular bone than in the compact bone.

The trabeculae are thin and consist of irregular lamellae of bone with lacunae containing osteocytes. The trabeculae are covered by a thin layer of connective tissue called *endosteum*, which contains osteoblasts, osteoclasts and osteoprogenitor (stem) cells (Fig. 8.4.6).

Cells of Bone

Osteoprogenitor cells These are stem cells of mesenchymal origin that can proliferate and convert themselves into osteoblasts whenever there is need for bone formation. They resemble fibroblasts in appearance.

- *In the fetus*, osteoprogenitor cells are numerous at sites where bone formation is to take place.
- *In the adults*, these cells are present over the periosteum as well as endosteum.

Osteoblasts Bone-forming cells are called osteoblasts. These are derived from the osteoprogenitor cells. Being concerned with bone formation, they are situated in the outer surface of bone (Fig. 8.4.7), the marrow cavity and epiphyseal plate cells. The differentiation of osteoprogenitor cells into osteoblast is by a specific ossification transcription factor, such as Cbfa/RunX2, bone morphogenetic proteins (BMPs) and Indian hedgehog (Ihh).

- Run X2 regulates the expression of various osteoblast, osteoprotein, osteocalcin, bone sialoprotein, type I collagen and receptor activator of NF-κβ ligand (RANKL).

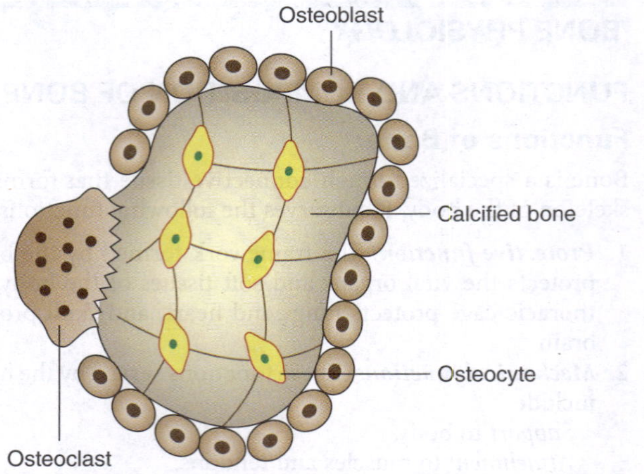

Fig. 8.4.7 Location of various bone cells.

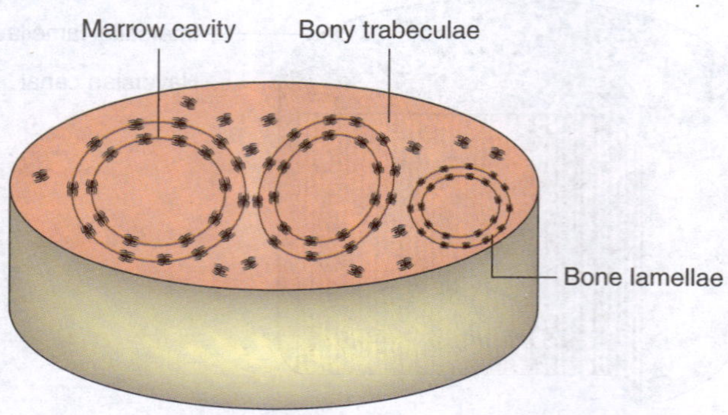

Fig. 8.4.6 Structure of trabecular bone.

> **Applied Aspects**
>
> Mutation of Run X2 causes cleidocranial dysplasia characterized by short stature and hypoplasia/aplasia of clavicles.

Functions Functions of osteoblast cells include:

Role in laying down of the organic matrix of bone: Osteoblasts are responsible for synthesis of bone matrix by secreting type I collagen and a protein called matrix gla protein (MGP), and other proteins involved in the matrix formation are albumin, thrombospondin, osteopontin and fibronectin.

Role in calcification: Enzyme alkaline phosphatase present in the cell membranes of osteoblasts plays important role in the calcification of bone matrix. Osteoblasts are believed to shed off matrix vesicles which possibly serve as points around which formation of hydroxyapatite crystals takes place.

Role in bone resorption: Osteoblasts may indirectly influence the resorption of bone by inhibiting or stimulating the activity of osteoclasts.

Fate of osteoblasts After taking part in bone formation, the osteoblasts are converted into osteocytes which are trapped inside the lacunae of calcified bone.

Osteocytes Cells of mature (or developed) bone are called osteocytes. As mentioned above, they represent osteoblasts, which during bone formation are 'imprisoned' in the lacunae between the bone lamellae (Fig. 8.4.7). The cytoplasmic processes from the osteocytes run into canaliculi and ramify throughout the bone matrix. The processes from neighbouring cells have contact with each other forming tight junction.

Functions Functions of osteocytes are as follows:

- Metabolic activity of osteocytes helps to maintain the bone as living tissue.
- Maintain the integrity of lacunae and canaliculi, and thus keep open the channels for diffusion of nutrients through bone.

- Play an important role in maintaining the exchange of calcium between the bone and ECF.
- Osteocytes are the major source of fibroblast growth factor 23 (FGF23), the main regulator of serum phosphate levels.
- Osteocytes produce sclerostin (SOST) that inhibits the differentiation of osteoblasts, thus inhibiting bone formation.

Applied Aspect

Mutation in sclerostin gene causes sclerosteosis, which is characterized by excessive bone mass.

Osteoclasts Bone-removing cells are called osteoclasts. These are giant multinucleated cells found in relation to surfaces where bone removal is taking place. At such locations, these cells occupy pits called *resorption bays* or *lacunae of Howship*. At sites of bone resorption, the surface of an osteoclast shows many folds which are described as a *ruffled membrane* (Fig. 8.4.7).

Osteoclasts are derived from haematopoietic stem cells via monocytes. Probably they are formed by fusion of many monocytes. The bone marrow stromal cells express RANKL on their surface. When these cells come in contact with monocytes expressing RANK (i.e. RANKL receptor), two signalling pathways get initiated (Fig. 8.4.8).

Differentiation of osteoclasts is facilitated by osteoblasts by secreting macrophage colony-stimulating factor (M-CSF) and RANKL and inhibited by osteoprotegerin (OPG).

Note: Osteoprotegerin (OPG) secreted by the precursor cells controls differentiation of monocytes into osteoclasts by competing with RANK for binding of RANKL.

Function Osteoclasts are responsible for bone resorption during bone remodelling. The lysosomal enzymes required for bone resorption are synthesized and released into the bone-resorbing compartment of osteoclasts.

Bone lining cells Bone lining cells are flattened cells which form a continuous epithelium-like layer on bony surfaces where active bone deposition or removal is not taking place. They are present on the periosteal surface as well as endosteal surface.

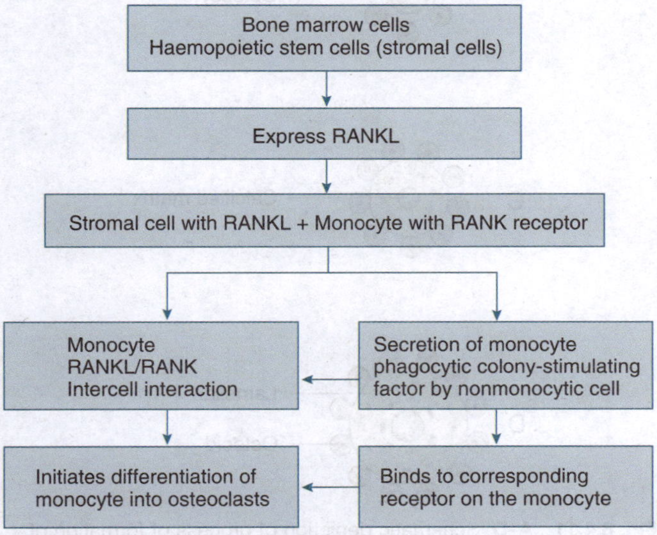

Fig. 8.4.8 Differentiation of monocytes into osteoclasts.

PHYSIOLOGICAL CONSIDERATIONS

The main physiological considerations which need emphasis are as follows:

- Bone growth
- Bone remodelling

Bone Growth

All bone is of mesenchymal origin. The process of bone formation is called ossification. There are two mechanisms of bone formation: endochondral bone formation and intramembranous bone formation.

Endochondral bone formation During fetal development, formation of most of the bones is preceded by the formation of a cartilaginous model which is subsequently replaced by bone. This kind of ossification is called endochondral bone formation.

Intramembranous bone formation Formation of some bones, e.g. clavicle, vault of skull and mandibles, is not preceded by formation of a cartilage model, but they are formed directly in a fibrous membrane. This kind of ossification is called intramembranous bone formation.

Steps of Growth of a Long Bone

1. Formation of a cartilage model In the region where a long bone is to be formed, the mesenchyme first lays down a cartilaginous model of bone.

2. Ossification and calcification The ossification is carried out by osteoblasts which enter the central part of the cartilaginous model. This area is called *primary centre of ossification* (Fig. 8.4.9A). Gradually, bone formation extends from the primary centre towards the ends of shaft (Fig. 8.4.9B). Process of formation of bony lamellae from osteoblasts is described separately.

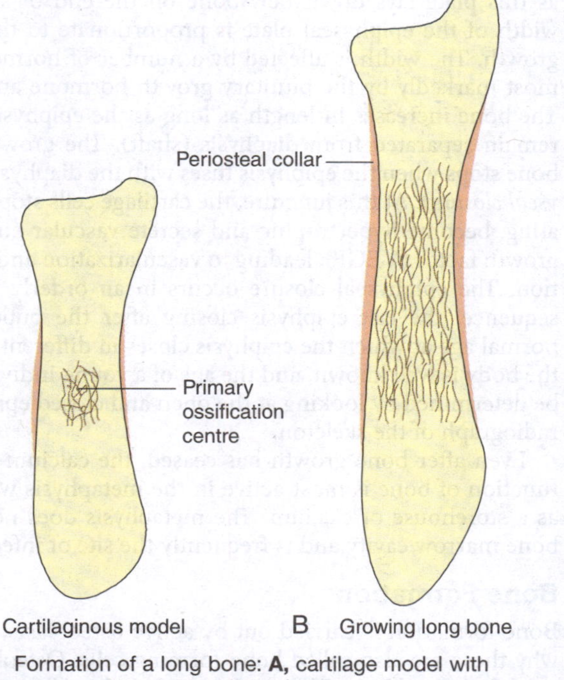

Fig. 8.4.9 Formation of a long bone: **A,** cartilage model with primary centre for ossification; and **B,** bone growth by extension of primary centre for ossification.

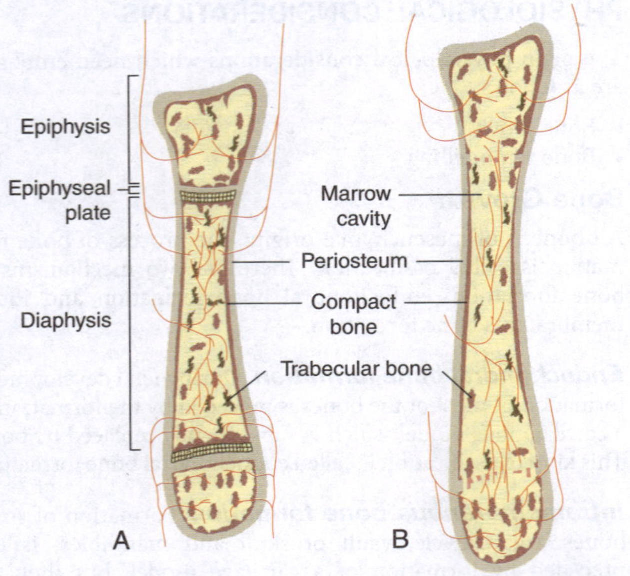

Fig. 8.4.10 Structure of a typical long bone before **(A)** and after **(B)** ossification.

3. Growth in length and girth At about the time of birth, developing bone consists of the bony diaphysis formed by extension of primary centre for ossification and cartilaginous ends. At varying times after birth, *secondary centres* of endochondral ossification appear in the cartilages forming the ends of bones. These centres enlarge and convert the cartilaginous ends into bone. The portion of the bone formed from one secondary centre is called *epiphysis*. During growth, the bone of diaphysis and the bone of epiphysis are separated by a plate of actively proliferating cartilage, the *epiphyseal plate* (Fig. 8.4.10). The portion of the diaphysis adjoining the epiphyseal plate is called metaphysis. It is highly vascular and a region of active bone formation. The bone increases in length as this plate lays down new bone on the end of shaft. The width of the epiphyseal plate is proportionate to the rate of growth. The width is affected by a number of hormones, but most markedly by the pituitary growth hormone and IGF-1. The bone increases in length as long as the epiphyseal plates remain separated from diaphysis (shaft). The growth of the bone stops when the epiphysis fuses with the diaphysis *(epiphyseal closure)*. At this juncture, the cartilage cells stop proliferating, become hypertrophic and secrete vascular endothelial growth factor (VEGF), leading to vascularization and ossification. The epiphyseal closure occurs in an orderly temporal sequence, the last epiphysis closing after the puberty. The normal age at which the epiphysis closes in different bones of the body is well known, and the age of a young individual can be determined by looking at the open and closed epiphysis in radiograph of the skeleton.

Even after bone growth has ceased, the calcium turnover function of bone is most active in the metaphysis which acts as a storehouse of calcium. The metaphysis does not have a bone marrow cavity and is frequently the site of infection.

Bone Formation

Bone formation is carried out by active osteoblasts, which is why these are also called bone-forming cells. Osteoblasts are modified fibroblasts. These cells are found in the periosteum and endosteum. Bone is continuously deposited by these cells.

The process of bone formation can be considered in the following steps:

- Formation of bone lamellae
- Formation of trabecular bone
- Formation of compact bone

It includes two main processes: osteoid formation and mineralization of bone matrix.

1. Osteoid Formation

The osteoblasts synthesize and lay down the type I procollagen molecules into the adjacent extracellular space (Fig. 8.4.11). These cells also secrete a gelatinous matrix in which the fibres get embedded. The collagen polymerizes to form collagen fibres which then swell up and can no longer be seen distinctly. The resultant mass of swollen fibres and matrix is called osteoid (Fig. 8.4.11).

Factors affecting process of osteoid formation include protein intake and a number of growth factors such as TGF-β, IGF-I, IGF-II, PDGF, and acidic and basic fibroblast growth factors. Besides these growth factors, insulin, GH, sex hormones (oestrogens, androgen), thyroid hormones, calcitriol and calcitonin also affect the process of osteoid formation.

2. Bone Matrix Mineralization

Soon after formation of osteoid, the process of bone matrix mineralization starts. It occurs in two phases: an initial slow process of initiation of mineralization followed by rapid mineralization process.

Initiation of mineralization or nucleation The bone matrix is surrounded by a metastatic solution of calcium and phosphate ions (solution in which concentration of Ca^{2+} and PO_4^{3-} exceeds the solubility product of the salt but precipitation is inhibited by certain inhibitors like pyrophosphate). For

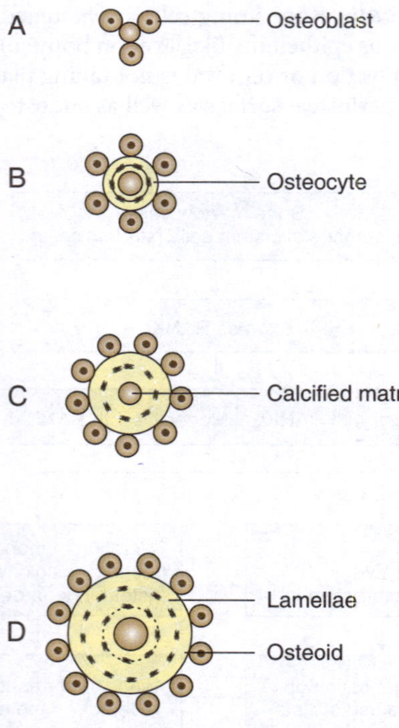

Fig. 8.4.11 **A–D**, Schematic depiction of process of formation of bony lamellae. For explanation, see text.

enucleation to take place, pyrophosphate has to be cleaved into inorganic phosphate by alkaline phosphatase which also has activity of pyrophosphatase. The process of mineralization greatly depends on the *calcium* × *phosphate* ion product in ECF. This product must be above 30/dL for this process to occur.

Rapid calcification after enucleation Approximately 10 days elapse between osteoid formation and initiation of mineralization. However, once mineralization is initiated, i.e. after nucleation, most of the calcium phosphate is deposited within 6–12 hours. Thereafter, hydroxide and bicarbonate ions are gradually added to the mineral mixture, and mature hydroxyapatite crystals are slowly formed. After the process of mineralization of bone matrix is completed, the osteoid is converted into a bone lamella (Fig. 8.4.11C).

Formation of a Trabecular Bone

After the formation of one bone lamella (as described above; Fig. 8.4.11A–C), another layer of osteoid is laid down by osteoblast. The osteoblasts move away from the bone lamella to line the new layer of osteoid. However, some osteoblasts are caught between the lamella and the osteoid (Fig. 8.4.11D). The osteoid is now ossified to form another lamella. The cells trapped between the two lamellae become osteocytes. In this way, a number of lamellae are laid down one over another and these lamellae together form a trabecula of bone, but many such trabeculae constitute the trabecular or cancellous bone. Within each lamella, mineral fluid-containing channels, called *canaliculi*, traverse the mineralized bone. Through these channels, the interior osteocytes remain connected with surface lining cells and with other osteocytes via syncytial cell processes. This system of interconnected cells formed by osteocytes and osteoblasts spreads over all the bone surfaces except small surface area adjacent to osteoclasts. This extensive system of osteocytes and osteoblasts constitutes an osteocytic membrane system which separates bone from ECF. A small amount of fluid called the bone fluid is present between the bone and osteocytic membrane. This arrangement permits transfer of calcium from the enormous surface area of the interior to the exterior of the bone units, and then into the ECF. This transfer process, which is carried out by the osteocytes, is known as *osteocytic osteolysis*. It probably does not actually decrease bone mass, but it simply removes calcium from the most recently formed crystals.

Conversion of Trabecular Bone to Compact Bone

All newly formed bone is cancellous. It is converted into compact bone (Fig. 8.4.12):

- Each space between the trabeculae of cancellous bone comes to be lined by osteoblasts (Fig. 8.4.12A and B).
- The osteoblasts lay down lamellae of bone as already described. The first lamella is formed over the inner wall of the original space and is therefore shaped like a ring (Fig. 8.4.12C).
- Subsequently, concentric lamellae are laid down inside this ring, thus forming an *osteon*. The original space becomes smaller and smaller and persists as a *Haversian canal* (Fig. 8.4.12D).

Bone Resorption

Bone resorption, like bone formation, is a continuous process. In bone resorption, destruction of entire matrix of bone occurs resulting in diminished bone mass.

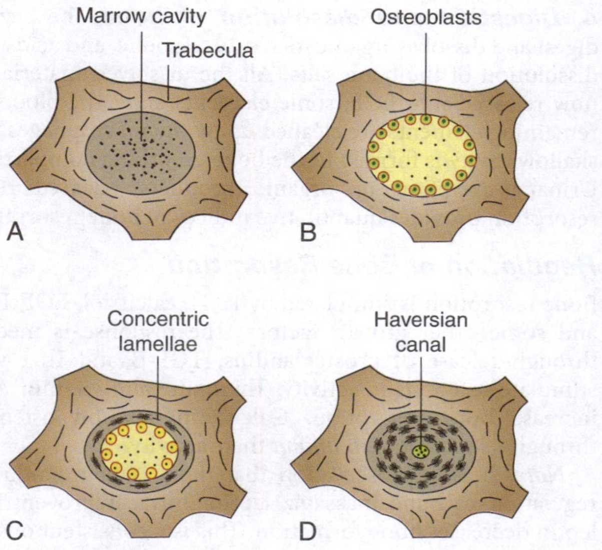

Fig. 8.4.12 A–D, Steps in the conversion of trabecular bone into compact bone.

Osteoclasts are the cells responsible for bone resorption. As mentioned earlier, these are giant multinucleated cells formed probably by fusion of circulating monocytes (or bone marrow monocyte precursor cells). These cells contain a large number of mitochondria and lysosomes. Process of bone resorption involves the following steps.

1. Removal of unmineralized osteoid layers Before osteoclastic resorption can begin, a thin 1–2 μm outer layer of unmineralized osteoid must be removed. This is achieved by collagenase released from lining cells. The lining cells also secrete a molecule that attracts osteoclasts to the site of new denuded bone.

2. Attachment of osteoclast Attachment of osteoclast on denuded bone surface (periosteum or endosteum) is the second step of bone resorption. This is mediated by the surface receptors called *integrins*. At the point of attachment, a ruffled border is created by infolding of the osteoclast's plasma membrane (villi formation). The part of the bone to be resorbed is called bone resorption compartment.

3. Release of proteolytic enzymes and acids At the site of attachment, the osteoclasts release proteolytic enzymes like cathepsin K and lysosomal enzyme and acid from the villi-like projections and facilitation of resorption process. Proton pump (i.e. H^+-dependent ATPase) moves from endosomes into the resorption compartment through the cell membrane and acidifies the area (pH ~4.0). Carbonic anhydrase II (CA-II) present inside the osteoclasts provides necessary H^+ ions.

Applied Aspects

Mutation in cathepsin K leads to **pyknodysostosis** (the condition in which osteoclasts are present but do not function properly).

4. Digestion and dissolution of bone The enzymes digest and dissolve organic matrix of the bone, and acids cause dissolution of the bone salts. All the dissolved materials are now released into ECF; some elements enter the blood. The remaining elements are cleaned up by the macrophages and a shallow cavity is formed in the bone-resorbing compartment. Urinary excretion of organic products released during resorption provides quantitative indices of bone resorption.

Regulation of Bone Resorption

Bone resorption is stimulated by PTH, calcitriol, EGF, PDGF and some other growth factors. The response is mediated through release of prostaglandins, TGF-β and IL-1 which stimulate osteoclastic activity. Thyroxine and vitamin A also increase bone resorption. Calcitonin acts on osteoclasts through its receptors to *inhibit* their activity.

Note. It is an observation that there is neuroendocrinal regulation of bone mass via leptin. Intracerebroventricular leptin decreases bone formation. This is a consistent observation that obesity protects against bone loss because obese persons are resistant to the effect of leptin.

Bone Remodelling

Bone remodelling refers to a process of bone resorption followed by bone formation which keeps on occurring throughout life in a cyclic manner.

Bone remodelling unit The bone remodelling appears to be the result of coordinated activity of groups of interacting osteoclast and osteoblast cells which make up the bone remodelling unit. A single remodelling unit creates approximately 0.025 mm^3 of bone.

Approximately 5% of the bone mass is being remodelled by approximately 2 million bone remodelling units in the human skeleton at any one time. The removal rate for bone is approximately 4% per year for compact bone and 20% per year for trabecular bone.

Phases of bone remodelling cycle A bone remodelling cycle takes approximately 100 days and consists of two phases: the resorption phase and the succeeding formation phase.

1. ***Resorption phase*** lasts for initial 10 days. In this phase, mineralized bone is reabsorbed by osteoclasts releasing calcium and phosphate.
2. ***Formation phase*** lasts for next 90 days and is characterized by reformation of bone by osteoblasts (assimilating calcium and phosphate).

Initiation of bone remodelling cycle Remodelling occurs in areas of bone that have been structurally weakened by fatigue, by having unusual mechanical stress placed on them or by disease. The osteocytes embedded deep within mineralized bone act as mechanoreceptors that pick up mechanical signals transmitted via interstitial fluid and respond by increasing phospholipase C, Ca^{2+} and protein kinase C activity. These lead to a stimulation of phospholipase A_2 and production of prostaglandins (PGE_2). PGE_2 in turn reaches the lining cells via the syncytial processes or the canaliculi. The lining cells then initiate recruitment differentiation of osteoclast cells via communication with stromal precursors in the bone marrow. Thus, resorption is the initial process carried out by osteoclast cells, but it is triggered by signals from the osteoblast cells.

Table 8.4.2 Factors regulating bone remodelling

Event	Stimulatory factors	Inhibiting factors
Bone resorption	Parathyroid hormone (constant)	Oestrogen
	Vitamin D, cortisol	Androgen
	Thyroxine	Calcitonin
	Prostaglandins	Transforming growth factor-β
	Interleukin-1	Interferon
	Interleukin-6	Nitric oxide
	• TNF	• $BMP_{2/4}$
	• PTHrP	• Thrombospondin (TPO)
	• Prolactin	• Interleukin-17
	• Oncostatin	• PGDF
	• Leukaemia inhibitory factor (LIF)	• Calcium
Bone formation	Growth hormone (constant)	
	Insulin-like growth factor	Cortisol
	Testosterone	
	Oestrogen	
	Transforming growth factor-β	
	Skeletal growth factor	
	Bone-derived growth factor	
	Calcitonin	
	Parathyroid hormone (intermittent)	

Regulation of bone remodelling The paired activity of osteoclast and osteoblast cells in bone remodelling is well regulated. All aspects of the remodelling cycle are influenced by a large number of hormones and growth factors, as well as cytokines from immune cells (Table 8.4.2). The process of bone remodelling is one example of coordinated function of the endocrine and immune systems.

Physiological significance of continuous bone remodelling includes:

- *Bone adjusts its strength* in proportion to the degree of bone stress. For example, in athletes, soldiers and others in whom the bone stress is more, the bones become heavy and strong.
- *Shape of bone can be rearranged* for proper support of mechanical force in accordance with the stress.
- *Old bone becomes relatively weak and brittle.* The development of new bone matrix maintains the toughness of bone.

CALCITROPIC HORMONES

PARATHYROID HORMONE

Functional Anatomy of Parathyroid Glands

Gross Anatomy

The parathyroid glands are two pairs of small endocrine glands closely applied to the back of the thyroid gland embedded within its fibrous capsule at the superior and inferior poles. Each gland is slightly oval in shape and is about the size of a split pea, measuring 6 × 4 × 2 mm. The total weight of four normal glands is approximately 140 mg. Normally, there are four parathyroid glands, but rarely they may be more (six or even eight).

Histological Structure

The parenchyma of the parathyroid gland is made up of cells that are arranged in cords. Numerous sinusoids lie in close relationship to the cells. The cells of the parathyroid glands are of two main types: chief cells and oxyphil cells.

Chief cells, also called principal cells, are much more numerous than the oxyphil cells. These are small round cells having clear (agranular) cytoplasm and vesicular nuclei. Chief cells secrete the PTH or parathormone.

Oxyphil cells, in contrast to chief cells, are much larger and contain granules that stain strongly with acidic dyes. These cells first appear at puberty and their function is still not clear.

Structure, Synthesis and Secretion of Parathyroid Hormone

Structure PTH is a single-chain polypeptide, containing 84 amino acids and having molecular weight 9500.

Synthesis PTH is synthesized from a precursor molecule called prepro-PTH, which contains 115 amino acids. The prepro-PTH is degraded to pro-PTH, and finally to active PTH.

Secretion PTH is released from chief cells by exocytosis in response to decrease in plasma ionized calcium concentration that is sensed by the calcium receptors in the parathyroid cells.

Regulation of Parathyroid Hormone Secretion

1. Role of plasma ionized calcium The secretion of PTH is mainly regulated by circulating levels of ionized calcium which act directly on the parathyroid glands in a feedback fashion. The secretion of PTH is inversely related to the plasma calcium concentration in a sigmoidal fashion (Fig. 8.4.13) indicating that:

- Maximum secretion occurs when plasma ionized calcium levels fall below 3.5 mg%.
- As the plasma ionized calcium concentration rises, PTH secretion progressively diminishes and reaches a persistent low basal rate when ionized calcium reaches up to 5.5 mg%. Rise in plasma ionized calcium levels does not further decrease PTH secretion.
- Calcium regulates PTH secretion by acting on its receptors called calcium-sensing receptors (CaSRs). The CaSRs are G-protein–coupled receptors present on the chief cells of parathyroids.

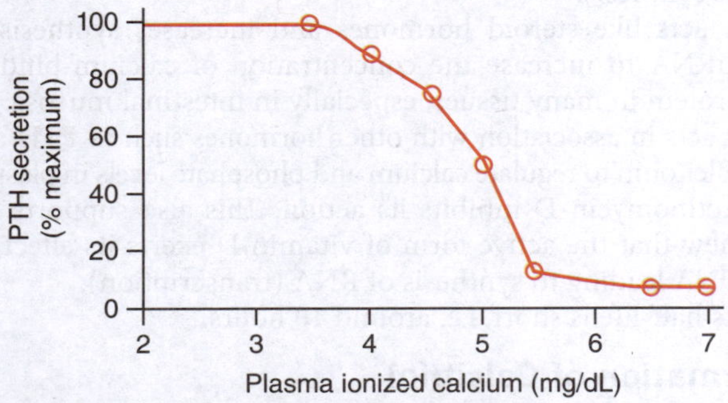

Fig. 8.4.13 The inverse relationship between parathormone (PTH) and plasma ionized calcium.

Applied Aspects

- Cinacalcet is the calcimimetic drug that activates CaSRs.
- Cinacalcet is useful in treatment of hyperparathyroidism in chronic renal disease and parathyroid carcinoma.
- Mutation of CaSR is the cause for familial hypocalciuric hypercalcaemia.

Important Note

- It is important to note that PTH secretion responds to a small alteration in the concentration of ionized plasma calcium within seconds, even if total calcium concentration is kept constant.

2. Role of serum magnesium concentration

- *Mild decrease* in serum Mg^{2+} concentration stimulates PTH secretion.
- *Severe decrease* in serum Mg^{2+} concentration inhibits PTH secretion and produces symptoms of hypoparathyroidism (e.g. hypocalcaemia).

3. Role of plasma phosphate concentration A rise in plasma concentration of phosphate causes an immediate fall in ionized calcium concentration, which in turn stimulates PTH secretion. In addition, high phosphate levels directly increase PTH secretion when ionized calcium concentration is kept constant.

4. Role of vitamin 1,25-$(OH)_2D_3$ It inhibits transcription of the PTH gene and decreases PTH secretion. It also inhibits proliferation of parathyroid cells and upregulates the Ca^{2+} receptors in parathyroid cells.

Plasma Levels, Half-life and Degradation of Parathyroid Hormone

Plasma level of PTH is approximately 130 pg/mL (approximately 3×10^{-12} M).

Half-life of PTH in plasma is 5–8 minutes.

Degradation of PTH occurs rapidly in the peripheral tissues. PTH is predominantly split in the liver. The major product is the circulating (6000 molecular weight) carboxy-terminal fragment that is further acted on in the kidney.

Mechanism of Action and Actions of Parathyroid Hormone

Mechanism of Action of Parathyroid Hormone

PTH acts through its receptors.

PTH receptors There are three different types of PTH receptors:

- hPTH/PTHrP receptors.
- PTH_2 (hPTH-R) is second type of receptors found in brain, placenta and pancreas which does not bind to PHTrP.
- CPTH, a third type of receptor, which reacts with carboxyl terminal of PTH rather than with amino terminal.

First two types of receptors (PTHrP and PTH_2) are coupled to Gs proteins.

PTH binds to a membrane receptor protein on the target cells (in bones, kidney and intestine) and activates adenylyl cyclase to liberate cAMP. The cAMP in turn increases intracellular calcium that promotes the phosphorylation of proteins (by kinases).

Actions of Parathyroid Hormone

The prime function of PTH is to elevate plasma calcium concentration and to decrease the plasma phosphate concentration by acting on three major target organs: directly on bone and kidney, and indirectly on the gastrointestinal tract (Fig. 8.4.14).

1. Actions on the bone PTH stimulates calcium and phosphate resorption from bones, i.e. causes decalcification or demineralization of bone by two processes which constitute the rapid and slow phases of demineralization.

i. ***Rapid phase of demineralization:*** This phase is also called *osteocytic osteolysis*. In this process, the calcium is transferred from the bone canalicular fluid into osteocytes and then into the ECF. In this process, phosphate is not mobilized along with calcium.
ii. ***Slow phase of demineralization:*** This effect requires several days of exposure to PTH. PTH stimulates formation of new osteoclasts from osteoprogenitor cells and causes activation of the osteoclasts already present in the bone to initiate the process of bone resorption in which both calcium and phosphate are released from bone and are transferred to ECF. For details about bone resorption, see page 709.

2. Actions on kidney On kidney, PTH causes:

Increase in calcium reabsorption PTH increases the reabsorption of calcium from the ascending limb of loop of Henle and the distal tubules of kidney and helps to prevent hypocalcaemia. However, hyperparathyroidism is characterized by hypercalciuria. This paradoxical effect can be explained by the fact that in hyperparathyroidism, hypercalcaemia produces such a large load of filtered calcium in glomerular filtrate that in spite of increased distal tubular calcium reabsorption, the net excretion of urinary calcium is increased. PTH increases calcium resorption from distal tubules through transient receptor potential cation channels or TRPV5 receptors.

Stimulation of renal 1-α- hydroxylase enzyme activity.

Inhibition of phosphate reabsorption in the proximal tubule is the most dramatic effect of PTH on the kidney. This effect produces phosphaturia and hypophosphataemia. This effect of PTH allows disposition of the extra phosphate released by PTH-stimulated bone resorption. PTH increases phosphate excretion by inhibiting the sodium–phosphate cotransporter (NaP_{i-11}) present in the proximal convoluted tubules.

i. ***Inhibition of reabsorption of Na^+ and HCO_3^- in the proximal tubule and stimulation of Na^+–H^+ exchanger*** by PTH cause acidification which may prevent the occurrence of metabolic alkalosis, which could result from the release of HCO_3^- during the dissolution of hydroxyapatite crystals in bone.
ii. ***Stimulation of reabsorption of Mg^{2+} by the renal tubules*** caused by PTH helps to conserve this important cation.
iii. ***Stimulation of synthesis of 1,25-dihydroxycholecalciferol*** is a very important action of PTH in the kidney.

3. Actions on intestines Parathormone greatly enhances both calcium and phosphate absorption from intestine indirectly by increasing synthesis of 1,25-dihydroxycholecalciferol in the kidney.

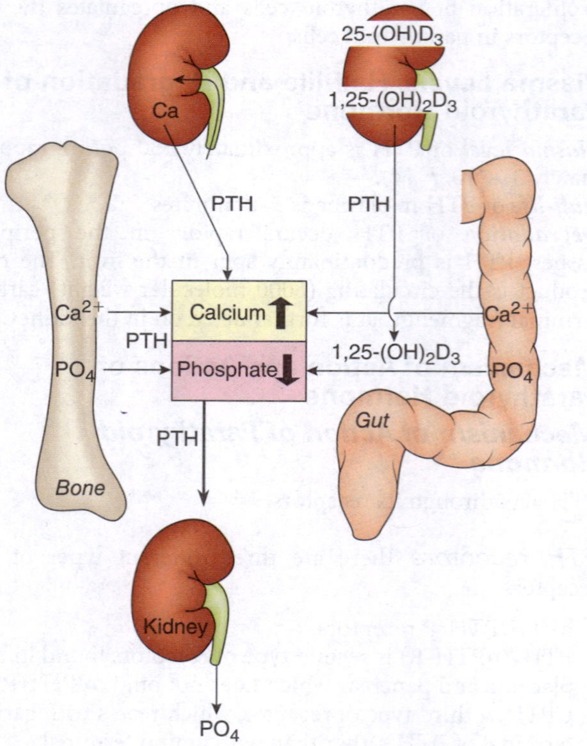

Fig. 8.4.14 Actions of PTH on bones (stimulation of calcium and phosphate resorption), kidneys (stimulation of calcium reabsorption but inhibition of phosphate reabsorption) and intestine (increase in absorption of both calcium and phosphate). PTH action leads to direct increase in calcium and decrease in serum phosphate level.

VITAMIN D

The term vitamin D refers to group of closely related steroids produced by the action of ultraviolet (UV) light on certain provitamins. There are various forms of vitamin D, such as D_2 and D_3 (most important). The active form of vitamin D, i.e. 1,25-dihydroxycholecalciferol, also called calcitriol, is now considered a hormone because of its following characteristics:

- Site of action is away from site of production. It is produced in the kidney and acts on intestine and bone.
- It acts through receptors present in the specific target organs which include intestine, bone and kidney.
- Feedback control mechanism is used for self-regulation of its synthesis.
- It acts like steroid hormones and increases synthesis of mRNA to increase the concentration of calcium-binding protein in many tissues, especially in intestinal mucosa.
- It acts in association with other hormones such as PTH and calcitonin to regulate calcium and phosphate levels in plasma.
- Actinomycin D inhibits its action. This also supports the view that the active form of vitamin D exerts its effect on DNA leading to synthesis of RNA (transcription).
- Its half-life is short, i.e. around 10 hours.

Formation of Calcitriol

Calcitriol, 1,25-$(OH)_2D_3$, is the active form of vitamin D_3. Steps involved in its formation are summarized next.

Source and Synthesis of Vitamin D_3

Vitamin D_3, the precursor (prohormone) of the hormone 1,25-dihydroxycholecalciferol, reaches the blood from two sources (Fig. 8.4.15):

Dietary Source Good dietary sources of vitamin D include fish, fish liver oils and egg yolk. Milk is not a good source of vitamin D. The daily requirement of vitamin D is 400 IU or 10 µg of cholecalciferol. In countries with good sunlight (like India), the recommended dietary allowance for vitamin D is 200 IU (or 5 µg cholecalciferol). Because of its fat solubility, vitamin D absorption from the intestine is mediated by the bile salts.

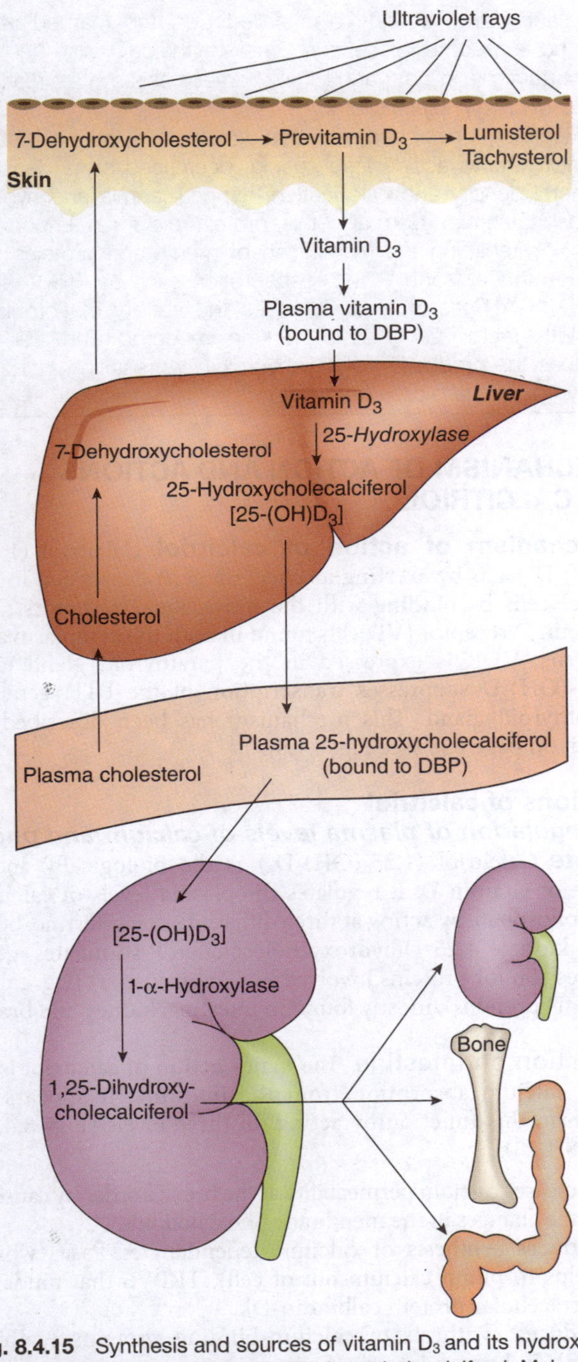

Fig. 8.4.15 Synthesis and sources of vitamin D_3 and its hydroxylation to form the hormone 1,25-dihydroxycholecalciferol. Main sites of actions of 1,25-dihydroxycholecalciferol are also shown.

Note. The plant sources provide vitamin D_2, whereas animal sources provide vitamin D_3.

Cutaneous Synthesis Besides dietary intake, cutaneous synthesis is the other more important source of vitamin D_3 (cholecalciferol) in the body. Vitamin D_3 is synthesized primarily in the specialized skin cells, called *keratinocytes*, which are located in the inner layers (Malpighian layer) of epidermis. The synthesis occurs by the action of UV rays on 7-dehydroxycholesterol (an intermediate in the synthesis of cholesterol). First, previtamin D_3 is formed which is then converted spontaneously over 3 days to vitamin D_3, in a reaction that is driven by thermal energy from sunshine (Fig. 8.4.15).

> **Important Note**
>
> Although cutaneous synthesis of vitamin D_3 is related in exponential fashion to exposure to UV rays (UV-B of wavelength 280–320 nm), excessive exposure to the sun, e.g. in fishermen, does not produce vitamin D toxicity, because continuous exposure to sunlight also causes photodegradation of previtamin D_3 to inactive (inert) products like lumisterol and tachysterol (Fig. 8.4.15).

Vitamin D_3 is the major storage and circulatory form of vitamin D. It is transported in the plasma bound to specific globulin called vitamin D–binding protein (DBP). DBP is also known as Gc protein and binds G-actin.

Synthesis of hormone 1,25-dihydroxycholecalciferol (1,25-$(OH)_2D_3$) Synthesis of hormone 1,25-dihydroxycholecalciferol (1,25-$(OH)_2D_3$) from vitamin D_3 is accomplished by two steps: first step takes place in the liver and second in the kidney.

In the liver, vitamin D_3 is converted to 25-hydroxycholecalciferol (25-$(OH)D_3$) or calcidiol by the enzyme 25-hydroxylase (Fig. 8.4.15), which through circulation reaches the kidney (bound to DBP).

In the kidneys, the enzyme 1-α-hydroxylase converts 25-$(OH)D_3$ to 1,25-$(OH)_2D_3$, i.e. 1,25-dihydroxycholecalciferol or calcitriol, in the cells of proximal convoluted tubules.

- Formation of calcitriol by enzyme 1-α-hydroxylase is the rate-limiting step in the synthesis of vitamin D.
- In the kidneys, the less active metabolite 24,25-dihydroxycholecalciferol is also formed.

Plasma Levels and Circulation of Hydroxylation Products of Vitamin D

Vitamin D_3, 25-$(OH)D_3$, 1,25-$(OH)_2D_3$ and 24,25-$(OH)_2D_3$ all circulate bound to DBP. The DBP has a half-life of only 3 days. It binds 25-$(OH)D_3$ with high affinity, and binds D_3 and 1,25-$(OH)_2D_3$ with much lower affinities. The concentrations, approximate half-lives and estimated daily production rates for the three key vitamin D metabolites in humans are shown in Table 8.4.3.

Regulation of Synthesis of 1,25-Dihydroxycholecalciferol

The formation of 25-$(OH)D_3$ from vitamin D_3 in liver does not appear to be strictly regulated. However, the activity of 1-α-hydroxylase enzyme which converts 25-$(OH)D_3$ into 1,25-$(OH)_2D_3$ in kidney is regulated (Fig. 8.4.16) as:

Table 8.4.3 Status of vitamin D metabolites in humans

Metabolite of vitamin D	Plasma concentration (ng/mL)	Plasma half-life (days)	Estimated production rate (μg/day)
$1,25\text{-}(OH)_2D_3$	0.03	0.25	1
$24,25\text{-}(OH)_2D_3$	2.00	15–40	1
$25\text{-}(OH)D_3$	30.00	15	10

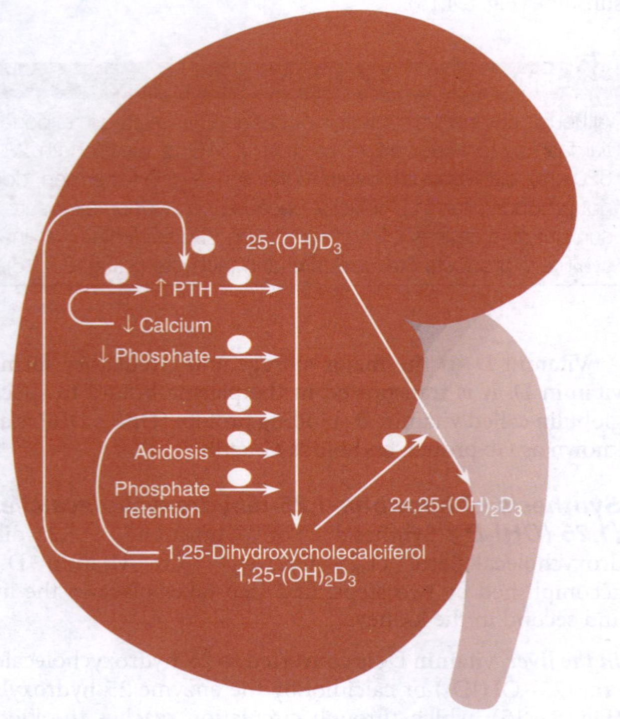

Fig. 8.4.16 Regulation of synthesis of calcitriol ($1,25\text{-}(OH_2)D_3$) from $25\text{-}(OH)D_3$ in the kidney.

1. Plasma calcium Plasma calcium levels regulate synthesis of $1,25\text{-}(OH)_2D_3$ by a feedback mechanism indirectly through PTH.

- ↓ Calcium → ↑ PTH → ↑ $1,25\text{-}(OH)_2D_3$
- ↑ Calcium → ↓ PTH → ↓ $1,25\text{-}(OH)_2D_3$

This effect is responsible for adaptative mechanism of intestinal absorption of calcium. When plasma calcium is little high, $1,25\text{-}(OH)_2D_3$ is produced and the kidneys mainly convert $25\text{-}(OH)_2D_3$ into the inactive metabolite $24,25\text{-}(OH)_2D_3$.

2. Plasma phosphate Plasma phosphate level regulates synthesis of $1,25\text{-}(OH)_2D_3$ by a feedback mechanism by its direct effect on the enzyme 1-α-hydroxylase.

- ↓ Phosphate → ↑ 1-α-hydroxylase → ↑ $1,25\text{-}(OH)_2D_3$ activity
- ↑ Phosphate → ↓ 1-α-hydroxylase → ↓ $1,25\text{-}(OH)_2D_3$ activity

3. $1,25\text{-}(OH)_2D_3$ $1,25\text{-}(OH)_2D_3$ level itself has:

- A direct negative feedback effect on its formation
- A positive feedback effect on the formation of $24,25\text{-}(OH)_2D_3$
- A direct action on the parathyroid gland to inhibit the production of mRNA for PTH

4. Other factors Other factors regarding $1,25\text{-}(OH)_2D_3$ synthesis are as follows:

- *Prolactin* increases $1,25\text{-}(OH)_2D_3$ synthesis.
- *Oestrogen* increases total circulatory $1,25\text{-}(OH)_2D_3$, but this effect is probably due to an increase in the secretion of binding protein (DBP).
- *Hyperthyroidism* is associated with decreased circulating $1,25\text{-}(OH)_2D_3$ and an increased incidence of osteoporosis.
- *Metabolic acidosis* depresses the synthesis.
- *Growth hormone*, hCS and calcitonin stimulate the formation of $1,25\text{-}(OH)_2D_3$.

Important Note

An 'antiageing protein', also called α-*Klotho* (named after Klotho – daughter of Zeus in Greek mythology), also has an important role in Ca^{2+} and PO_4^{3-} homeostasis by its effect on 1,25-hydroxycholecalciferol.

Recently, it has been seen that a mice deficient in α-Klotho protein shows accelerated ageing, decreased bone density, mineral density and calcification, hypocalcaemia and hyperphosphataemia. Normally, this protein plays an important role in stabilizing the localization of membrane proteins involved in Ca^{2+} and PO_4^{3-} reabsorption such as $TRPV_5$ and Na^+–K^+-ATPase. It also enhances the activity of fibroblast growth factor 23 (FGF23) at the receptor. The FGF23 inhibits the production of 1-α-hydroxylase, resulting in 1,25-dihydroxycholecalciferol reduction.

MECHANISM OF ACTION AND ACTIONS OF CALCITRIOL

Mechanism of action of calcitriol Calcitriol ($1,25\text{-}(OH)_2D_3$) acts by exerting its effect on gene expression in the target cells by binding with the intracellular receptors. The vitamin D receptor (VDR) is found in both the cytoplasm and nucleus. VDR is expressed in the parathyroid gland, and $1,25\text{-}(OH)_2D$ suppresses transcription of the PTH gene in parathyroid gland. This mechanism has been described in detail on page 658 (see Fig. 8.1.8).

Actions of calcitriol

I. Regulation of plasma levels of calcium and phosphate Calcitriol ($1,25\text{-}(OH)_2D_3$) is the biologically active form of vitamin D. It regulates the plasma levels of calcium and phosphate by acting at three different sites: intestine, bone and kidney. 1,25-Dihydroxycholecalciferol stimulates gene expression for proteins involved in Ca^{2+} transport (e.g. calbindin-D proteins), mostly found in intestine, kidney and brain.

1\. Action on intestine The major action of calcitriol is to help calcium absorption from the intestine. It appears to perform this function by acting on three levels (Figs 8.4.17 and 8.4.18):

- Increases calcium permeability at the brush border by causing some changes in the membrane phospholipids.
- Induces synthesis of calcium-dependent ATPase (which helps to pump calcium out of cell), TRPV6 that binds to intracellular protein calbindin-Dk.
- Induces synthesis of calcium-binding proteins (calbindin). In human intestinal epithelium, two types of calbindins are induced (calbindin-D_9k and calbindin 28k). These

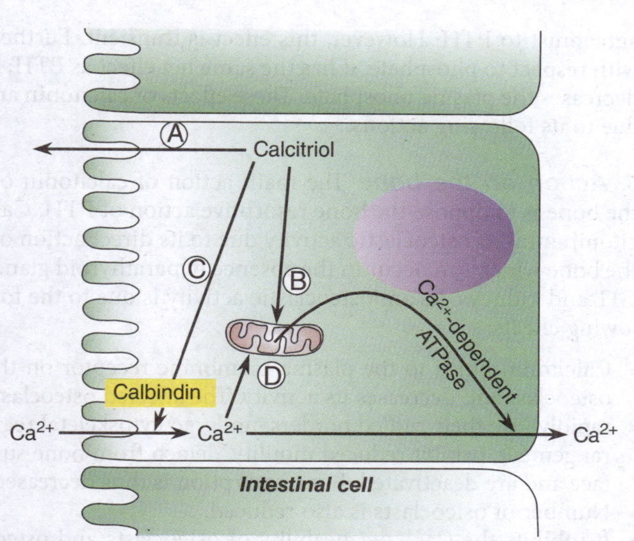

Fig. 8.4.17 Modes of action of calcitriol in increasing intestinal absorption of calcium: (**A**) action at brush borders; (**B**) induction of calcium-dependent ATPase; (**C**) increased synthesis of calcium-binding proteins, calbindins; and (**D**) promotion of entry of calcium into subcellular organelles.

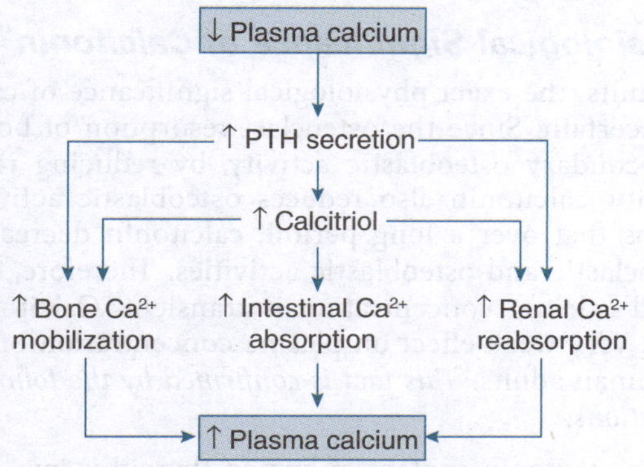

Fig. 8.4.18 Summary of actions of calcitriol in elevating plasma calcium.

molecules may carry calcium across the intestinal cell or they may be important for keeping concentration of free intracellular calcium low (when calcium is being absorbed from the food). The rate of calcium absorption across the duodenum is proportional to the cell content of calbindin.

- Calcitriol also promotes entry of calcium from cell cytoplasm into subcellular organelles (mitochondria).
- 1,25-$(OH)_2$D also increases phosphate absorption.

2. Actions on bone Calcitriol increases bone resorption as well as bone mineralization.

- *Bone resorption:* Calcitriol helps bone resorption by PTH. Calcitriol receptors are present in osteoblasts and not in osteoclasts. The formation of receptor–calcitriol complex in osteoblasts originates cytokine signal that stimulates recruitment, differentiation and fusion of precursors into osteoclasts. The osteoclasts cause bone resorption for which PTH is also required.
- *Osteocytic osteolysis* is also increased by calcitriol.
- *Bone mineralization:* Calcitriol maintains levels of calcium and phosphate, and calcium phosphate ion product in the normal range by causing bone resorption (as above). The ion product is important in the process of bone calcification. It also causes direct effect on bone formation by increasing osteoblastic proliferation, alkaline phosphatase secretion and osteocalcin synthesis. Lack of vitamin D is associated with defective mineralization of cartilage as well as bones.

3. Action on kidneys Calcitriol increases renal reabsorption of calcium and phosphate by increasing the number of calcium pump. Approximately 98%–99% of filtered calcium is absorbed (60% in the proximal tubule and rest in ascending limb of loop of Henle and distal tubule). The distal tubular Ca^{2+} reabsorption occurs via $TRPV_5$ channels.

II. Other actions of calcitriol Besides the abovementioned well-known sites of action (intestine, bone and kidney) of vitamin D, the calcitriol receptors have also been found on the cells in a number of tissues. The possible actions of calcitriol in such tissues are summarized:

1. ***Calcium transport into skeletal and cardiac muscles*** is stimulated by calcitriol. Therefore, vitamin D deficiency can result in muscle weakness and cardiac dysfunction.
2. ***Stimulation of differentiation of keratinocytes and inhibition of their proliferation*** is thought to be caused by calcitriol by its paracrine and autocrine function. Thus, formation of the outer cornified layer of the epidermis, with its appropriate content of enzymes and structural proteins, is regulated by vitamin D. Probably, because of this action, calcitriol has shown promise in the treatment of psoriasis.
3. ***Stimulation of differentiation of immune cells*** is caused by calcitriol. Therefore, an increased incidence of infections is noted in patients with deficiency of vitamin D. The role of vitamin D in immunoregulation is evidenced by the fact that macrophages, monocytes and transformed lymphocytes can synthesize 1,25-$(OH)_2D_3$ from 25-$(OH)D_3$, and that calcitriol receptors are expressed by promyelocytes, monocytes and activated T lymphocytes. The possible roles of vitamin D in immune modulation are as follows:
   - Calcitriol stimulates T-helper-2 cells to secrete interleukin-4 (IL-4), and TGF-β and T-helper-1 cells to decrease their production of interleukin-2, γ-interferon and tumour necrosis factor-α (TNF-α).
   - Calcitriol decreases the proliferation of T and B lymphocytes as well as immunoglobulin synthesis by B lymphocytes.
4. ***Calcitriol appears to be involved in regulation of growth and production of growth factors*** as the VDRs are also found in pancreatic islets, anterior pituitary, hypothalamus, placenta, ovary, aortic endothelium and skin fibroblasts.

CALCITONIN

Synthesis and Structure

Synthesis Calcitonin is synthesized in the C-cells or parafollicular cells of the thyroid gland. These cells are of neural crest origin, which during development migrate to the last ectodermal cleft and from these enter the developing thyroid gland. These cells constitute 0.1% of the epithelial cells of the thyroid gland and can be distinguished from ordinary thyroid hormone–producing cells by their large size, pale cytoplasm and small secretory granules.

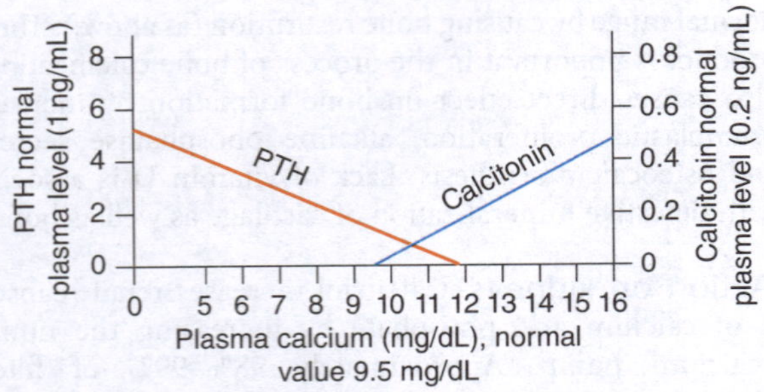

Fig. 8.4.19 Relationship of plasma calcium concentration with release of calcitonin and parathyroid hormone.

Calcitonin synthesis proceeds from a large molecule, the preprocalcitonin. In some cells, the primary RNA transcript encodes preprocalcitonin and directs synthesis of calcitonin.

The gene for producing calcitonin also produces another protein called calcitonin gene-related peptide (CGRP).

Structure Calcitonin is a straight-chain polypeptide with 32 amino acids. Its molecular weight is 3500.

Secretion Calcitonin is secreted in response to rise in plasma calcium level. The cAMP prompts exocytosis of calcitonin-containing granules.

Regulation of Secretion

1. ***Increase in plasma calcium concentration*** is the major regulator of calcitonin secretion. It is important to note that calcitonin is not secreted until the plasma Ca^{2+} concentration reaches 9.5 mg% and that above this calcium level, plasma calcitonin is directly proportional to plasma calcium. This provides a feedback mechanism for regulating serum calcium concentration which works exactly opposite to that of PTH (Fig. 8.4.19).
2. ***Gastrointestinal hormones*** such as gastrin, CCK, glucagon and secretin have all been reported to stimulate calcitonin secretion, with gastrin being the most potent stimulus. The elevated gastrin levels in patients with Zollinger–Ellison syndrome and in pernicious anaemia may account for raised plasma calcium levels by secreting calcitonin. However, it is important to note that the dose of gastrin required to secrete calcitonin is much more than the amount of gastrin secreted by food intake. Therefore, it is premature to conclude that calcium in the intestine initiates secretion of a calcium-lowering hormone before calcium is absorbed.
3. ***Other factors*** like β-adrenergic agonist, dopamine and oestrogen also stimulate calcitonin secretion.

Plasma Levels, Half-life and Degradation

Plasma levels of circulating calcitonin range from 10 to 20 pg/mL, which increase 2- to 10-fold after an acute increase in the plasma concentration of as little as 1 mg/dL.
Half-life of calcitonin is very short, i.e. less than 10 minutes.
Degradation: Circulating calcitonin is heterogeneous, and it is largely degraded and cleared by the kidney.

Actions and Physiological Role of Calcitonin

Actions

The major effect of calcitonin is to rapidly lower the plasma calcium level. This effect of calcitonin is clearly a physiological antagonist to PTH. However, this effect is transient. Further, with respect to phosphate, it has the same net effect as PTH; it decreases the plasma phosphate. These effects of calcitonin are due to its following actions:

1. Action on the bone The main action of calcitonin on the bone is to oppose the bone resorptive action of PTH. Calcitonin inhibits osteoclastic activity due to its direct action on the bone which can occur in the absence of parathyroid gland, GIT and kidneys. Its antiosteoclastic activity is due to the following effects:

- Calcitonin binds to the plasma membrane receptor on the osteoclast and decreases its activity. The affected osteoclasts rapidly lose their ruffled borders, undergo cytoskeletal rearrangement, exhibit reduced motility, detach from bone surface and are deactivated. Bone resorption is thus decreased.
- Number of osteoclasts is also reduced.
- It inhibits the Ca^{2+} permeability of osteoclasts and osteoblast cells and thereby inhibits the active transport of Ca^{2+} from bone cells into the ECF.

2. Action on kidney Calcitonin increases loss of calcium and phosphate in the urine. This effect also contributes in producing hypocalcaemia and hypophosphataemia.

Physiological Significance of Calcitonin

In adults, the exact physiological significance of calcitonin is uncertain. Since the osteoclast resorption of bone leads to secondary osteoblastic activity, by reducing resorptive activity, calcitonin also reduces osteoblastic activity. This means that over a long period, calcitonin decreases both osteoclastic and osteoblastic activities. Therefore, effect on blood calcium concentration is transient. Calcitonin thus has a very weak effect on plasma concentration of calcium in human adults. *This fact is confirmed by the following observations*:

- The calcitonin content of human thyroid is low, and after thyroidectomy, bone density and plasma calcium levels are normal as long as the parathyroid glands are intact.
- When a calcium load is injected after thyroidectomy, there occurs only transient abnormalities in calcium metabolism.
- Patients with medullary carcinoma of the thyroid have a very high circulatory calcitonin level but no symptoms directly attributable to the hormone are present. Further, their bones are also normal.
- No syndrome due to calcitonin deficiency has been described.
- From the above-stated observations, it can be concluded that any effect of calcitonin deficiency or excess is easily offset by appropriate adjustments of PTH and vitamin D concentrations.

The possible physiological roles of calcitonin are as follows:

In children, in whom bone turnover is high, calcitonin may play a role in skeletal development by promoting calcium storage in bones.
Postprandial hypercalcaemia may be prevented by calcitonin.
Protects the bones of mother from excess calcium loss during pregnancy and lactation when demand for calcium to be used elsewhere dramatically increases.

Calcitonin could participate in fetal skeletal development.
Calcitonin may have a functional role in the development of accelerated bone loss after menopause. This appears possible because of the fact that plasma calcitonin is lower in women than in men and that it declines with ageing.
Calcitonin is useful in the acute treatment of hypercalcaemia and in certain bone diseases in which a sustained reduction in osteoclastic resorption is therapeutically beneficial.
Calcitonin and CGRP may also have paracrine and neurotransmitter function. This function seems to be possible because of the discovery of calcitonin and CGRP in a number of locations throughout the body such as pituitary gland, hypothalamus and within cells of neural crest origin. In this regard, calcitonin does exhibit analgesic properties independent of the opioid system.

PARATHYROID HORMONE–RELATED PROTEIN

Origin and Structure

Sites of origin The PTHrP is produced by many different tissues in the body such as skin keratinocytes, lactating mammary epithelium, placenta and fetal parathyroid glands.

Structure PTHrP has 140 amino acid residues compared with 84 in PTH. The genes for PTHrP and PTH are on paired chromosomes 12 and 11, respectively. However, PTHrP and PTH have marked homology at their amino terminal ends, with 8 of the first 13 amino acid residues being in the same positions. Because of striking homology between PTHrP and PTH, the PTHrP binds to PTH receptors.

Physiological roles of Parathyroid Hormone–Related Protein

PTHrP is found in many tissues and may play a physiological role during intrauterine life and early infancy and later during development of different tissues.

1. Regulation of endochondral bone formation PTHrP is important for endochondral skeletal development. Without PTHrP or functional PTHrP/PTH receptors, the process of orderly progression of the growth plates at either end of the bone is severely disorganized, and the resulting bone becomes very abnormal. At puberty, the sex steroids stop the operation of PTHrP system and the epiphyseal growth plate permanently closes.

2. Role in the breast development PTHrP is produced in large amounts in breast and is involved in breast development and lactation. It is also secreted in large amounts in the milk. The PTHrP swallowed by the infant may thus react with its receptor present in the intestine or it may be absorbed in the infant's bloodstream to fulfil a systemic role.

3. Role in tooth development PTHrP allows normal tooth development and eruption by resorbing alveolar bone.

4. Role in skin development PTHrP acts as a growth factor for the development of skin and hair follicle.

5. Protective role in central nervous system The PTHrP is found in the brain (cerebral cortex, hippocampus and granular layer of the cerebellar cortex) where it protects the neurons from toxic overstimulation by glutamate receptors that activate voltage-dependent calcium channels.

Applied Aspects

PTHrP is responsible for hypercalcaemia in conditions like breast cancer, renal cell carcinoma and carcinoma of the lung.

OTHER HORMONES AND HUMORAL FACTORS AFFECTING CALCIUM METABOLISM

Certain hormones, other than the calcitropic hormones described above, that also have some effect on calcium metabolism are as follows.

1. Growth hormone This increases calcium excretion in urine, but it also increases intestinal absorption of calcium, and this effect seems to be greater than the effect on excretion, with a resultant positive calcium balance. Growth hormone also generates IGF-1 which stimulates protein synthesis in bone.

2. Glucocorticoids These inhibit bone formation and increase bone resorption by several actions, resulting in osteoporosis.

Glucocorticoids inhibit bone formation Glucocorticoids inhibit bone formation by the following effects:

- Decrease collagen synthesis and formation of mature osteoblasts from their undifferentiated precursors
- Increase apoptosis of osteoblasts and osteocytes which are the functional cells in bone formation
- Decrease the systemic and local generation of IGF-1 molecules

Glucocorticoids increase bone resorption Glucocorticoids increase bone resorption by their following effects:

- Increase the levels of immune and inflammatory cytokines that stimulate osteoclast formation and bone resorption by osteoclasts.
- Increase mRNA of collagenase, the enzyme essential for destroying the organic matrix of bone.
- Decrease the absorption of calcium and phosphate from the intestine and also increase the renal excretion of these ions. The resulting hypocalcaemia increases the secretion of PTH, which adds to the bone-resorbing effect of glucocorticoids.

3. Thyroid hormones Normal plasma levels of thyroxine are essential for proper skeletal development.

- Congenital hypothyroidism is associated with depressed skeletal development (see page 695).
- Hyperthyroidism may be associated with hypercalcaemia, hypercalciuria and in some instances osteoporosis.

4. Insulin This is required for bone formation and there is significant bone loss in untreated diabetics.

5. Oestrogens These prevent osteoporosis, probably by direct effects on osteoblasts. Therefore, incidence of osteoporosis in females increases after menopause.

- FGF23 is an important regulator of phosphate metabolism. It is primarily synthesized by osteocytes; its main action is to inhibit production of $1,25-(OH)_2D$ and phosphate reabsorption. The levels of FGF23 increase with high-phosphate diet.

Applied Aspects

Some of the important applied aspects with respect to endocrinal control of calcium metabolism and bone physiology are as follows:

- Hyperparathyroidism and hypercalcaemia
- Hypoparathyroidism and hypocalcaemia
- Metabolic bone diseases

Hyperparathyroidism and Hypercalcaemia

I. Hyperparathyroidism

Hyperparathyroidism is a clinical condition characterized by excessive secretion of PTH. It is of three types: primary, secondary and tertiary.

Primary Hyperparathyroidism

Aetiology Primary hyperparathyroidism occurs due to excessive secretion of PTH by:

- Single autonomous parathyroid adenoma of chief cells (most common) as part of hereditary syndromes like: multiple endocrine neoplasia (MEN) syndrome and hyperparathyroid jaw tumour (HPT-JT) syndrome
- Parathyroid carcinoma (rare)

Clinicobiochemical features are as follows:

- *Typical manifestations* are hypercalcaemia, hypophosphataemia, hypercalciuria and renal calculi (kidney stones).
- *Features of bone disease* are rarely seen in primary hyperparathyroidism. However, radiographic evidence of subperiosteal bone resorption may be seen in 20% of cases.
- *Hypercalcaemia* may produce muscle weakness, lethargy and constipation. Since calcium can stimulate release of gastrin, there may occur hyperchlorhydria and peptic ulceration. Hypercalcaemia may also cause hypertension, cardiac arrhythmias and ECG changes.
- Neuropsychiatric manifestations called psychiatric moans are depression, memory loss, poor concentration and fatigue.

Treatment of primary hyperparathyroidism consists of:

- Drugs like biphosphates (to reduce phosphate levels), D analogues and calcimimetics (cinacalcet), but
- Surgical resection of the adenoma is definitive treatment of choice.

Secondary Hyperparathyroidism. In this condition, excessive PTH secretion occurs secondary to persistent hypocalcaemia which causes continued stimulation of parathyroid gland. It is actually a compensatory mechanism to restore calcium levels at the expense of bones. Due to continuous stimulation, there occurs hyperplasia of all the parathyroid glands.

Aetiology Secondary hyperparathyroidism is typically seen in slowly developing renal failure. The plasma calcium level is low in chronic renal failure primarily because the diseased kidneys lose the ability to form 1,25-dihydroxycholecalciferol (calcitriol). However, phosphate retention with resulting hyperphosphataemia also contributes to the decreased plasma calcium in chronic renal failure.

Clinicobiochemical features are:

Increased PTH secretion may not always normalize serum calcium level (not to speak of hypercalcaemia). The main characteristic feature of secondary hyperparathyroidism is involvement of bones. Areas of osteoclastic hyperactivity and rampant bone resorption are present next to areas of excessive and disorganized trabecular bone formation. Bone pains, fractures and deformity may result. Alkaline phosphatase and osteocalcin levels are elevated.

Tertiary Hyperparathyroidism. It develops after a long period of secondary hyperparathyroidism due to unregulated parathyroid function, leading to high level of PTH and hypercalcaemia. This condition does not respond to medical therapy, so surgical treatment is recommended.

II. Hypercalcaemia

Causes. Causes of hypercalcaemia depending on the levels of PTH can be divided into two groups:

1. ***Conditions associated with hypercalcaemia and raised PTH level*** are:
   - Primary hyperparathyroidism
   - Chronic renal failure (tertiary hyperparathyroidism)
2. ***Conditions associated with hypercalcaemia and low or undetectable PTH level*** are:
   - Hypercalcaemia of malignancy
   - Multiple myeloma
   - Familial hypercalcaemia
   - Sarcoidosis
   - Hyperthyroidism
   - Thiazide diuretics
   - Milk alkali syndrome

i. Hypercalcaemia of malignancy is not uncommon. Tumours produce hypercalcaemia by two mechanisms:

Local osteolytic hypercalcaemia is seen in 20% of the patients who have bone metastasis. The osteolytic factors act locally by eroding the bone. These factors include prostaglandins, IL-1, TNF, TGF-β and vitamin D–like sterols.

Humoral hypercalcaemia of malignancy is seen in 91% of the patients who do not have bone metastasis. Hypercalcaemia in these patients with cancers of the breast, kidney, ovary, skin, etc., is caused by raised levels of PTHrP. The gene encoding for PTHrP is different from the one coding for PTH. There is, however, marked homology at N-terminal and between PTHrP and PTH.

ii. Familial hypercalcaemia occurs due to mutations in the gene for Ca^{2+} receptor (CaR). It occurs in two forms:

- Familial benign hypocalciuric hypercalcaemia is seen in individuals heterozygous for inactivating mutations. It is characterized by a chronic moderate elevation in plasma Ca^{2+} and normal or even raised plasma PTH levels.
- Neonatal severe primary hyperparathyroidism is seen in individuals who are homozygous for inactivating mutations.

Management include:

Surgery: Subtotal parathyroidectomy becomes necessary in patients experiencing life-threatening complication of hypercalcaemia, who develop parathyroid adenoma/hyperplasia.

III. Hypoparathyroidism and Hypocalcaemia

i. Hypoparathyroidism

Hypoparathyroidism refers to a clinical condition characterized by low level of plasma calcium due to either deficient production of PTH or its unresponsiveness. It can be classified into two main groups:

- True hypoparathyroidism
- Pseudohypoparathyroidism

A. True hypoparathyroidism In true hypoparathyroidism, there is deficient production of PTH due to heritable or acquired causes. Depending on the cause, true hypoparathyroidism may be:

1. *Postablative or postoperative hypoparathyroidism:* The most common cause of hypoparathyroidism is either damage to glands or their blood supply or their inadvertent removal during thyroidectomy operation. The incidence is 1% of all the thyroidectomies.
2. *Infantile hypoparathyroidism:* It is of two types: transient and persistent.
   - *Transient infantile hypoparathyroidism* occurs in infants born to mothers who were suffering from hyperparathyroidism or hypocalcaemia during pregnancy.
   - *Persistent infantile hypoparathyroidism* is seen in Di-George syndrome, a congenital immune deficiency disorder associated with parathyroid hypoplasia.
3. *Idiopathic hypoparathyroidism:* The exact cause is not known. But it is being considered as an acquired autoimmune disorder of parathyroid gland. It may occur at any age, but is more common in young individuals.

B. Pseudohypoparathyroidism This is a congenital condition in which PTH production is normal but the target tissues are resistant to its effects. The defect may lie in parathyroid receptors or there may be postreceptor defect. The clinical and biochemical features are similar to those of hypoparathyroidism, but PTH levels are elevated (since hypocalcaemia leads to more production of PTH). Pseudohypoparathyroidism occurs in two forms:

1. The common form in which PTH fails to produce normal increase in cAMP concentration due to congenital reduction of Gs protein
2. Other less common form in which cAMP production is normal, but phosphaturic action of PTH is defective

Characteristic features of hypoparathyroidism include:

Hypocalcaemia: Total serum calcium may be decreased to 4–8 mg% and the ionized calcium to 3 mg%. A 50% fall in the levels of ionized calcium leads to a clinical condition called *tetany* (described in the subsequent text).

Hyperphosphataemia, i.e. an increase in serum inorganic phosphate levels to 6–16 mg%.

Tetany

Tetany refers to a clinical condition resulting from increased neuromuscular excitability.

Causes The causes of tetany include:

1. ***Hypocalcaemia:*** Extracellular calcium plays an important role in membrane integrity and excitability. Thus, when concentration of ionic calcium is reduced to <50% of normal in ECF, cell membrane of neurons becomes more permeable resulting in series of action potentials. Thus, hypocalcaemia is the most common cause of increased neuromuscular irritability leading to tetany.
2. ***Hypomagnesaemia*** also causes tetany, because magnesium ions are also associated with neuromuscular irritability.
3. ***Alkalosis*** which reduces ionic calcium can also produce tetany.

Clinical features Tetany may be latent or manifest. In manifest tetany, symptoms and signs depend on the age of the patient.

In children, a characteristic triad of the following symptoms may be seen:

- *Carpopedal spasm:* The hands in carpopedal spasm adapt a peculiar posture in which there occurs flexion at metacarpophalangeal joints, extension at interphalangeal and apposition of thumb (Fig. 8.4.20). This peculiar posture of hand is called *obstetric hand* or *main d'accoucheur hand*. Pedal spasm is less frequent. In it, the toes are plantar flexed and feet are drawn up.
- *Laryngeal stridor* (loud sound): It results from spasm of laryngeal muscles. It may produce asphyxia.
- *Convulsions:* Convulsions and even death may result from the associated asphyxia.
- *Visceral features:* Visceral features of tetany include intestinal cramps, biliary spasm, bronchospasm, profuse sweating, etc. These features are due to increased excitability of autonomic ganglia.

Adult patients have the following features:

- *Paraesthesias*, i.e. tingling sensations in the peripheral parts of limbs or around the mouth, are a common feature.
- *Carpopedal spasms* are less common.
- *Laryngeal stridor and convulsions* are very rare.

Latent tetany

In latent or subclinical tetany, the above-described typical symptoms and signs of tetany are absent, but can be unmasked by the following provocative tests:

Trousseau's sign (pronounced as 'Troosoz's sign'): Occluding the blood supply to a limb for approximately 3 minutes by inflation of a sphygmomanometer cuff (above the systolic blood pressure level) produces characteristic carpal spasm (Fig. 8.4.21) or pedal spasm depending on the limb tested.

Chvostek's sign: It refers to the twitching of facial muscles produced by tapping the facial nerve at the angle of jaw. This occurs due to increased excitability of nerves to mechanical stimulation.

- Hypocalcaemia: It can cause prolongation of QT interval, which may predispose to ventricular arrhythmias.
- Prolonged hypocalcaemia and hyperphosphataemia: These may cause calcification of basal ganglia, epilepsy, psychosis and cataract.

Management of tetany include:

Treatment of hypocalcaemia: An intravenous injection of 20 mL of 10% calcium gluconate is given to correct hypocalcaemia and relieve tetany.

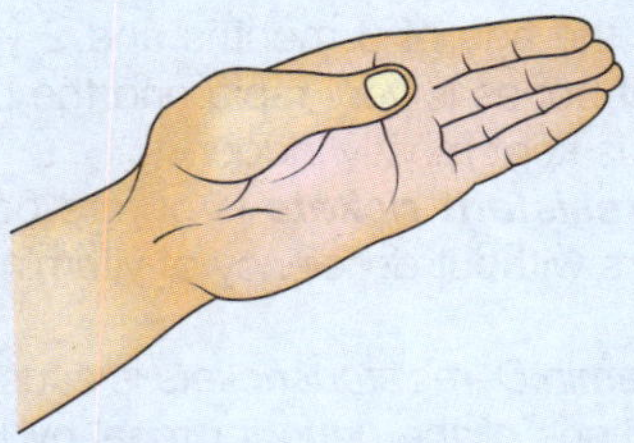

Fig. 8.4.20 Carpal spasm in a patient with tetany.

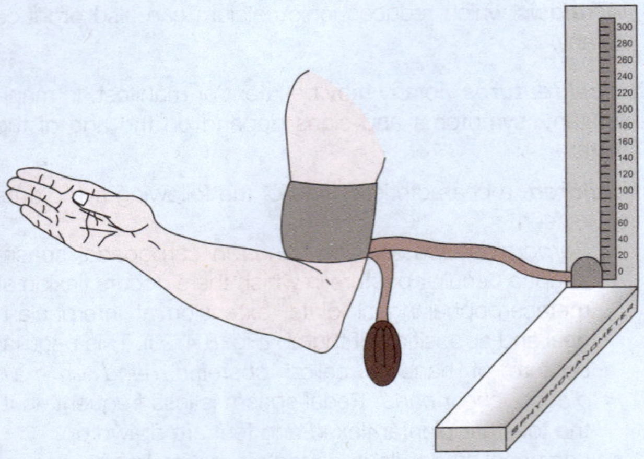

Fig. 8.4.21 Trousseau's sign to unmask tetany.

For persistent hypoparathyroidism: The patients are treated with oral calcium salt and vitamin D analogues (1-α-cholecalciferol or 1,25-cholecalciferol).

For osteoporosis: Recombinant PTH is given subcutaneously to treat osteoporosis.

Treatment of alkalosis: When the alkalosis is present, the treatment is must.

Treatment of the underlying cause: Treatment of the underlying cause of hypocalcaemia if found will cure the condition.

III. Metabolic Bone Diseases

The term metabolic bone disease is used for the bone diseases such as rickets, osteomalacia and osteoporosis.

i. Rickets and Osteomalacia

Rickets (occurring in children) and osteomalacia (occurring in adults) are metabolic bone diseases produced due to deficiency of vitamin D in which there is defective calcification of bone matrix.

Rickets

As mentioned above, in rickets, mineralization of organic bone matrix in growing children is defective. It may also involve cartilaginous matrix of growing end plates of bones.

Causes and types of rickets Depending on the cause, rickets is of the following types:

A. ***Vitamin D–deficiency rickets*** is the most common variety. It may occur because of the following:
   1. ***Nutritional rickets*** is caused by dietary deficiency of vitamin D, due to either poor intake or poor absorption due to high phytate in diet. Vegetarian diet is a poor source of vitamin D.
   2. ***Deficient synthesis through skin*** due to inadequate exposure to the sunlight in smoggy cities is particularly known to cause rickets. This disorder usually manifests between the age of 6 months and 2 years, when the growth of bones is very rapid and the baby is fed only milk and is kept mostly indoor.

B. ***Vitamin D–resistant rickets*** is of rare occurrence. In it, rickets occurs without deficiency of vitamin D. It can be of two types:
   1. *Type I vitamin D–resistant rickets* is caused by inactivating mutations of the gene for renal hydroxylase resulting in nonformation of 1,25-dihydroxycholecalciferol from vitamin D_3. In such cases, there occurs no response to vitamin D, but a normal response to 1,25-dihydroxycholecalciferol is seen.
   2. *Type II vitamin D–resistant rickets* occurs due to inactivating mutations of the gene for the 1,25-dihydroxycholecalciferol receptor. In such cases, there is deficient response to both vitamin D and 1,25-dihydroxycholecalciferol.

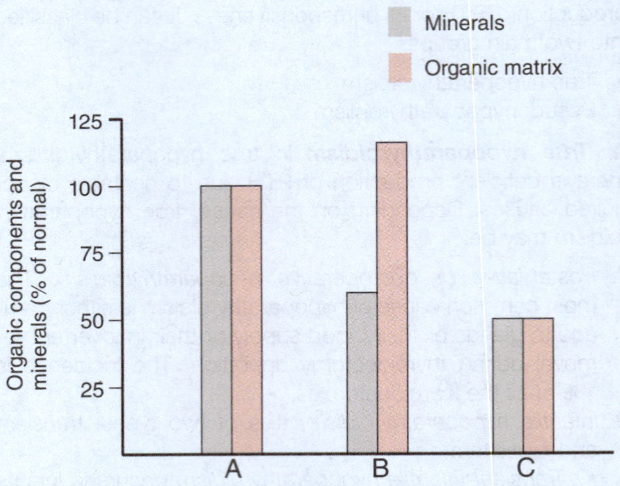

Fig. 8.4.22 Organic components and mineral contents of bone in: **(A)** normal; **(B)** osteomalacia; and **(C)** osteoporosis.

Pathogenesis of defective bone mineralization in rickets

Vitamin D deficiency leads to poor intestinal absorption of calcium and decreased reabsorption of calcium and phosphates from renal tubules. As a consequence, there is failure of mineralization of organic bone matrix. It is important to note that organic component of bone is normal or somewhat excessive (Fig. 8.4.22). Due to involvement of epiphyseal growth plate in growing bones, the process of ossification at the epiphyseal line is abnormal. Normally, the epiphyseal line is a well-defined narrow strip, 2 mm deep, behind which regular ossification occurs. Further, under normal circumstances, the older cartilage cells degenerate and disappear leaving many spaces into which the blood vessels and osteoblasts of the shaft can penetrate. In rickets, this apparently essential preliminary degeneration does not occur and so ossification is retarded. The cartilage cells persist and go on multiplying and give rise to broad irregular cartilaginous zone which can be felt as a marked project on the surface. The matrix between the cartilage cells and that of new bone itself does not become adequately mineralized resulting in softness of bones.

Clinical features of rickets are:

1. ***Bony defects*** seen in children with rickets are as follows (Fig. 8.4.23):
   - *Craniotabes* is the earliest lesion seen in an infant with rickets. It refers to small rounded areas in the membranous bones of skull which yield under pressure of finger.
   - *Widening of wrist* occurs due to epiphyseal widening of lower end of radius bone.
   - *Collapse of chest wall* occurs due to flattening of sides of thorax with prominent sternum.
   - *Rachitic rosary* refers to beading of costochondral junction of ribs.

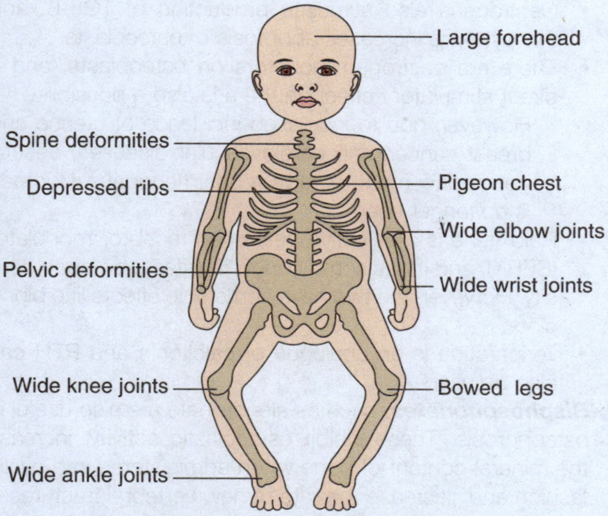

Fig. 8.4.23 Important clinical features of rickets.

- *Frontal bossing* and posterior flattening of skull.
- *Harrison's sulcus* refers to indentation of lower ribs at the site of attachment of diaphragm.
- *Bowing of legs* or knock-knee occurs when child starts walking.
- *Kyphosis and pelvic deformities* are also known.

2. ***General features*** include:
   - Infants with rickets are more prone to respiratory and gastrointestinal infections.
   - Developmental milestones are delayed.
3. ***Tetany and convulsions*** may occur in cases with marked hypocalcaemia.
4. ***Biochemical changes*** in rickets due to vitamin D deficiency are as follows:
   - Low levels of plasma calcium and phosphate.
   - Product of plasma Ca^{2+} and PO_4^{3-} is decreased to 30 (normal is 60).
   - Serum alkaline phosphatase levels are high due to increased osteoblastic activity.
   - Plasma 1,25-dihydroxycholecalciferol is also low or absent.

Management Adequate supply of calcium and vitamin D should be ensured. Therapeutic dose of vitamin D varies from 25 to 125 µg (1000–5000 IU) daily for 6–8 weeks followed by 200–400 IU daily.

Osteomalacia can be thought of as an adult counterpart of rickets. It is characterized by defective mineralization of the adult bones in which epiphyseal growth plates are already closed.

Aetiology Osteomalacia occurs due to:

1. ***Vitamin D deficiency*** is the main cause. The condition is more common in women in childbearing age, especially in Muslim women who use *purdah* and whose diet mainly consists of cereals and devoid of milk. These women confine themselves to indoors and seldom see the sun. Repeated pregnancy is an important contributory factor.
2. ***Other causes*** of osteomalacia with normal levels of calcium, phosphate and vitamin D include:
   i. *Primary nonmineralization defect:*
      - *Hereditary*
      - *Fluoride treatment*

   ii. Defective matrix synthesis:
      - Fibrogenesis imperfecta

   iii. Miscellaneous:
      - Aluminium bone disease

Pathogenesis of osteomalacia It is similar to rickets.

Clinical features Clinical features of osteomalacia are almost similar to those of rickets.

1. ***Skeletal abnormalities*** are dominant features and include:
   - *Diffuse skeletal pain* and bony tenderness are common complaints. Pain may vary from mild backache to severe pain around hip.
   - *Muscle weakness* is also common. A waddling gait may be present due to proximal muscle weakness.
   - *Bone becomes soft;* especially involved are pelvic girdle, ribs and femurs.
   - *Pseudofractures* are seen in flat bones (ribs, scapulae and pelvic rami) or in ends of long bones (e.g. femur).
2. ***Tetany*** may occur in few cases with carpopedal spasm.
3. ***Biochemical features*** are similar to those of rickets.

Treatment It is similar to that of rickets.

ii. Osteoporosis

Osteoporosis is characterized by a reduction of bone mass per unit volume with normal ratio of bone matrix and minerals, i.e. there occurs loss of both bone matrix and mineral component (Fig. 8.4.22).

Pathogenesis Osteoporosis develops due to a mismatch between bone resorption and bone remodelling process, the bone resorption being in excess.

Aetiology Senile osteoporosis is common disease and has become a major public health problem of elderly. All normal humans gain bone mass during adolescence. After a plateau between 20 and 45 years of age, all begin to lose bone mass progressively as they grow older (Fig. 8.4.24). In males, bone

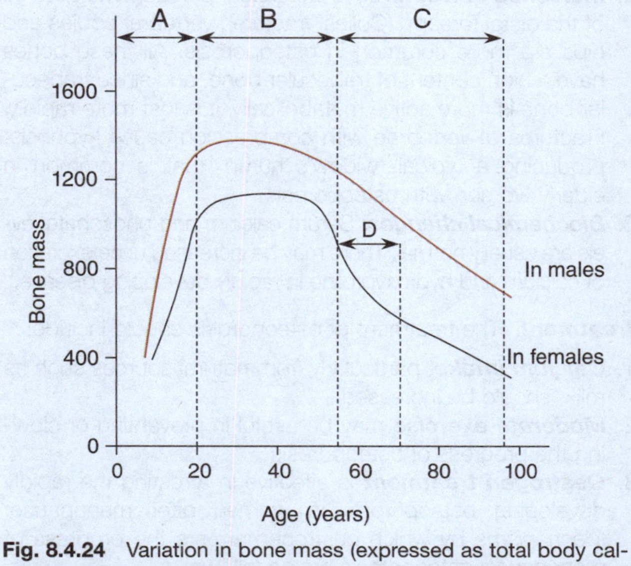

Fig. 8.4.24 Variation in bone mass (expressed as total body calcium) with age in males and females: **(A)** phase of rapid increase in bone mass; **(B)** plateau phase; **(C)** phase of steady bone loss with advancing age; and **(D)** phase of rapid bone loss in women after menopause.

loss is usually less significant than in females. Further, after menopause, women initially have more rapid bone loss because of additional factor of oestrogen deficiency.

Factors contributing to development of osteoporosis include:

- *Postmenopausal females* are more prone to osteoporosis due to deficiency of oestrogen. The low level of oestrogen leads to more bone resorption than formation resulting in osteoporosis.
  - *Immobilization:* Osteoporosis of immobilization occurs if bones are not subjected to the stress of walking.
  - *Weightlessness:* Weight-bearing is essential for maintenance of bone mass. Weightlessness in space travel produces significant osteoporosis within few months.
  - *Hyperthyroidism:* It is associated with more increased osteoclastic activity vis-à-vis bone formation activity, resulting in bone loss.
  - *Cushing syndrome:* It is also associated with increased osteoclastic activity and secondary osteoporosis.
  - *Bone secondaries:* These are associated with local release of certain osteoclastic factors which cause osteoporosis.
  - *Chronic renal failure:* It is associated with osteomalacia, but in severe cases, osteoporotic bone lesions due to tertiary hyperparathyroidism may also be present.
  - *Drugs:* Use of drugs like glucocorticoids, immunosuppressants (cyclosporin and tacrolimus), certain serotonin reuptake inhibitors, aromatase inhibitors and proton pump inhibitors also cause osteoporosis.
- *Increased alcohol intake* and smoking lead to decreased osteoblastic activity.

Characteristic features of osteoporosis are:

1. **Bone density** is reduced. In radiographs, the affected bones show clear glass appearance (e.g. ground glass appearance seen in osteomalacia). In severe cases, excessive bone resorption may lead to cyst formation (osteitis fibrosa cystica).
2. **Incidence of fractures** is increased; particularly, fractures of the distal forearm (Colles' fracture), vertebral bodies and hips are more common in osteoporosis. All these bones have a high content of trabecular bone, and since trabecular bone is more active metabolically, it is lost more rapidly. Fractures of vertebrae with compression cause kyphosis, producing a typical 'widow's hump' that is common in elderly women with osteoporosis.
3. **Biochemical changes:** Serum calcium and phosphate levels are usually normal. There may be increased urine excretion of calcium and hydroxyproline in rapidly developing disease.

Treatment. The treatment of osteoporosis should include:

1. **Calcium intake**, particularly from natural sources such as milk, should be increased.
2. **Moderate exercise** may be useful in preventing or slowing the progress of osteoporosis.
3. **Oestrogen treatment** is effective in arresting the rapidly developing osteoporosis in women after menopause. *Mechanisms* by which oestrogen arrests the progress of menopausal osteoporosis are as follows:
   - Oestrogens inhibit secretion of cytokines such as IL-1, IL-6 and TNF-α, and these cytokines foster the development of osteoclasts.
   - Oestrogens also stimulate production of TGF-β, and this cytokine increases apoptosis of osteoclasts.
   - There are oestrogen receptors on osteoblasts, and a direct stimulatory effect on them is also a possibility.

     However, due to increased incidence of uterine and breast cancer, and cardiovascular diseases, oestrogen replacement therapy in postmenopausal women is no longer used.
   - Raloxifene is a selective oestrogen receptor modulator (SERM) and it has some beneficial effects on bone density. However, the two have some side effects like blood clots.
   - Teriparatide is an analogue of calcitonin and PTH can also be used.
4. **Bisphosphonates**, such as alendronate are also useful in osteoporosis. These inhibit osteoclastic activity, increase the mineral content of bone when administered in a cyclic fashion and decrease the rate of new vertebral fractures.
5. **Fluoride which stimulates osteoblasts**, making bone more dense, has proved to be of little value in the treatment of osteoporosis.
6. **Denosumab** is the human monoclonal, an inhibitor of RANKL. It is useful in treatment of postmenopausal osteoporosis.
7. **Strontium ranelate** promotes bone formation and inhibits bone resorption.

Osteopetrosis

Osteopetrosis, also called marble bone disease or Albers–Schönberg disease, is a rare but severe bone disease, and occurs due to defective osteoclast activity. In this disease, osteoclasts are unable to resorb bone; therefore, osteoblastic activity unopposedly increases leading to steady increase in bone density resulting in narrowing and distortion of bony foramina.

Pathogenesis It occurs due to lack of a protein encoded by early gene c-Fos and PU-1 transcription factor. The hallmark of osteopetrosis is overexpression of osteoprotegerin (OPG). OPG is an inhibitor of RANKL, which is the main factor that regulates differentiation of osteoclasts.

- Another important cause of osteopetrosis is mutation in CA-II and proton pump gene (TCIR-I).

Characteristic features include:

- *Neurological defects* due to compression of nerves when passing through narrowed foramina.
- *Haematological abnormalities* due to crowding of bone marrow cavities.

Self-Assessment

1. Discuss the calcium metabolism and its balance.
2. Discuss the role of various calcitropic hormones in body calcium regulation.
3. Discuss the role of parathyroid hormone in bone physiology.
4. Discuss the physiological functions, distribution and mechanism of phosphorus balance.
5. Describe briefly the process of bone formation and role of RANKL-RNKL.

Clinical Cases

Case 1

A 2-year-old male child is brought to the paediatric department by his mother because she had observed that when her son walks, his legs bend and he cannot walk without support.

The personal and family history revealed that the child was born by emergency caesarean section due to previous multiple caesarean deliveries. Child was exclusively on breastfeeding for approximately 9 months.

Examination showed marked widening of the wrists and bowing of legs, and it was suspected as a case of rickets.

Q1. What is the causative reason of this condition in this case?
Q2. What are other clinical features of this condition?
Q3. What further investigations should be done to reach the final diagnosis?
Q4. What should be the plan of treatment?

Case 2

A 63-year-old woman fell in the bathroom and had fracture of distal end of the arm. She was brought in the orthopaedic department. History revealed that the patient is diabetic and also had hyperthyroidism.

X-ray findings revealed Colles' fracture, decreased bone density and a probable diagnosis of osteoporosis was made.

Q1. What are the risk factors of osteoporosis?
Q2. What are the biochemical findings in this condition?
Q3. How can the condition be prevented?
Q4. What should be the treatment in this case?
Q5. What is the role of oestrogen therapy in this condition?

Case 3

A young woman underwent thyroidectomy, subsequently developed twitching of facial muscles and tingling sensations in the hands.

Q1. What is the cause for these symptoms?
Q2. What are the biochemical findings in this condition?
Q3. What changes will occur in the ECG in this condition?
Q4. What should be the treatment plan for this condition?v

8.5 Adrenal Glands

CHAPTER OUTLINE

FUNCTIONAL ANATOMY

GENERAL CONSIDERATIONS

- There are two adrenal glands, one on either side, situated extraperitoneally at the upper pole of the kidney, hence also called 'suprarenal gland' (Fig. 8.5.1).
- These are also known as 'glands of emergency', as they secrete most vital hormones needed during an emergency.
- Normally, each gland weighs approximately 5 g and consists of two parts, the adrenal cortex and the medulla, which are absolutely distinct from each other structurally, functionally and developmentally (Fig. 8.5.1).
- The cortex (outer zone) makes up to 80%–90% of the gland and is a source of the cortisol hormone.
- The medulla (inner zone) makes up 10%–20% of the adrenal gland and is a source of the catecholamine hormones.
- Morphologically and physiologically, the fetal adrenal gland differs strikingly from that of the adult. The adrenal gland is larger at birth than it is during adulthood.

DEVELOPMENT

Adrenal Cortex

Adrenal cortex is a mesodermal derivative. During fetal life and in a newborn, the adrenal cortex comprises the outer *neocortex* (15% in volume), which is the progenitor of the adult cortex, and the inner *fetal cortex* (85% in volume). The fetal cortex or fetal zone undergoes rapid involution during the first few months of extrauterine life and completely disappears by 3–12 months postpartum. At the same time, the thin outer zone of the neocortex enlarges and differentiates permanently into the three-layered adrenal cortex of the mature human. It is a nuclear receptor with a currently uncertain ligand steroidogenic factor-1 (SF-1), which is essential for the development of the adrenal cortex and expression of the enzymes and steroid hormone biosynthesis. It is axiomatic that all endocrine glands derived from the mesoderm synthesize and secrete steroid hormones.

Adrenal Medulla

The adrenal medulla essentially represents an enlarged and specialized sympathetic ganglion derived from the neuroectodermal cells giving rise to sympathetic ganglia. The neural crest gives rise to neuroblasts, which eventually give rise to the autonomic postganglionic neurons, the adrenal medulla and the spinal ganglia. In early fetal life, the adrenal medulla contains only norepinephrine (NE).

HISTOLOGICAL STRUCTURE

Adrenal Cortex

The adrenal gland is covered by a connective tissue capsule from which septa extend into the gland substance. The mature

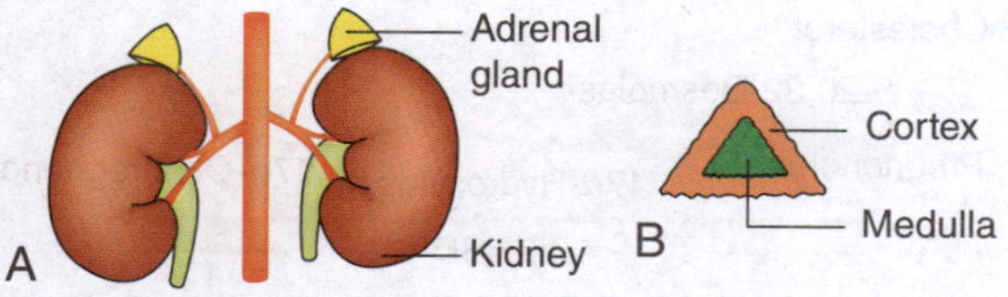

Fig. 8.5.1 Location (**A**) and divisions (**B**) of adrenal glands.

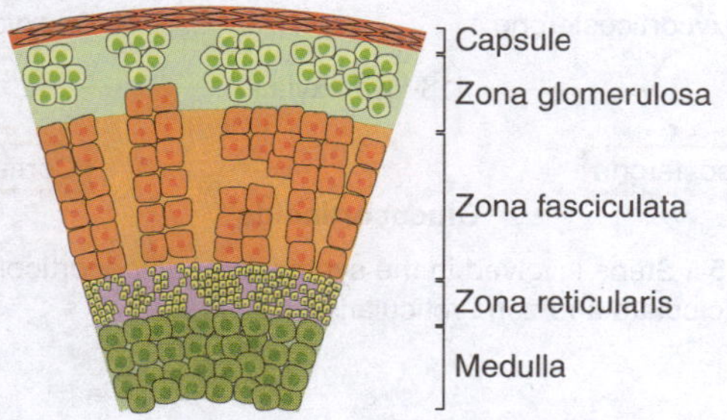

Fig. 8.5.2 Histological structure of adrenal gland.

human adrenal cortex consists of three distinct layers or zones of cells (Fig. 8.5.2).

1. ***Zona glomerulosa***, constituting outer one-fifth of the cortex, is a small zone present under the capsule. It consists of cells that are arranged as inverted U-shaped formations, or acinus-like groups. It is the site of *aldosterone* and *corticosterone* synthesis. Aldosterone is the principal mineral corticoid of the human adrenal cortex.
2. ***Zona fasciculata*** is the widest zone forming middle three-fifths of the cortex. It is made up of cells that are arranged in two-cell–thick straight columns. Sinusoids intervene between the columns and cells appear clear or vacuolated in stained sections because of high lipid (cholesterol) content.
3. ***Zona reticularis*** forms the inner one-fifth of the cortex. It is made up of a network of compactly arranged cords of cells that branch and anastomose with each other to form a kind of network (hence the name zona reticularis). These cells contain fewer lipids.

Zona fasciculata and zona reticularis constitute a single functional unit where mainly cortisol (and some corticosterone) and androgen (dehydroepiandrosterone [DHEA]) are synthesized.

Adrenal Medulla

The adrenal medulla essentially represents an enlarged and specialized sympathetic ganglion. Histologically, it is made up of chromaffin cells, also called pheochromocytes, innervated by preganglionic sympathetic neurons.

Chromaffin cells The cells forming adrenal medulla show yellow granules in their cytoplasm (i.e. *chromaffin reaction*) and hence called chromaffin cells.

- These cells are columnar or polyhedral and are arranged in all groups or columns that are separated by wide *sinusoids*.
- Functionally, these cells are considered to be modified postganglionic neurons, which do not have axons.
- There are two types of adrenomedullary chromaffin cells; one type of cells constitute 80% of the total cells and synthesize epinephrine (adrenaline), and the second type (remaining 20%) cells synthesize NE (noradrenaline).

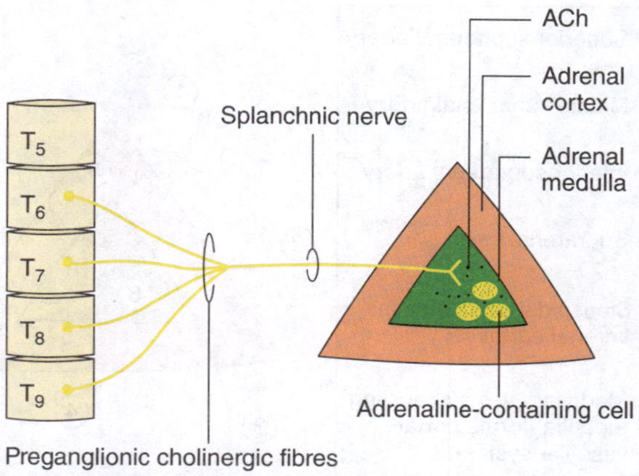

Fig. 8.5.3 Preganglionic sympathetic fibres synapsing directly on chromaffin cells in the adrenal medulla.

- The epinephrine and NE are largely stored in the subcellular particles called *chromaffin granules*. These granules are osmophilic, electron-dense, membrane-bound vesicles. In addition to the catecholamines, the chromaffin granules also contain proteins, lipids and adenine nucleotides (mainly ATP). One of the proteins localized in the particulate fraction is the enzyme, *dopamine* β-hydroxylase (DBH). Soluble acidic proteins found in the granules are called chromogranins.
- The adrenal medulla is now included in the amine precursor uptake and decarboxylation (APUD) cell system or the so-called *diffuse neuroendocrine system*.
- The chromaffin cells present in locations other than adrenal medulla are para-aortic bodies present along the sides of abdominal aorta, also termed *organ of Zuckerkandl*.

Nerve endings Nerve endings present in the adrenal medulla, are the *cholinergic preganglionic* sympathetic fibres that synapse directly on chromaffin cells. These fibres traverse the splanchnic nerve and are myelinated (type B) secretomotor fibres emanating mainly from the lower thoracic segments (T_5 and T_9) of the ipsilateral intermediolateral grey column of the spinal cord (Fig. 8.5.3).

BLOOD SUPPLY (FIG. 8.5.4)

Arterial blood supply The adrenal glands have one of the body's highest rates of blood flow per gram of tissue. The arterial blood to the gland reaches the outer capsule from the superior suprarenal artery (a branch of the inferior phrenic artery), middle suprarenal artery (a branch of the abdominal aorta) and the inferior suprarenal artery (a branch of the renal artery). The arterial blood enters sinusoidal capillaries in the cortex and then drains into medullary veins, which supply blood to the medulla and thus form a *portal system*. This arrangement of portal circulation exposes the medulla to relatively high concentrations of corticosteroids from the cortex. As most of the blood perfusing the medulla is derived from the portal system, it is, therefore, partly deoxygenated. There also exists a direct arterial blood supply to the medulla via the *medullary arteries*, which traverse the cortex.

Venous drainage The venous blood drains via single central vein, which passes along the longitudinal axis of the gland. The right suprarenal vein drains into the inferior vena cava and left suprarenal vein into the left renal vein.

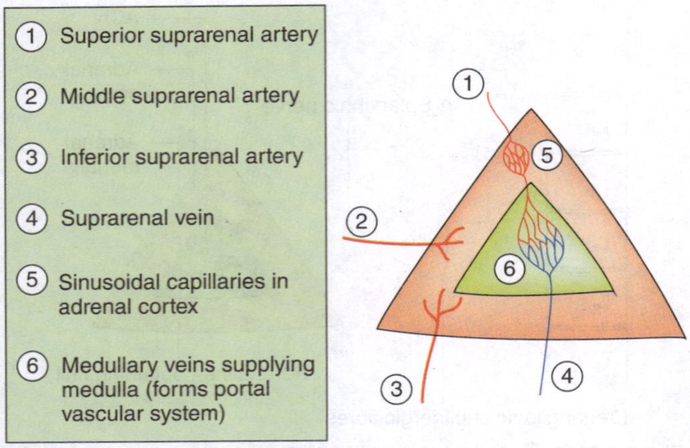

Fig. 8.5.4 Schematic diagram showing arterial blood supply and venous drainage of adrenal gland. The portal vascular system which exposes the medulla to high concentration constitutes a functional connection between the cortex and medulla.

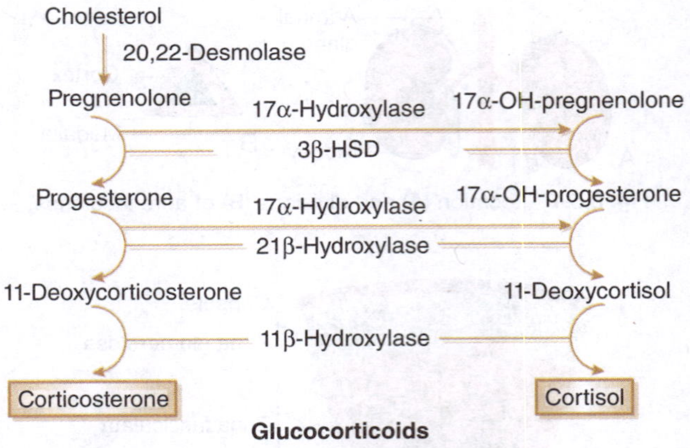

Fig. 8.5.5 Steps involved in the synthesis of glucocorticoids in the zona fasciculata and zona reticularis.

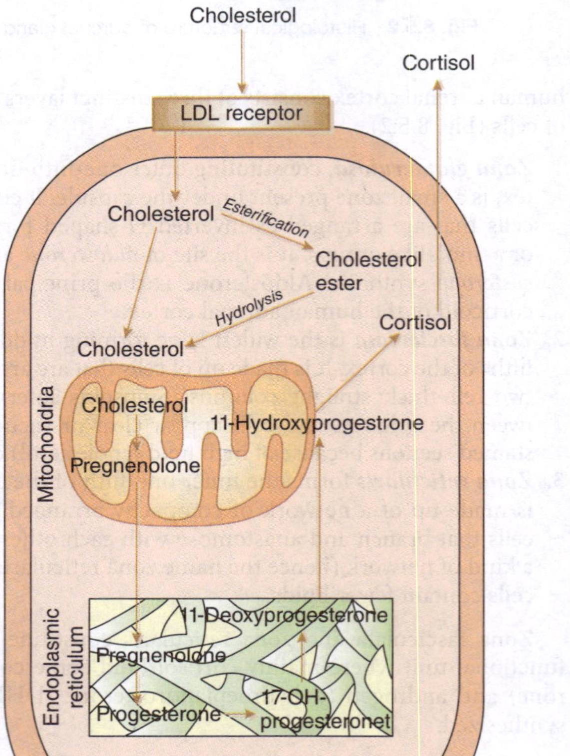

Fig. 8.5.6 Intracellular localization of steps involved in the synthesis of cortisol.

HORMONES OF ADRENAL CORTEX

Hormones secreted by adrenal cortex, called *corticosteroids*, can be grouped as:

Glucocorticoids: These include *cortisol* and *corticosterone*, which have a widespread effect on glucose and protein metabolism.

Mineral corticoids: Aldosterone is the chief mineralocorticoid. It regulates the sodium balance and extracellular fluid (ECF) volume in the body.

Adrenal sex steroids: These include androgenic substances such as DHEA and its sulphate ester.

In addition, adrenal cortex also secretes *biosynthetic precursors* of three end products – progesterone, 11-deoxycorticosterone and 11-deoxycortisol.

> **Important Note**
>
> It is important to note that the normal human adrenal cortex does not secrete physiologically effective amounts of testosterone or oestradiol.

GLUCOCORTICOIDS

Synthesis

The glucocorticoids are synthesized largely by the cells forming zona fasciculata with a small contribution by the cells of zona reticularis of adrenal cortex. The steps involved in the synthesis of glucocorticoids are summarized in Fig. 8.5.5 and their intracellular localization is depicted in Fig. 8.5.6.

Uptake of cholesterol The corticosteroid hormones are synthesized from cholesterol, which is actively taken up by the adrenal cells from low-density lipoprotein (LDL) of the blood. Cells of the adrenal cortex are rich in LDL receptors. After entry into the cell by endocytosis, microtubules move the cholesterol to cytoplasmic vacuoles, within which most of the cholesterol is stored as cholesterol ester. A small amount of cholesterol is also synthesized in the adrenal cells from acetyl-coenzyme A (acetyl-CoA). Under basal conditions, corticosteroids are synthesized from free plasma cholesterol but when the production is stimulated by adrenocorticotropic hormone (ACTH), the stored esterified cholesterol becomes the most important precursor which is hydrolysed by cholesterol esterase. The free cholesterol enters the mitochondria through steroidogenic acute regulatory protein (STAR).

Five oxidative CYP (formerly P450) enzymes (Table 8.5.1) act on various ring carbons of cholesterol to form corticosteroid hormones. As shown in Fig. 8.5.7, the basic steroid structure ring consists of four rings designated as A, B, C and D.

Table 8.5.1 Nomenclature and location of enzymes involved in synthesis of glucocorticoids

Trivial name	Code: Past	Code: Current	Location	Action
20,22-Desmolase	$P450_{SCC}$	CYP-11-A1	Mitochondria	Cleaves the side chain between carbons 20 and 22 of cholesterol
3β-OH-dehydrogenase	3β-HSD	3β-HSD	Endoplasmic reticulum microsome	Catalyses conversion of pregnenolone to progesterone
17α-Hydroxylase	$P450_{C17}$	CYP-17	Endoplasmic reticulum microsome	Catalyses the hydroxylation of C-17
21-Hydroxylase	$P450_{C21}$	CYP-21-A2	Endoplasmic reticulum microsome	Catalyses the hydroxylation of C-21
11β-Hydroxylase	$P450_{C11}$	CYP-11-B1	Mitochondria	Catalyses the hydroxylation at C-11

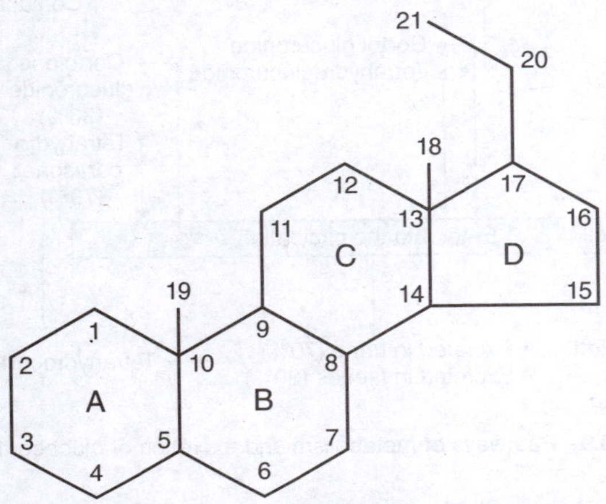

Fig. 8.5.7 Basic structure of steroid ring. Note that the four rings are designated **A, B, C and D.**

The individual carbon atoms comprising the steroid ring are numbered 1–21 (Fig. 8.5.7). Substituent groups in derivative steroid molecules are designated by the number of carbon ring atoms to which they are attached.

Side-chain cleavage of cholesterol This is caused by the mitochondrial enzyme 20,22-desmolase (also known as side-chain cleavage enzyme P450scc). As a result, the cholesterol is converted to pregnenolone, which is a common precursor of all steroid hormones. This is the *rate-limiting step* in the synthesis of corticosteroids.

Conversion of pregnenolone to 11-deoxycortisol and 11-deoxycorticosterone This occurs by hydroxylation reactions. These reactions subsequently follow after the formation of pregnenolone and progesterone and occur within the *endoplasmic reticulum* (Fig. 8.5.6). These reactions are catalysed by 17α-hydroxylase, 3β-1-dehydrogenase and 21-hydroxylase, and convert pregnenolone into 11-deoxycortisol and 11-deoxycorticosterone (Fig. 8.5.5).

Conversion of 11-deoxycortisol to cortisol The 11-deoxycortisol is transferred back into the mitochondria (Fig. 8.5.5). This step is very efficient in humans; 95% of the 11-deoxycortisol formed is converted into cortisol. The cortisol so formed rapidly diffuses out of the cell and is not stored appreciably in the adrenocortical cell. Hence, during acute need for increased amounts of circulating cortisol, the rapid activation of the entire synthetic sequence from cholesterol is activated by ACTH.

Conversion of 11-deoxycorticosterone to corticosterone Under normal circumstances, little corticosterone is formed and cortisol is the dominant glucocorticoid in humans. However, when cortisol synthesis is blocked, the pathway to corticosterone is opened and increased synthesis of corticosterone can provide the glucocorticoid activity necessary for maintaining health. The 11-deoxycorticosterone is converted to corticosterone by the enzyme 11β-hydroxylase.

Plasma Levels, Transport, Metabolism and Excretion of Glucocorticoids

Plasma Levels

Plasma levels of glucocorticoids and other corticosteroids are shown in Table 8.5.2. The plasma levels of total cortisol show diurnal fluctuation and range from 10 to 25 μg% with an average of 14 μg%. The rate of secretion of cortisol, which is approximately 15 mg/day under normal conditions, may increase to 300–400 mg/day under conditions of severe stress.

Transport

Cortisol In the plasma, cortisol circulates in two forms: bound (90%) and free (10%).

Bound form: Most of the plasma cortisol is bound to specific corticosteroid-binding α_2-globulin (CBG), which is a glycoprotein and is also called transcortin. A small amount (15%) is bound to albumin. The protein binding of the cortisol not only protects it from urinary excretion and degradation but also serves as a circulatory reserve of the hormone.

Free form: This form of cortisol constitutes only 5%–10% of the total plasma cortisol. However, it is the free form which is responsible for the physiological actions of the hormone including the feedback regulation of ACTH.

Table 8.5.2 Average 8 a.m. plasma levels and secretion rate of corticosteroids in adult humans

Corticosteroid	Plasma concentration (μg/dL)	Secretion rate ↑ (mg/day)
Cortisol	14.0	15
Corticosterone	1.0	3
Aldosterone	0.0006	0.15
Deoxycorticosterone	0.0006	0.20
Dehydroepiandrosterone (DHEA) sulphate	175	20

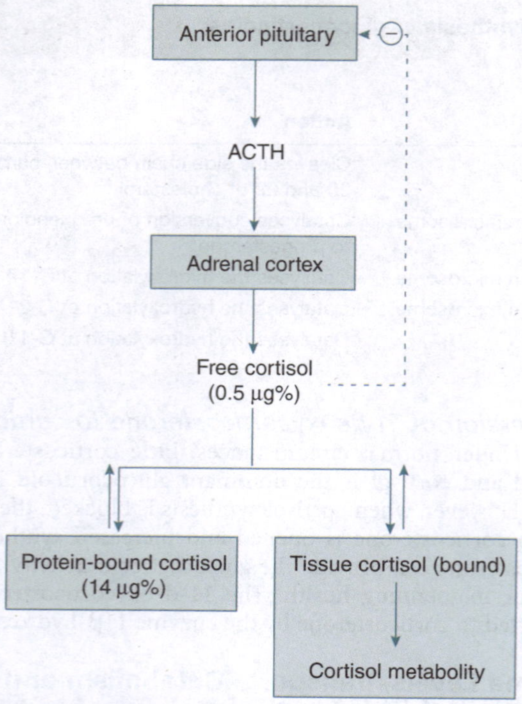

Fig. 8.5.8 Maintenance of interrelationship between free and bound plasma cortisol.

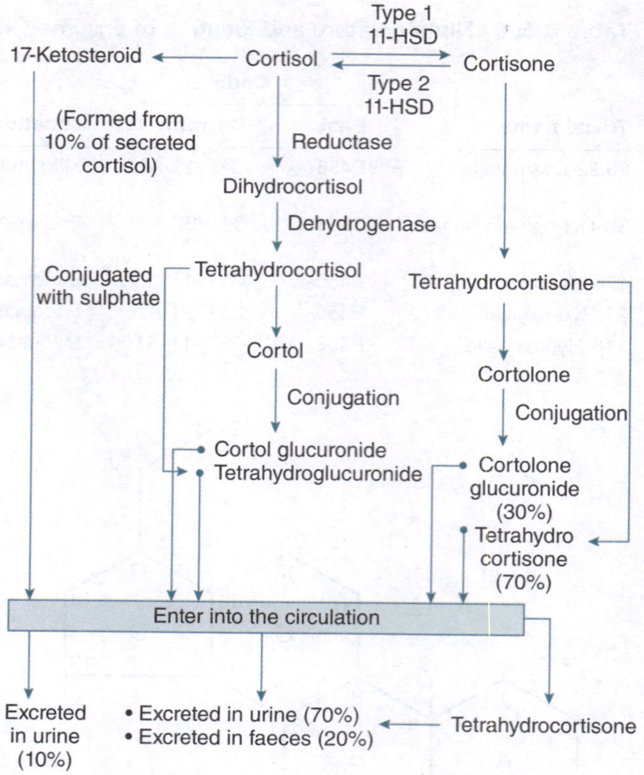

Fig. 8.5.9 Pathways of metabolism and excretion of glucocorticoids.

Interrelationship of free and bound forms (Fig. 8.5.8)

At the normal levels (average 14 µg/dL), the free form is less than 10% of total plasma cortisol. When the total plasma cortisol increases beyond 20 µg%, the binding sites on transcortin are saturated and there occurs some increase in albumin binding, but the main increase is in the free form.

Transcortin The normal plasma concentration of transcortin is 3 mg%, and its binding capacity is 20 µg cortisol/dL. It is synthesized in the liver, where its rate of production is increased by the oestrogen.

> **Important Note**
>
> The concentration of transcortin, and therefore of total cortisol, is increased during pregnancy and by oestrogen administration. In the third trimester of pregnancy, transcortin levels are twice those in nonpregnant state.

The increased total cortisol is, however, not associated with symptoms of excess cortisol as the levels of (physiologically active) free form of cortisol are normal.

> **Applied Aspects**
>
> ***Transcortin levels in plasma*** are decreased in cirrhosis liver (decreased synthesis), nephrosis (more loss in urine) and multiple myeloma. Decreased levels of plasma transcortin are associated with decreased total plasma cortisol levels but with no symptoms of cortisol insufficiency, as the levels of free form are normal.

Corticosterone Like cortisol, it also exists mainly in bound form, but to a lesser degree. That is why its half-life is slightly shorter than that of cortisol.

Interrelationship between cortisol and cortisone The cortisol is in equilibrium with cortisone via the enzyme 11β-hydroxysteroid dehydrogenase (HSD). Cortisol is converted to cortisone in the kidney by type 2,11-hydroxysteroid dehydrogenase (type 2,11-HSD) and the cortisone is returned to the plasma, from which it enters cortisol target cells. There cortisone is reconverted to cortisol by type 1,11-HSD (Fig. 8.5.9). The plasma ratio of total cortisone to total cortisol is 0.1:0.2, but because cortisone binds only weakly to transcortin, the plasma ratio of free cortisone to free cortisol is close to 1.0. Further, there is little diurnal variation in plasma cortisone levels.

> **Important Note**
>
> It is important to note that in effect, circulating cortisone is something of a prohormone for cortisol, and exogenous cortisone is an effective, though not ideal, replacement in cortisol-deficient individuals.

Metabolism and Excretion

Corticosteroids are degraded in the liver and conjugated with glucuronic acid.

Major pathway: This pathway of cortisol and cortisone metabolism is shown in Fig. 8.5.9. The reduced metabolites of cortisol and cortisone (the cortol and cortolone) are conjugated and excreted in the urine as cortol glucuronide and cortolone glucuronide, respectively.

Minor pathway: This pathway of cortisol metabolism includes its conversion to 17-ketosteroid derivatives, which are conjugated to sulphates and are rapidly excreted in urine. Approximately 10% of the secreted cortisol is metabolized by this pathway (Fig. 8.5.9).

Excretion: There is enterohepatic circulation of glucocorticoids. Approximately 70% of the conjugated steroids are excreted in the urine and approximately 20% in the faeces.

A total of approximately 22 mg of glucocorticoid derivatives is excreted in urine per day. The average amount of different derivatives excreted in the urine in 24 hours is

- 0.03 mg only as free cortisol (because of protein binding)
- 5 mg as tetrahydrocortisol glucuronide and cortol glucuronide
- 3 mg as tetrahydrocortisone glucuronide and cortolone glucuronide
- 6.0 mg as 17-ketosteroids derived from cortisol and cortisone (mostly sulphate conjugate)
- 7.0 mg as unidentified metabolites

Important Note

The rate of inactivation and conjugation of glucocorticoids is decreased in liver diseases and during surgery or other stresses. Therefore, in such conditions, the plasma free cortisol level rises higher than it does with maximum ACTH stimulation in the absence of stress.

Mechanism of Action of Glucocorticoids

Like other steroid hormones, the glucocorticoids act through effect on gene expression by binding with specific intracellular receptors called glucocorticoid receptors (GRs). For details of mechanism of action, see page 658 and Fig. 8.1.8. GRs are of two types: GR-I and GR-II, and are found in many tissues. Most cortisol effects in peripheral tissues are exerted through type II GR, while in the brain the effects are exerted mainly through type I GR. Glucocorticoids, after combining with the GR, alter the protein-synthesizing machinery of the target cells through transcription and translation effect. Altered synthesis of different enzymes in different tissues produces the multiple effects. In addition, glucocorticoids also have nongenomic actions.

Actions of Glucocorticoids

Glucocorticoids are essential for survival.

I. Metabolic effects of glucocorticoids Cortisol has major effects on protein, glucose and fat metabolism. By their metabolic effects, the glucocorticoids help to provide fuel molecules in circulation (Fig. 8.5.10). This effect is particularly useful during fasting, exercise and many other stresses. The nocturnal increase in plasma cortisol levels supports the enhancement of gluconeogenesis, lipolysis and ketogenesis, which are necessary for overnight metabolic stability. The different metabolic effects of glucocorticoids are as follows.

1. Effects on carbohydrate metabolism Glucocorticoids exert an anti-insulin effect, which leads to hyperglycaemia by the following actions (Fig. 8.5.10):

i. ***Increased gluconeogenesis:*** Glucocorticoids increase the rate of glucose production from noncarbohydrate sources by as much as 6- to 10-fold by the following mechanisms:
- Accelerating the synthesis of hepatic enzymes (e.g. glucose-6-phosphatase) involved in gluconeogenesis
- Providing more amino acids to the liver for gluconeogenesis by their catabolic effect on muscle protein and inhibitory effect on protein synthesis

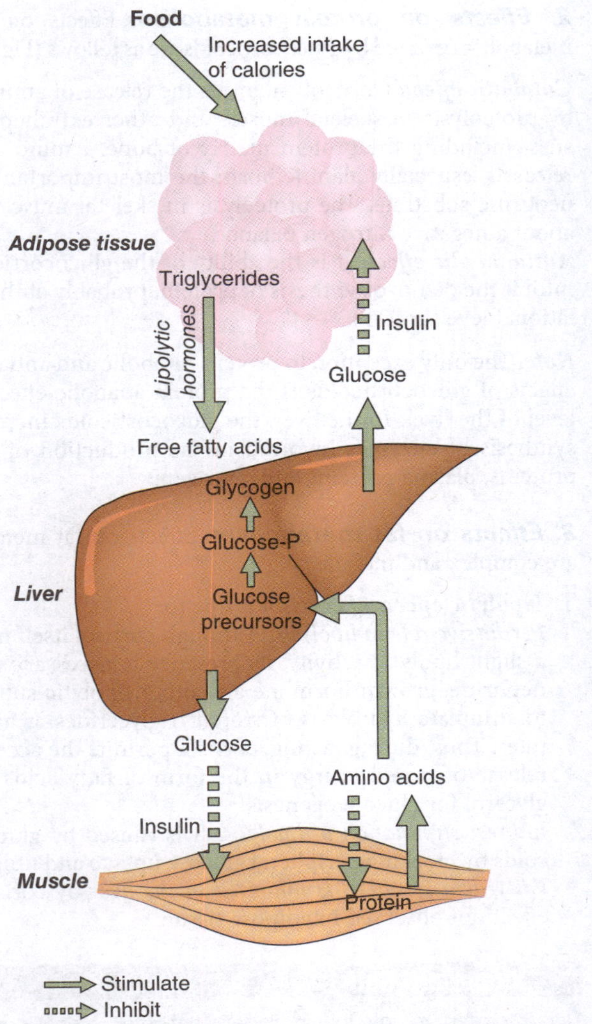

Fig. 8.5.10 Metabolic effects of cortisol. Note: Cortisol increases intake of calories by increasing appetite, facilitates release of amino acids from the muscle and their use for gluconeogenesis in liver and storage as glycogen, inhibits peripheral utilization of glucose and synthesis of proteins from amino acids and facilitates release of free fatty acids from the adipose tissues.

- Providing more glycerol to the liver for gluconeogenesis by increasing lipolysis

Important Note

It is important to note that normally increased glucose synthesis is associated with glycogen breakdown. But glucocorticoids promote gluconeogenesis, as well as the storage of carbohydrates as hepatic glycogens. Glycogen synthesis is increased by increasing glycogen synthetase.

ii. ***Decreased utilization of glucose in peripheral tissues:*** Glucocorticoids inhibit glucose uptake by peripheral tissues like the muscle, skin and connective tissue, lymphoid tissue, bone and adipose tissue. The heart, brain, liver and erythrocytes are spared from this action. In fact, glucose spared by the former group of tissues may be used by the latter group of tissues. This can be valuable in states of stress.

2. Effects on protein metabolism Effects on protein metabolism exerted by glucocorticoids are as follows (Fig. 8.5.10):

Catabolic effect: Cortisol enhances the release of amino acids by proteolysis in skeletal muscle and other extrahepatic tissues, including the protein matrix of bone. Amino acids so released, especially alanine, form the most important gluconeogenic substrate. The proteolysis in skeletal muscle brings about a negative nitrogen balance.

Antianabolic effect: It is the ability of the glucocorticoids to inhibit the de novo synthesis of protein, probably at the translational level.

Note. The only exception to protein catabolic and antianabolic effects of glucocorticoids is the protein anabolic effect at the level of the liver. In the liver, the glucocorticoids increase the synthesis of enzymes involved in the production of hepatic proteins, plasma proteins and glycogen.

3. Effects on fat metabolism Effects on fat metabolism are complex and include:

i. ***Lipolytic effects of cortisol*** is due to:
Permissive role in lipolysis: Although cortisol itself has only a slight lipolytic activity, its presence is necessary for epinephrine, growth hormone and other lipolytic substances to stimulate hydrolysis of stored triglycerides at maximal rates. Thus, during fasting, cortisol permits the accelerated release of stored energy in the form of fatty acids and of glycerol for gluconeogenesis.
Indirect stimulation of lipolysis: It is caused by glucocorticoids by blocking peripheral glucose uptake and utilization.
Fatty acid synthesis is inhibited in the liver by cortisol, an effect not observed in adipose tissue.

Important Note

It is important to note that in diabetic patients, cortisol increases plasma lipid levels and increases ketone body formation, which worsens diabetes. But in normal subjects, insulin secretion is increased by raised blood glucose levels and the insulin decreases lipase activity and counterbalances hyperglycaemia.

ii. ***Lipogenic role:*** Glucocorticoids increase differentiation of adipose tissue cells from preadipocytes to adipocytes and stimulate lipogenesis by increasing adipocyte lipoprotein lipase and glucose-6-phosphate dehydrogenase activity. The lipogenic effect varies in different regions of the body.

Note therefore, in cortisol excess, there occurs a selective accumulation of fat in the abdomen, trunk and above (trunked obesity), sparing the extremities which become thin due to loss of muscle mass. The deposition of fat in the face is called 'moon face' and in the suprascapular region it is referred to as '*buffalo hump*' or 'dowager's hump' (features Cushing syndrome).

Important Notes

It is important to note that the fat deposition observed in hypercortisolism reflects increased food intake rather than a change in the rate of lipid metabolism.
- Glucocorticoids increase appetite and food intake by:
  - Inducing neuropeptide Y (NPY) synthesis and NPY receptors in the hypothalamus
  - Suppressing CRH release
- Since cortisol also induces leptin synthesis in adipocytes, the gain in fat mass is eventually limited by the negative feedback of action of leptin on the appetite centre in the hypothalamus.

4. Effects on electrolyte and water metabolism Glucocorticoids control distribution of body water and electrolytes by their opposing actions:

i. ***Retention of sodium and water*** by the following actions:
Mineralocorticoid activity of glucocorticoids is mild but becomes of physiological importance because of the large quantity of cortisol secreted every day. By aldosterone-like activity, the glucocorticoids increase sodium and chloride retention and potassium excretion by the kidney.
Aldosterone secretion is increased by glucocorticoids by increasing the synthesis of angiotensinogens from the liver. The increased aldosterone secretion, in turn, causes excessive retention of sodium and water.

ii. ***Promotion of diuresis:*** Glucocorticoids promote diuresis by increasing the inactivation of ADH by liver and by antagonizing the action of ADH at the level of distal convoluted tubules of the kidney.

Applied Aspects

In cortisol insufficiency, be cautious while infusing saline/glucose because these patients cannot excrete water load (due to adrenocortical deficiency) and leads to water intoxication.

II. Physiological actions on various organs and systems In addition to the metabolic effects noted above, the glucocorticoids affect various organs and systems throughout the body (Fig. 8.5.11).

1. Effects on muscle

i. ***Contractility and work performance*** of skeletal and cardiac muscle is maintained by the cortisol. The effect on skeletal muscle is exerted at the myoneural junction, by an increase in acetylcholine synthesis. In cardiac muscle, cortisol increases Na^+–K^+-ATPase and β-adrenergic receptors.

ii. ***Decrease in muscle mass and strength*** is caused by an excess of cortisol. This occurs due to decrease in muscle protein synthesis and increase in muscle catabolism.

2. Effects on bone

i. ***Increased bone resorption:*** Glucocorticoids increase bone resorption transiently by increasing:
- Osteoclastic activity
- Activity of enzyme collagenase, which is essential for destroying the organic matrix of bone

ii. ***Inhibition of bone formation*** is the most profound effect of glucocorticoids caused by:
- Decreasing collagen synthesis
- Inhibiting formation of mature osteoblasts from the undifferentiated cells
- Increasing rate of apoptosis of osteoblasts and osteocytes
- Impeding calcium absorption from the intestinal tract by antagonizing the action of 1,25-$(OH)_2$-vitamin D and inhibiting its synthesis
- Increasing calcium excretion in urine, as glomerular filtration rate (GFR) increases

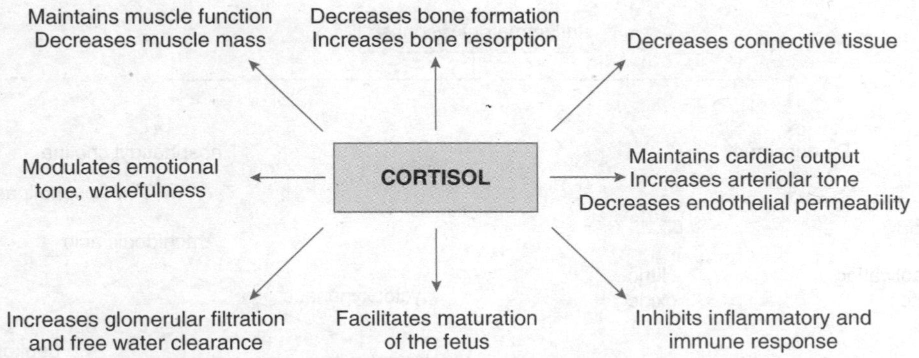

Fig. 8.5.11 Effects of glucocorticoids on various tissues and organs and systems of the body.

Note. Because of the above-mentioned effects on bone, *osteoporosis* (which results in skeletal deformity) is a feared and sometimes devastating complication of glucocorticoid therapy that lasts more than a few weeks.

3. Effects on connective tissue Cortisol decreases collagen synthesis, producing thereby:

Thinning of the skin
Thinning of walls of capillaries, which leads to their easy rupture and to intracutaneous haemorrhage

4. Effects on vascular system Cortisol is essential for maintaining normal blood pressure by:

- Sustaining myocardial performance
- Enhancing the vasopressure effect (responsiveness of arterioles to constrictive effect) of catecholamines (especially NE) and angiotensin II
- Decreasing production of vasodilator prostaglandins
- Maintaining normal blood volume by decreasing the permeability of the vascular endothelium

Therefore, in the absence of cortisol, the vasopressor action of catecholamines is diminished and hypotension ensues.

5. Effects on kidney are:
- Increase in GFR by increasing glomerular plasma flow
- Rapid excretion of water load
- Increase in calcium and phosphate excretion by decreasing their reabsorption in the proximal tubules

In the absence of cortisol, free water clearance is diminished, because the activity of ADH is not antagonized (also see effect on water and electrolyte metabolism, see page 730).

6. Effects on central nervous system GRs are present in various parts of the brain, especially in the limbic system. Through these receptors, the glucocorticoids modulate excitability behaviour and mood. Therefore, in the *absence of cortisol (Addison disease),* there occurs:

- Mood changes in the form of irritability, apprehension and inability to concentrate
- Increased sensitivity to olfactory and gustatory stimuli (especially salty taste)
- EEG waves slower than normal rhythm

Excess of cortisol is associated with:
- Increased brain excitability and insomnia
- Decreased memory function
- Decreased threshold for convulsive activity: Because of this reason, glucocorticoids are contraindicated in epilepsy

7. Effects on gastrointestinal tract The glucocorticoids increase gastric acid secretion and decrease proliferation of gastric mucosal cells. These effects can lead to peptic ulceration following long-term use of cortisol.

8. Effects on blood cells and lymphatic organs The excess of glucocorticoids leads to:

Eosinopenia and basopenia, due to their increased destruction and increased sequestration in lungs and spleen. The changes in eosinophilic count have been used as an index of change in ACTH secretion.
Lymphopenia, i.e. decrease in the number of lymphocytes, is caused by inhibiting their proliferation and increasing their destruction in the circulation. This leads to decreased size of lymph nodes, thymus, spleen and other lymphoid tissues.
Neutrophilia, i.e. increase in neutrophil count, occurs due to their increased release from bone marrow and decreased migration into tissues from the vascular spaces.
Polycythaemia, i.e. increased red blood cell (RBC) count, occurs due to stimulation of erythropoiesis.
Thrombocytosis, i.e. increased platelet count.

III. Anti-inflammatory and antiallergic effects These effects are not produced by the glucocorticoids, which are normally secreted physiologically, but are produced in large doses when administered therapeutically and are thus called the pharmacological actions of glucocorticoids.

1. Anti-inflammatory effects Anti-inflammatory effects of glucocorticoids are produced by the following actions (Fig. 8.5.12):

i. ***Glucocorticoids inhibit activation of nuclear factor-kappa B*** by increasing production of IkBa. NF-κB normally exists in the cytosol in bound form with IkBa (accelator protein), which makes it inactive. Inflammation stimuli such as virus, bacteria, cytokines and oxidant-induced signals dissociate NF-κB from IkBa. NF-κB then moves into the nucleus and binds to DNA of the genes to transcript numerous inflammatory mediators resulting in their increased production.
ii. ***Cortisol inhibits the activity of phospholipase A_2,*** which is responsible for arachidonic acid products (such as prostacyclins, prostaglandins and thromboxanes) that

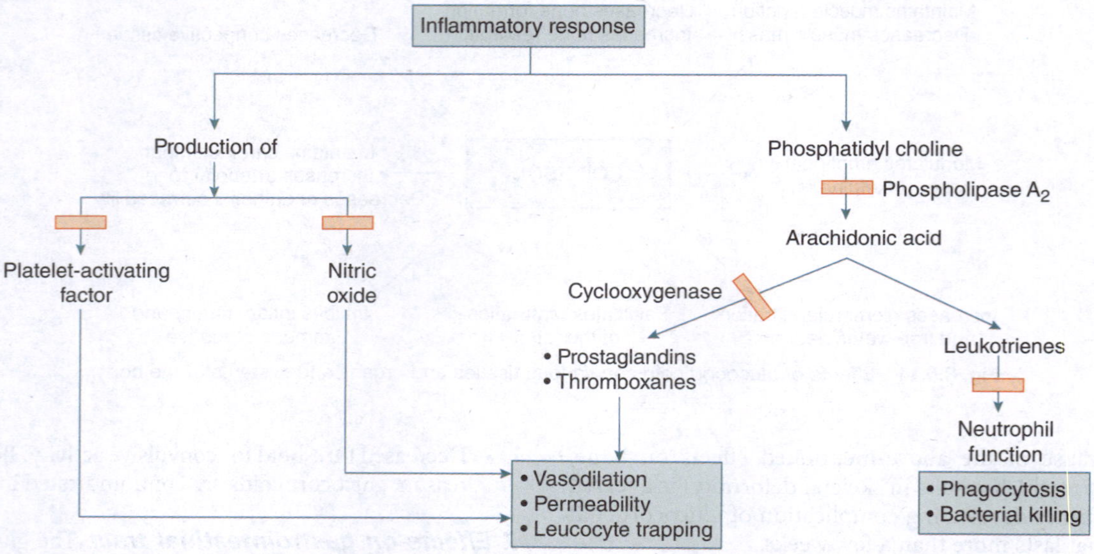

Fig. 8.5.12 Sites ( ) of action of cortisol in inhibiting inflammatory response.

may be involved in mediating vascular components of the inflammation, and thus reduce the severity of inflammation by decreasing hyperaemia and capillary permeability and thereby preventing exudation, migration and infiltration of leucocytes at the site of injury.

iii. ***Cortisol stabilizes the lysosomal membrane***, probably by inhibiting the phospholipase A_2, thereby preventing the release of proteolytic enzymes and hyaluronidase, which contribute to tissue damage and swelling.

iv. ***Cortisol inhibits migration of circulating*** leucocytes to the site of inflammation by blocking the leucocyte receptors for chemotactic agents.

v. ***Cortisol inhibits leukotriene*** and thus impairs neutrophil phagocytosis and bactericidal abilities.

vi. ***Cortisol decreases collagen formation*** and the proliferation of fibroblasts and thus impedes the chronic inflammatory responses.

2. Anti-immunity effect Cortisol inhibits both cellular and humoral immunity by decreasing the proliferation of T cells (involved in cellular immunity) and B cells (involved in humoral immunity) by producing antibodies. The sites of actions of cortisol in inhibiting immune response are shown in Fig. 8.5.13.

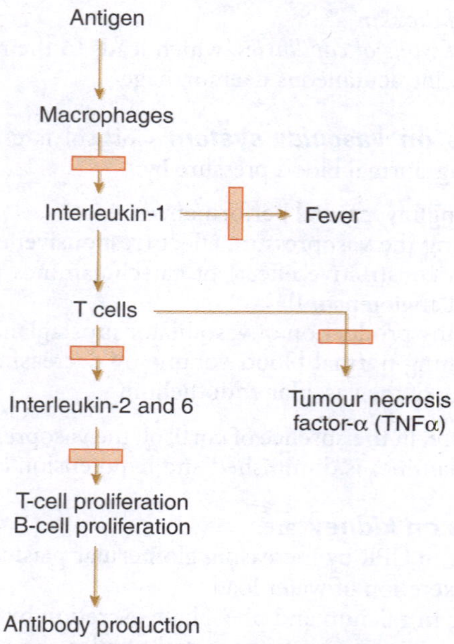

Fig. 8.5.13 Sites ( ) of action of cortisol in inhibiting immune response.

3. Antiallergic effect Cortisol reduces the number of circulating basophils and protects against the release of secretory products of granulocytes, mast cells and macrophages, which have vesicles containing serotonin, histamine and hydrolases. This accounts for the fall in blood levels of histamine and histamine-like substances, thereby reducing the histamine-induced features of allergy or hypersensitivity in response to antigen–antibody reaction. It is important to note that cortisol does not affect the combination of antigen with antibodies and has no influence on the effect of histamine once it is released, though it inhibits the intracellular synthesis of histamine.

IV. Role of glucocorticoids in fetal life

Maturation of CNS, retina and skin: It is facilitated by the cortisol in utero.

Maturation of lungs: During fetal life, oxygen is transferred from the maternal blood through the placenta. In the last weeks of gestation, preparation of the fetal lungs to permit satisfactory breathing immediately after birth is facilitated by cortisol by increasing the activity of key enzymes, such as phosphatidic acid phosphatase and choline phosphotransferase, which are involved in the biosynthesis of pulmonary surfactants. The pulmonary surfactant lowers the surface tension in pulmonary alveoli and thus permits proper inflation of lungs immediately after birth.

Applied Aspects

In infants, deficient secretion of glucocorticoids leads to infant respiratory distress syndrome.

Maturation of gastrointestinal tract: In fetal life, maternal glucose is transferred to the fetus through the placenta. The digestive enzyme capacity of the intestinal mucosa changes from a fetal pattern to a mature adult pattern under the influence of cortisol. This maturation process allows the newborn to digest disaccharides present in the milk.

V. Role of glucocorticoids in stress Various stresses, e.g. trauma, cold, illness and starvation, are associated with activation of the hypothalamic–hypophyseal–adrenal axis. Increased secretion of glucocorticoids is one of the various mechanisms involved in adaptation to various stresses (see page 750). A variety of stimuli, during stress, act on the hypothalamus and cause release of ACTH from the anterior pituitary via release of corticotropin-releasing hormone (CRH), which in turn increases glucocorticoid secretion to as much as 20-fold depending on the type of stress.

Important Note

It is important to note that resistance to stress is not increased by the administration of glucocorticoids. How cortisol helps against the stressful conditions is not exactly clear.

Regulation of Glucocorticoid Secretion

The glucocorticoid secretion is regulated by hypothalamic–anterior pituitary–adrenal cortex axis, which exerts its effect through (Fig. 8.5.14):

- Corticotropin-releasing hormone (CRH)
- ACTH
- Glucocorticoid negative feedback effect

Note. Since CRH and ACTH are related to regulation of glucocorticoid release, they are described in detail here, rather than along with other hormones of the hypothalamus and anterior pituitary, respectively.

1. Role of Corticotropin-Releasing Hormone

CRH is secreted by the small cells of the paraventricular nucleus of hypothalamus (the cells which also secrete ADH). It is the important and final mediator of the regulatory inputs of glucocorticoids. CRH is a polypeptide with 41 amino acids.

Control of CRH secretion is by:

i. ***Stressful stimuli*** (e.g. pain, anaesthesia, surgery and haemorrhage): These ultimately increase cortisol secretion within minutes to as much as 20-fold, and primarily act on the hypothalamus to increase the secretion of CRH via the reticular activating system (RAS). The tracts from RAS are *cholinergic* and those from the raphe nuclei and the locus coeruleus are catecholaminergic and serotonergic.

ii. ***Circadian rhythm:*** The CRH secretion, and thus ACTH and cortisol secretions, shows circadian rhythm (Fig. 8.5.15). If the serotonergic and cholinergic connections between the limbic system and hypothalamus are cut, the circadian rhythm is abolished but the responses to stress are still retained.

iii. ***ACTH:*** It acts on the hypothalamus to reduce the secretion of ACTH by short-loop negative feedback mechanism.

iv. ***Glucocorticoids:*** These exert a long-loop negative feedback effect on CRH secretion (Fig. 8.5.14).

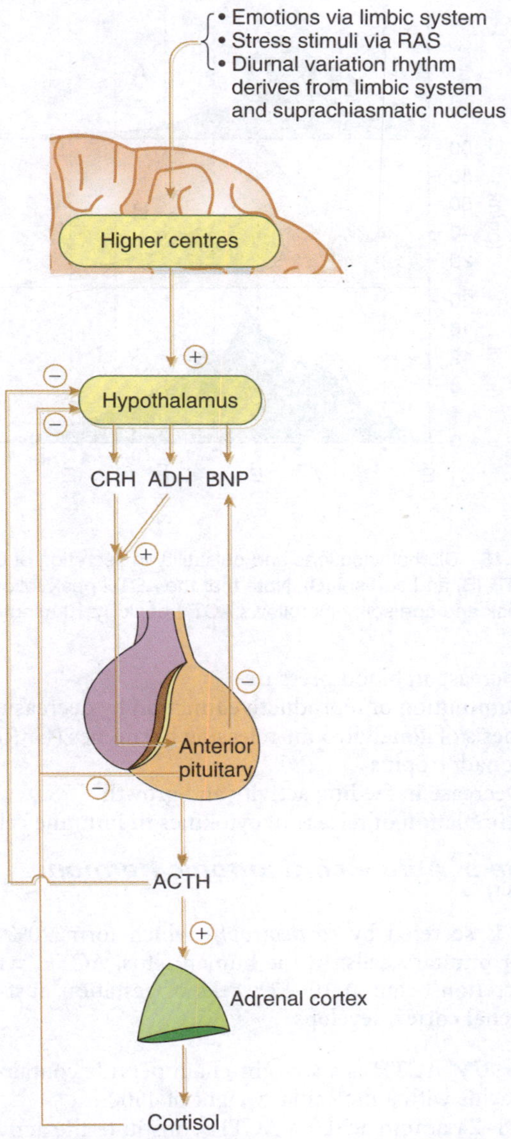

Fig. 8.5.14 Hypothalamic–anterior pituitary–adrenal cortex axis and negative feedback mechanism controlling glucocorticoid secretion.

Mechanism of action of CRH The CRH reaches the anterior pituitary through the hypothalamic–hypophyseal portal system and acts by cAMP mechanism through the CRH receptors. CRH receptors are G-protein–coupled receptors termed hCRH-RI and hCRH-RII.

Actions of CRH are:

i. ***Stimulation of synthesis and release of ACTH,*** by acting on the *corticotrophs*, is the *main function*. A lack of CRH (as in a CRH knockout model) greatly impairs the ACTH diurnal rhythm and its response to stress.

ii. ***Stimulation of synthesis and release of pro-opiomelanocortin (POMC) products*** by acting on corticotrophs of anterior pituitary via cAMP mechanism.

iii. ***Other actions of CRH:*** CRH receptors are also found throughout the brain and spinal cord and CRH is also synthesized in many peripheral cells including immune cells and cells in the skin. Other actions of CRH related to or independent of ACTH include:

- Central arousal

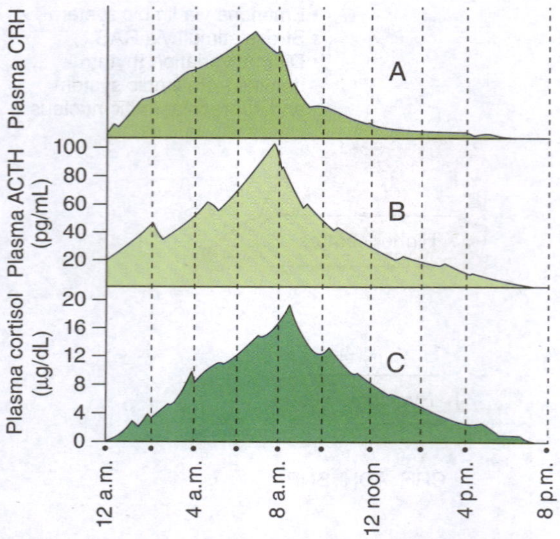

Fig. 8.5.15 Diurnal variations and pulsatility in secretion of CRH (**A**), ACTH (**B**) and cortisol (**C**). Note that the ACTH peak follows CRH peak and cortisol peak follows ACTH peak by 10 minutes.

- Increase in blood pressure
- Diminution of reproductive function by decreasing synthesis of gonadotropin-releasing hormones (GnRH) and gonadotropins
- Decrease in feeding activity and growth
- Stimulation of release of cytokines in immune cells

2. Role of Adrenocorticotropic Hormone (ACTH)

ACTH is secreted by *corticotrophs* which form 20% of the anterior pituitary cells. In the human fetus, ACTH synthesis and secretion begin at 10–12 weeks of gestation, just before the adrenal cortex develops.

Chemistry ACTH is a straight-chain peptide containing 39 amino acids with a molecular weight of 4500.

The 1–24 amino acids in ACTH constitute the active portion of the hormone, which contains full biological activity, and the remaining 15 amino acids constitute the tail, which serves the function of stabilization.

Synthesis ACTH, along with other peptides cosecreted in plasma, is derived from the single precursor pro-opiomelanocortin (POMC) consisting of 241 amino acids. The hormone of this group thus includes (see Fig. 8.2.6):

- ACTH.
- Melanocyte-stimulating hormone (MSH): The α- and β-MSH are produced in the intermediary lobe (which is rudimentary in humans).
- β-Lipotropin (LPH).
- β-Endorphin.
- Metenkephalin.
- Corticotropin-like intermediate lobe protein (CLIP).

Mechanism of action ACTH acts by combining with the ACTH receptors present on the surface of adrenal cortical tissue cells. ACTH receptors are termed melanocortin 2 receptors (MC_2R).

The receptor–hormone complex in the presence of calcium activates the cAMP, which is the principal second messenger. The cAMP leads to phosphorylation of key enzymes and histones which result in its biological action.

Actions of ACTH include:

i. ***Actions on adrenal cortex:*** ACTH is primarily concerned with the growth and functions of the adrenal cortex:
   - It promotes conversion of cholesterol to pregnenolone, which is the precursor of synthesis of all the hormones of the adrenal cortex.
   - It stimulates the secretion of glucocorticoids and the adrenal androgens. But it does not exert direct control on the secretion of mineralocorticoids (aldosterone) from the adrenal cortex.
   - It enhances RNA and protein synthesis in the adrenal glands and thus promotes adrenal cortex growth. ACTH increases the size rather than the number of adrenal cells and in the absence of ACTH, the relevant adrenal zones atrophy.

ii. ***Extra-adrenal actions*** of ACTH occur only with very high levels, which are seen in abnormal conditions. The extra-adrenal actions include:
   - *Lipolysis* in the adipose tissue is promoted by ACTH by activating the enzyme lipase.
   - *Stimulation of β-cells of pancreas* to increase the release of insulin.
   - *Stimulation of growth hormone–secreting* cells.
   - *MSH-like effect on the melanocytes* of skin resulting in increased pigmentation.

iii. ***Other actions of ACTH:*** ACTH synthesis and receptors for ACTH are also located in some other structures, where its possible roles are as follows:
   - Neuromodulatory or paracrine functions in brain and gastrointestinal tract.
   - ACTH receptor and ACTH secretion occur in lymphocytes, suggesting an important relationship between ACTH and the immune system.

Regulation of ACTH secretion occurred through:

i. Hypothalamic control on ACTH secretion is mainly exerted through CRH (see above). The hypothalamic control is responsible for the following characteristics of ACTH secretion:

Diurnal variation in the levels of ACTH (and thus of cortisol) is due to variation in CRH release. As shown in Fig. 8.5.15, a large peak in the levels of ACTH and cortisol occurs in the morning (6–8 a.m.) during awakening (plasma level of ACTH range between 20 and 100 pg/mL with an average of 50 pg/mL). Thereafter, the average level decreases markedly (5 pg/mL), just before or after the subject falls asleep. In night workers, the rhythm is reversed. The biological clock responsible for diurnal variation in CRH, ACTH and cortisol levels is located in either the limbic system or suprachiasmatic nucleus of the hypothalamus; destruction of any or both of them abolishes the circadian rhythm. The circadian rhythm is diminished or abolished by loss of consciousness, blindness or constant exposure to either dark or light.

Pulsatile release of ACTH is also due to pulsatile release of CRH. Three pulses occur per hour, and each pulse lasts approximately 20 minutes. Cortisol pulses follow the ACTH pulses. Both frequency and amplitude of ACTH pulses are greater in men than in women. Age has little effect on secretion of ACTH.

Release of ACTH in response to stress is mediated by CRH release (see above) and ADH release. During stress, ADH significantly augments the effect of CRH. In severe stress, the stress-induced hypersecretion of ACTH completely overrides the negative feedback. This hypersecretion cannot be suppressed even if the adrenal cortex secretes cortisol at its maximum levels. Stress may even abolish the diurnal variation of ACTH levels, but pulsatility always persists.

Brain natriuretic peptide (BNP), an analogue of the atrial natriuretic hormone (ANH), also inhibits the ACTH release and the ACTH responses to CRH stimulation in humans. BNP is synthesized in the hypothalamus and thus can be considered a corticotroph release–inhibiting hormone.

ii. Negative feedback inhibition of ACTH is caused by (Fig. 8.5.14):

- Plasma cortisol levels (long-loop negative feedback)
- Plasma ACTH levels (short-loop negative feedback)

3. Negative Feedback Control of Glucocorticoid Secretion

Chronically elevated plasma levels of free cortisol (and not the total cortisol, i.e. free plus bound forms) exert a direct negative feedback action on its own secretion. This effect is exerted at two levels (Fig. 8.5.14):

- On hypothalamus to decrease formation of CRH
- On anterior pituitary to decrease formation of ACTH

Applied Aspects

Two important clinical applications of the negative feedback control of glucocorticoid secretion which need to be considered are as follows:

i. ***Therapeutic administration of exogenous glucocorticoids*** for a long period suppresses the secretion of CRH and ACTH by negative feedback mechanism. This leads to a marked decrease or near absence of secretion of endogenous glucocorticoids from the adrenal cortex. However, the absence is not noticed because the pharmacological doses of exogenous glucocorticoids continue to perform the physiological functions of glucocorticoids as well. But when the exogenous glucocorticoids are stopped suddenly, the hypothalamus, pituitary and adrenal cortex cannot recover equally suddenly, leading to *acute adrenal deficiency* characterized by a sudden fall in blood pressure. The individual may even die of *adrenal crisis*. Therefore, to avoid this complication, exogenous steroids should never be stopped suddenly but their doses should be tapered off slowly over a long period.

ii. ***Dexamethasone suppression test:*** This test is based on the ability of dexamethasone (a potent synthetic glucocorticoid) to inhibit ACTH secretion. When the hypothalamic–pituitary–adrenocortical axis is normal, the administration of dexamethasone inhibits the secretion of ACTH and cortisol.

MINERALOCORTICOIDS

The mineralocorticoids include:

Aldosterone: It is the chief mineralocorticoid.
Deoxycorticosterone (DOC).
18-Hydroxy-deoxycorticosterone (18-OH-DOC) is secreted in small amounts and has some mineralocorticoid activity.

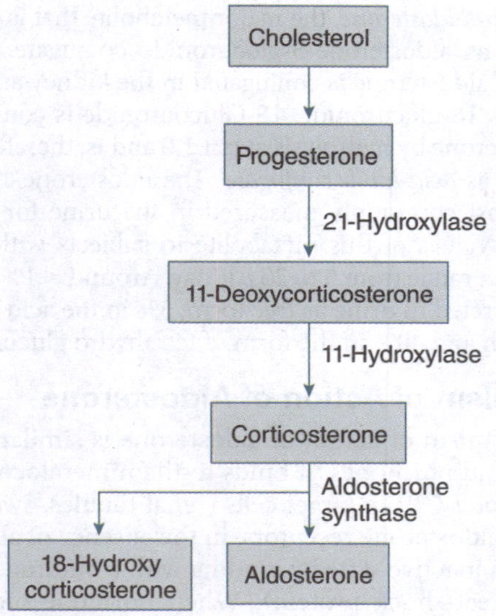

Fig. 8.5.16 Steps involved in the synthesis of aldosterone.

Since aldosterone is the major mineralocorticoid, discussion in this section is limited to it.

Synthesis

Aldosterone, the chief mineralocorticoid, is synthesized exclusively by the *zona glomerulosa cells*. The steps involved in the synthesis, summarized in Fig. 8.5.16, include the following.

Uptake of cholesterol for formation of corticosterone
This involves the same steps as in the synthesis of glucocorticoids in zona fasciculata (for details, see page 726 and Fig. 8.5.5).

Formation of aldosterone Some of the corticosterone is hydroxylated and converted to an aldehyde by aldosterone synthase, a mitochondrial P_{450} mixed oxygenase to yield aldosterone, which is rapidly released. The 18-hydroxycorticosterone is not a direct intermediate but a by-product of this enzyme reaction (Fig. 8.5.16).

Plasma Levels, Transport, Metabolism and Excretion

Plasma levels Depending on the dietary intake of sodium, the aldosterone secretion ranges from 50 μg/day (with dietary sodium intake of 150 mEq) to 250 μg/day (with dietary sodium intake of 10 mEq). Plasma levels of aldosterone show diurnal variation with a highest concentration at 8 a.m. (0.0006 μg/dL) and lowest at 11 p.m.

The diurnal variation The diurnal variation in aldosterone levels is not affected by variation in sodium intake, posture, ACTH suppression by exogenous glucocorticoids or plasma potassium levels.

Transport In the plasma, 40% aldosterone circulates in free form and 60% in bound form. Aldosterone is weakly bound to the specific aldosterone-binding globulin, to transcortin and to albumin. Because of the weaker binding of aldosterone as compared to cortisol, its plasma half-life is only 20 minutes.

Metabolism and excretion A total of 90% of aldosterone, like the glucocorticoids, is degraded in the liver and is reduced to *tetrahydroaldosterone*, the major metabolite that is excreted in the urine as aldosterone-3-glucuronide conjugate. A smaller amount of aldosterone is conjugated in the kidney and excreted in urine as 18-glucuronide. 18-Glucouronide is converted into free aldosterone by hydrolysis at pH 1.0 and is, therefore, usually referred to as *'acid-labile conjugate'*. The aldosterone-18-glucuronide is most commonly measured in the urine for diagnostic purposes. Values of this metabolite in subjects with a normal sodium diet range from 5 to 20 μg/day. Around <1% of aldosterone is excreted in urine as free form, 5% in the acid-labile conjugate form and 40% in the form of tetrahydro glucuronide.

Mechanism of Action of Aldosterone

The mechanism of action of aldosterone is similar to that of other steroid hormones. It binds to the mineralocorticoid receptor (*type I GR*) in target cells (renal tubules, sweat glands, etc.). The aldosterone receptors, in the absence of aldosterone, are kept in inactive state by binding with a binding chaperone protein (heat-shock protein). When hormone binds to the receptor, then these receptors get activated and the hormone–receptor complex migrates to the nucleus, which increases mRNA synthesis and induces or suppresses various proteins described below that mediate the hormone's effects. The aldosterone-stimulated proteins have two types of effects:

The rapid effect is by activating the serum/glucuronide-regulated kinase (SGK).

The slower effect is by increasing the activity of epithelial sodium channels (ENaCs). Aldosterone increases the insertion of ENaCs from the cytosolic pool into the cell membrane and also by increasing the synthesis of ENaCs. The aldosterone does not have an immediate effect. Approximately 1–2 hours is required between exposure to aldosterone and the onset of its action.

Aldosterone also increases the activity of Na^+–K^+ exchanger at cell membrane by rapid nongenomic action.

Actions of Aldosterone

A. Primary Actions of Aldosterone

1. Effects on renal tubules Aldosterone acts on late distal tubules and principal cells of collecting ducts of kidney and causes the following effects (Fig. 8.5.17):

i. ***Sodium reabsorption*** from the tubular fluid into the renal tubular epithelial cells: The Na^+–K^+ pump operates at the basolateral border and not at the luminal border of tubular epithelial cells and transports Na^+ into blood capillaries. Thus, under the influence of aldosterone, the urinary excretion of Na^+ is decreased and the amount of Na^+ in ECF is increased.

ii. ***Potassium excretion:*** In the kidney, the active reabsorption of Na^+ occurs in exchange of K^+ and H^+. Thus, aldosterone causes not only reabsorption of Na^+ but also excretion of K^+ by renal tubular epithelial cells (Fig. 8.5.17). The extent of K^+ excretion is parallel with the rate of delivery of Na^+ to the distal tubule. Thus, a high Na^+ intake will greatly exacerbate urinary K^+ losses caused by aldosterone.

iii. ***H^+ excretion:*** In addition to excretion of K^+, aldosterone also enhances the tubular secretion of H^+ as Na^+ is reabsorbed. Therefore, in aldosterone excess, there occurs mild systemic metabolic alkalosis.

iv. ***Ammonium and magnesium*** excretion: It is also increased by aldosterone.

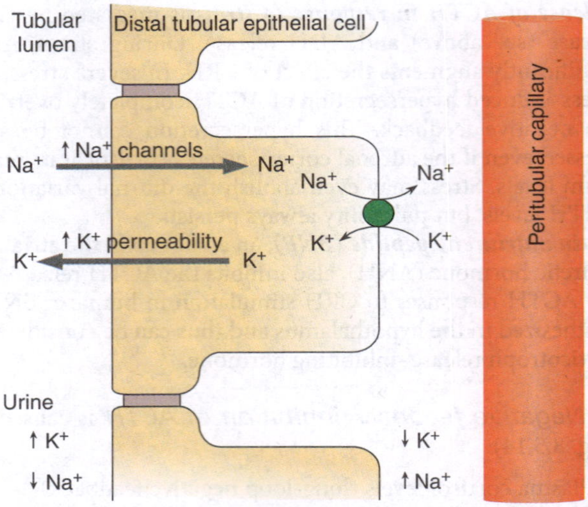

Fig. 8.5.17 Action of aldosterone on the distal renal tubule.

Mechanism of action As mentioned above, aldosterone acts by promoting specific protein synthesis. The *aldosterone-induced protein (AIP) synthesis* increases Na^+ reabsorption by the following effects:

Membrane permeability of tubular cells is increased by AIP, increasing passive Na^+ absorption along the electrical and concentration gradients.

Increase in number of thiazide-sensitive NaCl cotransporter is caused by aldosterone in the apical membrane of the distal convoluted tubular (DCT) cells. The NaCl cotransporter increases the inflow of Na^+ from the tubular urine to the renal cells.

Increase in the content of Na^+–K^+-ATPase at the basal (capillary) surface of the renal tubular cells is caused by aldosterone, which pumps the sodium out and then back into the plasma.

Increase in the Krebs cycle enzyme activity in the mitochondria caused by aldosterone helps to generate energy required for extrusion of Na^+ into the interstitial fluid and capillary blood.

Increase in phospholipase activity caused by aldosterone in the cytosol of cells leads to increased synthesis of fatty acids, which are used in membrane generation.

2. Effects on sweat glands, salivary glands and colon

Sweat glands and salivary glands produce primary secretions which contain large amounts of sodium chloride. The sodium chloride is absorbed as the secretion passes through the ducts, and, in turn, K^+ and HCO_3^- are excreted. Thus, aldosterone decreases the loss of Na^+ and Cl^- in sweat and salivary secretion.

Colon: The aldosterone stimulates sodium reabsorption from the colon while enhancing potassium excretion in the faeces.

Important Note

Relation of mineralocorticoid to glucocorticoid receptors: It is important to note that mineralocorticoid receptors have higher affinity to glucocorticoids than glucocorticoid receptors to glucocorticoids. Therefore, it raises a question: why do glucocorticoids not produce the mineralocorticoid effect in kidney and other target tissue having mineralocorticoid receptors? Because these mineralocorticoid-sensitive tissues contain the enzyme 11β-hydroxysteroid dehydrogenase type 2 (11β-HSD type 2) that converts cortisol to cortisone and corticosterone to its

11-oxy derivatives, and these derivatives do not bind to mineralocorticoid receptors.
Apparent mineralocorticoid excess (AME) syndrome occurs due to congenital absence or inhibition of enzyme 11β-HSD type 2. In this condition, cortisol has a marked mineralocorticoid effect resulting in a condition like hyperaldosteronism.
Hyponatraemia, due to salt wasting and hypotension, may develop.

B. Secondary Effects of Aldosterone

Secondary effects are produced in aldosterone excess or deficiency as a consequence of the described primary action of aldosterone. The secondary effects include those given next.

1. Effects on plasma potassium concentration include:

i. ***Hypokalaemia***, i.e. decrease in plasma K^+ levels, may occur in aldosterone excess due to increased urinary excretion of K^+. When plasma K^+ levels fall below 2.5 mEq/L, the hypokalaemia may produce:
Muscular weakness due to decreased excitability of nerves and muscles.
Hypokalaemic alkalosis may occur due to associated increased HCO_3^- reabsorption. Due to metabolic alkalosis, free ionized Ca^{2+} may be decreased leading to *tetany*.
Hypokalaemic nephropathy may occur in prolonged hyperaldosteronism producing polyuria, polydipsia and disturbance in concentrating ability of kidney.

ii. ***Hyperkalaemia*** may occur in aldosterone deficiency, which may lead to:
Dehydration and circulating collapse.
Cardiac toxicity, in the form of weakness of heart contraction and arrhythmia, may even result in death.

2. Effects on plasma sodium levels are:

i. ***Hypernatraemia***, which may occur in aldosterone excess, could lead to:
Increase in ECF volume: Absorption of Na^+ from renal tubules causes simultaneous osmotic absorption of water. This increases the ECF volume.
Hypertension: It may occur due to Na^+ and water retention.

ii. ***Hyponatraemia***, which could occur due to excess Na^+ loss in aldosterone insufficiency, may be associated with:
Decrease in ECF volume due to excessive Na^+ and water loss in urine.
Hypotension, i.e. decreased blood pressure.
Hypovolaemic shock.
Death may occur.

Therefore, *aldosterone is essential for life.*

Important Note

Aldosterone escape: As mentioned above, in hyperaldosteronism or when aldosterone is administered for several days to normal individuals, the increased sodium and water absorption by renal tubules leads to an increase in ECF volume and hypertension. However, after 10%–15% increase in ECF, *pressure diuresis occurs*, i.e. excretion of sodium and water in urine is increased, in spite of continued action of aldosterone. This phenomenon is called *aldosterone escape* and is probably due to increased secretion of *atrial natriuretic peptide* (ANP).

Regulation of Aldosterone Secretion

Aldosterone secretion is controlled by the following factors (Fig. 8.5.18).

1. Renin–Angiotensin System

The principal function of aldosterone is to maintain ECF volume by conserving body sodium. Hence, secretion of aldosterone is influenced by changes in the circulating fluid volume which are sensed in the kidney. The signals arising from the kidney increase aldosterone secretion when ECF volume is decreased and vice versa.

Conditions associated with decreased ECF

- Sodium deprivation (e.g. dietary restriction)
- Haemorrhage
- Upright posture for several hours
- Acute diuresis

Steps involved in the secretion of aldosterone by renin–angiotensin system

Decrease in ECF volume leads to decrease in renal arterial blood flow and pressure.
Decrease in renal perfusion pressure causes the juxtaglomerular cells of the afferent arterioles to secrete renin.
Renin catalyses the conversion of angiotensinogen (α-2-globulin substrate present in the plasma) to angiotensin I.

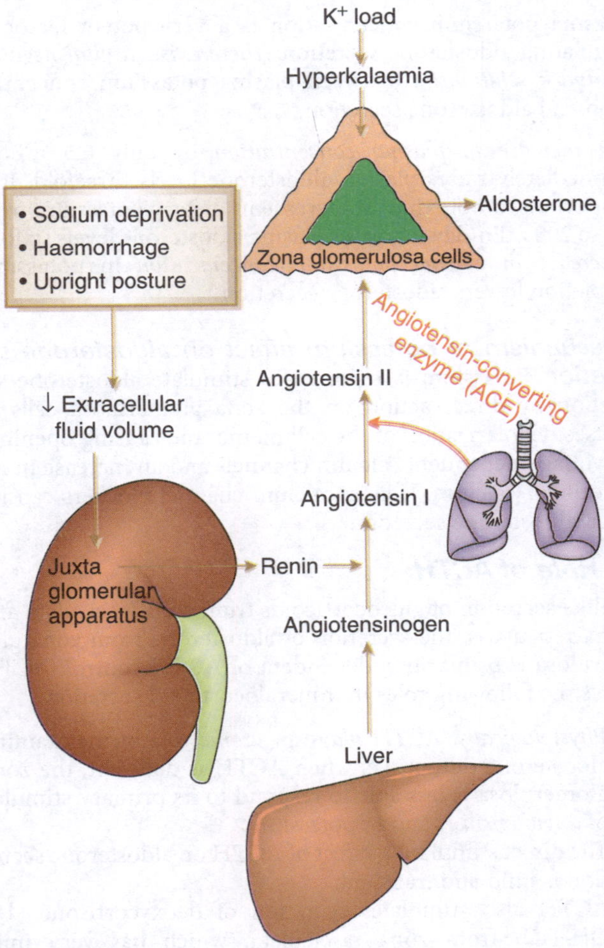

Fig. 8.5.18 Regulation of aldosterone secretion.

Angiotensin I is converted into angiotensin II by the action of angiotensin-converting enzyme (ACE) present in the endothelium of blood vessels, especially in the lungs.

Angiotensin II binds to specific plasma membrane receptors in the adrenal's zona glomerulosa cells and increases the secretion of aldosterone by action on the conversion of cholesterol to pregnenolone and on the conversion of corticoids to aldosterone.

Note. In addition to increasing secretion of aldosterone, angiotensin II also exerts other effects in controlling ECF volume and blood pressure (see page 337).

Aldosterone secretion may be increased fourfold to eightfold by the renin–angiotensin system. The daily aldosterone secretion by this mechanism may vary from 50 mg (with a dietary sodium intake of 150 mEq) to 250 mg (with a dietary sodium intake of 10 mEq).

Factors affecting aldosterone secretion by renin–angiotensin system:

- *Sympathetic neural activity* enhances renin release in response to hypovolaemia.
- *Local prostaglandins* also stimulate renin release; therefore, antiprostaglandin drugs can reduce aldosterone response.
- *Atrial natriuretic peptide* (ANP) reinforces the effects of the renin–angiotensin system on aldosterone secretion.

2. Plasma Potassium Concentration

Plasma potassium concentration is a very potent factor in regulating aldosterone secretion. *There exists a vital negative feedback relationship* between plasma potassium concentration and aldosterone secretion, i.e.:

An increase in plasma concentration by only 0.5 mEq/L immediately raises plasma aldosterone levels threefold. It is important to note that an increase in dietary potassium from 40 to 200 mEq/day increases plasma aldosterone levels sixfold. *Decrease in plasma potassium concentration* in potassium depletion lowers aldosterone secretion.

Mechanism of potassium effect on aldosterone secretion Potassium is reported to stimulate aldosterone secretion by direct action on the zona glomerulosa cells. It causes depolarization of the cell membrane causing openings of voltage-dependent calcium channels and an increase in intracellular calcium. Hence, calcium channel blockers can inhibit aldosterone secretion.

3. Role of ACTH

Unlike secretion of glucocorticoids from zona fasciculata and zona reticularis, the secretion of aldosterone from zona glomerulosa is primarily independent of ACTH control. ACTH plays the following roles in mineralocorticoid secretion:

- *Physiologically, ACTH plays an atonic role* in maintaining aldosterone output, i.e. when ACTH is deficient, the zona glomerulosa is less able to respond to its primary stimulus of *angiotensin II* and of potassium.
- The direct stimulating effect of ACTH on aldosterone secretion is mild and transient.
- ACTH also stimulates secretion of deoxycortisone (18-OH-DC) from zona fasciculata, which has very mild mineralocorticoid activity.

Applied Aspects

- ***Glucocorticoid-remediable aldosteronism (GRA)*** is a recently described syndrome which occurs due to autosomal dominant disorder. In this condition, there is increased aldosterone secretion and hypertension produced by ACTH. The gene encoding aldosterone synthase and 11β-hydroxylase are 95% identical. In patients with GRA, genes for 11β-hydroxylase and genes for aldosterone synthase get fused. An ACTH-sensitive aldosterone synthase is the product of the hybrid gene. The hyperaldosterone and hypertension in GRA can be remedied by suppressing ACTH secretion with administering glucocorticoids.

ADRENAL SEX STEROIDS

Adrenal sex steroids include:

Dehydroepiandrosterone (DHEA), its sulphate ester (DHEA-S) and *androstenedione* are the major androgenic precursor products of the adrenal cortex. They themselves are weak androgens but are converted to the more potent androgen testosterone in peripheral tissues.

Oestrogen and progesterone are produced in very small amounts.

Important Note

It is important to note that normal human adrenal cortex does not secrete physiologically effective amounts of testosterone and oestrogen.

Synthesis

The adrenal sex steroid precursors are synthesized in the *zona reticularis.*

The steps involved in the synthesis of androgen precursors are summarized in Fig. 8.5.19. The 17-hydroxylated derivatives of pregnenolone and progesterone are the starting points for synthesis of androgen precursors. Composite synthesis of adrenal cortex hormones is depicted in Fig. 8.5.20; 17-hydroxylation

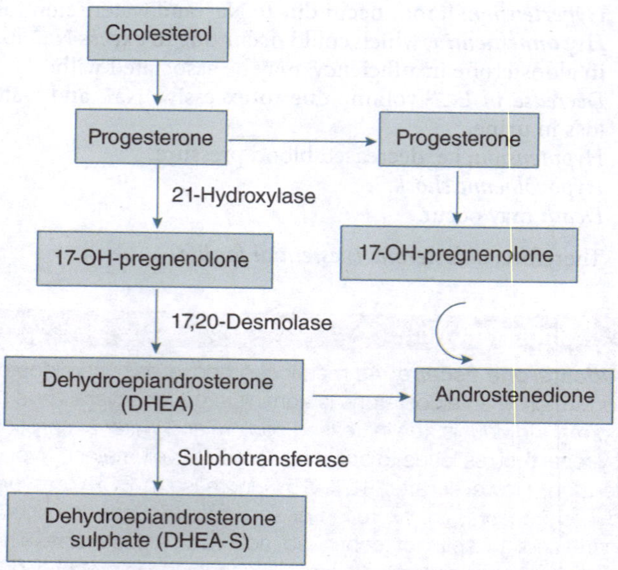

Fig. 8.5.19 Steps involved in the synthesis of androgen precursors in the zona reticularis.

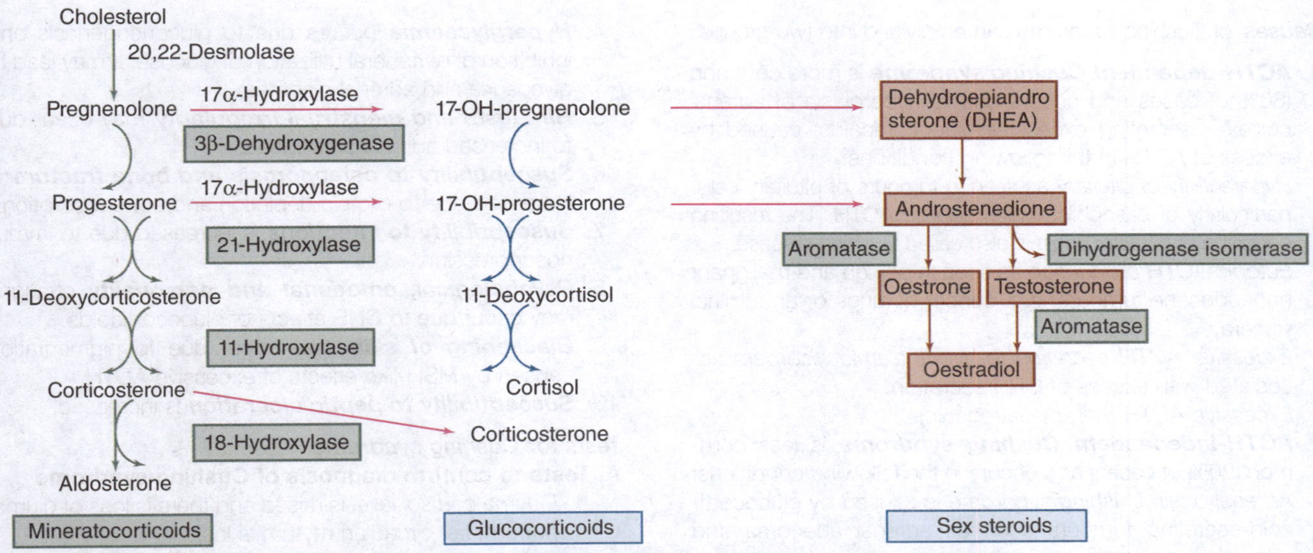

Fig. 8.5.20 Summary of synthesis of mineralocorticoids, glucocorticoids and sex steroids in adrenal cortex.

is the last reaction common to the synthesis of cortisol and the adrenal androgens. The circumstances that lead to impairment of cortisol synthesis at any point beyond this step cause accumulation of 17-hydroxypregnenolone and 17-hydroxyprogesterone leading to greatly increased androgen synthesis.

Plasma levels, contribution towards sex steroids, metabolism and excretion

Plasma levels: Normal plasma level of DHEA is 150–200 μg% at 25 years of age in both sexes.

Contribution of adrenal glands towards sex steroids and their functions are as follows:

During fetal life, the adrenal cortex is hyperplastic and secretes large amounts of DHEA which acts as the main precursor for synthesis of oestrogen by the placenta.

In adult women, the adrenal glands supply 50%–60% of the androgenic hormone requirement. DHEA-S contributes to increased muscle mass, growth of pubic and axillary hair and libido.

- The further conversion of androgen precursors to oestrogens in the adrenal cortex is not significant before menopause.
- After menopause, the oestrogen activity is provided by the oestrogen secreted from adrenal cortex and that arising from conversion of androgen precursors in peripheral tissues.

In adult males, since testes produce a large quantity of testosterone, the adrenal androgen precursors are of little biological importance. However, they may be partly responsible for development of male sex organs in childhood.

Applied Aspects

Tumours of adrenal cortex are associated with excessive secretion of adrenal androgens. In prepubertal males, occurrence of such tumours produces precocious pseudopuberty. In prepubertal or in adult females, they cause development of secondary male sexual characteristics (e.g. beard, muscular body and breaking of voice).

Metabolism and excretion The metabolism of androgens, in general, involves reduction of the 3-ketone group and the A-ring in the liver.

- Androsterone and etiocholanolone, the two isomers that are formed as end results of metabolism, are excreted in the urine. These metabolites are not specific for the adrenal gland, as they also arise from the gonadal androgens.
- DHEA-S is entirely excreted directly in the urine and is virtually adrenal-specific.
- Androsterone, etiocholanolone and DHEA-S are together known as *17-ketosteroids* and constitute the major part of a urinary fraction. Their normal values range from 5 to 14 ng/day in women and 8 to 20 ng/day in men.
- Normally, two-thirds of the urinary 17-ketosteroids are derived from the adrenal secretions and one-third from gonadal androgen secretions.
- In virilized children or adult women, a large increase in urinary 17-ketosteroid excretion almost always indicates an adrenal abnormality.
- Increased plasma and urinary levels of DHEA-S specifically indicate adrenal abnormality.

Applied Aspects

The important applied aspects in relation to the adrenal gland which need mention include:

- Hyperactivity of adrenal cortex
- Hypoactivity of adrenal cortex

Hyperactivity of Adrenal Cortex

Disorders of hyperactivity of adrenal cortex include:

- Cushing syndrome (hypercortisol state)
- Conn syndrome (hyperaldosteronism)
- Adrenogenital syndrome (excessive secretion of adrenal androgens)

1. Cushing Syndrome is described by Harvey Cushing. Is refers to the group of clinical conditions occurring due to prolonged excessive levels of glucocorticoids.

Causes of Cushing syndrome can be divided into two groups:

I. ***ACTH-dependent Cushing syndrome*** is more common (80% of cases and occurs due to hyperplasia of adrenal cortex – secreting excessive glucocorticoids) caused by excess of ACTH in the following conditions:
Hyperactivity of pituitary as seen in tumours of pituitary cells, particularly of basophils, which secrete ACTH. The resulting condition of pituitary origin is also called Cushing disease.
Ectopic ACTH production as seen in benign and malignant nonendocrine tumours, e.g. cancer of lungs or abdominal viscera.
Excessive ACTH secretion in hypothalamic disorders associated with excess of CRH secretion.
Excessive ACTH therapy (iatrogenic).

II. ***ACTH-independent Cushing syndrome*** is less common (20% of cases) and occurs in the following conditions:
Adrenal origin Cushing syndrome is caused by glucocorticoid-secreting tumours such as adrenal adenoma and adrenal carcinoma.
Excessive glucocorticoid administration (i.e. iatrogenic) for diseases such as rheumatoid arthritis.
Abnormal expression of receptors by adrenocortical cells for:
- Gastric inhibitory peptide (GIP)
- β-Adrenergic agonists
- Interleukin-1 (IL-1)
- GnRH

Characteristic features of Cushing syndrome are as follows (Fig. 8.5.21):

1. ***Truncal or centripetal obesity:*** It occurs due to redistribution of body fat from extremities (which is in the abdominal wall, back and face) producing the following characteristic features:
   - *Buffalo hump*, due to collection of fat at upper back.
   - *Moon face*, due to fat collection on the face.
   - *Purple striae or cutaneous abdominal striae or livid stretch marks:* The skin and subcutaneous tissue becomes thin due to protein catabolism. The stretching of abdominal skin due to excessive subcutaneous fat deposition causes rupture of subdermal tissues producing reddish-purple striae.
2. ***Muscle weakness and backache*** due to protein catabolism.
3. ***Sodium and water retention*** may cause weight gain, oedema and hypertension.
4. ***Hyperglycaemia*** occurs due to gluconeogenesis and inhibition of peripheral utilization of glucose. It may lead to glycosuria and adrenal diabetes.
5. ***Hirsutism and menstrual irregularity*** may occur due to increased adrenal androgens.
6. ***Susceptibility to osteoporosis and bone fracture*** is increased due to protein depletion and bone resorption.
7. ***Susceptibility to infections*** is increased due to immunosuppression.
8. ***Psychological, emotional and personality*** changes may occur due to CNS effects of glucocorticoids.
9. ***Blackening of skin*** may occur due to pigmentation caused by MSH-like effects of excessive ACTH.
10. ***Susceptibility to peptic ulceration*** is increased.

Tests for Cushing syndrome

A. Tests to confirm diagnosis of Cushing syndrome
- *Plasma cortisol level* is raised and there is loss of diurnal pattern, i.e. circadian rhythm is lost.
- *Dexamethasone suppression test* is not able to suppress plasma cortisol level.
- *Insulin-induced hypoglycaemia*, which raises plasma cortisol in normal persons, fails to raise it in Cushing syndrome.

The *24-hour urinary free cortisol* levels are raised.

B. Tests to differentiate between ACTH-dependent and ACTH-independent Cushing syndrome are shown in Table 8.5.3.

Treatment: The drugs inhibiting the synthesis of steroids from the adrenals used for treating Cushing syndrome are aminoglutethimide (inhibits conversion of cholesterol to pregnenolone), mitotane and metyrapone.

2. Hyperaldosteronism

Hyperaldosteronism refers to overproduction of the hormone aldosterone, a major sodium-retaining hormone.

Causes. Depending on the cause, hyperaldosteronism may be:

1. ***Primary hyperaldosteronism*** or ***Conn disease*** occurs due to tumour or hyperplasia of zona glomerulosa of adrenal cortex and glucocorticoid remediable hyperaldosteronism.
   The *aldosterone-secreting adrenocortical adenoma* is the most common cause.
   Glucocorticoid remediable hyperaldosteronism is another important cause, also occurs due to hybrid enzyme (i.e.

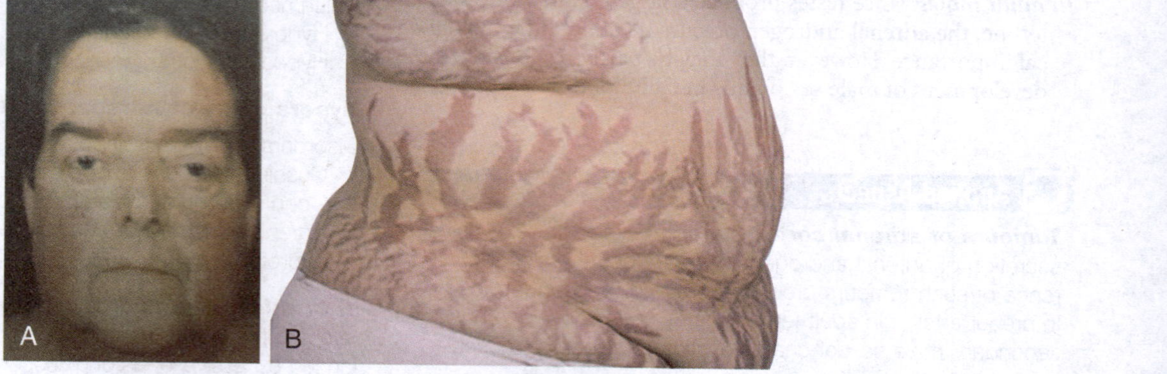

Fig. 8.5.21 Photograph of a patient with Cushing syndrome showing moon face (**A**) and truncal obesity and purple striae on the abdomen (**B**).

Table 8.5.3 Tests to differentiate between ACTH-dependent and ACTH-independent Cushing syndrome

Tests	ACTH dependent (pituitary causes)	ACTH independent (adrenal causes)
• *Plasma ACTH level* at 8 a.m.	Increased	Undetectable
• *ACTH level following* CRH stimulation	Increased	No change
• *Metyrapone test.* Levels of 11-deoxycortisol after 24 h of administration of metyrapone	Decreased	No change

fusion of aldosterone synthase and 11β-hydroxylase) leading to continuous elevation of aldosterone levels.

2. ***Secondary hyperaldosteronism*** occurs due to some extra-adrenal cause, which stimulates renin–angiotensin–aldosterone system, e.g. nephrotic syndrome, cirrhosis of liver, congestive heart failure and toxaemia of pregnancy.

Characteristic Features. The characteristic features of hyperaldosteronism are as follows:

Sodium and water retention leading to hypertension and oedema. It is important to note that marked hypernatraemia and oedema do not occur because Na^+ excretion is soon normalized despite hypersecretion of aldosterone (escape phenomenon, see page 757).

Hypokalaemia may occur due to increased potassium excretion producing muscle weakness and periodic muscle paralysis, whereas prolonged depletion of potassium may cause renal damage producing polyuria.

Metabolic alkalosis may occur due to secretion of more amount of H^+ into renal tubules and metabolic alkalosis may produce hypocalcaemia causing tetany.

Treatment. The treatment of hyperaldosteronism includes:

- Adrenalectomy if the lesions are unilateral.
- For bilateral adrenal hyperplasia, drugs like aldosterone receptor antagonists such as spironolactone and eplerenone are used.
- Low doses of dexamethasone – inhibit ACTH and ultimately secretion of aldosterone.

3. Adrenogenital syndrome

As mentioned earlier, the androgen precursors secreted by the adrenal cortex are of little biological importance under normal circumstances. However, when secreted in large amounts as in *tumour of zona reticularis* of adrenal cortex.

Causes. Adrenogenital syndrome usually occurs due to adrenocorticoid tumour and congenital adrenal hyperplasia (see page 742).

Characteristic features: The following abnormal features may be produced:

In prepubertal males, the excessive androgens produce precocious pseudopuberty (see page 800).

In males, the oestrogen-producing cells may produce female-like secondary sexual characters such as enlargement of breasts (gynaecomastia), atrophy of testes, loss of libido and feminine body.

In females, the prominent feature is virilization (i.e. hirsutism), development of male secondary sexual characteristics, such as beard, muscular body, breaking of voice, male-type hair growth, enlargement of clitoris and amenorrhoea.

Hypoactivity of Adrenal Cortex

Adrenocortical deficiency (insufficiency), depending on the site of lesion, can be divided into three types:

i. ***Primary adrenocortical deficiency*** occurs due to involvement of adrenal cortex and is associated with high ACTH levels due to feedback mechanism. The conditions producing primary adrenocortical deficiency include:
   - Addison disease
   - Congenital adrenal hyperplasia

ii. ***Secondary adrenocortical deficiency*** occurs due to involvement of pituitary or due to exogenous glucocorticoid administration and is associated with *low ACTH level* due to less production.

iii. ***Tertiary adrenal deficiency*** is caused by hypothalamic disorders.

1. Addison disease

Causes: Addison disease is an important condition of primary adrenocortical deficiency, occurring due to the following causes:

Autoimmune disease causing adrenal cortex atrophy

Tuberculosis, fungal and *cytomegalovirus* infections producing adrenal cortex destruction, an uncommon but well-recognized complication in patients with AIDS

Bilateral adrenalectomy, but failure to take hormone therapy

Malignant tumours producing destruction of hormone-producing cells in adrenal cortex

It also occurs as a part of autoimmune polyglandular syndromes (APSs). There are two types of APSs (APS-1 and APS-2). APS-1 is caused by mutation in the autoimmune regulator gene (AIRG) and APS-2 is associated with human leucocyte antigen-DR isotype 3 ($HLA\text{-}DR_3$).

Characteristic features occur due to chronic deficiency of hormones secreted by all the three zones of the adrenal cortex:

1. ***Glucocorticoid insufficiency*** produces weight loss, malaise, anorexia, nausea, vomiting, weakness and diarrhoea. Since glucocorticoids are essential for adaptation to stress, in Addison disease, exposure to any type of stress, e.g. even mild infection, may be fatal.
2. ***Mineralocorticoid deficiency*** produces hyponatraemia, hyperkalaemia, acidosis and decreased ECF volume with hypotension.
3. ***Loss of androgens*** causes sparse hair in females, dry and itchy skin.
4. ***Increased ACTH secretion*** occurs due to feedback mechanism and causes diffuse pigmentation of the skin and mucous membranes (because of its MSH-like actions).

Diagnosis of adrenal insufficiency: Tests for Addison disease:

i. ***Tests to diagnose hypoadrenalism:***
   - Plasma cortisol levels are low.
   - Plasma aldosterone levels are low or normal.
   - Serum sodium levels are low.
   - Serum potassium level is high or normal.
   - Blood glucose level is low in severe disease.
   - Plasma renin activity is high.

ii. ***Tests to differentiate between primary (Addison disease) and secondary hypoadrenalism:***
- *Basal ACTH level:* High in Addison disease and low in pituitary or hypothalamic disease
- *ACTH stimulation test:* 0.25 mg cosyntropin (ACTH 1-25) is given intravenously and blood samples are tested after 30 and 60 minutes. In Addison disease, plasma cortisol level does not rise, while in pituitary or hypothalamic disease there occurs a subnormal rise.

iii. ***Computerized tomography*** for adrenal imaging to find out the cause: metastatic or haemorrhagic

Treatment of Addison disease consists of replacement therapy:
- *Glucocorticoid replacement:* Oral prednisolone 20 mg in the morning and 10 mg in the evening is the drug of choice.
- *Mineralocorticoid replacement:* Fludrocortisone 0.05–0.1 mg/day is adequate to maintain blood pressure, electrolytes and renin activity.
- *Adrenal androgen replacement:* 20–25 mg DHEA is indicated mainly in women.

Addisonian Crisis or Adrenal Crisis. It refers to acute adrenal insufficiency characterized by sudden collapse. The condition becomes fatal if not treated in time.

Causes: Acute adrenal insufficiency may occur in the following conditions:
- *Acute precipitation of Addison disease* under the effect of any stress, e.g. infection and haemorrhage
- *Major surgical operation or trauma*
- *Sudden withdrawal of glucocorticoid treatment*

Treatment: It is a medical emergency requiring immediate treatment.

For acute adrenal insufficiency:
- Immediate rehydration by infusion of normal saline
- Glucocorticoid replacement by 100–200 mg hydrocortisone to provide stimulation of mineralocorticoid receptors
- Mineralocorticoids
- Treatment of precipitating factor

Secondary and Tertiary Adrenal Insufficiency

Secondary and tertiary hypoaldosteronism is usually milder than primary adrenal insufficiency. The plasma ACTH level is low; therefore, skin pigmentation does not occur.

2. Congenital Adrenal Hyperplasia

Causes: Congenital adrenal hyperplasia is caused by congenital deficiency of one of the enzymes involved in the biosynthesis of glucocorticoids, particularly *21-hydroxylase deficiency* and deficiency of 11-hydroxylase (Fig. 8.5.20).

Pathophysiological features include:
- *Cortisol and 11-deoxycortisol levels* are decreased due to reduced synthesis.
- *17-Hydroxyprogesterone*, which is substrate for 21-hydroxylase, is raised.
- *ACTH levels are raised* due to feedback mechanism excited by low cortisol levels. ACTH leads to hyperplasia of adrenal cortex.
- *Adrenal androgen (e.g. DHEA) levels* are increased because deficiency of 21-hydroxylase causes excess of 17-hydroxyprogesterone, which serves as a major precursor for adrenal androgens (see Fig. 8.5.19). The increased androgen levels cause sexual abnormalities.

Characteristic features occurring because of above-mentioned pathophysiological changes are virilism and excessive body growth.

In boys, adrenal hyperplasia leads to a congenital condition known as *macrogenitosomia praecox*. It is characterized by:
- Precocious body growth leading to stocky appearance called *infant Hercules*
- Precocious sexual development with enlarged penis even at age of 4 years

In female fetus, high plasma androgen levels cause *masculinized pattern* of development (*virilism*). Sometimes, the female fetus may be born with male-type external genitalia. This condition is called *pseudohermaphroditism*. For details, see page 795.

Hypoaldosteronism: Isolated cases of aldosterone deficiency have also been reported in patients with renal disorders and low circulating renin. This condition is also referred to as *hyporeninaemic hypoaldosteronism*.

Pseudohypoaldosteronism: It occurs when aldosterone secretion is normal but there is resistance to its action.

Characteristic features: The patients of hypoaldosteronism have marked hyperkalaemia.

HORMONES OF ADRENAL MEDULLA

The adrenal medulla secretes *catecholamines*, which include epinephrine, norepinephrine (NE) and dopamine (DA). Approximately 80% of adrenal medullary catecholamine is epinephrine and the rest is NE. Apart from catecholamines, the adrenal medulla also contains small amounts of *dynorphins, neurotensin, encephalin, somatostatin*, adrenomedullin (a vasodilator substance) and *substance P*.

Epinephrine circulating in the blood is almost exclusively produced in the medulla, with smaller amounts synthesized in the brain. Humans who have undergone bilateral adrenalectomy excrete practically no epinephrine in the urine, confirming the fact that the medulla is the sole source of circulating epinephrine.

NE is secreted by the medulla in small amounts. It is normally a neurotransmitter, but in select circumstances may also function as a hormone. It is widely distributed in neural tissues, which in addition to the medulla include sympathetic postganglionic fibres and central nervous system.

In the brain, the concentration of NE is the highest in the hypothalamus. The NE content of tissue reflects the density of its sympathetic innervation. Except for the placenta, which is devoid of nerve fibres, NE has been demonstrated in almost all tissues. Urinary levels of NE remain within normal limits even after bilateral adrenalectomy, indicating thereby that the NE originates from extra-adrenal sources (i.e. the terminals of the postganglionic sympathetic fibres and the brain).

SYNTHESIS AND STORAGE OF CATECHOLAMINE HORMONES

Synthesis of Catecholamines

Epinephrine and NE are synthesized in different cells. The biosynthetic pathway originates with l-tyrosine, which is derived from the diet or from the hepatic hydroxylation of

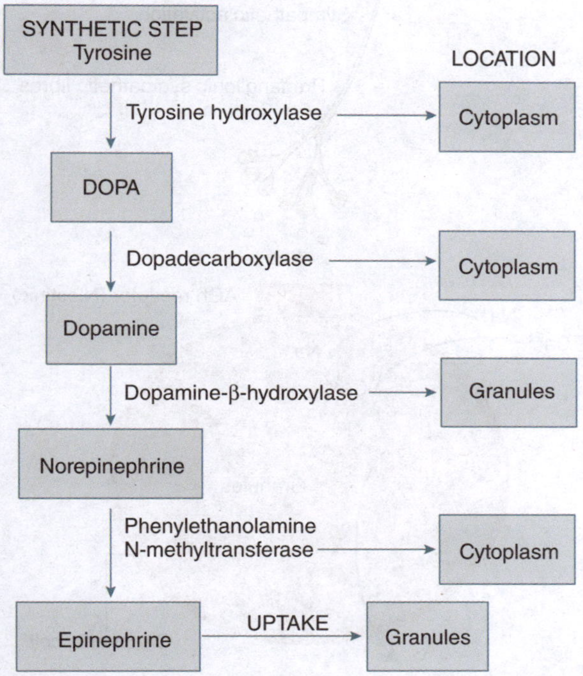

Fig. 8.5.22 Steps of catecholamine synthesis in the adrenal medulla.

l-phenylalanine by phenylalanine hydroxylase. Conversion of tyrosine to epinephrine occurs in four steps (Fig. 8.5.22):

1. ***Conversion of tyrosine to dihydroxyphenylalanine (DOPA):*** The conversion of tyrosine to DOPA is catalysed by the enzyme *tyrosine hydroxylase.* This reaction occurs in the chromaffin cell cytoplasm and requires the cofactor tetrahydrobiopterin, molecular oxygen and NADH. This is a rate-*limiting step* in catecholamine synthesis. The subsequent catecholamine products, i.e. DOPA, NE and DA, all inhibit this initial reaction. The enzyme tyrosine hydroxylase is found only in those tissues which synthesize catecholamines. Nerve impulses increase activity of this enzyme.
2. ***Conversion of DOPA to DA*** in the cytosol is catalysed by the enzyme *DOPA decarboxylase,* which requires pyridoxal phosphate as a cofactor. This enzyme is not confined only to catecholamine-synthesizing tissue.
   DA is a naturally occurring precursor of NE. It is a weak agonist of α- and β-adrenergic receptors. DA acts through two types of dopaminergic receptors D_1 and D_2.
   Effects of DA:
   - The main function of DA is in the central nervous system. For details, see page 983.
   - The physiological function of circulating DA is unknown, but injected DA produces vasodilation of renal and mesentery by acting on specific dopaminergic receptors.
   - On the heart, it has a positive ionotropic effect probably by releasing NE by its action on β-adrenergic receptors. Moderate doses of DA result in rise in systolic blood pressure (SBP) but there is no effect on diastolic pressure.

Important Note

DA is useful in treatment of traumatic and cardiogenic shock, because it causes renal vasoconstriction and relaxes mesangial cells and thus maintains glomerular filtration rate.

3. ***Conversion of DA to NE:*** DA from the cytosol enters the chromaffin granules by vesicular monoamine transport (VMAT), which can be blocked by the drug reserpine, where it is converted to L-epinephrine by the enzyme dopamine-β-hydroxylase (DBH). This reaction requires molecular oxygen and uses ascorbate as hydrogen donor. This enzyme is exclusively present in the granules of these tissues which synthesize catecholamines, e.g. in the granulated vesicles of sympathetic nerve endings and the chromaffin granules of the chromaffin cells of adrenal medulla.
4. ***Conversion of NE to epinephrine:*** In approximately 20% of chromaffin cells, the NE is the end product and the sequence ends here with its storage. In approximately 80% of chromaffin cells, NE diffuses back into the cytoplasm, where it is converted to epinephrine by the enzyme *phenylethanolamine N-methyltransferase (PNMT)* using *S*-adenosylmethionine as a methyl donor. The enzyme PNMT exists in significant concentration only in the adrenal medulla. Its activity is induced by glucocorticoids (cortisol), which are found in high concentration only in the adrenal portal blood draining the adrenal cortex and supplying the medulla.

Storage of Catecholamines in Storage Granules (Fig. 8.5.23)

The epinephrine formed in the cytoplasm is then taken back by the chromaffin granules, in which it is stored as the predominant adrenomedullary hormone. The uptake of DA, NE and epinephrine (E) by the secretory granules is an active process that requires ATP and magnesium. The catecholamines are stored complexed to calcium, ATP (1 mol of ATP with 4 mol of catecholamine), chromogranins and other factors to prevent excessive increase of intragranular osmotic pressure due to a high concentration of intragranular catecholamines and other molecules. It appears that DA, NE and epinephrine are protected in the granules from the oxidative activity of monoamine oxidase (MAO). Of the three, DA is most vulnerable.

Factors regulating catecholamine synthesis:

Acute sympathetic stimulation activates the enzyme tyrosine hydroxylase, possibly by decreasing cytoplasmic catecholamine levels and relieving product inhibition.

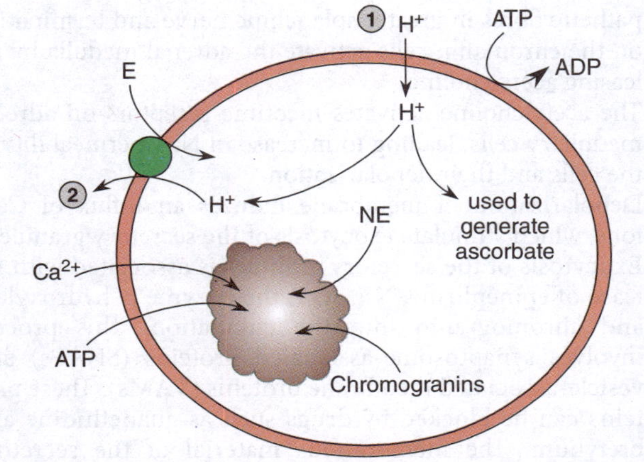

Fig. 8.5.23 Storage of catecholamines in chromaffin granules (for details, see text).

Chronic stimulation of preganglionic fibres increases the concentrations of both tyrosine hydroxylase and DBH, and thus helps to ensure maintenance of the output of both catecholamines when the demand is continuous. The mechanism of induction may involve a cAMP-dependent protein kinase.

ACTH acts directly and helps to sustain the levels of the enzymes tyrosine hydroxylase and dopamine-hydroxylase under stressful conditions.

Cortisol specifically induces the enzyme *N*-methyltransferase, and, therefore, selectively stimulates epinephrine synthesis. The portal circulation system subserves this action, because blood from the cortex has a high concentration of cortisol and it directly perfuses the chromaffin cells.

Epinephrine stimulates its own synthesis. From the medulla, epinephrine diffuses into the cortex, where it stimulates cortisol synthesis by activating the expression of the STAR gene.

Important Note

- After hypophysectomy, there is decreased synthesis of epinephrine due to decreased plasma levels of glucocorticoids.
- Glucocorticoids are necessary for the development of adrenal medulla. In deficiency of 21β-hydroxylase enzyme, reduction of glucocorticoids will result in dysplasia of the adrenal medulla. The babies born with 21β-hydroxylase deficiency have a low circulating level of catecholamines.

SECRETION OF CATECHOLAMINE HORMONES

Mechanism of secretion Secretion from the adrenal medulla is an integral part of the *flight-or-fight reaction* that is evoked by stimulation of the sympathetic nervous system as a response to stress. In other words, adrenal medulla is often activated in association with the rest of the sympathetic nervous system and acts in concert with this system during states of emergency.

Steps involved in the secretion of catecholamines from adrenal medulla (Fig. 8.5.24)

- Activation of sympathetic nervous system is caused by various stimuli (enumerated above), which are sensed at various higher levels.
- The nerve impulses travelling across the preganglionic sympathetic fibres in greater splanchnic nerve and terminating on the chromaffin cells activate the adrenal medulla by releasing acetylcholine.
- The acetylcholine activates nicotinic receptors on adrenal medullary cells, leading to increase in Na^+ permeability of the cells and their depolarization.
- Depolarization of membrane induces an influx of Ca^{2+} ions, which stimulate exocytosis of the secretory granules.
- Exocytosis of the secretory granules is associated with release of epinephrine, NE, ATP, the enzyme β-hydroxylase and chromogranin into the circulation. This process involves synaptosome-associated proteins (SNAPs) and vesicle-associated membrane proteins (VAMs). These proteins can be blocked by drugs such as guanethidine and bretylium. The membranous material of the secretory granules is retained in the chromaffin cells and probably recycled.

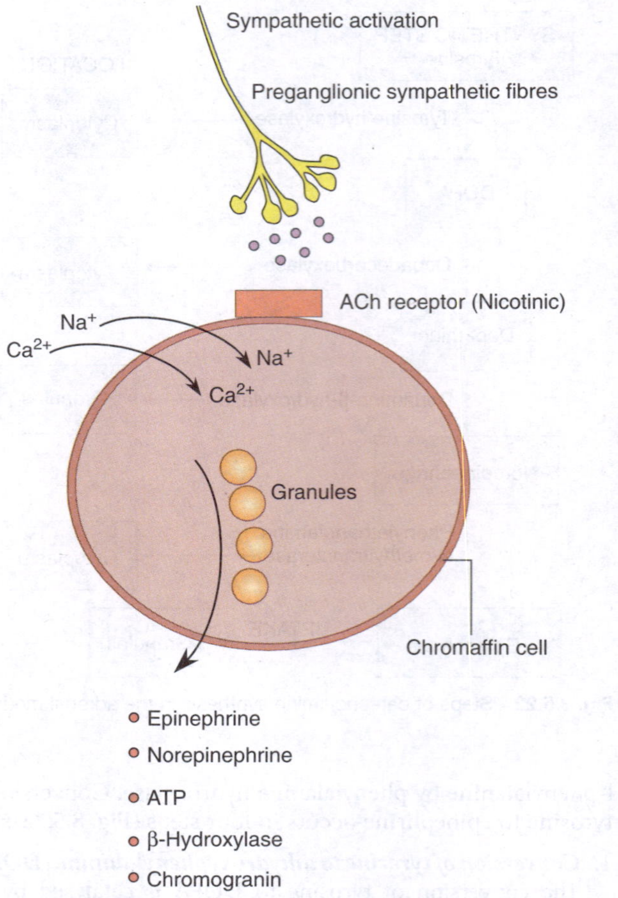

Fig. 8.5.24 Process of release of catecholamines by cells of adrenal medulla.

Nervous control of secretion The catecholamine secretion is entirely controlled by the splanchnic nerves supplying the medulla. These nerves comprise preganglionic sympathetic fibres emerging mainly from lower thoracic segments (T_5–T_9) of ipsilateral intermediolateral grey column of the spinal cord. These fibres, when stimulated, act by releasing acetylcholine close to the adrenal medullary chromaffin cells.

Therefore, the main physiological stimulus for release of catecholamines is acetylcholine. The mechanism of action of acetylcholine is described as above (Fig. 8.5.24).

Physiological and psychological stimuli for release

As mentioned in the beginning, the adrenal medullary activation occurs as a part of a generalized sympathetic response to any emergency situation. Therefore, this has also been called *sympathetic alarm* reaction. The various sensory stimuli associated with rapid release of epinephrine (and probably NE) from adrenal medulla include (Fig. 8.5.25):

- Perception or even anticipation of danger or harm (anxiety)
- Pain, trauma
- Hypovolaemia from haemorrhage or fluid loss
- Hypotension
- Anoxia
- Exposure to extremes of temperature
- Hypoglycaemia
- Severe exercise

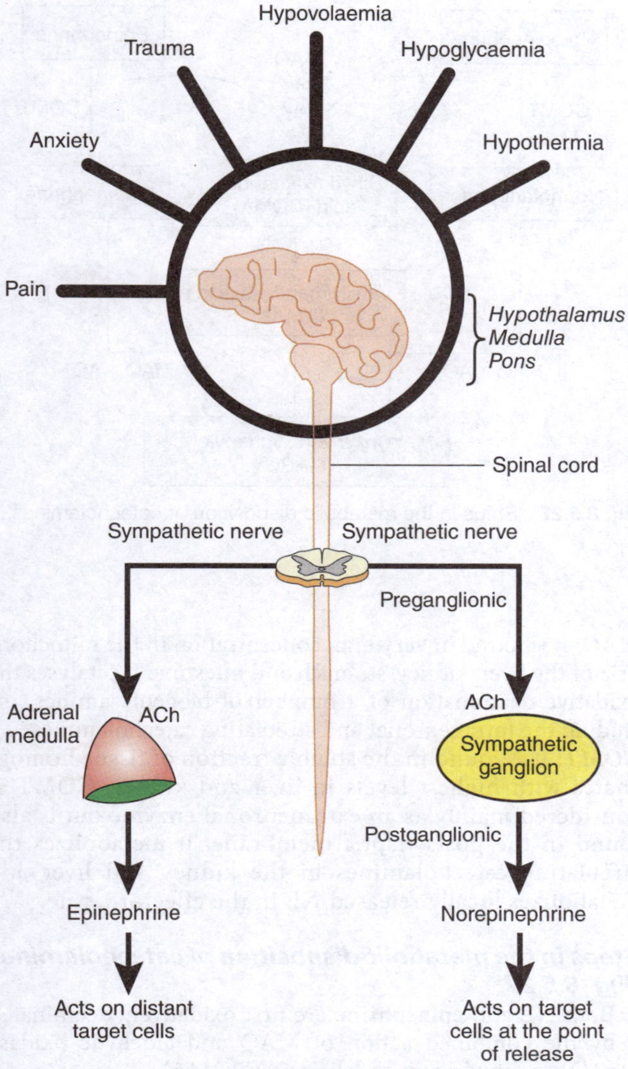

Fig. 8.5.25 Stimuli associated with secretion of catecholamines from adrenal medulla and sympathetic nervous system. Note that adrenal medulla releases primarily epinephrine into the bloodstream where it acts on distant targets. The sympathetic ganglia release norepinephrine into the synaptic cleft which acts on the target cell at point of release.

Selective secretion of catecholamines in response to specific stimuli In humans, epinephrine and NE appear to be released independently by specific stimuli:

Anger and aggressive states, which are associated with active and appropriate anticipatory behavioural responses to the challenge, i.e. the situations with which the individual is familiar, are associated with increased *NE secretion*.
States of anxiety, tense but passive emotional displays or threatening situations of unpredictable nature are associated with increased epinephrine secretion. Stimulation of adrenal medulla also occurs independently of the sympathetic system.

Adrenal medullary stimulation does not always occur as a part of a generalized sympathetic response, e.g. *hypoglycaemia* activates adrenal medulla producing marked increase in catecholamine secretion without any significant increase in sympathetic neural discharge. Conversely, in baroreceptor-mediated cardiovascular reflexes, sympathetic neural system is predominantly involved without activation of the adrenal medulla.

Circulation, Metabolism and Excretion

Circulation

Secreted epinephrine and NE from the adrenal medulla are in the ratio of 4:1. In plasma, approximately 95% of DA and 70% of NE and epinephrine are conjugated to sulphate. Sulphate conjugates are inactive and their function is unsettled.
Basal plasma levels (in recumbent humans) of free epinephrine are 30 pg/mL and those of free NE are 300 pg/mL.
After bilateral adrenalectomy, plasma epinephrine levels fall to almost zero but NE levels remain unchanged.
Variation in plasma levels of catecholamines according to physiological or pathological states is quite common. When adrenal medullary secretion increases, the secretion of epinephrine and NE usually increases in the same proportion. However, the threshold levels at which circulating NE can produce physiological effects is approximately six times its basal levels, while the threshold level at which epinephrine produces its effects is well achieved during that physiological state (Table 8.5.4; Fig. 8.5.26). Hence, in most of the physiological and pathological conditions, increased adrenal medullary secretion results in selective epinephrine-mediated effects, in spite of increased secretion of both catecholamines.

Table 8.5.4 Plasma concentration of catecholamines compared with their biological effective concentration in different physiological and pathological states

		Plasma epinephrine (pg/mL)		Plasma norepinephrine (pg/mL)	
Physiological/ pathological state	**Relevant biological action**	**Mean value**	**Effective range for relevant biological action**	**Mean value**	**Effective range for relevant biological action**
Basal (recumbent) position	–	30	–	300	–
Upright position	↑ Heart rate and blood pressure	70	50–125	500	+800
Hypoglycaemia	↑ Plasma glucose	230	150–200	260	+1800
Severe hypoglycaemia	–	1500	–	750	–
Diabetic ketoacidosis	↑ Lipolysis and ketosis ↑ Insulin	500	100–400	1200	1800

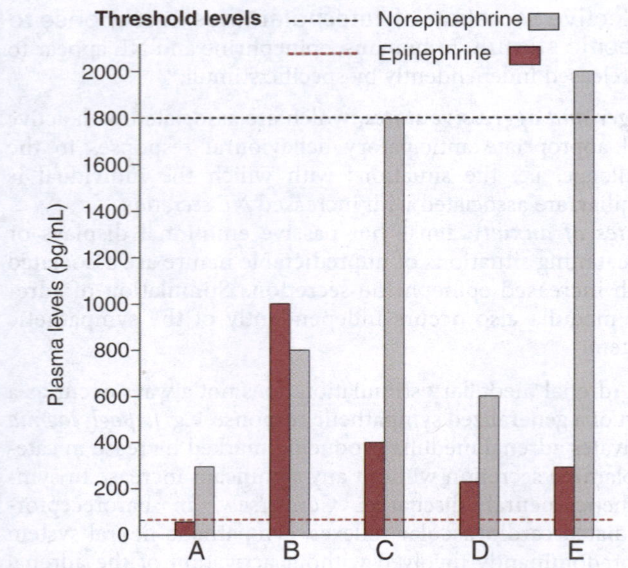

Fig. 8.5.26 Plasma concentration of epinephrine and norepinephrine in different physiological and pathological states with their threshold levels: **(A)** basal levels; **(B)** hypoglycaemia; **(C)** severe exercise; **(D)** surgical stress; and **(E)** pheochromocytoma.

Metabolism and Inactivation of Circulating Catecholamines

Plasma half-life of epinephrine (E) and NE is extremely short (1–3 minutes) and their metabolic clearance rates range from 2 to 6 L/min. The short half-life of catecholamines allows for a rapid turn of their dramatic effects.

Inactivation of catecholamines released by the sympathetic nerve endings at the synaptic clefts differs from that of the catecholamines released into circulation by the adrenal medulla.

Catecholamines released at sympathetic neuroeffector junction are inactivated by the following mechanisms:

Active neuronal reuptake into the presynaptic nerve terminals is the most important mechanism of termination of action of NE in the junctional space. This specific reuptake accounts for inactivation of approximately 85% of released NE. Transportation back into the nerve terminal is carried by specific norepinephrine transporter (NET). The NE reuptaken is either stored in the vesicles (*nonenzymatic inactivation*) or oxidized by the enzyme MAO present in the nerve endings (*enzymatic inactivation*).

Dilution by diffusion out of the junctional cleft.

Extraneural uptake: It accounts for removing the 15% of NE released from adrenergic nerve endings. It is mediated by postsynaptic cells and is followed by intracellular metabolic inactivation by the enzyme monoamine oxidase (MAO) and catechol-*O*-methyltransferase (COMT).

Circulating catecholamines (epinephrine and NE) are metabolized predominantly in the liver and kidney by the enzymes MAO and COMT.

Metabolic Disposition of Catecholamines

Enzymes involved in the metabolic disposition of catecholamines:

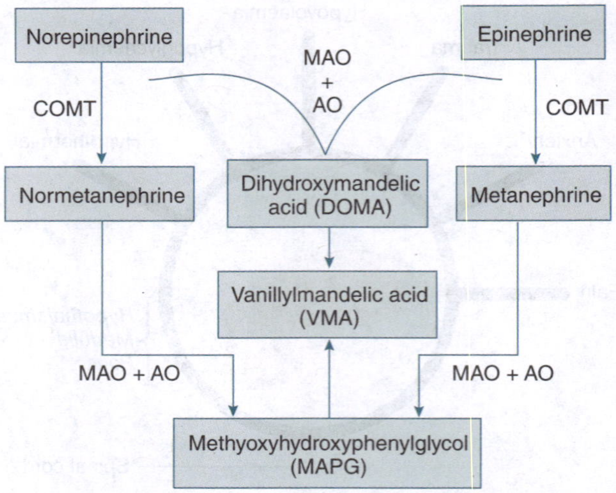

Fig. 8.5.27 Steps in the metabolic disposition of catecholamines.

MAO: It is found in very high concentration in the mitochondria of the liver, kidney, stomach and intestine. It catalyses the oxidative deamination of a number of biogenic amines, including the intraneuronal and circulating catecholamines.

COMT: It is found in the soluble fraction of tissue homogenates with highest levels in liver and kidney. COMT is considered mainly as an extraneuronal enzyme but is also found in the postsynaptic membrane. It metabolizes the circulating catecholamines in the kidney and liver and metabolizes locally released NE in the effector tissue.

Steps in the metabolic disposition of catecholamines (Fig. 8.5.27)

- Both NE and epinephrine are first oxidatively deaminated by the combined action of MAO and aldehyde oxidase (AO) to dihydroxymandelic acid (DOMA).
- DOMA is then O-methylated by the enzyme COMT to vanillylmandelic acid (VMA).
- Alternatively, the NE and epinephrine can be first O-methylated by COMT to produce normetanephrine and metanephrine, respectively.
- The normetanephrine and metanephrine are then oxidatively deaminated by the combined action of MAO and AO to methoxyhydroxyphenylglycol (MHPG) and then to VMA.
- VMA and MHPG are excreted in the urine and bile. These are conjugated to form glucuronides and sulphates.

Fate of circulating catecholamines It can be now summarized as:

- Only 2%–3% of catecholamines are directly excreted in urine mostly as conjugates.
- Approximately 50% of secreted catecholamines appear in the urine as free conjugated metanephrine and normetanephrine.
- Approximately 35% of secreted catecholamines appear in the urine as VMA and approximately 12%–13% as MHPG.
- In normal humans, approximately 30 μg of NE, 6 μg of epinephrine and 700 μg VMA are excreted per day.

Important Note

It is important to note that:

- Under normal circumstances, epinephrine accounts for a very small fraction of urinary VMA and MOPG; the majority is derived from the NE and thus reflects the activity of the nerve terminals of sympathetic nervous system rather than that of the medulla.
- Activity of the medulla can be assessed specifically only by the measurement of plasma epinephrine levels or of urinary free epinephrine excretion.

Adrenergic Receptors and Mechanism of Action of Catecholamines

Adrenergic Receptors

Like other amino acids and peptide hormones, catecholamines act through cell membrane and receptors known as adrenergic receptors. Based on their pharmacological properties, adrenergic receptors are of two types.

α-Receptors These are further of two types (α_1 and α_2). α-Adrenergic receptors are sensitive to both epinephrine and NE. α-Receptors have multiple subtypes (α_{1A}, α_{1B}, α_{1D}, α_{2A}, α_{2B} and α_{2C}). These receptors are associated with most of the excitatory functions of the body but have one major inhibitory function (i.e. inhibition of intestinal motility).

β-Receptors These are further of three types, β_1, β_2 and β_3. β-Adrenergic receptors respond to epinephrine and in general are relatively insensitive to NE. These receptors are associated with most of the inhibitory functions of the body but have an important excitatory function (i.e. excitation of myocardium).

Relative potency of two catecholamines varies with each receptor type. In general, epinephrine tends to react more strongly with β-receptors and NE with α-receptors but overlap is considerable.

Specific agonists and antagonists have been developed for each receptor type (Table 8.5.5).

Structurally, β_1-, β_2- and α_2-receptors are similar. All three of these receptors are single-unit transmembrane glycoproteins.

Table 8.5.5 Agonists and antagonists of adrenergic receptors

Type of adrenergic receptors	Agonist	Antagonist
α_1	Norepinephrine Phenylephrine Methoxamine	Phenoxybenzamine Phentolamine Prazosin
α_2	Clonidine Apraclonidine Brimonidine	Yohimbine Phentolamine
β_1	Norepinephrine Isoproterenol Dobutamine	Metoprolol Atenolol Betaxolol
β_2	Isoproterenol Albuterol	Propranolol Butaxamine Metaproterenol Salmeterol

α_1-Receptors differ from these receptors and have a higher molecular weight.

Mechanism of action and second messenger involved are as follows:

- α_1-Receptors are coupled to Gq proteins to phospholipase C, leading to the phosphatidylinositol membrane system, and diacylglycerol (DAG), which mobilizes calcium along with protein kinase C, to mediate the hormone effects.
- α_2-Receptors are coupled to an inhibitory G-protein; thus, hormone binding decreases cAMP levels and protein kinase A activity.
- β_1-, β_2- and β_3-receptors are coupled to and stimulate adenylyl cyclase; thus, cAMP is the second messenger for their biological effects.

Regulation of adrenergic receptors: A reciprocal relationship exists between catecholamine concentration and the number and function of adrenergic receptors.

Downregulation: Continuous stimulation of catecholamine release or exposure to catecholamine agonists is associated with a decreased number of adrenergic receptors in target cells and a decreased responsiveness to catecholamines. This phenomenon is called downregulation of receptors.

Upregulation: A sustained decrease in catecholamine secretion (e.g. following sympathectomy) increases the number of receptors and enhances sensitivity to catecholamines. This phenomenon is called upregulation and may account for the *denervation hypersensitivity*, which is observed in sympathetic neuroeffectors following autonomic fibre denervation.

Rapid desensitization to subsequent doses is produced by acute exposure to catecholamine hormones. This effect is caused by phosphorylation of the various receptors by the hormone-activated protein kinase A or C. Phosphorylation renders the receptors inaccessible to further hormone binding. Receptor desensitization is a form of rapid intracellular negative feedback, which limits hormone actions.

Note. For further details about adrenergic receptors, see page 957.

ACTIONS OF CATECHOLAMINES

General Considerations

- The catecholamines exert their effects by binding with adrenergic receptors as described above.
- Actions of catecholamines on individual organs and systems are similar to those resulting from stimulation of sympathetic nervous system and are summarized in Table 10.5.2.
- In general, the effects produced by adrenomedullary stimulation last (approximately 10 times) longer than those produced by sympathetic stimulation, and the effects on metabolism are more pronounced.
- Adrenal medullary stimulation releases predominantly epinephrine (and small amounts of NE), while sympathetic stimulation mainly releases NE. So, their effects are different in some tissues owing to the differential existence of two types of adrenergic receptors (α and β).

I. Metabolic Actions of Catecholamines

Epinephrine affects metabolic functions more than NE, via α- and β-receptors.

1. General metabolic effects of epinephrine These include:

- Increased O_2 consumption (by 20%–40%) and increased CO_2 output
- Raised basal metabolic rate (BMR) and respiratory quotient (RQ)
- Increased heat production due to stimulation of cellular oxidative processes

2. Effect on carbohydrate metabolism Epinephrine produces hyperglycaemia and makes the glucose available for the brain and other tissues to meet the emergency by its following effects:

Glycogenolysis is stimulated in the liver (releasing glucose in circulation) and in the muscle (providing lactate for hepatic gluconeogenesis).
Glycogenesis is reduced in the liver by inhibition of the enzyme glycogen synthase.
Gluconeogenesis, i.e. hepatic production of glucose from lactate, amino acids and glycerol, is increased.
Insulin secretion is inhibited. This ensures that glucose will be used mostly by the brain since most of the tissues except brain require insulin for glucose utilization.
Glucagon secretion is stimulated. This amplifies the hyperglycaemic effects of epinephrine.
ACTH secretion is stimulated, which then stimulates cortisol secretion. Cortisol is a potent gluconeogenic hormone, via the hepatic conversion of alanine to glucose.

3. Effects on fat metabolism NE has a more potent action on the lipid metabolism than epinephrine, which has a predominant effect on carbohydrate metabolism.

Catecholamines cause increase in lipolysis by stimulating hormone-sensitive lipase (via β-receptor, i.e. cAMP) in adipose tissue and muscles. This results in increase in free fatty acids in the circulation which are effectively utilized by the heart and muscle as fuel source.

II. Physiological Actions of Catecholamines

1. Effects on cardiovascular system are:

i. In an isolated heart, both epinephrine and NE stimulate β_1-receptors and produce:

- Increase in heart rate by action on SA node.
- Increase in conduction velocity and shortening of functional refractory period by action on AV node.
- Increase in force of contraction by direct effect on ventricular and atrial myocardium.
- In high doses, catecholamines produce multiple pacemaker activity especially in Purkinje fibres and can produce fibrillation, which is why epinephrine and NE are never administered intravenously.

ii. In intact heart and blood vessels, the net effects of epinephrine and NE are depicted in Table 8.5.6.

Table 8.5.6 Cardiovascular effects of epinephrine and norepinephrine

Parameter	Epinephrine	Norepinephrine
Heart rate	↑	↓
Cardiac output	↑	↓
Peripheral resistance	↓	↑
Systolic blood pressure	↑	↑
Diastolic blood pressure	↓	↑
Mean arterial pressure	↓ or N	↑

Explanation of the differential effects of epinephrine and NE

Epinephrine causes:

- Increased heart rate and force of contraction via β_1-receptors results in increased cardiac output and rise in systolic blood pressure (SBP).
- Causes vasoconstriction in renal, splanchnic and cutaneous vascular bed via β_1-receptors and vasodilation in muscle and liver vessels via β_2-receptors. The net effect is decrease in peripheral resistance, therefore fall in diastolic blood pressure (DBP).
- As a result of rise in SBP and fall in DBP, the pulse pressure (PP) is widened but mean arterial pressure, i.e. MAP (DBP + 1/3 PP), remains unchanged or slightly decreases. Thus, reflex effect on baroreceptors is negligible.

Norepinephrine causes:

- Increased heart rate and force of contraction via β_1-receptors results in increased cardiac output and rise in SBP.
- Causes vasoconstriction via α_1-receptors resulting in increased peripheral resistance and increased DBP.
  - As a result of increased SBP and DBP, mean blood pressure (MBP) is markedly increased, which reflexly by stimulation of baroreceptors (aortic and carotid sinus) decreases heart rate, force of contraction and cardiac output.
  - The net result of NE effect is decreased heart rate, decreased cardiac output, increased peripheral resistance and increased MBP. Because of this, NE and not epinephrine is useful in patients with shock.

2. Effects on other systems are:

On CNS Catecholamines via β-receptors activate RAS by lowering its threshold and thus lead to arousal and alerting responses producing anxiety, apprehension and coarse tremors of extremities.

On GIT Epinephrine via β-receptors causes relaxation of smooth muscles of wall of the gut decreasing its tone and motility. Via α-receptors, epinephrine causes contraction of sphincters of gut; the net result is production of constipation.

On urinary bladder Epinephrine produces circumstances conducive for retention of urine by relaxing the detrusor muscles via β-receptors and by contracting trigone and sphincters via α-receptors.

On skin Catecholamines via α-receptors act on the pilomotor muscle producing piloerection of hair and by acting on sweat glands of palm and sole, producing localized sweating called adrenergic sweating (e.g. generalized sweating, which is cholinergic).

On skeletal muscle During exercise, epinephrine via β_2-receptors increases blood supply (by causing vasodilation) producing severe contraction and quick fatigue of the skeletal muscles. It also increases glycogenolysis in muscle and releases glucose into circulation.

On eyes Epinephrine via α-receptors causes dilation of the pupil (mydriasis) by contracting dilator pupillae (radial) muscle, and via β-receptors causes relaxation of the ciliary muscle producing flattening of the lens. These effects provide better far vision benefit to the endangered individual.

On respiration Epinephrine via β_2-receptors relaxes smooth muscles of bronchioles producing bronchodilation. It also increases rate and force of respiration.

On blood Epinephrine produces the following effects:

- *Reduces blood coagulation time* by increasing activity of factor V.
- *Increases RBC count*, haemoglobin content and PCV due to release of RBCs in circulation by causing contraction of spleen.
- *Increases plasma protein concentration* by movement of fluid out of circulation.
- *Neutrophilia* occurs due to release of sequestrated neutrophils into the circulation.

On secretion of other hormones Catecholamines regulate secretion of a number of hormones:

- *Insulin and somatostatin* secretion is decreased via α_2-receptors (by decreasing cAMP).
- *Glucagon and pancreatic peptide* secretion is increased via β_2-receptors (by increasing cAMP).
- *TRH-induced secretion of TSH* from thyrotrophs is decreased via α_2-receptors (by decreasing cAMP).
- *Thyroid hormone* secretion is enhanced by catecholamines under certain circumstances and peripheral conversion of T_4 to T_3 is stimulated via β_2-receptors.

On glandular secretion Catecholamines cause slight increase in the secretion of *salivary glands* (via α- and β_2-receptors), apocrine sweat glands (via β_2-receptors) and lacrimal glands (via α-receptors).

On renin secretion and Na^+ and K^+ movement Catecholamines increase renin secretion by stimulation of β-receptors in the kidney. The increase in renin, in turn, increases aldosterone secretion, which, in turn, enhances sodium retention. This action is augmented by the local catecholamine effects in the kidney on the distribution of blood flow and on renal tubular function.

Influx of potassium into the muscle is stimulated by epinephrine via β_2-receptors. The movement of K^+ into the intracellular space helps to prevent hyperkalaemia.

On nerve fibres Epinephrine, via α-receptors, decreases the latency of action potential in the nerve fibres.

III. Role of Sympathoadrenal System in Various Physiological States

1. Role during exercise During mild to moderate exercise, mainly the sympathetic nervous system is activated. However, during severe exercise, the adrenal medullary secretion is also increased. Increased sympathoadrenal discharge during exercise plays the following physiological roles:

i. ***Mobilization of stored fuel***: Catecholamines stimulate:
   - *Glycogenolysis* in muscle for use of glycogen
   - *Gluconeogenesis* in liver from the lactate that is released by the exercising muscle
   - *Lipolysis* to provide FFA as alternative fuel which may be required during exercise

ii. ***Cardiovascular adjustments:*** These are caused by increased sympathoadrenal discharge, and lead to massive blood flow to the actively contracting muscles, while maintaining coronary and cerebral blood flow. Increased blood flow is necessary for providing oxygen and fuel (glucose, FFA) for increased muscle metabolism. Adrenergic blockade or autonomic neuropathy impairs cardiovascular responses to exercise and diminishes exercise tolerance.

2. Role during exposure to cold Sympathoadrenal system is essential for maintenance of body temperature during exposure to cold. Experimentally, it has been proven that the animals in which both sympathetic nervous system and adrenal glands have been knocked down die because of hypothermia when exposed to cold. However, either the sympathetic nervous system or adrenal medulla is alone incapable of sustaining life. The epinephrine maintains body temperature by conserving body heat, as well as by producing heat:

Heat conservation: During exposure to cold, epinephrine produces constriction of cutaneous vessels and helps to conserve heat. The skin becomes more or less a bloodless sheet of tissue insulating the deeper warmer tissue from the cold environment. Piloerection occurring during exposure to cold in animals with fur or feathers is also mediated through the sympathoadrenal system.

Thermogenesis: The sympathoadrenal system plays an important role in thermogenesis, i.e. heat production, by the following mechanisms:

- *BMR* is mainly regulated by thyroxine; but epinephrine increases BMR by 7%–15%.
- *Nonshivering thermogenesis* is increased by epinephrine. Brown adipose tissue is the site of nonshivering thermogenesis.
- *Chemical thermogenesis* is increased by catecholamines, which, in general, stimulates various chemical metabolic processes. For example, catecholamines increase the oxygen consumption beyond that induced by muscular activity. The additional substrate (glucose and FFA) for increased tissue metabolism is provided by catecholamine-induced glycogenolytic and lipolytic actions.

3. Role during hypoglycaemia Hypoglycaemia is a very potent stimulator of epinephrine secretion from the adrenal medulla, while it does not increase sympathetic neural activity to any significant degree. Plasma epinephrine levels may rise 10- to 50-fold depending on the severity of hypoglycaemia. By its effects on metabolism described above (page 748), the epinephrine restores plasma glucose levels and glucose delivery to the central nervous system.

AN INTEGRATED RESPONSE TO STRESS

Stress, may it be emotional, physical or biological, evokes an integrated response of the sympathoadrenal medullary system and hypothalamic–pituitary–adrenal cortex axis.

Steps involved in stress adaptation Steps involved in stress adaptation by an integrated response of the above-mentioned system are as follows (Fig. 8.5.28).

Perception of stress signals Stress is perceived by many areas of the brain, from the cortex down to the brainstem including limbic system and RAS.

Stimulation of hypothalamus Major stresses activate the CRH and ADH neurons in the paraventricular nucleus and adrenergic neurons.

Activation of hypothalamic–pituitary–adrenal axis CRH and ADH release stimulates ACTH release and ultimately elevates plasma cortisol levels.

Activation of sympathoadrenal medullary system Sudden exposure to any type of stress initially produces the sympathetic alarm reaction. Stimulation of adrenergic neurons of hypothalamus ultimately leads to release of epinephrine from adrenal medulla and NE from the sympathetic ganglia.

Integrated role of hormones released by hypothalamic–pituitary–adrenal axis and sympathoadrenal medullary system in stress adaptation Together, these hormones help in adaptation to stress by their following actions:

Increase in glucose production: Catecholamines rapidly raise plasma glucose by activating glycogenolysis, and cortisol acts

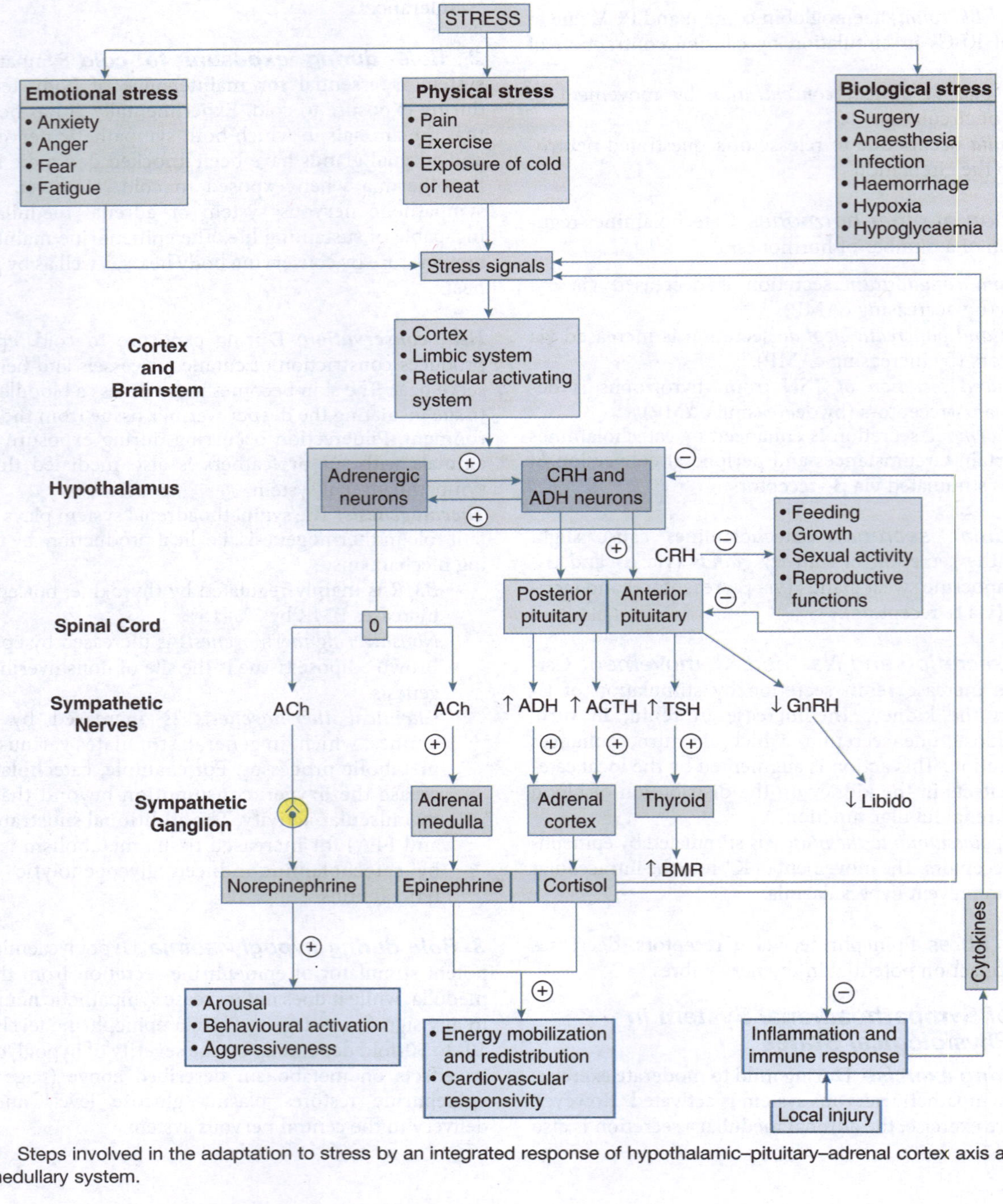

Fig. 8.5.28 Steps involved in the adaptation to stress by an integrated response of hypothalamic–pituitary–adrenal cortex axis and sympathoadrenal medullary system.

more slowly by providing amino acid substrate for gluconeogenesis. Together, they shift glucose utilization towards the central nervous system away from peripheral tissues.

Free fatty acid supply: Epinephrine rapidly augments the supply of free fatty acids to the heart and the muscles, and cortisol facilitates the lipolytic role.

Cardiovascular adjustments: Catecholamines and cortisol raise blood pressure and cardiac output, and they improve the delivery of substrates to tissues that are critical to the immediate defence of the organism.

Arousal, defensively useful behavioural activation and focussed attention result from the adrenergic stimuli to the pertinent brain centres.

Inhibition of activities that are not useful during stress and divert individuals and their resources from defensive responses to danger is an important part of adaptation to stress. For example, CRH input to hypothalamic neurons inhibits growth hormone, gonadotropin release and sexual activity. These actions are reinforced by excess of cortisol. In addition, CRH inhibits appetite and feeding behaviour, which are also inappropriate when the individual is facing immediate danger.

Important Note

Interaction with immune system: The hormones produced during stress interact with the immune system to produce a balance between useful local cytokine production at threatened or impenled sites and potentially dangerous systemic effects of these immune system products.

Applied Aspects

Diseases of Adrenal Medulla

Phaeochromocytoma

Phaeochromocytoma is a rare benign tumour arising from the epinephrine- and NE-secreting chromaffin cells of adrenal medulla. It derives its name because of black staining of chromaffin due to oxidation of catecholamines. Approximately 25%–30% of pheochromocytomas are usually associated with other inherited syndromes such as:

- Multiple endocrine neoplasia type 2 (MEN 2)
- von Hippel–Lindau syndrome (VHL), an autosomal dominant disorder associated with increased expression of vascular endothelial growth factor (VEGF) leading to angiogenesis
- Neurofibromatosis type 1 (NF1)
- Preganglioma syndrome

Clinical Features. The clinical features are produced by the excess of epinephrine and NE and include:

- Episodic or nonepisodic hypertension with postural drop
- Attacks of tachycardia, palpitation, sweating, pallor, headache and chest discomfort
- Abdominal pain, vomiting, constipation and glucose intolerance
- Weight loss and weakness
- Hypercalcaemia
- Erythrocytosis
- Anxiety, panic attacks and fear of death (angor animi)

Tests. The tests for diagnosis of phaeochromocytoma include:

- *24-Hour urinary excretion* of VMA, metanephrines and catecholamines are increased.
- *Plasma epinephrine* and NE levels are elevated.
- *Phentolamine suppression test*, i.e. 2.5 mg of phentolamine does not suppress plasma catecholamine at 10-minute sample.
- Imaging tests like contrast-enhanced *CT scan*, MRI *and radionuclide studies* to localize any tumour.
- Metaiodobenzylguanidine (MiBG) scintigraphy.
- Somatostatin scintigraphy.
- Fluoro-DOPA PET/CT.

Treatment. The treatment of phaeochromocytoma is surgical excision. However, medical treatment is necessary before and after the surgery, as well as in inoperable cases. Both α- and β-adrenoreceptor blockers, e.g. labetalol, or combination of phenoxybenzamine and propranolol is used to control hypertension.

Self-Assessment

1. Discuss the hormonal functions of adrenal cortex and explain how glucocorticoids are essential for survival.
2. Describe the anti-inflammatory and anti-allergic effect of glucocorticoids.
3. Discuss the role of mineralocorticoids.
4. Write briefly about:
   - Pathophysiology of Cushing syndrome
   - Hyperaldosteronism
   - Hormonal adaptation to stress
5. Write notes on:
   - Escape phenomenon
   - Pheochromocytoma
   - Adrenal sex steroids

Clinical Cases

Case 1

A 35-year-old female presented with complaints of rapid weight gain, irregular menstruation, excessive sweating, reddish marks on the body, feeling of weakness, tiredness and sleepiness for 3–4 months.

On examination from facial features and sign and symptoms, it was suspected to be a case of Cushing syndrome and referred to endocrinology department.

Q1. What is the cause of this condition?

Q2. What are the typical features of this condition and their physiological basis?

Q3. What investigations should be carried out to confirm the diagnosis?

Q4. What is the treatment plan for this condition?

Case 2

A 60-year-old male presented in medicine department with complaints of generalized weakness, tingling sensation in hands and feet, feeling of excessive thirst and increased urinary frequency. The personal history revealed that he is a case of hypertension for which he was taking antihypertensive treatment.

Examination showed the following: BP 184/110 mm Hg and pulse 88/min.

Laboratory investigations showed the following: serum electrolyte – Na^+ i22 mEq/L, K^+ 5.8 mEq/L; raised levels of aldosterone and renin

Q1. What is the probable diagnosis?

Q2. What is the cause of persistent high blood pressure in this case not even controlled with antihypertensive drugs?

Q3. What is the cause for raised aldosterone level in this case?

Case 3

A 45-year-old woman admitted with history of weight loss, generalized weakness, loss of appetite, change in skin colour from light to dark, nausea and sometimes vomiting.

Examination revealed patchy darkening of skin in the back, scanty axillary and pubic hair, BP 118/76 mm Hg and pulse 100/min

Laboratory investigations showed:

- Serum electrolyte: Na^+ 120 mEq/L, K^+ 5.8 mEq/L; decreased blood glucose level (fasting)
- Urine Na^+ raised and K^+ low, osmolality of urine >400 m Osmol/L

Q1. On the basis of history and signs and symptoms, what is the probable diagnosis?

Q2. Which further tests should be carried out to confirm the diagnosis?

8.6 Pancreatic and Gastrointestinal Hormones

CHAPTER OUTLINE

ENDOCRINE PANCREAS

FUNCTIONAL ANATOMY

The endocrine part of the pancreas comprises numerous rounded collections of cells known as *pancreatic islets* or the *islets of Langerhans*. These are embedded within the exocrine part. There are approximately 1 million islets in the pancreas, most numerous in the tail, and they constitute 1%–1.5% of the human pancreatic mass.

Islets of Langerhans

The islets are very richly supplied with blood through dense capillary plexus (as in all ductless glands) and innervated by vagal and sympathetic fibres.

Cellular structure Each islet contains, on average, 2500 cells which are of four types and arranged as (Fig. 8.6.1):

β-Cells or B cells make up 60%–70% of the total cells, and constitute the central core of the islet. These cells secrete insulin, amylin and C-peptide.
α-Cells or A cells form approximately 20% of the total cells and constitute the outer rim of the islet. These cells secrete glucagon.
δ-Cells or D cells form approximately 10% of total cells and are intermixed. These are source of somatostatin.
PP cells or F cells are also peripherally placed scattered among the α-cells. These are source of pancreatic peptide.
Epsilon (ϵ) cells, which secrete ghrelin.

Gap junctions These link β-cells to each other, α-cells to each other and β-cells to α-cells for rapid communication.

Vascular arrangement Small arterioles enter the core of each islet and break up into a network of capillaries with fenestrated endothelium. These capillaries then converge into venules, which carry blood to the mantle of the islet. This portal arrangement allows a high concentration of insulin from β-cell core, so bathe the α-, δ- and PP cells of the respective mantles. This type of vascular pattern also suggests the possible paracrine effects of insulin on the other islet cell types.

Pancreatic islets have strategic location The proximity of islets to pancreatic acini (of exocrine part) permits them to have local effects on exocrine pancreatic function. Islet hormones are secreted into the pancreatic vein and then into the portal vein, where they join the nutrient stream after meals. This arrangement preferentially exposes the liver, which is the central organ in substrate traffic, to islet hormone concentrations higher than those the peripheral tissues receive. In addition, the liver can extract variable amounts of insulin and glucagon on their first pass through this organ. In this manner, the liver can modulate the hormone's availability to other tissues.

INSULIN

Insulin is a polypeptide hormone secreted by the β-cells of islets of Langerhans of pancreas. Historically, insulin has several firsts to its credit.

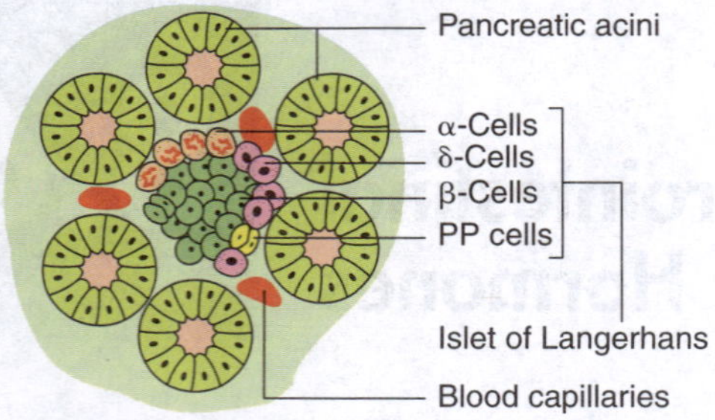

Fig. 8.6.1 Schematic histological structure of pancreas showing an islet of Langerhans surrounded by exocrine pancreatic acini.

Discovered by Banting and Best, but Nobel Prize in physiology and medicine was awarded to Banting and Macleod in 1923 for discovery of insulin.

- It was the first hormone to be isolated, purified, crystallized and synthesized.
- The first protein detected to possess hormonal activity.
- The first protein sequences for amino acids to determine the structure.
- The first protein estimated by radioimmunoassay.
- The first protein produced by recombinant DNA technology.

Structure and Biosynthesis

Structure The human insulin is a protein containing 51 amino acids, arranged in two polypeptide chains: A (having 21 amino acids) and B (having 30 amino acids). These chains are connected to each other by two interchain disulphide linkages, connecting A_7 to B_7 and A_{20} to B_{19}. In addition, there is an intrachain disulphide link in chain A between amino acids 6 and 11 (Fig. 8.6.2). If the two chains are split apart, functional activity of insulin is lost.

Biosynthesis of insulin β-Cells of islets of Langerhans synthesize insulin by the usual protein synthetic machinery. The steps involved are as follows (Fig. 8.6.3):

- The insulin genes for synthesis of insulin (located on chromosome 11) transcription factors that are essential during synthesis are hepatocyte nuclear factor (HNF) and insulin promoter factor-1 (IPF-1). They direct the synthesis of *preproinsulin*, an insulin precursor consisting of 86 amino acids.
- Preproinsulin is cleaved to form *proinsulin*.
- The *proinsulin molecule*, containing the A and B chains of insulin and connecting peptide (C-peptide), is guided to Golgi apparatus, disulphide linkages are established to yield the *folded proinsulin* molecule.
- Proinsulin is further cleaved in Golgi apparatus to form the *active hormone insulin* and a connecting peptide (C-peptide).

Insulin becomes associated with zinc as the secretory granules mature. The zinc–insulin crystals form the dense central core of the granules, whereas C-peptide is present in the clean space between the granule membrane and the core. The β-cell secretory granules contain insulin, C-peptide and amylin. The insulin molecule along with the C-peptide molecule is retained in the granules and released by exocytosis in equimolar amounts.

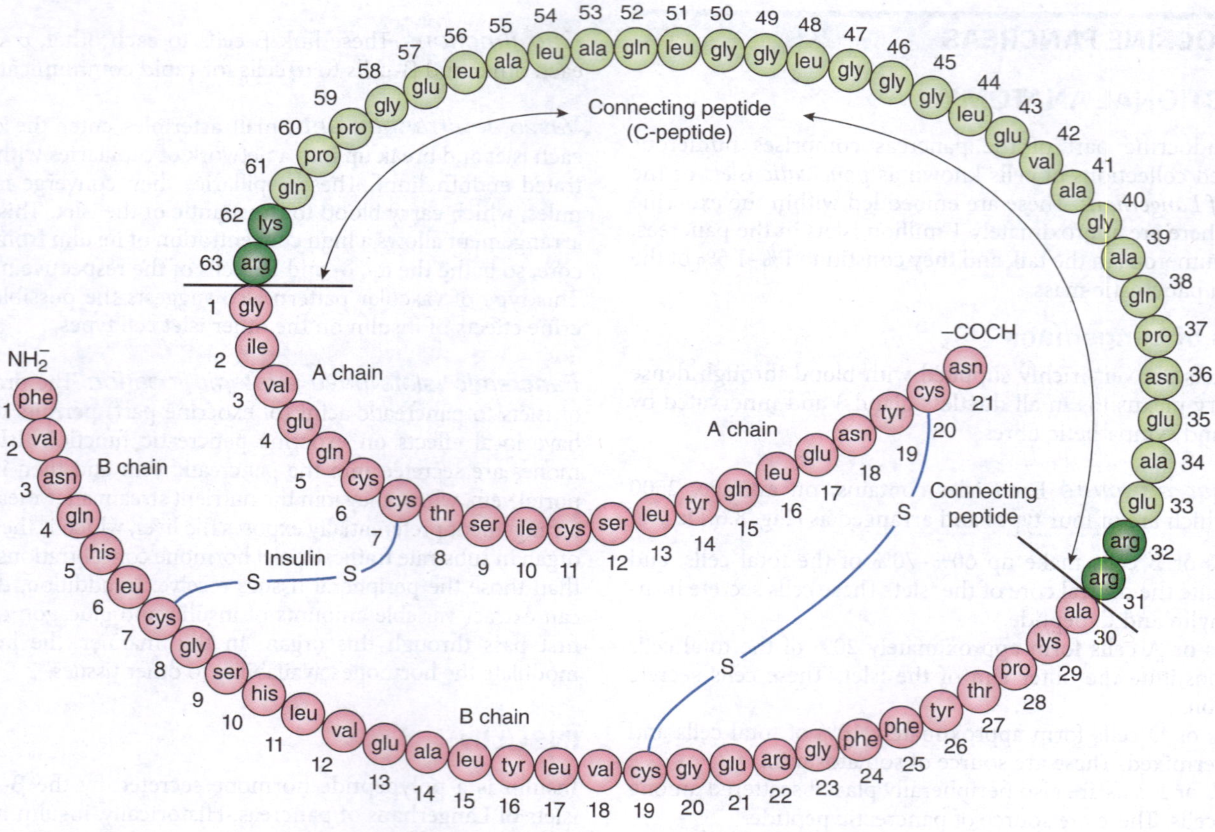

Fig. 8.6.2 Structure of an insulin molecule.

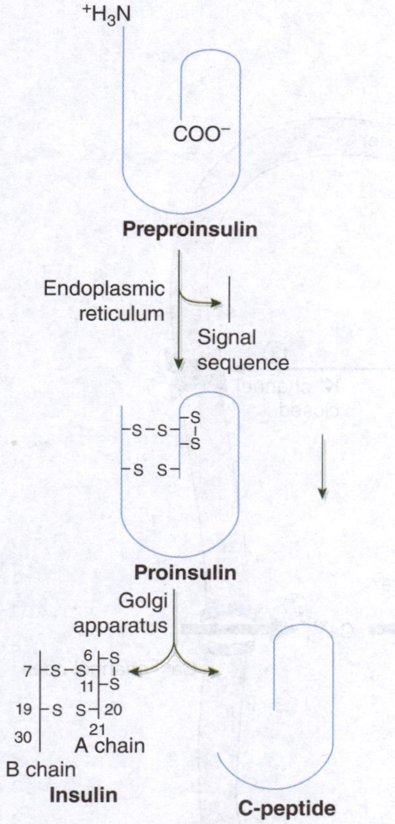

Fig. 8.6.3 Steps in the synthesis of insulin.

Important Note

- C-peptide has no biological activity; however, its estimation in the plasma and by radioimmunoassay serves as a useful index for the endogenous production of insulin.
- Zinc in the insulin structure stabilizes the structure of insulin.
- The zinc deficiency plays an important role in aetiology of diabetes mellitus.

Mechanism of Insulin Secretion

Mechanism of insulin secretion by blood glucose Blood glucose is the major stimulant for insulin secretion. The steps involved in the secretion of insulin from the β-cells are depicted in Fig. 8.6.4:

- Glucose diffuses into the β-cells by binding with the glucose transporter 2 (GLUT2) receptors (a specific transporter) on the β-cell membrane (Step 1, Fig. 8.6.4).
- Inside the β-cells, glucose is phosphorylated and metabolized to pyruvate. The pyruvate enters the mitochondria and is metabolized to CO_2 and H_2O via the citric acid cycle with formation of ATP (Step 2, Fig. 8.6.4). The enzyme glucokinase appears to function as the fundamental glucose sensor that controls the subsequent β-cell response.
- The increased ATP levels close the ATP-sensitive K^+ channels and suppress K^+ efflux from the cell causing depolarization of the β-cells (Step 3, Fig. 8.6.4).
- Depolarization opens voltage-regulated Ca^{2+} channels, leading to an increase in the intracellular Ca^{2+} (Step 4, Fig. 8.6.4).
- The elevated Ca^{2+} concentration activates the mechanism for insulin release from the secretory granules by exocytosis (Step 5, Fig. 8.6.4).
- Via the citric acid cycle, pyruvate metabolism also causes an increase in intracellular glutamate. Glutamate also causes release of insulin from secretory granules; this is reason for prolonged second phase of release of insulin in response to glucose.

Mechanism of insulin secretion by fuels other than glucose

- A sequence similar to glucose, with specific transporters and enzymatic steps, probably underlies the less prominent stimulation action of other fuels, such as amino acids, ketoacids and fatty acids (Step 6, Fig. 8.6.4).

Mechanism of insulin secretion by glucagon Glucagon mediates insulin-releasing effect by stimulatory G (G_s) protein via cyclic AMP. In contrast, inhibitory G_i proteins mediate the insulin-suppressive effects like peptides such as somatostatin (Step 7, Fig. 8.6.4).

Mechanism of insulin secretion by acetylcholine G-protein linked to phospholipase C mediates the ability of acetylcholine (ACh) to stimulate insulin release via generation of phosphatidylinositol (IP_3), second messenger and increased protein kinase activity (Step 8, Fig. 8.6.4).

Regulation of Insulin Secretion

I. Role of Exogenous Nutrients

Exogenous nutrients (glucose, amino acids, free fatty acids [FFAs], ketoacids and potassium) control insulin secretion by a feedback mechanism (Fig. 8.6.5). When substrate supply is abundant, insulin is secreted in response. Insulin then stimulates the use of these incoming nutrients and simultaneously inhibits the mobilization of analogous endogenous substrates. When nutrient supply is low or absent, insulin secretion is dampened and mobilization of endogenous fuels is enhanced.

1. Role of blood glucose Insulin secretion is mainly controlled by the level of blood glucose by feedback relationship.

The relationship between plasma glucose and plasma insulin is sigmoidal (Fig. 8.6.6). As shown in Fig. 8.6.6:

- Below 50 mg/dL levels of plasma glucose, virtually no insulin is secreted.
- Above 100 mg/dL levels of plasma glucose, rate of insulin secretion rises rapidly.
- At approximately 150 mg/dL levels of plasma glucose, a half-maximal insulin secretory response is obtained.
- At a level of approximately 300 mg/dL, a maximal insulin response occurs.

The rapidly increased insulin secretion above 100 mg/dL levels of plasma glucose in turn reduces blood glucose concentration to fasting level. Reduction of blood glucose causes rapid turning off of insulin secretion (feedback relationship).

Biphasic response of insulin secretion occurs in response to a continuous glucose stimulation (Fig. 8.6.7):

- *An immediate pulse of insulin* is released, within seconds of exposure to glucose, that peaks at 1 minute (approximately 10-fold rise) and then returns towards baseline in another 5–10 minutes.

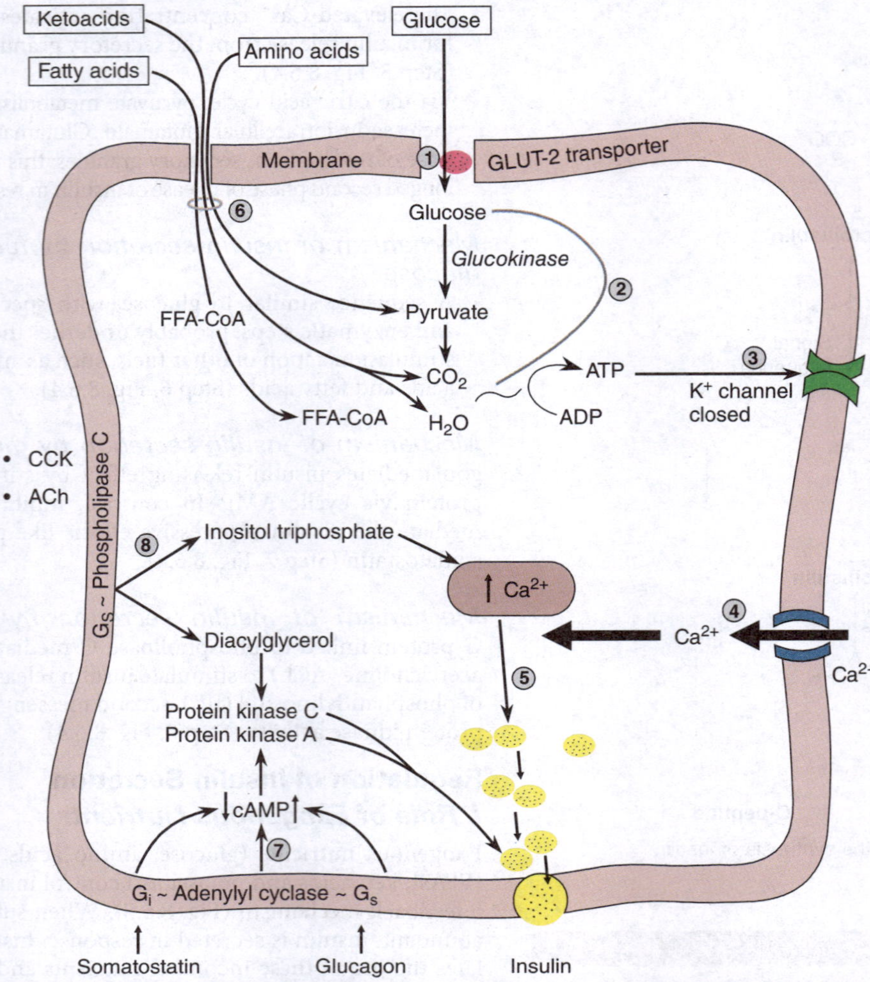

Fig. 8.6.4 Steps of mechanism of insulin secretion by different stimulants such as glucose (Steps 1–5), other fuels (Step 6), peptides such as glucagon (Step 7) and acetylcholine (Step 8).

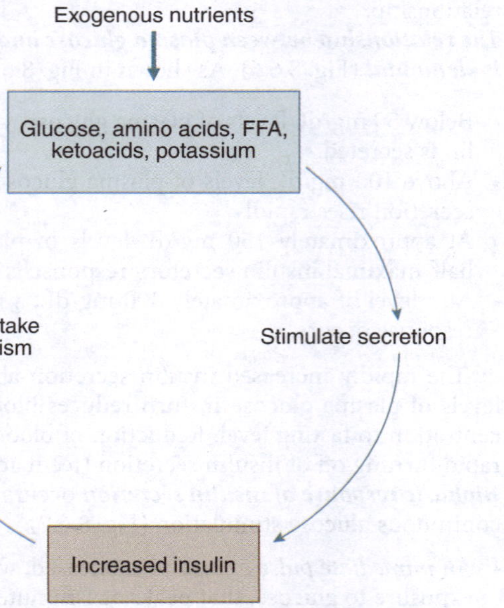

Fig. 8.6.5 Feedback control of insulin release by exogenous nutrients.

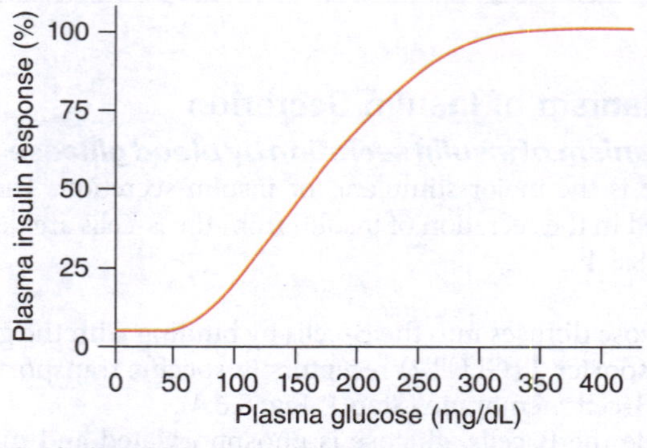

Fig. 8.6.6 A sigmoidal relationship between levels of plasma glucose and insulin secretion response.

- *A second phase of insulin secretion* begins after approximately 10 minutes of continuous stimulation. During this phase, plasma levels of insulin rise more slowly and reach a second plateau, which can be maintained for many hours in normal individuals.

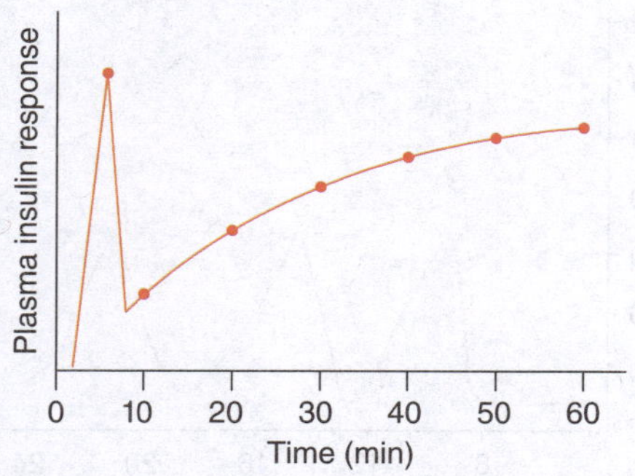

Fig. 8.6.7 Biphasic insulin response to glucose infusion consists of first phase of rapid release and fall followed by second phase of slow rise.

Factors responsible for biphasic response:

- Initial peak occurs due to release of preformed insulin.
- Second phase occurs due to glucose stimulation of insulin synthesis that sustains the secretory phase.
- Granules with different sensitivity also contribute to the biphasic response.

When glucose is given orally, a greater insulin response is elicited than when plasma glucose is elevated comparably by intravenous administration. This augmented response to oral glucose is attributed to the gastrointestinal (GIT) hormones like gastrin, secretin, cholecystokinin and gastric inhibitory polypeptide, i.e. gastric inhibitory peptide (GIP, most potent), that cause moderate increase in insulin secretion. Since these hormones are released immediately after meals, they cause anticipatory rise of insulin before actual absorption of glucose and amino acids.

2. Role of amino acids Amino acids also induce the secretion of insulin. This is particularly observed after the ingestion of protein-rich meal that causes transient rise in plasma amino acid concentration. The basic amino acids, arginine and lysine, are the most potent stimulants; leucine, alanine and other amino acids contribute modestly to this effect.

Important Note

As compared to glucose, amino acids cause only slight rise in insulin secretion. However, glucose and amino acids are synergistic stimulators of insulin release, so the plasma insulin rise that follows a meal represents more than the additive effects of its carbohydrate and protein content.

3. Role of triglyceride, ketoacid, free fatty acids, potassium, calcium and magnesium

Triglycerides exert only a small stimulatory effect on insulin release in humans. This small effect may be mostly indirect and exerted by means of GIP.

Ketoacids at concentrations that prevail during prolonged fasting modestly stimulate insulin secretion; this effect may help to sustain a critical low level of insulin when β-cell stimulation by ingested nutrients is absent.

FFAs, especially the longer chain and more saturated molecules, such as stearate, enhance insulin response to glucose during total fasting when plasma FFA rises and the β-cell content of FFA-CoA increases.

However, long-term exposure of β-cells to elevated FFA can have deleterious effects on insulin secretion. This occurs because FFA also stimulates apoptosis of β-cells.

Potassium and calcium *both* are essential for normal insulin response to glucose. Thus, relative insulin deficiency occurs in subjects depleted of potassium, calcium or the calcitropic hormone, vitamin D.

II. Role of Gastrointestinal and Other Hormones

Incretins are a group of metabolic hormones that stimulate fall in blood glucose level. Incretins are released after meals and increase the secretion of insulin from β-cells of pancreas. The two most important incretin hormones are glucagon-like polypeptide-1 (GLP-1) and GIP or glucose-dependent insulinotropic peptide.

- GLP-1 [7–36] or GLP-[7–36] that stimulates insulin secretion. β-Cells of islets have receptors for GLP-1 [7–36] as well as for GIP. Recently, GLP-1 [7–36] is considered to be more insulinotropic hormone than GIP. It acts by increasing Ca^{2+} influx through voltage-gated Ca^{2+} channels.

Important Note

GLP-1 is rapidly degraded by an enzyme dipeptidyl peptidase-4 (DDP-4). Therefore, blockers of DDP-4 prolong the action of GLP-1. Thus, they are used for treatment of diabetes mellitus.

- Glucagon also stimulates insulin secretion and pancreatic somatostatin.
- Pancreatic somatostatin, secreted from D cells of pancreatic islets, acts locally by paracrine fashion through its receptors and inhibits insulin secretion. For details, see page 769.

Other hormones, such as growth hormone, cortisol, glucagon and, to a lesser extent, progesterone and oestrogen, also stimulate insulin secretion. Prolonged secretion of any of these hormones can cause burning out of the islets of Langerhans, thereby causing diabetes mellitus.

III. Role of Sympathetic and Parasympathetic Nervous System

Sympathetic nerves and epinephrine These inhibit insulin secretion via α-adrenergic receptors (they stimulate insulin secretion via β-adrenergic receptors, but this effect is negligible). As a net result, the increased sympathetic discharge to pancreas causes inhibition of insulin release and stimulation of glucagon release resulting in rise in blood sugar level.

Epinephrine is the most predominant inhibitor of insulin release. In emergency situations like stress, extreme exercise and trauma, the nervous system stimulates the adrenal medulla to release epinephrine. The epinephrine suppresses insulin release and promotes energy-yielding compounds – glucose from liver and fatty acids from adipose tissue.

Parasympathetic nerves to pancreas and acetylcholine. These increase insulin secretion to some extent; ACh stimulates insulin release via generation of phosphatidylinositol second messenger (Step 8 in Fig. 8.6.4). Some of the important factors stimulating and inhibiting insulin secretion are depicted in Table 8.6.1.

Table 8.6.1 Factors stimulating and inhibiting insulin secretion

Factors stimulating insulin secretion	Factors inhibiting insulin secretion
• ↑ Blood glucose	• ↓ Blood glucose
• ↑ Amino acids (leucine and arginine)	• Somatostatin
• ↑ Fatty acids (long chain)	• Norepinephrine, epinephrine (α-adrenergic stimulation)
• Glucagon	• Galanin
• Intestinal hormones (GIP, GLP-1 [7–36], gastrin, secretin, CCK and others)	• K^+ depletion
• ACh	• Alloxan, streptozocin
• Growth hormones, cortisol	• Thiazide diuretic
• Theophylline	• Phenytoin
• Sympathetic discharge (β-adrenergic stimulation)	• Diazoxide

Plasma Insulin Levels, Circulation and Degradation

Plasma levels of insulin

Average basal peripheral plasma insulin level is 10 μU/mL.

- After several days of fasting, basal plasma levels of insulin decline over 50%, i.e. become less than 5 μU/mL.
- After prolonged exercise, the plasma insulin levels fall.
- Three- to fourfold increase in plasma insulin level is noted after a typical meal. The peak occurs after 30–60 minutes of initiating the meal.

Important Note

Although C-peptide is secreted in amounts that are equimolar to insulin, its basal peripheral plasma levels are approximately fivefold higher (averaging 1 ng/mL). This difference is caused by a lower rate of metabolic clearance for C-peptide.

Rate and total amount of insulin secretion per day

Basal insulin delivery rates to the peripheral circulation in humans are approximately 0.5–1.25 units/h (20–40 μg/h).

- During meals, the delivery rate increases up to 10-fold.
- Total daily peripheral delivery of insulin is approximately 30 units.
- If the amount of insulin removed during its first pass through the liver is accounted for (~50% of portal vein insulin), the actual β-cell secretory rate becomes approximately 2.5 units/h (60 units/day).

Cycles of insulin secretion In addition to the intrinsic low level, 15-minute cycles and the brush-off insulin secretion stimulated by meals, a higher amplitude insulin cycle exists. This cycle has pulses lasting 2 hours that are entrained by glucose and that represent feedback regulation.

The β-cell cyclic response (represented by fluctuations in insulin and C-peptide plasma levels) is exaggerated in obesity (Fig. 8.6.8).

Circulation and degradation of insulin

- *Insulin circulates* unbound to any carrier protein.
- *Half-life of insulin* in plasma is 5–18 minutes.

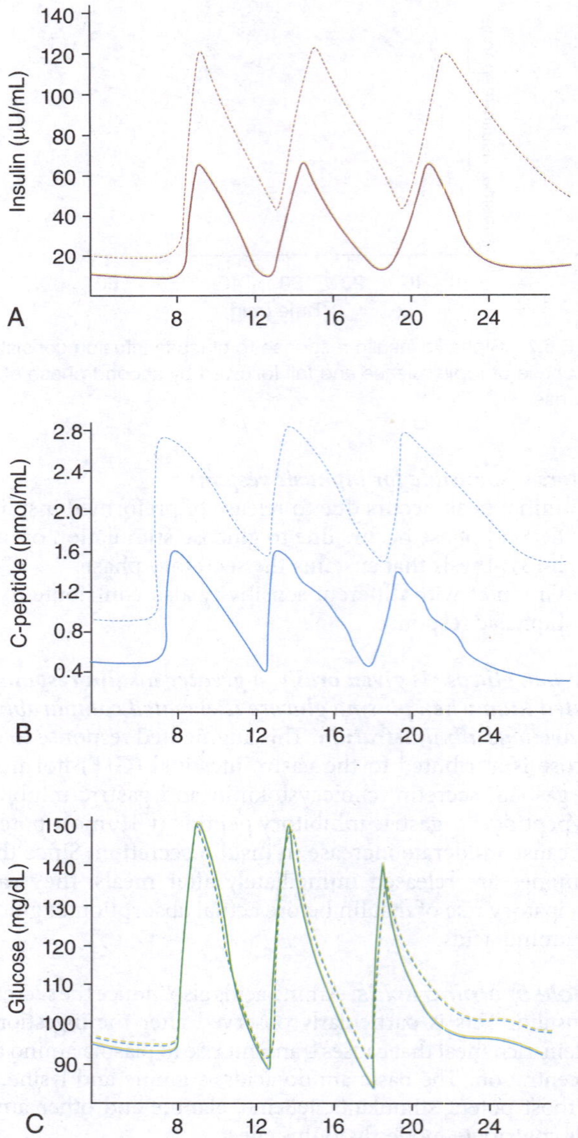

Fig. 8.6.8 Cyclic response of insulin (**A**), C-peptide (**B**) and fluctuations of blood glucose level (**C**) observed during 24-hour profile in a normal weight (solid lines) and in an obese (dotted line) human.

Short half-life permits rapid metabolic changes in accordance with the alterations in the circulating level of insulin. This is advantageous for the therapeutic purposes.

- *Metabolic clearance rate* of insulin is approximately 1000 mL/min.
- A protease enzyme, namely *insulinase* (mainly found in the kidneys and liver), degrades insulin. It splits the disulphide bonds and separates the A and B chains.
- Degradation of insulin also occurs in association with its plasma membrane receptors after it is internalized by target cells.
- Very little insulin is excreted unchanged in the urine.

Mechanism of Action of Insulin

Before discussing the steps involved in the mechanism of action of insulin, it will be worth to know about the insulin receptors.

Insulin Receptors

Insulin receptor is a protein kinase receptor that contains enzyme activity. Approximately 2–3 lakh insulin receptors are present on the cell membrane of target tissues for insulin.

Structure (Fig. 8.6.9) The insulin receptor is a tetramer having two identical α-subunits and two β-subunits. One α-subunit is bound with β-subunit by a disulphide bond to form a dimer. Two such identical dimers are joined extracellularly by another disulphide bond.

- *α-Subunits* (chains) are located on the outer surface of the plasma membrane and contain the insulin-binding domain.
- *β-Subunits* (chains) span across the plasma membrane and reside largely within the cytoplasm. These have tyrosine kinase domain.

Downregulation Downregulation of insulin receptors in target tissues is caused by insulin itself. Therefore, the number

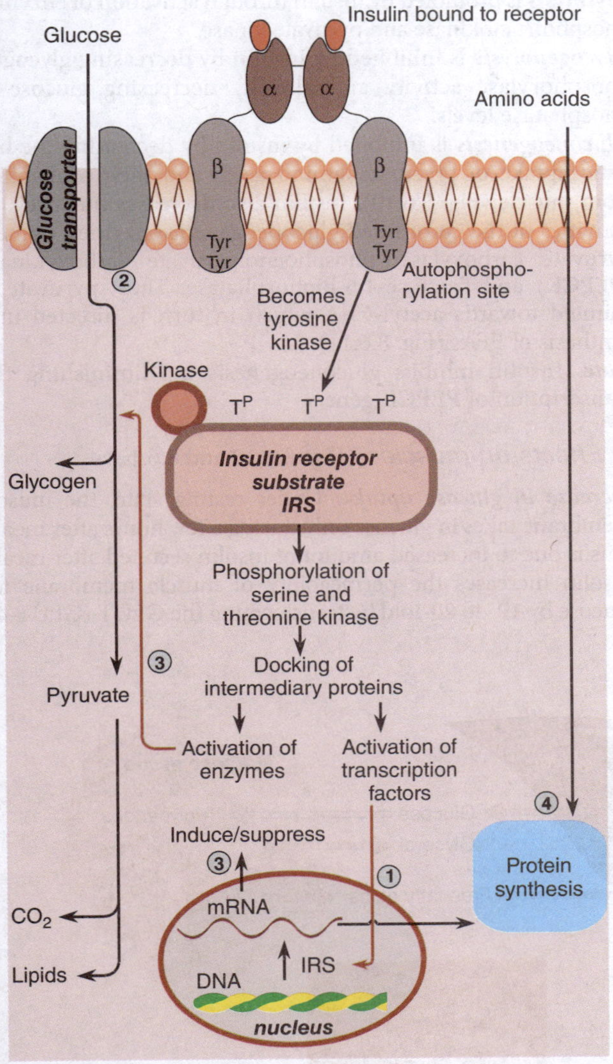

Fig. 8.6.9 Structure of insulin receptor and mechanism of insulin action on target cell. Note the activity of insulin receptor which ultimately produces the following effects of insulin on target cell: (1) gene expression; (2) translocation of glucose transporters from cytoplasm to plasma membrane; (3) activation or deactivation of various enzymes of glucose and fatty acid metabolism; and (4) protein synthesis through increased mRNAs.

of insulin receptors is increased in starvation and decreased in obesity.

Steps Involved in the Mechanism of Action of Insulin (Fig. 8.6.9)

- The first and overall rate-limiting step in insulin action is transport of insulin through the capillary wall to the target tissues, such as muscle and adipose tissue.
- Once insulin arrives at the target cell, it binds with the insulin receptor (on the insulin-binding domain present on the α-subunits).
- Binding of insulin to the α-chain activates the tyrosine kinase activity of the β-chains. The activated tyrosine kinase then autophosphorylates the β-chains.
- The phosphorylated receptor then phosphorylates tyrosine residues on intracellular protein substrate or insulin receptor substrate (IRS).
- The IRS tyrosine phosphorylations are followed by various cascades of events that ultimately produce the following effects:
  1. ***Gene expression*** in the nucleus of target cell leading to biological action.
  2. ***Translocation of glucose transport proteins to the plasma membrane:*** IRS recruits phosphatidylinositol-3 kinase (PI-3 kinase) pathway that mediates translocation of GLUT-4 transporter to cell membrane.
     The GLUTs are responsible for the insulin-mediated uptake of glucose by the cells. As the insulin levels fall, the GLUTs move away from the membrane to the intracellular pool for storage and recycle.
  3. ***Activation or deactivation of numerous enzymes*** in glucose and fatty acid metabolism is brought about by increased mRNAs.
  4. ***Protein synthesis:*** Increased mRNA synthesis (transcription) is followed by translation (protein synthesis). In this way, insulin promotes synthesis of enzymes such as glucokinase, phosphofructokinase and pyruvate kinase.
     Note. Individuals with 'insulin-resistant' diabetes secrete insulin normally, but their tissues do not respond to their own insulin or the injected insulin. In some of these cases, there is a mutation in the tyrosine kinase domain of the insulin receptor. Insulin binds normally to the mutant receptors, but the tyrosine kinase is inactive, and the downstream consequences of insulin binding do not occur.
  5. ***Growth-promoting and mitogenic function*** is through recruitment of 3 mitogen-activated protein (MAP) kinase pathway of insulin.

Actions of Insulin

The physiological effects of insulin are divided into rapid, intermediate and delayed actions (Table 8.6.2). The main effects include:

A. Metabolic effects
B. Effects on ion transport
C. Role in cell growth and development

A. Metabolic Effects of Insulin

Insulin plays a key role in the metabolism of carbohydrate, lipids and proteins. The major targets for insulin action are the muscle mass, the liver and adipose tissue.

1. Effects on carbohydrate metabolism In a normal individual, approximately half (50%) of the ingested glucose is utilized to meet the energy demands of the body (mainly

Table 8.6.2 Principal effects of insulin

Rapid effects of insulin occurs within second:
Transportation of glucose, amino acids and fatty acids into the insulin-sensitive cells
Intermediate effects of insulin occurs within minute:
(i) Protein synthesis/stimulation
(ii) Inhibition of protein degradation
(iii) Activation of glycolytic enzymes
(iv) Inhibition of phosphorylase and gluconeogenesis
Delayed effects in late hours:
Increased mRNA for lipogenic enzyme

through glycolysis). The other half is converted to either fat (~40%) or glycogen (~10%). This relation is maintained by insulin and is thus severely impaired in insulin deficiency.

As a net effect, insulin decreases blood glucose concentration by the following mechanisms:

1. ***Insulin increases uptake of glucose in target cells*** by translocating the GLUT into the cell membranes.
   - Insulin is required for the uptake of glucose by muscles (skeletal, cardiac and smooth), adipose tissue, leucocytes and mammary glands.
   - Tissues in which glucose transport is not insulin dependent include nervous tissue, kidney, RBC, retina, blood vessels and intestinal mucosa. This property is of critical importance in the nervous system because glucose is the only source of energy and insulin is presented in the blood for approximately 2 hours after each meal. Since transport of glucose into nervous tissue depends on blood glucose level only, severe hypoglycaemia results in convulsion, coma or even death.
   - Insulin is not required for entry of glucose in hepatocytes (liver); however, insulin-mediated increased utilization indirectly promotes its uptake.
2. ***Insulin promotes glucose utilization:***
   - *Glycolysis* (oxidation of glucose) is increased in muscle and liver by insulin.
   - *Glycogen* formation from glucose in muscle and liver is promoted by insulin.
3. ***Insulin decreases glucose production*** by inhibiting:
   - Gluconeogenesis
   - Glycogenolysis

Effects of insulin on carbohydrate metabolism in target tissues: Liver, muscle and adipose tissue

i. Effects on liver (Figs 8.6.10 and 8.6.11):

Increase in glucose uptake: Insulin increases the activity of enzyme *glucokinase* which enhances glucose utilization by catalysing its phosphorylation (Fig. 8.6.11). Thus, indirectly, insulin increases glucose uptake by increasing its utilization. In the liver, extracellular glucose levels equilibrate rapidly with intracellular levels by means of GLUT-2 transporter (Fig. 8.6.11).
Promotion of glycogen synthesis: Insulin promotes storage of glucose as glycogen by activating the *glycogen synthase enzyme* complex.
Glycolysis is promoted by insulin through activation of enzymes phosphofructokinase and pyruvate kinase.
Glycogenolysis is inhibited by insulin by decreasing glycogen phosphorylase activity and also by decreasing glucose-6-phosphatase levels.
Gluconeogenesis is inhibited by insulin by decreasing the hepatic uptake of precursor amino acids and their availability from muscle (Fig. 8.6.10). Insulin also decreases the levels or activities of the committed gluconeogenetic enzymes, namely pyruvate carboxylase, phosphoenolpyruvate carboxykinase (PEPCK) and fructose-1,6-biphosphatase. Thus, pyruvate is shunted towards acetyl-CoA which in turn is directed into synthesis of FFAs (Fig. 8.6.11).
Note. Insulin inhibits gluconeogenesis by diminishing the transcription of PEPCK gene.

ii. Effects on muscles (Figs 8.6.10 and 8.6.12):

Increase in glucose uptake: Under resting state, the muscle membrane takes in glucose only during a few hours after meals. This is due to increased amount of insulin secreted after meals. Insulin increases the permeability of muscle membrane for glucose by 10- to 20-fold by translocating the GLUT (GLUT-4).

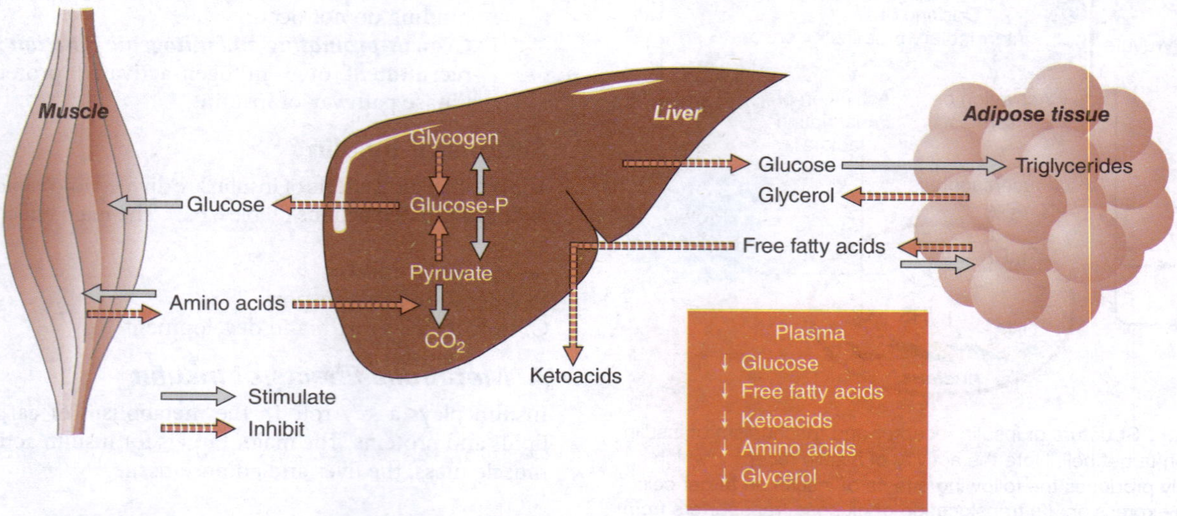

Fig. 8.6.10 Schematic diagram to illustrate metabolic effects of insulin on carbohydrate (glucose), fats (free fatty acids) and protein (amino acids) resulting in tissue uptake and decrease in plasma levels of substrates.

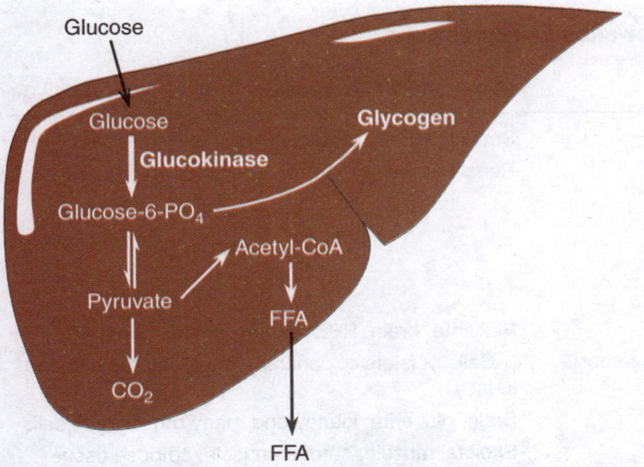

Fig. 8.6.11 Effects of insulin on carbohydrate metabolism in liver.

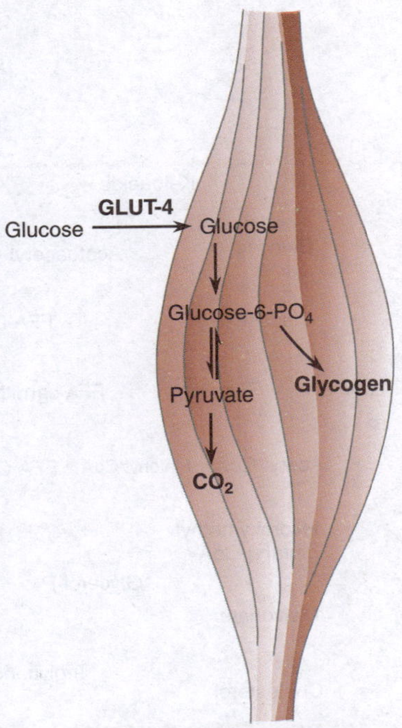

Fig. 8.6.12 Effects of insulin on carbohydrate metabolism in muscle.

However, during exercise, permeability of muscle membrane to glucose increases even in the absence of insulin. This is the reason that diabetics are advised regular moderate exercise.

Increase in glycolysis: Depending on the insulin concentration, 20%–50% of glucose that enters the muscle cell undergoes oxidation, mainly caused by the activation of pyruvate dehydrogenase (Fig. 8.6.12).

Increase in glycogen synthesis: The remainder glucose is deposited as muscle glycogen by insulin activation of glycogen synthase (Fig. 8.6.12).

iii. Effects on adipose tissue (Figs 8.6.10 and 8.6.13):

- Glucose transport into the adipose tissue cells is stimulated by insulin by translocating the GLUT (GLUT-4).
- Much of the glucose entering the cells is converted into α-glycerophosphate, which is used in the esterification of fatty acids and permits their storage as triglycerides (Fig. 8.6.13).

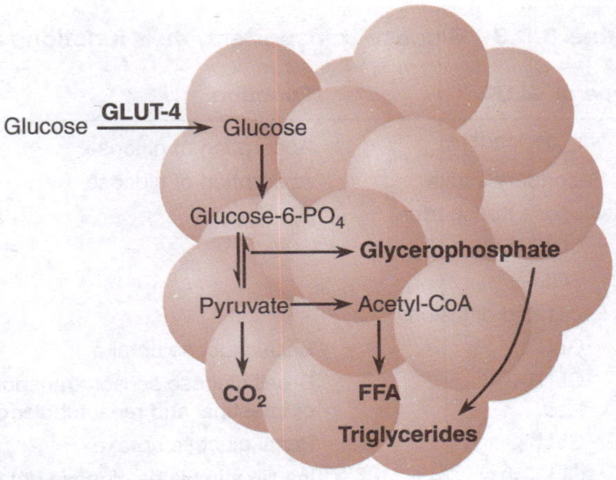

Fig. 8.6.13 Effects of insulin on carbohydrate metabolism in adipose tissue.

- To a minor extent, glucose can also be converted to fatty acids (Fig. 8.6.13).

GLUTs: Depending on the transport mechanisms, GLUTs are of two types:

Sodium-dependent glucose transporters (SGLT-1 and SGLT-2) are responsible for secondary active transport of glucose with sodium ions mainly in the intestine and renal tubules (for details, see pages 635 and 500).

GLUTs by which glucose enters the cell by facilitated diffusion are further of seven different types named GLUT 1–7 in order of their discovery. Each transporter has been assigned for a special task. Depending on insulin sensitivity of the cells, these GLUTs are as follows:

- Insulin-sensitive GLUTs (e.g. GLUT-4).
- Noninsulin-sensitive GLUTs: Other GLUTs are not insulin sensitive.

Mechanism of action. Insulin acts through:

- GLUT-4 transporter, present in the muscle and adipose tissue, is stimulated by insulin.
- The molecules of GLUT-4 are present in the cytoplasmic vesicles of insulin-sensitive cells.
  - When insulin receptors of these cells get activated, the vesicles containing GLUT-4 move rapidly towards plasma membrane and fuse with it (insertion of transporter).
  - Activation of insulin receptors causes movement of vesicles to cell membrane by activating PI-3 kinase.
  - On cessation of insulin activity, the cell membrane patches containing GLUT are endocytosed and ready for next exposure to insulin.
  - Insulin-sensitive tissues also contain GLUT-4 vesicles that move towards cell membrane in response to exercise (insulin-independent GLUT-4). The action of these receptors is triggered by A-5′-AMP-activated kinase protein.
  - The specific functions and major sites of expression of GLUT have been summarized in Table 8.6.3.

2. Effects on lipid metabolism

The metabolism of both endogenous and exogenous fat is profoundly influenced by insulin.

The net overall effect is to enhance storage and to block mobilization and oxidation of fatty acids by:

- Favouring lipogenesis
- Decreasing lipolysis
- Reducing ketogenesis

Table 8.6.3 Glucose transporters, their functions and major sites of expression

Type of GLUT	Function	Major site of expression
1. Na^+ dependent Secondary active Glucose transporter		
• SGLT-1	Absorption of glucose	Small intestine, renal tubules
• SGLT-2	Absorption of glucose	Renal tubules
2. Facilitated diffusion		
• GLUT-1	Basal glucose uptake	Placenta, brain, RBC, kidney, colon, retina
• GLUT-2	B-cell glucose sensor, transport of glucose out of intestinal and renal tubular cells	β-Cells of islets of pancreas, liver, enterocytes and kidney
• GLUT-3	Basal glucose uptake	Brain, placenta, kidney and many other organ cells
• GLUT-4	Insulin stimulates glucose uptake	Skeletal muscle, cardiac muscle, adipose tissue
• GLUT-5	Exercise-stimulated glucose uptake	Skeletal muscle
• GLUT-6	Fructose transport	Jejunum, sperms, brain, leucocytes, spleen
• GLUT-7	Glucose-6-phosphate transporter in endoplasmic reticulum	Liver

Effects of insulin on lipid metabolism in target tissues: liver, adipose tissue and muscle

i. Insulin increases lipogenesis by it effects on:

a. Lipogenic effects on liver (Figs 8.6.10 and 8.6.14):

Triglyceride synthesis: When insulin and carbohydrates are available, liver is quantitatively a more important site of fat synthesis than the adipose tissue. As described in the Effects of Insulin on Carbohydrate Metabolism (page 760), insulin promotes storage of glucose as glycogen in the liver cells. However, when glycogen concentration increases to 5%–6%, glycogenesis is inhibited and the additional glucose entering is converted to fat in the liver cells.

- First, glucose is split to pyruvate (in glycolytic pathway) and pyruvate is converted to acetyl-CoA which is a substrate for fatty acid synthesis.
- Increased citrate and isocitrate formed by citric acid cycle (when excess glucose is being used for energy) activate acetyl-CoA carboxylase to form malonyl-CoA, which is the first stage of fatty acid synthesis.
- Insulin favours synthesis of triglycerides from FFAs, glycerol-3-phosphate (from glycolysis) and NADPH (from hexose monophosphate [HMP] shunt).
- Triglycerides formed in liver cells are released to the blood.

Synthesis of cholesterol: Insulin also favours hepatic synthesis of cholesterol from acetyl-CoA by activating the rate-limiting enzyme hydroxymethylglutaryl-CoA reductase.

b. Lipogenic effects on adipose tissue (Fig. 8.6.15): ***Insulin activity promotes deposition of circulating fat into adipose tissue*** by activating the key enzyme *lipoprotein lipase* in the capillary wall of adipose tissue. This enzyme favours the uptake of very low density lipoprotein (VLDL) and chylomicrons into the adipose tissue from circulation by splitting them into FFAs. The FFAs are absorbed by fat cells and converted to triglyceride. The α-glycerophosphate required for esterification of FFA is obtained from the glucose in fat cells (whose uptake is also increased by insulin).

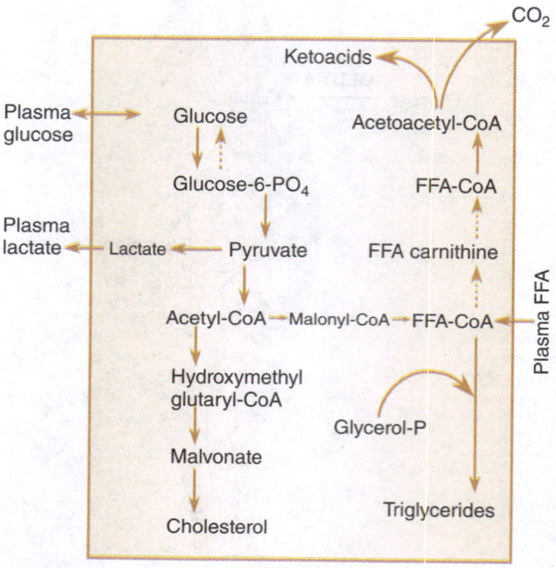

Fig. 8.6.14 Effect of insulin on lipogenesis in liver.

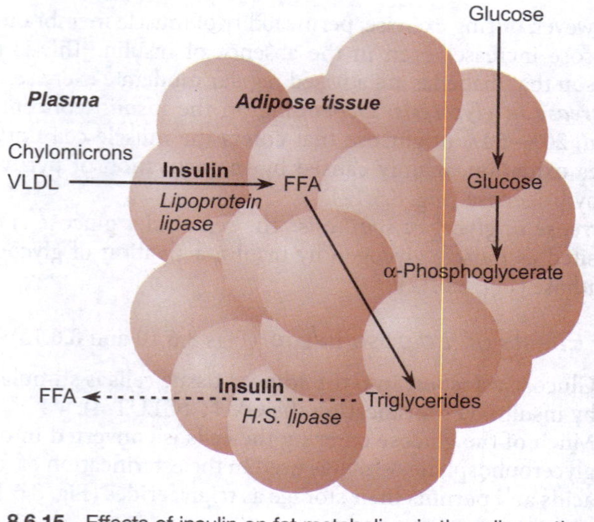

Fig. 8.6.15 Effects of insulin on fat metabolism in the adipose tissue.

c. Lipogenic effects of insulin in muscle Within muscle, insulin suppresses the enzyme lipoprotein lipase in inverse proportion to its stimulation of glucose uptake.

ii. Insulin decreases lipolysis

a. In adipose tissue, insulin profoundly inhibits *hormone-sensitive lipase activity*. By suppressing lipolysis and the release of stored fatty acids and glycerol, insulin diminishes their delivery to liver and peripheral tissues.

> **Important Note**
>
> It is noteworthy that abdominal visceral fat is less sensitive to insulin than is subcutaneous fat.
>
> ***Note.*** The hormones which promote lipolysis by activating hormone-sensitive lipase are epinephrine, norepinephrine, glucagon, growth hormone, cortisol and thyroid hormone.

b. In liver also, the mobilization of FFA to peripheral circulation.

c. In muscle also, the insulin inhibits lipolysis of triglyceride stores.

iii. Insulin reduces ketogenesis Insulin is the major and perhaps the sole antiketogenic hormone. Its antiketogenic effects are as follows:

- Insulin leads to decreased FFA flow to the liver from adipose tissue. As a consequence, there is marked reduction in the generation of ketoacids.
- Insulin also stimulates the use of ketoacids by the peripheral tissue.
- Under the influence of insulin, FFAs that enter the liver from circulation are shunted away from β-oxidation and ketogenesis.
- Antiketogenic action of insulin in the liver may also be mediated by stimulation of malonyl-CoA formation, because malonyl-CoA inhibits the enzyme carnitine acyltransferase. The latter enzyme is responsible for transferring FFAs from cytoplasm into the mitochondria for oxidation and conversion to ketoacids (Fig. 8.6.14).

iv. Effect of insulin on lipoprotein metabolism It appears that insulin is required for the utilization of VLDL and LDL. The levels of VLDL and LDL and consequently the concentration of cholesterol are elevated in diabetics, which has been implicated in the pathogenesis of atherosclerosis.

Insulin regulates use of glucose and FFA for energy production. From the effects of insulin on carbohydrate and fat metabolism described above, it is obvious that insulin regulates use of glucose and FFA for energy production.

- After a carbohydrate-rich meal, blood insulin level rises and consequently glucose becomes the chief fuel in the muscle. FFA is not used at this time because of low plasma FFA concentration induced by insulin.
- In between the meals, when the blood glucose level tends to fall, insulin secretion also decreases, resulting in greater lipolysis and increased production of FFA. Consequently, FFA becomes the chief fuel.

3. Effects of insulin on protein metabolism Insulin is an anabolic hormone; it stimulates protein synthesis and inhibits protein degradation.

i. Insulin stimulates protein synthesis Although insulin stimulates the general rate of protein synthesis in vitro, this stimulation is evident in vivo mostly, when amino acids are in abundance after a meal (in the basal state, insulin limits the availability of endogenous amino acids for new protein synthesis). The role of insulin in protein synthesis is as follows:

- It increases the transport of many amino acids (especially valine, leucine, isoleucine, tyrosine and phenylalanine) into the cells by increasing membrane permeability. Thus, plasma amino acids are lowered.
- Insulin increases the translation of messenger RNA on the ribosomes forming new proteins. In the absence of insulin, ribosomes stop working.
- Over a longer period, insulin also increases the rate of transcription of selected DNA genetic sequences in cell nuclei. This results in formation of increased quantities of mRNA causing still more protein synthesis, mainly enzymes for storage of fats, proteins and carbohydrates.
- In the liver, insulin decreases the rate of gluconeogenesis and thus conserves amino acids for protein synthesis.

ii. Insulin inhibits protein metabolism Insulin inhibits proteolysis. This action is manifested by suppression of the branched-chain and aromatic amino acids from muscle and inhibition of their oxidation.

B. Effects of Insulin on Ion Transport

Insulin increases K^+, PO_4^{3-} and Mg^{2+} uptake into the skeletal muscle cell and of K^+ and PO_4^{3-} into hepatic cells from ECF by increasing membrane permeability. Therefore, insulin secreted in response to a carbohydrate load lowers serum K^+, PO_4^{3-} and Mg^{2+} levels, and this hormone is considered to be one of the normal regulators of K^+ balance. This effect of insulin explains the occurrence of hypokalaemia in patients of diabetic acidosis treated with large doses of insulin.

The exact mechanism of hypokalaemia is not yet clear. However, insulin may increase the activity of Na^+–K^+-ATPase so that more K^+ is pumped into the cell. Insulin is very effectively used for temporary relief of hyperkalaemia in patients with renal failure.

Another effect of insulin on electrolytic balance is to increase reabsorption of K^+, PO_4^{3-} and Na^+ by the tubules of the kidney.

C. Role of Insulin in Cell Growth and Development

Insulin is an important factor for growth and development with the following roles:

Anabolic action: Anabolic action of insulin is as important as that of growth hormone for promotion of normal growth. Proper growth and development require the presence of both the hormones because anabolic action of one hormone cannot compensate for the other (because of their different modes of action).

Direct stimulatory effect on macromolecules: Insulin not only is a general anabolic hormone but also stimulates the synthesis of macromolecules in tissues such as cartilage and bone and thereby directly contributes to body growth.

Stimulation of other growth factors: The genes for insulin and its receptor are related to genes that encode a variety of tissue growth factors. These growth factors include somatomedins (insulin-like growth factors 1 and 2, i.e. IGF-1 and IGF-2), epidermal growth factor (EGF), nerve growth factor (NGF)

Table 8.6.4 Effects of insulin on body tissues

Liver
- Increases protein synthesis
- Increases lipid synthesis
- Decreases ketogenesis
- Decreases glucose output due to:
  - Decreased neoglucogenesis
  - Increased glycogenesis
  - Increased glycolysis

Muscle
- Increases glucose intake
- Increases glycogenesis
- Increases amino acid uptake
- Increases protein synthesis in ribosomes
- Decreases protein catabolism
- Decreases release of gluconeogenic amino acid
- Increases ketone uptake
- Increases K^+ uptake

Adipose tissue
- Increases glucose entry
- Increases fatty acid synthesis
- Increases glycerol phosphate synthesis
- Increases triglyceride deposition
- Increases activation of lipoprotein lipase
- Inhibition of hormone-sensitive lipase
- Increases K^+ uptake

General: Increases growth and development

and relaxin. Thus, insulin indirectly contributes to growth by stimulating the transcription of other related gene growth factors, such as IGF-1, and by suppressing the gene for one of the IGF-1-binding proteins.

Note. An insulin-deprived young animal or human has a reduced lean body and bone mass, and it may be profoundly retarded in height and maturation.

The effects of insulin are summarized in Table 8.6.4.

GLUCAGON

Structure and Synthesis

Structure Glucagon is secreted by A cells of islets of Langerhans and L cells of lower intestinal tract. It is a polypeptide composed of 29 amino acids in a single chain and has a molecular weight of 3500. The N-terminal residues 1–6 are essential for receptor binding and for biological activity. Unlike insulin, the amino acid sequence of glucagon is the same in all mammalian species.

Synthesis Glucagon is synthesized from a preproglucagon precursor by islet α-cells. It is actually synthesized as proglucagon (molecular weight 9000) which on sequential degradation releases active glucagon. In α-cells, human preproglucagon is processed to glucagon and major proglucagon fragment (MPGF). In L cells of lower intestinal tract, it is processed primarily to *glicentin* (a polypeptide consisting of glucagon with additional amino acid residues on either end) and *GLP-1* and *GLP-2*. Some oxyntomodulin also formed and glicentin-related polypeptide (GRPP) is left (Fig. 8.6.16).

- Glicentin has some glucagon-like activity, whereas GLP-1 and GLP-2 have no biological activity, but when GLP-1 is further processed to form GLP-1 [7–36], it is a potent stimulator of insulin (see page 757).
- GLP-2 is a mediator in a pathway from NTS to hypothalamus, and an injection of GLP-2 lowers food intake.
- Oxyntomodulin inhibits gastric acid secretion.
- GRPP does not have any established physiological effect.

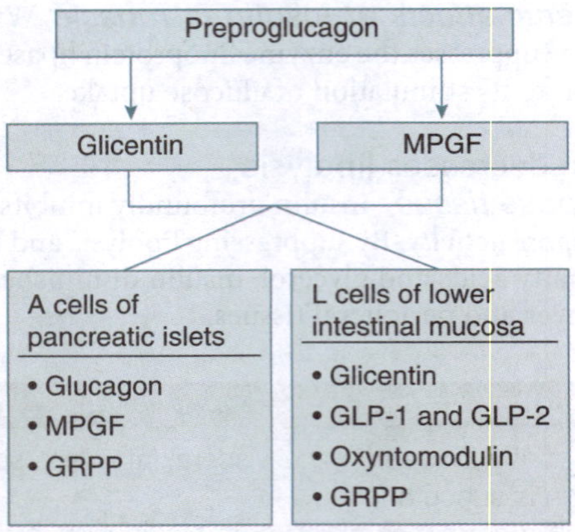

Fig. 8.6.16 Post-translational processing of preproglucagon in A and L cells. GLP, glucagon-like polypeptide; GRPP, glicentin-related polypeptide; MPGF, major proglucagon fragment.

Secretion Glucagon is stored in dense granules and is released by exocytosis. This process is inhibited if α-cell Ca^{2+} levels are decreased.

Plasma Levels, Circulation and Degradation

- *Circulation of glucagon* in plasma is in unbound form.
- *Basal levels* of glucagon in a normal fasting individual are 100–150 pg/mL.
- *Half-life* of this hormone is 6 minutes (range 5–9 minutes).
- *Secretion rate* of glucagon is estimated to be 100–150 μg/day.
- *Ratio of portal vein to peripheral vein* glucagon concentration is approximately 1.5 in the basal state. This is because glucagon enters the portal vein in relatively high concentration, approximately 50% of which is removed by the liver in a single passage through this organ.
- *Degradation* mainly occurs in the liver. Therefore, in cirrhosis of liver, peripheral blood level of glucagon increases. It is also degraded in tissues and plasma by an aminopeptide. The kidney is the other major site of glucagon degradation. Less than 1% of glucagon filtered by the glomerulus is excreted in the urine.

Mechanism of Action of Glucagon

Glucagon is glycogenolytic, gluconeogenic, lipolytic and ketogenic, and acts on G-protein–coupled receptors. It binds to the specific receptor on the plasma membrane of target cells and acts through the mediation of cyclic AMP as second messenger. Covalent modification of enzyme activities by phosphorylation is the main mechanism of action (for detail of mechanism, see page 659). Glucagon receptors have been identified in a variety of tissues. It mostly acts on liver and adipose tissue. It acts competitively at similar points in the liver as insulin. Glucagon may even be viewed as the primary hormone that regulates hepatic glucose production and ketogenesis, and insulin's role may be that of a glucagon antagonist.

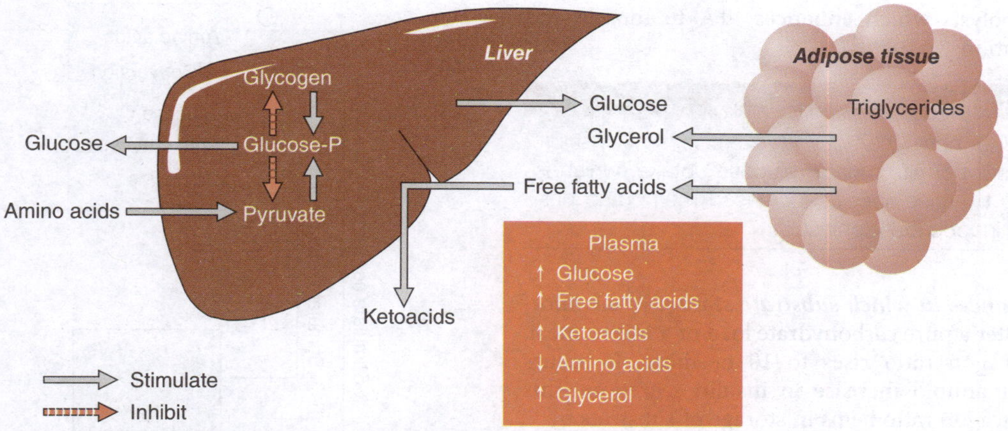

Fig. 8.6.17 Glucagon causes mobilization of stored energy fuels (glucose, fatty acids and ketoacids) into circulation and hepatic uptake of amino acids for gluconeogenesis; consequently, plasma levels of energy fuels increase and levels of amino acids decrease.

Actions of Glucagon

As mentioned above, the actions of glucagon, in almost all respects, are exactly opposite to those of insulin. It promotes mobilization of stored nutrients such as glucose, fatty acids and ketoacids (Fig. 8.6.17) and thus is a hormone of energy release. Its metabolic effects are as follows.

1. Effects on carbohydrate metabolism Glucagon predominately acts on the liver and increases the blood sugar level by the following actions:

Increased glycogenolysis: In the liver, glucagon exerts an immediate and profound glycogenolytic effect (breaking down of glycogens through activation of enzyme *glycogen phosphorylase* by cAMP-mediated mechanism). The glucose-1-phosphate released as a result of glycogen phosphorylase activation is prevented from undergoing resynthesis to glycogen by simultaneous inhibition of glycogen synthase. The glucose-1-phosphate is dephosphorylated and glucose is formed.

Increased gluconeogenesis: After the glycogen in liver is exhausted, glucagon increases the rate of gluconeogenesis, i.e. formation of glucose from lactate, pyruvate, glycerol and amino acids. Gluconeogenesis causes a slow but more sustained rise in blood glucose which lasts for hours and days. Glucagon activates multiple enzymes involved in gluconeogenesis, especially the enzyme system converting pyruvate to phosphopyruvate (rate-limiting step in gluconeogenesis). It also increases the entry of amino acids from blood to liver cells and makes them available for gluconeogenesis.

2. Effects on lipid metabolism Glucagon is a powerful *lipolytic agent*. It acts via stimulating cAMP system to activate lipase in adipose tissue which releases FFA and glycerol into the circulation. In the liver, excess of FFAs are oxidized resulting in energy production and ketone body synthesis (ketogenesis). In addition, glucagon also prevents synthesis of triglyceride from FFA by inhibiting the enzyme acetyl-CoA carboxylase. The spared FFAs are directed towards β-oxidation resulting in production of ketoacids. Thus, glucagon is a ketogenic as well as a hyperglycaemic hormone.

3. Effects on protein metabolism Glucagon increases the amino acid uptake of liver, which in turn promotes gluconeogenesis. Thus, glucagon *lowers plasma amino acids*.

4. Calorigenic effect Glucagon also has a calorigenic effect. This is not due to hyperglycaemia, but this action requires the presence of glucocorticoids and T_4. It is probably related to increased hepatic deamination of amino acids.

5. Other actions of glucagon Other miscellaneous actions of glucagon include:

- Inhibition of renal tubular sodium reabsorption, resulting in natriuresis.
- Modest increase in force of contraction of the heart by activation of myocardial adenylyl cyclase.
- The action of glucagon is useful in treatment of cardiac shock and as antidote for overdose of β-blocker.
- Stimulation of secretion of growth hormone, insulin and pancreatic somatostatin.
- It may also be synthesized in the central nervous system, and it may act locally in the regulation of appetite.
- It is also produced in the gastric and intestinal mucosa by certain cells resembling the α-cells of pancreatic islets. The physiological role of the extrapancreatic glucagon secretion is not clear.

Insulin–Glucagon Ratio

Insulin and glucagon are often secreted and act in a reciprocal fashion; when one is needed, the other usually is not. Therefore, the ratio of their concentrations may be more critical than their actual concentration. Together, they coordinate the flow and metabolic fate of endogenous glucose, FFAs, amino acids and other substrates to ensure that energy needs are met in the basal state and during exercise. In addition, they coordinate the efficient disposition of the nutrient input from the meals. They accomplish these functions by maintaining a critical ratio.

Under basal conditions, the usual molar ratio of insulin to glucagon in plasma is approximately 2.0.

Under circumstances that require mobilization and increased use of endogenous substrate such as fasting and prolonged exercise, the insulin–glucagon ratio drops to 0.5 or less. This decreased insulin–glucagon ratio results from both the decreased insulin secretion and increased glucagon secretion. Low insulin–glucagon ratio is helpful in maintaining glucose supply to CNS and energy requirement needs of the body by:

- Increasing glycogenolysis
- Increasing amino acid mobilization and promoting gluconeogenesis

- Increasing lipolysis which enhances FFA to muscle and liver for oxidation

Important Note

It is important to note that during exercise, low insulin–glucagon ratio still permits muscle glucose uptake, which is possible due to exercise-specific increased membrane permeability that is independent of insulin.

Under circumstances in which substrate storage is advantageous, such as after a pure carbohydrate load or a mixed meal, the insulin–glucagon ratio rises to 10 or more. It occurs mainly due to manifold increase in insulin secretion. This high insulin–glucagon ratio helps in storage of substrate by:

- Increasing glucose uptake, oxidation and conversion to liver and muscle glycogen
- Suppressing unneeded proteolysis and lipolysis
- Facilitating clearance of chylomicrons by activation of adipose tissue lipoprotein lipase

After a pure protein meal, interestingly, only a small change in insulin–glucagon ratio occurs; however, secretion of insulin as well as that of glucagon is increased.

- *Increased insulin secretion* prevents unneeded proteolysis and facilitates muscle uptake of some amino acids and their incorporation into proteins.
- *Increased glucagon secretion* is useful in preventing the decrease in hepatic glucose output and hypoglycaemia that would occur if the extra insulin action were completely unopposed.

Applied Aspects

Macrosomia and GLUT-1 Deficiency

Macrosomia refers to a condition of an infant born with low birthweight and large organ size, born to diabetic mother. The condition is caused by:

- Excess circulating antibodies against insulin in the fetus, resulting in pancreatic islet stimulation by raised blood glucose level and raised amino acids in the diabetic mother.
- Fetal macrosomia also occurs when in a pregnant woman antibodies develop against insulin or she is on bovine insulin therapy during pregnancy. Normally, free insulin in the maternal blood is destroyed by protease in the placenta, but antibody-bound insulin is protected and reaches the fetal blood.

The infant with GLUT-1 deficiency has defective glucose transportation across the blood–brain barrier; therefore, there is low CSF glucose, even in the presence of high blood glucose. These individuals develop seizure or severe development growth retardation.

Regulation of Glucagon Secretion

I. Role of blood levels of nutrients There exists a feedback relationship between blood levels of glucagon and nutrients (Fig. 8.6.18).

The most important principle is the maintenance of normoglycaemia in the face of increased nutrients in the control of glucagon discussed briefly, governing glucagon secretion tissue demands.

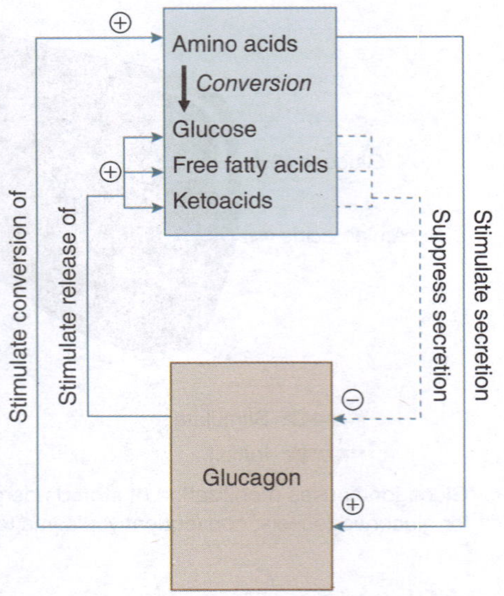

Fig. 8.6.18 Feedback relationship between glucagon and nutrients. Glucagon stimulates production and release of glucose, free fatty acids and ketoacids, which in turn suppress glucagon secretion, and glucagon in turn stimulates the conversion of amino acids to glucose.

1. Blood glucose level It affects glucagon secretion as follows:

Low blood glucose concentration is the most potent stimulus for secretion of glucagon. Hypoglycaemia causes a two- to four-fold increase in plasma levels of glucagon which acts to increase circulating glucose levels (Fig. 8.6.18). Glucagon secretion by α-cells increases even when blood sugar falls to just below 70 mg% (normal range 70–110 mg%). Glucagon secretion is stimulated much more by low glucose levels if insulin is absent. ***High blood glucose concentration*** inhibits glucagon secretion (Fig. 8.6.18). Hyperglycaemia lowers glucagon secretion by 50%. The presence of insulin greatly potentiates the suppressive effect of high glucose levels on α-cells.

Important Note

The pancreatic β-cells also contain GABA; it is suggested that hyperglycaemia induces insulin secretion as well as releases GABA; GABA in turn acts paracrinally on α-cells by activating $GABA_A$ receptors and inhibits glucagon secretion. The $GABA_A$ receptors are Cl^- channels; their activation causes Cl^- influx leading to hyperpolarization of α-cells.

Secretory pattern of glucagon in response to blood glucose levels is just opposite to that of insulin. Therefore, during starvation, glucagon secretion increases while that of insulin decreases, and conversely, after a carbohydrate-rich meal, glucagon secretion decreases while that of insulin increases.

2. Plasma amino acids Secretion of glucagon is increased by a protein-rich meal and, most effectively, by amino acids such as arginine and alanine. Since the amino acids increase insulin secretion also, the simultaneous release of glucagon along with insulin prevents the risk of hypoglycaemia, which otherwise would occur after a high-protein meal.

There exists a feedback relationship, i.e. amino acids stimulate glucagon secretion, and glucagon in turn stimulates the conversion of amino acids to glucose (Fig. 8.6.18).

3. Free fatty acids and ketoacids Glucagon stimulates production and release of FFAs and ketoacids, which in turn suppress glucagon secretion, i.e. there is a feedback relationship (Fig. 8.6.18).

II. Role of gastrointestinal hormones GT hormones such as CCK, gastrin and GIP increase glucagon secretion. This accounts for the enhanced glucagon response to orally ingested nutrients as opposed to the responses to intravenously delivered nutrients.

III. Role of nervous system *Sympathetic nerve stimulation* to pancreas increases glucagon secretion. The effect is mediated via β-adrenergic receptors and cAMP. Various stresses, fasting, exercise and infection increase the glucagon secretion in part by their stimulatory effect on sympathetic nervous system and partly by release of glucocorticoids.

- Vagal stimulation and ACh also acutely increase glucagon secretion.
- Neurohormone somatostatin inhibits the secretion of glucagon, probably by paracrine or neurocrine effects made possible by the islet microarchitecture.

The principle factors affecting glucagon secretion are summarized in Table 8.6.5.

HORMONAL REGULATION OF BLOOD GLUCOSE LEVEL

Normal Blood Glucose Levels and Body Glucose Reserves

Normal Blood Glucose Levels

A healthy individual is capable of maintaining the blood glucose level within a narrow range.

- Fasting blood glucose level in a postabsorptive state varies between 70 and 110 mg%.
- Postprandial blood glucose level, i.e. after a large carbohydrate meal or following oral administration of glucose in the dose of 1 g/kg body weight, the blood glucose level increases to approximately 140 mg% (<150 mg%) in a period of less than 1 hour. However, a prompt increase in insulin secretion brings it back to baseline value within 2 hours. This response to oral administration of carbohydrate, when

Table 8.6.5 Factors affecting glucagon secretion

Stimulators	Inhibitors
• Hypoglycaemia	• Insulin • Hyperglycaemia
• Glucogenic amino acids, alanine, serine, glycine, cysteine and threonine	• Neurohormones (somatostatins)
• GIT hormones (CCK, gastrin, GIP)	• Secretin
• Stresses: infection, exercise, cortisol, β-adrenergic stimulator, acetylcholine	• FFA, ketoacids
	• GABA, α-adrenergics, phenytoin

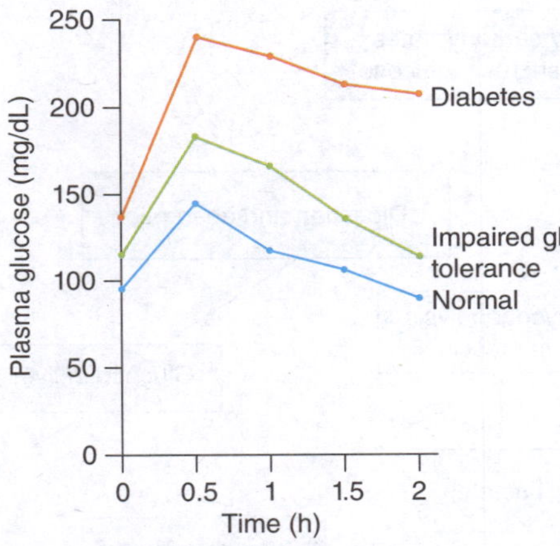

Fig. 8.6.19 Glucose tolerance curve.

plotted on a time scale, is called *glucose tolerance curve* (Fig. 8.6.19) and is used clinically as a test to study the maintenance of blood glucose levels.

Normal Body Reserves of Glucose

Free glucose is carbohydrate currency of the body. Approximately 18 g of free glucose is present in an adult human body. This amount is just sufficient to meet the basal energy requirements of the body for 1 hour.

Stored glucose is present in the form of glycogen in liver and muscles.

Liver has approximately 100 g stored glycogen. An adult liver (weighing approximately 1.5 kg) can provide only 40–50 g of blood glucose from glycogen that can last only for a few hours to meet the body requirement. However, liver is also capable of producing approximately 125–150 mg glucose/min or 180–220 g/2 h. Therefore, during an overnight fast, the glycogen stores of liver are not totally noncarbohydrate sources (gluconeogenesis).

Muscle glycogen store is much more than of liver. However, degradation of glycogen in muscle does not directly produce glucose but produces lactate which is used for gluconeogenesis.

Sources and Utilization of Blood Glucose

Sources of Blood Glucose (Fig. 8.6.20)

1. ***Dietary sources:*** The dietary carbohydrates are digested and absorbed as monosaccharides (glucose, fructose, galactose, etc.). The liver is capable of converting fructose and galactose into glucose, which can readily enter the blood.
2. ***Gluconeogenesis:*** The glucose is synthesized in the liver and kidney. Precursors for gluconeogenesis include lactate, glycerol, propionate and some amino acids.
   - Lactate is formed by degradation of glycogen stored in the muscle.
   - Free glycerol and propionate are formed by breakdown of fat in adipose tissue.
   - Amino acids may be derived from dietary sources or from protein breakdown.
3. ***Glycogenolysis:*** Stored glycogen in liver is degraded to glucose, while muscle glycogen after degradation produces lactate which is used for gluconeogenesis as described above.

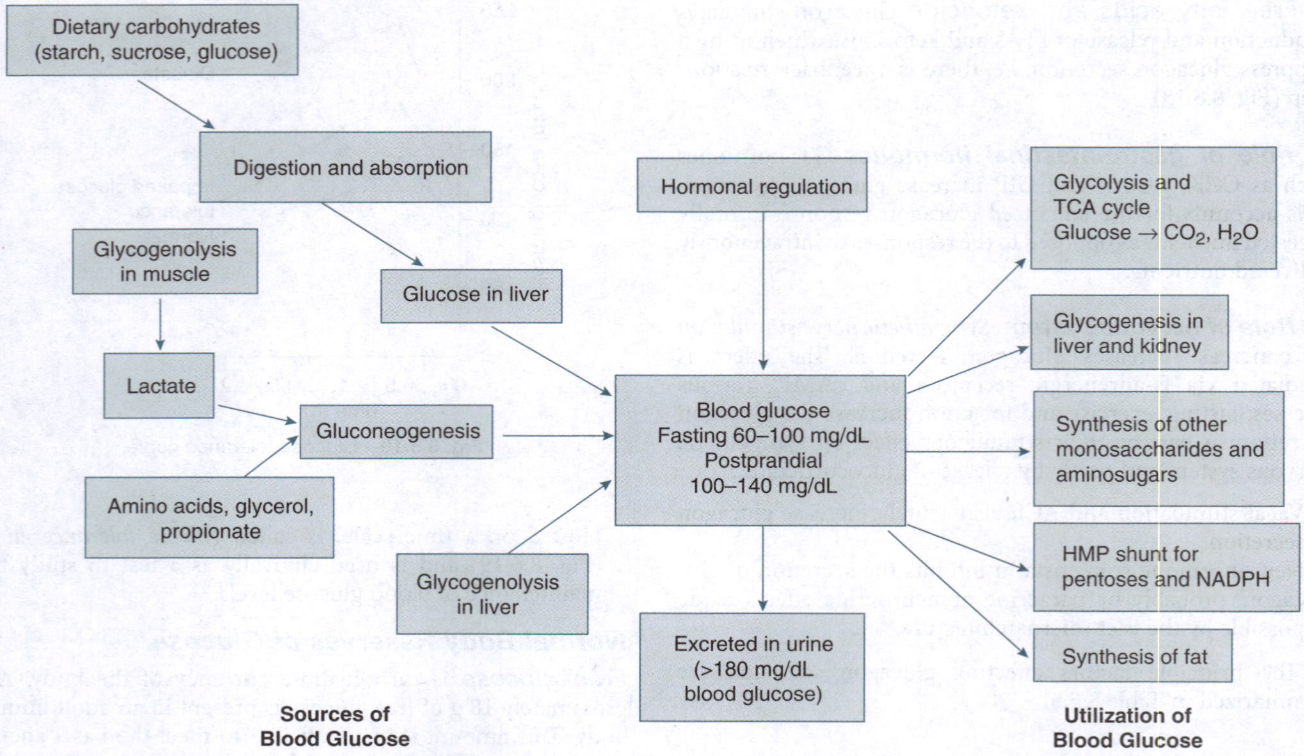

Fig. 8.6.20 Sources and utilization of glucose.

Utilization of Blood Glucose

The glucose present in the blood is utilized for:

1. ***Provision of energy needs to body tissues:*** The oxidative pathways in which glucose is used include:
   - Glycolysis and tricarboxylic acid (TCA) cycle
   - HMP shunt for pentoses and NADPH
   - Uronic acid pathway
2. ***Glycogenesis***, i.e. synthesis of glycogen in liver and kidney
3. ***Synthesis of other monosaccharides and amino sugar***
4. ***Synthesis of fat***

Role of Hormones in Regulation of Blood Glucose

Under normal circumstances, various hormones play a significant role in maintaining the blood glucose levels within normal physiological range. This is accomplished by preventing the occurrence of hyperglycaemia and hypoglycaemia.

Prevention of occurrence of hyperglycaemia The occurrence of hyperglycaemia after a pure carbohydrate load or a mixed meal in a healthy individual is prevented by a manifold (four to five times) increase in insulin secretion. Insulin normalizes the blood glucose levels by:

- Increasing uptake and utilization as chief fuel in the muscles
- Promoting storage of glucose as glycogen in liver and as triglycerides in the adipose tissue
- Decreasing glucose production by inhibiting gluconeogenesis and glycogenolysis (for details, see the section 'Actions of Insulin' on page 759)

Prevention of occurrence of hypoglycaemia Hypoglycaemia, which may occur due to fasting or prolonged exercise, is prevented in a healthy individual by a number of hormones, which include glucagon, epinephrine, growth hormone and glucocorticoids. It is obvious that there is only one hormone, insulin, which prevents hyperglycaemia, whereas at least four hormones are available for prevention of hypoglycaemia. This may be correlated with the fact that moderate and transient hyperglycaemia is harmless and occurs after every meal. However, even moderate hypoglycaemia may lead to serious complications. The brain, retina and germinal epithelium of the gonads are particularly vulnerable to the effects of hypoglycaemia, since they cannot use any fuel other than glucose.

The roles played by different hormones in preventing hypoglycaemia are described:

1. ***Role of glucagon:*** During normal pattern of food intake (consisting of two to three meals per day), in between the meals when glucose level tends to decrease, the insulin secretion stops and instead glucagon is poured into the bloodstream under these circumstances.
   - Glucagon promotes hepatic glycogenolysis and gluconeogenesis and, thus, glucose is poured into the circulation from the liver (Fig. 8.6.20).
   - At the same time, due to absence of insulin, glucose utilization by muscles is stopped and instead lipolysis in adipose tissue is promoted, and therefore FFAs become the chief fuel for muscles.
2. ***Role of epinephrine:*** When starvation period further increases (say many hours), even in the presence of glucagon, blood glucose levels begin to fall. The resulting hypoglycaemia stimulates the sympathetic nervous system through hypothalamus to promote the release of epinephrine from the adrenal medulla. Epinephrine so produced:
   - Increases blood glucose by supplementing the glycogenolytic and gluconeogenic effect of glucagon

- Increases FFA production (fuel for muscles) by promoting lipolysis

3. ***Role of growth hormone and glucocorticoids:*** When starvation is more prolonged (say for a few days), along with glucagon and epinephrine, secretion of growth hormone and glucocorticoids is also increased. These hormones, in addition to promoting glycogenolysis, gluconeogenesis and lipolysis, also decrease the peripheral utilization of glucose, thereby sparing glucose for nervous tissue, especially brain.

Important Note

Somogyi phenomenon is the classical hypoglycaemia followed by rebound hyperglycaemia, and occurs when level of insulin is high leading to hypoglycaemia. The hypoglycaemia evokes a compensatory response by hyperglycaemic hormones (cortisol, growth hormone, glucagon, ACTH, thyroid and epinephrine) leading to rebound hyperglycaemia.

Dawn phenomenon is early morning hyperglycaemia due to growth hormone. It differs from Somogyi phenomenon having low levels of insulin, whereas in Somogyi phenomenon hyperglycaemia is due to compensatory response to preceding hypoglycaemia.

SOMATOSTATIN AND PANCREATIC POLYPEPTIDE

Somatostatin

Structure and synthesis Pancreatic somatostatin is a neuropeptide containing 14 amino acids, synthesized by δ-cells. It is also synthesized by intestinal cells and was originally discovered as a hypothalamic neuropeptide that inhibits growth hormone secretion.

The two forms of pancreatic somatostatin are somatostatin-14 (SS-14) and somatostatin-28 (SS-28).The half-life of somatostatin is 1–3 minutes.

Regulation of secretion Somatostatin secretion is increased after ingestion of food, because increased blood glucose, amino acids, fatty acids and GT tract hormones stimulate its secretion. Glucagon, β-adrenergic and cholinergic neurotransmitters also stimulate somatostatin secretion. Insulin and α-adrenergic neurotransmitters inhibit somatostatin secretion.

Mechanism of action Somatostatin acts through its receptors; five different types of somatostatin receptors have been identified ($SSTR_1$–$SSTR_5$). Mostly these receptors are GPCR that inhibit adenylyl cyclase activity and exert various effects.

Actions Somatostatin has the following effects:

- Acts on the islets of Langerhans and inhibits secretion of insulin and glucagon via $SSTR_5$.
- Increases the motility of stomach, duodenum and gall bladder.
- Decreases secretion of hydrochloric acid, pepsin, gastrin, secretin, intestinal juices and pancreatic juice.
- Inhibits the absorption of glucose, xylose and triglycerides across the mucosal membrane.
- *Brain:* Somatostatin is found in various parts of the brain, where it functions as a neurotransmitter with effects on sensory inputs, locomotive activity and cognitive functions (see page 1004). In hypothalamus, it is secreted into portal–hypophyseal vessel and inhibits growth hormone secretion. $SSTR_2$ mediates cognitive and growth hormone inhibition effect.

In a nutshell, actions of somatostatin along with those of insulin and glucagon probably coordinate nutrient input with substrate disposal.

Important Note

Somatostatin analogues like octreotide and lanreotide are now used therapeutically to alleviate diarrhoea caused by unregulated GIT hormone secretion. They are also employed to inhibit unregulated release of various peptides and protein hormones in conditions such as neoplasms and acromegaly.

Pancreatic Polypeptide

Structure and synthesis Pancreatic polypeptide has 36 amino acids and belongs to a family of similar molecules including neuropeptide Y in the hypothalamus and GT polypeptide Y. It is synthesized by F cells of islets of Langerhans.

Regulation of secretion Pancreatic polypeptide is secreted in response to food ingestion via GT secretagogues and cholinergic stimulation. Its secretion is also stimulated by hypoglycaemia and inhibited by glucose administration.

Actions and physiological importance Its best known action is to inhibit exocrine pancreatic secretion and slows the absorption of food in humans. Its true physiological importance is not known except that:

- Increased plasma levels of PP serve as markers for the presence of islet cell tumours and their response to treatment.
- A failure of plasma pancreatic polypeptide to increase when plasma glucose is sharply reduced suggests loss of cholinergic pancreatic islet innervation.

Applied Aspects

Important applied aspects of endocrine pancreas which need mention are as follows:

- Diabetes mellitus
- Hypoglycaemia

I. Diabetes Mellitus

Diabetes mellitus, commonly called just diabetes, refers to a clinical syndrome of hyperglycaemia occurring due to deficiency of insulin.

Types and Stages of Diabetes Mellitus

Diabetes mellitus can be classified into the following types:

1. ***Primary diabetes mellitus*** in which the cause is not known. It is of further two types:
   - *Insulin-dependent diabetes mellitus* (IDDM) or type I
   - *Noninsulin-dependent diabetes mellitus* (NIDDM) or type II
2. ***Secondary diabetes mellitus:*** It is associated with certain pathological conditions such as pancreatitis, cystic fibrosis, acromegaly and Cushing syndrome.

Stages in the development of diabetes mellitus:

- *Prediabetics or potential diabetics:* These are the persons with normal blood glucose level but are potential candidates to develop diabetes due to strong genetic predispositions, e.g. first-degree relatives of diabetics.

- *Latent diabetics and chemical diabetics:* These persons have normal fasting and postprandial blood glucose levels and normal glucose tolerance test (GTT). But their blood glucose becomes abnormally high during stress or after administration of glucocorticoids.
- *Clinical diabetics:* They have hyperglycaemia, glycosuria and typical symptoms but without complications.
- *Complicated diabetics:* These are the patients with long-standing neglected diabetes with multiple complications.

Insulin-Dependent Diabetes Mellitus or Type I

- IDDM, or type I diabetes, is considered an autoimmune disorder in which antibodies destroy the β-cells of islets causing an absolute deficiency of insulin.
- Genetic susceptibility is a major determinant while environmental factors act as a trigger.
- The current view regarding type I diabetes is that this is a T-cell–mediated disease. The main genetic abnormality is in major histocompatibility complex (MHC) gene located on chromosome 6, though other genes are also involved.

Characteristic features of IDDM:

- It manifests before 40 years of age (usually between 12 and 15 years) and is also called juvenile-onset diabetes. It accounts for 5%–10% of cases of diabetes.
- Patients are usually lean.
- Classical triad of presenting symptoms consisting of polyuria, polydipsia and polyphagia is associated with weight loss.
- Ketosis and acidosis are common complications of this diabetes mellitus.
- Plasma insulin levels are very low or undetectable.

Noninsulin-Dependent Diabetes Mellitus or Type II. NIDDM or type II diabetes is also a genetic disorder. Overeating coupled with underactivity leading to obesity acts as a diabetogenic factor in genetically predisposed individuals. It is supposed to occur due to decrease in insulin receptors on the insulin-responsive (target) cells.

In type II diabetes, the genetic component is stronger compared to that in type I. Defects in individual genes have been identified; these include defect in glucokinase (1% of cases), insulin molecule (0.5% of cases), insulin receptors (1% of cases), GLUT-4 (1% of cases) and insulin receptor-1 (15% of cases), but the actual genes involved are still not known.

Characteristic features of NIDDM:

- It manifests after 40 years of age and so is also called *adult-onset diabetes or maturity-onset diabetes in young (MODY)*.
- It is most common and accounts for 80%–90% of diabetic population.
- Most of the patients are obese.
- Symptoms begin gradually and may be ignored and many a time diagnosis is made on urine examination which shows glycosuria.
- Plasma insulin levels are often normal or even elevated.
- Ketoacidosis is not very common.

Obesity (the Metabolic Syndrome). The incidence of obesity is increasing; it relates to the discrepancy between energy consumption and energy expenditure. The risk of type II diabetes increases 10-fold with body mass index (BMI) >30 kg/m^2 (normal BMI 18.5–24.9 kg/m^2). The susceptibility to obesity and its adverse consequences vary. Metabolic syndrome is mainly a glucose metabolism disorder; therefore, it has special relation with diabetes mellitus. As the body weight increases, there is increase in insulin resistance leading to decreasing ability of insulin to move glucose into muscle and adipose tissues, and glucose release from liver. Hence, obesity is associated with hyperinsulinaemia, dyslipidaemia (increased level of circulating triglycerides and HDL) and development of atherosclerosis. The combination of these findings is commonly referred to as metabolic syndrome or syndrome X. The patients with this syndrome may present as prediabetic or full-fledged type II diabetes.

IDDM versus NIDDM. The comparison between IDDM and NIDDM is given in Table 8.6.6.

Pathophysiology of Diabetes Mellitus

Pathophysiology of diabetes mellitus revolves around the metabolic alterations associated with insulin deficiency. Most important among them are hyperglycaemia, ketoacidosis, hypertriglyceridaemia and protein catabolism (Fig. 8.6.21).

1. Hyperglycaemia and its Consequences. Hyperglycaemia (elevation of blood glucose concentration) is the characteristic feature of uncontrolled diabetes mellitus. It occurs due to lack of insulin resulting in:

- Decreased peripheral utilization of glucose
- Increased hepatic output of glucose (owing to glycogenolysis and gluconeogenesis) into the circulation

Consequences of hyperglycaemia:

- Glycosuria and its consequences
- Impaired phagocytic function
- Hyperosmolar effects
- Glycosylation of haemoglobin

i. Glycosuria and its consequences

Glycosuria, i.e. excretion of glucose into the urine, occurs when the blood glucose level rises above the renal threshold point, i.e. above 180 mg/100 mL.

Polyuria refers to the passage of large amount of urine frequently. It is the result of osmotic diuresis caused by renal excretion of osmotically active glucose molecules.

Loss of electrolytes (sodium, potassium and phosphate) in urine also occurs as a side effect of osmotic diuresis.

Cellular dehydration: High glucose concentration increases osmotic pressure of extracellular fluid and osmotic transfer of water from cells to extracellular fluid leading to dehydration of cells. In addition to it, osmotic diuresis causes increased loss of water from the body, thereby reducing extracellular fluid volume which also causes compensatory dehydration of cells.

Polydipsia, i.e. excessive drinking of water, results from activation of thirst mechanism caused by cellular dehydration.

Increased caloric loss is the result of loss of glucose in urine.

Polyphagia, i.e. excessive eating, occurs due to stimulation of satiety centre caused by deficient utilization of glucose in the hypothalamic ventromedial nuclei. Increased caloric loss also results in compensatory polyphagia.

Loss of body weight occurs because of loss of calories in the urine and mobilization of fats and proteins for energy production. Since loss of body weight occurs in spite of excessive food intake, diabetes is called a *condition of starvation in the midst of plenty*.

ii. Impaired phagocytic function

Hyperglycaemia impairs all aspects of leucocytic phagocytic function, i.e. adherence, diapedesis, phagocytosis and

Table 8.6.6 IDDM versus NIDDM

Feature	IDDM	NIDDM
General features		
Defect	Insulin deficiency due to β-cell destruction	Resistance of target tissues to insulin
Prevalence	10%–20% of diabetic population	80%–90% of diabetic population
Age of onset	<40 years	>40 years
Body weight	Low (thin and lean)	High (obese or normal)
Gene locus	Chromosome 6	Chromosome 1
Family history	Mild or moderate	Very strong
Clinical features		
Duration of symptoms	Weeks (rapid)	Months to year (slow)
Presenting symptoms	Polyuria, polydipsia, polyphagia	Usually patients present with different complications
Complication at the time of diagnosis	Absent	Present (in 10%–20% of cases)
Acute complication	Ketoacidosis	Hyperosmolar coma
Biochemical features		
Plasma insulin	Decreased or absent	Normal or increased
Autoantibodies	Frequently found	Rare
Ketonuria	Present	Absent
Treatment		
Treatment of choice	Insulin (oral hypoglycaemics not useful)	Oral hypoglycaemics (insulin usually not required)
Mortality if not treated	High	Low

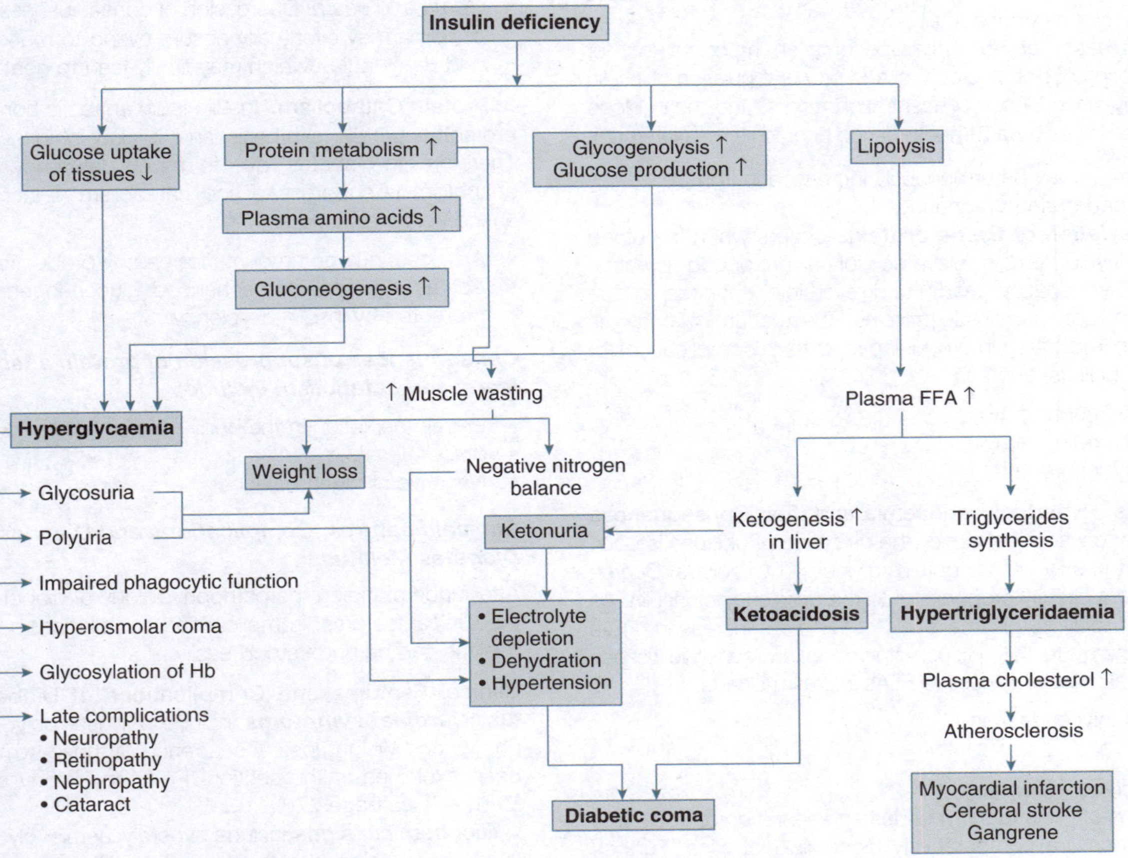

Fig. 8.6.21 Pathophysiology of diabetes mellitus and its complications.

intracellular killing. Because of impaired phagocytic function, diabetics are more prone to infections compared with the nondiabetics.

iii. Hyperosmolar effects

Osmolarity of the blood goes on increasing with the increasing blood sugar levels. With the passage of time, a stage may come when glucose production is increased and urinary excretion is decreased, and the plasma glucose level may increase up to 1000 mg%. Under such circumstances, the plasma osmolality may be over 375 mOsm/kg. Such a high hyperosmolality may cause dehydration in central nervous system leading to impairment of cerebral functions. Ultimately, a condition called nonketotic hyperosmolar coma may result, which may be even fatal.

iv. Glycosylation of proteins

Glycosylation of proteins refers to post-translation, nonenzymatic addition of sugar residues to amino acids of proteins.

Glycosylation of haemoglobin: Glycosylated haemoglobin refers to the glucose-derived products of normal haemoglobin (haemoglobin A [HbA]). Among the glycosylated haemoglobins, the most abundant form is HbA_{1C}, which is produced by condensation of glucose with N-terminal valine of each β-chain of HbA.

- *The rate of production of HbA_{1C}* is directly related to the exposure of RBC to glucose. Thus, the concentration of HbA_{1C} serves as an indicator of the blood glucose concentration over a period equal approximately to half-life of RBC haemoglobin (i.e. 6–8 weeks).
- *Normally, HbA_{1C}* concentration is approximately 3%–5% of the total haemoglobin.
- *During sustained hyperglycaemia*, as in diabetes mellitus, the concentration of HbA_{1C} may be elevated to 10%–20% of the total haemoglobin.
- *Determination of HbA_{1C}* has become an important tool for monitoring of diabetes control and proper regulation of insulin therapy since HbA_{1C} concentration reflects the mean blood glucose level over a 2-month period prior to its measurement.

Note. HbA_{1C} may be erroneously increased in iron-deficiency anaemia and during pregnancy.

Glycosylation of tissue proteins occurs when the blood glucose levels remain elevated for a prolonged duration (years). Glycosylation leads to irreversible changes in the chemical structure of tissue proteins. These chemical changes have been implicated in producing long-term complications of diabetes mellitus, such as:

- Diabetic nephropathy
- Diabetic retinopathy
- Diabetic neuropathy

2. Ketosis, Hypertriglyceridaemia and their Consequences

Since due to insulin deficiency the utilization of glucose is poor, the body turns to fats for obtaining energy by lipolysis. Degree of lipolysis is directly proportional to the deficiency of insulin. As a result of lipolysis, plasma levels of FFAs are increased. FFAs provide energy to the glucose-starved insulin-sensitive tissues like skeletal muscle. Excessive FFAs in plasma leads to:

- Hypertriglyceridaemia
- Ketosis

Hypertriglyceridaemia

Conversion of FFAs to triglycerides and secretion of VLDL and chylomicrons are comparatively higher in diabetics. Further, the activity of enzyme lipoprotein lipase is low in diabetic patients. Consequently, the plasma levels of VLDL, and chylomicrons and triglycerides are increased. Hypercholesterolaemia is also frequently seen in diabetics.

Ketosis

Utilization of fats beyond a certain point in the face of impaired carbohydrate utilization leads to formation of ketone bodies in excess. Ketone bodies act as metabolic fuel in the liver. If production of ketone bodies is more than their destruction, there occurs *ketosis* or *ketonaemia*.

Consequences of ketosis:

- *Cellular dehydration:* Ketone bodies being hyperosmolar remove water from the cells producing cellular dehydration.
- *Ketoacidosis:* Ketone bodies being strong acids dissociate readily and release H^+ ions. In the blood, these H^+ ions are buffered by bicarbonate ions (HCO_3^-) to form carbonic acid. Fall in bicarbonate level in blood leads to acidosis called ketoacidosis. Ketoacidosis develops rapidly in IDDM due to an absolute lack of insulin. This is not commonly seen in NIDDM where there is partial or no loss of insulin (but there is insulin resistance).

Features of ketoacidosis:

- Rapid, deep respiration (dyspnoea, Kussmaul breathing).
- Acetone smell in patient's breath.
- Urine becomes highly acidic.
- *Electrolyte loss:* When capacity of kidney to replace plasma cations accompanying the organic anions with H^+ and NH_4^+ is exceeded, Na^+ and K^+ are lost in the urine. The electrolyte and water loss further adds to cellular dehydration.
- *Hypovolaemia and hypotension:* These may ultimately result from water and electrolytic loss and cellular dehydration.
- *Coma and death:* Depression of consciousness to the level of coma may eventually ensure owing to marked acidosis and dehydration which may finally lead to death.

3. Protein Catabolism. Insulin is an anabolic hormone, i.e. it promotes protein synthesis and it also inhibits proteolysis. Therefore, in diabetes, due to insulin deficiency, the protein anabolism is suppressed and catabolism is increased. The amino acids released so:

- Are used in large amounts for energy production
- Act as substrate for enhanced gluconeogenesis in liver promoted by insulin deficiency

Consequences of suppression of protein anabolism and increased catabolism include:

- Protein depletion in the body
- Muscle wasting
- Negative nitrogen balance

Clinical Features, Complications and Diagnosis of Diabetes Mellitus

After understanding the pathophysiology of diabetes mellitus, the clinical features, complications and diagnosis of diabetes mellitus can be understood easily.

Clinical Features and Complications of Diabetes Mellitus. ***Cardinal symptoms*** include polyuria, polydipsia, polyphagia and weight loss. Occurrence of these symptoms has been explained in the section 'Pathophysiology of Diabetes Mellitus' (see page 770).

Biochemical signs include hyperglycaemia, glycosuria, ketosis, ketonuria and ketoacidosis. These have been fully elucidated in the section 'Pathophysiology of Diabetes Mellitus'.

Complications include:

Predisposition to infections due to impaired phagocytic function and protein depletion.

Acute complications include ketotic coma and nonketotic hyperosmolar coma (for details, see the section 'Pathophysiology of Diabetes Mellitus', see page 770).

Chronic complications include:

Atherosclerosis, i.e. deposition of lipids underneath the tunica intima of blood vessels. The common sites are coronary, cerebral and peripheral arteries. It occurs due to long-standing hyperlipidaemia and hypercholesterolaemia.

Microangiopathy, a vascular lesion in which the capillary basement membrane is thicker, probably due to structural changes caused in tissue proteins by their glycosylation. It is responsible for common complications of long-standing diabetes, which include:

Diabetic retinopathy leading to blindness.

Diabetic nephropathy leading to renal failure.

Diabetic neuropathy involves autonomic nervous system and peripheral nerves. Prolonged neuropathy and vasculopathy results in nonhealing of trivial injuries of the foot, ultimately leading to ulceration and gangrene known as diabetic foot.

Diagnosis of Diabetes Mellitus. In clinically suspected cases, diagnosis is confirmed by the following investigations:

1. Urine examination for glycosuria

This is a rapid, simple and easy test for diagnosis of diabetes mellitus. Amount of glucose excreted in urine depends on the severity of disease.

Disadvantage: Glycosuria depends on the renal threshold level which itself is variable; hence, both overdiagnosis (false-positive) and underdiagnosis (false-negative) of diabetes are possible. For example, a nondiabetic individual with low renal threshold may pass glucose in the urine (renal glycosuria), while a diabetic with raised renal threshold will have a negative urine test for glucose.

2. Urine examination for ketone bodies

Presence of ketone bodies (acetone) in urine along with glycosuria is almost diagnostic of diabetes mellitus. Other causes of ketonuria are starvation, prolonged fasting, following high-fat diet and after repeated vomiting.

3. Fasting and postprandial blood glucose levels

Samples for estimation of fasting blood glucose are taken after overnight fast and those for postprandial are taken after 2 hours of normal diet.

Normal values of plasma glucose are as follows:

- Fasting: 70–110 mg%
- Postprandial (after 2 hours of meals): <140 mg%

4. Glucose tolerance test

To perform this test, the patient is advised to have normal (unrestricted) carbohydrate diet at least 3 days prior to test. In the early morning, after an overnight fast, the fasting samples of blood and urine are taken. Then 75.0 g of glucose dissolved in 300 mL (a glass) of water is given orally, and blood and urine samples are collected every half an hour for 2.5–3 hours. Plasma glucose levels are plotted against the time scale and the graph so obtained is known as glucose tolerance curve. The results are interpreted as follows (Table 8.6.7):

Table 8.6.7 Interpretation of results of glucose tolerance test

	Plasma glucose concentration (mg%)		
	Normal	Impaired glucose tolerance	Diabetes mellitus
Fasting level	<110	110–126	≥126
Peak postprandial level	<140	>140 to <200	≥200

In a normal person, fasting plasma glucose levels range between 70 and 110 mg%, after glucose intake. The peak value of approximately 140 mg% is reached in an hour or so which returns to fasting level within 2–2.5 hours (Fig. 8.6.19). Urine does not show the presence of glucose.

In diabetes mellitus, glucose tolerance curve is abnormal. Fasting glucose level is high (≥126 mg%) after glucose intake peak is also high (≥200 mg%), and does not return to fasting level for a long time (4–6 hours) (Fig. 8.6.19). This slow fall of glucose level indicates failure to control due to lack of insulin secretion following sugar ingestion.

Impaired glucose tolerance: The fasting plasma levels between 110 and 126 mg% and peak values (after glucose ingestion) between 140 and 200 mg% are classified as impaired glucose tolerance (Fig. 8.6.19). Such patients are potential candidates to develop diabetes later on. Therefore, they need further supervision and repeated blood sugar estimations at frequent intervals to detect development of diabetes mellitus.

Glycosylated haemoglobin: The rate of formation of HbA_{1C} is directly proportional to ambient blood glucose concentration; a rise of 1% HbA_{1C} fraction indicates an average increase of 2 mmol/L (36 g%) plasma glucose. For details, see page 143.

Management of Diabetes Mellitus

Goals of therapy

Goals of therapy of diabetes mellitus, irrespective of the type of diabetes, are as follows:

- To maintain blood glucose to normal or near normal
- To maintain ideal body weight as far as possible
- To keep the patient symptom-free
- To prevent or retard the onset of complications

Treatment modalities

Patients with type II diabetes mellitus are initially treated with diet and exercise.

1. ***Dietary management*** may be required alone or in association with drug therapy.

   Total energy intake should be specified to keep ideal body weight:

   - *Low-energy and weight-reducing diet* is recommended for obese patients with NIDDM.
   - *Weight maintenance diet* is prescribed to nonobese patients with NIDDM.

   Dietary constituents recommended for allocation of calories are as follows:

• Carbohydrates	50%–60% of calories
• Proteins	10%–15% of calories
• Fats	30%–35% of calories
• Vitamins and minerals	Adequate

   Frequent small meals should be advised to prevent glycaemic peaks and troughs.

2. ***Exercise*** lowers blood glucose level by activation of cAMP kinase pathway that mediates insertion of GLUT-4 in the skeletal muscles. If these measures are not sufficient to control hyperglycaemia, then:
3. ***Oral antihyperglycaemic drugs,*** injectable glucagon-like peptide-1 (GLP-1) receptor agonists, insulin or combinations of these drugs are prescribed.

   Oral hypoglycaemic agents (OHA) includes:
   - *Biguanides* act by decreasing hepatic gluconeogenesis and release of the entry of glucose in muscles and adipose tissue by stimulation of GLUT-1 transporter.
   - *Sulphonylurea* acts on sulphonylurea receptors present on the membrane of β-cells, leading to depolarization of the membrane by decreasing conductance of ATP-sensitive K^+ channels, resulting in Ca^{2+} influx, thus increasing insulin secretion.
   - *Meglitinide* is used to control postprandial hyperglycaemia by acting on sulphonylurea receptors.
   - *Thiazolidinediones* stimulate transcription of insulin-responsive genes, which causes expression and translocation of GLUT-4, thus lowering blood glucose level.
   - *Glucosidase inhibitors* ***(Acarbose)*** cause inhibition of enzyme α-glucosidase resulting in decreased breakdown, digestion and absorption of polysaccharides.
   - *Dipeptidyl-4 (DDP-4)* inhibitors inactivate GLP-1 and GIP which potentiate insulin secretion from β-cells and inhibit glucagon release from α-cells of pancreas.
4. ***Insulin along with dietary management:*** Insulin is delivered by injections with a very fine and sharp needle.

   Indications of insulin use include:
   - All patients with IDDM (juvenile-onset diabetes)
   - Newly detected diabetes with ketoacidosis
   - Emergencies associated with IDDM and NIDDM
   - Patients with NIDDM not controlled by OHA

   Types of insulin: Three types of insulin preparations (ultrashort, short acting and long acting) are commercially available (Table 8.6.8).
   - *Conventional insulin* is prepared from the pancreas of beef or pork. The preparations include regular insulin, isophane and protamine zinc insulin (PZI).
   - *Recombinant insulin* is highly purified form of insulin produced by recombinant DNA technology in *E. coli* and yeast. It has higher stability and used to treat diabetics who are allergic to conventional insulin.
   - *Insulin analogues* include lispro insulin, aspartate insulin and glulisine insulin.

   Regimens of insulin therapy include:
   - *Conventional regimen* (single or two injections daily).
   - *Multiple subcutaneous injection regimen* (three to four injections daily covering the major meals and snacks).
   - Continuous subcutaneous insulin is delivered by insulin pump.

Table 8.6.8 Type of insulin

	Type of insulin	Available as (name)	Action period
1	Ultra-short acting	• Lispro insulin • Aspart insulin • Insulin glulisine	• Acts within 30 min • Peak occurs at 1–2 h • Effect lasts for 2–5 h
2	Short acting	• Regular insulin	• Acts within 1–7.5 h • Peak occurs in 2–4 h • Effect lasts for 6–8 h
3	Long acting	• Protamine zinc insulin • Insulin glargine	• Action starts within 1–2 h of administration • Peak occurs in 8–10 h • Effect lasts for 20–24 h
4	Long acting	• Protaminc zinc insulin • Insulin glargine	• Action starts within 4–6 h of administration • Peak occurs in 14–20 h • Effect lasts for 20–36 h

Awareness

It is essential to educate the patients to understand the disorder and learn to handle all aspects of their management comprehensively. Ideally, this can be achieved by multidisciplinary team of doctor, dietician and nurse in the outpatient department.

- Patients requiring insulin need to learn how to measure dose of insulin accurately with insulin syringe or pen, how to inject and how to adjust the dose of blood glucose level.
- Patients on insulin or on OHA should carry a card stating name, address, type of insulin/or antidiabetic drugs and their doses, and name and address details of treating physician.
- Self-assessment of glycaemic control particularly in patients with IDDM treated with insulin should be taught to perform capillary blood glucose measurements.
- Lifestyle advice should be recommended to type II diabetics to reduce the risk of progression.

Gestational Diabetes. During pregnancy, maternal glucose metabolism changes to meet nutritional demand of developing fetus. In second trimester of pregnancy, insulin resistance decreases and at the same time renal threshold for glucose lowers.

The risk factors include obesity and family history of type II diabetes.

- Gestational diabetes develops when pancreas is unable to secrete insulin to compensate insulin resistance.
- During pregnancy, placental hormones impair the action of insulin on body tissue, thus causing hyperglycaemia.
- The extra amount of glucose is transferred to the fetus through placenta and activates fetal pancreas to secrete more insulin. Excess insulin in fetus leads to macrosomia (baby to grow big size), characterized by increased tissue fat, hypoglycaemia and jaundice.

Treatment includes the following: strict glycaemic control is required by dietary modification, particularly reducing consumption of refined carbohydrates.

In patients with established diabetes, during pregnancy:

- Insulin doses must be increased.
- Monitoring is very essential which includes:
  - Frequent estimation of blood glucose including postprandial measurements
  - HbA_{1C}
  - Checks of blood glucose periodically during night
- Regular monitoring of fetus size and screening of fetal abnormalities.

ii. Hypoglycaemia

Hypoglycaemia refers to a clinical condition caused by blood glucose levels below 45 mg% (2.5 mmol/L). The human body has developed a well-regulated system for an efficient maintenance of blood glucose concentration (see the section 'Hormonal Regulation of Blood Glucose Level', page 766). However, still hypoglycaemia (though not common) is observed under some circumstances.

Types and Causes of Hypoglycaemia

Broadly, hypoglycaemia may be divided into two types:

- Hypoglycaemia in nondiabetics
- Hypoglycaemia in diabetics (more common)

A. Hypoglycaemia in Nondiabetics

1. ***Postprandial hypoglycaemia,*** also known as *reactive hypoglycaemia*, occurs typically after meals within 4 hours after ingestion of food. It is caused by transient rise in insulin levels, and symptoms are short lasting. It is more common in patients who have undergone gastric resection. In such patients, rapid movement of swallowed food into the intestine leads to sudden and marked increase in insulin secretion. The patients are advised to eat frequently rather than the three usual meals.
2. ***Postabsorption or fasting hypoglycaemia*** usually does not occur in normal fasting patients. It is seen in patients with:
   - *Insulin-secreting tumours* (adenomas) of pancreatic islets causing *hyperinsulinism, which* is a rare condition. Some adenomas (15%) may be malignant.
   - In some malignant tumours which do not involve pancreatic islets but hypoglycaemia occurs because of increased secretion of IGF-II.
   - *In hepatic failure*, degradation of insulin is less which may result in raised levels of insulin and hypoglycaemia.
   - Hypoglycaemia also occurs in hyperthyroidism and patients who have undergone gastrectomy. Gastrectomy leads to rapid passage of food into the intestine resulting in rapid absorption of glucose, though the plasma glucose level rises rapidly but is followed by a rapid fall (hypoglycaemia) due to rise in insulin secretion.
3. ***Hypoglycaemia due to alcohol intake:*** In some individuals who are starved or engaged in prolonged exercise, alcohol consumption may cause hypoglycaemia due to decreased gluconeogenesis.

B. Hypoglycaemia in Diabetics. Hypoglycaemia in diabetics is more common than in nondiabetics. Approximately 4% of deaths of IDDM are said to be due to hypoglycaemia.

Causes of hypoglycaemia in diabetics include:

- Overdose of antidiabetic drugs, especially insulin, is comparatively a common cause of hypoglycaemia. This occurs due to difficulty in adjusting the requirement of antidiabetic agents. This is particularly observed in patients who are on an intensive treatment regimen.

Other factors responsible for hypoglycaemia in patients on regular antidiabetic treatment:

- Intake of too little or no food
- Heavy exercise
- Mismatch between insulin administration and food habits
- Alcohol intake, etc.

Symptoms and Signs of Hypoglycaemia

Symptoms and signs of hypoglycaemia occur due to effects of low levels of glucose per se (mainly on nervous system, especially brain) and because of sympathetic stimulation (mainly on CVS, GIT and skin).

1. ***CNS*** symptoms are called ***neuroglycopaenic symptoms***. Since metabolism of brain mainly depends on blood glucose level, it is depressed when glucose level falls below 50–70 mg%. CNS becomes quite excitable (due to facilitation of neuronal activity by hypoglycaemia) which results in hallucinations, extreme nervousness, tremors, confusion, difficulty in concentration, incoordination, convulsions, drowsiness and cognitive dysfunctions. When blood glucose levels fall further (<30 mg%), hypoglycaemic coma may develop, which needs to be differentiated from hyperglycaemic coma in diabetics (Table 8.6.9), and needs an emergency treatment by immediate administration of large quantity of glucose intravenously.
2. ***CVS symptoms*** in hypoglycaemia are palpitation, tachycardia and cardiac arrhythmias.
3. ***GIT symptoms*** include nausea and vomiting.
4. ***Skin symptoms*** are sweating and hypothermia.

Table 8.6.9 Hypoglycaemic versus hyperglycaemic coma in diabetics

S. no.	Feature	Hypoglycaemic coma	Hyperglycaemic coma
1.	*Cause*	Regular dose of insulin and no food leading to fall in blood glucose level	Too little or no insulin with regular food intake leading to high blood glucose level
2.	*Precipitating factor*	Severe unaccustomed exercise	Untreated/hidden infection
3.	*Rate of onset*	Rapid, develops within minutes	Invariably slow, takes hours or days to develop
4.	*Symptoms and signs*		
	• Vomiting	• No or occasional vomiting	• Frequent vomiting with abdominal pain
	• Breathing	• Laboured breathing	• Rapid and shallow breathing (Kussmaul)
		• No abnormal smell in breath	• Air hunger present
	• Pulse	• Bounding	• Weak/feeble
	• Skin and tongue	• Moist as no dehydration	• Dry due to dehydration
	• CNS sign	• Tendon reflexes brisk	• Diminished
		• Plantar is extensor	• Plantar is normal (flexor)
5.	*Investigations*		
	i) Urine	• No glucose	• Glycosuria marked
		• No ketone bodies	• Ketonuria marked
	ii) Blood	• Low blood glucose (usually <30 mg%)	• High blood glucose (usually >400 mg%)
		• Bicarbonate level normal	• Low bicarbonate
		• pH normal	• Low pH

Management

Treatment of acute hypoglycaemia depends on its severity and whether the patient is conscious and able to swallow. The emergency treatment of hypoglycaemia includes:

In mild cases: The subject can be self-treated by fast-acting oral carbohydrate (10–15 g) taken as glucose drink or tablet followed by snack containing complex carbohydrates.

In severe cases: External help is required. If the patient is semiconscious/unconscious, parenteral treatment is required as follows:

- Intravenous 75 mL 20% dextrose or intramuscular glucagon (1 mg).
- If the patient is conscious and able to swallow, give oral refined glucose as drink or sweets (25 g) or supply glucose gel/jam/honey to buccal mucosa.

Prevention of Hypoglycaemia

- Patient's education regarding potential causes and risk factors inducing hypoglycaemia, its treatment (accessible supply of glucose) and regular blood glucose monitoring is fundamental to prevent potentially diagnosed side effect of treatment.
- Relatives and friends should also need to be familiar with signs and symptoms of hypoglycaemia and also instructed as to how a situation is to be managed.

Compensatory Mechanisms to Fight Hypoglycaemia. See regulation of blood sugar level on page 768.

GASTROINTESTINAL HORMONES

The glandular cells secreting GIT hormones are individually scattered in the epithelium of stomach and small intestine and not in the form of clusters of cells as in the endocrine glands. Hence, GIT may be considered as the largest mass of cells that secretes hormones.

The GIT hormones based on their physioanatomical similarities can be broadly classified into three groups:

1. Gastrin family of hormones
2. Secretin family of hormones
3. Other GIT hormones

For details, see page 564.

Self-Assessment

1. Discuss the structure, biosynthesis, mechanism of secretion and regulation of secretion of insulin.
2. Discuss the mechanism of action and actions of insulin.
3. Describe the following:
   - Structure, synthesis, mechanism of action and actions of glucagon
   - Hormonal regulation of blood glucose maintenance
4. Discuss the pathophysiology of signs and symptoms related to diabetes mellitus.
5. Describe the pathophysiology of hypoglycaemia, its consequences and management.
6. Write Notes on:
   - Glucose tolerance test
   - Macrosomia
   - Glucose transporters
   - Glucose–glucagon ratio and its significance
   - Pancreatic polypeptide
   - Somatostatin

Clinical Cases

Case 1

A 52-year-old obese male was admitted for cataract surgery. The routine examination and investigations showed the following: BP, 160/110 mm Hg; pulse, 86/min; random blood sugar, 290 mg/dL.

A probable diagnosis of diabetes mellitus was made, and the surgery was postponed.

Q1. What further investigations are advised to confirm the diagnosis?
Q2. What is the cause for raised BP in this case?
Q3. What complications can occur due to diabetes mellitus if not treated properly?
Q4. What is the pathophysiology of diabetes mellitus?

Case 2

A 30-year-old pregnant female in second trimester on routine investigation showed hyperglycaemia (300 mg/dL) and glycosuria.

Q1. What is this condition known as?
Q2. What are the risk factors of this condition?
Q3. What will be the effect on the fetus?
Q4. What is the pathophysiology for this condition?

Case 3

A 16-year-old thin, lean boy was admitted with complaints of increased urinary frequency, increased appetite and thirst, and was diagnosed as a case of diabetes mellitus.

Q1. Which type of diabetes mellitus is the patient suffering from?
Q2. What is the main cause of this disease?
Q3. What is predicted in biochemical investigations to confirm the diagnosis?
Q4. What is the treatment plan for this case?

Case 4

A 65-year-old known diabetic patient brought in the emergency department in a state of drowsiness and not responding properly.

Examination revealed the following: hypotension (BP 60/40 mm Hg); heart rate, 120/min; skin, cold and moist.

Q1. What is the diagnosis?
Q2. What biochemical and urine test will reveal in this condition?
Q3. What is the management plan for this condition?
Q4. What are the preventive measures for this condition?

8.7

Endocrinal Functions of Other Organs and Local Hormones

CHAPTER OUTLINE

In addition to the main endocrinal glands described in previous chapters, the other organs which have endocrinal functions are heart, kidney, pineal gland, thymus and others.

HORMONES OF THE HEART

The heart also acts as an endocrine organ. The muscle cells in the atria, and, to a much lesser extent, in the ventricle, contain secretory granules.

The hormones secreted by heart include:

- Atrial natriuretic peptide (ANP)
- Brain natriuretic peptide (BNP)
- C-type natriuretic peptide (CNP)

STRUCTURE

Atrial natriuretic peptide (ANP) It was the first natriuretic hormone isolated from the heart. It is a polypeptide and has 28 amino acid residues. It is formed from a large precursor molecule containing 151 amino acid residues.

Brain natriuretic peptide (BND) It was the second natriuretic hormone, first isolated from the porcine brain and hence named BNP. In humans, it is present in the heart and to a lesser extent in brain also. It is a polypeptide having 32 amino acid residues.

C-type natriuretic peptide (CNP) It was the third natriuretic hormone to be isolated in a sequence and so named CNP.

In the heart, it is present in a very small amount. It is mainly present in the brain, the pituitary, the kidneys and the vascular endothelial cells. It appears to be primarily a paracrine hormone, as very little amount is present in circulation.

SECRETION

ANP secretion is proportionate to the degree to which atria are stretched by increase in central venous pressure. Therefore, ANP secretion is affected by the following conditions:

Increase in ECF volume, following infusion of isotonic saline or ingestion of a high-sodium diet, increases ANP secretion.
Immersion of body in water up to neck increases central venous pressure by counteracting the effect of gravity on the circulation, and thus increases ANP secretion.
Rising from the supine to the standing position lowers the central venous pressure and thus decreases the ANP secretion.

PLASMA LEVELS, HALF-LIFE AND METABOLISM

Plasma levels Plasma levels of ANP in normal humans ingesting moderate amounts of sodium are approximately 5 fmol/mL.

Half-life Half-life of circulating ANP is very short.

Metabolism ANP is metabolized by the enzyme neural endopeptidase (NEP). Thiorphan inhibits the enzyme NEP, and thus when administered, it increases circulating ANP.

ACTIONS

1. Increase in sodium excretion by kidneys ANP and BNP increase excretion of sodium ion in urine by their following effects:

- Increasing glomerular filtration by dilating afferent arterioles and relaxing mesangial cells
- Inhibiting Na^+ reabsorption at the level of renal tubules

2. Role in escape phenomenon See page 737.

3. Lowering of blood pressure ANP lowers the blood pressure by their peripheral and central effects.

i. ***Peripheral blood pressure-lowering effects include:***
   - Increase the capillary permeability leading to extravasation of fluid and a decline in blood pressure.
   - Relax vascular smooth muscle (VSM) in arterioles and venules. CNP has a greater dilator effect on veins than ANP and BNP.
   - Inhibit renin secretion and thus counteract the pressor effects of catecholamines and angiotensin II.

ii. ***Central blood pressure-lowering effect*** is exerted through the ANP-containing neural circuits in the brain which project from the anteromedial part of the hypothalamus to the areas in the lower brainstem that are concerned with neural regulation of cardiovascular system. In general, the effects of ANP in the brain are opposite to those of angiotensin II. CNP and BNP in the brain probably have functions similar to those of ANP, but have not been elucidated in detail.

NATRIURETIC PEPTIDE RECEPTORS

Three types of natriuretic peptide receptors (NPRs) are known.

1. NPR-A It has an intracellular guanylyl cyclase domain (Fig. 8.7.1). ANP has greatest affinity for this receptor.

2. NPR-B It also has an intracellular guanylyl cyclase domain (Fig. 8.7.1). CNP has the greatest affinity for this receptor.

3. NPR-C It has only a small cytoplasmic domain (Fig. 8.7.1). It probably does not trigger any intracellular change. It removes natriuretic peptides from the bloodstream and then releases them later, helping to maintain a steady blood level of the hormones, and is thus also called *clearance receptor*.

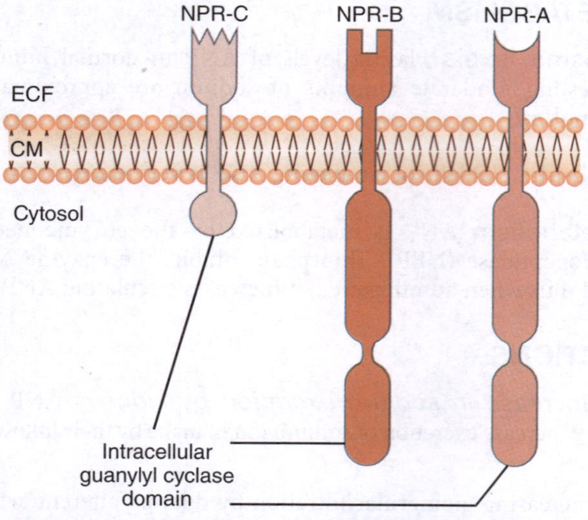

Fig. 8.7.1 Three types of natriuretic peptide receptors: NPR-A, NPR-B and NPR-C.

HORMONES OF THE KIDNEY

The kidneys secrete three hormones:

- Renin
- 1,25-Dihydroxycholecalciferol (see page 712)
- Erythropoietin (EPO)

RENIN

Renin is an aspartyl protease secreted by the granular cells of juxtaglomerular apparatus of the kidneys into the bloodstream. It acts in concert with angiotensin-converting enzyme (ACE) to form angiotensin II from the angiotensinogen, and constitutes the so-called *renin–angiotensin system.*

Structure Renin is a glycoprotein with a molecular weight of 37,326 in humans. Its molecule consists of two lobes, or domains. The active site of the enzyme is located in a deep cleft between the two lobes.

Synthesis Renin is synthesized as a large preprohormone. Stages in the synthesis are as follows:

- *Preprorenin:* It contains 406 amino acid residues.
- *Prorenin:* It contains 383 amino acid residues and is formed after the removal of a leader sequence of 23 amino acids from the amino terminal of preprorenin. Some prorenin is converted into renin in the kidneys and some is secreted in the circulation. In addition to the kidney, some other organs such as ovaries also secrete prorenin.
- *Renin:* The active renin contains 340 amino acid residues. It is formed after removal of the prosequence of 43 amino acids from the amino terminal of prorenin. It is important to note that prorenin is secreted by many organs, but the active renin is produced primarily in the kidneys.

Regulation The factors that affect renin secretion are as follows:

Stimulatory factors include:
- Increased sympathetic activity via renal nerves
- Increased circulating catecholamines
- Prostaglandins
- Conditions which decrease central venous pressure, such as Na^+ depletion, diuretics, hypotension, haemorrhage, upright posture, dehydration, cardiac failure, constriction of renal artery or aorta, cirrhosis and various psychological stimuli

Inhibitory factors include:
- Increased absorption of Na^+ and Cl^- across macula densa cells
- Angiotensin II
- Vasopressin
- Increased afferent arteriolar pressure

Actions Active renin has plasma half-life of 80 minutes or less. Its only action is to convert angiotensinogen (renin substrate) into angiotensin I. For further details about renin-angiotensin system, see pages 523 and 737.

ERYTHROPOIETIN

Structure EPO is glycoprotein with 165 amino acid residues and four oligosaccharide chains that are necessary for its activity in vivo. The gene encoding EPO is located on chromosome 7.

Source In the fetus and neonate, the major site of production of EPO is liver, but in adults, EPO is mainly (85%) secreted by the juxtaglomerular apparatus of the kidneys with some contribution (15%) from the perivenous hepatocytes in the liver. It is important to note that when renal mass is reduced in adults by renal disease or nephrectomy, the liver cannot compensate and anaemia develops.

Actions The main role of EPO is to stimulate the bone marrow and cause erythropoiesis (for details, see page 135).

Erythropoietin receptors and mechanism of action The *receptor for EPO* is a linear protein with a single transmembrane domain that is a member of the cytokine receptor superfamily. The gene encoding EPO receptors is located on chromosome 19q. The EPO receptor has three domains (extracellular, transcellular and intracellular).

Mechanism of action Renal tissue hypoxia leads to increased release of hypoxia-inducible factor-1 (HIF-1), which serves as a transcription factor. HIF-1 binds to hypoxia-response element (HRE) of EPO gene to induce transcription of mRNA for increased synthesis of EPO. EPO binds to the receptors on the target cells. The receptor has tyrosine kinase activity and it activates a cascade of serine and threonine kinases, resulting in the growth and development of target cells. Thus, EPO increases the number of EPO-sensitive committed stem cells in the bone marrow that are converted to red blood cell precursors and subsequently to mature erythrocytes.

For further details of mechanism of action, see page 136.

Plasma levels, half-life and metabolism Normal plasma levels of EPO are 50 U/L. Its plasma half-life is approximately 5 hours. It is mainly inactivated in the liver. Loss of even a small portion of the sialic acid residues in the carbohydrate moieties that are part of the EPO molecule shortens its half-life to 5 minutes, making it biologically ineffective.

Human recombinant erythropoietin (rHEPO) *Epoetin alfa* is a rEPO, which is produced in animal cells. Clinically, it has the following uses:

- In treatment of chronic anaemia, which occurs due to EPO deficiency in patients with renal failure
- To stimulate red cell production in individuals who are banking a supply of their own blood in preparation for autologous transfusions during elective surgery

Regulation of secretion of erythropoietin

1. ***Hypoxia*** is the main factor regulating EPO secretion. For example, occurrence of hypoxia following haemorrhage stimulates EPO secretion which in turn increases erythropoiesis to compensate hypoxia. Conversely, when the RBC volume is increased above normal by blood transfusion, the erythropoietic activity of the bone marrow decreases.

Mechanism: It has been suggested that the O_2 sensor-regulating EPO secretion in the kidney and liver is a haem protein that in the dioxy form stimulates and in the oxy form inhibits transcription of the EPO gene to form EPO mRNA.

2. ***Other factors*** that affect EPO secretion are as follows:
   - *Cobalt salt and androgens* stimulate EPO secretion.
   - *Alkalosis* that develops at high altitude facilitates EPO secretion.
   - *Catecholamines* via a β-adrenergic mechanism also facilitate EPO secretion.
   - *Adenosine* stimulates and adenosine antagonist (theophylline) inhibits EPO secretion.

PINEAL GLAND

FUNCTIONAL ANATOMY

Gross anatomy and location Pineal gland, also known as epiphysis, is a small structure (5 mm × 7 mm) shaped like a pine cone. It is situated in the groove between the two superior colliculi in diencephalic area of brain above the hypothalamus (Fig. 8.7.2). It forms the posterior boundary of the third ventricle and lies under the posterior end of corpus callosum (Fig. 8.7.3). It has a stalk which divides anteriorly into two laminae. The superior lamina contains the habenular commissure while the inferior lamina has the posterior commissure.

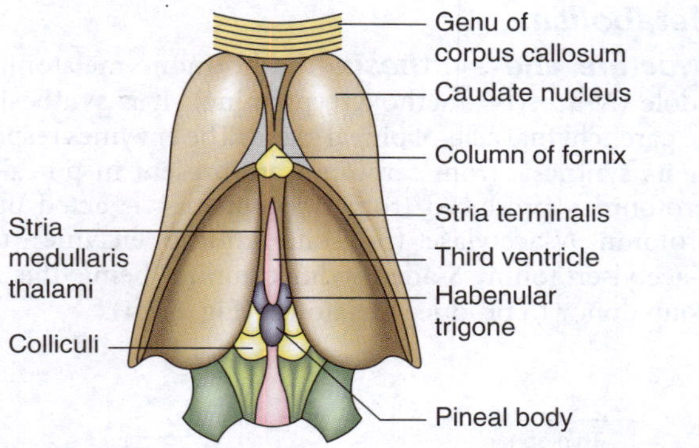

Fig. 8.7.2 Location of pineal body in the groove between the two superior colliculi.

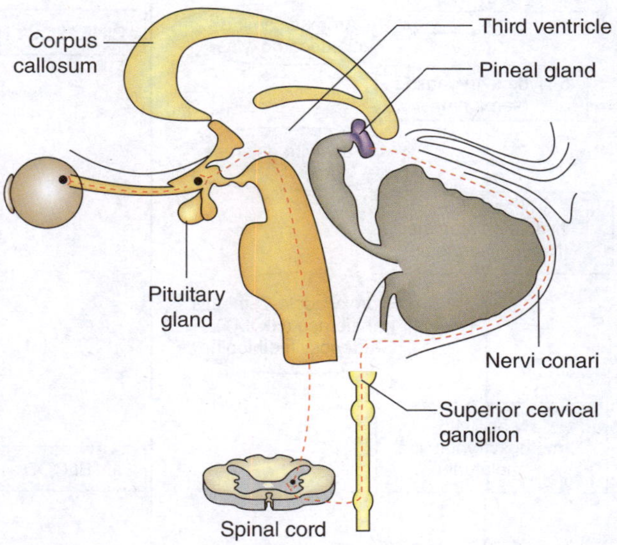

Fig. 8.7.3 Sagittal section of human brainstem showing pineal gland, its innervation (dotted line). Note that the pineal body forms the posterior boundary of third ventricle and lies under the posterior end of corpus callosum.

Structure The salient features are as follows:

The pineal stroma has two types of cells: neuroglial and parenchymal.

Parenchymal cells These are large epithelial cells (pinealocytes) with features suggesting that they have a secretory function.

- Like other endocrine glands, the pineal gland has highly permeable fenestrated capillaries.
- *In infants*, the pineal gland is large, and the cells tend to be arranged in alveoli.
- *In adults*, the pineal gland gets calcified, i.e. small concretions of calcium phosphate and carbonate (*pineal sand*) appear in the tissue. But the epithelial cells exist and secrete some hormonal substance. Because of calcification, the normal pineal gland is often visible on radiographic films of the skull in adults, and a shift of the pineal shadow to one side may indicate a space-occupying intracranial lesion on the other side.

MELATONIN

Structure, Synthesis, Plasma Levels and Metabolism

Structure and synthesis The hormone melatonin is an indole (*N*-acetyl-5-methoxytryptamine). It is synthesized by the parenchymal cells of pineal gland. The enzymes responsible for its synthesis from serotonin are present in pinealocytes. Serotonin – produced from tryptophan – is acted upon by serotonin *N*-acetylase (the rate-limiting enzyme) to give *N*-acetylserotonin, *S*-adenosylmethionine being the methyl group donor to produce melatonin (Fig. 8.7.4).

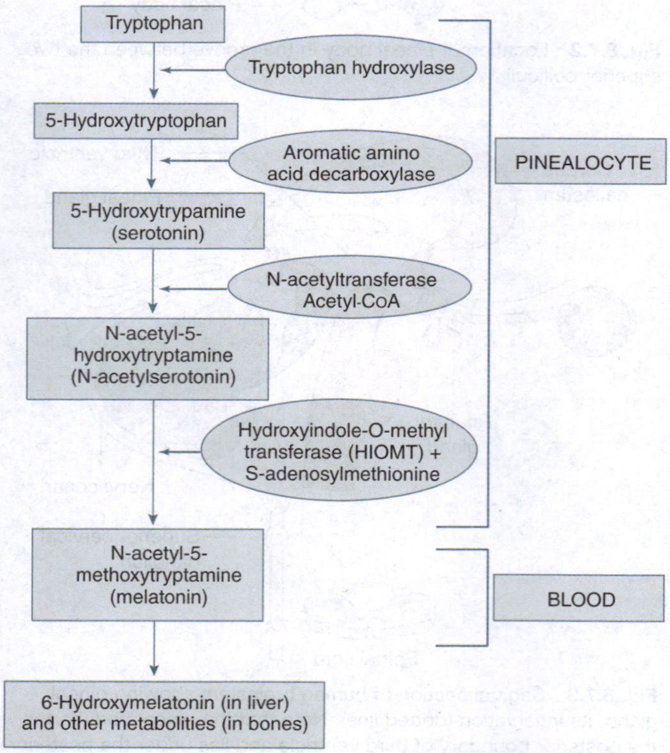

Fig. 8.7.4 Synthesis and metabolism of melatonin.

Plasma levels of melatonin These show fluctuations with night-time rise. The nocturnal plasma levels of melatonin are much higher in children than in adults and they decline with age. The average plasma levels of melatonin at various age groups are as follows:

- 1–3 years of age 250 pg/mL (1080 pmol/L)
- 8–15 years of age 120 pg/mL
- 20–27 years of age 70 pg/mL
- 67–84 years of age 30 pg/mL

Metabolism In the liver, circulating melatonin is rapidly metabolized by 6-hydroxylation followed by conjugation. More than 90% of melatonin that appears in the urine is in the form of 6-hydroxy conjugates and 6-sulphatoxymelatonin. The exact pathway for melatonin metabolism in brain is not known; perhaps it involves the cleavage of indole nucleus.

Melatonin Receptors and Functions of Melatonin

Melatonin receptors Melatonin acts through G-coupled receptors. Two types of melatonin receptors have been identified: MT-1 and MT-2.

- MT-1 receptors possess a high-affinity melatonin-binding site compared with MT-2 receptors and are of two subtypes: MT-1a and MT-1b.
- MT-1 receptors inhibit adenylyl cyclase, and MT-2 receptors stimulate phosphoinositol hydrolysis.

Functions of melatonin include:

1. ***Role in circadian rhythm of the body:*** The dark–light cycle through suprachiasmatic nuclei (SCN) of hypothalamus initiates neural and humoral signals that entrain a wide variety of well-known circadian rhythms, including diurnal variation in melatonin secretion. The nocturnal peaks in secretion of melatonin in turn appear to be an important hormonal signal entraining other cells in the body for circadian rhythm.
2. ***Effects on the gonads:*** Both inhibitory and facilitatory effects of melatonin on the gonads are described depending on the species and time of injection of melatonin. This variability in the effect has led to the hypothesis that it is not the melatonin per se but the diurnal change in melatonin secretion that functions as some sort of timing signal which coordinates internal events with the light–dark cycle in the environment.
3. ***Effect on MSH and ACTH secretion:*** An inhibitory effect of melatonin on MSH and ACTH secretion has been reported.
4. ***Other actions of melatonin: These*** include induction of sleep, and inhibition of puberty.

Regulation of Melatonin Secretion

Melatonin secretion shows diurnal variation Melatonin secretion shows diurnal variation in humans and all other species studied to date. It is secreted more during dark period of the day than during the daylight hours. This correlates with various internal activities in different periods of the day, i.e. circadian rhythm.

Hypothalamus is responsible for circadian fluctuations of melatonin secretion Hypothalamus exerts its effect through the norepinephrine secreted by postganglionic sympathetic nerves (nervi conari) that innervate the pineal gland. The neural pathway involved is as follows (Fig. 8.7.3):

Retinohypothalamic fibres involved in light–dark cycle synapse in SCN of hypothalamus.

Descending pathways from SCN of hypothalamus converge on the intermediolateral grey column of the thoracic spinal cord and end on the preganglionic sympathetic neurons.

Preganglionic fibres pass from the spinal cord to superior cervical ganglion.

Postganglionic neurons from the superior cervical ganglion project to the pineal in the nervi conari (Fig. 8.7.3).

Applied Aspects

The reduced melatonin levels are observed in diseases such as:

- Certain types of dementia
- Mood disorders
- Severe pain
- Cancer
- Type II diabetes

THYMUS

FUNCTIONAL ANATOMY

Thymus is a small lymphoid structure located in the lower part of neck in front of the trachea, below the thyroid gland. At birth, it is small (weighing 10–12 g), gradually enlarges till puberty when it weighs 20–30 g, and then it starts decreasing in size and in old age weighs approximately 3–6 g. The sex glands exert a depressant effect on the thymus; therefore, castration (removal of gonads) prolongs the period of persistence of the thymus.

Histologically, thymus consists of the inner medulla and outer cortex.

- *Medulla:* It comprises reticular epithelial cells, a few lymphocytes and concentric corpuscles of Hassall.
- *Cortex:* It includes actively multiplying, closely packed lymphocytes and contains no Hassall's corpuscles.

FUNCTIONS

Thymus has two functions:

- Immunological functions
- Endocrinal functions

1. Immunological functions of thymus

i. ***Development of immunologically competent T lymphocytes*** is an essential function of the thymus. The lymphocytes produced in bone marrow are processed in the thymus into T lymphocytes, which pass on to the lymph nodes. The hormone thymosin produced by reticuloepithelial tissue in the thymus stimulates lymphopoiesis. It mainly promotes proliferation of T lymphocytes. This occurs during the period between 3 months before and 3 months after the birth. Because of this reason, removal of thymus 3 months after birth will not affect the cell-mediated immunity. However, thymectomy in a newborn animal produces:
   - Lymphopenia and atrophy of all lymphoid tissue
   - Failure to produce circulating antibodies against the antigens entering the body (e.g. bacteria, viruses, red blood cells)
   - Suppression of delayed hypersensitivity reaction
   - Failure to produce graft rejection

ii. ***Maintenance of adequate pool of T lymphocytes:*** The hormone thymosin produced by thymus also stimulates lymphopoiesis in the peripheral lymphoid tissue and thus plays a role in maintenance of an adequate pool of T lymphocytes in adult life. Therefore, removal of thymus in adult animals causes decline of immunological capacity, but only after a few months during which the existing pool of competent lymphocytes becomes gradually depleted.

2. Endocrine function of thymus

Thymus tissue secretes two hormones, thymosin and thymin.

i. ***Thymosin:*** It is a peptide, which, as described above, promotes proliferation of T lymphocytes in the thymus and peripheral lymphoid tissue.
ii. ***Thymin***: It is also called thymopoietin, and inhibits acetylcholine release at motor nerve endings and thus suppresses neuromuscular activity. Therefore, in hyperactivity of thymus, myasthenia gravis occurs (see page 79).

LOCAL HORMONES

As described earlier, the endocrine glands secrete hormones into the bloodstream which show their actions at some distant places. In contrast, the local hormones are the substances which are produced in many tissues, and when activated in certain circumstances, execute their actions in the same area or in immediate neighbourhood. Commonly produced local hormones are as follows:

- Prostaglandins and related substances, such as thromboxanes, prostacyclin, leukotrienes and lipoxins.
- Other local hormones include acetylcholine; serotonin (5-HT); histamine; adenosine derivatives, e.g. AMP, ADP and ATP; and plasma polypeptides, e.g. angiotensin and plasma kinins.
- Local hormones produced in the blood, such as bradykinin, serotonin and angiotensinogen.

PROSTAGLANDINS AND RELATED SUBSTANCES

Prostaglandins and related substances include thromboxanes, prostacyclin, leukotriene and lipoxin. These substances are called *eicosanoids*, reflecting their origin from the 20-carbon (eicosa) polyunsaturated fatty acids *arachidonic acid*, linoleic acid and linolenic acid.

Prostaglandins

These were so named by Von Euler in 1937, because they were first isolated from prostatic secretion in semen. However, now they are known to be synthesized in almost all tissues of the body.

Structure

Prostaglandins are thus a series of 20-carbon unsaturated fatty acids containing a cyclopentane ring. On the basis of the configuration of this ring, prostaglandins are divided into various

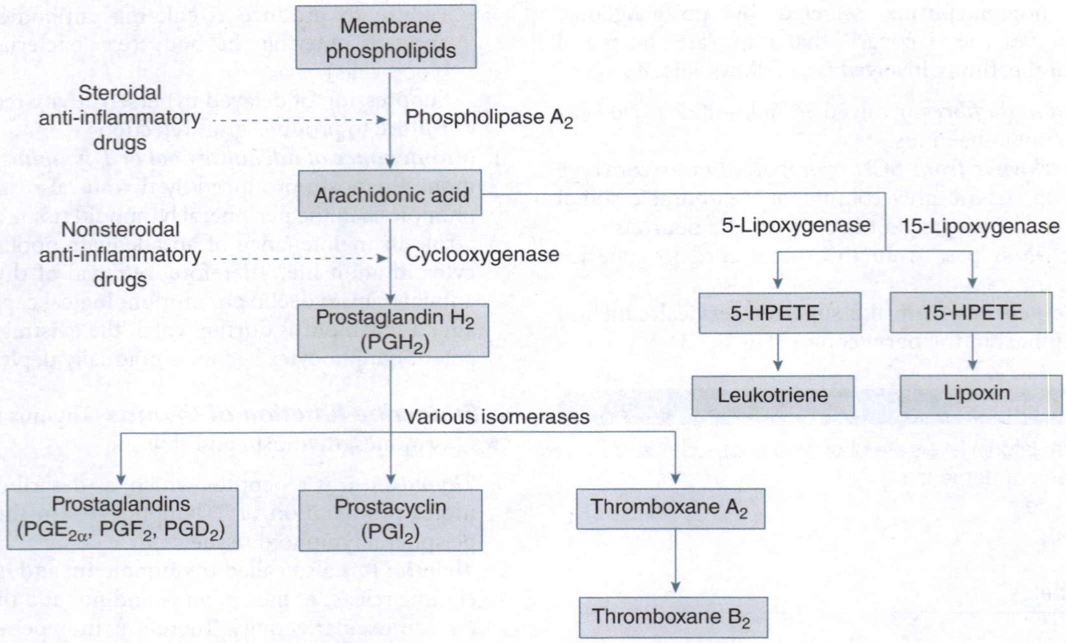

Fig. 8.7.5 Synthesis of prostaglandins and related substances.

groups, e.g. PGA, PGD, PGE and PGF. The number of double bonds in the side chain is indicated by subscript numbers, e.g. PGE_1 and PGE_2. Presently, a variety of prostaglandins are identified, but the active forms are PGD_2, PGE_2 and PGF_2.

Synthesis of prostaglandins and related substances

Steps involved in the synthesis of prostaglandins and the related substances are as follows (Fig. 8.7.5):

- *Phospholipids* of the cell membrane are released by the action of phospholipase A_2 and converted into arachidonic acid.
- *Arachidonic acid* is converted into prostaglandin H_2 (PGH_2) by the action of enzymes cyclooxygenase 1 and 2 (COX-1 and COX-2).
- *PGH_2* is converted into various other prostaglandins, thromboxanes and prostacyclin by various tissue isomerases (Fig. 8.7.5).

Note. In addition to the above-mentioned hormones, arachidonic acid is converted into two more hormones:

- By the action of 5-lipoxygenase into 5-hydroperoxyeicosatetraenoic acid (5-HPETE), which is converted into *leukotrienes*
- By the action of 15-lipoxygenase into 15-HPETE, which is then converted into *lipoxins*

Actions of Prostaglandins and Related Substances

Mechanism of action The nonvascular actions of PGs are related to cAMP but vascular actions are independent of cAMP. Thus, the actions of PGs are mediated at least in large part by the serpentine receptors coupled to G proteins (Table 8.7.1). The examples of the tissues in which the effects of the prostaglandins and related substances are predominant are also shown in Table 8.7.1.

Table 8.7.1 Prostaglandins and related substances, their receptors and tissues in which their effects are prominent

Substance	Receptors	Tissue
PGD_2	DP_1 and DP_2	Mast cells, airways and brain
PGE_2	EP_1, EP_2, EP_3 and EP_4	Vascular smooth muscle, kidney, platelets and brain
PGF	FP_α and FP_β	Vascular smooth muscle, uterus and airways
Thromboxanes	TP_α and TP_β	Platelets, vascular smooth muscle, macrophages and kidney
Prostacyclin	IP	Endothelium, kidneys, brain and platelets
Leukotriene	Cys LT_1, Cys LT_2 and BLT	Vascular smooth muscle, airways and leucocytes
Lipoxins	LP_α and LP_β	Vascular smooth muscle and lymphocytes

Actions of prostaglandins PGs have multitudinous and varied actions on almost all tissues of the body. Many of them are discussed in the chapters on the systems in which they play an important role. Some important actions of PGs are as follows:

1. ***Actions on cardiovascular system:***
   - Peripheral arteriolar dilatation, especially in splanchnic and muscular bed, is caused by PGA_1 and PGA_2.
   - Local vasodilatation, when given into an artery, is caused by PGE_2.
2. ***Actions on kidneys:*** PGA_2 increases renal cortical blood flow and increases urinary excretion of sodium, potassium and water.
3. ***Actions on female reproductive system:***
   - PGF_{2a} is reported to initiate labour by stimulating contraction of gravid uterus.

- PGF_{2a} is also reported to be responsible for painful uterine contractions during menstruation (dysmenorrhoea).
- PGEs and PGFs promote secretion of hypothalamic gonadotropin-releasing hormone (GnRH).

4. ***Role of prostaglandins in inflammation:*** Prostaglandins are reported to mediate the following effects of inflammation:
   - Histamine-induced vascular permeability
   - Pain-producing effect of bradykinin by sensitizing cutaneous nerves
   - Can produce pain by their direct action in higher concentration
   - Increased vascular permeability and cellular infiltration
5. ***Actions on blood platelets***:
   - PGE_1 inhibits platelet aggregation through activation of adenylyl cyclase.
   - PGE_2, PGG_2 and PGH_2 promote the aggregation of platelets. Nonsteroidal anti-inflammatory drugs (e.g. aspirin and indomethacin) inhibit this effect by preventing formation of PGG_2 and PGH_2 from arachidonic acid.
6. ***Action on bronchial musculature:***
   - PGE_{2a} causes contraction of bronchial smooth muscles and may precipitate bronchial asthma.
   - PGE_3, on the other hand, relaxes bronchial smooth muscles.
7. ***Actions on GIT:***
   - PGE_1, PGEs and PGA_1 inhibit the secretion of gastric HCl.
   - PGEs and PGF_{2a} cause inhibition of sodium and water absorption producing profuse watery, cholera-like diarrhoea.
   - PGE and PGF increase intestinal motility.
8. ***Metabolic actions of PGs:*** Metabolic actions of PGs in vivo are variable. In vitro, PGE_1 inhibits the ACTH, GH, glucagon and epinephrine-induced lipolysis.
9. ***Actions on nervous system:***
   - On CNS, the PGs function as transmitters or modulators of neuron activity.
   - In the ANS, the PGEs stimulate cholinergic neuroeffector junctions and inhibit the release and response to norepinephrine.
10. ***Actions on the eye:*** PGE_2 and PGF_{2a} occur in the iris and produce miosis. Therefore, nonsteroidal anti-inflammatory drugs are used to prevent occurrence of miosis during cataract operation.

Actions of Thromboxane A_2

Thromboxane A_2 is synthesized by platelets. It promotes:

- Vasoconstriction
- Platelet aggregation

Actions of Prostacyclin

Prostacyclin is produced in vascular endothelium. It produces vasodilatation. The important balance between thromboxane A_2 and prostacyclin in haemostasis is discussed in Chapter 3.5, see page 208.

Actions of Leukotrienes

Leukotrienes include C_4 (LTC_4), LTD_4, LTE_4 and LTF_4. They are mediators of allergic responses and inflammation. Their release is provoked when specific allergens combine with IgE antibodies on the surfaces of mast cells. They produce:

- Bronchoconstriction
- Arteriolar constriction
- Increased vascular permeability
- Attract neutrophils and eosinophils

Receptors for leukotrienes are as follows:

- Cys LT_1: It mediates bronchoconstriction, chemotaxis and increased vascular permeability.
- Cys LT_2: It mediates constriction of pulmonary VSM.
- BLT: It predominantly mediates chemotaxis.

Actions of Lipoxins

Physiological role of lipoxins is uncertain. Their actions include:

- Dilatation of microvasculature (by lipoxin A)
- Inhibition of cytotoxic effects of natural killer cells (by lipoxin A and lipoxin B)

OTHER LOCAL HORMONES SYNTHESIZED IN TISSUES

In addition to prostaglandins and related substances, the other local hormones synthesized in the tissues are as follows:

- Acetylcholine (see page 980)
- Serotonin (see page 339)
- Histamine (see pages 583 and 339)
- Substance P (see page 987)
- Heparin (see page 208)
- Gastrointestinal hormones (see page 565)

LOCAL HORMONES PRODUCED IN BLOOD

Local hormones produced in blood are as follows:

- Serotonin (see pages 339 and 524)
- Angiotensinogen (see page 337)
- Bradykinin (see page 337)

Self-Assessment

1. Discuss the endocrinal role of kidney.
2. Discuss the synthesis and regulation of melatonin secretion.
3. Discuss the synthesis of prostaglandins and their actions.
4. Write notes on:
   - Leukotrienes
   - Endocrine functions of thymus
   - Role of thromboxane A_2

Clinical Case

Case 1

A 67-year-old male consulted the physician for sleeplessness and feeling of tiredness, lack of interest, mood swings and remaining irritable throughout the daytime. The treating physician prescribe the drug melatonin.

Q1. How does melatonin help in induction of sleep?

Q2. What are other disorders which are associated with low levels of melatonin?

REPRODUCTIVE SYSTEM

SECTION 9

SECTION OUTLINE

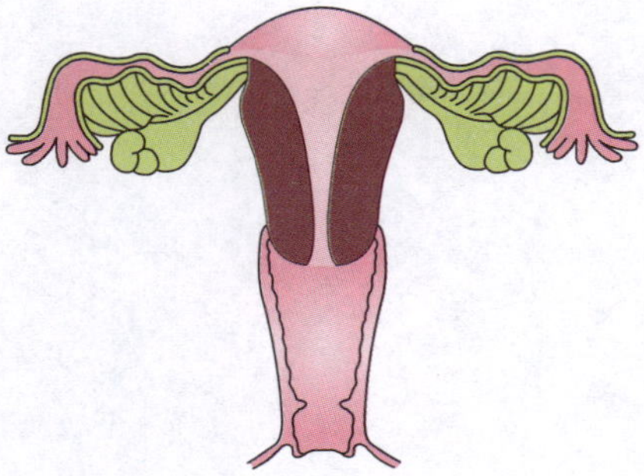

INTRODUCTION

Reproduction is a multidimensional subject with physiological, biochemical, genetic, psychological, emotional, social, economic, moral and many other aspects. The physiology of the reproductive system begins with *sex determination*, i.e. genetic differentiation, which occurs during fertilization (penetration of the ovum by the sperm). An ovum always contains 22+X chromosomes, whereas a sperm may contain either 22+X or 22+Y chromosomes. Therefore, after fertilization, the zygote's chromosomal patterns can be either 44+XX (i.e. female genotype) or 44+XY (i.e. male genotype). The next step in reproductive physiology is *sex differentiation* which begins at about 7–8 weeks of intrauterine life when the primitive, bipotential sex gland or gonad (gone = seed) differentiates into either testis or ovary depending on the genotype (gonadal differentiation). From this point onwards, depending on whether the embryo has a pair of testes or ovaries, there will occur development of male or female accessory sex organs (*genital differentiation or phenotype*). After remaining quiescent during childhood, the gonads suddenly awaken into vigorous activity for a period of 3–4 years during which gonadal development and maturation reaches the point where reproduction is possible for the first time. During this phase, there also occurs a sudden spurt of physical growth and the child grows into an adult. This transitional period between the childhood and the adulthood is called the period of *puberty*, during which the secondary sex characters develop.

The adult *male reproductive physiology* and *female reproductive physiology* involve gametogenic and endocrinal functions of testes and ovaries, respectively. In a sexually active female, the *physiology of pregnancy* involves fertilization at a proper time and place (fallopian tube), development of the fetus in the mother's womb and finally birth of a new human being, either male or female. After childbirth, the mother continues to provide nourishment by breastfeeding for a further period of 6–9 months (*physiology of lactation*).

The understanding of reproductive physiology is important not only for the promotion of conception and normal fetal growth but also for the prevention of conception (*physiology of contraception*) for population control which is of global concern.

The point when reproductive physiology ends is called *climacteric* (literally meaning a major turning point). In females, it is *menopause*, but in males, there is no sharp point.

Sexual Growth and Development

9.1

CHAPTER OUTLINE

PREPUBERTAL SEXUAL GROWTH AND DEVELOPMENT

In a human embryo, sexual growth involves two processes:

- Sex determination
- Sex differentiation

SEX DETERMINATION

Sex determination, also known as *genetic differentiation*, refers to the genotype of the fetus, whether male or female. The genotype is determined by the presence of sex chromosomes, hence also known as *chromosomal sex differentiation*.

Human chromosomes: Each cell (except ovum and sperm) in a normal adult male and female possesses 46 chromosomes (44 autosomes + 2 sex chromosomes) usually arranged in an arbitrary pattern (karyotype).

- These chromosomes exist in pairs (22 pairs of autosomes + 1 pair of sex chromosomes) and are referred to as diploid (or double number) *chromosomes*.
- *Autosome pairs* are identified by the numbers 1–22 on the basis of their morphological characteristics.
- *Sex chromosomes* are called X and Y chromosomes.
- *The females* possess 44 autosomes plus 2X chromosomes (44+XX).
- The males possess 44 autosomes plus an X chromosome and a Y chromosome (44+XY).

Human gametes: The mature male gametes are called sperms and the mature female gametes are called ova. During gametogenesis, there occurs meiosis (*reduction division*); therefore, the mature sperm and ovum contain half the number of chromosomes, i.e. 23 (22 autosomes + 1 sex chromosome). This is called *haploid* number.

- Since the primitive female germ cells (*oogonia*) from which mature ova are formed contain 44+XX chromosomes, each ovum will contain 22+X chromosomes (Fig. 9.1.1).
- The primitive male germ cells (spermatogonia) from which mature sperms are formed contain 44+XY chromosomes, so half of the normal sperms will contain 22+X and other half will have 22+Y chromosomes (Fig. 9.1.1).

Genetic sex determination of the embryo occurs during fertilization, i.e. penetration of the ovum by the sperm, as:

- When an ovum (22+X) is fertilized by a sperm containing 22+X chromosomes, the resultant zygote's chromosomal pattern will be 44+XX (*female genotype*).
- When an ovum (22+X) is fertilized by a sperm containing 22+Y chromosomes, the resultant zygote's chromosomal pattern will be 44+XY (male genotype).
- The human Y chromosome is smaller than the X chromosomes. The sperms containing the Y chromosomes are lighter and able to swim faster up in the female genital tract, thus reaching the ovum rapidly. This probably accounts for the fact that the number of males born is slightly greater than the number of females.

Formation of Barr Body

During embryonic development, the somatic cells start multiplying immediately after fertilization. It has been seen that one of X chromosomes of somatic cells in the female embryo becomes inactive, whereas the other remains active. The exact details about the inactivation process of X chromosomes are not known, but it may probably be due to the presence of a gene called *Xist* (X-inactivation centre) in the chromosome

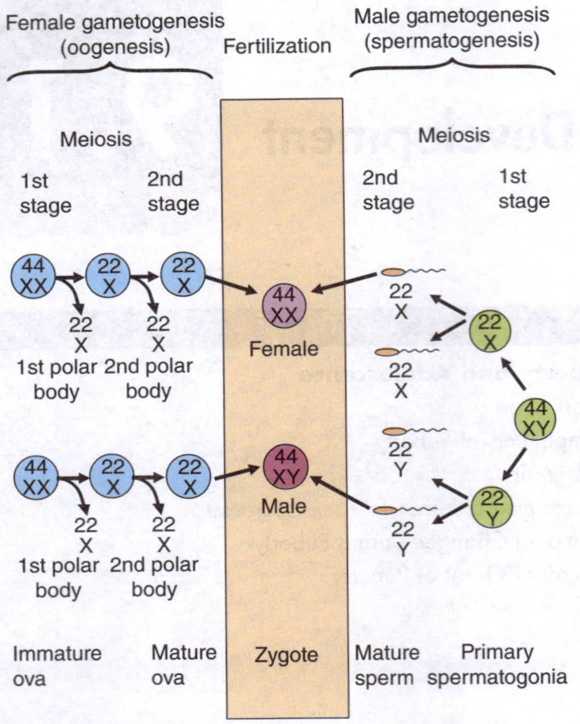

Fig. 9.1.1 Basis of genetic sex determination.

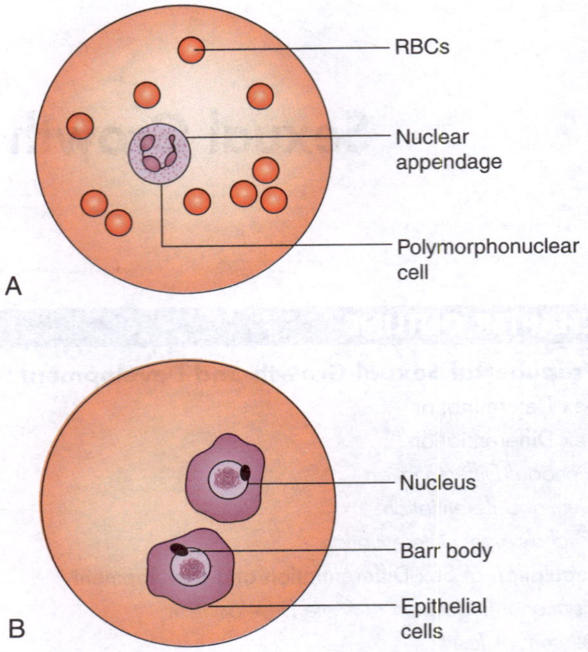

Fig. 9.1.2 Sex chromatins (Barr body) seen in: **A**, polymorphonuclear cell; and **B**, epithelial cells of epidermal spinous layer.

that produces noncoding mRNA. Formation of *noncoding mRNA* starts inactivation process in the centre of X chromosomes which continues in the subsequent divisions of the cells. The choice to be inactive of one of the X chromosomes is random. Therefore, in an adult female, about half of the somatic cells contain an active X chromosome of paternal origin and other half of maternal origin.

The inactive X chromosome of each somatic cell forms a condensed mass called *sex chromatin* or *Barr body*. The Barr body can be seen near the nuclear membrane of the cells (Fig. 9.1.2).

Significance of barr body includes:

1. ***Identification of sex genotype:*** Since Barr bodies are present in the somatic cells of females only, the sex genotype can be identified by a cytological test. The most suitable cells for this test are as follows:
   - Epithelial cells of epidermal spinous layer
   - Buccal mucosal cells
   - Mucosal cells of vagina
   - Polymorphonuclear cells (in about 15% of the polymorphonuclear cells, the Barr bodies are seen as drumsticks projecting from the nuclei)
2. ***Identification of abnormal genotypes:*** In the abnormal cells with three or more X chromosomes, there are two or more Barr bodies.

SEX DIFFERENTIATION

After the sex determination (genotype sex) during fertilization, the normal sex differentiation in the embryo proceeds sequentially. The stages of sex differentiation are as follows:

- Gonadal differentiation
- Genital differentiation
- Psychological differentiation

Gonadal Differentiation

Gonadal differentiation or *gonadogenesis* refers to formation of gonads, i.e. testes in males and ovaries in females. Gonadal sex differentiation is dependent on the genotype of the embryo.

Genital ridge or the urogenital ridge (the condensation of mesenchymal tissue present on each side near the adrenal glands) is the site where gonads develop. The primordial germ cells migrate into the genital ridge, where proliferation of both germinal and nongerminal cells leads to formation of bipotential gonads.

Bipotential gonads are also known as primordial or primitive or indifferent or ambisexual gonads. In a human embryo, these can be identified after 30 days of fertilization. Up to 6 weeks of gestation, the bipotential gonads are identical in both sexes and have the rudiments of both male and female gonads.

Structure: The bipotential gonad consists of a medulla, a cortex and primordial germ cells. The germ cells are embedded in the layer of cortical epithelium surrounding a core of medullary mesenchymal tissue (Fig. 9.1.3A and B).

Testicular Differentiation

In a genetic male (44+XY) embryo, the bipotential gonads begin to differentiate into testes at approximately sixth week. The Y chromosome plays a key role in the process of testicular differentiation.

Role of Y chromosome in testicular differentiation

Two transcription genes, one for testicular differentiation and another for formation of Müllerian inhibitory substance (MIS), also called anti-Müllerian hormone (AMH), are present on the Y chromosome.

- The gene responsible for testicular differentiation is located near the tip of the short arm of Y chromosome and is called SRY gene (SRY, sex-determining region of the Y chromosome).

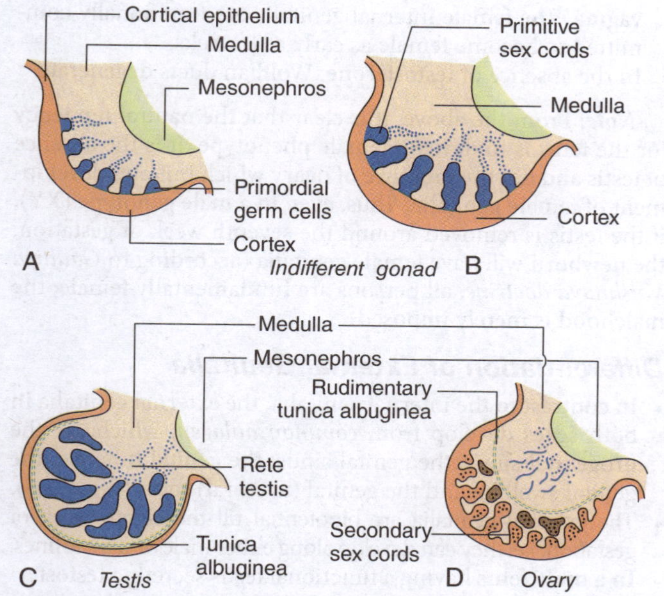

Fig. 9.1.3 Diagrammatic structure of human bipotential gonad (**A and B**), and development of testis from the medulla (**C**) and ovary from the cortex (**D**).

- The SRY gene encodes the *testis-determining factor* (TDF) which triggers the testicular differentiation.
- The TDF gene product causes Sertoli cell differentiation. Sertoli cell activity is critically important for all subsequent events in male sexual differentiation.

Other important genes involved in testicular development are as follows:

- SOX9 – for increasing AMH secretion
- Fibroblast growth factor-9 (FGF-9)
- Wilms tumour–related gene (WT-1)
- Steroidogenesis factor-1 (SF-1) which increases synthesis of testosterone
- DAX-1. ADX-1 gene is involved in dosage-sensitive sex reversal phenotype. It plays an important role in normal embryonic development.

Important Note

The ***PC-PNDT Act*** was acted on 20 September1994 with the intent to prohibit the prenatal diagnostic techniques for determination of fetal sex leading to female feticide and to correct declining sex ratio in India. The salient features of this Act are as follows:

1. It regulates the use of prenatal diagnostic techniques like ultrasound machine allowing only for the use of genetic abnormalities, congenital malformations, hemoglobinopathies and sex-linked disorders.
2. The Central Supervisory Board (CSB) was constituted by the government under Section 7 of the PC-PNDT Act (1994).
3. The violation of the Act is a punishable crime. The punishment of violation of the PC-PNDT Act is imprisonment for 3 years and fine.
4. As per rule 3 of the PC-PNDT Act, no medical geneticist, gynaecologist, paediatrician and registered medical practitioner can conduct/help in conducting herself/himself or through any other person any prenatal diagnostic technique at a place other than a place registered under this Act.

Process of Testicular Differentiation is as follows:

At about sixth week of gestation, the testicular differentiation begins with the appearance of primitive seminiferous cords (sex cords) from the germinal epithelium covering the medulla of bipotential gonad (Fig. 9.1.3).

At about seventh week of gestation:

- The solid sex cords are canalized to form seminiferous tubules.
- Meanwhile, a large number of Sertoli cells appear and get organized along the seminiferous tubules.
- The cortical region (from which female gonad develops) undergoes regression.

At about eighth week of gestation, Leydig (interstitial) cells appear in the interstitial spaces of seminiferous tubules and continue to proliferate. The Leydig cells are derived from the sex cords that are not canalized. The membrane of Leydig cells has receptors for human chorionic gonadotropins (hCG) and for luteinizing hormone (LH).

At about ninth week of gestation, the Leydig cells synthesize and secrete testosterone in response to hCG secreted by placenta.

At about 14th week of gestation, the number of Leydig cells is so much increased that they form more than half of the volume of the testes.

At the end of 16th week (4 months), the number of fetal Leydig cells decreases and at term only a few are present.

At about the 35th week of gestation, there occurs descent of testes through inguinal canal into scrotum. This marks the final stage of testicular differentiation.

Ovarian Differentiation

- In a genetic female (44+XX) embryo, by about 10th week of gestation, ovarian differentiation can be identified histologically. Since development of ovary requires the presence of XX chromosomes, with XO chromosomal constitution, there may be no ovarian tissue.
- Ovarian differentiation occurs in the absence of TDF.
- The ovaries develop on each side from the cortical region of the bipotential gonad (Fig. 9.1.3D).
- The coelomic epithelial cells (cortical cells) proliferate and form granulosa cells which surround the germ cells and commit them to oocyte formation. The hilar cells form later during the development.
- Meanwhile, the medulla, from which the testes develop, regresses.
- During 11–12 weeks of gestation, oogonia undergo meiotic division to form oocyte which is the end point of ovarian differentiation.
- Embryonic ovary, like testis, does not secrete any hormone.
- Hormonal treatment of the mother has no effect on gonadal (as opposed to ductal and genital) differentiation in humans, although it does in some experimental animals.

Note: Important genes involved during development of ovaries are as follows:

- WNT-4 that inhibits functions of SOX-9
- R-spondin-1

Genital Differentiation

Genital sex differentiation, also known as *phenotypic sex* differentiation, refers to the differentiation of internal genitalia, urethra and external genitalia.

Differentiation of Internal Genitalia

- The internal genitalia differentiate from the *neutral sex anlagen* which develop during the sixth week of gestation along with the development of bipotential gonad.
- The primordia of internal genitalia are a paired set of Wolffian (male) ducts and a paired set of Müllerian (female) ducts. By the seventh week of gestation, the embryo has both male and female primordial ducts (Fig. 9.1.4).

Differentiation of male internal genitalia In the genetic male fetus (44+XY) with functioning testes, testosterone and MIS are secreted which result in differentiation of male internal genitalia (Fig. 9.1.4B):

- The testosterone secreted by the Leydig cells stimulates the Wolffian ducts to form the epididymis, vas deferens and seminal vesicles.
- The MIS secreted by Sertoli cells causes regression of the Müllerian ducts by apoptosis on the side on which it is secreted.

Differentiation of female internal genitalia (Fig. 9.1.4C)

- In the genetic female fetus (44+XX), in the absence of MIS, the female ducts (Müllerian ducts) proliferate and form oviduct (uterine tubes), uterus and upper two-thirds of vagina. The female internal genitalia are functionally committed to become female as early as 8 weeks.
- In the absence of testosterone, Wolffian ducts degenerate.

Note: From the above, it is clear that the natural tendency for the fetus is to develop female phenotype. It is the absence of testis and not the presence of ovary which initiates development of female genitalia. Thus, even in a male genotype (XY), if the testis is removed around the seventh week of gestation, the newborn will have female genitalia (according to *Gaudiya Vaishnava doctrine*, all persons are fundamentally female; the malehood is merely imposed).

Differentiation of External Genitalia

- In contrast to the internal genitalia, the external genitalia in both sexes develop from *common anlagen*, which are the urogenital sinus, the genital sinus, the genital tubercle, the genital swelling and the genital (urethral) folds (Fig. 9.1.5).
- The external genitalia are bipotential till the eighth week of gestation, i.e. they can develop along either male or female lines.
- **In a male fetus** having a functional testis secreting testosterone and dihydrotestosterone (DHT), the external genitalia acquire male characteristics by the fifth month of gestation.
- **In a female fetus**, in the absence of any hormone, external genitalia differentiation occurs along the female line.

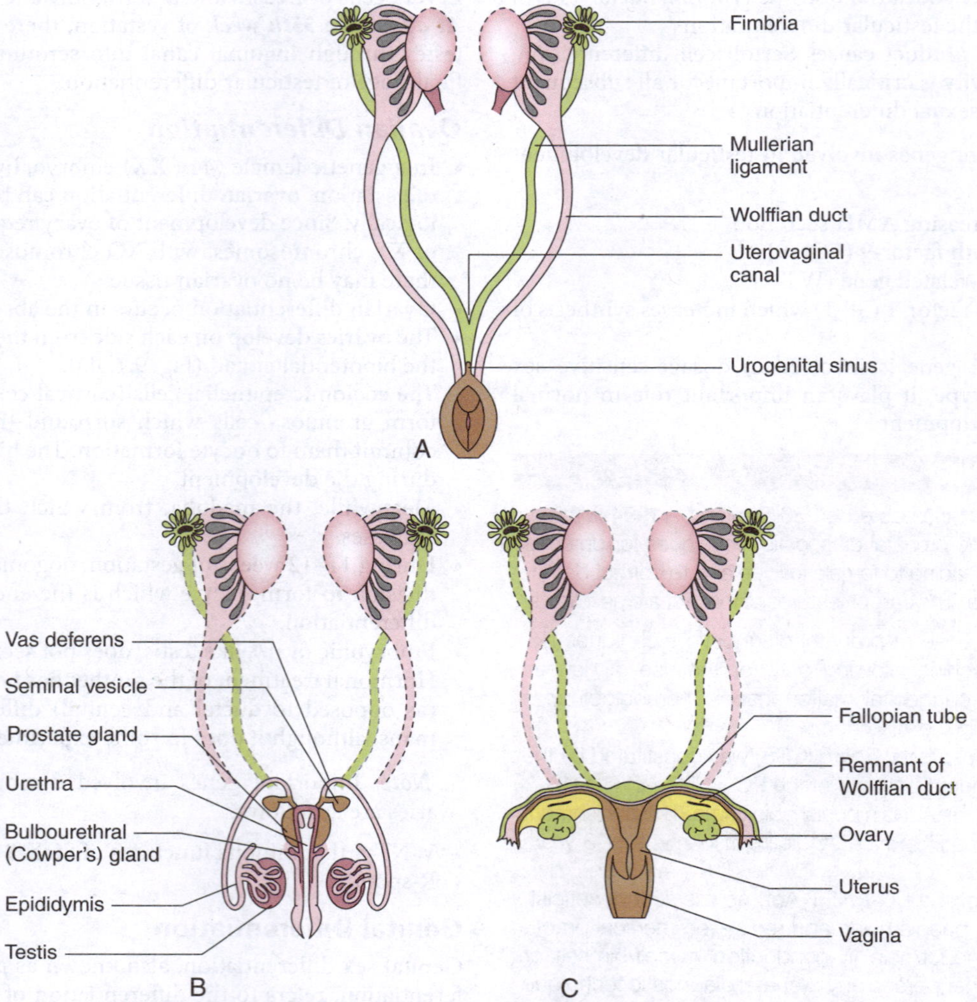

Fig. 9.1.4 Development of male (**B**) and female (**C**) internal genitalia from primordial genital ducts (**A**).

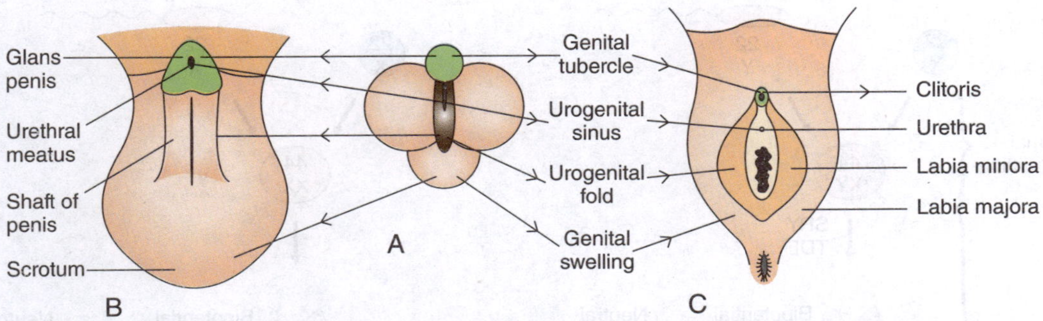

Fig. 9.1.5 Differentiation of external genitalia in male (**B**) and female (**C**) from common anlagen (**A**).

Table 9.1.1 Male and female external genitalia derived from the common anlagen

Anlagen part	Male derivative	Female derivative
Urogenital sinus	Prostate and prostatic urethra	Urethra
Urethral fold	Penile urethra and shaft of penis	Labia minora
Genital swelling	Scrotum	Labia majora
Genital tubercle	Glans penis	Clitoris

The external genitalia derived from the common anlagen in males and females are shown in Table 9.1.1.

Psychological Differentiation

Psychological sex differentiation refers to normal sexual behaviour in an adult male and female. The difference in male and female behaviour is due to some anatomical and functional differences in certain areas of the brain of two sexes. It is determined by the effect of androgens on the development of the brain in the embryonic stage. It has been studied that:

- A brief exposure of fetal hypothalamus to androgens (from its own testis) during early embryonic period causes male pattern of sexual behaviour during puberty. It occurs due to constant secretion of pituitary gonadotropins.
- Absence of androgenic exposure of fetal hypothalamus in female embryo causes it to stimulate the anterior pituitary in a cyclic way as in adult females.
- Early exposure of female fetus to androgens also produces significant masculinizing effect on sex behaviour in adulthood.

REGULATION OF SEX DIFFERENTIATION AND DEVELOPMENT

From the above discussion, it is apparent that the normal sex differentiation and sexual development proceeds sequentially: first, chromosomal sex is established at fertilization that determines *gonadal differentiation*. The *genital differentiation* (phenotypic sex) is dependent on *gonadal differentiation*. It is quite obvious that *Y chromosome* plays key role in testicular differentiation or male development. The absence of testicular differentiation results in ovarian differentiation or female-like development. The fetal functional testis by secreting MIS and testosterone regulates the activity.

Hormonal Regulation of Male Development

The two principal components of male (phenotypic) development (*Wolffian duct differentiation* and the *virilization of urogenital sinus*) and the development of external genitalia are under control of testosterone and DHT (Fig. 9.1.6). *Virilization of male embryo* is mediated by three hormones – MIS, testosterone and DHT.

1. *MIS* also called the Müllerian duct regression factor (MRF) or AMH, is produced by Sertoli cells of fetal testis. It is polypeptide in nature belonging to the family of *tissue growth factors* (TGF).

Plasma levels: The mean plasma level in a male child is 4 ng/mL and is reached by 1–2 years of age. Then the level starts declining, and by the age of puberty and afterwards, it is very low.
Note: MIS is also detected in girls, in very low quantity. It is probably secreted by *granulosa cells* of the ovarian follicles.
Functions: By local paracrine action, MIS causes:

- *Regression (involution) of Müllerian duct* occurs by apoptosis and thus prevents development of uterus, oviduct and upper vagina.
- *Continued growth of Wolffian duct* helps the testosterone in virilization of Wolffian duct and its derivatives.
- In later embryonic period, it helps in *descent of testis.*

2. *Testosterone* is secreted by the Leydig cells of the fetal testis in response to hCG.

Functions: Testosterone causes unilateral virilization of the Wolffian duct into vas efferens, epididymis, vas deferens, ejaculatory ducts and seminal vesicles by its local paracrine action (by maintaining local high concentrations). The local high concentration of testosterone is maintained because testosterone has a great affinity for androgen-binding protein released from Sertoli cells. In the bound form, testosterone flows along the Wolffian duct and released from the binding protein at its site of action.

- In other target organs (prostate and external genitalia), testosterone is first converted into DHT to produce all androgenic effects.

3. *DHT* is formed at its site of action from testosterone. The target organs contain an active enzyme 5α-reductase, which converts testosterone into DHT.

Functions: It causes masculinization of prostate and external genitalia.
Mechanism of action of androgens: As shown in Fig. 9.1.7, testosterone binds to androgen receptors in the nucleus of target

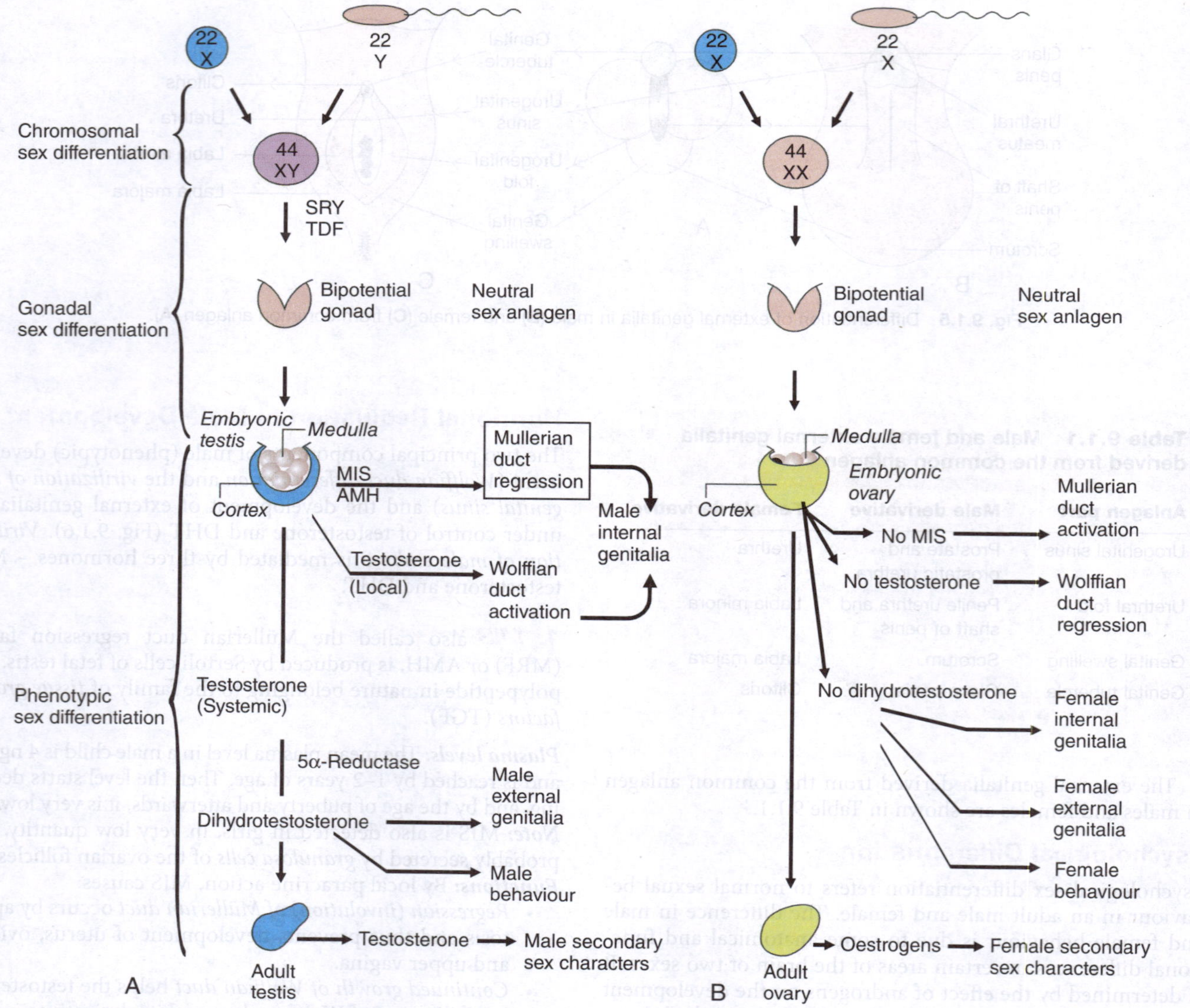

Fig. 9.1.6 Diagrammatic summary of regulation of normal sex determination, differentiation and development in male (A) and female (B).

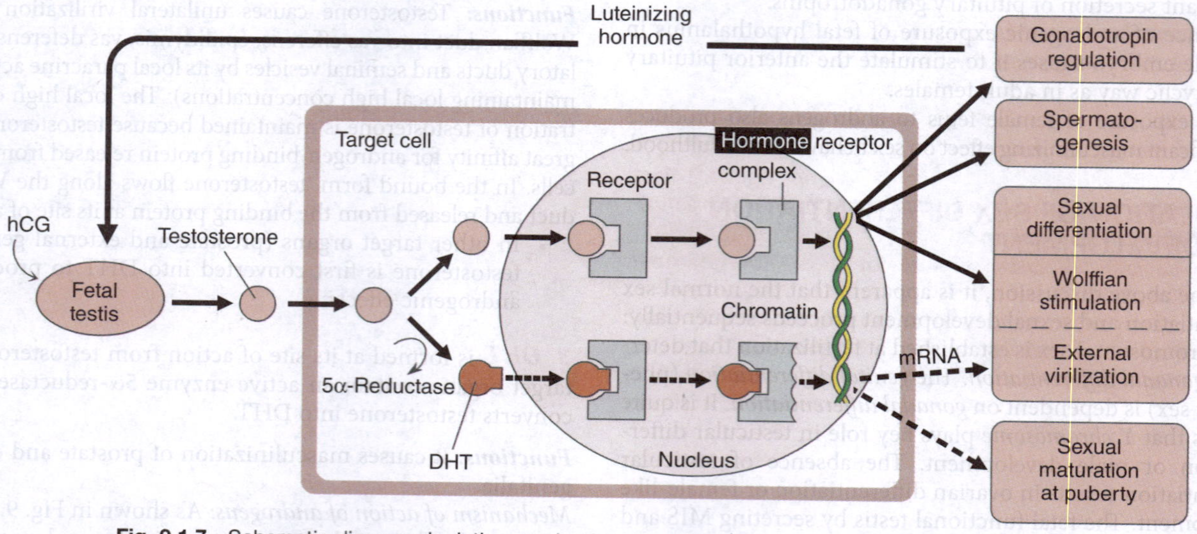

Fig. 9.1.7 Schematic diagram depicting mechanism of action of androgens secreted by fetal testis.

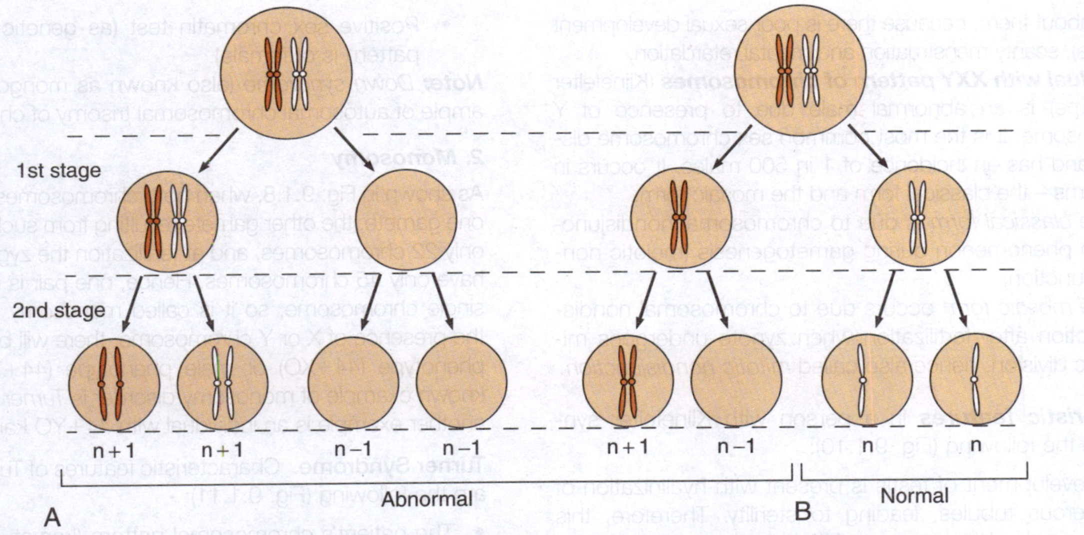

Fig. 9.1.8 Nondisjunction of sex chromosomes during meiotic division: **A**, in first stage; and **B**, in second stage.

organ either directly or following testosterone conversion to DHT. The receptor is common for both (testosterone and DHT), thus resulting in the formation of *hormone receptor complex*, which interacts with chromatin.

DHT is the most potent natural androgen and, therefore, it is necessary for virilization.

Note: *Castration* (removal of fetal testis) in an early embryonic stage prevents the formation of male genitalia and thus results in female-like development. However, castration of male fetus at a later stage does not affect male differentiation.

Descent of Testis

The descent of testis from its origin (near kidney) into the scrotum occurs in two phases – transabdominal phase and inguinoscrotal phase. Gubernaculum is a mesenchymal condensation of extracellular matrix that helps in descent of testis.

Transabdominal phase: The descent of testis depends on insulin-like growth factor-3 (INSL-3) produced by Leydig cells. INSL-3 acts through G-protein-coupled receptors and MIS.

Inguinoscrotal phase is androgen dependent. Androgens cause release of calcitonin gene–related protein (CGRP), and provide the chemotactic gradient for the descent of testis.

Applied Aspects

Disorders of Sexual Development

Abnormalities of sexual development occur due to:

- Defect in sex chromosomes leading to genetic abnormalities
- Hormonal abnormalities leading to defect in gonadal and genital differentiation

I. Chromosomal Abnormalities

Chromosomal abnormalities include:

- Trisomy
- Monosomy
- Chromosomal abnormality with more than three chromosomes
- Triploidy
- Abnormalities in number of chromosomes during crossing-over process
- Mosaicism

1. Trisomy

Chromosomal abnormalities usually arise during gametogenesis due to *nondisjunction* of sex chromosomes. Nondisjunction is a phenomenon in which a pair of chromosomes could not be separated during meiotic division and may go to same pole (Fig. 9.1.8). The resulting gamete then has 24 chromosomes instead of normal 23. At fertilization by this gamete (with 24 chromosomes), the zygote will, therefore, have 47 chromosomes (Fig. 9.1.9), there being 3 sex chromosomes instead of 1 of the normal pair (XY or XY). The presence of extra X or Y chromosome gives rise to many syndromes, associated with abnormal development, mental retardation and abnormal growth. Trisomy is presented as:

a. ***Individual with XXX (genotype) pattern of chromosomes*** is referred to as a 'superfemale'. However, there is nothing

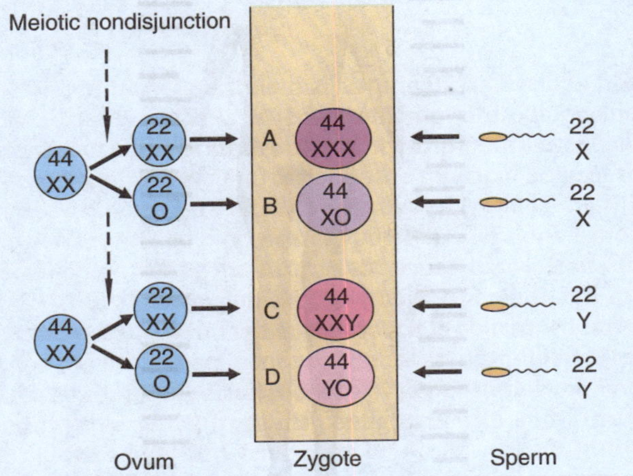

Fig. 9.1.9 Defects due to maternal nondisjunction of sex chromosomes at the time of meiosis: **A**, superfemale; **B**, gonadal dysgenesis (Turner syndrome); **C**, seminiferous dysgenesis (Klinefelter syndrome); and **D**, lethal monosomy.

super about them, because there is poor sexual development (infantile), scanty menstruation and mental retardation.

b. ***Individual with XXY pattern of chromosomes*** (Klinefelter syndrome) is an abnormal male due to presence of Y chromosome. It is the most common sex chromosome disorder, and has an incidence of 1 in 500 males. It occurs in two forms – the classical form and the mosaic form.
   i. *The classical form* is due to chromosomal nondisjunction phenomenon during gametogenesis (meiotic nondisjunction).
   ii. *The mosaic form* occurs due to chromosomal nondisjunction after fertilization when zygote undergoes mitotic division, hence also called *mitotic nondisjunction*.

Characteristic features in a person with Klinefelter syndrome are the following (Fig. 9.1.10):

- Poor development of testis is present with hyalinization of seminiferous tubules, leading to sterility. Therefore, this disorder is also known as *seminiferous dysgenesis*.
- Patients have normal male internal and external genitalia.
- Patients are usually tall (due to growth of lower body segment) and obese.
- Gynaecomastia (development of breast in male) is present.
- At the time of puberty and afterwards, the patient has signs of sexual immaturity, i.e. the secondary sex characters are poorly developed:
  - Sparse body and pubic hair are present.
  - Penis tends to be small.
  - Testes are very small (peanut size).
- Other associated features include:
  - Low or normal plasma testosterone level
  - High plasma level of gonadotropins (LH and follicle-stimulating hormone [FSH])
  - High plasma level of oestradiol

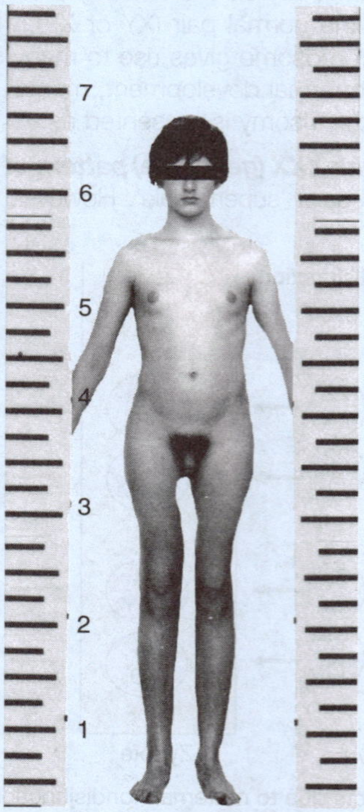

Fig. 9.1.10 Photograph of a patient with Klinefelter syndrome showing tall stature, famine stigmata, bilateral gynaecomastia and small-sized external genitalia.

- Positive sex chromatin test (as genetic chromosomal pattern is of female)

Note: *Down syndrome* (also known as mongolism) is an example of autosomal chromosomal trisomy of chromosome 21.

2. Monosomy

As shown in Fig. 9.1.8, when both chromosomes of a pair go to one gamete, the other gamete resulting from such a division has only 22 chromosomes, and at fertilization the zygote formed will have only 45 chromosomes. Hence, one pair is represented by single chromosome, so it is called monosomy. Depending on the presence of X or Y chromosome, there will be either female phenotype (44+XO) or male phenotype (44+YO). The best known example of monosomy disorder is *Turner syndrome* and another example is an individual with 44+YO karyotype.

Turner Syndrome. Characteristic features of Turner syndrome are the following (Fig. 9.1.11):

- The patient's chromosomal pattern (karyotype) is 44+XO; Y chromosome is absent; hence, the patient is phenotypically female.
- The incidence of Turner syndrome is 1 in 2500 females.
- There is ovarian dysgenesis because of XO karyotype.
- Normal female internal and external genitalia are present (female phenotype).
- Puberty is delayed. Although there is female type of sexual development, it is characterized by scanty menstruation, amenorrhoea (no menstruation), primary infertility and amastia.
- Another important associated feature is mental retardation.
- Among skeletal abnormalities, dwarfism is very common. The characteristic features are webbed neck (folds of skin on the side of the neck present), peculiar face with low hairline, ptosis (drooping of eyelids), epicanthus (low-set ears), micrognathia (small jaw) and co*arctation* of aorta.

Individual with karyotype 44+YO: The condition of monosomy is very lethal and leads to intrauterine death of the fetus.

Swyer Syndrome. Swyer syndrome is a rare genetic disorder leading to gonadal dysgenesis due to 46 XY karyotype.

The signs and symptoms **of Swyer syndrome include:**

- The woman with this syndrome is tall, and usually has small uterus and large clitoris.
- The patient lacks ovaries.

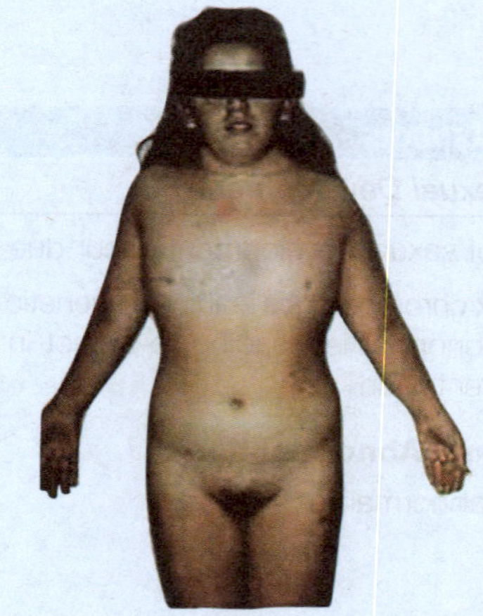

Fig. 9.1.11 Photograph of a patient with Turner syndrome (ovarian dysgenesis) showing short stature, webbed neck and underdeveloped secondary sexual characters (sexual infantilism).

Treatment: Replacement hormonal therapy (HRT) is the common option in these cases. However, in some severe cases, surgical procedures to repair external genitalia are required.

3. Chromosomal Abnormalities with More than Three Sex Chromosomes

Such abnormalities are present with XXXY, XXXXY, XXYY or XXXX chromosomal pattern. The disorders with these chromosomal patterns are recognized by severe mental retardation.

4. Triploidy

Sometimes gametes have diploid number of chromosomes; therefore, the zygotes so formed at the time of fertilization will have $46 + 23 = 69$ chromosomes. This condition is called triploidy. Such fetuses are generally born dead.

5. Abnormalities in Number of Chromosomes in Crossing-over Process

Abnormalities in the number of chromosomes in the crossing-over process are as follows:

- Translocation (part of chromosome may get attached to chromosome of different pair)
- Deletion (part of chromosome may be lost)
- Duplication (one chromosome is longer than the normal having duplication of genes and the other is shorter than the normal with some missing genes)
- Inversion

6. Mosaicism

During cell division, normally the centromere splits longitudinally so that each chromatid splits longitudinally and becomes separate chromosome, but sometimes centromere splits transversely, thus producing two dissimilar chromosomes (i.e. one chromosome is made up of only short arm of chromatid and the other chromosome is made up of only long arm). Such types of chromosomes are also called isochromosomes (mosaicism) and individuals with such chromosomal defects show various types of abnormalities.

Diagnosis of Chromosomal Abnormalities. Early diagnosis (in utero) of these types of disorders is very important. It is made possible by the techniques described next.

1. Amniocentesis In this procedure, amniotic fluid is collected by inserting a needle into the amniotic cavity through the anterior abdominal wall. The fetal cells present in the amniotic fluid are examined.

2. Chorionic Villus Sampling (CVS) In early pregnancy, the fetal cells are obtained by a needle biopsy of chorionic villi.

The cells obtained by amniocentesis or by CVS are grown in the laboratory and then chromosomes are examined under a microscope, and the picture of all the chromosomes arranged in order of longest to smallest, known as karyotype, shows number, size and shape of the chromosome, and helps genetic experts to identify any abnormality.

Hormonal Abnormalities

As discussed in hormonal regulation of sexual development (see page 791), androgens secreted by fetal testes are essential for male development in genetic male fetus, but genetic female when exposed to androgens during 8th to 13th weeks of gestation shows male-like development. The most common developmental disorder due to hormonal abnormalities is pseudohermaphroditism.

Pseudohermaphroditism

Pseudohermaphroditism means an individual having genotype (gonads) of one sex (either testes or ovaries) and genitalia of other sex. It occurs in two forms:

- Female pseudohermaphroditism
- Male pseudohermaphroditism

A. Female pseudohermaphroditism.

The conditions associated with female pseudohermaphroditism are as follows:

- *Congenital virilizing adrenal hyperplasia* of fetal adrenal glands
- *Excess of maternal androgens*
- *Iatrogenic*, i.e. following treatment with androgens or with synthetic progestational drugs

In all the above-mentioned conditions, there is exposure to increased levels of androgens to the genetic female fetus.

Characteristic features of female pseudohermaphroditism are the following (Fig. 9.1.12):

- Genotypically, the individual is female (XX).
- Gonads and internal genitalia are feminine-like (ovaries, oviduct and uterus are present), but at prepubertal age, masculinization occurs in the form of diamond-shaped pubic hair growth and development of penis.
- Increased plasma levels of testosterone and androgens are present.

B. Male Pseudohermaphroditism.

In this condition, the person is genetically male (XY) but has feminization (female internal and external genitalia). Male pseudohermaphroditism results in the following conditions:

- *Androgen resistance*
- *Defective testicular development*
- *Congenital* 17α-hydroxylase deficiency

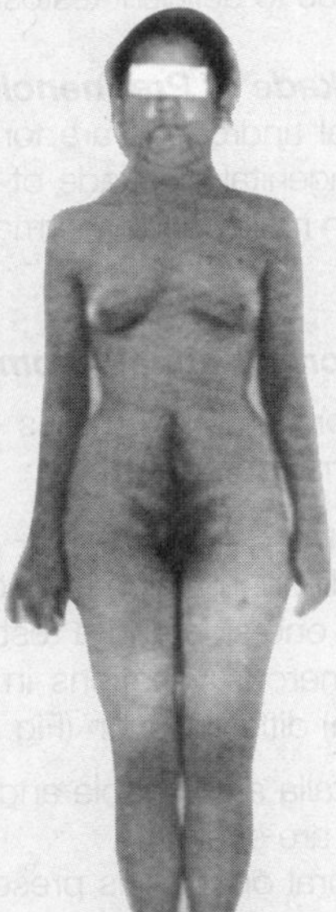

Fig. 9.1.12 Photograph of a patient with female pseudohermaphroditism due to congenital virilizing adrenal hyperplasia showing partial masculinization (diamond-shaped pubic hair).

- *Congenital blockade of pregnenolone formation*
- *Various other nonhormonal anomalies*

1. Androgen Resistance means that androgen levels are normal but cannot exert their full effect on the target tissue. It develops in the following circumstances: *when there is deficiency of enzyme* α-reductase in the target tissue (testosterone cannot be converted into DHT [natural potent androgen] and *when there is mutation of androgenic receptor genes*. The effect varies from mild defect to complete loss of responsiveness of receptors to androgens.

In mild defect, the patient is infertile and may or may not be associated with gynaecomastia.

In case of complete loss of responsiveness of androgen receptors to androgens, the patient presents with *testicular feminizing syndrome*. In this condition, MIS is present and testosterone is secreted at normal or at high rate. The patient presents with the following features:

- The external genitalia are of female type but the vagina ends blindly.
- There are no female internal genitalia because testicular hormone suppresses Müllerian duct derivatives (no uterus and oviducts); thus, at puberty:
  - Nervous system and hypothalamus develop as in a normal female (both physically and psychologically).
  - There occurs primary amenorrhoea due to lack of uterus.

This condition cannot be diagnosed until the patient seeks consultation for primary amenorrhoea.

2. Defective Testicular Development It leads to deficiency of MIS or MRF, which is responsible for feminization in a genetic male individual.

3. Congenital 17α-Hydroxylase Deficiency This enzyme converts adrenal androgens into testosterone. Thus, its deficiency causes feminization due to deficient testosterone.

4. Congenital Blockade of Pregnenolone Formation The testicular and adrenal androgens are formed from pregnenolone; hence, this congenital blockade of pregnenolone formation is associated with male pseudohermaphroditism. For detail see page 813.

5. Various Other Nonhormonal Anomalies

Various other nonhormonal anomalies are also associated with male pseudohermaphroditism.

True Hermaphroditism.

It is a very rare condition in which gonads of both sexes are present (an ovary on one side and a testis on the other side), thus resulting in numerous variations in phenotypic (internal and external genitalia) differentiation (Fig. 9.1.13).

- The external genitalia are variable and predominantly male and female forms are seen.
- The external urethral opening is present on the underside of the penis in predominantly male and in the vagina in predominantly female (hypospadias).
- The gonads may be located at variable sites, i.e. in the labiosacral fold, in the inguinal canal or in the abdomen.
- Breast development occurs in 60%–70% of these patients.

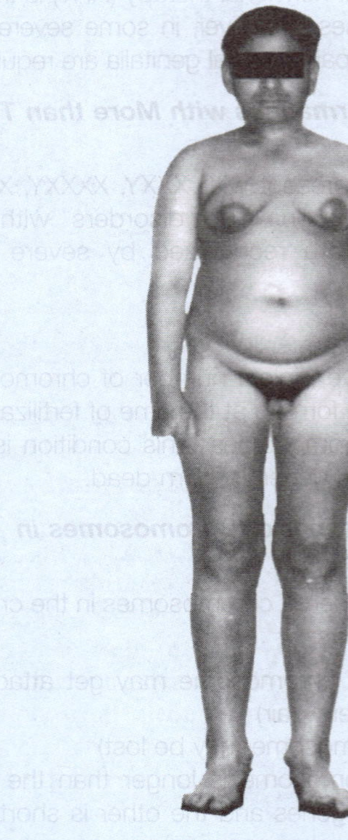

Fig. 9.1.13 Photograph of a patient with true hermaphroditism showing breast development and underdeveloped male genitalia.

- Chromosomal examination shows mixture of 46XX and 46XY constitution.
- Sex chromatin test may or may not be positive.

The true hermaphroditism results due to combined abnormalities.

PUBERTY AND ADOLESCENCE

INTRODUCTION

Puberty and adolescence are the phases of growth between childhood and adulthood.

- Puberty refers to the stage of gonadal development and maturation to the point where reproduction is possible for the first time.
- Adolescence refers to the period of sudden spurt of physical growth between childhood and adulthood.

Since these two phases (adolescence and puberty) of growth are overlapping, the terms are interchangeable. The total period of growth spurt ranges between 3 and 5 years. It starts from the age of 8 years. The average age of onset of puberty is 12 years in girls and 14 years in boys. The age at which puberty occurs varies. In Europe and the United States, the age of onset of puberty is declining.

COMPONENTS OF PUBERTY

The two principal components of puberty are sudden spurt of physical growth and appearance of secondary sex characters.

1. Sudden Spurt of Physical Growth

During sudden spurt of physical growth, there is increase in height, muscle mass and muscle strength of an individual. The height increases by 7–12 cm in boys and about 6–11 cm in girls (Fig. 9.1.14). The increase in height is mainly of the trunk part rather than of limbs.

The muscle mass and muscle strength also increase in both the sexes but the increase is far greater in boys as compared with that in girls.

2. Appearance of Secondary Sex Characters

Stages of development of secondary sex characters

The sequence of events of puberty which occurs in 3- to 5-year period has been discussed in five stages (Table 9.1.2).

Types of secondary sex characters The secondary sex characters are almost fully developed by the stage 5 of the puberty in both male and females. These can be grouped as (Table 9.1.3):

- Structural
- Functional
- Psychological

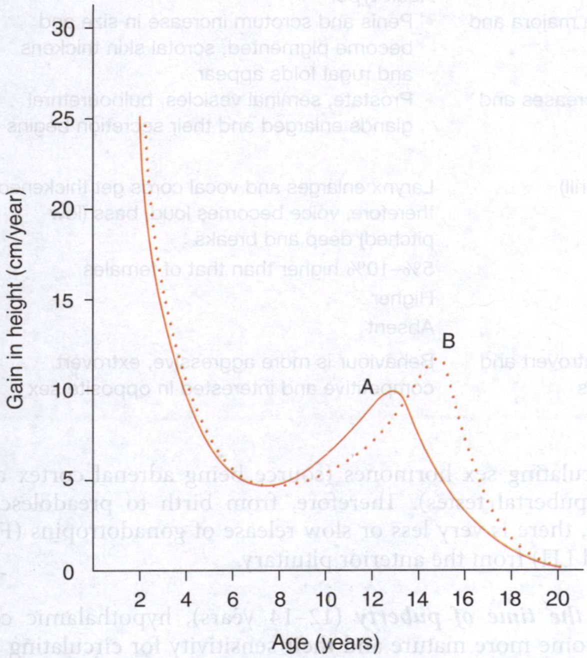

Fig. 9.1.14 Rate of linear growth from birth onwards. Note spurt of growth during adolescence in females (**A**) and males (**B**).

HORMONAL CHANGES DURING PUBERTY

Besides ovaries and testes, other endocrinal glands (adrenal, thyroid and anterior pituitary) also grow in size and their activity increases at the onset of puberty. The hormonal changes noticed at the time of puberty are given next.

1. Gonadotropins In both sexes, the levels of *gonadotropins*, follicle-stimulating hormone (FSH) and LH, secreted from the *anterior pituitary gland* rise slowly from birth of the child up to preadolescent age (Fig. 9.1.15), but at the time of puberty (early teenage), they suddenly increase (Fig. 9.1.15). In prepubertal stage, the gonadrotropin secretion is not under the check of gonadal hormones (oestrogen and testosterone). However, the natural mechanism operating to inhibit gonadotropin-releasing hormone (GnRH) pulse generator is not clearly understood. There may be a possibility that different genes are involved for inhibitory effect in prepubertal stage and stimulatory effects during pubertal stage.

2. Adrenal androgens There is an increase in the secretion of adrenal androgens at puberty. The onset of this stage of increase or activation is called adrenarche. It occurs at 8–10 years of age in girls and at 10–12 years of age in boys. *Adrenarche* is not associated with other adrenal cortex hormones like cortisol, and also there is no increase in ACTH from the anterior pituitary.

Mechanisms involved in increased production of adrenal androgen are as follows:

- More pregnenolone is diverted to androgen pathway (see page 738) due to changes in enzyme system in the adrenals.
- Adrenal androgen-stimulating hormone (AASH) is released from the anterior pituitary.

Functions subserved by adrenal androgens at puberty are as follows:

- Growth of pubic and axillary hair in both sexes
- Growth of muscle mass and its strength

Table 9.1.2 Sequence of events during puberty in males and females

	In females		In males	
Stage of puberty	**Bone age (years)**	**Characteristics**	**Bone age (years)**	**Characteristics**
Stage 1	Up to 7.5	Preadolescent age	7.5	Preadolescent age
Stage 2	10.5	Appearance of breast buds (thelarche)	12	Genital development begins (enlargement of testis)
Stage 3	11.5	(i) Axillary and pubic hair appear (pubarche) (ii) Enlargement of breast (elevation) (iii) Sudden increase in height (height spurt)	14	(i) Axillary and pubic hair start appearing (ii) Enlargement of penis
Stage 4	13	(i) Menstruation starts (menarche) (ii) Breast areola begins to elevate and project	15	(i) Further growth of testis, penis and genitalia (ii) Sudden increase in height (height spurt)
Stage 5	14	(i) Adult genitalia (ii) Secondary sex characters	16.5	Adult genitalia and secondary sex characters

Table 9.1.3 Secondary sex characters in females and males

Group	In females	In males
A. Structural		
i) *Body configuration*	Narrow shoulders, broad hips (broad pelvis) Thighs converge Arms diverge (wide carrying angle)	Shoulders are broader than pelvis
ii) *Skin*	Skin is smooth and light	Skin is thick, dark and oily (sebaceous gland secretion thickens and predisposing to acne)
iii) *Hair growth on:* • Body • Face • Scalp • Pubic region	Body hair fine and scanty • Thick growth, frontal hairline rounded Concave	Body hair rough and dark • Moustaches and beard appeared • Frontal hairline indented at the side Convex and extends towards umbilicus (triangle with apex up)
iv) *Muscularity*	Muscles are soft (+)	Muscle bulk and strength is far greater (+++)
v) *Subcutaneous fat*	Female distribution of fat due to deposition of fat in breast and hips which gives characteristic curves and contours to the body	
vi) *Genitalia and accessory sex organs*	Adult type: • Clitoris increases in size, labia majora and minora get enlarged • Breasts are developed • Uterus and vaginal growth increases and their activity starts	Adult type: • Penis and scrotum increase in size and become pigmented, scrotal skin thickens and rugal folds appear • Prostate, seminal vesicles, bulbourethral glands enlarged and their secretion begins
B. Functional		
i) *Voice*	No change (remains soft and shrill)	Larynx enlarges and vocal cords get thickened; therefore, voice becomes loud, bass (low pitched) deep and breaks
ii) *Basal metabolic rate (BMR)*	Lower	5%–10% higher than that of females
iii) *RBC count and Hb concentration*	Lower	Higher
iv) *Menstrual cycle*	Begins	Absent
C. Psychological	Girls are more emotional, shy, introvert and sexually attracted towards males	Behaviour is more aggressive, extrovert, competitive and interested in opposite sex

3. Growth hormone Normally from birth up to prepubertal stage, the growth hormone secretion is intermittent (a few peaks every 24 hours) but at the time of puberty, although basal level of growth hormone does not rise, there is an increase in the frequency and amplitude of the peaks. It is responsible for generalized growth spurt at adolescence (see page 677).

4. Thyroid gland secretions Thyroid gland secretions (thyroxine) also increase during puberty. Thyroxine is necessary for normal growth and development (see page 690).

5. Gonadal hormones (sex hormones) There is a slow increase in secretion of sex hormones in children between the age of 7 and 10 years. But there is a rapid rise in oestrogen secretion (in girls) and testosterone in boys in early teenage (Fig. 9.1.15).

CONTROL OF ONSET OF PUBERTY

The exact mechanism of onset of puberty is still not fully understood, but experimental and clinical observations support that the *hypothalamus* is intimately involved in this process, being a nodal point between nervous and hormonal circuits. The plausible mechanism involved is given next (Fig. 9.1.16).

Role of Hypothalamus

From birth to preadolescent age: GnRH secretion from the hypothalamus is highly sensitive to feedback inhibition by circulating sex hormones (source being adrenal cortex and prepubertal testes). Therefore, from birth to preadolescent age, there is very less or slow release of gonadotropins (FSH and LH) from the anterior pituitary.

At the time of puberty (12–14 years), hypothalamic cells become more mature and their sensitivity for circulating sex hormones (for negative feedback) decreases so much that there is pulsatile release of GnRH from the hypothalamus. As a result, there occurs an increase in secretion of pituitary gonadotropins (FSH and LH). They act on gonads to release gonadal sex hormones.

At the time of puberty, the pulsatile release of GnRH is initiated by excitatory neurotransmitters like kisspeptin. Kisspeptin, also called metastin, initiates pulsatile release of GnRH neurons. The gene that encodes kisspeptin is called KISS-1 gene.

Applied Aspects

Individuals with mutation of GPR-54 have hypogonadotropic hypogonadism. They fail to enter puberty due to absence of sexual maturation.

Awakening of hypothalamus: The hypothalamus at puberty is also positively stimulated (awakening of the hypothalamus) by the critical body mass and visual, olfactory and other sensory stimuli.

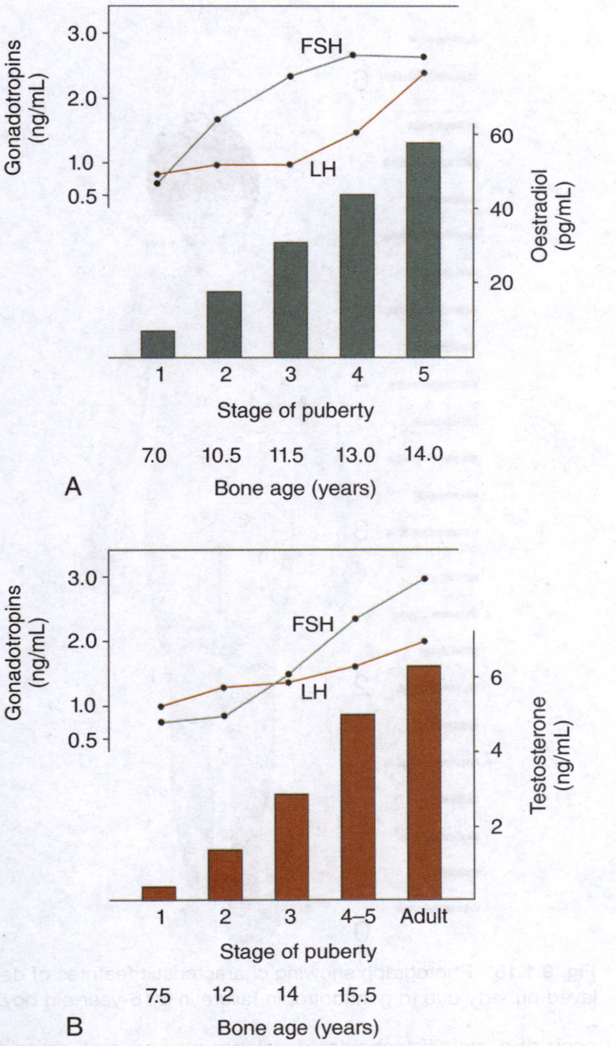

Fig. 9.1.15 Changes in plasma concentration of gonadotropins and gonadal hormones during different stages of puberty: **A**, in girls; and **B**, in boys.

Role of Leptin

Leptin (a Greek word meaning thin) is a circulating protein, formed in the fat cells. It is under the influence of Ob gene, hence called product of Ob gene. It acts on the hypothalamus by feedback control mechanism leading to decreased food intake and increased energy consumption (satiety) and thus controls the body weight (see page 932). Therefore, leptin acts as a link between critical body weight and onset of puberty. Certain observations in favour of this fact are as follows:

- Girls suffering from anorexia nervosa (loss of appetite) stop menstruation, and if they start eating and gain weight, they menstruate again.
- It has been observed in mice that having low plasma leptin levels (produced by fasting) is associated with inhibition of onset of puberty.
- The obese mice (due to defective Ob gene) that cannot produce leptin are infertile.

In both of the above-mentioned cases, injection of leptin restores fertility. Also, when leptin treatment is given to immature female mice, there is onset of puberty.

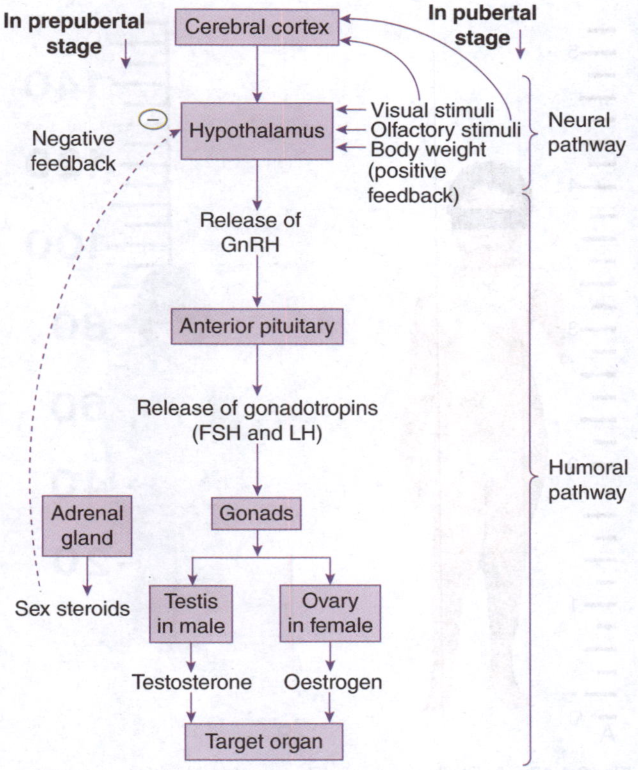

Fig. 9.1.16 Neurohormonal mechanism of onset of puberty.

Applied Aspects

Disorders of Puberty

Disorders of puberty are related to the time of its onset, e.g.:

- Early onset of puberty (precocious puberty)
- Late onset of puberty (delayed or absent puberty)

1. Precocious Puberty

Precocious puberty refers to onset of puberty in a child before 8 years of age. It is more commonly seen in girls. Precocious puberty is of two types – true precocious puberty and pseudoprecocious puberty.

i. True Precocious Puberty. *In the case of true precocious puberty*, there is early development of secondary sex characters and gametogenesis also starts earlier (Fig. 9.1.17). It operates through normal hypothalamic–pituitary–gonadal axis functioning (early but otherwise normal pubertal secretion of gonadotropins from the anterior pituitary) without any other endocrinal disorder. It proceeds isosexually, i.e. there are no disturbing signs of virilization in girls and no feminizing signs in boys.

Causes: A clear cause of precocious puberty may not be found in most of the cases. However, certain conditions related to the disorder are as follows:

- Constitutional or idiopathic, i.e. no cause is known. It is more common in girls.
- Conditions which disrupt the neural pathway for feedback inhibition of GnRH release from the hypothalamus. For example:
  - *Cerebral disorders* involving the posterior ventral hypothalamus near the infundibulum which may be tumour, infections and developmental abnormalities
  - *Pineal gland tumours* involving the hypothalamus

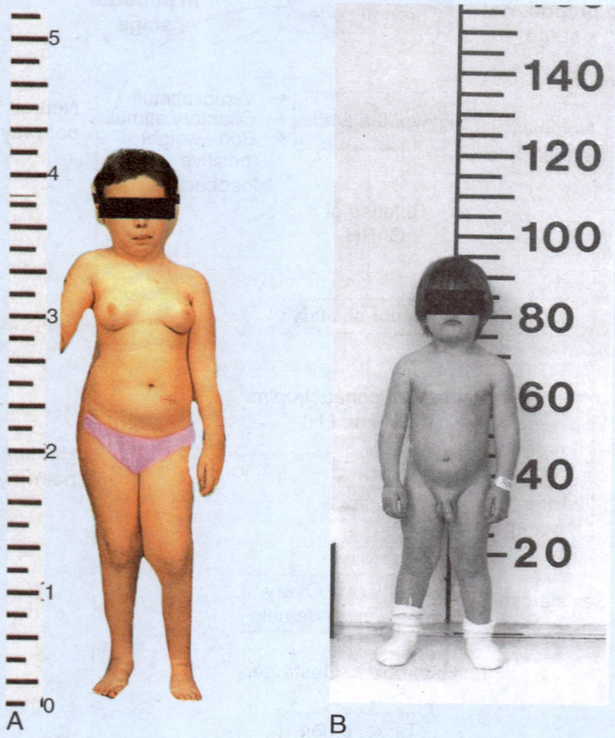

Fig. 9.1.17 **A**, Photograph of a 7-year-old girl with true precocious puberty (well-developed secondary sex characters). **B**, Photograph showing precocious puberty in a male child.

In all the above-mentioned conditions, there is early increased secretion of gonadotropins either due to *decreased inhibition of release of GnRH from the pulse generator* (hypothalamus) or due to chronic stimulation of hypothalamic cells by some irritative focus. Hence, the condition is also called *gonadotropin-dependent precocious puberty*.

- Precocious puberty also occurs with low or normal gonadotropin levels (hence known as gonadotropin-independent precocious puberty), for example, in case when there is insensitivity of LH receptors to gonadotropins due to mutations of G-proteins which couple receptors to adenylyl cyclase.

ii. Pseudoprecocious Puberty.

In pseudoprecocious puberty, there occurs early development of secondary sex characters without gametogenesis. It occurs due to abnormal exposure of sex hormones to an immature child. In this type of precocious puberty, the child may not remain isosexual and the normal sequence of events of puberty is also altered.

Causes: The following conditions involving adrenal or gonads result in pseudoprecocious puberty:

Adrenal conditions are:

- Congenital virilizing hyperplasia (see page 742)
- Androgen-secreting tumours in males
- Oestrogen-secreting tumours in females

Gonadal conditions are:

- Leydig cell tumour of the testis (in males)
- Granulosa cell tumour of the ovary (in females)

2. Delayed or Absent Puberty

Puberty is considered to be pathologically delayed in case of a female if menarche does not occur by 17 years of age, or in case of a male if testicular development and maturation fails to occur by the age of 20 years.

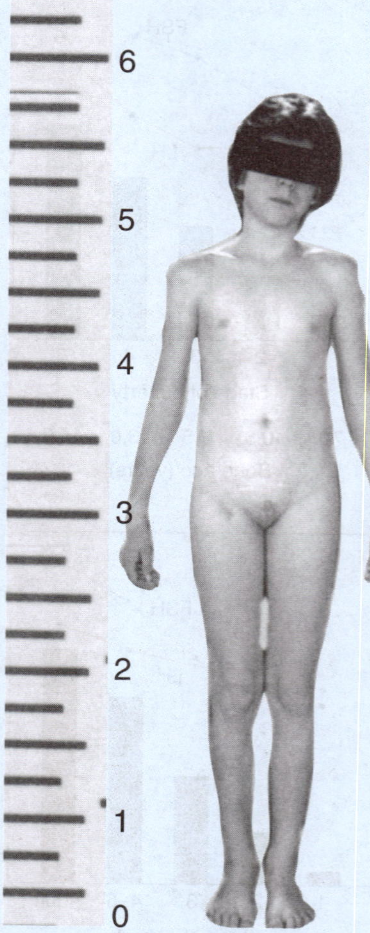

Fig. 9.1.18 Photograph showing characteristic features of delayed puberty due to gonadotropin failure in a 16-year-old boy.

Delayed puberty is more commonly observed in boys than in girls. Usually, it is constitutional or physiological delay and ultimately the child catches up. Delayed or absent puberty is a matter of great concern when it occurs in the following conditions (Fig. 9.1.18):

Failure of hypothalamus/pituitary to secrete gonadotropins, as in panhypopituitarism or isolated gonadotropin deficiency

Primary gonadal failure that refers to developmental failure or gonadal dysgenesis which occurs in Klinefelter syndrome in males and Turner syndrome in females (see page 794)

Deficiency of enzymes which are essential for steroid synthesis

Deficiency of specific receptors in the target tissue

Features of delayed or absent puberty are as follows:

- Lack of pubertal development
- Short stature (dwarf)
- Presence of associated features of other endocrinal abnormalities
- Low levels of gonadotropins

Note: In some cases, puberty is absent even when gonads are present and other endocrines are functioning normally. In males, this condition is known as *eunuchoidism*, and in females, it is called *primary amenorrhoea*.

Self-Assessment

1. Discuss the sex determination and sex differentiation.
2. Discuss the stages of puberty and its regulation.
3. Describe the following:
   - Male hermaphroditism
   - Hormonal changes at puberty in a female
   - Development of genitalia in a male
   - Karyotyping in sex determination
   - Delayed puberty
   - Role of leptin in puberty
4. Write notes on the following:
   - PC-PNDT Act

Clinical Cases

Case 1

A 30-year-old male visited a physician with the complaint of having small size of penis and testis and scanty hair on the body and parents forcing him for marriage.

On examination, the patient had obvious gynaecomastia, sparse pubic and axillary hair, and small-sized genitalia. From signs and symptoms, the probable diagnosis made was Klinefelter syndrome.

Q1. What is the genetic pattern of this condition?
Q2. What is the cause of type of pattern in this condition?
Q3. What biochemical tests should be done to confirm the diagnosis?
Q4. The patient should get married (Yes/No). Explain the reason.

Case 2

A 20-year-old female was brought to the gynaecologist by her mother for not starting of periods.

The examination revealed normal internal and external genitalia; the patient's height was only 3 feet 2 inches, and she had drooping eyes and webbed neck.

Q1. On the basis of physical findings, what is the probable diagnosis?
Q2. What is the genetic pattern of this condition?
Q3. What are the other associated features in this condition?
Q4. What biochemical tests should be done to conclude the final diagnosis?

Case 3

The mother of a 7-year-old female child brought her to the gynaecologist for development of an adult-sized breast and starting of periods 2 months back.

Q1. What is this condition known as?
Q2. What is the cause of this condition?
Q3. What tests should be advised to reach the conclusion?

9.2 Male Reproductive Physiology

CHAPTER OUTLINE

AN OVERVIEW OF MALE REPRODUCTIVE SYSTEM

The male reproductive system comprises the internal and external genital organs which can be functionally organized as given next (Fig. 9.2.1).

I. Gonads or Primary Male Sex Glands are a Pair of Testes

Gonads or primary male sex glands are a pair of testes which correspond with ovaries in females. The main functions of the testes are to produce sperms and secrete testosterone (male sex hormones).

II. Accessory Sex Glands of Male Reproductive System

Accessory sex glands of the male reproductive system are the following:

1. ***Seminal vesicles*** are two lobulated glands situated on either side of the prostate between the urinary bladder and the rectum.
   - They do not store sperms as their name implies.
   - They secrete a thick alkaline fluid that mixes with the sperms as they pass into the ejaculatory ducts and urethra.
   - The duct of each seminal vesicle joins the ductus deferens to form the ejaculatory duct.
2. ***Bulbourethral (Cowper's) glands*** are two pea-sized glands. Their mucus-like secretion enters the anterior (penile) urethra during sexual arousal.
3. ***Prostate gland*** is the largest accessory gland of the male reproductive system.
   - It lies just below the urinary bladder and the urethra passes through a small hole in the centre of the prostate.
   - It secretes a thin milky fluid which forms 30% of the volume of semen (a mixture of secretions produced by the testes, seminal vesicles, prostate and bulbourethral glands).
   - Composition and functions of prostatic fluid are described as a component of semen (page 809).

III. Ducts of the Male Reproductive System

These include:

1. ***Epididymis:*** It is formed by minute convolutions of the duct of the epididymis, so tightly compacted that they appear solid.
   - The efferent ductus transports the sperms from the rete testis to the epididymis where they are stored. The sperms can remain viable for a month in the epididymis.
   - Secretions of the epididymis provide nourishment to the spermatozoa and help them to mature.
   - Nonmotile spermatozoa become motile after passing through the epididymis.
2. ***Ductus deferens*** or ***vas deferens:*** It is the continuation of the tail of the epididymis. It ends by joining to the duct of seminal vesicle.
   - It serves as a secondary storehouse for spermatozoa which will be released at the time of ejaculation.
   - In vasectomy operation for sterilization in males, the vas deferens is ligated and sectioned.
3. ***Ejaculatory ducts:*** Each ejaculatory duct is a slender tube that arises by the union of the ductus deferens with the duct of seminal vesicle. The ejaculatory ducts open as a minute slit-like opening into the prostatic urethra which forms a part of the prostatic urethra.
4. ***Urethra:*** The male urethra is a muscular tube (18–20 cm long) that conveys urine from the internal urethral orifice of the urinary bladder to the external urethral orifice at the

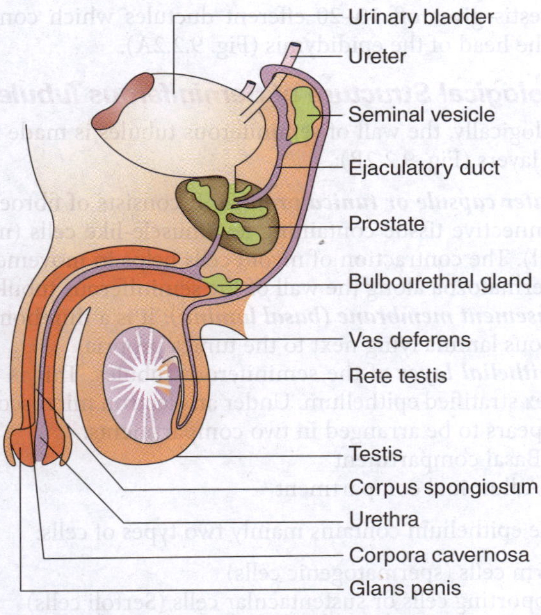

Fig. 9.2.1 Male reproductive system.

tip of the glans penis. The urethra also provides an exit for semen (sperms and glandular secretions) which is passed by the ejaculatory ducts in its prostatic part.

IV. Supporting Structures of the Male Reproductive System

1. ***Spermatic cord:*** It suspends the testes in the scrotum and contains structures that pass through the inguinal canal to and from the testis, i.e. ductus deferens, vessels and nerves of the testis.
   - Its coverings are internal spermatic fascia, cremasteric fascia and external spermatic fascia.
2. ***Scrotum:*** It is a cutaneous fibromuscular sac (can be considered an outpouching of the lower part of the anterior abdominal wall) which houses the testes, epididymis and lower ends of the spermatic cords.
   - Internally, the scrotum is divided into right and left compartments by the septum of the scrotum.
   - The scrotum maintains the temperature lower than the normal body temperature (about 32°C) which is necessary for normal spermatogenesis.
   - Exposure to cold also inhibits spermatogenesis; when exposure to cold occurs, the dartos muscle present in the scrotum contracts and puts up a thicker cover around the testes and thus keeps them warm.
3. ***Penis:*** It is the male copulatory organ and the common outlet for urine and semen. The penis can be divided into three parts – root, body and glans penis. It is composed of three cylindrical bodies of erectile cavernous tissue – the corpora cavernosa and corpus spongiosum.

FUNCTIONAL ANATOMY OF TESTES

GROSS ANATOMY

Location The testes are ovoid bodies suspended by spermatic cords into the scrotum, where they are maintained at a temperature lower than the normal body temperature (32°C) necessary for normal spermatogenesis.

Weight In an adult male, the average weight of each testis is 25 g (range 10–40 g). Ninety per cent of the volume of testis is due to the presence of seminiferous tubules. Weight of the testis decreases in old age.

Coverings Each testis from interior to exterior is covered by the following three layers (Fig. 9.2.2):

i. ***Tunica vasculosa:*** It is the innermost covering made up of loose connective tissue rich in blood vessels.
ii. ***Tunica albuginea:*** It is also called capsule of the testis and consists of closely packed collagen fibres intermingling with many elastic fibres.
   The tunica albuginea, on the posterior part of the testis, expands into a thick mass called *mediastinal testis*. Numerous septa from the mediastinal testis project into

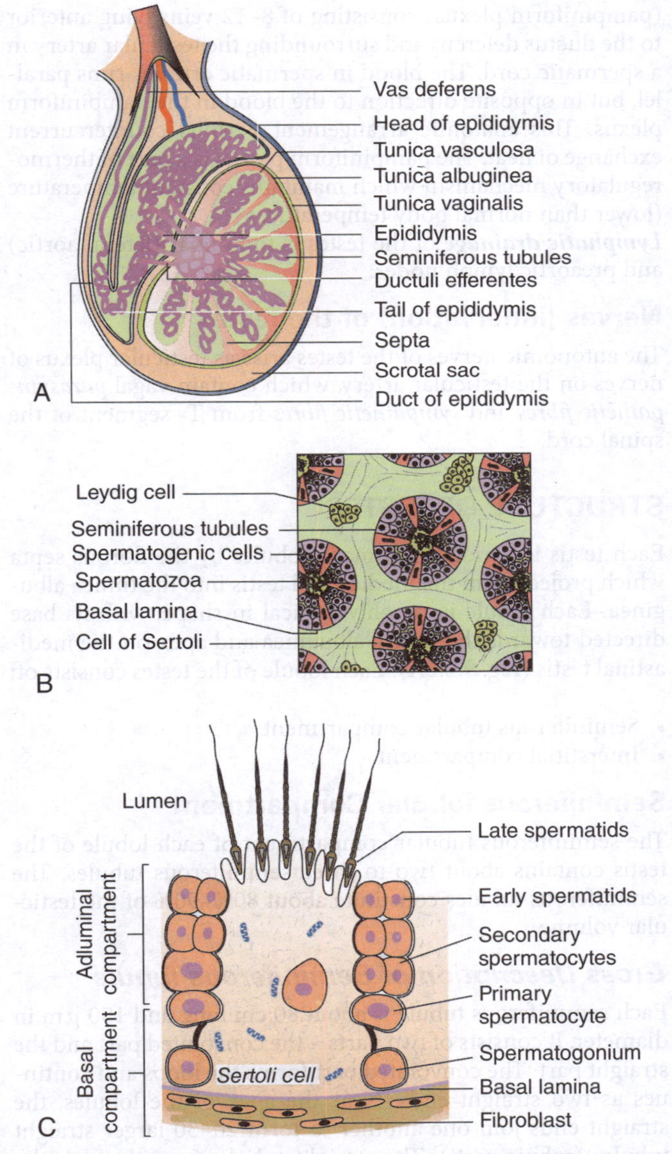

Fig. 9.2.2 Structure of testis: **A**, lateral view showing the cut section of testis, epididymis and distal part of spermatic cord; **B**, histology of testis; and **C**, electron microscopic structure of seminiferous epithelium.

the tunica albuginea and thus divide the substance of the testis into a large number of lobules.

iii. ***Tunica vaginalis*** is the outermost covering composed of mesothelial cells. It is a closed sac, partially surrounding the testis. It consists of two layers: the inner visceral layer of the tunica vaginalis which adheres to the tunica albuginea and the outer parietal layer of the tunica vaginalis which lies in close contact with the inner surface of the scrotum. A small space between these two layers (cavity of tunica vaginalis) is occupied by a small amount of fluid.

Coverings of the testis provide protection from trauma and allow free movement of the testis in the scrotum.

Blood Supply

The arterial blood supply to the testes is by testicular arteries (arise from the abdominal aorta). The testicular artery or one of its branches anastomoses with the artery of ductus deferens. **The *venous blood*** is drained by testicular veins emerging from the testes and epididymis and join to form a venous network (pampiniform plexus) consisting of 8–12 veins lying anterior to the ductus deferens and surrounding the testicular artery in a spermatic cord. The blood in spermatic arteries runs parallel, but in opposite direction to the blood in the pampiniform plexus. This anatomic arrangement permits countercurrent exchange of heat. The pampiniform plexus is a part of thermoregulatory mechanism which maintains constant temperature (lower than normal body temperature).

Lymphatic drainage of the testes is to lumbar (lateral aortic) and preaortic lymph nodes.

Nerves (innervation) of the Testes

The autonomic nerves of the testes arise as testicular plexus of nerves on the testicular artery, which contain vagal *parasympathetic fibres* and *sympathetic fibres* from T_7 segment of the spinal cord.

STRUCTURE OF TESTES

Each testis is divided into many lobules by the fibrous septa which project from the mediastinal testis into the tunica albuginea. Each lobule is roughly conical in shape, with its base directed towards the tunica albuginea and apex on the mediastinal testis (Fig. 9.2.2A). Each lobule of the testes consists of:

- Seminiferous tubular compartment
- Interstitial compartment

Seminiferous Tubular Compartment

The seminiferous tubular compartment of each lobule of the testis contains about two to three seminiferous tubules. The seminiferous tubules constitute about 80%–90% of the testicular volume.

Gross Description of Seminiferous Tubule

Each seminiferous tubule is about 80 cm long and 150 μm in diameter. It consists of two parts – the convoluted part and the straight part. The convoluted part forms the loops and continues as two straight ends. Near the apex of the lobules, the straight ends join one another to form 20–30 larger straight tubules (tubule recti). The straight tubules pass through the fibrous tissue of the mediastinal testis and unite to form a network called rete testis. At the upper end of each testis, the rete testis gives off 10–20 efferent ductules which continue into the head of the epididymis (Fig. 9.2.2A).

Histological Structure of Seminiferous Tubule

Histologically, the wall of seminiferous tubules is made up of three layers (Fig. 9.2.2B):

1. ***Outer capsule or tunica propria:*** It consists of fibroelastic connective tissue containing few muscle-like cells (myoid cell). The contraction of myoid cells helps in movement of spermatozoa along the wall of the seminiferous tubules.
2. ***Basement membrane (basal lamina):*** It is a thin homogeneous lamina lying next to the tunica propria.
3. ***Epithelial layer*** of the seminiferous tubules: This is complex stratified epithelium. Under an electron microscope, it appears to be arranged in two compartments:
   - Basal compartment
   - Adluminal compartment

   The epithelium contains mainly two types of cells:

- Germ cells (spermatogenic cells)
- Supporting cells or sustentacular cells (Sertoli cells)

Spermatogenic cells The spermatogenic cells lie in between the Sertoli cells. These are arranged in an orderly manner in four to eight layers, which extend from the basal lamina to the lumen of seminiferous tubule.

In children, the testis is not fully developed. So, only the primitive germ cells (spermatogonia) are present.

In a sexually mature individual, the spermatogenic cells of all stages of differentiation are seen, arranged in an orderly manner (Fig. 9.2.2C).

- Basal compartment or deep part of epithelium is occupied by cells of early stages of spermatogenesis (spermatogonia and primary spermatocytes).
- Adluminal compartment or superficial compartment contains cells of later stages of spermatogenesis; from periphery to lumen, these cells are secondary spermatocytes, early spermatid, late spermatid and spermatozoa.

Sertoli cells Under an electron microscope, each Sertoli cell appears as a slender cell having an irregular pyramidal shape. The base of Sertoli cells rests on the basal lamina and each cell stretches from the basal lamina to the lumen of tubule. Thus, each Sertoli cell occupies both the basal and adluminal compartments (Fig. 9.2.2C). Characteristic features of Sertoli cells are the following:

Nucleus lies near the base and has a prominent nucleolus.

Recesses: The sides and the apices of the cells are marked by recesses, which are occupied by developing cells of different stages of spermatogenesis (spermatogonia, spermatocytes, spermatids and spermatozoa) from basal to luminal region.

Tight junctions: There is no cytoplasmic continuity between the two adjacent Sertoli cells, but plasma membranes of two adjoining cells are connected by tight junctions in the basal region. Hence, the wall of seminiferous tubule is divided into two compartments.

The tight junction forms an effective permeability barrier within the seminiferous epithelium, which is defined in man as the *blood–testis barrier*.

Significance of blood–testis barrier: It limits the transport of many substances from blood to seminiferous lumen:

- This barrier maintains germ cells in a privileged location, because mature sperm cells are very immunogenic when introduced into the systemic circulation. Thus, the blood–testis barrier protects the cells of different stages of spermatogenesis from blood-borne toxic substances and from circulating antibodies.

- It prevents the entry of by-products of gametogenesis into the blood (that is why autoimmune reactions do not occur). Sometimes breakdown of this barrier leads to autoimmune response against germ cells.
- The maturing germ cells can pass through this barrier as they move from basal lamina to lumen (from basal compartment to adluminal compartment) of seminiferous tubule. This occurs due to disruption (breakdown) of tight junctions when maturing cell is passing through it and then a new tight junction is formed.
- Maintenance of luminal fluid composition: The blood–testis barrier helps in maintenance of seminiferous luminal fluid concentration, which contains:
  - Glucose and proteins in very low amount as compared with plasma
  - Androgens (testosterone) and potassium (K^+) in high concentration
  - Oestrogen, glutamic acid and inositol
- The blood–testis barrier helps in establishing an osmotic gradient that facilitates the movement of fluid and testosterone into the tubular lumen.
- Certain substances like steroids can easily cross through this barrier.

Cytoplasm: The cytoplasm of the Sertoli cells contains abundant mitochondria, endoplasmic reticulum and other organelles. The microfilaments and microtubules form cytoskeleton that is important for cohesive functions of these cells.

Functions of sertoli cells: Several functions have been attributed to Sertoli cells. These are the following:

1. ***Physical support and nutrition:*** The Sertoli cells provide physical support to maturing germ cells (the germ cells are present in the recesses on the side walls of the cells), nourish them (being rich in glycogen contents) and also remove waste products from the germ cells.
2. ***Phagocytic function:*** The residual cytoplasmic organelles are cast off from the spermatozoa during conversion of spermatids into sperms. These cytoplasmic by-products or residues are phagocytized by the Sertoli cells.
3. ***Maintenance of blood–testis barrier*** (see page 804): Sertoli cells maintain the blood–testis barrier, as described earlier.
4. ***Secretory functions:*** Sertoli cells secrete the following hormones and substances:
   - *Müllerian inhibitory substance (MIS)* or Müllerian duct inhibition factor (MIF) is secreted by Sertoli cells which helps in regression of Müllerian duct in fetus and male sexual development.
   - *Inhibin* is a substance that inhibits spermatogenesis before the onset of puberty by regulating follicle-stimulating hormone (FSH) secretion by negative feedback at anterior pituitary level.
   - *Androgen-binding protein (ABP)* or androgen-binding globulin is secreted by Sertoli cells. It has a high affinity for testosterone as well as for hydroxytestosterone, thus maintaining high concentration of androgens in the lumen of seminiferous tubules.
   - *Oestrogen:* A small amount of oestrogen is secreted by the testis due to conversion of androgenic precursors to oestradiol. An enzyme aromatase (CYP19) involved in this reaction is formed by the Sertoli cells.
   - *Transport proteins,* such as transferrins (the iron-transporting protein) and ceruloplasmin (copper-binding protein), are formed by Sertoli cells which help in transferring iron and copper to tubular cells.
   - *Plasminogen activator:* It is required for proteolytic activity for the disruption of tight junctions during migration of maturing germ cells from basal to luminal compartment, and is formed by Sertoli cells.
   - *Seminiferous tubular luminal fluid:* Sertoli cells secrete watery, solute-rich (K^+ and HCO_3^-) fluid into the lumen of seminiferous tubules. These cells pump ions into intercellular spaces to create an osmotic gradient that moves water from basal part of Sertoli cells to free luminal surface. This fluid movement provides a driving force for nonmotile spermatozoa.

Applied Aspects

Sertoli-cell-only (SCO) syndrome, also called germ cell aplasia or Del Castillo syndrome. In this condition seminiferous tubules are devoid of germ cell and only Sertoli cells are present.

Sertoli–Leydig cell tumour is a tumour of the ovary, usually seen in females of 20–30 years of age. It occurs due to mutation in DICER-1 gene that encodes an endonuclease, which is essential for processing of microRNAs.

MicroRNA dysregulation causes development of male-directed stromal cells in the females leading to excessive secretion of androgens. The main features of this tumour are virilization features like hirsutism, hypertrophy of cords and voice changes.

Interstitial Compartment

The interstitial spaces between the seminiferous tubules constitute about 10%–20% of volume of the testis. The interstitial compartment of each lobule is filled by loose connective tissue containing:

- Blood vessels
- Lymphatics
- *Leydig cells* (the Leydig cells or the so-called interstitial cells are present in groups; they have endocrine function of secretion of male sex hormone [testosterone])

FUNCTIONS OF TESTES

The two principal functions of testes are the following:

- Gametogenic function (spermatogenesis)
- Endocrine function

SPERMATOGENESIS

Spermatogenesis refers to the process of formation of spermatozoa from the primitive germ cells (spermatogonia).

Characteristic Features of Spermatogenesis

- Spermatogenesis begins at puberty and continues throughout adult life to decline in old age.
- The majority of the spermatogonia undergo continuous mitotic division to provide additional stem cells.

- Only a minority of the spermatogonia undergo further differentiation by meiosis, a process unique to germinal epithelium.
- Each differentiating spermatogonium develops into 512 spermatids.
- Spermatogenesis does not occur simultaneously in all the parts of testes. At any one moment, some areas of the seminiferous tubules are active, whereas others are in resting state.
- In humans, it takes an average of 74 days to form a mature sperm from a primitive germ cell.
- The spermatozoa formed in the seminiferous tubules are nonmotile structures.
- The spermatozoa undergo the process of maturation while passing through the male genital tract and acquire the ability of fertilization of an ovum (capacitation) in the female genital tract.

Phases of Spermatogenesis

The phases of spermatogenesis are given next (Fig. 9.2.3).

1. Phase of mitotic division of spermatogonia Spermatogonia or the primitive germ cells (44+XY) serve as a pool of undifferentiated stem cells from which develop the spermatozoa. These cells lie near the basal lamina of seminiferous tubules. Three main types of spermatogonia are described:

Dark type A (AD) spermatogonia (also called type A1) represent a reserve of resting stem cells. They have dark-staining oval nuclei. They divide to form more dark type A cells and also some light type A cells (or A2 cells).

Light or pale type A (AP) spermatogonia have light-staining oval nucleus. They divide to form more light type A spermatogonia and also some spermatogonia of type B.

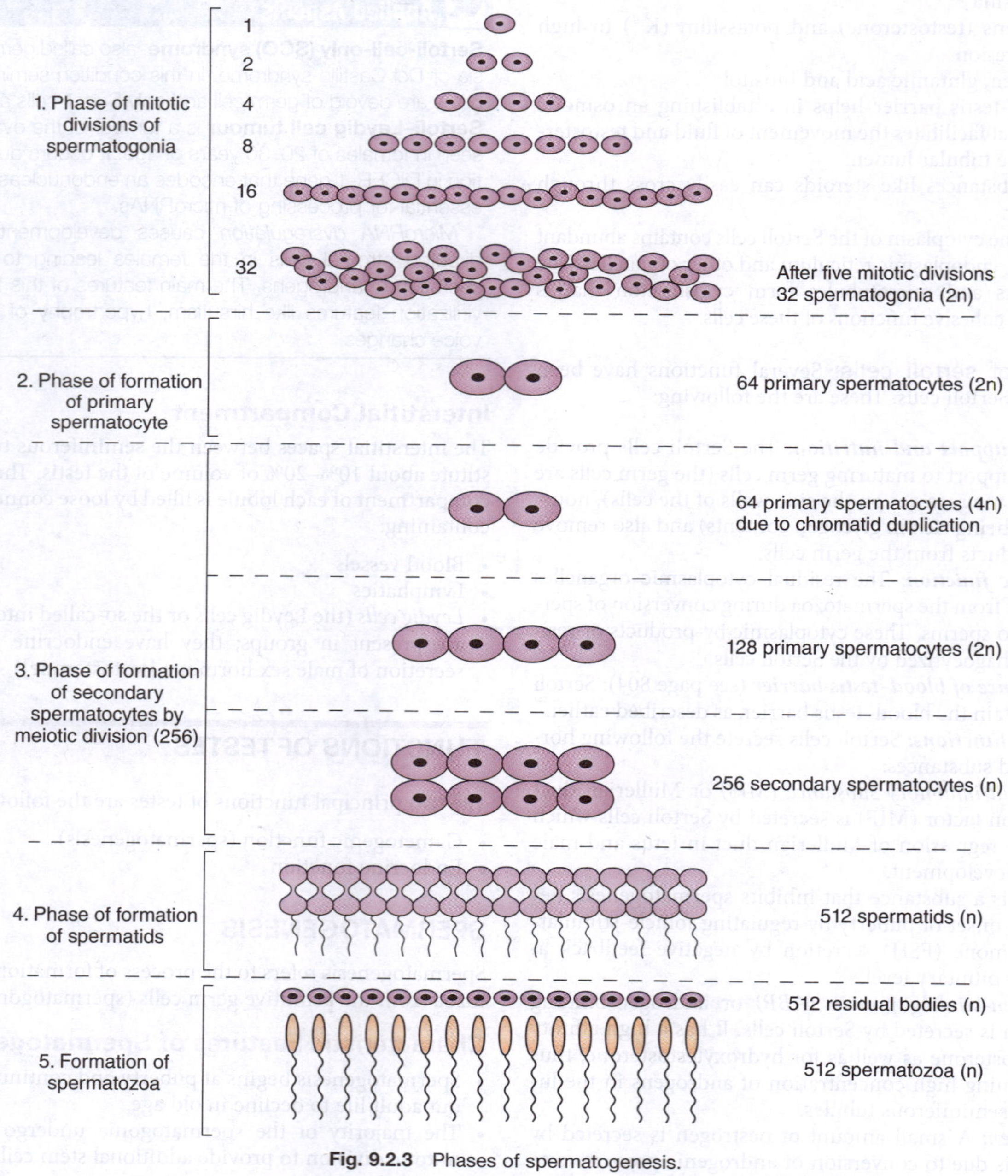

Fig. 9.2.3 Phases of spermatogenesis.

Type B spermatogonia have a spherical nucleus. Each type of spermatogonium divides mitotically 5 times to form 32 type B spermatogonia. The division occurs in the basal compartment of the seminiferous tubule. Due to incomplete cytokinesis, all cells derived from a single spermatogonium remain connected through cytoplasmic bridges and are synchronized in subsequent cell divisions. The connections remain throughout till the formation of individual spermatozoa.

2. Phase of formation of primary spermatocytes by mitotic division The 32 type B spermatogonia (44+X+Y) undergo mitosis to form 64 primary spermatocytes (44+X+Y). Primary spermatocytes are large cells with a large nucleus having diploid number of chromosomes (2n).

Formation of primary spermatocytes from spermatogonia occurs in 25 days.

3. Phase of formation of secondary spermatocyte by meiotic division Each primary spermatocyte undergoes meiotic division:

- In the prophase of meiotic division (when chromatids duplicate), each primary spermatocyte is represented as tetraploid number of chromosomes (4n). In this phase, they remain for about 22 days.
- After first reduction division (meiosis), the 64 tetraploid primary spermatocytes (4n) are converted into 128 primary spermatocytes with diploid number of chromosomes (2n).
- The 128 primary spermatocytes (meiosis) form 256 secondary spermatocytes having haploid number of chromosomes (n), i.e. either 22+X or 22+Y. Therefore, 50% of sperms will have X chromosome and other 50% will have Y chromosome.
- Size of secondary spermatocyte is quite small as compared with that of primary spermatocyte.
- This phase is completed within 9 days.
- From secondary spermatocytes, formation of spermatids occurs in the next 19 days.

4. Phase of formation of spermatid Each secondary spermatocyte divides mitotically to give rise to two spermatids. Thus, a total of 512 spermatids are formed from a single spermatogonium.

- *Early spermatid* is a small round cell with a spherical nucleus containing haploid number of chromosomes.
- *Late spermatids* are formed when the early spermatids undergo changes in the shape and orientation of organelles.

5. Phase of formation of spermatozoon (spermiogenesis) The spermatids do not divide further but undergo morphological changes to form sperms or spermatozoa. The spermatid undergoes changes in the shape and orientation of its organelles. The spermatids mature into spermatozoa in the deep folds of the cytoplasm of the Sertoli cells. During this process, the components of spermatid which take part in forming a spermatozoon are as follows (Fig. 9.2.4):

Nucleus undergoes condensation and changes its shape to form the head of the spermatozoon.

Nuclear proteins are replaced by protamine which surround the chromatins and thus protect them from mutagenic factors.

Centriole divides into two parts; the distal part forms the axial filament and the proximal part forms the basal body. In the beginning, both the parts lie close to each other but later they migrate away. The region earlier occupied by the centriole later on forms the neck of a spermatozoon.

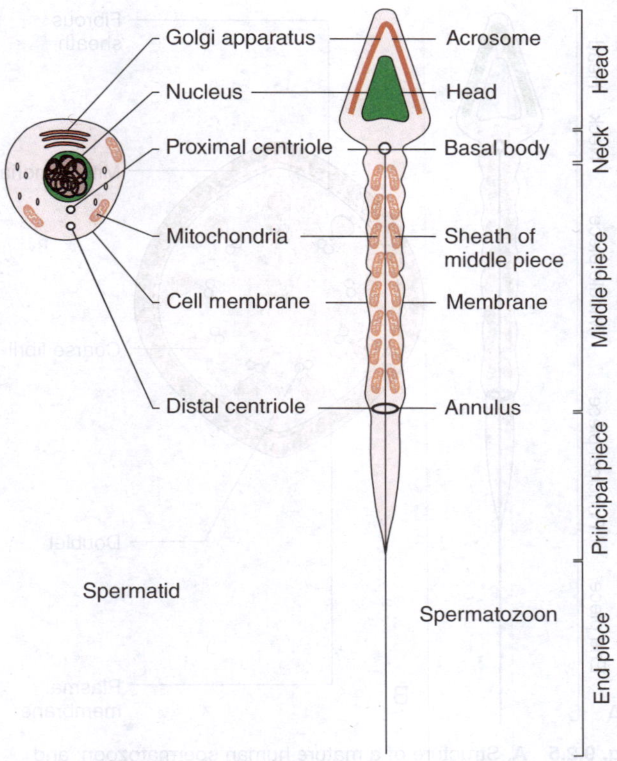

Fig. 9.2.4 Diagrammatic depiction of derivatives of different parts of spermatozoon from that of spermatid.

The Golgi apparatus forms the cap-like structure covering anterior two-thirds of the head (acrosome). It contains proteolytic enzyme (hyaluronidase) and other proteases, which help the sperm in penetration of an ovum during fertilization.

Mitochondria surround the tail part of the sperm lying wrapped in a sheath and provide energy for movements of the spermatozoon.

Cell membrane of the spermatid persists as covering of the spermatozoon. The membranes of late spermatids and of sperms contain germinal angiotensin-converting enzyme (gACE). The specific function of gACE enzyme has yet to be elicited.

The cytoplasm and other organelles (like lipids, ribosomes) shed off as residual bodies and are phagocytosed by Sertoli cells.

- The mature spermatozoa are released from the Sertoli cells and become free in the lumen of the seminiferous tubules.
- Mature spermatozoa are formed in 21 days from the spermatids.

The gametogenic function of testis is maintained by FSH and androgens. The stages from spermatogonium to spermatid are androgen independent. However, the maturation of spermatids to spermatozoa is androgen dependent acting on Sertoli cells. FSH acts on Sertoli cells and facilitates the last stage of maturation of spermatids and also promotes ABP.

Structure of Spermatozoon

A fully formed spermatozoon is an intricate motile cell about 55–65 μm in length. It comprises the following parts (Figs 9.2.4 and 9.2.5A):

- Head
- Neck
- Tail

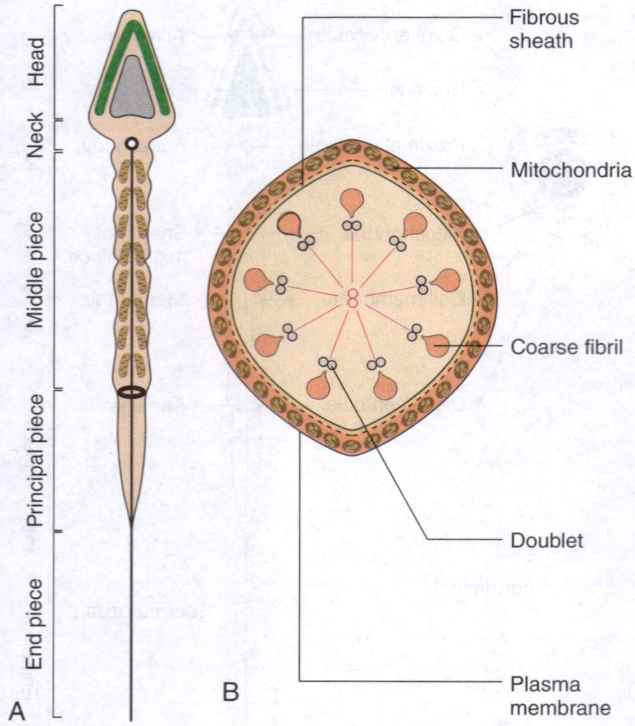

Fig. 9.2.5 **A**, Structure of a mature human spermatozoon; and **B**, transverse section of the middle piece of tail part showing its detailed structure.

1. Head The head is about 4–5 μm long, flattened from anterior to posterior. It is oval when seen from the front, but appears to be pointed (somewhat like a spearhead) when seen from one side. It is mainly composed of condensed nucleus with a very thin cytoplasmic cell membrane layer around it. It is surrounded by acrosome.

Acrosome is a thick cap-like structure which covers the anterior two-third part of the head. It is formed mainly from lysosome-like organelle containing a number of enzymes (hyaluronidase, proteolytic enzymes and acid phosphatase) which help the sperm in penetrating the ovum during fertilization.

2. Neck It is a narrow constricted part. It contains a funnel-shaped basal body and a spherical centriole.

- *Basal body* is also called *connecting piece*, because it helps to establish an intimate union between the head and the remainder of the spermatozoon through its convex articular surface which fits into a depression called the *implantation* fossa present in the head.

The basal body is made up of nine segmented rod-like structures which become continuous with the axial filaments present in the tail.

3. Tail The tail of the sperm is the motile portion and is also called the flagellum. It can be divided into three parts:

- Middle piece
- Principal piece
- End piece

The tail of the sperm consists of the following components:

Axoneme or axial filament: It forms the central skeleton of the tail. The axoneme begins just behind in the neck and extends through the entire length of the tail. It is made up of nine pairs (doublets) of microtubules arranged in a circle, surrounding the central pair (Fig. 9.2.5B). This structure is similar to that of a cilium. To-and-fro movements of the tail result due to rhythmic longitudinal sliding motion between the anterior and posterior tubules that make up axoneme.

Coarse fibrils: The nine petal-shaped coarse fibrils are present, one each just outside each doublet of microtubules (Fig. 9.5.5B). These coarse fibrils are present in the *middle piece* and principal piece, but do not extend into the end piece of the tail.

Fibrous sheath is present outside the coarse fibrils.

Mitochondria: In the region of the middle piece, i.e. proximal part of the tail, the fibrous sheath is surrounded by spirally arranged mitochondria in abundance. The mitochondria synthesize ATP which supplies energy for the motility of the tail.

Plasma membrane encloses the entire sperm.

Storage of Spermatozoa

About 120 million sperms are formed each day. A small quantity of them is stored in the epididymis but most of them are stored in the vas deferens and ampulla of vas deferens. They can remain stored maintaining their fertility for about a month.

Maturation and Capacitation of Spermatozoa

Role of epididymis The fully formed spermatozoa are released into the lumen of seminiferous tubules, from where they reach the epididymis after traversing the rete testis and efferent ducts of testes. Epididymis is the site of extratesticular maturation of spermatozoa. When the sperms arrive in the epididymis, they are nonmotile. They acquire some motility only after passing through the epididymis.

Mechanism: A special set of Ca^{2+} channels (belonging to CatSper family) located on the principal piece of the spermatozoal tail gets activated. The epididymal secretions required for this maturation are androgen dependent.

Role of seminal vesicles and prostate gland The secretions of seminal vesicles and the prostate have a stimulating effect on sperm motility, but the spermatozoa become fully motile only after ejaculation. In the female genital tract, Ca^{2+} channels present on the sperm tail become more sensitive to vaginal acidic pH (~5).

Role of female genital tract When introduced into the vagina, spermatozoa reach the uterine tubes much sooner than their own motility would allow, suggesting that contractions of uterine and tubal musculature exert a sucking effect.

Spermatozoa acquire ability to fertilize the ovum only after they have been in the female genital tract for some time (1–10 hours). This final step in their maturation is called capacitation.

Factors affecting spermatogenesis are:

1. ***Effect of temperature:*** The proper spermatogenesis occurs at a temperature lower than the normal body temperature (32°C), which is ensured by the following mechanisms:
   - Location of the testis outside the body cavity in the scrotum
   - Evaporative cooling in the scrotum
   - Countercurrent heat exchanger mechanism operating between the spermatic artery and the vein

Evidence which highlight the importance of proper temperature during spermatogenesis are the following:

Hot bath at a temperature of 43–45°C for 30 minutes daily results in sterility.

In athletes, use of insulated athletic supporters can reduce sperm count due to increased heat around the testis.

Cryptorchidism is a condition in which testes are undescended (remain in the abdominal cavity). Such individuals are usually sterile because of thermal damage to spermatogonia.

Varicocele (dilatation of veins of the pampiniform plexus) occurs due to incompetence of venous valves resulting in retrograde blood flow. In such cases, heat exchanger mechanism is disturbed. Such patients are usually sterile.

2. ***Seasonal variation*** in sperm count has been reported. It has been observed that sperm count is greater in the winter season than in the summer season, irrespective of the temperature to which the scrotum is exposed.
3. ***Infectious diseases*** such as mumps cause degeneration of seminiferous tubules, thereby decreasing spermatogenesis.
4. ***Hormonal control of spermatogenesis*** (see page 813).

Semen

Semen or the seminal fluid refers to the fluid ejaculated during the orgasm at the time of male sexual act.

Characteristic Features

Volume: The average volume of semen per ejaculation is 2.5–3.5 mL after an abstinence of 2 days. Volume of semen decreases with repeated ejaculations.

Appearance of semen is milky due to prostatic secretions.

Specific gravity is about 1.028.

Reaction is alkaline with a pH of 7.5. The alkalinity is due to prostatic secretions. The alkaline semen brings the vaginal pH from 3.5–4 to 6–6.5, the pH at which sperms show optimum motility.

Nature of the semen when ejaculated is liquid but soon it coagulates in vitro or in the vagina, and finally undergoes secondary liquefaction after about 15–30 minutes. The clotting of semen soon after ejaculation helps to retain it in the vagina for some time. Lysis later on would release the sperms for their free movement into the uterine cavity for fertilization. Mechanism of these changes is as follows:

- *Mechanism of coagulation of semen:* The fibrinogen present in the semen (contributed by seminal vesicles) is converted into a weak coagulum by the clotting enzyme contributed by the prostatic secretion.
- *Mechanism of liquefaction:* The coagulum is liquefied after 15–30 minutes by the enzyme fibrinolysin (plasmin). Fibrinolysin is the activated form of profibrinolysin produced in the prostate gland (about 2 mL of prostatic fluid at body temperature can liquefy 100–1000 mL of clotted plasma in 18 hours).

Components of semen and their characteristics

The semen comprises the components given next.

1. Spermatozoa The normal sperm count varies from 35 to 200 million/mL of semen with an average of 100 million/mL.

- Fifty per cent or more with counts of 200 million/mL and essentially all of those with counts less than 20 million/mL are sterile (although only one sperm is ultimately required for the fertilization of ovum).
- The sperms move at a speed of about 3 mm/min through the female genital tract. They reach the fallopian tubes 30–60 minutes after copulation. The uterine contraction during sexual act facilitates movement of sperms. The sperms remain capable of fertilizing an ovum for 28–48 hours after ejaculation in the female genital tract.

Applied Aspects

1. ***Azoospermia*** refers to complete absence of sperms ejaculated during orgasm. It may occur because of obstruction in the genital tract or due to inadequate sperm production.

   Obstructive azoospermia occurs due to:
   - Congenital bilateral absence of vas deferens
   - Young syndrome (combination of bronchiectasis, rhinosinusitis and infertility)
   - Cystic fibrosis
   - Post-vasectomy fibrosis

   Non obstructive azoospermia occurs due to endocrinal abnormalities.
2. ***Asthenospermia*** refers to reduced sperm motility. It is a common cause of male infertility.
3. ***Globozoospermia,*** also called round-headed spermatozoa, occurs due to malformation of the acrosome. In severe cases, acrosome is totally absent. This condition is also known as human infertility syndrome caused by defective spermatogenesis.

2. Secretions of seminal vesicles Secretions of seminal vesicles contribute 60% of the semen volume:

- The secretion from seminal vesicles is mucoid and viscous fluid.
- It is neutral or slightly alkaline in nature.
- It contains fructose, phosphorylcholine, ergothioneine, ascorbic acid, flavins and prostaglandins.

Functions subserved by seminal vesicle secretions are the following:

Nutrition to sperms after being ejaculated into the female genital tract is provided by the fructose and other nutritive substances from seminal vesicle secretions.

Clotting of semen soon after ejaculation into the female genital tract occurs due to fibrinogen present in the seminal vesicle secretions.

Fertilization of ovum may be enhanced by the prostaglandins present in seminal vesicle secretion by the following mechanisms:

- Increasing the receptive capacity of cervical mucosa for sperms
- Increasing the rate of transport of sperms in the female genital tract by inducing reverse peristaltic movement of the uterus and fallopian tubes

3. Secretion of prostate gland Secretion of the prostate gland forms about 10% of the total semen bulk:

- It contributes milky and alkaline fluid part of the semen.
- It contains spermine, citric acid, cholesterol, phospholipids, fibrinolysin, fibrinogenase, zinc, acid phosphatase, phosphate, bicarbonates and hyaluronidase.

Functions subserved by prostatic fluid component of semen are the following:

Maintenance of optimum pH for fertilization (6–6.5) is the function of alkaline prostate fluid, which neutralizes the acidity of vaginal secretion. At this pH, the sperms become motile and the chances of fertilization are enhanced.

Clotting of semen by converting fibrinogen (from seminal vesicles) into a coagulum is caused by the clotting enzymes present in the prostatic fluid.

Lysis of coagulum is caused by fibrinolysin present in prostatic secretions. The sperms become motile after the lysis of coagulum.

> **Important Note**
>
> *Prostate-specific antigen* (PSA) is a protease secreted by prostate. It hydrolyses the sperm motility inhibitor (semenogelin) in the semen, thus increasing sperm motility.
>
> Elevated plasma level of PSA is an effective screening tool in diagnosis of prostate carcinoma.

4. Secretion of bulbourethral gland Secretion of the bulbourethral gland and other mucous glands accounts for only a small amount of the semen volume. These secretions provide mucoid consistency to the semen after puberty.

ENDOCRINE FUNCTIONS TF TESTES

- The Leydig cells of testes produce male sex hormones known as androgen.
- The Sertoli cells of testes secrete oestrogen, *inhibin* and *activin*.
- The most important testicular hormone is testosterone. Therefore, if not stated otherwise, testicular hormone means testosterone.

Secretion and Transport of Androgens

Testes secrete the androgens (male sex hormones) given next.

1. Testosterone It is a steroid secreted by the Leydig cells. The Leydig cells are large polyhedral cells lying as cords or groups of cells around large blood capillaries in the interstitial connective tissue between the seminiferous tubules.

- Leydig cells are numerous in newborn male infants and in adult males. So, the androgens are secreted in infancy and after puberty.
- In childhood, Leydig cells are scanty or nonexisting. So in childhood, practically no testosterone is secreted approximately until 10–12 years of age.
- The androgen secretion starts decreasing after 40 years and becomes almost zero by the age of 80 years.
- A normal man secretes 300–1000 ng/dL (4–9 mg/day) of testosterone. Plasma testosterone level in adult males is about 0.65 µg%. More than 98% of secreted testosterone is bound to plasma proteins; 65% is bound to albumin, and 33% is bound to testosterone-binding globulin, also called sex steroid-binding globulin (SSBG) or gonadal steroid-binding globulin (GBG) (because it binds oestradiol as well). A very small percentage of the plasma testosterone is unbound. The free fraction of testosterone alone is physiologically active in the target tissues and testosterone, and acts as a final hormone (for the hypothalamus and anterior pituitary) and as prohormone for the skin and male reproductive tract.

2. Androstenedione Androstenedione is an important steroid precursor for blood oestrogens in men.

- It is secreted by the testes at a rate of about 2.5 mg/day.

> **Important Note**
>
> It is important to note that the major portions of blood oestradiol and oestrone in normal men are derived from blood testosterone and androstenedione, respectively. Only a small amount of oestradiol is secreted by the Sertoli and Leydig cells of testes.

3. Dihydrotestosterone Dihydrotestosterone (DHT) is another important androgen present in the blood.

- Only 20% of the plasma DHT is formed in the testes by the action of 5α-reductase (from the Sertoli cells) on the testosterone (secreted by Leydig cells).
- About 80% of the plasma DHT is derived from the peripheral conversion of testosterone. In the target tissues such as the skin and male reproductive tract (prostate glands, seminal vesicles and epididymis), the testosterone is converted (by 5α-reductase) into DHT.

> **Important Note**
>
> In tissues, therefore, DHT is the final hormone and testosterone is the *prohormone*.
>
> - DHT has more than twice the biological activity of testosterone.

Adrenal cortex also secretes androgens, normally testosterone, androstenedione and dehydroepiandrosterone (DHEA) (of these, the last one is more important). The action of adrenal androgens is unimportant under normal physiological conditions, because their quantity is insignificant. Under abnormal conditions, the excessive secretions of adrenal androgens, especially DHEA, may produce masculinizing effects in prepubertal or in adult females and precocious puberty in prepubertal boys (precocious pseudopuberty).

Synthesis of Androgens

Salient points about synthesis of androgens are as follows:

- Androgens (C-19 structure) are synthesized in Leydig cells from the cholesterol (C-27 structure).
- The key step in the synthesis of androgens is the conversion of cholesterol to pregnenolone.
- The CYP11Al enzyme is the rate-limiting enzyme for steroid synthesis in all steroid-producing tissues.
- In the developing male fetus, the stimulus for testosterone synthesis is human chorionic gonadotropin (hCG), which is the placental hormone secreted in highest amounts during the first trimester of pregnancy.

Biochemical pathways of synthesis of androgens The enzymatic processes involved in the conversion of cholesterol to androgens are shown in Fig. 9.2.6.

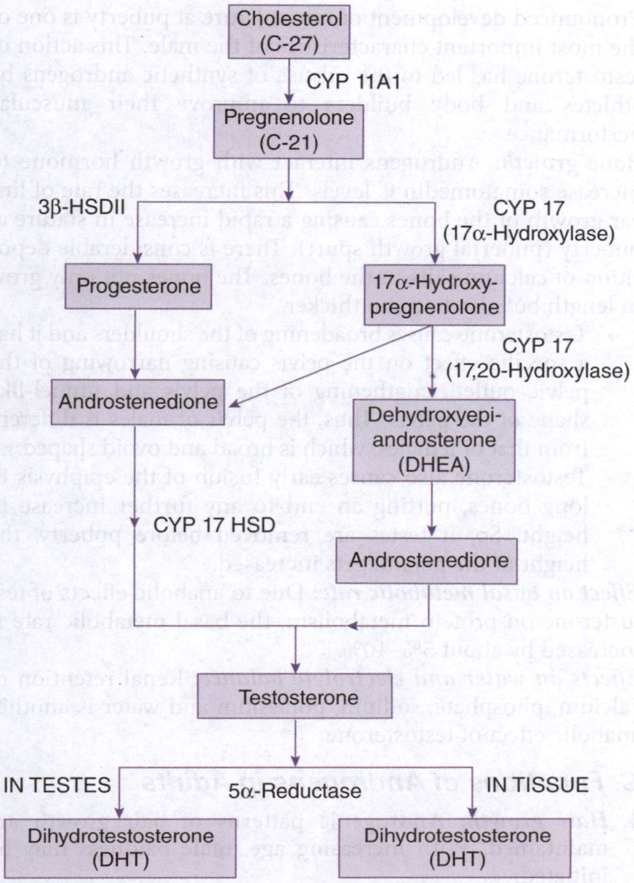

Fig. 9.2.6 Pathway of formation of androgens from cholesterol.

Metabolic Degradation and Excretion of Androgens

Within 25–30 minutes of entry of testosterone into circulation, it is either fixed to the target tissues or degraded in the liver. Testosterone can have one of the fates given next.

1. Conversion into DHT Conversion into DHT occurs in the skin and male reproductive tract (prostate gland, seminal vesicles and epididymis) by the enzyme 5α-reductase. DHT crosses the cell membrane of the target cells and produces its effects.

2. Conversion into oestradiol and oestrone Circulating testosterone and androstenedione can be converted to oestradiol and oestrone, respectively, by the action of aromatase (Fig. 9.2.7). Aromatases are membrane-bound enzymes found in the brain, skin, liver, mammary tissues and most significantly adipose tissue. Aromatization of circulating androgens is the major pathway for oestrogen formation in the male, although some oestrogens in males are derived from direct secretion by the testes.

3. Conversion into 17-ketosteroid The degradation products of testosterone include androsterone, epiandrosterone and etiocholanolone. These three products are grouped together as 17-ketosteroids.

These are conjugated with glucuronic acid or sulphuric acid in the liver and excreted in the bile and urine.

- The excretory rate of urinary 17-ketosteroids in normal men is 15–20 mg/day.

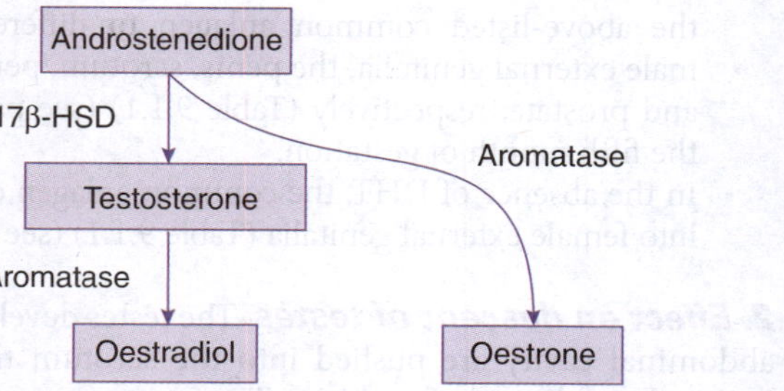

Fig. 9.2.7 Conversion of androgens to oestradiol and oestrone.

- About two-thirds of the urinary 17-ketosteroids are of adrenal origin (derived from DHEA) and only one-third are of testicular origin.

Important Note

Excessive secretion of 17-ketosteroids in the urine is an important sign of masculinizing tumours of the adrenal cortex. Because the urinary 17-ketosteroid pool reflects mainly adrenocortical activity, a measurement of the 17-ketosteroid secretion is not a good index of testicular function. The main test for assessing Leydig cell function is measurement of plasma testosterone.

Functions of Androgens

A. Functions of Androgens in Fetal Period (in Utero)

The testosterone is secreted by the fetal testes at about second to fourth months of embryonic life. The functions of androgens in fetal period are given next.

1. Effects on sex differentiation in fetus Effects on sex differentiation in fetus are the following:

Gonadal sex differentiation (as discussed on page 788) is dependent on the genotype of the embryo. In a genetic male embryo (44+XY), the bipotential gonads begin to differentiate into testes at approximately sixth week of gestation. The Y chromosome plays a key role in the testicular differentiation. In the genetic female (44+XX) embryo, the bipotential gonads differentiate into ovaries by about 10th week of gestation in the absence of testis-determining factor (see page 789).

Genital differentiation: *Differentiation of internal genitalia* occurs from the primordia which are a paired set of Wolffian (male) ducts and a paired set of Müllerian (female) ducts. By the ninth week of gestation, the embryo has both male and female primordial ducts (Fig. 9.1.4).

- The testosterone secreted by the Leydig cells of fetal testes (at about seventh week of intrauterine life) stimulates differentiation of the Wolffian ducts into the epididymis, vas deferens and seminal vesicles.
- In the absence of testosterone, Wolffian ducts degenerate and female sex organs develop from the Müllerian ducts in the absence of MIS.

Differentiation of external genitalia:

- The external genitalia develop from common anlagen, which are the genital tubercles, genital swelling, genital fold and urogenital sinus (Fig. 9.1.5) (see page 790). The hormone DHT produced by testes in male fetus stimulates the above-listed common anlagen to differentiate into male external genitalia, the penis, scrotum, penile urethra and prostate, respectively (Table 9.1.1) (see page 791) by the fifth month of gestation.

- In the absence of DHT, the common anlagen differentiate into female external genitalia (Table 9.1.1) (see page 791).

2. Effect on descent of testes The testes developed in the abdominal cavity are pushed into the scrotum through the inguinal canal just before birth. Testosterone is necessary for this descent of testes. In a child born with undescended testes (cryptorchidism), administration of testosterone or even gonadotropic hormones (which stimulate the Leydig cells) can cause the testes to descend if the inguinal canal is large enough to allow the passage of testes.

B. Functions of Androgens at Puberty

1. Effects on External Genitalia Testosterone (with or without DHT) causes pubertal enlargement of the penis.

- DHT promotes growth. The scrotum increases in size and becomes pigmented. Rugal folds appear in the scrotal skin.

2. Effects on accessory sex organs Testosterone (with or without DHT) causes enlargement of seminal vesicles.

- DHT promotes growth of prostate and stimulates prostatic secretions.

3. Development of male secondary sexual characters Development of male secondary sexual characters progresses as follows:

Body hair: DHT stimulates the hair follicles and produces the male pattern of hair growth characterized by beard growth, diamond-shaped pubic escutcheon, relatively large amount of body hair and the recession of the temporal hairline (which in some men culminates in baldness).

Voice: The testosterone causes enlargement of the larynx and thickening of vocal cords resulting in a deeper low-pitched voice (characteristically masculine).

Muscle mass and shoulder girdle: Testosterone causes enlargement of the muscle mass (especially shoulder and pectoral muscles) at puberty.

Changes in skin: The skin becomes thicker all over the body. DHT increases production of sebum by the sebaceous glands with consequent development of acne, especially during puberty.

4. Effects on psyche Androgens play the following roles:

Psychological differentiation: A brief exposure of the fetal hypothalamus to androgens (from its own testes) during early embryonic period causes male pattern of sexual behaviour during puberty. It occurs due to constant secretion of pituitary gonadotropins.

Libido: During puberty, testosterone initiates sexual drive (libido) and erectile function (potency).

Aggressive behaviour: Testosterone produces aggressive behaviour and interest in the opposite sex.

5. Anabolic and general growth-promoting effects Testosterone causes nitrogen retention in the body (positive nitrogen balance) and causes increased synthesis and decreased breakdown of tissue proteins resulting in accelerated growth of the body and skeletal muscles in particular. Pronounced development of musculature at puberty is one of the most important characteristics of the male. This action of testosterone has led to the misuse of synthetic androgens by athletes and body builders to improve their muscular performance.

Bone growth: Androgens interact with growth hormone to increase somatomedin C levels. This increases the rate of linear growth of the bones causing a rapid increase in stature at puberty (pubertal growth spurt). There is considerable deposition of calcium salts in the bones. The bones not only grow in length but also become thicker.

- Testosterone causes broadening of the shoulders and it has a specific effect on the pelvis causing narrowing of the pelvic outlet, lengthening of the pelvis and funnel-like shape of the pelvis. Thus, the pelvis of males is different from that of females, which is broad and ovoid shaped.
- Testosterone also causes early fusion of the epiphysis in long bones, putting an end to any further increase in height. So, if testes are removed before puberty, the height of the person gets increased.

Effect on basal metabolic rate: Due to anabolic effects of testosterone on protein metabolism, the basal metabolic rate is increased by about 5%–10%.

Effects on water and electrolyte balance: Renal retention of calcium, phosphate, sodium, potassium and water is another anabolic effect of testosterone.

C. Functions of Androgens in Adults

1. ***Hair growth:*** Androgenic patterns of hair growth are maintained. With increasing age, male baldness may be initiated.
2. ***Psyche:*** Behavioural attitudes and sexual potency are maintained in postpubertal adults.
3. ***Bone:*** Bone loss and osteoporosis are prevented by the androgens in adult males.
4. ***Spermatogenesis:*** It is maintained in adulthood by testosterone along with FSH. The testosterone, by paracrine effect, diffuses into seminiferous tubules and acts on both Sertoli cells and germ cells and thus maintains spermatogenesis.

Important Note

It is important to note that within the seminiferous tubules, the testosterone concentration, because of the paracrine effect, is tremendously high and that such a high concentration in the local region cannot be achieved by exogenous testosterone therapy by parenteral route. Lack of spermatogenesis due to pituitary failure therefore cannot be corrected by parenteral testosterone therapy.

5. ***Haematopoiesis:*** Testosterone stimulates the production of erythropoietin and also has a direct massive effect on erythropoiesis. These effects account for the greater haemoglobin concentration and RBC count in males.
6. ***Effects on circulating and stored body fats:*** Testosterone increases circulating levels of low-density lipoprotein cholesterol and decreases plasma high-density lipoprotein cholesterol.
   - Testosterone favours accumulation of upper body, abdominal and visceral fat.
7. ***Regulation of gonadotropin secretion:*** Androgen suppression of luteinizing hormone–releasing hormone (LHRH)

and LH by negative feedback is largely a function of testosterone.

Mode of Action of Androgens

The testosterone may act as the final hormone or prohormone in the target tissues. In the skin and male reproductive tract, the testosterone is converted into DHT by 5α-reductase. Humans have two types of 5α-reductase encoded by two different genes:

- Type 1: 5α-Reductase is present in the skin throughout the body, predominantly in the scalp.
- Type 2: 5α-Reductase is mainly present in the genital skin, prostate and other genital tissues.

The testosterone and DHT, like other steroid hormones, cross the cell membrane of the target tissues and bind with the cytoplasmic androgen receptor (R) to form the androgen–R complex. The androgen–R complex moves to the nucleus to promote greater transcription of mRNA leading to greater synthesis of proteins in the ribosomes. Thus, the testosterone primarily results in increased synthesis of specific proteins required for development of accessory sex organs and muscular growth.

Applied Aspects

Congenital 5α-reductase deficiency occurs when there is mutation of gene for 5α-reductase, leading to male pseudohermaphroditism. The characteristic features of this condition are as follows:

- Persons are born with male internal genitalia (with testis) but have external genitalia of a female.
- These individuals are usually raised as a girl, but at puberty, there is increased secretion of LH and testosterone. Therefore, consequently, they develop male body contours and male libido.
- It change the gender identity as a boy. The clitoris gets enlarged. The enlargement of the penis may occur because of high circulating level of LH and testosterone.

Inhibin and Activins

In males, inhibin is a testicular factor produced by Sertoli cells that inhibits FSH secretion by direct action at the pituitary. Inhibin consists of three polypeptide subunits – one α-subunit which is glycosylated and other two nonglycosylated β-subunits (β_A and β_B). The α-subunit combines with the β_A-subunit by disulphide bond to form heterodimer. There are two types of inhibin – inhibin A (ab_A) and inhibin B (ab_B).

- In women, inhibins are produced by granulosa cells of ovarian follicles.
- The heterodimers and homodimers of inhibin stimulate FSH secretion rather than inhibiting it; therefore, these are called activins.
- Both inhibins and activins belong to TGF-β superfamily and act through activin receptors, located at the gonads, brain and bone marrow. In embryonic period, activins are involved in formation of mesoderm.
- Inhibins and activins bind to α_2-macroglobulin in the plasma and in the tissue bind to glycoprotein known as follistatin. In bound form, the physiological activity of both activin and inhibin decreases.

Control of Androgen Secretion

See page 814.

Control of Testicular Functions

The two main functions of testes, i.e. spermatogenesis and secretion of testosterone, are controlled by the hypothalamic–hypophyseal–testicular axis.

Control of spermatogenesis The hypothalamic–hypophyseal–testicular (seminiferous tubular) axis controlling the spermatogenesis is given next.

I. Stimulatory control

1. Role of hypothalamus Spermatogenesis begins at puberty and continues throughout adult life to decline in old age. It is believed that at puberty, hypothalamic cells become more mature and their sensitivity for circulating sex hormones (negative feedback) decreases so much that there is a pulsatile release (8–14 pulses/day) of gonadotropin-releasing hormone (GnRH) from the *parvocellular-peptidergic neurons of the hypothalamus*. The GnRH is a decapeptide. It stimulates the anterior pituitary to secrete LH and FSH.

2. Role of anterior pituitary The anterior pituitary controls spermatogenesis through the gonadotropic hormones (FSH and LH) and growth hormones. Neither FSH nor LH acts on the spermatogonia. Yet, normal spermatogenesis requires both FSH and LH, described as follows:

FSH stimulates cells of Sertoli which play the following roles during spermatogenesis:

- Sertoli cells help in conversion of spermatids to sperms.
- They secrete ABP which stabilizes the high supply of testosterone to the developing germ cells in the seminiferous tubular lumen.
- FSH also promotes the synthesis of inhibin by Sertoli cells.

FSH indirectly affects testosterone synthesis by increasing the number of LH receptors on the Leydig cells.

Role of LH (also called interstitial cell–stimulating hormone [ICSH]): The LH stimulates Leydig cells to cause testosterone secretion. The testosterone is required for normal spermatogenesis.

Role of growth hormone: Growth hormone specifically promotes early division of the spermatogonia themselves. In its absence, as in pituitary dwarfs, spermatogenesis is severely deficient or absent.

3. Role of testicular hormones Testosterone secreted by Leydig cells by paracrine effect diffuses into seminiferous tubules, where its high local concentration is maintained by ABP. The testosterone acts on both Sertoli cells and germ cells and thus maintains spermatogenesis.

Important Note

- Exogenous testosterone cannot promote spermatogenesis in men lacking Leydig cells, because it is not possible to achieve the required high concentration by parenteral therapy.
- DHT is not required for normal spermatogenesis; therefore, normal sperm development occurs in men with × α-reductase deficiency.

Oestrogen formed from testosterone by Sertoli cells (when stimulated by FSH) is probably also essential for spermatogenesis.

II. Feedback inhibitory control The rapid speed of spermatogenesis is controlled by the following negative feedback mechanisms (Fig. 9.2.8):

Inhibin secreted by Sertoli cells acts directly on the anterior pituitary and inhibits the secretion of FSH.

Testosterone and oestradiol inhibit LH secretion by negative feedback mechanism:

- *Oestradiol* exerts the negative feedback effect at both the hypothalamic (GnRH) and pituitary (LH) levels.
- *Testosterone* has its feedback effect mainly at the hypothalamic (GnRH) level.

Note: Plasma physiological level of testosterone does not produce significant feedback inhibition of FSH secretion.

Control of Testosterone Secretion

In fetus During fetal life, hCG secreted by the placenta stimulates the development of Leydig cells in the testes of fetus and causes testosterone secretion.

In adults Testosterone secretion is regulated by:

I. Stimulatory control The hypothalamic–hypophyseal–testicular (Leydig cell) axis controls the secretion of testosterone in adults as (Fig. 9.2.9):

Hypothalamus produces GnRH which stimulates the anterior pituitary to secrete FSH and LH.

Anterior pituitary controls secretion of testosterone (steroidogenesis) primarily through LH.

- The secretion of LH has been shown to be concordant with the frequency of hypothalamic pulse generator.
- In experimental animals, it has been observed that hypophysectomy produces atrophy of Leydig cells which can be restored to normal by administration of LH.

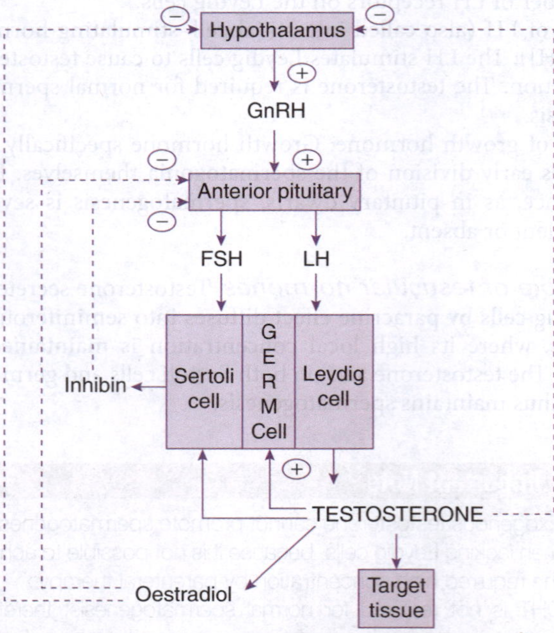

Fig. 9.2.8 Stimulatory and feedback inhibitory control of spermatogenesis.

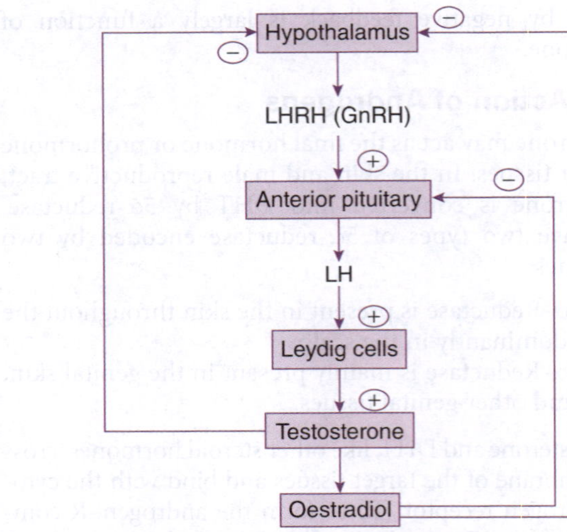

Fig. 9.2.9 Stimulatory and feedback inhibitory control of secretion of testosterone.

Leydig cells of testes have LH receptors located on their plasma membrane. LH binds to these receptors to activate cyclic AMP synthesis which triggers testosterone synthesis and its secretion.

II. Feedback inhibitory control Plasma testosterone level is maintained at a constant level by a feedback control exerted by testosterone and oestradiol independently to control LH (Fig. 9.2.9):

Testosterone negative feedback is exerted mainly on the opioidergic neurons that project to GnRH (LHRH) neurons.

Testosterone plays a minor role in the inhibition of LH secretion at the level of the pituitary.

Oestradiol exerts negative feedback effects at both hypothalamic and pituitary levels.

- Oestradiol, in contrast to testosterone, exerts a significant direct inhibitory effect on LH secretion at the pituitary level.
- Oestradiol formed by local hypothalamic conversion of testosterone also inhibits LHRH (GnRH).

Applied Aspects

Some of the important applied aspects in relation to male reproductive physiology are as follows:

- Cryptorchidism
- Extirpation
- Hypogonadism in males
- Hypergonadism in males
- Male infertility
- Vasectomy

1. Cryptorchidism

The testes develop in relation to the lumbar region of the posterior abdominal wall. During fetal life, they gradually descend to the scrotum by the end of the eighth month of gestation (see page 789). Cryptorchidism refers to a condition in which the descent of the testes may fail to occur or may be incomplete.

- In some cases, the testes may complete their descent after birth.
- The incidence of an undescended testis is 2% at the age of 1 year and falls to 0.3% after the age of puberty.

Causes: An undescended testis may occur due to the following reasons:

- *Prematurity*, which is the leading cause
- Hormonal disorders
- Spina bifida
- Defective genital development and conditions of fetus that can restrict growth, such as Down syndrome

Characteristic features of cryptorchidism are as follows:

- The undescended testes may lie in the lumbar region, in the iliac fossa, in the inguinal canal or in the upper part of the scrotum.
- Spermatogenesis often fails to occur in cryptorchidism (due to high temperature of the abdominal cavity) resulting in sterility.
- Androgen secretion from the Leydig cells of testes is unaffected, so male secondary sexual characters develop normally.
- An undescended testis is more likely to develop malignant tumour than a normal testis.

Treatment: Cryptorchidism should be treated as early as possible to prevent male sterility. Surgical correction is advised for correction of undescended testes. However, in some children, administration of testosterone or gonadotropic hormone (which stimulates the Leydig cells) can cause the testis to descend provided the inguinal canal is large enough to allow passage of the testis.

2. Extirpation

Extirpation or castration refers to the removal of testes. It will produce the effects given next.

Effects of Extirpation of Testes Before Puberty

The removal of testes before puberty results in a clinical condition which is known as *eunuchoidism*. It is characterized by:

Permanent sterility occurs as there is no testis, so there are no sperms.

Underdevelopment of external genitalia (i.e. penis and scrotum) and accessory sex organs (i.e. seminal vesicles and prostate gland) is present.

Underdevelopment of secondary sexual characters is present, that is:

- *Hair growth* on the face and trunk and in axilla is scanty.
- *Voice is high pitched* like that of a child due to underdevelopment of the larynx.
- *Muscle mass and shoulder girdle* development is poor.
- *Female-like body configuration* occurs due to abnormal deposition of fat on buttocks, hips, pubis and breasts.

Abnormal bone growth due to delay in the union of epiphysis may lead to *increase in height* of the individual, but the bones are weak and thin.

Effects of Extirpation of Testes After Puberty

Under such circumstances, some of the male secondary sexual characters and accessory organs (which depend on testosterone) are depressed not only for development but also for maintenance, whereas some of the masculine features are retained as:

Accessory sex organs are depressed, i.e. seminal vesicles and prostate undergo atrophy.

Penis remains normal in size.

Sexual desire and sexual activity are slightly impaired. Erection occurs but ejaculation is rare because of atrophy of accessory sex organs and lack of sperm.

Voice usually remains masculine as the growth of the larynx is completed during adolescence.

Other secondary sexual characters are not lost.

Other body functions including life span, senility, intelligence, etc., are not affected.

3. Hypogonadism in Males

Causes: Hypogonadism in males results from absent or deficient testicular functions which may occur in the following conditions:

- Congenital nonfunctioning of testes
- Underdeveloped testes due to absence of hCG in fetal life
- Cryptorchidism (undescended testes) associated with partial or total degeneration of seminiferous tubules
- Extirpation of testes
- Absence of androgen receptors in testes

Effects of male hypogonadism depend on whether the testicular deficiency occurs before or after puberty and are similar to those occurring after extirpation before or after puberty, respectively.

Fröhlich Syndrome

Fröhlich syndrome, also known as adipose genital syndrome or dystrophy, is a rare childhood metabolic disorder characterized by obesity, growth retardation and hypothyroidism.

Causes are as follows:

- Hypothalamic disorders
- Pituitary disorders
- Genetic inability of hypothalamus to secrete LHRH, i.e. GnRH

Features: Under this condition, hypogonadism is often associated with delayed physical growth and the development of secondary sex characters. Therefore, children with this syndrome tend to have a short stature and may develop intellectual difficulties, defective vision, diabetes insipidus and hypothermia due to tumour growth.

Diagnosis of Fröhlich syndrome is performed by:

- *Blood tests* including TSH, FSH and LH
- *Imaging studies* including X-ray skull, CT scan of the head and neck region or MRI

Treatment: Pituitary extracts or specific missing hormone may be administered.

- *For males*, administration of hCG to reach puberty followed by testosterone with androgen and progesterone
- *For females*, hormonal replacement therapy with oestrogen and progesterone
- *Surgical removal of tumour*
- *Weight control through appetite*

4. Hypergonadism in Males

Causes: Hypergonadism in males results from excessive secretion of male sex hormones (androgens) as occurs in tumours of Leydig cell.

Features: The occurrence of tumour of Leydig cell is common in prepubertal boys who develop precocious pseudopuberty which is characterized by:

- Rapid growth of musculature and bones, but height is less due to early closure of epiphysis
- Excessive development of sex organs and secondary sexual characters at an early age
- Gynaecomastia because the tumours can also secrete oestrogenic hormones which can cause overgrowth of breasts

5. Male Infertility

Male infertility refers to the inability of sperm to fertilize the ovum.

Causes of male infertility can be grouped as:

1. ***Androgen dysfunction with normal sperm count*** is seen in:
   - Hypothalamic pituitary defects
   - Leydig cell defects
   - Androgen resistance
2. ***Isolated dysfunction of sperm cell production with normal androgen levels*** may occur due to:
   - Infection or trauma
   - Congenital deformation of passages
   - Formation of nonmotile or otherwise abnormal sperms
3. ***Combined androgen and sperm cell production defects*** are as follows:
   - Developmental defects such as Klinefelter syndrome
   - Abnormal testicular descent which is associated with degeneration of developing sperm cells in the seminiferous tubules due to higher temperature of abdominal cavity or inguinal canal
   - Acquired testicular defects, such as infections (mumps orchitis) and autoimmune orchitis
   - Systemic diseases (e.g. chronic liver and kidney diseases)
4. ***Failure of deposition of sperms in the female genital tract*** as occurs in:
   - Obstruction of the vas deferens
   - Failure of ejaculation during intercourse
   - Failure of erection during intercourse
   - Following vasectomy operation

Diagnosis: To find out the cause of infertility, the following tests are carried out:

1. ***Semen analysis*** is always the first step to investigate about infertility. The World Health Organization has accepted certain lower limit values of semen analysis for infertility as:
   - Ejaculation volume: It is 1.5 mL (normal 2.5–3.5 mL).
   - pH: It is <7.0 or >7.6 (normal 7.2–7.5).
   - Sperm count: It is 15 million/mL (35–200 million/mL).
   - Normal morphology: It is $<50\%$.
   - Sperm liquefaction: Normally after ejaculation, semen liquifies within 15–30 minutes. If liquefaction time is more than 30 minutes, then fertility could be affected.
   - Sperm motility: By automated system analyser, the scale ranges between 0 and 4. Score of 0 means that sperms are not moving and score of 3 or 4 represents good movement. Scale score <3 represents infertility.
2. ***Hormonal test*** evaluates levels of testosterone and FSH to determine the overall state of sperm production.
3. ***Seminal fructose test*** identifies whether fructose is properly added to the semen or not.
4. ***Postejaculate urinalysis*** determines obstruction or retrograde ejaculation.
5. ***Semen leukocyte analysis*** helps to know whether there are WBCs in the semen.
6. ***Antisperm antibody test*** identifies the presence of antibodies that may contribute to infertility.
7. ***Sperm penetration assay (SPA)*** confirms sperm's ability for fertilization.
8. ***Ultrasonography*** detects varicose veins or duct obstruction.
9. ***Testicular biopsy*** helps to know whether sperm production is impaired.
10. ***Genetic testing*** rules out underlying mutation of one or more regions of Y chromosome.

6. Impotence

Impotence refers to inability to achieve or maintain erection during sexual activity.

It may be:

- *Primary impotence*, which is of rare occurrence
- *Secondary impotence*, which may have organic causes or may be followed by drugs or alcohol (stress and depression are also possible causes)

7. Vasectomy

Vasectomy is a surgical procedure for male sterilization (see page 870).

8. Male menopause

The term male menopause has been used to describe decreasing testosterone levels related with ageing. In men, testosterone levels decline on an average about 1%/year after the age of 40 years. The signs and symptoms of low testosterone level include are as follows:

- Reduced sexual desire and activity
- Decreased spontaneous erection
- Swelling of breasts/discomfort
- Low bone density causing increased risks of fracture
- Hot flushes or night sweats
- Decreased energy, lack of motivation and confidence, mood swings, poor concentration and insomnia

Treatment

The suggestive treatment for male menopause includes:

- Lifestyle changes which include regular exercise and consuming zinc and vitamin D
- Reducing alcohol consumption
- Replacement therapy also advised in severe cases

Self-Assessment

Q1. Discuss the process of spermatogenesis and its control?

Q2. Discuss the synthesis, storage, mechanism of action and functions of testicles?

Q3. Describe the following:
- Functions of Sertoli cells
- Significance of blood testis barrier
- Effects of extirpation of testes

Q4. Write notes on:
- Cryptorchidism
- Male infertility
- Male menopause
- Azoospermia

Clinical Cases

Case 1

A male baby born with absence of testis in the scrotum was referred to pediatrician.

Q1. What is this condition called as?
Q2. Normally at what stage of fetal life testes are descended into the scrotum?
Q3. What is the effective treatment for this condition?
Q4. What are the after effects if this condition is not treated timely?

Case 2

A 22-year-athlete. Now he got married and his wife is not conceiving even when the couple is not having taking any contraceptive measure. The couple referred to infertility clinic for testing.

History revealed that the husband, during athletic practice was using high dose of testosterone. The examination and tests showed no sign of infertility in the wife but male is infertile.

Q1. What is the cause of infertility in this case?
Q2. What is the physiological basis for this condition?

9.3 Female Reproductive Physiology

AN OVERVIEW OF FEMALE REPRODUCTIVE SYSTEM

The female reproductive system comprises internal and external genitalia which can be organized as given next (Fig. 9.3.1).

I. PRIMARY SEX ORGANS OR OVARIES

The primary sex organs are a pair of ovaries which correspond with testes in males. The main functions of ovaries are as follows:

- To produce ova
- To secrete female sex hormones
  For details, see page 822.

II. ACCESSORY SEX ORGANS

The accessory sex organs of females include internal genital organs and external genitalia.

Female Internal Genitalia

The internal genital organs include the uterus, fallopian tubes and vagina.

I. Uterus

The uterus is a hollow, thick-walled muscular organ, situated between the urinary bladder and the rectum. It can be divided into two parts (Figs 9.3.1 and 9.3.2).

1. Body of the uterus It forms the upper two-third part of the uterus. Its lower limit is marked by a constriction which corresponds to narrowing of the uterine cavity at *internal os*. The body of the uterus can be divided into two parts:

Fundus is the rounded part of the body that lies superior to the opening of the fallopian tubes.
Isthmus is the relatively constricted region of the body (approximately 1 cm long) just above the cervix.

2. Cervix of the uterus It is the cylindrical lower part which protrudes into the uppermost vagina. It is approximately 2.5 cm long in an adult nonpregnant woman. Its cavity extends from the *internal os* to the *external os* which opens into the vagina.

Structure of uterus The wall of the body of the uterus consists of three layers (Fig. 9.3.3):

1. Perimetrium is the external serosal layer.

2. Myometrium is the middle muscular layer comprising bundles of smooth muscles among which there is a connective tissue.

- The muscle fibres run in various directions and distinct layers are difficult to define. However, three layers – external, middle and internal – are usually described.
- The muscle cells of the uterus are capable of undergoing great elongation in association with the great enlargement of organ in pregnancy.

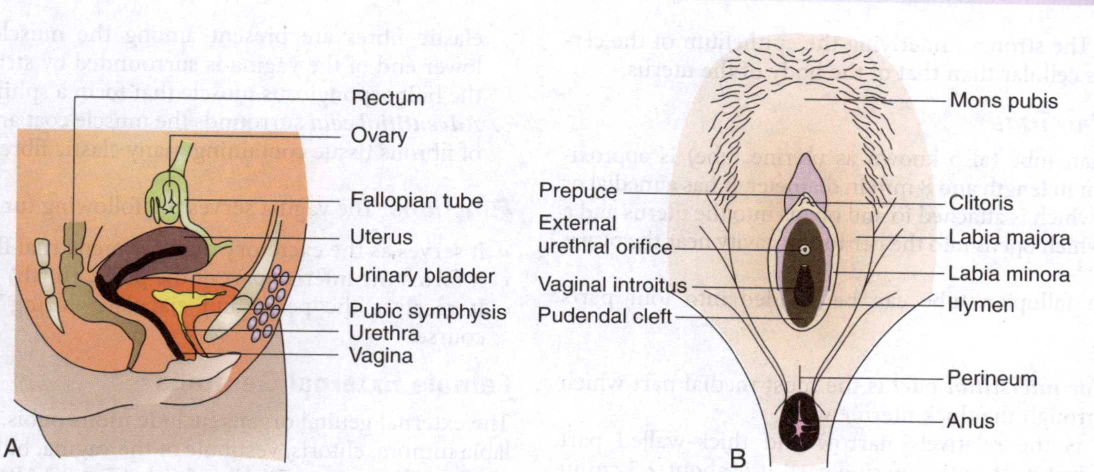

Fig. 9.3.1 Female reproductive organs: **A**, lateral view showing position of internal reproductive organs in relation to pelvic viscera; **B**, female external genitalia.

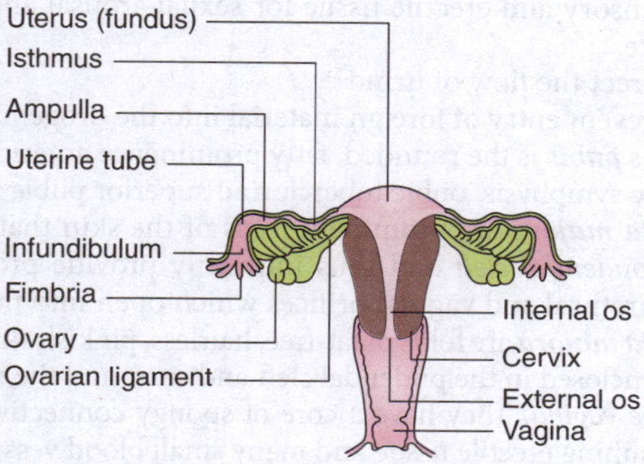

Fig. 9.3.2 Parts of the uterus and fallopian tube.

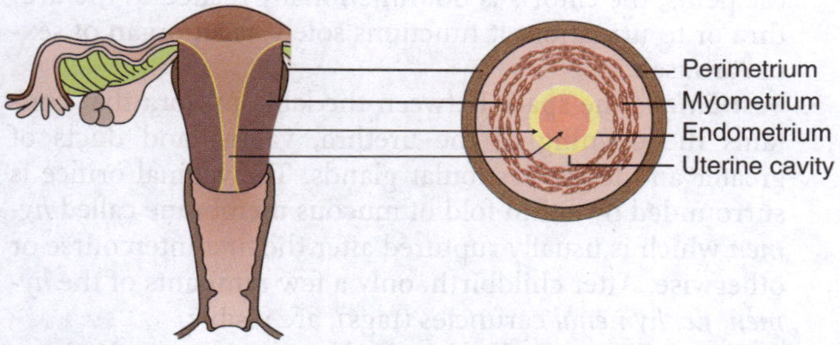

Fig. 9.3.3 Histological structure of the body of the uterus.

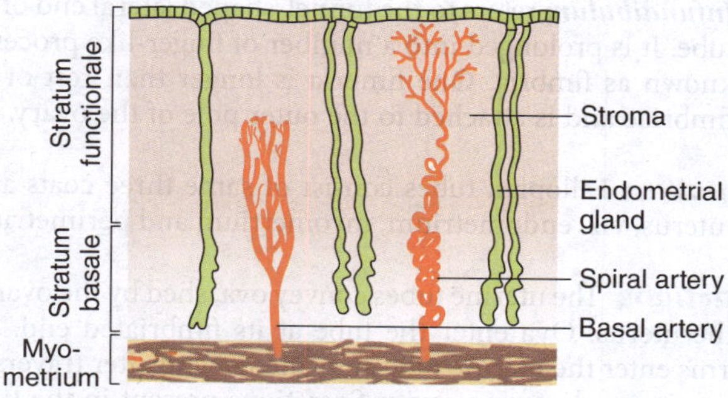

Fig. 9.3.4 Histological structure of the endometrium.

- Contractions of myometrium are responsible for the expulsion of the fetus at the time of childbirth.

3. Endometrium is the inner layer of the uterus which consists of epithelial lining and the stroma (Fig. 9.3.4):

- *Epithelial lining* is made up of columnar cells. Before menarche (i.e. the age of onset of menstruation), the cells are ciliated, but thereafter, most of the cells may not have cilia.
- *Stroma* of the endometrium, on which the epithelium rests, is highly cellular and contains numerous blood vessels and numerous simple tubular uterine glands which are lined by columnar epithelium.

Functional divisions of endometrium: Functionally, the endometrium of the body of the uterus can be divided into two strata:

1. *Stratum functionale* includes superficial two-third thickness of endometrium which undergoes monthly cyclic changes in preparation for the implantation of fertilized ovum and is shed during menstruation. This portion of endometrium is supplied by long and spiral (coiled) arteries.
2. *Stratum basale* is the deeper one-third layer of endometrium. It does not participate in cyclic changes but functions as a regenerative layer. This part of endometrium is supplied by short and straight *basal arteries*.

Structure of cervix The structure of the cervix of the uterus is somewhat different from that of the body.

1. Perimetrium is the outermost serous layer.

2. Myometrium layer of the cervix is much less muscular as compared with the body of the uterus, and contains more connective tissue. During childbirth, when the myometrium of the body of the uterus contracts, the myometrium of the cervix dilates; consequently, the cervical canal becomes large enough for the fetal head to pass through.

3. Endocervix refers to the innermost mucosal layer of the cervix in contrast to endometrium of the body of the uterus. It is not shed at the time of menstruation. Endocervix consists of:

Epithelium: The mucous membrane of the upper two-thirds of the cervical canal is lined by *ciliated columnar epithelium*, but its lower one-third epithelium is nonciliated columnar. Near the external os, the canal is lined by stratified squamous epithelium which is continuous over the external surface of the part of the cervix projecting into the vagina and with the vaginal epithelium.

Stroma: The stroma underlying the epithelium of the cervix is less cellular than that of the body of the uterus.

II. Fallopian Tubes

Each fallopian tube (also known as uterine tube) is approximately 10 cm in length and 8 mm in diameter. It has a medial or *uterine end* which is attached to and opens into the uterus and a *lateral end* which opens into the peritoneal cavity near the ovary.

Parts Each fallopian tube can be divided into four parts (Fig. 9.3.2):

1. ***Uterine or interstitial part*** is the most medial part which passes through the thick uterine wall.
2. ***Isthmus*** is the relatively narrow and thick-walled part which is just next to the uterine part. It is about 2.5 cm in length.
3. ***Ampulla*** is the next thin-walled and dilated part of the uterine tube. It is the largest part (7 cm) of the uterine tube.
4. ***Infundibulum*** refers to the funnel-shaped lateral end of the tube. It is prolonged into a number of finger-like processes known as fimbria. One fimbria is longer than rest of the fimbriae and is attached to the outer pole of the ovary.

Structure Fallopian tubes consist of same three coats as of the uterus, viz. endometrium, myometrium and perimetrium.

Functions The uterine tubes convey ova, shed by the ovaries, to the uterus. Ova enter the tube at its fimbriated end. The sperms enter the uterine tube at its medial end after traversing the vagina and uterine cavity. Secretions present in the tubes provide nutrition, oxygen and other requirements for ova and spermatozoa passing through the tube. Fertilization takes place in the ampulla and the fertilized ovum travels towards the uterus through the tube. The ciliated epithelial cells lining the tube help to move ova towards the uterus.

III. Vagina

- The vagina is a musculomembranous tube (about 8–10 cm long) located anterior to the rectum and posterior to the urethra and urinary bladder.
- Its upper end surrounds the lower part of the cervix and its lower end, i.e. vaginal orifice, opens into the vestibule of the vagina (the cleft between the labia minora).
- No glands open into the vagina. The small amount of secretion present in the vagina is derived partly from the mucous discharge from the cervix and partly from the transudation of fluid from the vaginal epithelium which contains glycogen. Action of bacteria on the glycogen present in the vaginal secretion produces lactic acid which maintains the vaginal pH around 4.5. Acidic environment of the vagina prevents the growth of pathogenic organisms.

Structure The wall of the vagina consists of a mucous membrane, a muscle coat and an outer fibrous coat or adventitia.

1. ***Mucous membrane*** shows numerous longitudinal folds and is firmly fixed to the underlying muscle layer. In an adult female, the vaginal mucosa is lined by stratified squamous epithelium. The epithelial cells are rich in glycogen and this property is oestrogen dependent.
2. ***Muscle coat*** is made up of an outer layer of longitudinal fibres and a much thinner layer of circular fibres. Many elastic fibres are present among the muscle fibres. The lower end of the vagina is surrounded by striated fibres of the bulbospongiosus muscle that form a sphincter for it.
3. ***Adventitial coat*** surrounds the muscle coat and is made up of fibrous tissue containing many elastic fibres.

Functions The vagina serves the following functions:

- It serves as the excretory duct for menstrual fluid.
- It forms the inferior part of the pelvic (birth) canal.
- It receives the penis and ejaculate during sexual intercourse.

Female External Genitalia

The external genital organs include mons pubis, labia majora, labia minora, clitoris, vestibule of the vagina, bulbs of the vestibule and greater vestibular glands (Fig. 9.3.1B).

The synonymous terms vulva and pudendum include all these parts. The vulva serves:

- As sensory and erectile tissue for sexual arousal and intercourse
- To direct the flow of urine
- To prevent entry of foreign material into the urogenital tract

1. ***Mons pubis*** is the rounded, fatty prominence anterior to the pubic symphysis, pubic tubercle and superior pubic rami.
2. ***Labia majora*** are prominent folds of the skin that bound the *pudendal cleft* and thus indirectly provide protection for urethral and vaginal orifices which open into this cleft.
3. ***Labia minora*** are folds of fat-free, hairless, pinkish skin. They are enclosed in the pudendal cleft and surround the *vestibule of the vagina*. They have a core of spongy connective tissue containing erectile tissue and many small blood vessels.
4. ***Clitoris*** is an erectile organ located where the labia minora meet anteriorly. It is analogous to male penis, but unlike the penis, the clitoris is not functionally related to the urethra or to urination. It functions solely as an organ of sexual arousal.
5. ***Vestibule*** is the space between the labia minora that contains the opening of the urethra, vagina and ducts of greater and lesser vestibular glands. The vaginal orifice is surrounded by a thin fold of mucous membrane called *hymen* which is usually ruptured after the first intercourse or otherwise. After childbirth, only a few remnants of the *hymen, i.e. hymenal* caruncles (tags), are visible.
6. ***Bulbs of the vestibule*** are paired masses of erectile tissue which lie along the sides of vaginal orifice under cover of bulbospongiosus muscles. These are homologous with the bulb of the penis and corpus spongiosum.
7. ***Vestibular glands*** include a pair each of greater vestibular and lesser vestibular glands. These glands secrete mucus into the vestibule during arousal.

OVARIES

FUNCTIONAL ANATOMY

A pair of ovaries, forming the female gonads, is located (one on each side) behind and below the fallopian tubes. The ovaries are ovoid glands with a combined weight of 10–20 g during reproductive years, which decreases with increasing age. Each ovary is about 3–5 cm in length and is attached to the uterus by the broad ligament and round ligament of the ovary.

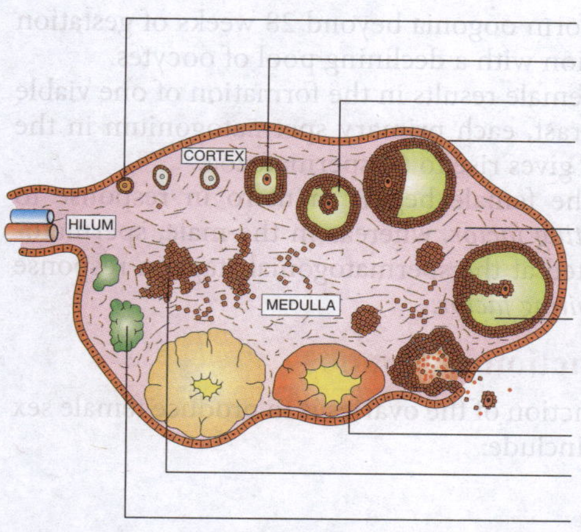

Fig. 9.3.5 Schematic diagram of the histology of ovary depicting various stages of development of follicles and corpus luteum.

Structure

Histologically, each ovary consists of the parts given next (Fig. 9.3.5).

1. Germinal epithelium Germinal epithelium refers to the epithelium lining the outer surface of the ovary and consists of a single layer of cuboidal cells. This epithelium is continuous with the mesothelium lining the peritoneum, and represents a modification of the latter. The term germinal epithelium is a misnomer, as it does not produce germ cells. The cells of this epithelium bear microvilli and contain numerous mitochondria. They become larger in pregnancy.

2. Cortex The cortex is the outer thick main part of the substance of the ovary. It consists of the following tissues:

Tunica albuginea is the outer condensation of the connective tissue present immediately below the germinal epithelium. The tunica albuginea of the ovary is much thinner and less dense than that of the testis.

Stroma of the cortex, present deep to the tunica albuginea, is made up of reticular fibres and numerous fusiform cells that resemble mesenchymal cells.

Ovarian follicles at various stages of development are scattered in the stroma. Each follicle contains a developing ovum. The formation of ova and the development and fate of ovarian follicles are described in 'Oogenesis'.

3. Medulla The medulla is the inner small part of the substance of the ovary. It consists of connective tissue in which numerous blood vessels (mostly veins), smooth muscles and elastic fibres are present.

4. Hilum The hilum refers to the area where the ovary attaches to the mesentery. It is the site for entry of blood vessels and lymphatic. It also contains some remnants of the mesonephric ducts, and hilus cells that are similar to interstitial cells of the testis. The hilum is continuous with the medulla of the ovary.

FUNCTIONS OF OVARIES

The two principal functions of ovaries are as follows:

- Gametogenic function, i.e. oogenesis
- Endocrine function, i.e. secretion of female hormones called ovarian hormones

Oogenesis

Oogenesis refers to the process of formation of ova from the primitive germ cells.

Phases of oogenesis include:

- Fetal oogenesis
- Postnatal oogenesis
- Prepubertal oogenesis
- Pubertal oogenesis

1. Fetal Oogenesis

Unlike the fetal testis (in which spermatogenesis begins at puberty), the fetal ovary begins oogenesis by 10 weeks of gestation.

Primitive germ cells When the bipotential gonads differentiate into ovaries in genetic female (44+XX) embryo (in the absence of testis-determining factor [TDF]) by the 10th week of gestation, the primitive germ cells increase in number by mitosis to form oogonia.

Oogonia are the stem cells from which ova are derived. They proliferate by mitosis to form primary oocytes. The process begins at the 15th week and reaches a peak between 20 and 28 weeks of gestation.

- The oogonium is unique in that it is the only female cell in which both X chromosomes are active.

Primary oocytes formed from the oogonia enter a prolonged prophase (*diplotene stage*) of the first meiotic division and remain in this state until ovulation occurs after puberty.

Primordial follicles The *diploid primary oocytes* become enveloped by a single layer of flat granulosa cells and in this form are called *primordial follicles.* (The granulosa cells are formed by proliferation of coelomic epithelium, i.e. cortical cells.) Each primordial follicle is enveloped in a thin membrane called the *basal lamina.* The follicles lack a direct blood supply.

- The primordial follicle is fundamental in the reproductive unit of the ovary.
- During the peak of development (between 20 and 28 weeks of gestation), the two ovaries contain about 7 million germ cells in the form of oogonia, primary oocytes and primordial follicles.
- Many germ cells undergo atresia (involution) and at term only 2 million germ cells are present, most of which have developed into primordial follicles, and some are as oogonia and primary oocytes.

2. Postnatal and Prepubertal Oogenesis

- The number of primordial follicles present in the ovaries at birth rapidly diminishes thereafter.
- By 6 months postpartum, all of the oogonia have been converted into primary oocytes and primordial follicles.
- No new ova are formed after birth.
- By the onset of puberty (at about 12–13 years of age), the two ovaries contain about 300,000 primordial follicles.

3. Pubertal Oogenesis

- After puberty, the oogenesis or formation of ovum occurs in a highly cyclic fashion, once every 28 days till menopause.
- Every month, in each ovary, more than one primordial follicle starts undergoing maturation process but only one reaches maturity and the rest undergo atresia at different

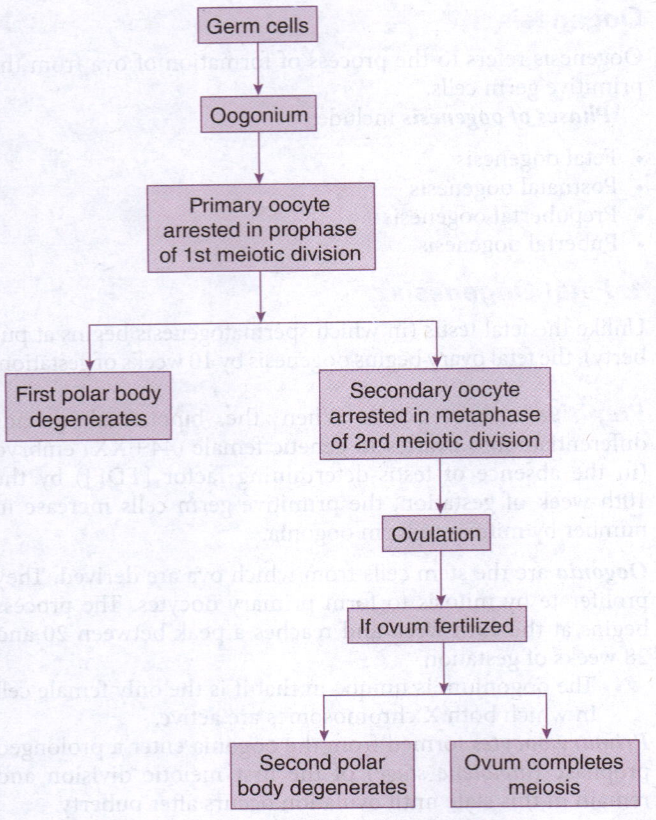

Fig. 9.3.6 Oogenesis.

stages of development. Thus, throughout the whole normal reproductive life of about 30 years (from 13 to 42 years), about 450 ova are expelled and the remainder degenerate.

- The different stages of maturation of primordial follicle into Graafian follicle (*folliculogenesis*) are described in 'Ovarian Cycle' (see page 828).

The primary oocytes which are in the prophase of the first meiotic division since fetal life complete the first meiotic division just before ovulation. The granulosa cells secrete oocyte maturation inhibiting factor (OMIF) that keeps the ovum arrested in prophase of the first meiotic division.

- As a result, *secondary oocyte* containing most of the cytoplasm and *first polar body* are formed. The first polar body soon fragments and disappears (Fig. 9.3.6).
- The *secondary oocyte* (haploid cell) immediately begins the *second meiotic division* but this division stops at metaphase and is completed only if the mature ovum (ootid) is fertilized by a sperm. In some species, the arrest in metaphase is due to formation of a protein in the ovum known as $PP^{3q\ mos}$ encoded by proto-oncogene (C-mos). On fertilization, $PP^{3q\ mos}$ is destroyed within 30 minutes by calpain (a Ca^{2+}-dependent protease). At that time, the *second polar body (polocyte)* is extruded and the fertilized ovum proceeds to form a new individual. Fertilization normally occurs in the ampulla of the fallopian tube.

Pubertal Oogenesis Versus Spermatogenesis

From the above-given description of pubertal oogenesis and spermatogenesis (page 805), the following can be concluded:

- In contrast to the male who produces spermatogonia and primary spermatocytes continuously throughout life, the female cannot form oogonia beyond 28 weeks of gestation and must function with a declining pool of oocytes.
- Meiosis in the female results in the formation of one viable oocyte. In contrast, each primary spermatogonium in the male ultimately gives rise to 64 spermatozoa.
- Oogenesis in the female begins in utero in response to *meiosis-stimulating factor*, whereas in the male, spermatogenesis is arrested at the spermatogonial stage in response to *meiosis-inhibiting factor*.

Endocrine Function of Ovaries

The endocrine function of the ovaries is to produce female sex hormones which include:

- Oestrogens
- Progesterone
- Activin
- Inhibin
- Relaxin

Oestrogens

Oestrogens are C-18 steroids. The naturally occurring oestrogens include:

- *Oestradiol (E_2):* It is the principal and physiologically most potent oestrogen. Ovarian oestradiol accounts for more than 90% of the circulating oestrogens.
- *Oestrone (E_1):* It is a weak ovarian oestrogen.
- *Oestriol (E_3):* It is the degradation product of oestradiol and oestrone. It is the weakest of all naturally occurring oestrogens.

Synthesis, plasma levels and transport of oestrogens

Sites In the normal nonpregnant female, oestrogens are mainly secreted by theca interna and granulosa cells of the ovarian follicles. A small quantity is also produced by the adrenal cortex and breast, some areas of the brain and placenta (during pregnancy), and Sertoli cells (in males).

Biosynthesis The salient points of oestrogen synthesis are as follows:

- Oestrogens are mainly synthesized from cholesterol derived from blood and to a slight extent from acetyl *coenzyme A*.
- During synthesis, progesterone and testosterone are synthesized first and then these are converted into oestrogens.
- The biochemical steps for synthesis of oestrogen are shown in Fig. 9.3.7. There are two pathways (Δ5 pathway and Δ4 pathway) for oestrogen synthesis. The first step, i.e. the conversion of cholesterol into pregnenolone, is common in both the pathways. This reaction is stimulated by gonadotropins (follicle-stimulating hormone [FSH] and luteinizing hormone [LH]).

Δ5 pathway This pathway involves:

- Synthesis of 17α-hydroxypregnenolone and dihydroxyepiandrosterone (DHEA). The reactions are catalysed by enzymes 17α-hydroxylase and 17,20-hydroxylase, respectively (CYP-17).

Note: CYP-17 is an enzyme which catalyses hydroxylation of C-17 and cleavage of two carbon side chains at C-17 of pregnenolone and progesterone.

- Then DHEA (17-ketosteroid) is converted to androstenedione (another androgenic 17-ketosteroid) by an enzyme 3β-hydroxysteroid dehydrogenase (3βHSD) and Δ5-reductase.

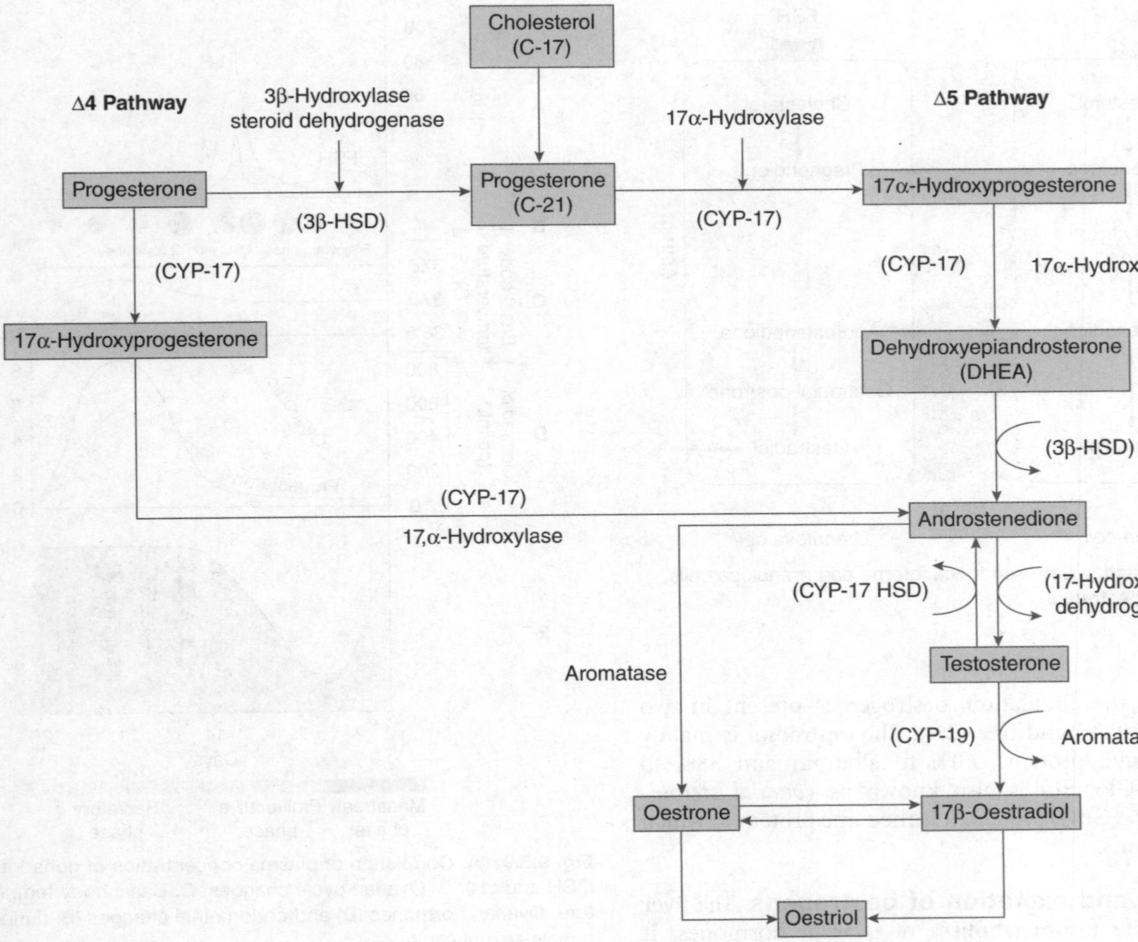

Fig. 9.3.7 Biosynthesis and metabolism of oestrogen.

- Androstenedione is then converted into *testosterone* by 17-hydroxysteroid dehydrogenase. This reaction is reversible.
- Testosterone is a precursor for oestradiol formation by aromatase (CYP-19) enzyme.

Δ4 pathway In this pathway, progesterone is the initial compound which is formed from pregnenolone by 3βHSD and Δ5 isomerase.

- Then progesterone is converted to 17α-hydroxyprogesterone by 17α-hydroxylase (CYP-17). 17α-Hydroxyprogesterone is another precursor for androstenedione via 17α-hydroxylase.
- Then both androstenedione and testosterone are converted to oestradiol and oestrone by aromatases (CYP-19).

Mechanism of biosynthesis of oestrogen Gonadotropins (FSH and LH) from the anterior pituitary stimulate the synthesis of female sex hormones by acting on the receptors.

- Theca interna cells have many LH receptors. The LH therefore increases the conversion of cholesterol to androstenedione via cyclic AMP.
- The granulosa cells also possess many FSH receptors. FSH, therefore, facilitates the secretion of oestradiol by acting on these receptors through activation of cyclic AMP, which increases the activity of aromatase enzyme. The mature granulosa cells also acquire LH receptors; therefore, LH stimulates the oestradiol production from granulosa cells also.
- There exists an interaction between theca interna and granulosa cells for oestrogen synthesis (Fig. 9.3.8). The granulosa cells can synthesize oestradiol only when androstenedione is provided to them. The theca interna cells provide supply of androstenedione to granulosa cells.
- In primates, it seems that the oestradiol present in the follicular fluid comes from the granulosa cells.
- The stromal tissue of the ovaries can also synthesize androgens and oestrogens in insignificant amounts.

Plasma levels In a normal adult woman, the plasma levels of oestrogen vary in different phases of the ovarian cycle (Fig. 9.3.9; Table 9.3.1). As shown in Fig. 9.3.9D, there are two peaks of oestrogen secretion. The first occurs just before the ovulation (12th to 13th day of a sexual cycle) and is called *oestrogen surge*, and the second peak occurs in the mid-luteal phase. The secretion rate of oestrogen in different phases is as follows:

- In early follicular phase : 36 μg/day
- Just before ovulation : 380 μg/day
- During mid-luteal phase : 250 μg/day

After menopause, the oestrogen level falls to minimum of 50 μg/day.

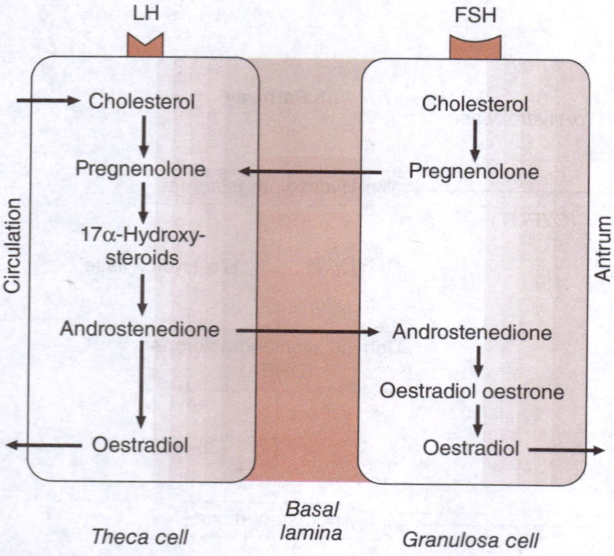

Fig. 9.3.8 Interaction between theca interna and granulosa cells for synthesis of oestradiol.

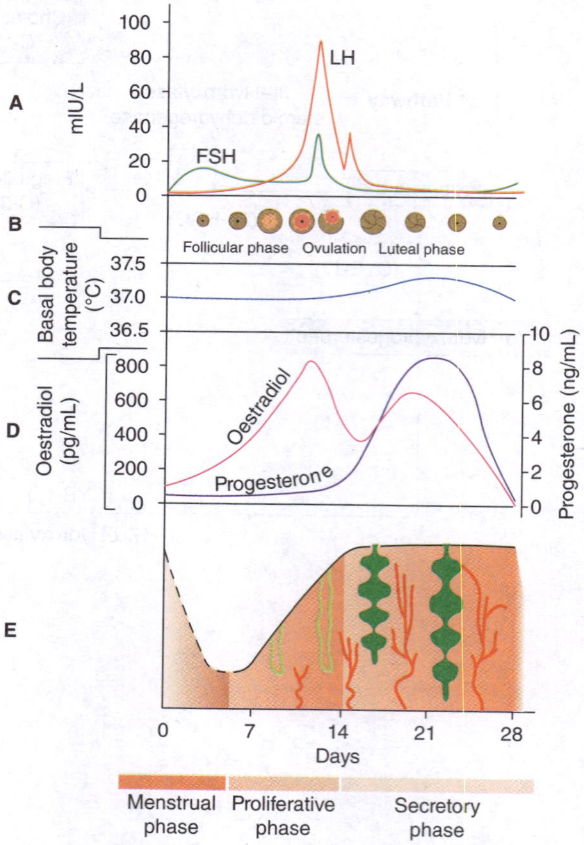

Fig. 9.3.9 **A**, Correlation of plasma concentration of gonadotropins (FSH and LH). **B**, Ovarian cycle changes. **C**, Basal body temperature. Ovarian hormones (**D**) and endometrial changes (**E**) during female sexual cycle.

Transport In the circulation, oestrogen is present in two forms, bound (98%) and free (2%). The oestradiol is mainly bound to plasma proteins: 60% to albumin and 38% to β-globulin. β-Globulin is also known as *gonadal steroid-binding globulin* (GBG) *protein*. It is the same protein to which testosterone binds.

Metabolism and excretion of oestrogens The liver is the main site for metabolism of ovarian hormones. It involves the steps given next.

Catabolism Large quantities of oestrogens (oestradiol and oestrone) are hydroxylated at C-16 position to form *oestriol*. A small quantity of oestrogens is catabolized by hydroxylation at C-2 and C-4 positions to form *catechol oestrogens*.

Conjugation In the liver, the degradation metabolites are conjugated with glucuronic acid and sulphuric acid to form water-soluble compounds (glucuronides and sulphates of oestriol and catecholestriole).

Excretion Most (four-fifth) of the water-soluble compounds of oestrogens are excreted by the kidney into the urine and a small amount (one-fifth part) of them is secreted into the bile and gets reabsorbed into the blood by enterohepatic circulation.

Table 9.3.1 Plasma levels and production rate of ovarian hormones

Hormone	Early follicular phase: Plasma concentration (ng/dL)	Early follicular phase: Production rate (μg/day)	Preovulatory phase: Plasma concentration (ng/dL)	Preovulatory phase: Production rate (μg/day)	Mid-luteal phase: Plasma concentration (ng/dL)	Mid-luteal phase: Production rate (μg/day)
Oestrogens (C-18)						
• Oestradiol	6	36	50	380	20	250
• Oestrone	5	50	20	350	10	250
• Progesterone (C-21)	9	1000	100	2000	1000	25,000
• 17α-Hydroxyprogesterone	30	600	200	4000	200	4000
Androgens (C-19)						
• Testosterone	40	144	40	171	40	126
• Androstenedione	150	2600	150	4700	150	3400
• Dehydroepiandrosterone	500	7000	500	7000	500	7000

Functions of Oestrogens

The functions of oestrogen for descriptive purposes can be grouped as reproductive actions and other actions.

I. Reproductive actions are:

A. During Embryonic Life During embryonic life, like testosterone (in males), oestrogen has no effect on sex differentiation (gonadal and genital sex).

B. During prepubertal stage During girlhood period, the oestrogens are secreted in a very small amount which have little physiological actions.

C. At puberty At puberty, oestradiol is secreted in larger amounts which cause the following changes:

1. Growth and development of genital organs:

i. ***Ovaries*** increase in size and complete ovarian cycles start which are characterized by folliculosis, ovulation and corpus luteum formation.
ii. ***Fallopian tubes*** become functional and show certain changes such as epithelium becoming more ciliated; motility of fallopian tubes also increases at ovulation to transport shedded gametes.
iii. ***Uterus:*** The following changes occur in the uterus:
   - *Size:* It enlarges in size, the smooth muscle fibres in myometrial coat increase in number and in size, the contractile protein contents also increase and the muscle fibres become active and excitable.
   - *Endometrium* gets thickened due to increase in stroma and blood flow. The rhythmic cyclic changes (proliferative and secretory) occur with the onset of menstrual cycle.
iv. ***Cervix*** also enlarges and with the onset of menstrual cycle, endocervix undergoes cyclic changes (see page 832).
v. ***Vagina*** increases in size. Its epithelial lining increases in height (from 2- to 3-layer cuboidal epithelium to 10- to 12-layer cornified squamous epithelium). Vaginal epithelium is quite sensitive to oestrogen and thus shows cyclic changes during sexual cycle (see page 832).
vi. ***External genitalia:*** The following changes occur in external genitalia:
   - *Clitoris increases in size.*
   - *Labia majora and labia minora* increase in size and get widened.

2. Appearance of secondary sex characters: Oestrogen is responsible for appearance of secondary sex characters (see page 798):

- In an adult woman, oestrogens along with progesterone regulate the ovarian cycle, menstrual cycle and cyclic changes in the cervix, vagina and fallopian tubes (see page 833) in a nonpregnant state.
- Oestrogen plays an important role in maintenance of pregnancy and then during parturition (see page 855).
- It is important for breast development (see page 859).

II. Other actions are:

The other functions of oestrogens include the effects on the following:

1. Effects on bones are:

i. Oestradiol accelerates the linear growth of bones at puberty by its osteoblastic activity. The epiphyseal centres are more sensitive to oestrogen than to testosterone; therefore, average height of females is little less than that of the males.
ii. Oestradiol enlarges the hip and widens the inlet of the pelvic bone to facilitate childbirth.
iii. Oestrogen maintains balance between bone formation and bone resorption by the following ways:
   - It promotes bone formation by deposition of bone matrix by causing Ca^{2+} and HPO_4^{2-} retention.
   - It inhibits bone resorption by inhibiting the production of osteoclasts and their activity. These effects are achieved by inhibiting the production of lymphokines such as interleukin-1 (IL-1), TNF-α and granulocyte–macrophage colony-stimulating factor which promote proliferation of osteoclasts.

Note: Loss of oestrogen actions after menopause shifts the bone balance towards bone resorption, thus causing osteoporosis (see page 721).

2. Effects on metabolism are:

i. ***Protein metabolism:***
- Oestrogens cause positive nitrogen balance due to growth-promoting effect which causes slight increase in the total body proteins.
- Oestrogens also increase the hepatic synthesis of certain circulating proteins, such as thyroxine-binding globulin, cortisol-binding globulins, renin substrate, angiotensinogens, very low-density lipoproteins (VLDL) and high-density lipoproteins.

ii. ***Fat metabolism:***
- Oestrogens cause fat deposition in subcutaneous tissues, breasts and thighs.
- They lower the plasma cholesterol level and low-density lipids due to increase in the number of LDL receptors.

3. Water and electrolyte balance: Oestrogens, like other steroids in general, cause salt and water retention in the body and produce premenstrual tension in some women.

4. Effects on vasculature: In general, oestrogens have vasodilator and antivasoconstrictor effects.

- The vasodilator effect is through local release of vasodilator substances like nitric oxide (NO), prostaglandins E_2 and prostacyclin.
- The antivasoconstrictor effect is through inhibition of endothelin-1 release (a vasoconstrictor agent).

Important Notes

- At the end of luteal phase of menstrual cycle, there is sudden fall in plasma concentration of oestrogen which results in alterations in the balance of vasodilatation and antivasoconstriction and thus initiates ischaemic necrosis during menstrual phase.
- Loss of vasodilator effect in postmenopausal women leads to increased risk of coronary heart disease.

5. Effects on CNS: Oestrogens are responsible for oestrous behaviour in animals and also increase the libido in human females.

- Oestrogens also act on other areas of the brain and affect the neuronal discharge and thus affect the brain functioning. It has been observed that in mice, oestrogen improves the memory and learning. Therefore, deficiency of oestrogen in postmenopausal women is associated with defects in declarative memory and development of Alzheimer disease (see page 1091).

6. Effects on skin include:

- Oestrogens make the skin soft and more vascular.
- They make the sebaceous gland secretions thin and inhibit formation of blackheads (comedones) and acne. Therefore, synthetic oestrogens are used as a part of treatment in acne.

Mechanism of Action of Oestrogens Oestrogens act by entering into the cell and then binding with cytoplasmic receptors.

Oestrogen receptors Oestrogen receptors are of two types (oestrogen receptor α [ERα] and oestrogen receptor β [ERβ]) and are coded by two different genes located on separate chromosomes.

ERα are mainly present in the endometrium, breasts, pituitary gland and adrenal glands, and in the testes and epididymis in males, whereas *ERβ* are located in the ovaries (granulosa cells), bones (osteoclasts), lungs and some areas of the brain, and in prostate gland and urinary bladder in males.

It has been suggested that the actions of oestrogen which are carried out by circulatory oestrogens and through the hypothalamo–pituitary–gonadal axis are mainly mediated through ERα receptors and the actions of oestrogen present in the follicular antrum are mediated through ERβ receptors.

- The receptors contain a heat shock protein (HSP). When oestrogen binds to the receptor, the HSP gets displaced and *oestrogen receptor complex* so formed is transferred onto the nucleus of the target cell.
- Then the oestrogen receptor gets bound to oestrogen response element present on the DNA molecule, and promotes the synthesis of new mRNA and that in turn directs the synthesis of new proteins which modify the target cell activity.

Note: Most of the actions of oestrogens are mediated via genomic receptors (ERα and ERβ). However, some of their effects are so rapid (e.g. effect on brain neuronal discharge and feedback effect on gonadotropin release) that they might be mediated through nongenomic receptors present on the plasma membrane.

Synthetic Oestrogens Various types of synthetic preparations of oestrogen available are as follows:

1. ***Ethinyl derivatives*** of oestradiol such as *diethylstilbestrol* and *ethinyloestradiol* are the potent oestrogens when given orally (because these are not metabolized in the liver like natural oestrogens).
2. ***Plant oestrogens:*** Oestrogenic substances are present in plants, which rarely cause adverse effects in human beings.
3. ***Nonsteroidal*** preparations also have oestrogenic activity.
   - Selective oestrogen receptor modulators (SERMs) are the partial agonists and antagonists of oestrogen. These drugs are clomiphene, tamoxifen, raloxifene, etc. These drugs are mainly used for treatment of cancer and menopausal osteoporosis.

Therapeutic uses The oestrogenic preparations are used under the following conditions:

- To reduce menopausal symptoms like hot flushes
- To prevent postmenopausal osteoporosis
- To prevent progression to atherosclerosis and incidence of heart attacks and strokes
- As a contraceptive when used along with progesterone

Side effects (adverse effects) They stimulate growth of the endometrium and breast and thus increase the incidence of carcinoma of the breast and of the uterus. The compounds like *tamoxifen* and *raloxifene* are under trial. It has been suggested that these compounds are effective to check osteoporosis and have cardiovascular effects as those of oestradiol but do not have growth-promoting effect on the uterus and cervix.

Progesterone

Progesterone is C-21 steroid meant for maintenance of pregnancy and biologically called prostagen or gestagen.

Synthesis, plasma levels and transport of progesterone

Sites In a normal adult nonpregnant woman, progesterone is mainly secreted by the corpus luteum and during pregnancy by the placenta. A small amount is also secreted by the adrenal cortex and by testes in case of males.

Biosynthesis Progesterone is synthesized from cholesterol. Progesterone itself is an important intermediary compound formed during biosynthesis of steroids (oestrogens and androgens). For biosynthesis pathways and steps involved, see page 823 and Fig. 9.3.7.

Plasma levels In a normal adult woman, the plasma levels of progesterone vary with different phases of sexual cycle (Table 9.3.1; Fig. 9.3.9D).

In early follicular phase, plasma concentration of progesterone is very low (about 0.9 ng/mL or 9 ng/dL). About 80%–90% of the progesterone is derived from the conversion of adrenal DHEA and androstenedione. But a large amount is also present in the follicular antrum.

In midcycle (late follicular phase), its level starts rising due to secretion from the granulosa cells and it is mainly 17α-hydroxyprogesterone.

In luteal phase, it reaches its peak value, i.e. 18 ng/mL.

At the end of cycle, its levels fall to its minimum value.

During pregnancy, the levels of progesterone further rise (see page 844).

After menopause: Progesterone levels fall to their minimum (0.2 ng/mL) or are even not detectable.

Transport In the plasma, progesterone is present in two forms:

Bound form: About 98% of progesterone in the blood is present in bound form with plasma proteins – 80% with albumin and 18% with corticoid-binding protein (CBP), also known as *transcortin*. Hence, progesterone is mostly present in loosely bound form with albumin.

Unbound form or free form: Only 2% of circulating progesterone is present in this form.

Metabolism and excretion of progesterone

Metabolism In the liver, progesterone is metabolized to form pregnanediol and 17α-hydroxyprogesterone to pregnanetriol.

The metabolites then conjugate with glucuronic acid and sulphuric acid to form water-soluble substances.

Excretion The water-soluble substances (glucuronides and sulphates) of pregnanediol and pregnanetriol are excreted by the kidney into the urine and a small amount is also secreted into the bile.

Functions of progesterone The physiological actions of progesterone can be grouped as reproductive actions and other actions.

I. Reproductive actions Reproductive actions are mainly on the reproductive organs primed by oestrogens and these include those given next.

1. Action on uterus Under the influence of progesterone, uterus shows the following changes:

Endometrium changes are:

- Progesterone slows the proliferation of endometrial cells by decreasing mitotic activity of the cells.
- The thickness of endometrium also increases.
- The endometrial glands become tortuous and contain fluid containing glycogen, glycoproteins and glycolipids which provide nutrition to blastula if fertilization occurs.
- The glandular cells show vacuolation near their bases and the vacuolations move from peripheral part towards the lumen of the gland.
- The spiral arteries become more coiled.
- The stroma of endometrium becomes oedematous.

Thus, progesterone is responsible for secretory phase of the endometrial cycle and prepares the endometrium to receive the zygote.

Uterine motility: Progesterone decreases the uterine motility by the following ways:

- It has antioestrogenic effect on the myometrial cells, decreasing the excitability sensitivity to oxytocin and spontaneous electrical activity and increasing membrane potential.
- It decreases the synthesis of voltage-dependent Ca^{2+} channel proteins; therefore, Ca^{2+} uptake decreases.
- It decreases the number of oestrogen receptors on the myometrium.

2. Endocervix The cervical secretions become thick and viscid, and ferning pattern disappears.

3. Vagina Vaginal epithelium becomes thickened, cornified and infiltrated with leucocytes.

4. Fallopian tubes Progesterone increases the beating rate of cilia of fallopian tubes towards the uterus. The epithelial cell secretions also increase in amount and are rich in nutritive materials to provide nutrition to a shedded ovum, incoming sperm or zygote if fertilization occurs.

5. Breast Progesterone causes lobular and alveolar growth (see page 859) of the breast.

6. During pregnancy During pregnancy, the main function of progesterone is to maintain the pregnancy (see page 845).

II. Other actions The other systemic effects of progesterone are those given next.

1. Thermogenic effect Progesterone is known as a thermogenic steroid which increases the basal body temperature by 0.5°C in the postovulatory phase.

2. Effect on CNS Progesterone alters the secretion and release of various neurotransmitters in the hypothalamus and other areas of the brain and thereby decreases the appetite and produces *somnolence*.

3. Effect on respiration Progesterone increases the sensitivity of the respiratory centre to carbon dioxide stimulation. Due to this fact, the $pACO_2$ is slightly less in woman during luteal phase of sexual cycle. Therefore, progesterone is used in *Pickwickian syndrome*.

4. Effect on fat metabolism Progesterone (particularly C-19 progesterone) decreases the serum HDL. Thus, it acts as a proatherogenic agent.

5. Effect on kidney Large dose of progesterone produces natriuresis, by blocking action of aldosterone on the kidney.

Mechanism of action The effect of the progesterone on its target cell is achieved by acting through its receptors.

- The progesterone receptors are present in the cytoplasm of the target cells and contain a protein called HSP.
- Being lipid, progesterone easily enters through bilayer lipid membrane and combines with its receptors.
- Then the HSP displaces and thus exposes the DNA binding site.
- Then the receptor–progesterone complex gets transferred onto the nucleus and binds to a specific site on the DNA molecule, and initiates encoding of gene expression to form new mRNA. The mRNA then directs the apparatus to form new proteins (enzymes and structural proteins) which modify the activities of the target cells.

Important Note

A synthetic steroid mifepristone (RU-486) binds to progesterone receptors and blocks the DNA binding site. Therefore, this drug acts as an antiprogesterone drug.

Synthetic preparations of progesterone Various synthetic preparations are available under the name *prostagens* and gestagens. Therapeutically, these drugs are used:

- In inevitable abortion
- As contraceptives when used along with oestrogens

Other Ovarian Hormones

Besides female sex steroids (oestrogen and progesterone), ovaries also secrete peptide hormones as given next.

1. Inhibin Structurally, it is a polypeptide; it inhibits the FSH release. For details, see page 813.

2. Activin Structurally, it is also a polypeptide; its action is to activate FSH secretion from the anterior pituitary (see page 813).

3. Relaxin Relaxin is a polypeptide hormone produced by the corpus luteum and other sites include the uterus, placenta and mammary glands, and the prostate gland in males.

Its main role is during pregnancy, mentioned as follows:

- It relaxes pubic symphysis and pelvic joints, softens and dilates the uterine cervix and facilitates delivery.

In nonpregnant state, it releases from the corpus luteum and endometrium; during secretory phase, its function is not known.

In males, relaxin is present in the semen and helps in sperm motility and penetration of ovum by the sperm.

4. Ovarian androgens A small amount of testosterone is also secreted by the ovaries during biosynthesis of oestrogen and progesterone, but the main source of androgens in a female is adrenal cortex.

These androgens are responsible for acne vulgaris, libido and pubic hair.

FEMALE SEXUAL CYCLE

The sexual life span of a female can be divided into three periods.

1. Birth to puberty During this period, primary and accessory female sex organs remain quiescent. Puberty occurs between 12 and 14 years of age.

2. Puberty to menopause With the onset of puberty, the female sexual cycle starts, which repeats every 28 days. The occurrence of the first menstrual cycle is called *menarche*. The permanent stoppage of menstrual cycle is called *menopause*, which occurs at the age of about 45–50 years. The period between menarche and menopause is called *reproductive period*. During this period, females have rhythmical sexual cycles.

3. Postmenopausal period The postmenopausal period extends after menopause (45–50 years) to rest of the life. During this period, the female sexual cycle ceases.

Female sexual cycle refers to monthly rhythmic sexual cycle occurring in females during the normal reproductive period.

Components of human female sexual cycle: During each female sexual cycle, rhythmical changes occur in ovaries and accessory sex organs – uterus, cervix and vagina. The components of female sexual cycle are as follows:

- Ovarian cycle
- Endometrial cycle
- Changes in the cervix uteri
- Changes in the vagina
- Other changes during sexual cycle
- Changes in gonadotropin secretion, i.e. hormonal control of female sexual cycle

Duration of the female sexual cycle is usually 28 days. But under physiological conditions, it may vary between 20 and 40 days. Traditionally the first day of the menstrual bleeding is taken as the first day to each component of female sexual cycle.

I. OVARIAN CYCLE

Ovarian cycle refers to rhythmic changes occurring in ovaries during each female sexual cycle of about 28 days (range 20–40 days). During each cycle, a single mature ovum is released from the ovary. Ovarian changes occurring during the female sexual life completely depend on the gonadotropic hormones (FSH and LH) which are secreted by the anterior pituitary. Both FSH and LH stimulate ovarian target cells by combining with highly specific FSH and LH receptors (G-coupled receptors) present on their membranes. FSH and LH activate cyclic adenosine monophosphate (cAMP). However, some effects of hormones cannot be attributed entirely to the cAMP system. The ovarian cycle can be divided into three phases:

- Preovulatory phase or follicular phase
- Ovulation
- Postovulatory phase or luteal phase

A. Preovulatory Phase

Preovulatory or follicular phase of the ovarian cycle extends from the 5th day of the cycle till the time of ovulation (which takes place at about 14th day of the cycle). Thus, this phase generally lasts for 8–9 days (but may vary from 10 to 25 days).

Changes in the ovary during preovulatory phase or follicular phase are mostly under the influence of FSH from the anterior pituitary. LH also helps in maturation of the follicle in the latter part of follicular phase (for details, see 'Hormonal Control of Female Sexual Cycle'; page 834).

During this phase of each cycle (of about 28 days), approximately 10–15 primordial follicles start maturing, but only 1 follicle matures fully, which is the dominant follicle and the rest undergo atresia (atrophy) at different stages of development. The process of maturation of follicle is called folliculogenesis.

Phases of Folliculogenesis

The follicles at different stages of maturation are given next (Fig. 9.3.10).

1. Primordial follicles Primordial follicles are the fundamental reproductive units of the ovary. At the time of puberty, both ovaries contain about 300,000 primordial follicles.

- Primordial follicles are formed in fetal life. Each primordial follicle consists of the primary oocyte in prophase of the first meiotic division surrounded by a single layer of spindle-shaped (flat) cells called the granulosa cells.
- Both the granulosa cells and the primary oocyte are enveloped in a thin membrane called basal lamina (Fig. 9.3.10A).
- The primordial follicles lack a direct blood supply.
- The granulosa cells of the primordial follicle are believed to provide nutrition to the ovum (primary oocyte) throughout the childhood (from birth to puberty). These cells also secrete *OMIF* which keeps the ovum in immature stage till puberty. At the onset of puberty, under the influence of FSH and LH, the primordial follicles start growing and convert into primary follicles.

2. Primary follicle The primary follicle is formed when the primordial follicle undergoes the following developmental changes (Fig. 9.3.10B):

Granulosa cells, which are flat (spindle-shaped) in primordial follicle, become columnar and undergo mitotic division to form a multilayered stratum granulosum.

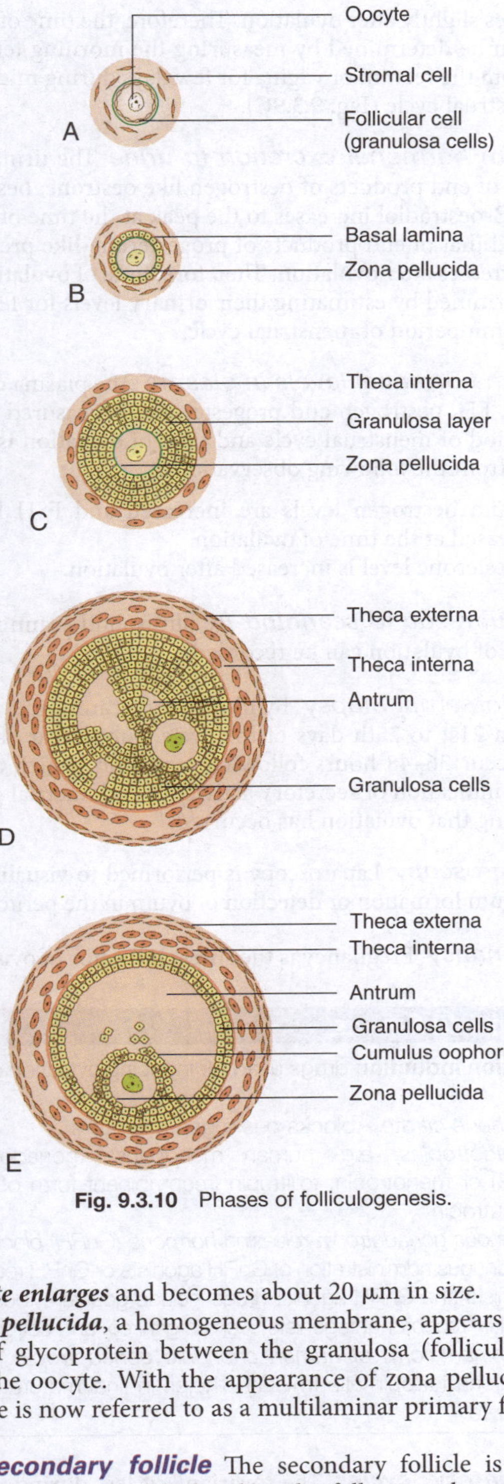

Fig. 9.3.10 Phases of folliculogenesis.

Oocyte enlarges and becomes about 20 μm in size.

Zona pellucida, a homogeneous membrane, appears consisting of glycoprotein between the granulosa (follicular) cells and the oocyte. With the appearance of zona pellucida, the follicle is now referred to as a multilaminar primary follicle.

3. Secondary follicle The secondary follicle is formed from the primary follicle when the following changes occur (Fig. 9.3.10C):

Granulosa cells undergo further proliferation.

Oocyte further increases in size up to 100 μm. Its nucleus becomes larger and vesicular, forming germinal spots.

Theca folliculi or follicular sheath is formed outside the basal lamina from the spindle-shaped cells from the stroma of the cortex in the ovary. The theca folliculi consist of an inner rim of secretory cells called *theca interna* and an outer rim of thickly packed fibres and spindle-shaped cells called *theca externa* (which merges with the surrounding stroma).

Independent blood supply consisting of arterioles that do not penetrate the basal lamina is acquired by the secondary follicles.

- The dominant follicle starts growing rapidly and is characterized by a large number of FSH receptors, highest concentration of oestrogen, inhibin and high activity of enzyme aromatase.

4. Tertiary follicle The tertiary follicle is characterized by the following features:

Formation of antrum: After proliferation, the granulosa cells start secreting follicular fluid; this causes cavity to be formed in the stratum granulosum (cavitation), which is called antrum or follicular cavity. The fluid filled in the antrum is called liquor folliculi which also contains oestrogen. The granulosa cells continue to proliferate and the size of follicle is increased (Fig. 9.3.10D).

Changes in theca folliculi: The theca cells proliferate more rapidly. The theca interna is transformed into theca interstitial cells which will become steroidogenic cells which synthesize and secrete androgens (androstenedione) in response to gonadotropins (FSH and LH).

Blood vessels of the follicle do not penetrate the zona pellucida and thus the oocyte and the granulosa remain avascular.

Up to this stage, follicular growth is mainly stimulated by FSH alone.

5. Graafian (antral) follicle After about the seventh day of sexual cycle, one of the tertiary follicles increases in size in response to gonadotropins (both FSH and LH) and forms the mature follicle called Graafian or antral or vesicular follicle (Fig. 9.3.10E). It is uncertain how one follicle is selected to become the mature Graafian follicle in this follicular phase of the cycle, but it seems to be related to the ability of the follicle to secrete the oestrogen inside it that is needed for final maturation. Rest of the follicles degenerate and become atrophied by apoptosis. A fully matured Graafian follicle is characterized by the following features:

Size of the follicle increases markedly to about 2–5 mm. The growth of the Graafian follicle is accomplished by granulosa and theca proliferation. It extends through the whole thickness of the cortex of the ovary. At one place, it encroaches upon the tunica albuginea and bulges out of the surface of the ovary into the peritoneal cavity.

Antrum becomes larger and distended with fluid. With the enlargement of follicles, the follicular fluid collects in such a large amount that it surrounds the ovum all around except at one point. As a result, the ovum covered by a layer of cells called *corona radiata* remains in contact with granulosa cells only at a hill-like area called *cumulus oophorus*.

Theca interna becomes more prominent. The thickness of theca interna becomes double with a rich network of capillaries. The oestrogen-secreting cells of theca interna increase and are called the cells of theca glands.

Formation of secondary oocyte: Just prior to ovulation, the primary oocyte of the fully matured Graafian follicle completes the first meiotic division (which began in fetal life at about 20th and 28th weeks of gestation, i.e. before birth), and forms the secondary oocyte with a haploid nucleus and the first polar body.

B. Ovulation

Ovulation refers to release of secondary oocyte from the ovary (following rupture of Graafian follicle) into the peritoneal cavity. It usually occurs *14 days after the onset* of menstruation, i.e. *early on day 15* in a normal 28-day cycle (Fig. 9.3.9B).

Process of ovulation involves the following sequence of events:

LH surge and ovulatory peak of FSH: The ovulation is caused by an LH surge at midcycle in response to an elevation in plasma oestradiol concentration (150 pg/mL).

Onset of LH surge (a relatively precise indicator of ovulation) occurs 34–36 hours before ovulation.

Peak of the LH surge occurs 12–24 hours before ovulation (secretion of LH increases 6- to 10-fold).

Immediately before the LH peak, oestradiol levels in the plasma fall.

Ovulatory peak of FSH (twofold to threefold increase in secretion) occurring 2 days prior to ovulation is thought to be stimulated by progesterone. FSH increases the granulosa cell LH receptors. LH surge causes:

- Rapid secretion of progesterone
- Completion of meiosis-1 phase and formation of secondary oocyte (haploid) and first polar body
- Induction of cyclooxygenase-2 (COX-2) and prostaglandin synthesis
- Epidermal growth factors (EGFs) such as amphiregulin, epiregulin, betacellulin and neuregulin (all these factors are required for ovulation)

The FSH surge around ovulation is responsible for increasing plasmin, proteolytic enzymes and prostaglandins which cause follicular rupture and release of secondary oocyte.

Changes in Graafian follicle The LH and FSH produce the following changes in Graafian follicle before ovulation:

Rapid swelling of the follicle is caused by FSH and LH a few days before ovulation. There occurs a rapid growth of new blood vessels into the follicle wall and prostaglandins are secreted into the follicular tissue. Both these cause diffusion of plasma into the follicular fluid and further swelling of the follicle.

Formation of stigma: Due to rapid swelling of the follicle, its outer wall is stretched forming a very thin avascular area (stigma) over the most convex point of the follicle which protrudes like a nipple in the peritoneal cavity.

Release of proteolytic enzymes from the lysosomes in the theca externa cells is activated by the progesterone.

Dissolution of capsular wall and its further weakening is caused by the proteolytic enzymes.

Rupture of Graafian follicle: The simultaneous stretching and enzymatic dissolution of the follicular wall leads to degeneration of *the stigma*. Within 30 minutes of protrusion, fluid begins to ooze from the stigma followed soon by rupture of follicle with release of ovum (secondary oocyte) surrounded by corona radiata into the peritoneal cavity near the fimbriated end of the fallopian tube. Thus, usually only one ovum is released from any one of two ovaries during each sexual cycle. The released ovum enters the fallopian tube through its fimbriated end.

Determination of Ovulation Time

Ovulation usually occurs 14 days after the onset of menstruation, i.e. early on day 15 in a normal 28-day cycle. The ovulation time can be determined by the indirect methods given next.

1. From basal body temperature The basal body temperature falls slightly (0.3–0.5°C) just prior to ovulation and increases slightly after ovulation. Therefore, the time of ovulation can be determined by measuring the morning temperature from the rectum or vagina for few days during midperiod of menstrual cycle (Fig. 9.3.9C).

2. From hormonal excretion in urine The urinary excretion of end products of oestrogen like oestrone, oestradiol and 17β-oestradiol increases to the peak at the time of ovulation and that of end products of progesterone-like pregnanediol increases after ovulation. Therefore, time of ovulation can be determined by estimating their urinary levels for few days during midperiod of menstrual cycle.

3. From hormonal levels in plasma The plasma content of FSH, LH, oestrogen and progesterone is measured during midperiod of menstrual cycle and time of ovulation is determined from the following observations:

- LH and oestrogen levels are increased and FSH level is decreased at the time of ovulation.
- Progesterone level is increased after ovulation.

4. By ultrasound scanning By ultrasound scanning, the process of ovulation can be recorded.

5. Endometrial biopsy By ultrasound scanning is usually done on 21st to 25th days of the cycle. Subnuclear vacuolations occur 36–48 hours following ovulation, which are the earliest indication of secretory activity of endometrial glands, indicating that ovulation has occurred.

6. Laparoscopy Laparoscopy is performed to visualize corpus luteum formation or detection of ovum in the peritoneum.

7. Pregnancy Pregnancy is the surest indicator of ovulation.

Applied Aspects

Ovulation induction drugs used for inducing ovulation are as follows:

Clomiphene citrate – blocks oestrogen receptors

Gonadotropins, e.g. human menopausal gonadotropin (hMG) or menotropin, follitropin (recombinant form of FSH) and lutropin

Endogenous gonadotropin-releasing hormone (GnRH) blockers – i.e. continuous administration of GnRH agonists or GnRH receptor antagonists (the GnRH agonist drugs include goserelin, buserelin and GnRH receptor antagonists such as ganirelix and cetrorelix)

Recombinant form of human chorionic gonadotropin (hCG) (choriogonadotropin alfa [rhCG]) – helps in final maturation of the oocyte.

Anovulatory cycles The ovarian cycles during which ovulation does not occur are called unovulatory cycles. If LH surge occurring prior to ovulation is not of sufficient magnitude, ovulation does not occur. First few cycles after puberty may be unovulatory.

C. Postovulatory Phase

The postovulatory phase, also called luteal phase, of ovarian cycle is of remarkably constant period of about 14 days. Therefore, retrospectively, the time of ovulation can be estimated by subtracting 14 days from the total duration of the menstrual cycle. This phase is characterized by the events given next (Fig. 9.3.5).

Formation of corpus haemorrhagicum Following ovulation, the outer wall of the Graafian follicle collapses and promptly fills with blood forming the so-called corpus haemorrhagicum. Minor bleeding from the follicle into the abdominal cavity may cause peritoneal irritation and fleeting lower abdominal pain (mittelschmerz).

Formation of corpus luteum Soon, the granulosa cells and theca cells of the follicle lining begin to proliferate, and the clotted blood is rapidly replaced with yellowish lipid-rich *luteal cells, also called K cells*. The yellow colour is due to pigment carotene. This process is called *luteinization* and the total mass of the cells is now called *corpus luteum*. LH is responsible for luteinization. The lutein cells secrete a large amount of progesterone and also oestrogen to a lesser extent. Seven days after ovulation, i.e. by the 22nd day of menstrual cycle, the corpus luteum attains a diameter of about 1.5 cm. Growth of corpus luteum depends on its developing blood supply and vascular endothelial growth factor (VEGF), the key component responsible for vasculogenesis. The progesterone secreted by these has a strong negative feedback effect on the anterior pituitary gland to decrease secretion of both LH and FSH. The fate of the corpus luteum depends on whether or not pregnancy occurs.

Formation of corpus albicans If there is no fertilization and pregnancy does not occur, the corpus luteum begins to involute (regress) after the 24th day of the sexual cycle and is eventually replaced by a whitish scar tissue, called the corpus albicans. This involution occurs due to falling levels of FSH and LH and also the hormone *inhibin* secreted by the lutein cells. With the involution of the corpus luteum, on the 26th day of the normal female sexual cycle, levels of oestrogen, progesterone and inhibin fall. This removes the feedback inhibition of the anterior pituitary; consequently, the FSH and within a few days LH secretion begins and the next ovarian cycle is initiated.

Corpus luteum of pregnancy However, if the ovum released is fertilized and pregnancy occurs, then the corpus luteum formed during postovulatory phase persists and serves as the major source of oestrogen and progesterone till the third month of pregnancy when the placenta takes over its endocrine function.

Applied Aspects

Luteal phase defect (LPD): It is an important cause of female infertility due to inadequate growth and function of corpus luteum. Causes of LPD are hyperprolactaemia, hypothyroidism and pelvic endometriosis.

- *Treatment:* Luteotropic hormone, human chorionic gonadotropin (hCG) and progesterone vaginal suppositories are effective.
- ***Luteinized unruptured follicular syndrome (LUF):*** In this condition, the ovum is trapped inside the follicle and gets luteinized. This condition is also associated with hyperprolactaemia and pelvic endometriosis.

II. ENDOMETRIAL CYCLE (UTERINE CYCLE)

The endometrial cycle refers to the cyclic changes occurring in the endometrium during active reproductive period (menarche to menopause) in females leading to recurrent monthly bleeding per vaginum (menstruation). These cyclic changes in the endometrium are brought about by the cyclic production of oestrogens and progesterone by the ovaries. Strictly speaking, the menstrual cycle is synonymous with the female sexual cycle and includes cyclic changes in all the female reproductive organs. However, in day-to-day practice, the term menstrual cycle is used for cyclic changes in the endometrium. Menstrual is a Latin word meaning mensis, i.e. lunar month of 28 days. Although the menstrual cycle for description purposes is considered to be of 28 days, the cycle is by no means as regular as the name suggests. The menstrual cycles of 25–35 days are also regarded as normal cycles.

Phases of Endometrial Cycle

Conventionally, the first day of the bleeding is considered to be the first day of the endometrial cycle. The endometrial cycle of 28 days can be divided into three phases (Fig. 9.3.9E):

- Menstrual phase (1st to 5th days)
- Proliferative phase (6th to 14th days)
- Secretory phase (15th to 28th days)

For the purpose of better understanding, the menstrual phase is described last of all.

A. Proliferative phase The extent of proliferative phase, also known as preovulatory phase, of endometrial cycle is from day 6th to 14th. It follows the phase of menstruation, after which only a thin basal layer of the original endometrium is left.

Hormone responsible for changes in the endometrium during this phase is oestrogen secreted by the developing Graafian follicle in the ovary. Thus, the proliferative phase of endometrial cycle coincides with the follicular phase of ovarian cycle.

Changes in endometrium, which occur under the influence of oestrogens during proliferative phase, are as follows:

1. Epithelial cells are stimulated to grow and reepithelialize the endometrial surface.
2. Thickness of endometrium, which is less than 1 mm at the end of the menstrual phase, increases to 3–4 mm at the end of the proliferative phase.
3. Mitosis of the stratum basale regenerates the stroma of the stratum functionale.
4. Angiogenesis in the stratum functionale leads to proliferation of blood vessels which become the spiral arterioles that profuse the stratum functionale.
5. Endometrial glands are stimulated to grow. The glands contain glycogen but they are nonsecretory.
6. Ovulation occurs at the end of this phase.

B. Secretory phase The extent of secretory phase (also known as postovulatory phase of endometrial cycle) is from day 15th to 28th.

Hormones responsible for changes in the endometrium during this phase are both oestrogens and progesterone secreted by the *corpus luteum* formed after ovulation. Thus, the secretory phase of endometrial cycle coincides with the luteal phase of ovarian cycle.

Changes in the endometrium, which occur under the influence of oestrogen and progesterone during this phase, are as follows:

Additional proliferation of cellular stroma is caused by oestrogens.

Differentiation of the endometrium is promoted by progesterone causing elongation and coiling of endometrial mucous glands. These glands become secretory and secrete thick viscous fluid containing glycogen.
Blood supply of endometrium further increases as progesterone promotes spiralling of blood vessels.
Two characteristic features of endometrium in secretory phase thus are prominent corkscrew-shaped glands and increased vascularity.
Thickness of endometrium increases to 5–6 mm at the end of secretory phase. Thus, the thickened endometrium with large amounts of nutrients is ready to provide appropriate conditions for implantation of ovum during this phase.
If fertilization does not occur and there is no pregnancy, the corpus luteum in the ovary involutes to form corpus albicans and on day 26th of the menstrual cycle, the levels of oestrogen and progesterone fall suddenly and mark the end of secretory phase of endometrial cycle.

C. Menstrual phase The menstrual phase of the endometrial cycle is also called the bleeding phase. The average duration of this phase is 3–5 days, but it may be as short as 1 day and as long as 8 days in a normal woman.

Cause of bleeding and sequence of events: About 24 hours before the end of the menstrual cycle, there is a sharp decline in the plasma levels of oestrogen and progesterone, which is responsible for menstrual bleeding. The sequence of events is as follows:

Intense spasm of spiral arteries occurs leading to hypoxia and ischaemia. This effect is mediated via local production of *leukotrienes* and *prostaglandins* (PGF2α).
Necrosis of stratum functionale of the endometrium and of the walls of the spiral arteries occurs as a result of ischaemia.
Blood vessels get opened up due to necrosis of their wall resulting in seepage of blood into the surrounding endometrial necrotic tissue.
Separation of necrotic tissue starts gradually from the underlying basal viable tissue and ultimately it is sloughed off. The necrosis and sloughing does not occur simultaneously in whole of the uterus; rather, it occurs in patches and is completed in 3–5 days.
Endometrial debris contains necrosed sloughed-off tissue, blood, serous fluid and a large amount of prostaglandins and fibrinolysins.
Average amount of blood loss during each menstrual cycle is 30 mL. Normally, it may vary from slight spotting to about 80 mL and is affected by factors like endometrial thickness and the conditions which affect clotting mechanism. The menstrual blood is predominantly arterial, with only 25% being of venous origin.
Menstrual blood immediately gets clotted inside the uterine cavity but soon gets liquefied by fibrolysins present in endometrial debris. This is the reason that menstrual blood does not normally contain blood clots unless the flow is excessive.
The prostaglandins of the endometrial debris cause further spasm of spiral arteries and also produce contractions of myometrium.
During the menstrual phase, about two-thirds of the superficial endometrium is sloughed off and only a thin basal layer (2 mm thick) is left behind.

III. CYCLIC CHANGES IN CERVIX

The uterine cervix (cervix uteri) is continuous with the body of the uterus. The mucosal lining of the cervix (endocervix) also shows certain cyclic changes during the sexual cycle. These are as follows:

During menstruation phase, the mucosa of the cervix does not undergo desquamation (shedding off) like that of the endometrium.

During proliferative phase (oestrogen phase), the secretions of the mucosal cells of the endocervix become thin, watery and alkaline. At the time of ovulation (14th day of sexual cycle), the cervical mucus is the thinnest and its elasticity is maximum. It can be stretched like a long, thin elastic thread up to 8–12 cm (spinnbarkeit effect). The mucus also produces a characteristic fern-like pattern when a drop of mucus is spread on the glass slide and allowed to dry (*fern test*) (Fig. 9.3.11B).

This characteristic nature of cervical mucus favours the transport of sperms in the female genital tract and makes the conditions favourable for fertilization.

During secretory phase, under the influence of progesterone, cervical secretions decrease in quantity and become thick, tenacious and cellular, and fern pattern is not seen (Fig. 9.3.11C). These changes make a plug and prevent the entry of sperm through the cervical canal.

Important Note

Fern test: The fern pattern of cervical mucus in proliferative phase and its disappearance in secretory phase is indicative of ovulatory cycle, whereas persistence of the fern pattern (Fig. 9.3.11D) throughout the cycle indicates unovulatory cycle.

IV. CYCLIC CHANGES IN VAGINA

The vaginal canal is lined by stratified squamous epithelium which is highly sensitive to oestrogens (oestradiol). Vaginal epithelium undergoes the following cyclic changes in endometrial cycle:

In the proliferative phase, vaginal epithelium becomes thickened (by adding up more and more layers of epithelium) and cornified. The cornified cells and maturing cells accumulate glycogen. Vaginal smear at this time shows many large eosinophilic cornified cells having a small pyknotic nucleus or it may be absent (Fig. 9.3.12A).

In the secretory phase, under the influence of progesterone, vaginal epithelium proliferates and gets infiltrated with leucocytes (Fig. 9.3.12B) and the vaginal secretions become thick and viscid.

V. OTHER CHANGES DURING SEXUAL CYCLE

Although hormonal oscillations during sexual cycle mainly affect the ovaries, uterus, cervix and vagina, some changes have also been observed in the fallopian tubes, breast and the body weight.

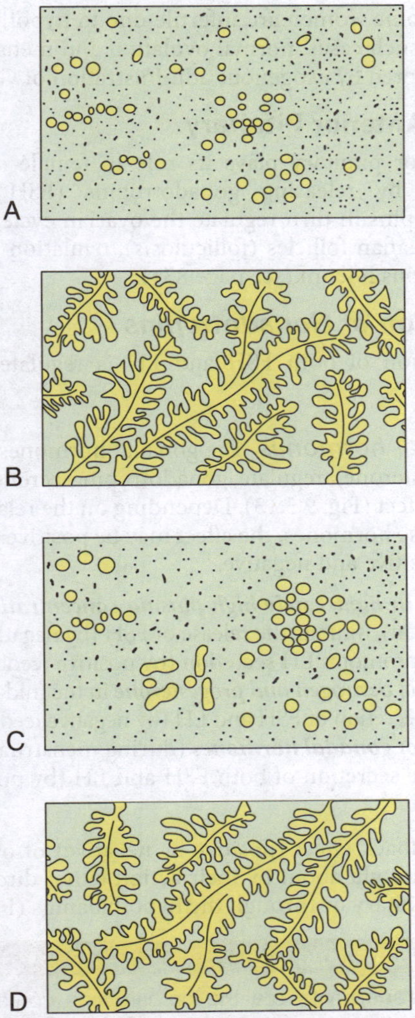

Fig. 9.3.11 Characteristics of cervical mucus as seen on smear examination during various phases of normal menstrual cycle: **A**, on 7th day (no fern pattern); **B**, on 14th day (typical fern pattern); **C**, on 21st day (fern pattern disappears); and **D**, on 21st day of an unovulatory cycle (fern pattern persists).

1. Changes in fallopian tubes Changes in fallopian tubes are as follows:

i. ***During follicular phase***, under the influence of oestrogen, there occurs:
   - Increase in the number of cilia of epithelial cells and their rate of beating
   - Increase in the number of secretory epithelial cells
   - An increase in the vascularization of fimbria

ii. ***At the time of ovulation***, the motility of fallopian tubes increases.

iii. ***During the luteal phase***, under the influence of progesterone, there occurs an increase in the secretion of epithelial cells. This provides nutrition to the ovum, incoming sperm and zygote if fertilization occurs.

2. Changes in breast Some women complain of feeling of fullness and tenderness in the breasts. These symptoms have been related to the proliferation of lobules and duct system under the influence of oestrogen and progesterone. All these symptoms regress during the menstrual phase.

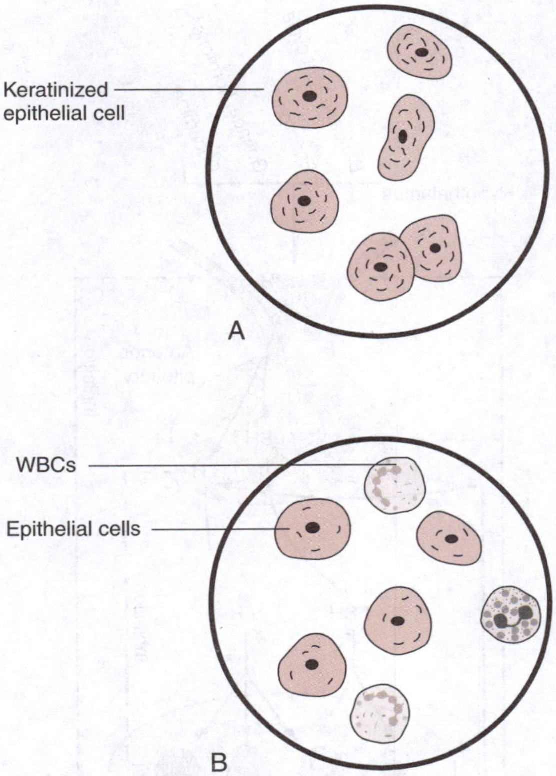

Fig. 9.3.12 Characteristic features of vaginal epithelium seen on vaginal smear examination during (**A**) proliferative phase and (**B**) secretory phase of menstrual cycle.

3. Premenstrual weight gain Many women experience a feeling of heaviness (premenstrual tension) near the end of cycle. This effect is due to salt and water retention caused by the oestrogen. The feeling of heaviness disappears during the menstruation phase.

OESTROUS CYCLE

Except primates, in all other mammals, the sexual cycle is called *oestrous cycle*. It has derived its name from the word oestrous meaning 'heat'. This is the only period when sexual interest is aroused in the female animals. It happens at the time of ovulation and coincides with the male's sexual desire. In oestrous cycle, the underlying endocrinal changes are similar to those in menstrual cycle in primates but bleeding per vaginum does not occur and the duration of cycle also varies from species to species. For example:

- In rat and mouse: 4–6 days
- In sheep and guinea pig: 14 days
- In cow: 20 days
- In bitches: Twice in a year

Two different patterns of oestrous cycles are known in different species:

Spontaneous ovulation occurs in some species such as the dog, rat, guinea pig and cow.

Reflex ovulation is known to occur in some species such as rabbit, ferret and cats; in these species, ovulation is brought about by *neuroendocrinal reflex* which is aroused by copulation.

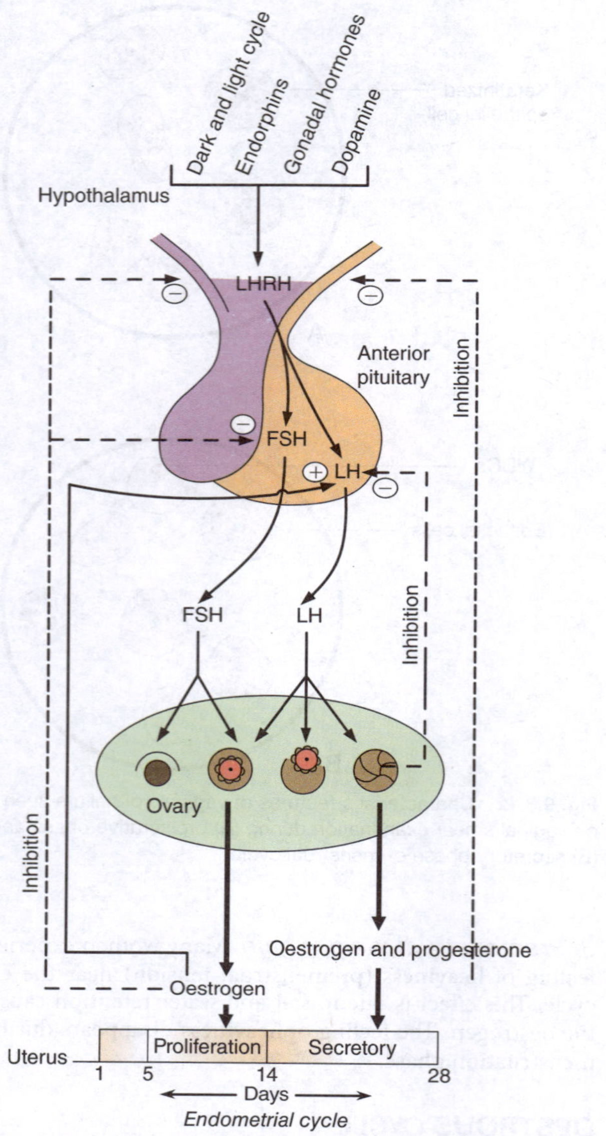

Fig. 9.3.13 Hypothalamo–hypophyseal ovarian axis regulating the female sexual cycle through positive and negative feedback mechanisms.

HORMONAL CONTROL OF FEMALE SEXUAL CYCLE

The hypothalamic–hypophyseal–gonadal axis regulates the cyclic changes occurring during female sexual cycle. The role of each component of the axis is given next (Fig. 9.3.13).

Role of Hypothalamus

The hypothalamus regulates the secretions of gonadotropins (both FSH and LH) through the GnRH. The GnRH, also known as luteinizing hormone–releasing hormone (LHRH), is predominantly secreted from the cells of arcuate nucleus and preoptic area. It reaches the anterior pituitary through hypothalamic–hypophyseal portal system where it is stored as small granules. It stimulates the anterior pituitary cells to release gonadotropins. The release of GnRH is influenced by various factors, such as dopamine, endorphins, ratio of FSH and LH, gonadal hormones (oestrogen and progesterone), and dark and light cycles operating through melatonin (released from the pineal gland).

Note: Some women are infertile due to hypothalamic disorders. In such cases, normal ovulation and menstrual cycles can be restored by exogenous administration of GnRH.

Role of Anterior Pituitary

The anterior pituitary plays its role in female sexual cycle regulation by releasing gonadotropins (FSH and LH). Gonadotropins in turn regulate the ovarian cycle, i.e. formation of Graafian follicles (folliculosis), ovulation and formation of corpus luteum (see page 831).

Regulation of Gonadotropins

The secretion of both FSH and LH is regulated by those given next.

1. Gonadal hormones The gonadal hormones (oestrogen and progesterone) regulate gonadotropin secretion by their feedback effect (Fig. 9.3.13). Depending on the relative plasma level of these hormones, the effect may be positive or negative, or both positive and negative.

Oestrogen, in moderately high plasma concentration (just before ovulation), inhibits the release of FSH (by negative feedback effect) and promotes LH secretion (by positive feedback effect). ***High levels of oestrogen and progesterone*** in the mid-luteal phase inhibit the secretion of FSH and LH (by negative feedback effect). ***Low levels of gonadal hormones*** (during menstruation phase) increase the secretion of both FSH and LH (by positive feedback effect).

The feedback effect (positive or negative) of ovarian hormones is brought about by their action either directly on the anterior pituitary or through the hypothalamus (Fig. 9.3.13).

Important Note

Oral contraceptives are the preparations containing high concentration of oestrogen and progesterone. These drugs inhibit gonadotropin release by negative feedback effect and prevent ovulation.

2. Human chorionic gonadotropin Human chorionic gonadotropin (hCG) is a glycoprotein secreted by syncytiotrophoblasts during early pregnancy (12–16 weeks of gestation). Like LH, hCG also maintains the functional state of the corpus luteum and thus elevates gonadal hormones resulting in inhibition of gonadotropin release.

3. Prolactin It is a mammotropic hormone secreted from the anterior pituitary during lactation. It inhibits GnRH release and thus lowers the basal secretion of FSH and LH (cause for lactation amenorrhoea).

4. Activin It is structurally quite similar to inhibin (secreted from the ovary). It is synthesized in the cells of the anterior pituitary. It stimulates the synthesis and release of FSH by autocrine and paracrine actions.

Role of Ovaries

Ovaries play an important role in the regulation of ovarian cycle and endometrial cycle by secreting gonadal hormones (oestrogen and progesterone) (Fig. 9.3.9).

Oestrogen In each sexual cycle, the plasma concentration of oestrogen starts rising from the first day of the cycle and reaches its peak just before ovulation (at the 12th or 13th day), called *oestrogen surge*.

- Then within 24 hours, burst of LH secretion (LH surge) takes place at midcycle, leading to sudden rise in plasma concentration of LH (Fig. 9.3.9A). Thus, oestrogen surge has a positive feedback effect.
- Oestrogen increases the sensitivity and responsiveness of gonadotrophs to GnRH.
- The LH surge is followed (after about 9 hours) by ovulation. Therefore, oestrogen through its positive feedback effect is responsible for *ovulation* due to LH surge.
- Oestrogen is responsible for the proliferative phase of endometrial cycle.

Progesterone After ovulation, there occurs formation of the corpus luteum and the progesterone concentration starts rising. Therefore, in the luteal phase of the ovarian cycle, levels of both oestrogen and progesterone are high, but progesterone rises markedly.

- The high levels of gonadal hormones inhibit gonadotropin release by negative feedback effect. Therefore, the levels of FSH and LH are low.
- Progesterone prepares the oestrogen-primed endometrium for implantation. Thus, it is responsible for the secretory phase of endometrial cycle.
- *If fertilization does not occur*, the corpus luteum involutes and levels of oestrogen and progesterone decline.
- Withdrawal of hormonal support results in menstruation; at the same time, negative feedback effect on the anterior pituitary and hypothalamus is also abolished, leading to further increase in gonadotropin, and the next ovarian and endometrial cycle starts.
  If fertilization occurs, then the hCG level rises, which maintain the corpus luteum. Therefore, the levels of oestrogen and progesterone remain high, and by negative feedback effect, gonadotropin levels (FSH and LH) remain low.

MENOPAUSE

With advancing age, the human ovaries become unresponsive to gonadotropins and secretion of ovarian hormone declines, resulting in permanent stoppage of menstrual cycle, which is called menopause. The usual age of menopause is 45–55 years (average 50 years).

- The unresponsiveness of the ovary to gonadotropin occurs due to decrease in the number of primordial follicles. Therefore, the ovaries no longer secrete progesterone, and the oestrogen level also declines.
- Due to the gonadal hormone negative feedback mechanism, there is a high plasma level of FSH and LH.
- During premenopausal period, FSH level increases before a rise in LH; therefore, irregular menstrual cycle occurs due to decrease in oestrogen, progesterone and inhibin.
- The loss of ovarian functions leads to the following symptoms:
  Hot flashes are the sensation of warmth spreading from the trunk region to the face and night sweats. They occur in 75% of menopausal women. The exact cause of hot flushes is not known, but they are associated with surge of LH secretion. In menopausal women, due to absence of gonadal hormone, the peaks of episodic burst of LH secretion increase.
  - It is observed that with removal of the anterior pituitary, the hot flushes continue that indicates that LH itself is not responsible for hot flushes; instead, it appears that some oestrogen-sensitive event in the hypothalamus may initiate both release of LH and episode of flushing.
  - With the onset of menopause, risk of diseases such as osteoporosis, ischaemic heart disease and renal disease also increases.

Treatment includes:

Hormonal replacement therapy (HRT): In postmenopausal women, HRT is given to relieve the symptom and to prevent osteoporosis but is associated with side effects. The typical regimen of HRT is oestrogen 1–21 days, and progesterone is added from days 14 to 21 as oral contraceptives.
  - The side effects of HRT – fluid retention, weight gain, hypertension and thrombosis – are a matter of concern.
- Transdermal HRT may be a more appropriate alternative.
- The time of discontinuation of HRT and duration of therapy is still a matter of debate.

ABNORMALITIES OF FEMALE SEXUAL CYCLE

The abnormalities of female sexual cycle are grouped as:

- Abnormalities of ovarian functions
- Abnormalities of menstruation

Applied Aspects

A. Abnormalities of Ovarian Functions

1. ***Hypogonadism*** (hyposecretion of ovarian hormones) means less than normal secretions by the ovaries. It occurs when the ovaries are poorly developed or absent since birth or genetically become abnormal and nonfunctional.
   A number of gene mutations cause reproductive abnormalities in women such as:
   - *Kallmann syndrome* causes hypogonadotropic hypogonadism.
   - *GnRH resistance (FSH and LH resistance)* occurs due to defect in FSH and LH receptors.
   - *Aromatase deficiency* due to gene mutation 'prevents' oestrogen synthesis.

   Hypogonadism results in female eunuchoidism (see page 700).
2. ***Ovariectomy:*** When ovaries are removed surgically in a sexually mature female, it leads to the following effects:
   - Atrophy of the genital apparatus (i.e. uterus, vagina and external genitalia)
   - *Stoppage of menstruation*
   - *Breast changes* (breasts may enlarge or get atrophied)
   - *Vasomotor changes*, such as flushing of the skin of the face, neck and chest (hot flushes)
   - Emotional disturbances such as irritability and depression
3. ***Hypersecretion by the ovaries:*** The ovarian secretions are well regulated by the hypothalamo–hypophyseal ovarian axis. Hence, extreme hypersecretion by the ovaries is a rare condition but it can occur in ovarian tumours. The

effects of hypersecretion (mainly oestrogen) depend on the age of an individual. If it occurs in:

- *Prepubertal stage*, then precocious puberty results (see page 799).
- *Postmenopausal stage*, then hypertrophy of the endometrium and irregular bleeding are the common features.

4. ***McCune–Albright syndrome (MAS)*** is a complex genetic defect in which somatic mutation occurs after initial cell division in the embryo that leads to activation of certain cells. It is a complex genetic disorder. It mainly affects the bone, skin and endocrine system, and is clinically defined by triad: fibrous dysplasia of bone, skin spots and precocious puberty.

B. Abnormalities of Menstruation

1. ***Anovulatory cycle*** means that menstrual cycles occur at normal intervals, but ovulation does not occur. Anovulatory cycles are the normal entity up to 1–2 years after the menarche and few years before menopause. An anovulatory cycle in the fertile period of womanhood is the main cause of female infertility.
2. ***Amenorrhoea:*** The term amenorrhoea refers to absence of menstrual bleeding or periods. It is of two types:
   - *Primary amenorrhoea* means that menstrual bleeding has never occurred and this condition is because of failure of sexual maturation.
   - *Secondary amenorrhoea* means cessation of menstrual cycles in a woman who previously had normal and regular cycles. Pregnancy is the most common cause of secondary amenorrhoea. Other conditions which result in secondary amenorrhoea are emotional disturbances, environmental changes, hypothalamic and pituitary disorders, and certain systemic diseases.
3. ***Hypomenorrhoea:*** The term refers to scanty menstruation.
4. ***Menorrhoea:*** It refers to abnormally profuse bleeding during normal regular cycles.
5. ***Metrorrhagia:*** This condition refers to occurrence of uterine bleeding in between the periods.
6. ***Oligomenorrhoea*** means infrequent and reduced frequency of menstruation.
7. ***Dysmenorrhoea*** is the term related to discomfort menstruation (or painful menstruation). It is very common in young women and it disappears after the first pregnancy.
8. ***Premenstrual syndrome (PMS):*** About 7–10 days before the end of cycle, some women experience symptoms like irritability, lack of concentration, feeling of depression, heaviness, headache and constipation which is called PMS (see page 833).

Self-Assessment

1. Discuss the ovarian and endometrial changes during female sexual cycle.
2. Discuss the hormonal control of menstrual cycle.
3. Describe the following:
   - Functions of ovarian hormones
   - Amenorrhoea
4. Write notes on the following:
   - Indicators of ovulation
   - Menopause
   - Role of pituitary in menstrual cycle
   - Functions of fallopian tubes

Clinical Cases

Case 1

A 30-year-old woman married for 7 years consulted an infertility expert for having no issue. History revealed that the couple was not using any contraceptive measures. The advised test reports indicated no abnormality in the husband. However, in the female, ultrasound showed multiple small cysts in both the ovaries.

Q1. What is the probable diagnosis?
Q2. What is the reason of infertility in this case?

Case 2

A 32-year-old female was having carcinoma breast; as a part of treatment, both of her ovaries were removed.

Q1. What are the effects of ovariectomy?
Q2. What is treatment to relieve symptoms due to ovariectomy?

Case 3

A 24-year-old female consulted the gynaecologist for headache, feeling of heaviness and tenderness in the breast, and remaining irritable few days before the periods.

Q1. What is this condition known as?
Q2. What is the pathophysiology for these symptoms?

Case 4

A 46-year-old female consulted the gynaecologist for complaints of irregular periods, sensation of warmth spreading from the trunk to the face and lot of sweating at night even in an air-conditioned room.

Q1. What is the diagnosis?
Q2. What is the pathophysiology of the signs and symptoms?
Q3. Which hormone is responsible for this condition?
Q4. What is the treatment to relieve symptoms?

9.4 Physiology of Coitus, Pregnancy and Parturition

CHAPTER OUTLINE

PHYSIOLOGY OF COITUS

Coitus refers to the process of sexual intercourse by which sperms are deposited into the vagina. Physiologically, coitus involves both male and female sexual acts or sexual arousal.

MALE SEXUAL ACT OR MALE SEXUAL AROUSAL

The male sexual act is reflexogenic in nature and involves both psychological and physiological components. It consists of the following sequence of events:

- Erection of penis
- Emission of seminal fluid
- Ejaculation

I. Erection of Penis or Stage of Excitement

In this stage, the penis becomes hard, stiff and an elongated structure. Erection of the penis is brought about by integrity of the reflex arc, which comprises:

- Sexual stimulation
- Afferents to the integrating centres
- Integrating centres
- Efferents
- Response

1. Sexual stimulation Sexual stimulation has two components:

Psychological component: It is in the form of thought, feeling, watching movie or book picture, etc. The psychological component arises in the cerebral cortex or from the limbic system. The impulses from psychic stimulations are carried or descend to the integrating centres located in the spinal cord. The psychic component can *reinforce* or inhibit the integrating centres.

Physical components of sexual sensations involve:

i. ***Sensations from genitalia*** (mainly from the glans penis; the glans penis contains highly sensitive sensory end organs, which are activated by massaging action of the intercourse)
ii. ***Sensations from adjacent*** areas like the scrotum, epithelium of the anus and perineal structures
iii. ***Sensations from internal structures*** like the urethra, bladder, prostate, seminal vesicles, testes and vas deferens particularly when these structures are filled with the secretions

2. Afferents to integrating centres From genitalia and other structures, the afferent impulses are carried by *pudendal nerve* and *sacral plexus* to the sacral part of the spinal cord.

3. Integrating centres Integrating centres for reflexogenic erection are located in lumbar segments (L_2–L_3) and sacral segments (S_2–S_4) of the spinal cord. The lumbar centres are in turn connected to sacral centres.

4. Efferent pathway The efferent pathway for erection is carried through sacral parasympathetic fibres via nervi erigentes to the:

- Smooth muscle fibres of the penile arterioles
- Erectile tissue (corpora cavernosa and corpora spongiosum of the penis)
- Bulbourethral glands

- The efferent parasympathetic fibres in pelvic splanchnic nerves (nervi erigentes) release acetylcholine and vasoactive intestinal peptide (VIP) as cotransmitter.
- Nervi erigentes also carry noncholinergic and nonadrenergic fibres, which contain a large amount of enzyme *NO synthase* which causes formation of nitric oxide (NO). NO is another potent vasodilator. It activates soluble guanylyl cyclase resulting in increased production of cyclic GMP (cGMP), which is a potent vasodilator.
- Therefore, the substances (neurotransmitters) released are ACh, VIP and NO.

5. Response By acting on the effector structures, there occurs:

- Vasodilation of the penile arterioles leads to increased blood flow under pressure resulting in filling of the erectile tissue with blood.
- The blood-filled erectile tissue compresses the central vein of the penis (blocking the venous flow from the penis), which further increases the pressure within the sinusoids of erectile tissue, and thus the penis becomes a hard, rigid structure.
- *Lubrication:* Parasympathetic activity during sexual stimulation causes secretion of mucus from the urethral and bulbourethral glands.

Important Note

Drugs like sildenafil, tadalafil and vardenafil all inhibit breakdown of cGMP, thus are used as treatment for erectile dysfunction.

II. Emission of Seminal Fluid

In this stage, semen moves into the urethra. Emission is a sympathetic response integrated at upper lumbar spinal segment centres (L_1 and L_2).

- When sexual stimulus becomes very strong, reflexly emission and ejaculation occur. The afferent fibres are mostly from touch receptors present on the glans penis (which are stimulated by friction of the glans penis and vaginal wall) and are carried by internal pudendal nerve to the spinal cord (lumbar segment L_1–L_2). Efferents are then carried along sympathetic fibres through hypogastric and pelvic sympathetic plexus to initiate emission.
- Emission is carried out by contraction of vas deferens.

III. Ejaculation

Ejaculation means deposition of seminal fluid into the vagina of female.

Applied Aspects

Erectile dysfunction (impotence) is the inability of men to get and maintain the erection sufficient for intercourse. It occurs because of vasculogenic, neurogenic, hormonal or psychogenic factors.

Premature ejaculation is a disorder characterized by ejaculation that occurs with minimal sexual stimulation after penetration.

Retrograde ejaculation is a disorder in which semen travels backwards into the urinary bladder rather than out of the penile shaft during ejaculation. For neurological dysfunction, the most common cause is damage to penile innervations during prostate surgery.

FEMALE SEXUAL ACT

Female sexual act, similar to male sexual act, is reflexogenic and involves psychological and physical components. The three phases of female sexual act are as follows:

- Sexual excitement
- Orgasm
- Resolution

I. Phase of Sexual Excitement

The phase of sexual excitement is also called phase of female erection and lubrication. It corresponds to erection of the penis in males. This phase is brought about by integrity of the reflex arc which comprises the components given next.

1. Sexual stimulation Sexual stimulation in females like that of males has two components – psychological and physical.

Psychological stimulation: The sexual desire in females is aroused by erotic thoughts which originate from the cerebral cortex or limbic system (amygdala). The sexual desire is believed to be increased at the time of ovulation (may be because of high levels of oestrogen). It is also believed that sexual desire in females is produced partly by oestrogen.

Physical component of the sexual stimulation consists of sexual sensations aroused from massaging/irritation of external genitalia (vulva, clitoris, labia minora and labia majora) and perineal region. The clitoris is highly sensitive and is responsible for initiation of sexual sensations. Massaging of the breasts and even kissing enforce the sexual sensations.

2. Afferents to the integrating centres The sensory signals are transmitted via the pudendal nerve to the spinal cord. The impulses are then transmitted to the cerebral cortex and also to the integrating centres for local reflex responses.

3. Integrating centres The local reflexes are integrated in sacral segments (S_2, S_3 and S_4) and lumbar segments (L_1 and L_2) of the spinal cord. These integrating centres are also influenced by psychological components.

4. Efferent pathway The parasympathetic signals for female erection and lubrication travel by nervi erigentes from the sacral plexus to the arteries of external genitalia and Bartholin glands and mucosal epithelial cells of the vagina.

5. Response During sexual intercourse, the erectile tissue (located around the introitus and clitoris) is activated by parasympathetic impulses producing:

- Increase in blood flow and accumulation of blood in erectile tissue resulting in increase in the size of external genitalia and vaginal congestion. Congestion of the vagina occurs due to transudation of fluid from the vaginal epithelium.
- Vaginal lubrication facilitates the penile insertion. Further vaginal congestion leads to tightening of the vaginal opening around the penis.

- Stimulation also results in copious secretion from Bartholin glands (situated beneath labia minora) and mucous cells in the vagina. These secretions further lubricate the vagina and help in producing massaging effect on the penis.
- With increasing excitement, blood flow further increases resulting in deepening of colour of labia majora. Along with local response, systemic effects (as increase in heart rate, respiratory rate and blood pressure) and in general increase in the muscle tone also occur.

II. Orgasm

The orgasm results when the intensity of sexual stimulation reaches its peak. It is analogous to emission and ejaculation in males.

During orgasm, there occurs rhythmic contractions of peroneal muscles, uterus and vagina, and dilatation of the cervical canal. The intense sexual sensation perceived during orgasm is called climax. This stage lasts for about 15–30 seconds.

It has been observed that in lower animals, oxytocin released from the posterior pituitary via the amygdala (limbic system–hypothalamus–posterior pituitary stimulation) is responsible for uterine contractions.

III. Resolution Phase

Orgasm is immediately followed by resolution phase. This phase is characterized by a sense of satisfaction followed by the relaxed state of mental peacefulness called resolution. The heart rate, blood pressure, respiration and all other parameters come to their normal level and there occurs relaxation of the muscles.

Applied Aspects

Dyspareunia refers to recurrent/persistent genital pain before, during (most common) or after sexual intercourse. This problem is more common in females than in males, and is more of a physical or psychogenic problem.

PHYSIOLOGY OF PREGNANCY

Physiology of pregnancy is mainly concerned with maternal adaptations to provide ideal atmosphere for fertilization, nutrition to the growing fetus, safe childbirth and thereafter to fulfil nutritional needs of the newborn. Although mainly the reproductive system is involved in pregnancy, other body systems also undergo adjustments. The physiology of pregnancy, for convenience of description, can be discussed under the following headings:

- Fertilization and implantation
- Formation of placenta and its functions
- Physiological changes during pregnancy
- Applied aspects

FERTILIZATION AND IMPLANTATION

Fertilization

Fertilization refers to fusion of male and female gametes (i.e. spermatozoon and ovum). It takes place in the middle segment (ampulla) of the fallopian tube. It involves the events given next.

1. Transport of Gametes

Before fertilization, the ovum and sperms reach the ampulla for fertilization.

Transport of ovum At the time of ovulation, the ovum is directly expelled into the peritoneal cavity and then enters the fallopian tube.

Mechanism: The fimbriae of the fallopian tube are internally lined by ciliated epithelium. When ovulation occurs, the fimbriae of the infundibulum encircle the surface of the ovary, rub it, pick up the ovum and then direct it towards the ostium by continuous beating of cilia. The contractions of smooth muscle fibres present in the wall of the fallopian tube also help in transport of the ovum. These contractions are increased at the time of ovulation under the influence of oestrogen.

Structure of ovum: The released mature ovum (Fig. 9.4.1) consists of oocyte (containing 23 unpaired chromosomes) surrounded by the inner membranous layer called zona pellucida consisting of glycoproteins and on its outer side surrounded by corona radiata consisting of granulosa cells arranged in multilayers. These cells are held together by a matrix composed of hyaluronic acid.

Fate of ovum: The ovum is held up at the ampullary–isthmic junction for 12–24 hours. It remains viable for 12–24 hours after ovulation for fertilization. During this period, if a viable sperm penetrates it, then fertilization takes place, leading to pregnancy. On the other hand, if fertilization does not occur, the ovum dies out and degenerates.

Transport of sperms in the female genital tract After ejaculation, several million sperms (average 200 million sperms per ejaculation) get deposited in the vagina. Out of these, about 50–100 sperms manage to reach ovum and only one is able to penetrate it. This is because of several factors that affect the transportation and accessibility of the sperm to ovum.

Motility of sperms: After ejaculation, normal sperm shows flagellar movements in the fluid medium at a rate of 1–4 mm/min. Therefore, in 30–60 minutes, it is able to reach the fallopian tube. The motility of sperms in turn depends on:

- pH of the fluid medium
- Cervical mucus secretions

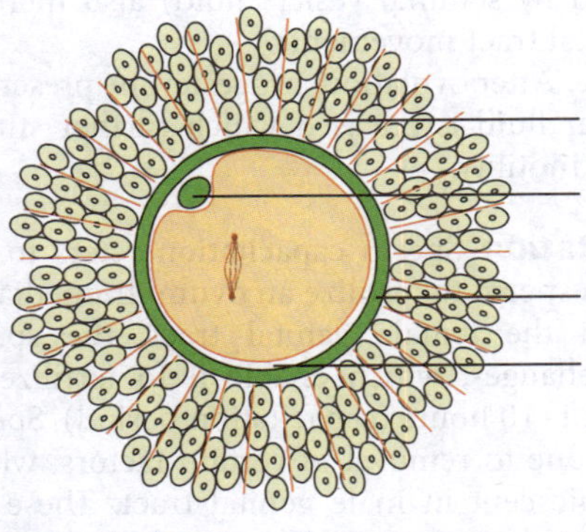

Fig. 9.4.1 Structure of a mature ovum at the time of ovulation.

- Fluid currents
- Temperature
- Hormones

i. ***pH of medium:*** Neutral and alkaline pH enhances the activity of sperms, but it is greatly depressed in even mild acidic medium. The vaginal fluid is acidic; hence, immediately sperm activity is inhibited and sperms become nonmotile. The alkaline semen (pH 7.5) neutralizes the vaginal acidic fluid. Therefore, in less than 60 minutes after ejaculation, sperms again become active and their activity increases in the cervix and in the body of uterus for the next 25–40 hours.

Mechanism: The principal piece of sperm tail possesses a special set of proteins (CatSper family) which are alkaline-sensitive Ca^{2+} channels. Therefore, the sperms become most active as they pass from vaginal acidic pH (~5) to cervical mucus pH (~8).

ii. ***Cervical secretion:*** The cervical secretion acts as a mechanical barrier for sperms. The nature of cervical secretion depends on the hormonal concentrations in the plasma. During proliferative phase of menstrual cycle and at the time of ovulation (under the influence of high level of oestrogen), cervical secretion becomes thin and watery, which favours the passage of the sperms. The morphologically abnormal sperms cannot pass through cervical mucus barrier and get entrapped within the fluid.

iii. ***Fluid currents:*** The vaginal and uterine cavity represent a vast sea in which currents are set up by ciliary movements towards exterior (antagonistic direction), which further resists sperm motility.

iv. ***Temperature:*** With rising temperature, the activity of sperms increases but their life span is shortened. In ejaculated semen, the maximum life span of sperm is 24–48 hours at body temperature. At lower temperature, however, semen can be stored for several weeks, and at −100°C, sperms can be preserved for many years.

v. ***Hormones:*** Local release of hormones as well as high concentration of certain hormones in the blood affects sperm transport. These include:

- *Oxytocin:* During coitus, stimulation of female genitalia leads to reflex release of oxytocin from the neurohypophysis; oxytocin causes propulsive movements of the uterus, which help to aspirate seminal fluid from the vagina into the fallopian tube.
- *Oestrogen:* It makes the cervical secretion thin and watery, thus favouring transport of sperms.
- *Prostaglandins:* Prostaglandins present in the semen (contributed by seminal vesicle fluid) also increase female genital tract movements.
- *Progesterone:* After ovulation, progesterone present in the follicular fluid is released which further stimulates sperm motility.

2. Sperm capacitation Sperm capacitation refers to the process that makes a sperm to fertilize an ovum. Immediately after ejaculation in the female genital tract, the sperm undergoes certain changes, which enable it to fertilize an ovum. It takes about 1–10 hours (capacitation period). Sperm capacitation occurs due to removal of certain factors, which normally remain quiescent in male genital tract. These are as follows:

Cholesterol contents of acrosomal membrane: In the male genital tract, the acrosomal membrane remains very tough because of high cholesterol contents. In contrast, in the female genital tract, the cholesterol contents of acrosomal membrane decrease and it becomes weak leading to easy release of enzymes from the head.

Calcium ions: The membrane of sperm becomes permeable to calcium ions. The influx of Ca^{2+} acts by two ways: it makes the flagellar movements of the sperms more strong and whipish (hyperactivation of sperms) and, second, it triggers the release of enzymes from the acrosome.

3. Fusion of gametes The fusion of ovum and sperm involves the steps given next.

i. Chemoattraction Chemoattraction of the sperms to ovum occurs by substances produced by the ovum. Certain olfactory receptors are expressed by the spermatozoa. A recent view is that ovaries produce certain odorant molecules that interact with these olfactory receptors present on the sperm and are the cause of motility (chemotaxis).

ii. Penetration of sperm through ovum coverings

The sperm passes through two layers (corona radiata and zona pellucida) before it reaches the oocyte.

Penetration of corona radiata (Fig. 9.4.2A): It is made possible by release of enzyme hyaluronidase and other proteolytic enzymes present on the acrosome of the sperm and hyperactivation of the sperm.

- The hyaluronidase polymerizes the hyaluronic acid present in the intercellular matrix holding granulosa cells.
- The proteolytic enzymes digest away the proteins of the structural tissues.

Hyperactivation of sperms (increased flagellar movements) produces penetrating thrust on the ovum due to vigorous lashing of sperm's tail.

Binding of sperm to zona pellucida: After passing through multilayered granulosa cells (corona radiata), many sperms make contact with zona pellucida by binding to receptor protein called *zona pellucida glycoprotein* (ZP_3) (Fig. 9.4.2B). The binding of sperm to ZP_3 triggers acrosomal reaction.

Acrosomal reaction (Fig. 9.4.2C): It involves release of acrosin (protease enzyme) from anterior membrane of acrosome of the sperm. Acrosin opens the penetrating pathway for passage of the sperm head into the perivitelline space (space between zona pellucida and oocyte membrane). For effective penetration by the sperm, the acrosomal reaction should take place at the zona pellucida because the life span of acrosomal-reacted sperm is very short. If it takes place outside zona pellucida, the sperm cannot pass through this membrane.

The acrosomal reaction is also important for actual fusion of sperm cell with oocyte membrane.

iii. Fusion of sperm with oocyte (Fig. 9.4.2D) The equatorial region of acrosome is considered to be the site of initial contact between sperm and oocyte membrane (vitelline membrane). *Fertilin* is a protein present on acrosomal-reacted sperm which interacts with the protein present on vitelline membrane and within 30 minutes the membranes of sperm and oocyte fuse, and genetic material of sperm enters the oocyte and causes fertilization and embryo begins to develop.

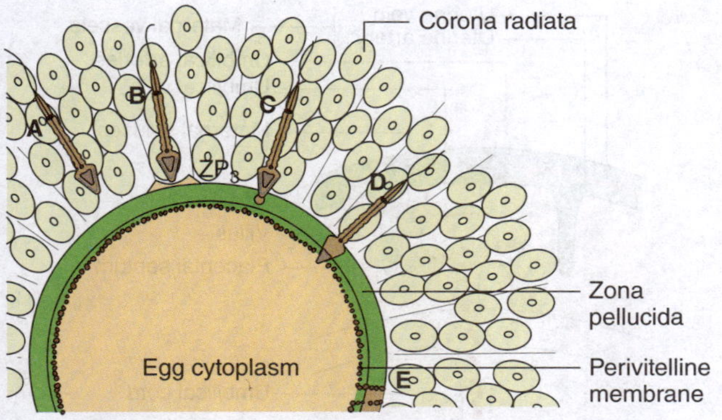

Fig. 9.4.2 Sequential events of fertilization of an ovum by the sperm: **A**, penetration of corona radiata; **B**, binding of sperm to zona pellucida; **C**, acrosomal reaction; **D**, fusion of sperm with oocyte; and **E**, discharge of cortical granules into the perivitelline space producing vitelline block to polyspermy.

Only one sperm can enter the oocyte, and further entry of sperms is prevented by the activation of ovum.

iv. Ovum activation Fusion of membranes of the gametes leads to ovum activation, which involves the following events:

The membrane potential of the ovum decreases (depolarization), which is followed by some structural changes in the zona pellucida.

Release of calcium from intracellular egg reserve leads to exocytosis of the cortical granules (situated near the oocyte membrane) into the perivitelline space (Fig. 9.4.2E).

Vitelline block to polyspermy: The spread of cortical granules along the perivitelline membrane prevents further entry of sperm into the ovum. This is called vitelline block to polyspermy.

Zona blockade to polyspermy: The cortical granules contain certain substances like glycosidases and proteases. Glycosidases cause alterations in the ZP_3 receptor protein of the zona pellucida and proteases degrade the ZP_3. Both of these mechanisms cause loss of affinity of sperm for zona pellucida and thus prevent polyspermy. This is called zona block to polyspermy.

Implantation

Implantation of a fertilized ovum involves the steps given next.

1. Formation of blastocyst The fertilized ovum starts dividing immediately and is called morula (16-cell stage) and blastocyst (100-cell stage). On cut section, it shows inner cell mass surrounded by a layer of cells called trophoblast which is covered by zona pellucida (Fig. 9.4.3). Trophoblast cells layer has a great sticking property to the epithelial cells of the fallopian tube. As the blastocyst is covered by zona pellucida, the trophoblasts are not exposed and hence the blastocyst is usually not implanted in the fallopian tube. Thus, the presence of zona pellucida layer prevents its implantation in the fallopian tube.

2. Transportation of blastocyst in uterine cavity In the next 3–4 days, blastocyst is transported into the cavity of the uterus. The transportation is assisted by fluid currents and ciliary movements of the epithelial cells of the fallopian tube and uterus.

In the cavity of the uterus, blastocyst floats for some time and by this time the zona pellucida layer disappears and trophoblast cell layer is exposed.

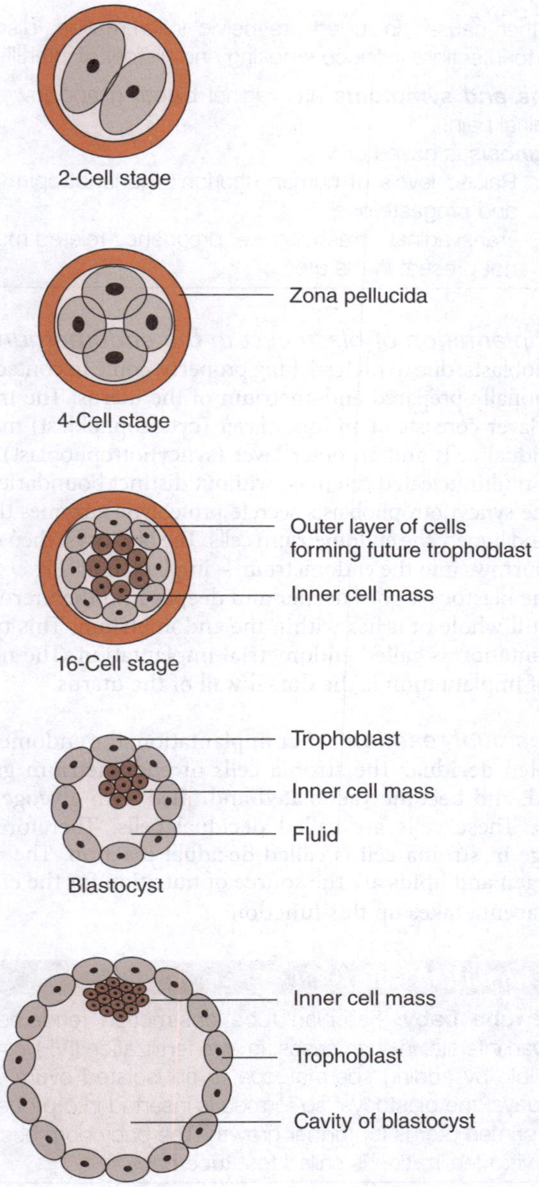

Fig. 9.4.3 Stages of formation of blastocyst.

Applied Aspects

Ectopic pregnancy: When the cilia of the uterine tube are injured or incapable of movement, embryo may implant within the fallopian tube itself called ectopic pregnancy. The risk factors for ectopic pregnancy are as follows:

- Chromosomal abnormalities of the conceptus which are the most frequent cause of overt miscarriage (increasing maternal age is associated with an increased frequency of chromosomal abnormalities)
- Congenital or acquired anatomical defects in the uterus
- Endocrine abnormalities leading to alteration of maturation of ova before ovulation, and during development and maturation of embryo

A high oestrogen/progesterone ratio may also cause ectopic pregnancy by felicitating retention of ovum in the uterine tube.

Other causes included are pelvic inflammation, diseases due to infection, tobacco smoking and history of infertility.

Signs and symptoms are vaginal bleeding and lower abdominal pain.

Diagnosis is based on:

- Raised levels of human chorionic gonadotropin (hCG) and progesterone
- Transvaginal ultrasound, i.e. pregnancy-related material not present in the uterus

3. Implantation of blastocyst in the endometrium The trophoblasts, due to high sticking property, come in contact with hormonally prepared endometrium of the uterus. The trophoblast layer consists of an inner layer (cytotrophoblast) made of individual cells and an outer layer (syncytiotrophoblast) made up of multinucleated cell mass without distinct boundaries.

The syncytiotrophoblasts secrete proteolytic enzymes that digest and liquefy the endometrium cells. The blastocyst then erodes and burrows into the endometrium – implantation (Fig. 9.4.4).

The blastocyst goes deeper and deeper into the uterus mucosa till whole of it lies within the endometrium. This type of implantation is called endometrial implantation. The normal site of implantation is the dorsal wall of the uterus.

4. Decidual reaction After implantation, the endometrium is called decidua. The stroma cells of endometrium get enlarged, and become vacuolated and filled with glycogen and lipids. These cells are called decidual cells. Therefore, this change in stroma cell is called decidual reaction. The stored glycogen and lipids are the source of nutrition for the embryo till placenta takes up this function.

Important Note

Test tube baby: Fallopian tube obstruction rendered the woman infertile. In such cases, in vitro fertilization (IVF) is made possible by adding spermatozoa to an isolated ovum. After few days, the blastocyst so formed is inserted into progesterone-primed uterus for further growth. The baby born because of in vitro fertilization is called test tube baby.

PLACENTA AND PREGNANCY TESTS

Placenta

Placenta is a temporary organ formed during pregnancy. It is an important link between the mother and the fetus.

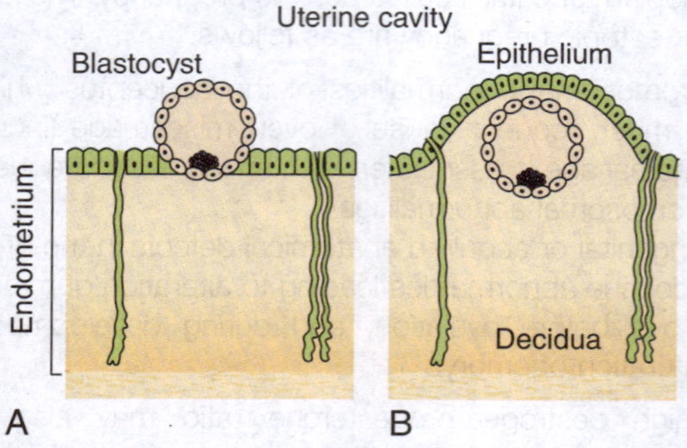

Fig. 9.4.4 Implantation of blastocyst in the (**A**) endometrium and (**B**) decidual reaction.

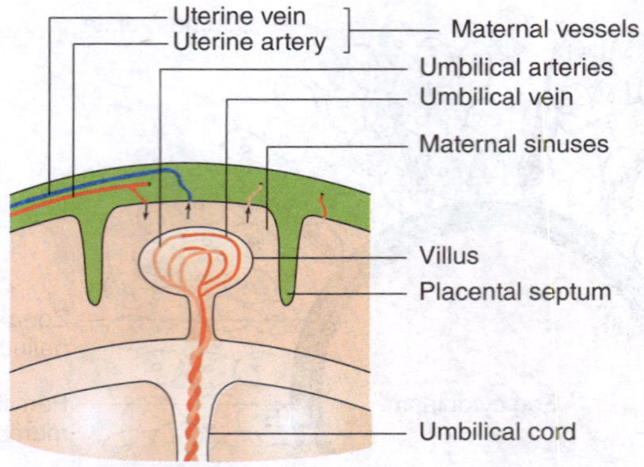

Fig. 9.4.5 Schematic diagram showing structure of placenta.

Formation of Placenta

The decidual part where placenta is to develop is called *decidua basalis* or *decidual plate*. The part of the decidua that separates the embryo from the uterine cavity is called the *decidua capsularis*, whereas the part lining the rest of the uterine cavity is called *decidua parietalis*. In the region of decidua basalis, the maternal blood vessels proliferate and grow. The syncytiotrophoblast sends cords into the decidua basalis. These cords further grow and send more projections to form *placental villi*. In the placental villi, the blood capillaries grow from the vascular system of the embryo. The capillaries are covered by thin endothelial cells which are surrounded by mesenchymal tissue (Fig. 9.4.5).

The placental villi are surrounded by blood-filled maternal sinuses (intervillus spaces). The maternal blood flows through uterine arteries into the maternal sinuses and back through the uterine veins of the mother. The fetal blood flows through umbilical arteries into the capillaries of placental villi and back through an umbilical vein into the fetus.

- When fully formed, the placenta is a disc-shaped structure, has a diameter of 15–20 cm and weighs about 500 g.
- After birth of the baby, the placenta is shed off along with the decidua.

Placental Membrane

The maternal and fetal blood do not mix with each other. They are separated by a placental membrane, made up of the layers of the wall of the villus. From the fetal side, these are as follows (Fig. 9.4.6):

- *Endothelium* of fetal blood vessels and its basement membrane
- Surrounding mesenchymal tissue (connective tissue)

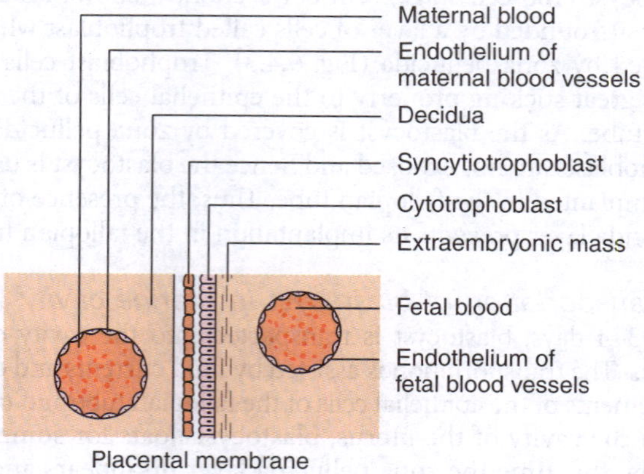

Fig. 9.4.6 Structure of the placental membrane.

- Cytotrophoblast and its basement membrane
- *Syncytiotrophoblast*

All interchanges of oxygen, nutrition and waste products between the maternal blood and the fetal blood take place through the placental membrane barrier. The total area of the membrane varies from 4 to 14 m^2. Its thickness is 0.025 mm in the beginning and in the later part of pregnancy it is reduced to 0.002 mm, because the cytotrophoblastic layer disappears and also there is considerable thinning of the connective tissue. Thinning of the placental membrane increases its efficiency.

Important Notes

It is important to note that the fetus and the mother are two genetically different individuals and the fetus is like a foreign tissue (transplant) in the mother. However, the transplant is well tolerated and not rejected. The possible reasons are as follows:

i. Placental trophoblast which separates maternal and fetal tissues does not express polymorphic MHC class I and II genes; rather it expresses HLA-G (monomorphic) genes. Therefore, antibodies against fetal proteins do not develop (see page 178).
ii. Furthermore, production of maternal antibodies during pregnancy is reduced in general. Moreover, on the surface of placenta, Fos ligand is present which binds to T cells and leads to their apoptosis. For example, a woman with Graves disease usually becomes euthyroid during pregnancy and shows a decreased level of antithyroid antibodies.

Functions of Placenta

The fully functional placenta develops by the end of the third month (12 weeks) of pregnancy. Placenta serves mainly three functions:

- Hormone secretion (endocrinal functions of placenta)
- Transport of substances between the mother and the fetus
- Protection of the fetus

A. Hormone secretion The syncytiotrophoblast of the placenta serves as an endocrine gland. The hormones secreted by the placenta are as follows:

- hCG
- Human chorionic somatomammotropins (hCS):
  - Pregnancy-specific β-glycoprotein-1 (PS-β-1G)
  - Early pregnancy factor (EPF)
- Pregnancy-associated plasma protein-A (PAPP-A)
- Human chorionic thyrotropin (hCT)

The placental steroid hormones are as follows:

- Placental progesterone
- Placental oestrogens
- Relaxin

1. Human chorionic gonadotropins hCG is a polypeptide hormone containing 236 amino acid residues (largest active peptide). It is secreted by syncytiotrophoblast soon after fertilization. It is made up of two subunits – hCG-α (molecular weight 18,000) and hCG-β (molecular weight 28,000). hCG-α is quite similar to α-subunit of luteinizing hormone (LH), follicle-stimulating hormone (FSH) and thyroid-stimulating hormone (TSH).

Plasma concentration: hCG is produced soon after fertilization and is detected in the maternal blood as early as 6–8 days after conception, and reaches its peak between 60 and 90 days of gestation. After this, the concentration falls to a very low level and just before labour, its level falls to zero (Fig. 9.4.7A). Its approximate peak value in human maternal blood during normal pregnancy ranges from 100 to 200 IU/mL. It can be measured by using radioimmunoassay technique.

Physiological effects of hCG are as follows:

- hCG is a luteotropic hormone. Its actions are similar to those of LH of the anterior pituitary; hence, it is also called second *luteotropic hormone*. It maintains the functions of the corpus luteum up to 7 weeks after conception until the fetoplacental unit is able to synthesize its own oestrogen and progesterone.
- hCG converts corpus luteum of menstruation into corpus luteum of pregnancy and stimulates it to secrete 17α-hydroxyprogesterone and lesser amount of progesterone.

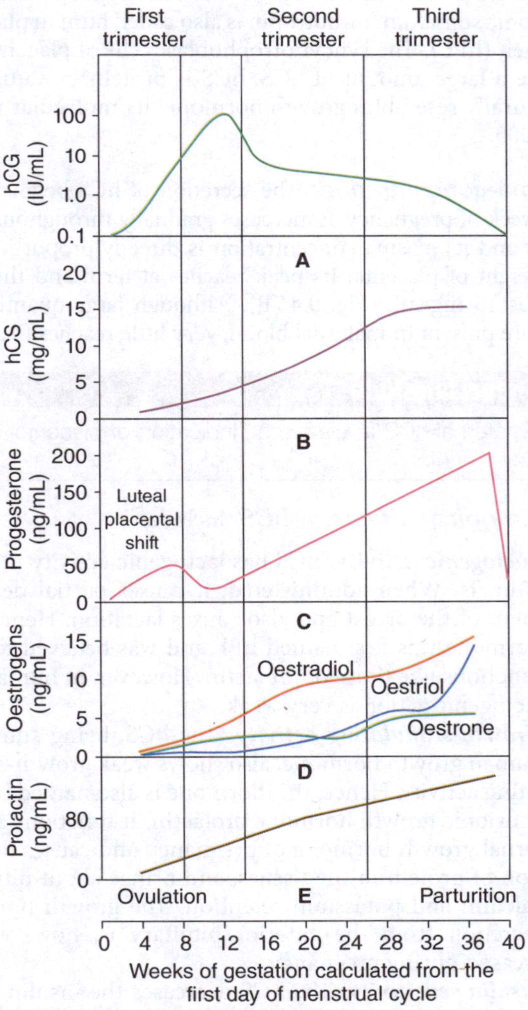

Fig. 9.4.7 Profile of plasma concentration of hormones during normal pregnancy: **A**, human chorionic gonadotropin (hCG); **B**, human chorionic somatomammotropin (hCS); **C**, progesterone; **D**, oestrogen; and **E**, prolactin.

Blood 17α-hydroxyprogesterone level is an excellent indicator of the activity of corpus luteum of pregnancy. Its peak level is reached 3–4 weeks after conception.

- hCG stimulates fetal testes in male fetus to secrete testosterone prior to fetal pituitary LH secretion. This testosterone and MRF secreted by fetal testes are responsible for development of male genital organs and descent of testes during intrauterine life.
- hCG may also serve as a tropic agent for the adrenal cortex fetal zone to secrete dehydroepiandrosterone (DHEA).

Clinical importance (application) of hCG:

The presence of hCG in the urine forms the basis of all the pregnancy tests (see page 847). hCG appears in the urine as early as 10 days after gestation with 99% accuracy. Even though it is not absolutely specific for pregnancy because small amounts are also secreted by various gastrointestinal and other tumours in both sexes. Therefore, hCG has been measured as a tumour marker in an individual with a suspected tumour.

If fetus dies early, then hCG disappears from the blood as well as from the urine.

2. Human chorionic somatomammotropin Human chorionic somatomammotropin is also called human placental lactogen (hPL). The syncytiotrophoblast cells of placenta also secrete a large amount of hCS. hCS is protein in nature and structurally resembles growth hormone. Its molecular weight is 38,000.

Plasma concentration: The secretion of hCS begins at the fifth week of pregnancy. It increases gradually throughout pregnancy and its plasma concentration is directly proportional to the weight of placenta. Its peak reaches at term and the peak value is 15 mg/mL (Fig. 9.4.7B). Although large quantities of hCG are present in maternal blood, very little reaches the fetus.

Important Note

Low maternal hCS levels are an indication of placental insufficiency.

Physiological effects of hCS include:

i. ***Lactogenic activity:*** hCS has lactogenic activity in lower animals. When administered, it causes partial development of the breast and also causes lactation. Hence, this hormone was first named hPL and was believed to have functions like those of prolactin. However, in humans, its lactogenic action is very weak.

ii. ***Growth-stimulating activity:*** The hCS, being similar to human growth hormone, also shows weak growth-stimulating activity. Hence, this hormone is also named human chorionic growth hormone prolactin. It functions as maternal growth hormone of pregnancy and causes deposition of protein in the tissues, and brings about nitrogen, calcium and potassium retention. The growth hormone secretion from the anterior pituitary is, however, decreased during pregnancy.

iii. ***Insulin sensitivity:*** The hCS decreases the insulin sensitivity, thus leading to decreased utilization of glucose by the mother. Therefore, a larger quantity of glucose is made available to the growing fetus. Glucose is the main substrate used by the fetus.

iv. ***Lipolysis:*** The hCS promotes release of fatty acids from fat stores of the mother and thus provides an alternate source of energy for metabolism in the mother. Human chorionic somatomammotropic hormone is now considered to be a general metabolic hormone that has specific nutritional implications for both the mother and the fetus.

v. ***Angiogenic activity:*** It is a potent angiogenic hormone and plays an important role in development of fetal vasculature.

3. Human chorionic thyrotropin hCT secreted by the placenta has properties quite similar to those of TSH. The physiological role of this substance is not very clear but its plasma concentration curve is like that of hCG.

4. Pregnancy-specific β-1 glycoproteins PS-β-1G are a group of molecules mainly produced by placental syncytiophore and play immunomodulatory role during pregnancy.

5. Pregnancy-associated plasma protein-A PAPP-A are immune-suppressors; therefore, they prevent rejection of the fetus.

6. Placental progesterone Progesterone is C-21 steroid hormone.

Synthesis: During early pregnancy, it is synthesized by corpus luteum of pregnancy and then by syncytiotrophoblasts of placenta (85% of total contribution). The various facts regarding synthesis of progesterone in placenta are as follows:

- Placental syncytiotrophoblasts do not synthesize cholesterol from acetate which is the main substrate for progesterone synthesis. Therefore, cholesterol is mainly derived from maternal circulation and very little is contributed by the fetus.
- The fetus, placenta and mother, though being independent, constitute a functional unit called the *fetoplacental maternal unit*.
- The pathways of progesterone synthesis in the fetoplacental maternal unit are shown in Fig. 9.4.8.
- In the syncytiotrophoblasts of placenta, pregnenolone is formed from maternal cholesterol.

Pregnenolone is then oxidized by 3β-hydroxysteroid dehydrogenase (3β-HSD) to progesterone.

Plasma concentration: During pregnancy, plasma concentration of progesterone rises steadily throughout gestation (Fig. 9.4.7C) reaching a maximum plateau at 30–40 weeks of gestation and its level does not fall to zero like other placental hormones. Just before the onset of labour, its level decreases.

The initial rise in concentration of progesterone is mainly due to *hydroxyprogesterone* secreted by the corpus luteum and its peak is reached at 3–4 weeks of gestation in response to hCG secretion. Then the level of hydroxyprogesterone starts declining, but plasma concentration as such starts rising in the later part of pregnancy. Therefore, the significance of 17α-hydroxyprogesterone level in plasma as well as in urine reflects corpus luteum activity and second steady rise in plasma concentration of progesterone reflects placental trophoblast secretion and is referred to as *luteal placental shift*. It occurs at the seventh week of gestation. The peak plasma concentration value of progesterone is 190 ng/mL at term.

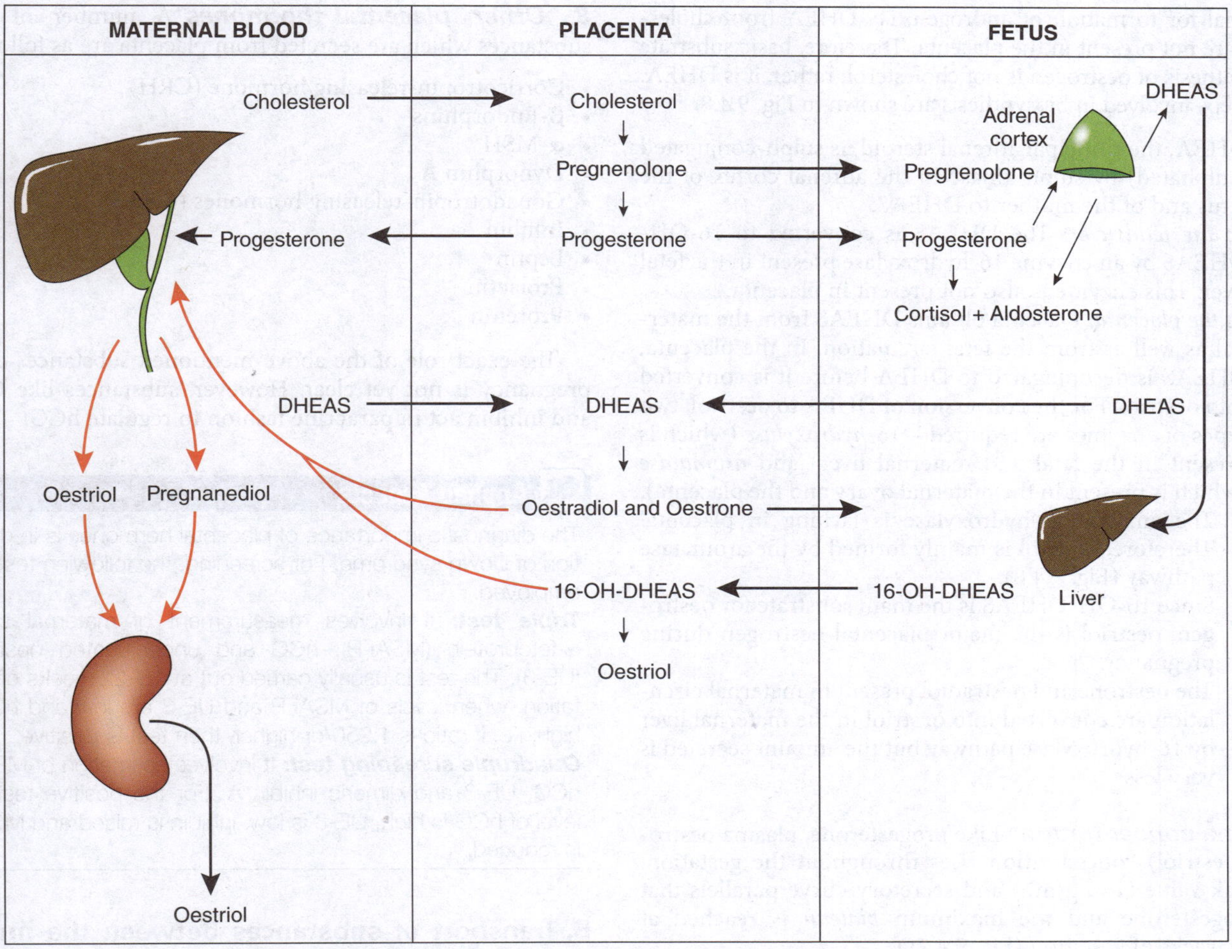

Fig. 9.4.8 Fetoplacental maternal unit for steroid hormone synthesis.

Fate and metabolism of progesterone: Progesterone synthesized by placenta diffuses back into the maternal circulation and also in the fetal circulation.

In the maternal circulation: The progesterone exerts its physiological effects and is then metabolized in the liver. The principal metabolite of progesterone is *pregnanediol* which is glucuronized and secreted by kidneys into the urine.

In the fetal circulation: Up to the 10th week of gestation, the fetal adrenal cortex (inner zone or fetal zone) cannot synthesize its corticosteroids (cortisol) because 3β-HSD enzyme system is blocked. Therefore, it requires placental progesterone, which circulates into the fetal adrenal cortex and gets hydroxylated at C-17, C-21 and C-11 positions to form aldosterone, cortisol and corticosterone (Fig. 9.4.8).

After the 10th week of gestation, the fetal adrenal cortex no longer depends on placental progesterone for synthesis of corticosteroids.

Some of pregnenolone entering fetus from placenta along with the pregnenolone synthesized in the fetal liver is a substrate for the formation of dehydroepiandrosterone sulphate (DHEAS) and 16-hydroxydehydroepiandrosterone (16-OH-DHEAS).

Physiological effects of placental progesterone:

i. It helps to preserve the pregnancy by promoting the growth of endometrium. It converts secretory endometrium of luteal phase of menstrual cycle to decidua during pregnancy.
ii. Progesterone has a marked inhibitory effect on the contractions of the uterus. It is important to note that if progesterone is not secreted in adequate amount, there is likelihood of threatened abortion.
iii. It causes development of the alveolar system of the mother's breast. Its synergic action with oestrogen prepares the breast for lactation after the birth of the baby.
iv. Progesterone has an immunosuppressive role in protecting the fetus.
v. By acting as a precursor for corticosteroid synthesis by the fetal adrenal cortex, it helps in growth and development of the fetus.
vi. Progesterone antagonizes the effect of aldosterone and thus promotes renal excretion of Na^+ during pregnancy.

7. Placental oestrogens Placental oestrogens are C-21 steroid hormones; quantitatively, oestriol is the major oestrogen of pregnancy with a smaller amount of oestradiol and oestrone.

Synthesis: During early pregnancy, like progesterone, it is synthesized by corpus luteum and then by the placental syncytiotrophoblasts (90%). However, oestrogen production is different in the placenta than that in the ovary because the enzymes 17-hydroxylase and 17,20-desmolase (CYP-17, 20) which are essential for formation of androgen, i.e. DHEA from cholesterol, are not present in the placenta. Therefore, basic substrate for synthesis of oestrogen is not cholesterol; rather, it is DHEA. The steps involved in biosynthesis are shown in Fig. 9.4.8.

i. DHEA, the principal adrenal steroid, is sulph-conjugated (sulphated) by sulph kinase in the adrenal cortex of the fetus and of the mother to DHEAS.
ii. *In the fetal liver:* The DHEAS is converted to 16-OH-DHEAS by an enzyme 16-hydroxylase present in the fetal liver. This enzyme is also not present in placenta.
iii. *In the placenta:* Placenta obtains DHEAS from the maternal as well as from the fetal circulation. In the placenta, DHEAS is deconjugated to DHEA before it is converted into oestriol. For the conversion of DHEA to oestriol, two types of enzymes are required – 16-*hydroxylase* (which is present in the fetal and maternal liver) and *aromatase* (which is present in the maternal ovary and the placenta).
   The enzyme 16-hydroxylase is lacking in placenta. Therefore, oestriol is mainly formed by the aromatase pathway (Fig. 9.4.8).
   Since 16-OH-DHEAS is the main substrate for oestrogen, oestriol is the major placental oestrogen during pregnancy.
   The oestrone and oestradiol present in maternal circulation are converted into oestriol in the maternal liver by 16-hydroxylase pathway but the amount secreted is very less.

Plasma concentration: Like progesterone, plasma oestrogen (oestriol) concentration rises throughout the gestation. Its peak value (14 ng/mL) and secretory curve parallels that of progesterone and the maximum *plateau* is reached at 30–40 weeks of gestation (Fig. 9.4.7D).

Important Note

The plasma concentration of oestriol reflects the functional status of the fetoplacental maternal unit activity.

Metabolism: Oestrogens are metabolized in the liver and excreted in urine as soluble conjugates (glucuronides and sulphates).

Important Note

Monitoring of urinary oestriol excretion of the mother is an index of fetus status.

Physiological effects: Oestrogenic effects of pregnancy are primarily caused by oestradiol, which is the most potent oestrogen. It mediates the following effects:

i. It causes growth and development of maternal reproductive organs (the uterus increases in size, weight, length and volume by both hypertrophy and stretching of the myometrium).
ii. Oestrogen stimulates development of the lactiferous ductal system in mammary glands.
iii. It stimulates hepatic synthesis of thyroxine-binding globulins, steroid-binding globulins and angiotensinogens. It also stimulates renin secretion.
iv. Just before term, oestrogen to progesterone ratio increases and the uterus is dominated by oestrogen.

8. Other placental hormones A number of other substances which are secreted from placenta are as follows:

- Corticotropin-releasing hormone (CRH)
- β-Endorphins
- α-MSH
- Dynorphin A
- Gonadotropin-releasing hormones (GnRH)
- Inhibin
- Leptin
- Prolactin
- Prorenin

The exact role of the above-mentioned substances during pregnancy is not yet clear. However, substances like GnRH and inhibin act in paracrine fashion to regulate hCG.

Applied Aspects

The diagnostic importance of placental hormones is in detection of Down syndrome. For screening, the following tests are employed:

Triple test: It involves measurement of maternal serum α-fetoprotein (MSAFP), hCG and unconjugated oestriol-3 (UE-3). The test is usually carried out at 15–22 weeks of gestation, when levels of MSAFP and UE-3 are low and hCG is high, i.e. if ratio is 1:250/or higher, then test is positive.

Quadruple screening test: It involves estimation of MSAFP, hCG, UE-3 and dimeric inhibin A. For the positive test, the level of hCG is high, UE-3 is low, inhibin is raised and MSAFP is reduced.

B. Transport of substances between the mother and the fetus

1. Transport of nutrients The major function of placenta is to provide foodstuffs from the mother's blood into the fetus.

During the first few weeks after implantation, the nutrients are derived from the plasma into the oedematous decidua and from endometrial glandular secretions containing glycogen.

By the fourth week of pregnancy, the placenta takes up the nutritive functions. The nutritive materials which are transported from the mother's blood into the fetus are as follows:

Glucose: Glucose passes by facilitated diffusion through a carrier molecule present on the trophoblast cells. Glucose level in fetal blood is 20%–30% lower than that in maternal blood.

Note: Fructose and sucrose are synthesized in the placenta itself.

Fats: Fetal fat is derived from transfer of free fatty acids and cholesterol across the placenta and is also synthesized from the carbohydrates.

The solubility of fatty acids is high in the cell membranes; therefore, they are transferred by simple diffusion method, but more slowly as compared with glucose.

Amino acids, calcium and inorganic phosphates are actively absorbed by the placental membrane.

Potassium, sodium and chloride ions and substances with molecular weight less than 1000 can cross readily by simple diffusion.

2. Excretion of waste products through placenta Excretory products, especially urea, uric acid, creatinines, etc., formed in the fetus are transported into the mother's blood and then excreted by the mother's kidneys. Thus, placenta also acts as fetal kidney.

3. Diffusion of respiratory gases

i. ***Oxygen transport*** through the placental membrane follows the same principle as the diffusion of oxygen through the pulmonary membrane. It occurs as follows:
   - Dissolved oxygen from the maternal sinuses of placenta diffuses into the fetal blood along the pressure gradient (mean pO_2 in the mother's blood is 50 mm Hg, whereas in the fetal blood, mean pO_2 is 30 mm Hg).
   - The low pO_2 of fetal arterial blood would have been a serious problem but presence of fetal haemoglobin in the RBCs which has a higher affinity for oxygen than for adult haemoglobin, and higher haemoglobin concentration in the fetal blood (50% greater than that in the mother's blood), shifts the oxygen–haemoglobin dissociation curve to the left.
   - The fetal blood coming to placenta carries more of CO_2 which is released into maternal blood. Therefore, the pH of maternal blood is slightly acidic as compared with that of fetal blood. The haemoglobin–oxygen dissociation curve of fetal blood shifts to the left and of maternal blood to the right (double Bohr's effect). All the above-mentioned factors help the fetus to receive sufficient oxygen (Fig. 9.4.9).

ii. ***Transport of CO_2:*** Transport of CO_2 from fetus occurs by diffusion along the pressure gradient. The pCO_2 of fetal blood is 2–3 mm Hg higher than that of maternal blood (as CO_2 is continuously being formed in the fetus and eliminated only through placenta). Thus, placenta acts as fetal lungs.

4. Transport of antibodies

Maternal immunoglobulins are transferred by receptor-mediated endocytosis into the fetus and are responsible for innate immunity.

Rh agglutinins are easily transported as compared with ABO agglutinins; that is why the effects of Rh incompatibility are more severe.

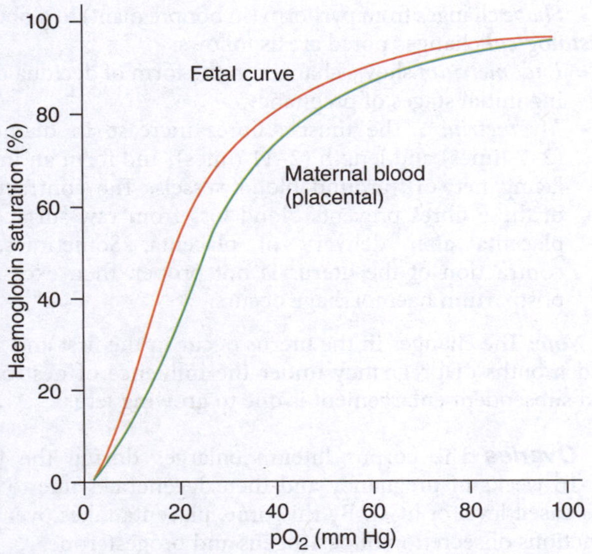

Fig. 9.4.9 Oxygen–haemoglobin dissociation curve for maternal and fetal blood.

5. Transport of harmful substances

Certain viruses and many drugs (like nicotine and barbiturates) can easily cross the placental barrier and may produce harmful effect on the fetus. Therefore, as far as possible, one should avoid these drugs and smoking during pregnancy. One should also try to remain away from viral infections. HIV virus is also transmitted from the mother to the fetus.

C. Protection of the fetus

Placenta protects the fetus in many ways:

- It acts as a barrier for certain harmful substances.
- It provides nutrition to the fetus.
- Its hormonal secretion is responsible for proper growth of the fetus.
- Placental progesterone decreases uterine contractions and thus protects the fetus from being expelled.

Pregnancy Tests

In an adult healthy woman, amenorrhoea is the first sign of pregnancy, but it occurs in many other conditions as well. Therefore, detection of early pregnancy is made possible by certain pregnancy tests. The pregnancy detection tests are based on presence of hCG in the urine of a pregnant lady. The sensitivity of these tests varies, but usually concentration required to obtain a positive test is about 2500 IU/L and this occurs at about 10–12 days after a missed period. There are two types of pregnancy detection test.

A. Biological Tests

The biological pregnancy tests are based on the luteinizing activity of hCG. The urine of the pregnant woman is injected by either intraperitoneal or subcutaneous route into the female virgin animal; there occurs ovulation which is detected as haemorrhagic spots on the corpora lutea. Various biological pregnancy tests are summarized in Table 9.4.1.

Note: Although biological tests are very sensitive, nowadays, they are replaced by immunological tests of pregnancy because of convenience and immediate results.

B. Immunological Tests

Immunological pregnancy tests are based on antigenic properties of hCG.

Gravindex test:

For Gravindex test:

- The kit for this test consists of Gravindex antigen (latex particles coated with hCG), Gravindex antibodies (serum containing antibodies against hCG) and a dark-coloured slide.
- The antibodies are prepared by injecting urine of a pregnant woman containing hCG into the rabbits. Then after few weeks, blood from the rabbit is withdrawn and serum is separated (containing anti-hCG antibodies).

Procedure

This test is performed on the control and test samples of urine.

Control sample: A drop of urine sample from a nonpregnant subject (containing no hCG) is mixed with a drop of antiserum containing hCG antibodies. Then it is mixed with hCG-coated latex particles. There will be agglutination, because urine of a nonpregnant subject does not contain antigen; therefore, antibodies are not neutralized. Thus, occurrence of agglutination indicates no pregnancy or pregnancy test is negative.

Table 9.4.1 Biological tests of pregnancy

Test	Criteria for positive test
1. Aschheim–Zondek test	
Urine (2–5 mL) from pregnant woman is injected (intraperitoneal/subcutaneous) into an immature mouse two to three times in a day for 2–3 days	On the third day, abdomen is opened and ovaries are examined; haemorrhagic spots on corpora lutea indicate that ovulation has occurred
2. Friedman's test	
Urine of pregnant woman is injected into an immature female rabbit or into a mature adult female rabbit (isolated from male rabbits for a week)	Abdomen is opened after 24 h; detection of haemorrhagic spots on corpora lutea indicates positive test
3. Hogben's test	
5 mL urine from pregnant woman is injected into the large dorsal lymph sac of the female toad	After 2–3 h, shedding of ova is observed which indicates positive pregnancy test
4. Kupperman's test	
3–5 mL of urine of a pregnant woman is injected subcutaneously into an immature rat	After 6 h, ovaries show hyperaemia
5. Galli–Mainini test	
3–5 mL urine is injected into lymph sac of male frog (*Xenopus*)	After 2 h, urine is withdrawn from cloaca of male frog and presence of sperms in the urine indicates +ve pregnancy test

Test sample: A drop of urine of a suspected pregnant lady (containing hCG) is mixed with a drop of antiserum (containing hCG antibodies). Then it is mixed with hCG-coated latex particles. There will be no agglutination, because antibodies have been neutralized by the hCG present in the urine. Therefore, occurrence of no agglutination means positive pregnancy test. The procedure can be summarized as:

Control	Test
A drop of urine of nonpregnant woman (no hCG)	A drop of urine of pregnant woman (hCG)
+	+
A drop of hCG antiserum	A drop of hCG antiserum
+	+
hCG-coated latex particles	hCG-coated latex particles
↓	↓
Agglutination (–ve pregnancy test)	No agglutination (+ve pregnancy test)

Important Note

It is important to note that:

- This test is not absolutely specific for pregnancy. It is positive in the presence of certain tumours which secrete hCG.
- Proteinuria may give false-positive results.
- The test becomes negative in later months of pregnancy when hCG level falls.

C. Blood Tests

Blood tests for pregnancy are of two types:

- *Qualitative blood/serum test:* This test confirms the pregnancy on the basis of whether hormone hCG is present or not. The test is quite similar to urine pregnancy test; however, chances of false-negative are present.
- *Quantitative blood/serum test:* It is also known as beta-hCG (β-hCG) test. This test measures the exact amount of hCG and is the most accurate.

PHYSIOLOGICAL CHANGES IN MOTHER DURING PREGNANCY

The normal average duration of pregnancy in human beings is 280 days (40 weeks) and is calculated from the first day of the last menstrual period (LMP), or 256–270 days from the time of ovulation. As pregnancy progresses, growing fetus imposes various types of extra demands on the mother's body, which are met with by certain adaptations in almost all the organ systems of the body. These physiological changes include those given next.

I. Changes in Genital Organs

1. Uterus To accommodate the growing fetus, marked increase in the size of the uterus takes place. The enlargement is mainly due to hypertrophy and to some extent hyperplasia of the myometrial smooth muscle fibres. The amount of connective tissue and elastic tissue in between muscle fibres also increases.

Gross changes occurring in the uterus are summarized as follows:

- *Weight* increases from 30–50 to 1000–1200 g at full term.
- *Length* increases from 7.5 cm (in nonparous state) to 35 cm at term.
- *Thickness* of the wall of the uterus decreases from 1.25 cm to only 5 mm at term, and fetus can be palpated through it.
- *Volume* of the uterus increases from few millilitres to about 5–7 L at term and mainly due to fetus (50%), placenta, amniotic fluids, etc.
- *Shape* changes from pyriform (in nonpregnant) to globular.

Histological changes noted are as follows:

- *Endometrium* shows changes in the form of decidua during initial stages of pregnancy.
- *Myometrium:* The muscle fibres increase in diameter (2–7 times) and length (2–11 times), and form an interlacing network around blood vessels. The contraction of these fibres prevents blood loss from raw surface of placenta after delivery of placenta. Sometimes, if contraction of the uterus is not proper, then excessive postpartum haemorrhage occurs.

Note: The changes in the uterus occur in the first and second months of pregnancy under the influence of oestrogen and subsequent enlargement is due to growing fetus.

2. Ovaries The corpus luteum enlarges during the first 12–16 weeks of pregnancy and then degenerates due to the decreased level of hCG. By this time, placenta takes over the functions of secretion of oestrogens and progesterone.

The follicular changes and ovulation do not occur because FSH and LH of the anterior pituitary are inhibited.

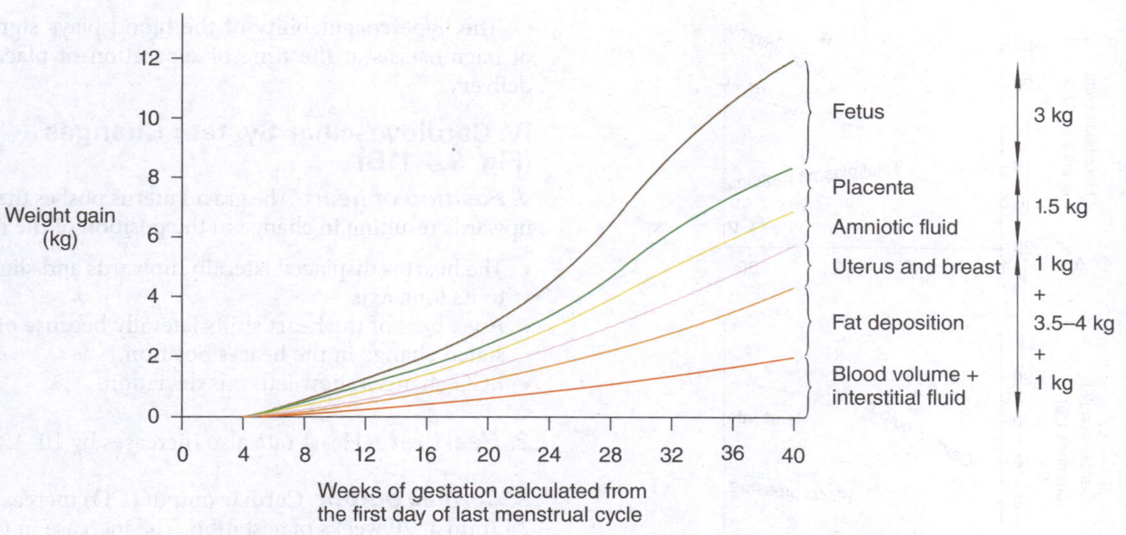

Fig. 9.4.10 Pattern and components of weight gain during normal pregnancy.

3. Cervix The changes in the cervix include:

- Endocervix gets hypertrophied.
- The cervical glands increase in number and their secretions form a plug that closes the cervical canal.
- The tough cervix becomes soft.

4. Fallopian tubes The fallopian tubes are pushed upwards due to increase in the size of the uterus. There occurs hyperplasia of the epithelial cells and blood supply also increases.

5. Mammary glands Under the influence of various hormones, the breast enlarges in early pregnancy. Hyperplasia of ductal and alveolar tissue occurs, the areola becomes pigmented and many sebaceous glands become prominent in the areola. Nipples also become larger and pigmented.

II. Weight Gain

A woman may gain total of 10–12 kg of weight during normal pregnancy, which is contributed by (Fig. 9.4.10):

- Fetus: 3 kg
- Placenta and amniotic fluid: 1.5 kg
- Uterus and breast enlargement: 1.0 kg
- Increase in blood volume and interstitial fluid: 1.5 kg
- Fat deposition: 3.5–4 kg

Important Note

Important points about the weight gain are as follows:

- During antenatal examination, regular monitoring of body weight is very important. Absence of weight gain in the second or third trimester is a sign of fetal growth retardation and fetal death.
- During early pregnancy, weight loss may be observed because of excessive vomiting.
- Due to increased secretion of oestrogen, progesterone, aldosterone and antidiuretic hormone (ADH) during pregnancy, Na^+ and H_2O retention occurs.
- Oedema is common, particularly in the lower limbs which is because of pressure of gravid uterus on the femoral vein and also because of Na^+ and water retention.
- Rapid and excessive weight gain raises the suspicion of toxaemia of pregnancy due to excessive fluid retention.

III. Haematological Changes (Fig. 9.4.11A)

1. Blood volume The blood volume increases during pregnancy to increase the blood supply to:

(i) Uterus (to meet its demands)
(ii) Skin to dissipate heat generated in the body
(iii) Kidney for excretion of extra waste products

The total blood volume increases by 30%. It begins to increase by the 12th week of pregnancy and continues till delivery.

Important Note

The plasma volume increases relatively more than red cell volume which causes haemodilution; thus, there is physiological anaemia of pregnancy.

2. Haemataological indices The haemataological indices show the following changes:

- RBC count decreases.
- Hb concentration decreases.
- PCV decreases.
- ESR increases.
- Reticulocyte count increases.

3. Plasma proteins Plasma proteins show the following changes:

- The total concentration of plasma proteins decreases from 7.5 to 6 g% due to haemodilution.
- The fibrinogen level increases to 300–400 from 200–300 mg/dL.
- Serum albumin is markedly decreased.
- Globulins (α and β) are increased.

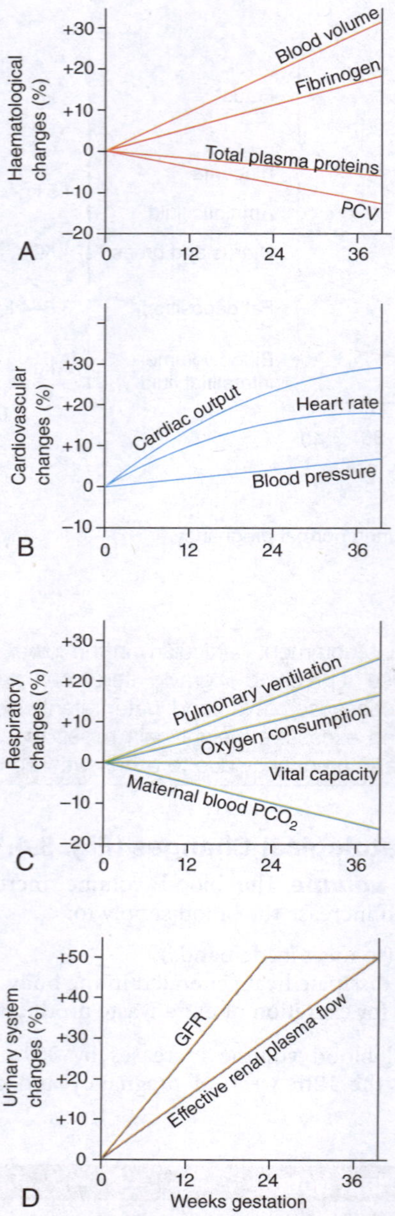

Fig. 9.4.11 Some physiological changes in the mother during pregnancy: **A**, haematological changes; **B**, cardiovascular changes; **C**, respiratory changes; and **D**, urinary system changes.

4. Leucocytes Total leucocyte count (TLC) increases and may reach up to 20,000/mm^3.

- DLC: Polymorphonuclear cells are predominantly increased with little change in monocytes, eosinophils and basophils and no change in number of lymphocytes.

5. Platelets There occurs slight decrease in platelet count.

6. Coagulation factors Pregnancy seems to be a hypercoagulable state due to increase in the following coagulation factors:

- Fibrinogen
- Factors VII, VIII, IX and X

The hypercoagulability of the blood plays significant role of haemostasis at the time of separation of placenta during delivery.

IV. Cardiovascular System Changes (Fig. 9.4.11B)

1. Position of heart The gravid uterus pushes the diaphragm upwards resulting in change in the position of the heart as:

- The heart is displaced laterally, upwards and slightly rotated to its long axis.
- Apex beat of the heart shifts laterally because of the above-stated change in the heart's position.
- ECG changes show left-axis deviation.

2. Heart rate Heart rate also increases by 10–12 beats/min.

3. Cardiac output Cardiac output (CO) increases from 5 to 7 L/min at 20 weeks of gestation. The increase in CO is due to increase in both stroke volume and heart rate during pregnancy. Increase in stroke volume is mainly due to increase in the total blood volume.

4. Blood pressure Blood pressure may show the following changes:

- *Systolic blood pressure:* In normal pregnancy, either there is no change in systolic pressure or some fall may occur.
- Diastolic pressure decreases and by 16–20 weeks of pregnancy, its value is the lowest. Then it starts rising and comes back to normal. Vasodilatation due to the effect of vasoactive substances (like kinins, endothelium-derived releasing factor, NO) is the main cause of fall in diastolic pressure.

5. Blood flow Blood flow to the skin, uterus and kidneys increases to meet the demands.

6. Venous pressure The gravid uterus exerts pressure on the pelvic veins, abdominal veins and femoral veins, thus increasing the venous pressure. The rise in femoral venous pressure results in oedema in feet (common occurrence), and the increased abdominal venous pressure predisposes to varicose veins, piles and peripheral venous thrombosis.

V. Respiratory System Changes (Fig. 9.4.11C)

1. Anatomical changes Anatomical changes in the respiratory system occur due to elevation of the diaphragm by the enlarged uterus. It causes increase in transverse diameter of the thoracic cage and subcostal angle. These two changes in turn increase the air flow across the bronchial tree.

2. Hyperventilation High levels of plasma progesterone during pregnancy increase the sensitivity of respiratory neurons to CO_2 resulting in hyperventilation. As a result of the maternal blood, pCO_2 decreases by 10%–15% and pCO_2 becomes about 30 mm Hg (normal, 40 mm Hg).

3. Ventilatory functions The anatomical changes and hyperventilation during pregnancy result in some changes in the parameters of ventilatory functions:

- *Tidal volume* increases.
- *Vital capacity* shows no changes.
- *Inspiratory capacity* increases.

- *Residual volume* decreases.
- *Functional residual capacity* decreases.
- *Forced expiratory volume* (FEV_1) and peak flow rate do not change.

4. Gas exchange Gas exchange across the alveoli is greatly enhanced due to marked increase in the pulmonary blood flow.

5. Oxygen consumption Oxygen consumption of body increases by 15% to meet the demands of growing fetus and for the extra work of the heart, uterus and other tissues.

VI. Urinary System Changes (Fig. 9.4.11D)

Kidney functions show the changes given next.

1. Renal blood flow There is marked increase in renal blood flow due to increase in CO and vasodilatation.

2. Effective renal plasma flow Effective renal plasma flow (ERPF) increases by 60% during pregnancy.

3. Glomerular filtration rate Glomerular filtration rate (GFR) increases by 50% due to increase in renal blood flow and solute load.

4. Renal tubular absorptive capacity Renal tubular absorptive capacity for sodium and chloride ions also increases by 50% due to high level of steroid hormones secreted by the placenta and the adrenal cortex.

5. Clearance rate Clearance rate of substances like creatinine and urea increases; therefore, the plasma creatinine and plasma urea values decrease during pregnancy.

6. Glycosuria Glycosuria is a common physiological phenomenon during pregnancy.

7. Proteinuria Proteinuria occurs due to increase in excretion of proteins.

8. Water balance During later months of pregnancy, excess of water is retained due to:

- *Decreased protein concentration*, especially albumin (proteinuria), leading to decreased colloidal osmotic pressure
- Retention of sodium

9. Acid–base balance Hyperventilation during pregnancy results in respiratory alkalosis. Kidneys, therefore, compensate for it by excreting more HCO_3^- ions in the urine.

- Respiratory alkalosis (slight rise in pH) shifts the haemoglobin–oxygen dissociation curve of maternal blood to left.
- Slight rise in pH of blood stimulates the formation of 2,3-DPG, which shifts the Hb–oxygen dissociation curve to the right and facilitates oxygen transfer to the fetus.
- Decreased pCO_2 of maternal blood facilitates transfer of CO_2 from the fetus to the mother.

VII. Gastrointestinal System Changes

1. GIT secretions Hypochlorhydria is very common due to decreased gastric secretion.

2. GIT motility GIT motility decreases under the influence of hormones resulting in delayed gastric emptying.

3. Gall bladder functions The gall bladder increases in size and empties its contents at a very slow rate.

4. Liver functions Liver functions are also altered during pregnancy. The fibrinogen synthesis increases and albumin decreases; thus, plasma A:G ratio is also altered.

5. Morning sickness Anorexia, nausea and vomiting are very common in early pregnancy (first trimester), especially in the morning hours, hence known as morning sickness. The cause for the morning sickness is not known. But the most common theory is that morning sickness is the body reaction to the pregnancy hormone hCG, which is produced at a higher level during the first trimester.

6. Glucose tolerance curve Glucose tolerance curve also shows disturbances. It becomes diabetic type due to glucose being rapidly absorbed from the intestine. For details, see page 767.

VIII. Metabolic Changes

1. The basal metabolic rate The basal metabolic rate (BMR) of the pregnant woman increases by about 15% during later half of the pregnancy.

2. Protein metabolism When the diet is balanced and adequate, there is nitrogen retention and positive nitrogen balance. The proteins are deposited in the uterus, breast, fetus and placenta.

3. Carbohydrate metabolism Carbohydrate metabolism shows the following changes:

- Blood glucose level increases due to rapid absorption from the gut.
- *Glycosuria* is of common occurrence due to increase in GFR and decrease in renal threshold for glucose.
- *Hepatic glycogen* level decreases.
- Ketosis may occur due to anorexia and excessive vomiting.
- Hyperplasia of β cells of islets of Langerhans of the pancreas occurs leading to increased level of insulin.

4. Fat metabolism About 3–4 kg of fat is deposited in the body during pregnancy. There occurs an increase in plasma concentration of cholesterol, phospholipids and triglycerides.

5. Mineral metabolism Mineral metabolism depicts the following changes:

Calcium and phosphorus: In normal pregnancy, the mother retains about 50 g of extra calcium and 30–40 g of phosphorus. These are deposited in the fetus and also retained in the mother stores (skeleton). These stores act as reservoir for extra demand of Ca^{2+} during lactation. During pregnancy, deficiency of calcium occurs, because normally its absorption is poor. Therefore, dietary supplementation of calcium is very important along with that of vitamin D.

Iron metabolism: Iron requirement tremendously increases during pregnancy and lactation as:

- About 375 mg of iron is needed for fetal blood formation, and 600 mg (extra) is needed to form the mother's own blood and cell mass.

- During pregnancy, nonhaemoglobin store of iron varies from 100 to 700 mg.
- Vitamin K should be supplemented to the mother's diet to prevent excessive haemorrhage at the time of delivery.

IX. Endocrine System Changes

The endocrine glands of the mother react substantially during pregnancy: first, due to increased metabolic load on the mother and, second, in response to the hormones produced by the placenta and fetus.

1. Anterior pituitary The anterior pituitary gland increases in size by 50% and shows hyperplasia of lactotropes. The anterior pituitary hormones show the following changes:

Prolactin: Maternal prolactin level increases progressively throughout the pregnancy under the influence of high level of oestrogen (Fig. 9.4.7E).
ACTH: The plasma concentration of ACTH increases.
Human growth hormone by the maternal anterior pituitary decreases. This is due to suppression by the chorionic isoform (hCS) of growth hormone.
Gonadotropins and sex hormones: Under the influence of high concentration of oestrogen and progesterone during pregnancy, the secretion of FSH and LH from the maternal anterior pituitary is suppressed. Therefore, low concentration of FSH and LH inhibits the maturation of Graafian follicles in the ovaries.
TSH concentration also rises.

2. Posterior pituitary ***Oxytocin*** secretion is inhibited during pregnancy due to high levels of oestrogen and progesterone, but its levels increase during labour.

Antidiuretic hormone (ADH) level also increases during pregnancy. For details, see page 777.

3. Thyroid The size and secretory activity of the thyroid gland increases during pregnancy.

Thyroid-binding globulin increases which in turn increases the bound fraction of T_3 and T_4. Plasma level of free T_4 remains unchanged. Increased iodide uptake, BMR and resting pulse during pregnancy are indicators of increased thyroid activity.

4. Parathyroid functions

- Parathyroid glands show an increase in their size and parathyroid hormone (PTH) secretion.
- Raised level of PTH increases the active form of vitamin D_3 (1,25[OH]$_2$-cholecalciferol) and vitamin D_3–binding protein.
- Increased PTH helps in absorption of calcium from the gut and decreases excretion through kidneys, and thereby fulfils the increased requirement of calcium during pregnancy.
- The fetal calcium concentration is more than the maternal levels.

5. Adrenal cortex The maternal adrenal glands get enlarged during pregnancy and also there is increase in the width of zona fasciculata. It serves the following functions:

- Increased concentration of glucocorticoids is responsible for fat deposition in the adipose tissue and appearance of stria.
- Aldosterone secretion increases progressively and reaches up to sixfold to eightfold at term. This occurs due to natriuretic effect of progesterone and atrial natriuretic peptide (ANP).
- Normal pregnancy is also associated with increased levels of angiotensinogen, renin and several angiotensins including angiotensin II.
- Other mineral corticoids and deoxycorticosteroid are increased several thousandfold to maintain Na^+ balance and plasma volume.

6. Pancreas As already mentioned in the section 'Carbohydrate Metabolism', there is β-cell hyperplasia leading to increased level of insulin. However, maternal tissue sensitivity to insulin is variable during pregnancy. It increases in the first half and decreases in the second half of pregnancy (insulin resistance).

X. Changes in The Skin

1. Hyperpigmentation Hyperpigmentation occurs on the face (butterfly pattern known as chloasma), areola, nipple and midline of the abdomen (linea alba) extending from the pubic symphysis to the xiphisternum. The hyperpigmentation is related to increased secretion of ACTH and MSH during pregnancy.

2. Striae gravidarum These are linear scars present on the lower abdomen due to stretching of the skin.

XI. Psychological Changes

The nervous system shows mild changes in the form of craving for particular types of food item and alterations in the behaviour, emotions and mood. In few cases, true psychosis may also develop but cause is not known.

PHYSIOLOGY OF PARTURITION

Parturition is the process by which a baby is born. It involves preparation for childbirth, act of childbirth and recovery from childbirth. The uterine myometrium and cervix play an important role in this process. Therefore, knowledge about the functional anatomy of these structures is mandatory to understand the physiology of parturition.

FUNCTIONAL ANATOMY

Uterine myometrium The characteristic feature of myometrium is that it consists of two layers of smooth muscle fibres, which are arranged in closely interwoven bundles embedded in the matrix surrounding the blood vessels. The smooth muscle cells are linked with adjacent muscle cells through gap junctions. The number of gap junctions determines the excitability state of the myometrium. The matrix mainly consists of collagen fibres.

Cervix It predominantly consists of collagen fibres and ground substance. The ground substance is composed of glucosans such as hyaluronic acid, dermatan sulphate and chondroitin sulphate.

MECHANICS OF PARTURITION

From the functional point of view, mechanics of parturition mainly involves:

- Uterine contractions
- Cervical dilatation

Uterine Contractions

The uterus, which remains quiescent during the period of pregnancy, becomes progressively more and more excitable towards the end of pregnancy, until finally it begins strong rhythmical contractions with such a force that the fetus is expelled.

The uterine activity in a pregnant woman can be studied by recording amniotic fluid pressure changes and intrauterine pressure changes during pregnancy and labour. The characteristic features of uterine activity are as follows:

Up to the 30th week (7 months) of pregnancy, there is very little uterine activity. The uterus undergoes periodic episodes of weak and slow rhythmic contractions called *Braxton Hicks contractions*.

After the 30th week, the activity gradually increases. The characteristics of these contractions are as follows:

Start of contraction: The uterine contractions during labour start at the top of the fundus of the uterus and spread on to the body part.
Force of contractions is high in the fundus and body part of the uterus and comparatively weak in the lower segment near the cervix.
Frequency of contractions in early labour is only once in 30 minutes (1/30 minutes) and as labour progresses, it increases to one in 3 minutes (1/3 minutes).
Pressure during contractions may rise up to 30–35 mm Hg.
Period of relaxation follows each contraction.
Type of contraction: Uterine contractions are intermittent and are beneficial for the fetus; otherwise, strong and continuous contractions sometimes impede blood supply through placenta and would cause fetal death.

Control or Regulation of Uterine Contractility

The exact cause of increased uterine activity is not known, but few factors which lead towards parturition are progressive hormonal changes that cause increased excitability of uterine musculature and progressive mechanical changes (for details, see page 855).

Cervical Dilatation

Throughout pregnancy, the cervix remains as a rigid structure, but at the time of parturition, certain structural and biochemical changes occur and the cervix becomes soft. This is known as cervical ripening. It allows the cervix to stretch when uterine contractions start.

The changes in the cervix which are responsible for its dilatation are as follows:

- Breakdown of collagen fibres
- Increase in amount of hyaluronic acid, having high water-retaining capacity
- Decrease in amount of dermatan sulphate

These changes are mainly under the influence of prostaglandins.

PHASES OF PARTURITION

The period of parturition extends from conception to restoration of fertility for the next conception.

For successful childbirth, the myometrium and cervix show an ordered sequence of events, as discussed in the section 'Mechanics of Parturition'. These changes have been divided into four phases – phases 0, 1, 2 and 3 (Fig. 9.4.12).

Phase 0 of Parturition

This phase corresponds to the period of pregnancy, i.e. it extends from conception to initiation of the process of childbirth. The average duration of human pregnancy is 270 days from the day of fertilization of the ovum. Since this day cannot be accurately determined, the first day (date) of the LMP is the day from which the duration of pregnancy and expected date of delivery is conventionally calculated and when counted in this way, the average period of gestation is 284 days.

- Throughout this phase, the uterus is quiescent and the cervix remains rigid.
- This phase is under the control of progesterone.
- Myometrial tranquillity during this phase is attributed to:
  - Depressed uterine smooth muscle contractile response due to decreased intracellular calcium in myometrial smooth muscle cells
  - Increased degradation of endogenously produced uterotonics by enzymes, e.g. prostaglandins by prostaglandin dehydrogenase, oxytocin by oxytocinase and histamine by diamine oxidase
  - Inhibition of myometrial cell contractile signal propagation due to sparse oxytocin receptors and paucity of gap junctions between the myometrial cells

Phase I of Parturition

This phase is the period of preparation for the labour. It commences in the final days of gestation and extends up to the onset of labour. It is difficult to predict the exact date of onset of labour. It may occur any time between the 37th and the 40th week of gestation. During this phase, the myometrium becomes responsive to oxytocin and the cervix undergoes a biochemical remodelling called cervical ripening. Thus, in this phase, uterine quiescence is suspended and contractile competency of the uterus is increased and the cervix is made ready for dilatation.

Increased myometrial excitability to oxytocin near term Increased myometrial excitability to oxytocin near term is attributed to:

- An increase in the number of oxytocin receptors on the cells of the uterine smooth muscle during the final weeks of pregnancy
- An increase in the number and size of gap junctions between the myometrial cells
- Increased synthesis of contractile proteins in the myometrial cells

Cervical ripening Cervical ripening occurs, i.e. the cervix becomes soft and yielding, due to the following biochemical changes:

- *Breakdown and rearrangement of collagen fibres*
- Alteration in relative amounts of glycosaminoglycans, i.e. an increase in the content of the hyaluronic acid and decrease in dermatan sulphate content

The above-mentioned changes in the cervix are mediated by the prostaglandins under the influence of oestrogen.

Onset of labour The onset of labour marks the end of phase I and beginning of phase II of parturition. The exact

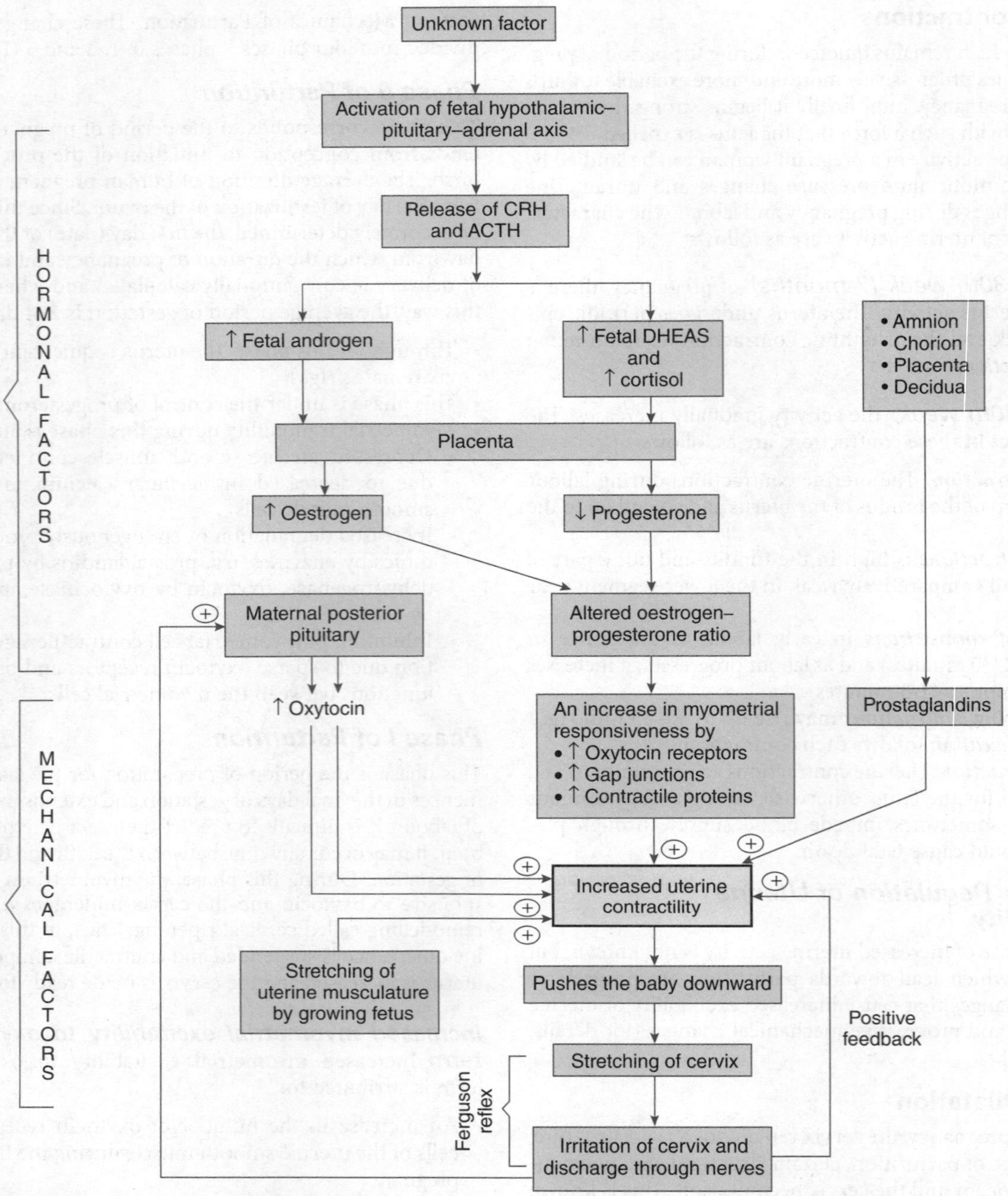

Fig. 9.4.12 Summary of control of parturition depicting role of hormonal and mechanical factors.

cause of onset of labour in humans is still not certain. The possible hypothesis is discussed (see page 855).

Phase II of Parturition

This is a phase of active labour. It extends from the onset of labour to the delivery of conceptus. It is characterized by powerful uterine contractions which bring about progressive cervical dilatation, fetal descent and finally expulsion of fetus and placenta. This phase is further divided into three stages of labour – stages first, second and third.

First stage The first stage of labour is characterized by:

- Strong contractions of the upper uterine segment which drive the fetus downwards with each contraction
- Cervical effacement and progressive dilatation, until it is fully dilated to form a birth canal by merging with the lower uterine segment

This stage is said to be over when the diameter of external os of the cervix is large enough (about 10 cm) to allow the head of fetus to pass into the vagina.

This stage lasts for 8–24 hours in the first pregnancy, but its duration decreases in multipara.

Second stage The second stage of labour is characterized by:

- Fully dilated cervix
- Rupture of amniotic membranes and loss of amniotic fluid through the vagina

- Strong and more frequent uterine contractions which in association with abdominal muscle contractions (bearing-down pains due to neurogenic reflexes from the spinal cord to the abdominal muscle) lead to expulsion of fetus through the dilated vagina

Duration of this stage varies from 1 minute (in multipara) to about 1 hour (in the first pregnancy).

Third stage The third stage is the stage of separation and expulsion of placenta.

- During the next 10–45 minutes after the birth of baby, the uterus contracts to a small size resulting in separation of placenta from its implantation site. Separation of placenta causes bleeding due to opening up of maternal sinuses. The arrangement of smooth muscle fibres in the myometrium is such (form figure of 8 around uterine vessels) that their contraction causes constriction of blood vessels and bleeding stops. The prostaglandins released also have some vasoconstrictor effect.

Applied Aspects

On an average, about 350 mL of blood is lost in normal pregnancy. In some women, the uterus fails to contract strongly causing risk of severe bleeding. In such cases, the uterus can be induced to contract by injection of synthetic oxytocin and ergometrine.

Postpartum haemorrhage (PPH) refers to excessive bleeding after childbirth (>500 mL).

Causes are as follows:
- Loss of tone of uterine musculature
- Bleeding disorder
- Placenta failing to come out or tearing of placenta

Signs and symptoms of PPH include vaginal bleeding that does not slow/stop and associated symptoms due to blood loss (hypotension, tachycardia).

Treatment: The conservative treatment is in the form of:
- Uterotonic medication which causes the uterus to contract
- External uterine massage
- Depending on cause and severity of symptoms blood transfusion, may require removal of residual placenta/uterus (hysterectomy)

Phase III of Parturition

This is the phase of parturient recovery. It begins after the delivery of conceptus and extends till fertility is restored. Oxytocin and endothelin are important hormones regulating the processes which occur during this phase. This phase is characterized by:

- Uterine contraction and retraction occur to prevent puerperal haemorrhage.
- Lactation and milk ejection are initiated to facilitate breast-feeding.
- Involution of the uterus (i.e. decrease in size and weight) takes place during the first 4–5 weeks after parturition. Lactation hastens this process.
- The raw surface of the endothelium is re-epithelialized and fertility is restored to normal.

Control of Parturition

The mechanisms responsible for onset of labour in humans are still not understood exactly. However, it has been postulated that parturition in human beings closely mimics bovine parturition which is seen reasonably clear in the form of sheep model of parturition. Although the fundamental biomolecular processes of parturition are expected to be similar in all mammalian species, a few important endocrinal differences exist between human and sheep pregnancy before the initiation of parturition. The control of parturition includes the role of (Fig. 9.4.12):

- Hormonal factors
- Mechanical factors

A. Hormonal factors The hormonal changes that initiate the parturition and that cause increased excitability of uterine musculature are given next.

1. Activation of fetal hypothalamic–pituitary–adrenal axis Recently it has been hypothesized that the initial signals for the onset of labour come from the fetus only. Experimental destruction of fetal pituitary in sheep has been shown to delay the onset of labour.

From sheep model of parturition, it has been postulated that in humans, some unknown factors are involved in CRH secretion in the fetus resulting in an increase in ACTH secretion few days before parturition. ACTH causes fetal adrenal cortex to secrete a large amount of androgens which are converted to oestrogen in the placenta, and DHEAS and cortisol, which may inhibit the conversion of fetal pregnenolone to progesterone.

The above changes lead to an altered oestrogen–progesterone ratio.

2. Role of altered oestrogen–progesterone ratio The oestrogen and progesterone are secreted progressively in increasing amounts by the placenta during pregnancy. In the third trimester, the rate of progesterone secretion remains constant, whereas the rate of oestrogen secretion continues to rise as described in the section 'Activation of fetal hypothalamic–pituitary–adrenal axis'. The progesterone reduces whereas the oestrogen increases the contractility of the uterine smooth muscle. Therefore, it has been suggested that as the ratio of oestrogen to progesterone is increased during the final week of pregnancy, the uterus begins to contract. The altered oestrogen–progesterone ratio also causes:

- An increase in release of oxytocin from the maternal posterior pituitary
- An increase in the number of oxytocin receptors in the myometrium
- An increase in prostaglandin synthesis
- An increase in synthesis of myometrial contractile proteins

3. Role of oxytocin and prostaglandins The altered ratio of oestrogen–progesterone in late gestation seems to be responsible for increase in the number of oxytocin receptors and also for more release of oxytocin from the posterior pituitary of the mother. As discussed above, the uterine excitability to oxytocin is increased in late gestation due to increase in oxytocin receptors, increase in gap junctions and increase in synthesis of contractile proteins in the myometrial cells.

It has been suggested that the altered oestrogen–progesterone ratio leads to prostaglandin synthesis in human pregnancy from the placenta, amnion, chorion and decidua. The prostaglandins enhance the force of oxytocin-induced uterine contractions. Administration of drugs like aspirin or indomethacin, which inhibit prostaglandin synthesis, may interfere with the process of labour.

B. Mechanical factors Mechanical factors that increase the contractility of uterus include those given next.

1. Stretch of uterine musculature Stretch of uterine musculature usually increases its own contractility (myogenic theory). During pregnancy, movements of the fetus cause stretching. As the pregnancy advances, with growing fetus, stretch further increases leading to uterine contractility.

2. Positive feedback effect Stretching and irritation of the cervix is particularly important in eliciting uterine contractions. The exact mechanism is not known but possibly may be because of positive feedback effect through initiation of the reflex increase in uterine contractility as depicted in Fig. 9.4.12.

The positive feedback mechanism continues until the baby is expelled.

3. Role of Ferguson reflex Once labour is started, the uterine contractions dilate the ripened cervix. The cervical dilatation in turn sets off signals in afferent nerves that increase oxytocin secretion from the posterior pituitary. This is called Ferguson reflex.

Spinal reflexes and abdominal muscle contractions help in labour and delivery; however, delivery is possible even without reflex release of oxytocin. Since paraplegic women can go into labour and normal parturition take place.

Applied Aspects

The obstetricians frequently induce labour by rupturing the membrane so that the head of the baby stretches the cervix more forcefully than usual and thus initiates it, leading to initiation of positive feedback effect and Ferguson reflex.

SUMMARY

The control of parturition is summarized in Fig. 9.4.12.

Applied Aspects

1. Miscarriage

Miscarriage is defined as pregnancy loss before 20 weeks of gestation, and the medical term is spontaneous abortion. The cause of pregnancy loss may occur in conceptus or in the microenvironment of the maternal reproductive tract at the time of conception. The causes of recurrent pregnancy loss include:

- Parental chromosome translocations
- Structural uterine abnormalities such as longitudinal septa and uterine adhesions
- Endocrinal disorders
- Polycystic ovary syndrome
- Thyroid dysfunctions, poorly controlled diabetes
- Autoimmune conditions

Signs and symptoms

The most common sign is vaginal bleeding which may vary from mild (spotting) to heavy.

Lower back pain varies from mild to severe (cramping).

Treatment: Dilatation and curettage (D&C)

2. Preterm Labour

Preterm labour is onset of labour before 37 weeks of gestation. The risk factors and potential mechanism of preterm labour include:

- Multiple gestations may occur.
- Excessive amniotic fluid volume stretches the myometrium and may stimulate muscle activity.
- Intrauterine infection is associated with a high level of cytokine, interleukin-1β, interleukin-6, TNF-α and prostaglandins. All these substances stimulate the myometrium.
- Thrombin has been recently considered to be an extremely potent uterotonic agent responsible for preterm labour. The increased production of thrombin accompanying bleeding in pregnancy is associated with preterm labour.

3. Preeclampsia

Preeclampsia has been defined as triad of hypertension, proteinuria and oedema in pregnant women. It typically occurs in the third trimester of pregnancy. The presentation of this disorder occurs as:

- *Central nervous system* involvement can manifest as severe headache, visual changes, seizers, stroke and blindness.
- *Renal involvement* occurs in almost all cases and can manifest as proteinuria, oliguria or renal failure.
- *Oedema fluid* can accumulate in many sites including hands and feet, face and lungs.
- *Hepatic dysfunction* results in haemolysis, deranged liver function tests and low platelet count.

Mechanism of Pathogenesis of Preeclampsia It was observed that the cytotrophoblast fails to properly invade the maternal blood vessels in preeclampsia. No single mechanism has proven to be wholly responsible for this condition; there are several initiating factors for endothelial dysfunction.

Recently it is found that soluble vascular endothelial growth factor (sVEGF) and placental growth factor are markedly elevated in the serum a few weeks before the symptoms. The explanation is that placenta in preeclamptic pregnancies secretes increased amount of δFLt-1 (the soluble antagonist to VEGF) which inhibits the development of small blood vessels.

Treatment The ultimate treatment of this condition is delivery of pregnancy. If the mother is medically supported through timely delivery and postpartum recovery, all deranged physiology will revert back to the normal provided no permanent tissue damage has occurred.

Self-Assessment

1. Discuss the process of fertilization and implantation.
2. Discuss the endocrinal functions of placenta.
3. Describe the following:
   - Cardiovascular changes in the mother during pregnancy
   - Process of parturition
4. Write notes on the following:
   - Fetoplacental unit
   - Corpus luteum of pregnancy
   - Sperm capacitation
   - Polyspermy blockage
   - Acrosomal reaction

Clinical Cases

Case 1

An 8-week pregnant lady was brought to the emergency with complaints of severe pain in the lower back and vaginal bleeding. On the basis of examination and ultrasound report, she was diagnosed a case of miscarriage.

Q1. What are the causes of miscarriage?
Q2. What is the treatment plan in this case?
Q3. How can miscarriage be prevented?

Case 2

A 26-year-old married woman who missed her periods and was diagnosed pregnant on positive pregnancy test was brought to emergency with complaints of vaginal bleeding and severe pain in lower back and suspected a case of abortion/ectopic pregnancy. Physical examination revealed hypotension and tachycardia.

Q1. What tests should be done to diagnose ectopic pregnancy?
Q2. What is the pathophysiology?
Q3. What are the risk factors?

Case 3

A 20-week pregnant lady was brought to the emergency with complaints of severe headache, blurring of vision and vomiting. On examination, there was swelling of the face, hands, feet and ankles.

Q1. What is the probable diagnosis?
Q2. What is the pathophysiology of this condition?
Q3. What are the risk factors?
Q4. What complications can occur if not treated?

9.5 Physiology of Lactation

CHAPTER OUTLINE

DEVELOPMENT AND FUNCTIONAL ANATOMY OF BREAST

Breastfeeding is the characteristic feature of all the mammals, including human beings. It has evolved as the best method of nourishing the newborn. The mammary glands (the secondary sex organs) play an important role in lactation process.

DEVELOPMENT OF BREAST

Mammary glands are present in both the sexes; in males, they remain rudimentary, but in females, they are well developed after puberty. The different phases of its development are described next.

Breasts in intrauterine life (embryogenesis) At 18–19 weeks of gestation, mammary glands develop from a thickened mass of epithelium of the epidermis known as mammary bud (Fig. 9.5.1A).

- From this thickened mass, about 16–20 solid outgrowths arise and project into the dermis (Fig. 9.5.1B).
- Then the thickened mass as well as these outgrowths is canalized (Fig. 9.5.1C) to form the rudimentary duct system.
- The secretory element of the gland is formed by proliferation of the terminal part of the outgrowths. It occurs at puberty only.
- The proximal end of each duct opens into a common pit formed by cavitation of the thickened mass (Fig. 9.5.1D); later on, growth of underlying mesodermal tissue pushes the wall of the pit outwards as nipple (Fig. 9.5.1E).

Breasts at birth At birth, the mammary glands are rudimentary consisting of a tiny nipple and few ducts radiating from it.

Breasts at puberty From birth to puberty, the mammary glands remain quiescent. During puberty, the following changes occur:

At thelarche, i.e. at the time of puberty (9–11 years of age), before the start of menses, the breasts start developing and get enlarged. During this stage, only duct system proliferates and shows branching.
At menarche, i.e. after the onset of menses, cyclic growth of mammary glands (period of growth followed by quiescence) occurs in each menstrual cycle. The growth period further corresponds to phases of menstrual cycle.
In proliferative phase (or oestrogen phase), the duct cells proliferate and continue throughout the rest of the cycle.
In luteal phase (progestational phase), progesterone stimulates the proliferation of terminal ductules, so there is formation of glandular tissue.
At menstruation (bleeding phase), there occurs no proliferation of duct cells as well as of glandular tissue, because levels of both oestrogen and progesterone are lowered. Hence, this period is called quiescence period.

With the onset of the next menstrual cycle, further growth occurs. Thus, there is a progressive growth of breast in successive cycles, along with modelling of the breast by fat deposition in the adipose tissue.

Breasts in pregnancy During pregnancy, remarkable growth of both ductal and glandular systems occurs. It is only during first pregnancy that glandular tissue develops fully.

In the first half of pregnancy, the duct system proliferates and shows extensive sprouting and branching along with the growth of stroma and deposition of fat.

In the second half of pregnancy, there is enormous growth of glandular tissue.

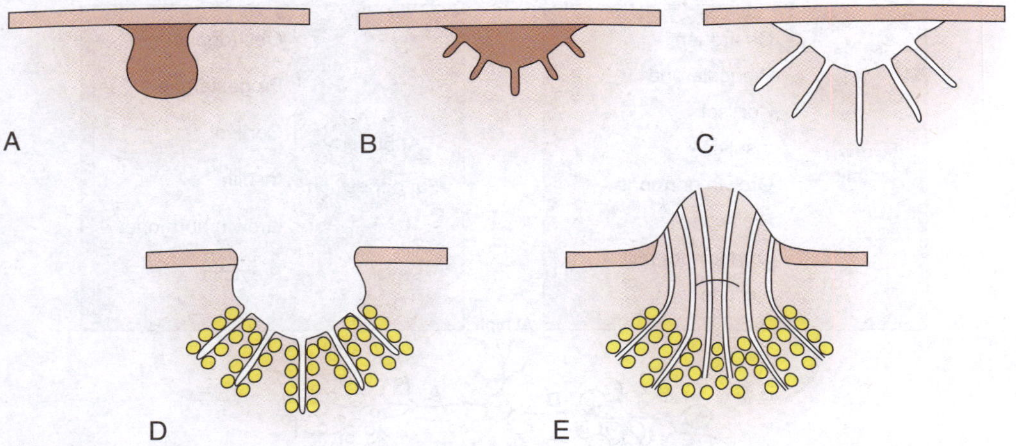

Fig. 9.5.1 Stages of development of breast in intrauterine life: **A**, formation of mammary bud; **B**, outgrowths of mammary bud; **C**, canalization of outgrowths; **D**, formation of secretory element and formation of common pit; and **E**, formation of nipple.

The extensive growth of mammary glands during pregnancy is known as *mammogenesis* or preparation of the breast for lactation.

Breasts during lactation After childbirth, the alveolar cells get enlarged and distended and start forming milk (lactogenesis).

Involution of breast After a normal period of lactation (7–9 months), the alveolar epithelium undergoes apoptosis and glands revert back to prepregnant stage.

FUNCTIONAL ANATOMY OF BREAST

Gross anatomy The fully developed breast is a soft, rounded, elevated structure present over the pectoral region, having a central dark pigmented area (areola). The central part of the areola, projected above the surface, is called nipple.

Histological structure Each mammary gland is covered by overlying skin and underlying it discrete masses of glandular tissue are present in the connective tissue consisting of stroma and adipose tissue (Fig. 9.5.2).

The fascia covering the mammary gland is connected by suspensory ligaments to overlying skin and underlying muscle.
The mammary glands consist of 15–20 lobes and each lobe has a number of lobules.
The glandular tissue mainly consists of alveoli having secretory cells.
The secretions from these cells are poured by apocrine manner and by exocytosis into the ducts (lactiferous ducts). About 15–20 ducts open at the summit of the nipple, and just before the opening, lactiferous ducts show a dilatation called lactiferous sinus.
The smaller ductules are lined by single layer of columnar epithelial cells, whereas large ducts are lined by one or two layers of cells and near the opening at the nipple, these are lined by squamous cells.
Around the alveoli, ductules and lobules are present in myoepithelial cells (Fig. 9.5.2). They squeeze the contents and pour their secretions into the ductules.
Electron microscopically, the secretory cells contain both rough and smooth surface endoplasmic reticulum, numerous mitochondria, prominent Golgi apparatus and lysosomes. The proteins are present in the cytoplasm as membrane-bound vesicles and fat is stored as large globules.

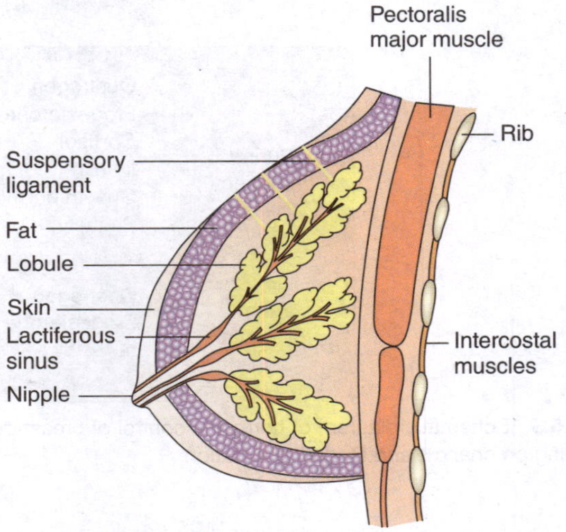

Fig. 9.5.2 Structure of mammary gland.

CONTROL OF BREAST DEVELOPMENT AND GROWTH

Various hormones necessary for full growth and development of mammary glands at various stages are given next (Fig. 9.5.3).

1. Oestrogen It is primarily responsible for ductal growth and fat deposition. It also causes thickening of nipples.

2. Progesterone The development of glandular tissue mainly depends on progesterone. Both oestrogen and progesterone work best with cooperation of the hypothalamopituitary–adrenal cortex axis.

3. Other hormones Other hormones including growth hormone, thyroxine, cortisol and insulin enhance overall growth and development of mammary glands at all stages.

4. Corpus luteal and placental hormones Corpus luteal and placental hormones, particularly oestrogen, progesterone and

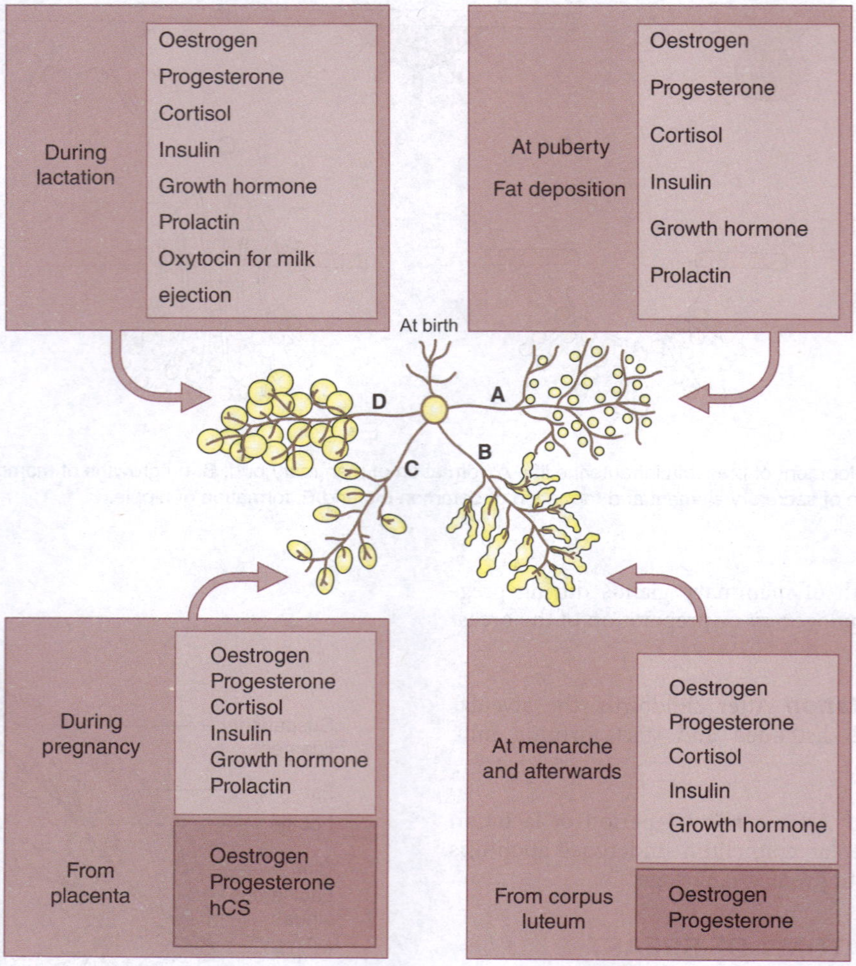

Fig. 9.5.3 Schematic diagram of hormonal control of breast development during different stages: **A**, at puberty; **B**, at menarche and afterwards; **C**, during pregnancy; and **D**, during lactation.

human chorionic somatomammotropic (hCS, or hPL) hormone, are essential for further growth of the breast during pregnancy.

5. Prolactin It is another very important hormone for development of breasts during pregnancy and lactation. It acts on mammary gland tissue which has already grown under the influence of oestrogen and progesterone. It needs to be discussed in detail.

HUMAN PROLACTIN

Structure, Secretion and Plasma Concentration

Structure and secretion Human prolactin is a single peptide chain, secreted by acidophilic cells of the anterior pituitary gland.

Plasma concentration The prolactin secretion is pulsatile, and shows diurnal variations (secretion increases about 1 hour after the onset of sleep and continues throughout the sleep period). Its basal average value varies in different conditions (Table 9.5.1).

During pregnancy, prolactin secretion starts rising from the eighth week onwards and the peak value (200–400 ng/mL) is reached at term. The sources of prolactin during pregnancy are the placenta, amniotic fluid and maternal anterior pituitary gland. The prolactin secretion during pregnancy and during lactation is affected by *oestrogen*. Prolactin secretion parallels with secretion of oestrogen, i.e. seventh to eighth weeks of gestation onwards, prolactin secretion rises along with oestrogen (Fig. 9.4.7). This is due to oestrogen inhibition of hypothalamic prolactin inhibitory factor (PIF) (Fig. 9.5.4).

Table 9.5.1 Range of plasma concentration of prolactin

Condition	Plasma concentration (ng/mL)
• Prepubertal period and after menopause	2–8
• Fertile period (16–45 years)	9–14
• Early pregnancy (8 weeks)	10–25
• Late pregnancy (at term)	200–500
• Lactation period	
• Immediately after birth to 10 days	200–400
• 10–90 days (first week to 3 months)	70–200
• 90–180 days (3–6 months)	100–250
• 6 months to 1 year	30–40

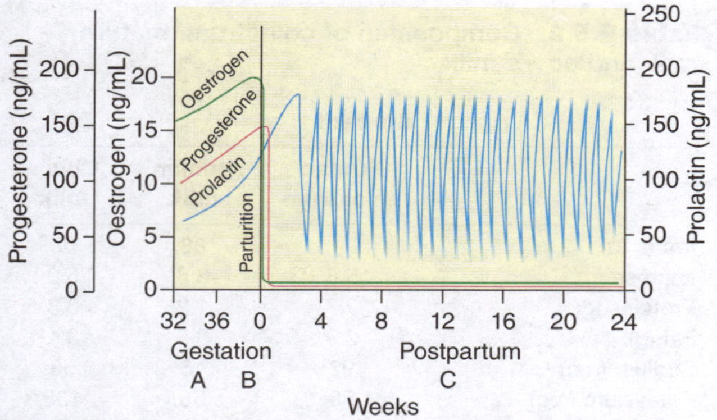

Fig. 9.5.4 Changes in rate of secretion of oestrogen, progesterone and prolactin: **A**, in late pregnancy; **B**, before parturition; and **C**, during postpartum period.

Control of Prolactin Secretion

Hypothalamic control Secretion of prolactin from the anterior pituitary is controlled by the hypothalamus. A PIF formed in the arcuate nucleus of the hypothalamus is transported through the hypothalamohypophyseal portal system to the anterior pituitary where it checks the synthesis and release of prolactin.

PIF has been identified as dopamine. Therefore, the substances like dopamine agonists (bromocriptine) and serotonin antagonists block the secretion of prolactin. Therapeutically, bromocriptine is used during postpartum period for reducing prolactin level to inhibit lactation.

Factors enhancing the release of prolactin:

Thyrotropin-releasing hormone (TRH): There is prolactin-releasing factor for prolactin, but TRH also causes release of prolactin from the anterior pituitary.

Stress: Psychological stress, physiological stress (exercise, pregnancy and lactation) and pathological stress increase prolactin secretion.

Substances like dopamine antagonists (phenothiazine and tranquilizers), adrenergic blockers and serotonin agonists stimulate prolactin release.

Oxytocin: Oxytocin acts directly on the acidophilic cells of the anterior pituitary to stimulate prolactin release.

Sectioning of pituitary stalk or lesion which interferes with pituitary portal circulation also increases prolactin secretion (because secretion is tonically inhibited by hypothalamus).

Factors that decrease the release of prolactin are dopamine agonists.

Physiological Effects of Prolactin

1. Breast growth During pregnancy, it increases the breast growth particularly of alveolar tissue in the form of alveolar distension, dilatation of mammary vessels and formation of new capillaries.

2. Lactogenic effect Prolactin acts on the alveolar epithelium and stimulates the secretory activity. For lactogenic effect, prolactin acts by two ways:

- Directly by attaching on the surface of the alveolar epithelial cells
- By binding onto the receptors on the membrane of epithelial cells

During pregnancy, the lactogenic effect is suppressed by high concentration of oestrogen and progesterone. The exact mechanism involved in suppressing the lactogenic effect is not known but it occurs probably by inhibiting the binding of prolactin to its receptors and onto the surface of the cell or by inhibiting the translocation of prolactin into the nucleus of the cell.

After parturition, the lactogenic effect of prolactin is enhanced because of the following reasons:

- The inhibitory factors are withdrawn.
- Oxytocin level is increased.

Important Note

After parturition when the women do not wish to feed their babies or when the baby dies immediately after birth, oestrogen is administered to stop lactation.

3. Suppression of ovarian cycle in nursing mothers Prolactin inhibits the secretion of gonadotropin-releasing hormone from the hypothalamus. Therefore, gonadotropin (FSH and LH) secretion from the anterior pituitary also decreases. Thus, in nursing mothers, due to low levels of gonadotropins, the ovarian cyclic changes do not occur.

Applied Aspects

Chiari–Frommel syndrome: Although this is a rare condition, it is associated with: (i) persistence of lactation (galactorrhoea) and (ii) amenorrhoea in women who do not nurse their babies after delivery. Sometimes it is also associated with genital atrophy. The reason is persistent release of prolactin causing suppression of FSH and LH.

Galactorrhoea refers to secretion of breast milk in states not associated with nursing. It occurs due to hyperprolactinaemia or hypersensitivity of the breast to normal circulating levels of prolactin. The common causes of hyperprolactinaemia are as follows:

- Some antipsychotic drugs
- Antihypertensive drugs
- Certain antiemetic drugs
- Analgesics
- Medication interfering with dopamine action
- Hyperthyroidism

Treatment: Galactorrhoea can be suppressed by the use of dopamine agonist.

Chromophobe cell tumour of the pituitary gland is characterized by galactorrhoea and high level of prolactin in non-pregnant women.

Signs and symptoms of hyperprolactinaemia are as follows:

- Milky discharge from the nipples
- Irregular menstruation
- Infertility
- Vaginal dryness
- Mood disturbances

Diagnosis is based on the blood tests and imaging.

Treatment: The most common treatment for prolactinomas is medication which can shrink the tumour and regulate prolactin levels. The commonly used medication is bromocriptine (dopamine agonist). If medication is not effective, then surgical removal of prolactinoma is performed.

PHYSIOLOGY OF LACTATION

PHASES OF LACTATION

The physiology of lactation can be divided into four phases:

- Preparation of the breast for milk secretion (mammogenesis)
- Synthesis and secretion of milk (lactogenesis)
- Expulsion of milk (galactokinesis)
- Maintenance of lactation (galactopoiesis)

Mammogenesis

During pregnancy: The breast develops fully and is prepared for milk secretion after delivery (see page 849).

Lactogenesis

Stages of Lactogenesis

The process of milk secretion occurs in two stages.

Stage I In later few weeks of pregnancy, a small amount of fluid is secreted in the alveolar cells. It is called colostrum. Its rate of secretion is only 1/100th that of milk secretion in the postpartum period. Its composition is the same as that of human milk except that fats are absent. The stage I secretion occurs due to high plasma levels of prolactin and placental hCS. But due to suppressive lactogenic action of oestrogen and progesterone, free flow of milk never occurs during pregnancy (Fig. 9.5.4).

Stage II It is the initiation of lactation after childbirth. Immediately after the baby is born, sudden loss of oestrogen and progesterone secretion by the placenta allows the lactogenic effect of prolactin. In this stage:

- The secretion rate increases to 500–750 mL/day.
- In the next 1–7 days, the breasts begin to secrete milk instead of colostrum.

Human milk

Types of human milk It is the secretion of mammary glands. Its nature and composition vary with the postpartum period. Therefore, the human milk is of three types – colostrum, transition milk and mature milk.

1. ***Colostrum*** is a deep yellow-coloured fluid secreted by the mammary glands during the first few days of the postpartum period; it contains:
   - High protein contents (8.5 g%), rich in immunoglobulins and lactoferrin
   - Granular bodies (colostrum corpuscles) – consisting of alveolar cells and leucocytes loaded with fats

   The colostrum is easily coagulated into solid masses.
2. ***Transition milk or intermediate milk:*** It is secreted from the 6th to the 15th day of the postpartum period. The nature and composition of the secretion changes from colostrum to mature milk. Hence, it is called transition milk.
3. ***Mature milk*** is formed from the 15th day of postpartum onwards and continues during the whole lactation period (7–9 months).

Composition of human milk Human milk contains 88.5% water and about 11.5% solids. The solids include both organic and inorganic constituents. The composition of mature human milk, colostrum and cow's milk is shown in Table 9.5.2.

Table 9.5.2 Composition of colostrum, mature milk and cow's milk

Content	Human colostrum	Human milk	Cow's milk
Water (g)	–	88	88
Lactose (g)	5.3	6.8	5.0
Proteins (g)	2.7	1.2	3.3
Fat (g)	2.9	3.8	3.1
Sodium (mg)	92	15	58
Potassium (mg)	55	55	138
Chloride (mg)	117	43	103
Calcium (mg)	31	33	125
Magnesium (mg)	4	4	12
Phosphorus (mg)	14	15	100
Vitamin A (μg)	89	53	34
Thiamine (μg)	15	16	42
Riboflavin (μg)	30	43	157
Nicotinic acid (μg)	75	172	85
Ascorbic acid (mg)	4.4	4.3	1.6

Note: Human milk is balanced diet as it contains first-class proteins (caseinogen and lactalbumin), carbohydrates, fat, mineral salts and vitamins. Therefore, it is an ideal food for the baby.

Formation of milk During lactation, the mammary glands are metabolically very active. The milk-specific substances amino acids, fatty acids, glucose, Ca^{2+}, etc., are derived from plasma into the alveolar cells. The various secretory processes involved in milk synthesis include: (i) fat synthesis and its secretion, (ii) ion and water secretion, (iii) transcytosis of immunoglobulins and other substances from interstitial spaces, and (iv) exocytosis. The hormones like growth hormone, thyroid hormone, parathyroid hormone, insulin and cortisol of the mother increase the capacity of the breast to secrete milk by providing necessary raw materials.

Expulsion of Milk or Galactokinesis

Although milk is secreted continuously into the alveoli of the breast, it does not flow continuously from the alveoli into the duct system. It depends on the suckling reflex and some local mechanisms acting within the breast.

Suckling Reflex

It is a neuroendocrinal reflex. The characteristic features and mechanism of suckling reflex (Fig. 9.5.5) are as follows.

- When the baby suckles, the sensory nerve endings or receptors located in the skin of the areola and nipple get stimulated.
- The sensory impulses are transmitted to the hypothalamus through somatic nerves (from the nipple and areola to the spinal cord and then to the hypothalamus). The activation of the hypothalamus causes release of oxytocin and prolactin from the pituitary gland.
- The oxytocin is carried to the breasts through blood, where it causes contraction of myoepithelial cells that surround the outer wall of the alveoli; thereby, the milk is expressed from alveoli into the ducts at a pressure 10–20 mm Hg. It is also aided by positive pressure applied by the baby by

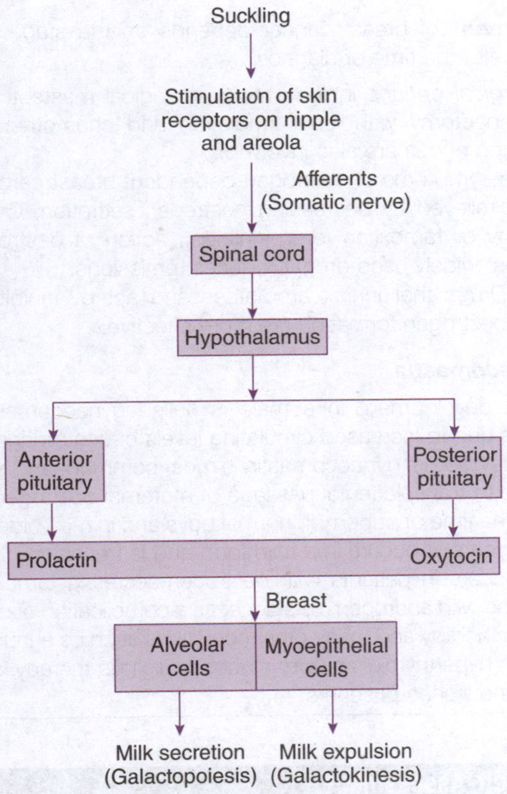

Fig. 9.5.5 Mechanism of suckling reflex.

making an airtight connection around the nipple and then blowing his/her cheeks. Therefore, when the baby suckles first, he/she virtually receives no milk; then within 30 seconds to 1 minute, suckling becomes effective and milk begins to flow. This process is called *milk ejection* or *milk expulsion* or *milk let-down*.

Important Note

- Another important observation is that suckling of one breast causes milk flow in the other breast also.
- Stimuli such as sight, sound or crying and thought of their infants also cause milk ejection, indicating the psychological component in the neuroendocrine reflex.
- Engorgement of breasts is a very painful condition that occurs after delivery. In this situation, suckling becomes difficult, so oxytocin administration leads to free flow of the milk.

Applied Aspects

Inhibition of Milk Ejection

Many psychogenic factors in the form of psychological stress, pain, etc., inhibit milk ejection by inhibiting oxytocin release.

- Alcohol is also a potent inhibitor of oxytocin.

Maintenance of Milk Secretion or Galactopoiesis

Maintenance of milk secretion or galactopoiesis depends on the surge in prolactin secretion. After few weeks of childbirth, prolactin level falls to its basal value; however, in nursing mothers, neuroendocrine reflex causes 10- to 20-fold surge in prolactin secretion that lasts for 1 hour (Fig. 9.5.4). Each time when the baby suckles, the impulses from the nipple and areolar receptors are transmitted by somatic nerves up to the hypothalamus, which cause 1- to 20-fold surge in prolactin secretion.

The amount of milk production is related to the infant's demand.

IMPORTANCE OF LACTATION

Breastfeeding is being advocated all over the world because of its advantages both for the baby and for the mother.

Advantages of Breastfeeding to the Baby

1. Balanced diet Human milk contains proteins, carbohydrates, fat, mineral salts (calcium and phosphorus) and vitamins. So, it is a natural balanced food for the newborn.

2. Protection against infections Human milk has high count of lymphocytes, neutrophils and macrophages and high content of lysozymes and immunoglobulins. All these substances due to anti-infection property confer nonspecific as well as specific immunity.

3. Easily digestible Human milk because of its following digestive properties can be easily digested by the newborn babies:

- Casein is easily digestible.
- Lactoferrin prevents iron overloading.
- Folate- and cobalamin-binding proteins assist in absorption of corresponding vitamins.
- Higher concentration of lactose promotes calcium absorption.
- Lipases assist in lipid digestion, because lipid digestion is poor in newborn babies.

4. Growth factors Growth-promoting factors, like epidermal growth factor, insulin and somatomedin-C, are present in the human milk.

5. Other advantages of breastfeeding Other advantages of breastfeeding to the baby are as follows:

- It is sterile.
- It is convenient to give at right temperature.
- It is inexpensive.
- Chances of allergy to breast milk are rare.

Psychological effects of breastfeeding in children are as follows:

- It provides skin-to-skin contact between the mother and the infant.
- It encourages early mother–child social exchange.
- It triggers the suckling reflex in the baby early.
- It calms the infant easily.

For the above-mentioned reasons, kangaroo mother care (KMC) is recommended.

KMC method involves the baby being carried by the mother for skin-to-skin contact, especially a newborn baby with low birth weight or born preterm. The benefits of KMC are both ways, to the mother and to the newborn.

- The mother makes more milk and has a better chance of breastfeeding.

- The baby stays warm and his/her body temperature is maintained properly.
- The baby's vital signs (heart rate and breathing) improve.
- The baby gains weight and has improved sleep.
- The baby cries less and has a lower stress level.

Advantages of Breastfeeding to the Mother

1. Lactational amenorrhoea Due to high plasma level of prolactin during lactation, there occurs suppression of FSH and LH. Therefore, after birth of the baby, menstruation and ovulation do not start. The period of lactational amenorrhoea is variable (3 months to 3 years). This is the natural way of contraception and birth spacing.

2. Involution of uterus The oxytocin released during each session of breastfeeding also acts on the uterine myometrium, and helps it to involute during the postpartum period. The proper involution of the uterus protects it against infections.

3. Protection against breast engorgement Breastfeeding does not allow the milk to stagnate, thus preventing the breast engorgement, which is a highly painful condition. The stagnant milk acts as a favourable medium for bacterial growth. Therefore, breastfeeding protects against infection.

4. Protection against obesity Body fat is used for milk synthesis; therefore, there are less chances of becoming obese after pregnancy.

5. Emotional bonding Emotional bonding and psychological satisfaction are enhanced by breastfeeding.

6. Protection against cancer The chances of breast cancer are more in those women who have never borne children. This is related to the hormone oestrogen which is responsible for aetiology of breast cancer. Therefore, prolonged lactation provides protection against breast cancer.

Psychological factors affecting breastfeeding. The main psychological factors that affect breastfeeding include:

- Postnatal depression
- Stress
- Breastfeeding intention
- Mental outlook towards the breastfeeding process
- Social approval

Applied Aspects

Hormones and Carcinoma Breast

Breast Cancer

Breast cancer is the most common malignancy in women. About 35% of carcinomas of the breast are oestrogen-dependent. The risk of breast cancer is higher in prolonged ovarian hormonal exposure in the form of postmenopausal hormonal replacement therapy.

- About 10% of breast cancer is familial, and occurs due to mutation involving BRCA-1 and BRCA-2 tumour suppressor genes.
- In nonfamilial breast cancers, molecular studies have identified abnormalities that involve oncogenes, ERBBZ and c-myc, the tumour suppressor gene TP53 and telomerase.
- Environmental factors include delayed childbearing among better educated women, alcohol intake and smoking.

Treatment of breast cancer depends on the stage of the disease at the time of diagnosis.

- *Surgical options* include modified radical mastectomy or lumpectomy with local irradiation and chemotherapy (if lymph nodes are also involved).
- The symptoms of oestrogen-dependent breast carcinoma are relieved by decreasing oestrogen secretion. Ovariectomy or tamoxifen (drug-inhibiting action of oestrogen – most widely used drug) produces remissions.
  - *Drugs* that inhibit aromatase and act by inhibition of oestrogen formation are more effective.

Gynaecomastia

Breast development in a male is called gynaecomastia. It occurs due to increased circulating levels of oestrogens.

- In newborns, gynaecomastia is most common, and occurs due to transplacental passage of maternal oestrogens.
- At the time of puberty in normal boys and in men older than 50 years, it occurs in a mild form and is transient.
- It occurs in patients with oestrogen-secreting tumours, in those with androgen resistance, as a complication of oestrogen therapy and many other conditions such as eunuchoidism, hyperthyroidism, liver cirrhosis, digitalis therapy, and in malnourished prisoners.

Self-Assessment

Q1. Discuss the hormonal control of mammary glands.
Q2. Discuss the regulation of different phases of lactation.
Q3. Write notes on the following:
- Suckling reflex
- Galactorrhoea
- Importance of breastfeeding
- Significance of kangaroo mother care

Clinical Cases

Case 1

A 28-year-old woman married for the last 5 years visited a gynaecologist for milky discharge from the nipples, irregular periods, discomfort during sex and not conceiving. The personal history of the patient revealed that she was stressed and very apprehensive. Physical and gynaecological examinations were normal. Blood tests and MRI of the brain showed:

- High levels of prolactin
- Low levels of LH and FSH
- Growth in the pituitary region

On these findings, it was suspected a case of prolactinoma.
Q1. What are the causes of high prolactin?
Q2. What is the pathophysiology related to signs and symptoms in this case?

Case 2

A 40-year-old female was suffering with breast cancer. Before starting the treatment, the oncologist advised tests to know the type and cause of cancer and it was concluded as oestrogen-dependent breast cancer.
Q1. What is the pathophysiology of high oestrogen level related to breast cancer?
Q2. What are other causes of breast cancer?
Q3. What is the treatment plan for this case?

Physiology of Contraception

9.6

CHAPTER OUTLINE

INTRODUCTION

Aims of contraception: Contraception refers to prevention of pregnancy. The aims of contraception are as follows:

- The main aim of contraception is family planning to check the enormous increase in population growth, which is the root cause of socioeconomic problems of poor and developing countries, like India.
- Certain contraceptive measures are important to prevent the sexually transmitted diseases like AIDS.
- Contraceptives are also recommended on medical grounds to control the stress of pregnancy, labour and lactation in women suffering from heart diseases, etc.

Methods of contraceptions can be broadly grouped as:

- Spacing methods
- Terminal methods

Both types of contraceptive measures are available for use by females as well as by males; therefore, these can be described as:

- Contraceptive methods in females
- Contraceptive methods in males

CONTRACEPTIVE METHODS IN FEMALES

SPACING METHODS

The spacing methods increase the gap between two pregnancies. These include:

- Rhythm method
- Barrier methods
- Chemical methods
- Intrauterine contraceptive devices (IUCDs)

Rhythm Method

Rhythm method is also known as *calendar method* or *safe period method* or natural method. This method of contraception depends on the time of ovulation. In a woman having a regular menstrual cycle, ovulation occurs on the 14th day of the cycle. After ovulation, ovum remains viable for 48–72 hours. Similarly, after ejaculation, sperms remain alive for 24–48 hours. Thus, pregnancy occurs only if coitus is performed during this period. This is the period of high fertility and is called *dangerous period*.

Therefore, to avoid pregnancy, intercourse should be avoided in the dangerous period. Rest of the cycle, i.e. 5–6 days after bleeding phase of menstrual cycle and 5–6 days before the next cycle, is the *safe period* (period of least fertility). This method of contraception is successful only if menstrual cycles are regular and the woman knows the exact time of ovulation by keeping a record of basal body temperature.

Disadvantage of this method is that it is the most unreliable method when the menstrual cycles are irregular and time of ovulation is variable.

Barrier Methods

Barrier methods of contraception prevent the meeting of ovum and sperms after coitus. These include:

- Mechanical barriers
- Chemical barriers
- Combined (mechanical and chemical barriers)

1. Mechanical barriers Mechanical barriers used as contraceptive are diaphragm and cervical caps.

Diaphragm: It consists of a flexible rim, made up of a spring to which is attached a cup-shaped synthetic rubber or plastic (Fig. 9.6.1A). The diaphragm is available in different sizes. It is inserted into the vagina over the cervix.

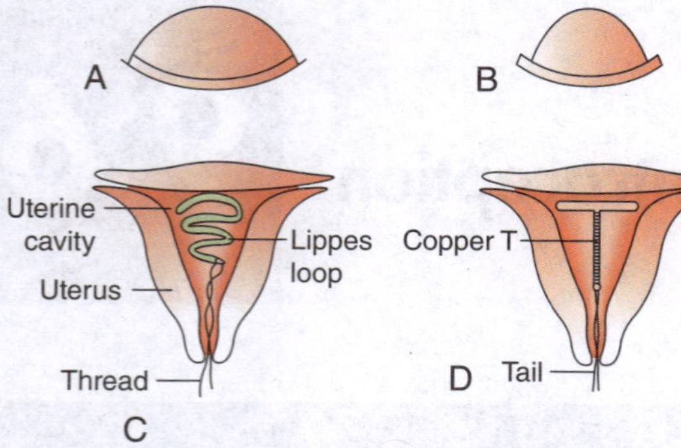

Fig. 9.6.1 Female contraceptive devices: **A**, vaginal diaphragm; **B**, cervical cap; **C**, Lippes loop; and **D**, copper T.

Cervical cap: It is smaller as compared with a diaphragm (Fig. 9.6.1B) and is applied onto the cervix itself.
Note: For proper use of mechanical barriers, some spermicidal cream or jelly should be applied in the centre of the device.
Advantages: These devices are inexpensive and usually do not require any medical consultation.
Disadvantages of mechanical barriers include:

- Demonstration by a trained person is needed for the proper use.
- Failures are quite common because chances of displacement of the device are very high.
- Some women get cervicitis (inflammation of the cervix) and local irritation.

2. Chemical barriers Chemical barriers refer to spermicidal agents which can destroy the sperms when applied in the female genital tract before coitus. The common spermicidal agents used are as follows:

- Ricinoleic acid (oldest)
- Nanoxynol-9
- Octoxynol-3

These spermicidal agents are available in various forms such as foam tablets, pastes, creams, jellies and vaginal sponges. Vaginal sponge is a polyurethane sponge impregnated with nanoxynol-9. It is available by the trade name 'TODAY'.

Advantages: Chemical barriers are inexpensive, are well tolerated and provide good protection.
Disadvantages are that the chemical barriers cause *messiness* and also sometimes may lead to *local irritation* and burning sensation.

3. Combined methods As mentioned above, mechanical barriers (diaphragm and cervical caps) along with spermicidal agents give good protection.

Chemical Methods

Chemical methods for contraceptions are used in various forms like locally applied chemicals (in the form of cream, jellies, etc.) and taken as drugs (orally or in injectable form or as implants). The drugs are further of two types – steroidal drugs (oestrogen and progesterone) and nonsteroidal drugs.

I. Steroidal Drugs

A. Oral contraceptives Oral contraceptives are the most widely used contraceptive measure by the women all over the globe. These are recommended in women of younger age group (up to 35 years).

Mechanism of action: In general, oral contraceptives contain synthetic preparation of oestrogen and progesterone and when taken orally, the plasma concentration of these hormones rises. The raised levels of these hormones by their negative feedback effect act on the anterior pituitary to inhibit the release of gonadotropins (FSH and LH) and thus inhibit ovulation.
Types of pills: The oral contraceptives are available in different types of pills:

- Combined pill (classical pill)
- Sequential pill
- Minipill
- Postcoital (morning-after) pill

1. Combined pill or classical pill It contains both oestrogen and progesterone. Oestrogen (20–50 μg) in combined pills is usually *ethyloestradiol* or mestranol (methoxy derivative of ethyloestradiol) and progesterone (0.5–2 mg) like norethisterone, norgestrel or levonorgestrel.

Availability The combined pills are available under two brand names: **Mala-N** (packet of 21 tablets) and **Mala-D** (packet of 28 pills, out of which 21 are white coloured of hormones and 7 are brown coloured containing *ferrous fumarate*).

Dosage The combined pills are taken orally every day at a fixed time (preferably at night before going to bed) for 21 days, starting from the 5th day of menstrual cycle to the 25th day followed by a gap of 7 days in case of Mala-N. During this gap period, bleeding occurs. This bleeding is not a menstrual bleeding as it occurs due to withdrawal of the hormones; therefore, it is called *withdrawal bleeding*.

Mechanism of action Combined pill acts by three ways:

i. It prevents ovulation.
ii. It prevents implantation if ovulation occurs and ovum is fertilized by a sperm.
iii. It makes the cervical secretion thick and viscid and thus prevents entry of sperms in the female genital tract.

Note: In combined pills, these days, *phase regimens* (biphasic or triphasic) are preferred, because they are more physiological than fixed-dose preparations.

2. Sequential pill These pills contain a high dose of oestrogen along with a moderate dose of progesterone.

Dosage Only oestrogen is given starting from the 5th day of menstrual cycle to the 15th day and then followed by both (oestrogen + progesterone) for the next 5 days.
Note: Nowadays, the sequential pill is not used because of high incidence of *endometrial carcinoma*.

3. Minipill Minipill (progesterone only) or *micropill*.

Composition These preparations contain low doses of progesterone (norethisterone, 0.35 mg; or norgestrel, 0.075 mg).

Dosage The regimen of these pills is that the pill should be taken daily through whole of menstrual cycle.

Mechanism of action Minipill prevents fertility without inhibiting ovulation. It acts on cervical mucosa (makes it thick), and also decreases motility of fallopian tubes.

4. Postcoital pill (morning-after pill) As the name indicates, it is recommended within 72 hours of the unprotected intercourse.

Dosage Double dose of combined pill (two pills) should be taken immediately followed by another double dose (two pills) after 12 hours.

Indications This method of contraception should be used only in emergency cases like rape, contraceptive failure and unprotected sex.

Mechanism of action Possible mechanisms involved are as follows:

- It causes hypermotility of the fallopian tubes and of the uterus and thus prevents fertilization and implantation.
- If ovulation and fertilization have occurred, then it prevents implantation of the blastocyst.

Disadvantages This method of contraception is not practised routinely because of various side effects like nausea and vomiting.

Advantages and Disadvantages of Oral Contraceptives

Advantages Oral contraceptives have 100% effectivity.

Disadvantages Although oral contraceptives are extensively used, their prolonged use leads to certain adverse effects such as:

- Hypertension
- Risk of thromboembolism
- Metabolic effects like diabetes and obesity
- Carcinogenic effects (carcinoma breast and carcinoma cervix)

Contraindications There are two types of contraindications:

Absolute contraindications for the use of oral contraceptives are as follows:
- Woman having carcinoma of the breast or of the uterus
- Liver diseases
- Hyperlipidaemia

Relative contraindications: Oral contraceptive should not be given to women older than 35 years.

B. Depot preparations Depot preparations are long-acting drugs and are highly effective. These are available in three forms:

- Injectable preparations
- Subdermal implants
- Vaginal rings

1. Injectable preparations Injectable preparations are oily solutions injected intramuscularly. They are of the following types:

i. ***Oily progestin preparations:*** These are available as:
   - *Medroxyprogesterone acetate (DMPA)* is injected intramuscularly every 3–6 months. Its dose is 150–400 mg.
   - *Norethindrone enanthate (NET-EN)* is injected intramuscularly every 3 months. Its dose is 200 mg.

   Note: These preparations should be injected in the first 5 days of menstrual cycle (bleeding phase) to rule out pregnancy.

ii. ***Combined injectable preparations:*** These preparations contain both oestrogen and progesterone. These are given intramuscularly at monthly interval.

   Mechanism of action: These preparations prevent ovulation and alter cervical mucosal secretions.

2. Subdermal implants The Population Council of New York has developed subdermal implants. These are of two types:

i. ***Norplant:*** It consists of six flexible silastic (made of silicon) tubes, each containing 35 mg progesterone (levonorgestrel).
ii. ***Norplant (R)2:*** It consists of two rods of levonorgestrel.

The subdermal implants are implanted beneath the skin of the arm or forearm. Effective contraception is achieved within 24 hours and lasts for 5–6 years.

3. Vaginal rings Vaginal rings containing norgestrel are implanted intravaginally. The progesterone is absorbed slowly through vaginal mucosa.

Advantages and disadvantages of depot preparations

Advantages As depot preparations are long-acting drugs, to avoid daily intake of oral pill, these preparations are preferred, and also:

- The contraceptive effectivity lasts for a longer period.

Disadvantages Disadvantages of depot preparation are that sometimes they lead to sterility and alterations in menstrual bleeding pattern.

II. Nonsteroidal Contraceptive Drugs

Centchroman It is a nonsteroidal oral contraceptive drug developed by the Central Drug Research Institute (CDRI), Lucknow. It is marketed under the trade name ***Saheli***.

Dose is 30 mg twice in a week for 12 weeks followed by once in a week.

Mechanism of action: It causes:
- Suppression of corpus luteum functions
- Interference with motility of fallopian tubes

Both these effects interfere with implantation.

Advantages of the use of centchroman are as follows:
- Menstrual cycle remains normal.
- There is complete reversibility on its withdrawal.

Intrauterine Contraceptive Devices

IUCDs are inserted into the uterine cavity for long-term contraception. The devices are usually made up of inert materials like plastic, polythene and metal.

Types of IUCDs

Basically, two types of intrauterine devices are available – nonmedicated and medicated.

a. Nonmedicated IUCDs: These are also known as *first-generation IUCDs*. Lippes loop is included in this category.

Lippes loop (Fig. 9.6.1C): It is a serpentine or S-shaped device made up of plastic to which is attached a fine nylon tail. The plastic used is nontoxic and nontissue reactive. A small amount of *barium sulphate* is also present in the plastic material to allow its radiographic observation. Lippes loop is available in different sizes.

b. Medicated IUCDs:
These are of two types:

Second-generation IUCDs: These are made up of metal (copper). The copper ions are released slowly and have a strong antifertility effect. This group includes:

- Copper T-200
- Copper T
- Some variants of copper T
- Newer devices like NOVA-7, NOVA-T and multiload devices

Third-generation IUCDs: These are hormone-releasing intrauterine devices. These are filled with progesterone (progesterone reservoir) which is released continuously for 1 year.

Copper T: Copper T is the most commonly used IUCD in India. As the name indicates, it is made up of copper and its shape resembles the letter T. Like Lippes loop, it is also attached with a nylon thread (tail) (Fig. 9.6.1D).

Insertion: Copper T can be inserted into the uterus with the help of a plunger (inserter) any time during a woman's reproductive period except during pregnancy. The most ideal time for its insertion is during menstruation or within 10 days of the beginning of menstruation, because the diameter of the cervical cavity at this time is greater. It can also be inserted during the first week after the delivery.

Ideal candidate for IUCDs is the one who:

- Has borne one child
- Has a normal menstrual cycle
- Has no pelvic inflammation
- Is ready to check the tail of the device

Mechanism of action: Copper T acts by the following ways:

- It *prevents implantation* and growth of fertilized ovum by evoking aseptic inflammation and thus making the endometrium unsuitable for implantation.
- *Sperm phagocytization:* During aseptic inflammatory reaction, a large number of neutrophils, macrophages and leucocytes migrate. The sperms get phagocytosed by these cells.
- Copper ions also affect the enzymes of the endometrium, sperm motility and its capacitation.
- IUCDs filled with progesterone alter the mucous composition of the cervix and make it thick and viscid and thus prevent the entry of sperm through the cervical canal.

Advantages, Disadvantages and Contraindications of IUCDs

Advantages Advantages of IUCDs are as follows:

- This method of contraception is quite safe, effective and reversible. IUCDs can be easily pulled out or removed when contraception is not required.
- It provides long-term contraception without adverse effects.

Disadvantages Disadvantages of IUCDs are as follows:

- In some cases, they may cause heavy bleeding.
- The IUCD may come out accidentally when not inserted properly.
- Risks of ectopic pregnancy are present.

Contraindications The use of IUCD is contraindicated in the following conditions:

- In case of suspected pregnancy
- In women having pelvic inflammation
- In case of heavy bleeding during menstruation
- In case of women suffering from carcinoma cervix

TERMINAL METHODS

Terminal method of contraception means permanent sterilization, which can be achieved either surgically or laparoscopically. The methods given next have been employed.

Surgical Methods

1. Tubectomy Tubectomy is the permanent method of sterilization in females and is recommended only when the family is completed.

Procedure: In tubectomy operation, fallopian tubes are cut and then cut ends are ligated and buried as shown in Fig. 9.6.2.

2. Laparoscopic occlusion In this procedure, the fallopian tubes are occluded using silicon rubber bands, Falope rings or Hulka-Clemens clips. This method is much quicker and simple and hospitalization is not required.

Note: Although tubectomy is a permanent method of sterilization, if necessary, recanalization can be done using plastic tubes. The chances of successful canalization are only 55%.

Medical Termination of Pregnancy

Medical termination of pregnancy (MTP or abortion) is allowed under the MTP Act (1971). The MTP Act has laid down the following criteria:

- Conditions in which pregnancy can be terminated
- The person who can do termination
- The place where it should be performed

Indications Conditions in which pregnancy can be terminated are as follows:

- *Medical:* When continuation of pregnancy is hazardous to the mother
- *Eugenic:* When there is substantial risk to the child if born from that pregnancy
- *Humanitarian grounds:* When pregnancy is the result of rape
- *Failure of contraceptive measure*

Methods MTP is possible only in the first few months of pregnancy (from the seventh week to the beginning of the second trimester). The procedures given next have been employed depending on the duration of pregnancy.

1. Dilatation and curettage (D and C) In this procedure, the cervix is dilated with dilators and the implanted ovum is removed by doing curettage of the endometrium.

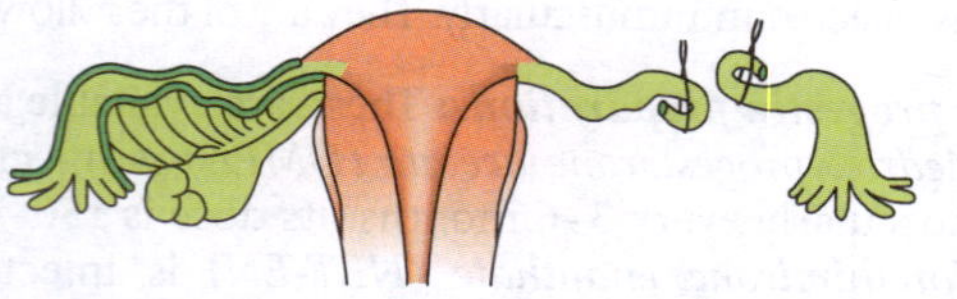

Fig. 9.6.2 Procedure of tubectomy (female sterilization).

2. Vacuum aspiration Like D and C, in this procedure, the cervix is dilated and then the implanted ovum is removed (aspirated) by applying suction. This method is employed only up to 12 weeks of gestation.

3. Administration of prostaglandins In this method, prostaglandins are administered into the vagina (intravaginally) which causes uterine contractions resulting in expulsion of the products of conception.

PREGNANCY VACCINES

Pregnancy vaccines are under experimental trial. These have not yet been tried in women. Two types of vaccines under considerations are as follows:

Active immunization** by **injecting β-subunit of hCG and tetanus toxoid: Tetanus toxoid increases the antigenicity capacity. The antibodies produced against β-hCG destroy hCG produced by syncytiotrophoblast cells of the fetus.

Vaccine against zona pellucida protein is also under trial.

CONTRACEPTIVE METHODS IN MALES

SPACING METHODS

The spacing methods of contraception used in males are as follows:

- Natural method
- Barrier method
- Chemical methods

Natural Method or Coitus Interruptus

It is the oldest method of voluntary fertility control. In this method, the male withdraws the penis before ejaculation into the vagina and tries to prevent deposition of semen into the vagina. This method needs practice and discipline. The failure rate is high because of the following reasons:

- Precoital secretions of the male may contain sperms and even a drop of semen is sufficient to cause pregnancy.
- Slightest mistake in timings of withdrawal may lead to deposition of a certain amount of semen.

Barrier Method

Condom: Condom is the most widely used barrier by the males all around the world. In India, it is known by its trade name *Nirodh* (Fig. 9.6.3). It consists of a fine latex sheath and is electronically tested. Various types of condoms available in the market are dry type, lubricated and deluxe.

Instructions: Instructions to be followed while using a condom are as follows:

- Condom should be worn on an erect penis before intercourse.
- Air must be expelled from the teat of the condom.

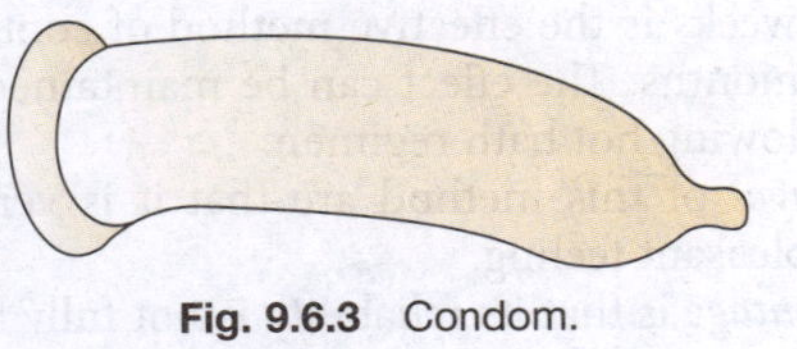

Fig. 9.6.3 Condom.

- It should be held carefully when withdrawing from the vagina to avoid spilling of semen in the vagina.
- A new condom should be used for each sexual act.

Mechanism of action Condom prevents deposition of semen into the vagina, thus does not allow the sperms and the ovum to meet.

Advantages

- They are easily available, safe and inexpensive.
- Their use does not require any medical supervision.
- They also provide protection against sexually transmitted diseases.

Disadvantages Disadvantages are as follows:

- It may slip off or tear off during coitus due to its incorrect use.
- It interferes with sexual sensations.

Chemical Methods

Antispermatogenic Drugs

Few drugs which inhibit spermatogenesis have been available. These include those given next.

1. Male pill (gossypol) Male pill contains gossypol, a phenolic derivative of cottonseed oil.

Dose: The recommended dose is 200 mg/day for 2 months and followed by 60 mg/week. The drug is taken by oral route.

Mechanism of action: Gossypol acts as an effective azoospermic agent. Its exact mechanism of action is not yet known. In 99.9% of cases, sperm count decreases to 4 million/mL.

Advantages: Male pill neither contains any hormone nor has antihormonal activity; therefore, there is no change in libido and potency of the male.

Disadvantages:

- Men may become permanently azoospermic after constant use for 6 months.
- It also has toxic effects.

2. Hormonal preparations Various hormonal preparations which can be used as contraceptive measures in males are as follows:

Testosterone: Testosterone (400 mg) when given orally produces azoospermia.

Testosterone with danazol (17α-ethyltestosterone): This preparation is better tolerated and is more effective.

Cyproterone acetate: Chemically, this drug is related to progesterone. It acts as a potent antiandrogenic agent. It produces oligospermia but also causes loss of libido.

3. Tripterygium wilfordii This is a special type of vine used in Chinese medicine. The extract from the Chinese herb contains many active compounds (triptolide, triptiolide, 16-hydroxytriplide and T7/19) which reduce the sperm count, but mechanism of action is not yet known.

4. Calcium channel blockers Calcium channel blockers (e.g. nifedipine) block the Ca^{2+} channels on the cell membrane of the sperms (see page 840), thus preventing the influx of Ca^{2+}. As a result, the sperm membrane becomes rigid and loaded with cholesterol. The rigid membrane of sperm prevents its binding to the zona pellucida of the ovum. Because of this effect, the patients who are suffering from hypertension and are on nifedipine treatment become sterile.

Terminal Methods

The permanent methods employed for sterilization in males are as follows:

- Vasectomy
- Vas occlusion using no-scalpel technique

1. Vasectomy Vasectomy is a simple operation in which about 1 cm piece of vas deferens is removed after clamping. Then both the ends are ligated and sutured so that they face away from each other (Fig. 9.6.4). This procedure reduces the risk of recanalization later on.

Mechanism of action: After vasectomy, sperm production and hormones are not affected but entry of the sperms into the semen is prevented.

Postoperative instructions: Subjects should be advised to follow certain instructions postoperatively. Immediately after vasectomy, he is not sterile because the sperms already formed are stored. After about 30 ejaculations, semen becomes free from sperms. Therefore, he must use a contraceptive measure (condom) postoperatively before he becomes azoospermic.

Advantages Advantages of vasectomy are that it is a simpler, faster and less expensive procedure and no hospitalization is required. It is 100% effective.

Disadvantages Disadvantages are as follows:

- *Failure rate* of vasectomy is only 0.15% and that too because of wrong identification of the vas.
- *Complications:* Few complications that may occur following vasectomy are as follows:
  - *Spontaneous* recanalization
  - Autoimmune response

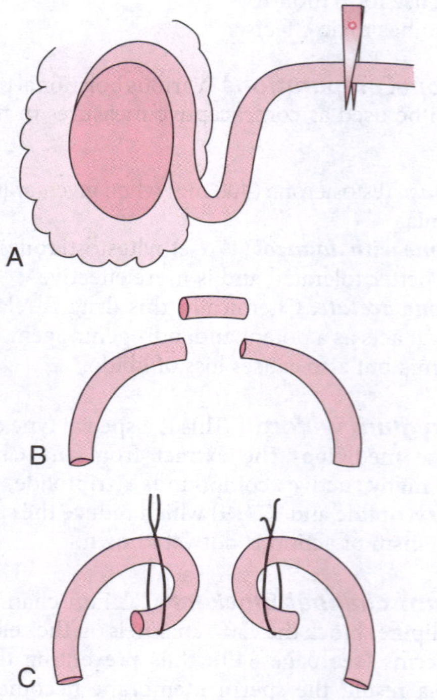

Fig. 9.6.4 Procedure of vasectomy (male sterilization).

- Psychological effects like diminution of sexual vigour, impotence and headache

2. No-scalpel vas occlusion No-scalpel vas occlusion is a newer technique, which is quite safe, convenient and acceptable to males.

Principle of occlusion An elastomer is injected into the vas deferens; it gets hardened in situ within 20 minutes and plugs the vas (occludes it).

Methods of vas occlusion The vas is occluded by using various types of materials:

- Elastomer plugs
- Shug
- Reversible inhibition of sperm under guidance (RISUG)

i. ***Elastomer plugs*** are of two types:
   - Medical grade polyurethane (MPU)
   - Medical grade silicon rubber (MSR)

   MPU and MSR are injected into the vas, which gets hardened within 25 minutes forming a plug which acts as a barrier for sperms.
   Advantages: It is an easy procedure and reversal is possible with 100% efficacy.

ii. ***Shug:*** It is a preformed, flexible silicon rubber plug which can be inserted into the vas deferens using no-scalpel technique.
   Advantages: It is a preformed plug; therefore, the effect is immediate as the time required for hardening of the material (as in MPU and MSR) is not wasted.

iii. ***RISUG*** is the latest technology. As the name indicates, it is a noninvasive and reversible technique. In this method, *styrene maleic anhydride* (SMA) is used. SMA is a copolymer when injected along with dimethyl sulphoxide into the vas deferens; it forms a coating along the inner wall of the vas deferens.
   Mechanism of action: SMA acts by three ways:
   - It blocks the lumen of the vas deferens.
   - Its pH is alkaline; therefore, it interferes with acidic pH of the sperms.
   - It ruptures the membrane of sperms and destroys them.

   Advantages: It can be easily removed by flushing the vas deferens with a *solvent* or by manually squeezing the vas deferens. RISUG has completed phase I and phase II trial stages. Therefore, it seems to be a method of male contraception with 100% efficacy, reversibility and safety.

MISCELLANEOUS METHODS

Miscellaneous methods of contraception which can be used in males are given next.

Thermal method It is based on the fact that sperms are destroyed by heat (above body temperature). Therefore, the following methods are employed:

i. ***Hot baths:*** Daily immersion of testes in hot water (46°C) for few weeks is the effective method of contraception for several months. The effect can be maintained by periodically following hot bath regimen.
   Advantages of this method are that it is very cheap and gives a pleasant feeling.
   Disadvantage is that its reliability is not fully known.

ii. ***Suspensories:*** Men are advised to wear a specifically fitted set of briefs (which hold the testes close to the body) during day time.

iii. ***Insulated scrotal sack:*** It consists of a heating element, a thermometer and a control unit (comprising power source and timer). The sack is worn on the waist. In this method, external heat is used for a short period. Reliability of this method has not yet been proved.

Self-Assessment

1. Discuss the contraceptive measures in females.
2. Discuss the methods of contraception in males.
3. Describe the following:
   - Mechanism of action of oral contraceptives
   - Medical termination of pregnancy
4. Write notes on the following:
   - Antispermatogenic drugs
   - Contraindications of IUCD
   - Vasectomy

Clinical Cases

Case 1

A 30-year-old female got copper T inserted 1 month after delivery. After 3 months, she is complaining of heavy bleeding during periods and abdominal pain. Examination revealed that the CuT has been properly inserted.

Q1. What are the side effects of CuT?
Q2. What are the contraindications of IUCDs?
Q3. How does CuT cause contraception?

Case 2

A 24-year-old newly married female consulted a gynaecologist for irregular periods, tenderness in the breast, nausea and mood irritability. History revealed that the woman was taking oral contraceptive pills.

Q1. What is reason for symptoms?
Q2. What are the disadvantages of oral contraceptives?
Q3. What are the contraindications?

NERVOUS SYSTEM

SECTION 10

SECTION OUTLINE

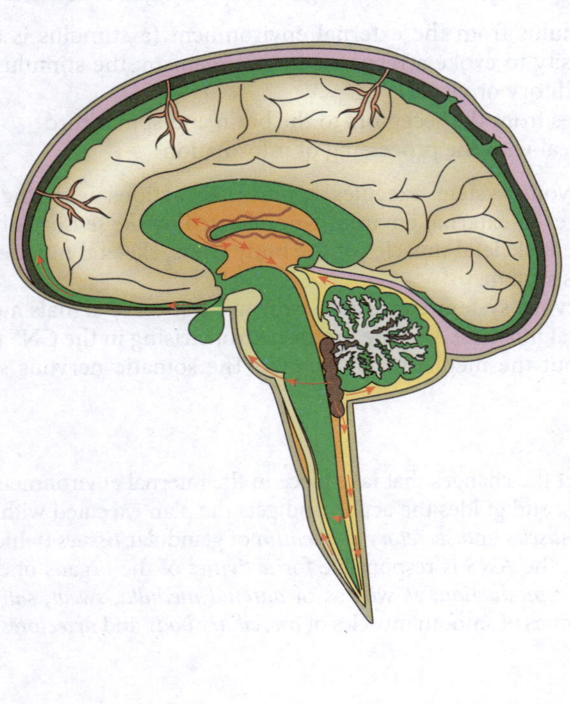

INTRODUCTION

ORGANIZATION OF NERVOUS SYSTEM

The nervous system, through sophisticated signalling, acts as a control network within the body. The specialized cells that constitute the functional units of the nervous system are called *neurons*. The neurons are responsible for the reception and response to changes in the internal and external environment. It is estimated that the human nervous system is composed of more than 100 billion neurons which are linked together in a highly intricate manner. Thus, the various parts of the nervous system are interconnected, but for convenience of description, the nervous system can be divided anatomically and functionally into different divisions.

ANATOMICAL DIVISIONS OF THE NERVOUS SYSTEM

The nervous system is broadly classified into two anatomical divisions – the central nervous system (CNS) and the peripheral nervous system (PNS).

1. **CNS**, which occupies the central axis of the body, includes the brain and spinal cord. The brain has three parts:
   - *Forebrain* that comprises telencephalon, i.e. central hemispheres (cerebrum) or anterior part of the forebrain, and diencephalon or posterior part of the forebrain (the upper two-thirds of diencephalon is called thalamus and the lower one-third is called hypothalamus)
   - *Midbrain* or mesencephalon
   - *Hindbrain* or rhombencephalon that comprises pons, medulla oblongata and cerebellum
2. **PNS** is the part of nervous system which lies outside the CNS. It consists of peripheral nerves and the ganglia associated with them. Peripheral nerves attached to the brain are called *cranial nerves* (12 pairs), and those attached with the spinal cord are called *spinal nerves* (31 pairs).

FUNCTIONAL DIVISIONS OF THE NERVOUS SYSTEM

Functionally, the nervous system can be divided into two parts:

- Somatic nervous system
- Autonomic nervous system (ANS)

Both somatic nervous system and ANS have two divisions:

- Sensory division (for collecting information)
- Motor division (for executing the action)

1. Somatic nervous system

Sensory division of the somatic nervous system collects the information about the changes that take place in the external environment and interprets the meaning of these changes. It consists of:

- *Sensory receptors* that receive stimulus from the external environment (a stimulus is a change of environment of sufficient intensity to evoke a response in an organism; the stimulus may be mechanical, chemical, thermal, auditory or visual)
- *Afferent neurons* that carry impulses from the receptors to the brain and spinal cord
- *Parts of the brains* that primarily deal with the processing of information

Motor division of the somatic nervous system executes appropriate actions with the help of skeletal muscles in response to changes in external environment detected by *the sensory* division. It also coordinates the actions of different skeletal muscles of the body. Thus, skeletal muscles are the *effector organs* of the somatic nervous system.

Motor division of the somatic nervous system consists of neurons that carry signals away from the brain and spinal cord to the skeletal muscles. A single motor neuron arising in the CNS traverses directly to the skeletal muscle without the mediation of ganglia. The somatic nervous system is under voluntary control.

2. Autonomic nervous system

The ANS collects the information about the changes that take place in the internal environment (i.e. internal viscera), interprets these changes, and guides the action and gets the plan executed with the help of smooth muscles of viscera, *cardiac muscles* and *secretory epithelium* of glandular *tissues* (which are effector organs of ANS). In other words, the ANS is responsible for *activities* of the organs of digestion, circulation, excretion, respiration and *reproduction*, as well as of *adrenal medulla*, *sweat*, *salivary* and *lacrimal glands*. It also controls the activities of smooth muscles of *iris*, *ciliary body* and *arrectores pilorum*.

The word autonomous is taken from the Greek words '*autos*' meaning self and '*nomos*' meaning control. Thus, ANS is an involuntary system.

Divisions of ANS: The ANS has two main divisions – sympathetic and parasympathetic, each having a central and a peripheral component.

- *Sympathetic division*, also called *thoracolumbar division*, consists of thoracic and lumbar chains of sympathetic ganglia.
- *Parasympathetic division*, also called *craniosacral division*, consists of the ganglia associated with cranial nerves III, VII, IX and X.

UNDERSTANDING THE NERVOUS SYSTEM

For the purpose of understanding, this section on nervous system has been divided into two subsections:

Subsection 10A

Physiological anatomy and functions of nervous system. This subsection deals with the anatomy and functions of various parts of the nervous system.

Subsection 10B

Neurophysiology. Neurophysiology or neurophysiological processes include the study of sensory, motor, autonomic and higher functions of the nervous system. Neurophysiology, though a very complex subject, primarily involves the following processes:

- *Reception of changes in internal and external environment.* It is a function of receptors which are of various types.
- *Transmission of impulses from the receptors to the brain* is the function of afferent neurons. Specialized junctions called synapses are present to transmit impulses from one nerve cell to another. This process is known as *synaptic transmission*. The sensations ascend along the *sensory tracts*.
- *Relay of sensory impulses* occurs in the thalamus, which is a large cluster of nuclei that serves as a relay station.
- *Processing of the sensation* occurs in the cerebral cortex. The part of the brain that deals primarily with processing of *somatic* sensations is called the *somatosensory cortex*. Similarly, the part of the brain which is involved in processing visual sensation is called *visual cortex*.
- *Initiation of the response* to a sensation occurs from the concerned area of the cerebral cortex. For example, the somatic motor commands are initiated from the motor cortex.
- *Modulation and coordination of the response* occurs in subcortical centres. For example, the commands from motor cortex are coordinated and refined by the *basal ganglia loop system* as well as by the cerebellum.
- *Execution of response:* The response to a sensation is ultimately conveyed to the effector organs by the efferent nerves. The *efferent nerves* to the skeletal muscles are called *somatic motor nerves*. The response invoked may be involuntary, i.e. in the form of reflexes or voluntary movements.
- *Storage of information* occurs in the nervous system in the form of memory for future plans.
- *Emotional and instinctual behaviour* is controlled by the hypothalamus and limbic system.
- *Consciousness and sleep* are special functions of the brain. These include activity of reticular activating system and other systems.
- *Higher functions of the nervous system* include learning, memory, judgement, language and other functions of the mind.

10.1

Physiological Anatomy, Functions and Lesions of Spinal Cord and Brainstem

CHAPTER OUTLINE

PHYSIOLOGICAL ANATOMY AND FUNCTIONS OF SPINAL CORD

GROSS ANATOMY

- The spinal cord (Fig. 10.1.1) extends from the upper border of the first cervical vertebra to the lower border of the first lumbar vertebra.
- Its upper end becomes continuous with the medulla oblongata and its lower end called *conus medullaris* becomes continuous with a fibrous cord called *filum terminale.*
- The spinal cord is cylindrical in shape and presents two fusiform-shaped enlargements: the *cervical enlargement* for innervation of upper limbs and the *lumbar enlargement* for innervation of lower limbs.
- The cord possesses in the midline anteriorly a deep longitudinal fissure, the *anterior median fissure,* and on the posterior surface a shallow furrow, the *posterior median sulcus.*
- The spinal cord, like the brain, is surrounded by three meninges – the dura mater, the arachnoid mater and the pia mater.

INTERNAL STRUCTURE

As seen on cross-section (Fig. 10.1.2), the neural tissue of the spinal cord presents inner grey matter and outer white matter. Grey matter is constituted by the nerve cell bodies, dendrites and parts of axons, whereas white matter is formed by the myelinated and unmyelinated nerve fibres.

A. Spinal Grey Matter

In transverse section, the grey matter of the spinal cord forms an H-shaped mass in the centre of which is present a canal called the spinal canal. The *spinal grey* matter exhibits the following parts:

Dorsal horn or posterior grey column refers to the posterior horn-like projection of the H-shaped grey matter in each lateral half of the cord. The dorsal grey column has been subdivided (from anterior to posterior side) into a base, a neck and a head. ***Ventral horn*** or anterior grey column refers to the anterior projection of the grey matter in each lateral half of the cord. The ventral grey column has been subdivided into an anterior part (the head) and a posterior part (the base).

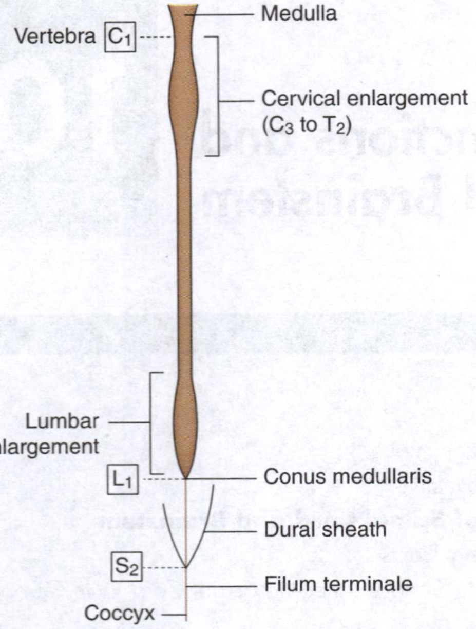

Fig. 10.1.1 Gross appearance of the spinal cord and its relation with vertebrae.

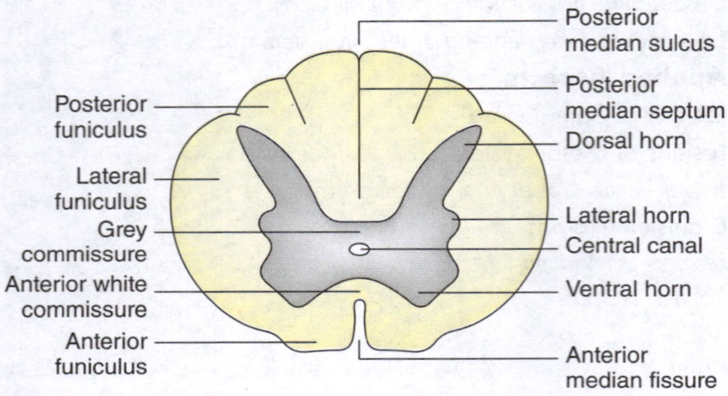

Fig. 10.1.2 Cross-section of thoracic segment of the spinal cord.

Lateral horn or intermediate horn or lateral column refers to small lateral projection between the ventral and dorsal grey columns, present in the thoracic segments and first two lumbar segments only.

Grey commissure is the part of the grey matter which connects the two (right and left) symmetrical halves of spinal grey matter across the midline. It is traversed by the central canal.

Neurons in Spinal Grey Matter

Neurons in ventral horn The ventral horn neurons of spinal grey matter are involved in motor functions and send motor nerve fibres to the muscles and other effector organs. Functionally, the motor neurons are of four types.

Groups of ventral horn neurons (nuclei in ventral horn grey matter): The above-described neurons of the ventral horn are arranged in three mediolateral columns:

1. Medial group
2. Lateral group
3. Central group (for details, see Chapter 10.9, page 1017)

Neurons in dorsal horn The dorsal horn neurons of spinal grey matter are involved in sensory functions. They are of two types.

1. Internuncial neurons These are located between the sensory fibres terminating in the dorsal horn and the motor neurons originating in the ventral horn.

2. Tract cells These cells receive impulses from the various receptors of the body through dorsal nerve root fibres. Axons of these cells enter the white matter of the spinal cord on the same or opposite side and constitute either intersegmental tracts or ascending tracts which terminate in various masses of grey matter in the brain. These tracts form a considerable part of white matter of the spinal cord.

Groups of dorsal horn neurons (nuclei in dorsal horn grey matter): The above-described neurons of the dorsal horn are arranged in four sets of longitudinal neuronal columns. From the apex to the base of the dorsal horn, these groups are given next (Fig. 10.1.3).

1. Substantia gelatinosa of Rolando It is a column of small cells which caps the apex of the dorsal horn as gelatinous material along the entire length of the spinal cord. It is continuous above with the nucleus of the spinal tract of the trigeminal nerve. The substantia gelatinosa (SG) is traversed by the fibres of the lateral division of the dorsal nerve roots which convey primarily pain and thermal sensations. The SG cell has a role in the 'gate control' of pain.

2. Nucleus proprius It extends along the entire length of the spinal cord and is composed of internuncial cells and tract cells whose axons form the ascending tracts which occupy the anterolateral white funiculi of white matter of the spinal cord.

3. Dorsal nucleus Dorsal nucleus, also called the thoracic nucleus or Clarke's column, extends from C_8 to L_2 segments of the spinal cord. It is composed of tract cells which receive proprioceptive, touch and pressure sensations from the trunk and lower limbs. Axons of these cells form the ipsilateral posterior spinocerebellar tract.

4. Posteromarginal nucleus It is formed by the marginal cells which cover the SG at the very tip of the dorsal horn.

Neurons in the lateral horn The lateral horn cells of spinal grey matter are also called neurons of the intermediolateral group of visceral efferent neurons which extends from T_1 to L_2 segments and from S_2 to S_4 segments of the spinal cord.

Neurons present in T_1 to L_2 lateral horn: These are preganglionic neurons of the sympathetic nervous system. Their axons terminate in relation to postganglionic neurons in sympathetic ganglia.

Neurons present in S_2 to S_4 lateral horn: These are preganglionic neurons of the sacral component of the parasympathetic nervous system. Their axons leave the spinal cord through the ventral nerve roots to reach the spinal nerves. They leave the spinal nerves as the pelvic splanchnic nerves which are distributed to some viscera in the pelvis and abdomen.

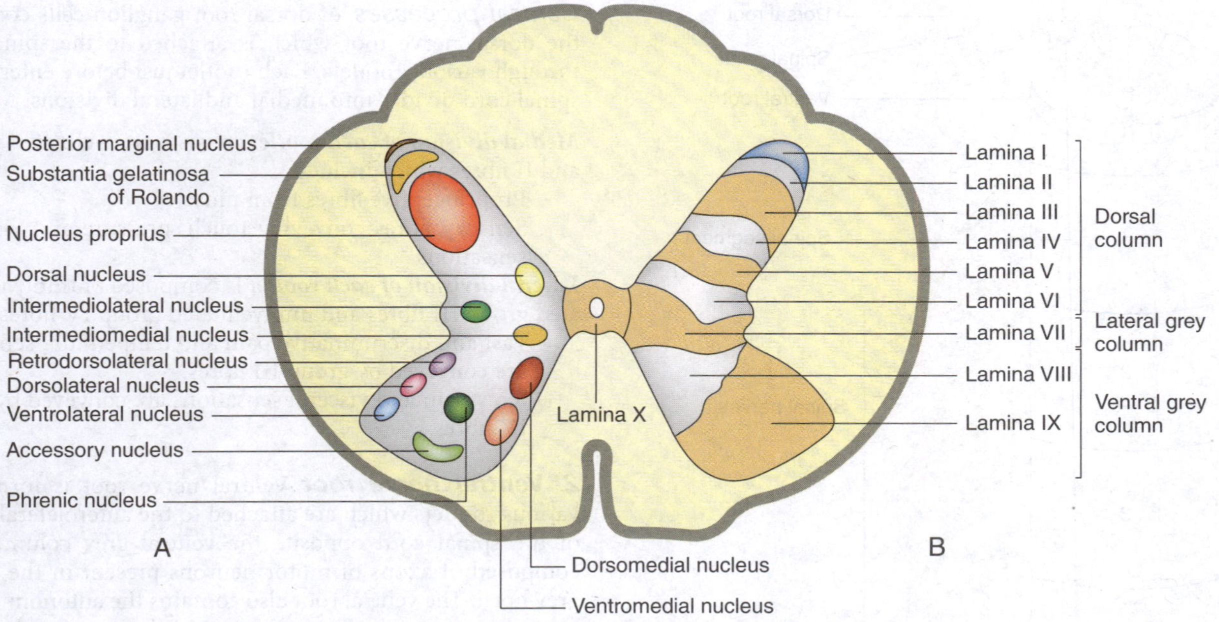

Fig. 10.1.3 Subdivisions of the grey matter of the spinal cord: **A**, into nuclei; and **B**, into laminae.

Divisions of Spinal Grey Matter into Laminae

From the point of view of neuronal connections, the spinal grey matter (which has been divided into ventral, lateral and dorsal columns and grey commissure as described above) can be divided into 10 laminae (I–X) called Rexed laminae (Fig. 10.1.3).

Laminae I–VI are confined to the dorsal grey column.

- *Lamina I* corresponds to posteromarginal nucleus.
- *Lamina II* corresponds to the SG.
- *Laminae III and IV* correspond to nucleus proprius.
- *Lamina V* corresponds to the neck of the dorsal grey column.
- *Lamina VI* corresponds to dorsal nucleus in the base of the dorsal grey column.

> **Important Note**
>
> Afferent fibres carrying cutaneous sensations end predominantly in laminae I–VI. Proprioceptive impulses reach laminae V and VI. These also receive numerous fibres from the cerebral cortex.

Lamina VII is confined to the lateral grey column (lateral or intermediate horns). It is composed of autonomic preganglionic neurons.

Laminae VIII** and **IX are confined to the ventral grey horn.

Lamina VIII occupies most of the ventral horn in the thoracic region. It is made of interneurons that receive terminals of vestibulospinal and reticulospinal tracts. Its efferent fibres are projected to lamina IX.

Lamina IX contains alpha and gamma motor neurons (that give off efferent fibres to skeletal muscles) and several internuncial neurons.

Lamina X forms the grey matter around the central canal and consists mostly of neuroglial cells.

B. White Matter of Spinal Cord

White matter is formed by the nerve fibres which are arranged as ascending and descending tracts (described later). In general, the white matter of the spinal cord is divided into right and left halves, in front by a deep *anterior median fissure* and behind by the *posterior median septum* (Fig. 10.1.2). In each half, the spinal white matter exhibits the following parts:

Posterior funiculus or posterior white column is formed by the white matter present medial to the dorsal grey horn.

Anterior funiculus or anterior white column refers to the white matter present anterior and medial to the ventral grey horn.

Lateral funiculus is formed by the white matter present lateral to the ventral and dorsal grey columns.

Anterolateral funiculus refers to the anterior and lateral funiculi collectively.

Ventral (anterior) white commissure refers to the white matter which is present anterior to the anterior grey commissure and joins the right and left halves of white matter.

Dorsal (posterior) white commissure refers to some myelinated fibres running transversely in the grey commissure, posterior to the central canal.

> **Important Note**
>
> Tracts of the spinal cord are described along with the tracts of the brainstem (see page 885).

SPINAL SEGMENTS AND SPINAL NERVES

Spinal Segments

The spinal cord, though a continuous structure, can be considered to consist of 31 spinal segments, each giving attachment to rootlets of the ventral and dorsal roots, of each spinal nerve (Fig. 10.1.4). The 31 segments of the spinal cord correspond symmetrically to 31 spinal nerves and are named as:

Eight cervical segments give attachment to eight cervical nerves.

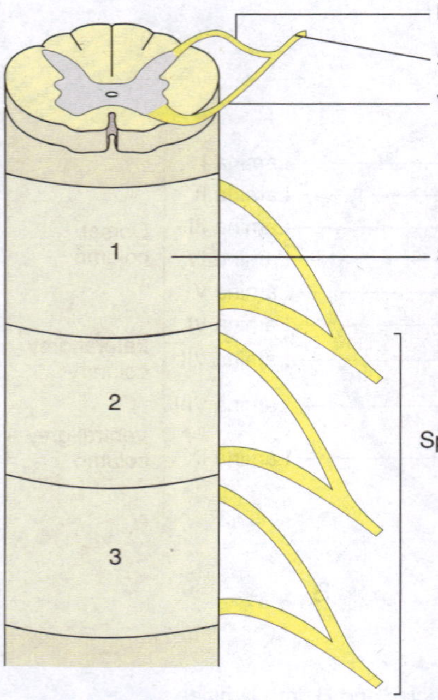

Fig. 10.1.4 Scheme to illustrate the concept of spinal segments and roots of spinal nerve.

Twelve thoracic segments give attachment to 12 thoracic nerves.
Five lumbar segments give attachment to five lumbar nerves.
Five sacral segments give attachment to five sacral nerves.
One coccygeal segment gives attachment to one coccygeal nerve.

Spinal Nerves

Each spinal nerve is a mixed nerve formed by union of two roots – a dorsal (sensory) root and a ventral (motor) root (Fig. 10.1.5).

1. Dorsal nerve root The dorsal nerve root is formed by several rootlets which are attached to the surface of the spinal cord along a vertical groove called the posterolateral sulcus. All sensory fibres reach the spinal cord through dorsal nerve roots. Each dorsal nerve root is marked by a swelling called dorsal nerve root ganglion or spinal ganglion. Dorsal root ganglion is composed of T-shaped unipolar neurons with peripheral and central processes.

Peripheral processes of dorsal root ganglion cells extend up to sensory receptors in the skin. The area of the skin supplied by a spinal nerve is called dermatome.

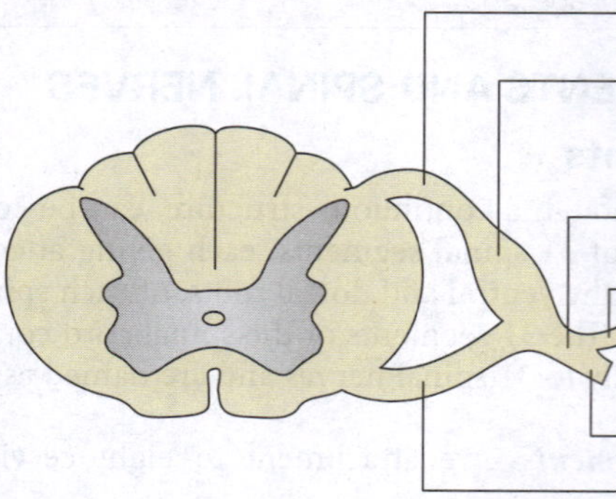

Fig. 10.1.5 Beginning of spinal nerve and its roots.

Central processes of dorsal root ganglion cells constitute the dorsal nerve root which is attached to the spinal cord through various rootlets. Each rootlet just before entering the spinal cord divides into medial and lateral divisions.

Medial division of each rootlet consists of myelinated group I and II fibres which include:
- Proprioceptive fibres from muscles
- Sensory fibres conveying touch, pressure and vibratory sensations

Lateral division of each rootlet is composed of thinly myelinated group III fibres and unmyelinated group IV fibres:
- Fast and discriminative pain and temperature sensations are conveyed by group III fibres.
- Slow pain and visceral sensations are conveyed by group IV fibres.

2. Ventral nerve root Ventral nerve root is formed by various rootlets which are attached to the anterolateral aspect of the spinal cord opposite the ventral grey column. It is composed of axons of motor neurons present in the ventral grey horn. The ventral root also contains the autonomic fibres originating from the lateral (intermediate) horn of the spinal grey matter (lamina VII).

FUNCTIONS OF SPINAL CORD

The spinal cord serves three groups of functions:
- Sensory functions
- Motor functions
- Autonomic functions

1. Sensory Functions

Entry of somatic sensations in spinal cord All the somatic afferent impulses enter the spinal cord through the dorsal nerve root as:

- The fibres mediating *thermal and pain sensations* enter the spinal cord through the lateral division of dorsal nerve root.
- The fibres conveying all *other sensory impulses* and proprioceptive impulses (touch, deep pressure, joint sense, vibration sense) from muscles, tendons and joints enter the spinal cord through the medial division of the dorsal nerve root.

Onward transmission of somatic sensations After entering the spinal cord, all the somatic sensations are conveyed to the brain (postcentral gyrus) by the following ascending tracts:

Spinothalamic tracts convey sensations from the opposite side as:
- *Ventral spinothalamic tract* conveys gross (crude) touch and tactile sensations.
- *Lateral spinothalamic tract* conveys pain and temperature.

Dorsal column tract sensations: These occupy the dorsal column of the white matter of the cord. These are upward continuation of the fibres of the medial division of the dorsal nerve roots of the same side. These tracts mediate sensations of fine touch, tactile localization and discrimination, pressure, vibration sense, sense of position and sense of movement.

2. Motor Functions

The spinal cord performs motor functions through:

Pyramidal tracts which include corticospinal (ventral and lateral) tracts

Extrapyramidal tracts which include vestibulospinal tract, tectospinal tract, rubrospinal tract, olivospinal tract and reticulospinal tract

Motor functions served by the spinal cord are as follows:

- Control of tone and power of muscles
- Control of movement of muscles and joints
- Control of deep (tendon) reflexes
- Control of superficial reflexes

3. Autonomic Functions

Visceral afferent impulses in the spinal cord travel through dorsal nerve roots to lateral horns of T_1 to L_2 and S_2 to S_4 spinal segments.

Autonomic efferents travelling through the spinal cord supply the visceral organs and control the activity of smooth muscles, heart, glands of GIT, sweat glands and adrenals. The spinal cord also regulates the body temperature. In other words, the spinal cord helps in maintaining the optimal internal environment of the body through its autonomic function.

PHYSIOLOGICAL ANATOMY AND FUNCTIONS OF BRAINSTEM

The brainstem consists (from below upwards) of the medulla oblongata, pons and midbrain (Fig. 10.1.6).

MEDULLA OBLONGATA

Gross Anatomy

The medulla oblongata is conical in shape and connects the pons above to the spinal cord below.

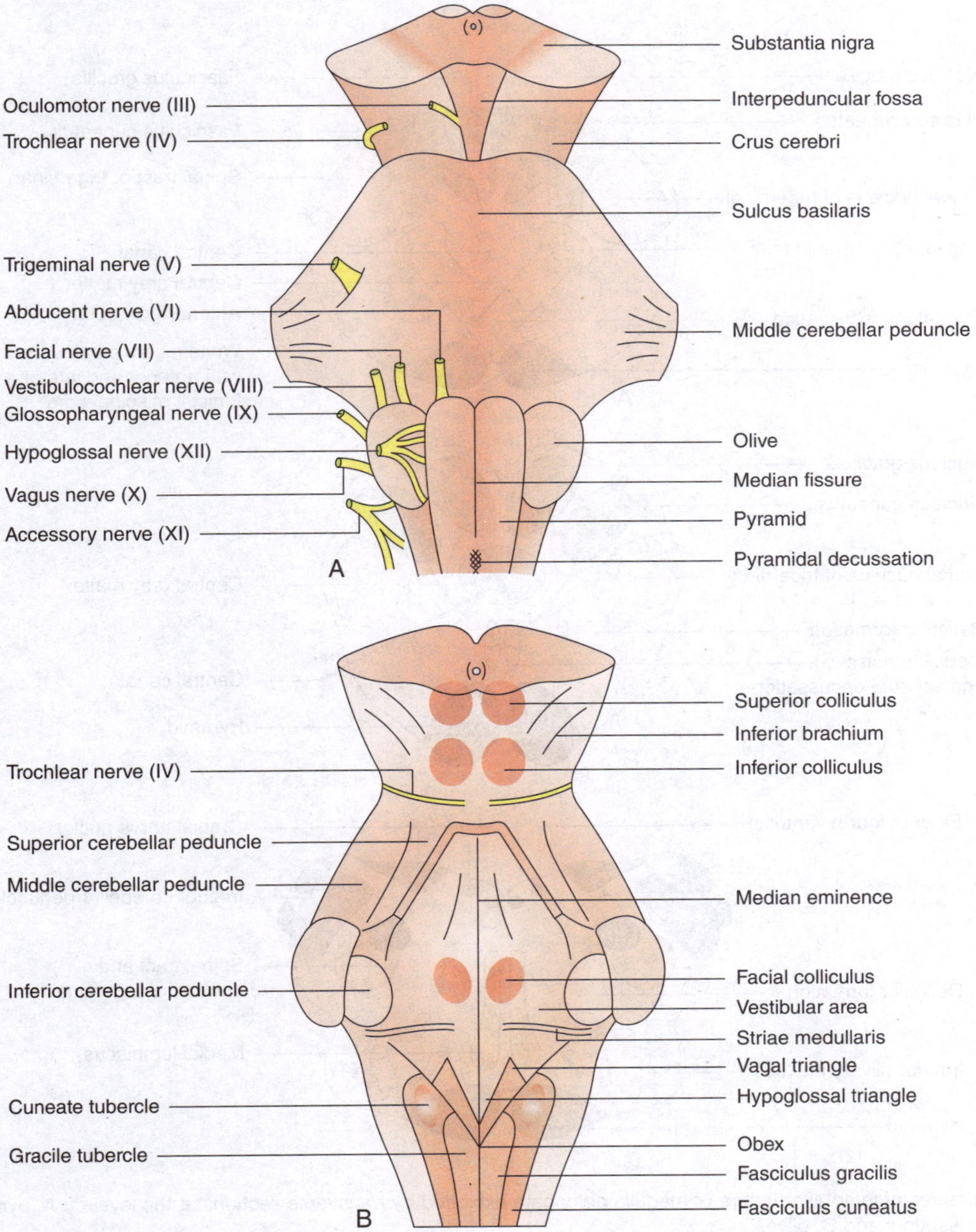

Fig. 10.1.6 Gross anatomy of brainstem: **A**, ventral aspect; and **B**, dorsal aspect.

Surface of Medulla

Surface of the medulla (Fig. 10.1.6) exhibits:

Median fissure, present in the centre of anterior surface of the medulla, is continuous below with the anterior median fissure of the spinal cord.

Pyramids are two swellings, one each present on either side of median fissure. These are composed of bundles of nerve fibres that originate in large nerve cells in the precentral gyrus of the cerebral cortex. The pyramids taper below, and have most of the descending fibres which cross over to the opposite side, forming the *decussation of pyramids*.

Olives are oval-shaped elevations, present one on each side just posterior to the pyramids. These are produced by the underlying olivary nuclei.

Inferior cerebellar peduncles, which connect the medulla to the cerebellum, are present behind the olives.

Gracilis and cuneatus tubercles (produced by the medially placed underlying nucleus gracilis and the laterally placed underlying nucleus cuneatus, respectively) are present on the posterior surface of the inferior part of the medulla oblongata.

Cranial nerves – IX, X, XI and XII – emerge from the surface of the medulla.

Internal Structure

The main features of the internal structure of the medulla oblongata are most easily reviewed by examining cross-sections at the following levels:

- Transverse section at the level of pyramidal decussation (Fig. 10.1.7A)
- Transverse section at the level of sensory decussation (Fig. 10.1.7B)
- Transverse section at the level of olive (Fig. 10.1.7C)

Note: For detailed description, refer any standard textbook of neuroanatomy.

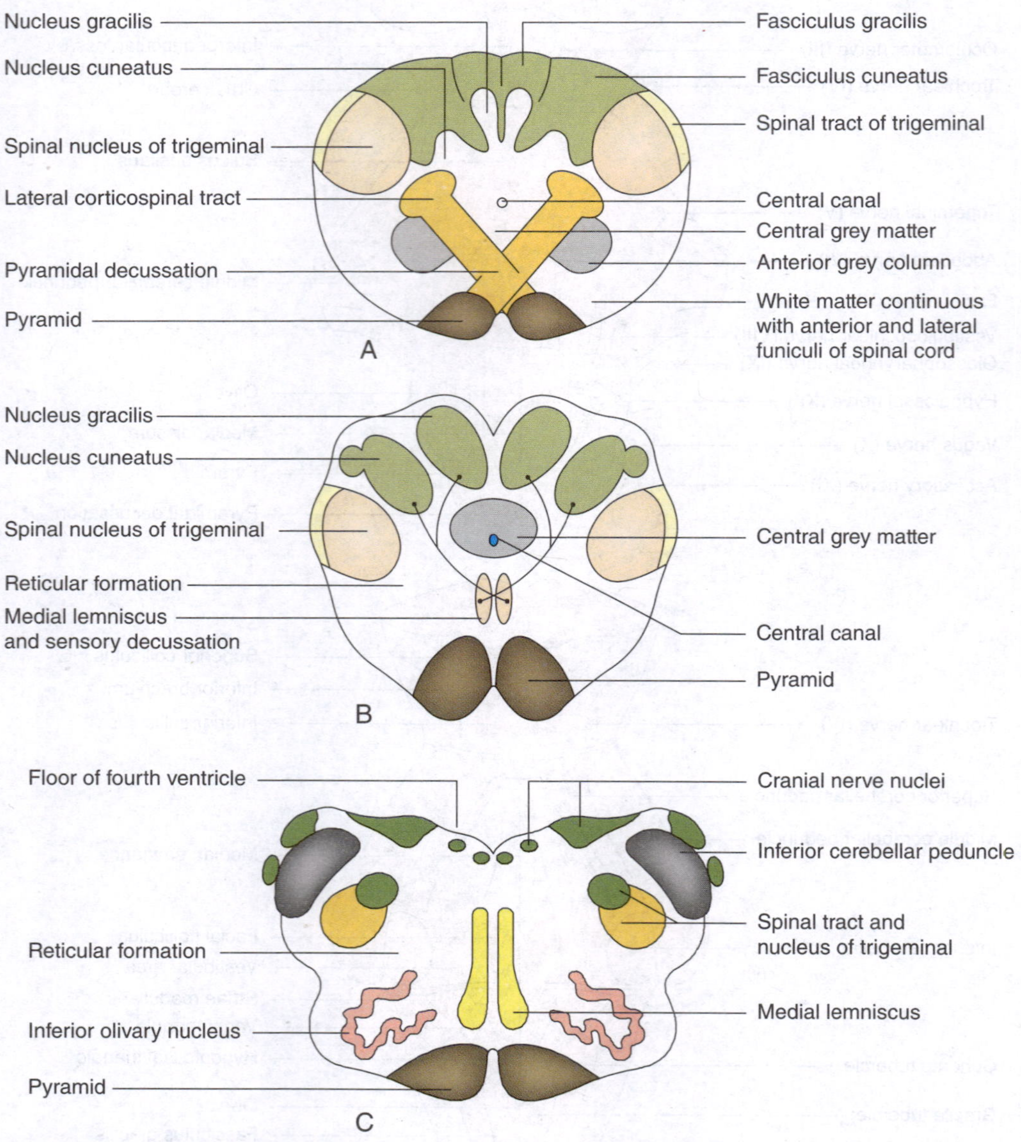

Fig. 10.1.7 Main features of internal structure of medulla oblongata exhibited by transverse sections at the level of: **A**, pyramidal decussation; **B**, sensory decussation; and **C**, olive.

Functions

1. Pathway for ascending and descending tracts: The medulla oblongata forms the main pathway for the ascending and descending tracts of the spinal cord.

2. House of vital centres: The medulla oblongata houses many important centres which control the vital functions of the body:

Respiratory centres (inspiratory and expiratory) control the normal rhythmic respiration (page 430).
Vasomotor and cardiac centres control the blood pressure and functions of the heart and vascular system (page 325).
Deglutition centre controls the pharyngeal and oesophageal phase of deglutition (page 572).
Vomiting centre is responsible for inducing vomiting in disorders of the gastrointestinal tract.
Superior and inferior salivary nuclei, located in the medulla, control the salivary secretion (page 570).

3. Cranial nerve nuclei located in the medulla control the following functions:

Twelfth cranial (hypoglossal) nerve controls the movements of the tongue.
Eleventh cranial (accessory) nerve controls the movements of the shoulder.
Tenth cranial (vagus) nerve controls the functions of important viscera, i.e. heart, lungs and GIT.
Eighth cranial nerve controls the auditory function (cochlear division of the nerve has the relay in the medulla oblongata) and vestibular function (medial and inferior vestibular nuclei extend through much of the medulla).

PONS

Gross Anatomy

The pons is situated on the anterior surface of the cerebellum below the midbrain and above the medulla oblongata.

Gross features of the pons (Fig. 10.1.6) are as follows:

Anterior surface of the pons is convex, exhibits prominent transversely running fibres and is marked in the midline by a shallow groove, the *sulcus basilaris*, which lodges the basilar artery.
Middle cerebellar peduncles, present laterally, connect the pons with the cerebellum.
Junction between the pons and the medulla is marked by a groove through which emerge the cranial nerves VI, VII and VIII.
Posterior aspect of pons forms the upper part of the floor of the fourth ventricle.

Internal Structure

The main features of internal structure of the pons can be best studied by transverse sections at the level of facial colliculus, i.e. through the lower part of the pons (Fig. 10.1.8A) and through the upper part of the pons (Fig. 10.1.8B). Internally, the pons is divisible into two parts:

1. Ventral (basilar) part of the pons contains:

Transverse fibres form the middle cerebellar peduncle when traced laterally.

Vertical fibres, present in the pons, are of two types:
- Corticopontine fibres, which end in pontine nuclei
- Corticospinal fibres that descend through the pons into the medulla where they form pyramids

Pontine nuclei are the groups of neurons which are scattered among the nerve fibres.

2. Dorsal (tegmental) part of the pons contains:

- Decussations of the trapezoid body
- Nuclei of cranial nerves V, VI, VII and VIII
- Pontine reticular formation
- A number of descending and ascending tracts

The most prominent ascending tracts are the four lemnisci: medial, trigeminal, spinal and lateral.

Functions

The pons subserves the following functions:

1. ***Connecting pathway between the cerebral cortex and the cerebellum*** (the pontine nuclei receive corticopontine fibres and their axons from the middle cerebellar peduncles which serve as a connecting pathway between the cerebral cortex and the cerebellum)
2. ***Pathway for ascending and descending tracts*** of the spinal cord and medulla oblongata
3. ***Houses the nuclei*** of cranial nerves V, VI, VII and VIII
4. ***Joining station*** for medial lemniscus with fibres of cranial nerves V, VII, IX and X
5. ***Contains pneumotaxic and apneustic centres*** for regulation of respiration (page 432)

MIDBRAIN

Gross Anatomy

The midbrain is a narrow part of the brain that connects the forebrain to the hindbrain. Gross anatomical features of the midbrain are as follows (Fig. 10.1.6):

Anterior surface of the midbrain exhibits (Fig. 10.1.6A):

Crura cerebri: These are two large bundles of fibres, one on each side of the middle line.
Interpeduncular fossa is present in the triangular space between the two crura.
***Oculomotor** nerve* emerges from the medial aspect of the crus of the same side.

Posterior surface of the midbrain exhibits (Fig. 10.1.6B):

Superior colliculi are two rounded swellings, one on each side of midline. Each superior colliculus acts as subcortical centre for visual reflexes and is connected to the lateral geniculate body by a raised band known as superior brachium.
Inferior colliculi are two rounded swellings, one on each side of the midline located below the superior colliculi. Each inferior colliculus acts as subcortical centre for auditory reflexes and is connected to the medial geniculate body by an elevated band known as the *inferior brachium.*

Internal Structure

The main features of the internal structure of the midbrain can be studied by making two transverse sections – one at the rostral level through the superior colliculi, and the other at the caudal level through the inferior colliculi.

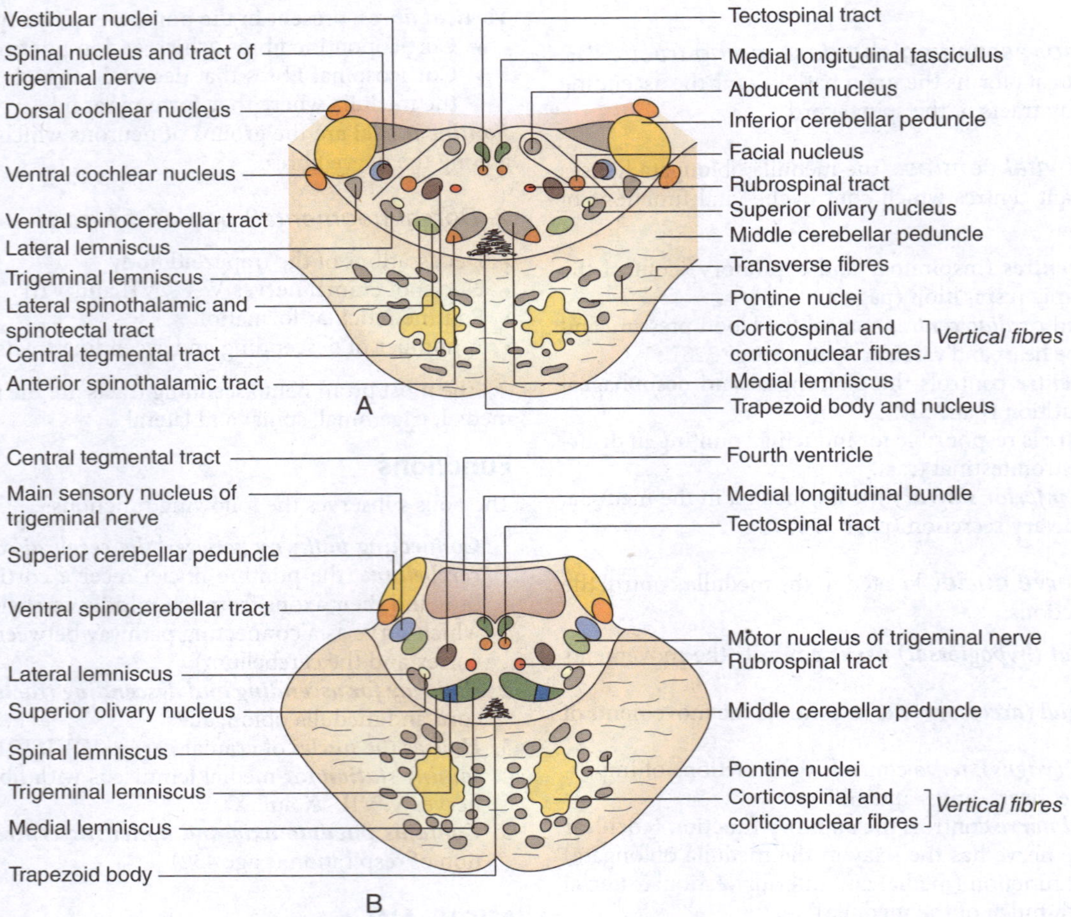

Fig. 10.1.8 Main features of internal structure of pons exhibited by transverse sections at the level of: **A**, lower part of pons; and **B**, upper part of pons.

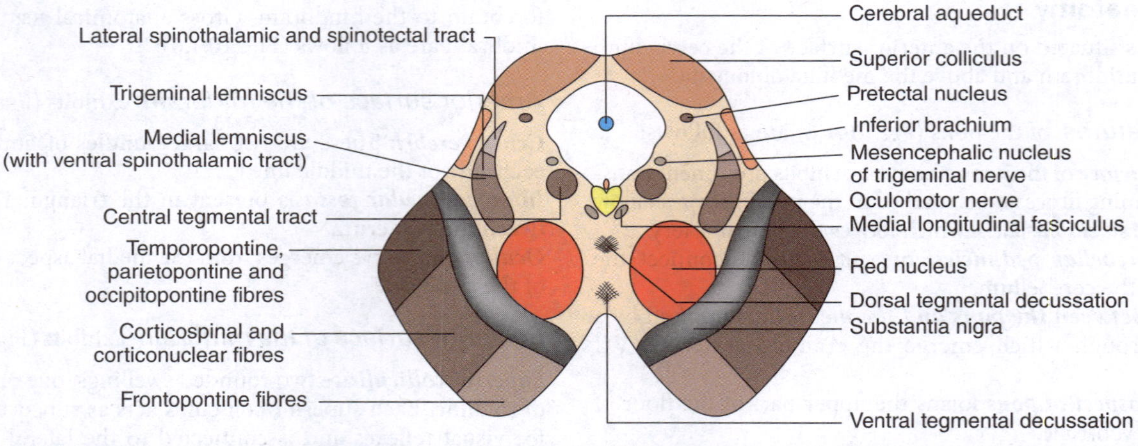

Fig. 10.1.9 Main features of internal structure of midbrain exhibited by transverse section at the level of superior colliculi.

Internally, for convenience of description, the midbrain can be divided into two parts (Fig. 10.1.9).

i. Tectum Tectum refers to the part of the midbrain lying behind a transverse line drawn through the cerebral aqueduct. It consists of superior and inferior colliculi of two sides.

ii. Cerebral peduncles Cerebral peduncles (right and left) constitute the part of the midbrain lying in front of the line passing through the cerebral aqueduct. Each cerebral peduncle in turn consists of three parts, which from anterior to posterior side are as follows:

Crus cerebri (or basis pedunculi): It consists of large mass of vertically running descending fibres from the cerebral cortex which include frontopontine fibres (occupying the medial one-sixth of the crus), corticospinal and corticonuclear fibres (occupying intermediate two-thirds of the crus) and temporopontine, parietopontine and occipitopontine fibres (occupying the lateral one-sixth of the crus).

Substantia nigra is a mass of pigmented grey matter (therefore appears dark in colour). Physically, it is considered part of basal ganglia. The connection and functions of substantia nigra are discussed on page 915.

Tegmentum of the two sides is continuous across the midline. It contains the following important masses of grey matter and nerve fibres:

Red nucleus is the biggest nucleus present in the upper part of the midbrain. Physiologically, the red nucleus is a part of basal ganglia and is involved in regulation of posture (see page 1035).
Nuclei of cranial nerves III, IV and V are present in the tegmentum.
Reticular formation of the midbrain is continuous below with the reticular formation of the pons and medulla.
Fibre bundles of the tegmentum include medial lemniscus, trigeminal lemniscus, lateral lemniscus, and tectospinal and rubrospinal tracts.
Three decussations take place in the tegmentum due to crossing of fibres of the superior cerebellar peduncle, rubrospinal tracts (Forel's decussation) and fibres of the medial longitudinal bundle (Meynert decussation).

TRACTS OF SPINAL CORD AND BRAINSTEM

The tracts that transmit sensory impulses to the brain are termed *ascending tracts*, and the tracts which are responsible for transmission of motor impulses from the brain to motor neurons reaching muscles and glands are termed *descending tracts*. There are numerous ascending and descending tracts in the spinal cord and brainstem.

ASCENDING TRACTS

Ascending tracts convey impulses arising in various parts of the body to different parts of the brain. The ascending tracts present in the spinal cord (Figs 10.1.10 and 10.1.11) can be grouped as:

- Ascending tracts connecting the spinal cord with the cerebral cortex
- Ascending tracts ending in the brainstem
- Spinocerebellar pathways

I. Ascending Tracts Connecting Spinal Cord with Cerebral Cortex

1. Posterior Column–Medial Lemniscus Pathway

Fasciculus gracilis and fasciculus cuneatus Fasciculus gracilis and fasciculus cuneatus occupy the posterior white funiculus of the spinal cord, and are, therefore, often referred to as the *posterior column tracts*. Fasciculus gracilis is situated medial to fasciculus cuneatus. The posterior intermediate septum separates the two in the cervical and upper thoracic segments (Fig. 10.1.10).

Origin These tracts are unique in that they are formed predominantly by the axons of the first-order sensory neurons located in dorsal root ganglia (Fig. 10.1.12).

- Recently, it has been shown that these tracts also contain some fibres that originate in the dorsal grey column (laminae III and IV), i.e. sensory neurons of second order.

Arrangement of fibres The fibres derived from the lowest ganglia are situated most medially, whereas those from the highest ganglia are most lateral. Therefore:

Fasciculus gracilis, which lies medially, is composed of fibres from the coccygeal, sacral, lumbar and lower thoracic ganglia.
Fasciculus cuneatus, which lies laterally, consists of fibres from the upper thoracic and cervical ganglia.

Course After entering the spinal cord, the fibres ascend through the posterior white funiculus and reach the medulla (Fig. 10.1.12). These fibres do not synapse in the spinal cord. Some fibres of the medial division of the posterior nerve root descend through the posterior white funiculus in the form of fasciculus interfasciculi or comma tract of Schultze.

- Some afferents from spinal ganglia pass through the posterior funiculus to reach the dorsal nucleus and other areas of spinal grey matter.

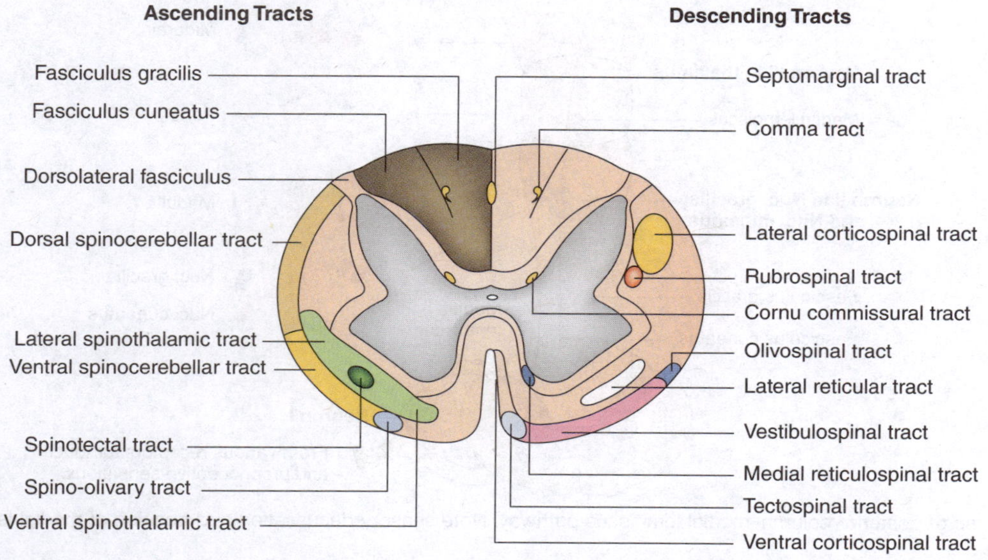

Fig. 10.1.10 Schematic diagram to show the position of the main ascending and descending tracts of the spinal cord and brainstem.

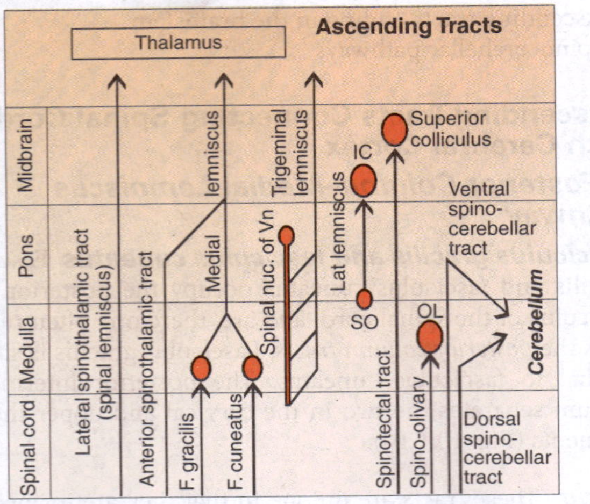

Fig. 10.1.11 Schematic diagram to show the various ascending tracts of spinal cord and brainstem. IC, inferior colliculus; OL, olivary nucleus; SC, superior colliculus; SO, superior olivary nucleus; VN, vestibular nucleus.

Termination After reaching the medulla, the fibres of gracilis and cuneatus fasciculi terminate by synapsing with neurons in the nucleus gracilis and nucleus cuneatus, respectively (Fig. 10.1.12).

Medial lemniscus The neurons of nucleus gracilis and nucleus cuneatus form the *second-order sensory neurons*. Their axons form the *internal arcuate fibres* which run forwards and medially to cross the midline. The crossing fibres of the two sides constitute the *sensory decussation* or *lemniscus* decussation and then ascend through the medulla, pons and midbrain as *medial lemniscus* (Fig. 10.1.12). The fibres of medial lemniscus terminate in ventral posterolateral nucleus of the thalamus.

Third-order sensory neurons The fibres of medial lemniscus synapse with the third-order sensory neurons located in the thalamus. Axons of the third-order neurons pass through the internal capsule and corona radiata to reach the somatosensory areas of the cerebral cortex.

Functions of posterior column–medial lemniscus pathway These fibres carry sensations of some components of touch, vibration and proprioception to the cortex and thus help in the following functions:

1. ***Components of sense of touch*** include:
   - Deep touch and pressure
   - Fine touch, i.e. epicritic tactile sensations
   - Tactile localization, i.e. the ability to localize exactly the part of the skin touched
   - Tactile discrimination, i.e. the ability to recognize as separate two points on the skin that are touched simultaneously
   - Stereognosis, i.e. the ability to recognize the shape of known objects by touch with closed eyes
2. ***Proprioceptive impulses*** help in conscious kinaesthetic sensations, i.e. the sense of position of different parts of the body under static conditions as well as rate of change of movement of different parts during body movements.
3. ***Sense of vibrations***, i.e. ability to detect rapidly changing peripheral conditions. This is the ability to perceive the vibrations conducted to deep tissues through the skin.

2. Spinothalamic Pathways

Anterior and lateral spinothalamic tracts The spinothalamic tracts are formed by the axons of the second-order sensory neurons of the pathway of crude touch and pressure (anterior spinothalamic tract) and pain and temperature (lateral spinothalamic tract) (Fig. 10.1.13).

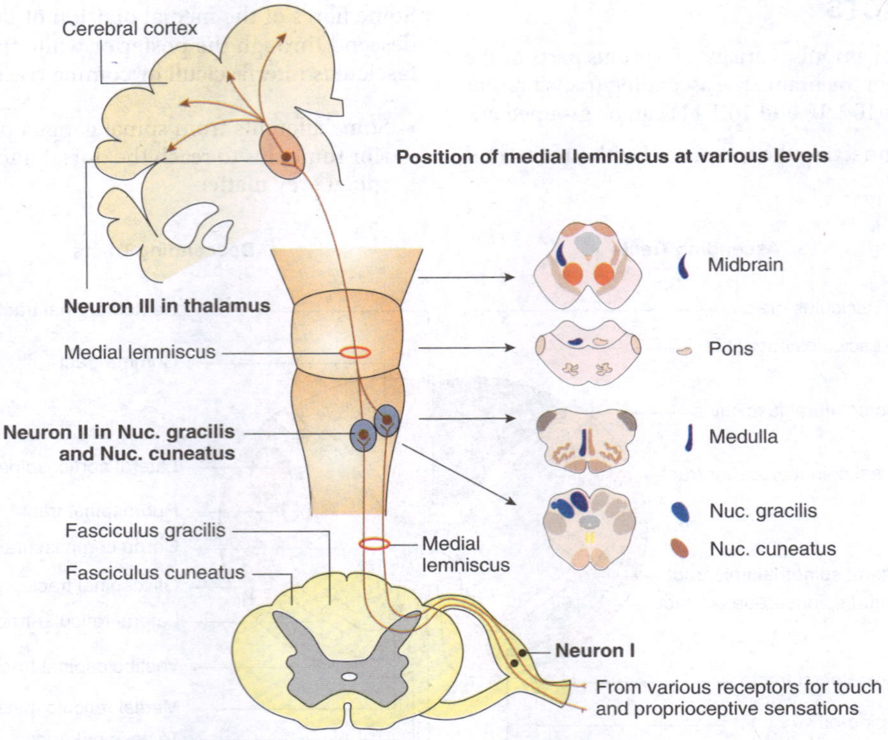

Fig. 10.1.12 Course of posterior column–medial lemniscus pathway. Note sensory decussation and position of medial lemniscus at various levels of brainstem.

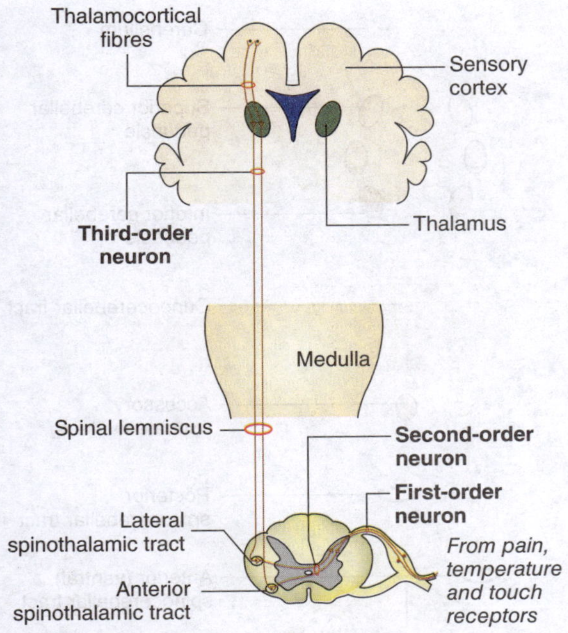

Fig. 10.1.13 Course of anterior and lateral spinothalamic tracts.

Location The anterior spinothalamic tract is located in the anterior white funiculus near the periphery, whereas the lateral spinothalamic tract is located in the lateral funiculus towards the medial side, i.e. near the grey matter (Fig. 10.1.10).

Origin The spinothalamic tracts are formed by the axons of chief sensory cells of posterior grey horn which form the second-order sensory neurons. The first-order neurons of this pathway are located in spinal ganglia. These neurons receive the impulses from the cutaneous receptors. Central processes of these neurons enter the spinal cord and terminate in relation to chief sensory cells of spinal grey matter. They may ascend in the dorsolateral tract (situated near the tip of dorsal grey column, Fig. 10.1.10) for one or more segments before ending in grey matter.

Course After taking origin from the chief sensory cells, the fibres of the anterior spinothalamic tract ascend in posterior grey horn for two to three segments on the same side. Then, they cross obliquely to the opposite side of the spinal cord in the white commissure (but some fibres may remain uncrossed).

The fibres of the lateral spinothalamic tract cross within the same segment of the spinal cord and reach the lateral column of the same segment.

The two tracts also carry about 10% of uncrossed fibres and run up in the spinal cord, medulla, pons and midbrain and reach the thalamus. In the brainstem, they form the so-called spinal lemniscus.

Termination All the spinothalamic fibres running in spinal lemniscus terminate in the ventral posterolateral nucleus of the thalamus. The neurons of this thalamic nucleus form the *third-order neurons* of this sensory pathway and relay the impulses to the somaesthetic area of the cerebral cortex.

Functions Traditionally, it has been said that the anterior spinothalamic tracts carry sensations for *crude touch and pressure*, whereas the lateral tracts have been said to carry sensations of *pain and temperature*. However, it is now realized that although different fibres within the spinothalamic tracts carry different types of sensations, the anterior and lateral spinothalamic tracts constitute a single functional unit.

Dorsolateral spinothalamic tract The dorsolateral spinothalamic tract is also called *fasciculus dorsolateralis* or *tract of Lissauer*.

Origin This is formed by the fibres arising from the neurons of the posterior root ganglia which form the *first-order neurons*.

Location It is located in the lateral white column between the periphery of the spinal cord and the tip of the posterior grey horn (Fig. 10.1.10).

Course These fibres enter the spinal cord through the lateral division of posterior nerve root and pass upwards or downwards for few segments on the same side and synapse with cells of SG of Ronaldo situated in the posterior grey column. The processes of these cells (*second-order neurons*) cross to the opposite side and ascend in the dorsolateral fasciculus to reach the ventral posterolateral nucleus of the thalamus where they synapse.

Functions This tract carries impulses arising in the skin (mainly pain and temperature). Relief of pain after dorsolateral cordotomy may be a result of the cutting of these fibres.

Spinocervicothalamic pathway It is another pathway through which cutaneous sensations (touch, pressure, pain and temperature) reach the thalamus.

Origin This tract is formed by the axons arising from neurons located in laminae III–V of spinal grey matter.

Course and termination After origin, the fibres ascend through the dorsolateral fasciculus and end in the *lateral cervical nucleus* (which is a small collection of neurons lying among the fibres of the lateral funiculus in spinal segments C_1 and C_2). New fibres arising here project to the ventral posterolateral nucleus of the thalamus.

II. Ascending Tracts Ending in Brainstem

The ascending tracts arising in spinal grey matter and ending in masses of grey matter in different parts of the brainstem are (Fig. 10.1.11) given next.

1. Spinoreticular Tract

Location This tract is located in anterolateral white funiculus (Fig. 10.1.10).

Origin The spinoreticular fibres begin from spinal neurons mainly in lamina VII (also V and VIII).

Course The fibres are partly crossed and partly uncrossed, and ascend in the ventrolateral part of the spinal cord, intermingling with the spinothalamic tracts.

Termination These fibres end in reticular formation of the medulla and pons:

- In the medulla, the fibres end in nucleus reticularis gigantocellularis and lateral reticular nucleus of same side; some fibres terminate in the opposite side.

- In the pons, these fibres terminate in the nucleus reticularis pontis caudalis of the same side or opposite side.
- Very few fibres terminate in midbrain.

Functions The fibres of the spinoreticular tract are the components of the ascending reticular activating system (RAS) and are concerned with arousing consciousness or alertness.

2. Spinotectal Tract

Location This tract is located in the lateral side of lateral white funiculus anterior to the lateral spinothalamic tract. It is bounded anteriorly by the anterior nerve root (Fig. 10.1.10).

Origin Fibres of this tract arise from the chief sensory cells of posterior grey column. The first appearance of the fibres is in upper lumbar segments. This tract is very prominent.

Course and termination After origin from the spinal grey matter, the fibres cross to the opposite side through the anterior white commissure to the lateral funiculus. Then the fibres ascend up to the midbrain along with the anterior spinothalamic tract and end in the superior colliculus and midbrain reticular nuclei.

Functions These fibres form an alternate route for conduction of *slow pain* and are also concerned with *spinovisual reflexes*.

3. Spino-Olivary Tract

Location This tract is located in the anterolateral part of white funiculus and occupies mostly the anterior white funiculus (Fig. 10.1.10).

Origin, course and termination The origin of the fibres of this tract is not specific. It is also a crossed tract. Its fibres terminate into the olivary nucleus of the medulla oblongata, from where the neurons project into the cerebellum.

Function This tract is concerned with proprioception.

III. Spinocerebellar Tracts

The spinocerebellar tracts carry proprioceptive impulses arising in the lower part of the body to the cerebellum. Recent investigations have shown that some exteroceptive sensations (e.g. touch) may reach the cerebellum through these pathways. Thus, the spinocerebellar tracts are constituted by the fibres of second-order neurons of the pathway for subconscious kinaesthetic sensation (Fig. 10.1.14). The spinocerebellar pathway is organized into the ventral and dorsal tracts.

1. Ventral Spinocerebellar Tract

Location It is located in lateral white funiculus of the spinal cord along the lateral periphery (Fig. 10.1.10).

Origin The ventral (anterior) spinocerebellar tract, also known as *Gower's tract*, is constituted by the second-order neurons (of proprioceptive pathway) located in the junctional area between the ventral and the dorsal grey column (laminae V, VI, VII) in the lumbar and sacral segments of the cord. These neurons receive impulses from the first-order neurons located in the posterior root ganglia. The peripheral processes of first-order neurons receive impulses from muscle spindles, Golgi tendon organs and other proprioceptive receptors. Some fibres are related to end organs concerned with exteroceptive sensations (touch, pressure).

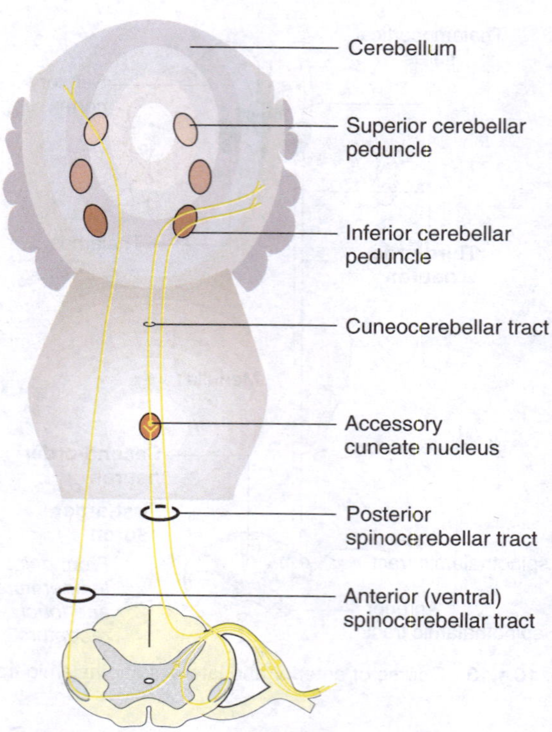

Fig. 10.1.14 Spinocerebellar tracts.

Course After origin from the junctional (marginal) cells, the majority of fibres of the ventral spinocerebellar tract cross to the opposite side and ascend in the lateral funiculus, anterior to the fibres of the dorsal spinocerebellar tract (Fig. 10.1.10) (some fibres ascend in the lateral funiculus of the same side also). Then these fibres ascend through the spinal cord, medulla, pons and midbrain. Finally, these fibres reach the cerebellum through the superior cerebellar peduncle (Fig. 10.1.14).

Termination These fibres terminate in the lower limb area of the cerebellar cortex.

2. Dorsal (posterior) Spinocerebellar Tract

Location This tract is located in the lateral funiculus along the posterolateral periphery of the spinal cord. It is situated posterior to the ventral spinocerebellar tract and anterior to the entry of the posterior nerve root (Fig. 10.1.10).

Origin The first-order neurons are located in the posterior nerve root ganglia. The peripheral processes of *first-order neurons* receive impulses from the muscle spindles, Golgi tendon organs and other proprioceptive receptors.

Course Unlike the ventral spinocerebellar tract, the dorsal spinocerebellar tract is *uncrossed*. The fibres of this tract after originating reach the lateral funiculus of the same side and ascend through other spinal segments and reach the medulla oblongata. From here, the fibres reach the cerebellum through the inferior cerebellar peduncle.

Termination Most of the fibres of this tract terminate in the cortex of the anterior lobe of the cerebellum.

Functions This tract transmits proprioceptive information from the thoracic region and lower limb.

3. Cuneocerebellar Tract

The central processes of some first-order neurons (related to cervical segments) reach the *accessory cuneate nucleus* in the medulla. The central processes of the second-order neurons located in the accessory cuneate nucleus form the cuneocerebellar tract (posterior external arcuate fibres), which enter the inferior cerebellar peduncle of the same side to reach the cerebellum.

Functions This tract brings the *conscious proprioception* impulses from the upper limb. Thus, it may be regarded as the forelimb equivalent of the dorsal spinocerebellar tract.

4. Rostral Spinocerebellar Tract

Origin, course and termination This tract is believed to arise from spinal grey matter in lower four cervical segments (lamina VII) from the neurons which constitute the *nucleus centrobasalis*.

Most of the fibres of this tract are uncrossed. They reach the cerebellum through the inferior and superior cerebellar peduncles.

Functions This pathway is regarded, functionally, as the forelimb equivalent of the ventral spinocerebellar tract.

The major ascending tracts of the spinal cord are summarized in Table 10.1.1.

DESCENDING TRACTS

The descending tracts, concerned with the various motor activities of the body, are formed by the motor nerve fibres arising from the brain and descending into the spinal cord and brainstem (Fig. 10.1.15).

Descending Tracts Ending in Spinal Cord

Traditionally, the descending tracts ending in the spinal cord have been divided into two groups:

- Pyramidal tracts
- Extrapyramidal tracts

I. Pyramidal Tracts

The pyramidal tracts refer to the corticospinal tracts which are constituted by the axons that transmit motor signals directly from the cortex to the spinal cord (Fig. 10.1.16).

Origin Corticospinal tract fibres originate from the following nerve cells in the cerebral cortex:

- Primary motor cortex (area 4): 31%
- Premotor area (area 8) and supplementary motor area: 29%
- Somatic sensory areas (areas 3, 1, 2): 40%

All the above-stated fibres form the fibres of upper motor neurons (UMNs) of the motor pathway.

Course and termination After originating from the cerebral cortex, the corticospinal tract fibres descend as part of the corona radiata and then pass through the posterior limb of the internal capsule and then downwards through the brainstem, forming pyramids in the medulla (hence the name pyramidal tracts).

In the lower part of the medulla, about 90% of fibres of each pyramid decussate in the midline to reach the opposite side. From here downwards, the fibres of corticospinal tracts are divided into two separate tracts:

1. ***Lateral corticospinal tract*** is constituted by 80% of fibres which have crossed to the opposite side. The lateral corticospinal tract fibres descend the full length of the spinal cord through the posterior part of lateral white funiculus (Figs 10.1.10 and 10.1.16). Most of these fibres terminate in the internuncial neurons of the spinal grey matter. The

Table 10.1.1 Major ascending tracts in the spinal cord

Tract	Location	Origin[a]	Termination	Functions
Fasciculus gracilis and fasciculus cuneatus (tracts of Goll and Burdach)	Posterior white column of spinal cord	Dorsal root ganglia of spinal nerves of the same side	Nucleus gracilis and nucleus cuneatus in medulla of the same side	Joint sense, vibration sense, two-point discrimination, stereognosis, conscious kinaesthesia
Spinothalamic tracts				
• Lateral spinothalamic tract	Lateral white column	Posterior horn cells of spinal cord of opposite side	Ventral posterolateral (VPL) nucleus of thalamus	Carry pain and temperature from opposite side of the body
• Anterior spinothalamic tract	Anterior white column	Posterior horn cells of spinal cord of opposite side	VPL nucleus of thalamus	Carry light touch, pressure, tickle and itch sensation from opposite side of the body
Spinotectal tract	Lateral white column	Posterior horn cells of spinal cord of opposite side	Superior colliculus of tectum of midbrain	Visuomotor reflexes, i.e. head and eye movements, towards the source of stimulation
Spinocerebellar (anterior and posterior) ***tracts***	Lateral white column (superficially)	Posterior horn cells of spinal cord of same side	Cerebellum	Unconscious kinaesthesia (proprioception)

[a]Location of cell bodies of neurons from which the axons of tract arise.

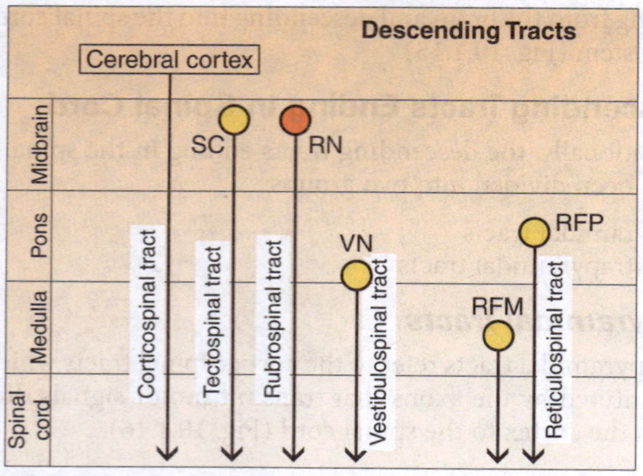

Fig. 10.1.15 Schematic drawing to show the various descending tracts ending in spinal cord and brainstem. RFM, reticular formation of medulla; RFP, reticular formation of pons; RN, red nucleus; SC, superior colliculus; VN, vestibular nucleus.

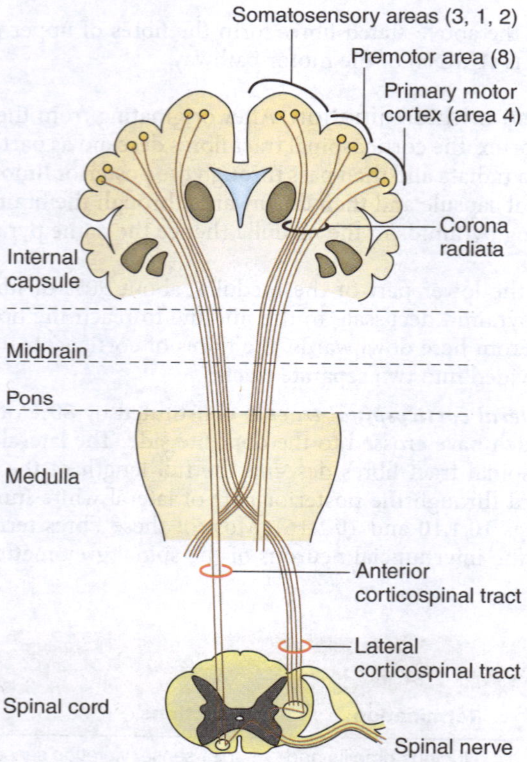

Fig. 10.1.16 Pathway of corticospinal tracts.

internuncial neurons carry the impulses to motor neurons situated in the ventral grey horn. Some fibres of the tract terminate directly on ventral horn cells. The axons of the ventral motor neurons supply the skeletal muscles directly by passing through the ventral nerve root. The neurons giving origin to the fibres of the pyramidal tract along with their axons constitute the *UMNs*. The ventral motor neurons in the spinal cord along with their axons constitute the *lower motor* neurons (LMNs).

2. ***Anterior corticospinal tract*** is formed by 20% of uncrossed pyramidal fibres. These fibres descend down through the anterior white funiculus of the same side. The anterior corticospinal tract fibres do not reach further than the mid-thoracic region. On reaching the appropriate level of the spinal cord, the fibres of this tract cross the midline (through the anterior white commissure) to reach grey matter on the opposite side of the cord and terminate in a manner similar to that of the fibres of the lateral corticospinal tract. Thus, the corticospinal fibres of both the lateral and anterior tracts ultimately connect the cerebral cortex of one side with ventral horn cells in the opposite half of the spinal cord.

Salient features of nerve fibres of corticospinal tracts

- Fibres of the corticospinal tract are unmyelinated at birth. Myelination begins in the second postnatal week and is completed by 2 years.
- Most (80%) of the fibres of corticospinal tracts are of a small diameter (1–4 μm), whereas about 20% of fibres are of a large diameter (11–22 μm).
- The large-diameter fibres originate from the giant pyramidal neurons (cells of Betz) present in the primary motor cortex (area 4). These fibres transmit impulse at the rate of 70 m/s.
- The large fibres of pyramidal tracts have the tendency to disappear at old age causing automatic shaking movements of old age.

Functions The cerebral cortex controls voluntary fine-skilled movements of the body through the corticospinal tracts. Interruption of the tract anywhere in its course leads to paralysis of the muscles concerned. As the fibres are closely packed in their course through the internal capsule and brainstem, small lesions here can cause widespread paralysis.

- The pyramidal tract fibres also send collaterals to other areas of motor control systems, thus communicating motor command to the basal ganglia, cerebellum and brainstem.
- In their course through the brainstem, some of the fibres (corticonuclear fibres) terminate directly on the motor nuclei of cranial neurons controlling facial muscles. Since these fibres perform the same function as pyramidal tracts, they are also considered part of the pyramidal system.

II. Extrapyramidal Tracts

The descending tracts of the spinal cord other than the pyramidal tracts are collectively called extrapyramidal tracts. These include:

- Rubrospinal tract
- Vestibulospinal tract
- Reticulospinal tract
- Tectospinal tract
- Olivospinal tract
- Medial longitudinal fasciculus (MLF)

1. Rubrospinal tract This tract arises from the large cells (nucleus magnocellularis) or red nucleus in the midbrain.

Course After arising from the red nucleus, the fibres of this tract cross to the opposite side in the lower part of segmental decussation of the midbrain (ventral segmental decussation). Then, the tract descends through the pons and medulla and follows a course similar to that of the lateral corticospinal tract in the lateral funiculus of the spinal cord (Figs 10.1.10 and 10.9.3; see page 1035).

Termination The fibres terminate mainly on interneurons along with corticospinal fibres.

Functions This tract exhibits facilitatory influence on the flexor muscles and inhibitory influence on the extensor muscles of the body.

- The red nucleus also receives the corticorubral fibres from the ipsilateral motor cortex. The corticorubrospinal tract thus formed may act as an alternate route of the pyramidal system to exert influence on LMNs.
- The rubrospinal tract is the most important and much better developed in some animals than in humans. In humans, the red nucleus is relatively small and the rubrospinal tract reaches only the upper three cervical segments of the spinal cord.

2. Vestibulospinal tracts There are two vestibulospinal tracts – lateral and medial.

i. Lateral vestibulospinal tract Fibres of this tract arise from the lateral vestibular (Deiters') nucleus. These fibres are somatotopically arranged. Fibres to cervical segments arise from the cranioventral part, those to thoracic segments from the central part and those to lumbosacral segments from the dorsocaudal part of lateral vestibular nucleus.

Location and course This tract is uncrossed and lies in the anterior funiculus of the spinal cord (Fig. 10.1.10), shifting medially as it descends.

Termination The fibres extend up to caudal segments of the cord and terminate into neurons of ventral grey column (laminae VII and VIII). Through the interneurons, these are projected to the alpha and gamma neurons of lamina IX; some fibres directly reach the alpha neurons.

Functions Vestibular nucleus receives afferents from the vestibular apparatus, mainly from the utricles. This pathway is principally concerned with adjustment of postural muscles to linear acceleratory displacements of the body. The lateral vestibulospinal tract mainly facilitates the activity of extensor muscles and inhibits the activity of flexor muscles in association with the maintenance of balance.

ii. Medial vestibulospinal tract The fibres of this tract arise from the medial vestibular nucleus.

Location and course This tract descends through the anterior funiculus (within the sulcomarginal fasciculus). The fibres are mostly uncrossed but some fibres are crossed.

Termination The fibres end in the anterior motor neurons directly or through internuncial neurons (laminae VII and VIII) of the cervical segments of the spinal cord.

Functions This part of the vestibular nucleus receives signals from the vestibular apparatus, mainly from the semicircular canals. Functionally, the medial vestibulospinal tract is the donor connection of MLF. This tract provides a reflex pathway for movements of the head, neck and eyes in response to visual and auditory stimuli.

3. Reticulospinal tracts There are two reticulospinal tracts – the medial (pontine) reticulospinal tract and the lateral (medullary) reticulospinal tract.

i. Medial (pontine) reticulospinal tract It arises in the medial pontine reticular formation.

Course The tract descends, mostly uncrossed, in the anterior funiculus of the spinal cord.

Termination The fibres terminate in the laminae VII and VIII of spinal grey matter and through internuncial neurons influence alpha and gamma neurons of lamina IX.

ii. Lateral (medullary) reticulospinal tract The fibres of this tract originate from the gigantocellular component of medullary reticular formation.

Course These fibres are mostly uncrossed and a few crossed. This tract descends in the lateral funiculus medial to the lateral corticospinal and rubrospinal tracts (Fig. 10.1.10).

Termination The fibres terminate in the internuncial neurons of laminae VII, VIII and IX of the spinal cord.

Functions of reticulospinal tracts The reticular formation of the brainstem receives input mostly from the motor cortex through the corticoreticular fibres which accompany the corticospinal tracts. Thus, the corticoreticulospinal tracts form additional polysynaptic pathways from the motor cortex to the spinal cord. These tracts are concerned with control of movements and maintenance of muscle tone. The reticulospinal tracts, probably, also convey autonomic information from the higher centres to the intermediate region of spinal grey matter and regulate respiration, circulation and sweating.

The pontine and medullary reticular nuclei mostly function antagonistic to each other as:

- Pontine nuclei are excitatory to antigravity muscles and medullary nuclei are inhibitory.
- Pontine nuclei facilitate whereas medullary nuclei inhibit the control of voluntary and reflex movements and control of muscle tone through gamma neurons.
- Pontine reticular formation favours expiration, whereas medullary reticular formation favours inspiration.
- Pontine nuclei cause vasoconstriction and medullary nuclei cause vasodilatation.

4. Tectospinal tract Fibres of this tract arise from superior colliculi.

Course In contrast to other tracts of the extrapyramidal system, the fibres cross the midline in the lower part of segmental of the midbrain forming dorsal segmental decussation. Then the tract descends through the pons and medulla into the anterior white funiculus of the spinal cord (Fig. 10.1.10).

Termination The fibres terminate in upper cervical levels by synapsing on the anterior horn cells through internuncial neurons located in laminae V and VII of the spinal grey matter.

Function This tract forms the motor limb of the reflex pathway for turning the head and moving the arms in response to visual, hearing or other exteroceptive stimuli.

5. *Olivospinal tract* The origin of this tract is of doubtful existence, originating from the inferior olivary nucleus.

Course and termination The tract fibres descend and terminate ipsilaterally in the anterior horn cells of the spinal cord.

Functions Exact connections are unknown. The inferior olivary nucleus receives afferent fibres from the cerebral cortex, corpus striatum, red nucleus and spinal cord. It influences muscle activity. Probably, it is involved in reflex movements arising from the proprioceptors.

6. *Medial longitudinal fasciculus* The MLF extends from the midbrain downwards. The fibres of this tract take origin from different areas of the brainstem, namely:

- Vestibular nuclei
- Reticular formation
- Superior colliculus
- Interstitial nucleus of Cajal
- Nucleus of posterior commissure
- Nucleus of Darkschewitsch

Course The MLF (Fig. 10.1.17) in the brainstem is closely related to the nuclei of cranial nerves III, IV, VI and XII. It is also related to the fibres of nerve VII (as they wind around the abducens nucleus), and to some fibres arising from the cochlear nuclei. Below, the MLF becomes continuous with the anterior intersegmental tract of the spinal cord (Fig. 10.1.10) which descends through the posterior part of anterior white funiculus. This tract is well defined only in the upper cervical segments. Below this level, the fibres run along with the fibres of the medial vestibulospinal tract.

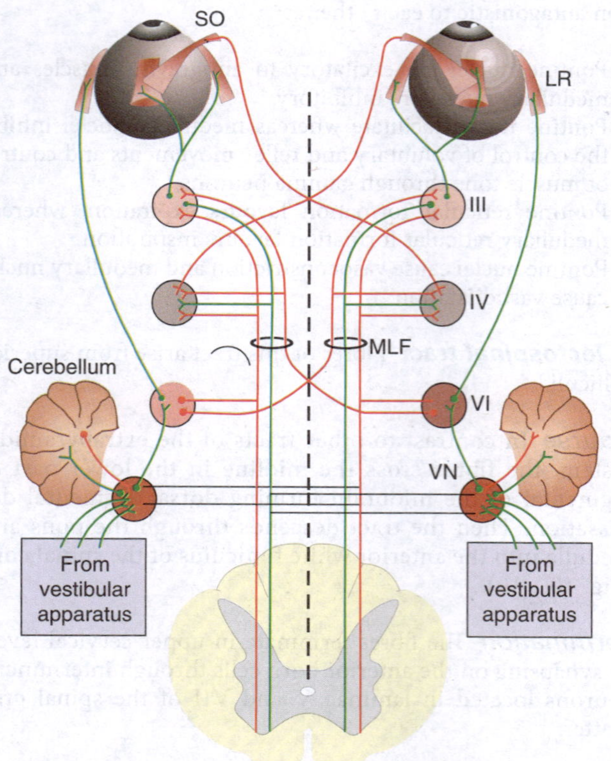

Fig. 10.1.17 Connections of medial longitudinal fasciculus. LR, lateral rectus, III, IV and VI (nuclei of cranial nerves III, IV and VI); SO, superior oblique; VN, vestibular nuclei.

Termination Along with the fibres of the medial vestibulospinal tract, the fibres of this tract make connections with ventral horn cells that innervate the muscles of the neck.

Functions MLF plays an important role in the pathway of ocular movements. Its function can be summarized as:

- It ensures harmonious movements of the eyes and neck (head) in response to vestibular stimulation and auditory stimuli.
- It facilitates simultaneous movements of the lips and tongue as in speech.

Descending Tracts Ending in the Brainstem

1. *Corticonuclear tracts* These arise from the cerebral cortex along with the corticospinal tracts (see page 889).

Course and termination These fibres descend along with corticospinal tract fibres as part of corona radiata and then pass through the posterior limb of the internal capsule. In the brainstem, they cross to the opposite side at various levels and end by synapsing with cells of the cranial nerve nuclei, either directly or through interneurons.

Functions The nuclei of cranial nerves that supply skeletal muscles are functionally equivalent to ventral horn cells of the spinal cord. These are controlled by corticonuclear fibres.

2. *Corticopontocerebellar pathway* This pathway consists of the fibres arising in the cerebral cortex of the frontal, temporal, parietal and occipital lobes.

Course After originating from the cerebral cortex, the fibres descend through the corona radiata and internal capsule to reach the crus cerebri (Fig. 10.1.10). These fibres synapse with the pontine nuclei of the same side. Axons of the neurons in the pontine nuclei form the transverse fibres of the pons. These fibres cross the midline and pass into the middle cerebellar peduncle of the opposite side and reach the cerebellar cortex.

Functions This pathway forms the anatomical basis for control of cerebellar activity of the cerebral cortex.

3. *Other fibres ending in the brainstem* Other fibres arising from the cerebral cortex end in the following masses of grey matter of the brainstem:

- Red nucleus (corticorubral fibres)
- Tectum (corticotectal fibres)
- Substantia nigra
- Inferior olivary nucleus (cortico-olivary fibres)
- Reticular formation (corticoreticular fibres)

The above-stated fibres ultimately form part of the extrapyramidal system.

The major descending tracts in the spinal cord are summarized in Table 10.1.2.

Table 10.1.2 Major descending tracts of the spinal cord

Tract	Location	Origin[a]	Termination	Functions
Pyramidal tracts				
• Lateral corticospinal (crossed pyramidal) tract	Lateral white column of spinal cord	Primary motor cortex (area 4), premotor cortex (area 6) of the opposite cerebral hemisphere *(upper motor neurons)*	Anterior horn cells of the spinal cord *(lower motor neurons)*	Controls conscious skilled movements especially of hands (contraction of individual or small group of muscles particularly those which move hands, fingers, feet and toes)
• Anterior corticospinal (uncrossed pyramidal) tract	Anterior white column	Primary motor cortex (area 4), premotor cortex (area 6) of the opposite cerebral hemisphere *(upper motor neurons)*	Anterior horn cells of the spinal cord *(lower motor neurons)*	Same as that of lateral corticospinal tracts
Extrapyramidal tracts				
• Rubrospinal tract	Lateral white column	Red nucleus of the opposite side located in midbrain	Anterior horn cells of the spinal cord	Unconscious coordination of movements (controls muscle tone and synergy)
• Vestibulospinal tract	Anterior white column	Vestibular nucleus	Anterior horn cells of the spinal cord	Unconscious maintenance of posture and balance
Reticulospinal tracts				
• Medial reticulospinal tract	Anterior white column	Reticular formation in medulla	Anterior horn cells of the spinal cord	Mainly responsible for inhibitory influence on the motor neurons to the skeletal muscles
• Lateral reticulospinal tract	Lateral white column	Reticular formation in midbrain, pons and medulla	Anterior horn cells of the spinal cord	Mainly responsible for facilitatory influence on the motor neurons to the skeletal muscles
Tectospinal tract	Anterior white column	Superior colliculus of the opposite side	Cranial nerve nuclei in medulla and anterior horn cells of the upper spinal segments	Controls movements of head, neck and arms in response to the visual stimuli

[a]Location of cell bodies of neurons from which the axons of tract arise.

Applied Aspects

Lesions of Spinal Cord and Brainstem

I. Transection of the Spinal Cord

Transection of the spinal cord can be divided into three types:

- Complete transection
- Incomplete transection
- Hemisection

1. Complete Transection of Spinal Cord

Common causes of complete transection are as follows:

- Gunshot injuries
- Dislocation of the spine
- Occlusion of the blood vessels

Common site of involvement is at the mid-thoracic level.

Clinical Stages The effects (symptoms and signs) produced by complete transection of the spinal cord occur in the following three stages:

- Stage of spinal shock
- Stage of reflex activity
- Stage of reflex failure

A. Stage of Spinal Shock. Spinal shock refers to cessation of all the functions and activity below the level of the section immediately after injury.

- *Effects depend on the site of injury*; complete transection in the cervical region (above C_5) is usually fatal, because of cutting of connections between the respiratory centre and the respiratory muscles leading to paralysis of respiratory muscles.
- *In quick transection of the spinal cord*, the patient feels as if it has been cut into two portions; the upper portion (higher centres and mind) is unaffected, but the whole body below the level of injury is deprived of all the sensations and motor activity.
- *Cause of stage of spinal shock* (also called stage of flaccidity) is not known, but it is related to cessation of tonic neuronal discharge from the upper brainstem or supraspinal pathway.
- *Duration and severity* of spinal shock depends on the evolution of animal. Higher the animal, more profound and longer lasting is the spinal shock. This is probably due to encephalization, i.e. greater dependence of the spinal cord on higher centres. Therefore, spinal shock lasts for few minutes in frogs, for few hours in cats and dogs, for days in monkeys and for about 3 weeks in humans.

In higher animals, the entire nervous system is integrated as a functional unit; therefore, damage to any part of the nervous system disturbs its smoothness of working and the functional failure is more severe. This is called *diaschisis*.

Characteristic effects during spinal shock can be summarized:

1. ***Motor effects*** include:
   - *Paralysis of the muscles* occurs below the level of section. Depending on the site of lesion, when both lower limbs are paralysed (transection between cervical and lumbosacral enlargements), it is called paraplegia, and when all the four limbs are affected (transection below C_5), it is called quadriplegia.
   - *Loss of tone* occurs in the paralysed muscles. So the muscles become atonic or flaccid. This is called the state of flaccid paralysis.
   - *Areflexia,* i.e. all the superficial and deep reflexes are markedly decreased or lost.
2. ***Sensory effects:*** All the sensations are lost below the level of transections.
3. ***Vasomotor effects:*** The sympathetic vasoconstrictor fibres leave the spinal cord between T_1 and L_2. Therefore, depending on the site of lesion, the vasomotor effects produced are as follows:
   - *Transection of the cord below L_2 segment* will produce no effect or very little fall in blood pressure.
   - *Transection at the level of T_1 segment* cuts off all the thoracolumbar sympathetic neurons from the medullary cardiovascular centre. As a result, there occurs loss of sympathetic tonic discharge causing arteriolar dilatation leading to a sharp fall in blood pressure (MBP may fall from a normal resting value of 100 mm Hg to about 40 mm Hg). Fall in blood pressure is less marked as the section shifts more distally towards L_2 segment.

     Absence of movements due to paralysis of muscles further retards the circulation and also the venous return producing cold and blue (cyanotic) extremities. The skin becomes dry and scaly and bed sores may develop.

Important Note

It is important to note that after paralysis of the muscles, the body temperature becomes subnormal (as muscular contraction is a major source of heat production). When hot bottles are given to raise the body temperature, under such circumstances, bed sores develop.

4. ***Visceral effects*** produced are as follows:
   - *Urinary bladder* is paralysed; however, the sphincter vesicae regain tone early leading to retention of urine.
   - *Rectum* is also paralysed. Since the bowels become hypotonic, there occurs constipation.
   - *Penis* becomes flaccid and erection becomes impossible.
   - When lesion is at T_6 level, all impulses coming in from the abdominal viscera are cut off from the brain; therefore, gripping sensations or distension of viscera are not appreciated.

B. Stage of Reflex Activity. If the patient survives the stage of spinal shock, gradually he/she gains few functions. That is why this is also called the stage of recovery. After about a 3-week period, depending largely on the general health of the patient, the reflex activity begins to return to the isolated segments of the spinal cord below the level of lesion. Various developments which take place, in a chronological order, in this stage are as follows:

1. ***Smooth muscles regain functional activity first of all***, and the urinary bladder becomes automatic, i.e. reflex evacuation is gradually established in a perfectly normal manner. Similarly, reflex defaecation is also established.
2. ***Sympathetic tone of the blood vessels is regained***, next to smooth muscles, when connector cells in the spinal cord begin to act independently of the vasomotor center (VMC). As a result:
   - *Blood pressure* is restored to normal.
   - *Skin*, which has become dry and scaly, now shows sweating again and becomes more healthy. Bed sores, if any, heal up rapidly.
3. ***Skeletal muscle tone then recovers slowly after 3–4 weeks.*** Recovery of muscle tone is reflex in character and is produced by impulses entering the spinal cord from the muscles.
   - Tone of flexor muscles returns first; therefore, flexors become less hypotonic than extensors leading to '*paraplegia in flexion*' (both lower limbs are in state of flexion).
   - In 'spinal man', the limbs cannot support the weight of the body.

Important Note

No wasting of muscles is seen, because although the muscles are paralysed for voluntary movements, they are in constant reflex activity.

4. ***Reflex activity begins to return after few weeks of recovery of muscle tone.*** Recovery of reflex excitability is due to the development of *denervation hypersensitivity* to the mediators released by the remaining spinal excitatory endings and the growing of collaterals from existing neurons with the formation of additional excitatory ending on interneurons and motor neurons.
   - *Flexor reflexes* return first, and to elicit flexor reflex, a painful stimulus is required. The first reflex which usually appears is Babinski reflex (i.e. *Babinski* sign is positive).
   - *Extensor reflexes* return after a variable period of 1–5 weeks of the appearance of flexor reflexes. Initially, the *knee jerk* appears, and then the *ankle jerk* may return still later. Generally, about 6 months after the occurrence of transection, marked activity appears in the extensor arcs. This results in exaggerated extensor reflexes with the appearance of extensor spasms.
   - *Mass reflex* can be elicited in some cases by scratching the skin over the lower limbs or the anterior abdominal wall, depending on the level of lesion. It is characterized by spasm of flexor muscles of both the limbs, evacuation of the bladder and profuse sweating below the level of the lesion.

Important Note

The mass reflex can be utilized to provide paraplegic patients a degree of bladder and bowel control. Patients can be trained to initiate urination and defaecation by intentionally producing mass reflex with the help of a stroke or a pinch on their thighs.

C. Stage of Reflex Failure. The failure of reflex activity may occur when the general condition of the patient starts deteriorating due to malnutrition, infections or toxaemia; under such circumstances:

- Reflexes become more difficult to elicit.
- The threshold for stimulus increases.
- Mass reflex is abolished.
- The muscles become extremely flaccid and undergo wasting.

2. *Incomplete Transection of Spinal Cord*

In incomplete transection, the spinal cord is gravely injured but does not suffer from complete transection (i.e. a few tracts are intact).

Effects of incomplete transection can be divided into three clinical stages:

- Stage of spinal shock
- Stage of reflex activity
- Stage of reflex failure

A. Stage of Spinal Shock. Features of this stage are similar to those described in the stage of spinal shock of complete transection of the spinal cord (see page 893).

B. Stage of reflex activity. Features of this stage differ remarkably from those of the stage of reflex activity of complete transection of the spinal cord:

1. ***Tone appears in extensor muscles first*** (cf. complete transection in which tone appears in flexor muscles first). This is because of the fact that in incomplete transection, some of the descending fibres in the lateral column of the cord, especially the vestibulospinal and reticulospinal tracts, may escape injury, and both these tracts mainly reinforce activity of extensor motor neurons. Because of comparatively higher tone in extensor muscles, a condition called 'paraplegia in extension' results (cf. complete transection in which paraplegia in flexion is seen).
2. ***Extensor reflexes (stretch reflexes) return first*** and flexor reflexes reappear later (cf. complete transection in which flexor reflexes return first). Extensor reflexes which can be elicited in this stage in incomplete transection and not in complete transection are as follows:
   - *Phillipson reflex:* It refers to extension of the opposite limb produced by gentle flexion of one limb. The flexed limb then becomes extended and the opposite one flexed, i.e. the response alternates in each limb producing a steppage movement.
   - *Extensor thrust reflex:* It refers to physiological extensor response (i.e. active contraction of quadriceps, and posterior calf muscles with straightening of limb) obtained by pressing the foot upward with the palm of the hand in a patient in whom the lower limb has been passively flexed and allowed to rest on the bed.
   - *Crossed extensor reflex:* It refers to occurrence of forcible extension of the opposite limb associated with withdrawal (flexor) reflex produced by noxious stimulus to the sole of the foot of one limb.
3. ***Mass reflex is not elicited*** in incomplete transection (cf. complete transection in which mass reflex is elicited). This is because the controlling effect of the brainstem persists through motor fibres (vestibulospinal and reticulospinal) which have escaped injury.

C. Stage of Reflex Failure. Features of this stage are similar to those of the stage of reflex failure with complete transection of the spinal cord.

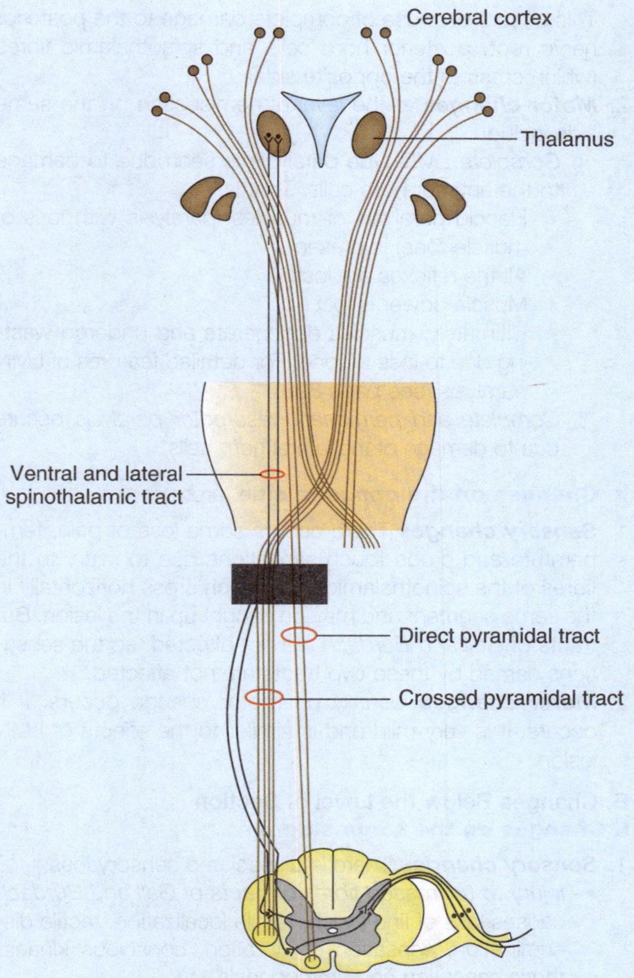

Fig. 10.1.18 Hemisection of the spinal cord.

3. *Hemisection of the Spinal Cord (Brown-Séquard Syndrome)*

Hemisection of the spinal cord refers to a lesion involving one lateral half of the spinal cord (Fig. 10.1.18). It can occur following accidental injuries. It can also be produced for experimental studies in the animals.

The effects of hemisection of the spinal cord can be described in two stages:

- Immediate effects
- Late effects

Immediate effects: *Immediate effects following hemisection of the spinal cord are those of 'spinal shock' (see page 893).*

Late effects: *If the patient survives, typical motor and sensory changes develop after recovery from the spinal shock. These changes constitute the* Brown-Séquard syndrome *and can be described as:*

- Changes at the level of section
- Changes below the level of section
- Changes above the level of section

A. Changes at the Level of Hemisection

I. Changes on the same side are:

1. ***Sensory changes*** All the sensations are lost (complete anaesthesia) at the level of hemisection on the same side.

This occurs because of complete damage to the posterior nerve root, posterior horn cells and spinothalamic fibres (which cross to the opposite side).

2. ***Motor changes*** at the level of hemisection on the same side include:
   i. *Complete LMN*-type paralysis is seen due to damage to the anterior horn cells. That is:
      - Flaccid paralysis of muscles (paralysis with loss of muscle tone) is present.
      - All the reflexes are lost.
      - Muscle power is lost.
      - Ultimately, muscles degenerate and undergo wasting due to loss of tone. For detailed features of LMN paralysis, see page 898.

   ii. *Complete and permanent vasomotor paralysis* occurs due to damage of the lateral horn cells.

II. Changes on the opposite side are:

1. ***Sensory changes*** There occurs some loss of pain, temperature and crude touch sensations due to injury to the fibres of the spinothalamic tract which cross horizontally in the same segment and may be caught up in the lesion. But tracts of *Goll and Burdach* are not affected, so the sensations carried by these two tracts are not affected.
2. ***Motor changes*** Usually no motor change occurs. If it occurs, it is very mild and is similar to the effects of LMN lesion.

B. Changes Below the Level of Section

I. Changes on the same side are:

1. ***Sensory changes*** There is dissociated sensory loss:
   - *Injury to uncrossed fibres of tracts of Gall and Burdach* causes loss of fine touch, tactile localization, tactile discrimination, sensation of vibration, conscious kinaesthetic sensation and stereognosis.
   - *No injury occurs to spinothalamic tracts* which cross to the opposite side, so crude touch, pain and temperature sensations are not lost.
2. ***Motor changes*** There occurs UMN type of paralysis due to injury to the pyramidal tracts. Features of UMN paralysis include:
   - Increased muscle tone, leading to spastic paralysis
   - Loss of superficial reflexes
   - Exaggeration of deep reflexes
   - Positive Babinski sign
   - Rigidity of limbs
   - No degeneration and wasting of muscles
3. ***Vasomotor changes*** There occurs temporary loss of vasomotor tone due to damage to the descending fibres from the VMC in the medulla to the lateral horn cells. This leads to:
   - Dilatation of blood vessels
   - Fall in blood pressure

   However, soon the intact lateral horn cells start acting as supplementary VMC and vasomotor tone returns leading to normalization of blood pressure.

II. Changes on the opposite side are:

1. ***Sensory changes*** Dissociated sensory loss occurs as:
   - *Injury to crossed spinothalamic tracts* causes loss of the following sensations on the opposite side below the level of lesion: crude touch, pain and temperature.
   - *No injury occurs to uncrossed tracts of Gall and Burdach*, so the following sensations on the opposite side below the level of lesion are not lost: fine touch, tactile localization, tactile discrimination, vibratory sense, conscious kinaesthetic sensation and stereognosis.
2. ***Motor changes*** Usually, no motor change on the opposite side below the level of lesion occurs. UMN lesion-type paralysis of a few muscles, however, may occur sometimes due to possible damage to some fibres of direct pyramidal tracts of the same side when these fibres cross.

   In a nutshell, below the level of lesion, there occurs:
   - Extensive motor loss but little sensory loss on the same side
   - Extensive sensory loss but little motor loss on the opposite side

C. Changes Above the Level of Lesion

I. Changes on the same side are:

1. ***Sensory changes*** A band of hyperaesthesia, i.e. increased cutaneous sensations, is present in one or two segments above the level of section on the same side. This occurs due to irritation of the neighbouring posterior nerve roots above the level of section.
2. ***Motor changes*** Twitching of muscle in upper one or two segments on the same side may occur due to irritation of the neighbouring anterior nerve roots above the level of section.

II. Changes on the opposite side are:

1. ***Sensory changes*** Either no sensory change or referred hyperaesthesia may be seen one or two segments above the lesion on the opposite side.
2. ***Motor changes*** No motor change occurs on the opposite side above the level of section.

Regional Peculiarities in Hemisection of Spinal Cord

1. Hemisection in Cervical Region shows the following peculiar changes:

- *Constriction of pupil occurs on the same side*, due to damage to dilator fibres passing via T_1, T_2 and T_3 anterior nerve roots.
- *Loss of the following jerks* occurs if the lesion involves C_4, C_5 and C_6 segments: biceps, triceps, supinator and pronator jerks.
- *Paralysis of diaphragm* on the same side occurs due to involvement of phrenic nerve (C_3, C_4 and C_5).

2. Hemisection in Lumbar Region may show the following peculiarities:

- Loss of knee jerk
- Disturbances in the micturition due to involvement of L_3 and L_4

3. Hemisection in Lumbosacral Region is associated with loss of control over the sphincters of:

- Urinary bladder
- Anus

Complications in Patients With Spinal Cord Transection

Patients with spinal cord transection get immobilized due to paraplegia or quadriplegia and thus may develop the following complications:

1. ***Decubitus (postural) ulcers*** occur due to compression of circulation to the skin over bony prominences in bed-ridden patients by the body weight. These ulcers heal very poorly and are prone to secondary infections.
2. ***Hypercalcaemia, hypercalciuria and calcium stone formation in the urinary tract*** may occur due to breakdown of proteins from the bone matrix.
3. ***Urinary tract infections*** are very common owing to urinary stasis associated with paralysis of the urinary bladder.
4. ***Septicaemia, uraemia, coma and even death*** may occur as a complication of severe urinary tract infection.

   Treatment: High dose of corticosteroid if administered immediately after spinal cord injury has some value, because steroids decrease the inflammatory reaction by suppressing neutrophil activity, and improving capillary permeability.

II. Lesions of Sensory System in Spinal Cord

A. Deafferentation (Dorsal Nerve Root Lesion).

Injury to the dorsal nerve root (afferent nerve) produces the following effects:

1. ***Loss of all sensations*** occurs, i.e.:
   - Loss of exteroceptive senses with anaesthesia and analgesia
   - Loss of conscious muscle sense, producing ataxia
   - Loss of unconscious muscle sense from stretch receptors of muscle spindle, with hypotonia or atonia
   - Loss of visceral senses
2. ***Loss of all reflexes*** All the reflexes, superficial as well as deep, are lost.
3. ***Muscle tone*** is lost.
4. ***Marked weakness in the movements of parts*** occurs because the higher centres concerned with reflex control of posture are deprived of afferent impulses from joints and muscles.

B. Syringomyelia.

Syringomyelia is a rare disease in which there occurs excessive overgrowth of neuroglial tissue accompanied by cavitation in the grey matter around the central canal of the spinal cord. This disease involves the cervical enlargement of the cord more frequently.

Characteristic Features include:

I. ***Sensory features*** are predominant and occur in the form of dissociated anaesthesia, i.e. loss of pain and temperature with retention of touch sensation as:
   - *Loss of pain, temperature and crude touch* sensation occurs due to destruction of the fibres which carry these sensations and are decussating in the grey commissure.
   - *Fine touch sensation* is not lost because the fibres carrying this sensation ascend in the dorsal column and escape damage.

   Note: The symptoms are bilateral and usually occur in the hands and arms due to the *predilection* of syringomyelin for the cervical enlargement of the cord.

II. ***Motor features*** may also occur due to further spread of gliosis and cavitations:
   - *Flaccid paralysis of the upper limb muscle* (LMN-type paralysis) may occur initially due to involvement of anterior horn cells.
   - *Progressive spastic paralysis of the legs* (UMN-type paralysis) may occur later on due to involvement of pyramidal and extrapyramidal tracts.

C. Tabes Dorsalis.

Tabes dorsalis is a disease, usually caused by syphilis, in which there occurs bilateral degeneration of posterior nerve roots and posterior funiculi, especially fasciculus gracilis.

Characteristic Features include:

1. ***Lightening pains*** occur in intermittent attacks due to stimulation of pain fibres in dorsal nerve roots in the initial stages.
2. ***Loss or decrease*** of pain sensibility occurs after some time producing the following features:
   - *Trophic disturbances* in the form of perforating ulcers of the skin at pressure points. *Charcot joint refers* to deformed joints produced by repeated trauma due to loss of pain sensations. There is no proper support and movements of the joints of the body become uncontrolled.
   - Anaesthesia of the central part of the face occurs due to involvement of cranial nerve V.
   - Anaesthesia at the upper chest, inner border of the hands, around the anus and over the legs occurs due to involvement of dorsal nerve roots in cervicothoracic and lumbosacral regions.
3. ***Loss of deep sensations:*** The following sensations are lost on the same side at and below the level of lesion: position sense, vibratory sense, sense of stereognosis and discriminative touch.
4. ***Loss of reflexes:*** Both superficial and deep reflexes are lost in tabes dorsalis mostly because of loss of sensations.
5. ***Sensory ataxia*** occurs due to lack of coordination of voluntary involvement. In it, the patient walks on a broad base with the legs apart and eyes fixed to the ground for correcting the steps. Typically, the patient raises the legs excessively high and slopes the feet on the ground. *Romberg sign* is positive.

D. Multiple Sclerosis.

Multiple sclerosis (MS) is a demyelinating disorder having widespread disseminated involvement of white matter of the central nervous system (CNS). Because of this, it was also called disseminated sclerosis. It is currently considered to be an autoimmune disease, pathologically characterized by focal inflammation, demyelination and gliosis or scarring. A remitting and relapsing course is the most common, with either complete recovery or residual damage with each attack.

Manifestations of MS depend on the area of CNS involved. The commonest symptoms reported are as follows:

- Limb weakness (75%)
- Sensory loss (37%)
- Paraesthesia (24%)

- Optic neuritis (37%)
- Diplopia, vertigo and ataxia – comparatively less common

E. Subacute Combined Degeneration of the Spinal Cord. Subacute combined degeneration of the spinal cord is usually associated with pernicious anaemia, due to lack of intrinsic factor which is essential for the absorption of vitamin B_{12}.

In this condition, bilateral degeneration of white fibres of the dorsal column and lateral column of the spinal cord occurs, especially involving the lumbosacral segments. Its manifestations include:

- Loss of position and vibrating senses of the lower extremities
- Signs of UMN lesions such as bilateral spasticity, exaggerated tendon reflexes and positive Babinski sign

III. Lesions of Motor System

Lower Versus Upper Motor Neuron Lesion

Differences between LMN lesions and UMN lesions are shown in Table 10.1.3.

IV. Brainstem Lesions

Lesions of Medulla

1. ***Medial medullary syndrome*** Medial medullary syndrome results from occlusion of the blood supply (anterior spinal artery and its paramedian branches) to medial zone of the medulla. It is characterized by:

- LMN paralysis of ipsilateral tongue muscles due to involvement of the hypoglossal nerve
- UMN paralysis on the contralateral side due to involvement of the corticospinal tract
- Contralateral loss of discriminative senses of the body due to interruption of the medial lemniscus rostral to the decussation

2. ***Lateral medullary syndrome*** Lateral medullary syndrome results from the occlusion of the posterior inferior cerebellar artery supplying the posterolateral part of the medulla.

Characteristic Features Characteristic features of this syndrome are as follows:

Ipsilateral loss of pain and temperature sensations in the face and forehead area due to interruption of the spinal tract of the trigeminal nerve

Contralateral loss of pain and temperature in the rest of the body due to involvement of spinal lemniscus

Paralysis of the muscles of the soft palate, pharynx and larynx on the side of lesion due to destruction of the nucleus ambiguus

Table 10.1.3 Lower versus upper motor neuron lesions

Lower motor neuron lesion (LMNL)	Upper motor neuron lesion (UMNL)
1. LMNL refers to involvement of neurons (α and γ) of anterior horn of spinal cord and neurons of cranial nerve nuclei.	1. UMNL refers to involvement of motor neurons that influence the activity of LMN of spinal cord or cranial nerve nuclei located in brainstem. Thus, in UMNL, the pyramidal and extrapyramidal descending tracts are involved.
2. LMN paralysis is typically observed in poliomyelitis, when the poliovirus selectively affects the lower motor neurons of spinal cord and brainstem.	2. UMN paralysis occurs commonly in vascular accidents or space-occupying lesions.
3. Usually a single or individual muscle is affected.	3. Usually a group of muscles is affected.
4. Flaccid paralysis of the involved muscle as muscle tone is lost due to involvement of stretch reflex arc.	4. Spastic paralysis of the involved muscles as the inhibitory higher control is lost and stretch reflex arc is intact.
5. Muscle power is lost and ultimately muscles degenerate and undergo wasting due to disuse (disuse atrophy).	5. No degeneration and wasting of muscles as they are constantly involved in reflex activity (although the voluntary movements are lost).
6. Areflexia, i.e. all the superficial as well as deep reflexes are lost.	6. Superficial reflexes (abdominal, cremasteric, anal are lost but deep reflexes are exaggerated [because of increased gamma-motor discharge]).
7. Babinski sign is negative, i.e. on stroking the outer edge of the sole of the foot with firm tactile stimulus, there occurs plantar flexion (downward movement). It is called floor response (withdrawal reflex) and is considered a normal response.	7. Babinski sign is positive, i.e. on stroking the outer edge of the sole of the foot with firm stimulus, there occurs dorsiflexion of the great toe and fanning out (abduction) of small toes. It is also called extensor response. Positive Babinski sign indicates involvement of corticospinal tract. In normal infants, this sign is positive prior to myelination of the corticospinal tract (i.e. younger than 1 year).
8. Clonus is absent.	8. Clonus is present. It refers to a sustained series of rhythmic muscle jerks when a quick stretch is applied to a tendon. Ankle clonus is usually observed in UMNL by sudden dorsiflexion of the foot.
9. Clasp knife reflex is absent.	9. Clasp knife reflex is present, i.e. muscular resistance to passive movement is exaggerated; this resistance is strong at the beginning of movement, but yields suddenly in a clasp knife fashion as more force against resistance is applied. The initial resistance is offered because of the stretch reflex developed in extensor muscles, e.g. triceps of the elbow. The sudden relax of resistance is due to the activation of inverse stretch reflex.

LMN, lower motor neuron; UMN, upper motor neuron.

Cerebellar asynergia and hypotonia when the inferior cerebellar peduncle is also affected
Nystagmus when vestibular nucleus is also affected

3. ***Cerebellopontine syndrome*** Cerebellopontine syndrome refers to the lesions produced by a tumour in the cerebellopontine angle compressing on the neighbouring structures.

Characteristic Features Characteristic features of this syndrome are as follows:

Involvement of the cranial nerve VII produces:
- Ipsilateral LMN paralysis of facial muscles of expression
- Hyperacusis due to paralysis of stapedius muscle
- Loss of taste sensation from the anterior two-thirds of the tongue

Involvement of cranial nerve VIII causes:
- Persistent tinnitus
- Progressive deafness on the affected side
- Vertigo

Cerebellar dysfunctions may occur in the forms of:
- Intention tremors
- Dysmetria
- Adiadochokinesis
- Ataxia on the affected side

Involvement of the spinal tract of trigeminal causes:
- Ipsilateral loss of pain and temperature of the face and forehead

Involvement of the spinal lemniscus produces:
- Contralateral loss of pain and temperature of the body

V. Pontine Lesions

1. Alternative trigeminal hemiplegia Alternating trigeminal hemiplegia is seen in lesions involving the lateral part of mid-pons.

Characteristic Features Characteristic features include:

1. ***Damage to trigeminal nerve*** results in:
   - Ipsilateral absence of all general senses of the face and the forehead
   - Ipsilateral LMN paralysis of the muscles of mastication
2. ***Damage to pyramidal tracts*** causes:
   - Contralateral hemiplegia

2. Raymond syndrome Raymond syndrome, also known as alternating abducent hemiplegia, is characterized by:

1. ***Damage to nerve VI*** causing:
   - Paralytic convergent squint (esotropia) due to paralysis of lateral rectus muscles
2. ***Damage to pyramidal tracts*** causing:
   - Contralateral hemiplegia

3. Millard–Gubler syndrome Millard–Gubler syndrome results due to lesions of the ventral pons involving sixth nerve fasciculus as it passes through pyramidal tracts and is characterized by:

- Ipsilateral sixth nerve palsy
- Contralateral hemiplegia
- Ipsilateral facial nerve palsy

4. Foville syndrome Foville syndrome results due to lesions of the lower part of the pons and is characterized by the same features as those of Millard–Gubler syndrome except that sixth nerve palsy is replaced by loss of conjugate movement to the same side.

VI. Midbrain Lesions

1. ***Weber syndrome*** Weber syndrome occurs in lesions of the midbrain involving fascicular part of the third nerve while passing through cerebral peduncle. It is characterized by:

- Ipsilateral third nerve palsy
- Contralateral hemiplegia due to damage to corticospinal tracts
- Facial palsy of UMN type

Features of third nerve palsy Features of third nerve palsy are as follows:

Ptosis occurs due to paralysis of lateral palpebral superioris (LPS) muscle.
Deviation: Eyeball is turned down and out due to unopposed action of superior oblique and lateral rectus muscles.
Ocular movements are restricted due to paralysis of the muscles supplied by the third nerve as:
- Adduction: Due to paralysis of medial rectus
- Elevation: Due to paralysis of superior rectus and inferior oblique
- Depression: Due to paralysis of inferior rectus
- Extension: Due to paralysis of inferior rectus and inferior oblique

Pupil is fixed and dilated due to paralysis of the sphincter pupillae muscle.
Accommodation is completely lost due to paralysis of ciliary muscles.
Crossed diplopia, elicited on manually raising the eyelid, occurs due to paralytic divergent squint.
Head posture: If the pupillary area is uncovered, the head takes a position consistent with the directions of actions of the paralysed muscles, i.e. the head is turned on the opposite side and is tilted towards the same side and the chin is slightly raised.

2. ***Benedikt syndrome*** Benedikt syndrome results when the lesion involves the intermediate part of the midbrain. It is characterized by:

- Ipsilateral third cranial nerve palsy
- Contralateral loss of pain, touch, temperature, vibratory and proprioceptive senses due to involvement of medial lemniscus
- Contralateral jerky movements and tremors due to involvement of the red nucleus and superior cerebellar peduncle

Self-Assessment

1. Discuss the functional anatomy, functions and sensory disturbances associated with spinal cord lesion.
2. Discuss the role of pyramidal and extrapyramidal tracts.
3. Describe the following:
   - Brown-Séquard Syndrome
   - Spinal shock
   - Significance of Babinski sign
4. Write notes on the following:
   - Clonus
   - Syringomyelia
   - Spastic paralysis

Clinical Cases

Case 1

A 65-year-old male hypertensive patient developed inability to speak and understand, bolŁ numbness in the face, left arm and leg, and unable to move them. History revealed that he had stopped taking medicine for hypertension for the last 3 months.

Examination observations showed positive Babinski sign, reduced sensations and exaggerated deep tendon reflexes (biceps, triceps).

Q1. What is the cause for observed signs and symptoms?
Q2. The patient is suffering from which type of lesion?
Q3. Why are the deep reflexes exaggerated?
Q4. What are the other causes for this lesion?

Case 2

A 40-year-old male while travelling on bike was injured in a road accident and brought to the trauma centre. Examination showed BP 100/60 mm Hg, pulse 100/min, muscle twitching, decreased muscle tone of lower limbs, superficial reflexes and deep tendon reflexes not elicited.

Q1. What is this neurological condition called?
Q2. Why are superficial reflexes not elicited?
Q3. What is the status of plantar reflex in this state?
Q4. How can the site of lesion be determined?

Case 3

In a road accident, a 30-year-old male had head injury and developed drooping of the left eye, turning of the left eyeball downwards, and a fixed and dilated pupil.

Q1. What is the probable diagnosis?
Q2. This condition occurs due to lesion of which part of the brain?

10.2

Physiological Anatomy, Functions and Lesions of Cerebellum and Basal Ganglia

CHAPTER OUTLINE

CEREBELLUM

PHYSIOLOGICAL ANATOMY

Cerebellum, the largest part of the hindbrain, consists of two lateral parts called the *cerebellar hemispheres* connected in the midline by a narrow central region called the *vermis*.

External Features (Fig. 10.2.1)

Surfaces The cerebellum has two surfaces:

- *Superior surface* is related to the tentorium cerebelli.
- *Inferior surface* is related to the *hollow* of occipital bone.

Folia The surfaces of the cerebellum are thrown into numerous transverse folds called folia.

Fissures The surface of the cerebellum presents three main fissures (Fig. 10.2.1):

1. ***Primary fissure*** lies on the anterosuperior aspect of the cerebellum. It is V shaped, with open being forwards. It forms the posterior limit of the anterior lobe.
2. ***Horizontal fissure*** separates the superior surface of the cerebellum from its inferior surface and thus follows the convex posterior and anterolateral border of the cerebellar hemisphere. It is of no functional significance.
3. ***Posterolateral fissure*** is situated anteriorly on the inferior surface of the cerebellar hemisphere and separates the posterior lobe from the flocculonodular lobe.

Anatomical Parts of Cerebellum

The cerebellum consists of two cerebellar hemispheres, and a median vermis has been divided into many parts which have functional and morphological significance. To show the various parts of the cerebellum in a single illustration, it is usual to represent the organ as if it has been opened out (flattened) so that both the superior and inferior aspects can be seen (Fig. 10.2.1).

Parts of vermis Vermis is so named because it resembles a worm, which is bent on itself to form a complete circle. Superior and inferior surfaces of the vermis are termed superior vermis and inferior vermis. Proceeding from above downwards, the opened-up vermis (as seen in Fig. 10.2.1) consists of the following parts: lingula, central lobule, culmen, declive, folium, tuber, pyramis, uvula and nodule.

Parts of hemisphere With the exception of the lingula, each part of the vermis is related laterally to a part of hemisphere as shown in Fig. 10.2.1.

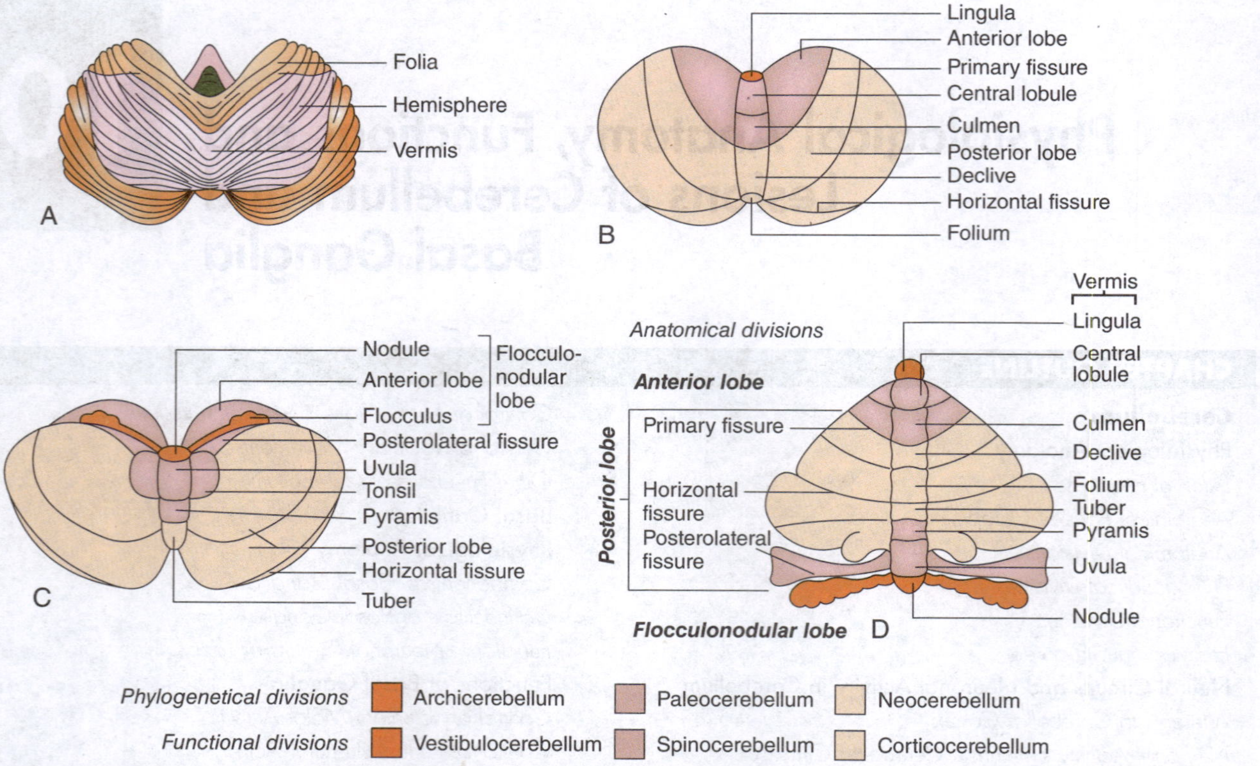

Fig. 10.2.1 Gross anatomy of cerebellum: **A**, superior surface showing folia; **B** and **C**, superior and inferior surfaces showing fissures, lobes and parts of vermis; and **D**, schematic diagram showing the parts of vermis and hemisphere in an opened-up (unrolled) cerebellum.

Anatomical Divisions

Anatomically, the cerebellum has been divided into three lobes:

1. ***Anterior lobe*** is that part of the cerebellum which lies in front of the primary fissure on the superior surface (Fig. 10.2.1). The parts of the vermis and hemisphere forming the anterior lobe are shown in Fig. 10.2.1 and Table 10.2.1.
2. ***Posterior lobe*** is that part of the cerebellum which lies between the primary fissure and the posterolateral fissure. Thus, it includes both surfaces of the cerebellum (the superior surface rostral to the horizontal fissure and the inferior surface caudal to the horizontal fissure); parts of the vermis and hemisphere forming the posterior lobe are shown in Fig. 10.2.1 and Table 10.2.1.
3. ***Flocculonodular lobe*** is that part of the cerebellum which lies anterior to the posterolateral fissure on the inferior surface. It consists of (Fig. 10.2.1; Table 10.2.1):
   - *Nodule*, which is the rostral part of the vermis
   - *Flocculi*, which are irregular-shaped masses attached to nodule on each side (they are almost completely separated from the rest of the cerebellum)

Table 10.2.1 Lobes of cerebellum and parts of vermis and hemisphere forming them

Lobes of cerebellum	Part of vermis	Part of hemisphere
Anterior lobe	Lingula	No lateral projection
	Central lobule	Alae
	Culmen	Anterior quadrangular lobule
Primary fissure	Declive	Posterior quadrangular lobule
Posterior lobe		
	Folium	Superior semilunar lobule
Horizontal fissure	Tuber	Inferior semilunar lobule
	Pyramis	Biventral lobule
	Uvula	Tonsil
Posterolateral fissure	Nodule	Flocculus
Flocculonodular lobe		

Phylogenetical Divisions

Phylogenetically, i.e. according to evolutionary stages, the cerebellum consists of three subdivisions.

1. Archicerebellum It is the oldest part to develop. It consists of (Fig. 10.2.1):

- Flocculonodular lobe
- Lingula

2. Palaeocerebellum Phylogenetically, it is the next part to appear. It consists of (Fig. 10.2.1):

- Entire anterior lobe except lingula, and the following parts of the posterior lobe: pyramis, uvula and paraflocculus

3. Neocerebellum It is the latest part to develop. It consists of whole of the posterior lobe except pyramis and uvula (Fig. 10.2.1).

Functional Divisions

Functionally, the cerebellum is divided into three divisions.

1. Vestibulocerebellum It includes the flocculonodular lobe, which is its principal component and has vestibular connections only.

- Fastigial nucleus is its effector nucleus.
- It is concerned with control of body posture and equilibrium.

2. Spinocerebellum It includes the parts forming the palaeocerebellum, i.e. entire anterior lobe except lingula, and some parts of the posterior lobe (pyramis, uvula and paraflocculus).

- *Interpositus nucleus*, i.e. nucleus globosus and nucleus emboliformis, is its effector nucleus.
- It receives proprioceptive inputs from the spinal cord and is concerned with control of axial (trunk) and limb muscle postural reflexes.

3. Corticocerebellum Corticocerebellum, also called central cerebellum, includes whole of the posterior lobe except pyramis and uvula.

- Nucleus dentatus is its effector nucleus.
- It occupies the more lateral regions of the cerebellar cortex and receives information from the cerebral cortex and pons.
- It is concerned with smooth performance of highly skilled voluntary movements.

Histological Structure

Histologically, cerebellum consists of (Fig. 10.2.2):

- Cerebellar cortex (outer grey matter layer)
- White matter (formed by afferent and efferent nerve fibres of the cerebellum) forming the medullary core
- Deep cerebellar nuclei (masses of grey matter embedded in the medullary core)

I. Cerebellar Cortex

Grossly in cut section, the cerebellar cortex is seen as extensively folded on itself constituting the *folia*, i.e. leaf-like parts which are marked off from one another by fissures. In striking contrast to the cortex of the cerebral hemisphere, the cerebellar cortex has a uniform structure in all parts of the cerebellum. ***Microscopically,*** the grey matter of the cerebellar cortex consists of five main types of neurons (stellate cells, basket cells, Purkinje cells, granule cells and Golgi cells) which are arranged in three layers:

- Molecular layer (most superficial)
- Purkinje cell layer (middle layer)
- Granule cell layer (inner layer)

1. Molecular layer is composed of two types of neurons (stellate and basket cells) and unmyelinated nerve fibres.

i. ***Stellate cells*** are star shaped and more superficially located. Their *dendrites* synapse with parallel fibres of granule cells, and their *axons* synapse with dendrites of Purkinje cells.

ii. ***Basket cells*** are located deep in the molecular layer.
   - They receive inputs from the parallel fibres.
   - Their axons branch and form basket around the cell bodies of Purkinje cells (hence the name).
   - Each basket cell may synapse with about 70 Purkinje cells.

Nerve fibres present in the molecular layer are parallel fibres (axon of granule cells), dendrites of Purkinje cells and climbing fibres from the inferior olivary nucleus.

2. Purkinje cell layer: It is composed of a single layer of large flask-shaped Purkinje cells (biggest neurons in the body).

- Dendrites of Purkinje cells extend into the molecular layer and provide a huge surface area for axodendritic synapses.
- Axons of these cells make synaptic connection with the deep cerebellar nuclei in the medullary core. They act as the

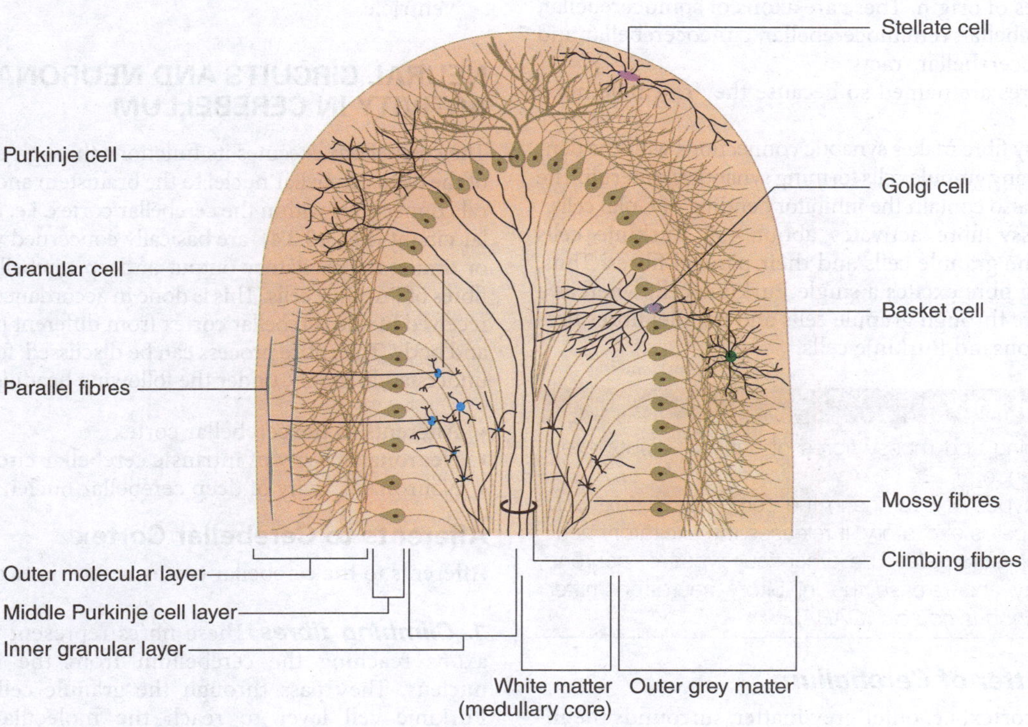

Fig. 10.2.2 Histology of cerebellar cortex.

sole output neurons from the cerebellar cortex, and exert an inhibitory influence to the deep cerebellar and lateral vestibular nuclei.

3. Granule cell layer consists of granule and Golgi cells, with their processes, and sensory mossy fibres with their synaptic glomeruli.

i. ***Granule cells*** are very small, numerous (about 10 billion) spherical neurons. Axons of the granule cells ascend into the molecular layer, and form the parallel fibres that make excitatory synapses with dendrites of Purkinje cells, stellate cells, basket cells and Golgi cells.
ii. ***Golgi cells*** are large cells and less numerous than the granule cells.
   - Their dendrites project into the molecular layer and receive inputs from the parallel fibres.
   - Their cell bodies receive inputs via collaterals from the incoming climbing fibres and Purkinje cells.
   - Their axons branch extensively and make inhibitory synaptic connection with the dendrites of granule cells.

Sensory inputs to cerebellar cortex The cerebellar cortex receives sensory inputs (afferent fibres) from other parts of the brain by two types of sensory fibres – the climbing fibres and mossy fibres. Both sets of fibres reach the cerebellum through the peduncles, and are excitatory in nature.

1. ***Climbing fibres*** arise from the neurons of the inferior olivary nucleus situated in the medulla and reach the cerebellum via the olivocerebellar tract.
   - Climbing fibres establish 'one-to-one' connection with the Purkinje cell dendrites and excite them to discharge.
   - Collaterals of climbing fibres synapse with all other types of neurons in the cerebellar cortex and also the deep cerebellar nuclei.
2. ***Mossy fibres:*** Unlike climbing fibres, the mossy fibres have many sources of origin. These are axons of spinocerebellar, vestibulocerebellar, reticulocerebellar, cuneocerebellar and corticopontocerebellar tracts.
   - Mossy fibres are named so because they resemble moss plant.
   - Each mossy fibre makes synaptic connections with the dendrites of many granule cells forming synaptic glomeruli. The glomeruli also contain the inhibitory ending of Golgi cells.
   - Each mossy fibre activates about 450 Purkinje cells through the granule cells and their parallel fibres. Thus, a climbing fibre excites a single Purkinje cell, whereas a mossy fibre through granule cells and parallel fibres fires several thousand Purkinje cells.

Important Note

Both the climbing and mossy fibres of sensory inputs exert excitatory influence.
- Out of five types of neurons in the cerebellar cortex, only the granule cell is excitatory; it releases the excitatory neurotransmitter *glutamate*. The other four types of neurons are inhibitory and release the inhibitory neurotransmitter *gamma-aminobutyric acid (GABA)*.

II. White Matter of Cerebellum

The cerebellar cortex, i.e. outer grey matter, surrounds the inner medullary core of white matter (an arrangement opposite to what is seen in the spinal cord). White matter is formed by both afferent and efferent fibres. These fibres can be classified into three groups:

1. ***Projection fibres*** of the cerebellum leave or enter the cerebellum and connect it with other parts of the central nervous system. These are arranged in three bundles:
   - *Inferior cerebellar peduncle* consists of fibres connecting the cerebellum with the medulla.
   - *Middle cerebellar peduncle* contains the fibres which connect the cerebellum with the pons.
   - *Superior cerebellar peduncle* connects the cerebellum with the midbrain.
2. ***Association fibres*** connect different regions of the same cerebellar hemisphere.
3. ***Commissural fibres*** connect the areas of two halves of the cerebellar cortex with each other.

III. Deep Cerebellar Nuclei

Within the white matter of the medullary core of the cerebellum are embedded four pairs of masses of grey matter called deep cerebellar nuclei. They lie in close relationship with the roof of the fourth ventricle, and therefore are known as roof nuclei (Fig. 10.2.3).

1. ***Dentate nucleus*** or nucleus dentatus is the largest cerebellar nucleus. Shaped like a purse and made up of a crenated lamina of grey matter, it has an open anteromedian hilum to receive the fibres of the superior cerebellar peduncle.
2. ***Emboliform nucleus*** or nucleus emboliformis is an oval mass of grey matter, located just anteromedian to the hilum of dentate nucleus.
3. ***Globosus nucleus*** lies medial to the nucleus emboliformis, and therefore together they are referred to as nucleus interpositus.
4. ***Fastigial nucleus*** or nucleus fastigii is nearly spherical and lies close to the midline just over the roof of the fourth ventricle.

NEURAL CIRCUITS AND NEURONAL ACTIVITY IN CEREBELLUM

The cerebellum executes its functions through excitatory output of the deep cerebellar nuclei to the brainstem and thalamus. Neural connections within the cerebellar cortex, i.e. intrinsic cerebellar circuit (Fig. 10.2.4), are basically concerned with modulating or timing the excitatory output of deep cerebellar nuclei via the fibres of Purkinje cells. This is done in accordance with the signals received by the cerebellar cortex from different parts of the brain and body. The entire process can be discussed, for the purpose of understanding only, under the following headings:

- Afferents to the cerebellar cortex
- Neuronal activity of intrinsic cerebellar circuitry
- Neuronal activity of deep cerebellar nuclei

Afferents to Cerebellar Cortex

Afferents to the cerebellar cortex reach via two types of fibres.

1. Climbing fibres These fibres represent terminations of axons reaching the cerebellum from the inferior olivary nucleus. They pass through the granule cell layer, and the Purkinje cell layer to reach the molecular layer. In the molecular layer, each climbing fibre ends on dendrites of

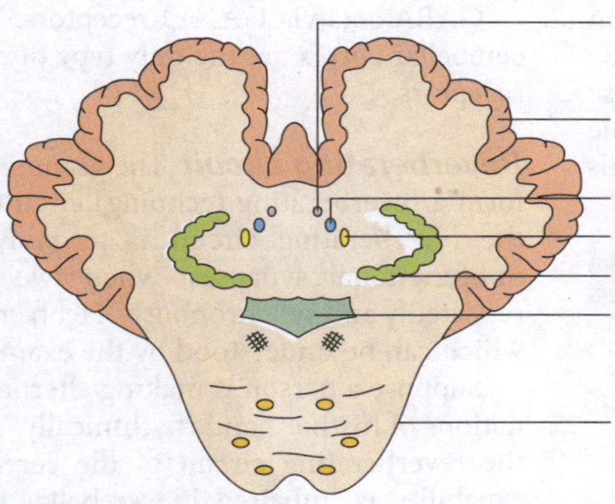

Fig. 10.2.3 Diagrammatic view of nuclei of cerebellum in relation to roof of fourth ventricle.

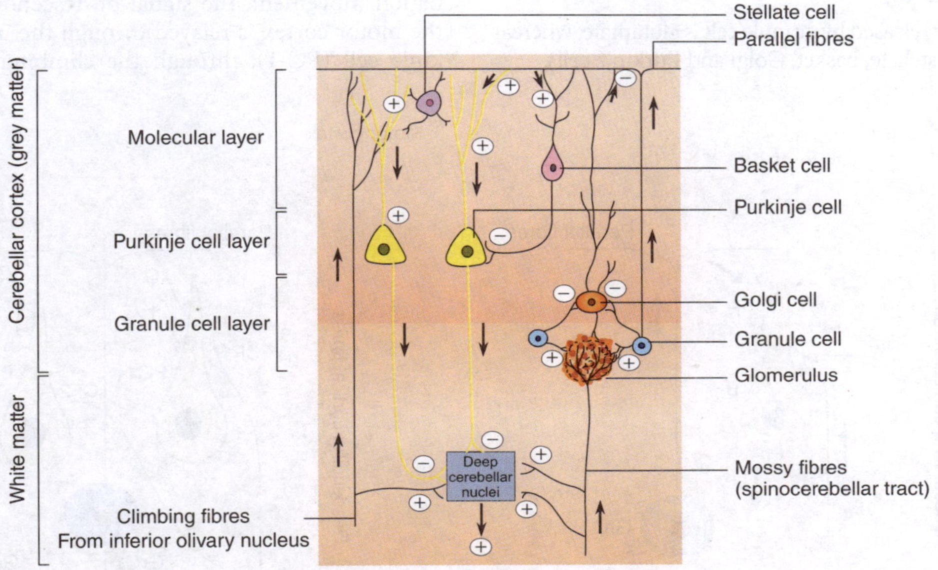

Fig. 10.2.4 Intrinsic cerebellar circuitry.

single Purkinje cell (Fig. 10.2.4). Because of this, the excitatory effect of climbing fibres on Purkinje cell is very strong. The climbing fibres thus excite the Purkinje cells directly and the deep cerebellar nuclei via the collaterals by releasing the excitatory neurotransmitter aspartate.

2. Mossy fibres All the afferent fibres entering the cerebellum, other than the olivocerebellar, are called mossy fibres. These fibres after reaching the granular layer of the cerebellar cortex branch profusely and then each branch terminates within a glomerulus (Fig. 10.2.4). The core of each glomerulus is formed by the expanded termination of a mossy fibre called the rosette. About 20 dendrites of granule cells synapse with a rosette in a glomerulus. These synapses are axodendritic. The glomerulus also receives axon terminals of Golgi cells (Fig. 10.2.4).

- In the glomeruli, the mossy fibres release excitatory neurotransmitter glutamate and excite the granule cells and Golgi cells.
- The mossy fibres excite the Purkinje cells indirectly through the granule cells.
- The collaterals of mossy fibres excite the deep cerebellar nuclei directly.

Neuronal Activity of Intrinsic Cerebellar Circuitry

As a result of excitatory input from the climbing fibres or mossy fibres, the activity given next is set up in the intrinsic cerebellar circuitry.

Feed-forward inhibition of Purkinje cells Granule cells, which are activated by mossy fibres, in turn excite the Purkinje cells. However, this excitation is extremely short lasting. This is because the granule cell also excites basket cell, which in turn produces IPSP in the Purkinje cells, shortly after stimulation (Fig. 10.2.4). Since Purkinje cell and basket cell are excited by the same excitatory input, this arrangement is called feed-forward inhibition. This mechanism helps to limit the duration of excitation produced by given afferent impulses.

Feed-forward inhibition of granule cells As shown in Fig. 10.2.4, the mossy fibres stimulate the granule cells. However, this excitation is short lasting. This is because the mossy fibre also excites Golgi cell, which in turn inhibits the granule cell. Since the granule cell and Golgi cells are excited by the same excitatory input (from mossy fibres), this arrangement is said to produce feed-forward inhibition of the granule cells.

Feedback inhibition of granule cells As shown in Fig. 10.2.4, the granule cell is excited by the mossy fibres. The axon of granule cell excites the Golgi cell dendrites, whose axon inhibits the granule cell. Thus, excitation of the granule cell is rapidly extinguished by a negative feedback loop. This arrangement is called feedback inhibition of granule cells.

Important Note

From the above description, it is clear that at least three of the identifiable neural circuits inside the cerebellum are meant for ensuring that discharges of the granule cells and Purkinje cells are extremely precise and short lasting (neural sharpening). This helps in accurate timing of action potentials.

Neurotransmitters Affecting Intrinsic Cerebellar Circuitry

The neurotransmitter released by granule cell is glutamate, whereas GABA is released by stellate, basket, Golgi and Purkinje cells. GABA acts via GABA^{A} receptors. The granule cells of the cerebellar cortex are the only type of neuron that has GABA^{A} receptors.

Reverberating circuit The granule cells and Purkinje cells form a reverberating (echoing) circuit. The main function of the reverberating circuit is to revive and strengthen the nonfunctional synapses, when two neurons discharge by repeatedly and synchronously. Hebb enunciated this principle, which can be understood by the example given next.

Suppose a person is making alternate supinations and pronations of his/her hand rhythmically. This is made possible by the reverberating circuit of the cerebellum. Therefore, this capability is impaired in cerebellar disorders and is called adiadochokinesis. This can be explained as given next.

As shown in the Fig. 10.2.5, when the person makes supination movement, the signal of descending command from the motor cortex is relayed through the inferior olive to Purkinje cell (PC-1), through the climbing fibres (CF-1). The

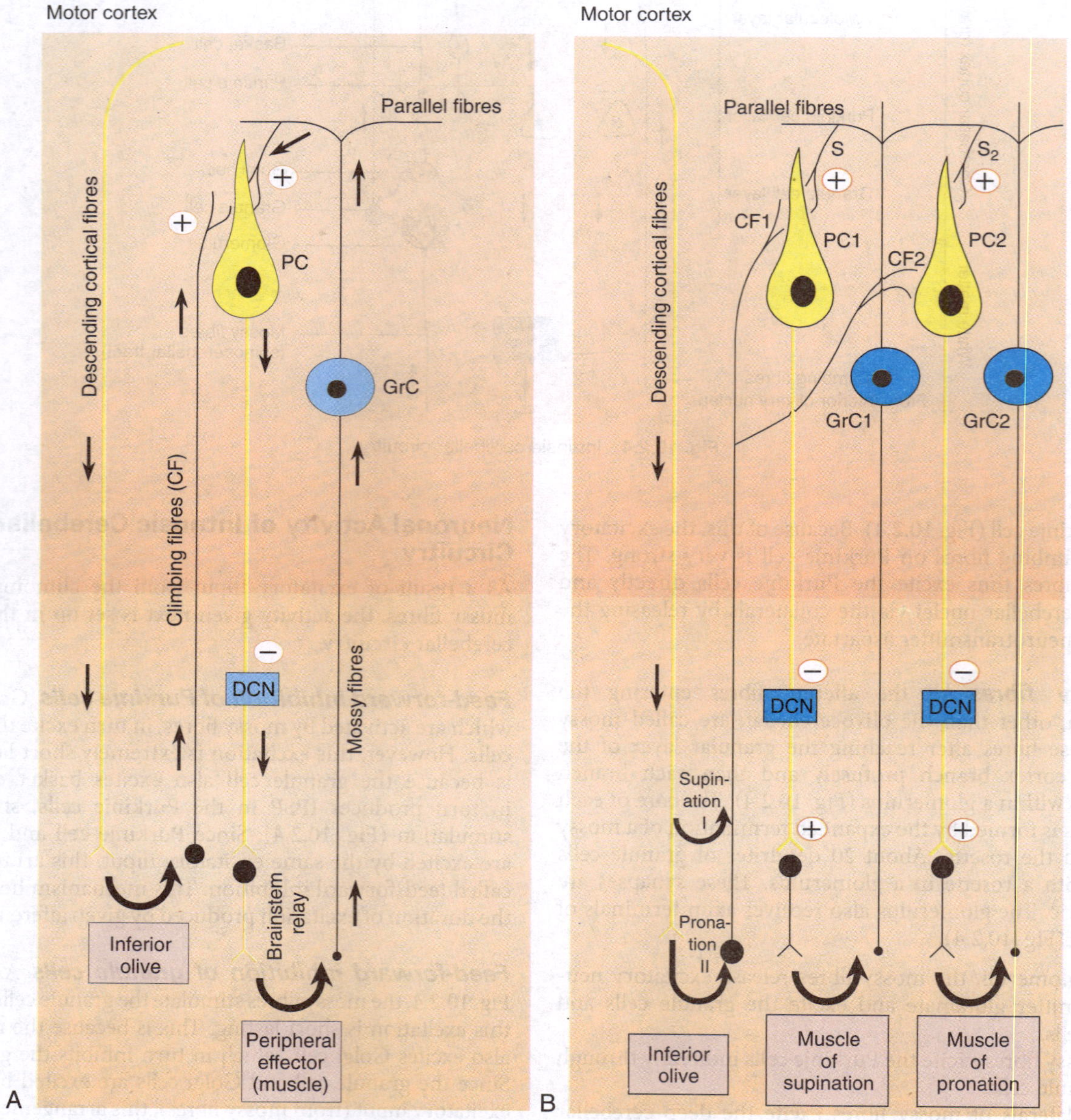

Fig. 10.2.5 Reverberating circuit: **A**, basic elements; and **B**, two sets of reverberating circuits are shown to illustrate their functioning in supination and pronation movements. CF, climbing fibre; DCN, deep cerebellar nuclei; GrC, granule cell; PC, Purkinje cell.

stimulated Purkinje cell (PC-1) sends a signal to the muscles of supination.

When the muscles of supination contract, a set of proprioceptive receptors is stimulated, from where the sensory information is conveyed through the mossy fibre to the granule cell (GrC-1) of the cerebellum. The stimulation of granule cell (GrC-1) sets up excitation in the parallel fibres. Although parallel fibres make synaptic connection with Purkinje cells, most of these are not functional. Therefore, excitation of parallel fibres initially does not cause excitation of Purkinje cells. It is important to note that excitation of parallel fibres occurs a little while after the excitation of Purkinje cell (PC-1), which has already been explained above, and is extremely short lived. Excitation of parallel fibres, a little while after the excitation of Purkinje cell, can be compared with an echo, which is heard moments after the original sound stops. Because of this similarity, this circuit is called reverberating (echoing) circuit.

Pronation movement (which follows supination) will lead to stimulation of another Purkinje cell (PC-2) through another climbing fibre (CF-2). If the pronation is appropriately timed, the stimulation of PC-2 coincides with the echo of PC-1, i.e. stimulation of parallel fibres of GrC-1.

When supination occurs again, the stimulation of PC-1 coincides with the echo of PC-2, i.e. stimulation of parallel fibres of GrC-2.

When the rhythmic supination and pronation are practised repeatedly, the synaptic connections between PC-1 and parallel fibres of GrC-2, and between PC-2 and parallel fibres of GrC-1 get strengthened. Once this happens, the Purkinje cells PC-1 and PC-2 get automatically stimulated, rhythmically through each other's echo. Under such circumstances, stimulation of Purkinje cell through the climbing fibres is needed only to trigger off the rhythmic sequence.

Neuronal Activity of Deep Cerebellar Nuclei

- The deep cerebellar nuclei are made of excitatory neurons. These nuclei receive excitatory inputs via collaterals from the mossy fibres, climbing fibres and also other excitatory inputs.
- These sensory inputs maintain the deep cerebellar nuclei in a continuously excitatory state.
- In turn, these nuclei send excitatory impulses to thalamus and brainstem nuclei.
- However, Purkinje cell output is inhibitory to deep cerebellar nuclei via inhibitory neurotransmitter GABA. Purkinje cells inhibit the activities of vestibular nuclei also.

Thus, from the above discussion, it is clear that neuronal activity in the cerebellar cortex plays an important role in modulating the excitatory signals of the following pathways:

- From deep cerebellar nuclei to thalamus and then to cerebral cortex, and motor pathway to spinal cord
- From deep cerebellar nuclei to brainstem nuclei

Because of this modulating or timing effect, the cerebellar cortex is able to well organize and coordinate the different movements of the body.

CONNECTIONS OF THE CEREBELLUM

Cerebellar Peduncles

The cerebellum receives afferents from various sources and sends efferents to different targets. The afferents enter and the efferents leave the cerebellum through three pairs of cerebellar peduncles.

1. Inferior cerebellar peduncle The inferior cerebellar peduncle, also called restiform bodies, connects the cerebellum to the dorsolateral aspect of the medulla. These constitute the main entrance gates of the cerebellum as they contain predominantly afferent fibres.

Afferent fibres passing through the inferior cerebellar peduncle are as follows:

- Dorsospinocerebellar tract
- External arcuate fibres
- Reticulocerebellar tract
- Olivocerebellar tract
- Vestibulocerebellar tract

Efferent fibres leaving through the inferior cerebellar peduncle are as follows:

- Cerebellovestibular pathway
- Cerebelloreticular pathway
- Cerebello-olivary pathway

2. Middle cerebellar peduncle The middle cerebellar peduncle, also known as brachium pontis, connects the cerebellum to the dorsum of the pons. Most of the fibres of the middle cerebellar peduncle are commissural fibres, which connect the area of both the halves of the cerebellar cortex.

Afferent fibres which enter through this peduncle are the cerebro-ponto-cerebellar fibres.

3. Superior cerebellar peduncle The superior cerebellar peduncle, also called brachium conjunctiva, connects the cerebellum to the back of the midbrain. Since most of efferent fibres travel through this peduncle, it is also called the exit gate of the cerebellum.

Afferent fibres passing through the superior cerebellar peduncle include (Fig. 10.2.6):

- Ventral spinocerebellar tract
- Tectocerebellar tract

Efferent fibres leaving through the superior cerebellar peduncle are as follows:

- Dentatorubral fibres
- Dentatothalamic fibres
- Cerebellar reticular fibres to the midbrain

Afferent and Efferent Connections

Salient points of afferent and efferent connections of the cerebellum are summarized next.

Afferent Connections

1. Dorsal spinocerebellar tract It is an uncrossed tract, which arises from the ipsilateral Clarke's column of cells and carries proprioceptive information from the limbs of the same side. It enters through the ipsilateral inferior cerebellar peduncle and is distributed to the spinocerebellum (for details, see page 888).

2. Ventral spinocerebellar tract The fibres of this tract arise from the marginal cells in the dorsal grey horn of the spinal cord. After taking origin, the fibres cross the midline and ascend in the opposite side. This tract carries the proprioceptive information from the limbs of the opposite side. It enters the cerebellum through the superior cerebellar peduncle, and is distributed to the lower limb area of the cortex of the spinocerebellum (details on page 888).

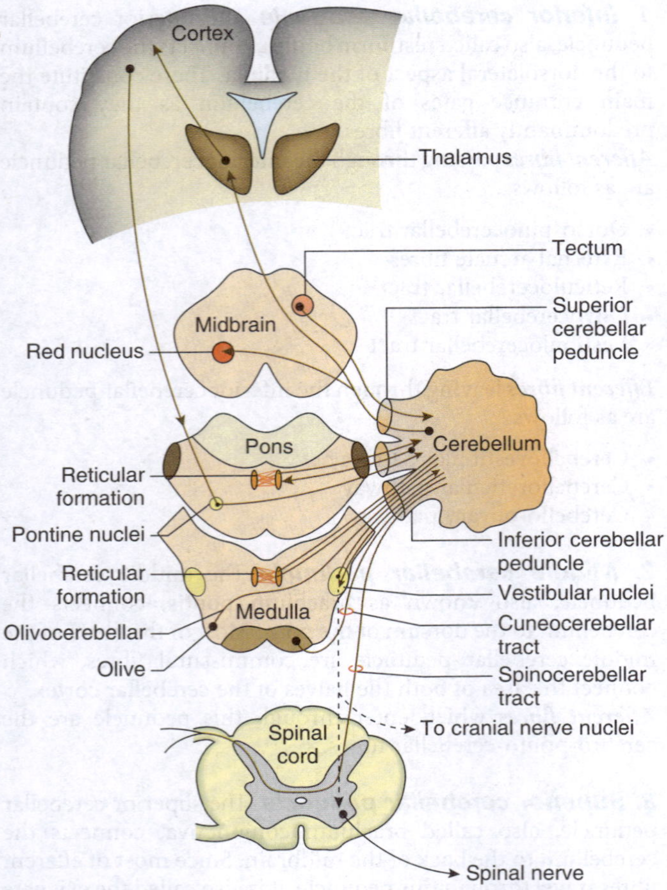

Fig. 10.2.6 Diagrammatic depiction of main connections of cerebellum.

3. *Cuneocerebellar tract* It arises from the accessory cuneate nucleus and carries proprioceptive impulses from the upper limb, upper trunk and neck. It enters through the ipsilateral inferior cerebellar peduncle and is distributed to the spinocerebellum.

4. *Olivocerebellar tract* This tract arises from the olivary nucleus and crosses to the opposite side. The olivary nucleus receives afferents from three sources:

- Brainstem nuclei of the same side
- Spinal cord through spino-olivary tract of the same side
- Cerebral cortex of the opposite side

It carries proprioceptive impulses from the whole body and output signals from the cerebral cortex. It enters the cerebellum through the inferior cerebellar peduncle of the opposite side and is distributed to all parts of the cerebellar cortex and the deep cerebellar nuclei (for details, see page 888).

5. *Corticopontocerebellar tract* The corticopontine fibres arise from the cerebral cortex and end in pontine nuclei from where the pontocerebellar fibres cross to enter the opposite side through the middle cerebellar peduncle. The cortex of each cerebral hemisphere is connected with the opposite half of the cerebellum through this tract. This tract conveys the information to the spinocerebellum, about the major signals discharged from the cerebral cortex. The cerebral cortex and the cerebellum work in close cooperation in order to affect the proper coordination of muscular action in voluntary movements (see page 892).

6. *Tectocerebellar tract* It arises from the superior and inferior colliculi of the tectum of the midbrain, and enters the cerebellum via the superior cerebellar peduncle. It carries visual impulses from the superior colliculi and auditory impulses from the inferior colliculi (see page 907).

7. *Vestibulocerebellar tract* It arises from the ipsilateral vestibular nuclei and carries information concerning the position and the movements of the head. It enters through the inferior cerebellar peduncle and conveys impulses to the vestibulocerebellum (flocculonodular lobe) via deep cerebellar nuclei (nucleus globosus, nucleus emboliformis and nucleus fastigii).

8. *Rubrocerebellar tract* It arises from the red nucleus, and is both crossed and uncrossed. It enters through the superior cerebellar peduncle and is distributed mainly to the dentate nucleus. It transmits impulses which have originated from the motor cortex and relayed in red nucleus.

9. *Reticulocerebellar tract* It arises from the lateral reticular nucleus, enters through the ipsilateral inferior cerebellar peduncle and is distributed to the whole of the cerebellar cortex.

Localization of the sensory impulses to the cerebellum The cerebellar cortex, like sensory and motor cerebral cortex, exhibits point-to-point representation of sensory impulses (tactile, proprioceptive, visual and auditory) from the whole body. For the purpose of representation, the cerebellar cortex has been divided into three zones:

Vermal zone, i.e. cortex of vermis area (a narrow band in the centre of the cerebellum)
Paravermal or intermediate zone, i.e. cortex of medial halves of the cerebellar hemisphere
Lateral zone, i.e. cortex of lateral halves of the cerebellar hemisphere (Fig. 10.2.7)

Areas of representation There is a double representation on the superior surface (anterior area) and on the inferior surface (posterior area).

Anterior area encloses the entire anterior lobe and lobulus simplex. In the anterior area, the body representation is an inverted ipsilateral projection. Axial parts of the body lie in the vermis, whereas limbs and facial region lie in the intermediate zone of the cerebellar cortex.
Posterior area is located primarily in the paramedian lobule. In this area, the body representation is a bilateral projection, less defined and erect.

- There is same topographical representation of motor areas in the cerebellum as is for the sensory areas. Stimulation of these areas produces movements in parts of the body that correspond roughly to those from which sensory impulses are received.
- In addition to the proprioceptive impulses, the cerebellum also receives auditory and visual impulses. The auditory and visual areas lie primarily in the lobulus simplex, folium and tuber vermis (Fig. 10.2.7).

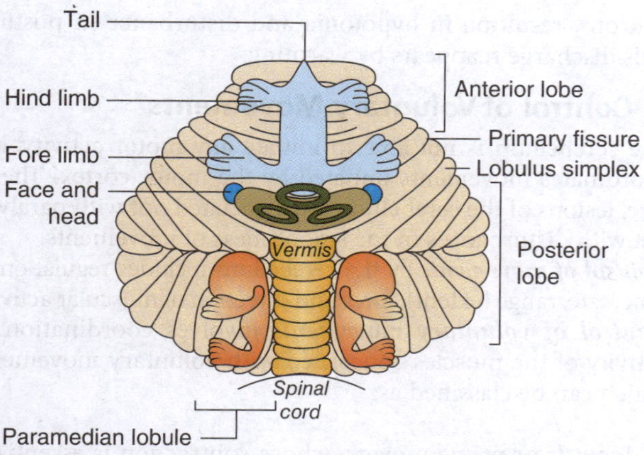

Fig. 10.2.7 Localization of sensory projection areas on the cerebellar cortex.

- The large lateral zones of the cerebellar cortex do not have topographical representations of the body. These areas receive signals entirely and exclusively from the cerebral cortex, and premotor areas of the frontal cortex, somatosensory and sensory association areas of the parietal cortex. These connections play an important role in planning and coordinating rapid sequential muscular activities of the body.

The main afferents that converge to form mossy fibres and climbing fibres to the cerebellum are summarized in Table 10.2.2.

Efferent Connections (Fig. 10.2.6)

1. Dentato-rubro-thalamo-cortical path It is a multisynaptic path, synapsing at least in the red nucleus and thalamus. The fibres originate from the dentate nucleus, which is recent in origin and most well developed in humans and so the red nucleus, thalamus and cerebral cortex of the opposite side.

2. Cerebello-thalamo-cortical path It has also the same function, i.e. controlling or influence over the opposite motor cortex.

3. Cerebelloreticular path Anterior horn cells of the spinal cord are controlled by the cerebellum through reticulospinal tracts (direct fibres from the cerebellum to the anterior horn cells do not exist).

4. Cerebellovestibular fibres Cerebellovestibular fibres pass through the inferior cerebellar peduncle to the vestibular nuclei. These efferents control anterior horn cells of the spinal cord through the vestibulospinal tract.

5. Cerebello-olivary fibres Cerebello-olivary fibres reach the inferior olivary nucleus.

6. Some fibres from the cerebellum Some fibres from the cerebellum also reach the nucleus of the oculomotor nerve and the tectum.

FUNCTIONS OF CEREBELLUM

Functionally, the cerebellum has been divided into three divisions:

- Vestibulocerebellum
- Spinocerebellum
- Corticocerebellum

These three functional divisions play important role in the different functions given next.

A. Control of Body Posture and Equilibrium

Vestibulocerebellum Vestibulocerebellum, which includes flocculonodular lobe as its principal component and nucleus fastigii (as its effector nucleus) and vermal region of the cerebellum, is concerned with control of body posture and equilibrium.

Afferents to cerebellum Afferents to the cerebellum concerned with the control of body posture and equilibrium include:

Vestibulocerebellar tracts, which carry input from vestibular nuclei, convey afferents from the macula of saccule and utricle for

Table 10.2.2 Principal afferent system to the cerebellum

Afferent tracts	Impulses transmitted	Via	Distributed to
1. Dorsospinocerebellar tract	Proprioceptive information from limbs of same side	Inferior cerebellar peduncle	Spinocerebellum
2. Ventrospinocerebellar tract	Proprioceptive information from limbs of opposite side	Superior cerebellar peduncle	Spinocerebellum
3. Cuneocerebellar tract	Proprioceptive information from upper limb, trunk and neck	Ipsilateral inferior cerebellar peduncle	Spinocerebellum
4. Olivocerebellar tract	Proprioceptive information from whole body and signals from cerebral cortex	Contralateral inferior cerebellar peduncle	Whole cerebellar cortex and deep cerebellar nuclei
5. Tectocerebellar tract	Auditory and visual impulses through superior and inferior colliculi of midbrain	Superior cerebellar peduncle	Spinocerebellar
6. Vestibulocerebellar tract	Vestibular (position and movement of head) information	Inferior cerebellar peduncle	Vestibulocerebellum (flocculonodular lobe)
7. Pontocerebellar tract	Signals from contralateral cerebral cortex	Middle cerebellar peduncle	Spinocerebellum
8. Rubrocerebellar tract	Signals originated from motor cortex	Middle cerebellar peduncle	Dentate nuclei
9. Reticulocerebellar tract	Lateral reticular nuclei	Ipsilateral cerebellar peduncle	Whole of cerebellar cortex

static equilibrium and from the ampullary crests of semicircular ducts for kinetic equilibrium.

Spinocerebellar and cuneocerebellar tracts carry feedback about the tone of muscles or position of the limbs in space.

Reticulocerebellar tracts bring feedback about activities of extrapyramidal tracts.

Efferents The flocculonodular lobe and fastigial nuclei project output fibres through the inferior peduncle to vestibular and reticular nuclei of the brainstem. The vermal cerebellum sends back the information to the spinal cord indirectly through fastigial nuclei.

Mechanism of action The efferents from the cerebellum influence the spinal motor neurons to keep the body posture upright through the vestibulospinal and reticulospinal tracts, and regulate the position of eyes in relation to movements of the head by connecting motor nuclei of extraocular muscles (third, fourth and sixth cranial nerves) via medial longitudinal fasciculus.

Important Note

It is important to note that the cerebellum does necessary corrections for maintaining posture and equilibrium, without participation of conscious will, and that the corrections made are highly smooth and precise.

B. Control of Muscle Tone and Stretch Reflexes

Spinocerebellum, which includes the entire anterior lobe except the lingula and some parts of the posterior lobe (pyramis, uvula and paraflocculus) as its principal components and nucleus globosus and nucleus emboliformis as its effector nuclei, is mainly concerned with control of muscle tone and anticipatory adjustment of muscle contraction during movement.

Afferents Spinocerebellar, cuneocerebellar and olivocerebellar tracts carry proprioceptive and tactile inputs from the limbs, trunk, neck and other parts of the body. These give feedback about tone of muscles or position of limbs and body. The spinocerebellum also receives auditory and visual impulses through the tectocerebellar tract. It also receives the cortical impulses via pontine nuclei.

Efferents The spinocerebellum is projected into the cerebellar nuclei – fastigii, emboliformis and globosus. Fibres from these nuclei pass through fastigiobulbar, cerebelloreticular and cerebello-olivary tracts and, ultimately, relay to the α- and γ-motor neurons through the reticulospinal and olivospinal tracts.

Mechanism of action The spinocerebellum regulates the postural reflexes by modifying muscle tone. It facilitates the gamma motor neurons in the spinal cord via cerebello-vestibulo-spinal and cerebello-reticulo-spinal tracts. The γ-motor neurons reflexly modify the activity of α-motor neurons and thus regulate the muscle tone. Thus, the cerebellum forms an important site of linkage of α–γ systems responsible for muscle tone.

Proofs Temporary suppression of anterior lobe activity by surface cooling abolishes discharge from the γ-motor neurons, resulting in hypotonia and disturbance in posture. This discharge reappears by warming.

C. Control of Voluntary Movements

The cerebellum is not able to initiate any motor activity, but coordinates movements initiated by the motor cortex. Therefore, lesions of the cerebellum are associated not with paralysis but with disturbances in the smoothness of movements.

Control of movements by the cerebellum includes regulation of time, rate, range (extent), force and direction of muscular activity.

Control of voluntary movements involves coordination of activity of the muscles concerned with voluntary movements which can be classified as:

- *Agonists* or prime movers, whose contraction is essentially responsible for the movement of the part
- *Antagonists*, which oppose the prime movers
- *Synergists*, which assist the prime movers and reduce unnecessary involvements to a minimum
- *Fixation muscles*, whose contraction causes the fixation of neighbouring joints and maintains the limbs or body in a position appropriate for carrying out the particular movement

Pathway of Control of Voluntary Movements

Corticocerebellum, also called cerebrocerebellum, is mainly concerned with integration and regulation of well-coordinated muscular activity (though other parts of the cerebellum also work in close cooperation in this task). It includes whole of the posterior lobe, except pyramis and uvula, with dentate nucleus as its effector nucleus. Corticocerebellum takes part in smooth performance of highly skilled voluntary movements because of its afferent and efferent connections which form two feedback loops – open and close.

1. Open feedback loop Open feedback loop, also known as cerebro-cerebello-cerebral connection or *afferent–efferent circuit*, consists of the following fibres (Fig. 10.2.8):

1. Cerebro-ponto-cerebellar tract which is formed by:

Corticopontine fibres: These arise from the association areas of the cerebral cortex and project to ipsilateral pontine nuclei. Pontocerebellar fibres from the pontine nuclei pass through the middle cerebellar peduncle of the opposite side and terminate in the cerebellar cortex of the hemisphere zone (lateral). Thus, the whole pathway is called the cerebro-ponto-cerebellar tract. This part of the cerebellum does not receive significant proprioceptive input from the spinal cord. The cerebellar cortex in turn connects to the effector nucleus, the dentate nucleus.

2. Dentato-rubro-thalamic cortical tract which includes the following fibres:

- *Dentatorubral fibres* start from the dentate nucleus and pass via the superior cerebellar peduncle to end in the red nucleus of the opposite side.
- *Rubrothalamic fibres* start from the red nucleus and go to the thalamus.
- *Thalamocortical fibres* connect the thalamus to areas 4 and 6 of the motor cortex of the cerebrum.

Functions: The cerebro-cerebello-cerebral circuit modulates the motor command of the pyramidal tract with a programming of movement.

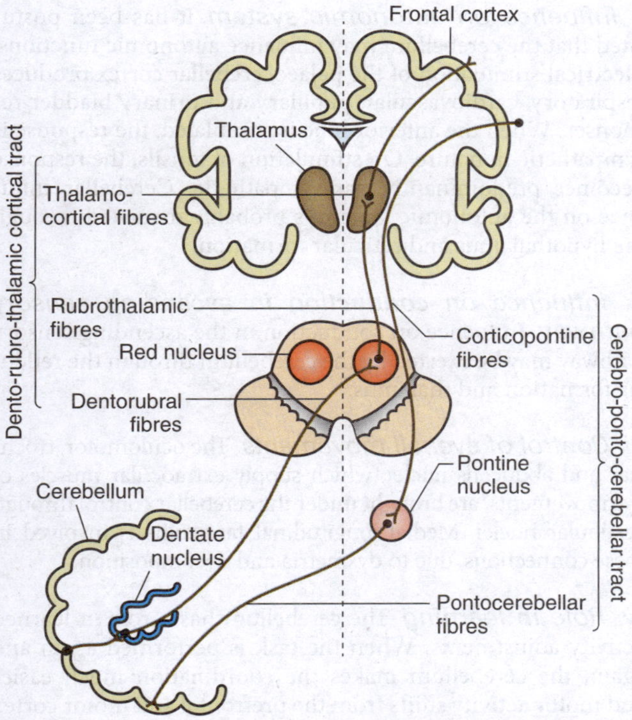

Fig. 10.2.8 Cerebro-cerebello-cerebral circuit (open-feedback loop).

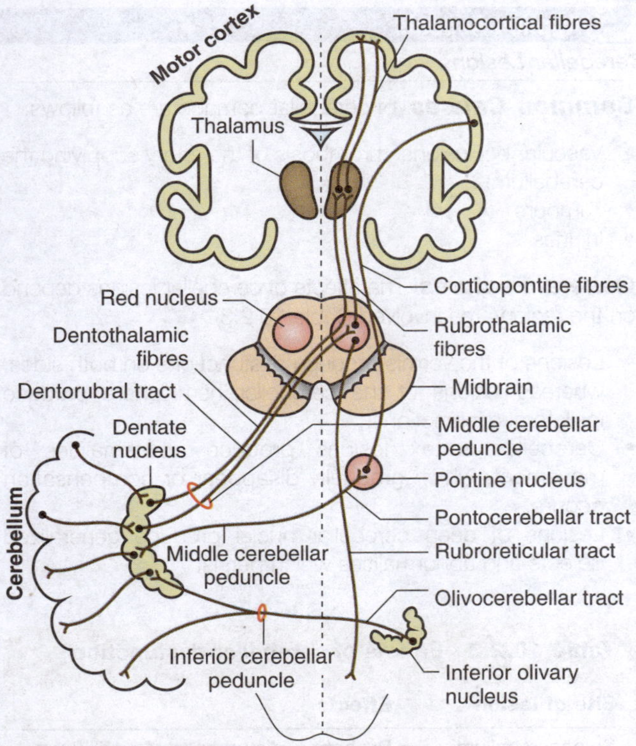

Fig. 10.2.9 Connections of corticocerebellum (closed circuit).

2. Closed feedback loop It is formed by the fibres from the cerebral motor cortex to the paravermal cerebellum to the cerebral motor cortex as (Fig. 10.2.9):

Afferent limb is formed by collaterals of corticospinal tracts (which influence the contralateral lower motor neuron of the spinal cord), which while descending through the brainstem synapse with the ipsilateral pontine nuclei, inferior olivary nucleus and contralateral reticular nucleus of the medulla.

i. *Pontocerebellar fibres* from the pontine nucleus and *olivocerebellar* fibres from the inferior olivary nucleus reach the contralateral cerebellar cortex; *reticulocerebellar fibres* from the lateral reticular nucleus are projected to the ipsilateral cortex. All the aforesaid fibres are connected to the paravermal (intermediate) region of the cerebellum and provide on their way collaterals to the deep cerebellar nuclei.
ii. *Paravermal cerebellar cortex* is in turn connected to the nucleus interpositus and partly to the dentate nucleus.

Efferents from dentate nucleus pass through the superior cerebellar peduncle, cross the midline and form decussation with the fibres of the opposite side. After forming the decussation, these fibres divide into two groups:

i. *Dentatothalamic fibres:* Some fibres arising from the dentate nucleus pass through the red nucleus, without having any synapse, and terminate in the thalamus. The thalamus in turn projects into the motor cortex via thalamocortical fibres.
ii. *Dentatorubral fibres:* The remaining fibres terminate in the red nucleus of the opposite side. From the red nucleus, the following tracts arise:
   - *Rubrothalamic tract* terminates in the thalamus, from where thalamocortical fibres arise and reach the cerebral cortex.
   - *Rubroreticular tract* terminates into reticular formation which projects into the spinal cord via the reticulospinal tract.
   - *Rubrospinal tract:* The red nucleus also projects directly into the spinal cord through the rubrospinal tract.

Mechanism of Action

The cerebellum controls the voluntary movements by the actions given next.

i. Comparator function The cerebellum integrates and coordinates the patterns of movement involving mostly the distal parts of limbs, especially the hands, fingers and feet, by its comparator function.

- When the motor cortex sends impulses through the corticospinal tracts to the lower motor neurons for commanding movements of exploratory nature, it sends messages on way to the paravermal cerebellum about the sequential intended plan of movements for the next fraction of second.
- The cerebellum also gets feedback from the proprioceptive endings of muscles, tendons and joints about what actual movements result.

The paravermal cerebellum (intermediate zone of the cerebellar cortex) then compares the intended movement with the actual movement, and through nucleus interpositus sends corrective signals to the motor cortex through the thalamus and red nucleus. This system of cerebellar *comment* on every command of the motor cortex is completed within 10–20 milliseconds.

Thus, the exploratory movement initiated in the motor cortex is corrected by the paracerebellum via the closed-loop circuit (Fig. 10.2.9).

ii. Damping action By its comparator action, the cerebellum provides smooth coordinate movements of agonist and antagonist muscles of the limbs for the performance of acute purposeful patterned movements. However, all the movements are pendular and have a tendency to overshoot. The corticocerebellum sends impulses to the cerebral cortex to discharge appropriate signals to the muscles so that any extra or exaggeration of muscular activity does not occur and thus prevents the overshooting. In this way, the movements become smooth and accurate. This action of the corticocerebellum is called damping action.

iii. Timing and programming the movements When the perfection of movements is fully assured, the planning of sequence of movements and the timing of the learned movements is then maintained from the association cortex to the motor cortex, through the lateral zone of the cerebellar cortex along with the associated dentate nucleus forming an open-loop circuit (Fig. 10.2.8).

Planning of sequence of movements: Lateral parts of the cerebellar hemisphere communicate with the premotor and sensory portion of the cerebral cortex and there is two-way communication between these areas. Plan is transmitted from the cerebral cortex to the cerebellum and two-way traffic between two areas provides appropriate transition from one movement to the next. This plan is stored in the cerebral cortex in the form of memory. So, after the learning process is over, these activities are executed easily and smoothly in sequence.

Timing function: The lateral cerebellar hemisphere also provides appropriate timing for each movement, without which succeeding movements may begin far early or too late.

Predicting events: The cerebellum also plays a role in predicting events, e.g. rate of progression of auditory and visual phenomena. From the changing visual scene, a person can predict how rapidly he/she can approach an object.

Important Note

It is important to note that all fast-skilled movements such as typing, writing and playing of music instruments are possible because of timing and programming of movements by the cerebellum.

iv. Control of ballistic movements The rapid alternate movements, which take place in different parts of the body, while doing any skilled work like dancing are called ballistic movements. The cerebellum coordinates the action of agonist and antagonist muscles, especially when they occur rhythmically. This is explained in 'Reverberating Circuit' (see page 906).

v. Servomechanism From the above discussion, it is clear that the cerebellum plays an important role in learning of motor skills. Once the skilled works are learnt, the sequential movements could be executed without any interruption. The cerebellum lets the cerebral cortex discharge the signals, which are already programmed and stored at the sensory motor cortex, and does not interfere much. However, if there is any disturbance or interference, the corticocerebellum immediately influences the cerebral cortex and corrects the movements. This action of the corticocerebellum is known as servomechanism.

D. Other Functions of Cerebellum

Recent studies have shown that the importance of the cerebellum may extend beyond control of motor activity as given next.

i. Influence on autonomic system It has been postulated that the cerebellum may influence autonomic functions. Electrical stimulation of the palaeocerebellar cortex produces respiratory, cardiovascular, pupillary and urinary bladder responses. When the anterior lobe is stimulated, the response is sympathetic in nature. On stimulation of tonsils, the response becomes predominantly parasympathetic. Cerebellar influence on the autonomic system is probably mediated through the hypothalamus and reticular formation.

ii. Influence on conduction in ascending sensory pathway Influence on conduction in the ascending sensory pathway may be exerted by the cerebellum through the reticular formation and thalamus.

iii. Control of eyeball movements The oculomotor, trochlear and abducens nuclei, which supply extraocular muscles of eye movements, are brought under the cerebellar control through vestibular nuclei. Medial longitudinal fasciculus is involved in these connections, due to dysmetria and decomposition.

iv. Role in learning The cerebellum has a role in learned activity adjustments. When the task is performed again and again, the cerebellum makes the coordination much easier and motor activity shifts from the prefrontal and motor cortex to the cerebellum. The olivary nucleus inputs to the cerebellum are the basis for learned activity.

Applied Aspects

Cerebellar Lesions

Common Causes of cerebellar damage are as follows:

- Vascular occlusions (thrombosis of the artery supplying the cerebellum)
- Tumours
- Injuries

General Features The effects of cerebellar lesions depend on the region/area involved (Table 10.2.3).

- Lesions of the vermis produce dysfunctions on both sides, whereas lesions of the cerebellar hemisphere produce ipsilateral dysfunctions.
- Cerebellar cortex lesions produce abnormalities of movement, which gradually disappear or compensation occurs.
- Lesions of deep cerebellar nuclei produce generalized defects and abnormalities which persist.

Table 10.2.3 Effects of cerebellar dysfunction

Site of lesion	Effects
Spinocerebellum	Dysarthria, disturbance of equilibrium (unable to maintain upright posture against gravity)
Cerebrocerebellum	Delay in initiation of movements and composition of movements, i.e. movements occur in stages at different joints
Vestibulocerebellum	Ataxia, nystagmus and dysequilibrium

Signs of Cerebellar Dysfunctions Common signs observed in patients with cerebellar dysfunction due to lesions of the cerebellum are given next.

I. Disturbances in Tone and Posture include:

1. ***Atonia or hypotonia:*** Hypotonia refers to reduction and atonia to loss of tone in muscles. It occurs due to reduction of the facilitatory neocerebellar output to the descending inhibitory reticular formation.
2. ***Attitude changes*** in unilateral lesions of the cerebellum are as follows:
   - *Rotation of the face towards the opposite side* (pulled by the healthy muscles)
   - Lowering of the shoulder on the affected side
   - Outward rotation and abduction of the leg on the involved side
   - Trunk bent with concavity towards the affected side (this is because the weight of the body is thrown on the unaffected leg)
3. ***Deviation movement:*** The arm held straight out in front of the body deviates laterally when the eyes are closed. In bilateral lesions, both arms deviate.
4. ***Effect on deep reflexes:*** The deep or tendon reflexes become weak and pendular, for example, *pendular knee jerk* in which after the initial reflex response the leg shakes several times (to-and-fro movements) before it comes to rest. It occurs due to hypotonia of the quadriceps muscle.

II. Disturbances in Equilibrium. It appears when the flocculonodular lobe is affected, e.g. by the tumour medulloblastoma in children. The patient suffering from disturbance of equilibrium, walking on a wide base, sways from side to side (drunken-like gait), and is unable to maintain the upright posture due to involvement of the vestibular system.

III. Disturbances in Movements. Disturbances in movements include:

1. ***Ataxia***, i.e. lack of coordination of movements, is the hallmark of cerebellar disorder. It is characterized by:
   - *Decomposition of movements,* i.e. the movements seem to occur in stages at different joints.
   - *Asynergia,* i.e. there is lack of coordination between the protagonist, synergist and antagonist muscles.
   - *Dysmetria,* i.e. movements are incorrect in range, direction and force. The movements may overshoot their intended mark (hypermetria) or fall short of it (hypometria).

Important Note

Ataxia also occurs in certain hereditary conditions; examples are Friedrich's ataxia (an autosomal recessive condition occurring below the age of 25 years) and Machado–Joseph disease.

2. ***Intention tremors*** become evident during purposeful movements, and diminish or disappear with rest. These tremors become more marked as the hand approaches the object, i.e. are observed at the end of movement and are coarse, oscillating, to-and-fro and rhythmic. These are significantly observed when the efferent pathways of superior cerebellar peduncles are involved.
3. ***Nystagmus*** refers to regular and rhythmic, to-and-fro involuntary oscillatory movements of the eyes, occurring due to incoordination of extraocular muscles. Cerebellar nystagmus occurs during damage to flocculonodular lobes and occurs at rest (when neither the person nor the visual scene is moving).
4. ***Dysarthria*** or scanning speech occurs due to incoordination of various muscles and structures involved in speech. The speech is slurred, prolonged and explosive, with pauses at wrong places.
5. ***Astasia or abasia*** refers to unsteady voluntary movements across multiple joints and abasia refers to loss of ability to maintain upright stance against gravity.

Clinical Tests for Cerebellar Dysfunctions Clinically, cerebellar dysfunctions can be demonstrated by the tests given next.

1. Finger–Nose Test. The patient has great difficulty in promptly bringing the finger of the outstretched arm to touch the tip of his/her nose. This is because the intention tremors become more severe as the hand approaches the face.

2. Adiadochokinesia/dysdiadochokinesia. Adiadochokinesia/dysdiadochokinesia occurs, i.e. the patient is unable to rapidly perform alternating movements, e.g. supination and pronation of the forearm.

3. Rebound Phenomenon. It refers to inability of agonist and antagonist muscles to adapt to rapid changes in load, i.e. when the patient attempts to do a movement against a resistance, and if the resistance is suddenly removed, the limb moves forcibly in the direction towards which the effect was made. This is called rebound phenomenon. It is due to the absence of breaking action of antagonistic muscles.

4. Gait Test. When the patient is asked to walk on a straight line, he/she is unable to do so (even with eyes open); he/she follows a zigzag path due to disturbance of equilibrium.

5. Past Pointing. Past pointing occurs, i.e. the movement goes beyond the intended point. This is called overshooting and is a manifestation of dysmetria.

6. Heel-to-shin Test. Lying in a supine position, the patient is asked to place his/her heel on the opposite knee, and then slide his/her heel up and down the shin between the knee and the ankle. The test is abnormal if the heel waves away from the line of the shin.

7. Romberg Sign. The patient is asked to stand erect with closed eyes. If swaying occurs, then Romberg sign is positive. This sign is not specific for cerebellar ataxia, because it is positive for ataxia due to other reasons also.

Treatment: Ataxia in cerebellar dysfunction can be managed by:

- *Supportive therapy* includes physical, occupational and speech therapy.
- *Deep brain stimulation (DBS)* of ventral intermediate nucleus of the thalamus may be effective in ataxia.
- Coenzyme Q-10 replacement is beneficial to some extent in familial ataxia (due to low level of CoQ-10).

BASAL GANGLIA

PHYSIOLOGICAL ANATOMY

Components of Basal Ganglia

According to anatomic definition, basal ganglia are subcortical nuclear masses which include corpus striatum (amygdaloid body and claustrum). They are so named as they develop in the

basal part the of cerebral hemisphere. However, from the physiological viewpoint, the term basal ganglia includes:
- Corpus striatum
- Subthalamic nucleus (STN) (body of Luys)
- Substantia nigra

Corpus Striatum

Corpus striatum (Fig. 10.2.10) comprises subcortical masses of grey matter, which are situated in the white core of each cerebral hemisphere. It is divided almost completely by the fibres of the internal capsule into two parts:

i. Caudate nucleus (medial part)
ii. Lenticular nucleus (lateral part), which is further subdivided into two parts:
   - Putamen (outer part)
   - Globus pallidus (inner part)

Phylogenetically and functionally, the corpus striatum can be divided into two parts:
- Neostriatum or striatum
- Palaeostriatum or pallidum

1. ***Neostriatum or striatum:*** Phylogenetically, the caudate nucleus and putamen are of more recent origin and hence called neostriatum or striatum in short. Functionally and structurally also, the caudate nucleus and putamen are similar. The striatum is divided into:
   - Dorsal striatum
   - Ventral striatum
2. ***Palaeostriatum*** refers to globus pallidus, which is an older and primitive part. It is also called pallidum, as it is pale (pallid). The pallidum is subdivided into:
   - Dorsal pallidum
   - Ventral pallidum

Salient features of nuclei of corpus striatum (Fig. 10.2.10)

Caudate nucleus It is a highly curved, comma-shaped band of grey matter. It consists of a head, body and tail. Caudate nucleus is separated from the lentiform nucleus almost completely by the fibres of the internal capsule, except the lower part of its head where it is continuous with putamen nucleus (part of lentiform nucleus). This area of continuity is known as *fundus striati*. The tail of caudate nucleus ends by becoming continuous with putamen and lies in close relation to the amygdaloid body.

Lenticular nucleus It is shaped like a biconvex lens and is triangular in both coronal and horizontal sections. It is divided into two parts by an external lamina of white matter:

Putamen is the outer part of lentiform nucleus. It is dark in colour and is roughly quadrilateral.

Globus pallidus is the inner small part which is paler in appearance. It is further divided by an internal lamina of white matter into:
- External segment (globus pallidus externa [GPe])
- Internal segment (globus pallidus interna [GPi])

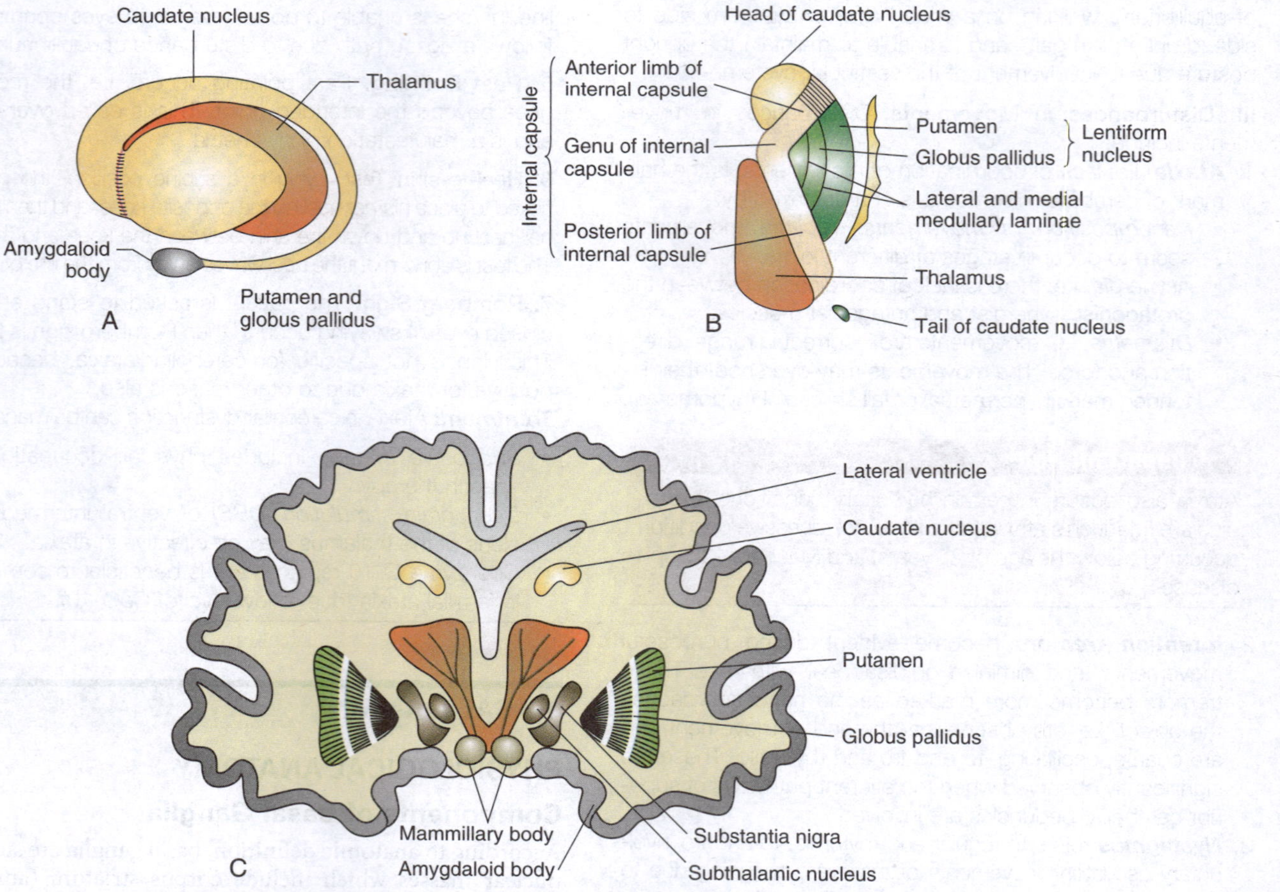

Fig. 10.2.10 Anatomy of basal ganglia: **A**, lateral view; **B**, horizontal section; and **C**, frontal section.

The striatum has four types of neurons; 95% are GABAergic medium spiny neurons, and remaining 5% striatal neurons are nonspiny, which include large (cholinergic), medium (somatostatinergic) and small (GABAergic).

Subthalamic Nucleus

STN (body of Luys) is a biconvex mass of grey matter, which is situated lateral to red nucleus and dorsal to substantia nigra in the mesencephalon.

STN is separated from the ventral nuclei of the thalamus by a thin sheet of grey matter known as *zona incerta*.

Substantia Nigra

Substantia nigra is a sheet made up of small unpigmented and large pigmented nerve cells. It appears dark in unstained sections as neurons within it contain the pigment neuromelanin. It extends along the entire length of the midbrain. Its cranial end reaches close to the STN. Substantia nigra is divisible into two parts:

1. ***Pars compacta*** is the dorsal part of substantia nigra. Pars compacta of the two sides are continuous with each other across the ventral tegmentum. It contains two types of neurons:
   - Dopaminergic neurons constitute about 75%.
   - Cholinergic neurons are about 25%.
2. ***Pars reticularis*** is the ventral part of substantia nigra. Superiorly, it becomes continuous with the globus pallidus. Most of the neurons in the pars reticularis are GABAergic.

Connections of Basal Ganglia

- Striatum (caudate nucleus and putamen) forms the main input side of the basal ganglia.
- Striatum in turn projects mainly to globus pallidus and substantia nigra.
- Pallidum (globus pallidus) is the main output side of the basal ganglia.

Therefore, connections of the basal ganglia (Fig. 10.2.11) can be considered under the following three headings:

i. Afferents or input to striatum
ii. Projections from striatum
iii. Efferents or output from globus pallidus

Afferents or input to striatum The striatum (caudate nucleus and putamen) is regarded as the input side of the basal ganglia receiving the following afferents:

1. ***Corticostriate projections:*** These originate from all parts of the cerebral cortex (premotor, supplementary motor cortex and primary somatosensory) and terminate in the striatum. These fibres are glutamatergic.
2. ***Thalamostriate fibres:*** These originate from centromedian nucleus of the thalamus and terminate in the striatum.
3. ***Nigrostriate fibres:*** These originate from the pars compacta, part of substantia nigra, and terminate in the striatum. These are dopaminergic fibres. They are distributed in a typically ordered manner.
4. ***Raphe striate fibres*** are serotoninergic fibres received by the striatum from raphe nuclei in the reticular formation of brainstem.
5. ***Locus coeruleus striate fibres*** are noradrenergic fibres received by the striatum from the locus coeruleus.

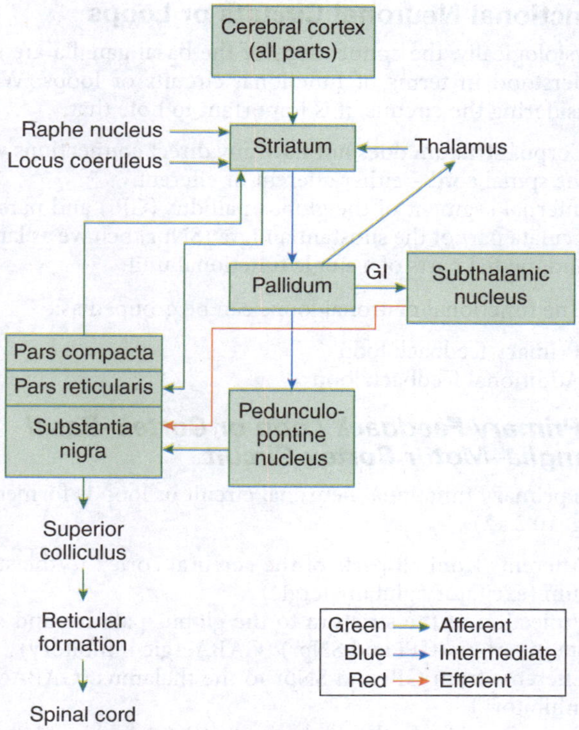

Fig. 10.2.11 Connections of basal ganglia.

Projections from striatum

1. ***Striatum to globus pallidus:*** The striatum (caudate nucleus and putamen) which receives most of the afferents gives robust projection to both segments of the globus pallidus. These are GABAergic inhibitory projections.
2. ***Striatum to substantia nigra:*** The striatum also gives GABAergic inhibitory impulses to pars reticulata of the substantia nigra.

Efferents or output from globus pallidus The pallidum (globus pallidus) is the output side of the basal ganglia. The efferents of the pallidum are as follows:

1. ***Efferents to thalamus:*** These fibres are called thalamic fasciculus or ansa fascicularis. They arise from the internal segment of the globus pallidus (GP_1) and go to ventroanterior (VA), ventrolateral and centromedian nuclei of the thalamus. From the thalamus, fibres project on to the prefrontal and premotor cortex.
2. ***Efferents to STN:*** These in turn project to the substantia nigra.
3. ***Efferents to substantia nigra:*** The pallidum projects to the substantia nigra. These fibres take three routes:
   - Some reach the substantia nigra directly.
   - Others go via STN.
   - Still others go via pedunculopontine nucleus.

Substantia nigra, in turn, sends the following descending projections:

i. Substantia nigra brainstem reticular formation: Reticulospinal tract pathway
ii. Substantia nigra superior colliculus: Tectospinal tract pathway
iii. Substantia nigra: Habenula

4. ***Efferents to red nucleus:*** This pathway includes fibres from the globus pallidus–red nucleus–rubrospinal tract pathway.

Functional Neuronal Circuits or Loops

Physiologically, the connections of the basal ganglia are best understood in terms of functional circuits or loops. While considering the circuits, it is important to note that:

- Corpus striatum does not have any direct connections with the spinal cord – either afferent or efferent.
- Internal segment of the globus pallidus (GPi) and pars reticulata part of the substantia nigra (SNpr) behave as lateral and medial parts of a single functional unit.

The functional neuronal loops can be grouped as:

1. Primary feedback loop
2. Additional feedback loop

1. Primary Feedback Loop or Cortex–Basal Ganglia–Motor Cortex Circuit

The primary functional neuronal circuit or loop is formed by (Fig. 10.2.12):

- Afferents from all parts of the cerebral cortex to the striatum (excitatory glutamatergic)
- Projection of the striatum to the globus pallidus and substantia nigra (GPi and SNpr) (GABAergic inhibitory)
- Efferents from GPi and SNpr to the thalamus (GABAergic inhibitory)
- Projections from the thalamus to the motor cortex and striatum

Functions The cortex–basal ganglia–cortex neuronal circuit provides a negative feedback loop to control the activity of the motor cortex.

Parts The primary feedback loop (cortex–basal ganglia–cortex neuronal circuit) consists of two parts, i.e. two distinct loops built into it:

- Caudate loop
- Putamen loop

i. Caudate loop or circuit is shown in Fig. 10.2.13A. This loop passes through the caudate part of the pallidum (GPi) and the caudal part of the substantia nigra (SNpr) and ventrolateral parts of the thalamus.

Functions: The caudate loop plays a role in cognitive control of motor activity (thinking process of the brain). It also plays a role in the control of eye movements.

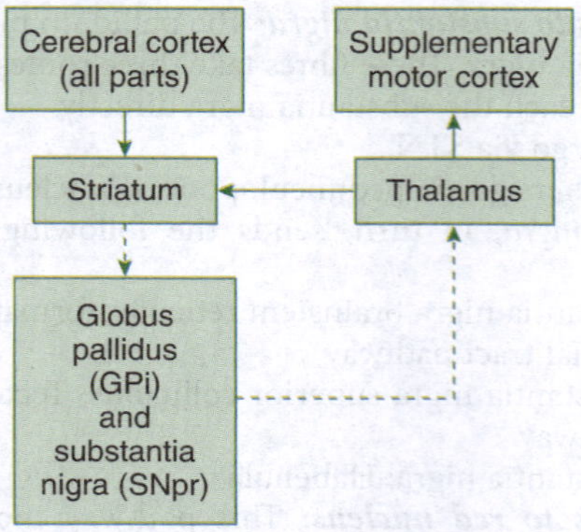

Fig. 10.2.12 Pathway of primary feedback loop (cortex–basal ganglia–cortex neuronal circuit).

ii. Putamen loop or circuit: As shown in Fig. 10.2.13B, the putamen loop passes through the rostral part of GPi and SNpr, and VA part of the thalamus.

Function: The putamen loop is mainly responsible for motor control of body movements.

Initiation of voluntary movements:

- To initiate voluntary movement, the motor cortex must inhibit the basal ganglia. The motor cortex does this by activating the striatum.
- The striatum then inhibits GPi by releasing neurotransmitter (GABA).
- Inhibition of GPi results in disinhibition of *VA* nucleus of the thalamus, which in turn activates the motor cortex to initiate voluntary movements

2. Additional Feedback Loop

In the primary feedback loop, the connections between the striatum and the globus pallidus are direct. However, there are two additional indirect feedback loops:

I. Indirect pathway via STN: As shown in Fig. 10.2.14, this pathway contains three inhibitory neurons:

- One from the striatum to the external segment of the globus pallidus (GPe)
- Another from GPe to STN
- The third from the internal segment of the globus pallidus (GPi) to the thalamus

As shown in Fig. 10.2.14, the striatum disinhibits the STN. The STN in turn stimulates GPi, which then releases its inhibitory output to the thalamus. The overall effect of this circuit is therefore inhibitory.

II. Indirect pathway involving pars compacta, part of substantia nigra: As shown in Fig. 10.2.15, in this pathway, the pars compacta part of the substantia nigra (SNpc) projects to the striatum (nigrostriatal pathway). The nigrostriatal pathway utilizes dopamine as a neurotransmitter. The SNpc is inhibited by the striatum through the striatonigral pathway. The SNpc in turn exerts both, facilitatory and inhibitory, effects on the striatum through the dopamine as:

- *Dopamine exerts an excitatory effect* when it acts through D_1 dopamine receptors present as the excitatory cholinergic interneuron of the striatum.
- *Dopamine exerts inhibitory effect* when it acts through D_2 receptors present on the excitatory cholinergic interneuron.

Function: As mentioned above, the main function of the indirect pathway is inhibitory; therefore, it is involved in termination of voluntary movements initiated by the primary feedback loop (basal ganglia–thalamic–cortex loop).

- For termination of voluntary movement, the GPi has to be activated again, which takes place by the STN.
- The STN is tonically inhibited by GPe. Therefore, the motor cortex activates the striatum to inhibit GPe leading to activation of STN.
- The STN in turn activates GPi. Once GPi is activated, it further inhibits VA nucleus of the thalamus to inhibit the cortex to terminate the voluntary movement.

The entire process of termination of voluntary movement is through the indirect pathway.

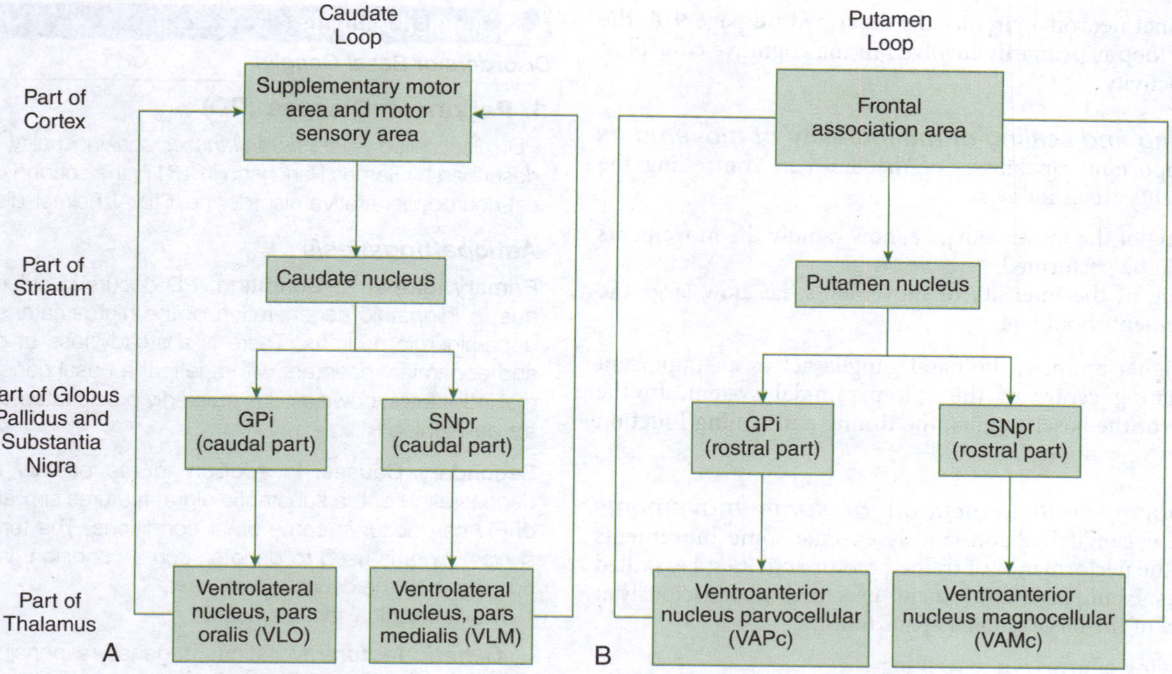

Fig. 10.2.13 A, Pathway of caudate loop; and B, pathway of putamen loop.

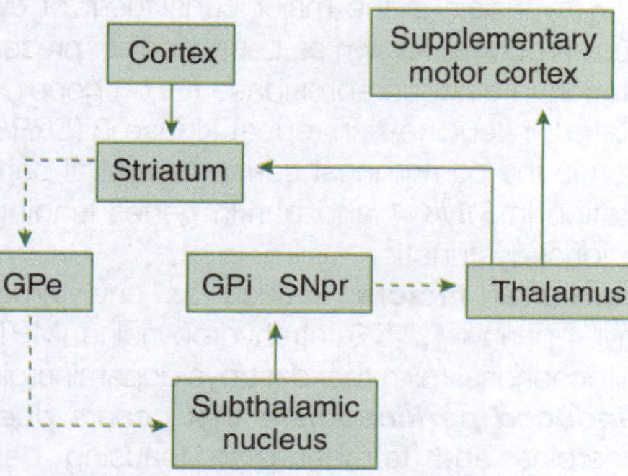

Fig. 10.2.14 Indirect pathway of feedback loop involving subthalamic nucleus.

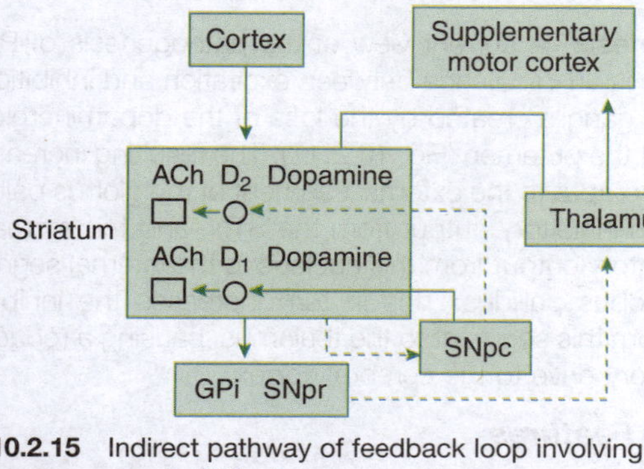

Fig. 10.2.15 Indirect pathway of feedback loop involving substantia nigra pars compacta (SNpc).

Important Note

In essence, the primary or direct pathway is mainly for initiation of the voluntary movement by inhibition of GPi, and the indirect pathway is for termination of initiated movement by activation of GPe.

FUNCTIONS OF BASAL GANGLIA

I. Control of Voluntary Motor Activity

The basal ganglia control the voluntary movements, which are initiated by the motor cortex. During lesions of the basal ganglia, the controlling mechanism is lost and so movements become inaccurate and awkward.

Role of the basal ganglia in control of voluntary motor activity includes:

- Cognitive control of motor activity
- Timing and scaling of intensity of movements
- Subconscious execution of some movements

i. Cognitive control of motor activity Physiological studies have shown that neural discharge in the basal ganglia, like that in the cerebellum, begins well before the movements begin. Therefore, it is believed that the basal ganglia, like the cerebellum, are involved in the planning and programming of the movement (Fig. 10.2.16).

Most of the motor actions occur as a consequence of thoughts generated in the mind. This process is known as cognitive control of motor activity.

Pathway: The cognitive control of motor activity is executed by the basal ganglia through the feedback loops

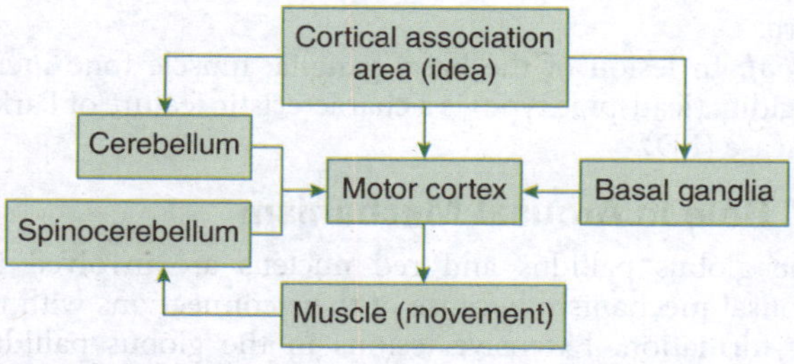

Fig. 10.2.16 Planning and programming of movement.

(functional neuronal circuit). As described on page 916, the caudate loop is primarily involved in the cognitive control of motor activity.

ii. Timing and scaling of the intensity of movements

Two important capabilities of the brain in controlling the movements are as follows:

- Timing of the movements, i.e. how rapidly the movements should be performed
- Scaling of the intensity of movements, i.e. how large the movement should be

In higher animals, the basal ganglia act as an important coordinating centre of the extrapyramidal system. In the absence of the basal ganglia, the timing and scaling function becomes very poor.

iii. Subconscious execution of some movements

The basal ganglia subconsciously execute some movements during the performance of trained motor activities, i.e. skilled activities. Examples of movements executed subconsciously at the level of the basal ganglia are as follows:

- Swinging of arms while walking
- Crude movements of facial expression that accompany emotions
- Movements of limbs while swimming
- Control of clutch and brake while driving (constant attention is required during initial stages; however, they are carried out subconsciously by the basal ganglia as they become routine)

Importance: By subconscious control of activities, the basal ganglia relieve the cortex from routine acts so that the cortex can be free to plan its actions.

Pathway: As described on page 916, the putamen feedback circuit is concerned with control of subconscious execution of some movements, during the performance of trained motor activities as listed above.

II. Control of Reflex Muscular Activity

The basal ganglia exert inhibitory effect on spinal reflexes and regulate activity of muscles, which maintain posture. Visual and labyrinthine reflexes are important in the maintenance of posture. The coordination and integration of impulses for these activities depend on the basal ganglia.

III. Control of Muscle Tone

Muscle spindles and the gamma motor neurons of the spinal cord (which are responsible for maintaining the tone of the muscles) are controlled by the basal ganglia, especially the substantia nigra.

Pathway includes projection from the cortical inhibitory area–striatum–pallidum–substantia nigra–reticular formation–spinal cord.

Proof: In lesion of the basal ganglia, muscle tone increases. Rigidity (lead-pipe type) is a characteristic feature of Parkinson disease (PD).

IV. Role in Arousal Mechanism

The globus pallidus and red nucleus are involved in the arousal mechanism because of their connections with reticular formation. Extensive lesions in the globus pallidus are associated with drowsiness, leading to sleep.

Applied Aspects

Disorders of Basal Ganglia

I. Parkinson Disease (PD)

PD, also called *paralysis agitans* or shaking palsy, was first described by James Parkinson in 1817, the second commonest neurodegenerative disorder next to Alzheimer disease.

Aetiopathogenesis

Primary Idiopathic Condition. PD occurs in elderly people due to idiopathic degeneration of the nigrostriatal system of dopaminergic neurons. There is a steady loss of dopamine and dopamine receptors with age in the basal ganglia in normal individuals; however, it is markedly precipitated in individuals developing PD.

Secondary Causes. In addition to the primary idiopathic degeneration of the substantia nigra, features similar to those of PD can occur in some other conditions. The term *parkinsonism nigra* is used to denote such a condition, which may occur due to the causes given next.

The aetiological factors include:

i. ***Genetic factors:*** Mutations in genes responsible for PD are as follows:
   - *α-Synuclein*, which is a prion protein and mutation in α-synuclein gene is considered to be the cause of parkinsonism (α-synuclein is the major constituent of cytoplasmic inclusion bodies, known as Lewy bodies, present in PD)
   - Mutation in glucocerebrosidase (*GBA*) gene
   - Mutation in leucine-rich repeat kinase-2 (*LRRK-2*) gene, which is the commonest cause of familial parkinsonism
   - Mutation in *PINK-1* and parkin genes leading to mitochondrial dysfunction

ii. ***Environmental factors*** – such as environmental toxin 1-methyl-4-phenyl-1,2,5,6-tetrahydropyridine (MPTP) (MPTP is as mitochondrial toxin that destroys dopaminergic neurons)

iii. ***Drug-induced parkinsonism*** that occurs due to drugs like reserpine and tetrabenazine (causing depletion of dopamine) and haloperidol

iv. ***Viral infections*** – influenza virus and viral hepatitis

v. Viral encephalitis

vi. Cerebral arteriosclerosis

Pathogenesis. A current view of the pathogenesis of PD is that there is an imbalance between excitation and inhibition in the basal ganglia created by the loss of the dopaminergic inhibition of the putamen (Fig. 10.2.17). The resulting increase in inhibitory output to the external segment of the globus pallidus decreases inhibitory output from the STN, and this increases the excitatory output from this nucleus to the internal segment of the globus pallidus. This in turn increases the inhibitory output from this segment to the thalamus, causing a reduction in excitatory drive to the cerebral cortex.

Clinical Features

PD has both hypokinetic and hyperkinetic features. Its cardinal features are a triad of akinesia, rigidity and tremor, of which akinesia is a hypokinetic feature, whereas rigidity and tremors are hyperkinetic features.

1. Akinesia or Hypokinesia. The patient is unable to initiate the voluntary movements (akinesia) or the voluntary movements are decreased (hypokinesia).

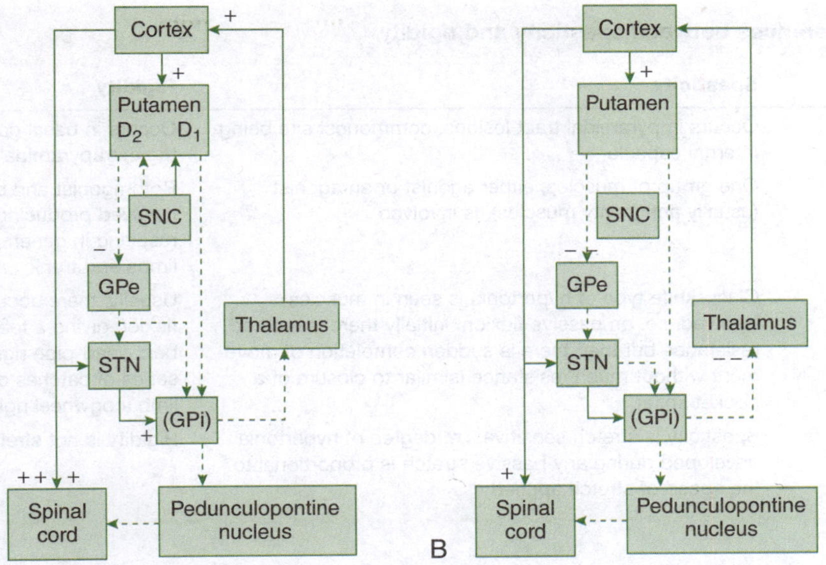

Fig. 10.2.17 Basal ganglia–thalamocortical circuitry: **A**, in normal; and **B**, in Parkinson disease. Solid arrows indicate excitatory output and dashed arrows inhibitory output. Number of plus (+) and minus (−) signs indicate relative increase and decrease in excitation and inhibition of outputs. GPe, external segment of globus pallidus; GPi, internal segment of globus pallidus; SNC, substantia nigra compacta; STN, subthalamic nucleus.

Causes: Akinesia is not due to any paralysis or decrease in muscle power; the sensory system is also normal. Difficulty in initiating voluntary movements is because of hypertonicity of the muscles.

Manifestations of akinesia or hypokinesia include:

- Delayed motor initiative, as evidenced by prolonged reaction time
- Slow performance of voluntary movements (bradykinesia)
- Mask-like facial expression due to decrease in movements of facial muscles
- Absence of normal associated movements, e.g. swinging of arms during walking
- Shuffling or festinant-type gait, in which the patient is bent forward and walks quickly with short steps as if trying to catch up the centre of gravity or preventing himself/herself from falling
- Retropulsion, i.e. when a walking patient is suddenly pulled backwards, he/she begins to walk backwards and is unable to stop

2. Rigidity. Rigidity refers to increase in tone of the muscles.

Characteristic features of rigidity occurring in PD are as follows (Fig. 10.2.18):

- It occurs due to increased tone in both the protagonist and antagonist muscles.
- Mainly, the large proximal group of muscles of limbs, e.g. biceps and knee flexors, is affected.
- Usually, there occurs uniform resistance to flexion giving a feeling as if a lead pipe is being bent (lead-pipe rigidity).
- Sometimes, there is a series of catches during passive motion of the limbs (cogwheel rigidity).
- Due to rigidity, posture becomes that of flexion attitude in which the back is flexed, the arms are abducted and flexed, and the knees are bent.
- In advanced cases, the rigidity may increase to such an extent that a statue-like appearance is produced with complete absence of movements.
- Rigidity differs from spasticity seen in lesions of pyramidal tracts (see Table 10.2.4).

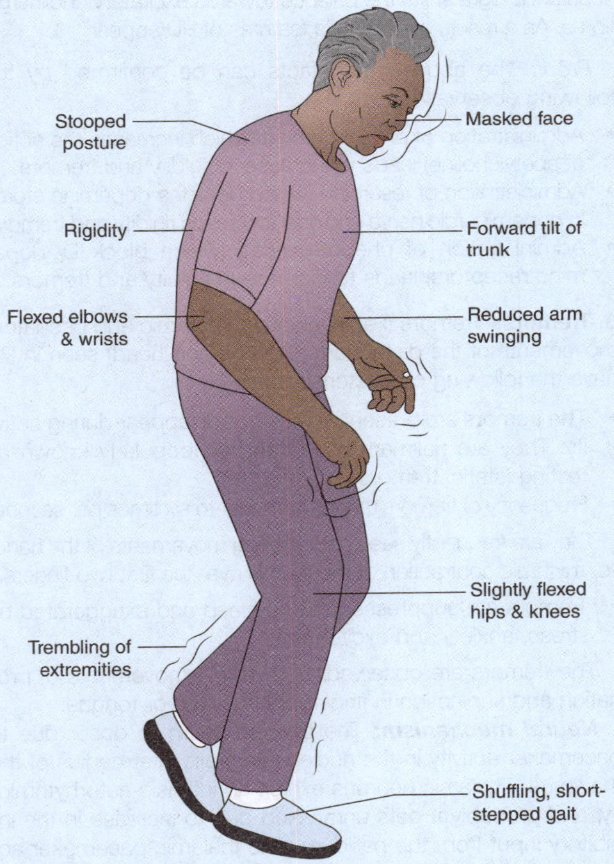

Fig. 10.2.18 Characteristic features of Parkinson disease.

Cause of rigidity: An increased discharge of γ-efferents supplying the muscle spindle causes rigidity. This fact is confirmed by the observation that local injection of 1% procaine solution into the affected muscles decreases rigidity by abolishing the γ-discharge.

Neural mechanism: As described on page 916, the striatum (caudate nucleus and putamen) is under the influence of both

Table 10.2.4 Differences between spasticity and rigidity

Feature	Spasticity	Rigidity
1. Lesion	Occurs in pyramidal tract lesions, commonest site being internal capsule	Occurs in basal ganglia lesion, therefore called the extrapyramidal rigidity
2. Muscles involved	One group of muscles, either agonist or antagonist (usually antigravity muscles), is involved	Both agonist and antagonist muscles are involved producing a uniform hypertonia often resulting in general attitude of flexion of the limbs and trunk
3. Characteristics of hypertonia	Clasp-knife type of hypertonia is seen in muscles involved, i.e. on passive flexion, initially there is marked resistance but then there is sudden completion of movement without much resistance (similar to closure of a pocket knife)	Usually, there occurs a uniform resistance to flexion giving a feeling as if lead pipe is being bent (lead-pipe rigidity); sometimes there is a series of catches during passive motion of the limb (cogwheel rigidity)
4. Relation of hypertonia to stretch	Spasticity is stretch sensitive, i.e. degree of hypertonia developed during any passive stretch is proportional to the speed of stretch applied	Rigidity is not stretch sensitive

excitatory (cholinergic) fibres and inhibitory (dopaminergic) fibres. Under normal circumstances, there exists a balance between the excitatory and inhibitory influences. In patients with PD, lack of dopaminergic activity due to degeneration of neurons in the substantia nigra shifts the balance towards excitatory cholinergic fibres. As a result, hyperkinetic features of PD appear.

Proof: The above-stated facts can be confirmed by the following observations:

- Administration of physostigmine (which increases the action of acetylcholine) leads to increase in rigidity and tremors.
- Administration of reserpine (which depletes dopamine stores in dopaminergic nerve endings) increases rigidity and tremors.
- Administration of phenothiazines (which block D_2 dopamine receptors) leads to increase in rigidity and tremors.

3. Tremors. Tremors (i.e. involuntary, rhythmic and oscillatory movements of the distal parts of limbs and head) seen in PD have the following characteristics:

- The tremors are present at rest, but disappear during activity. They are hallmark of PD and so popularly known as resting (static) tremors.
- Frequency of tremors ranges from four to six times per second.

They are frequently seen as pill-rolling movements of the hand, i.e. rhythmic contraction of the thumb over the first two fingers.

- Tremors are suppressed during sleep and exaggerated by stress, anxiety and excitement.

The tremors are observed as rhythmic movements of pronation and supination in fingers, hands, lips or tongue.

Neural mechanism: The tremors seem to occur due to pacemaker activity in the nucleus ventralis intermedius of the thalamus. Thalamic neurons exhibit an intrinsic autorhythmicity, and probably it gets unmasked due to increase in the inhibitory input from the pallidum. The thalamic pacemaker activity induces oscillation in the long-loop reflex pathways, which originate from muscle spindle. The reflex path runs through the thalamus up to the cortex and then loops back to extrafusal muscle fibres along the corticospinal tract.

4. Other Associated Features. Other associated features of PD are as follows:

- *Sleep disturbances* – such as daytime sleepiness, early awakening and restless sleep
- *Cognitive disturbances* – such as amnesia, confusion in evening hours, dementia or difficulty in thinking and understanding
- *Speech* – difficulty in speaking and speech becoming soft
- *Mood changes* – anxiety and depression
- *Urinary control* disturbed, i.e. dribbling of urine or leaking of urine
- *Constipation*, difficulty in swallowing, blank stare, loss of contrast sensitivity, neck stiffness, small handwriting and loss of smell
- *General fatigue and weight loss*

Stages of PD

The staging system of PD is of two types:

Braak staging – which depends on the degree of pathological changes

Clinical staging – which depends on the rating scale, which is assessed by motor symptoms (such as movements and tremors) and nonmotor symptoms like loss of smell (there are five stages)

Braak staging is useful to assess the spread of Lewy bodies in brain areas in PD. There are the following five stages:

Stage	Brain areas
Stage 1	Olfactory nucleus and brainstem
Stage 2	Higher brainstem
Stage 3	Substantia nigra
Stage 4	Mesocortex and thalamus
Stage 5	Whole of neocortex

Clinical staging of PD is as follows:

- Stage 1: Mild symptoms such as tremors on one side of the body are present.
- Stage 2: Both sides of the body may be affected by tremors/rigidity; therefore, posture and walking become noticeable.
- Stage 3: Motor symptoms worsen and the patient experiences loss of balance leading to fall, and movements get slow.
- Stage 4: In this stage, the normal activity is limited because of symptoms and the patient needs assistance.

- Stage 5: It is the most advanced stage of PD. In this stage, the patient cannot stand and walk. Skilled activity is highly impaired; patients also suffer from hallucinations.

Treatment

Drug treatment: The drugs used in PD are as follows:

1. ***Levodopa (l-DOPA)*** is used in the treatment of PD. It can cross the blood–brain barrier and reaches the brain tissue, where it is concentrated into dopamine and thus compensates its deficiency.
   - Drug dopamine is not used as it cannot cross the blood–brain barrier.
   - Along with L-DOPA, carbidopa (Sinemet) is also used. Carbidopa prevents the conversion of L-DOPA into dopamine in the liver and thus prevents side effects, which can occur due to excessive dopamine content in the liver.
   - Carbidopa cannot cross the blood–brain barrier and thus in the brain L-DOPA is converted into dopamine.
   - L-DOPA in low doses diminishes rigidity and in high doses reduces tremors.
2. ***Dopamine receptor agonists***, such as apomorphine, bromocriptine, pramipexole and ropinirole, also have an effective role in some patients with PD.
3. ***Catechol-O-methyltransferase (COMT) inhibitors*** such as entacapone, when given along with L-DOPA, act by blocking the breakdown of L-DOPA and increase its concentration in the brain.
   - *Monoamine oxidase-B (MAO-B) inhibitors* (e.g. selegiline) and rasagiline also prevent breakdown of dopamine.

Surgical Treatment. Surgical treatment is indicated in PD when the patient suffers disability due to tremors or due to L-DOPA-induced motor complications. The surgical treatment includes:

- *DBS* – i.e. electrical stimulation of STN or GPi – is done.
- Pallidotomy – surgical destruction of GPi or of STN (thalamotomy) – is done.
- Ventrolateral nucleus of the thalamus can also ameliorate the symptoms of PD by restoring the output balance towards normal.
- Implantation of dopamine-secreting tissue in or near the basal ganglia is done.
- Transplant of adrenomedullary tissue of the patient's own also works effectively for some time.
- Fetal striatal tissue transplantation is better taken up and makes connections with the host basal ganglia.

II. Chorea and Athetosis

Chorea and athetosis are abnormal involuntary movements due to a neurological disorder called dyskinesis. Chorea is derived from the Greek word 'dance', and primarily affects the face, mouth, trunk and limbs.

Chorea is characterized by rapid, jerky and involuntary movements (dancing movements). It occurs due to damage to caudate nucleus. Chorea is seen frequently in children as a complication of rheumatic fever.

Athetosis is a movement dysfunction that may occur in children following birth injuries.

Choreoathetosis: Chorea and athetosis are very similar. In fact, they can occur together; then this condition is called choreoathetosis, characterized by slow, rhythmic, twisting, worm-like and confluent writhing movements of the extremities, affecting chiefly the fingers and the wrists. It occurs due to damage to the putamen.

III. Huntington Disease

Cause

It is a genetic disease of the nervous system, characterized by CAG trinucleotide repeat expansion. It is inherited as an autosomal dominant disorder, usually occurring between 30 and 50 years of age. The abnormal gene responsible for the disease is located near the end of short arm of chromosome 4. The abnormal gene codes for a protein called huntingtin, which is comparatively less soluble and forms toxic aggregates in the nuclei of the cell. Huntington disease is also related to increased activity of tissue caspase-1 in the brain, due to mutation or knocked-out gene for apoptosis-regulating enzyme.

Site of Lesion

There occurs damage to GABAergic and cholinergic neurons of the striatum (caudate and putamen) that project to the pallidum. The loss of GABAergic pathway to the external pallidum releases inhibition, permitting the hyperkinetic features of the disease to develop.

Characteristic Features

Characteristic features of Huntington disease are as follows:

- An early sign is jerky trajectory of the hand when reaching to touch a spot.
- Later, hyperkinetic choreiform movements appear, and gradually increase until they incapacitate the patient.
- Speech becomes slurred and then incomprehensible.
- There occurs progressive loss of memory (dementia).

It is a gradually progressive disease, with no effective treatment, which ultimately leads to death.

Treatment

Treatment consists of supportive help, but the following drug is also used:

1. *Tetrabenazine:* Administration of tetrabenazine is efficiently used to reduce choreiform movements (the characteristics of Huntington disease). This drug binds with vesicular monoamine transporters (VMAT), and thus inhibits uptake of monoamines into the synaptic vesicles and also acts as dopamine receptor antagonist.

IV. Hemiballism

Cause

It is a rare disease caused by damage of STN. The common cause of damage is haemorrhage in the nucleus. Damage to the STN reduces inhibitory output from GPi SNpc to the thalamus (Fig. 10.2.14). This leads to disinhibition of thalamic output, resulting in hyperkinetic movements, mediated by corticospinal tracts.

Characteristic Features

The most important feature of hemiballism is spontaneous attacks of flail-like, intense and violent movements affecting whole of the opposite half of the body.

V. Wilson Disease

Wilson disease, also known as hepatolenticular degeneration, is caused by copper toxicity, resulting from impaired biliary excretion of dietary copper. It is a genetic autosomal recessive disorder occurring due to mutation of copper-transporting ATPase gene (ATP7β) located on the long arm of chromosome 13q.

Characteristic features of Wilson disease are due to involvement of different body parts.

Liver involvement is in the form of cirrhosis, hepatitis and haemolytic anaemia.

Ophthalmic manifestations: Copper accumulates in the periphery of the cornea and causes characteristic yellow rings (Kayser–Fleischer rings). Deposition of copper in the lens leads to opacification (sunflower cataract).

- *In the brain*, the lesions are widespread. However, the changes are more marked in lenticular nucleus, particularly putamen, resulting in symptoms of parkinsonism, i.e. muscular rigidity, tremors and akinesia.

Diagnosis

In this condition, the copper content of substantia nigra is high and the plasma level of ceruloplasmin (copper-binding protein) is low.

Liver biopsy is the gold standard for diagnosis of Wilson disease.

Treatment

Chelating agents such as penicillamine and trientine are used to decrease copper in the body in Wilson disease.

Zinc therapy has a significant role in Wilson disease.

VI. Kernicterus

Kernicterus refers to damage of globus pallidus caused by indirect bilirubin, which crosses the blood–brain barrier. It occurs in haemolytic disease of newborn, which results due to Rh antibodies. In this condition, death is very common. However, if the child survives, he/she may show rigidity, chorea, athetosis and mental deficiency (also see page 149).

VII. Tardive Dyskinesia

Tardive dyskinesia is another basal ganglia disease, caused by neuroleptic drugs such as phenothiazide or haloperidol, used as medical treatment for psychiatric disorders. Prolonged use of these drugs produces biochemical abnormalities in the striatum by blocking dopaminergic transmission.

Characteristic features are as follows:

- Involuntary movements of the face and tongue
- Cogwheel rigidity

Treatment

Clozapine is an atypical effective neuroleptic drug used as a substitute for traditional neuroleptic drugs to avoid risk of development of tardive dyskinesia.

Self-Assessment

1. Discuss the significance of intrinsic circuitry of cerebellum.
2. Discuss the components of basal ganglia and role in control of motor activity.
3. Describe the following:
   - Role of cerebellum in regulating motor activity
   - Significance of feed-forward and feedback inhibition
4. Write notes on the following:
   - Tests for cerebellum dysfunction
   - Chorea
   - Parkinsonism
   - Servo mechanism of cerebellum

Clinical Cases

Case 1

A 42-year-old male, a diagnosed case of epilepsy, developed disturbances in speech and gait, and also developed tremors and was referred to the neurologist. The history revealed that the patient was on antiepileptic drugs for the last 4 years.

The examination observations showed nystagmus and dysmetria.

Q1. From the signs and symptoms, what is the probable diagnosis?

Q2. What further tests should be carried out to reach the conclusion?

Q3. What is the treatment plan?

Case 2

A 60-year-old male was referred to neurology OPD with symptoms of tremors, difficulty in walking, slowness of body movements and tendency to fall. History revealed sleep disturbance, constipation and weight loss

Examination showed resting tremors, masked face and lead-pipe rigidity.

From signs and symptoms, the probable diagnosis was Parkinson disease.

Q1. What is the pathophysiology?

Q2. What is the stage of this condition?

Q3. What is the cause for rigidity and tremors?

Q4. What is the treatment plan?

Case 3

A 19-year-old male patient was referred to the neurologist due to the following symptoms:

- Depression
- Inability to concentrate
- Memory lapses
- Abnormal limb movements
- Difficulty in swallowing and speaking

The probable diagnosis made was Huntington disease.

Q1. What is the type of this disease?

Q2. What is site of lesion in the brain?

Q3. What is the pathophysiology of the disease?

Q4. What is the best treatment for this disease?

10.3

Physiological Anatomy, Functions and Lesions of Thalamus and Hypothalamus

CHAPTER OUTLINE

THALAMUS

PHYSIOLOGICAL ANATOMY

The thalamus proper (i.e. dorsal thalamus) along with ventral thalamus (old name subthalamus), epithalamus and hypothalamus constitutes the diencephalon. The diencephalon along with the cerebral hemispheres forms the so-called forebrain. It is important to note that:

- The thalamus proper is now called *dorsal thalamus*.
- The *ventral thalamus* is the new name for the subthalamus.
- The *reticular nucleus*, earlier included in the dorsal thalamus, is now considered a part of ventral thalamus (on functional grounds).
- The *subthalamic nucleus* is now included among the basal ganglia (page 915) to which it is closely related functionally. It is not included in the ventral thalamus (old name, subthalamus).
- The *medial geniculate bodies (MGB) and lateral geniculate bodies* (LGB) are now considered as an integral part of dorsal thalamus.

Earlier, they have been considered distinct from the other regions of the thalamus and have been grouped together as metathalamus.

External Features

The dorsal thalamus is a large ovoid structure placed immediately lateral to the third ventricle. It has an anterior and a posterior end and four surfaces, i.e. dorsal, ventral, medial and lateral.

Anterior end (or pole) lies just behind the interventricular foramen.

Posterior end (or pole) is expanded and is called pulvinar. It lies just above and lateral to the superior colliculus.

Dorsal or superior surface of the thalamus is convex and triangular in outline. It forms the part of floor of the central part of the lateral ventricle (Figs 10.3.1 and 10.3.2).

Ventral or inferior surface of the thalamus is related to the hypothalamus anteriorly (Fig. 10.3.1) and to the ventral thalamus posteriorly (Fig. 10.3.2).

Medial surface forms the greater part of the lateral wall of the third ventricle and is lined by the ependyma. The medial surfaces of the two thalami are connected by a short bar of grey matter called the *interthalamic adhesion*. Inferiorly, the medial surface is separated from the hypothalamus by *hypothalamic sulcus* (Fig. 10.3.1).

Lateral surface of the thalamus is related to the posterior limbs of the internal capsule.

Internal Structure

Like other parts of the brain, the thalamus consists of grey matter (mainly) and white matter (Fig. 10.3.3).

White matter The white matter is scanty in the thalamus and includes:

Stratum zonale is a thin layer of white matter covering the superior surface of the thalamus.

External medullary lamina is a thin layer of white matter covering the lateral surface of the thalamus. It consists of thalamocortical and corticothalamic fibres.

Internal medullary lamina is a Y-shaped sheet of white matter placed vertically in the grey matter of the thalamus. It consists mainly of internuclear thalamic connections.

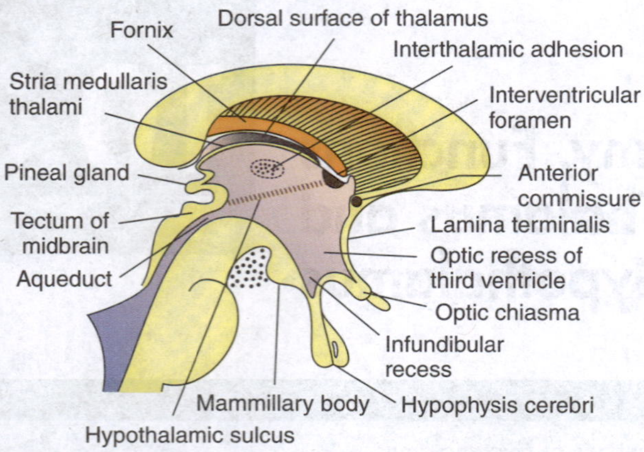

Fig. 10.3.1 Median section through the brain showing medial surface of thalamus and hypothalamus.

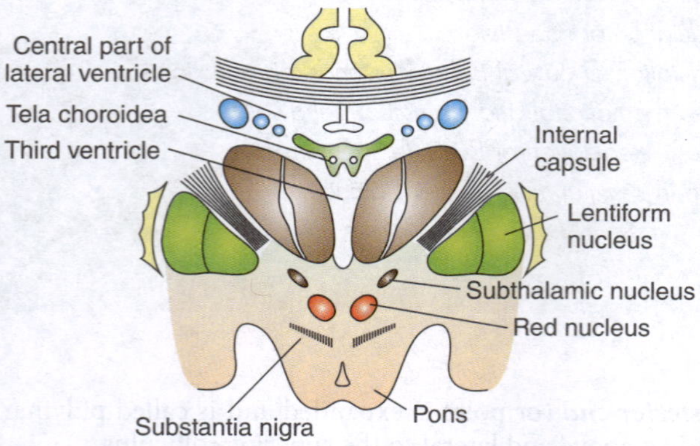

Fig. 10.3.2 Coronal section through the brain passing through the basilar part of pons showing the relations of ventral surface of thalamus and subthalamic structures.

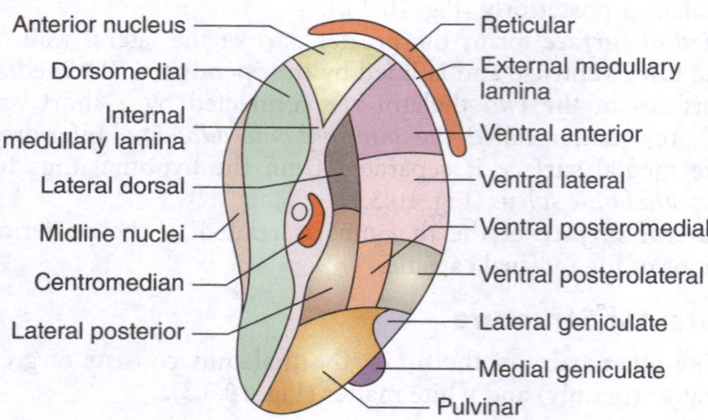

Fig. 10.3.3 Horizontal section of right thalamus (superior aspect) showing nuclear subdivisions.

Grey matter The grey matter of the thalamus is divided into three masses of nuclei by the Y-shaped internal medullary lamina (Fig. 10.3.3):

- Anterior part
- Lateral part
- Medial part

Classification of Thalamic Nuclei

Anatomical Classification of Thalamic Nuclei

Anatomically, thalamic nuclei can be classified as given next (Fig. 10.3.3).

1. Anterior group of nuclei The mass of grey matter enclosed within the bifurcation of the internal medullary lamina is called *anterior nucleus.*

2. Lateral group of nuclei The mass of grey matter present in the lateral part of the thalamus is subdivided into ventral and dorsal groups of nuclei, each containing three nuclei:

(i) ***Ventral group of nuclei*** includes:
- *Ventral anterior (VA) nucleus*
- *Ventral lateral (lateroventral) nucleus*
- *Ventral posterior (posteroventral) nucleus which is further divided into two parts:*
  - Ventral posterolateral nucleus
  - Ventral posteromedial nucleus
- *MGB and LGB* present in the posterior zone of ventral groups of nuclei

(ii) ***Dorsal group of nuclei*** is as follows:
- *Lateral dorsal nucleus*
- *Lateral posterior nucleus*
- *Pulvinar*

3. Medial group of nuclei The medial group of nuclei includes:

- *Dorsomedial nuclei,* present in the medial part of the thalamus
- *Centromedian nucleus* and other interlaminar nuclei present within the internal medullary lamina
- *Midline nuclei* that lie between the medial part of the thalamus and the ependyma of the third ventricle

Functional Classification of Thalamic Nuclei

Functionally, the thalamic nuclei can be grouped under two divisions:

- Nonspecific projection nuclei
- Specific projection nuclei

A. Nonspecific projection nuclei Nonspecific projection nuclei are those which receive impulses for diffuse secondary responses from the reticular activating system (RAS) and project diffusely to the whole of the neocortex. These include:

- Midline nuclei
- Centromedian nucleus

B. Specific projection nuclei Specific projection nuclei receive specific sensations and project to specific portions of the neocortex and limbic system. Depending on the type of sensation, the specific projection nuclei can be divided into four groups.

I. Specific sensory relay nuclei These include:

1. MGB
2. LGB
3. Posteroventral group of nuclei

II. Motor control nuclei These include:

1. Ventrolateral (VL) group of nuclei
2. VA nucleus

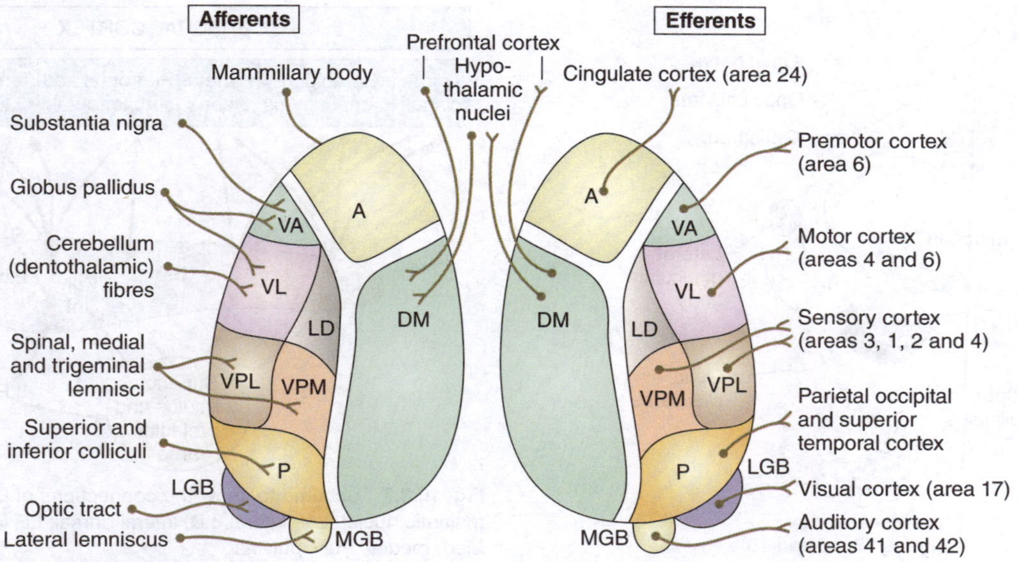

Fig. 10.3.4 Afferent and efferent connections of some of thalamic nuclei. A, anterior; LGB, lateral geniculate body; MGB, medial geniculate body; P, pulvinar; VA, ventral anterior; VL, ventral lateral; VP, ventral posterior.

III. Visceral efferent control nuclei These include:

1. Anterior group of nuclei
2. Dorsomedial nucleus

IV. Integrative and perceptual function control nuclei

1. Pulvinar nucleus
2. Lateral posterior nucleus
3. Dorsal lateral nucleus

Connections of Thalamus

Afferent and efferent connections of the various thalamic nuclei based on their functional classification are given next (Fig. 10.3.4).

Connections of Nonspecific Projection Nuclei

These are functionally associated with *diffuse thalamic projection* which produces marked changes in the electrical activity of the cerebral cortex when it is stimulated.

Nonspecific projection nuclei include:

- Centromedian nucleus and other intralaminar nuclei
- Midline nuclei

Afferents to these nuclei come from RAS, basal ganglia and other thalamic nuclei.

Efferents from these nuclei project to the stratum and the entire neocortex.

Connections of Specific Projection Nuclei

These nuclei receive specific sensations and project to specific portion of the neocortex and limbic system. Depending on the type of sensation, the specific projection nuclei can be divided into four groups.

I. Specific sensory relay nuclei include:

1. Medial geniculate bodies (Fig. 10.3.5)

Afferents: MGB receive a 'topically' organized projection of auditory fibres from the cochlear nerve, lateral lemniscus and also inferior colliculi.

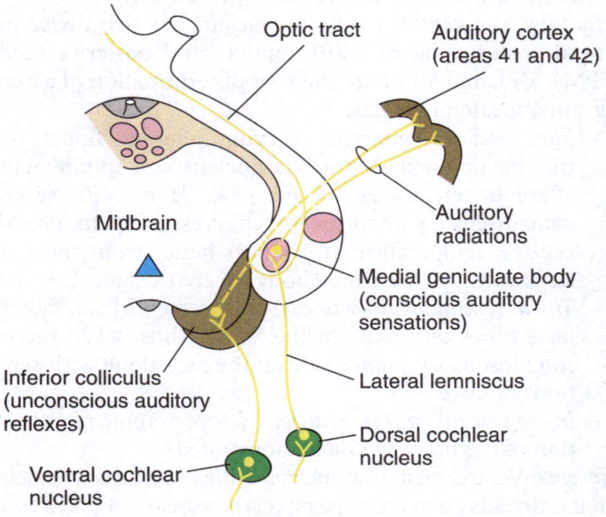

Fig. 10.3.5 Connections of medial geniculate body.

Efferents: The MGB project onto the auditory area of the cerebral cortex (areas 41 and 42).

Applied Aspects

Destruction of a small part of MGB produces deafness of a particular band of sound frequency.

2. Lateral geniculate bodies (Fig. 10.3.6)

Afferents: LGB show an orderly organized representation of the retina. They receive projections from the optic tracts from both eyes (temporal fibres of the same side and nasal fibres of the opposite side). They also receive projections from the superior colliculi. In the LGB, the macula is represented in the caudal two-thirds, whereas the remaining retina is represented in the rostral one-third (see page 947).

Efferents from LGB (optic radiations) project topographically on the visual cortex of the occipital lobe (areas 17, 18 and 19).

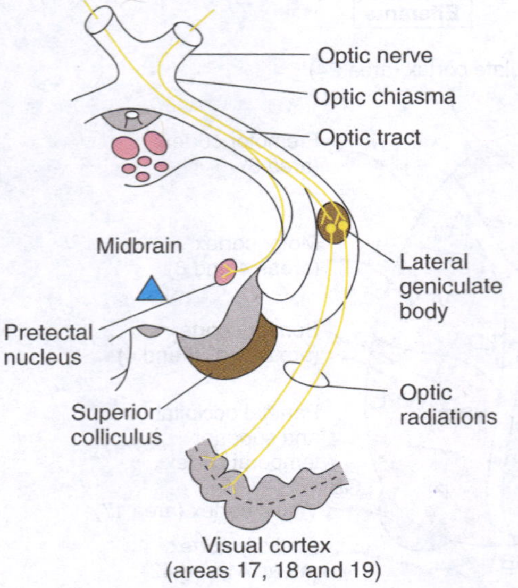

Fig. 10.3.6 Connections of lateral geniculate body.

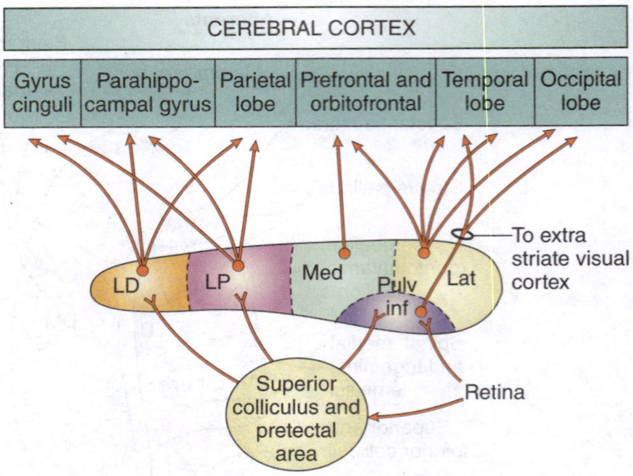

Fig. 10.3.7 Scheme to show the connections of lateral group of thalamic nuclei. Lat, lateral; LD, lateral dorsal; LP, lateral posterior; Med, medial; Pulv, pulvinar.

3. Ventral posterior nucleus (Fig. 10.3.4)

Afferents: The ventral posterior nucleus has two divisions – ventral posterior lateral (VPL) and ventral posterior medial (VPM). VPL and VPM are the sites of termination of ascending somatic afferent tracts.

- *The medial lemniscus* carrying afferent fibres from the gracile nucleus, cuneate nucleus and spinothalamic afferents terminates in the VPL. Thus, VPL receives somatosensory impulses (touch, pressure, pain, proprioceptive, temperature and kinaesthetic) from the trunk and limbs, i.e. the whole body except the face.
- *The trigeminal lemniscus* carrying afferents from face and taste fibres terminate in the VPM. Thus, VPM receives somatosensory impulses from the face along with sensations of taste.
- *In the ventral posterior nucleus,* a topographic representation of the body can be demonstrated.

Efferents: Ventral posterior nucleus is the main sensory nucleus and its efferents go to the sensory cortex – areas 3, 1 and 2 (postcentral gyrus) – via the posterior limb of the internal capsule.

II. Motor control nuclei include:

1. Ventral lateral nucleus (Fig. 10.3.4)

Afferents: VL nucleus is the chief motor nucleus of the thalamus. It acts as a relay station for cerebellar impulses. It receives the dentatothalamic fibres from the dentate nucleus of the opposite cerebellar hemisphere. It also receives fibres from the globus pallidus via the thalamic fasciculus.

Efferents from VL nucleus project on the primary motor cortex and premotor cortex (areas 4 and 6), via the posterior limb of the internal capsule.

These relay proprioceptive information and voluntary motor functions.

2. Ventral anterior nucleus (Fig. 10.3.4)

Afferents: The VA nucleus is involved in the programming of movements controlled by the basal ganglia. Its afferents come from the globus pallidus, cerebellum and substantia nigra.

Efferents from VA go to the premotor cortex (area 6).

III. Visceral efferent control nuclei The nuclei concerned with visceral efferent control mechanism are given next.

1. Anterior nucleus (Fig. 10.3.4)

Afferents: Anterior (A) nucleus belongs to the Papez circuit of the limbic system (see page 1048). It is concerned with recent memory and emotions. It receives afferents from the hippocampus directly via the fornix and relayed through the mammillary body (mammillothalamic tract).

Efferents from the anterior nucleus go to the cingulate gyrus (area 24) of the cerebral cortex.

2. Dorsal medial nucleus

The dorsal medial nucleus has reciprocal connections with the prefrontal cortex and hypothalamus. Its point-to-point interconnections with the prefrontal cortex imply important functions in thinking, memory, judgement and emotional behaviour.

IV. Integrative and perceptual function control nuclei

1. Pulvinar nucleus (Fig. 10.3.7)

Afferents: Pulvinar nucleus is concerned with integration of visual, auditory and other sensations. It receives afferents from the superior and inferior colliculi.

Efferents go to the parietal, occipital and superior temporal cortex (auditory and visual association areas).

2. Lateral posterior nucleus (Fig. 10.3.7)

Afferents: It receives fibres from the superior colliculus.

Efferents from the lateral posterior nucleus reach the cerebral cortex of the superior parietal lobule. They also reach the cingulate and parahippocampal area.

3. Dorsal lateral nucleus (Fig. 10.3.7)

Afferents: It receives afferents from the superior colliculus.

Efferents: Projections reach the cingulate gyrus, the parahippocampal gyrus and parts of the hippocampal formation. Some fibres reach the cortex of the parietal lobe.

Functions of Thalamus

1. Sensory relay centre

Almost all the sensory impulses (except olfactory) reach the thalamic nuclei, which relay them to the cerebral cortex by a series of projection fibres collectively termed the thalamic radiations (ascending thalamocortical system). Because of this, the thalamus is usually considered the head ganglion of all the sensory system.

2. Centre for integration of sensory impulses The thalamus not only is a great relay station for all sensations but also forms a major centre for integration and modification of peripheral sensory impulses before the impulses are projected to specific areas of the cerebral cortex. This function of the thalamus is called processing of sensory information. Because of this, the thalamus is usually considered as a functional gateway of the cerebral cortex.

3. Crude centre for perception of sensations In addition to processing and relaying of sensations, the thalamus also acts as a crude centre for sense perception. Pain sensation is perceived in the thalamus itself. Usually, the sensations have two qualities – the discriminative nature and the affective nature.

The discriminative nature is the ability to recognize type, location and other details of the sensation. It is the function of the cerebral cortex.

The affective nature is the capacity to determine whether a sensation is pleasant or unpleasant and agreeable or disagreeable. It is the function of the thalamus.

4. Centre for integration of motor function The thalamus receives the output from the basal ganglia and the cerebellum before projecting it to the motor cortex, thereby helping in integration of motor functions by unconscious regulation of muscle tone.

5. Role in arousal and alertness reaction Majority of nonspecific ascending impulses from RAS are relayed to the thalamus before proceeding to the cortex. Through these fibres, the thalamus is involved in controlling the level of consciousness and maintaining a state of alertness and wakefulness.

6. Role in emotional aspect of behaviour Because of intimate connections between the thalamus and the frontal cortex and hypothalamus, the thalamus is involved in subjective feeling of various emotions. Thus, it acts as a part of the limbic system. It also forms a part of the Papez circuit and is concerned with recent memory and emotions.

7. Role in language The thalamus is also concerned with language (speech) function. Integration between different cortical parts by subcortical connections in the thalamus helps to achieve speech.

8. Role in synchronization of electroencephalogram The thalamus also plays an important role in the genesis of synchronization of electroencephalogram (EEG).

9. Centre for integration of visceral and somatic function The thalamus receives somatic as well as autonomic sensations, and is also connected with the hypothalamus. Because of this, it also acts as a centre for integration of visceral and somatic functions.

10. Centre for sexual sensations The thalamus also acts as a centre for perception of sexual sensations.

11. Centre for reflex activity All the sensory fibres relay in the thalamus, so it forms the centre for many reflex activities.

Applied Aspects

1. Thalamic Syndrome

The thalamic syndrome is a disturbance of emotional responses to sensory experience.

Cause Thalamic syndrome is produced by damage to posteroventral and posterolateral nuclei as a result of thrombotic blockage of the thalamogeniculate branch of the posterior cerebral artery.

Symptoms and Signs Symptoms and signs in thalamic syndrome occur on the opposite side of the body. These include:

I. ***Sensory symptoms*** due to involvement of posteroventral nucleus are as follows:
   - *Contralateral hemianaesthesia* occurs due to damage to VPL and VPM (sensory nuclei of the thalamus).
   - *Astereognosis* occurs due to loss of tactile localization, tactile discrimination and stereognosis.
   - *Thalamic phantom limb:* The patient is unable to locate the position of limbs with closed eyes and searches for the limb in air. This occurs due to loss of kinaesthetic sensations.
   - *Thalamic overreaction:* The threshold for pain, touch and temperature is decreased and the sensations become exaggerated and disagreeable.
   - *Amelognosis:* It is illusion felt by the patient that his/her limb is absent.
   - *Contralateral homonymous hemianopia* occurs due to involvement of LGB.

II. ***Motor symptoms*** due to involvement of posterolateral nucleus are as follows:
   - *Ataxia, decreased muscle* tone and profound muscular weakness occur due to damage to cerebellar afferents.
   - *Involuntary movements:* Any of the following may be associated:
     - Involvement of fibres coming from the globus pallidus leads to chorea (quick jerky movements) or athetosis (slow writhing and twisting movements).
     - Intention tremors are usually associated with thalamic syndrome.
   - *Thalamic hand or athetoid hand* refers to the abnormal posture of the hand occurring in patients with thalamic syndrome. It is characterized by moderate flexion of the wrist with hyperextended fingers.

Frontal Lobotomy

For relief of intractable pain, connections of the dorsal nuclei of the thalamus with the frontal lobe are divided surgically especially by an operation called *frontal lobotomy*, after which the patient feels the pain, but does not show a disagreeable response.

2. Korsakoff Syndrome

Korsakoff syndrome refers to lesions of mediodorsal nucleus of the thalamus characterized by difficulty in remembering new information.

HYPOTHALAMUS

PHYSIOLOGICAL ANATOMY

External Features

The hypothalamus, though a very small part of the brain (a few cubic centimetres in size and weighing about 10 g), plays a very important role of regulating all vegetative and most endocrine processes in the body. It is the most important organ of integration in the homeostatic control of internal environment. It is a bilateral diencephalic structure, with diffuse nuclear mass situated below the thalamus.

Boundaries of the hypothalamus are as follows (Fig. 10.3.1):

- *Superiorly*, the hypothalamic sulcus separates it from the thalamus.
- *Inferiorly*, it is related to the structures in the floor of the third ventricle, i.e. tuber cinereum, infundibulum and mammillary bodies, which are considered its parts.
- *Medially*, it forms part of the wall of the third ventricle.
- *Laterally*, it is in contact with the internal capsule.
- *Anteriorly*, it extends up to the anterior commissure and lamina terminalis.
- *Posteriorly*, the hypothalamus merges with the ventral thalamus at a vertical plane just caudal to the mammillary bodies.

Subdivisions and Nuclei of Hypothalamus

For convenience of description, the hypothalamus can be divided as:

From medial to lateral, into two zones:

- Medial zone
- Lateral zone

From anterior to posterior, the hypothalamic nuclear mass is arranged in four regions:

- Preoptic region
- Supraoptic region
- Tuberal region
- Mammillary region

Hypothalamic Nuclei

Nuclear masses of the hypothalamus present in different regions of the hypothalamus are as follows (Fig. 10.3.8):

1. ***Preoptic region:*** It is located behind the lamina terminalis. It contains preoptic nucleus.
2. ***Supraoptic region:*** It lies above the optic chiasma and is rostrally continuous with the preoptic area. It forms the anterior nucleus group which includes:
   - Suprachiasmatic
   - Supraoptic anterior
   - Paraventricular nucleus
3. ***Tuberal region:*** It is the widest region of the hypothalamus and forms the middle nuclear group which includes dorsomedial, lateral, tuberal, ventromedial and arcuate (infundibular or tuberal) nucleus.
4. ***Mammillary region:*** It forms the *posterior nuclear* group, which includes the posterior and mammillary nucleus.

Connections of Hypothalamus

The hypothalamus serves as the main integrator of the autonomic nervous system and is concerned with visceral functions, and is, therefore, connected to other areas having a similar function. These include the various parts of the limbic system, the reticular formation and autonomic centres in the brainstem and spinal cord.

Apart from its neural connections, the hypothalamus also acts by releasing secretions into the bloodstream and into the CSF.

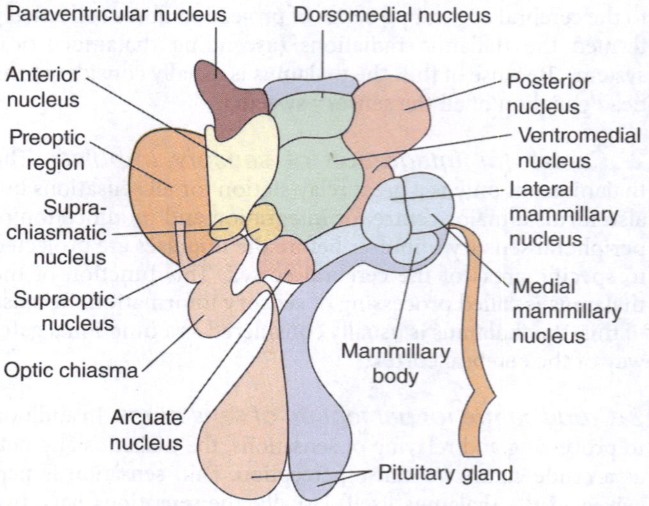

Fig. 10.3.8 Nuclei of hypothalamus.

Afferent Connections

1. From other parts of limbic system The hypothalamus receives afferents from other parts of the limbic system in the form of the following nerve fibre bundles (Figs 10.3.9 and 10.3.10):

Medial forebrain bundle forms the major pathway of the hypothalamus. It consists of both ascending and descending fibres. The descending fibres begin in the anterior olfactory areas (anterior perforated substance, olfactory tubercle and pyriform cortex) and run through the lateral zone of the hypothalamus, to reach the tegmentum of the midbrain. These fibres end in hypothalamic nuclei and raphe nuclei of the reticular formation of the midbrain. These fibres are related to basic emotional drives and to the sense of smell.

Fornix is the main projection for the hippocampal formation and ends in the mammillary body, and on the arcuate nucleus, some hippocampal fibres are carried to the medial forebrain bundle which relays them in septal nuclei.

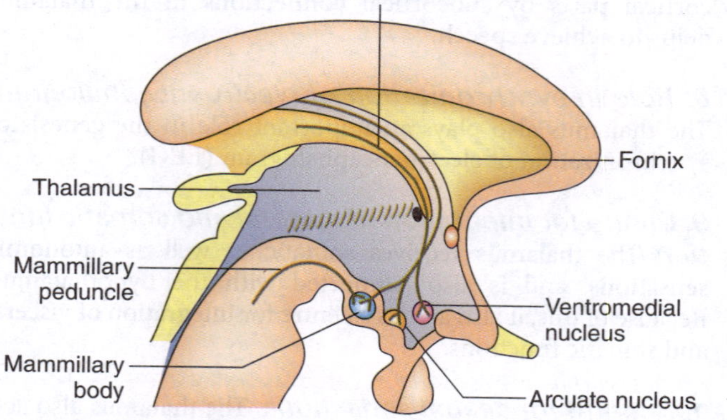

Fig. 10.3.9 Some afferent connections of hypothalamus.

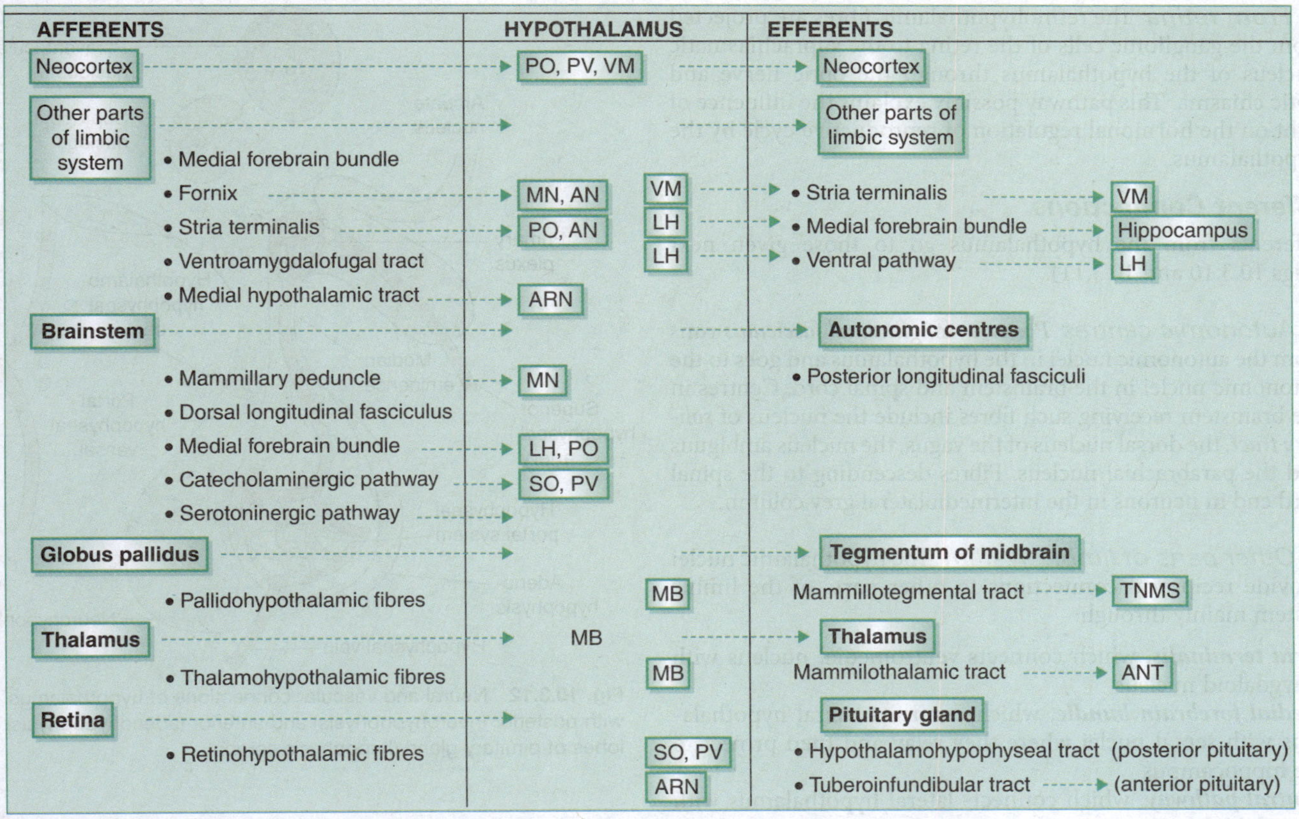

Fig. 10.3.10 Simplified scheme of main afferent and efferent connections of hypothalamus. AN, anterior nucleus; ARN, arcuate nucleus; LH, lateral hypothalamus; MB, mammillary body; MN, medial nucleus; PO, preoptic; PV, paraventricular; SO, supraoptic; VM, ventromedial.

Stria terminalis arises from the amygdaloid body, reaches over the thalamus and terminates in the preoptic area and anterior nucleus of the hypothalamus. Some fibres from the amygdaloid body also pass the hypothalamus through the ventral amygdalofugal tract.

Medial hypothalamic tract runs from the restricted region of the hippocampus to the arcuate nucleus. This pathway and stria terminalis are the only two major afferent pathways running directly to the medial hypothalamus. Other afferent fibres take an indirect route in the medial forebrain bundle and lateral hypothalamus to reach the medial hypothalamus.

Cingulate gyrus establishes connections with the hypothalamus through its projections to the hippocampus.

2. From brainstem From brainstem, the afferents reach the hypothalamus via the following nerve bundles:

Mammillary peduncle: It is a bundle of fibres that connects the tegmentum of the midbrain to the mammillary body. The fibres in it carry gustatory and general visceral impulses from the spinal cord and brainstem centres (nucleus of tractus solitarius and dorsal nucleus of vagus) to the hypothalamus.

Dorsal longitudinal fasciculus of Schutz arises from the periaqueductal grey matter and spreads over dorsal and caudal region of the hypothalamus. These fibres also carry visceral impulses to hypothalamus.

Medial forebrain bundle: As mentioned above, the medial forebrain bundle consists of both descending and ascending fibres. The ascending fibres arise from the midbrain and project to the lateral hypothalamic and preoptic nuclei. These fibres also carry visceral impulses to the hypothalamus.

Catecholaminergic pathways from the locus coeruleus ascend monosynaptically to the cerebrum and cerebellum. On way to the cerebellum, they project fibres to the thalamic nuclei, hypothalamus, septal area, amygdaloid body and hippocampus. These projections modify the degree of alertness. Ascending catecholaminergic fibres are distributed to supraoptic and paraventricular nuclei, and possibly regulate the output of the releasing hormones of the hypothalamus.

Serotoninergic pathways ascending from the raphe nuclei of the pons and lower midbrain terminate in the hypothalamus, septal nuclei, amygdaloid body and neocortex. Presumably, they regulate the sleep–wake cycle, because total insomnia develops when the serotonin stores are depleted by the use of the drug reserpine.

3. From neocortex Corticohypothalamic fibres have been described to exist in humans that interconnect the prefrontal and posterior orbitofrontal regions with preoptic, paraventricular and ventromedial nuclei of hypothalamus. Some authors, however, deny such neocortical projections to the hypothalamus.

4. From globus pallidus The pallidohypothalamic fibres from the globus pallidus go to the diffused area of the hypothalamus.

5. From thalamus The thalamohypothalamic fibres from the dorsomedial and midline nuclei of the thalamus go to the diffused area of the hypothalamus.

6. From retina The retinohypothalamic fibres are projected from the ganglionic cells of the retina to the suprachiasmatic nucleus of the hypothalamus through the optic nerve and optic chiasma. This pathway possibly explains the influence of light on the hormonal regulation of reproductive cycle by the hypothalamus.

Efferent Connections

Efferents from the hypothalamus go to those given next (Figs 10.3.10 and 10.3.11).

1. Autonomic centres *Posterior longitudinal fasciculus* runs from the autonomic nuclei in the hypothalamus and goes to the autonomic nuclei in the brainstem and spinal cord. Centres in the brainstem receiving such fibres include the nucleus of *solitary tract*, the dorsal nucleus of the vagus, the nucleus ambiguus and the parabrachial nucleus. Fibres descending to the spinal cord end in neurons in the intermediolateral grey column.

2. Other parts of limbic system The hypothalamic nuclei provide reciprocal connections to other parts of the limbic system mainly through:

Stria terminalis, which connects ventromedial nucleus with amygdaloid nucleus
Medial forebrain bundle, which connects lateral hypothalamus with septal nuclei where they relay and then project to the hippocampus
Ventral pathway, which connects lateral hypothalamus with amygdaloid nucleus

3. Thalamus The *mammillothalamic tract* (bundle of Vicq d'Azyr) connects the mammillary body to the anterior nucleus of the thalamus which in turn is connected with gyrus cinguli, thus forming a component of Papez circuit of the limbic system. These fibres are responsible for those emotions and aspects of behaviour that are related to preservation of the individual and species.

4. Tegmentum of midbrain The mammillotegmental tract arises from the mammillary body and terminates in the ventral and dorsal tegmental nuclei of the midbrain.

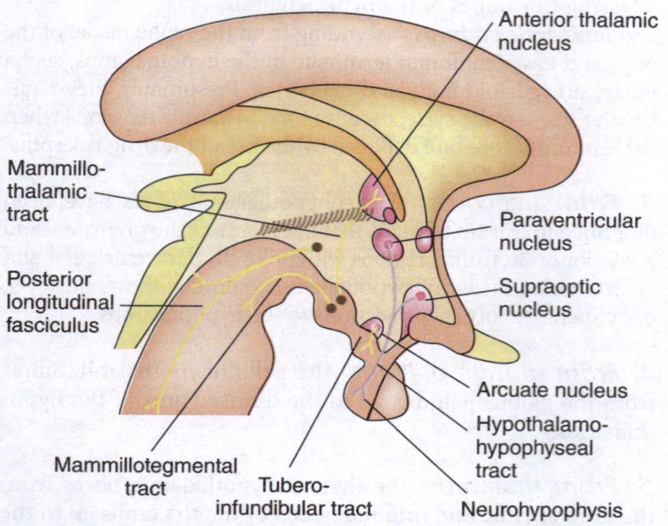

Fig. 10.3.11 Some efferent connections of hypothalamus.

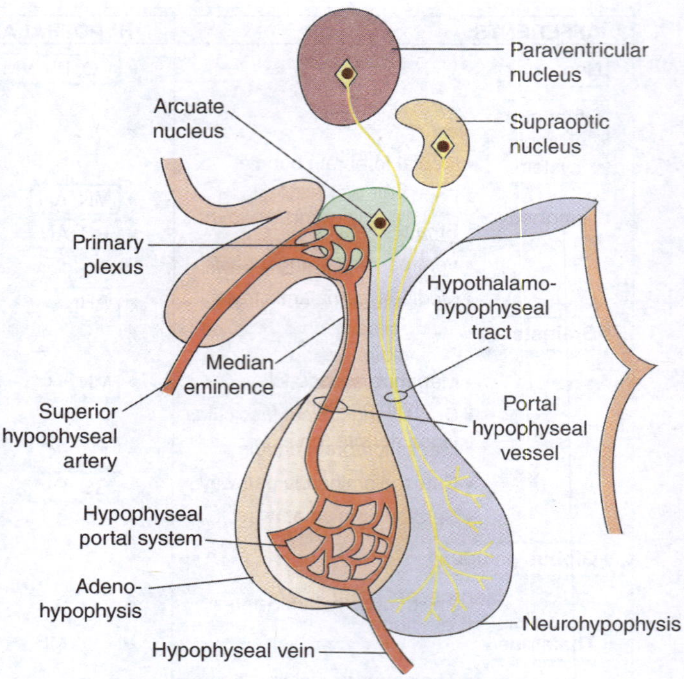

Fig. 10.3.12 Neural and vascular connections of hypothalamus with posterior (neurohypophysis) and anterior (adenohypophysis) lobes of pituitary gland (hypophysis cerebri).

5. Neocortex Fibres from the hypothalamus project widely to the neocortex. They play a role in maintaining the cortical arousal.

6. Pituitary gland Influences from the hypothalamus are conveyed to the pituitary gland (hypophysis cerebri) in two different forms:

i. ***Hypothalamohypophyseal tract*** (Fig. 10.3.12): It is composed of axons of the large neurosecretory cells of the supraoptic and paraventricular nuclei of the hypothalamus. The fibres of this tract are unmyelinated and pass to the posterior lobe of the pituitary (neurohypophysis) through the infundibular stem of the hypothalamus and form a series of dilated terminals known as *Herring bodies* which come in contact with the capillary bed of the neurohypophysis. The neurosecretory cells of supraoptic and paraventricular nuclei secrete *vasopressin* (antidiuretic hormone [ADH]) and *oxytocin*.
The neurons producing vasopressin and oxytocin are distinct. Although both types of neurons are found in each nucleus, the supraoptic nucleus is believed to mainly produce vasopressin, and the paraventricular nucleus is believed to mainly produce oxytocin.

Important Note

Afferents from the nipple of the breast, stimulated by suckling by the baby, increase the discharge rate of neurons in the paraventricular nuclei leading to release of oxytocin from the posterior pituitary. For details, see page 862.

ii. ***Tuberoinfundibular tract*** (tuberohypophyseal tract): It consists of fibres arising from the arcuate nuclei of the tuberal region of the hypothalamus, and extends to the median eminence and infundibular stem where the fibres come in close contact with the capillary plexus of the *hypophyseal portal system* (Fig. 10.3.12). The neurons of hypothalamic nuclei synthesize certain *releasing* or *inhibiting factors* (or hormones) which are conveyed as membrane-bound vesicles by the tuberoinfundibular tract to the hypophyseal portal vessels. These hormones are carried by the portal vessels to the anterior pituitary (adenohypophysis) where they regulate the secretion of anterior pituitary hormones.

FUNCTIONS OF HYPOTHALAMUS

1. Autonomic Functions

Sherrington described the hypothalamus as the *head ganglion* of the autonomic nervous system.

Anterior hypothalamus is the parasympathetic area. It has an excitatory effect on this system.
Posterior hypothalamus is the sympathetic area and has an excitatory effect on it.

Autonomic functions subserved by the hypothalamus are given next.

i. Cardiovascular Regulation

The hypothalamus regulates the cardiovascular system through cardiovascular control centres in the reticular regions of the medulla and pons.

- Stimulation of posterior and lateral nuclei of the hypothalamus increases the heart rate and arterial blood pressure and produces cutaneous vasoconstriction.
- Stimulation of the preoptic area decreases the heart rate and arterial blood pressure and produces cutaneous vasodilatation.

ii. Regulation of Pupil Size

- Stimulation of the posterior and lateral hypothalamus causes dilatation of the pupil.
- Stimulation of anterior and medial parts of preoptic and supraoptic areas produces constriction of the pupil.

iii. Regulation of Peristaltic and Secretomotor Functions of Alimentary Tract

- *Stimulation of the posterior and lateral hypothalamus* diminishes the secretion and motility of the gastrointestinal tract (GIT) (ergotropic function).
- *Stimulation of the anterior and medial hypothalamus* increases peristalsis and secretomotor functions of the alimentary tract (trophotropic function).

2. Endocrinal Functions

i. Control of Anterior Pituitary The hypothalamus controls the functions of the anterior pituitary by secreting certain 'releasing' and 'inhibiting' hormones which reach the anterior pituitary by a neurovascular link through the tuberoinfundibular tract and hypophyseal portal vessels as described on page 866.

Functions through the releasing hormones The hypothalamus performs the following functions:

- Controls the metabolism by controlling the thyroid gland (see page 688)
- Controls the metabolism of different foodstuffs and maintains electrolyte balance through its influence over the adrenal cortex (see page 730)
- Keeps the gonads inhibited till the physical growth is complete (after physical growth is complete, this inhibition is removed so that gonads start functioning and gametes are produced [propagation of species]; gonadal hormones acting on the brain bring about physiological changes for mating of male and female)
- Controls the formation of milk by the breasts by controlling prolactin secretion (see page 861).

ii. Regulation of posterior pituitary functions The hypothalamus regulates the posterior pituitary functions through the hypothalamic–hypophyseal tract (for details, see page 665).

Neural control of the posterior pituitary with the secretion of ADH by the supraoptic and paraventricular nuclei helps in regulation of water balance by controlling water excretion by kidneys (see page 678).

iii. Regulation of uterine contractility and regulation of milk ejection from the breast Stimulation of paraventricular nucleus of the hypothalamus causes its cells to secrete the hormone oxytocin. Oxytocin increases the contractility of the uterus. It also contracts the myoepithelial cells that surround the alveoli of the breast and cause milk ejection. At the end of pregnancy, especially large quantities of oxytocin are secreted. Oxytocin helps to promote labour contractions.

When the baby suckles the breast, signals from the nipple to the hypothalamus cause reflex oxytocin release which causes expulsion of milk through the nipples. For details, see page 861.

3. Regulation of Sleep–Wake Cycle

The hypothalamus plays an important role in sleep–wake cycle:

Anterior hypothalamus is considered a *sleep facilitatory centre*, as its stimulation leads to sleep.
Posterior hypothalamus acts as a *waking centre*, as its stimulation causes wakefulness.
Sleep is also considered to occur as a negative phenomenon, i.e. inhibition of wakefulness centre in the posterior hypothalamus by the anterior hypothalamus also contributes to occurrence of sleep. Lesions in the posterior hypothalamus produce severe coma (for details, see page 1069).

4. Control of Circadian Rhythm

Circadian rhythm refers to rhythmic fluctuations in certain physiological parameters of the body. These are called circadian rhythms because they often show 24-hour cycles (circadian around a day). Many of the rhythms are coordinated with each other.

Common rhythmic variations in homeostatic regulatory mechanism are as follows:

- Rhythmic secretion of ACTH (see page 734)
- Rhythmic secretion of growth hormone (see page 670)
- Rhythmic secretion of melatonin (see page 780)
- Sleep–wake cycles (as described above)
- Body temperature rhythm (see page 933)
- Rhythmic gonadotropin secretion (see pages 797 and 834)

Basis of circadian rhythm: The circadian rhythms are *internally driven*. The *suprachiasmatic nucleus* of the hypothalamus is the main site of most circadian rhythms in the body. These are believed to contain the 'biological clock', which regulates the circadian rhythm according to the 24-hour light–dark cycles. The suprachiasmatic nuclei receive important inputs from:

- The eyes via retinohypothalamic fibres (page 831)
- The lateral geniculate nuclei

Effect of environmental factors on circadian rhythm: Environmental factors such as light–dark cycles, temperature and meal timing provide only *hints* and are required only to set a circadian rhythm cycle of 24 hours. Otherwise, the circadian rhythms are internally driven and can occur in the absence of environmental factors evidenced as follows:

- Normally, rats show locomotor activity in the dark (at night) and inactivity in the daytime. These cycles of activity and inactivity continue even when the rats are put permanently in a darkened laboratory for a few days with no exposure to light.
- The cycles of activity and inactivity can be disrupted by bilateral lesions of suprachiasmatic nuclei.

Physiological significance of circadian rhythm:

- The circadian rhythm enables *homeostatic mechanism* to be utilized immediately and automatically. For example, there is a rhythm in the urinary excretion of ACTH.
- The circadian rhythms have effects on the body's resistance to various drugs. For example, difference in the sensitivity of dose of a potentially lethal drug depends markedly on the time the drug is given.

Applied Aspects

Disturbances of circadian rhythm can occur during high-speed jet travel. One may travel several thousand kilometres within a few hours. As a result, the traveller's external clock (day or night) does not coincide with the internal biological clock. That is, the body may be in rest (night) phase while it is daytime in the country of destination. It results in irritability, mental depression or even physical illness. The symptoms subside in a few days. The condition is called jet lag.

5. Regulation of Food Intake

The regulation of food intake is an essential vegetative function of the hypothalamus which maintains the body weight of an individual relatively constant over a long period. To regulate the food intake, the hypothalamus has two centres, namely the *feeding centre* and the *satiety centre* located in the tuberal region.

Feeding Centre

The lateral hypothalamic nucleus subserves as the feeding centre or hunger centre. When this is stimulated in animals, it creates a sensation of hunger and leads to increased food intake (hyperphagic). This causes obesity. The destruction of the feeding centre leads to loss of appetite (anorexia).

Normally, the feeding centre is always active and its activity is inhibited by the satiety centre after food intake.

Satiety Centre

Satiety is opposite to hunger, i.e. it is a feeling of fulfilment after food intake. The *ventromedial nucleus* of the hypothalamus acts as the satiety centre. Stimulation of this in animals causes sensation of food intake (fulfilment). Destruction of the satiety centre leads to hyperphagia.

There are the following hypotheses regarding regulation of food intake:

- Glucostatic theory
- Lipostatic theory
- Gut peptide theory
- Thermostatic theory

Glucostatic theory: The cells of the satiety centre act as glucoreceptors (also called glucostats); therefore, the activity of the satiety centre is governed by glucose utilization of these cells. The satiety centre activity decreases when the glucose supply is inadequate leading to less or no inhibition of the feeding centre, resulting in its inactivation, and the individual feels hungry. On the other hand, when there is adequate supply of glucose, the satiety centre cells' activity increases leading to inhibition of the feeding centre and there is feeling of fulfilment.

Important Note

Polyphagia in diabetes mellitus is explained by the glucostatic theory. There is inadequate glucose utilization by glucoreceptors of the satiety centre (due to deficiency of insulin).

Lipostatic theory: The neurons of the feeding centre respond to levels of fatty acids and amino acids. The body fat depots initiate either neural or hormonal signals that are related to the hypothalamus and control the food intake:

- Leptin (Greek word, means thin) is a circulating protein hormone produced by the adipose cells. By its action on the hypothalamus, it decreases release of neuropeptide Y resulting in a decrease in food intake.

Important Note

Leptin acts through leptin receptors, mainly present in brown adipose tissue and brain microvasculature. It controls the size of body fat; therefore, obesity occurs due to defective leptin receptor gene (Ob gene).

Gut peptide theory: According to the gut peptide hypothesis, presence of food in GIT releases certain polypeptides and GIT hormones (like CCK, glucagon, GRP, peptide YY and somatostatin) that act on the hypothalamus to inhibit food intake. Circulating CCK plays a major role through its receptors (CCK_A and CCK_B) present in the hypothalamus.

Thermostatic theory: Body temperature (core) regulates food intake. Fall in body temperature increases and rise decreases the food intake.

The balanced activity of satiety and feeding centres is responsible for the normal food intake.

Role of neurotransmitters in food intake *Food intake is increased* by the stimulation of α_2-adrenergic receptors in the medial hypothalamus and centrally acting opioids.

Food intake is decreased by the stimulation of β-adrenergic and dopaminergic receptors in the lateral hypothalamus and by stimulation of serotonergic pathways (see page 984).

Role of hypothalamic peptides Principal hypothalamic polypeptides (neuropeptide Y, orexin-A and orexin-B, melanin-concentrating hormone [MCH], agouti-related peptide [AgRP] and ghrelin) increase the food intake, whereas α-MSH, cocaine- and amphetamine-regulated transcript (CART) and corticotropin-releasing hormone (CRH) decrease the food intake.

6. Regulation of Sexual Behaviour and Reproduction

In animals, the hypothalamus plays an important role in maintaining the sexual function, especially in females. A decorticate female animal will have regular oestrous cycle provided the hypothalamus is intact.

A pathway of sex regulation has been identified as amygdala–stria terminalis–preoptic area–tuberal region of the hypothalamus. The tuberal region of the hypothalamus maintains the basal secretion of gonadotropin-releasing hormone (GnRH), and its connection with the preoptic area is essential for the cyclical surge of gonadotropin before ovulation.

Proof: Electrical stimulation of the preoptic area produces ovulation in experimental animals, and destruction of neural links between the preoptic and the tuberal region prevents ovulation. For details, see page 833.

7. Role in Emotional and Instinctual Behaviour

The emotional and instinctual behaviour is mainly regulated by the limbic cortex (for details, see page 1051). The hypothalamus along with the limbic structures is concerned with affective nature of sensory impulses, i.e. whether the sensations are pleasant or unpleasant. These affective qualities are also called a reward and punishment. The two centres in the hypothalamus involved in such a behaviour and emotional changes are called reward centre and punishment centre.

Reward centre is located along the course of the medial forebrain bundle, especially in lateral and ventromedial nucleus of the hypothalamus. Electrical stimulation of this area encourages the animal to seek more of such stimulation.

Punishment centre is located in the medial hypothalamus (periventricular zone). The electrical stimulation of this area leads to pain, fear, defence, escape reactions and other elements of punishment. The experimental animal avoids further stimulation of this area.

Role of reward and punishment centres: Almost anything that we do is related in some way to reward and punishment. If we do something that is rewarding, we continue to do it. If we do something that is punishing, we cease to do it.

- Therefore, *reward and punishment centres constitute one of the most important of all the controllers of our bodily activities, our drives, our aversions and our motivation.*
- Sensory experience that is causing neither reward nor punishment is remembered hardly at all; the animal becomes habituated to such sensory experience and then ignores it.
- When the sensory experience causes either reward or punishment, the cortical response becomes progressively more and more intense. Thus, *reward and punishment centres help in selecting the information that we learn.*

Rage: Strong stimulation of punishment centres produces a violent and aggressive emotional state called rage. Normally, it is kept in check by counterbalancing activity of ventromedial nuclei of the hypothalamus, hippocampus, amygdala and anterior portion of the limbic cortex. *Rage* reaction is characterized by:

- Development of a defence posture
- Extension of limbs
- Lifting of tail
- Hissing and splitting
- Piloerection
- Wide opening of eyes
- Dilation of pupil
- Severe savage attack, even on mild provocation

Sham rage: Normally, animals and humans maintain a balance between the rage and the opposite state, i.e. calm emotion. This occurs due to reciprocal connections between the hypothalamus and the cerebral cortex. When the connection between the cerebral cortex and the hypothalamus is severed by decortication, the experimental animal exhibits an outburst of rage on mild peripheral stimulation. This is known as *sham rage*, because the emotions associated with rage are absent. Thus, sham rage is due to release of the hypothalamus from the cortical control, and it can be abolished by lessening the caudal hypothalamus.

8. Role in Regulation of Body Temperature

The hypothalamus acts as a principal integrating centre for heat regulation. By adjusting a balance between heat production and heat loss, it helps to maintain body temperature at 37°C. The hypothalamus accomplishes this function by two centres.

i. Heat loss centre The anterior hypothalamus, especially the preoptic area, acts as a heat loss centre.

- Increase in the temperature of blood flowing through this area increases the activity of temperature-sensitive neurons which results in cutaneous vasodilatation and increased sweating causing more heat loss.
- Lesions of the anterior hypothalamus abolish the physiological response to heat exposure.

ii. Heat gain centre The posterior hypothalamus acts as a heat gain centre. Electrical stimulation of the posterior hypothalamus results in cutaneous vasoconstriction and shivering.

A lesion of the posterior hypothalamus abolishes body response not only to cold but also to heat, because this area is the final integration centre for all thermoregulatory signals. Final efferent signals for heat production or heat loss emerge from the posterior hypothalamus.

Regulation of body temperature is discussed in detail in Chapter 12.4 (see page 1198).

9. Role in Regulation of Water Balance

The hypothalamus regulates the water balance of the body by two mechanisms (Fig. 10.3.13):

- *Through thirst centre* by controlling water intake
- *Through osmoreceptors* in supraoptic nucleus by controlling water loss

i. Through thirst centre Thirst centre located in the lateral nucleus of the hypothalamus is stimulated by plasma hypertonicity (which occurs when the water content of the body is reduced). This causes intense desire for water and the animal drinks large quantities of water. It has been observed that:

- Discrete lesions of the thirst centre abolish fluid intake and the animal dies of dehydration.
- Electrical stimulation of this area in conscious animals (through chronically implanted electrodes) causes the animal to drink water as long as the stimulation continues.

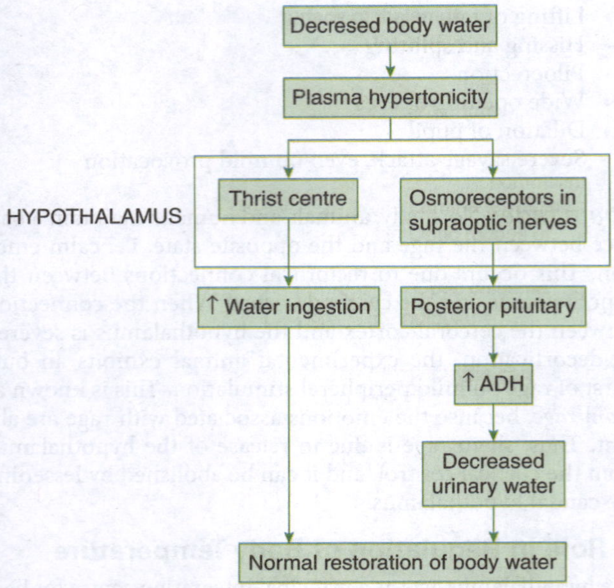

Fig. 10.3.13 Mechanism of regulation of water balance by hypothalamus.

- Injection of hypertonic saline in this area induces the animal to drink a large amount of water. However, injection of isotonic saline, distilled water and even hypertonic urea does not induce drinking. These experiments suggest that the thirst centre monitors plasma osmolality and is separate from the osmoreceptors involved in ADH release.

Furthermore, it has been observed that the sensation of thirst is satisfied simply by the act of drinking, even before sufficient water is absorbed from the GIT to correct the plasma osmolality. Oropharyngeal and upper gastrointestinal receptors appear to be involved in this response. However, relief of the thirst sensation via these receptors is short lived. Thirst is completely satisfied only when the plasma osmolality, blood volume and arterial pressure are corrected.

- Decrease in ECF volume also stimulates thirst by an independent pathway. Haemorrhage leads to increased drinking even when there is no increase in osmolality of plasma. The effect of decreased ECF volume on thirst is mediated via the renin–angiotensin system (see page 737). Renin secreted in response to hypovolaemia results in an increase in circulating angiotensin II that acts on the subfornical organ (a specialized receptor area in the diencephalon) and organum vasculosum of lamina terminalis (OVLT). Both the areas are highly permeable and are part of circumventricular organs and located outside the blood–brain barrier.
- Baroreceptors located in the heart and blood vessels also play a role in thirst mechanism.

ii. Through osmoreceptors in supraoptic nucleus

The increased plasma osmolality also stimulates osmoreceptors in supraoptic nucleus. The stimulated neurons of supraoptic nucleus in turn send impulses to the posterior pituitary gland to secrete hormone ADH. This hormone reaches the kidney tubules through blood and causes increased absorption of water from the collecting ducts of the kidneys. Thus, water loss is decreased. When body has excess water, exactly opposite events occur.

iii. Other factors regulating water intake

Prandial drinking: Increased intake of liquids during eating is considered to be learned or a habit, but it may be associated with:

- Increased plasma osmolality occurring due to absorption of food
- Action of certain GIT hormone

If protein intake is high, the metabolic products of protein cause osmotic diuresis; therefore, to maintain water balance, intake of water increases.

Psychological factors also play an important role in water intake. It has been observed that in patients with psychosis or some hypothalamic disease, dehydration causes hypernatraemia, but they cannot increase their water intake on stimulation of the thirst centre.

Local factors: Dryness of the pharyngeal mucous membrane causes sensation of thirst.

Dehydrated animals, such as dogs and cats, can drink lots of water to make up the water deficit but stop drinking even before the water is absorbed and plasma osmolality is still higher. This observation suggests that some gastrointestinal metering mechanism is also involved.

For further details of water balance control of body fluid osmolality, see page 522.

Applied Aspects

Lesions of Hypothalamus

Lesions of the hypothalamus include:

- Tumour
- Inflammation (or encephalitis)
- Ischaemia due to vascular disorder
- Damage due to surgical operations in this area

Disturbances in Hypothalamic Lesions

The lesions of the hypothalamus may result in a variety of disturbances:

- Autonomic disturbances
- Disturbances of body temperature regulation
- Sleep disturbances due to lesions in the mammillary body and anterior hypothalamus
- Endocrine abnormalities, e.g. hypogonadism and hypothyroidism
- Disturbance in sexual functions due to involvement of mid-hypothalamus
- Disturbance of body water balance due to damage to supraoptic nuclei or infundibular stalk, characterized by excessive thirst and polyuria
- Emotional disturbances leading to sham rage due to lesions in ventromedial and posterolateral parts

Clinical Conditions in Hypothalamic Lesions

Lesions of the hypothalamus may produce any of the specific clinical conditions given next.

1. Diabetes Insipidus

Diabetes insipidus occurs due to deficiency of ADH occurring in a tumour or sham lesions of the anterior hypothalamus in which supraoptic nuclei are damaged. It is characterized by excessive thirst and polydipsia. For details, see page 682.

2. Narcolepsy

It is a hypothalamic disorder with an abnormal sleep pattern. The patient gets sudden attacks of unresistable desire of sleep during daytime. The duration of sleep is usually short – from few seconds to about 20 minutes (see page 1076).

3. Cataplexy

Cataplexy refers to sudden emotional outburst of anger, fear or excitement associated with narcolepsy. The attack lasts for few minutes. In this, consciousness is not lost.

4. Wernicke–Korsakoff psychosis syndrome

Wernicke–Korsakoff psychosis syndrome occurs due to degeneration of mammillary bodies due to thiamine deficiency, which is mainly associated with alcoholism and is characterized by clinical triad, i.e. ophthalmoplegia, ataxia and global confusion.

Treatment: Wernicke–Korsakoff psychosis is an emergency condition and is treated by intramuscular injection of 100 mg thiamine.

5. Confabulations

Confabulation is a memory disorder defined as production of fabricated, distorted or misinterpreted memories about oneself or the word, i.e. synthesizing memory of an event that never occurred.

Self-Assessment

1. Discuss the principal nuclei of thalamus and their functional role.
2. Discuss the role of hypothalamus in regulation of hunger and feeding.
3. Describe the following:
   - Role of hypothalamus in thirst mechanism
   - Role of hypothalamus in circadian rhythm
4. Write notes on the following:
   - Hypothalamic dysfunction
   - Narcolepsy
   - Rage
   - Leptin

Clinical Cases

Case 1

A 50-year-old male was referred to the neurologist for presenting symptoms – flexion at the wrist joint and hyperextension of fingers with severe pain which was affecting his daily routine activities. The history revealed that he suffered from stroke in the past and was fully recovered.

Q1. The signs and symptoms depict which neurological condition?
Q2. What is the site of lesion?
Q3. What is the cause for severe pain?

Case 2

A 40-year-old male suffered from a brain tumour and fully recovered by surgical removal. After 1 year, he developed sudden attacks of sleepiness in daytime which lasted only for few minutes. He also had feeling of cold even in the extreme hot weather and sexual disturbances.

Q1. What is the cause for above-mentioned symptoms?
Q2. What is the lesion site for the symptoms?

10.4 Physiological Anatomy and Functions of Cerebral Cortex and White Matter of Cerebrum

CHAPTER OUTLINE

CEREBRAL CORTEX

EXTERNAL FEATURES

Poles, Surfaces and Borders of Cerebral Hemisphere

Cerebrum Cerebrum consists of two cerebral hemispheres which are separated from each other in the upper part by a median longitudinal fissure in which the *falx* cerebri (a fold of dura mater) invaginates. In the lower part, the two cerebral hemispheres are connected by the largest white commissure called *corpus callosum*.

Each cerebral hemisphere has three poles, three surfaces and three borders.

Poles Three poles of each hemisphere are as follows:

Frontal pole anteriorly
Occipital pole posteriorly
Temporal pole that lies between the frontal and occipital poles, and points forwards and somewhat downwards

Surfaces Three surfaces of each hemisphere are as follows:

- *Superolateral surface*
- *Medial surface*
- *Inferior surface* which is further subdivided into an anterior orbital part and a posterior tentorial part

Borders Three borders of each hemisphere are as follows:

- *Superomedial border* separates the superolateral surface from the medial surface.
- *Inferolateral border* intervenes between the superolateral surface and the inferior surface.
- *Medial border* separates the medial surface from the inferior surface. From front to backwards, it is divided into three parts – medial orbital border, hippocampal border and medial occipital border.

Sulci and Gyri

The surface of the cerebral hemisphere is covered by a thin layer (2–4 mm thick) of grey matter called the cerebral cortex. The entire surface of the cerebral hemisphere is folded with intervening grooves of fissures. The folds or convolutions are called gyri, and the intervening fissures are called sulci. The cerebral cortex follows the irregular contour of the sulci and gyri of the hemisphere and extends into depth of the sulci. As a result of the folding of the cerebral surface, the cerebral cortex acquires a much larger surface area (about 2200 cm^2) than the size of the hemisphere would otherwise alone.

Lobes of Cerebral Hemisphere

Each cerebral hemisphere is divided into four lobes. The boundaries separating one lobe from the other on the superolateral

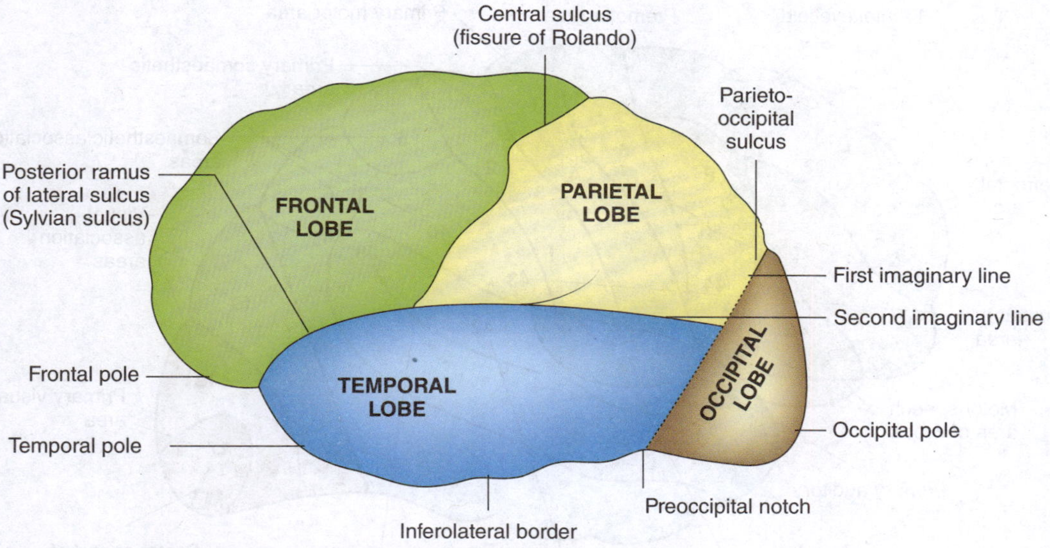

Fig. 10.4.1 Superolateral surface of cerebral hemisphere to show different lobes, poles and borders.

surface of the cerebral hemisphere are formed by three prominent sulci and two imaginary lines (Fig. 10.4.1).

Sulci, which separate the lobes, are as follows:

- Central sulcus or fissure of Rolando
- Posterior ramus of lateral or Sylvian sulcus
- Parieto-occipital sulcus

Imaginary lines which complete the subdivisions of the hemisphere into lobes are as follows:

- *First imaginary line* connects the upper end of the parieto-occipital sulcus to the parieto-occipital notch.
- *Second imaginary line* is a backward continuation of the posterior ramus of the lateral sulcus to meet the first imaginary line.

The four lobes of each cerebral hemisphere as seen on the superolateral surface (Fig. 10.4.1) are as follows:

Frontal lobe: It lies in front of the central sulcus and above the posterior ramus of the lateral sulcus. It is concerned with motor functions.

Parietal lobe: It lies between the central sulcus and the parieto-occipital sulcus and upper part of the first imaginary line. Below, it is separated from the temporal lobe by the posterior ramus of the lateral sulcus and its continuation (the second imaginary line). It is concerned with sensory functions.

Temporal lobe: It lies below the posterior ramus of the lateral sulcus and its continuation (the second imaginary line). Behind, it is separated from the occipital lobe by the lower part of the first imaginary line. It is concerned with hearing.

Occipital lobe: It lies behind the parieto-occipital sulcus and its continuation (the first imaginary line). It is concerned with vision.

CORTICAL FUNCTIONAL AREAS

On the basis of the number and thickness of cortical laminae and cell type (cytoarchitecture), Brodmann divided the cortex into 47 areas.

The concepts regarding the different functional areas of the cerebral cortex have undergone considerable modifications in recent years. It has been seen that motor and sensory functions are strictly not separated. Many motor fibres arise outside the motor cortex from areas which are regarded as partly sensory. However, in clinical work, reference continues to be made to classical subdivisions.

Classically, cortical functional areas are subdivided into (Fig. 10.4.2):

Motor areas include:

- Primary motor area (Brodmann's area 4)
- Premotor area (area 6)
- Frontal eye field (area 8)
- Supplementary motor area

Sensory areas include:

- Primary somaesthetic areas (areas 3, 1 and 2)
- Secondary (supplementary) somaesthetic area
- Somaesthetic association areas (areas 5, 7 and higher association area 40)

Auditory areas include:

- Primary auditory area (area 41) or auditory area I
- Auditory association area (area 42) or auditory area II
- Higher auditory association area (area 22)

Visual areas include:

- Primary visual area (area 17) or visuostriate area of visual area I
- Visual association area 18 (peristriate area)
- Visual association area 19 (parastriate area)

Speech areas include:

- *Motor speech* area comprises:
  - Anterior area (Broca's area) or areas 44 and 45
  - Superior area
- *Sensory speech areas* comprise:
  - Area 39 (or reading centre)
  - Area 40
  - Area 22 (Wernicke's area)

Smell area is the following:

- Area 28

Gustatory area is the following:

- Area 43

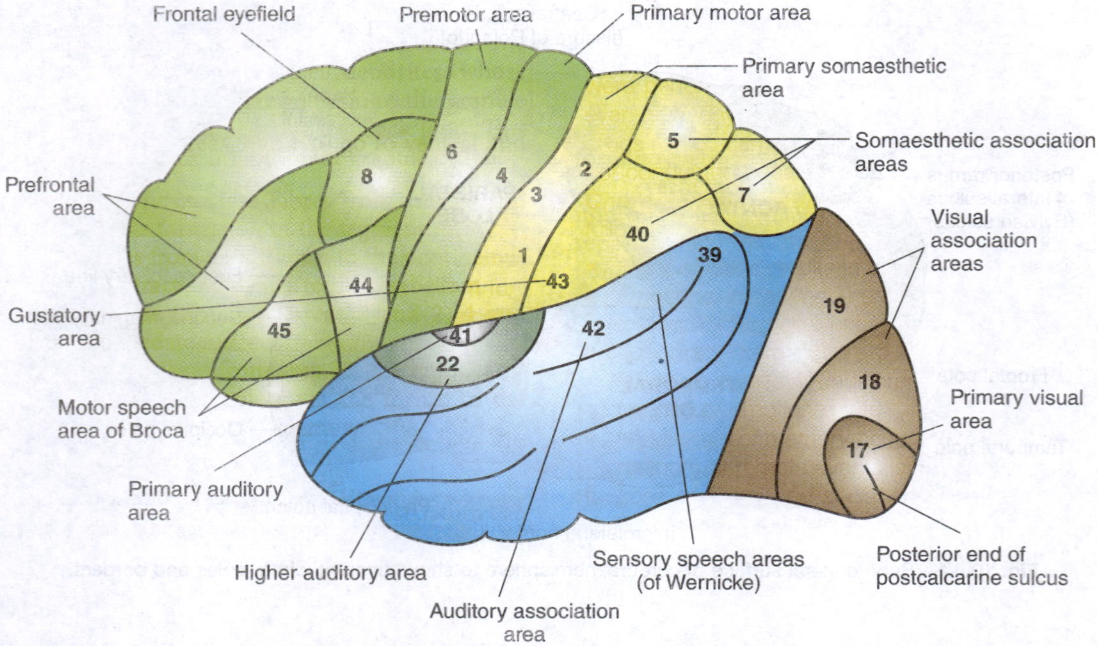

Fig. 10.4.2 Different areas on the lateral surface of the human cerebral cortex.

Important Note

The different cortical functional areas are described along with the description of various lobes of the cerebral cortex.

PHYLOGENETICAL DIVISIONS OF CEREBRAL CORTEX

The cerebral cortex, also known as pallium, is divided phylogenetically into three parts – allocortex, mesocortex and neocortex.

1. Allocortex Allocortex or old cortex forms about 10% of the entire cortex and can be further subdivided into:

Archipallium (ancient cortex) includes hippocampus and dentate gyrus.

Palaeopallium (old cortex) comprises uncus and part of parahippocampal gyrus, which belong to the piriform area of olfactory cortex.

Since most of the allocortex is located around the peripheral margin of the diencephalon in the form of a ring, it is also called *limbic cortex*. This ring of limbic cortex functions as a two-way communication linkage between the neocortex and the lower limbic structures. Along with the thalamus and hypothalamus, the limbic cortex is concerned with emotional and instinctive behaviour.

2. Mesocortex Mesocortex, which is the transitional zone between the allocortex and the neocortex, comprises the cingulate gyrus, part of parahippocampal gyrus and *subiculum*.

3. Neocortex Neocortex, also called an isocortex, comprises rest of 90% of the cerebral cortex in the human brain. The actual extent of the neocortex has increased with the evolution of mammals. The comparative ratio of the allocortex and neocortex in rat, cat, monkey and humans is shown in Fig. 10.4.3.

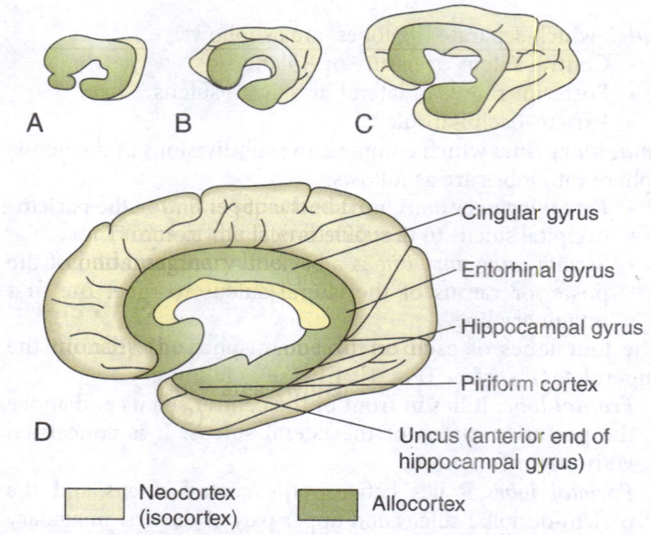

Fig. 10.4.3 Relative extent of allocortex and neocortex in different mammals: A, rat; B, cat; C, monkey; and D, human.

HISTOLOGICAL STRUCTURE OF CEREBRAL CORTEX

Histologically, the allocortex is composed of three distinctive layers, whereas the neocortex is composed of six layers named I–VI from outside to inside (Fig. 10.4.4).

Histologically, the cerebral cortex is composed of nerve cells and fibres.

Types of Cells

Three types of cells may be identified in the cerebral cortex.

1. Pyramidal cells About two-thirds of all cortical neurons are pyramidal cells. These cells have triangular cell bodies,

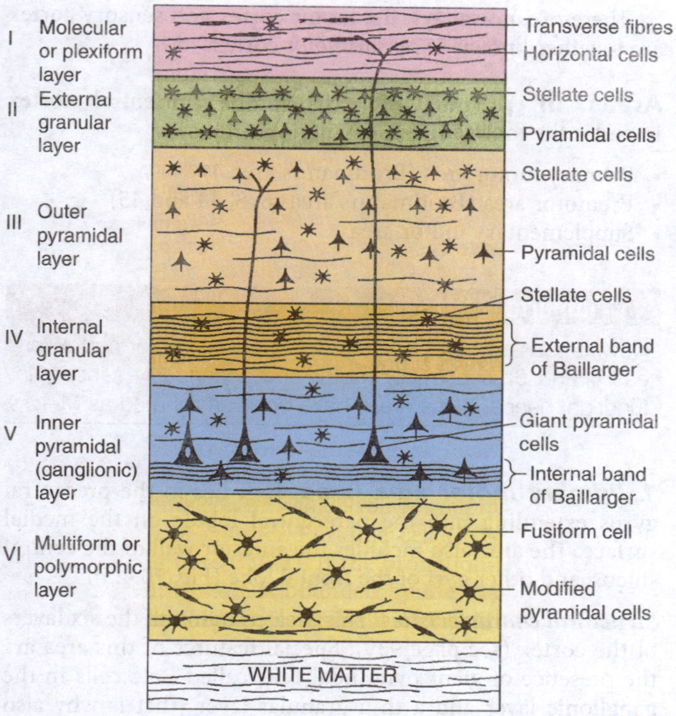

Fig. 10.4.4 Histological structure of neocortex.

with the apex generally directed towards the surface of the cortex. Axon arises from the base of the cell and a large dendrite arises from the apex, and other dendrites arise from the basal angles. The processes of pyramidal cells extend vertically through the entire thickness of the cortex. These cells are present in layers II, III and V of the neocortex.

2. Stellate or granule cells These cells form about one-third of the total neurons. These cells have small cell bodies from where the dendrites arise in all directions. Layer IV is packed with such cells and is best developed in the primary sensory cortex.

3. Fusiform cells These are comparatively few in number. Such cells have spindle-shaped cell bodies, and are present in layer VI.

Laminae of Neocortex

The six laminae of neocortex numbered I–VI are given next (Fig. 10.4.4).

I. Molecular or plexiform layer It mainly consists of transverse nerve fibres dispersed with occasional horizontal cells.

The transverse fibres are derived from the apical dendrites of pyramidal cells, axons of stellate and *Martinotti* cells (pyramidal cells with short axon) of the deeper layer which ascend and ramify horizontally in this layer.
The horizontal cells of Cajal are small pear-shaped or fusiform.

II. External granular layer It contains numerous stellate or granule cells, and a lesser number of small pyramidal cells. It is traversed by afferent and efferent projection fibres. Dendrites of cells of this layer pass into the molecular layer. The axons end in the deeper layer. Some axons enter the white substance of the hemisphere.

III. Outer pyramidal layer It consists mainly of pyramidal neurons and some stellate and basket cells. The pyramidal cells are of two types – the *small cells* lie in the superficial zone and the *medium-sized* cells occupy the deeper zone.

IV. Internal granular layer This layer consists of densely packed stellate cells. The inner zone of this layer is traversed by a prominent aggregation of transversely running fibres called external band of Baillarger.

V. Inner pyramidal (ganglionic) layer This layer consists of large pyramidal cells. It is specially developed in the motor cortex, where these cells are called giant cells or Betz cells. This layer is traversed by a prominent aggregation of transversely running fibres called *internal band of Baillarger*.

VI. Polymorphous or multiform layer This layer contains neurons of various sizes and shapes, many of which are probably modified pyramidal cells. Many spindle-shaped cells called fusiform cells are present in this layer. This layer also contains cells of Martinotti, whose axons project vertically towards the outer surface of the cortex to ramify in the molecular layer. This layer merges with the white matter of the cerebral cortex.

Important Notes

- Most of afferent fibres from the specific nuclei of the thalamus make synapses in laminae ***I–IV***.
- Afferent projections from the nonspecific thalamic nuclei and from the ascending reticular system terminate in all laminae of the cortex.
- Laminae II and IV are concerned with sensorial modalities.
- Laminae III–V are meant for somatomotor or visceromotor activities.
- Laminae I and VI are engaged for integration of association of sensorimotor behaviour.

Types of Neocortex

Depending on the local variations in the histological layers, the neocortex can be divided into five types.

Type 1 or agranular cortex It is characterized by:

- Granule cells or stellate cells are absent.
- Pyramidal cells in lamina V (inner pyramidal or ganglionic) are large and called giant cells or Betz cells.

Sites: Agranular cortex is seen in the motor cortex (area 4), Broca's area (area 44, motor speech area) and anterior part of the island of Reil.

Type 2 or frontal cortex Characteristic feature is the presence of triangular granule cells.

Sites: Frontal cortex is seen in anterior two-thirds of the frontal lobe.

Type 3 or parietal type Characteristic features are as follows:

- Depth and density of two granule layers II and III is increased.

- Granule cells are round in shape.
- Pyramidal cells are smaller, slender and more numerous.

Sites are parietal lobe and junctional region of parietal, occipital and temporal lobes.

Type 4 or polar type Characteristically, the cortex is narrow and all layers are reduced in depth, though the cells are more densely packed.

Sites are frontal and occipital poles.

Type 5 or granular cortex It is characterized by excess of granule cells which have largely replaced the pyramidal cells in layers III and V.

Sites are sensory cortex (postcentral gyrus), calcarine region (visual cortex) and *Heschl's* gyrus, i.e. superior temporal gyrus (hearing area 41).

AREAS, CONNECTIONS, FUNCTIONS AND APPLIED ASPECTS OF DIFFERENT LOBES

A. Frontal Lobe

The frontal lobe lies in front of the central sulcus and above the posterior ramus of the lateral sulcus (Fig. 10.4.2). It forms about one-third of the cortical surface. On the basis of function, the frontal lobe is subdivided into two main areas:

- Precentral cortex
- Prefrontal cortex

I. Precentral Cortex

Precentral cortex refers to the posterior part of the frontal lobe that includes the lip of the central sulcus, precentral gyrus and posterior part of superior, middle and inferior frontal gyri. Stimulation of different points in this area causes activity of discrete skeletal muscles. Therefore, the precentral cortex is also called excitomotor area of the cortex. Stimulation of motor area also causes some sensory perception.

Therefore, nowadays, the motor cortex and sensory cortex are together known as *sensorimotor* cortex.

Areas in precentral cortex The precentral cortex includes the following important areas:

- Primary motor area (Brodmann's area 4)
- Premotor area (Brodmann's areas 6, 8, 44 and 45)
- Supplementary motor area

Important Note

Now, it has been suggested that the sensorimotor cortex (areas 4 and 6) is primarily motor and secondarily sensory in function; hence, these areas have been designated as M-1.

1. Primary motor area (area 4) It lies in the precentral gyrus extending into the paracentral lobule on the medial surface. The area also includes the anterior wall of the central sulcus, and other gyri of the frontal lobe (Fig. 10.4.5).

Structural characteristics: This area contains all the six layers of the cortex (see page 939). Special features of this area are the presence of giant pyramidal cells called Betz cells in the ganglionic layer and a thin granular layer (that is why also called agranular cortex).

Topographic representation: Different parts of the contralateral half of the body are represented separately in more or less inverted order. Those parts of the body that carry out the most skilled movements, e.g. the fingers and thumb, have the largest areas of cortical representation. The areas for tongue, jaw and facial movements lie in the inferior part of the motor cortex; those for the arm, trunk and leg are arranged in sequence in the motor area, which extends to the vertex, and on to the medial surface of the cerebral hemisphere. The parts in the paracentral lobule are for the foot and perineum. Thus, the body is represented upside down (however, the face is not represented in an inverted manner) (Fig. 10.4.6A).

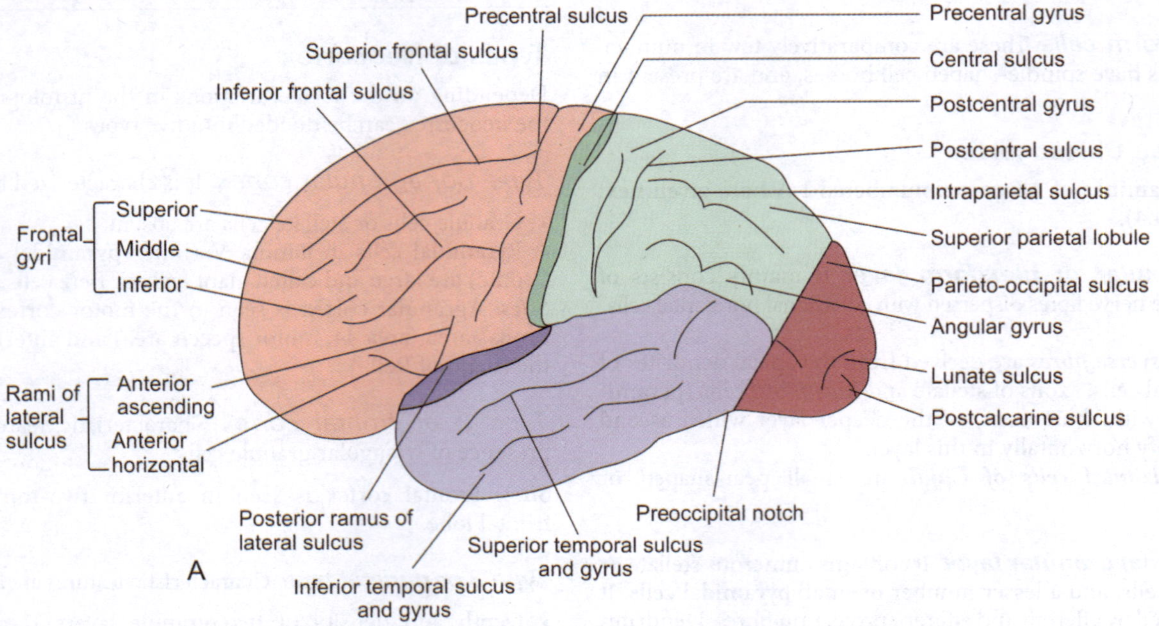

Fig. 10.4.5 Left cerebral hemisphere showing lobes, sulci and gyri: **A**, superolateral surface;

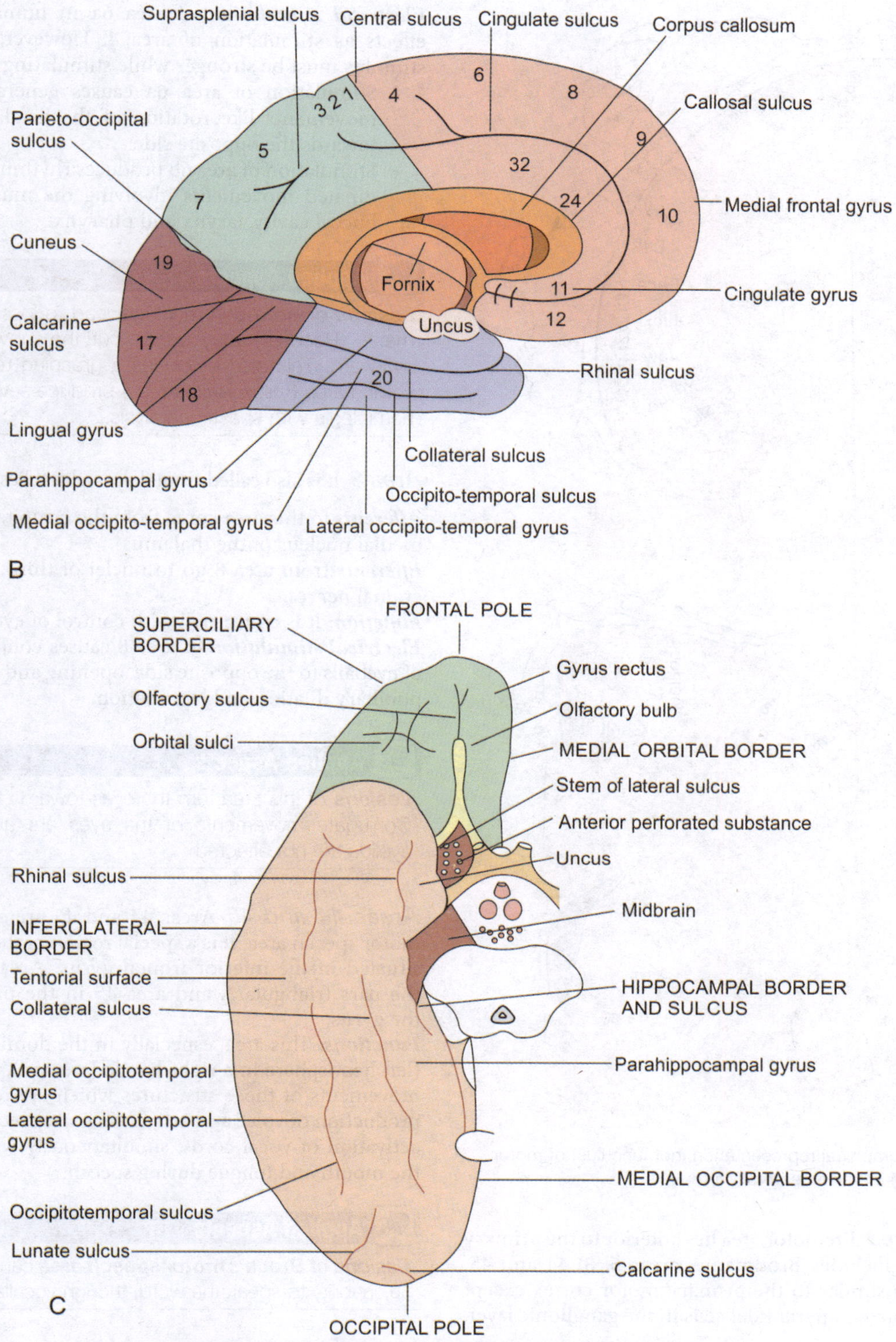

Fig. 10.4.5, cont'd **B**, medial surface; and **C**, inferior surface.

Electrical stimulation of this area reveals:

- Above-described motor homunculus (topographical representation) is revealed.
- Motor cortex is organized in terms of movements rather than individual muscles (i.e. stimulation reveals discrete isolated movements on the opposite side of the body).
- Stimulation of the points representing upper parts of the face, pharynx and vocal cords produces bilateral responses.

Functions: From the above, it is clear that this area is the centre for volition, i.e. it is concerned with initiation of voluntary movements of the contralateral half of the body and initiation of speech.

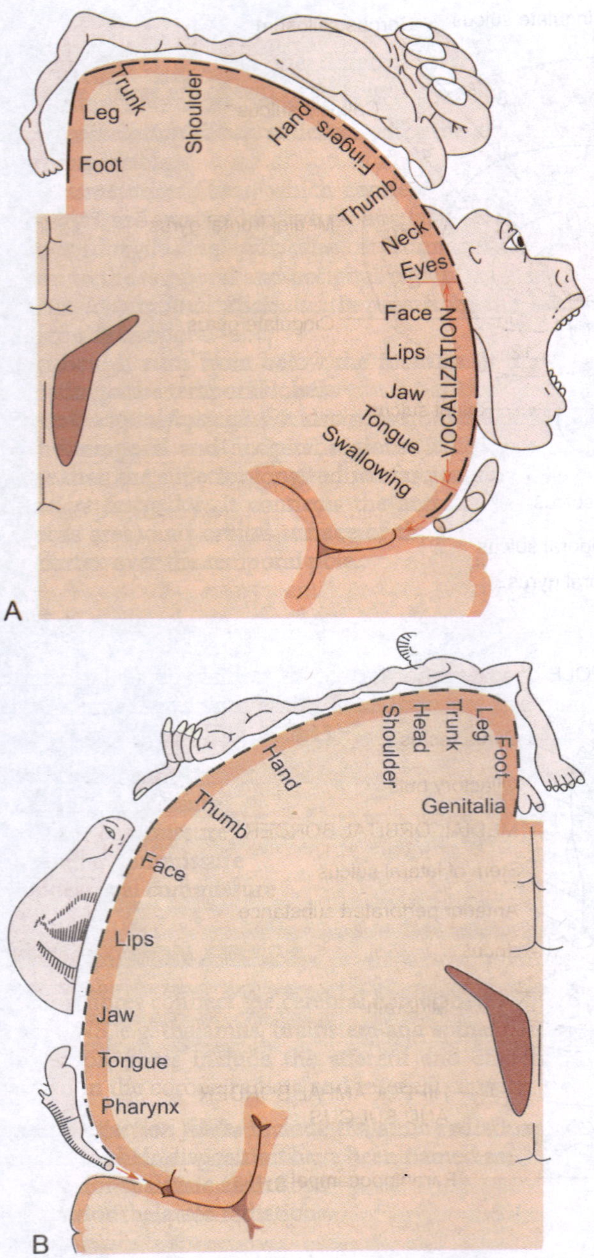

Fig. 10.4.6 Topographical representation (homunculus) of motor (**A**) and sensory (**B**) areas in cerebral cortex.

2. Premotor area Premotor area lies anterior to the primary motor area and includes Brodmann's areas 6, 8, 44 and 45. Structurally, it is similar to the primary motor cortex except for the absence of giant pyramidal cells in the ganglionic layer.

Area 6 It abuts on the primary motor cortex area both above and behind, and thereby includes the posterior parts of the superior, middle and inferior frontal gyri. This area is divided into two parts – upper 6a and lower 6b. Cells from this area contribute fibres to pyramidal tracts.

Topographical organization of this area is roughly the same as that of the primary motor cortex.

Functions: Area 6 coordinates the voluntary action of area 4 and extrapyramidal system and is, therefore, involved in the integration of voluntary movements. Thus, the skilled movements are accurate and smooth.

Electrical stimulation of area 6a in humans causes same effects as stimulation of area 4. However, the strength of stimulus must be stronger while stimulating area 6.

- Stimulation of area 6a causes generalized pattern of movements like rotation of the head, eyes and trunk towards the opposite side.
- Stimulation of area 6b produces rhythmic, complex coordinated movements involving the muscles of the face, buccal cavity, larynx and pharynx.

Applied Aspects

Lesions of area 6 in monkeys lead to loss of skilled movements. Recovery may occur, but the movements become awkward. This also produces a grasping reflex. Lesions involving area 6 along with area 4 produce severe symptoms of hemiplegia with spastic paralysis.

Area 8 It is also called frontal eye field. It lies anterior to area 6.

Afferents to this area come from the occipital lobe and dorsomedial nucleus of the thalamus.

Efferents from area 8 go to nuclei of third, fourth and sixth cranial nerves.

Function: It is concerned with control of eye movements.

Electrical stimulation of area 8 causes conjugate movements of eyeballs to the opposite side, opening and closure of eyelids, pupillary dilation and lacrimation.

Applied Aspects

Lesions of this area turn the eyes towards the affected side. Conjugate movements of the eyes are absent. Pupil and eyelids are not affected.

Areas 44 and 45 Areas 44 and 45 are also called Broca's motor speech area. It is a special region of the premotor cortex situated in the inferior frontal gyrus. Area 44 is situated in the pars triangularis and area 45 in the pars opercularis of the gyrus.

Functions: This area, especially in the dominated hemisphere (left hemisphere in a right-handed person), is concerned with movements of those structures which are responsible for the production of voice and articulation of speech, that is, it causes activation of vocal cords, simultaneously with movements of the mouth and tongue during speech.

Applied Aspects

Lesions of Broca's motor speech area cause motor aphasia, i.e. inability to speak the word, though vocalization is possible.

3. Supplementary motor area Supplementary motor area is located in the medial surface of the frontal lobe rostral to the primary motor area (Fig. 10.4.5).

Topographical organization: In this area, components of the upper body are located dorsal to those of the lower body.

Functions: This area in association with the premotor area provides attitudinal movements, fixation movement of different segments of the body and positional movements of the head and eyes.

Connections of precentral cortex includes Afferents and efferents:

Afferents to the precentral cortex come from the following sources:

1. ***Fibres from adjacent regions*** include those from:
   - Somatic sensory area of the parietal cortex
   - Adjacent areas of the frontal cortex anterior to the motor cortex
   - Subcortical fibres from auditory and visual cortices
2. ***From opposite hemisphere:*** Subcortical fibres passing through the corpus callosum connect corresponding areas of cortices in the two sides of the brain.
3. ***Fibres from thalamus*** include:
   - Tracts from ventrolateral and ventroanterior nuclei of the thalamus which in turn receive from the cerebellum and basal ganglia. They cause coordination between functions of the motor cortex, basal ganglia and cerebellum.
   - Fibres from intralaminar nuclei of the thalamus cause general level of excitability of the motor cortex.

Efferents from precentral cortex Efferents from the precentral cortex include:

1. Corticospinal tract (pyramidal tract) is the most important tract through which the motor cortex controls the activity of the anterior horn cells in the spinal cord. About 30% of fibres arise from the primary motor area, 30% from the premotor and supplementary motor areas and 40% from the somatic sensory area of the parietal lobe.

2. Collaterals from pyramidal tracts and large number of fibres from the motor cortex go to deeper regions of the cerebrum and brainstem as follows:

Adjacent areas of cortex: Axons of Betz cells send collaterals to adjacent areas of the cortex. These collaterals inhibit adjacent areas (lateral inhibition) and sharpen the boundaries of excitatory signals.
Basal ganglia: A large number of fibres go to caudate nucleus and putamen from where an additional pathway goes to the brainstem.
Red nucleus: Some fibres go to red nuclei and then to the spinal cord through rubrospinal tracts.
Reticular substance: Some fibres go to the reticular substance of the brainstem, from where fibres pass to the spinal cord through the reticulospinal tract.
Vestibular nuclei: Some fibres go to vestibular nuclei, from where through the vestibulospinal tract they reach the spinal cord.
Pontine nuclei: A large number of fibres synapse in pontine nuclei and pass to the cerebellum (pontocerebellar fibres).
Inferior olivary nuclei: Collaterals also go to inferior olivary nuclei and then to the cerebellum through the olivocerebellar tract.

II. Prefrontal Cortex

Location: Prefrontal cortex, also called prefrontal lobe or orbitofrontal cortex, is the anterior part of the frontal lobe lying anterior to areas 8 and 44 (Fig. 10.4.5).

Major areas: Prefrontal cortex has different Brodmann's areas such as 9–14, 23, 24, 29, 32 and 44–47 located as:

Areas 9–12 lie in the superior frontal gyrus and also extend onto the adjacent medial surface of the hemisphere.
Area 13 is located in the orbital part of the inferior surface of the frontal lobe.
Area 24 is situated in the pericallosal part of the cingulate gyrus on the medial surface.
Area 32 lies in the cingulate gyrus.
Areas 44–47 lie in the inferior frontal gyrus.

Connections of the prefrontal cortex shown in Fig. 10.4.7 are as follows:

Afferents to the prefrontal cortex come from:

i. ***Dorsomedial nucleus of the thalamus*** projects onto areas 9–12 on the lateral and adjacent medial surface and areas 44–47 in the inferior frontal gyrus. Since the dorsomedial nucleus of the thalamus in turn receives afferents from the posterior hypothalamus, the impulses which reach the prefrontal lobe via the medial nucleus represent a resultant of hypothalamic and thalamic activity.
ii. ***Anterior nuclei of the thalamus*** project onto the cingulate gyrus (areas 23, 24, 29 and 32). Since the anterior nucleus of the thalamus receives afferents from the mammillary bodies of the hypothalamus, they in turn receive the afferents from the hippocampus via the fornix. The hippocampus is thus ultimately projected to the inhibitory area 24.

The prefrontal lobe thus forms a closed circuit connection with the thalamus called *Papez* circuit (Fig. 10.10.4; see

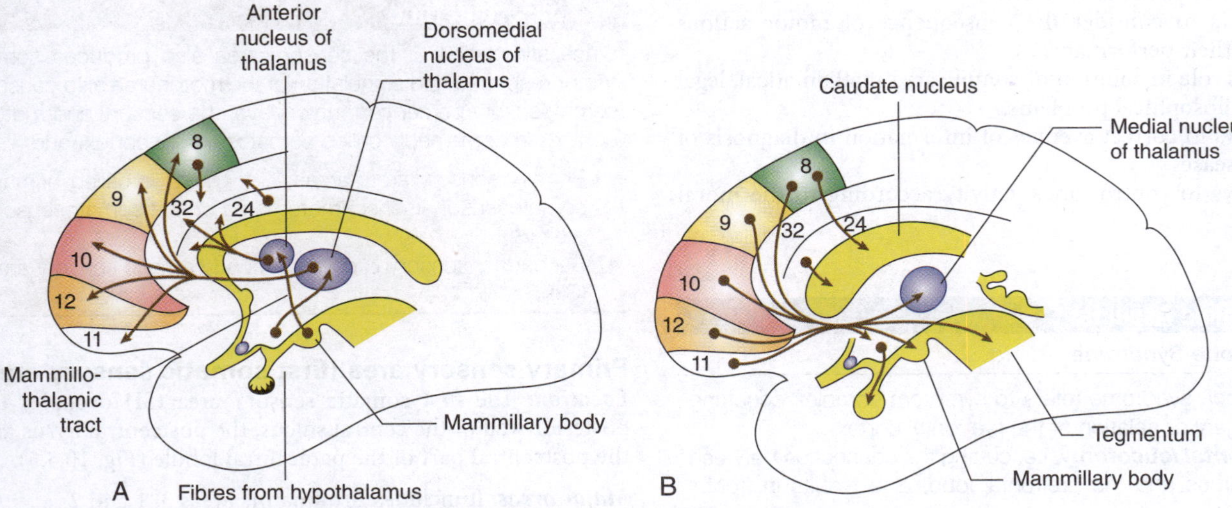

Fig. 10.4.7 Connections of prefrontal lobe: **A**, afferents; and **B**, efferents.

page 1049). This circuit is responsible for resting EEG and plays an important role in the genesis of emotions.

Efferents from the prefrontal cortex go to:

i. ***Thalamus:*** Fibres from areas 9 and 10 go to ventral and medial thalamic nuclei.
ii. ***Tegmental reticular formation:*** Fibres from areas 9 and 10 also go to reticular formation in the tegmentum.
iii. ***Pontine nuclei:*** Fibres from area 10 pass to the pontine nuclei as frontopontine tract and thence to the cerebellum.
iv. ***Caudate nucleus:*** The inhibitory areas 8 and 2, 4 and 5 discharge to the caudate nucleus.
v. ***Mammillary bodies:*** Fibres from area 13, the hippocampus, uncus and amygdala project via the fornix to the mammillary bodies of the hypothalamus.

Functions of prefrontal cortex include:

1. Centre for planned actions Prefrontal association areas in close association with the motor cortex plan complex patterns and sequence of motor movements.

2. Centre for higher functions This forms the centre for higher functions like emotions, learning, memory and social behaviour. It is responsible for various autonomic changes during emotional conditions because of its connections to the hypothalamus and brainstem.

3. Seat of intelligence Short-term memories are registered in the prefrontal cortex. It can keep track of many bits of information and also has ability to recall this information bit by bit for subsequent thoughts. It is therefore called the seat of intelligence or an organ of mind.

4. Control of intellectual activities The prefrontal cortex has the following intellectual abilities:

- It allows the person to prognosticate.
- It allows the person to plan the future.
- It allows the person to concentrate on the central theme of thought. It helps in depth and abstractness of thought and thereby in elaboration of thought.
- It allows to delay action in response to incoming sensory signals so that sensory information can be weighed until the best response is obtained.
- It allows to consider the consequence of motor actions before their performance.
- It plays role in solution of complicated mathematical, legal and philosophical problems.
- It allows to correct avenues of information in diagnosis of rare diseases.
- It allows to control one's activity according to the moral laws.

Applied Aspects

Frontal Lobe Syndrome

Frontal lobe syndrome refers to symptom complex occurring due to injury or ablation of the prefrontal cortex.

Prefrontal leucotomy, i.e. cutting the connection between the thalamus and the prefrontal lobe, also results in frontal lobe syndrome. Bilateral prefrontal lobectomy (extirpation) also results in a similar condition. In the past, these operations were performed in patients with severe mental illness. However, nowadays, due to availability of tranquilizers and other drugs (which can control mental illness), these operations are not conducted because of the associated complications.

Characteristic features of frontal lobe syndrome are as follows:

- *Flight of ideas* results in difficulty in planning.
- *Emotional instability:* There occurs lack of restraint leading to hostility, aggressiveness and restlessness.
- *Euphoria:* There occurs a false sense of well-being and failure to realize or indifference to seriousness of other's feelings or emotions.
- *Impairment of memory* occurs for recent memory only. The memory of remote events is not lost.
- *Loss of moral and social sense* is common and there is loss of love for family.
- *Lack of attention and power of concentration* associated with restlessness is a common feature.
- *Lack of initiative following marked depression* of intellectual activity leads to reduced mental drive.
- *Functional abnormalities* may occur in the form of:
  - Hyperphagia, i.e. increased appetite
  - Loss of control over urinary or rectal sphincters
  - Disturbances in orientation
  - Slight tremor

B. Parietal Lobe

Parietal lobe (Fig. 10.4.1) lies between the central sulcus and the parieto-occipital sulcus, and upper part of the first imaginary line. Below, it is separated from the temporal lobe by the posterior ramus of the lateral sulcus and in continuation of it the second imaginary line.

Areas of Parietal Lobe

Functionally, the parietal lobe can be divided into three parts:

- Primary sensory area (which corresponds to Brodmann's areas 3, 1 and 2)
- Secondary sensory area
- Sensory association areas (Brodmann's areas 5 and 7)

Important Note

Since stimulation of the sensory area also produces some motor response and stimulation of the motor area also causes some sensory perception, nowadays, the sensory and motor cortex are combinedly called somatosensory cortex, and:

- Primary sensory area (areas 3, 1 and 2) is called primary somatosensory (sensorimotor) area or first somatosensory area (SI).
- Secondary sensory is called second somatic sensory area (SII).

Primary sensory area (first somatic sensory area)

Location: The first somatic sensory area (SI) occupies the posterior wall of the central sulcus, the postcentral gyrus and the postcentral part of the paracentral lobule (Fig. 10.4.5).

Major areas: It includes Brodmann's areas 3, 1 and 2.

Structurally, the primary sensory cortex is granular cortex which is densely packed with stellate cells, with a few small and medium-sized pyramidal cells.

Topographical organization: The primary sensory cortex receives sensory inputs from the opposite half of the body. The representation of the body within this area is similar to that already noted in the primary motor cortex (page 942, Fig. 10.4.6B).

The sensations derived from the skin are appreciated in the anterior part of the area and proprioceptive sensations in the posterior part of the area.

Electrical stimulation of the primary sensory area (SI) produces vague sensations like numbness and tingling.

Applied Aspects

Lesions: If lesions occur only in the sensory cortex without involvement of the thalamus, the sensations are perceived but the discriminative functions are lost. If the thalamus is also affected by the lesion, there occurs loss of sensations in the opposite side of the body.

Secondary sensory area also called second somatic sensory area (SII).

Location: Secondary sensory area is situated in the postcentral gyrus below the area of the face of the first somatic sensory area. Most of it is buried in the superior wall of the Sylvian fissure (lateral cerebral sulcus).

Topographical representation: The secondary sensory area (SII) receives sensory impulses from the primary sensory area (SI) as well as from the thalamus directly. Like SI, the SII area also manifests a dermatomal (point-to-point) sequence of representation (although there is more overlap). Thus, the body is represented twice in the somatic sensory cortex, i.e. in area SI as well as in area SII.

- Neurons in the anterior part of area SII respond to touch, whereas neurons in the posterior part can be excited by touch, auditory, visual and nociceptive stimuli.

Applied Aspects

Lesions of SII produce deficits in discrimination power, whereas sensory processing in SI is not affected.

Sensory association areas The sensory association areas include areas 5 and 7. Area 40 is a higher association area.

Area 5: It lies posterior to area SI in the parietal lobe and contains neurons which react to passive or active rotation of a joint or joints. Few neurons respond to tactile stimuli like the other areas in SI and SII; area 5 also displays a columnar organization (point-to-point representation).

Area 7: It is located in the superior parietal lobule deep into the intraparietal sulcus extending close up to the occipital lobe. This area is concerned with the more elaborate process of discrimination between the stimuli.

Area 40: This is a higher association area, located in the supramarginal gyrus, and is concerned with stereognosis, i.e. recognition of common objects placed in the hand without looking at them. A lesion affecting area 40 produces tactile agnosia (astereognosis and tactile aphasia).

Connections of Parietal Lobe

Afferent connections of somatosensory area Afferent connections of the somatosensory area include:

First somatic sensory area (SI) receives afferent projections from posteromedial (VPM) and posterolateral (VPL) parts of the ventral posterior nucleus of the thalamus, which convey exteroceptive and proprioceptive impulses from the contralateral side but from both sides of the face.

Area 3 neurons respond to light touch and receive a dense input from the thalamus.

Area 1 and 2 neurons respond to deep stimuli such as pressure and joint movements and receive few thalamic fibres.

- None of the neurons of the primary sensory cortex are influenced by nociceptive (painful) stimuli.
- Sensory area in the paracentral lobule receives the sense of distension from the bladder and rectum.
- The lower part of the postcentral gyrus acts as a taste receptive centre.

Second somatic sensory area (SII) receives afferent projection from area SI as well as directly from the thalamus.

Sensory association area receives impulses from areas SI and SII.

Efferents from somatosensory area

- Pyramidal cells of the sensory area contribute fibres to corticospinal, corticobulbar and corticonuclear tracts. These fibres presumably modulate the sensory input at the root entry zone of the posterior grey column of the spinal cord, and nuclei gracilis and cuneatus of the lower medulla.
- All somatosensory areas (particularly SI) send fibres to the caudate nucleus and putamen.
- Area SI also sends efferent fibres:
  - Back to its own thalamic projection nuclei
  - To the tectum, pons and cerebellum

Association fibres from the sensory cortex

- Through association fibres, the sensory cortex is connected with other cortical areas.
- Association fibres interlinking the areas SI, SII, 5 and 4 are involved in somatic sensations (Fig. 10.4.8).

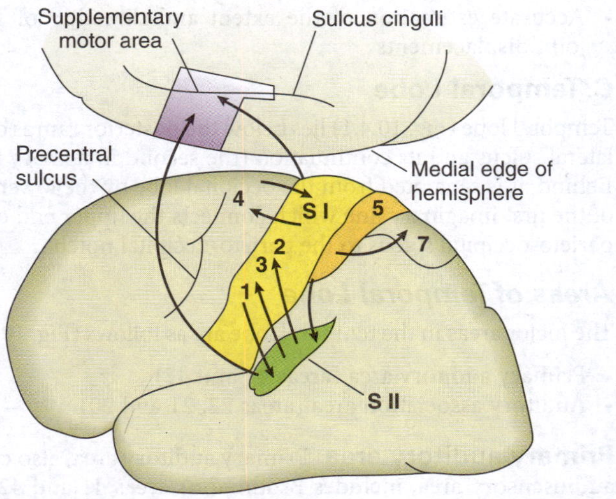

Fig. 10.4.8 Connections of parietal lobe areas involved in somatic sensations.

Commissural fibres from the sensory cortex

- Commissural fibres are mostly axons of pyramidal cells of layer III and connect the corresponding somatosensory areas with those of the opposite hemisphere.
- Area SI projects to the contralateral areas SI and SII.
- Area SII projects only to area SII of the opposite hemisphere.

Functions of Parietal Lobe

First somatic sensory area (SI) (areas 3, 1 and 2) localizes, analyses and discriminates different cutaneous and proprioceptive senses:

Area 3 receives cutaneous sensations of touch, pressure, position and vibratory senses (pain and temperature have a slight representation in the primary sensory area).
Area 1 receives projections from cutaneous and joint senses.
Area 2 is primarily concerned with deep senses from muscles and joints.

Second somatic sensory area (SII) receives sensory impulses from SI and from the thalamus directly. Though the exact role of this area is not clear, it is concerned with the perception of sensation. Thus, the sensory parts of the body have two representations in areas SI and SII.

Sensory association areas (areas 5 and 7) are associated with the more elaborate process of discrimination between the stimuli, thus helping in differentiating the relative intensity of different stimuli. Therefore, warm objects are distinguished from warmer, cold from colder, rough from rougher, etc.

Higher association area (area 40) helps in recognition of common familiar objects placed in the hand without looking at them (stereognosis).

Inferior part of the postcentral gyrus contains the centre for taste and general sensations from the tongue. Lesion of this part causes loss of taste and general sensations of the opposite half of the tongue.

Angular gyrus helps in recognition of spatial relationship by:

- Tactile localization, i.e. the precise point stimulated is accurately localized
- Tactile (two-point) discrimination, i.e. two points of a compass placed close together are recognized as two and not as one
- Accurate estimation of the extent and direction of small joint displacements

C. Temporal Lobe

Temporal lobe (Fig. 10.4.1) lies below the posterior ramus of the lateral sulcus and its continuation (the second imaginary line). Behind, it is separated from the occipital lobe by the lower part of the first imaginary line which connects the upper end of the parieto-occipital sulcus to the parieto-occipital notch.

Areas of Temporal Lobe

The major areas in the temporal lobe are as follows (Fig. 10.4.5):

- Primary auditory area (areas 41 and 42)
- Auditory association area (areas 22, 21 and 20)

Primary auditory area Primary auditory area, also called audiosensory area, includes Brodmann's areas 41 and 42 and forms the centre for hearing. It is situated in the middle of the superior temporal gyrus on the upper margin and on its deep or insular aspect (Heschl's or transverse temporal gyrus). Heschl's gyrus can be seen only when the lips of the lateral sulcus are widely separated (Fig. 10.4.2).

Connections of this area are as follows:

Afferents are received from:
- Medial geniculate body via auditory radiations
- Pulvinar of the thalamus

Efferents are sent to:
- Medial geniculate body
- Superior colliculus
- Pulvinar

Functions: This area perceives the nerve impulses as sound, i.e. auditory information such as loudness, pitch, source and direction of sound.

Auditory association area Auditory association area corresponds to Brodmann's areas 22, 21 and 20.

Area 22 Area 22, also called Wernicke's area, is a sensory speech centre situated in the posterior part of the superior temporal gyrus behind the areas 41 and 42 (Fig. 10.4.2), in the categorical hemisphere, i.e. dominant hemisphere.
Functions: It is concerned with:

- Interpretation of the meaning of what is heard
- Comprehension of spoken language and the formation of ideas that are to be articulated in speech (for detail, see page 1079)

Areas 21 and 20 Areas 21 and 20 are located in the middle and inferior temporal gyrus, respectively.
Functions: These areas receive impulses from the primary area and are concerned with interpretation and integration of auditory impulses.

> **Applied Aspects**
>
> **Unilateral Removal of Temporal Lobe**
>
> Unilateral removal of the temporal lobe causes no deafness. This is because each ear is bilaterally represented in the auditory pathway from the medulla upwards and projects about equally to the two cerebral hemispheres. Thus, the removal of one auditory cortex has only a slight effect on auditory acuity (sharpness of hearing).
>
> **Temporal Lobe Syndrome**
>
> Temporal lobe syndrome, also known as *Kluver–Bucy syndrome*, is produced in animals, particularly monkeys, after removal of the bilateral temporal lobe along with the amygdala and uncus.
>
> ***Characteristic features*** of this syndrome are as follows:
>
> **Aphasia:** Disturbances in speech occur.
> **Visual agnosia:** There occurs inability to recognize the objects in spite of good vision.
> **Auditory disturbances** occur in the form of frequent attacks of tinnitus and auditory hallucinations with sounds like buzzing, ringing or humming.
> **Hyperphagia and omniphagia:** The animal starts eating more and eating that diet which it was not eating previously.
> **Hypersexuality** is noted in male animals due to damage to amygdaloid nuclei and piriform cortex.

Increased oral activity: The animal starts repeatedly putting up in its mouth all the moveable objects present in the surrounding.

Hypermetamorphosis: The animal starts responding to every stimulus, whether it is experienced before or not.

Dreaming states: The animals are not aware of their own activities and have the feeling of unreality.

Clinical significance: In humans with bilateral temporal lobe diseases or lesions, various above-mentioned symptoms are seen.

Mesial Temporal Lobe

This condition occurs when the most sensitive limbic system is affected. Damage to this area causes mesial temporal lobe epilepsy (MTLE). The main features are as follows:

- Focal seizures occur.
- Olfactory or gustatory hallucinations occur.
- Unfamiliar environment seems familiar and familiar environment seems unfamiliar

D. Occipital Lobe

Occipital lobe lies behind the parieto-occipital sulcus and its continuation down an imaginary line (Fig. 10.4.1). It is concerned with vision.

Areas of Occipital Lobe

Occipital lobe is mostly formed of sensory and association areas and has only slight motor function. It contains the visual cortex having three areas (Figs 10.4.2 and 10.4.5):

- Primary visual cortex (area 17)
- Visual association area (area 18)
- Visual association area or occipital eye field (area 19)

Primary visual cortex is also called striate area (area 17). It lies on the medial surface of the occipital lobe in and near the calcarine sulcus occupying parts of the lingual gyrus and cuneus. It also extends to the superolateral surface of the occipital lobe limited in front by the lunate sulcus.

It receives the fibres of the optic radiations which bring impulses from parts of both retinae, and these parts are represented within the area in a specific orderly manner. It constitutes the centre of vision.

Peristriate area, also called visual association area (area 18), lies in the walls of the lunate sulcus.

Parastriate area (area 19) is also a visual association area. It lies in the cortex in front of the lunate sulcus.

Modified nomenclature of visual areas: Recently, a modified nomenclature recognizing five visual areas has been described:

V1: First visual area in area 17

V2: Second visual area occupying the greater part of area 18, but not the whole of it

V3: Third visual area occupying a narrow strip over the anterior part of area 18

V4: Fourth visual area within area 19

V5: Fifth visual area at the posterior end of the superior temporal gyrus

Connections

Afferents to the visual cortex come from the lateral geniculate body in the form of optic radiations. The right visual cortex receives impulses arising from the temporal half of the right retina and nasal half of the left retina, and the left visual cortex receives those arising from the temporal half of the left retina and nasal half of the right retina.

Thus, there is a point-to-point projection of the retina in the visual cortex in such a way that the right visual cortex is concerned with perception of objects situated to the left of the vertical median line in the visual fields and left visual cortex with the objects situated to the right half.

Efferents from visual cortex go to:

Various parts of the cerebral cortex in both hemispheres; in particular, they reach the frontal eye field which is concerned with eye movements.

Superior colliculus, the pretectal region and the nuclei of cranial nerves supplying muscles that move the eyeballs also receive efferents from the visual cortex.

Corticogeniculate projection has also been evidenced physiologically.

Thalamus (pulvinar) also receives efferents from the visual cortex.

Functions

Primary visual area (area 17) is concerned with perception of visual impulses.

Visual association areas (areas 18 and 19) are concerned with interpretation of visual impulses. These are involved in the recognition and identification of objects in the light of past experience.

Occipital eye field area (area 19) is concerned with the movements of the eyeball. Therefore, like other sensory areas, the visual area should also be regarded as partly motor in function. For details, see page 1129.

WHITE MATTER OF CEREBRUM

Passing through, between and around the subcortical masses of grey matter of the cerebrum are tracts of white fibres. The white fibres of the cerebrum are of three types (Fig. 10.4.9):

- Association fibres
- Commissural fibres
- Projection fibres

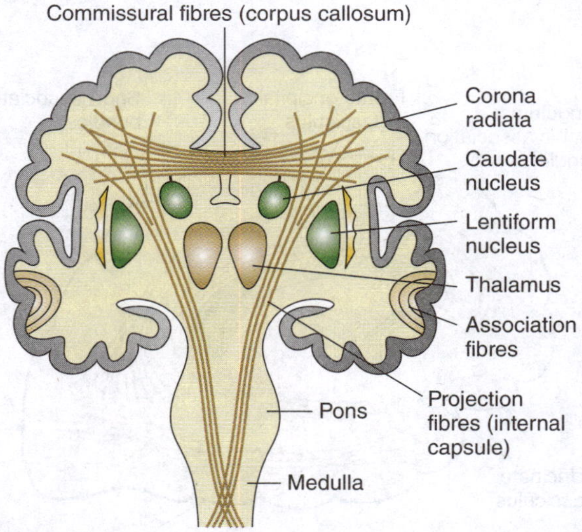

Fig. 10.4.9 Frontal view of coronal section of brain showing the position of the association, commissural and projection fibres.

I. ASSOCIATION FIBRES

Association fibres connect the different gyri of the same hemisphere. These are of two types (Fig. 10.4.10):

1. ***Short association fibres***, which connect the adjacent gyri, are innumerable.
2. ***Long association fibres***, which connect the widely separated gyri, are arranged in five groups:
   Superior longitudinal fasciculus: It connects the frontal region to the temporal and occipital region.
   Inferior longitudinal fasciculus: It runs from the occipital pole to the temporal lobe.
   Cingulum: It runs from below the rostrum of the corpus callosum to the temporal lobe.
   Fronto-occipital fasciculus: It also runs from the frontal pole to the temporal and occipital regions. It lies in a deeper plane than the superior longitudinal fasciculus.
   Uncinate fasciculus: It connects the anterior speech area (Broca's area) and orbital surface of the frontal lobe with the cortex over the temporal pole.

II. COMMISSURAL FIBRES

Commissural fibres connect the corresponding parts of two cerebral hemispheres with each other. There are five bundles of commissural fibres (Fig. 10.4.11):

- Corpus callosum
- Anterior commissure
- Posterior commissure
- Habenular commissure
- Hippocampal commissure

III. PROJECTION FIBRES

Projection fibres connect the cerebral hemispheres with other parts of CNS, e.g. thalamus, brainstem and spinal cord.

Projection fibres include the afferent and efferent tracts contained in the corona radiata and internal capsule.

Afferent projection fibres include thalamic radiations, which according to their disposition have been named as:

- Anterior thalamic radiations
- Superior thalamic radiations

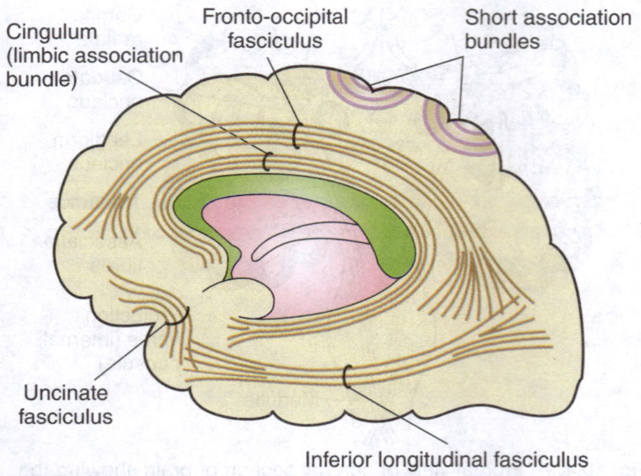

Fig. 10.4.10 Short and long association fibres.

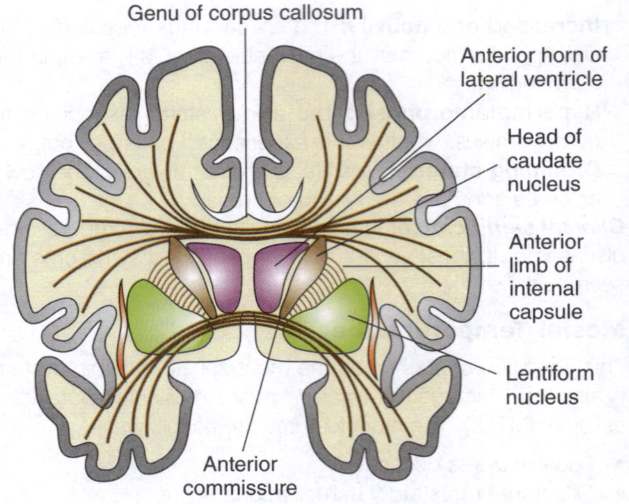

Fig. 10.4.11 Genu of corpus callosum and anterior commissure.

- Posterior thalamic radiation (including optic radiations)
- Inferior thalamic radiation (including auditory radiations)

Efferent or motor projection fibres include:

- Corticobulbar and corticospinal tracts (pyramidal system)
- Corticopontine fibres
- Corticorubral fibres
- Corticothalamic fibres

Corona Radiata

Corona radiata (fountain of fibres) refers to that part of projection fibres that radiates from the upper end of the internal capsule to the cerebral cortex (Fig. 10.4.9). It contains both the ascending and descending fibres.

Internal Capsule

Internal capsule is a thick curved band of projection fibres (ascending and descending) that occupy the space between the thalamus and the caudate nucleus medially, and the lentiform nucleus laterally. Superiorly, it fans out as corona radiata and inferiorly, the fibres descend into the crus cerebri.

Subdivisions of Internal Capsule (Fig. 10.4.12)

1. Anterior limb It is short and lies between the head of the caudate nucleus and the lentiform nucleus. It consists of:

Anterior thalamic radiations, containing reciprocal connections between the dorsomedial and anterior nuclei of the thalamus and prefrontal cortex and gyrus cinguli

Corticopontine (frontopontine) fibres from the frontal cortex to nuclei pontis

2. Genu It is the region of the band in the capsule situated medial to the apex of the lentiform nucleus. It connects the anterior and posterior limbs. It contains the following fibres:

Anterior part of superior thalamic radiations

Corticonuclear (corticobulbar) fibres which extend from the frontal eye field and motor area of the cortex to the motor nuclei of the cranial nerves of the opposite side

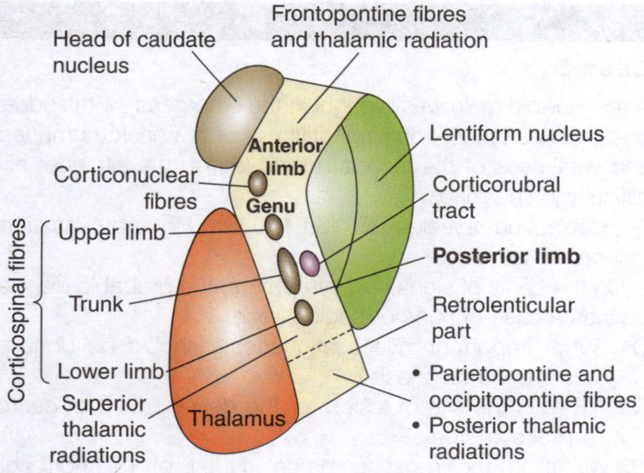

Fig. 10.4.12 Parts of internal capsule; disposition of motor fibres and thalamic radiations passing through it.

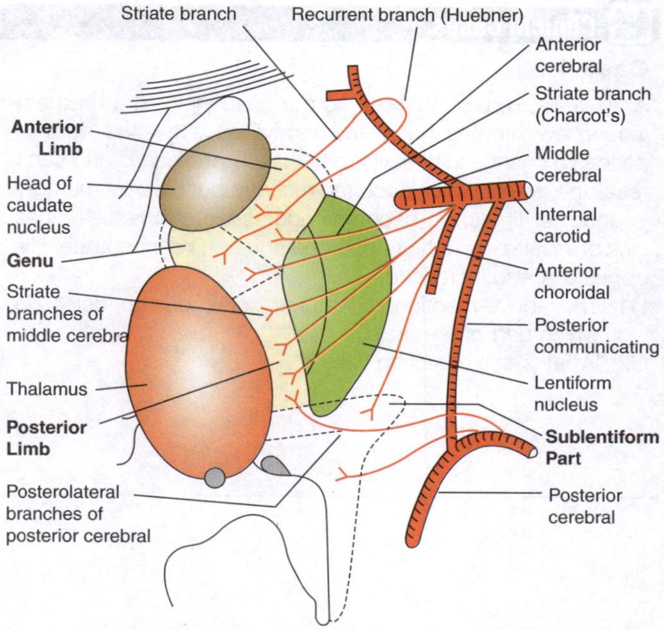

Fig. 10.4.13 Arterial supply of internal capsule (schematic).

3. Posterior limb

It is bounded by the thalamus medially and the lentiform nucleus laterally. It is longer than the anterior limb and contains:

Corticospinal tract: The anterior two-thirds of the posterior limb contains most of these fibres with the upper limb in the front, the trunk in the middle and the lower limb behind, i.e. the body is represented in the internal capsule in a fore-and-after manner with the head in front in the genu and the rest in the posterior limb. It contains:

- *Corticopontine (parietopontine) fibres*
- *Superior thalamic radiations* which comprise the fibres having reciprocal connections between the ventral nuclei of the thalamus and the parietal lobe

Corticorubral tract arises from the motor and premotor areas of the frontal cortex and end in the red nucleus.

4. Retrolenticular or caudal part

It occupies the region behind the lentiform nucleus and consists of:

Posterior thalamic radiations having fibres of reciprocal connections between the lateral geniculate body and the occipital lobe

Optic radiations (geniculocalcarine tract) extending from the lateral geniculate body to the visual cortex

Corticopontine (parietopontine, occipitopontine and temporopontine) fibres

5. Sublentiform part

It occupies the region beneath the posterior part of the lentiform nucleus and consists of:

Auditory radiations which originate in the medial geniculate body and terminate in the Heschl's convolutions on the superior surface of the superior temporal gyrus (auditory area)

Inferior thalamic radiations having fibres of reciprocal connections between the medial geniculate body and the temporal lobe

Corticopontine (parietotemporopontine) fibres

Blood Supply of Internal Capsule

The internal capsule is supplied by the branches of middle cerebral, anterior cerebral and posterior cerebral arteries (Fig. 10.4.13).

Applied Aspects

Internal capsule fibres are densely crowded in a narrow area. Pyramidal fibres being compressed in this little space are particularly vulnerable to effects of even a pinpoint vascular lesion.

- Damage to the internal capsule from infarction and haemorrhage is a common form or stroke, resulting in loss or decrease in sensations and movements of the opposite half of the body (hemianaesthesia and hemiplegia).
- The most common cause of hemiplegia is the thrombosis or rupture of one of the striate branches of the middle cerebral artery which passes through the anterior perforated substance to supply the internal capsule. One of the lateral striate arteries, which is the largest of the perforating branches, is said to be particularly prone to such pathological conditions and is commonly called the artery of the cerebral haemorrhage (Charcot's artery) (Fig. 10.4.12). Usually all tracts are involved causing complete contralateral hemiplegia with associated sensory loss.
- Thrombosis of the anterior choroidal artery (Fig. 10.4.13) involves the optic radiations producing contralateral hemianopia and hyperacusis.
- Thrombosis of the recurrent branch of the anterior cerebral artery (Huebner artery) (Fig. 10.4.13) results in contralateral paralysis of the face and upper limbs on account of the involvement of corticonuclear fibres and adjacent pyramidal fibres for the superior extremity.

Self-Assessment

1. Discuss the topographical representation of the body in the motor and sensory areas of the cerebral cortex.
2. Discuss the significance of prefrontal cortex.
3. Describe the following:
   - Characteristic features of frontal lobe syndrome
   - Characteristic features of temporal lobe syndrome
4. Write notes on the following:
   - Applied aspects of internal capsule
   - Histology of neocortex

Clinical Cases

Case 1

A 20-year-old male suffered from a head injury in a road accident few months back and recovered. Now the parents noticed a change in behaviour; he has flight of ideas and can't recall the events which occurred recently, but his past memory is good; at times, he becomes aggressive and restless, has lack of initiative, is not well oriented and can't concentrate. His appetite is also increased.

Q1. The above-mentioned features occur due to defect in which part of the brain?

Q2. What is this condition called?

Case 2

A 46-year-old male was brought in the emergency with sudden onset of headache; vomiting; stiffness of the neck; numbness and weakness of the face, arm and leg on the left side; and difficulty in speaking.

Examination revealed BP 180/120 mm Hg and sensations lost on the left side.

On the basis of signs and symptoms, the probable diagnosis was a case of haemorrhagic stroke.

Q1. What important investigations/tests should be done to confirm the diagnosis?

Q2. What is the site of lesion for the development of neurological symptoms?

Q3. What is the most common cause of haemorrhagic stroke?

Autonomic Nervous System

10.5

CHAPTER OUTLINE

ANATOMICAL CONSIDERATIONS

AUTONOMIC NERVOUS SYSTEM: DIVISIONS

The autonomic nervous system (ANS) collects the information about the changes that take place in the internal environment (i.e. internal viscera), interprets these changes, guides the actions and gets the plan executed with the help of smooth muscles of viscera, cardiac muscles and secretory epithelium of the glandular tissues (which are the effector organs of ANS). In other words, ANS is responsible for activities of the organs of digestion, circulation, excretion, respiration and reproduction, as well as of the adrenal medulla, sweat, lacrimal and salivary glands. It also controls the activity of smooth muscles of the iris, ciliary body and arrectores pilorum.

The word autonomous is taken from Greek words the *autos* meaning 'self' and the *nomos* meaning 'control'. Thus, ANS is an involuntary system. Since it controls the vegetative functions, it is also called vegetative system.

Divisions of ANS

ANS has two main physiological as well as anatomical divisions – sympathetic and parasympathetic – each having a central and a peripheral component.

Sympathetic division, also called thoracolumbar division, consists of thoracic and lumbar chains of sympathetic ganglia.

Parasympathetic division, also called craniosacral division, consists of the ganglia associated with cranial nerves III, VII, IX and X.

Somatic versus autonomic nervous system Sensory division of the somatic nervous system collects information about the changes that take place in the external environment, whereas that of ANS collects the information about the changes that take place in the internal environment (viscera).

Effector organs of the somatic nervous system are skeletal muscles, whereas that of ANS are smooth muscles, cardiac muscles and secretory glandular epithelium.

General arrangement of the somatic nervous system and ANS (Fig. 10.5.1) shows that:

Afferent (sensory) neuron of the somatic system having cell body in the dorsal root ganglion terminates in the dorsal horn, whereas that of ANS terminates in the intermediolateral horn.

- *The interneuron* (connector neuron) of the somatic system has cell body in the dorsal horn and terminates in the ventral horn, whereas that of ANS has cell body in the intermediolateral horn and terminates in the autonomic ganglia.

Efferent (motor) neuron has cell body in the ventral horn and its axon carries impulses of skeletal muscles (effector organ). The postganglionic neuron in ANS has cell body outside the

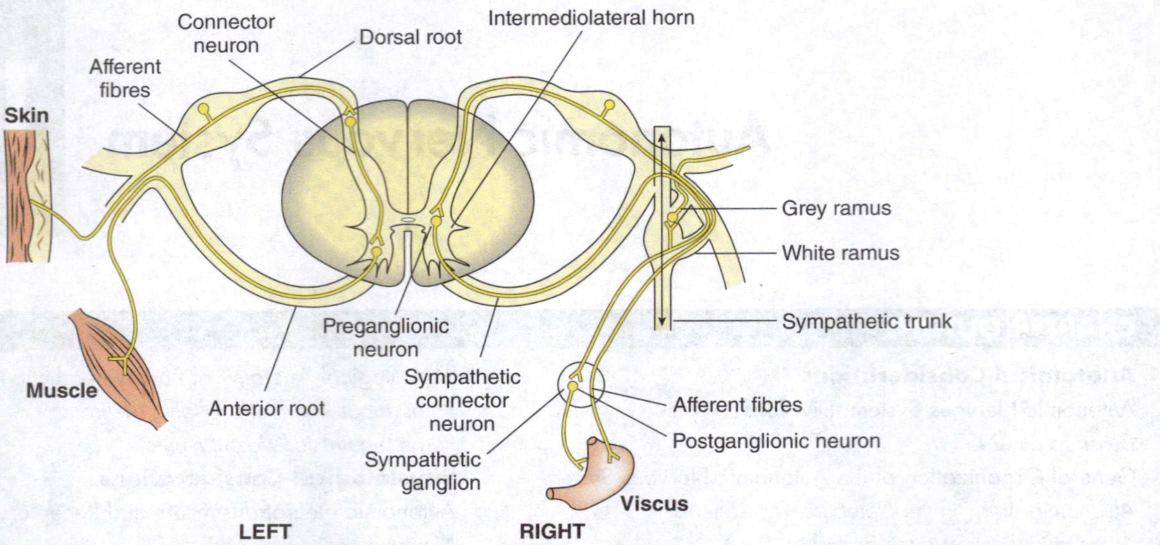

Fig. 10.5.1 General arrangement of somatic parts of nervous system (on the left) compared with autonomic parts of nervous system (on the right).

CNS in the autonomic ganglion and its axon terminates in visceral effector.

- There is a single efferent neuron in the somatic system, which extends from CNS to the effector organ, whereas in ANS there are two efferent neuron chains between CNS and the effector organ: the first efferent neuron (preganglionic neuron) has its cell body in CNS, and the second efferent neuron (postganglionic neuron) has its cell body outside CNS in the ganglion (Fig. 10.5.1).
- The somatic motor system innervates the skeletal muscles, whereas the ANS innervates the smooth muscles, cardiac muscles and secretory glandular epithelium.

Neurotransmitter released at efferent (motor) neuron ending in the somatic system is acetylcholine (ACh), whereas in ANS, the neurotransmitter released between preganglionic and postganglionic neurons is also ACh, but that between the postganglionic and the effector organ depends on the component of ANS (see page 956).

- Somatic system activity always causes muscle excitation, whereas ANS can cause both excitation and inhibition.
- Somatic motor activity is always voluntary, whereas ANS motor activity is usually involuntary.

GENERAL ORGANIZATION OF THE AUTONOMIC NERVOUS SYSTEM

The ANS is organized as given next.

I. Autonomic Areas in the Cerebral Hemispheres

The autonomic areas controlling visceral functions located in the cerebral hemisphere are as follows:

- Structures included in the limbic system (see page 1048)
- Prefrontal cortex
- Hypothalamus
- Part of thalamus

Higher brain centres, such as the limbic cortex and parts of the cerebral cortex, can influence the activity of ANS by sending signals to the hypothalamus and lower brain area.

Hypothalamus is the site of integration of somatic, autonomic and endocrine functions. Such an integration is essential for the maintenance of homeostasis during exposure to stresses like extreme hot, extreme cold, stress of surgical operation, stress of injuries and haemorrhage.

Since the hypothalamus plays an important role in the regulation of autonomic activity, it has been called the main ganglion of the ANS. However, it is now known that the limbic cortex is equally important in the regulation of the ANS.

II. Autonomic Centres in the Brainstem

These are located in the reticular formation and in the general visceral nuclei of cranial nerves.

Autonomic centres in reticular formation Autonomic centres in reticular formation include:

- *Gigantocellular* nucleus
- *Parvocellular nuclei*

Stimulation of the gigantocellular nucleus and the upper part of the ventral reticular nucleus causes depression of vasomotor activity, whereas stimulation of other areas has a pressure effect.

These effects are mediated through connections between the reticular formation and autonomic centres in the brainstem and spinal cord, but the pathways concerned are not well defined.

General visceral nuclei of cranial nerves These include both general visceral afferent and efferent nuclei.

General visceral afferent nucleus is represented by the nucleus of the solitary tract present in the medulla. It receives fibres carrying general visceral sensations through the vagus and glossopharyngeal nerves. Through these afferents and through connections with the reticular formation, the nucleus plays an important role in reflex control of respiratory and cardiovascular functions.

Fibres of taste (special visceral afferents) carried by the facial, glossopharyngeal and vagus nerves end in the upper part of the nucleus of the solitary tract which is sometimes called *gustatory nucleus.*

According to some authorities, some general visceral afferents end in the dorsal vagal nucleus.

General visceral efferent nuclei: These nuclei give origin to preganglionic fibres that constitute the cranial parasympathetic outflow. *The general visceral efferent nuclei* include:

- Edinger–Westphal nucleus (of oculomotor nerve) situated in the midbrain
- Salivary nucleus (superior and inferior) located in the pons
- Dorsal nucleus of the vagus, present in the medulla

III. Autonomic Centres in the Spinal Cord

These are located in the intermediolateral grey column of the spinal cord at two levels:

1. Neurons present in the thoracic and upper two or three lumbar segments of the spinal cord (T_1 to L_3) constitute the preganglionic neurons of the sympathetic nervous system (thoracolumbar outflow).
2. Neurons present in the second, third and fourth sacral segments of the spinal cord (S_2 to S_4) are the preganglionic neurons of the sacral part of the parasympathetic system, which along with the cranial part constitute the craniosacral outflow.

IV. Peripheral Part of ANS

This is made up of all autonomic nerves and ganglia throughout the body. It is important to stress here that there is no nerve in the body which is totally made of autonomic fibres. Hence, it is not possible to speak of autonomic nerves. In fact, autonomic fibres are intimately related to different cranial and spinal nerves.

NEURONS OF ANS

It is believed that ANS has both afferent and efferent components. The visceral afferents are sometimes called *autonomic afferents*; however, many disagree and consider the ANS essentially an efferent (motor) system for the visceral organs, blood vessels and secretory glands. Unlike in motor nerves, where a single motor neuron travels all the way from the spinal cord or cranial nuclei to the muscle, the autonomic efferent pathway from the spinal cord or cranial nuclei is made of two neurons – the preganglionic and the postganglionic.

Preganglionic neurons The cell body of the preganglionic neuron is located in either the brainstem or the spinal cord. The axon of this visceral motor neuron projects as a thinly myelinated preganglionic fibre to an autonomic ganglion.

Postganglionic neuron The body of the postganglionic neuron is located in the autonomic ganglion and sends an unmyelinated axon, the postganglionic fibre, to visceral effector cells.

In general, sympathetic ganglia are located close to the central nervous system, whereas parasympathetic ganglia are located close to the effector tissues. Therefore, the sympathetic pathway has short preganglionic fibres and long postganglionic fibres, whereas the parasympathetic pathway has long preganglionic fibres and short postganglionic fibres.

PHYSIOLOGICAL ANATOMY OF SYMPATHETIC NERVOUS SYSTEM

Sympathetic Preganglionic Neurons

The cell bodies of sympathetic preganglionic neurons are located in the intermediolateral horn of the spinal cord from level T_1 to L_2. The myelinated axons of these visceral motor neurons leave the spinal cord via the ventral root and then pass via the white rami communicantes to the paravertebral ganglia of the sympathetic trunk (Fig. 10.5.1). After reaching the sympathetic trunk, preganglionic fibres may pass to one of the following three destinations:

- They may terminate in the ganglion at the level of entrance by synapsing with an excitor cell in the ganglion (Fig. 10.5.2).
- They may travel up or down in the sympathetic trunk to terminate in the ganglia located at a higher or lower level (Fig. 10.5.2).
- They may travel through the sympathetic trunk, and exit without synapsing via the splanchnic nerve and terminate in a prevertebral ganglion (Fig. 10.5.2).

Preganglionic fibres that innervate the adrenal medulla travel through the sympathetic trunk exit without synapsing via the greater splanchnic nerve and end directly on the cells of the suprarenal medulla. These medullary cells may be regarded as modified sympathetic excitor cells that secrete epinephrine and norepinephrine (NE) into the bloodstream. These secretory cells of the adrenal medulla are derived embryologically from nervous tissue and are analogous to postganglionic neurons.

Sympathetic Ganglia

The sympathetic ganglia are of three types:

- Paravertebral ganglia
- Prevertebral or collateral ganglia
- Peripheral or terminal ganglia

1. Paravertebral ganglia Paravertebral ganglia are arranged as enlargements along the entire length of two sympathetic trunks (right and left placed on either side of the vertebral column throughout its length). Paravertebral ganglia of the sympathetic trunk are divided into:

- *Cervical ganglia* are three in number – superior, middle and inferior.
- *Thoracic ganglia* are 11–12 in number.
- *Lumbar ganglia* are four in number.

Important Note

In all, there are 22 or 23 ganglia on each trunk.

The inferior cervical ganglion and the first thoracic ganglion are often fused to form a large stellate ganglion.

The two sympathetic trunks end below by joining together to form a single ganglion, the ganglion impar.

2. Prevertebral or collateral ganglia Prevertebral or collateral ganglia are three in number (coeliac ganglion, inferior mesenteric ganglion and superior mesenteric ganglion).

3. Peripheral or terminal ganglia Peripheral or terminal ganglia are located within or close to structures innervated by them. Heart, bronchi, pancreas and urinary bladder are innervated by the terminal ganglia.

Postganglionic Sympathetic Neurons

The sympathetic postganglionic neurons are located primarily in ganglia on the sympathetic trunks. Some are located in the prevertebral ganglia and the peripheral autonomic plexus

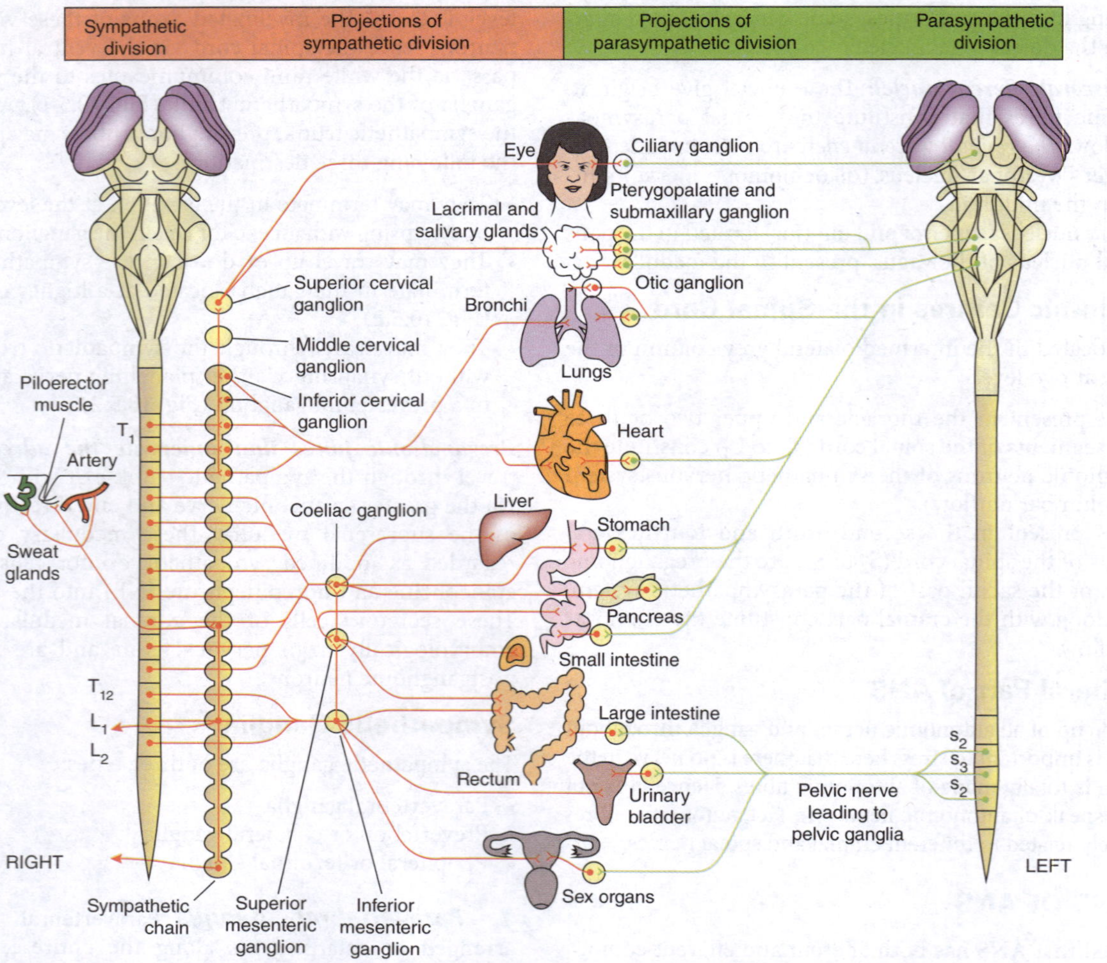

Fig. 10.5.2 Efferent parts of autonomic nervous system: parasympathetic (on the left) and sympathetic (on the right).

(Figs 10.5.1 and 10.5.2). Axons arising from these neurons behave in one of the following ways:

The axons may pass through a grey ramus communicantes and re-enter the ventral root to reach a spinal nerve (Fig. 10.5.1). The grey rami communicantes are grey in colour because the postganglionic fibres are unmyelinated fibres. In the spinal nerve, the postganglionic fibres travel through its branches to innervate sweat glands and arrectores pilorum muscles of the skin in the region to which the spinal nerve is distributed.

The axons may reach a cranial nerve through a communicating branch and may be distributed through it as in the case of the spinal nerve.

The axons may pass into a vascular branch and may be distributed to branches of the vessel.

Some fibres from these plexuses may pass to other structures in the neighbourhood of the vessel.

The axons of postganglionic neurons arising in sympathetic ganglia may travel through the vascular branches and through the autonomic plexus to reach some viscera (e.g. the heart).

The axons of postganglionic neurons located in the peripheral autonomic plexus innervate neighbouring viscera. These fibres often travel to the viscera in plexuses along blood vessels. For example, fibres for the gut travel along plexuses surrounding the branches of coeliac, superior mesenteric and inferior mesenteric arteries.

Sympathetic Afferent Fibres

The afferent myelinated fibres travel from the viscera through the sympathetic ganglia without synapsing (Fig. 10.5.1). They enter the spinal nerve via the white rami communicantes and reach their cell bodies in the posterior root ganglia of the corresponding spinal nerve. The central axons then enter the spinal cord and may form the afferent component of a local reflex arc. Others may pass up to higher autonomic centres in the brain.

Distribution of Sympathetic Preganglionic Neurons and Postganglionic Fibres

The distribution of preganglionic neurons and postganglionic fibres is shown in Table 10.5.1 and Fig. 10.5.2.

PHYSIOLOGICAL ANATOMY OF PARASYMPATHETIC NERVOUS SYSTEM

Parasympathetic Preganglionic Neurons

The parasympathetic fibres form the *craniosacral outflow*, consisting of cranial parasympathetic outflow and sacral parasympathetic outflow.

Table 10.5.1 Distribution of preganglionic neurons and postganglionic fibres

Segmental level of preganglionic neurons	Area of distribution	Final distribution of postganglionic fibres
T_1 and T_2	Head and neck	Dilator pupillae muscle, superior and inferior, Muller's muscles of eyelids, blood vessels and sweat glands
T_3 and T_4	Thoracic viscera	Heart, oesophagus, trachea, bronchi and lungs
T_5 to T_9	Upper limb	Blood vessels, sweat glands and arrectores pilorum muscles
T_{10} to L_2	Lower limb	Blood vessels, sweat glands and arrectores pilorum muscles
T_6 to T_{12}	Upper abdominal viscera	GIT, liver, spleen capsule, adrenal medulla and urinary tract
L_1 and L_2	Lower abdominal viscera	Bladder, uterus and fallopian tubes (or testis, vas deferens, seminal vesicles and prostate)
T_1 to T_{12}	Thoracic and abdominal parietes	Blood vessels, sweat glands and arrectores pilorum muscles

I. Cranial Parasympathetic Outflow

The cell bodies of the neurons which give rise to preganglionic parasympathetic fibres are located in the general visceral efferent nuclei. These preganglionic fibres end in peripheral ganglia associated with the branches of cranial nerves. Postganglionic fibres arising in these ganglia supply smooth muscles or glands. Cranial parasympathetic outflow can be further divided into:

- Midbrain or tectal outflow
- Bulbar outflow

1. Midbrain or tectal outflow The general visceral efferent nucleus associated with midbrain outflow is Edinger–Westphal nucleus.

Edinger–Westphal nucleus: It lies in the midbrain and is closely related to the oculomotor nucleus complex.

- *Preganglionic fibres* arising from Edinger–Westphal nucleus pass through the oculomotor (cranial III) nerve and relay in the ciliary ganglion.
- *Ciliary ganglion* is a peripheral parasympathetic ganglion placed in the course of the oculomotor nerve.
- *Postganglionic fibres* arising in the ciliary ganglion pass through the short ciliary nerves and supply the sphincter pupillae and the ciliary muscle.

2. Bulbar outflow The general visceral efferent nuclei associated with bulbar outflow are as follows:

- Superior salivary nucleus
- Lacrimal nucleus
- Inferior salivary nucleus
- Dorsal vagal nucleus

i. ***Superior salivary nucleus:*** *Preganglionic fibres* arising from superior salivary nucleus enter the facial (cranial VII) nerve and ultimately relay in the *submandibular ganglion*. Postganglionic fibres pass to submandibular and sublingual salivary glands to which they are secretomotor.

ii. ***Lacrimal nucleus*** of the cranial nerve VII sends preganglionic fibres to the *pterygopalatine* (sphenopalatine) ganglion. The postganglionic fibres reach the lacrimal gland to which they are secretomotor.

iii. ***Inferior salivary nucleus*** sends preganglionic fibres into the glossopharyngeal (cranial IX) nerve. These fibres relay in the otic ganglion, from where the postganglionic fibres go to the parotid gland to which they are secretomotor.

iv. ***Dorsal (motor) nucleus of the vagus:*** About 75% of all parasympathetic fibres arise from dorsal nucleus.
Preganglionic fibres travelling in the vagus nerve end in ganglia (or nerve plexuses) closely related to the visceral organs, such as the heart, lungs, bronchi, oesophagus, stomach, small intestine and large intestine up to two-thirds of the transverse colon.
Postganglionic fibres arise in these ganglia, and run a short course to supply smooth muscles and glands in these organs.

II. Sacral Parasympathetic Outflow

The cell bodies of the preganglionic neurons, which constitute the sacral parasympathetic outflow, are located in the intermediolateral grey horn of second, third and fourth sacral segments (S_2, S_3 and S_4) of the spinal cord (Fig. 10.5.2).

1. Preganglionic fibres Preganglionic fibres pass out through the ventral spinal root of corresponding nerves. These axons leave the spinal nerves to form the pelvic splanchnic nerves, which end in the pelvic autonomic plexuses.

2. Postganglionic fibres The postganglionic neurons are located in the pelvic autonomic plexuses close to or within the viscera. Their axons (postganglionic fibres) run a very short course to supply the concerned pelvic viscera. These fibres also supply the rectum, the sigmoid colon, the descending colon and the left one-third of the transverse colon.

Parasympathetic Afferent Fibres

The afferent myelinated fibres travel from viscera to their cell bodies located either in the sensory ganglia of the cranial nerves or in the posterior root ganglia of the sacrospinal nerves. The central axons then enter the central nervous system and take part in the formation of local reflex arc, or pass to higher centres of the ANS.

The afferent component of ANS is identical to the afferent component of somatic nerves and forms part of the general afferent segment of the entire nervous system. The nerve endings in the autonomic afferent component may not be activated by such sensations as heat or touch but instead by stretch or lack of oxygen. Once the afferent fibres gain entrance to the spinal cord or brain, they are thought to travel alongside or are mixed with the somatic afferent fibres.

PHYSIOLOGICAL CONSIDERATIONS

AUTONOMIC NEUROTRANSMITTERS AND RECEPTORS

Neurotransmitters of ANS (Fig. 10.5.3)

Parasympathetic fibres

1. Preganglionic fibres: ACh
2. Postganglionic fibres: ACh

Sympathetic fibres

1. Preganglionic fibres: ACh
2. Postganglionic fibres:

   Adrenergic fibres: NE (mainly) or epinephrine and all postganglionic sympathetic fibres other than cholinergic

> **Important Note**
>
> The catecholamines present in plasma are NE, epinephrine and dopamine and the source of dopamine comes from the adrenal medulla, whereas NE mainly releases from the nerve endings, which diffuses into the bloodstream. NE has a prolonged effect compared with ACh.

Cholinergic fibres: The postganglionic sympathetic cholinergic nerve fibres supplying sweat glands, blood vessels in the heart and skeletal muscles

Thus:

- All preganglionic fibres (sympathetic as well as parasympathetic) release ACh.
- All postganglionic parasympathetic fibres release ACh.
- Most postganglionic sympathetic (adrenergic) fibres release NE.
- A few postganglionic sympathetic (cholinergic) fibres release ACh.

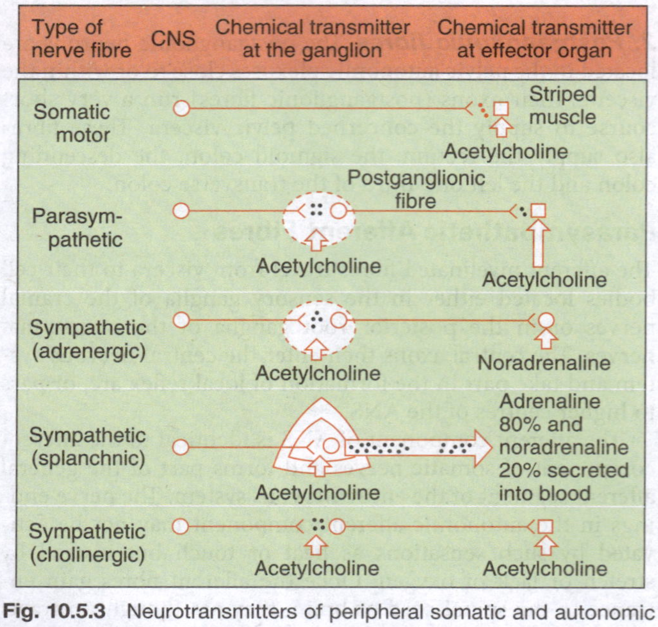

Fig. 10.5.3 Neurotransmitters of peripheral somatic and autonomic nervous system.

> **Important Note**
>
> ACh released from the nerve endings acts locally, and usually does not circulate in the blood. The effect of ACh is of short duration because of high concentration of ACh esterase at cholinergic nerve endings.

For details about neurotransmitters, see page 979.

Autonomic Receptors

The autonomic neurotransmitters (ACh and NE) produce their effects on the organs by combining with specific protein molecules known as receptors, which are of the types given next.

1. Cholinergic receptors On the basis of their pharmacological properties, these are of two types:

- Nicotinic receptors
- Muscarinic receptors

i. Nicotinic receptors (nAChR)

Location: These receptors are located in/at:

- Autonomic ganglia of sympathetic and parasympathetic nervous systems
- Neuromuscular junction
- Adrenal medulla

The receptors at these locations are similar but not identical. At the autonomic ganglia, the nicotinic cholinergic receptors are further of two types:

- *Nn type* which are blocked by hexamethonium
- *Nm type* which are located at the neuromuscular junction and are blocked by D-tubocurarine

Activation: Nicotinic receptors are activated by:

- ACh
- Nicotine

Effect: These receptors produce excitation.

Blockage: Ganglion blockers (e.g. hexamethonium and trimethaphan) block the nicotinic receptors for ACh in the autonomic ganglia, but not at the neuromuscular junction.

Mechanism of action: The nicotinic receptors are ion-gated protein channels for Na^+ and K^+; ACh binds to α-subunit of the nicotinic cholinergic receptors.

ii. Muscarinic receptors

Location: Muscarinic receptors are located in the:

- Heart
- Smooth muscles (except vascular smooth muscle)
- Glands

Types: The muscarinic receptors are divided into subtypes, i.e. M_1–M_5. M_2 and M_3 are the main subtypes; M_2 receptors are present mainly in the heart and M_3 are located on smooth muscles and glands.

Activation: These receptors are activated by:

- ACh
- Muscarine

Effect produced by their stimulation is as follows:

- *Inhibitory in the heart*, e.g. decreased heart rate and decreased conduction velocity in the atrioventricular (AV) node
- *Excitatory* in smooth muscle and glands (e.g. increased gastrointestinal motility and increased secretion)

Blockage: Muscarinic receptors for ACh are blocked by atropine.

Mechanism of action:

- *In the heart at the sinoatrial (SA) node*, these receptors cause inhibition of adenylyl cyclase, which leads to opening of K^+ channels, slowing of the rate of spontaneous depolarization and decreased heart rate.
- *In smooth muscle and glands*, these receptors act by formation of inositol 1,3,5-triphosphate (IP_3) and increase in intracellular Ca^{2+}.

2. Adrenergic receptors On the basis of their pharmacological properties, adrenergic receptors are of two types:

Alpha (α) adrenergic receptors (which are of further two types: α_1 and α_2)

Beta (β) adrenergic receptors (which are of further three types: β_1, β_2 and β_3)

i. α_1-Receptors

Location: α_1-Receptors are located on:

- Vascular smooth muscles of the skin and splanchnic regions
- Gastrointestinal and bladder sphincters
- Radial muscles of the iris

Effect: These receptors produce excitation, e.g. contraction or constriction.

Catecholamine sensitivity: α_1-Receptors are equally sensitive to NE and epinephrine, but only NE is present in concentrations that are high enough to activate α_1-receptors.

Mechanism of action: These receptors act by the formation of IP_3 and increase in intracellular Ca^{2+}.

ii. α_2-Receptors

Location: α_2-Receptors are located in:

- Presynaptic nerve terminals
- Platelets
- Fat cells
- Walls of the gastrointestinal tract

Effect: These receptors often produce inhibition (e.g. relaxation or dilatation).

Mechanism of action: α_2-Receptor causes inhibition of adenylyl cyclase and decrease in cyclic adenosine monophosphate (cAMP).

iii. β_1-Receptors

Location: β_1-Receptors are located in the:

- SA node
- AV node
- Ventricular muscles of the heart

Mechanism of action: β_1-Receptors are G-protein-coupled receptors, and act through cAMP and cAMP-dependent protein kinase.

Effect: These receptors produce excitation (e.g. increased heart rate, increased conduction velocity and increased contractility).

Catecholamine sensitivity: β_1-Receptors are sensitive to both NE and epinephrine, and are more sensitive than the α_1-receptors.

iv. β_2-Receptors

Location: β_2-Receptors are located on:

- Vascular smooth muscle of skeletal muscle
- Bronchial smooth muscle
- Walls of the gastrointestinal tract
- Bladder

Effect: These receptors produce relaxation (e.g. dilation of vascular smooth muscle, dilation of bronchioles and relaxation of the bladder wall).

Sensitivity to epinephrine is more than to NE. These are more sensitive to epinephrine than the α_1-receptors, e.g. when small amounts of epinephrine are released from the adrenal medulla, vasodilation (β_2-effect) occurs, and when larger amounts of epinephrine are released from the adrenal medulla, vasoconstriction (α_1-effect) occurs.

Mechanism of action: It is same as that for β_1-receptors.

v. β_3-Receptors

These receptors are located on the adipose tissue and cause lipolysis.

Mechanism of action: β_3-Receptors cause an increase in cAMP.

> **Important Note**
>
> The type of adrenergic receptors present in various organs and the effects produced by their stimulation are depicted in Table 10.5.2.

3. Nonadrenergic and noncholinergic transmitters

Some autonomic fibres release neuropeptide besides classical neurotransmitters. These include:

i. ***Adenosine triphosphate (ATP):*** The small vesicles of postganglionic noradrenergic fibres contain ATP. The low-frequency stimulation causes ATP release.

ii. ***Neuropeptide Y*** is another transmitter present in large vesicles of postganglionic sympathetic endings supplying to the vasculature of viscera, skin and skeletal muscles that releases on high-frequency stimulation in addition to NE.

iii. ***Galanin, vasoactive intestinal peptide (VIP), calcitonin gene-related peptide (CGRP) or substance P*** is released along with ACh on sympathetic stimulation to sweat glands.

FUNCTIONS OF AUTONOMIC NERVOUS SYSTEM: EFFECTS OF AUTONOMIC NERVE IMPULSES ON EFFECTOR ORGANS

General Principles

- ANS controls the various vegetative functions which are beyond voluntary control and thus plays an important role in maintaining the constant internal environment (homeostasis).
- Most of the visceral organs have dual innervation, i.e. are supplied by both sympathetic and parasympathetic divisions of ANS. The two divisions produce antagonistic effects on each organ and provide a very fine degree of control over the effector organ. When the fibres of one division supplying to an organ are sectioned or affected by a lesion, the effects of fibres from the other division on the organ become more prominent.
- Some of the visceral organs are innervated by one division of ANS only, e.g.:
  - Uterus, adrenal medulla and most of the arterioles are innervated by the sympathetic division only.
  - Glands of the stomach and pancreas are innervated by the parasympathetic division only.
- In the case of sphincter muscles, both adrenergic and cholinergic innervations are excitatory, but one supplies the constrictor component of the sphincter and the other the dilator.

Table 10.5.2 Responses of effector organs to sympathetic and parasympathetic stimulation

		Sympathetic effect	
Effector organ	**Parasympathetic effect**	**Receptor type**	**Response**
1. ***Eyes***	–	α_1	Contraction (mydriasis)
• Dilator pupillae muscle	Contraction (meiosis)	–	
• Sphincter pupillae muscle	Contraction (produces accommodation for near vision)	–	
• Ciliary muscle			
2. ***Heart***	↓Heart rate and vagal arrest	β_1	↑Heart rate
• SA node	↓Contractility,	β_1 and β_2	↑Contractility
• Atria	↓Conductivity	β_1 and β_2	↑Conductivity
• AV node and conduction system	↓Conduction velocity	β_1 and β_2	↑Conduction velocity
• Ventricles	↓Contractility		↑Contractility
3. ***Arterioles***	No supply	α_1 and α_2	Constriction
• Coronary	No supply	β_2	Dilatation
• Cutaneous and mucosal	Dilatation	α_1 and α_2	Constriction
• Skeletal muscle	Dilatation	α_1	Constriction
• Cerebral	No supply	β_2	Dilatation
• Pulmonary	No supply	α_1	Constriction
• Abdominal viscera	Dilatation	α_1	Constriction
• Renal		β_2	Dilatation
• Salivary glands		α_1	Constriction
		α_1 and α_2	Constriction
		β_1 and β_2	Dilatation
		α_1 and α_2	Constriction
4. ***Systemic veins***	No supply	α_1 and α_2	Constriction
		β_2	Dilatation
5. ***Lungs***	Contraction	β_2	Relaxation
• Bronchial muscles	Stimulation	α_1	Inhibition
• Bronchial glands		β_2	Stimulation
6. ***Salivary glands***	Stimulation (profuse watery secretion)	α_1	Stimulation (thick viscous secretion)
7. ***Stomach***	Increases	α_1, α_2 and β_2	Decreases
• Motility and tone	Relaxation	α_1	Contraction
• Sphincters	Stimulation	α_2	Inhibition
• Secretion			
8. ***Gall bladder***	Contraction	β_2	Relaxation
9. ***Liver***	–	α_1 and β_2	Glycogenolysis
10. ***Pancreas***	Stimulates secretion	α_1	Inhibits secretion
• Exocrine glands	–	α_2	Inhibits insulin secretion
• Endocrine glands		β_2	Stimulates glucagon
11. ***Spleen capsule***		α_1	Contraction
		β_2	Relaxation
12. ***Adrenal medulla***	Secretion of epinephrine and norepinephrine	–	–
13. ***Urinary bladder***	Contraction	β_2	Relaxation (usually)
• Detrusor muscle	Relaxation	α_1	Contraction
• Sphincter			
14. ***Uterus***	Variable	α_1	Contraction (pregnant)
		β_2	Relaxation (nonpregnant)
15. ***Male sex organ***	Erection	α_1	Ejaculation
16. ***Lacrimal glands***	Secretion		
17. ***Skin***	–	α_1	Contraction (erection of hair)
• Pilomotor muscle	Generalized (cholinergic sweating)	α_1	Localized (adrenergic) sweating
• Sweat glands			
18. ***Nasopharyngeal glands***	Secretion	–	–
19. ***Adipose tissue***	–	α_1 and β_1	Lipolysis, release of FFA
		β_3	
20. ***Juxtaglomerular cells***	–	β_1	Increased renin secretion

Table 10.5.2 Responses of effector organs to sympathetic and parasympathetic stimulation—(Continued)

Effector organ	Parasympathetic effect	Sympathetic effect: Receptor type	Sympathetic effect: Response
21. ***Pineal gland***	–	β_1	Increased melatonin synthesis
22. ***Skeletal muscles***	–	β_2	Increased glycogenolysis
23. ***Basal metabolic rate***	–	β_2	Increased
24. ***Mental activity***	–		Increased

AV, atrioventricular; SA, sinoatrial.

- *Effects of ACh,* i.e. of localized cholinergic discharge, are generally discrete and short lasting, because ACh is rapidly removed from the nerve endings, due to high concentration of ACh esterase at cholinergic nerve endings.
- *Effects of NE* are more prolonged than of ACh, as it spreads further. In the blood, epinephrine and dopamine come from the adrenal medulla, whereas NE diffuses from the adrenergic nerve endings.

Epinephrine versus NE (also see page 748):

- Epinephrine acts equally on α- and β-receptors, and has a special property of stimulating β_2-receptors, whereas NE acts mainly on α-receptors and on β_1-receptors but has no action on β_2-receptors.

Effects of Stimulation of Sympathetic and Parasympathetic Divisions of ANS

Responses of effector organs to autonomic nerve impulses are summarized in Table 10.5.2.

DIFFERENCES BETWEEN SYMPATHETIC AND PARASYMPATHETIC SYSTEMS

As summarized in Table 10.5.3, sympathetic and parasympathetic systems produce antagonistic effects on each organ of the body. The main differences between sympathetic and parasympathetic systems are depicted in Table 10.5.3.

Applied Aspects

A few important considerations about applied aspects of ANS are as follows:

- Diseases/syndromes due to dysfunction of ANS
- Autonomic failure
- Autonomic drugs
- Autonomic function tests

Diseases/Syndromes of Autonomic Dysfunctions

1. Organophosphate Poisoning

Organophosphates are cholinesterase inhibitors present in pesticides. Acute pesticide (organophosphate) poisoning occurs due to rapid absorption of organophosphates from the gut, lungs, skin and conjunctiva.

Mechanism: When an organophosphate pesticide, e.g. parathion, malathion and nerve gases (like soman, serine), binds to the enzyme, it undergoes hydrolysis and leads to the signs and symptoms given next.

Signs and symptoms of organophosphate poisoning occur due to excessive activation of autonomic/muscarinic activity. These include:

GIT: Excessive salivation, vomiting, gastric erosions and haematemesis

Respiration: Bronchial constriction, pulmonary haemorrhage, pulmonary oedema and ultimately respiratory failure

CNS: Cognitive disturbances, convulsions, seizures and even coma

CVS: Tachycardia and arrhythmia leading to cardiac failure

Renal system: Acute oliguria leading to renal failure

Management: As poison is most toxic and lethal, early diagnosis and management is mandatory. The treatment is mainly supportive as:

- *Maintenance of patent airway* by endotracheal intubation with assisted ventilation
- *Oxygen therapy* to overcome hypoxia only when there is respiratory failure
- *Fluids:* Intravenous fluid therapy under central venous pressure (CVP) monitoring to compensate fluid loss
- *Removal of poison* from GIT by gastric lavage
- *Haemodialysis* for renal failure
- *Specific treatment* includes:
  - Atropine (muscarinic cholinergic receptor antagonist) should be given parenterally to control the signs.
  - Cholinesterase regenerator (pralidoxime) can also be given.
  - Benzodiazepine can be used to control the seizures.

2. Mushroom Poisoning

There are many poisonous varieties of mushrooms which can be confused with edible fungi or mycelium and may be eaten by mistake resulting in mushroom poisoning. About 95% of mushroom poisoning is caused by the ingestion of *Amanita phalloides*. This variety of mushroom contains toxins (phallotoxin and amatoxins).

Signs and symptoms occur due to excessive activation of muscarinic cholinergic synapses. The major signs of mushroom poisoning occur within 2–3 hours and include:

- Nausea, vomiting, vasodilation, sweating, diarrhoea and urinary urgency occur within 2–3 hours.
- After about 12 hours, the stage is marked by severe hepatocellular and renal damage.

Table 10.5.3 Main differences between sympathetic and parasympathetic systems

Feature	Sympathetic system	Parasympathetic system
Location	Cell bodies of preganglionic neurons are located in intermediolateral horn of T_1–L_2 or L_3 spinal segments, so also called thoracolumbar outflow.	Cell bodies of preganglionic neurons are located in: • *Cranial nuclei* associated with cranial nerves III, VII, IX and X (cranial outflow) • Intermediolateral horn of S_2 to S_4 spinal segments (sacral outflow); so, it is also called craniosacral outflow
Components and ganglia	• Components are consolidated • Ganglia are linked up to form a chain	• Components are isolated • Ganglia remain isolated
Preganglionic fibres	Are short, myelinated and end in paravertebral or prevertebral ganglia.	Are long, myelinated and end on short postganglionic neurons located on or near the viscera.
Postganglionic fibres	• Long • Nonmyelinated	• Short • Myelinated
Neurotransmitter		
• Preganglionic fibres	• Mostly adrenergic	• Cholinergic
• Postganglionic fibres	• Cholinergic	• Cholinergic
Area of effect	Preganglionic fibres branch, enter several ganglia and transmit nerve impulse to many postganglionic fibres. So, sympathetic activity is spread over many segments.	Preganglionic fibres do not branch; each enters a single ganglion and transmits nerve impulses to a single postganglionic fibre. Therefore, parasympathetic activity is localized, i.e. target is usually a single organ or system.
Functions	Mass sympathetic discharge usually occurs in threatening situation, i.e. it prepares the individual to cope with the emergency. It causes flight-or-fight reactions characterized by: • Dilatation of pupil • Increased heart rate • Increased blood pressure (providing better perfusion of the vital organs and muscles) • Constriction of cutaneous arterioles (which limits blood loss from wounds, if any) • Increased alertness and arousal due to decreased threshold in the reticular formation • Increased blood glucose and FFA levels (supplying more energy) Because of these actions, sympathetic system is also sometimes called *catabolic nervous system*.	Unlike sympathetic nervous system, the functions of parasympathetic system are discrete and each function is separately regulated. This system is concerned with vegetative aspect of day-to-day living. For example, its action favours: • Digestion and absorption of food, increased activity of intestinal musculature and increased gastric secretion and pyloric relaxation • Micturition • Pupillary constriction • Bradycardia Since parasympathetic system decreases the rate of metabolism, it is also called *anabolic nervous system*.

- The final stage (after 72 hours) is characterized by acute renal failure, hepatic necrosis, sepsis and coma.

Antimuscarinic syndrome occurs due to ingestion of a separate variety of mushroom (*Amanita muscaria*). This variety of mushroom also contains an alkaloid that blocks muscarinic cholinergic receptors. The classical symptoms of antimuscarinic syndrome are as follows:

- Red as beet, i.e. flushed skin
- Hot as hare, i.e. hyperthermia
- Dry as bone, i.e. no sweating and dry mucous membrane
- Blind as bat, i.e. blurred vision and cycloplegia
- Mad as a hatter, i.e. confusion and delirium

Diagnosis of mushroom poisoning: The diagnosis is made on clinical history of ingestion, identification of mushroom (if possible) and measurement of amatoxin in blood by radioimmunoassay.

Management includes:

- Gastric lavage and activated charcoal may be given to absorb the poison.
- Supportive treatment is done by i.v. fluids.
- Antidotes of amatoxin such as penicillin G and silibinin inhibit uptake of amatoxin by the liver cells.
- Thioctic acid (a Krebs cycle coenzyme) also has a role.
- Atropine: Rapid onset of muscarinic poisoning can be effectively treated with atropine.
- Physostigmine (cholinesterase).
  - Antimuscarinic syndrome can be treated with physostigmine that acts peripherally and centrally.
- If the patient is agitated, then he/she is sedated with benzodiazepine or an antipsychotic drug treatment.

Autonomic Failure

Autonomic failure is of two types:

Primary autonomic failure from the unexplained (primary) autonomic neuronal degeneration: It was previously known as orthostatic hypotension because this is the chief presenting feature of the disorder.

Secondary autonomic failure occurs secondary to some general medical disorders. Diabetes mellitus is the most common cause of secondary autonomic dysfunction.

Features of autonomic failure (primary or secondary) are as follows:

- *Cardiovascular features* include tachycardia and orthostatic hypotension.
- *Sudomotor features* are anhidrosis and heat intolerance.
- *Gastrointestinal features* include constipation, occasional diarrhoea and dysphagia.
- *Urinary features* are nocturia, frequency, urgency, incontinence and retention of urine.
- *Reproductive organ problems* include erectile and ejaculation failure.
- *Ocular features* include miosis and enophthalmos.

Management: There is no specific treatment; however, to relieve symptoms, treatment includes:

I. Treatment of underlying disease
II. Management of specific symptoms, e.g.:
   - For GIT: Change in diet (more dietary fibre and fluids)
   - For heart rate and blood pressure problem: High-salt diet and fluids
   - BP and heart rate: Medication and beta-blockers to regulate BP

Horner Syndrome

Horner syndrome refers to ipsilateral *oculosympathetic paresis* due to any cause. Its common causes are Pancoast tumour of the lung and malignancy of cervical lymph nodes pressing on the cervical sympathetic chain.

Clinical features of Horner syndrome are as follows:

Ptosis (drooping down of upper eyelid) due to paralysis of Muller's muscle of the upper eyelid
Miosis (small pupil) due to paralysis of dilator pupillae muscle
Facial anhidrosis, i.e. reduced sweating on the ipsilateral face and neck

Autonomic Drugs

Autonomic drugs exert their effects by action on the autonomic receptors directly or indirectly. These include:

- Sympathomimetic drugs
- Sympatholytic drugs or sympathetic blockers
- Parasympathomimetic drugs
- Parasympatholytic drugs or parasympathetic blockers

Sympathomimetic Drugs. Sympathomimetic drugs, also called adrenaline-like drugs, when administered in the body produce effects similar to the effects of sympathetic nerve stimulation. These can be divided into two main groups:

Directly acting sympathomimetic drugs: These drugs act directly on the α- and/or β-adrenergic receptors. Examples of these drugs are adrenaline, noradrenaline, phenylephrine, isoproterenol and albuterol.

Indirectly acting sympathomimetic drugs: These drugs enhance the actions of naturally occurring NE in body by any of the following mechanisms:

- By displacing NE from the storage sites in the sympathetic nerve endings, e.g. amphetamine
- By inhibiting the reuptake of NE by noradrenergic nerve endings and hence increasing the NE concentration in sympathetic sites, e.g. imipramine
- By acting as monoamine oxidase (MAO) inhibitor agent and hence decreasing the catabolism of NE in sympathetic nerve terminals

Sympathetic Blockers. The sympathetic blockers or sympatholytic drugs block the actions of sympathetic neurotransmitters. Mechanisms by which sympatholytic drugs act are as follows:

- Prevention of synthesis and storage of NE, e.g. reserpine
- Prevention of release of NE, e.g. guanethidine
- Blockage of α-receptors, e.g. phentolamine
- Blockage of β-receptors, e.g. propranolol, metoprolol and timolol
- Blockage of transmission of nerve impulse through sympathetic ganglion (ganglion blockers), e.g. hexamethonium and pentolinium

Parasympathomimetic Drugs. The parasympathomimetic drugs, also known as ACh-like drugs, when administered in the body produce effects similar to the effect of parasympathetic nerve stimulation. Depending on their mechanism of action, parasympathomimetic drugs are of the following types:

Drugs acting on muscarinic receptors, e.g. pilocarpine and methacholine
Drugs prolonging the action of ACh, e.g. neostigmine and physostigmine, which inhibit the activity of ACh esterase

Parasympathetic Blockers. The parasympathetic blockers, also called parasympatholytic drugs, block the actions of parasympathetic neurotransmitters by blocking the muscarinic receptors. Examples of parasympathetic blockers are atropine, homatropine, scopolamine, cyclopentolate and tropicamide.

Autonomic Function Tests

The tests of autonomic functions are broadly divided into two categories – noninvasive and invasive tests.

Noninvasive Tests

A. Tests of cardiovascular autonomic function include:

1. Valsalva Manoeuvre After closing both the nostrils, the patient is made to blow into a tube connected to sphygmomanometer and maintain air pressure at 40 mm Hg for 15 seconds. The ECG recording is done during 15 seconds following the Valsalva manoeuvre. The normal response consists of tachycardia during strain and bradycardia after release (Fig. 10.5.4) (see page 367).

Valsalva ratio: The ratio between the longest R–R interval (after the strain) and the shortest R–R interval (during the strain) is known as the Valsalva ratio. The normal Valsalva ratio is >1.20. In autonomic neuropathy, Valsalva ratio is <1.20.

2. Heart Rate Variation During Deep Breathing

While recording ECG, the patient is asked to inhale deeply for 5 seconds followed by exhalation for 5 seconds alternately for six times. The ratio between the longest R–R interval during expiration and the shortest R–R interval during inspiration (E/1 ratio) in each respiratory cycle is calculated, and averaged for the total record. The normal ratio is >1.2 (Fig. 10.5.5). In autonomic dysfunction, E/1 ratio is <1.2.

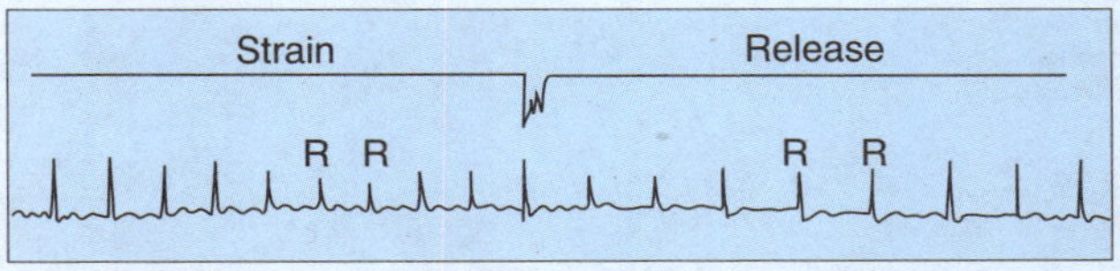

Fig. 10.5.4 Effect of Valsalva manoeuvre on heart rate.

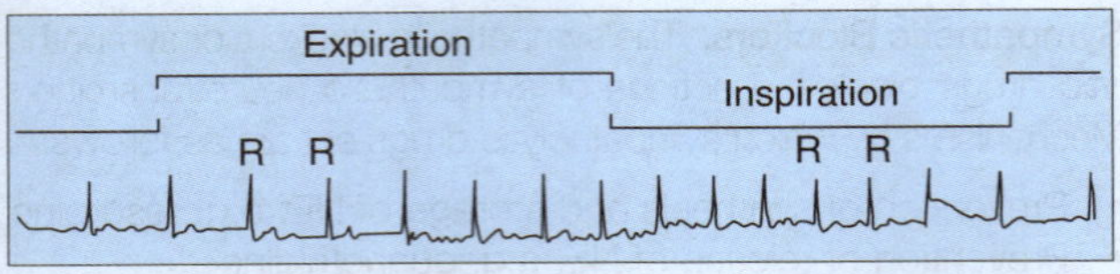

Fig. 10.5.5 Heart rate variations during deep breathing.

3. Heart Rate Response to Standing Normally, a change of posture from supine to standing results in a mild increase in HR. The change in heart rate is calculated by dividing the length of the maximum R–R interval (which occurred during 30-second ECG recording) by the length of the minimum R–R interval. An increase in standing heart rate <15% over supine is suggestive of autonomic neuropathy.

4. Heart Rate Variability Heart rate variability (HRV) refers to beat-to-beat variation of heart rate. The sympathetic and vagal discharges directed to the SA node are usually synchronous with each cardiac cycle. These discharges can be modulated by central and peripheral oscillators. These modulating effects of neural mechanism on heart rhythm are inferred with the help of HRV analysis.

5. Cold Pressor Test Cold pressor test (CPT) measures the function of sympathetic neural control of the cardiovascular system. Blood pressure is recorded while dipping the hand in cold water at temperature 8–10°C. Rise in blood pressure should be more than 15 mm Hg from the basal value, which is considered to be a normal response.

6. Blood Pressure Response to Standing Normally, a change of posture from supine to standing leads to a slight fall in systolic blood pressure (SBP), which is never more than 10 mm Hg. In autonomic dysfunction, this fall in SBP on change of posture is 10 mm Hg or even more. This is called *orthostatic hypotension*.

7. Blood Pressure Response to Sustained Hand Grip The patient is asked to maintain hand grip or a hand grip dynamometer at 30% of the maximum voluntary contraction for 5 minutes. Blood pressure is recorded just before and at the end of hand grip. Normally, the diastolic blood pressure (DBP) shows an increase by more than 15 mm Hg. In autonomic dysfunction, the rise in DBP is always less than 10 mm Hg.

B. Test of sudomotor function include:

1. Evaluation of Sweating Response to Heat Exposure Evaluation of sweating response to heat exposure tests the sudomotor functions. This test is performed by exposing the patient to electric heater till his/her body temperature is raised by 1°C, and the sweating response is studied by demarcating the area of sweating with the help of iodine starch or alizarin red, or quinizarin powders which change colour when moist.

2. Galvanic Skin Response (GSR) Galvanic skin response (GSR) is based on change in skin electrical resistance. It is an electrodermal response that determines change in the electrical conductivity of the skin, caused by increased activity of sweat glands. The sympathetic activity increases the conductance that is measured from the fingertips by placing electrodes on middle distal phalanges, and index and middle fingers. The wave-like increase in skin conductance begins 1–2 seconds after the onset of stimulus and the peak reaches within 5 seconds.

C. Tests of pupillary functions include:
Pupillary function tests are specifically useful in detecting sympathetic denervation of the iris (e.g. in Horner syndrome). Commonly performed tests are given next.

1. Cocaine Test Cocaine prevents the reuptake of NE at the adrenergic synapse and thus when 4% cocaine is instilled in both eyes, the normal pupil will dilate but the Horner's pupil will not.

2. Adrenaline Test When adrenaline 1 in 1000 strength or 1% noradrenaline is instilled in both the eyes, Horner's pupil dilates more than the normal due to denervation hypersensitivity in the involved eye.

D. Tests of bladder function include:
In autonomic dysfunction, a cystometrogram reveals:

- Absence of accommodation of the urinary bladder in response to bladder filling
- Absence or poor voluntary bladder contraction when asked to micturate (the bladder capacity may be increased to 1 L in advanced cases of autonomic neuropathy)

Invasive Tests

- Intravenous recording of postganglionic sympathetic activity
- Response of ANS to infusion of pressor agents
- Estimation of plasma catecholamine levels

Note: Noninvasive methods are commonly used due to their ease of performance.

Self-Assessment

1. Discuss the function tests to assess cardiovascular autonomic function.
2. Discuss the role of various autonomic neurotransmitters.
3. Describe the following:
   - Cholinergic receptors and their mode of action
   - Autonomic drugs
4. Write notes on the following:
   - Features of autonomic failure
   - Valsalva manoeuvre
   - Effects of stimulation of sympathetic division of ANS

Clinical Cases

Case 1

A 24-year-old male visited the fields in the village; after some time, he developed nausea, vomiting, abdominal pain and difficulty in breathing, and was brought to the emergency.

History revealed that pesticide spray was done in the fields 1 day before he went there and he had eaten raw tomatoes from the field.

Examination showed that the patient's sensorium was disturbed. The probable diagnosis kept in mind was a case of organophosphate poisoning.

Q1. What is the mechanism of action of organophosphate?
Q2. What is the specific treatment for this poisoning?
Q3. What are the supportive measures to relieve the symptoms?

Case 2

A 18-year-old boy on a trekking trip consumed mushroom soup; after 3 hours, he complained of a feeling of nausea, vomiting and extreme warmth, and was brought to the emergency. On examination, the body temperature was found to be raised, and redness of the skin, mouth dryness and blurring of vision were present; there was no sweating and the patient was in a confused state.

Q1. What is the probable diagnosis?
Q2. What tests should be done to confirm the diagnosis?
Q3. What are the complications if the case is not treated properly?
Q4. Which type of mushroom causes such symptoms?
Q5. What is the management plan?

Case 3

65-year-old male diabetic patient complained of dizziness while getting up from the bed, getting up five to six times during night for urgency of urination but expelling out only few drops of urine every time, and difficulty in swallowing.

Examination observations revealed orthostatic hypotension and tachycardia.

Q1. What is the probable diagnosis?
Q2. What tests should be carried out for confirmation of the diagnosis?
Q3. What is the cause for orthostatic hypotension?

Case 4

A 24-year-old female presented to the eye department with drooping down of the left upper eyelid. Examination revealed a small-sized pupil and reduced sweating of the left side of the face.

Q1. What is the diagnosis?
Q2. Why is there drooping of the upper eyelid and a small pupil?
Q3. Which nerve pathway is affected for above-observed signs and symptoms?

10.6 Meninges, Cerebrospinal Fluid, Blood–Brain Barrier and Cerebral Blood Flow

CHAPTER OUTLINE

MENINGES OF THE BRAIN

The brain is enclosed within the cranial cavity by three concentric connective tissue layers – pia mater, arachnoid mater and dura mater – which constitute the meninges of the brain (Fig. 10.6.1).

PIA MATER

Pia mater the delicate inner layer, is a thin and highly vascular membrane. Folds of the pia mater enclose tufts of capillaries called choroid plexuses to form tela choroidea in relation to ventricles of the brain.

ARACHNOID MATER

Arachnoid mater is connected to the pia mater by many filamentous fibres. Subarachnoid space between these two layers is filled with cerebrospinal fluid (CSF).

DURA MATER

Dura mater is composed of two layers – outer endosteal and inner meningeal. These are fused except where folds form (e.g. falx cerebri) or venous sinuses (e.g. superior sagittal sinus) are enclosed between them. *Subdural space* separates the dura mater from the arachnoid mater. The arachnoid mater has minute protrusions (*arachnoid villi*), which pass through fenestrae in the dura mater and project into the venous sinuses to allow escape of CSF into venous sinuses.

CEREBROSPINAL FLUID

Cerebrospinal fluid (CSF) cushions the brain and, along with the blood–brain barrier (BBB), the buffering function of neuroglia and the regulation of CNS circulation, controls the extracellular environment of neurons. Within the substance of brain in the *ventricular system*, there are series of spaces filled with CSF.

COMPOSITION, VOLUME AND PRESSURE OF CSF

Composition of CSF The extracellular fluid within the CNS communicates directly with the CSF. Thus, the composition of CSF indicates the composition of the extracellular environment of the neurons in the brain and spinal cord. The composition of CSF vis-à-vis blood is depicted in Table 10.6.1. The CSF differs from blood in having a lower concentration of K^+, glucose and protein, and a higher concentration of Na^+ and Cl^-. CSF normally lacks blood cells. The increased concentration of Na^+ and Cl^- enables the CSF to be isotonic to blood, despite the much lower concentration of proteins in the CSF.

CSF volume and pressure The cranial cavity contains about 140 mL CSF, 100 mL blood and 200 mL of extracellular fluid in the brain which weighs about 1350 g. Thus, the extracellular fluid space in the cranial cavity totals approximately 440 mL.

The volume of CSF within the cerebral ventricles is approximately 40 mL, and that in the subarachnoid space is about 100 mL. The pressure in the CSF column is about 18–20 cm H_2O when a person is recumbent. Rate of CSF formation (about 0.35 mL/min) is independent of CSF pressure as well as systemic blood pressure.

Important Notes

a. As compared with plasma, CSF has:
   - High concentrations of chloride and magnesium
   - Equal concentration of bicarbonate ions and osmolality
   - Low concentration of K^+, $Ca^{2}+$, glucose, protein and uric acid
b. β-2-Transferrin, which is a product of neuraminidase activity, is present only in CSF.

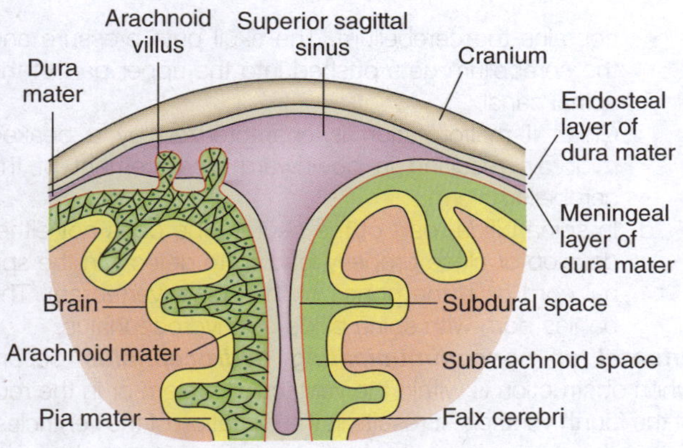

Fig. 10.6.1 Meninges of brain.

Table 10.6.1 Composition of CSF vis-à-vis blood

Constituent	Lumbar CSF	Blood
Na^+ (mEq/L)	148	136–145
K^+ (mEq/L)	2.9	3.5–5
Mg^{2+}	2.2	1.6
Ca^{2+}	2.3	4.7
HCO_3^-	25	24.8
Cl^- (mEq/L)	120–130	100–106
PCO_2 (mm Hg)	50	40
Osmolality (mOsm/kg H_2O)	289	289
Glucose (mg/dL)	50–75	70–100
Protein (mg/dL)	15–45	6.8×10^3
pH	7.3	7.4
Inorganic P (mg/dL)	3.4	4.7
Urea (mg/dL)	120	15.0
Creatinine (mg/dL)	1.5	1.2
Uric acid (mg/dL)	1.5	5.0
Cholesterol (mg/L)	0.2	175.0
Urea (mg/dL)	12.0	15

CSF, cerebrospinal fluid.

FORMATION, CIRCULATION AND ABSORPTION OF CSF

Formation of CSF The CSF is mainly formed by the choroidal plexuses, which are covered by specialized ependymal cells. The *choroidal plexuses* are located in the cerebral ventricles (lateral, third and fourth). About 500 mL of CSF is secreted per day.

Mechanism of formation of CSF: CSF is formed continuously by choroid plexus in two stages:

- *In the first stage*, plasma is passively filtered across the capillary endothelium of the choroid.
- *In the next stage*, ions and water are secreted actively across the choroid endothelium.
- HCO_3^-, Cl^- and K^+ enter the CSF via channels located on the apical membrane of the epithelial cells.
- Water is secreted through aquaporins to maintain osmotic gradient.

Circulation of CSF (Fig. 10.6.2) CSF formed in the lateral ventricles passes through the interventricular foramina (of Monro) into the third ventricle. Thence, the fluid flows through the cerebral aqueduct (aqueduct of Sylvius) into the fourth ventricle. From the fourth ventricle, some CSF passes into the central canal of the spinal cord, but most escapes into the subarachnoid space (surrounding the brain and spinal cord) through the median aperture (foramen of Magendie) of the fourth ventricle and the two lateral apertures of the fourth ventricle (foramina of Luschka).

Subarachnoid cistern refers to the regions where the subarachnoid space is distended to form pools of CSF. An example is the *lumbar cistern*, which surrounds the lumbar and sacral spinal roots below the level of termination of the spinal cord. The lumbar cistern is the target for lumbar puncture, a procedure used clinically to sample the CSF.

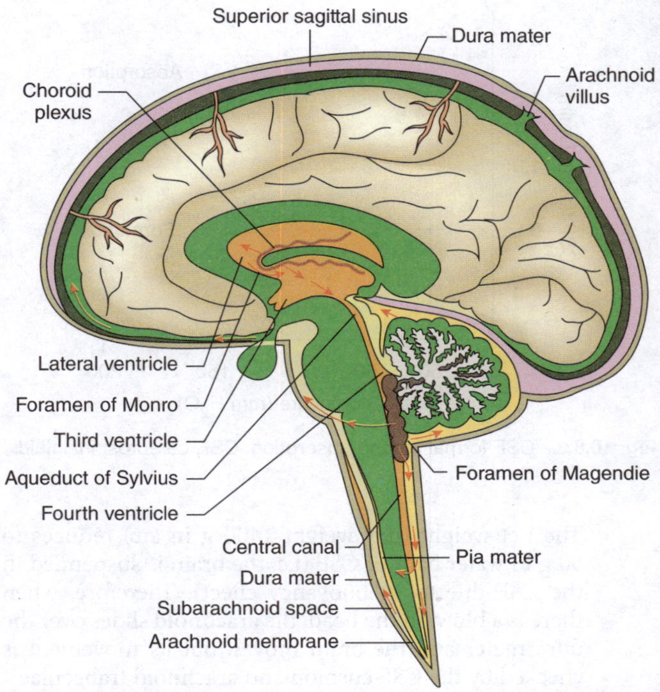

Fig. 10.6.2 Circulation of cerebrospinal fluid. Arrows indicate the direction of flow.

Absorption of CSF A large part of CSF is removed by bulk flow, through the valvular *arachnoid villi* into the dural venous sinuses in the cranium. Unlike rate of formation, the absorption rate of CSF is a direct function of the CSF pressure.

- At normal average CSF pressure (112 mm H_2O), the filtration and absorption are equal, and at pressure 68 mm H_2O, CSF absorption is zero (Fig. 10.6.3).

FUNCTIONS OF CSF

i. **Protects CNS** by acting as a 'water jacket', as it absorbs shock in the event of blow, due to the following effects:
   - The dura mater is attached to the cranial bone firmly and there is no subdural space.
   - The arachnoid mater is being held to the dura mater by surface tension of the thin layer of fluid present between two layers.
   - The brain within the arachnoid is supported by the blood vessels, fibrous arachnoid trabecular and various nerve roots.

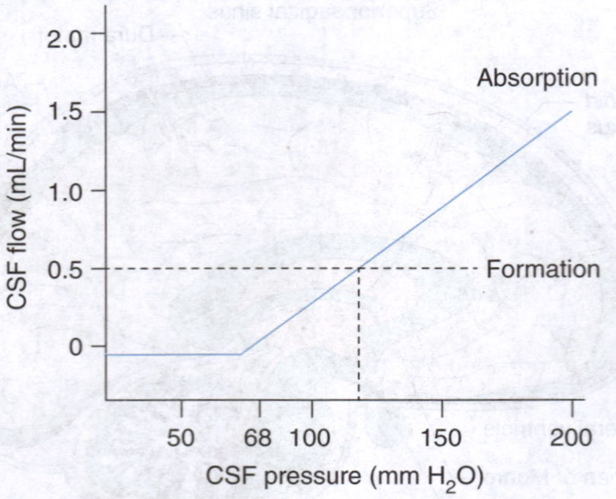

Fig. 10.6.3 CSF formation and absorption. CSF, cerebrospinal fluid.

- The net weight (dry weight 1400 g in air) reduces to 50 g in water bath of CSF (i.e. the brain is suspended in the CSF due to its buoyancy effect). Therefore, when there is a blow on the head, the arachnoid slides over the dura mater and the brain moves, but its movement is checked by the CSF cushion and arachnoid trabeculae.

ii. ***Removes waste products*** of brain metabolism
iii. ***Regulates extracellular environment*** for the neurons of the central nervous system
iv. ***Transports*** hormones and hormone-releasing factors

Applied Aspects

1. Head Injuries

The brain injury occurs most commonly:

- When the skull is fractured and bone is driven into the neural tissue (depressed fracture).
- Due to blow on the head (the brain is accelerated and driven against the skull or tentorium at the point just opposite to where the blow is struck [contrecoup injury])
- When movement of the brain is so strong as to tear the delicate bridging veins from the cortex to the bone

2. Hydrocephalus

Hydrocephalus refers to an abnormal accumulation of CSF in the cranium due to:

- Obstruction to CSF circulation
- Excessive production of CSF
- Interf erence with absorption of CSF

Types of hydrocephalus: The hydrocephalus is of the following types:

Congenital hydrocephalus, the causes of which are as follows:

a. Aqueductal stenosis is one of the known causes of hydrocephalus and the most common cause of congenital hydrocephalus
b. Dandy–Walker malformations an uncommon type of brain malformation in which there is agenesis or hypoplasia of the vermis, resulting in ventricular dilatation and hydrocephalus
c. Chiari I and Chiari II malformations occurs when part of the skull is too small or misshapen and this part contains the cerebellum. The skull puts pressure and the cerebellum gets pushed into the upper part of the spinal canal.
   Chiari II malformation is characterized by a beaked midbrain resulting in downward displacement of the cerebellum vermis.
d. In spina bifida, part of the neural tube does not either develop or close properly leading to defects in the spinal cord or in the bones of the spine (vertebrae). The babies born with spina bifida get hydrocephalus.

Internal or noncommunicating hydrocephalus occurs when obstruction is within the ventricular system or in the roof of the fourth ventricle. It results in the dilatation of the ventricles.

External or communicating hydrocephalus occurs when obstruction is in the subarachnoid space or arachnoid villi. In this, excess fluid is mainly in the subarachnoid space. It occurs mainly due to delay in CSF absorption.

The arachnoid granulations often suffer from moderate obstruction in patients suffering from cerebral meningitis or haemorrhage into the subarachnoid space.

In infants, there is a rapid increase in head size, sleepiness and vomiting.

Older people may have severe headache, double vision, urinary incontinence and personality changes.

Diagnosis. To diagnose hydrocephalus, ultrasound, MRI scan or CT scan help to confirm the enlargement of the ventricles.

Management of hydrocephalus:

- Ventriculostomy is performed for ventricular drainage for symptomatic relief.
- Ventricular CSF shunting is the best treatment for chronic hydrocephalus.

3. Pseudotumour Cerebri

Pseudotumour cerebri, also called benign intracranial hypertension, is characterized by elevated CSF pressure.

- It usually affects obese females in the age group of 30–45 years. The main cause of pseudotumour cerebri is drug toxicity like tetracycline, corticosteroids and nalidixic acid.
- The main presenting symptom is headache that worsens with Valsalva manoeuvre.
- On fundus examination, papilloedema is observed.

Treatment: Diuretics like acetazolamide and frusemide are effective in lowering the intracranial pressure.

4. CSF Rhinorrhoea

Leaking of clear CSF through nares occurs in facial trauma. The condition usually resolves within 7–14 days.

5. CSF Otorrhoea

Leakage of CSF from ear occurs due to temporal bone fracture.

Lumbar and Cisternal Puncture

Lumbar puncture refers to tapping of CSF from the lumbar cistern. CSF examination is required in many disorders of CNS. It is performed by inserting a needle in between the L_2 and L_3 or the L_3 and L_4 vertebrae.

Cisternal puncture refers to tapping of CSF from the cisterna magna. To do this, a needle is passed through the posterior atlanto-occipital membrane, forwards and upwards, to a depth of 4.5 cm from the surface.

CSF analysis reveals the following:

a. ***Colour:*** Yellow-coloured CSF (xanthochromic) indicates bleeding into the subarachnoid space.
b. ***Presence of leucocytes*** indicates infection of the meninges (meningitis). Predominant presence of different leucocytes in CSF indicates:
   - Neutrophils: Bacterial meningitis
   - Eosinophils: Parasitic meningitis
   - Lymphocytes: Viral meningitis
c. ***Presence of immunoglobulins (IgG)*** is suggestive of multiple sclerosis.
d. ***RBCs*** are suggestive of subarachnoid haemorrhage.

Important Note

Post–lumbar puncture headache: Headache after lumbar puncture is quite common. The exact pathophysiology is unclear. However, it may be related to the hole in the dura mater after withdrawal of the needle resulting in persistent leak of CSF from the subarachnoid space. The leakage results in fall in intracranial CSF volume and pressure. The low CSF volume depletes the cushion of fluid supporting the brain and meninges resulting in traction of pain-sensitive intracranial tissue.

Pain worsens in upright posture and reduces on lying down.

BLOOD–BRAIN BARRIER AND BLOOD–CSF BARRIER

BLOOD–BRAIN BARRIER (BBB)

BBB restricts the movement of large molecules and highly charged ions from the blood into the brain and spinal cord. It is formed by CNS capillary endothelial cells, their intercellular junctions (tight junctions) and astrocytic foot processes.

Most substances that must cross the BBB are not lipid soluble, and therefore cross by specific carrier-mediated transport system. Penetration of substances into the brain is as follows:

- *Water* crosses using carrier protein aquaporin-4.
- *CO_2, O_2, lipid-soluble substances and free form of steroid hormone* can penetrate the brain easily, whereas all proteins and polypeptides do not.
- *Glucose,* the main source of energy for neurons, crosses the BBB very slowly but can be transported into CSF rapidly by specific glucose transporters (GLUT-1). In the brain, two forms of GLUT-1 exist, i.e. GLUT-1 55K and GLUT-1 45K. Though both forms are encoded by the same gene, they differ due to the extent they are glycosylated. For details of glucose transporters, see page 635.
- *P-glycoprotein,* also called multidrug resistance protein-1 (MRP-1), is a nonspecific transporter present in the apical membrane of the endothelial cells. This multidrug nonspecific transporter transports a large number of drugs or peptides back into the blood which cross cerebral capillaries.

Important Notes

- In the absence of this transporter, the concentration of various chemotherapeutic agents, analgesic and opioid peptide is higher than in control. Therefore, the inhibitors of this transporter can be of great value for achieving proper concentration of therapeutic treatment of CNS disorders and tumours.
- Drugs like verapamil (Ca^{2+} channel blocker) and cyclosporine inhibit the function of P-glycoprotein. Therefore, these drugs are used along with protease inhibitors for controlling CNS infections.

Circumventricular organs (Fig. 10.6.4) Some areas of the brain do not have a BBB, e.g. posterior pituitary and circumventricular organs. The absence of BBB in these regions is consistent with their physiological functions. These leaky regions are isolated from the rest of the brain by specialized ependymal cells called *tanycytes*. These areas are as follows:

- Posterior pituitary (neurohypophysis) and ventral part of medial eminence
- Area postrema
- Organum vasculosum of lamina terminalis (OVLT)
- Subfornical organs (SFO)

Functions Being outside the BBB, they function as:

Neurohaemal organs: The secreted polypeptides (neurohormones) by the neurons enter the circulation.

Chemoreceptor zone: They also contain receptors for many different types of peptides and other substances. The circulating substances act on these receptors and thus trigger change in brain activity, e.g.:

- Area postrema, also called chemoreceptor trigger zone for emesis, induces vomiting by chemotherapy induced by chemotherapy.
- Angiotensin II acts on OVLT (osmoreceptor) to increase water intake.

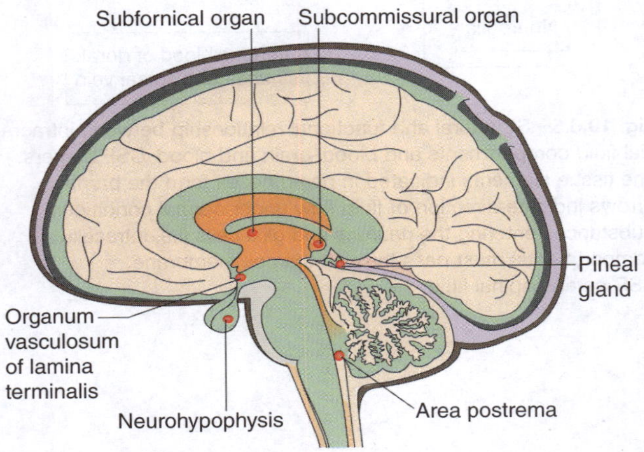

Fig. 10.6.4 Circumventricular organs.

Applied Aspects

Disruption of BBB occurs in a variety of pathological situations such as brain tumours and bacterial meningitis. This fact can be exploited radiologically by introducing into the circulation a substance that normally cannot penetrate the BBB. If the substance can be imaged, its leakage into the region occupied by the brain tumour can be used to demonstrate the distribution of tumour.

Kernicterus: The BBB is immature at birth; therefore, in severely jaundiced infants with high levels of bilirubin (due to hepatic-bilirubin-conjugating system immaturity), bilirubin enters the brain and damages the basal ganglia leading to kernicterus. For details, see page 922.

Crigler–Najjar syndrome: Congenital deficiency of glucuronyl transferase leading to high levels of free bilirubin in blood causes encephalopathy but does not cause brain damage.

Blood–CSF Barrier

The capillaries that traverse the choroidal plexuses are freely permeable to plasma solutes. However, a barrier (blood–CSF barrier) exists at the level of epithelial cells that make up the choroid plexuses. This barrier is responsible for carrier-mediated active transport.

Relationship between intracranial fluid compartments and the BBB and blood–CSF barrier is shown in Fig. 10.6.5.

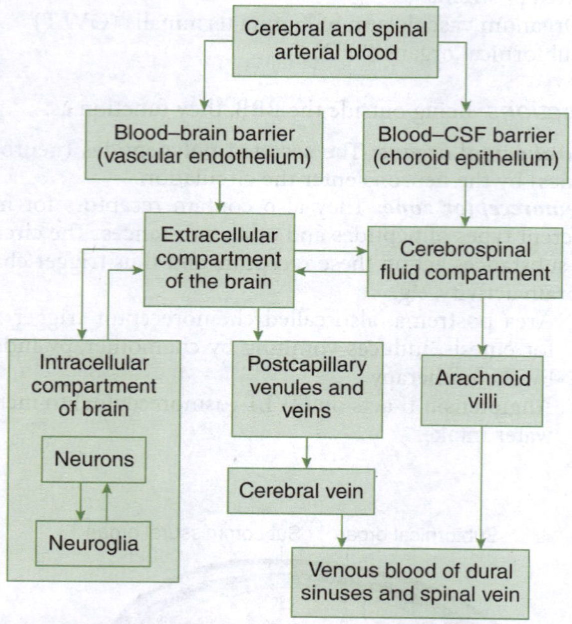

Fig. 10.6.5 Structural and functional relationship between intracranial fluid compartments and blood–brain and blood–CSF barriers. The tissue elements indicated in parentheses form the barrier. Arrows indicate direction of fluid flow under normal conditions. Substances entering the neurons and glial cells (i.e. intracellular compartments) must pass through the cell membrane. CSF, cerebrospinal fluid.

CEREBRAL BLOOD FLOW

Functioning of the brain is closely related to the level of cerebral blood flow. Total cessation of blood flow to the brain causes unconsciousness within 5–10 seconds because of the decrease in oxygen delivery and the resultant cessation of metabolic activity.

Normal cerebral blood flow in an adult averages 50–65 mL/100 g or 750–900 mL/min. Thus, the brain receives approximately 15% of the total resting cardiac output.

Details of cerebral blood flow are given on page 352.

Self-Assessment

1. Discuss the composition, formation, route of circulation and functions of cerebrospinal fluid.
2. Describe the following:
   - Significance of blood–brain barrier
   - Hydrocephalus
3. Write notes on the following:
   - Circumventricular organs
   - Significance of P glycoprotein

Clinical Cases

Case 1

The parents visited the paediatric department with their 4-month-old male baby. They had noticed an increase in the size of the head of the baby at 3 months of age and since then it was increasing gradually. There was no history of infection. On examination of other systems, no abnormality was detected. Cranial ultrasound scan showed bilateral ventriculomegaly.

Q1. What is the diagnosis?
Q2. What are the common causes for this condition?
Q3. What is the management plan for this condition?

Case 2

A 40-year-old female suffering from carcinoma breast is on chemotherapy. After chemotherapy infusion, she usually has nausea, vomiting, light-headedness and excessive salivation.

Q1. What is the pathophysiology of chemotherapy-induced nausea and vomiting?
Q2. Which area of the brain is responsible for induction of vomiting?

Synaptic Transmission 10.7

CHAPTER OUTLINE

SYNAPSE: DEFINITION AND TYPES

DEFINITION

The synapse is the anatomic site where the nerve cells communicate among themselves. The term synapse was coined by Sir Charles Sherrington – father of neurophysiology.

There is no anatomical connection or continuity between different neurons. They are connected only functionally. So, a synapse is the functional junction between two neurons.

TYPES OF SYNAPSES

A. Anatomical Types

Depending on the manner an axon terminates on the other neurons, the synapses can be of the types given next (Fig. 10.7.1).

1. Axodendritic synapse Axodendritic synapse (Fig. 10.7.1A) is the synapse between axon of a neuron and dendrite of another neuron. It is the most common type of synapse. Synapse on dendrites may be located on spines or on the smooth areas between spines (Fig. 10.7.2).

2. Axosomatic synapse Axosomatic synapse (Fig. 10.7.1B) refers to the synapse between axon of a neuron with the soma (body) of another neuron.

3. Axoaxonic synapse Axoaxonic synapse (Fig. 10.7.1C) is the synapse between axon of a neuron and axon of another neuron. It is a less common type of synapse. An axoaxonal synapse may be located either on the initial segment (of the receiving axon) or just proximal to an axon terminal.

In some parts of the brain (e.g. thalamus), some synapses are seen in which the presynaptic element is a dendrite instead of an axon. Such synapses may be *dendroaxonic* or *dendrodendritic*. In yet others, the soma of the neuron may synapse with the soma of a neuron (*somatosomatic synapse*) or with a dendrite (*somatodendritic synapse*).

B. Physiological Types

Depending on the process of transmission of impulse, the synapses can be classified as:

1. Chemical synapses are those in which transmission is carried out by a *neurotransmitter*. Most synapses in the human nervous system are of this type. Chemical synapses conduct information only in one direction. These synapses are more vulnerable to fatigue on repeated stimulation (*synaptic fatigue*) and to the effects of hypoxia and pH changes. Chemical synaptic transmission is definitely slower than the velocity of nerve conduction resulting in the synaptic delay.

Chemical synapses are of two types:

- Type I
- Type II

2. Electrical synapses are those in which transmission occurs through gap junctions. Transmission at electrical synapses is essentially an electronic conduction between two

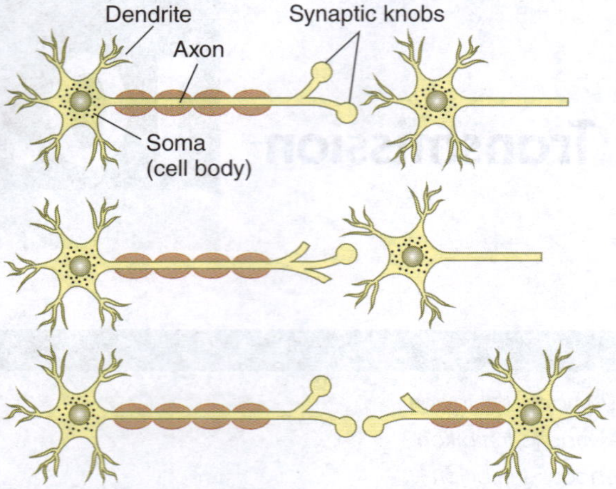

Fig. 10.7.1 Types of synapses depending on the manner an axon terminates on the other neuron: **A**, axodendritic synapse; **B**, axosomatic synapse; and **C**, axoaxonic synapse.

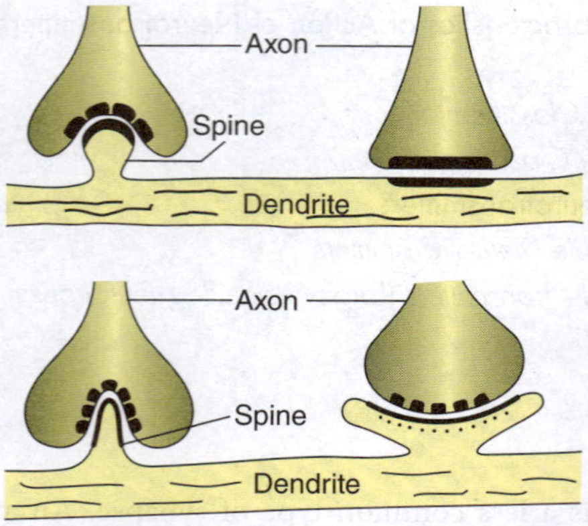

Fig. 10.7.2 Variations in the orientation of axodendritic synapses.

neurons. It is similar to the process of nerve conduction. The electrical synapses can conduct in both directions. The speed of transmission at electrical synapses is the same as that of nerve conduction.

Electrical transmission is seen in a few locations (e.g. within the retina and olfactory bulb) in the human nervous system. It is found mainly in invertebrates and lower vertebrates.

3. Conjoint synapse refers to a synapse in which both the chemical and the electrical transmissions coexist.

CHEMICAL SYNAPSE

STRUCTURE OF A CHEMICAL SYNAPSE

As mentioned earlier, the synapse is the functional junction between two neurons. A typical chemical synapse between the axon of one neuron and the dendrite of another neuron exhibits the characteristics given next (Fig. 10.7.3).

Synaptic knob or button As the axon of a neuron approaches the synapse, it loses the myelin sheath and divides into a number of fine branches which end in small swellings called the *synaptic knobs* or *synaptic buttons*, which make synapse with the soma or dendrite of the postsynaptic neuron. Each synaptic knob

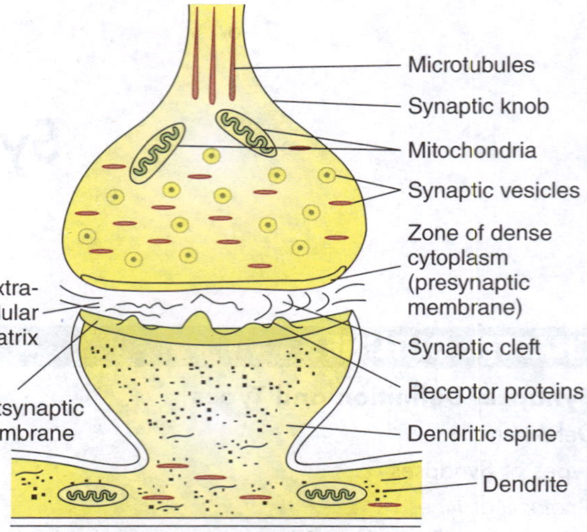

Fig. 10.7.3 Structure of a chemical synapse.

contains a large number of mitochondria and synaptic vesicles containing neurotransmitter. Mitochondria provide adenosine triphosphate (ATP) required for synthesis of neurotransmitter.

There are three types of synaptic vesicles:

Small clear vesicles contain acetylcholine (ACh), glycine or γ-aminobutyric acid (GABA).
Small vesicles with dense core contain catecholamines.
Large vesicles with dense core contain neuropeptides as transmitters.

Besides the neurotransmitter, the vesicles also contain other proteins to bind the neurotransmitter to the vesicle. The microtubules present in the synaptic knob transport the vesicles along the axons up to the presynaptic grid. Cross-bridges have been observed between the vesicles and the microtubules suggesting that the mechanism of transport of the vesicles along the microtubules may be similar to the sliding of actin on myosin filament.

Presynaptic membrane Presynaptic membrane refers to the axonal membrane lining the synaptic knobs. On the inner aspect of the presynaptic membrane are present *zones of dense cytoplasm*, which presumably form a *presynaptic vesicular grid* for organized channelling of the vesicles to the presynaptic membrane at a site opposite to the receptors on the postsynaptic membrane.

Synaptic cleft Synaptic cleft is a small gap (20–40 nm wide) between the pre- and postsynaptic membranes. It is filled by the extracellular fluid containing some glycoproteins. A neurotransmitter is released into this cleft from the presynaptic membranes. Enzymes present in the cleft destroy the neurotransmitter. The extracellular matrix may be acting as an adherent between synaptic neurons. Postsynaptic process is the name given to the region of the receiving neuron (e.g. dendritic spine) where the synaptic knob synapses.

Postsynaptic membrane Postsynaptic membrane is the membrane lining the postsynaptic process. On the inner aspect of the postsynaptic membrane is present a *zone of dense cytoplasm* which constitutes the active zone of a synapse. The postsynaptic membrane contains a large number of receptor proteins which protrude outwards in the synaptic cleft. A neurotransmitter released in the synaptic cleft binds with these receptor proteins to cause the effect.

Table 10.7.1 Features of type I and type II chemical synapses

Feature	Type I or asymmetric synapses	Type II or symmetric synapses
• Structure	Asymmetric	Symmetric
• Synaptic cleft	Wider (about 30 nm)	Narrower (about 20 nm)
• Thickening of postsynaptic membrane	Marked	Less marked
• Dense extracellular material in the synaptic cleft	Present	Absent
• Shape of vesicles	Small spherical and dense cored	Flat or elongated
• Neurotransmitters released	Acetylcholine, glutamate or serotonin is released by spherical vesicles; dense-core vesicles release noradrenaline, adrenaline or dopamine	GABA, glycine
• Type of effect	Mostly excitatory	Mostly inhibitory
• Type of synapse	Usually axodendritic	Usually axosomatic

GABA, γ-aminobutyric acid.

Receptor proteins are of two types:

1. ***Ion channel receptor proteins:*** These line the ion channels (Na^+, K^+, Cl^-, etc.) and the neurotransmitter released in the cleft causes opening of the channels by reacting with these receptor proteins.
2. ***Enzymatic type of receptor proteins:*** The neurotransmitter released in the cleft reacts with enzymatic type of receptor proteins and causes the following effects:
   - Activation of cellular gene for manufacture of additional receptor protein channels in the membrane
   - Activation of protein kinase which decreases the number of receptor protein channels in the membrane (thus, there occurs alteration in the reactivity of the neuron to the transmitter; such effects are called *synaptic modulator effects*)

Types of Chemical Synapses

On the basis of the ultrastructure and neurotransmitter present, two types of chemical synapses have been distinguished by Golgi – type I or asymmetric synapses and type II or symmetric synapses. Their features are summarized in Table 10.7.1.

PROCESS OF CHEMICAL SYNAPTIC TRANSMISSION

Most synapses within the central nervous system (CNS) use chemical transmitters. The sequence of events which occurs during chemical synaptic transmission is as follows:

- Release of neurotransmitter
- Development of the excitatory postsynaptic potential (EPSP) or inhibitory postsynaptic potential (IPSP)
- Removal of neurotransmitter from the synaptic cleft
- Development of action potential (AP)

A. Release of Neurotransmitter

The steps involved in release of neurotransmitter are as follows:

- When the nerve impulse (AP) travelling in a nerve fibre (axon) reaches the nerve terminal (synaptic knobs), there occurs depolarization of the presynaptic terminal.
- As a result of depolarization, the voltage-gated Ca^{2+} channels present on the presynaptic membrane open up, increasing its permeability to Ca^{2+} ions. Consequently, the Ca^{2+} ions present in the ECF of synaptic cleft enter the axon terminal.
- The elevated Ca^{2+} levels in the cytosol of axon terminal stimulate the sliding of synaptic vesicles along the presynaptic grid towards the presynaptic membrane, presumably by triggering the cross-bridge movements.
- Synaptic vesicles discharge their contents through a small hole in the cell membrane, and then the membrane reseals and the main vesicle remains inside the cell. This phenomenon of discharge of neurotransmitter is called *kiss-and-run discharge*.
- This results in marked increase in exocytosis of vesicles releasing neurotransmitter into the synaptic cleft (Fig. 10.7.4). Usually, only one type of neurotransmitter is released from all the terminals of a single neuron. This was first *propounded* by Dale, and is called *Dale's phenomenon*.

Important Note

Neurexins (NRXN) are proteins bound to the presynaptic membrane; these cell adhesion proteins present in the presynaptic terminals play an important role in neurotransmission. There are more than 1000 different types of neurexins that provide synapse specificity.

- The proteins involved during the process of vesicle docking and fusion with nerve endings are as follows:
  - V-snare protein (synaptosome-associated protein [SNAP]), responsible for fusion of vesicle to cell membrane
  - Synaptobrevin responsible for docking the vesicle membrane with t-SNARE protein (syntaxin) in the cell membrane
  - Multiprotein complex regulated by small GTPases such as Rab-3 (Fig. 10.7.5)
- After being released from the presynaptic terminal, the transmitter diffuses across the synaptic cleft and binds to the postsynaptic receptors. The time lapse (<1 millisecond) occurring between the arrival of nerve impulse at the presynaptic terminal and the effect of neurotransmitter on the postsynaptic membrane is called *synaptic delay*.

B. Development of Excitatory Postsynaptic Potential and Inhibitory Postsynaptic Potential

Binding of the neurotransmitter to the postsynaptic receptors causes the opening of channels through which ions can flow. Both excitatory and inhibitory receptors exist on the postsynaptic membrane.

Excitatory postsynaptic potential EPSP, i.e. depolarization of the postsynaptic membrane, is produced by the excitatory neurotransmitters. The most common excitatory neurotransmitter within the CNS is *glutamate*.

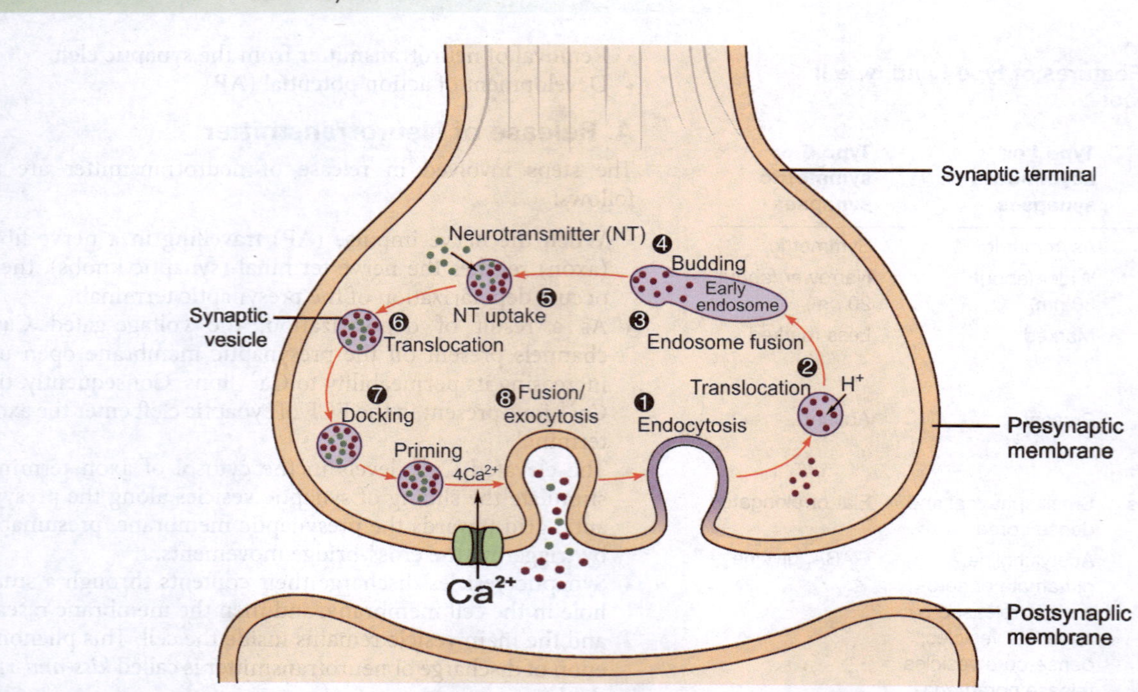

Fig. 10.7.4 Steps of release of neurotransmitter at synaptic cleft and synaptic vesicle cycle in the presynaptic terminal: 1, endocytosis; 2, vesicle formation; 3, endosomal fusion; 4, budding; 5, neurotransmitter uptake; 6, translocation; 7, docking; and 8, exocytosis.

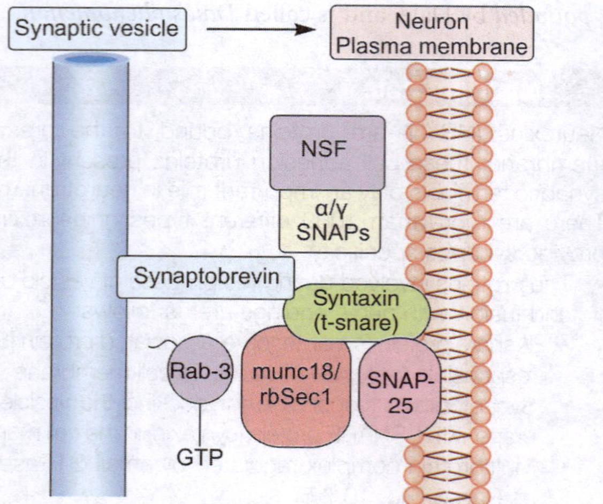

Fig. 10.7.5 Proteins involved during process of synaptic vesicle docking and fusion in nerve endings.

Recording of EPSP The EPSP is a local response. It can be studied by inserting a microelectrode into ventral horn cell of the spinal cord and stimulating the sensory nerve fibres in the dorsal root (Fig. 10.7.6A).

The magnitude of the EPSP is 8 mV. The depolarization starts with a latency of 0.5 millisecond, rises to its peak in 2.0 milliseconds and then declines with a half-life of 4.0 milliseconds (Fig. 10.7.6B).

Ionic basis of EPSP The excitatory neurotransmitter binds with a specific receptor protein and opens the ligand-gated Na^+ channels on the postsynaptic membrane. As a result, the Na^+ ions diffuse inward and depolarize the membrane. However, since a very small area of the postsynaptic membrane develops increased Na^+ permeability, the amount of Na^+ influx is able to produce only a brief depolarization followed by a slower decline to resting potential.

Conduction of EPSP The EPSP does not transmit over the cell. However, it can depolarize the adjacent membrane. This occurs passively due to local currents which are set up.

Summation of EPSP The EPSP is a graded response. It does not follow all-or-none law like AP. It shows temporal and spatial summation.

Temporal summation occurs when repeated stimuli are applied at very short intervals (i.e. before the EPSP due to previous stimulus having been decayed). The next stimulus adds to the previous postsynaptic potential producing a large response (Fig. 10.7.7A).

Spatial summation occurs when the postsynaptic membrane receives impulses from a large number of presynaptic terminals simultaneously. The effect of all the impulses is added up and enough transmitter substance is released to cause a greater response (Fig. 10.7.7B).

Both types of summations occur simultaneously in the neuronal pool. When the temporal or more commonly spatial summation brings the membrane potential of the cell to the firing level, an AP is fired and propagated in the postsynaptic neuron.

Inhibitory postsynaptic potential IPSP, i.e. hyperpolarization of the postsynaptic membrane, is produced by the inhibitory neurotransmitters released in the synaptic cleft. The most common inhibitory neurotransmitters within the CNS are *glycine* and GABA. IPSP is produced by stimulation of certain presynaptic fibres which regularly initiate a hyperpolarizing response in spinal motor neurons.

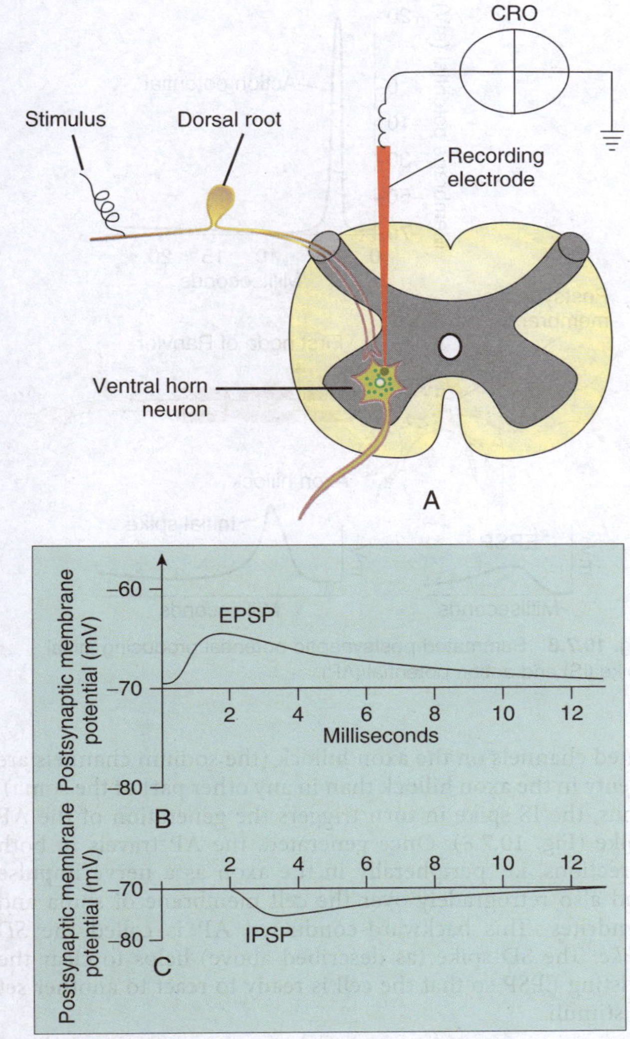

Fig. 10.7.6 Excitatory postsynaptic potential (EPSP) and inhibitory postsynaptic potential (IPSP): **A**, method of recording of EPSP and IPSP; **B**, the record of EPSP; and **C**, the record of IPSP.

Ionic basis of IPSP The inhibitory transmitter released at the synaptic cleft causes opening of either K^+ channels or Cl^- channels in the postsynaptic membrane, leading to diffusion of a large number of K^+ ions from the neuron to the extracellular fluid or diffusion of a large number of Cl^- ions to the interior of the neuron. This causes postsynaptic membrane potential to become more negative (*hyperpolarization*). This change in potential is called IPSP.

Value of IPSP The magnitude of IPSP is −2 mV. The hyperpolarization has a latency of 2.0 milliseconds, attaining its maximum at 4 milliseconds and then returning towards the resting membrane potential (RMP) with a half-life of 3 milliseconds (Fig. 10.7.6C).

Recording of IPSP Recording of IPSP can be made by a technique similar to that of recording of EPSP (Fig. 10.7.6A).

Summation of IPSP Spatial and temporal summation also occurs, as seen with EPSP (Fig. 10.7.7). This type of inhibition is called postsynaptic (or direct) inhibition.

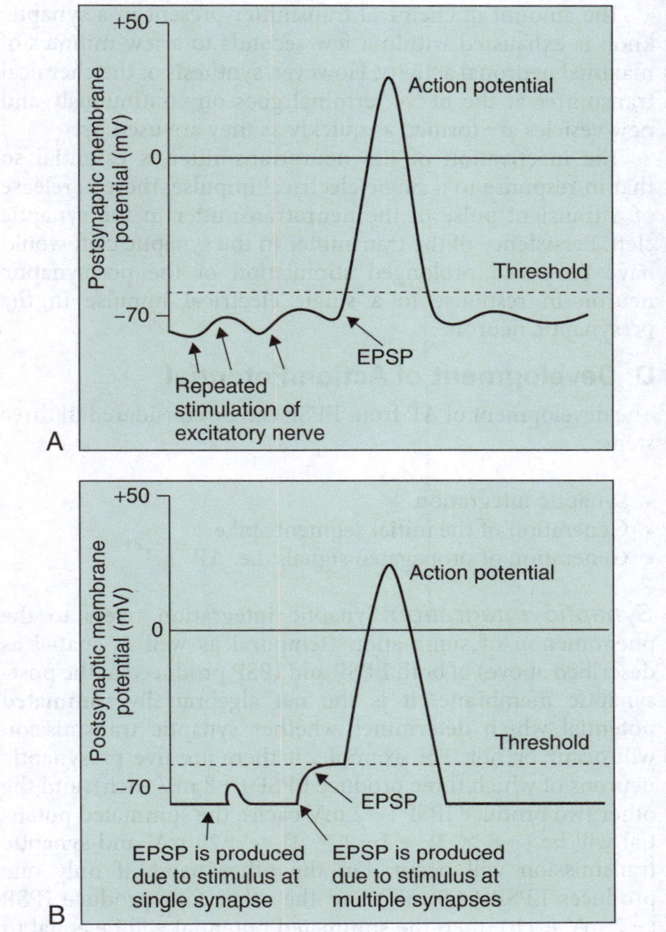

Fig. 10.7.7 Excitatory postsynaptic potential (EPSP) summation resulting in action potential (AP) when threshold is reached: **A**, temporal summation; and **B**, spatial summation.

Arrangement of Neurons Involved in Production of EPSP and IPSP

Afferent fibres in the dorsal nerve root mostly have EPSP-producing terminals (page 978, Fig. 10.7.18). Both afferents A and B release EPSP-producing neurotransmitter. Stimulation of afferent B produces IPSP because of the intervention of Golgi bottle neuron that releases an inhibitory chemical transmitter (glycine) near the ventral horn cells. The Golgi bottle neurons are small plump cells present in the grey matter of the spinal cord, inserted in the pathway between the dorsal root afferents and the ventral horn cells (an interneuron).

C. Inactivation of Neurotransmitter From the Synaptic Cleft

The neurotransmitter released in the synaptic cleft from the presynaptic terminal is soon inactivated in one of the following three ways:

- Diffusion of the transmitter out of the cleft
- Enzymatic degradation of the transmitter, e.g. dissociation of ACh by acetylcholinesterase
- Active transport back into the presynaptic terminal (transmitter reuptake), e.g. active reuptake of norepinephrine (NE) at sympathetic postganglionic nerve endings

The amount of chemical transmitter present in a synaptic knob is exhausted within a few seconds to a few minutes of maximal neuronal activity. However, synthesis of the chemical transmitter at the nerve terminal goes on continuously and new vesicles are formed as quickly as they are used up.

The inactivation of the neurotransmitter is essential so that in response to a single electrical impulse, there is release of a transient pulse of the neurotransmitter in the synaptic cleft. Persistence of the transmitter in the synaptic cleft would have produced prolonged stimulation of the postsynaptic neuron in response to a single electrical impulse in the presynaptic neuron.

D. Development of Action Potential

The development of AP from EPSP can be considered in three steps:

- Synaptic integration
- Generation of the initial segment spike
- Generation of propagated signals, i.e. AP

Synaptic integration Synaptic integration refers to the phenomenon of summation (temporal as well as spatial as described above) of both EPSP and IPSP produced at the post-synaptic membrane. It is the net algebraically summated potential which determines whether synaptic transmission will occur or not. For example, if there are five presynaptic neurons of which three produce EPSP (+8 mV each), and the other two produce IPSP (−2 mV each), the summated potential will be $(+8 \times 3) + (-2 \times 2) = +20$ mV and synaptic transmission will occur. On the other hand, if only one produces EPSP (+8 mV) and the other four produce IPSP (−2 mV each), then the summated potential will be equal to zero and no synaptic transmission will occur.

Important Note

It is important to note that after giving out the summated output (i.e. after synaptic integration), the entire somatodendritic (SD) tree is quickly resorted to its resting potential by the *SD spike*, i.e. the AP that travels retrogradely over the soma and dendrites (as described below). It allows fresh summation of subsequently generated EPSPs and IPSPs.

Generation of initial segment spike The summated potential (EPSP and IPSPs) produced by the excitatory and inhibitory neurotransmitters spreads passively to the initial segment which comprises axon hillock and the proximal part of the unmyelinated nerve fibres. If the summated potential is large enough to depolarize the initial segment of the neuron to the threshold level of about 6–10 mV (the threshold of the initial segment is the lowest as compared with that of the other parts of the nerve fibre), a spike potential called the *initial spike* (IS) is generated (Fig. 10.7.8). The magnitude of IS is 30–40 mV from the threshold level.

Generation of propagated signals, i.e. action potential The IS spike requires a relatively low degree of depolarization for its own production (due to low threshold value of the initial segment), but once initiated, it itself produces a further depolarization of 30–40 mV by opening the voltage-gated channels on the axon hillock (the sodium channels are plenty in the axon hillock than in any other part of the soma). Thus, the IS spike in turn triggers the generation of the AP spike (Fig. 10.7.8). Once generated, the AP travels in both directions, i.e. peripherally in the axon as a nerve impulse and also retrogradely over the cell membrane of soma and dendrites. This backward-conducted AP is called the *SD spike*. The SD spike (as described above) helps to clear the existing EPSP so that the cell is ready to react to another set of stimuli.

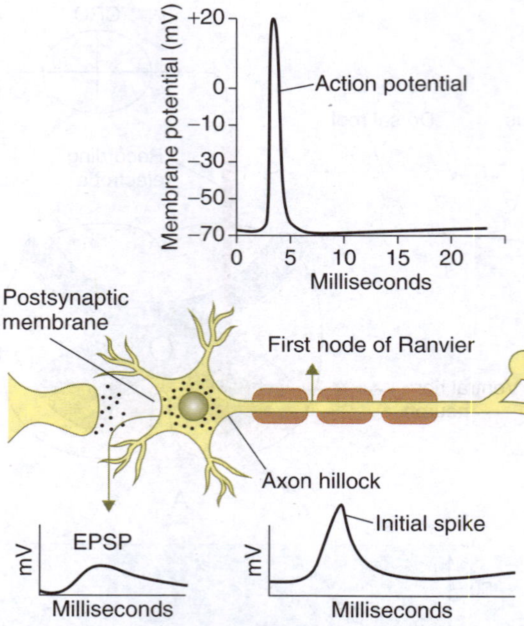

Fig. 10.7.8 Summated postsynaptic potential producing initial spike (IS) and action potential (AP).

INHIBITION AT SYNAPSES

Four different types of inhibitions known to occur at synapses in the CNS are as follows:

- Postsynaptic inhibition
- Presynaptic inhibition
- Feedback inhibition
- Feed-forward inhibition

1. Postsynaptic Inhibition

The postsynaptic inhibition, i.e. inhibition of the postsynaptic membrane, can occur by the mechanisms given next.

i. Direct postsynaptic inhibition by development of inhibitory postsynaptic potential Direct postsynaptic inhibition by development of IPSP occurs due to release of inhibitory neurotransmitters.

ii. Postsynaptic inhibition without development of IPSP Postsynaptic inhibition without development of IPSP can occur due to some short-circuiting mechanism as described next.

In some neurons, the concentration differences for K^+ and Cl^- ions are such that the Nernst potential of these ions is equal to the RMP of the neuron. Therefore, even if either K^+

or Cl^- channels open, there is no net transfer of ions in either direction and no EPSP can develop. But when the neuron is excited through other synapse causing inflow of Na^+ ions, the rapid flux of K^+ and Cl^- ions (because K^+ and Cl^- channels are open) would nullify EPSP produced. Greater influx of Na^+ is therefore required to overcome K^+ or Cl^- flux and cause excitation (may be 5–20 times the normal). This tendency of K^+ or Cl^- ions to maintain potential to RMP level (when channels are wide open) masks the effect of sodium current flow by excitatory synapse, thus causing inhibition.

iii. Postsynaptic inhibition due to refractory period

Sometimes, the postsynaptic membrane can be refractory to the excitation because it has just fired and is in its refractory period, i.e. existing EPSP has not been still cleared by the SD spike.

2. Presynaptic Inhibition

This is also known as indirect inhibition as IPSP is not produced. In presynaptic inhibition, the excitability of the postsynaptic cell is not diminished, whereas in postsynaptic inhibition, the IPSP reduces the effectiveness of all excitatory input to a cell. Presynaptic inhibition allows a particular excitatory input to be inhibited without affecting the ability of other excitatory synapses to fire the cells. It occurs because of the failure of the release of excitatory neurotransmitter substance from the presynaptic axon terminal. This occurs in synapses in which an inhibitory neuron (neuron C in Fig. 10.7.9) synapses with the afferent fibres of an excitatory neuron (neuron A in Fig. 10.7.9) before the latter synapses with the afferent neuron (neuron B in Fig. 10.7.9). In other words, the presynaptic inhibition occurs because of axoaxonic synapse. There are two mechanisms by which presynaptic release of neurotransmitter is decreased.

i. By opening Cl^- channels of presynaptic terminal

The inhibitory neuron (neuron C in Fig. 10.7.9) releases an inhibitory neurotransmitter (i.e. GABA) which binds to GABA-gated Cl^- channels on the presynaptic neuron terminal (neuron A in Fig. 10.7.9). Increase in Cl^- permeability results in hyperpolarization of the presynaptic axon terminal (neuron A). When an AP arrives at the presynaptic terminal, the size of AP is reduced because of the increased Cl^- conductance. Because of smaller size of AP, less Ca^{2+} enters the nerve terminal, and thus the amount of excitatory neurotransmitter released is markedly decreased.

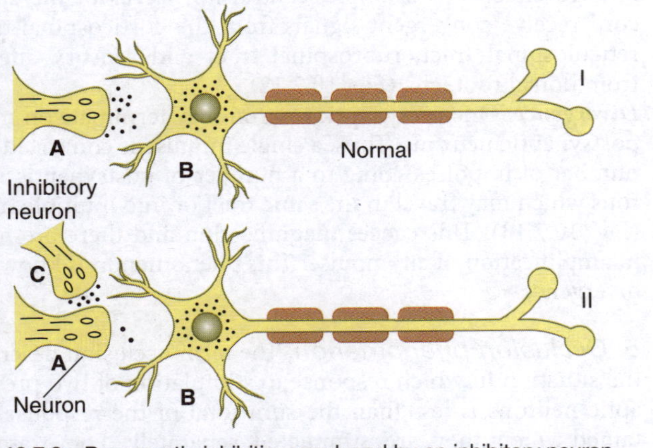

Fig. 10.7.9 Presynaptic inhibition produced by an inhibitory neuron (C) which synapses with presynaptic axon terminal (A), i.e. by axoaxonic synapse. **I**, Normal excitatory neurotransmitter released by presynaptic terminal (A); and **II**, reduced excitatory neurotransmitter released by presynaptic terminal (A) due to effect of inhibitory neuron (C).

ii. By activation of G protein

When the inhibitory transmitter GABA released from the inhibitory neuron (neuron C in Fig. 10.7.9) binds to a receptor called a *GABA receptor*, it activates a *G protein*. The G protein aids in reducing the amount of excitatory neurotransmitter released from the presynaptic terminal (neuron A) by acting in one of the following two ways:

By opening K^+ channels: The G proteins may open K^+ channels that reduce the size of AP reaching the nerve terminal by hyperpolarizing the presynaptic nerve terminal.

By directly blocking the Ca^{2+} channels: The G protein may directly block the opening of Ca^{2+} channels that normally occurs when the AP reaches the nerve terminal; consequently, less Ca^{2+} enters the presynaptic terminal and the amount of excitatory neurotransmitter release is diminished.

3. Feedback Inhibition

The feedback inhibition, also known as *Renshaw cell inhibition*, is known to occur in spinal α-motor neurons through an inhibitory interneuron (the Renshaw cell, Fig. 10.7.10). In feedback (or recurrent) inhibition, a neuron inhibits those very neuron(s) that excite it. In other words, a neuron is inhibited by its own output (that is why it is called negative feedback inhibition). In this way, firing of an AP by a motor neuron of the spinal cord is followed by a phase of hyperpolarization (inhibition) of not only the same motor neuron but also many others in the neighbourhood. The feedback inhibition is thus basically a postsynaptic inhibition but is classified separately because the inhibitor Renshaw cells are activated by a collateral of the ventral horn cell rather than an afferent neuron. This type of feedback inhibition is also seen in other parts of CNS. It serves to limit the excitability of the motor neurons.

4. Feed-Forward Inhibition

Feed-forward inhibition is seen in the cerebellum. In this type of inhibition, a neuron is connected through two pathways – one excitatory and other inhibitory. For example, in the cerebellum, the granule cell (GrC) excites Purkinje cells (PC),

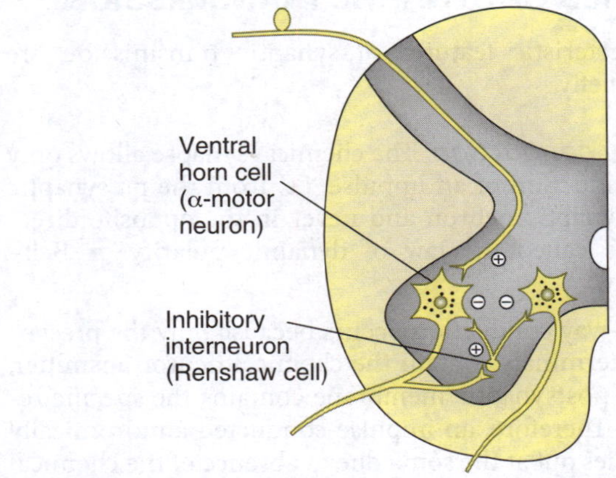

Fig. 10.7.10 Renshaw cell when excited by a recurrent branch of an α motor neuron produces feedback inhibition of the soma of the same and other motor neurons.

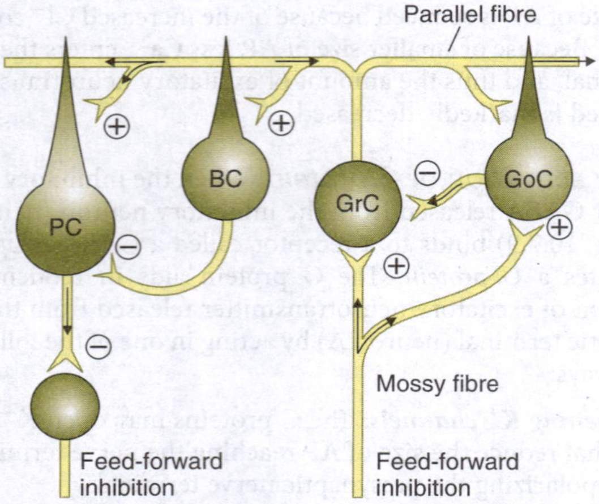

Fig. 10.7.11 Feed-forward inhibition of Purkinje cell (PC) by basket cell (BC). Note that both PC and BC are excited by the granule cell (GrC).

which is soon inhibited by the basket cell (BC), which in turn was also excited by the GrC (Fig. 10.7.11). This type of arrangement in the cerebellum limits the duration of excitation produced by any given afferent volley, i.e. allows a brief and precisely timed excitation. For details, see page 905.

Significance of Synaptic Inhibition

In CNS, the synaptic inhibition offers a type of restriction over neurons and muscles to react properly and appropriately. Thus, the inhibition helps to select the exact number of impulses and to omit or block the excess ones. When the inhibitory system at the synaptic level is destroyed, for example:

- By a poison like strychnine, there occurs continuous and convulsive activity even with slight stimulation. In the nervous disorders like parkinsonism, the inhibitory system is impaired resulting in rigidity.
- *Clostridium tetani* releases the toxin tetanospasmin that travels to the spinal cord and inhibits Renshaw cells to release neurotransmitter glycine (an inhibitory neurotransmitter). As a result, the α-motor neurons become hyperactive.
- Therefore, the muscles remain in the contracted state (spasticity).

PROPERTIES OF SYNAPTIC TRANSMISSION

Some characteristic features of synaptic transmission are described briefly.

1. One-way conduction The chemical synapse allows only one-way conduction of an impulse, i.e. from the presynaptic to the postsynaptic neuron and never in the opposite direction. This is called the law of dynamic polarity or Bell–Magendie law.

Cause: One-way conduction occurs because only the presynaptic nerve terminals contain the chemical neurotransmitter, whereas the postsynaptic membrane contains the specific receptor sites. Therefore, an impulse conducted antidromically in an axon dies out at the soma due to absence of the chemical transmitter in the cell body.

Significance: The axons can conduct impulse in either direction with equal ease. However, the synapses act like a valve and are responsible for the orderly conduction of impulse in one direction only.

2. Synaptic delay Synaptic delay refers to a time lapse which occurs between arrival of nerve impulse at the presynaptic terminal and its passage to the postsynaptic membrane. Normally, synaptic delay occurs by approximately 0.5 millisecond (almost always less than 1 millisecond).

Causes of synaptic delay include time taken for:

- Release of neurotransmitter
- Diffusion of transmitter through the synaptic cleft to the postsynaptic membrane
- Action of neurotransmitter to bind with receptors on the postsynaptic membrane and to cause the opening of ion channels
- Diffusion of ions causing changes in RMP (i.e. development of EPSP or IPSP)

Significance: When an impulse passes through a chain of neurons, it is delayed at every synapse. The synaptic delay is one of the causes for the latent period of the reflex activity. The number of neurons involved in the reflex can be estimated from the duration of reaction time of a reflex action.

3. Summation property of synapse A synapse exhibits property of both temporal and spatial summation of EPSP and IPSP (see page 972).

Significance: Excitation of a single presynaptic terminal almost never excites (or inhibits) the postsynaptic neuron as sufficient neurotransmitter is not released to raise the EPSP to a threshold level. Therefore, property of summation is essential for stimulation of the postsynaptic membrane either by simultaneous stimulation of a large number of presynaptic terminals on a postsynaptic neuron (spatial summation) or by repeated stimulation of a presynaptic terminal (temporal summation).

4. Convergence and divergence Convergence and divergence property is present in a chemical synapse.

Convergence refers to a phenomenon of termination of signals from many sources (i.e. many presynaptic neurons on a single postsynaptic neuron). Information coming from a large number of presynaptic neurons is integrated to decide the onward effect. For example, ventral horn cells of the spinal cord receive convergent signals from the corticospinal tract, reticulospinal tract, rubrospinal tract and sensory afferent from dorsal root, etc. (Fig. 10.7.12).

Divergence: One presynaptic neuron may terminate on many postsynaptic neurons. Thus, a single impulse is converted to a number of impulses going to a number of postsynaptic neurons which may travel in the same tract or into multiple tracts (Fig. 10.7.13). This causes magnification and therefore helps in amplification of an impulse. This phenomenon is known as divergence.

5. Occlusion phenomenon The term occlusion describes the situation in which response to stimulation of two presynaptic neurons is less than the sum total of the response obtained when they are stimulated separately. For example, when 2 presynaptic neurons (say A and B) are stimulated separately, each stimulates 10 postsynaptic neurons (making a total of 20), but when stimulated simultaneously, they stimulate less than 20 postsynaptic neurons (say 15). This happens

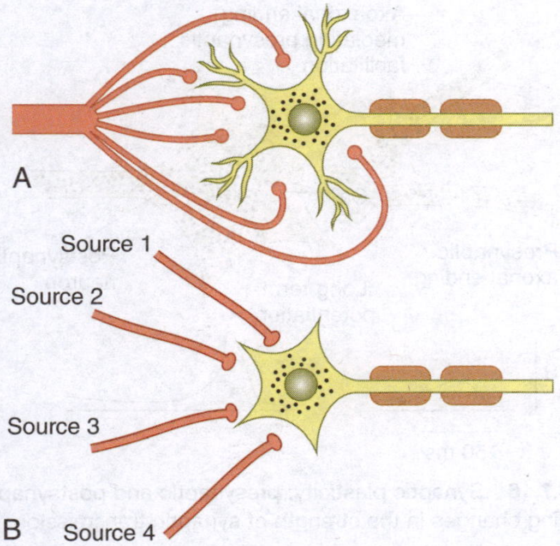

Fig. 10.7.12 Convergence of signals on a single neuron: **A**, convergence from a single source; and **B**, convergence from multiple sources (e.g. ventral horn cell of spinal cord).

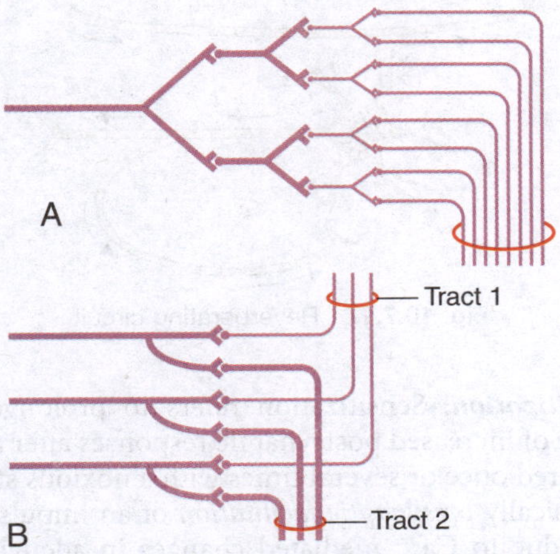

Fig. 10.7.13 Phenomenon of divergence: **A**, divergence in same tract; and **B**, divergence into multiple tracts.

because of the fact that some postsynaptic neurons are common to both the presynaptic neurons (Fig. 10.7.14). Thus, occlusion is due to overlapping of afferent fibres in their central distribution.

6. Subliminal fringe effect An afferent nerve fibre divides into many hundred branches. Of these, a large number may terminate on one efferent neuron, whereas a smaller number terminate on another efferent neuron lying nearby. When an afferent neuron is stimulated, the efferent (postsynaptic) neuron that has many presynaptic terminals is excited to the threshold level and AP is fired. Others in the peripheral zone (fringe area) are excited to the subthreshold level only, i.e. their excitability is increased but an AP is not fired. This is known as *subliminal fringe effect* (subliminal means below threshold and fringe means border). Thus, the postsynaptic neurons that are fired are said to be in the discharging zone and those which are not fired are said to be in the subliminal fringe (i.e. not in the discharging zone).

Because of subliminal fringe effect, the response obtained by the simultaneous stimulation of two presynaptic neurons is

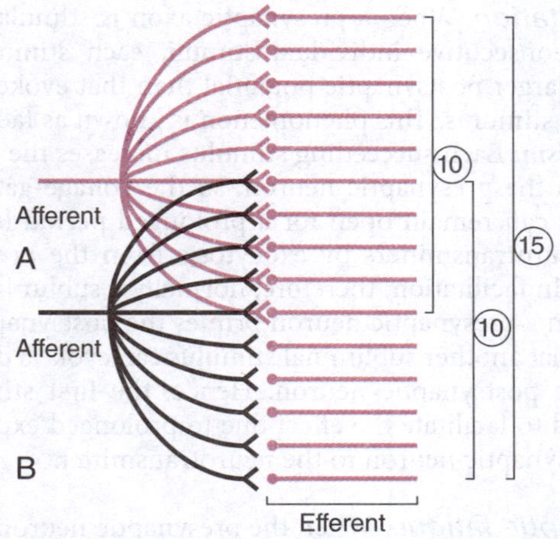

Fig. 10.7.14 Occlusion phenomenon: stimulation of afferent neurons **A** and **B** each excites 10 efferent neurons. Simultaneous stimulation of neurons **A** and **B** together excites 15 efferent neurons because 5 efferent neurons are common to both.

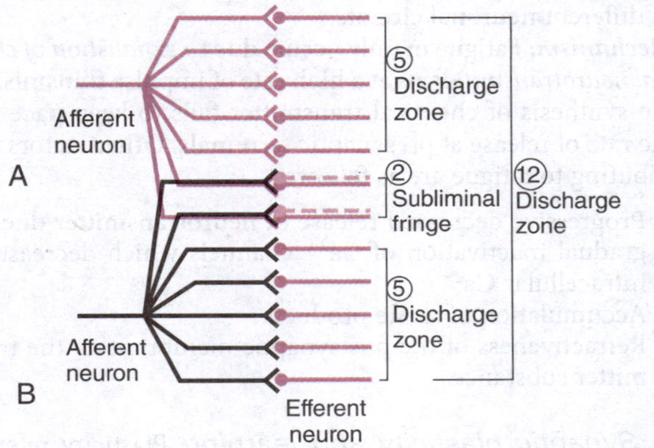

Fig. 10.7.15 Subliminal fringe effect: stimulation of afferent neurons **A** and **B** each excites five efferent neurons and subliminal fringe effect on two efferent neurons (which are common to both **A** and **B** neurons). Simultaneous stimulation of neurons **A** and **B** together excites 12 efferent neurons because the subliminal fringe effect on 2 neurons gets summated to produce threshold stimulation.

greater than the sum total response obtained when they are separately stimulated. This is exactly opposite to occlusion and can be explained as below. Suppose separate stimulation of afferent neurons 'A' and 'B' each causes depolarization of 5 efferent neurons and subliminal fringe effect in 2 efferent neurons; then a total of 10 efferent neurons are stimulated. But when neurons A and B are stimulated simultaneously, the number of postsynaptic neurons stimulated is more (say 12) (Fig. 10.7.15). This is because of the fact that two efferent neurons which are excited subliminally by both the neurons A and B summate to produce threshold stimulation. This is another example of spatial summation.

Physiological significance: As a result of summation, occlusion and subliminal fringe effect, the patterns of impulses in peripheral nerves are usually altered as they pass through synapses on the way to the brain. One such effect is the phenomenon of referred pain (see page 1002).

7. Facilitation When a presynaptic axon is stimulated with several consecutive individual stimuli, each stimulus may evoke a larger postsynaptic potential than that evoked by the previous stimulus. This phenomenon is known as facilitation. ***Mechanism:*** Each succeeding stimulus increases the duration of AP in the presynaptic neuron, so the voltage-gated Ca^{2+} channels can remain open for a prolonged period liberating more neurotransmitters by exocytosis from the presynaptic neuron. In facilitation, therefore, normally a subliminal stimulus from a presynaptic neuron primes the postsynaptic neuron, so that another subliminal stimulus can evoke a discharge from the postsynaptic neuron. Hence, the first stimulus is supposed to facilitate the effect due to prolonged exposure of the postsynaptic neuron to the neurotransmitter.

8. Synaptic fatigue When the presynaptic neuron is stimulated separately, the rate of impulse discharge in the postsynaptic neuron is initially high but within a few seconds there occurs a gradual decrease and finally disappearance of the postsynaptic response. This phenomenon is called *synaptic fatigue* or *habituation*. Fatigue is a temporary phenomenon. Therefore, fatigue and recovery from fatigue constitute an important short-term mechanism for modulating sensitivities of different neuronal circuits.
Mechanism: Fatigue mainly occurs due to *exhaustion of chemical neurotransmitter*, as at a high rate of impulse transmission, the synthesis of chemical transmitter fails to keep pace with the rate of release at presynaptic terminals. Other factors contributing to fatigue are as follows:

- Progressive decreased release of neurotransmitter due to a gradual inactivation of Ca^{2+} channels which decrease the intracellular Ca^{2+}
- Accumulation of waste products
- Refractiveness of the postsynaptic membrane to the transmitter substance

9. Synaptic plasticity and learning Plasticity refers to the capability of being easily moulded or changed. Synaptic transmission can be increased or decreased on the basis of past experience. The changes in synaptic transmission can occur due to alterations at the pre- or postsynaptic location. Plastic changes in synaptic transmission known are as follows:

- Post-tetanic potentiation
- Long-term potentiation
- Synaptic fatigue or habituation
- Sensitization
- Low-frequency depression

i. ***Post-tetanic potentiation:*** When a presynaptic neuron is stimulated with a single stimulus, followed by stimulation with a volley of stimuli (says 100/s) for 2 seconds and then again with a single stimulus, the second stimulus evokes a larger postsynaptic response than the first stimulus. The phenomenon is called post-tetanic potentiation. This occurs due to the fact that a brief tetanizing stimulus in the presynaptic neuron results in an increase in intracellular Ca^{2+} due to increased Ca^{2+} influx (Fig. 10.7.16).

ii. ***Long-term potentiation:*** When the post-tetanic potentiation gets much more prolonged and lasts for days, it is called long-term potentiation. It occurs due to an increase in the intracellular Ca^{2+} in the postsynaptic neuron rather than in the presynaptic neuron. This phenomenon commonly occurs in the hippocampus.

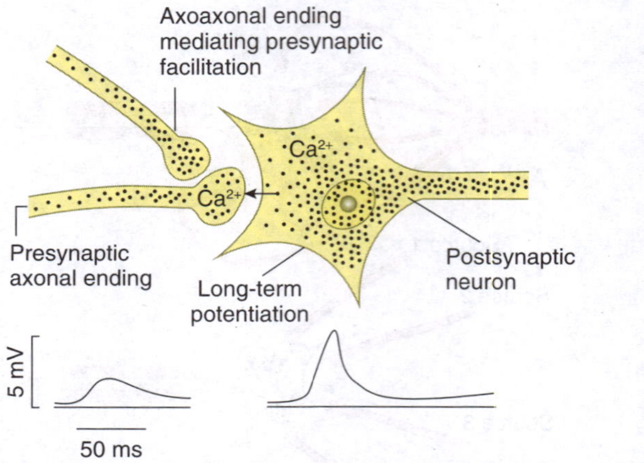

Fig. 10.7.16 Synaptic plasticity: presynaptic and postsynaptic sites producing changes in the strength of synaptic transmission.

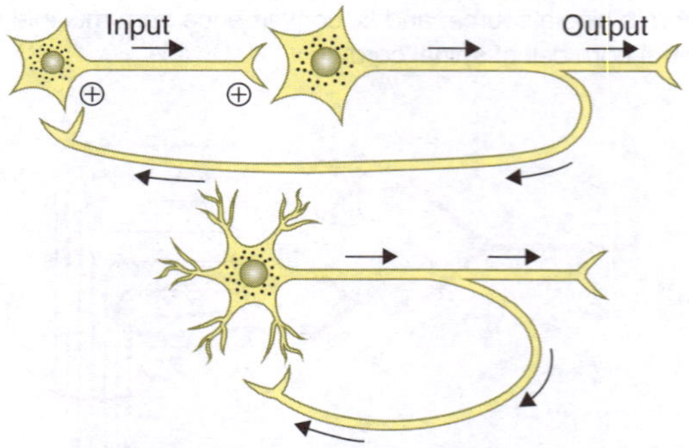

Fig. 10.7.17 Reverberating circuit.

iii. ***Sensitization:*** Sensitization refers to prolonged occurrence of increased postsynaptic responses after a stimulus is paired once or several times with a noxious stimulus. It is basically *presynaptic facilitation* of an impulse that occurs due to Ca^{2+}-mediated changes in adenylyl cyclase that results in greater production of cAMP.

10. Reverberation Reverberation refers to the phenomenon of passage of impulse from the presynaptic neuron and again back to the presynaptic neuron to cause a continuous stimulation of the presynaptic neuron. The nervous system is a network of fibres and in this network it is possible that a branch of axon of a neuron may establish connection with its own dendron. This causes reverberation of impulse through the same circuit again and again (Fig. 10.7.17). This is prevented to some extent by the phenomenon of fatigue.

11. Reciprocal inhibition Reciprocal inhibition refers to a phenomenon in which an afferent signal activates an excitatory neuron to a group of muscles and simultaneously activates inhibitory signals to another, usually antagonistic muscles. For example, during flexion of a joint, the afferent stimulus causes excitation of the neurons supplying the flexor muscles of the joint and at the same time a branch of afferent fibre excites an inhibitory interneuron which synapses with the motor neuron supplying the extensor muscles of the joint (Fig. 10.7.18).

12. Afterdischarge Afterdischarge of a synapse refers to a phenomenon in which a single instantaneous input results in sustained output signals (i.e. a series of repetitive discharges).

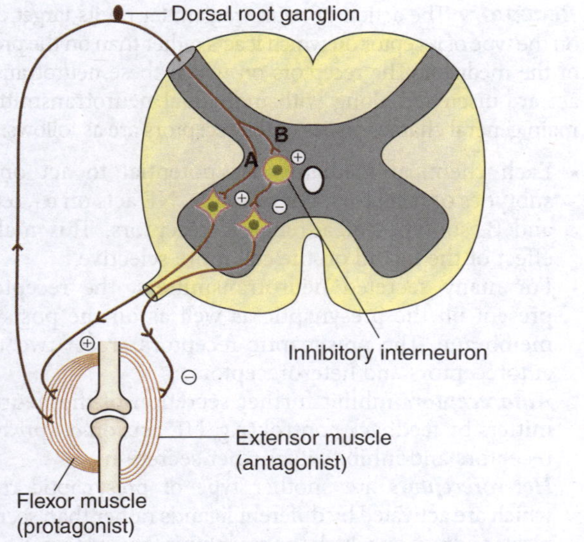

Fig. 10.7.18 Neuronal arrangement of reciprocal inhibition. An afferent stimulus producing contraction of flexors of a joint (through A) and causes inhibition of extensors (through B) by intervention of an inhibitory neuron.

Input signals last only for 1 millisecond and output signal lasts for many milliseconds.

13. Effect of acidosis and hypoxia The CNS neurons cannot sustain lack of oxygen. Synaptic transmission is particularly vulnerable to the effect of acidosis and hypoxia. This may explain why the first site of fatigue of the synaptic chain is located in the brain.

NEUROTRANSMITTERS

DEFINITION

Neurotransmitters are the chemical substances which are responsible for transmission of an impulse through a synapse.

Criteria for a neurotransmitter A chemical substance to be qualified as a neurotransmitter should fulfil the following criteria:

- A neurotransmitter should be synthesized by presynaptic neurons and stored in the vesicles which are present in the axon terminal. The synthesizing enzymes should be present in the nerve at the storage site.
- A neurotransmitter should be released on stimulation of a nerve.
- A neurotransmitter travels a very small distance between the presynaptic membrane and the postsynaptic membrane.
- A neurotransmitter is associated with an enzyme or enzyme system for its inactivation.
- A neurotransmitter when applied extrinsically should mimic the effects of the nerve stimulation.
- Drug, which modifies the response to nerve stimulation, should also modify the proposed transmitter action in a similar way.

Extended definition of neurotransmitter Extended definition of a neurotransmitter also includes, in addition to the principal neurotransmitters, the following chemical substances:

Neuromediators or ***neurohormones:*** These chemical substances are synthesized in neurons and poured into the bloodstream through terminals resembling synapses in structure. Similar chemical substances are also poured into the cerebrospinal fluid or into the intercellular spaces to influence other neurons in a diffuse manner.

Neuromodulators are the chemical substances which are associated with synapses but do not influence synaptic transmission directly, but influence the effects of transmitters or of neuromediators. Several peptides found in the nervous system probably act as neuromodulators. These include substance P, vasoactive intestinal polypeptide (VIP), somatostatin, cholecystokinin (CCK) and many others.

GENERAL CHARACTERISTICS OF ACTION OF NEUROTRANSMITTERS

- The neurotransmitter released from the presynaptic membrane diffuses through the synaptic cleft to the postsynaptic membrane. The postsynaptic cell may be a neuron, muscular cell or glandular cell.
- On the postsynaptic membrane, the neurotransmitter combines with a receptor protein. The receptor of the effector cell may be associated with:
  - Ion channels that alter the membrane potential of the cell
  - An enzyme that results in the formation of a second messenger in the effector cell
- Action of neurotransmitter occurs within milliseconds; therefore, changes induced are fast and direct.
- A neurotransmitter can activate both postsynaptic and presynaptic receptors.
- The neurons may release more than one transmitter which interact often both presynaptically and postsynaptically with specific receptors and produce effects. The balance between various transmitters released may vary under different conditions so that differential release of one or other mediator may result from varying impulse patterns.

CLASSIFICATION

At present, more than 50 substances have been reported to fulfil the criteria as a neurotransmitter. Generally, these substances can be classified in two ways.

Biochemical Classification

Biochemically, neurotransmitters can be divided into two groups.

A. Small-molecule neurotransmitters These act rapidly and cause acute response. These are synthesized and packed into synaptic vesicles in the axon terminal. Important small-molecule neurotransmitters with their site of release given in *parentheses* are as follows:

I. ***Acetylcholine (ACh):***
  - Neuromuscular junction
  - All preganglionic autonomic neurons
  - All postganglionic parasympathetic neurons
  - Postganglionic sympathetic neurons to sweat glands and skeletal muscle blood vessels
  - Some amacrine cells of the retina
  - Many parts of CNS

II. ***Biogenic amines:***
- Catecholamines: Epinephrine (EP), NE, dopamine (DA)
- Serotonin (5-hydroxytryptamine [5-HT])
- Histamine

III. ***Amino acid neurotransmitters:***
- Gamma-aminobutyric acid (GABA)
- Glycine
- Glutamic acid or glutamate
- Aspartic acid or aspartate
- ATP

B. Neuropeptide transmitters These are large molecules, are slowly acting and have a prolonged effect. These neurotransmitters include:

- Neuroactive peptides
- Pituitary peptides
- Peptides acting on the gut and brain
- Neuropeptides from other tissues

In general, neuropeptides are co-localized with one of the small-molecule neurotransmitters (Table 10.7.2).

Physiological Classification

Some of the neurotransmitters cause excitation of postsynaptic neurons, whereas others cause inhibition. Thus, physiologically, neurotransmitters can be divided into two groups:

- Excitatory neurotransmitters
- Inhibitory neurotransmitters

1. ***Excitatory neurotransmitters*** can cause an AP (if the target cell is another neuron), contraction (if the target cell is a muscle) or secretion (if the target cell is a gland).
   In the CNS, the excitatory neurotransmitters produce a depolarization of the postsynaptic membrane called the EPSP. The most common excitatory neurotransmitter within the CNS is glutamate. Other excitatory neurotransmitters are ACh, aspartic acid, etc.
2. ***Inhibitory neurotransmitters*** reduce or block the activity of the postsynaptic cell. They produce a hyperpolarization of the postsynaptic membrane called the IPSP. The most common inhibitory neurotransmitters within the CNS are *glycine* or *GABA*. Other inhibitory neurotransmitters include DA.

Table 10.7.2 Small-molecule neurotransmitters and their colocalization with various neuropeptides

Neurotransmitters	Neuropeptide
1. Acetylcholine	Substance P, vasoactive intestinal peptide (VIP), somatostatin, GnRH, enkephalin, calcitonin gene–related protein (CGRP) and neurotensin
2. GABA	Substance P, somatostatin, cholecystokinin and TRH
3. Glycine	Neurotensin
4. Glutamate	Substance P
5. Norepinephrine	Enkephalin, neuropeptide Y, somatostatin, vasopressin and neurotensin
6. Epinephrine	Enkephalin, neuropeptide Y, neurotensin and substance P
7. Dopamine	Enkephalin, somatostatin and cholecystokinin
8. Serotonin	Cholecystokinin, neuropeptide Y (NPY), substance P and VIP

Receptors The action of neurotransmitter on its target depends on the type of receptor on which it acts rather than on the properties of the mediator. The receptors on which these neurotransmitters act are discussed along with individual neurotransmitter. The main general characteristics of the receptors are as follows:

- Each chemical mediator has potential to act on many subtypes of receptors. For example, NE acts on α_1, α_2, β_1, β_2 and β_3 subtypes of adrenergic receptors. This makes the effect of the ligand on the cell more selective.
- For many secreted neurotransmitters, the receptors are present on the presynaptic as well as on the postsynaptic membrane. The presynaptic receptors are of two types – autoreceptors and heteroreceptors.
  Autoreceptors inhibit further secretion of the neurotransmitters by feedback control (e.g. NE acts on α_2-presynaptic receptors and inhibits its further secretion).
  Heteroreceptors are another type of presynaptic receptors which are activated by different ligands rather than secreted by nerve endings on which the receptor is located (e.g. NE acts on cholinergic nerve endings to inhibit the release of ACh).
- All the receptors and their subtypes are basically divided into two main groups – ionotropic and metabotropic receptors.
  Ionotropic receptors are ligand-gated membrane channels. When the ligand binds to the receptor, the membrane channel opens (activation) and increases the ion conductance. The activation is for a brief period (few milliseconds); therefore, these receptors are meant for fast synaptic transmission.
  Metabotropic receptors are G protein–coupled transmembrane receptors (GPCR). When the neurotransmitter binds to the receptors, the activated receptor initiates production of the second messenger that modulates the voltage-gated channels present on the neuronal membrane.

PRINCIPAL NEUROTRANSMITTERS

A. Small-Molecule Neurotransmitters

I. Acetylcholine

ACh is a principal neurotransmitter released by many neurons in the nervous system.

Cholinergic neurons Cholinergic neurons, i.e. neurons which secrete ACh at their nerve endings, include:

- Nerve endings at the neuromuscular junction
- Preganglionic parasympathetic nerves
- All preganglionic sympathetic nerves
- All postganglionic parasympathetic nerves
- Postganglionic sympathetic cholinergic nerves, those which innervate:
  - Sweat glands
  - Skeletal muscle blood vessels (sympathetic vasodilator nerves)
- Endings of some amacrine cells of the retina
- Many parts of the brain (especially cerebral cortex, thalamus and forebrain nuclei) (ACh is specifically released by large pyramidal cells and many neurons of the basal ganglia)

Cholinergic receptors ACh receptors are of two types – nicotinic and muscarinic (see page 956).

i. ***Nicotinic receptors*** (which respond to low doses of nicotine) are present on the postsynaptic membrane of:
   - All autonomic (sympathetic as well as parasympathetic) ganglia

- Postsynaptic membrane at neuromuscular junctions in skeletal muscle

The nicotinic receptors are of two types – N_M and N_N receptors. The N_N receptors are present at the neuromuscular junction and the N_M receptors at the autonomic ganglia and in many parts of CNS.

ii. ***Muscarinic receptors*** (which respond to mushroom poison muscarine) are present on postsynaptic membranes of:
- Smooth muscles
- Cardiac muscles
- Glandular cells

Various types of muscarinic receptors are M_1–M_5.
- The M_1, M_4 and M_5 receptors are present in the CNS.
- The M_2 receptors are present in the heart.
- The M_3 receptors are present in the smooth muscles and glands.

ACh synthesis, storage, release and removal

ACh synthesis and storage: ACh is synthesized within the mitochondria in the presynaptic terminal from acetyl coenzyme A (CoA) and choline by a reaction catalysed by the enzyme choline acetyltransferase (ChAT). After formation, ACh is stored temporarily in synaptic vesicles with ATP and proteoglycan for later release.

Release of ACh by the nerve terminal: See page 76.

Removal of ACh from synaptic cleft: See page 78.

Biochemical events at cholinergic synapse The biochemical events at cholinergic synapse are as follows (Fig. 10.7:19):

- Choline is transported into the presynaptic terminal by a Na^+-dependent choline transporter (CHT).
- ACh is synthesized from choline and acetyl-CoA by enzyme ChAT in the cytosol.
- ACh is then transported from the cytosol into the vesicles by vesicle-associated transporter (VAT) along with a peptide (P) and ATP.
- Release of ACh from the nerve terminal occurs on opening of voltage-gated Ca^{2+} channels.
- Influx of Ca^{2+} leads to fusion of vesicles containing ACh to the surface of the membrane (exocytosis).
- Expulsion of ACh and cotransmitter into the synaptic cleft involves SNAPs and vesicle-associated membrane protein (VAMPs).
- Released ACh acts on muscarinic G protein–coupled protein (GPCR) on the postsynaptic target (e.g. smooth muscles) and on nicotinic receptors (autonomic ganglia and neuromuscular junction).
- ACh is metabolized rapidly by enzyme acetylcholinesterase in the synaptic cleft.
- Presynaptic autoreceptors and heteroreceptors modulate ACh release.

Actions of ACh ACh is very quick in action and in most instances it is excitatory. It produces the excitatory function of synapse by opening the ligand-gated Na^+ channels. At very few places (vagus supplying the heart), ACh acts as an inhibitory transmitter.

Muscarinic versus nicotinic actions of ACh on the postsynaptic receptors are summarized in Table 10.7.3.

Role of ACh in function of brain: Both muscarinic and nicotinic receptors are found in the CNS; however, most of these are muscarinic. The cell bodies of cholinergic neurons in the

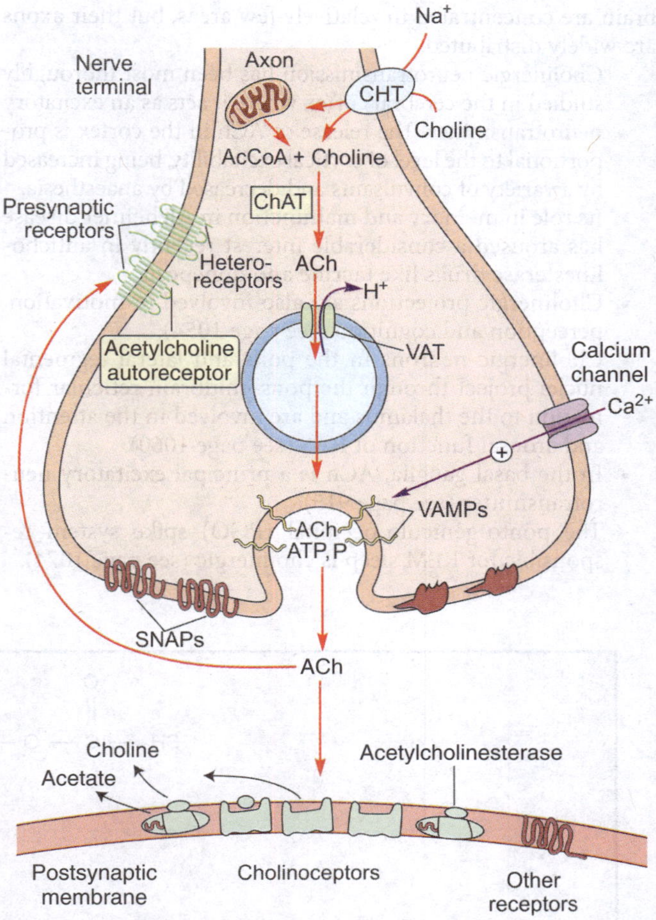

Fig. 10.7.19 Biochemical events at a cholinergic synapse.

Table 10.7.3 Muscarinic versus nicotinic actions of ACh

Features	Muscarinic action	Nicotinic action
1. Site of action	• Postsynaptic membranes in cardiac muscles, smooth muscles and glandular cells	• All autonomic ganglia • Neuromuscular junctions in skeletal muscles
2. Characteristics of action	• Actions resemble those of mushroom poison muscarine • Actions are slow in onset • Actions are prolonged	• Action resembles the drug nicotine • Actions are quick in onset • Actions are of brief duration
3. Actions are antagonized by	• Atropine which combines with ACh receptors at the sites of muscarinic action	• Hexamethonium at autonomic ganglia • Tubocurarine at skeletal muscles

ACh, acetylcholine.

brain are concentrated in relatively few areas, but their axons are widely distributed.

- Cholinergic neurotransmission has been most thoroughly studied in the cerebral cortex where it acts as an excitatory neurotransmitter. The release of ACh in the cortex is proportional to the level of cortical excitability, being increased by a variety of convulsants and decreased by anaesthesia.
- Its role in memory and malfunction in Alzheimer disease has aroused a considerable interest recently in anticholinesterase drugs like tacrine and donepezil.
- Cholinergic projections are also involved in motivation, perception and cognition (see page 1054).
- Cholinergic neurons in the pons and lateral tegmental nuclei project through the pons–midbrain reticular formation to the thalamus and are involved in the attention and arousal function of RAS (see page 1060).
- In the basal ganglia, ACh is a principal excitatory neurotransmitter (see page 915).
- The ponto-geniculo-occipital (PGO) spike system responsible for REM sleep is cholinergic (see page 1074).

Drugs which cause alteration in cholinergic transmission include:

- Hemicholinium: Blocks the CHT
- Vesamicol: Blocks the VAT
- Botulinum toxin: Prevents the release of ACh

II. Biogenic Amines

1. Catecholamines include EP (adrenaline), NE (noradrenaline) and DA.

- EP is not a common neurotransmitter in the brain or peripheral nervous system but is the major hormone secreted by the adrenal medulla.
- The biogenic amines are basic *by R-NH₂* group. Catecholamines contain a catechol ring (a six-sided carbon ring with adjacent hydroxyl group) and an amine ring (Fig. 10.7.20).

Biosynthesis, metabolism and excretion The three catecholamines – EP, NE and DA – are synthesized from

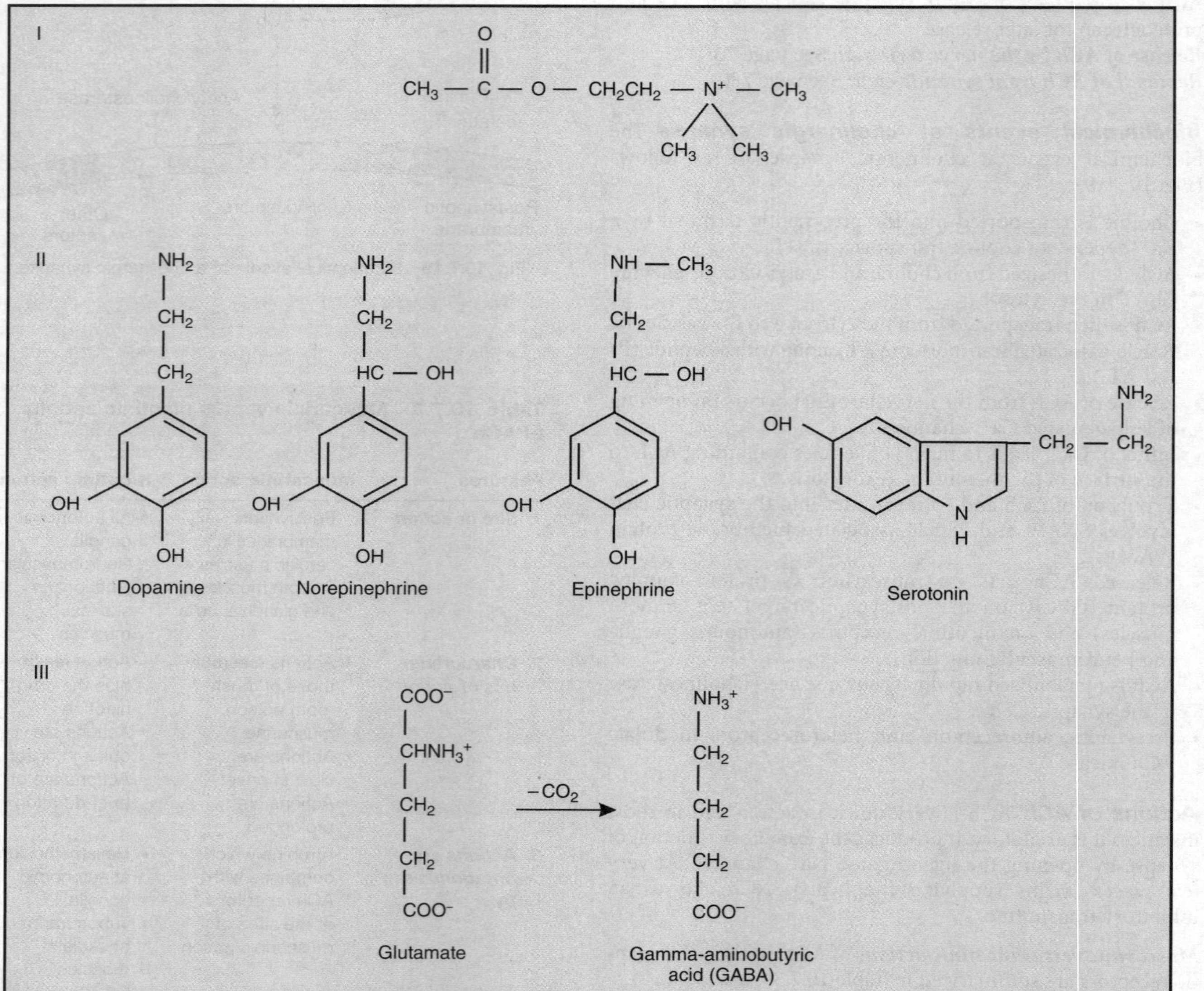

Fig. 10.7.20 Structures of various neurotransmitters: *I*, acetylcholine; *II*, biogenic amines; and *III*, amino acids.

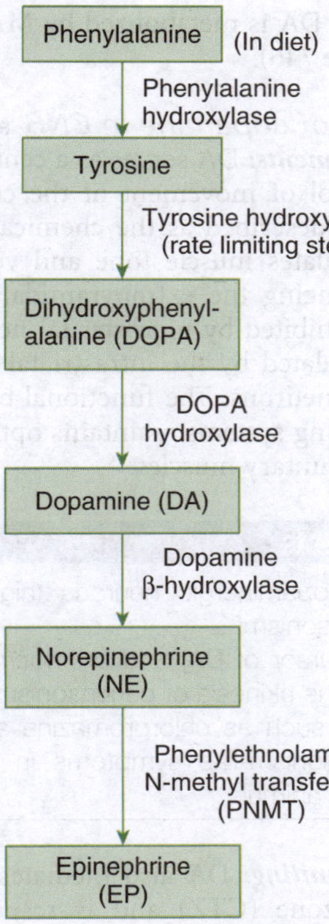

Fig. 10.7.21 Synthesis of catecholamines from the amino acid phenylalanine.

the amino acid phenylalanine (Fig. 10.7.21). For details, see page 742.

Norepinephrine and epinephrine Adrenergic neurons refer to those neurons which secrete either EP (adrenaline) or NE (noradrenaline) at their nerve endings.

EP is produced almost exclusively in the adrenal medulla, with a small amount being synthesized in the brain (see page 742). ***NE*** is released by the adrenal medulla and the following noradrenergic nerve endings in the peripheral nervous system and CNS:

- Postganglionic sympathetic neurons: It is the primary neurotransmitter released from postganglionic sympathetic neurons except those supplying the sweat glands and blood vessels of skeletal muscles.
- Neurons of the cerebral cortex and hypothalamus also release NE.
- Noradrenergic neurons of the pons and medulla oblongata constitute two major systems – locus coeruleus system and lateral tegmental system (Fig. 10.7.22A and B). From these neurons, the axons descend to the *spinal cord* and *cerebellum*, and ascend to innervate the nuclei of the hypothalamus (supraoptic, paraventricular and periventricular), thalamus and most of the neocortex. NE primarily acts as a modulator in these regions.

Regulation of NE release: There is a presynaptic regulation of NE release mediated by presynaptic α receptors and a positive feedback mechanism mediated by presynaptic β receptors. Such combined effects control the need-oriented release of neurotransmitter.

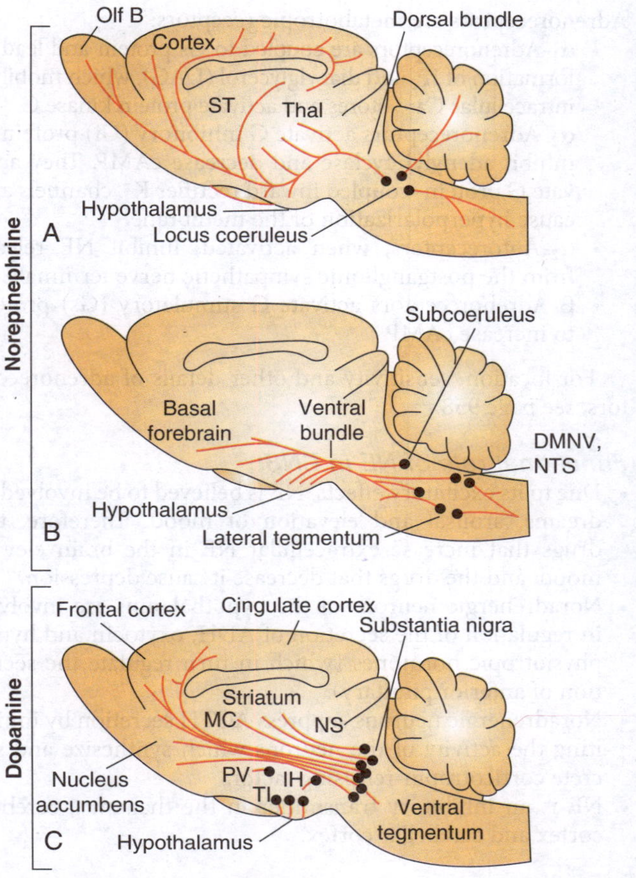

Fig. 10.7.22 Aminergic pathways in central nervous system. The principal noradrenergic systems. **A,** Locus coeruleus; **B,** lateral tegmental; and **C,** dopaminergic pathway. DMNV, dorsal motor nucleus of vagus; MC, mesocortical system; NS, nigrostriatal system; NTS, nucleus tractus solitarius (nucleus of solitary tract); Olf B, olfactory bulb; PV, periventricular system; ST, stria terminalis; Thal, thalamus.

Removal and metabolism of NE: NE is removed from the synapse by *reuptake* or is *metabolized* in the presynaptic terminal by monoamine oxidase (MAO) and catechol-*O*-methyltransferase (COMT). The metabolites are dihydroxymandelic acid (DOMA), normetanephrine (NMN) and 3-methoxy-4-hydroxyphenylglycol (MOPG). For details, see page 746 (Fig. 8.5.27).

Distribution of noradrenergic neurons in the CNS is shown in Fig. 10.7.22.

Actions: For detailed action of EP and NE on different systems of the body, see page 747.

- In general, NE is mainly an excitatory neurotransmitter; only at a few places, it is inhibitory.
- EP and NE produce different effects due to the existence of two types of adrenergic receptors – α and β, each further subdivided into α_1 and α_2, and β_1, β_2 and β_3, respectively.
- EP acts equally on both α and β receptors, whereas NE acts on α receptors (see page 747).
- Their receptor action is linked for the second messengers cAMP, cGMP, etc.

Adrenoreceptors: EP and NE act on both types (α and β) of adrenoreceptors. Both α and β receptors have subtypes – α_{1A}, α_{1B}, α_D, α_{2A}, α_{2B}, α_C, β_1 and β_2.

Adrenoreceptors are metabotropic receptors:

- α_1-Adrenoreceptors are coupled to Gs protein and lead to formation of IP_3 and diacylglycerol (DAG), which mobilize intracellular Ca^{2+} stores and activate protein kinase C.
- α_2-Adrenoreceptors activate G inhibitory (Gi) protein to inhibit adenylyl cyclase and decrease cAMP. They activate G protein–coupled inward rectifier K^+ channels and cause hyperpolarization of the membrane.
- α_2-Autoreceptors, when activated, inhibit NE release from the postganglionic sympathetic nerve terminals.
- β-Adrenoreceptors activate G stimulatory (Gs) protein to increase cAMP.

For location, sensitivity and other details of adrenoreceptors, see page 958.

Functional role of NE in CNS:

- Due to its excitatory effects, NE is believed to be involved in dreams, arousal and elevation of mood. Therefore, the drugs that increase extracellular NE in the brain elevate mood, and the drugs that decrease it cause depression.
- Noradrenergic neurons of the hypothalamus are involved in regulation of the secretion of ADH, oxytocin and hypophysiotropic hormones (which in turn regulate the secretion of anterior pituitary).
- Noradrenergic neurons suppress ACTH secretion by inhibiting the activity of the neurons which synthesize and secrete corticotropin-releasing factor.
- NE is an inhibitory transmitter in the thalamus, cerebral cortex and cerebellar cortex.

Drugs that cause alteration in noradrenergic transmission are as follows:

- Metyrosine: Blocks the action of tyrosine hydroxylase
- Reserpine: Blocks VMA, which transports DA into the synaptic vesicles
- Bretylium and guanethidine: Prevent the release of noradrenaline
- Cocaine and tricyclic antidepressants: Block the reuptake of noradrenaline

Dopamine (DA) DA is a naturally acting precursor of NE.

DA receptors: DA acts on two main classes of DA receptors – D_1 and D_2. Five different types of DA receptors have been cloned, but these basically fall into two major classes:

- D_1 receptors (D_1 and D_5)
- D_2 receptors (D_2, D_3 and D_4)

All DA receptors are metabotropic:

- *D_1* receptors activate adenylyl cyclase via Gs protein.
- *D_2* receptors inhibit adenylyl cyclase via Gi protein. The brain contains more of D_2 receptors.

Dopaminergic neurons have their cell bodies in the midbrain. They project from the substantia nigra to the (Fig. 10.7.22C):

- Striatum (nigrostriatal tract)
- Olfactory tubercle
- Nucleus accumbens
- Limbic system area

Important Note

The highest concentration of DA is present in the basal ganglia, limbic system and chemoreceptor trigger zone (CTZ) in the medulla. It does not cross the blood–brain barrier.

Metabolism of DA: DA is metabolized by MAO and COMT (for details, see page 746).

Functional roles of dopamine in CNS are:

1. ***Control of movements:*** DA serves as a central neurotransmitter for control of movement of the corpus striatum, which has been described as the chemical factory of the CNS, and modulates muscle tone and voluntary movements by influencing the extrapyramidal motor system, which can be inhibited by nigrostriatal neurons releasing DA and is stimulated by the intrastriatal release of ACh from excitatory neurons. The functional balance between these two opposing systems maintains optimum tone and movement of voluntary muscles.

Applied Aspects

- Deficiency of dopaminergic neurons (nigrostriatal tract) produces parkinsonism.
- Levodopa (precursor of DA) and *bromocriptine* (DA agonist) overcome the akinesia of parkinsonism.
- DA antagonists such as chlorpromazine and haloperidol produce parkinsonism-like symptoms in human beings and catalepsy in animals.

2. ***Induction of vomiting:*** DA also mediates the activity of chemoreceptor zone (CTZ) and is responsible for the induction of all types of vomiting other than that of vestibular origin (see page 592).
3. ***Inhibition of prolactin secretion and stimulation of GnRH:*** DA is released in the hypothalamus and causes:
   - Inhibition of prolactin secretion
   - Stimulation of GnRH release
4. ***Retina*** also contains some inhibitory dopaminergic neurons.

Applied Aspects

DA and schizophrenia: Schizophrenia type of psychosis involves increased levels of D_2 receptors.

- Amphetamine, which stimulates secretion of NE and DA, produces schizophrenia when administered in high doses.
- Several drugs used as tranquilizers reduce the content of DA in the brain neurons and are effective in relief of schizophrenia (see page 1056).

DA is involved in addiction and reward (see page 1055).

Important Note

It is possible that there exist different cotransmitters for DA in different areas which affect its activity differently.

2. Serotonin

Synthesis and metabolism Serotonin (5-HT) is synthesized from tryptophan (an essential amino acid). It is inactivated by MAO to form 5-hydroxyindoleacetic acid (5-HIAA), which is excreted in urine. In the pineal gland, 5-HT is converted into melatonin.

Sites of secretion 5-HT is present in the brain and non-neural cells.

In the brain, serotonergic neurons have their cell bodies in the brainstem and they project to portions of the hypothalamus, limbic system, neocortex and spinal cord.

Non-neural cells that contain serotonin are blood platelets (highest concentration), mast cells, GIT enterochromaffin cells and myenteric plexus.

Serotonergic receptors Serotonergic receptors have been classified into seven major types (5-HT_1–5-HT_7) and they are further of subtypes:

- 5-HT_1: 5-HT_{1A}, 5-HT_{1B}, 5-HT_{1C}, 5-HT_{1D}, 5-HT_{1E} and 5-HT_{1F}
- 5-HT_2: 5-HT_{2A}, 5-HT_{2B} and 5-HT_{2C}
- 5-HT_5: 5-HT_{5A} and 5-HT_{5B}

Location and main functions are as follows:

- 5-HT receptors are presynaptic as well as postsynaptic.
- 5-HT_{2A} cause smooth muscle contraction and platelet aggregation.
- 5-HT_{2C} regulates food intake in response to leptin.
- 5-HT_3 is present in GIT and area postrema, and is related to vomiting.
- 5-HT_4 receptors are present in GIT (responsible for peristalsis) and also in the brain.
- 5-HT_6 and 5-HT_7 are distributed in the limbic system.

Effects of 5-HT General considerations are as follows:

- Some 5-HT receptors are excitatory, whereas others are inhibitory. In general, 5-HT has an excitatory effect on the motor pathways and an inhibitory effect on the sensory pathways.
- Effects of 5-HT generally have a low onset indicating that it works as a neuromodulator (which often modifies the postsynaptic cell's response to specific neurotransmitters).
- The activity of serotonergic neurons is the lowest or absent in sleep and the highest during states of alert and wakefulness. The increased 5-HT activity causes increase in motor responsiveness and suppresses sensory systems to screen out distracting stimuli.

Functional roles of 5-HT in CNS Functional roles of 5-HT in CNS include:

1. ***Regulation of carbohydrate intake and hypothalamic-releasing hormones:*** Serotonergic pathways function in regulation of carbohydrate intake and hypothalamic-releasing hormones, and they have been implicated in alcoholism and other obsessive–compulsive disorders.
   Both NE and 5-HT are involved in food intake and control of body temperature.
2. ***Pain inhibition:*** Serotonin inhibits impulses of pain sensation in the posterior grey horn of the spinal cord. The presence of descending serotonergic neurons in the brainstem and spinal cord is essential for the analgesic action of morphine.
3. ***Hallucinations and 5-HT:*** Lysergic acid diethylamide (LSD), the most potent hallucinogenic drug known, activates the serotonergic neurons.
   Several chemical substances related to 5-HT, such as *psilocybin*, a hallucinogenic agent found in some mushrooms, have potent psychic effects.
4. ***Depression of mood*** (see page 1056):
   - *Drugs that modulate serotonergic transmission include* fluoxetine that belongs to selective serotonin uptake inhibitors (SSRIs).

3. Histamine

Synthesis Histamine is formed by decarboxylation of the amino acid histidine.

Sites of secretion Histamine is secreted in the brain and non-neural cells.

In the brain, histaminergic neurons have their cell bodies mainly in the posterior hypothalamus and their axons project to all parts of the brain, including the cerebral cortex and spinal cord.
Non-neural cells that contain histamine are of gastric mucosa and heparin-containing mast cells.

Histamine receptors Histamine receptors are of four types – H_1, H_2, H_3 and H_4. All types of receptors are found in the brain and peripheral tissues:

- H_1 receptors activate phospholipase C.
- H_2 receptors increase intracellular cAMP.
- H_3 receptors are presynaptic, and they mediate inhibition of the release of histamine via a protein.
- H_4 receptors are recently described receptors and they play a role in regulating cells of the immune system.

Functional role of histamine in CNS Histamine is an excitatory neurotransmitter. The exact function of diffuse histaminergic system is not known as yet. It is believed that histamine plays an important role in arousal and sexual behaviour, regulation of secretion of some anterior pituitary hormones, drinking and pain threshold.

4. Adenosine Triphosphate

ATP has recently been identified as a small-molecule neurotransmitter. It is colocalized and is coreleased from synaptic vesicles of noradrenergic postganglionic neurons.

Receptors The ATP receptors are **P** receptors and are further of three subtypes – $\mathbf{P_{2X}}$, $\mathbf{P_{2Y}}$ and $\mathbf{P_{2U}}$.

- $\mathbf{P_{2X}}$ receptors are ligand-gated ion channels involved in rapid synaptic responses in the autonomic nervous system. They are widely distributed throughout the body, but mainly in the dorsal horn cells; thus, ATP has a role in sensory transmission.
- $\mathbf{P_{2Y}}$ and $\mathbf{P_{2U}}$ receptors are metabotropic, which are G protein–coupled receptors (GPCR).

III. Amino Acid Neurotransmitters

Excitatory amino acid neurotransmitters that cause neuronal depolarization include glutamic acid (glutamate) and aspartic acid (aspartate).
Inhibitory amino acid neurotransmitters that cause neuronal hyperpolarization include GABA and glycine.

1. Glutamic acid Glutamic acid (glutamate) is the most prevalent *excitatory neurotransmitter* in the brain and dorsal sensory nerve terminals.

Synthesis, storage and release and removal In the CNS neurons, glutamate is mainly derived either from glucose, via the Krebs' cycle, or from glutamine which is synthesized by glial cells and taken up by the neurons.

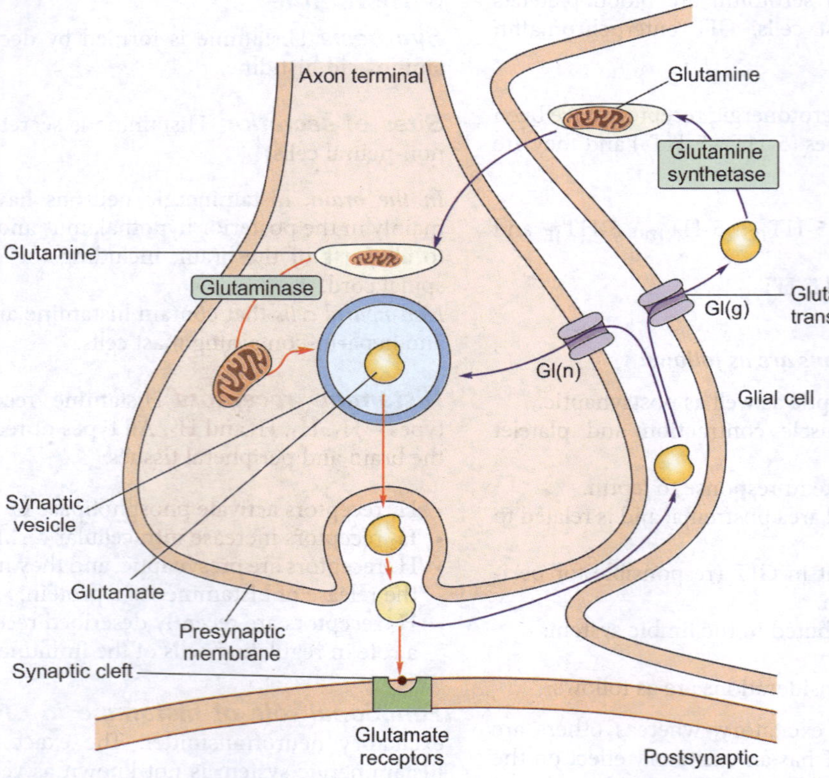

Fig. 10.7.23 Biochemical events at a glutamatergic synapse. Glutamate released into the synaptic cleft by Ca^{2+}-dependent exocytosis. Released Glu can act glutamate on ionotropic and G protein–coupled receptors on the postsynaptic neuron.

- *In the first pathway* (Fig. 10.7.23), the α-glutarate produced by Krebs cycle is converted into glutamate by enzyme GABA transaminase (GABA-T).
- *In the second pathway*, the glutamate released from the nerve terminal by exocytosis is transported into the glial tissue by a transporter (glutamate reuptake transporter), and converted into glutamine by the enzyme glutamine synthase. Glutamine then diffuses back into the nerve terminal and gets hydrolysed by the enzyme glutaminase. The released glutamate is also taken directly from the synaptic cleft into the nerve terminal by a membrane transporter.

It is stored in the synaptic vesicles. Vesicular glutamate transporter is responsible for maintaining its high concentration in the vesicles and released by calcium-dependent exocytosis. The action of glutamate is mainly terminated by Na^+ dependent glutamate-transporter (Gtg) located on the presynaptic membrane (carrier-mediated reuptake) into the nerve terminals and neighbouring glial cells by Gtg transporter.

Glutamate receptors Glutamate receptors present on the postsynaptic neurons are as follows:

Inotropic glutamate receptors which when stimulated increase the conductance of Na^+ and Ca^{2+} into the cell leading to depolarization

There are three subtypes of ionotropic glutamate receptors, each named after the specific agonists:

- α-Amino-3-hydroxy-5-methylisoxazole-4-propionate (AMPA)
- Kainate (kainati, a seaweed acid)
- *N*-Methyl-D-aspartate (NMDA)

Distribution The neurons of CNS have both AMPA and NMDA receptors. In contrast, kainate receptors are located on:

- Presynaptic GABA-secreting nerve endings
- Postsynaptically in the hippocampus, cerebellum and spinal cord

Action NMDA receptors are involved in memory and learning (see page 1087).

Metabotropic glutamate receptors Metabotropic glutamate receptors ($mGLuR_s$) stimulate the phosphoinositol turnover and DAG or decrease in intracellular cAMP. Eight different subtypes of $mGLuR_s$ are known (mGLuR1–8). These receptors are located on both presynaptic and postsynaptic sites and are widely distributed in the brain.
Action: $mGLuR_s$ are involved in synaptic plasticity.

Excitotoxicity occurs in conditions such as ischaemia, anoxia/hypoxia, hypoglycaemia and trauma due to excessive level of glutamate. The excitatory neurotransmitter glutamate increases Ca^{2+} influx that leads to neuronal death due to excitation.

2. Aspartic acid

Aspartic acid or aspartate seems to be the chief excitatory transmitter of cortical pyramidal cells.

3. Gamma-aminobutyric acid

GABA is the major inhibitory neurotransmitter in the whole CNS, i.e. spinal cord, brainstem, cerebral cortex and cerebellum.

Synthesis: It is formed by decarboxylation of glutamic acid by the enzyme glutamate decarboxylase (GAD), pyridoxal phosphate; a vitamin B-complex derivative is cofactor for GAD.

Removal of GABA from the synaptic cleft occurs chiefly by its reuptake via GABA transporter, and transported into the synaptic vesicles by vesicular GABA transporter.

GABA receptors: There are three subtypes of GABA receptors – $GABA_A$, $GABA_B$ and $GABA_C$.

- $GABA_A$ receptors are pentameric, made up of combination of α-, β-, γ-, δ- and ϵ-subunits.
- $GABA_A$ and $GABA_B$ are ionotropic receptors and allow entry of Cl^- into the neurons.
- $GABA_C$ receptors are metabotropic GPCR and act by:
  - Increasing conductance in K^+ channel
  - Inhibiting adenylyl cyclase
  - Inhibiting Ca^{2+} influx

GABA produces presynaptic inhibition, i.e. indirect inhibition (see page 975), by these types of receptors.

Thus, due to the effect of GABA on the postsynaptic membrane, K^+ comes out of synapse and Cl^- enters in. This leads to hyperpolarization which is known as IPSP (see page 972).

Drugs like benzodiazepine and barbiturates are GABA agonists.

Applied Aspects

Kleine–Levin syndrome (KLS) is caused by intoxication by γ-hydroxybutyric acid (a metabolite of GABA), the main inhibitory neurotransmitter in the brain. The relationship between GABA and glutamate (excitatory neurotransmitter) promotes excitation.

Clinical manifestations of KLS are mainly of excitatory type, e.g. insomnia, hyperphagia, anxiety and sexual disturbances.

GABA is also targeted in treatment of epilepsy and many other psychiatric diseases.

4. Glycine Glycine has inhibitory as well as excitatory effects:

- Glycine is an inhibitory neurotransmitter found primarily in the grey matter of the spinal cord and brainstem.
- It produces direct inhibition (postsynaptic inhibition) in the spinal cord and acts by increasing Cl^- conductance by acting on glycine receptor which functionally resembles GABA receptors.
- Agents, such as strychnine and tetanus toxin, that antagonize the postsynaptic inhibitory action of glycine produce convulsions and muscular hyperactivity.
- Glycine when binds to NMDA receptors makes them more sensitive to glutamate action. Therefore, it facilitates pain transmission by NMDA receptors.

In the CNS, glycine participates in processing of sensory and motor information that permits movements, vision and audition.

Applied Aspects

- Children with glycine deficiency may not gain weight and grow as per the expected rate and have a delayed development of motor skills such as sitting and walking.
- Glycine encephalopathy (GCE) is another inherited metabolic disorder that occurs due to deficient activity of glycine cleavage enzyme.

B. Neuropeptide Transmitters (Large-Molecule Neurotransmitter)

Neuropeptide transmitters are slowly acting and have a prolonged effect in contrast to small-molecule transmitters, which act rapidly and cause short-lasting acute response. These cannot be synthesized in the cytosol of the axon terminal but are typically synthesized in the soma as integral components of large proteins. These large molecules are cleaved in the cell body and packaged into vesicles in the Golgi apparatus either as an active peptidergic agent or as a precursor of the neuroactive substance. The vesicles are delivered to axon terminals, and the transmitter is released into the synaptic cleft.

Mechanism of Action

The peptides can alter ion channel function and modify cell metabolism or gene expression, and these actions can be sustained for minutes, hours, days or presumably even longer.

Types of Neuropeptides

Many of the peptides function in communication network within the neural, endocrine and immune systems. These are given next.

1. Neuroactive peptides These include releasing hormones from the hypothalamus such as TRH, LH-releasing hormone and somatostatin.

2. Pituitary peptides These include ACTH, β-endorphin, vasopressin and oxytocin.

Vasopressin (ADH) and oxytocin: Besides acting as hormones (see page 777), they are also present in the neurons that project to the brainstem and spinal cord. They appear to be involved in control of CVS.

3. Peptides acting on the gut and brain These include leucine, enkephalin, methionine, substance P, CCK, VIP, neurotensin, insulin, glucose and opioid polypeptides.

Opioid peptides:

- Enkephalins are peptides that bind to opioid receptors and are called opioid peptides.
- Enkephalins are two closely related pentapeptides – met-enkephalin and leu-enkephalin.
- Enkephalins are mainly found in nerve endings of GIT, many parts of the brain and substantia gelatinosa of the spinal cord.
- Endogenous opioid peptides are synthesized as large precursor molecules. For details, see page 1006.

Enkephalins act on three types of receptors which occur in discrete locations in CNS:

- In areas that contain the pathway which conveys pain information
- In parts of the brain involved in mood
- In parts of the brain involved in emotions

Opioid receptors:

- Opioid receptors are μ, κ and δ. They differ in their physiological effects and affinity for various opioid peptides. Opioid receptors are GPCR, and act by inhibiting adenylyl cyclase. μ receptors increase K^+ conductance; κ and δ receptors close the Ca^{2+} channels. By all these effects, they cause hyperpolarization of central neurons and primary afferents.

Substance P: Substance P is a polypeptide containing 11 amino acids, which belongs to tachykinin family of polypeptides. Other members of this family are neurokinin A and neurokinin B. It is the transmitter released by:

- Primary pain nerve endings in the spinal cord

- Hypothalamus
- Nigrostriatal system of the basal ganglia

Receptors: There are three types of neurokinin receptors – NK_1–NK_3. Substance P binds preferably to NK_1 receptors. Activation of these receptors leads to increased production of IP_3 and DAG.

The actions of substance P are as follows:

- It acts as a mediator for transmission of pain in the dorsal horn.
- In the hypothalamus, it may play a role in neuroendocrine regulation.
- In the skin, it acts as a mediator released by nerve endings and is responsible for axon reflex (see page 357).
- In the intestine, it is involved in peristalsis.
- NK_1 receptor antagonists have been used as antidepressants and antiemetics in patients undergoing chemotherapy.

CCK and VIP: These are also found in the brain, the former in the hypothalamus and the latter in the cerebral cortex. *Opioid polypeptides* have an important role in the inhibition of pain signals in the brain and spinal cord.

4. Neuropeptides from other tissues These include angiotensin II, bradykinin, bombesin and neuropeptide-α. *Neuropeptide Y* is closely related to pancreatic polypeptide and is present in many parts of the brain and ANS. It increases the vasoconstrictive effect of NE. Its level in the circulation from sympathetic nerves increases during severe exercise.

Self-Assessment

1. Discuss the process of chemical transmission.
2. Discuss the synaptic inhibition and its significance.
3. Describe the following:
   - Classification of principal neurotransmitters
   - Role of acetylcholine on CNS
4. Write notes on the following:
   - Functional role of dopamine on CNS
   - Synaptic delay
   - Subliminal fringe
   - Opioid peptides
   - EPSP

Clinical Case

Case 1

A 15-year-old girl was referred to the neurology department for attacks of convulsions. On the basis of history, symptoms and signs, and EEG report, she was diagnosed to be a case of epilepsy. The treatment prescribed was a GABA agonist.

Q1. Why is GABA agonist prescribed in this disease?

Q2. What is the mechanism of action of GABA in this case?

10.8

Somatosensory System

CHAPTER OUTLINE

GENERAL SENSORY MECHANISM

INTRODUCTION

Sensations

Sensory division of the human nervous system is concerned with collection of the information about the outside world, and changes occurring within the body itself. Sensation refers to conscious perception of sensory information reaching the brain. Sensations may be broadly classified into two groups.

1. Special senses These include visual sensations, auditory sensations, gustatory sensations (taste sensation) and olfactory (smell) sensations. These have been discussed in detail in different chapters of Section 11 (see page 1097).

2. Somaesthetic senses These, depending on their point of origin, can be classified into three types:

A. ***Exteroceptive sensations***, also known as cutaneous sensations, arise from the surface of the body and can be divided into two groups:
   i. *Epicritic sensations* are mild or light sensations, which are perceived more accurately. These include:
      - *Fine touch* or tactile sensation is the light touch sensation arising from the surface of the body.
      - *Tactile localization* is the ability to locate the area of the skin where tactile stimulus is applied.
      - *Tactile discrimination* is the ability to locate the two adjacent areas of the skin where tactile stimuli are applied.
      - *Temperature sensation is the sensation with fine range,* i.e. between 25°C and 40°C.
   ii. *Protopathic sensations* are primitive or crude type of exteroceptive sensations. These include:
      - Pressure sensation
      - Pain sensation
      - Temperature sensation with a wider range, i.e. below 25°C and above 40°C

B. ***Visceral sensations*** arise from the viscera, i.e. internal organs, and thus are called visceral sensations.

C. ***Proprioceptive and kinaesthetic sensations*** arise from the muscles, tendons and joints. These include:
   i. *Proprioceptive sensations:* These are concerned with the physical state of the body, i.e. the sense of position, tendon and muscle sensations, deep pressure and sense of equilibrium.
   ii. *Kinaesthetic sensations* or kinaesthesia: It is the conscious recognition of rate of movement of different parts of the body. Kinaesthetic sensations include both of the following:
      - Conscious kinaesthetic sensations
      - Unconscious kinaesthetic sensations

Components of Sensory System

The sensory division of the human nervous system includes the components given next (Fig. 10.8.1).

1. Sensory receptors These are specialized cells that transduce stimulus energy into neural signals.

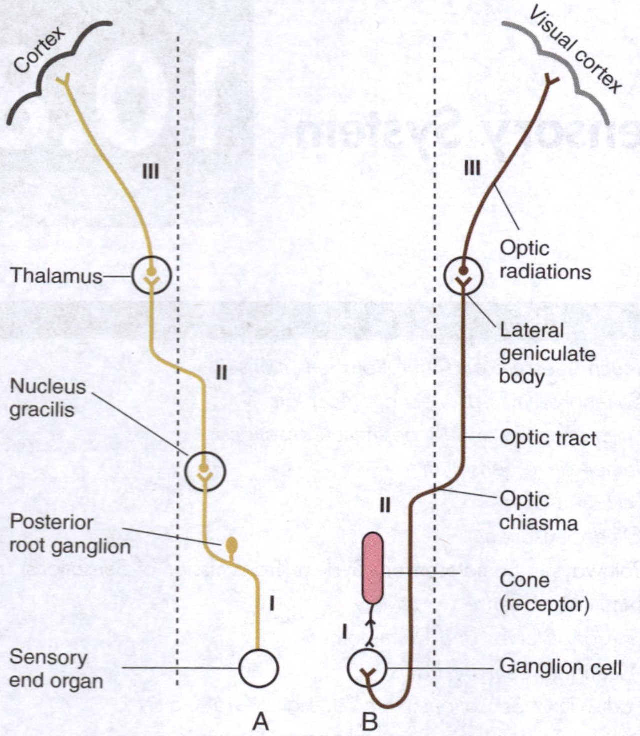

Fig. 10.8.1 Pathway of somatic (**A**) versus visual (**B**) sensations.

2. Afferent neurons These carry sensory impulses to the sensory cortex and constitute the neural pathway. Sensory neural pathway consists of:

- First-order neurons
- Second-order neurons
- Third-order neurons

3. Sensory cortex It includes the sensory areas of the cerebral cortex. It is formed by fourth-order sensory neurons. The information received in the sensory cortex results in a conscious perception of the stimulus, i.e. a sensation.

RECEPTORS

Sensory receptors are specialized cells that receive stimuli from the external or internal environment, and transduce these signals into neural signals. A *stimulus* is a change of environment of sufficient intensity to evoke a response in an organism. The external stimuli may be mechanical, chemical, thermal, auditory or visual.

Classification of Receptors

Receptors can be variously classified.

A. Depending on the Source of Stimulus (Sherrington's Classification)

1. ***Exteroceptors***, i.e. the receptors which receive stimuli from immediate surrounding outside the body, e.g.:
   Cutaneous receptors for pain, touch and temperature
2. ***Enteroceptors***, i.e. the receptors which receive stimuli from within the body. These include:
   - *Chemoreceptors* that measure blood gases
   - *Baroreceptors* that measure blood pressure
   - *Proprioceptors* that measure the position of the limbs or the force of muscle contraction
   - *Osmoreceptors* that respond to osmotic pressure of plasma
   - *Glucoreceptors* that respond to arteriovenous blood glucose difference
3. ***Telereceptors***, i.e. the receptors that receive stimuli from the distance, e.g.:
   - *Visual receptors*
   - *Cochlear receptors*
   - *Olfactory receptors*

B. Depending on Type of Stimulus Energy

1. Mechanoreceptors, i.e. those receptors which respond to mechanical stimuli. These include:

i. ***Cutaneous receptors (in epidermis and dermis)*** *for cutaneous tactile sensibility, e.g.:*
   - Free nerve endings
   - Merkel's discs (expanded nerve endings)
   - Ruffini's endings (spray endings)
   - Meissner's corpuscles (encapsulated nerve endings)
   - Krause's corpuscles (encapsulated nerve endings)
   - Hair end organs

ii. ***Cutaneous receptors for deep tissue sensibility, e.g.:***
   - Free nerve endings
   - Merkel's discs
   - Ruffini's endings
   - Pacinian corpuscles (encapsulated nerve endings)

iii. ***Muscle and joint receptors, e.g.:***
   - Muscle spindles or stretch receptors
   - Golgi tendon receptors
   - Joint receptors

iv. ***Hair cells, e.g.:***
   - Hair cells in organ of Corti (cochlear) or auditory receptors
   - Hair cells in vestibular apparatus or vestibuloreceptors for equilibrium

v. ***Baroreceptors*** of carotid sinus and aortic arch for detecting level of arterial blood pressure

2. Thermoreceptors, which detect environmental temperature, e.g.:

- Cold receptors
- Warm receptors

3. Photoreceptors or electromagnetic receptors, i.e. rods and cones of the retina that respond to light stimuli

4. Chemoreceptors which detect change in chemical composition of the environment in which they are located, e.g.:

- Taste receptors
- Olfactory receptors
- Osmoreceptors in supraoptic nuclei of the hypothalamus
- Aortic and carotid body receptors that detect the level of arterial pO_2, pCO_2 and pH
- Glucoreceptors
- Chemoreceptors on the surface of the medulla for detecting the level of blood pCO_2
- Chemoreceptors in the hypothalamus for detecting the levels of blood glucose, fatty acids and amino acids

5. Nociceptors, i.e. the receptors which respond to extremes of mechanical, thermal and chemical stimuli producing pain

C. Depending on the Type of Sensations

- Touch receptors
- Cold receptors
- Heat receptors
- Pain receptors
- Taste receptors
- Olfactory receptors
- Auditory receptors
- Light receptors

D. Depending on the Rate of Adaptation

1. ***Slowly adapting receptors***, i.e. tonic or static receptors that fire action potentials continuously during stimulus application, e.g. pain receptors, cold receptors and muscles and joint receptors
2. ***Rapidly adapting receptors***, i.e. phasic or dynamic receptors, which fire action potentials at a decreasing rate during stimulus application, e.g. Pacinian corpuscles and olfactory receptors

E. Clinical or Anatomical Classification of Receptors

1. ***Superficial receptors***, i.e. those present in the skin and mucous membrane
2. ***Deep receptors***, i.e. those present in muscles, tendons, joints and subcutaneous tissue
3. ***Visceral receptors***, which are present in the visceral organs

Sensory Transduction

Sensory transduction refers to the phenomenon of transduction of environmental signals into neural signals by the receptors. Steps of sensory transduction are as follows:

- Arrival of stimulus to receptor
- Production of generator or receptor potential
- Production of action potential in sensory nerve

Arrival of Stimulus to Receptor

The stimulus arriving at the given sensory receptor may be in the form of:

Mechanical force causing depression of the skin, which stimulates mechanoreceptors
Light or electromagnetic wave, which stimulates photoreceptors of the retina
Chemical, e.g. a molecule of NaCl on the tongue which stimulates chemoreceptors
Cold or warm temperature – stimulating thermoreceptors
Sound energy – stimulating auditory receptors, and so on and so forth

Production of Receptor Potential

When a stimulus excites the receptor, it changes the potential across the membrane of the receptors. This change in the potential is called receptor or generator potential.

Mechanism of development of receptor potential (Fig. 10.8.2) The change in membrane potential in a receptor is caused by a change in permeability of membrane of the unmyelinated terminals to Na^+. The resultant influx of Na^+ causes development of generator or receptor potential.

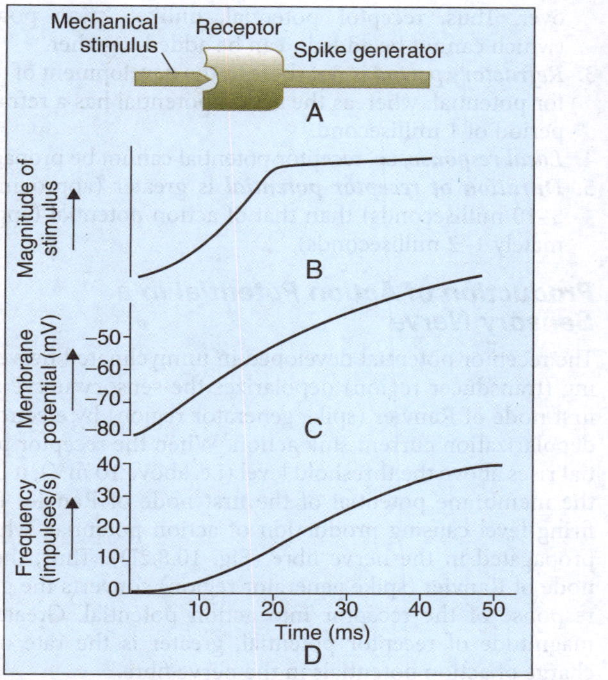

Fig. 10.8.2 Mechanism of development of generator potential, and its relationship with the intensity of stimulus: **A**, stimulus to mechanoreceptor causes its deformation which opens up channels which are permeable to Na^+ causing membrane depolarization; **B**, the magnitude of stimulus intensity; **C**, the receptor potential (generator potential) follows the time course; and **D**, the action potential. ***Note:*** The magnitude of generator potential and frequency of action potential are proportionate to the magnitude of the stimulus.

The different stimuli initiate change in the membrane permeability by the following mechanisms:

Mechanical deformation of the receptor causes its stretching and opens the ion channels (Fig. 10.8.2A).
Chemical stimulus opens the ion channels by direct effect on the membrane.
Change in temperature of the membrane changes the permeability of the membrane.
Effect of light on the photoreceptors changes the membrane permeability.

Opening up of ion channels in the sensory receptors allows current to flow. Usually the current is inward, which produces depolarization of the receptor. The exception is in the photoreceptors, where light causes hyperpolarization.

Properties of receptor potential The receptor potential is not action potential. It is similar to excitatory postsynaptic potential (EPSP) in synapse, end plate potential (EPP) in a neuromuscular junction and electrotonic potential in a nerve fibre. The important properties of receptor potential are as follows:

1. ***Graded response:*** Receptor potential is a graded response, i.e. its amplitude increases with the increasing velocity of stimulus application and increasing strength of stimulus. Thus, unlike action potential, it does not obey all-or-none law.
2. ***Summation***, i.e. receptor potential from two stimuli can be added if the second stimulus arrives before the receptor potential developed due to the first stimulus is

over. Thus, receptor potential, unlike action potential (which cannot be added), can be added together.

3. ***Refractory period*** is not there in the development of receptor potential, whereas the action potential has a refractory period of 1 millisecond.
4. ***Local response***, i.e. receptor potential cannot be propagated.
5. ***Duration of receptor potential*** is greater (approximately 5–10 milliseconds) than that of action potential (approximately 1–2 milliseconds).

Production of Action Potential in a Sensory Nerve

The receptor potential developed in unmyelinated nerve ending (transducer region) depolarizes the sensory nerve at the first node of Ranvier (spike generator region) by electrotonic depolarization current sink action. When the receptor potential rises above the threshold level (i.e. above 10 mV), it brings the membrane potential of the first node of Ranvier to the firing level causing production of action potential, which is propagated in the nerve fibre (Fig. 10.8.2D). Thus, the first node of Ranvier (spike generator region) converts the graded response of the receptor into action potential. Greater the magnitude of receptor potential, greater is the rate of discharge of action potentials in the nerve fibre.

Recording of Receptor Potential and Action Potential

For the purpose of demonstration, the receptor potential can be recorded from Pacinian corpuscles, because:

- It is a large-sized receptor.
- It can be easily dissected from the mesentery of experimental animals.
- Its anatomical configuration allows study with the microelectrode.

Structure of pacinian corpuscle A Pacinian corpuscle consists of concentric lamellae of connective tissue, surrounding an unmyelinated terminal portion of a nerve fibre. The myelin sheath of the sensory nerve fibre begins inside the corpuscle. Therefore, the first node of Ranvier is located inside the corpuscle but the second node of Ranvier is mostly outside the corpuscle (usually near the point at which the nerve fibre leaves the corpuscle) (Fig. 10.8.3A).

Technique of recording Recording electrodes (connected to a cathode ray oscilloscope [CRO]) are placed on the nerve fibre, one on the unmyelinated ending and other on the second node of Ranvier (Fig. 10.8.3A).

- When a mild pressure is applied on the corpuscle, a mild nonpropagated depolarizing potential called the generator or receptor potential can be recorded.
- When the pressure is increased in steps, the magnitude of receptor potential is increased (Fig. 10.8.3B).
- The depolarized segment of the unmyelinated nerve ending produces electrotonic depolarization (current sink action) in the first node of Ranvier.
- When the magnitude of receptor potential is sufficient (above 10 mV), an action potential is generated in the first node of Ranvier, which is propagated in the nerve fibre (Fig. 10.8.3B).

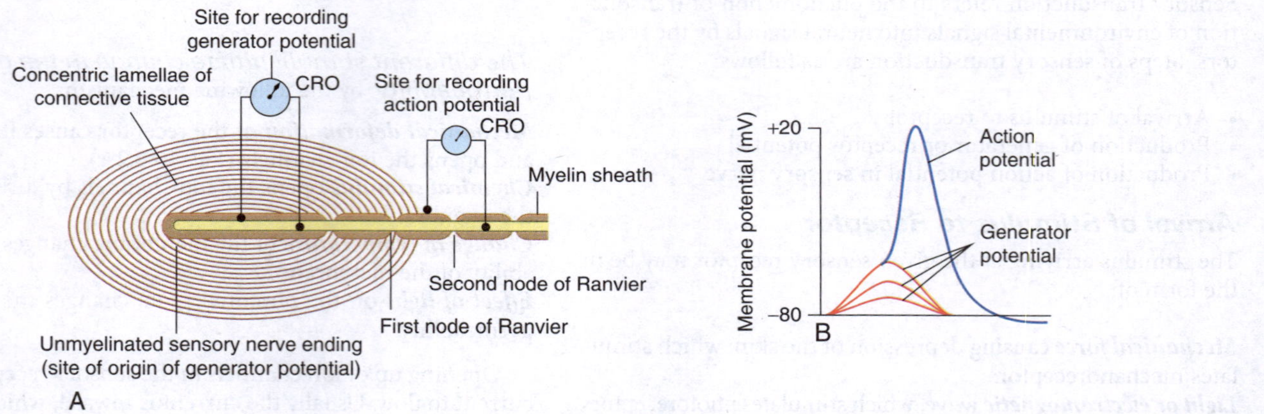

Fig. 10.8.3 Recording of receptor potential from Pacinian corpuscle: **A**, placement of recording electrodes; **B**, record of receptor potential and action potential produced by graded pressure to the Pacinian corpuscle; **C**, same response as in 'B' after the removal of connective tissue capsule indicates that receptor potential originates from the unmyelinated nerve endings, and not the capsule; **D**, blockage of first node of Ranvier abolishes conduction of receptor potentials produced; and **E**, no response is produced when sensory nerve is cut.

- If still greater pressure is applied on the receptor, the frequency of discharge is proportionately increased.

Demonstration of Site of Receptor Potential

The receptor potential originates from the unmyelinated nerve ending or from the first node of Ranvier which can be demonstrated experimentally as:

- When pressure is applied to the naked unmyelinated nerve ending after removal of the connective tissue of the corpuscle, the receptor potential is still produced but it decays more slowly (Fig. 10.8.3C).
- When pressure is applied to the naked unmyelinated nerve ending after blockage of the first node of Ranvier (by pressure or drug, e.g. narcotics), the receptor potential response persists but action potential cannot be recorded (Fig. 10.8.3D).
- When the sensory nerve is cut and allowed to degenerate, neither the receptor potential nor the action potential can be recorded (Fig. 10.8.3E).

Properties of Receptors

1. Specificity of response Each receptor is easily stimulated (has low threshold) by only one type of appropriate (adequate) specific stimulus. This specificity of response by a particular receptor is also called law of adequate stimulus. Although each receptor is exquisitely sensitive to its adequate stimulus, receptors can respond to other forms of energy if the intensity is high enough. For example:

Adequate stimulus for rod and cones of the retina is light. Therefore, the retina can detect the presence of a single photon of light. Pressure on the eyeball can also stimulate retinal receptors, but the threshold of these receptors to pressure is much higher than the threshold of the pressure receptors in the skin.
Adequate stimulus for Ruffini's receptors is warm water at low intensity of stimulus producing a specific response. The warm water at very high stimulus intensity can also stimulate naked nerve ending of pain, but the response produced is not complete.

2. Production of receptor potential on stimulation
As described in detail above, each receptor produces receptor or generator potential, when stimulated by adequate stimulus. When the receptor potential rises above the threshold, the action potential is produced in the nerve fibre attached to the receptor (for details, see page 991).

3. Adaptation When a receptor is continuously stimulated with the same strength of stimulus, the receptors respond at a very high impulse rate at first, but the frequency of action potential in its sensory nerve decreases progressively, till finally many of them no longer respond at all in some of the receptors (Fig. 10.8.4). This property is called adaptation. Depending on the rate of adaptation, the receptors are of two types:

Tonic receptors: These are slow and incompletely adapting receptors. These receptors keep on firing action potentials continuously during the stimulus application. Such receptors are important for life as they keep the brain constantly appraised of status of the body and its relation to its surroundings. Examples of such receptors are as follows:

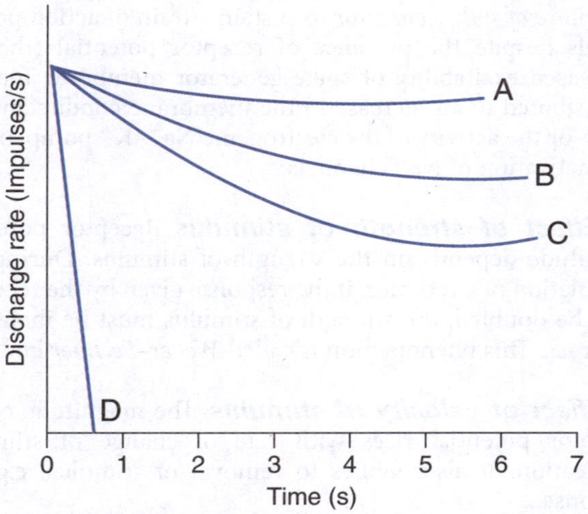

Fig. 10.8.4 Adaptation in sensory receptors with sustained stimulation: **A**, pain receptors; **B**, muscle spindles show minimal adaptation; **C**, thermoreceptors show moderate adaptation; and **D**, touch (Meissner's corpuscles) and pressure (Pacinian corpuscle) receptors show most rapid adaptation (phasic receptors).

Muscle spindles are tonic receptors which continue to discharge as long as the muscle is stretched and thus are helpful in prolonged postural adjustments.
Pain and cold receptors are tonic receptors which keep on giving warning to the brain about the noxious stimuli till they are present.
Baroreceptors and chemoreceptors are also tonic receptors that operate continuously in the regulation of blood pressure.

Important Note

Imagine, if the above-mentioned receptors would have showed marked adaptation, the life would have not been possible.

Phasic receptors: These are rapidly adapting receptors, which fire action potentials at a progressively decreasing rate, during stimulus application. These transmit signals only when the stimulus strength is changed. Therefore, the number of impulses transmitted is directly proportional to the rate at which the changes take place. Thus, the receptor potential in them is short and decays rapidly. Examples of phasic receptors are as follows:

- *Meissner's corpuscles*
- *Pacinian corpuscle*
- *Olfactory receptors*

Function of adaptation is to decrease the amount of sensory information reaching the brain.

Mechanism of adaptation varies in different receptors, for example:

- *Rods and cones* adapt by changing their chemical composition.
- *Mechanoreceptors* (Pacinian corpuscles) adapt due to redistribution of fluid.

Basically, sensory adaptation takes place via two major mechanisms:

- *Failure of transducer mechanism to maintain* a receptor potential despite continued stimulus application

- *Failure of spike generator* to sustain a train of action potentials despite the presence of receptor potential (the decreased excitability of spike generator membrane may be attributed to an increase in the membrane conductance to K^+ or the activity of the electrogenic Na^+–K^+ pump, or the inactivation of Na^+ channels)

4. *Effect of strength of stimulus* Receptor potential amplitude depends on the strength of stimulus. During the stimulation of a receptor, if the response given by the receptor is to be doubled, the strength of stimulus must be increased 10 times. This phenomenon is called *Weber–Fechner law*.

5. *Effect of velocity of stimulus* The magnitude of the receptor potential rises with rate of change of stimulus application. It also applies to removal of stimulus, e.g. off response.

6. *Projection* When any part of sensory path is stimulated, a conscious sensation referred to the location of receptor is produced. This is called *law of projection* (for details, see the section 'Encoding: Recognition of Type of Sensation', page 995).

ENCODING: RECOGNITION OF TYPE OF SENSATION

As discussed above, the sensory receptors transduce all forms of sensory stimuli into a common type of neural signal, i.e. action potentials which are carried by the peripheral nerves and sensory tracts in the spinal cord and brainstem to the sensory cortex. The question that arises is: how does the brain differentiate between the action potentials generated from a touch receptor and those from a pain receptor and interpret the sensation accordingly? It is believed that the sensory receptors themselves act as peripheral analysers. The intensity, location and quality of a stimulus are encoded as given next.

1. Encoding of Stimulus Intensity

The brain interprets different intensities of sensation (i.e. whether the touch is light or heavy; pain is mild, moderate or severe) by the following two mechanisms:

- By frequency of action potentials generated in the sensory fibres
- By the number of recruitments of sensory units

A. *By frequency of action potential generated in sensory nerve fibres* The encoding of intensity of stimulus is related to the rate of impulse discharge in the sensory nerve fibres as explained:

i. The magnitude of receptor potential is directly proportional to the logarithmic increase in the intensity of stimulus. For example, if the response given by a receptor is to be doubled, the strength of stimulus must be increased 100 times.
ii. The frequency of action potential produced in a sensory nerve is directly proportional to the magnitude of receptor potential (Fig. 10.8.5).
iii. From the above statements (i) and (ii), the frequency of action potential (S) in a sensory nerve is directly proportional to the logarithmic increase in intensity of stimulus (I), i.e.:

$$S = k \log I + C$$

where K and C are constants.

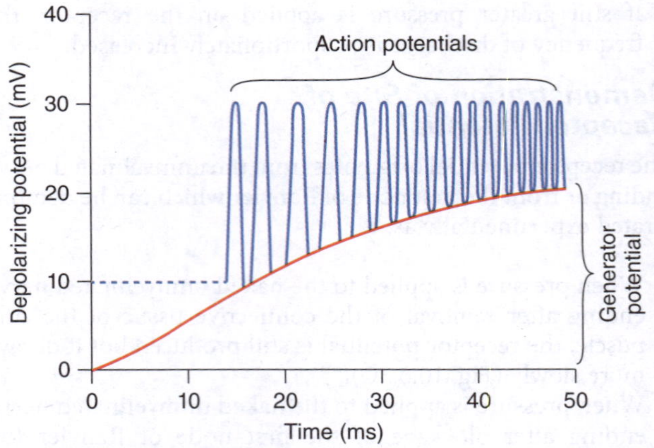

Fig. 10.8.5 Relationship between intensity of stimulus, magnitude of receptor potential and frequency of action potential.

The above-stated equation is called 'Weber–Fechner law', which states that the magnitude of sensation felt is directly proportional to the log of intensity of the stimulus.

B. *By number of recruitments of sensory units* A single afferent neuron with all its receptor endings makes up a *sensory unit* (Fig. 10.8.6). When the strength of stimulus is increased, it spreads over a large area activating more and more receptors in the neighbouring area and thus more and more *sensory units are recruited* to convey the impulse to the brain. This increase in the recruitment of sensory units is interpreted as increase in the intensity of the stimulus.

2. Encoding of Stimulus Location

The stimulus location is recognized accurately due to point-to-point representation of the body in the somatosensory cortex. Therefore, when the sensory fibres are experimentally stimulated anywhere in their course to the cortex, the conscious sensation produced is referred to the location of the receptor. This principle is called the *law of projection*. Because of this, after amputation of a limb, sometimes a patient complains of intense pain in the absent limb (*phantom limb*). These sensations are produced due to irritation of the damaged nociceptive and proprioceptive afferents at the stump of the amputated limb. The sensations evoked are projected to the area where receptors used to be located.

This mechanism of encoding, called *topographic representation*, is also used by visual sensation in addition to the

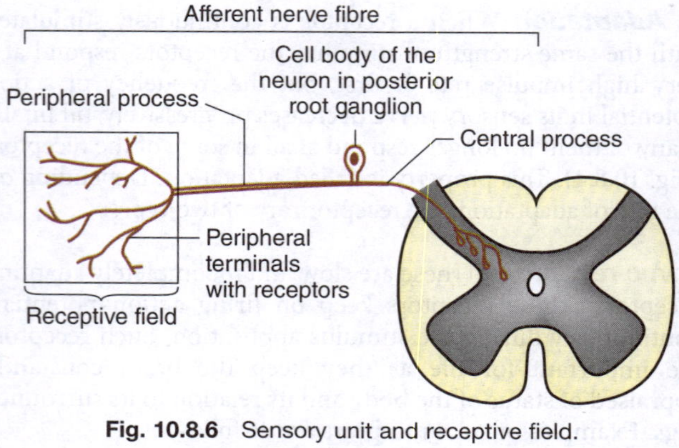

Fig. 10.8.6 Sensory unit and receptive field.

somatosensory system to localize the point of stimulus application. This mechanism of encoding by topographic representation is influenced by:

- Receptive field of neurons
- Phenomenon of lateral inhibition

Receptive field of neuron Each sensory neuron receives information from a particular sensory area called its receptive field (Fig. 10.8.6). Generally, the receptive fields of neighbouring neurons overlap and interdigitate with the areas supplied by others.

The smaller the receptive field, the more precise the encoding of stimulus localization is. For example, the ability to distinguish between two adjacent mechanical stimuli to the skin *(two-point discrimination)* is greater on the fingertips and lips where the receptive fields are much smaller and overlap considerably than on the hands and back where the receptive fields are large and widely separated.

Lateral inhibition Lateral inhibition is a phenomenon by which stronger inputs are enhanced and the weaker inputs of adjacent sensory units are simultaneously inhibited. Stimulus localization can be made more precise by lateral inhibition as explained: when two stimuli are applied to the skin, in the absence of lateral inhibition, they can be recognized as separate only if they are applied in receptive fields that are separated from each other by a nonstimulated receptive field (Fig. 10.8.7A); otherwise, the stimuli will produce an equal discharge in all these neurons (Fig. 10.8.7B).

- With lateral inhibition, the neuron with the receptive field in the centre is presynaptically inhibited by collaterals from the neurons with receptive fields located laterally. As a result, the receptive field in the centre does not fire and two stimuli are perceived (Fig. 10.8.7C).

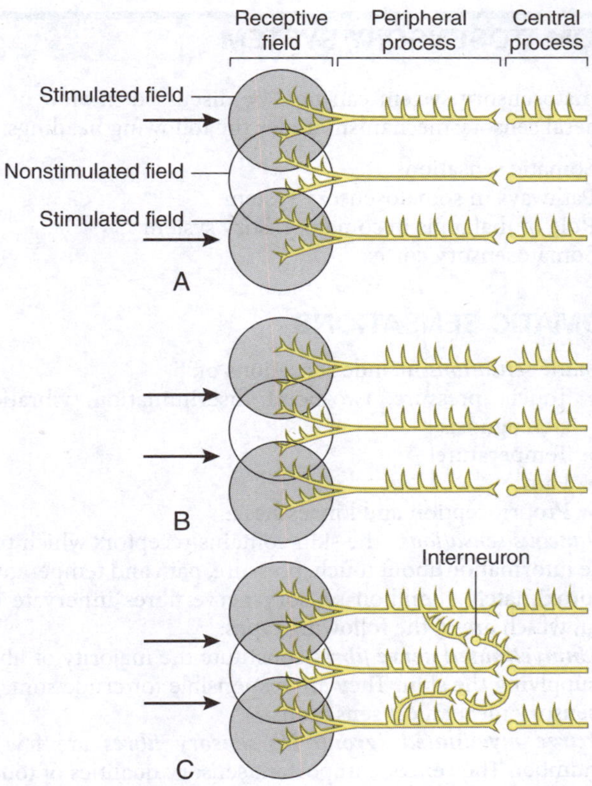

Fig. 10.8.7 Two stimuli can be perceived distinct in the absence of lateral inhibition if they stimulate receptive fields that are separated from each other by a nonstimulated receptive field (**A**). Otherwise the stimuli produced equal amount of discharge in all the three neurons (**B**). With lateral inhibition, the neurons with receptive field in the centre are presynaptically inhibited by collaterals from the neurons located laterally. As a result, the receptive field in the centre does not fire and two stimuli are perceived (**C**).

3. Encoding of Stimulus Quality

In general, since action potentials are similar in all nerves, why does stimulation of a touch receptor cause a sensation of touch and not of warmth? Similarly, stimulation of photoreceptors causes a sensation of light and not of hearing. Stimulus quality is encoded by the following mechanisms:

i. Labelled line mechanism: It is the mechanism in which the stimulus quality is encoded by the particular neural pathway that is stimulated. The basic sensory modalities are encoded by this mechanism. Each fibre or collection of neurons linked by related sensory fibres is referred to as a *labelled line*. For example, action potentials travelling along the fibres and neurons that comprise the anterolateral system (spinothalamic tract [STT]) are perceived as pain, whereas action potentials carried over the dorsal column–medial lemniscus system are distinguished as touch or pressure. Furthermore, (i) the sensation of touch is elicited whether the receptors on the skin are excited by mechanical deformation or by electrical stimulation, and (ii) the same type of sensation results no matter where along the sensory pathway the stimulus is applied.

The specificity of the sensory pathway from the receptors to the sensory cortex has been called *Muller's doctrine of specific nerve energies.*

ii. Pattern of activity within the neural pathway that carries information to the brain, which is used to encode stimulus quality, is a more complex mechanism. The two types of pattern coding are as follows:

In temporal pattern coding, the same neuron can carry two different types of sensory information depending on its pattern of activity. For example, cutaneous cold receptors indicate temperatures below or above 30°C by firing with or without bursts, respectively.

In spatial pattern coding, the activity of several neurons is required to elicit a sensation. For example, three neurons may be required to encode different taste sensations. A sour taste may result if all three neurons are activated, whereas a salty taste may result if only two neurons fire.

iii. Feature detectors are used in the sophisticated mechanism of sensory coding. They are neurons within the brain that integrate information from a variety of sensory fibres and fire to indicate the presence of a complex stimulus.

- For example, the location of an object in space can be encoded by cortical cells receiving information from a single eye. However, special feature detectors receiving information from both eyes are required to specify the depth of an object in the space.
- Similarly, the location of sound in space requires integration of information from both ears by feature detectors within the brainstem.

SOMATOSENSORY SYSTEM

Somatosensory system can now be discussed in view of the general sensory mechanism under the following headings:

- Somatic sensations
- Pathways in somatosensory system
- Role of thalamus in somatosensory system
- Somatosensory cortex

SOMATIC SENSATIONS

Somatic sensations include sensations of:

- Touch, pressure, two-point discrimination, vibration, stereognosis
- Temperature
- Pain
- Proprioception and kinaesthesia

Cutaneous sensations: The skin contains receptors which provide information about touch, pressure, pain and temperature. Approximately 1 million sensory nerve fibres innervate the skin, which are of the following types:

Unmyelinated nerve fibres constitute the majority of fibres supplying the skin. They are responsible for crude somatosensory mechanical sensations.

Large myelinated (group II) sensory fibres are few in number. They encode important sensory qualities of touch, vibration and pressure.

Small myelinated (Aδ) fibres and unmyelinated (C) fibres encode sensations of temperature and pain.

Cutaneous receptors can be grouped as:

- Mechanoreceptors
- Thermoreceptors
- Nociceptors

Touch, Pressure and Vibration Sensations

Mechanoreceptors

Mechanoreceptors provide information about touch, pressure and vibration stimuli to the skin. In general, these receptors consist of an unmyelinated axon surrounded by lamellated connective tissue corpuscles. These include those given next (Fig. 10.8.8).

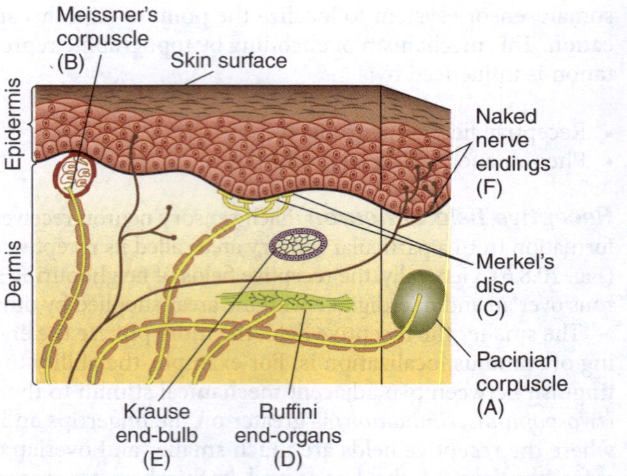

Fig. 10.8.8 Sensory receptors: **A**, Pacinian corpuscle; **B**, Meissner's corpuscle; **C**, Merkel's disc; **D**, Ruffini's end organs; **E**, Krause's end bulb; and **F**, free nerve endings.

1. Pacinian corpuscles Pacinian corpuscle, about 1 mm in diameter, consists of onion-like concentric lamellae of connective tissue surrounding an unmyelinated terminal portion of a nerve fibre. The myelin sheath of the sensory nerve fibre begins inside the corpuscle. Therefore, the first node of Ranvier is located inside the corpuscle but the second node of Ranvier is mostly outside the corpuscle (Figs 10.8.3A and 10.8.8A).

Location Pacinian corpuscles are located in the skin, subcutaneous tissue, mesentery and neighbourhood of tendons and joints.

Function They *detect tissue vibration* or other extremely rapid changes in the mechanical state of the tissue.

Receptive field, stimulus and adaptation Receptive field of Pacinian corpuscles is large. Pacinian corpuscles respond to deformation caused by mechanical pressure. The Pacinian corpuscle is a very *rapidly adapting* receptor, so only a few action potentials are generated, regardless of stimulus intensity. The deformation of the nerve terminal is not maintained during continuous stimulus application because the inner lamellae become rearranged. This is called adaptation. That is why we do not feel seat pressure when sitting. A *vibratory stimulus*, however, produces a steady discharge of the Pacinian corpuscle. Each time the stimulus is removed and applied, the Pacinian corpuscle discharges another action potential.

2. Meissner's corpuscles They are small encapsulated receptors supplied by Aβ type (group II) of myelinated nerve fibres (Fig. 10.8.8B).

Location They are present in nonhairy parts of the skin and are abundant at fingertips, lips, nipples and orifices of the body.

Receptive field, stimulus, function and adaptation These can be stimulated only by deformation of the small region of the skin lying just above the receptors; therefore, they have a *small receptive field*. They are used to detect rate of stimulus application. They are sensitive to movements of light objects over the surface of the skin. The ability to detect the rate of deformation when the skin is moved over an object is especially important to blind individuals using Braille. Meissner's corpuscles rapidly adapt to a maintained or slowly applied stimulus.

3. Merkel's discs Merkel's discs are unique because the transducer is not on the nerve terminal but on the epithelial cells that make up the disc (Fig. 10.8.8C). The epithelial sensory cells form synaptic connections with branches of a large single group II afferent myelinated fibre.

Location They are present in areas where Meissner's corpuscles are present, i.e. in abundance at fingertips, lips, nipples and orifices of the body.

Receptive field, stimulus, function and adaptation Merkel's discs are *slowly adapting* receptors with a *small receptive field* that is used to detect the *location of a stimulus*. They, along with Meissner's corpuscles, play an important role in localizing touch sensations and also in determining the texture of what is felt. Therefore, they are also called *tactile receptors*.

4. Ruffini's end organs Ruffini's end organs are multibranched encapsulated endings (Fig. 10.8.8D).

Location The receptor is located on the terminal of a group II axon that is covered by a liquid-filled collagen capsule. Collagen strands within the capsule make contact with the nerve fibres and overlying skin. They are present in the deeper layers of the skin and also in the deeper tissues.

Receptive field, stimulus, function and adaptation Ruffini's end organ is a *slowly adapting* receptor with a *large receptive field*, which is used to detect the *magnitude of stimulus*. Since Ruffini's end organs adapt very little, they continuously signal the state of deformation of the skin and deeper tissues. They are present in joint corpuscles where they detect the degree of joint rotation.

5. Hair end organs Each hair and its basal nerve fibre form the hair end organ.

Stimulus and function Hair end organ is stimulated by slight movement of hair. These receptors mainly detect the movement of objects on the surface of the body.

6. Krause's end bulbs They are spherical mechanoreceptors (Fig. 10.8.8E). Their afferent fibres belong to the Aδ group.

Location They are present in conjunctiva, in the papillae of lips and tongue, in the skin of genitalia and in the sheath of nerves.

Stimulus and function They detect touch and pressure.

7. Free nerve endings These are terminal branches of thin myelinated Aδ or unmyelinated C fibres (Fig. 10.8.8F).

Location They are present everywhere in the skin and in many other tissues.

Stimulus and function As mechanoreceptors, they detect touch and pressure.

Salient Features of Mechanoreceptors

Salient features of main mechanoreceptors are summarized in Table 10.8.1.

Functions of Touch and Pressure Mechanoreceptors

1. Detection of touch, pressure and vibration sensations by mechanoreceptors Touch, pressure and vibration are considered to be different forms of the same sensation.

Pressure is felt when the force applied on the skin is sufficient to reach the receptors located in the deeper layers of the skin.
Touch is felt when the force is insufficient to reach the deeper layers.
Vibrations are felt when there are rhythmic vibrations in the force.

Detection of touch, pressure or vibration sensation by a mechanoreceptor depends, among other factors, on whether it is a rapidly adapting or a slowly adapting receptor.

Slowly adapting mechanoreceptors, in general, are meant for sensing sustained pressure. They are of no use in detecting vibrations. These include Merkel's discs and Ruffini's end organs.

Rapidly adapting mechanoreceptors, in general, are meant for detecting rapid fluctuation in pressure (vibration). They are of not much use in signalling sustained pressure. These include Pacinian corpuscles, Meissner's corpuscles, Krause's end bulbs and hair end organs.

2. Two-point discrimination It is the ability to distinguish two touch stimuli separately. It depends on the interaction of touch sensibility and parietal lobe. The minimum distance by which two touch stimuli can be perceived as separate stimuli varies from 2–3 mm on the lips and fingertips to greater than 60 mm on the back of the trunk. The difference in the distance between the two points seems to be related to the density of touch receptors in different parts of the body.

3. Stereognosis Stereognosis refers to the ability to recognize familiar objects such as a key, coins, pen, pencil and spoons by merely handling them without looking at them. Touch and pressure receptors are involved in this sensation,

Table 10.8.1 Salient features of cutaneous mechanoreceptors

Receptors	Main descriptive feature	Receptive field size	Adaptation sensation	Encoded
Pacinian corpuscles	Onion-like capsule surrounding unmyelinated nerve ending	Large	Very rapid	Vibration, tapping
Meissner's corpuscles	Small, encapsulated, present in nonhairy skin	Small	Rapid	Speed of stimulus application
Merkel's disc	Transducer is on epithelial cells	Small	Slow	Location of stimulus
Ruffini's end organs	Multibranched Encapsulated Liquid-filled collagen corpuscle	Large	Slow	Magnitude and duration of stimulus (pressure)
Hair end organs	Hair and its basal nerve	Small	Rapid	Movement of object on the surface of body
Krause's end bulbs		Small	Rapid	Touch and pressure

but the cerebral cortex (somatic sensory association area) plays a major role.

> **Applied Aspects**
>
> ***Astereognosis***, i.e. loss of stereognosis, is an early sign of damage to the parietal lobe when the touch–pressure sensation is normal.

Neural Transmission

Type of nerve fibres The touch–pressure sensation from the mechanoreceptors is carried to CNS by:

- Aβ and Aδ sensory fibres
- Unmyelinated C fibres, which also conduct some touch impulses

Spinal cord tracts which carry touch–pressure sensations Spinal cord tracts which carry touch–pressure sensations are two lemniscus systems (dorsal column and ventral STT).

Dorsal column carries sensations of:

- Fine touch (touch with low threshold excitation)
- Detailed tactile localization
- Two-point discrimination
- Stereognosis

> **Applied Aspects**
>
> ***Lesions of the dorsal column*** are therefore associated with elevation of touch threshold and loss of above-mentioned sensations.

Ventral STT carries sensations concerned with gross tactile sensations of crude touch.

> **Applied Aspects**
>
> ***Lesions of ventral STT*** are therefore associated with slight touch deficit. The touch localization remains normal.

Proprioceptive and Kinaesthetic Sensations

Proprioceptive and kinaesthetic sensations arise from the muscles, tendons and joints. These include those given next.

1. Proprioceptive sensations These are concerned with the physical state of the body, i.e. sense of position, tendon and muscle sensations, deep pressure and sense of equilibrium.

2. Kinaesthetic sensations Kinaesthesia is the conscious recognition of rate of movement of different parts of the body. Kinaesthetic sensations include:

- Conscious kinaesthetic sensations
- Unconscious kinaesthetic sensations

Receptors Concerned

The receptors concerned are called *proprioceptors* and include:

- Muscle spindle or stretch receptors (see page 1017)
- Joint receptors located in the joint capsules and ligaments around the joints (Ruffini's end organs are the most important receptors for this function; a few Pacinian corpuscles are also involved)
- Golgi tendon organ (see page 1026)
- Vestibular receptors (see page 1040)

Neural Transmission

Type of nerve fibres Sensations from the above-mentioned receptors are carried by the myelinated nerve fibres (groups I and II) in the peripheral nerves. Neural pathway involved is:

Conscious sense of position, vibration and deep pressure is carried by axons from joint receptors and Pacinian corpuscles. These enter via the posterior root, branch and enter the *dorsal column* on the same side. From the spinal cord, ultimately these sensations reach the somatosensory cortex.

Unconscious proprioceptive information arising from the muscle spindles, Golgi tendon organs and joint receptors travels through group Ia and Ib fibres in peripheral nerves and through spinocerebellar tracts and dorsal column in the spinal cord. From the nuclei gracilis and cuneatus, fibres concerned with unconscious proprioception reach the cerebellum as external arcuate fibres. Spinocerebellar tracts enter the cerebellum through the inferior peduncle.

Temperature Sensation

Thermoreceptors

Thermoreceptors refer to a special type of free nerve endings, which are responsible for detecting temperature sensation. Separate receptors with discrete receptive fields exist for encoding warm and cold sensations and are called warm receptors and cold receptors, respectively. Free nerve endings of unmyelinated C fibres form the *warm receptors* and those of *small myelinated* Aδ fibres form the *cold receptors*.

Location Thermoreceptors are located in the skin of all parts of the body. However, density of thermoreceptors is greatest in the lips, moderate in the fingertips and least in the skin of the trunk.

Receptive fields The receptor fields of thermoreceptors (unlike those of mechanoreceptors) do not show any overlap, probably because precise localization of thermal stimulus is rarely important to the body. Because of the lack of overlap, it is possible to delineate distinct *hot spots* (areas having warm receptors) and *cold spots* (areas having cold receptors) on the skin that respond to warmth and cold, respectively. In any area of the body, the number of cold spots is about 4–10 times the number of hot spots.

Stimulus Thermoreceptors respond to the temperature of subcutaneous tissue surrounding them and not to the environmental temperature as such. Because of this reason, cold metal objects feel colder than wooden objects of the same temperature. The metal being a good conductor conducts heat away from the skin more rapidly and cools the subcutaneous tissue to a greater degree than the wood. Similarly, the alcohol-induced cutaneous vasodilatation gives a feeling of warmth, even when the person is exposed to extreme cold.

Salient features of response exhibited by warm and cold receptors are:

Warm receptors They are activated when skin temperature is between 30°C and 43°C (Fig. 10.8.9A).

- The steady-state firing rate of warm receptors reaches a peak at temperatures of approximately 42°C (Fig. 10.8.9A).

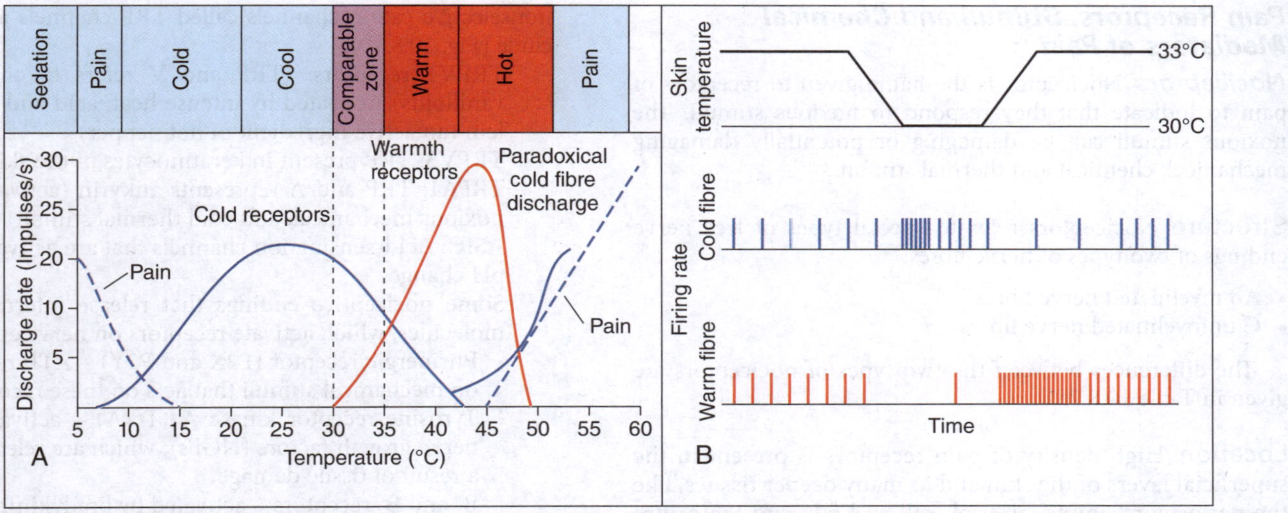

Fig. 10.8.9 **A**, Impulse discharge rate of cold and warm receptors as a function of temperature; and **B**, spike train illustrating the dynamic response of warm and cold receptors to a change in temperature. When the temperature decreases, cold fibres increase their firing rate transiently and then adapt to firing rate. Similarly, when temperature increases, warm fibres transiently increase their firing rate before adapting to rate indicated by the graph.

- Warm receptors transiently increase their firing rate when skin temperature increases, and decrease their firing rate when skin temperature decreases (Fig. 10.8.9B). This is because the sensation produced by a small change in temperature depends on the current skin temperature. For example, a stimulus of 35°C feels warm if the skin is at 30°C, and cool if the skin is at 40°C.

Cold receptors *They are activated when the skin temperature is between 10°C and 40°C* (Fig. 10.8.9A).

- The steady-state firing rate of cold receptors reaches a peak at temperatures between 25°C and 30°C (Fig. 10.8.9A).
- Cold fibres transiently increase their firing rate when temperature decreases, and transiently decrease their firing rate when skin temperature increases (Fig. 10.8.9B).
- Paradoxically, temperatures between 45°C and 50°C stimulate cold fibres as well as pain fibres producing mixed sensations of cold and pain (Fig. 10.8.9A).
- Cold temperature below 10°C stimulates only pain receptors (Fig. 10.8.9A).
- Thus, between 30°C and 40°C, both cold and warm receptors are stimulated, which help the person in fine gradation of temperature. Therefore, between 30°C and 40°C (neutral or comfort zone), complete perceptual adaptation occurs (i.e. awareness of temperature disappears).
- At moderate cold, the receptor activated is TRAM 8 (transient potential channel [TRP] and M signifies menthol ingredient present in mint that gives a cool taste).
- At temperature 34°C, TRPV4 (TRP and V refers to vanilloids) receptors activate a group of chemical complexes by heat, acid and chemical capsaicin (ingredient of hot pepper).
- At temperatures between 35°C and 39°C, TRPV3 (TRP vanilloid) are activated.

Adaptation Thermoreceptors show moderate degrees of adaptation (Fig. 10.8.4C). Therefore:

- On exposure to cold, when skin temperature begins to fall, initially the person feels much colder than at a later stage, even when exposed to the same cold environments. This is because when the temperature decreases, cold fibres increase their rate of firing and then adapt to the firing rate (Fig. 10.8.9B).
- Similarly, on sudden exposure to hot environment, the feeling of warmth is more intense in the beginning. This is because, when the temperature increases, warm receptors increase their firing rate before adapting to the rate indicated in the graph (Fig. 10.8.9B).

Neural Pathway

The impulses from cold receptors are carried by Aδ myelinated fibres, and those from the warm receptors are carried by unmyelinated fibres in the lateral STT. In the CNS, the lateral STT and the medial lemniscus carry impulses to the thalamus. Ultimately, impulses reach the somatosensory cortex.

Pain Sensation

Definition and Purpose

Definition Pain refers to an unpleasant sensory and emotional experience associated with actual or potential tissue damage. The word pain has been derived from a Greek word *Poena* meaning 'penalty or punishment'.

Purpose Pain sensation is different from other sensations because its purpose is not to inform the brain about the quality of a stimulus, but rather to indicate that the stimulus is physically damaging. Therefore, though the pain sensation is unpleasant, it is useful in the following ways:

- It makes one aware of a harmful agent in close contact with the body, and the body gives preferential treatment to this information.
- It causes the individual to react to remove the pain stimulus to prevent further damage to the tissues.
- Pain receptors are nonadaptable receptors; therefore, they keep the person apprised of the damaging stimulus as long as it persists. Thus, the pain sensation has a protective function.

Pain Receptors, Stimuli and Chemical Mediators of Pain

Nociceptors Nociceptor is the name given to receptors of pain to indicate that they respond to noxious stimuli. The noxious stimuli can be damaging or potentially damaging mechanical, chemical and thermal stimuli.

Structure Nociceptors refer to special types of free nerve endings of two types of nerve fibres:

- Aδ myelinated nerve fibres
- C unmyelinated nerve fibres

The differences between the two types of nociceptors are given in Table 10.8.2.

Location High density of pain receptors is present in the superficial layers of the skin and in many deeper tissues, like the periosteum, joints, arterial wall and falx and tentorium in the cranium. Parenchyma of the liver and alveoli of the lungs are insensitive to pain, but the liver capsule, bronchi and parietal pleura are very sensitive to pain. Most other deeper tissues have relatively sparse pain nerve endings, but widespread tissue damage always results in pain, even in these areas.

Types Nociceptors can be broadly grouped as somatic nociceptors and visceral nociceptors.

1. ***Somatic nociceptors*** are free nerve endings of Aδ and C fibres as mentioned above. Depending on the response to different noxious stimuli, the types of nociceptors are as follows:
   - *Unimodal nociceptors* respond exclusively to one modality, such as noxious chemical or heat stimulation.
   - *Polymodal nociceptors* are sensitive to several varieties of noxious stimuli.
   - *Silent nociceptors* are activated only in inflammation or tissue damage. Up to 40% of C fibres and 30% of Aδ fibres are silent nociceptors.

   Different varieties of receptors are located on the nociceptive nerve endings, activated by noxious, thermal, mechanical or chemical stimuli. These receptors mainly belong to nonselective cation channels called TRP channels and include (Fig. 10.8.10):
   - TRPV1 receptors: (TRP and V refers to chemical vanilloids) Activated by intense heat, acid and capsaicin (an active ingredient of hot pepper)
   - TRPV3: TRP present in keratinocytes of the skin
   - TRPA1: TRP and A represents ankyrin (activated by noxious mechanical, and cold thermal stimuli)
   - ASIC: Acid-sensing ion channels that are activated by pH changes
   - Some nociceptive endings that release intermediate molecules, which activate receptors on nerve endings:
     - Purinergic receptor (P2X and P2Y) – ATP released on mechanical stimuli that acts on these receptors
     - Tyrosine receptor kinase A (TrkA) – activated by nerve growth factors (NGFs), which are released as a result of tissue damage
     - B_1 and B_2 receptors – activated by bradykinin
     - Prostanoid receptors – activated by prostaglandins
     - Cytokine receptors

   All these receptors mediate inflammatory pain.
2. ***Visceral nociceptors:*** Visceral pain is not produced by many tissue-damaging stimuli such as localized cutting, clamping or burning. However, widespread inflammation, ischaemia, mesenteric stretching, or spasm or dilatation of hollow viscera produces pain. There is little evidence for specialized pain receptors in viscera. Visceral pain is often due to excessive tension on nerve endings in the smooth muscles, i.e. probably stretch receptors produce pain when stimulated to high firing rates by intense stimuli, e.g. pain due to uterine contractions during childbirth, or pain due to colic of alimentary, biliary or urinary tracts.

Pain stimuli Pain receptors are activated by three types of noxious stimuli – mechanical, thermal and chemical.

Mechanical and thermal stimuli tend to elicit fast pain. *Fast pain* is felt when a needle is stuck into the skin, when the skin is cut with a knife or when the skin is acutely burned. It is also felt when the skin is subjected to electric shock. Fast, sharp pain is not felt in most of the deeper tissues. Mechanical and thermal stimuli, however, can also elicit slow pain.

Table 10.8.2 Characteristic features of Aδ-fibre and C-fibre nociceptors

Feature	Aδ-fibre nociceptors	C-fibre nociceptors
1. Number	Less	More
2. Myelination	Myelinated	Unmyelinated
3. Diameter	2–5 m	0.4–1.2 μm
4. Conduction velocity	12–30 m/s	0.5–2 m/s
5. Specific stimulus	Most sensitive to pressure (mechanoreceptor)	Most sensitive to chemical agents like: Local anaesthetics Histamine Kinins Prostaglandins
6. Impulse conduction	Conduct impulses only in response to noxious stimuli (fast component of pain)	Conduct impulses in response to thermal and mechanical stimuli (slow component of pain)
7. Sensitivity to electrical stimulus	More	Less

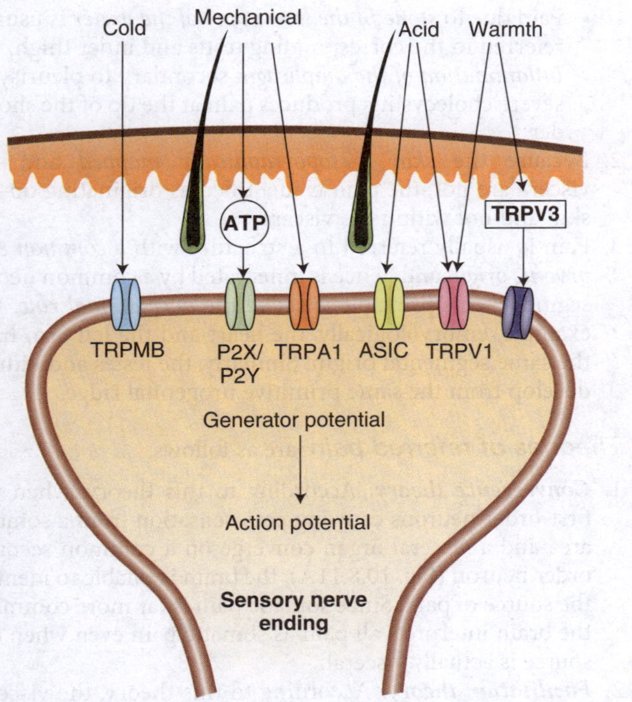

Fig. 10.8.10 Receptors on receptive unmyelinated nerve terminals in the skin.

Chemical stimuli usually tend to elicit slow suffering type of pain that occurs after tissue injury, although this is not always the cause.

As mentioned earlier, pain sensation is associated with actual or potential tissue damage caused by noxious stimuli. Damaged tissue releases certain chemicals which act on nociceptors and cause pain sensations. Chemical mediators of pain include:

- ***K^+, ATP and ADP*** are released following cell death.
- *Bradykinin* is formed by the reaction of certain circulating globulins with proteolytic enzymes released by dying cells. It is most powerful in causing tissue damage pain.
- *Leukotrienes* are released from mast cells.
- *Serotonin* is released from platelets.
- *Histamine* is released from mast cells.
- Accumulation of *lactic acid* in tissues due to anaerobic mechanism during ischaemia also stimulates nociceptors and causes pain.
- *Prostaglandins* are mediators of pain, fever and inflammation. These are synthesized by enzyme cyclooxygenase, which is induced in peripheral tissues by cytokines, growth factors and other inflammatory stimuli.
- Activation of a nociceptive nerve terminal stimulates the axon reflex and releases *substance P* and *calcitonin gene-related peptide* (CGRP) from other terminals of the same nociceptive nerve fibre.
- Prostaglandins and substance P enhance the sensitivity of pain endings but do not directly excite them.
- Nociceptin also causes pain.

Classification of Pain

Basically, pain is classified as physiological pain (acute pain) and pathological pain (chronic pain).

Physiological or acute pain has a sudden onset, recedes with healing process and is also termed *'good pain'* as it is an important protective mechanism. Withdrawal reflex is an example of protective role.

Pathological pain or chronic pain is also considered as *'bad pain'* because it persists for a long period. Chronic pain occurs due to injury (neuropathic pain), inflammation and ischaemia, and persists for a long time even after recovery and is usually unresponsive to analgesic agents.

Qualitative Types of Pain Sensations

Qualitatively pain sensations are of two types – fast pain and slow pain.

1. Fast pain Fast pain is a sharp, well-localized, pricking sensation that results from activation of the nociceptors on the Aδ fibres. The fast pain sensations travel faster and thus appear within 0.1 millisecond after the application of the stimulus. It is carried by Aδ fibres, which have a small receptive field and a topographic representation in the cortex.

Accompaniments of fast pain:

- *Withdrawal reflex*, which causes the individual to move the involved body part away from the source of painful stimulus
- *Sympathetic response*, i.e. increased blood pressure, tachycardia and mobilization of body energy supply

2. Slow pain Slow pain is a poorly localized, dull, throbbing, burning sensation that results from activation of nociceptors on the C fibres. It appears after 1 second or more following the application of stimulus. It is carried by C type of nerve fibres, which are unmyelinated fibres.

Accompaniments of slow pain:

- *Emotional perception* in the form of unpleasantness, and in long-standing cases irritation, frustration and depression
- *Autonomic symptoms* in the form of nausea, profuse sweating, vomiting and lowering of blood pressure
- *Generalized reduction in skeletal muscle tone*

Clinical Types of Pain

In clinical practice, pain sensations can be classified as:

- Somatic pain
- Visceral pain
- Referred pain
- Radiating pain
- Projected pain

1. Somatic pain Somatic pain, as the name indicates, arises from the tissues of the body other than viscera. It is of two types:

Superficial somatic pain arises from the skin and superficial tissues. Its features are usually similar to those of the *fast pain*.
Deep somatic pain arises from the muscles, joints, bones and fascia. Usually, its features are similar to those of *slow pain*.

Clinical conditions associated with somatic pain:

Common conditions that are associated with pain stimuli in day-to-day clinical practice are as follows:

- *Injuries:* These can be in the form of mechanical trauma, chemical injuries (e.g. those caused by acid burns) and thermal injuries.
- *Tissue ischaemia:* Blockage of the blood flow to the tissues causes severe pain. Pain is caused due to accumulation of lactic acid in the tissues due to anaerobic mechanisms

during tissue ischaemia. Other agents such as bradykinin and proteolytic enzymes released due to tissue damage caused by ischaemia may be more important causes of pain.

- *Inflammation* of the tissues caused by infecting agents (bacteria, virus and other organisms) is a very important cause of pain in clinical practice. Chemical mediators released due to tissue damage are responsible for eliciting pain.
- *Muscle spasm:* It causes pain due to direct stimulation of mechanosensitive pain receptors as well as indirectly by producing tissue ischaemia due to spasm of blood vessels.

2. Visceral pain The receptors for visceral pain are:

Visceral nociceptors: See page 1000.

Features of visceral pain are as follows:

- *Poorly localized,* because pain receptors in viscera are comparatively few
- *Unpleasant* because of emotional perception
- *Autonomic symptoms* in the form of nausea, vomiting, profuse sweating and lowering of blood pressure
- *Reflex contraction of skeletal muscle* of the abdominal wall, clinically known as guarding, which is a common association, especially when inflammation of viscera involves the peritoneum (it is a protective reflex which helps to protect the underlying inflamed structures from unintentional injury)
- *Radiates* or is referred to other site (see the section 'Referred Pain')

Common causes of visceral pain are as follows:

1. *Inflammation* of the viscera, e.g. appendicitis, cholecystitis and pancreatitis
2. *Overdistension of hollow viscera,* e.g. intestinal distension in intestinal obstruction and urinary bladder distension in urinary obstruction
3. *Spasm of hollow viscus* (pain is caused due to mechanical stimulation of pain endings and due to ischaemia, e.g. pain due to uterine contraction during childbirth and pain due to colics of alimentary, biliary or urinary tracts)
4. *Chemical stimuli* (damaging substances may leak from the gastrointestinal tract into the peritoneal cavity, e.g. gastric acid leaking through perforated gastric or duodenal ulcer)
5. *Ischaemia,* as occurring in tractions on the mesentery (pain is due to acidic metabolic end products or tissue degenerative products such as bradykinin and proteolytic enzymes)

Neural pathway Visceral pain sensation is carried by unmyelinated type C afferent fibres in the sympathetic (from most of the viscera) and in the parasympathetic (from many pelvic viscera) nerves. Their cell bodies are located in the dorsal roots and the homologous cranial nerve ganglion.

In the central nervous system, visceral pain fibres travel along with somatic pain fibres in the STT and medial lemniscus.

3. Referred pain Referred pain, as the name indicates, is that pain which originates due to irritation of a visceral organ and is felt not in the organ but in some other somatic structure (usually skin) supplied by the same neural segment.

Characteristic features of referred pain are as follows:

1. Such a pain is said to be referred to the second structure. For example:
   - In *myocardial ischaemia,* pain is referred to the left shoulder and arm.
   - Pain due to *stone in the lower part of the ureter* is usually referred to the corresponding testis and inner thigh.
   - *Inflammation of the diaphragm* secondary to pleurisy or severe cholecystitis produces pain at the tip of the shoulder.
2. Because the *skin is topographically mapped* and the viscera are not, the pain is identified as originating on the skin and not within the viscera.
3. Pain is usually referred to a structure with a *common embryonic origin* and hence is innervated by a common neural segment. This principle is called the *dermatomal rule.* For example, embryologically, the heart and the left arm have the same segmental origin. Similarly, the testes and kidney develop from the same primitive urogenital ridge.

Theories of referred pain are as follows:

1. ***Convergence theory:*** According to this theory, when the first-order neurons carrying pain sensation from a somatic area and a visceral organ converge on a common second-order neuron (Fig. 10.8.11A), the brain is unable to identify the source of pain. Since somatic pain is far more common, the brain interprets all pain as somatic pain even when the source is actually visceral.
2. ***Facilitation theory:*** According to this theory, the visceral irritation is inadequate for producing pain by itself. However, it facilitates pain fibres from somatic structures (Fig. 10.8.11B), so that even minor somatic irritation produces perceptible pain.

4. Radiating pain Sometimes, visceral pain is experienced both locally and at a distant point (referred pain). In fact, pain seems to spread from the local area to the distant site. This is called radiating pain. An example of radiating pain is as follows:

- In appendicitis, pain starts in the right iliac fossa and radiates towards the centre of the abdomen.

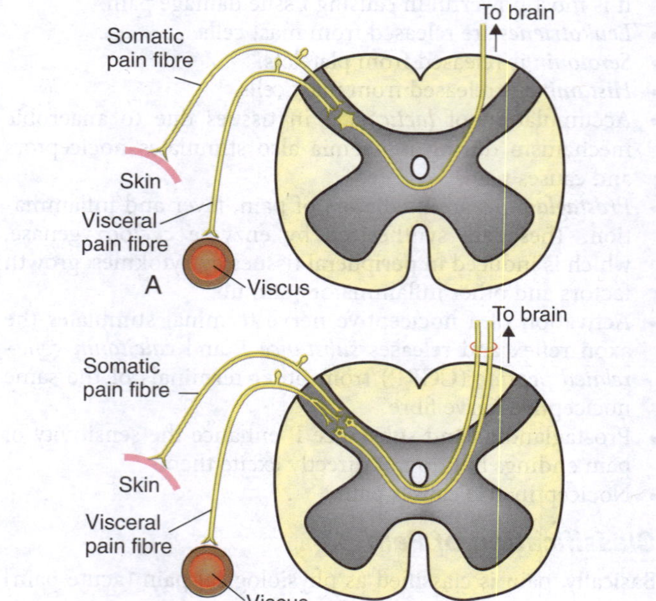

Fig. 10.8.11 Theories of referred pain: **A,** convergence theory; and **B,** facilitation theory.

5. Projected pain When the sensory fibres carrying pain sensations are stimulated anywhere in their course to the sensory cortex, the pain sensations evoked are projected to the area where receptors are located. This is called *projected pain*. It should not be confused with referred pain in which pain originating in visceral organs is referred to sites on the skin. Projected pain follows the *law of projection* (see page 994). Examples of projected pain are as follows:

- After amputation of a limb, sometimes the patient complains of intense pain in the absent limb (phantom limb). The pain sensations are produced due to irritation of nociceptive fibres at the stump but are projected to the area where receptors used to be located.
- Striking the elbow causes pain to be projected to the hand.

6. Hyperalgesia Hyperalgesia refers to enhanced painful response to a stimulus. It is of two types:

i. ***Primary hyperalgesia:*** In it, the noxious stimuli produce more severe pain than expected. It occurs over an area of tissue damage. The pain threshold is lowered, so that even non-noxious stimuli (e.g. touch) produce pain (*allodynia*). Both the movement-related symptoms of osteoarthritis and touch-evoked pain of herpetic neuralgia are examples of mechanical allodynia. Primary hyperalgesia is due to release of allogeneic pain-producing substances like histamine, 5-HT, plasma kinin and prostaglandins from the damaged tissues. Several other changes occurring that lead to chronic pain are as follows:
   - NGF released by damaged tissue is retrogradely transported to cell bodies of dorsal root ganglia and increases production of substance P, and also affects expression of tetrodotoxin-resistant voltage-gated Na^+ channels on dorsal root ganglia and increases their activity.

ii. ***Secondary hyperalgesia*** refers to occurrence of far more severe pain than expected in response to a noxious stimulus applied to the normal healthy skin. In this condition, there is no lowering of pain threshold. Secondary hyperalgesia has been explained to result due to the phenomenon of subliminal fringe. Primary pain afferents from an area of tissue damage not only stimulate the appropriate second-order neurons to the threshold level producing pain and primary hyperalgesia but also excite the second-order neurons belonging to the nearby area to the subthreshold level. Hence, application of noxious stimulus produces more intense pain in this area.

Important Note

Nociceptin is an opioid-like polypeptide, and has no binding affinity for opioid receptors. It causes hyperalgesia when injected intracranially in experimental animals. It probably has a role in pain transmission.

7. Causalgia Causalgia is a condition in which spontaneous burning pain sensation occurs after a long time in the area of even trivial injuries. It is also accompanied by *hyperalgesia* and reflex sympathetic dystrophy (RSD).

RSD, also known as complex regional pain syndrome (CRPS), means that sympathetic discharge reflexly causes pain in the injured skin area. The exact cause is not known, but research in the animals reveals that:

- In the affected area, the skin becomes thin, hair growth increases and nerve injuries lead to sprouting of the sympathetic nerve fibres. The overgrowth of sympathetic (noradrenergic) endings enters the dorsal root ganglia of the spinal nerves. Therefore, discharge of these noradrenergic endings stimulates the altered circuitry of nerve fibres in the skin.
- Use of α-adrenergic blocker helps in relief of causalgia-type pain.
- Excessive activation of NMDA receptors on spinal motor neurons leads to increased activity in pain pathways.
- Increased activation of neuroglia (microglia) near afferent nerve terminals by release of neurotransmitters from sensory afferents, in turn, leads to release of proinflammatory substances (cytokines) that act presynaptically on pain processing by PK_{2X} receptors and increase the excitability of postsynaptic neurons. Therefore, antagonists of PK_{2K} receptors may be used therapeutically to alleviate chronic pain.

Properties of Pain Sensations

In general, properties of pain sensation are as follows:

Threshold and intensity: Pain is not felt when the intensity of stimulation is low (i.e. subthreshold stimulus). However, when the intensity increases, more and more pain is felt according to Weber–Fechner law (page 994). When the intensity of stimulus is very high, pain even spreads to neighbouring areas.

Adaptation: Since pain receptors do not show any adaptation, pain continues as long as receptors are stimulated. In some instances, the activation of pain receptors becomes progressively greater as the pain stimulus continues; this is called *hyperalgesia*.

Localization of pain: In general, pain sensations are poorly localized. Superficial pain is comparatively better localized than deep pain. Visceral pain is most of the time referred to the area other than the area overlying the viscus.

Emotional accompaniment: Pain sensation is usually associated with unpleasantness. Long-standing pain causes irritation, frustration and even depression.

Influence of rate of damage on intensity: If rate of damage (extent of damage in time) is high, intensity of pain is high and vice versa. Therefore, slowly growing tissue-damaging agents, e.g. cancer, at early stage may not produce pain at all.

Qualitative types: Qualitatively pain sensation is of two types – fast and slow – each type having its typical features as described above (page 1001).

Muscular response: Acute pain may be associated with skeletal muscle spasm in the affected area, e.g. spasm of the muscles around the fractured area. This has a beneficial effect as it causes immobilization of the part and the part gets rested automatically.

Reflex response: Fast pain evokes a *withdrawal reflex* and a sympathetic response (see page 1026). Slow pain is associated with autonomic symptoms (see page 1024).

Neural Pathway and Perception of Pain Sensations

Two separate pathways exist for transmission of fast and slow pain to the brain.

Pathway for the fast pain

Pathway for the fast pain is as follows:

In peripheral nerves: Fast pain signals are transmitted from the Aδ fibres at velocities between 6 and 30 m/s to the dorsal root ganglion and then enter the spinal cord at the dorsal root

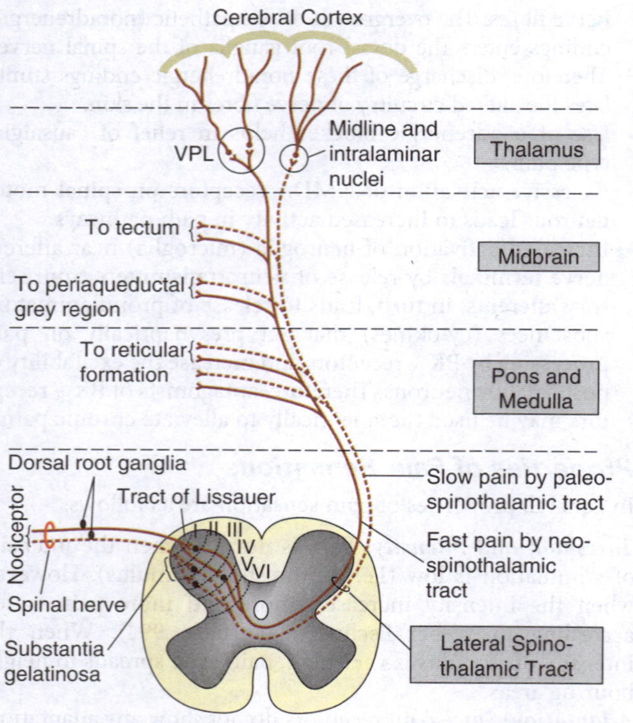

Fig. 10.8.12 Neural pathway of fast and slow pain.

of the spinal nerve (formed by axons of cells of the dorsal root ganglion) (Fig. 10.8.12).

In the spinal cord, Aδ fibres ascend or descend for one or two segments in the tract of Lissauer lying immediately posterior to the dorsal horn and then terminate into neurons of lamina I. These neurons give rise to fibres that immediately cross to the opposite side of the cord through the anterior commissure (Fig. 10.8.12) and then pass upwards to the brain in the anterolateral columns as the *neospinothalamic tract*.

In the brainstem, a few fibres from the neospinothalamic tract terminate in the reticular formation, but most of them pass upwards to the thalamus (Fig. 10.8.12).

In the thalamus, most of the fibres project to the ventral posterolateral (VPL) nucleus. From here, thalamic neurons project to the primary sensory cortex (Fig. 10.8.12).

Important Note

This system is primarily used in the localization of pain stimuli. When tactile receptors are also stimulated along with fast pain fibres, localization of fast pain is exact. If only pain receptors are stimulated, localization is poor.

Pathway for slow pain Pathway for slow pain is as follows:

In peripheral nerves, slow pain impulses are carried by slow-conducting unmyelinated fibres at velocities ranging from 0.5 to 2 m/s to the dorsal root ganglion and then enter the spinal cord at the dorsal root of the spinal nerve (formed by axons of cells of the dorsal root ganglion) (Fig. 10.8.12).

In the spinal cord, the C fibres terminate in the laminae II and III of the dorsal horn. Laminae II and III are together known as substantia gelatinosa.

From here, fibres go to lamina V of the dorsal horn. Axons of neurons of lamina I of the dorsal horn which receive impulses from C fibres cross the midline near their level of origin and form the palaeospinothalamic tract, which passes upwards to the brain in the anterolateral column along with the fibres of fast pain.

In the brainstem, these fibres terminate very widely, mainly in the reticular formation, and also in the superior colliculus and periaqueductal grey (PAG) region. A system of ascending fibres, mainly from the reticular formation, proceeds rostrally to the intralaminar nuclei and posterior nuclei of the thalamus, as well as to a portion of the hypothalamus. The intralaminar nuclei of the thalamus in turn relay activating signals to all parts of the brain (Fig. 10.8.12).

Important Notes

- Transmission of pain signals through two routes explains why a single prick with a sharp needle produces almost immediately sharp localized pain, followed about 1 second later by slowly increasing painful sensation that lasts many seconds and sometimes even minutes.
- The fact that the brainstem reticular areas and the intralaminar thalamic nuclei that receive input from the palaeospinothalamic pathway are part of the brainstem-activating or alerting systems may explain why individuals with chronic pain syndromes have difficulty in sleeping.

Perception of pain sensations Perception of pain is the phenomenon by which noxious stimuli reach consciousness. It involves two components:

- Nociceptive component
- Affective (cognition and attention) component

1. Nociceptive component of pain perception Nociceptive component of pain perception involves the neural pathway of pain as described above.

The role of somatic sensory cortex (SI) in pain perception is not entirely clear. Complete removal of SI cortex does not eliminate the perception of pain. Such lesions do, however, interfere with the ability to interpret the quality of pain and to determine its precise localization. Therefore, it is believed that pain perception occurs at subcortical levels, i.e. in the thalamus and in the reticular formation of the brainstem. However, the somatosensory cortex helps in exact and meaningful interpretation of quality and localization of pain.

2. Affective (cognitive and attention) component of pain perception Affective (cognitive and attention) component of pain perception is the psychological component. It involves the activity of the STT–limbic system pathway. *Cognitive perceptions* are those abilities that recognize, discriminate, memorize or judge afferent information. It involves the patient's ability to relate a painful experience to another event, e.g. pain experienced in a pleasant environment elicits a less intense response than that experienced in a setting of depression.

Attention plays role in the perception of pain on the basis that only a fixed number of afferent stimuli can reach cortical centres. Therefore, if a patient in pain concentrates on a separate and unrelated image, e.g. getting deeply involved in music or an interesting movie on television, it is possible that he/she will perceive lesser intensity of pain than otherwise. The biofeedback and hypnosis, for their positive impact on pain, operate on this principle.

Pain Suppression Systems in CNS

The degree of reaction to painful stimuli varies from individual to individual, mainly because of existence of pain suppression systems in the central nervous system. The pain suppression consists of two major components:

- Spinal pain suppression system
- Supraspinal pain suppression system

A. Spinal pain suppression system There exists a pain inhibitory complex in the dorsal horn of the spinal cord which blocks the pain signals at the initial entry point to the spinal cord.

Gate control hypothesis Gate control hypothesis has been put forward by Metzak and Wall in 1965 to explain the working of the spinal pain suppression system. According to this hypothesis, the dorsal grey horn acts as a gate for transmission of pain sensation and this gate can be partly or completely closed by:

- Segmental suppression
- Supraspinal suppression

1. ***Segmental suppression:*** It has been observed that activation of large myelinated touch fibres (Aβ) reduces pain. It is called the gating of pain and occurs because after entering the spinal cord, the Aβ fibres give collaterals that cause *presynaptic inhibition* (primary afferent depolarization) of pain carrying both type C and Aδ fibres, where they synapse in the dorsal horn (Fig. 10.8.13). This is done by blocking calcium channels in the membranes of nerve terminals. Although poorly understood, such circuitry probably explains the relief of pain achieved by the following manoeuvres:
   - Rubbing or massage or pressure in the vicinity of the painful area
   - Local application of warmth or cold
   - Local application of counterirritants, i.e. stimulation of the skin
   - Acupuncture
   - Transcutaneous electric nerve stimulation (TENS) in which the pain site or the nerves leading from it are stimulated by electrodes placed on the surface of the skin
2. ***Supraspinal suppression*** is caused by the supraspinal suppression system described below.

B. Supraspinal pain suppression system There exist three different supraspinal descending pain modulation pathways:

- Descending serotonergic and opioid inhibitory system
- Descending purinergic inhibitory system
- Descending adrenergic inhibitory system

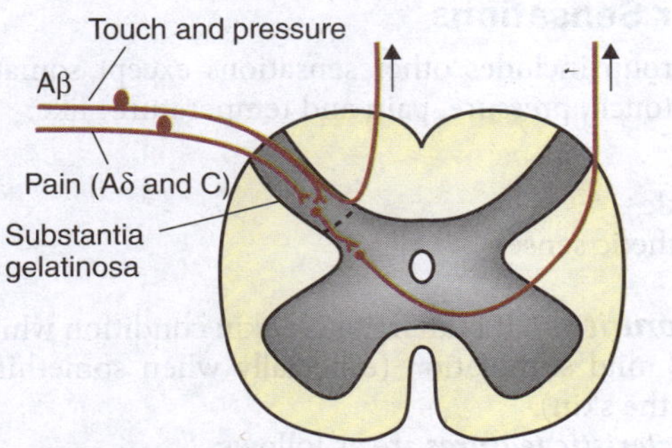

Fig. 10.8.13 Spinal pain suppression system. ***Note:*** The collateral from Aβ fibres from touch receptors causes presynaptic inhibition of pain afferent Aδ and C fibres.

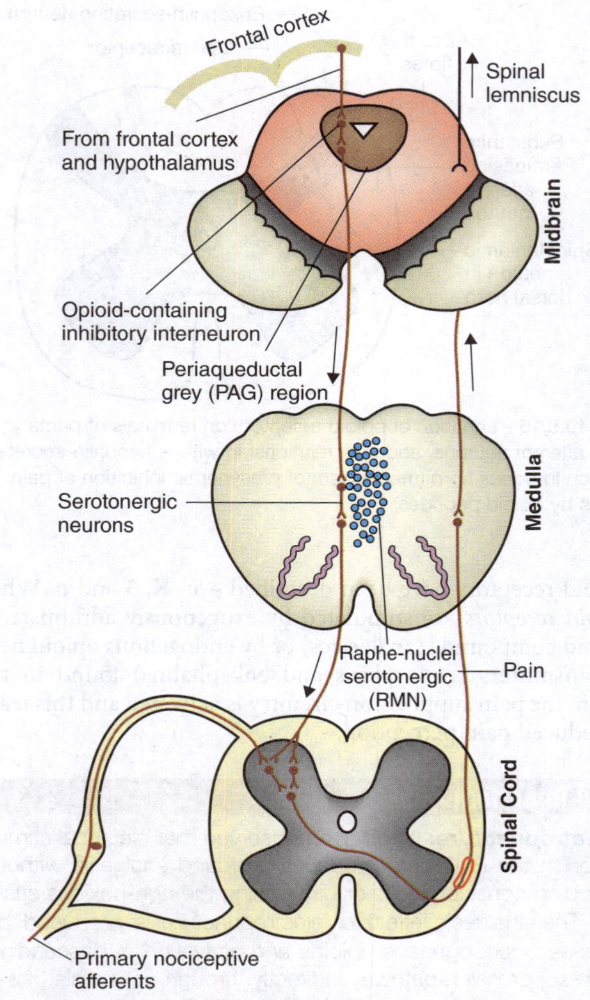

Fig. 10.8.14 Supraspinal serotonergic and opioid pain inhibitory system.

1. Descending serotonergic and opioid inhibitory system It is the most important supraspinal pain inhibitory system. Components of this system (Fig. 10.8.14) are as follows:

i. Raphe magnus nucleus (RMN): It is a thin midline nucleus located in the lower pons and upper medulla. Its neurons receive innervation from the PAG reticular formation, hypothalamus and frontal cortex. Neurons of RMN contain both serotonin (5-HT) and substance P. The *serotonergic neurons* of the RMN project down the dorsolateral column to influence the neurons in the dorsal horn of the spinal cord, which are excited by primary nociceptive afferents. The serotonergic fibres are believed to exert their effect by *postsynaptic inhibition*. The drug amitriptyline alleviates pain by increasing the levels of serotonin. The function of substance P in these neurons and their relationship with serotonin are uncertain. Inhibition of pain fibres in the spinal cord inhibits withdrawal reflex evoked by application of noxious stimuli. Other sensory modalities like touch and temperature are not affected.

ii. PAG area in the midbrain: It inhibits pain by stimulating the RMN (Fig. 10.8.15). Neurons of PAG have opioid receptors on their surface membranes. In general, four types of

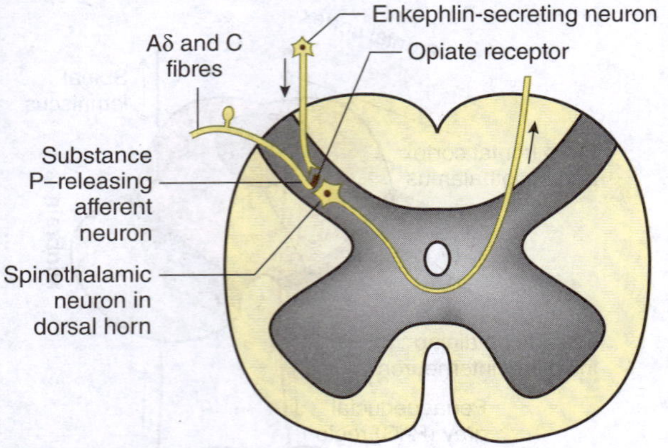

Fig. 10.8.15 Location of opioid receptors on terminals of primary pain afferent neurons, and their relationship with enkephalin-secreting neuron in dorsal horn (mechanism of presynaptic inhibition of pain fibres by opioid peptides).

opioid receptors have been described – **n**, **K**, **5** and **o**. When *opioid receptors* are stimulated by exogenously administered opioid compounds (analgesics) or by endogenous opioid neurotransmitters (endorphins and enkephalins) found in the brain, the pain suppression circuitry is activated and this leads to reduced pain perception.

Important Note

Electropuncture: It has been observed that electrical stimulation in the PAG area produces profound analgesia without clouding consciousness or diminishing the non-noxious stimuli. The analgesic effect of electropuncture is produced by release of endogenous opioids and activation of descending pain suppression pathway indirectly through collaterals of ascending pain transmission pathway to PAG, brainstem serotonergic and catecholaminergic region. Analgesia produced by electrical stimulation is reversed by *naloxone*, implicating endogenous opioid peptides as mediators.

Opioid receptors are also present on the membrane surface of the terminals of primary afferent pain-carrying fibres, which terminate in substantia gelatinosa of the dorsal horn. These neurons secrete *substance* P as a neurotransmitter. The opioid peptides (endorphin and enkephalin) released on stimulation of descending pain inhibitory pathway bind with opioid receptors and decrease the release of substance P from the primary afferent neurons terminating in the dorsal horn (Fig. 10.8.15), and thus inhibit the pain by presynaptic inhibition.

Physiological significance: Morphine relieves pain by two mechanisms:

- *At the spinal level* by binding to opioid receptors and thereby decreasing release of substance P
- *At the supraspinal level* by binding to opioid receptors in PAG and thus activating descending inhibitory pathway that produces inhibition of primary afferent transmission in the dorsal horn

Cannabinoid receptors: There are mainly two types of cannabinoid receptors – CB_1 present on the central neurons and CB_2 present on the peripheral neurons. Some non-neural cells also possess these receptors. An endogenous ligand analogous to these receptors (anandamide) exerts its analgesic effect by binding to these receptors.

iii. Hypothalamus and frontal cortex also play a role in pain suppression. Neurons descending from the hypothalamus and frontal cortex stimulate both the above-described brainstem centres of pain inhibition, i.e. PAG and RMN (Fig. 10.8.14).

The descending serotonergic and opioid pain inhibitory system is stimulated in the situations given next.

iv. Stress-induced analgesia occurs:

When limbic system is stimulated: The limbic system is the seat of emotions. Fibres from the limbic system supply the PAG. This explains why a soldier wounded in the battlefield may feel no pain during the heat of battle, also called stress-induced analgesia. In this condition:

- Release of norepinephrine from brainstem catecholaminergic neurons and amygdala (part of the limbic system) is involved in motivational–affective response to pain.

Release of cannabinoids, such as 2-archidonoylglycerol (2-AG) and anandamide, may have a role in stress-induced analgesia.

Autofeedback: When the STT is stimulated, the collaterals from STT stimulate the descending inhibitory pathway (Fig. 10.8.15).

2. Descending purinergic inhibitory system Descending purinergic inhibitory system, comprising specifically adenosine, has been recognized. Adenosine exhibits both presynaptic and postsynaptic actions and produces antinociception by indirect interaction with excitatory amino acid release. Role of adenosine in pain suppression system is corroborated by the following two observations:

- Significant decrease in circulating blood and CSF adenosine levels in patients with neuropathic pain
- Effective attenuation of neuropathic pain following low-dose infusion of adenosine

3. Descending noradrenergic inhibitory system Fibres of this system originate from the *locus coeruleus* and medullary reticular formation and descend in the dorsolateral fasciculus. Environmental factors, such as stress, may activate this descending inhibitory mechanism. Norepinephrine-depleting agents, including reserpine and α_2-antagonists, and lesions within the noradrenergic system, all interfere with morphine analgesia.

4. Acetylcholine Epibatidine, a cholinergic agonist, is a strong nonopioid analgesic agent. Its effect is blocked by cholinergic-blocking agents. This suggests that nicotinic cholinergic mechanism is also involved in regulation of pain but its exact role is not yet cleared.

Other Sensations

This group includes other sensations except somatic sensations (touch, pressure, pain and temperature) like:

- Itch
- Tickle
- Synthetic senses

Itch (pruritus) It is an irritative skin condition which occurs due to mild stimulation (especially when something moves across the skin).

Characteristic features are as follows:

1. It occurs only in the skin, eyes and certain mucous membranes but not in the deep tissue and viscera.

2. It originates due to stimulation of *itch receptors* which are naked nerve endings of unmyelinated C fibres. The receptors are stimulated by two ways:
   - By repeated local mechanical stimulation of the skin
   - By certain chemical agents, e.g.:
     - *Bile salts* (raised plasma concentration of bile salts during pregnancy)
     - *Histamine* (in urticaria, severe itching results due to release of a large quantity of histamine from antigen–antibody complex)
     - *Kinins*
       Kinins produce their effect by activation of GPCRs (B_1 and B_2). B_2 receptors are protease-activated receptor-2 (PAR-2) that produce both nociceptive and pruritogenic responses.
3. The pathway for itch sensation like pain is carried by fibres into the spinal cord and then conducted by lateral STT.
4. Scratching relieves the itching. The mechanism is the same as gate control hypothesis in pain sensation, i.e. scratching stimulates large, fast-conducting afferents which cause presynaptic inhibition of fibres in the dorsal horn cells.
   - Antihistaminics
   - β_2 antagonists – effective in reducing pruritus and reduce scratching behaviour (occurs in response to activation of PAR-2 receptors)

Tickle Tickle is another variable of touch sensation. It is regarded as a pleasurable feeling compared with itching (which gives an annoying feeling) and pain (which is an unpleasant feeling).

Synthetic sense The combinations of various cutaneous sensations produce different experiences that are entirely different from primary sensation. Therefore, the new experience is regarded as synthetic sense.

PATHWAYS IN SOMATOSENSORY SYSTEM (TRANSMISSION OF SENSATIONS)

Neurons of Sensory Pathway

Pathways in the somatosensory system are formed by a chain of three neurons, which ultimately reach the sensory cortex.

First-Order Neurons

These are the primary afferent neurons that receive the transduced signals from the sensory receptors and carry them to the spinal cord or brainstem. The cell bodies of the primary afferent neurons are located in *dorsal root ganglia*. These are T-shaped unipolar neurons with peripheral and central processes. The peripheral processes reach the sensory receptors and form the sensory part of *spinal nerves* (which are mixed nerves). Central processes constitute the *dorsal nerve root* of the spinal nerve (and also see page 880).

Type of sensory fibres The fibres of first-order neurons in the spinal nerves and dorsal nerve root comprise Aα, Aβ, Aδ and C-type fibres, and are often referred to as group I, II, III and IV, respectively, by the sensory physiologists (Table 10.8.3). Aα and β fibres are not present in sensory pathways. For further details about types of fibres, see page 70.

Table 10.8.3 Types of sensory fibres

Sensory group	Fibre type	Origin
Ia	Aα	Annulospinal endings on intrafusal muscle fibres
Ib	Aα	Golgi tendon organs
II	Aβ	Flower-spray endings on intrafusal muscle fibres; touch and pressure receptors
III	Aδ	Receptors for pain (fast), cold and crude touch receptors
IV	C	Pain (slow) and temperature receptors

Second-Order Neurons

The second-order neurons are located in the spinal cord or brainstem. They receive information from one or more primary afferent neurons and transmit it to the thalamus. *In the spinal cord*, the neurons involved in sensory functions are present in the dorsal horn of spinal grey matter. The grey matter of the *dorsal horn* is divided into laminae. For details, see page 879, before proceeding further. Axons of the second-order neurons form the *ascending sensory tracts* described in the subsequent text.

Third-Order Neurons

Third-order neurons of the sensory pathway are located in specific nuclei of the thalamus. From here, the encoded sensory information ascends to the sensory cortex through the thalamic radiations.

Sensory Nerves and Dermatomes

Sensory Nerves

All sensory fibres reach the CNS through their cranial equivalents.

Dorsal nerve roots in spinal cord (Fig. 10.1.5; see page 880) Different types of sensory fibres forming sensory part of spinal nerve carry different types of sensations (Table 10.8.3). Each dorsal nerve root is attached to the spinal cord through various rootlets. Each rootlet just before entering the spinal cord divides into medial and lateral divisions.

Medial divisions of each rootlet consist of myelinated group I and II fibres which include:
- Proprioceptive fibres from muscles
- Sensory fibres conveying touch, pressure and vibratory sensations

Lateral division of each rootlet comprises:
- Thinly myelinated group III (Aδ) fibres that carry fast and discriminative pain and temperature sensations
- Unmyelinated group IV (type C) fibres which carry slow pain and visceral sensations

Dermatomes

Dermatome refers to the area of the skin supplied by one dorsal root (spinal cord segment). It is important to note that dermatomes are quite different from the peripheral nerve fields, because fibres from one dermatome may be present in different peripheral nerves.

During the embryo stage, the body is divided into orderly metameres. In the postnatal life, owing to excessive growth of

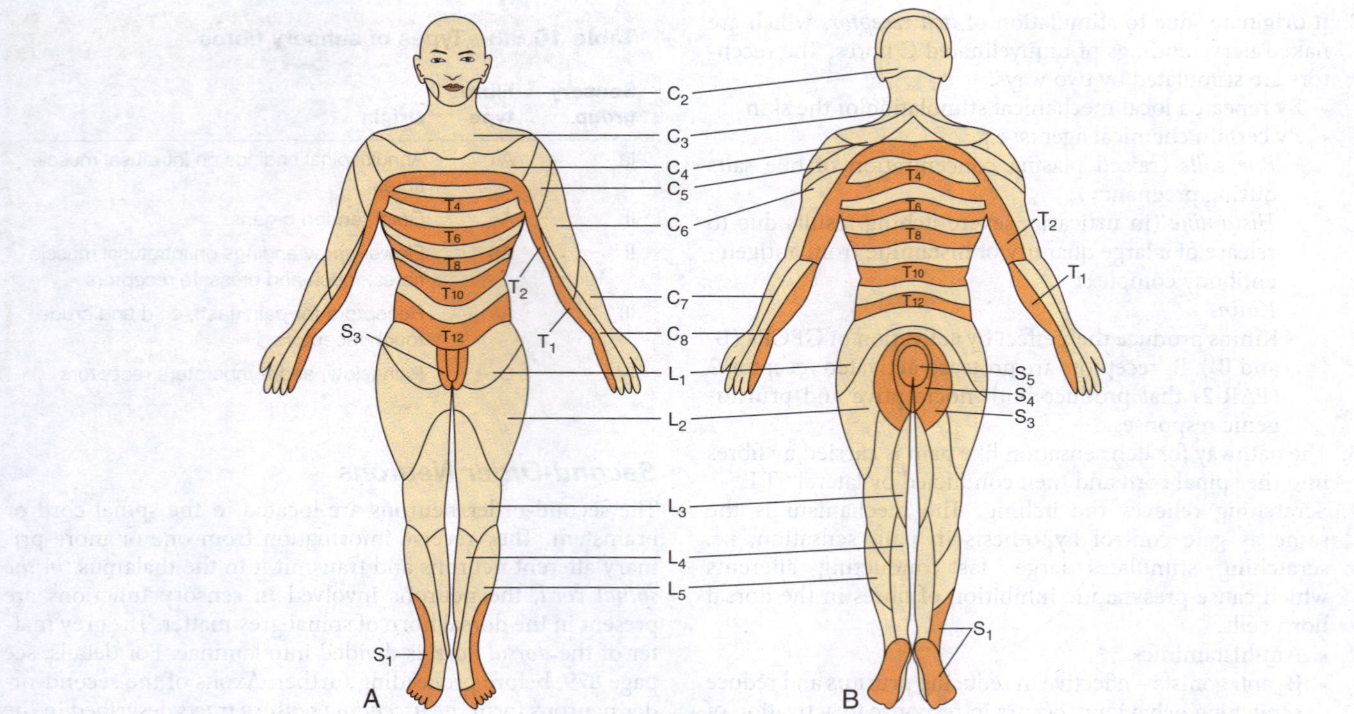

Fig. 10.8.16 Dermatomes as seen from front (**A**) and back (**B**).

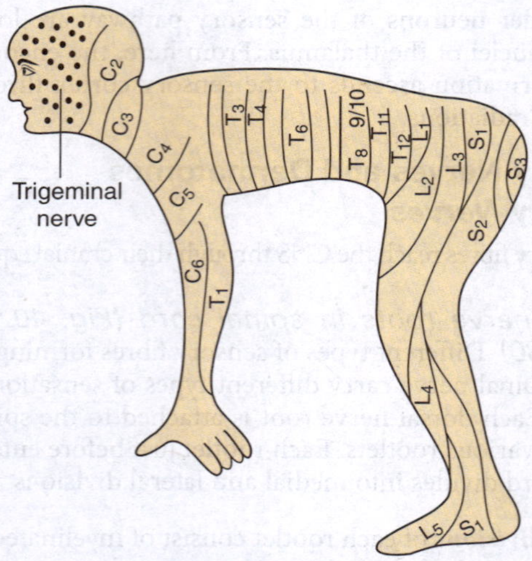

Fig. 10.8.17 Dermatomes in humans visualized as quadruped animal (like ancestors), to clarify the apparent complexity and to memorize the various dermatomes.

limbs, the metamere arrangement, except in the trunk, is no longer present. Therefore, dermatomes are remnants of an orderly metameric arrangement, which has survived only in the trunk, where the dermatomes consist of a series of 12 narrow overlapping bands running from the vertebral column to the midventral line (Fig. 10.8.16). The bands slope down as they pass around the body. Apparently, the dermatomes are not arranged in an orderly way, as the L_5 dermatome in the leg is at a more distal site than the S_4 dermatome, which is near the anus (Fig. 10.8.17). However, this apparent complexity of the dermatomes in humans is simplified if the human is visualized as a quadruped animal (like monkey, the ancestor of humans) (Fig. 10.8.17). The knowledge of dermatomes is utilized to know the level of spinal cord injury or the level of spinal tumour or other lesions by mapping the area of altered sensation produced.

Plasticity of dermatomes The dermatomes were originally marked by Sherrington in the later years of the nineteenth century. This is a landmark discovery for which Sherrington may be considered the father of neurology. Much later, Kirk and Denny Brown reported that under some conditions, dermatomes may alter their area of supply to a slight extent. This phenomenon is called plasticity of dermatomes.

Ascending Sensory Tracts

The major ascending sensory tracts in the spinal cord have been grouped as:

- Dorsal column sensory pathway
- Anterolateral sensory pathway
- Dorsolateral column sensory pathway

The ascending sensory tracts are summarized in the subsequent text (for details, see page 885).

Dorsal Column Sensory Pathway

Dorsal column sensory pathway (Fig. 10.1.12) in humans is well developed and wholly myelinated.

First-order neurons are formed by Aα(Ia) and Aβ(II) fibres that enter the spinal cord at the medial division of dorsal nerve roots. These carry sensations of fine touch, tactile localization, two-point discrimination, vibration, pressure with intensity discrimination and sense of position and proprioception. These fibres run in the spinal cord through the *dorsal column* as fasciculus gracilis and fasciculus cuneatus (Fig. 10.8.18) to end in the *nucleus gracilis* and *nucleus cuneatus*, respectively. Many fibres of the dorsal columns, on their way up, terminate or relay in the dorsal grey horn.

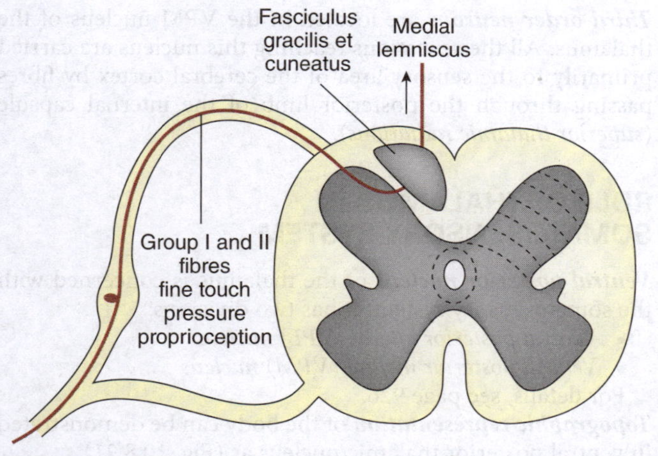

Fig. 10.8.18 Dorsal column sensory pathways. Fibres carrying touch, pressure and proprioceptive sensations are arranged as fasciculus gracilis and fasciculus cuneatus in dorsal column of spinal cord.

Second-order neurons arise from the nucleus gracilis and nucleus cuneatus located in the medulla oblongata. These decussate in the medulla as *internal arcuate fibres* and ascend up in the brainstem as medial lemniscus. The fibres of *medial lemnisci terminate* in the *ventroposterior lateral* (VPL) nucleus of the thalamus.

Third-order neurons are from the *ventroposterior lateral nucleus* of the thalamus. These ascend to the sensory cortex through the thalamic radiations.

Spatial orientation of nerve fibres in dorsal column In the dorsal column, fibres coming from lower parts of the body are in the centre, whereas those coming from progressively higher segmental level form successive layers laterally.

Functions of dorsal column pathway See page 886.

Applied Aspects

Effects of damage to dorsal column pathway: Sensations of fine touch, tactile discrimination, vibration sense, joint and position sense are carried by the dorsal column pathway. Therefore, damage to this pathway will produce the following effects:

Sensory ataxia, i.e. imbalance due to damage to the sensory pathway. In it, it is difficult for the person to detect the position without the help of visual apparatus in an erect position. If this person is asked to stand and close his/her eyes, the body cannot maintain balance properly and tends to fall in one direction (Romberg sign).

Loss of sensations of fine touch, tactile discrimination and vibration sense occurs on the affected side.

Anterolateral Pathway

First-order neurons of the anterolateral pathway are formed by Aδ fibres which enter the spinal cord as lateral division of the dorsal nerve root. These carry sensations of pain, temperature and crude touch. After entering the spinal cord, these fibres separate into short ascending and descending branches, which constitute the *dorsolateral tract of Lissauer*. They finally terminate on the *nucleus proprius* of the spinal cord, one or two segments rostral and caudal to the point of entry of the dorsal root. Some sensory afferents end on the short interneurons in the *substantia gelatinosa*, which connects them to nucleus proprius (Fig. 10.8.12).

Second-order neurons arise from the nucleus proprius and cross in the anterior commissure of the spinal cord to the opposite side in anterior and lateral white column in which they run upward to the brain as anterior and lateral STTs, respectively.

Anterior STT mainly carries the sensation of crude touch, tickle, itch, etc. Higher up in the brainstem, the anterior STT joins the medial lemniscus of the thalamus.

Lateral STT consists of the fibres carrying pain and temperature sensation, and higher up in the brainstem is called the spinal lemniscus (Fig. 10.8.12).

Important Note

In addition, there are spinoreticular (to the reticular system of the brainstem) and spinotectal (to the tectum) pathways.

Anterolateral pathways terminate in two areas:

- They terminate throughout *reticular nuclei* of the brainstem.
- Spinal and medial lemnisci terminate in the *ventrobasal complex* and *intralaminar* nuclei of the thalamus. Generally, tactile signals and temperature signals terminate in the ventrobasal complex. Pain signals only partly project to the ventrobasal complex of the thalamus. Instead, most of them enter the reticular nuclei of the brainstem and then to intralaminar nuclei of the thalamus.

Third-order neurons arise from the ventrobasal complex of the thalamus and carry tactile signals to the somatic sensory area of the cortex along with the fibres of the dorsal column.

Characteristics of transmission in anterolateral pathway In general, the anterolateral system is a crude type of transmission than the dorsal column system, as depicted by the following characteristics:

Velocity of transmission is about one-third compared with that of the dorsal column system (8–40 m/s).

Spatial organization in the pathway is poor, causing poor degree of localization of sensation.

Gradation of intensities judged is far less accurate compared with that by the dorsal column system.

Ability to transmit repetitive signals is also poor.

Dorsolateral Column Pathway

Dorsolateral column pathways carry proprioceptive impulses arising from the muscles and joint receptors of the lower part of the body to the cerebellum. Recent investigations have shown that some exteroceptive sensations, e.g. touch, may also reach the cerebellum through these pathways.

First-order neurons are located in the posterior root ganglia. Their peripheral processes receive impulses from muscle spindles, Golgi tendon organs and other proprioceptive receptors. Some fibres are related to end organs concerned with exteroceptive sensations (touch and pressure).

Second-order neurons are located in the junctional area between the ventral and the dorsal grey column (laminae V, VI and VII) in the lumbar and sacral segments of the spinal cord. Their axons form the:

- *Ventral spinocerebellar tract*
- *Dorsal spinocerebellar tract*

Note: For details, see page 888.

Pathway of Sensations from Face and Oral Cavity

The sensations of touch, pain and temperature from the face and oral cavity, including teeth, and proprioceptive information from the jaw muscles are carried by the trigeminal nerve.

First-order neurons are located in the *trigeminal ganglion*, which is equivalent to dorsal nerve root ganglia in the spinal cord. The peripheral processes of these neurons form three divisions of the trigeminal nerve – ophthalmic, maxillary and mandibular – which innervate different areas of the facial skin (Fig. 10.8.19). The central processes of these neurons of trigeminal ganglia terminate in different components of trigeminal sensory nucleus as (Fig. 10.8.20):

- *Principal sensory trigeminal nucleus*, located in the pons, receives fibres carrying *tactile* sensations.
- *Spinal nucleus* is elongated and extends down to the upper spinal cord. It receives fibres carrying *pain* and *temperature* sensations.
- *Mesencephalic nucleus*, which extends from the pons into the midbrain, receives fibres carrying *proprioceptive* information.

Second-order neurons are located in the above-described three components of the sensory trigeminal nucleus. Axons of these neurons cross to the opposite side and ascend as *trigeminal lemniscus* to the ventroposterior medial (VPM) nucleus of the thalamus.

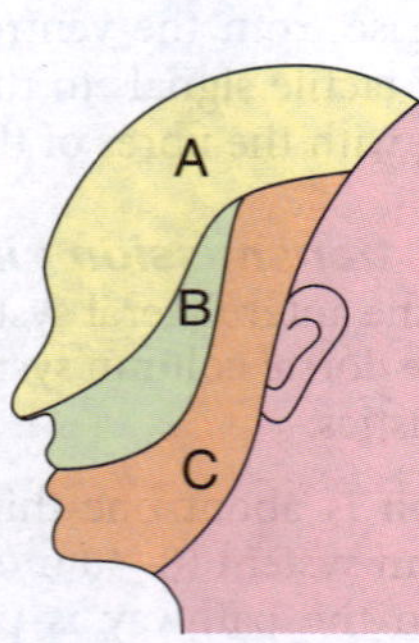

Fig. 10.8.19 The areas of face innervated by three divisions of trigeminal nerve: **A**, ophthalmic; **B**, maxillary; and **C**, mandibular.

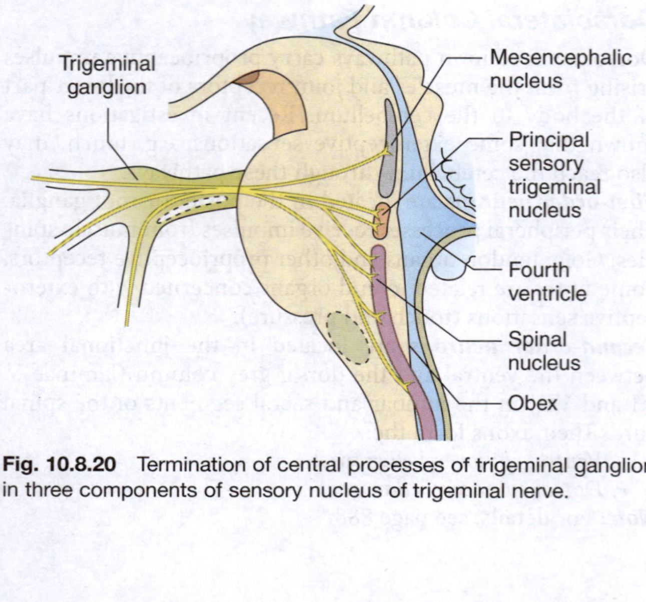

Fig. 10.8.20 Termination of central processes of trigeminal ganglion in three components of sensory nucleus of trigeminal nerve.

Third-order neurons are located in the VPM nucleus of the thalamus. All the sensations reaching this nucleus are carried primarily to the sensory area of the cerebral cortex by fibres passing through the posterior limb of the internal capsule (*superior thalamic radiations*).

ROLE OF THALAMUS IN SOMATOSENSORY SYSTEM

Ventral posterior nucleus of the thalamus is concerned with the somatosensory system. It has two divisions:

- *Ventral posterior lateral (VPL) nucleus*
- *Ventral posterior medial (VPM) nucleus*

For details, see page 926.

Topographic representation of the body can be demonstrated in ventral posterior thalamic nucleus as (Fig. 10.8.21):

- *Face region:* Fibres carrying sensations from the face terminate in the most medial part of the nucleus.
- *Arm region* is represented in the middle part of the nucleus.
- *Leg region* is represented in the most lateral part of the nucleus.

Somatosensory functions of thalamus: The thalamus acts as a:

- Sensory relay centre
- Centre for integration of sensory impulses
- Crude centre for perception of sensations

In short, pain sensations are perceived in the thalamus itself. All other sensations are transmitted to the cerebral cortex by third-order neurons arising from the thalamus (for details, see page 926).

SOMATIC SENSORY CORTEX

Somatic sensory cortex is described under the following headings:

- Areas
- Topographical organization of the body in the somatic sensory cortex
- Connections
- Functions

For details, see page 944.

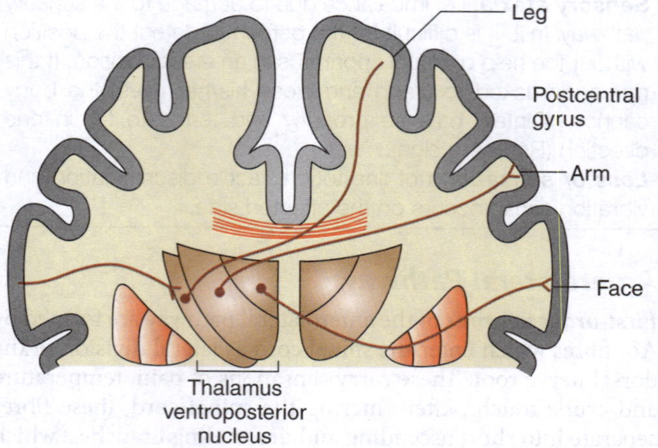

Fig. 10.8.21 Topographic representation of the body in ventral posterior nucleus of thalamus and thalamic projections to sensory cortex.

Self-Assessment

1. Discuss the components of the sensory system and their role.
2. Discuss the classification of sensory receptors and their characteristic features.
3. Discuss the electrochemical events during sensory transduction.
4. Describe the following:
   - Pain sensation, its receptors and types, and how it is perceived
   - Pain suppression pathway
5. Write notes on the following:
   - Weber–Fechner law
   - Muller's doctrine of specific nerve energies
   - Law of projection
   - Neutral zone
   - Referred pain

Clinical Cases

Case 1

A 35-year-old male had a crush injury of lower extremity few years back and was completely recovered. Presently, he has burning pain sensations in the extremity.

Q1. What is the diagnosis?
Q2. What is the cause for burning sensation?
Q3. Which type of pain receptors are involved in this case?
Q4. What is the treatment?

Case 2

A 60-year-old male patient visited the dentist for swelling and pain in the upper tooth. During examination, when the dentist touched the tooth, the patient experienced severe pain radiating to the lower jaw, ears and neck region.

Q1. What is the type of pain?
Q2. What is the pathophysiology of this type of pain?
Q3. What are the proposed theories about this pain?

10.9 Somatic Motor System

CHAPTER OUTLINE

INTRODUCTION

Effector organ The motor activity, be it in the form of walking, physical labour, skilled work like typing or even expression of thoughts and feelings through gesture of speech, is a result of highly coordinated movements produced by the skeletal muscles. The skeletal muscles thus form the *effector organ* of the somatic motor system.

Motor unit and motor neuronal pool The skeletal muscle activity basically depends on the pattern and rate of discharge of motor neurons supplying the muscles. A *motor unit* consists of single motor neuron and the muscle fibres that it innervates. For fine control (e.g. muscles of the eye), a single motor neuron innervates only a few muscle fibres. For larger movements (e.g. postural muscles), a single motor neuron may innervate thousands of muscle fibres. All the motor neurons for a given muscle make up the *motor neuron pool* for the muscle. The force of muscle contraction is graded by recruitment of additional motor units (size principle). The *size principle* states that as additional motor units are recruited, more motor neurons are involved and more tension is generated.

Lower motor neurons and final common pathway

Thus, the somatic motor activity depends ultimately on the pattern and rate of discharge from the α-motor neurons situated in the ventral (grey) horn of the spinal cord and its homologous neurons in the motor nuclei of the cranial nerves present in the brainstem. The *α-motor neurons* are also known as lower motor neurons. The lower motor neurons form the only pathway through which the signals from other parts of the nervous system reach the muscles. Therefore, the *lower motor neurons* constitute the so-called *final common pathway* of the motor system.

Somatic motor activity Somatic motor activity, in general, comprises voluntary movements, reflex responses, rhythmic motor activities and control of posture and equilibrium.

1. ***Voluntary movements***, like typing, playing musical instruments, writing, drawing and painting, represent the most complex motor activity. Such movements are characterized by being purposeful and initiated at will. These movements can improve with training and, once learned, they can be executed with minimal voluntary attention. In other words, the motor system 'learns by doing', and performance improves with repetition. This involves the *synaptic plasticity*.
2. ***Reflex responses*** are rapid, stereotyped and involuntary activities. They are purposeful but not under voluntary control. They are produced in response to specific stimuli, e.g. withdrawal reflex in response to a nociceptive stimulus.
3. ***Rhythmic motor activities*** like walking, running and chewing combine features of the voluntary as well as reflex responses. These movements are initiated and terminated voluntarily. However, once initiated, these relatively stereotyped repetitive movements may continue in almost reflex response–like pattern.
4. ***Control of posture and equilibrium:*** The maintenance of upright posture is a prerequisite for any goal- and direction-oriented phasic movement. It is impossible to separate postural adjustments from voluntary movement in any rigid way, but it is possible to differentiate a series of postural reflexes that not only maintain the body in an upright, balanced position but also provide the constant adjustments necessary to maintain a stable postural background for voluntary activity.

Medial versus lateral motor system The skeletal muscles, which are the effector organs for motor activity, have been organized into two groups – medial proximal and lateral distal. The *medial proximal group* comprises the axial and girdle muscles, whose actions involve the axis and proximal limbs. Their activity determines posture, progression and equilibrium. The *lateral distal group* of muscles is the muscles of digits and distal segments of limbs. They are responsible for skilled voluntary movements. There exists a topographical organization of these groups in the central nervous system as medial and lateral motor nervous systems.

Medial motor system: Phylogenetically, the medial motor system is old. It includes the following tracts:

- Anterior corticospinal tract
- Fibres of the corticobulbar tract other than those belonging to the lateral system
- Lateral and medial vestibulospinal tracts
- Reticulospinal tract
- Tectospinal tract

The fibres of the medial motor system terminate on the motor neurons situated in the medial part of the ventral grey horn of the spinal cord (via interneuron). Axons of the medial group of motor neurons of the spinal cord supply the axial and proximal limb muscles (medial proximal group of muscles), which are concerned with posture of the body. The corticobulbar fibres of the medial system innervate the axial muscles of the upper part of the trunk and are involved in the maintenance of posture and equilibrium. These fibres are also involved in the movements of chewing and movements of eyebrows.

Lateral motor system: Phylogenetically, the lateral motor system is new. It includes the following tracts:

- Lateral corticospinal tract
- Rubrospinal tract
- A part of corticobulbar tract

The fibres of the lateral motor system terminate in the motor neurons situated in the lateral part of the ventral grey horn in the spinal cord (directly or via interneurons) and on the equivalent motor neurons of cranial nerve nuclei in the brainstem. Axons of these motor neurons supply the muscles of digits and distal segments of the limbs and regulate the skilled voluntary movements.

The corticobulbar fibres of the lateral system are concerned with movements of expression in the lower part of the face and movements of the tongue.

Control of somatic motor activity The voluntary actions and postural movements are carried out by not only the simple contraction and relaxation of skeletal muscles but also the adjustment of tone in these muscles. The execution, planning, coordination and adjustments of the movements of the body are under the influence of different parts of the nervous system which together constitute the somatic motor system, which is organized as a three-tier system consisting of highest level of motor control, middle level of motor control and lowest level of motor control.

1. ***Highest level of motor control*** involves activities of various areas of the cerebral cortex. It is mainly concerned with generation of the idea of voluntary movements (motor plan) and issuing the motor commands for their execution.
2. ***Middle level of motor control*** involves activities of various subcortical centres such as basal ganglia, some brainstem nuclei and cerebellum. It is concerned with developing and perfecting each motor programme and subprogramme for bringing out a motor act. It also supervises the implementation of a motor programme.
3. ***Lowest level of motor control*** is exerted by cranial nerve nuclei in the brainstem and spinal cord. The spinal cord contains the final common pathway through which a movement is executed.

Role of sensory receptors in motor control activity

Feedback signals to CNS from the proprioceptors in muscles, joints, skin and other sensory receptors are used to adjust the motor commands during somatic motor activity.

Plan of study of somatic motor control system In view of the above-stated background, the somatic motor control system is discussed in detail under the following headings:

- Components of the somatic motor control system
- Skeletal muscles: The effect or organ of the somatic motor system
- Reflexes
- Regulation of posture and equilibrium

COMPONENTS OF SOMATIC MOTOR CONTROL SYSTEM

The somatic motor control system is organized as a three-tier system consisting of (Fig. 10.9.1):

- Highest level of motor control
- Middle level of motor control
- Lowest level of motor control

These components of the somatic motor control system work in concert to exert their control over skeletal muscles and their coordinated activity.

I. HIGHEST LEVEL OF MOTOR CONTROL

Cerebral Cortex

The highest level of motor control is exerted through the motor cortex and two major descending pathways emerging from the motor areas.

Motor Cortex

Areas of the motor cortex include (Fig. 10.9.2):

Primary motor cortex (Brodmann area 4): It is located in the frontal lobe within the precentral gyrus. It is somatotopically organized. It is organized in terms of movements rather than individual muscles, e.g. stimulation reveals discrete isolated movements on the opposite half of the body.

Premotor cortex: It is located immediately anterior to the lateral portion of the primary cortex. It includes Brodmann areas 6, 8, 44 and 45.

Supplementary motor cortex is located in the medial surface of the frontal lobe rostral to the primary motor area (Figs 10.4.5, see page 941, and 10.9.2).

Important Note

For details of motor cortex, see page 940.

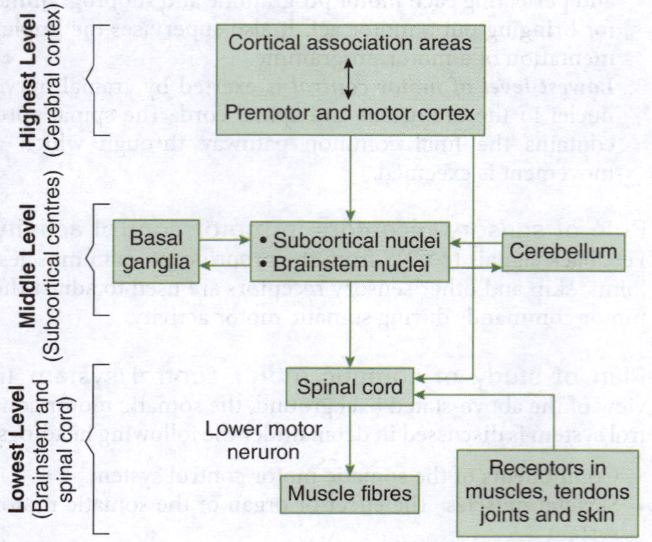

Fig. 10.9.1 Integration of highest, middle and lowest levels of somatic motor control system.

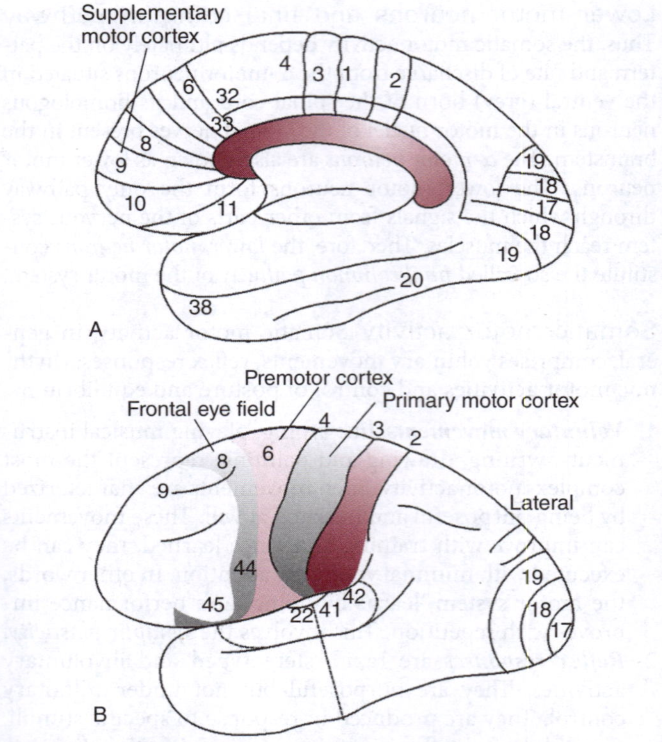

Fig. 10.9.2 Medial (above) and lateral (below) views of human cerebral cortex to show the motor cortex.

Functional role of the motor cortex in control of voluntary movements is summarized as follows:

Supplementary motor cortex is responsible for generating the idea for a movement. It plans the movements. Lateral cerebellum and basal ganglia are also involved in the planning and programming of movements. This is evidenced from the fact that all these areas involved in planning show electrical activity before the primary motor cortex. Basal ganglia play their cognitive role through the *caudate loop* (motor association → cortex → caudate nucleus → thalamus → cortex) (see page 917 and Fig. 10.2.13A).

Primary motor cortex is responsible for execution of movement. Programmed patterns of motor neurons are activated in the motor cortex. Excitation of upper motor neurons in the motor cortex is transferred in large part via the corticospinal tracts to the spinal cord and the corresponding corticobulbar tracts to motor neurons in the brainstem, where the lower motor neurons are activated and cause voluntary movement.

Premotor cortex coordinates the voluntary activity:

Area 6 coordinates the proximal and axial muscles during a motor task. Therefore, it is involved in the integration of voluntary movements. It ensures that the skilled movements are accurate and smooth.

Area 8, also called frontal eye field, is involved in coordination of eye movements.

Areas 44 and 45, also called Broca motor speech areas (especially in dominant hemisphere, e.g. left hemisphere in a right-handed person), are engaged in coordination of the activity of musculature involved in speech, e.g. activation of vocal cords simultaneously with movements of the mouth and tongue during speech.

A head rotation area associated with the frontal eye field is functionally linked to area 8 and serves to enable movements of the head correlated with eye movements.

An area related to the control of fine movements of the hand is located within the premotor cortex, just anterior to the hand region of area 4. When this area is damaged, the muscles of the hand are not paralysed, but certain hand movements are lost; this is called *motor apraxia*.

Plasticity property of motor cortex: The motor system 'learns by doing', and performance improves with repetition. This involves synaptic plasticity. The motor cortex shows plasticity. This has been confirmed by positron emission tomography (PET) and functional MRI (fMRI) in intact experimental animals and humans. For example, the finger areas of the contralateral motor cortex show enlargement as a pattern of rapid finger movement is learned with the fingers of one hand; this change is detectable at 1 week and maximal at 4 weeks.

Descending Motor Pathways from Motor Cortex

A. Pyramidal tracts include the tracts which are constituted by the axons that transmit motor signals directly from the cortex to the spinal cord (*corticospinal tracts*) and cranial nerve nucleus (*corticobulbar tracts*). *Corticospinal tracts* include 31% of fibres arising from the primary cortex (area 4), 29% from the premotor area (area 6) and supplementary cortex, and 40% arising from the somatic sensory cortex (areas 3, 1 and 2). Corticospinal fibres are divided into two tracts (Fig. 10.1.16, see page 889):

Lateral corticospinal tract is constituted by the 80% of fibres which cross the midline in the medullary pyramids. These fibres end directly in neurons in the ventral horn that innervate the distal limb muscles which are responsible for making skilled precision movements (e.g. the muscles that move the fingers and hands and the muscles that produce speech) (*lateral motor system*).

Anterior corticospinal tract is formed by 20% of uncrossed fibres which descend ipsilaterally in the ventral white column of the spinal cord. These fibres ultimately cross the midline but only at the level where they synapse. This pathway phylogenetically is the oldest and does not synapse directly with ventral horn cells, but an interneuron is always interposed in between. These interneurons synapse on neurons in the *medial portion of the ventral horn* that controls the axial (trunk muscles) and proximal limb muscles that are concerned with posture and equilibrium (*medial motor system*).

B. Extrapyramidal tracts: These are a large number of fibres arising from the motor cortex which do not enter the corticospinal tracts but relay in the various basal ganglia, red nucleus, reticular formation of the brainstem and vestibular nuclei. Ultimately, they constitute the reticulospinal (or corticoreticulospinal), vestibulospinal (or corticovestibulospinal), rubrospinal (or corticorubrospinal), tactospinal (or corticotactospinal) and olivospinal tracts. All these are combinedly called the extrapyramidal tracts. Thus, in contrast to pyramidal tracts, the extrapyramidal tracts constitute a multisynaptic pathway affecting the contralateral side of the spinal cord (Fig. 10.9.3).

Functions: Extrapyramidal pathways are chiefly concerned with regulation of muscle tone and posture and equilibrium.

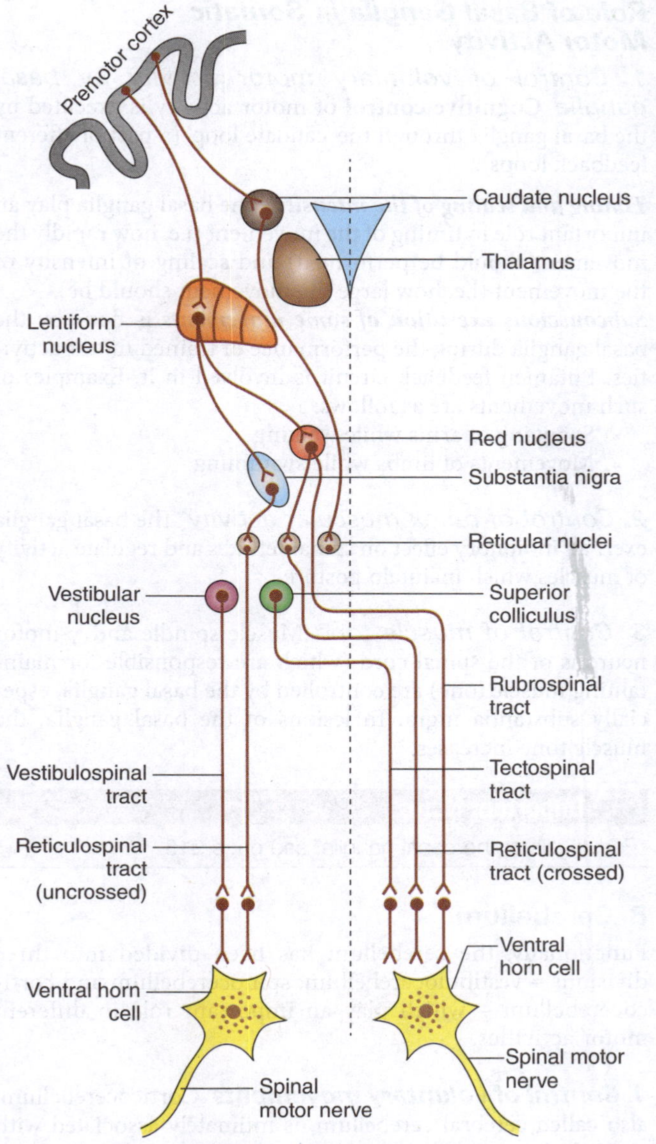

Fig. 10.9.3 The extrapyramidal tracts.

Important Note

For details of the corticospinal tract, see page 889, and for details of the extrapyramidal tracts, see page 890.

II. MIDDLE LEVEL OF MOTOR CONTROL

The middle level of motor control specifies the postures and movements necessary to carry out the desired acts. It is concerned with developing and perfecting each motor programme and subprogramme for bringing out a motor act. It also supervises the implementation of motor programmes.

The middle level of motor control involves activities of the basal ganglia, cerebellum and brainstem.

A. Basal Ganglia

Physiologically, the basal ganglia include corpus striatum (caudate nucleus and lenticular nucleus having two parts, e.g. putamen and globus pallidus), subthalamic nucleus and substantia nigra.

Role of Basal Ganglia in Somatic Motor Activity

1. Control of voluntary motor activity by basal ganglia **Cognitive control** of motor activity is executed by the basal ganglia through the 'caudate loop' (a part of afferent feedback loops).

Timing and scaling of the intensity: The basal ganglia play an important role in timing of the movement (i.e. how rapidly the movement should be performed) and scaling of intensity of the movement (i.e. how large the movement should be).

Subconscious execution of some movements is done by the basal ganglia during the performance of trained motor activities. Putamen feedback circuit is involved in it. Examples of such movements are as follows:

- Swinging of arms while walking
- Movements of limbs while swimming

2. Control of reflex muscular activity The basal ganglia exert an inhibitory effect on spinal reflexes and regulate activity of muscles which maintain posture.

3. Control of muscle tone Muscle spindle and γ-motor neurons of the spinal cord (which are responsible for maintaining muscle tone) are controlled by the basal ganglia, especially substantia nigra. In lesions of the basal ganglia, the muscle tone increases.

Important Note

For details of the basal ganglia, see page 913.

B. Cerebellum

Functionally, the cerebellum has been divided into three divisions – vestibulocerebellum, spinocerebellum and corticocerebellum – which play an important role in different motor activities.

1. Control of voluntary movements Corticocerebellum, also called cerebral cerebellum, is intimately associated with control of timing, rate, range (extent), duration, direction and strength of a movement. It performs this function through the following neuronal circuits:

- *Open feedback loop* or cerebro-cerebello-cerebral circuit (Fig. 10.2.8)
- *Closed feedback loop* formed by fibres from the cerebral motor cortex to the paravermal cerebellum to the cerebral cortex (Fig. 10.2.9)

Mechanism of action: The cerebellum controls the voluntary movements by the following actions:

i. ***Comparator function:*** The cerebellum receives inputs from the command neurons about the sequential intended plan of movements for the next fraction of second. It also gets feedback (afferents) from the proprioceptive endings of muscles, tendons and joints about what actual movements result. All this information is integrated and the corrective signals are sent to the motor cortex. This happens through the closed feedback loop.
ii. ***Damping action:*** Corticocerebellum sends impulses to the cerebral cortex to discharge appropriate signals to the muscles so that any extra or exaggeration of muscular activity does not occur and thus overshooting is prevented. This action of the corticocerebellum is called damping action.
iii. ***Timing and programming of the skilled movements*** is done by the corticocerebellum through open feedback loop (Fig. 10.2.8), which modulates the motor command of pyramidal tracts through two-way communication.
iv. ***Servomechanism:*** Cerebellum lets the cerebral cortex to discharge the signals which are already programmed and stored at the sensory motor cortex, and does not influence much. However, if there is any disturbance or interference, the corticocerebellum immediately influences the cerebral cortex and corrects the movements. This action of the corticocerebellum is known as servomechanism.

2. Control of body posture and equilibrium Control of body posture and equilibrium is done by the vestibulocerebellum (see page 1030).

3. Control of muscle tone and stretch reflex Control of muscle tone and stretch reflex is the function of the spinocerebellum (see page 910).

Important Note

For details about the cerebellum, see page 901.

C. Brainstem

Reticular formation and vestibular nuclei are important components of the motor control system present in the brainstem.

Reticular formation The *motor control centres* within the reticular formation are a relay station for all descending motor commands, except those requiring the greatest precision, which are transferred directly from the cortex to the spinal cord.

- The motor control centres receive and modify the motor commands to the proximal and axial muscles of the body responsible for maintaining normal posture tone.
- These neurons are prevented from firing too rapidly by inhibitory input derived from the cerebral and cerebellar components of the motor control system. The amount of inhibition is increased to reduce postural tone and is decreased to enhance postural tone. The withdrawal of inhibition, called release of inhibition, is frequently used to increase neuronal activity within the CNS.

Vestibular nuclei Vestibular nuclei, located within the brainstem and cerebellum, receive information from *vestibular receptors* via vestibular nerve fibres (cranial nerve VIII). Vestibular system reflexes:

- Maintain tone in antigravity muscles
- Coordinate the adjustments made by the limbs and trunk to maintain balance
- Adjust the position of the eyes to maintain visual fixation when the position of the head changes

III. LOWEST LEVEL OF MOTOR CONTROL

The lowest level of motor control is exerted by motor nuclei of cranial nerves and spinal cord. The spinal cord contains the *final common pathway* through which a movement is executed. Organized in the spinal cord are patterns of movements that involve nearly all muscles in the body. By selecting the proper motor neurons for a particular task and by reflexly adjusting the amount of motor neuron activity, the spinal cord contributes to the proper performance of a motor task. The spinal cord activity ranges from a simple withdrawal reflex to a coordinated movement of all four extremities.

Spinal Cord

Motor Neurons

Motor neurons of the spinal cord present in the ventral horn are given next.

1. α-Motor neurons These are the largest neurons which give rise to myelinated axons that average about 14 μm in diameter and conduct action potentials very rapidly. The axons of α-motor neurons leave the spinal cord through the ventral nerve roots of spinal nerves and innervate the extrafusal fibres of the skeletal muscles. These are responsible for contraction of muscles in upper limbs, trunk and lower part of the body.

2. γ-Motor neurons These are much smaller and give rise to smaller axons that average about 5 μm in diameter and conduct action potentials at a slower velocity than the α-motor neurons. These neurons innervate the intrafusal fibres of the muscle spindles and are responsible for maintenance of muscle tone.

3. Interneurons These are about 30 times more numerous than motor neurons, are highly excitable and may have a spontaneous firing rate as high as 1500/s. The interneurons actually receive the bulk of synaptic input that reaches the spinal cord, as either incoming sensory information or signals descending from higher centres in the brain.

4. Renshaw cells Renshaw cells are a particular variety of interneurons that receive input from collateral branches of the axons of α-motor neurons. Their axons carry the impulses back to the cell bodies of the same α-motor neurons. These are inhibitory neurons that play an important role in synaptic inhibition at the spinal cord.

Arrangement of Motor Neurons in Ventral Horn

The motor neurons responsible for the contraction of skeletal muscles are arranged topographically in the ventral grey horn of the spinal cord in three mediolateral column groups.

1. Medial group It extends along most of the length of the spinal cord. The neurons situated in the medial part of the ventral grey horn innervate the muscles near the midline of the body called *axial muscles and the muscles in the proximal portions of limbs*. These muscles are involved in the adjustment of posture and gross movements.

2. Lateral group This group of neurons is confined to the cervical and lumbosacral enlargements and supplies the muscles in distal portions of the limbs called distal muscles. These distal muscles are involved in the well-coordinated skilled voluntary movements.

3. Central group This group of neurons is represented by the phrenic and accessory nuclei (in the cervical region) and by the lumbosacral nucleus (in the lumbosacral region).

Motor Functions

Motor functions served by the spinal cord are as follows:

- Control of movement of muscles and joints
- Control of tone and power of muscles
- Control of deep (tendon) reflexes
- Control of superficial reflexes

SKELETAL MUSCLES: THE EFFECTOR ORGAN OF SOMATIC MOTOR SYSTEM

Motor activity, be it in the form of walking, physical labour, skilled work like typing, performing surgical operations or even expression of thoughts and feelings through gesture or speech, is a result of highly coordinated movements produced by the skeletal muscles. The skeletal muscles thus form the effector organ of the somatic motor system. The physiology of skeletal muscle has been discussed in Chapter 2.3; see page 81. However, certain aspects of skeletal muscle as an effector organ that need elaboration and are relevant to complete the study of the somatic motor system are as follows:

- Motor unit
- Muscle sensors (proprioceptors)
- Muscle tone

MOTOR UNIT

The motor unit is the functional module used by the motor control system to carry out a movement. The movement produced by a skeletal muscle basically depends on the pattern and ratio of discharge of motor neurons supplying the muscle. A *motor unit consists* of single motor neuron and the muscle fibres that it innervates.

Important Note

It is suggested that before proceeding further, details about the motor unit should be read (see page 90).

MUSCLE SENSORS

Muscle sensors refer to the proprioceptors present in the muscles, tendons of muscles, joints, ligaments and fasciae. Proprioceptors are the receptors which give information about change in position of different parts of the body in space, especially joints or tension of muscles at any given moment. The muscle sensors are as follows:

- Muscle spindle
- Golgi tendon organ
- Pacinian corpuscle
- Free nerve endings

In addition to the above-mentioned proprioceptors, the labyrinth also contains proprioceptors (see page 1041).

1. Muscle Spindle

Muscle spindles are *stretch receptors* present in the skeletal muscles, also called Kuhne spindles. These are meant for

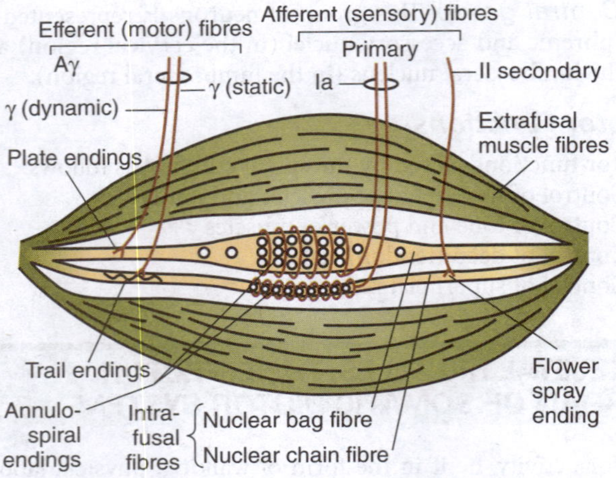

Fig. 10.9.4 Structure of a muscle spindle.

proprioceptive mechanism and so are a type of proprioceptors. Each skeletal muscle contains muscle spindles of variable number depending on the task performed. Muscles involved in precision movements contain many more spindles than muscles used to maintain posture. For example, hand muscles have approximately 80 spindles, which is 20% of the number of spindles contained in back muscles weighing 100 times as much.

Structure (Fig. 10.9.4): Each muscle spindle consists of 3–10 small muscle fibres (called intrafusal muscle fibres), encapsulated in a thin connective tissue capsule containing fluid. The muscle spindles are present in between and parallel to the extrafusal fibres (large force-generating muscle fibres). Either end of the muscle spindle is attached to the endomysium of the extrafusal muscle fibres.

Intrafusal muscle fibres consist of a central noncontractile portion which does not contain actin and myosin filaments and is thus devoid of striations. Portions on either side of the central part are contractile (as they contain actin and myosin filaments) and are called striated poles. The central part of each intrafusal fibre is the sensory portion. Stretching or contraction of the polar striated regions of the intrafusal fibre causes the stretching of this central noncontractile sensory portion. Intrafusal fibres are of two types:

Nuclear bag fibres: Each spindle contains about two to five nuclear bag fibres which are about 30 μm in diameter and 7 mm in length. In these fibres, many nuclei are congregated into an expanded bag in the central portion, hence the name.
Nuclear chain fibres are 15 μm in diameter and 4 mm in length. In these fibres, nuclei are arranged in a single file in the central part in the form of a chain, hence the name. Approximately 6–10 nuclear chain fibres exist in each typical spindle.

Nerve supply of the muscle spindle The muscle spindle is innervated by both sensory and motor nerve fibres. It is the only receptor in the body which has got motor nerve supply also.

i. Sensory nerve supply The central noncontractile portion of each intrafusal fibre is the receptor portion. Sensory fibres supply this area. There are two types of sensory fibres:

Group Ia fibres, also known as primary sensory endings, supply central receptor portions of both nuclear bag and nuclear chain fibres. Since these fibres spirally wind around the intrafusal fibres, these are also called annulospiral endings. They have diameter of about 17 μm and carry impulses at the rate of 70–120 m/s.

The primary endings supplying both the nuclear bag and nuclear chain intrafusal fibres are stimulated when the muscle spindle is stretched. But the pattern of response is different: a *dynamic response* is shown by nerve endings supplying the nuclear bag fibres and a static response is shown by the nerve endings supplying the nuclear chain fibres (see below).

Type II fibres, also known as secondary sensory endings, innervate the receptor portion of mainly nuclear chain fibres on one side of the primary endings. They are also known as flower spray endings. They have a diameter of about 8 μm. These nerve endings respond mainly to sustained stretching, and therefore measure the muscle length.

ii. Motor supply The efferent fibres to the muscle spindle are called *γ-fibres* because their axons belong to the Aγ group of fibres. γ-Efferent fibres control the sensitivity of the receptors to stretch. There are two types of γ-fibres:

Dynamic γ-fibres primarily innervate the striated poles of nuclear bag fibres where they end as motor end plate, hence also called *plate endings*. These fibres increase the sensitivity of the Ia afferent fibres to stretch. That is, the Ia afferent firing rate for a given *velocity of stretch* is increased by the discharge of the dynamic γ-fibres.
Static γ-fibres primarily innervate the striated poles of nuclear chain fibres where they end as a network of branches called *trail endings*. They increase the tonic activity in the Ia afferent fibres at any given muscle length. Sometimes, they also give a branch to some nuclear bag fibres which have characteristics similar to those of nuclear chain fibres (so-called static nuclear bag fibres).

Functions of Muscle Spindle

1. Role in stretch reflex Muscle spindle forms the receptor organ of stretch reflex and thus plays a key role in stretch reflex (for details, see page 1022).

2. Role in maintaining muscle tone Muscle spindle plays an important role in maintaining the muscle tone by controlling the discharge from γ-motor neurons (for details, see page 1025).

3. Role in maintaining skeletal muscle at a certain physiological length Most important function of the muscle spindle is to act as a comparator of the extrafusal fibre length. At a normal resting extrafusal fibre length, there is a slight discharge in the type Ia afferents. When the muscle length is passively increased (i.e. when muscle is stretched passively), type Ia discharge is increased. The reflex increase in α-motor neuron discharge causes contraction of the extrafusal fibres and restores their original length. Thus, the muscle spindles, through the stretch reflex, act as a feedback device to maintain the skeletal muscle at a certain physiologically useful length. This action of muscle spindles (particularly in the antigravity muscles) is of fundamental importance in the maintenance of standing posture.

4. Role as proprioceptor Muscle spindle plays the role of proprioceptor in the following sensations:

Unconscious proprioceptive sensations are carried from the muscle spindles to the spinal cord, where the second-order neurons constitute the dorsal and ventral spinocerebellar tracts.

Conscious kinaesthetic sensations are carried from the muscle spindles in the dorsal columns to ultimately reach the somatic sensory cortex. This function of the muscle spindle is similar to that of joint receptors.

2. Golgi Tendon Organ

The Golgi tendon organs are high-threshold stretch receptors present in the tendons. They are supplied by group Ib afferent fibres and detect muscle tension (for details, see page 1026).

3. Pacinian Corpuscle

Pacinian corpuscles are pressure receptors situated in fasciae throughout the muscles, tendons, joints and periosteum. They are supplied by *group II afferent fibres* and detect *vibration*.

4. Free Nerve Endings

Free nerve endings are basically pain receptors situated in the muscles, tendons, fasciae and joints. They are supplied by *group III and IV afferent fibres* and detect noxious stimuli.

MUSCLE TONE

Definition Muscle tone is defined as resistance offered to active or passive stretch. In other words, muscle tone refers to sustained partial state of contraction of the muscle under resting condition, i.e. a state of partial tetanus. The muscle tone is present in all the muscles, but is well pronounced in the extensor muscles, i.e. antigravity muscles.

Basis of muscle tone The muscle tone is purely a function of myotactic (stretch reflex), occurring due to low-frequency and asynchronous discharge of γ-motor neurons. The discharges are out of phase with each other which ultimately merge to produce smooth muscle contraction.

Applied Aspects

Anomalies of Muscle Tone

1. **Hypotonia** refers to decrease in muscle tone. The hypotonic or also called flaccid muscle offers little or no resistance to stretching. The muscles are generally hypotonic when the rate of γ-efferent discharge is low, i.e. when stretch reflex becomes hypoactive.

   Causes of hypotonia *include:*

   i. *Destruction of efferent or afferent pathway of stretch reflex:*
      - Destruction of efferent (motor) nerve to a muscle may occur by injury or poliomyelitis.
      - Destruction of afferent pathway may be seen in tabes dorsalis, a syphilitic affection of the dorsal nerve root of the spinal cord.

   ii. *Stimulation of inhibitory areas* of the brain located in the medulla

   iii. *Inhibition* or destruction of facilitatory areas of the brain located in the pons

   iv. *Decreased γ-motor discharge during sleep*

   v. *Effects of certain drugs* like barbiturates and tranquilizers in high doses

   vi. *Destruction of the cerebellum* that also produces hypotonia rather than hypertonia (see page 913)

   vii. *Hypothyroidism*

2. **Hypertonia** refers to increase in muscle tone. The hypertonic or spastic muscle offers high resistance to stretch. The muscles are generally hypertonic when the rate of γ-efferent discharge is high, i.e. when stretch reflex becomes hyperactive.

   Causes of hypertonia *include:*
   - *Stimulation of facilitatory area* of the brain
   - *Destruction of any of the inhibitory areas* of the brain
   - *Other factors* which increase the γ-efferent discharge including anxiety, unexpected movements and stimulation of the skin by noxious agents

   Types of hypertonia: Hypertonia is of two types:
   - *Spasticity* refers to hypertonia which is confined to only one group of muscles. For example, lesions of the internal capsule and upper motor neuron lesions (UMLs) produce spasticity.
   - *Rigidity* refers to hypertonia which involves both groups of muscles, i.e. extensor as well as flexors equally. For example, lesions of the basal ganglia produce rigidity.

REFLEX ACTIVITY

GENERAL CONSIDERATIONS

A reflex is an involuntary response to a peripheral nervous stimulation. In other words, it is a mechanism by which sensory impulse is automatically converted into a motor effect through the involvement of CNS. It is a type of protective mechanism which tries to protect the body from irreparable damage. For example, when the hand is placed inadvertently on a hot object, it is immediately withdrawn reflexly. Thus, the hand is protected from getting burnt.

ANATOMICAL ASPECTS

Reflex arc

The pathway for a reflex activity is called reflex arc. It forms the functional unit of the nervous system for a reflex and consists of (Fig. 10.9.5):

- Afferent limb
- Centre
- Efferent limb

1. Afferent limb of each reflex arc consists of a receptor and an afferent or sensory nerve.

Receptor is a modified nerve ending which receives the stimulus and after getting stimulated (depolarized) sends information to the CNS through the afferent neurons.

Afferent neuron carries sensory input from the receptor to the centre. The afferent neurons enter the CNS via the dorsal roots or cranial nerves and have their cell bodies in the dorsal root ganglia or in the homologous ganglia on the cranial nerves.

2. Centre: This is the part of CNS (spinal cord or brain) where the afferent limb ends and either synapses directly with the efferent motor neuron or establishes a connection with the efferent neuron via interneurons (internuncial or intercalated neurons). Thus, the number of synapses (connection between afferent and efferent neurons) may vary from one (in the simplest form of reflex) to many hundred.

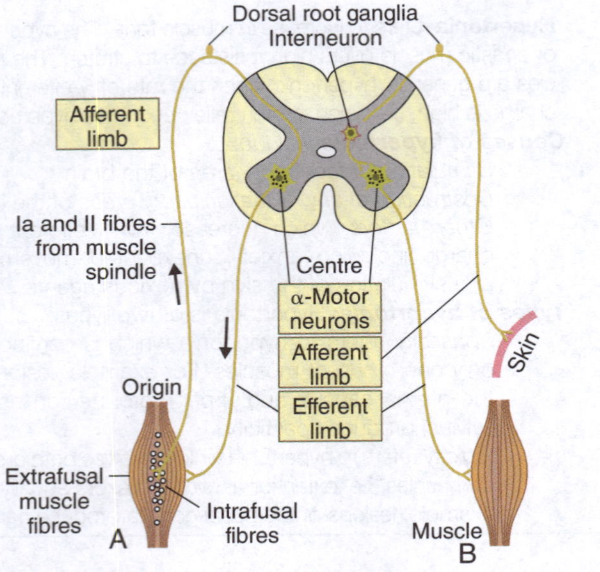

Fig. 10.9.5 Components of reflex arc in a monosynaptic (**A**) and a disynaptic (**B**) reflex.

3. Efferent limb of a reflex arc consists of an efferent or motor nerve and an effector organ.

Efferent nerve transmits motor impulses from the centre to the effector organ. Since the connection between afferent and efferent neurons is usually present in the CNS, activity in the reflex arc is modified by the multiple inputs converging on the efferent neuron.
Effector organ may be in the form of a muscle or a gland which shows the response to the stimulus.

Classification of Reflexes

Reflexes can be classified in different ways.

I. Depending on the Number of Synapses

1. ***Monosynaptic reflexes*** (MSRs) are those which contain only one synapse, e.g. stretch reflexes (biceps, triceps or knee jerk).
2. ***Disynaptic reflexes*** have two synapses, i.e. one interneuron is placed between afferent and efferent neurons of the reflex arc, e.g. inverse stretch reflex.
3. ***Polysynaptic reflexes*** are characterized by more than one interneuron placed between afferent and efferent neurons of the reflex arc, e.g. withdrawal reflex, crossed flexor reflex and crossed extensor reflex.

II. Anatomical Classification

Depending on the location of the reflex arc centre, the reflexes can be classified as:

1. ***Cortical reflexes:*** In these reflexes, the centre is located in the cerebral cortex.
2. ***Cerebellar reflexes*** have the centre of reflex arc in the cerebellum.
3. ***Midbrain reflexes:*** The centre of reflex arc in such a reflex is located in the midbrain.
4. ***Bulbar or medullary reflexes:*** In these reflexes, the centre is located in the medulla oblongata.
5. ***Spinal reflexes*** have the centre of reflex arc in the spinal cord. Depending on the segments involved, the spinal reflexes can be divided into three groups:
   - *Segmental reflexes:* In such reflexes, the efferent neuron begins in the same segment of the spinal cord where the afferent neuron ends.
   - *Intersegmental reflexes:* In these reflexes, the efferent neuron ends in a segment of the spinal cord and the efferent neuron begins in some other segment of the spinal cord.
   - *Suprasegmental reflexes:* The centre for such reflexes lies above the spinal cord.

III. Physiological Classification

1. ***Flexor reflexes:*** These reflexes occur in response to nociceptive (pain) stimuli and are characterized by flexion of the joints, e.g. thorn prick to the sole is immediately followed by reflex flexion of the knee and hip joints. These reflexes are also called *withdrawal reflexes.*
2. ***Extensor reflexes:*** Stretch reflexes are extensor reflexes. These are the basis of muscle tone and posture of the body. These are also called *antigravity reflexes.*

IV. Inborn Versus Acquired Reflexes

1. ***Inborn or unconditional reflexes*** are present since birth and do not require any previous learning or training, e.g. reflex salivation when any object is kept in the mouth.
2. ***Acquired or conditional reflexes*** develop after birth. Such reflexes are acquired after conditioning, i.e. after previous learning or training, e.g. reflex salivation by the sight, smell, thought or hearing of a known edible substance.

V. Clinical Classification

Clinically, reflexes are classified into:

- Superficial
- Deep
- Visceral
- Pathological reflexes

Animal Preparations for Study of Reflexes

The reflexes can be studied in:

- Spinal preparation
- Decerebrate preparation

1. Spinal preparation In it, the spinal cord is transected at the cervical region and respiration is maintained by respiratory pump. When the spinal cord is transected in the thoracic region, artificial respiration is not required since diaphragmatic breathing continues. Such preparation allows study of properties of spinal reflex.

2. Decerebrate preparation In decerebrate preparation, the transection is taken in the brainstem between superior and inferior colliculi.

Properties of Reflexes

1. Adequate stimulus Reflex response is obtained only when a precise stimulus for a given reflex activity is applied. The precise stimulus that involves a reflex response is called *adequate stimulus* for that particular reflex. For example, scratch reflex in a dog is initiated only by multiple linear touch stimuli. If multiple stimuli are widely separated, the reflex is not initiated.

2. Delay All reflex activity is associated with delay. Delay refers to the time interval between application of stimulus and starting of the response. It is attributed to synaptic delay and to time required for passage of impulse along the nerves. Therefore, delay is minimum in MSR.

3. One-way conduction During any reflex activity, the impulses are transmitted in only one direction through the reflex arc as per Bell–Magendie law. The impulses pass from the receptors to the centre and then from the centre to the effector organ.

4. Summation Summation of stimuli, both temporal and spatial, plays an important role in the facilitation of responses during the reflex activity as explained:

Temporal summation: Application of a subminimal (subthreshold) stimulus to a nerve fibre does not elicit reflex response. However, when the nerve fibre is stimulated repeatedly with subthreshold stimuli in quick succession (taking care of refractory period of the nerve), response does occur. This occurs due to summation of EPSPs produced by subthreshold stimuli, a phenomenon called temporal summation.
Spatial summation: When an efferent nerve fibre supplying a muscle is stimulated with subthreshold stimulus, a reflex response is not elicited. However, when two or more nerve fibres supplying the same muscle are stimulated simultaneously with subthreshold stimuli, a reflex contraction of the muscle is obtained due to the phenomenon of spatial summation.

5. Occlusion Occlusion refers to a phenomenon by which stimulation of two neighbouring nerves simultaneously evokes lesser response than sum total of the responses obtained when each nerve is separately stimulated. This can be demonstrated in a flexor reflex involving a muscle which is innervated by two motor nerves, say A and B. For example, electrical stimulation of nerve A causes development of tension of 8 T (an arbitrary unit). Stimulation of the nerve B with the same electric shock causes development of tension of 8 T. When both nerves, A and B, are stimulated simultaneously with the same electric shock, the tension developed is about 12 T, i.e. it is less than the sum of tensions produced (8 T + 8 T = 16 T) by the two nerves separately. This phenomenon is called occlusion. This occurs because of the fact that there is overlapping of the nerve fibres during the distribution, i.e. fibres are supplied by both A and B nerves (Fig. 10.9.6).

6. Subliminal fringe Subliminal fringe refers to a phenomenon by which simultaneous stimulation of two nerves (say A and B) with weak shock evokes greater response than the sum total of the responses when each nerve is separately stimulated with the weak shocks. Thus, a subliminal fringe phenomenon appears to produce opposite effect to that of occlusion phenomenon. Phenomenon of subliminal fringe can be explained as:

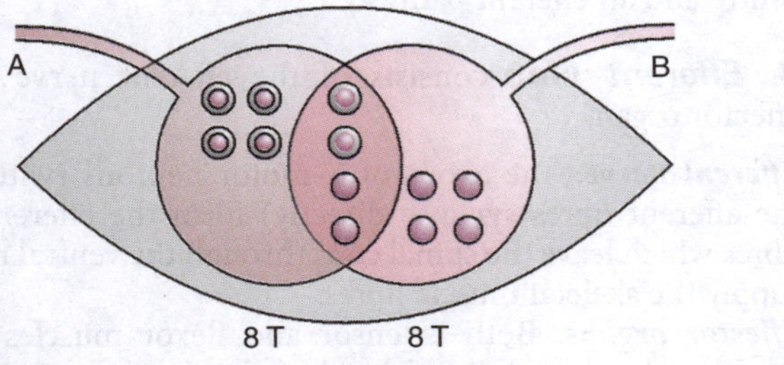

Fig. 10.9.6 Occlusion occurs due to overlapping in the distribution of nerve fibres.

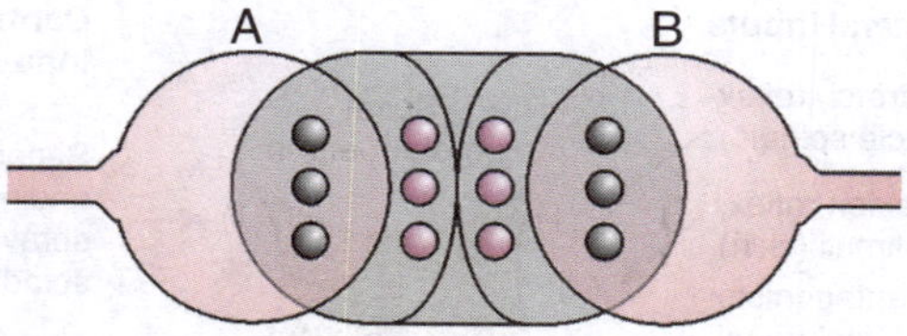

Fig. 10.9.7 Subliminal fringe.

Each afferent nerve on entering the spinal cord stimulates two groups of neurons – one group is stimulated adequately and the second group subminimally. Each weak stimulus, therefore, produces action potential in the nerves of group one neurons. The neurons belonging to the second group are also excited but only subminimally (so this group is common). When both A and B are simultaneously stimulated, the action potential also develops in the second group of neurons and therefore response obtained is greater (Fig. 10.9.7).

7. Recruitment When an excitatory nerve is stimulated with a stimulus of constant strength for a long time, there occurs a progressive increase in the response of reflex activity. This is due to the progressive increase in the number of motor neurons activated. This phenomenon is called recruitment. However, there is a limit to the number of motor neurons which can be recruited. So, beyond a certain limit, the prolongation of stimulation does not increase the response and a plateau is reached.

8. Irradiation When the sensory stimulus is too strong, impulse spreads to many neighbouring neurons in the centre and produces a wider response. It is due to transmission of impulse through a large number of collaterals of afferents and their interneurons.

9. Final common pathway Efferent pathway of the reflex arc is formed by α-motor neurons that supply the extrafusal muscle fibres. All neuronal influences (excitatory and inhibitory) affecting muscular contraction ultimately funnel through the motor neurons; therefore, they are called common final pathway. Numerous inputs converge on them and determine the activity in the final common path (Fig. 10.9.8). If an α-motor neuron is stimulated, skeletal muscle fibres contract; if the α-motor neuron is not stimulated, the skeletal muscle fibres relax. Thus, the α-motor neuron forming the final common pathway serves as both an integrating centre and an efferent pathway.

10. Facilitation When a reflex is elicited repeatedly at proper intervals, the response becomes progressively higher for first few occasions, i.e. each subsequent stimulus exerts a better effect than the previous one. This is due to facilitation occurring at the synapse.

11. Inhibition During a reflex activity, impulses through sensory fibres from protagonist muscles inhibit the action of antagonist muscles. For example, when flexor muscles of a joint are stimulated, extensor muscles are inhibited. The inhibitory

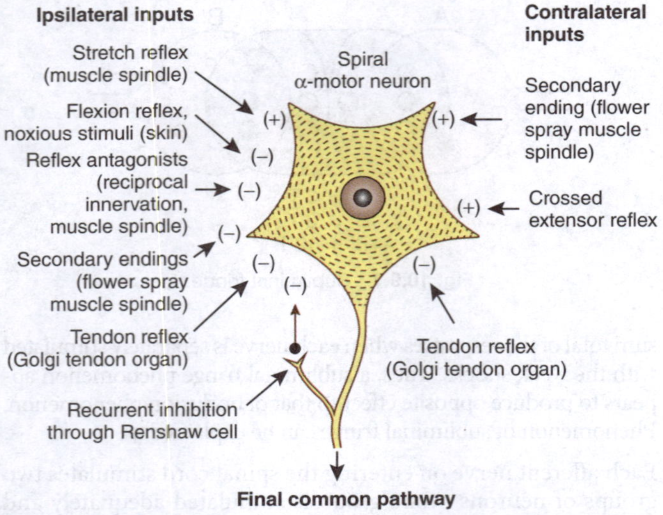

Fig. 10.9.8 The inputs converging on the body of α-motor neuron (final common pathway).

activity exerted by interneurons is responsible for such a reciprocal inhibitory effect.

12. Afterdischarge When a reflex action is elicited continuously for some time, and then the stimulation is stopped, the reflex response (contraction) may continue for some time even after cessation of the stimulus. This is called afterdischarge. This occurs because of the fact that the centre continues to discharge even after stoppage of stimulus. This is mainly because of the internuncial neurons which continue to transmit impulses to the centre even after cessation of stimulus. This happens because the motor neurons are stimulated through multiple internuncial pathways, and some of them take a longer time to reach the motor neurons.

13. Fatigue or habituation When a particular reflex is elicited repeatedly at frequent intervals, the response is reduced progressively and then disappears all together. This is called fatigue or habituation. The first site of fatigue is synapse, then the motor endings and lastly the muscle.

14. Rebound phenomenon The reflex activity can be inhibited for some time by some method. However, once the inhibitory effect is over, the reflex activity reappears and becomes more powerful. This is called rebound phenomenon. Its cause is still not known.

15. Fractionation The force of a muscle contraction is much higher when it is stimulated directly through a motor nerve compared with when it is stimulated reflexly through a sensory nerve. This is due to phenomenon of occlusion of the motor neurons when a sensory nerve is stimulated. Because of occlusion, the number of motor neurons stimulated is lesser.

16. Sensitization When an injurious stimulus is repeatedly applied, intensification of response occurs. This is known as sensitization. Sensitization, in fact, is the presynaptic facilitation of an impulse.

SPINAL CORD REFLEXES

Spinal cord reflexes enhance the ability of the motor control system to produce a coordinated movement. According to the receptors from which they originate, the spinal cord reflexes can be categorized into muscle reflexes and cutaneous reflexes.

Muscle reflexes: Two important reflexes which originate in muscles are as follows:

- Stretch reflex
- Lengthening reaction or Golgi tendon reflex

Cutaneous reflexes: The most important of the cutaneous reflexes is as follows:

- Withdrawal (flexor, pain) reflex

1. Stretch Reflex

Stretch reflex, also known as myotactic, refers to reflex contraction of a muscle that is stretched.

Type: It is the best known MSR in the body.

Stimulus that evokes the reflex response is 'stretch' to the muscle.

Reaction time, i.e. the time between the application of the stimulus and the response for a stretch reflex, is 19–24 milliseconds. Stretch reflex is the quickest of all the reflexes.

Central delay, i.e. the time taken for the reflex activity to traverse the spinal cord, in a stretch reflex (being monosynaptic) is only 0.6–0.9 millisecond.

***Stretch reflex** is well developed* in antigravity muscles such as extensor group of muscles of legs and flexor groups of muscles of arms.

Examples of stretch reflexes are knee jerk, ankle jerk, biceps jerk and triceps jerk (see page 1029).

Reflex Arc of Stretch Reflex (Fig. 10.9.5)

1. Afferent limb consists of receptor and afferent nerve.

Receptor for stretch reflex is muscle spindle. As a sensory receptor, the muscle spindle detects the degree and rate of muscle stretch. For detailed structure of the muscle spindle, see page 1018.

Afferent nerve: As described in 'Nerve Supply of the Muscle Spindle', two types of nerve fibres – group Ia fibre and group II fibres – supply the muscle spindle (see page 1018). The afferent nerve fibres emerging from the muscle spindle travel along the spinal nerve and enter the spinal cord through the dorsal root and send branches to every α-motor neuron that goes to the muscle from which the Ia originated.

2. Centre: The centre for stretch reflex is the ventral grey horn area where the afferent nerve ends and synapses directly with the α-motor neuron. Thus, an α-motor neuron is the final common pathway, serving as both an integrating centre and an efferent pathway.

3. Efferent limb consists of the efferent nerve and an effector organ.

Efferent nerve: The axons of α-motor neurons (with which the afferent fibres synapse directly) form the efferent nerve fibres which leave the spinal cord through the ventral root and supply the skeletal muscle fibres.

Effector organs: Both extensor and flexor muscles exhibit stretch reflexes, and thus form the effector organs.

Reciprocal Innervation in Stretch Reflex

The stretch reflex is characterized by reciprocal innervation, i.e. excitation of one group of muscles is associated with inhibition of the antagonistic group of muscles on the same side, allowing the agonistic muscles to contract without interference. Reciprocal innervation is one of the important features of both flexor and extensor reflexes.

Pathway of reciprocal innervation Pathway of reciprocal innervation is biphasic. A collateral from each Ia fibre passes in the spinal cord to an inhibitory interneuron (Golgi bottle neuron) that synapses directly on one of the motor neurons supplying the antagonist muscles. Thus, this is an example of postsynaptic inhibition (Fig. 10.7.18, see page 979).

Significance of reciprocal innervation Reciprocal innervation is very important in spinal reflexes, which are involved in locomotion. It helps in the forward movement of one limb while causing the backward movement of the other limb.

Dynamic Stretch Reflex Versus Static Stretch Reflex

Dynamic stretch reflex When the muscle is stretched suddenly, the length of spindle receptor also increases suddenly (as the intrafusal fibres forming the muscle spindle are attached in parallel with extrafusal fibres of the muscle). Sudden increase in length of spindle receptor stimulates the primary nerve ending powerfully. The primary nerve endings supplying the nuclear bag fibres show a dynamic response, i.e. they discharge most rapidly while the muscle is being stretched (Figs 10.9.9 and 10.9.10B) and transmit strong signals to the spinal cord, and it causes instantaneous, very strong reflex contraction of the same muscle from which the signals originated. This is called dynamic stretch reflex, the function of which is to oppose sudden change in length, e.g. knee jerk and ankle jerk. Dynamic stretch reflex is over within fraction of a second, because primary nerve endings supplying nuclear bag fibres are stimulated actively only when there is a rapid change of length, i.e. they are stimulated only when the length is actually increasing. As soon as the length stops increasing, the rate of impulse discharge through those endings returns back to normal. Furthermore, when the muscle contracts reflexly, the spindle receptors shorten, and the discharge through primary ending even decreases momentarily (Fig. 10.9.10C).

Static stretch reflex When the muscle is stretched slowly and kept stretched, signals are continuously sent through primary and secondary nerve endings supplying the nuclear chain fibres only (Fig. 10.9.29A) and cause reflex contraction of the muscle. This is because the nerves from the primary ending on the nuclear chain fibres show a static response, i.e. they discharge at an increased rate throughout the period when a muscle is stretched (Fig. 10.9.29b). This is called static stretch reflex. This static reflex therefore causes muscle contraction as long as the muscle is maintained at excessive length. The muscle contraction thus opposes the force that is causing the excess length. The static stretch reflex plays an important role in control of posture, e.g. when the person is standing, gravity causes continuous stretch on the antigravity muscles making them to remain in a contracted state as long as gravity is causing the stretch.

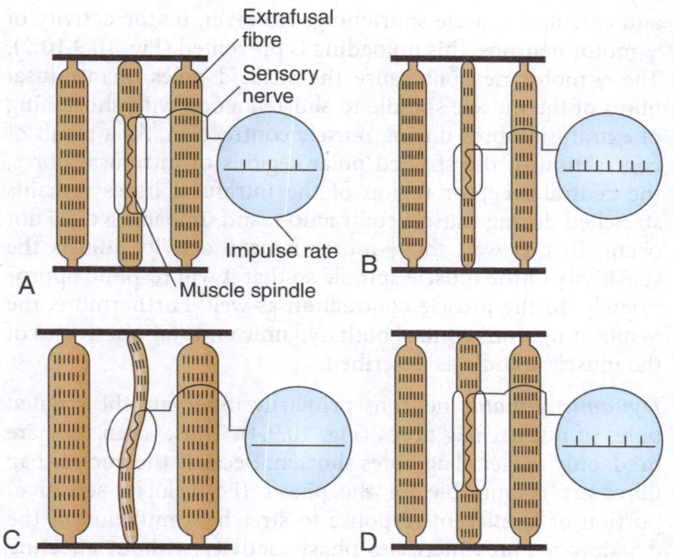

Fig. 10.9.10 Firing rate of primary nerve endings (Ia) under different conditions: **A**, muscle at rest; **B**, muscle stretched; **C**, muscle contracted; and **D**, muscle contracted with increased γ efferent discharge.

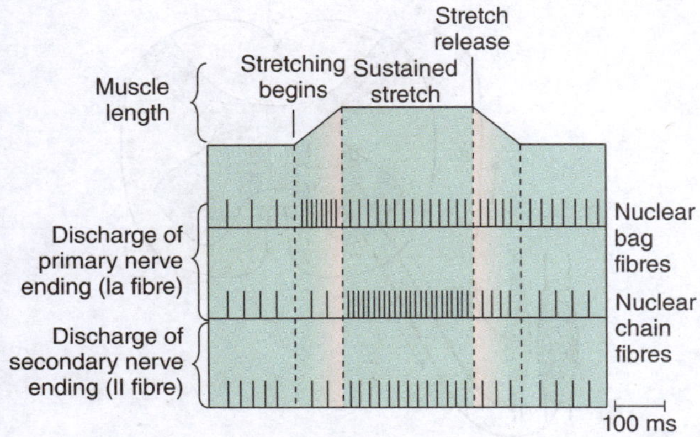

Fig. 10.9.9 Response of primary (Ia) and secondary (II) nerve endings of muscle spindles to muscle stretch.

Important Note

From the above, it is clear that a primary nerve ending responds to both changes in length (static stretch reflex) and changes in the rate of stretch (dynamic stretch reflex). The response of primary endings to the phasic as well as static events in the muscle is important because the prompt, marked phasic response helps to dampen oscillations caused by conduction delays in the feedback loop regulating the muscle length.

Role of γ-Motor Neurons

1. Role of γ-efferent discharge in adjusting the spindle sensitivity by preventing unloading As discussed above, the firing rate of primary nerve endings (Ia fibres) increases when the muscle is stretched (Fig. 10.9.10B), and causes reflex contraction of the muscle by increased α-motor neuron activity. Contraction of the extrafusal muscle fibres makes the muscle spindle slack and decreases the firing rate of Ia fibres (Fig. 10.9.10C). The decreased rate of Ia afferent discharge that occurs during muscle contraction is called *unloading of the muscle spindle*, and is functionally disadvantageous because the CNS stops receiving information about the rate and extent of muscle shortening. However, by the activity of γ-motor neurons, this unloading is prevented (Fig. 10.9.10D). The γ-motor neurons cause the striated poles of intrafusal fibres of the muscle spindle to shorten along with shortening of extrafusal fibres during muscle contraction. As a result of contraction of the striated polar regions of intrafusal fibres, the central receptor region of the intrafusal fibres remains stretched during muscle contraction, and unloading does not occur. In this way, the γ-motor neuron activity adjusts the sensitivity of the muscle spindle so that it will respond appropriately during muscle contraction as well. Furthermore, the γ-motor neurons control both dynamic and static activities of the muscle spindle as described.

Dynamic γ-motor neurons primarily innervate the striated poles of nuclear bag fibres (Fig. 10.9.4). Thus, when they are fired, only nuclear bag fibres shorten. Because the nuclear bag fibres are responsible for the phasic (i.e. velocity-sensitive) portion of Ia afferent response to stretch, stimulation of the dynamic γ-fibres increases phasic activity without affecting static activity.

Static γ-fibres primarily innervate the striated poles of nuclear chain fibres (Fig. 10.9.4). When they are fired, only the nuclear chain fibres shorten. Because the nuclear chain fibres are responsible for the static (i.e. length-sensitive) component of Ia afferent response to stretch, stimulation of the static γ-fibres increases static activity without affecting phasic activity.

Important Note

The above-described γ-motor neuron–mediated change in length of intrafusal fibres forms the so-called *length servomechanism*, which is a system of negative feedback device that operates to maintain muscle length during body movements and thus helps in regulation of posture (see page 1031).

2. Role of coactivation of α- and γ-motor neurons During a normal voluntary movement (e.g. *lifting a weight*), the active shortening of the extrafusal fibres would relieve tension on the muscle spindles (i.e. unload the spindle) and hence tend to decrease Ia discharge. However, during voluntary contraction, the motor control system causes α–γ *coactivation*, preventing the unloading of the muscle spindle that would occur during muscle contraction. Thus, increased γ-discharge along with the increased α-discharge during voluntary movement maintains constant Ia discharge. The constant level of Ia input to the CNS during a voluntary movement indicates that motor command is being carried out.

Important Note

The α–γ coactivation also forms the so-called *follow-up servomechanism* during voluntary movements.

For example, during voluntary movement of weightlifting, if the weight to be lifted is underestimated by the CNS, the motor command system does not activate a sufficient number of α-motor neurons to lift the weight and the extrafusal fibres fail to contract to the desired length. However, because of γ-motor neuron activity, the intrafusal fibres contract stretching the central receptor region of the intrafusal fibres, resulting in increased Ia afferent activity. This is called *loading of the muscle spindle*. The increased Ia activity indicates that the motor command is not being carried out. The CNS uses this information to readjust its command to the spinal cord. Even before the CNS responds to the information provided by the Ia fibres, the increased Ia activity directly stimulates the α-motor neurons of the spinal cord causing forceful muscle contraction sufficient to lift the unexpected weight. This change in α-motor neuron activity at the spinal cord level (without the higher motor command system) forms the 'follow-up servomechanism', which ensures that the extrafusal fibres contract to the desired length in spite of mismatched motor command.

3. Role of γ-loop It is theoretically possible that the CNS is capable of initiating movements directly by stimulating only γ-motor neurons, using a pathway called the γ-loop (Fig. 10.9.11). The loop begins with γ-motor neuron, which discharges to cause intrafusal muscle fibre contraction. This leads to an increase in Ia afferent fibre activity, which in turn causes increased γ-motor neuron discharge via an MSR causing muscle contraction.

Although the γ-loop can elicit movement on its own, it normally does not do so. However, because of coactivation, the γ-loop is activated during all movements and thus contributes to the excitability and firing rate of the α-motor neurons.

Higher Control of Stretch Reflex

From the above discussion, it is clear that stretch reflex involves three types of nerve fibres:

- Afferent fibres (Ia type)
- γ-Motor efferents
- α-Motor efferents

Though the stretch reflex is a spinal reflex, the activity in the reflex arc can be modified (inhibited or facilitated) by higher centres through their influence on the above-cited nerve fibres involved in stretch reflex.

1. Control of afferent (Ia type) discharge: The afferent fibres carry input arising from the activity of muscle spindle. The higher centres control it by presynaptic modulation of the sensory input (Fig. 10.9.12A).

2. Control of γ-efferent discharge:

i. ***Direct modulation of γ neuronal activity (centrifugal control):*** The motor neurons of the γ-efferent system are regulated to a large degree by descending tracts from a number of areas in the brain (Fig. 10.9.12C). Via these

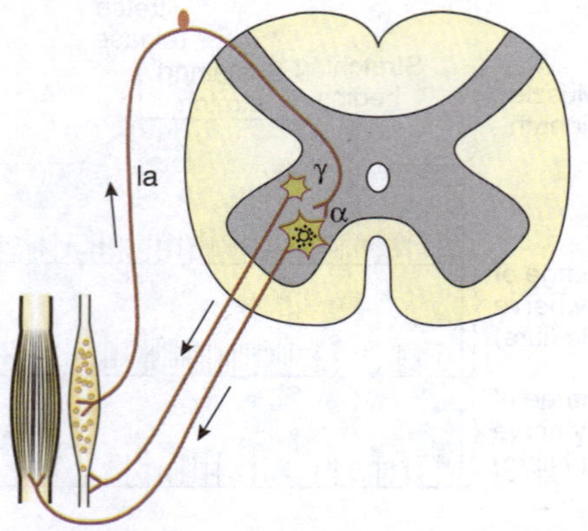

Fig. 10.9.11 The γ-loop system of initiating muscle contraction directly through stimulation of γ-motor neurons.

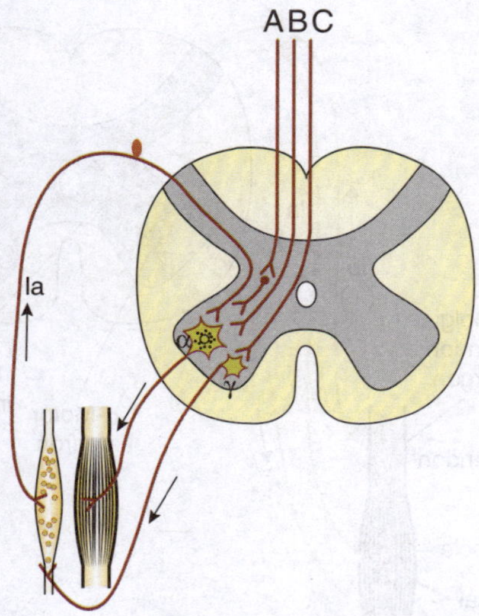

Fig. 10.9.12 Higher control of stretch reflex: **A**, presynaptic modulation of Ia sensory input; **B**, direct action on α-motor neurons; and **C**, modulation of γ-motor neuronal activity (centrifugal control).

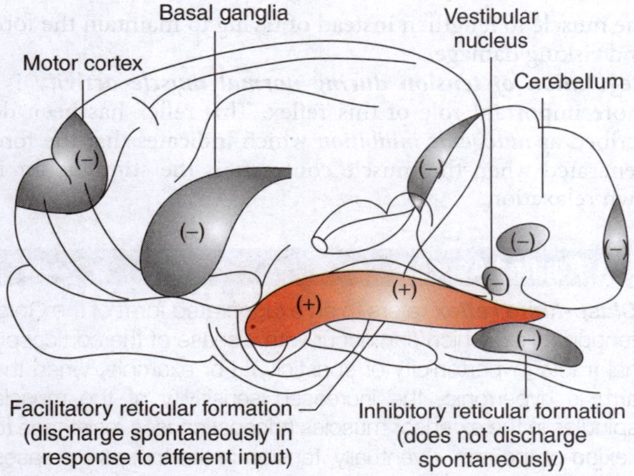

Fig. 10.9.13 Brain areas that have facilitatory (+) and inhibitory (–) effect on stretch reflex.

pathways, the sensitivity of the muscle spindles and hence the threshold of the stretch reflexes in various parts of the body can be adjusted and shifted to meet the needs of postural control. Some of the important brain areas that facilitate or inhibit the stretch reflex are as follows (Fig. 10.9.13):

Facilitatory reticular formation (FRF) is a large area in the brainstem which discharges spontaneously in response to afferent input. This increases discharge of γ-motor neurons and stretch reflex becomes hyperactive.

Inhibitory reticular formation (IRF) is a small area which does not discharge spontaneously. It acts by inhibiting γ-efferent neuron discharge, thereby decreasing the spindle sensitivity.

Cerebral motor cortex and cerebellum reflexly inhibit the stretch reflex by stimulating the IRF.

ii. ***Other factors which influence γ-efferent discharge:***

Anxiety causes an increased discharge, a fact that probably explains the hyperactive tendon reflexes sometimes seen in anxious patients.

Unexpected movement is also associated with a greater γ-efferent discharge.

Stimulation of the skin, especially by noxious agents, increases γ-efferent discharge to ipsilateral flexor muscle spindles and decreases that to extensors and produces the opposite pattern in the opposite limb.

> **Important Note**
>
> This fact is sometimes used as reinforcement to elicit deep tendon reflexes (such as knee jerk), which are not being elicited otherwise. For it, the individual is asked to pull the hands apart when the flexed fingers are hooked together; this facilitates the knee jerk (*Jendrassik* manoeuvre). It is contributed to increased γ-efferent discharge initiated by afferent impulses from the hands.

3. Control of α-motor efferent discharge: α-Motor neurons form the efferent pathway of stretch reflex. All neural influences (excitatory or inhibitory) affecting muscle contraction ultimately funnel through the α-motor neurons; therefore, they form the so-called *final common pathway*. Numerous inputs converge on them and determine the activity in final common path (Figs 10.9.8 and 10.9.12B).

Functions of Stretch Reflex

i. Role in Maintaining Muscle Tone The muscle tone refers to partial state of contraction of the muscle under resting condition. It is the function of stretch reflex, which is under the influence of discharge from the γ-motor neuron. In the brainstem, there are two areas – facilitatory area is the pons and inhibitory area is the lower part of the medulla. These areas send the impulses to γ-motor neurons. Facilitatory area is intrinsically active, so it continues to discharge facilitatory impulses causing constant activation of γ-motor neurons. This causes stretching of the muscle spindle fibres resulting in slight reflex contraction of the extrafusal fibres of muscle under resting state (producing muscle tone). Inhibitory area in the medulla becomes active only if it receives impulses from the cerebellum or cerebral cortex.

ii. Role in maintaining posture Static component of stretch reflex, the fundamental posture control mechanism, is especially prominent in medial extensor muscles and antigravity muscles. For example, when a person is standing upright, gravity tends to stretch the quadriceps muscle. This stretching elicits a stretch reflex resulting in sustained contraction of quadriceps as long as the stretch is there. This maintains the extension around the knee joint and upright posture.

iii. Role in control of voluntary movement A stretch reflex helps the motor command system in performing voluntary movements. During activity generated by the motor command system, the group Ia fibres from the muscle spindle inform the motor control system about the changes in muscle length. The constant level of Ia input to the CNS during a movement indicates that the motor command is being carried out. An increase in activity of Ia indicates that motor command is not being carried out. The CNS uses this information to readjust its command to the spinal cord. In addition, the Ia activity is also used at the spinal cord level to adjust the α-motor neuron activity as per need. Thus, the Ia activity provides the α-motor neuron with a source of excitatory input in addition to that coming from the higher centres.

2. Golgi Tendon Reflex (Disynaptic Reflex)

The Golgi tendon reflex, also called 'inverse stretch reflex', is a disynaptic reflex. The receptors involved are the Golgi tendon organs.

Golgi Tendon Organs

Golgi tendon organs (Fig. 10.9.14) are high-threshold stretch receptors located in the tendons and musculoaponeurotic junction. They are placed in series between the muscle fibres and the tendon (in contrast to muscle spindles which are located in parallel to muscle fibres) and are thus stretched whenever the muscle contracts. Usually, 10–15 muscle fibres are connected in series with 1 Golgi tendon organ. Each Golgi tendon organ basically consists of a group of nerve endings covered by a capsule of connective tissue. In a given muscle, the Golgi tendon organs are less numerous than muscle spindles.

- The Golgi tendon organs are supplied by *Ib-type sensory nerve fibres*. The nerve fibres supplying the Golgi tendon organ ramify into many branches. Each branch ends in the form of a knob.
- The Golgi tendon organs have neither muscle fibres nor an efferent innervation.

Pathway and Activity of Reflex (Fig. 10.9.15)

- When a muscle contracts, the muscle tension increases. The Golgi tendon organ detects the muscle tension and sends impulses through afferent (group Ib) fibres which enter the spinal cord through the dorsal root.
- In the spinal cord, the group Ib afferents stimulate the inhibitory interneurons.
- The inhibitory interneurons in turn release inhibitory mediator glycine which inhibits α-motor neurons and cause relaxation of the muscle that was originally contracted.
- At the same time, due to reciprocal innervation, the antagonistic muscles are excited.
- The Golgi tendon reflex thus displays reciprocal innervation but lacks afterdischarge and irradiation.

Physiological Role

The functions of Golgi tendon reflex are as follows:

Protective function: Historically, this reflex has been described as a protective reflex in which a strong and potentially damaging muscle force reflexively inhibits the muscle, causing

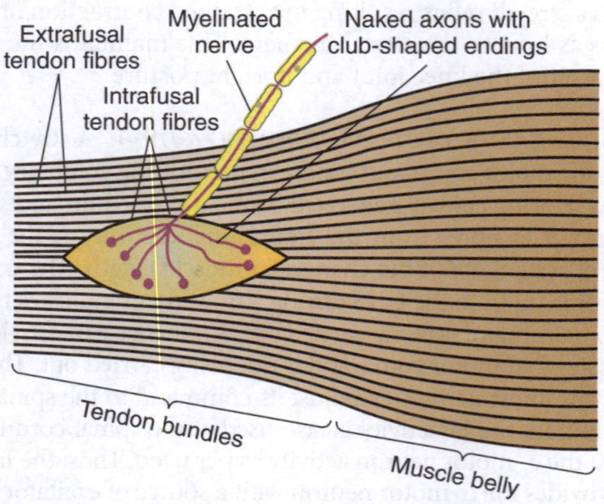

Fig. 10.9.14 Structure of Golgi tendon organ.

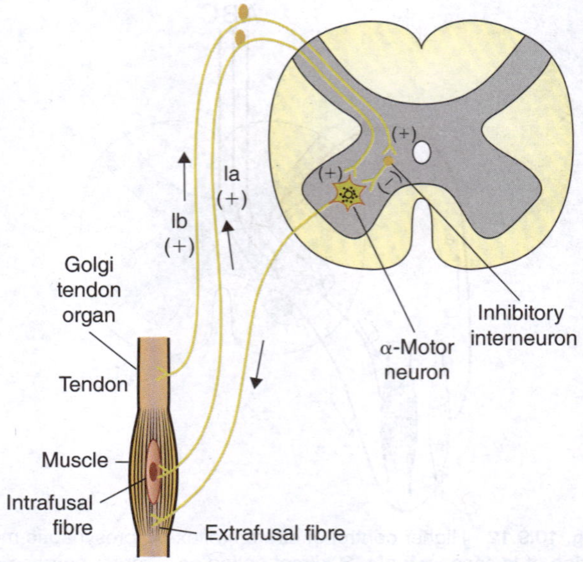

Fig. 10.9.15 Pathway of stretch and inverse stretch reflex.

the muscle to lengthen instead of trying to maintain the force and risking damage.

Regulation of tension during normal muscle activity is a more important role of this reflex. This reflex has been described as *autogenic inhibition* which indicates that the force generated when the muscle contracts is the stimulus for its own relaxation.

Applied Aspects

Clasp-knife reflex refers to an exaggerated form of the Golgi tendon reflex, which can occur with disease of the corticospinal tracts (hypertonicity or spasticity). For example, when the arm is hypertonic, the increased sensitivity of the muscle spindles in the extensor muscles (triceps) causes resistance to flexion of the arm. Eventually, tension in the triceps increases to the point at which it activates Golgi tendon reflex, causing triceps to relax and the arm to flex closed like a jack knife, hence the name clasp-knife reflex. The physiological name for it is *lengthening reaction*, because it is the response of a spastic muscle to lengthening.

3. Withdrawal Reflex (Polysynaptic Reflex)

Withdrawal reflex, also known as flexor reflex, is a cutaneous reflex that occurs in response to nociceptive (pain) stimuli and is characterized by removal of a body part from a painful stimulus.

Receptors

The receptor of withdrawal reflex are *nociceptors* located in free nerve endings of Aδ and C fibres.

Pathway (Reflex arc) of Withdrawal Reflex

Withdrawal reflex is a polysynaptic reflex consisting of the following pathways (Fig. 10.9.16):

- The pain fibres carrying impulses, on entering the spinal cord, synapse on many interneurons. Some of these also convey information to CNS. Others form several reflex pathways.

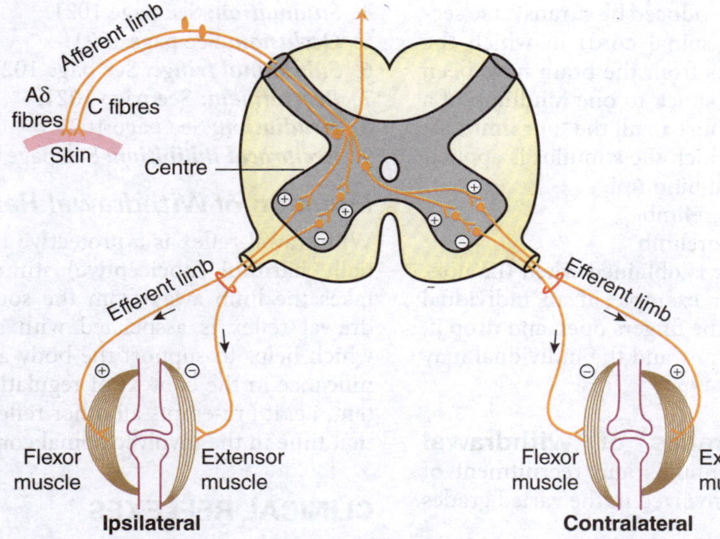

Fig. 10.9.16 Reflex arc of a polysynaptic reflex (withdrawal reflex or crossed extensor reflex).

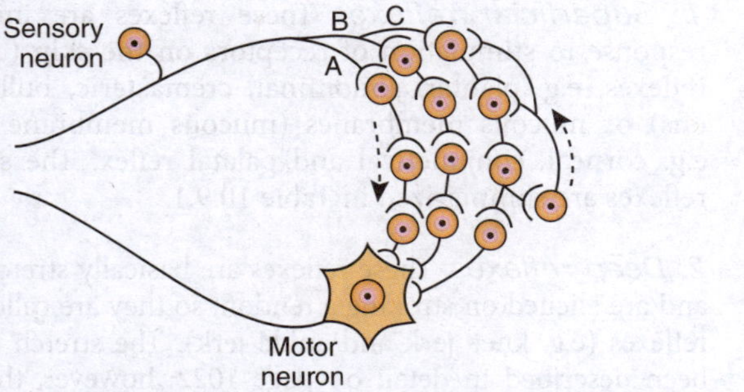

Fig. 10.9.17 Schematic depiction of connections between afferent and efferent neurons in the spinal cord. The dorsal root fibre has been shown to activate pathway **A** with three interneurons, pathway **B** with four interneurons and pathway **C** with four interneurons. **Note** that one of the interneurons in the pathway **C** connects to a neuron that feeds back on previously excited neuron forming reverberating circuits.

- Polysynaptic reflex paths branch in a complex fashion. The number of synapses in each of their branches is variable (Fig. 10.9.17).
- A branch from some of the axons of interneuron in the reflex pathway feeds back on themselves forming the *reverberating circuits*, which are responsible for afterdischarge (Fig. 10.9.17).
- The interneurons form several pathways of different lengths to ultimately end on α-motor neurons as follows (Fig. 10.9.17):
  - Some of the interneurons project onto α-motor neurons on the ipsilateral side and stimulate the flexors which withdraw the limbs.
  - Some of the interneurons form inhibitory pathway and terminate on α-motor neurons supplying the extensor muscles on the ipsilateral side producing their relaxation. This is called reciprocal innervation, which ensures that the flexion movement is not impeded by contraction of the extensors.
  - Some of the interneurons cross to the opposite side of the spinal cord and end on the α-motor neurons supplying the extensors on the contralateral side. In case of need, this pathway produces extension of the opposite limbs (crossed extensor reflex).

Effector organs The effector organs of the withdrawal reflex are the skeletal muscles that cause withdrawal of the limb. Although they are called flexors, these muscles are flexors in the physiological, not anatomic, sense. For example, the muscles that cause the fingers to open to drop a hot coal, although anatomically referred to as extensors, are considered flexors, because they are involved in the withdrawal reflex.

Response in Withdrawal Reflex

The reflex response to a painful stimulus varies from just withdrawal of the affected part to withdrawal of the whole body depending on the strength of the painful stimulus and location of the stimulus. The different types of responses observed in a withdrawal reflex are as follows:

Local sign refers to the ability of the reflex to confine to the portion of the body affected by the noxious stimulus. For example, if the medial surface of a limb is stimulated, the response will include some abduction, whereas stimulation of the lateral surface will produce adduction and flexion. The reflex response in each case generally serves to effectively remove the limb away from the irritating stimulus. Therefore, if an individual accidentally touches a hot stove, it is likely that he/she will jerk only the hand away from the stove (one-limb response).

Flexor response: When a noxious stimulus is applied to a limb, the typical response is in the form of contraction of flexors and inhibition of extensors leading to flexion of the stimulated limb and its withdrawal from the irritating stimulus.

Crossed extensor reflex response (two-limb response): When a strong stimulus is applied to a limb, the response includes not only flexion and withdrawal of the limb but also extension of the opposite limb. This crossed extensor response is produced by the interneuronal pathway that crosses to the opposite side of the spinal cord. In lower limbs, crossed extensor reflex allows one limb to support the body while the other is raised off the ground.

Shifting reaction (four-limb reflex response): It is difficult to demonstrate this response in normal animals but is easily demonstrated in spinal animals (produced by a transverse section in the lower region of the spinal cord) in which the modulating effects of the stimulus from the brain have been abolished. Application of electric shock to one hindlimb of a spinal animal will produce a response in all the four limbs as:

- Flexion of the hindlimb to which the stimulus is applied
- Extension of the contralateral hindlimb
- Extension of the ipsilateral forelimb
- Flexion of the contralateral forelimb

Widespread withdrawal response is obtained when the noxious stimulus is very strong. For example, if an individual picks up a hot coal, not only will the fingers open and drop it, but also the entire arm will withdraw and the individual may even leap away from the fire.

Mechanism of varied grades of withdrawal response Irradiation of the stimulus and recruitment of motor units are the mechanisms involved in the varied grades of response in withdrawal reflex.

Irradiation Irradiation refers to spread of excitatory impulses up and down the spinal cord to more and more motor units leading to activation of a large number of impulses. This occurs when the noxious stimulus is strong enough that impulses spread to many neighbouring neurons in the centre and produce a wider response.

Recruitment of motor units Recruitment of motor units refers to progressive increase in the number of motor units activated by spreading interneuronal activity. Of course, there is a limit to the number of motor units that can be recruited. So, beyond a certain limit, prolongation of stimulation does not increase the response and a plateau is reached.

Characteristics of Withdrawal Reflex

1. ***Long latency:*** The withdrawal reflex has a relatively long latency, i.e. has a higher reaction time. *Reaction time* is the interval between the application of a stimulus and the onset of response. It is determined in part by the time taken by the impulse transmission in afferent and efferent limbs of the reflex arc (*peripheral delay*) and in part by the time spent by the impulse in traversing the spinal cord (*central delay*). The long latency in withdrawal reflex is because of peripheral delay (as the afferent pathway uses small, slowly conducting fibres) as well as due to central delay (as it involves many synapses).
   It is important to note that in case of stretch reflex, the central delay is less than 1 millisecond, indicating that it is an MSR. In case of flexor reflex, the central delay is much longer.
   In crossed extensor response, the central delay may be longer than 20 milliseconds, reflecting the huge number of interneurons involved in the reflex.
2. ***Response outlasts stimulus,*** i.e. withdrawal reflex shows afterdischarge. *Afterdischarge* refers to the continuation of reflex withdrawal of the limb even after the sensory receptor has stopped firing. It is produced by *reverberating circuits* (i.e. a branch from the axon of one interneuron in the reflex pathway feeds back onto previously excited neurons, re-exciting them and prolonging α-motor neuron firing).
3. ***Patterned response:*** The crossed extensor reflex produces a patterned response, i.e. the affected limb always flexes, whereas the contralateral limb extends.
4. ***Summation:*** See page 1021.
5. ***Occlusion:*** See page 1021.
6. ***Subliminal fringe:*** See page 1021.
7. ***Recruitment:*** See page 1021.
8. ***Irradiation:*** See page 1021.
9. ***Reciprocal inhibition:*** See page 978.

Function of Withdrawal Reflex

Withdrawal reflex is a protective reflex initiated by a potentially harmful (nociceptive) stimulus. The flexor response takes the limb away from the source of irritation. A withdrawal reflex is associated with a crossed extensor reflex, which helps to support the body and is of physiological significance in the context of regulation of posture. It is prepotent, i.e. it pre-empts all other reflex activities taking place at that time in the involved spinal cord segment.

CLINICAL REFLEXES

Clinically, the reflexes can be grouped as given next.

I. Physiological Reflexes

1. Superficial reflexes These reflexes are initiated in response to stimulation of receptors on the skin (cutaneous reflexes, e.g. plantar, abdominal, cremasteric, bulbocavernous) or mucous membranes (mucous membrane reflexes), e.g. corneal, conjunctival and palatal reflex. The superficial reflexes are summarized in Table 10.9.1.

2. Deep reflexes These reflexes are basically stretch reflexes and are elicited on stroking a tendon, so they are called tendon reflexes (e.g. knee jerk and ankle jerk). The stretch reflex has been described in detail on page 1022; however, the various clinically known stretch reflexes are summarized in Table 10.9.1.

3. Visceral reflexes Visceral reflexes are elicited from the visceral organ or at least one part of the reflex arc is formed by autonomic nerve, e.g. carotid sinus reflex (see page 330), micturition reflex (see page 551) and occulocardiac reflex. A few of the clinically known visceral reflexes are summarized in Table 10.9.1.

II. Pathological Reflexes

The pathological reflexes are abnormal reflexes, which are not found normally. They are elicited in pathological conditions, e.g.:

- Babinski sign
- Mass reflex
- Clonus
- Pendular movements

1. Babinski sign It is the abnormal plantar reflex, i.e. instead of plantar flexion of the great toe, there occurs dorsiflexion of the great toe and abduction (fanning out) of the small toes and this is also accompanied with flexion of the knee and dorsiflexion at the ankle joint. The abnormal plantar response is called *extensor plantar or Babinski sign positive.*

Significance: Babinski sign is present in the following conditions:

- Upper motor neuron lesion (UML): It is the most important sign.
- Physiologically, it is present in infants (younger than 1 year) due to nonmyelination of pyramidal tracts and also during deep sleep.

Table 10.9.1 Characteristic features of clinical reflexes

Reflex	Method to elicit	Response	Spinal segment/cranial nerve and centre involved
I. Superficial reflexes			
(a) Cutaneous reflexes			
1. *Plantar reflex*	Strike the outer aspect of the sole of the foot with a blunt object (e.g. key) and move towards the ball of small toes.	Plantar flexion of the foot and toes	L_5 to S_1
2. *Abdominal reflex*	Lightly stimulate the wall of abdomen by stroking with key or some blunt object from outside to inside (parallel to costal margin) in upper quadrants and (parallel to inguinal ligament) in lower quadrants of the abdomen.	Contractions of the underlying abdominal muscle **Note:** The reflex is difficult to elicit in elderly individuals, obese persons and multipara	T_7 to T_{12}
3. *Cremasteric reflex*	Stimulate the skin of upper and inner part of the thigh.	Pulling upwards of scrotum and testicles due to contraction of cremasteric muscles; this reflex may not be elicited in elderly individuals	L_1 and L_2
4. *Scapular reflex*	Stroke the skin of interscapular region.	Contraction of supraspinatus and infraspinatus muscles	C_5 to T_1
5. *Anal reflex*	Gently stimulate the skin of perianal region.	Contraction of external and internal anal sphincters	S_2 to S_4
6. *Bulbocavernous reflex*	Gently pinch the dorsum of glans penis.	Contraction of bulbocavernous muscle	S_3 to S_4
(b) Mucous membrane reflexes			
7. *Corneal reflex*	Touch the cornea with wisp of cotton from lateral aspect.	Closure of eye of same and of opposite side	*Afferents:* Via ophthalmic division of (trigeminal) cranial nerve V *Centre:* In the pons *Efferents:* Via facial nerve to orbicularis oculi muscle
8. *Conjunctival reflex*	Touch the conjunctiva with wisp of cotton.	Closure of the eyes	Pathway is same as for corneal reflex
9. *Palate reflex*	Touch either side of posterior pharyngeal wall with a swab stick.	The contraction of the palate	*Afferents:* Cranial nerve IX *Centre:* Nucleus ambiguus *Efferents:* Cranial (vagus) nerve X
II. Deep reflexes (tendon reflexes)			
1. *Knee jerk*	The subject is in lying or in sitting position. Place the left hand under the knee (to be tested). Tap the tendon of the quadriceps midway between its origin and insertion with knee hammer.	Observe the extension of knee due to contraction of quadriceps femoris muscle; sometimes, if unable to elicit, then apply reinforcement (Jendrassik manoeuvre, page 1025)	Femoral nerve (L_2, L_3 and L_4)
2. *Ankle jerk*	With foot slightly everted and dorsiflexed, strike on the tendo-Achilles.	Plantar flexion of the foot occurs due to contraction of calf muscle	S_1 and S_2
3. *Triceps jerk*	Keep the forearm of the subject to rest across his/her chest; then tap the triceps tendon with broader side of the patellar hammer.	Contraction of triceps with extension of the elbow	C_6 and C_7
4. *Biceps jerk*	Keep the position of elbow at right angle with forearm and the forearm is semipronated; the examiner then places his/her thumb or index finger on the tendon of the biceps muscle and then strikes on the finger (kept on biceps tendon) with patellar hammer.	Contraction of biceps with flexion of elbow	C_5 and C_6
5. *Supinator*	Tap the lower end of the radius at styloid process, keeping the position of elbow same as for biceps jerk.	Supination of forearm and flexion of elbow	C_5 and C_6
6. *Jaw jerk*	Ask the subject to open the mouth slightly; then place one finger firmly below the lower lip and tap on the finger in a downward direction.	Contraction of masseter muscle causes closure of the jaw	Afferent and efferents are carried by trigeminal nerve; centre lies in the pons

2. Mass reflex This reflex can be elicited in patients with spinal cord lesions. When the skin (on any portion in the midline) is stimulated by gentle pinpricks, there occurs evacuation of the bowel or bladder, flexion of the lower limb and sweating of the skin below the level of lesion.

Significance: Patients suffering from spinal cord injuries are particularly trained to elicit mass reflex to evacuate the bowel and bladder.

3. Clonus Clonus means a series of rapid and jerky movements which occur due to involuntary contraction of the muscle in response to sudden rapid and constant stretch. It signifies hyperflexia and hypertonia associated with increased γ-efferent activity. Clonus is seen in calf muscles (producing ankle clonus) and quadriceps (patellar clonus).

Ankle clonus: To elicit ankle clonus, support the slightly bent knee on one hand and hold the foot and suddenly dorsiflex the ankle and maintain the stretch for some time. This causes a series of rhythmic plantar flexion at the ankle joint.

Patellar clonus: The patient's leg is extended, and then the patella is suddenly pushed downwards towards the foot. Repeated contraction of quadriceps results in rhythmic movements of the leg.

Clonus occurs due to:

- *The stretch reflex–inverse stretch reflex sequence:* The basis of this sequential event is synchronized discharging of motor neurons without involving Golgi tendon discharges.
- *The muscle spindles of the tested muscle* become hyperactive and their discharges lead to excitation of all the motor neurons supplying at one time and cause contraction of the muscle.
- *The muscle contractions* (extrafusal fibres) result in stoppage of spindle discharges (relaxation of muscle) but as the stretch on the muscle is maintained, there occurs spindle activation and again muscle contraction.

4. Pendular movements In patients with cerebellar dysfunctions, while eliciting tendon jerk, slow oscillatory movements develop instead of brisk movement. Such movements are called pendular movements and are a manifestation of hypotonia and lack of restrictive effect.

REGULATION OF POSTURE

- Physiologically, posture refers to subconscious adjustment of tone in different muscles so as to maintain balance during displacement of the body caused by gravity or acceleration.
- The erect posture is a prerequisite to most of the somatic motor activities of humans and other higher animals.
- In humans, maintenance of an erect posture is more difficult than in the quadruped animals, because the tall body has to be maintained in an erect posture over a small base provided by two feet.
- Largely, the posture is maintained through reflex adjustments of tone in proximal extensor muscles. As gravity is the main force tending to displace the body, the proximal extensor muscles are also called antigravity muscles. Since a standing human being can fall in any direction, the muscles which oppose the fall act as antigravity muscles, depending on the direction of the fall. Therefore, any of the muscles of the trunk and limbs can act as antigravity muscles.
- Maintenance of an erect posture during movements of the body and more so while performing physical work (*dynamic posture*) is more complicated than maintenance of posture while standing still (*static posture*). This uphill task is accomplished by a very complex and coordinated reflex activity occurring in response to afferent input from muscle joints and vestibular and visual receptors.
- For the purpose of understanding, the regulation of posture can be discussed under two main headings:
  - *Mechanisms involved in maintenance of posture*
  - *Role of different regions of nervous system in maintenance of posture*

MECHANISMS INVOLVED IN MAINTENANCE OF POSTURE

At any given moment, in any position of the body (static or dynamic), the posture is maintained by alteration in the tone of different muscles which is controlled by a stretch reflex. The stretch reflex is a spinal reflex influenced by supraspinal control. The input to higher centres involved in the control of muscle tone through certain reflexes (called postural reflexes) significantly contributes to the maintenance of tone and hence the posture. Thus, the two main mechanisms involved in maintenance of posture are as follows:

- *Muscle tone*
- *Postural reflexes*

Role of Muscle Tone

Largely, the posture is maintained through reflex adjustments of tone in the antigravity muscles. The basic postural reflex involved in the control of muscle tone is stretch reflex described in detail on page 1025.

- Posture control is required not only for holding the body in an erect position but also for fixation of the body parts over adjoining body segments. The centre of gravity of the head passes in front of the centre of gravity of the atlanto-occipital joint. Thus, the head has got always a tendency to roll forwards. To hold the head in an erect position, cervico-occipital muscles are to be maintained in a state of constant tension. A similar problem is encountered in maintaining the equilibrium of the body in an erect position.
- In the upright position, gravity tends to displace the body downward, stretching quadriceps muscles as the legs flex at the knees. The muscle stretch evokes discharge from the muscle spindles of the quadriceps leading to its reflex contraction. This ensures that the knee joints, i.e. the main weight-bearing joints, do not give way under the effect of gravity. This maintains the leg as a pillar of support and thus counteracts the gravitational displacement of the body.
  In general, the antigravity muscles of the body are endowed with a somewhat higher muscle tone than the other muscles of the body.
- In humans, flexors of upper extremity and extensors of lower extremity are the main antigravity muscles. Retractors of the neck, the elevators of joints, supraspinatus, the extensors of the back, rectal muscles of the abdominal wall, and extensors of the knee and ankle are the muscles that exhibit the greatest degree of tone. When these muscles completely relax (as in an unconscious person), the body collapses.

- Various postural reflexes (described below) influence the medial motor system and the motor neurons of antigravity muscles. The inputs to this system through the postural reflexes significantly contribute to the maintenance of tone. Thus, tone is the result of activity of various medial system pathways that descend to excite both α- and γ-motor neurons, which innervate antigravity muscles and their spindles. Spinal transection interrupts this activity in the descending medial system and hence abolishes tone of the antigravity muscles (proximal extensors) below the level of transection. The two pathways of the medial system that are most important in maintenance of tone are the *lateral vestibulospinal tract* and *pontine reticulospinal tract*. Thus, spinal shock can be produced by any transection caudal to the origin of the vestibulospinal tract from the lateral vestibular nucleus. However, if the transaction is just rostral to this nucleus, then in contrast to spinal shock, the tone of antigravity muscles is actually enhanced and an exaggerated antigravity muscle posture is obtained. This phenomenon is called decerebrate rigidity (see page 1037).

Maintenance of Muscle Tone

Stretch reflex, as mentioned earlier, plays the main role in maintenance of muscle tone (page 1025). Though the stretch reflex is a spinal reflex, supraspinal control modifies the reflex in an intact animal.

Centre for muscle tone: The centre for muscle tone lies in anterior motor neurons (α-motor neurons) of the spinal cord, which are stimulated through a constant γ-motor neuron discharge. Activity of γ- and α-motor neurons is modified by both extrapyramidal and pyramidal fibres which terminate on them (directly or through interneurons). Mainly, the extrapyramidal system is responsible for maintaining tone. It consists of the basal ganglia, motor nuclei of reticular formation of the brainstem, vestibular nuclei and descending fibres conveying impulses to the spinal cord. From the cerebral cortex (area 6), also some fibres descend and merge with the extrapyramidal nuclei.

Supraspinal control on muscle tone is (Fig. 10.9.18) exerted by facilitatory and inhibitory areas in the brainstem through γ-motor neurons.

Bulboreticular facilitatory area is located in the pons and discharges facilitatory impulses to spinal motor neurons. This area in turn receives facilitatory impulses from vestibular nuclei, facilitatory portion of the cerebral cortex, cerebellum and basal ganglia. The facilitatory area continues to discharge impulses causing constant activation of γ-motor neurons. This causes stretching of the muscle spindle fibres resulting in reflex partial contraction of the muscle under resting state, thus producing muscle tone.

Bulboreticular inhibitory area is located in the lower part of the medulla. This area has no intrinsic activity of its own. It becomes active only if it receives impulses from the cerebellum or cerebral cortex and in turn inhibits the bulboreticular facilitatory area to some extent. But without support from the cerebrum or cerebellum, this area cannot inhibit the activity of the facilitatory area.

Role of cerebellum: Cerebellum is the site of α–γ linkage. Therefore, in the presence of the cerebellum, the muscle tone is maintained through both the α (nonmyotatic) and the γ (myotatic) activity. However, in the absence of the cerebellum, muscle tone is maintained by α (nonmyotatic) activity only.

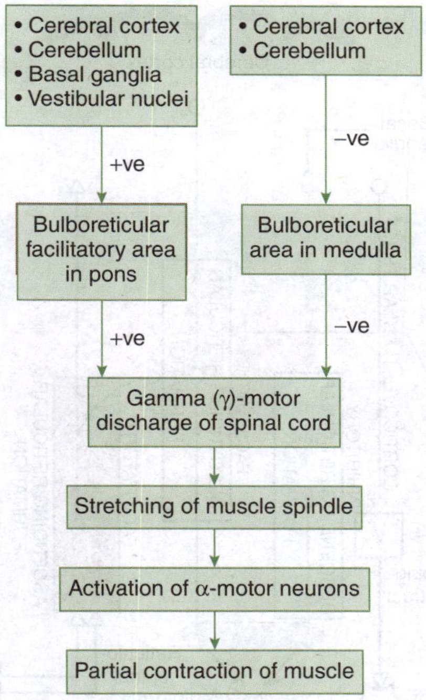

Fig. 10.9.18 Flowchart depicting control of muscle tone.

This can be demonstrated by classical and ischaemic decerebrate rigidity.

Important Note

Normally, the muscle tone is due to tonic discharge of γ-motor neurons to the muscles due to predominant effect of descending fibres of facilitatory reticular formation. Thus, muscle tone is normally not under the tonic control of α-motor neurons (tonic control of motor neurons should not be confused with the stimulation of α-motor neurons through corticospinal fibres during voluntary phasic contraction). It is important to note that tonic control of α-motor neurons is exerted almost entirely through the vestibulospinal pathway. However, the vestibular nucleus (especially the Deiters nucleus) is constantly inhibited by corticospinal fibres as well as fastigiovestibular fibres from the cerebellum (Fig. 10.9.19).

Under certain abnormal conditions and under experimental situation when the vestibular nucleus gets disinhibited, there occurs exaggeration of muscle tone that is α-led rather than γ-led.

Postural Reflexes

The postural reflexes help to maintain the body in an upright and balanced position. They also provide adjustments necessary to maintain a stable posture during voluntary activity.

Reflex arc of postural reflexes is as follows (Fig. 10.9.20):

- *Afferent pathways* of reflex arc come from the eyes, the vestibular apparatus and the proprioceptors.
- *Integrating centres* are formed by neuronal networks in the brainstem and spinal cord.
- *Efferent pathways* consist of α-motor neurons supplying the various skeletal muscles which form the effector organs.

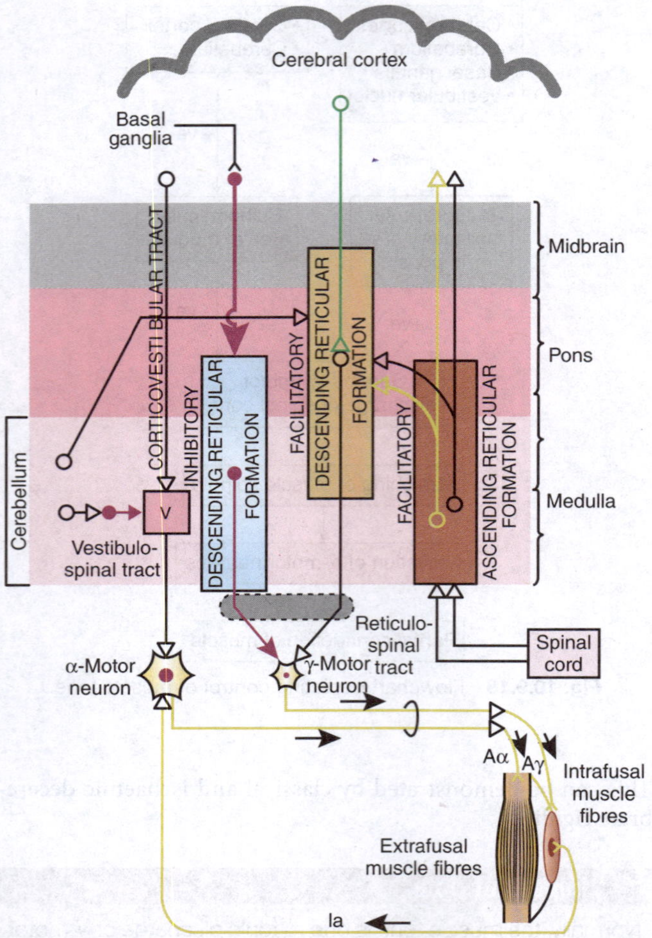

Fig. 10.9.19 Supraspinal control of muscle tone (solid circles and arrows indicate inhibitory signals and open circles and arrows indicate facilitation). V, vestibular nuclei.

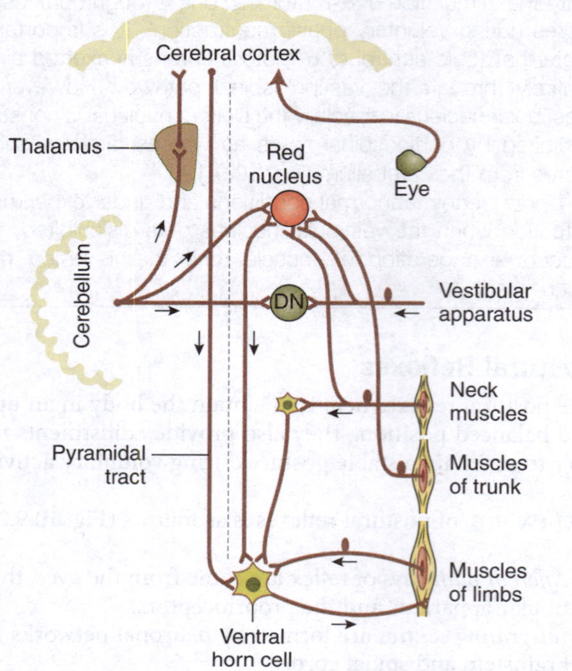

Fig. 10.9.20 Neuronal pathway of postural reflexes. DN, Deiters nucleus.

Types of postural reflexes: Broadly, postural reflexes are of two types:

Static reflexes: These are elicited by gravitational pull and involve sustained contraction of muscles.

Statokinetic reflexes: These reflexes, also called phasic reflexes, are elicited by acceleratory displacement of the body. They maintain a stable postural background for voluntary activity.

Both static and statokinetic postural reflexes are integrated at various levels in the CNS from the spinal cord to the cerebral cortex and are affected largely by pyramidal pathways.

A. Static Reflexes

Static reflexes are primarily involved in adjustments to displacements produced by gravity. These are of three types:

- Local static reflexes
- Segmental static reflexes
- General static reflexes

I. Local static reflexes

As the name indicates, the local static reflexes exert their effect on the same limb from which the stimulus was initiated. Some of the important local static reflexes include:

- Reflex control of antigravity muscle tone
- Positive supporting reaction
- Negative supporting reaction

1. Reflex control of antigravity muscle tone The most important of the local static reflexes is basic stretch reflexes (which have been described in detail on page 1025) controlling tone in those extensor muscles which keep the body upright (*antigravity muscles*).

Muscle tone in antigravity muscles is best illustrated in decerebrate preparations (see page 1037), where it produces decerebrate rigidity. The hypertonicity in decerebrate preparations has a characteristic extensor distribution, resulting in a caricature (i.e. exaggerated mimicry) of the normal posture.

2. Positive supporting reflexes Positive supporting reflex or reaction is characterized by simultaneous reflex contractions of both extensors and flexors of a limb (i.e. both the protagonists and the antagonists) converting it into a solid rigid pillar. The positive supporting reaction plays an important role of *steadying the ankle joint in standing position.* At the ankle joint, both dorsiflexion and plantar flexion are possible, but neither of them is desirable during standing position. The dorsiflexion of the foot would tip the body forward, whereas plantar flexion would throw the body backward (Fig. 10.9.21). The stabilization of the ankle joint in intermediate position is possible by simultaneous contraction of extensor and flexors of the foot brought about by the positive supporting reaction. Afferent impulses from the stimulated skin of the sole (touch–pressure receptors) and the muscles (proprioceptors) cause reflex contraction of both flexor and extensor muscles acting on the ankle joint, converting the leg and ankle joint into one solid pillar.

3. Negative supporting reaction Negative supporting reaction refers to disappearance of positive supporting reaction. It is also an active phenomenon initiated by stretch

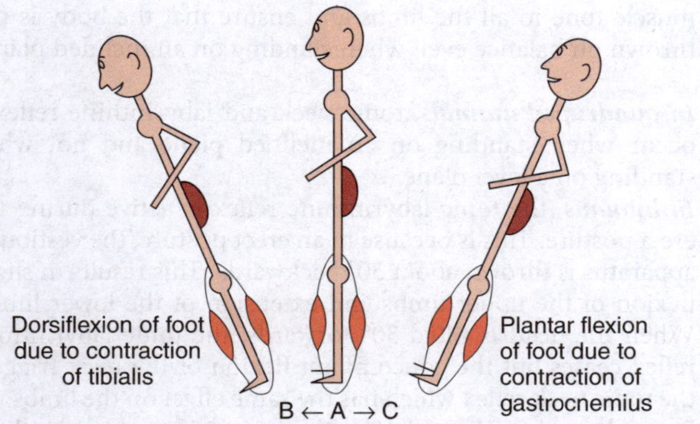

Fig. 10.9.21 Role of positive supporting reaction in stabilizing the ankle joint: **A**, simultaneous contraction of flexors and extensors of foot to stabilize ankle joint; **B**, dorsiflexion at foot produces forward fall; and **C**, plantar flexion at foot produces backward fall.

of the extensor muscles. This helps the limbs to be used for activities other than supporting the body weight.

Demonstration of local reflexes The centres of the local static reflex are located in the spinal cord. These can be demonstrated in a spinal animal (see page 1035).

II. Segmental static reflexes The segmental static reflexes are characterized by a bilateral reflex response when stimulus is applied to one limb. The best example of segmental static reflexes is crossed extensor reflex response component of withdrawal reflex. In this reflex, a strong stimulus to one limb produces flexion in the ipsilateral limb and extension in the contralateral limb (see page 1027).

Role of crossed extensor reflex in control of posture

- In the lower limb, this reflex allows one limb to support the body while the other is raised off the ground. For example, when one limb is flexed reflexly due to a painful stimulus, the extensor of the other limb compensates and sees to it that the body is not thrown off balance.
- The crossed extensor reflex also plays an important role during walking. During walking, the flexors are active and the extensors are inhibited on one side, whereas the reverse is seen on the other side.

Demonstration of static segmental reflex The centres for these reflexes are situated in the spinal cord. These can be best demonstrated in a *spinal animal* (see page 1035).

III. General static reflexes General static reflexes are characterized by a generalized effect from the many muscle groups in the body in response to a stimulus that arises at one side of the body. For example, numerous postural adjustments occur in response to changes in the head position. Broadly, general static reflexes can be divided into three groups:

- Attitudinal or statotonic reflexes
- Long-loop stretch reflexes
- Righting reflexes

a. Attitudinal reflexes Statotonic reflexes, also known as attitudinal reflexes, are initiated when the attitude of the body is changed, i.e. while standing on an inclined plane. These reflexes are of two types:

- Tonic labyrinthine reflexes
- Tonic neck reflexes

1. Tonic labyrinthine reflexes These reflexes are produced in response to *alteration in the position of the head relative to the horizontal plane*, e.g. while standing on an inclined plane. These reflexes decrease or increase the tone of the skeletal muscles of the limbs in accordance with the attitude of the head, e.g. while standing on an inclined plane.

Stimulus for tonic labyrinthine reflex is gravity.
Receptors for these reflexes are in the otolith organs, present in the labyrinthine apparatus.
Afferents: The afferent impulses generated from the receptors (present in otolith organs) travel along the vestibular nerves.
Centres for these reflexes are in the vestibular and reticular nuclei present in the medulla oblongata.
Efferents: The descending tracts employed are vestibulospinal and reticulospinal tracts which end on α-motor neurons of the spinal cord.
Reflex response: The labyrinthine reflexes are particularly effective in extensor muscles. The impulses from labyrinthine exert the same effect on all the four limbs.

Depending on the position of the head in relation to the horizontal plane, the reflex response produced is as follows:

- When a quadruped stands on an inclined plane in such a manner that its *head is tilted to the right*, the labyrinth (vestibular apparatus) is stimulated and the tonic labyrinthine reflex is evoked. The reflex causes flexion of the left limbs and extension of the right limbs, thereby lending some amount of postural stability on the inclined plane (Fig. 10.9.22A).
- When the quadruped stands on the inclined plane in such a manner that the *head is tilted backwards*, the tonic labyrinthine reflexes cause reflex flexion of the forelimbs and reflex extension of the hindlimbs (Fig. 10.9.22B).

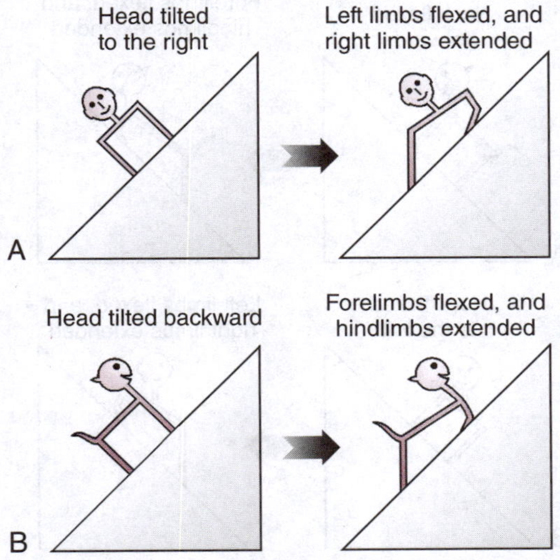

Fig. 10.9.22 Reflex response of tonic labyrinthine reflexes: **A**, when head is tilted to the right; and **B**, when head is tilted backwards.

2. Tonic neck reflexes These reflexes are produced in response to alteration in the position of the head relative to the body.

Stimulus for tonic neck reflexes is stretch of neck muscles.
Receptors of tonic neck reflexes are probably Pacinian corpuscles in the ligaments of the cervical joints, particularly atlanto-occipital joint and also *muscle spindles* of neck muscles.
Centre for these reflexes lies in the medulla oblongata.
Efferent paths are the long corticospinal tracts.
Reflex response obtained depending on the position of the head in relation to the body is as follows:

- *Ventroflexion (turning down) of the head* causes flexion of the forelimbs and extension of the hindlimbs (Fig. 10.9.23A).
- *Dorsiflexion (turning up) of the head* causes extension of the forelimbs and flexion of the hindlimbs.
- *Turning of the head sideways*, i.e. towards right or left, produces flexion of the ipsilateral limbs and extension of contralateral limbs (Fig. 10.9.23B).

Combined response of tonic neck and labyrinthine reflexes Under normal circumstances, when the position of the head is changed, the tonic neck and labyrinthine reflexes are simultaneously evoked such that they produce algebraic sum of separate responses:

On dorsiflexion of the head, labyrinthine impulses produce increased tone in extensors of all the four limbs, whereas impulses from the neck extend forelimbs and flex hindlimbs. Therefore, the actual result observed is extension of forelimbs (as both reflexes tend to increase extensor tone) and little change in hindlimbs (because two reflexes are exerting antagonistic influences).

On ventroflexion of the head, labyrinthine impulses produce increased tone in the flexors of all the four limbs, whereas impulses from the neck flex forelimbs and extend hindlimbs. Therefore, the actual result observed is flexion of the forelimbs (as both reflexes tend to increase flexor tone) and little change in the hindlimbs (because two reflexes are exerting antagonistic influences).

Role of tonic neck and labyrinthine reflexes The tonic neck and labyrinthine reflexes bring about a redistribution of muscle tone in all the limbs and ensure that the body is not thrown off balance even when standing on an inclined plane.

In quadruped animals, tonic neck and labyrinthine reflexes occur when standing on an inclined plane and not while standing on a level plane.
In humans, the tonic labyrinthine reflex is active during the erect posture. This is because in an erect posture, the vestibular apparatus is thrown about 30° backwards. This results in slight flexion of the upper limbs and extension of the lower limbs. When the head is tilted 30° forwards, the tonic labyrinthine reflex ceases but the concomitant flexion of the neck triggers the tonic neck reflex which has the same effect on the limbs. As in quadrupeds, in humans too, the tonic neck and labyrinthine reflexes are observed when the trunk is not upright.

However, similar to other postural reflexes, these reflexes too can be suppressed voluntarily.

b. Long-loop stretch reflexes The long-loop stretch reflexes, also called *functional stretch reflexes*, are polysynaptic reflexes with their reflex arc centred in the cerebral cortex. These reflexes are continuously active in the erect posture and bring about a continuous correction of the sways that occur from moment to moment during standing. The human body behaves like an inverted pendulum hinged at the ankle joint. For example, when the body sways forwards, there occurs stretching of the gastrocnemius muscle. This initiates monosynaptic stretch reflex as well as long-loop polysynaptic reflex which brings about reflex contraction in the gastrocnemius muscle resulting in correction of forward sway. In addition, the visual inputs which suggest that the body is swaying also initiate long-loop postural reflexes.

The two long-loop reflexes (one proprioceptive and the other visual) ensure that the body is not thrown off balance when tipped over its centre of gravity. The importance of these two reflexes can be realized in patients with lesions of the dorsal column such as tabes dorsalis. *Sensory ataxia* seen in such patients is accentuated on closing of the eyes (Romberg sign). The Romberg sign is pathognomonic of sensory ataxia and helps to differentiate it from cerebellar ataxia, in which this sign is absent.

c. Righting reflexes Righting reflexes help to correct the position of the body when it goes off balance and falls down. In other words, righting reflexes help to maintain the head and body in an erect position under all circumstances. For example, if an animal is laid on its side or back, the head at once rights itself, the body follows and the animal finally resumes the upright posture. Decerebrate animal, though, remains in the upright position, and can never actively resume the upright posture as it has no righting reflexes.

The righting reflexes consist of a chain of reactions following one another in an orderly sequence. Each reflex causes the development of the succeeding one as follows:

1. ***Head righting reflex***, also called labyrinthine righting reflex, is initiated when the animal's head is in lateral position. The impulses arising from the saccules reflexly stimulate the appropriate muscles to bring the head back to the upright position.
2. ***Body righting reflexes or body-on-head righting reflex:*** When an animal lies on the ground, the side in contact with the ground is constantly stimulated, whereas the other

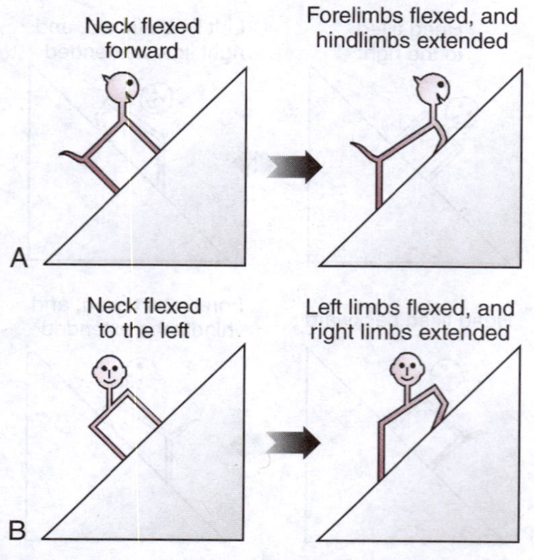

Fig. 10.9.23 Reflex response of tonic neck reflexes: **A**, when neck is flexed forward; and **B**, when neck is flexed to the left.

side is not. This differential stimulation of the deep structures in the body wall reflexly rights the head. The head can thus be righted even after bilateral labyrinthectomy.

3. ***Neck righting reflex or 'neck-on-body' righting reflex:*** As a result of labyrinthine righting reflex and body-on-head righting reflexes, the head is righted but the body remains in the lateral position. This leads to twisting of the neck, which in turn involves a further reaction, the neck righting reflex. This reflex brings the thorax and lumbar region successively into the upright position.
4. ***Body-on-body righting reflex:*** When the body is lying on the ground and the righting of the head is prevented, the differential stimulation of the body surfaces provides the necessary cues for righting the body directly. This is called body-on-body righting reflex.
5. ***Limb righting reflex:*** Impulses arising from the limb muscles are responsible for attainment of appropriate posture of limbs.
6. ***Optical righting reflexes:*** Optical impulses also cause righting of the head. This has been confirmed by the fact that in animals with visual cortex intact, righting of the head can take place with eyes open even after denervation of the labyrinths and neck muscles. In humans, optical righting reflexes are far more important than the labyrinthine righting reflex.

Centres of righting reflexes *Chief centre* for all the righting reflexes, except the optical righting reflexes, is *red nucleus* lying in the midbrain. Red nucleus controls these reflexes through the following tracts:

Rubrospinal tract: It arises from the small number of large nerve cells which form the *nucleus magnocellularis* part of the red nucleus.
Rubroreticular tract: It arises from the large number of small nerve cells forming the *nucleus parvocellularis* part of the red nucleus.
Centre for optical righting reflex lies in the visual cortex, from where impulses ultimately pass to neck muscles to right the head.

B. Statokinetic Reflexes

Statokinetic reflexes are elicited by angular (rotatory) and linear acceleratory (progressive) stimuli to the labyrinthine receptors of the vestibular apparatus.

These are programmed reflexes that depend on the motor cortex. Ultimately, these reflexes are mediated by lateral vestibulospinal tracts. These include those given next.

1. Vestibular placing reaction This reflex is evoked by linear acceleration through stimulation of receptors in the utricle and saccule. This reflex response is an adaptive reaction that prepares the animal for appropriate support by the limbs on surface contact. Thus, as soon as the foot comes in contact with any firm surface, the foot is reflexly placed on the surface and the leg muscles are adjusted so as to support the body.

2. Visual placing reaction The placing response as described above can be initiated by visual cues as well and is then labelled as visual placing reaction. Many postural reflexes mediated by the vestibular system can be stimulated by visual stimuli. Thus, the visual system frequently compensates for lesions of the vestibular apparatus or its central pathways.

3. Hopping reaction Hopping reactions occur in the form of hopping movements that keep the limbs in position to support the body when a standing animal is pushed laterally.

Thus, placing and hopping reactions, like the long-loop stretch reflex, ensure that the body is not thrown off balance when tipped over its centre of gravity.

Summary of postural reflexes The various postural reflexes are summarized in Table 10.9.2.

ROLE OF DIFFERENT REGIONS OF NERVOUS SYSTEM IN MAINTENANCE OF POSTURE

The role of different regions of the nervous system in the maintenance of posture can be experimentally investigated (usually in a cat) by producing transection in the neuraxis at various levels.

Role of Spinal Cord (Spinal Animal)

The role of the spinal cord in the maintenance of posture can be studied in a spinal animal.

The spinal animal can be produced by a transection in the spinal cord at the cervical region and respiration is maintained artificially by the respiratory pump. In this way, most of the cord functions can be studied in a spinal animal. If spinal cord is transected below the origin of the phrenic nerve in the midthoracic region, then diaphragmatic respiration continues and so the artificial respiration is not required.

Effects of spinal cord transection: As described earlier, the effects produced by complete spinal cord transection occur in three stages:

- *Stage of spinal shock*
- *Stage of reflex activity*
- *Stage of reflex failure*

For details, see page 893.

Posture in Spinal Animal During Stage of Reflex Activity

Except the basic stretch reflex and supporting reflexes which are integrated in the spinal cord (Table 10.9.2), all other postural reflexes are absent, as they require the integrity of upper motor neurons coming from various levels of neuraxis.

Postural characteristics of a spinal animal thus are as follows:

Stretch reflex (page 1022) and ***supporting reaction*** (page 1032), though present, are very weak and cannot support the weight of the animal. Therefore, the animal cannot stand on its legs.
Muscle tone returns first in flexor muscles; therefore, flexors become less hypotonic than extensors producing
Paraplegia in flexion (both lower limbs are in state of flexion).

Role of Brainstem: Bulbospinal Animal or Decerebrate Animal

Decerebrate Animal

The decerebrate animal is one in whom the brainstem is transected at the intercollicular level (between superior and inferior colliculi).

Table 10.9.2 Various postural reflexes

Reflex	Stimulus	Response	Receptors	Integrating centre in CNS
A. Static reflexes				
I. Local static reflexes				
i. Stretch reflex	Stretch	Contraction of antigravity muscles	Muscle spindles	Spinal cord and midbrain
ii. Positive supporting reflex	Contact of skin of the sole of foot with ground	Contraction of flexors and extensors of the limb	Touch and pressure receptors from skin of sole of foot; proprioceptors from distal flexors	Spinal cord
iii. Negative supporting reaction	Stretch of extensor muscles	Disappearance of positive supporting reaction	Proprioceptors in extensors	Spinal cord
II. Segmental static reflexes				
Crossed extensor reflex	Painful stimulus	Contraction of flexors of the ipsilateral limb and extensors of contralateral limb to support the body	Nociceptors	Spinal cord
III. General static reflexes				
1. Attitudinal reflexes				
i) Tonic labyrinthine reflex	Gravity (alteration of position of head relative to horizontal plane)	Extensor rigidity	Otolith organs	Vestibular and reticular nuclei present in the medulla oblongata
ii) Tonic neck reflex	Stretch of neck muscles due to alteration of position of head relative to body	Flexion of forelimbs and extension of hindlimbs on ventroflexion of head (turning down); extension of forelimbs and flexion of hindlimbs on upward turning of head; flexion of ipsilateral limbs and extension of contralateral limbs on turning the head sideways	Pacinian corpuscles in the ligaments of cervical joint (atlanto-occipital joint), and muscle spindles of neck muscles	Medulla
2. Long-loop stretch reflex	Stretch of the muscle due to swaying of body	Continuous moment-to-moment corrections of sways which occur during standing	Muscle spindles (monosynaptic reflex) Visual receptor (long-loop reflex)	Spinal cord Cerebral cortex
3. Righting reflexes				
i) Labyrinthine righting reflex	Gravity	Brings the head in upright level	Otolith organs in saccules of labyrinth	Midbrain
ii) Body righting reflex (body-on-head righting reflex)	Pressure on side of body (differential stimulation of deep structures of the body wall)	Righting of head	Exteroceptors	Midbrain
iii) Neck righting reflex (neck-on-body righting)	Stretch of neck muscles	Righting of thorax and shoulders and then pelvis	Muscle spindles	Midbrain
iv) Body on body righting reflex	Pressure on side of the body	Righting of body even when righting of head is prevented	Exteroceptors	Midbrain
v) Limb righting reflex	Stretch of limb muscles	Appropriate posture of limbs	Muscle spindles	Midbrain
vi) Optical righting reflex	Visual cues	Righting of head	Eyes	Cerebral cortex
B. Statokinetic reflexes				
i) Vestibular placing reaction	Linear acceleration	Foot placed on supporting surface in position to support body	Receptors in utricle and saccule	Cerebral cortex
ii) Visual placing reaction	Visual cues	Foot placed on supporting surface	Eyes	Cerebral cortex
iii) Hopping reactions	Lateral displacement while standing	Hops, maintains the limb in position to support the body	Muscle spindle	Cerebral cortex

Characteristic features Characteristic features of a decerebrate animal are as follows:

1. ***Decerebrate rigidity***, i.e. spasticity in all the antigravity muscles occurs immediately after decerebration. This will be discussed later.
2. ***No spinal shock:*** Spinal shock does not develop with lesion at this level or any other higher level.
3. ***Postural reflexes present in a decerebrate animal*** are those which have their integration centre in the spinal cord or medulla or pons. These include:
   - *Stretch reflexes:* These are strongly positive. Decerebrate rigidity is basically due to harmoniously operating group of stretch reflexes.
   - *Positive supporting reaction:* This can be elicited by application of pressure on the pads of fingers or toes. The afferent impulses from the skin and interossei muscles (which are stretched) cause reflex contraction of both extensors and flexors of the limb, converting the limb into a rigid pillar. All the joints are locked. Limbs support the weight of the body and the degree of tone is adequate to maintain the upright posture, but is not sufficient to take up upright position.
   - *Negative supporting reaction:* This can be elicited by passive plantar flexion which releases the limbs from positive reaction.
   - *Crossed extensor reflex:* This can also be demonstrated, i.e. when one forelimb is flexed, the other forelimb is adjusted (page 1028).
   - *Tonic neck and tonic labyrinthine* reflexes are also present (for details, see page 1033). Therefore, in decerebrate animals, posture of limbs and trunk can be adjusted accordingly with the help of these reflexes.
4. ***Righting reflexes are absent***; therefore, a decerebrate animal can stand on its four legs but slight displacement causes the decerebrate animal to topple over.

Decerebrate Rigidity

Decerebrate rigidity refers to marked increase in the tone (hypertonia) of extensors, i.e. antigravity muscles occurring immediately after decerebration of the animal.

Characteristic features of decerebrate rigidity Characteristic features of decerebrate rigidity (Fig. 10.9.24) are as follows:

- Hyperextension of all the four limbs is present.
- Dorsiflexion (hyperextension) of the tail and head is present.
- Extreme hyperextension of the spine (opisthotonus) produces concave configuration of the back.
- The animal can be made to stand on four limbs but is easily toppled by a slight push.
- Postural reflexes, which can be elicited in decerebrate rigidity, are described above.

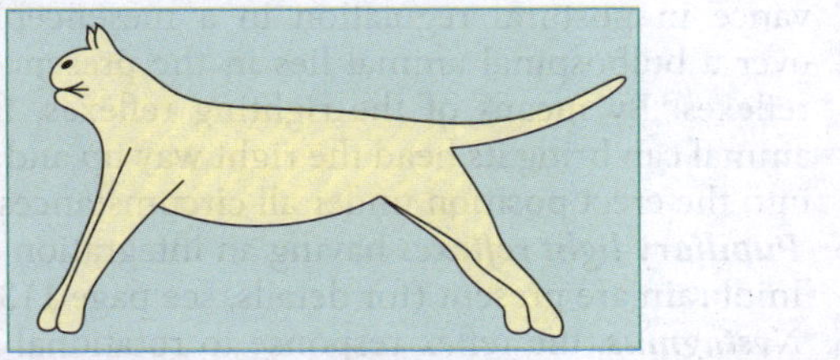

Fig. 10.9.24 Characteristic features of decerebrate rigidity in cat.

Mechanism of decerebrate rigidity Depending on the mode of production, the decerebrate rigidity is of two types:

- Classical decerebrate rigidity
- Ischaemic decerebrate rigidity

Mechanism of classical decerebrate rigidity Classical decerebrate rigidity refers to the decerebrate rigidity that occurs following transection of the brainstem at the intercollicular level. It is produced by exaggerated stretch reflex due to increased activity of γ-motor neurons as explained:

- As mentioned earlier (page 1031), the γ-motor drive to muscles is maintained by descending impulses from FRF as well as IRF with the former predominating.
- IRF or bulboreticular inhibitory arc has no intrinsic activity but is kept activated by descending supraspinal fibres mostly from the basal ganglia, cerebral cortex and cerebellum.
- FRF or bulboreticular facilitatory area, in contrast, gets facilitatory inputs mainly from the ascending sensory stimuli which relay through ascending reticular formation. It also receives facilitatory corticobulbar extrapyramidal projections.
- Transection at the midcollicular level cuts off all facilitatory and inhibitory corticobulbar extrapyramidal pathways. Hence, following decerebration, the IRF, having no intrinsic activity, becomes less active since none of it is driven by the cerebellum only. In contrast, FRF, which is mainly derived by ascending sensory stimuli, remains strongly active.
- Thus, the resulting release of spinal γ-motor neurons from the descending IRF and continued effect of FRF markedly increases muscle spindle sensitivity to stretch resulting in rigidity of muscles (Fig. 10.9.25).
- This rigidity is lost by deafferentation (cutting of afferents from muscle). This proves that decerebrate rigidity is due to increased activity of γ-motor neurons causing exaggerated stretch reflex.
- The rigidity observed after classical decerebration is actually a form of spasticity. When a spastic muscle is stretched passively, initially great resistance is offered by the muscles. However, if still more force is used, the resistance suddenly disappears. This type of response is called *clasp-knife* effect. The initial intense resistance is due to the exaggerated stretch reflex and the sudden decrease in resistance is due to activation of the Golgi tendon reflex.
- In humans, similar spasticity is observed in the extensors of the lower limb and flexors of the upper limb in patients with hemiplegia due to vascular lesions in the internal capsule leading to destruction of pyramidal and extrapyramidal tracts.

Mechanism of ischaemic decerebrate rigidity Ischaemic decerebration is obtained by ligating the common carotid artery and basilar arteries in which the cerebral cortex is rendered ischaemic and nonfunctional. This safer alternative method of decerebration was attempted as classical decerebration was frequently associated with the death of the experimental animal.

- The rigidity observed after ischaemic decerebration is different from that observed in classical decerebration and occurs due to an entirely different reason. The ischaemic decerebrate rigidity is in fact due to disinhibition of α-motor neurons, i.e. exaggerated α-motor neuron discharge. The increased α-motor neuron drive results in direct stimuation of extrafusal fibres (*α-rigidity*).

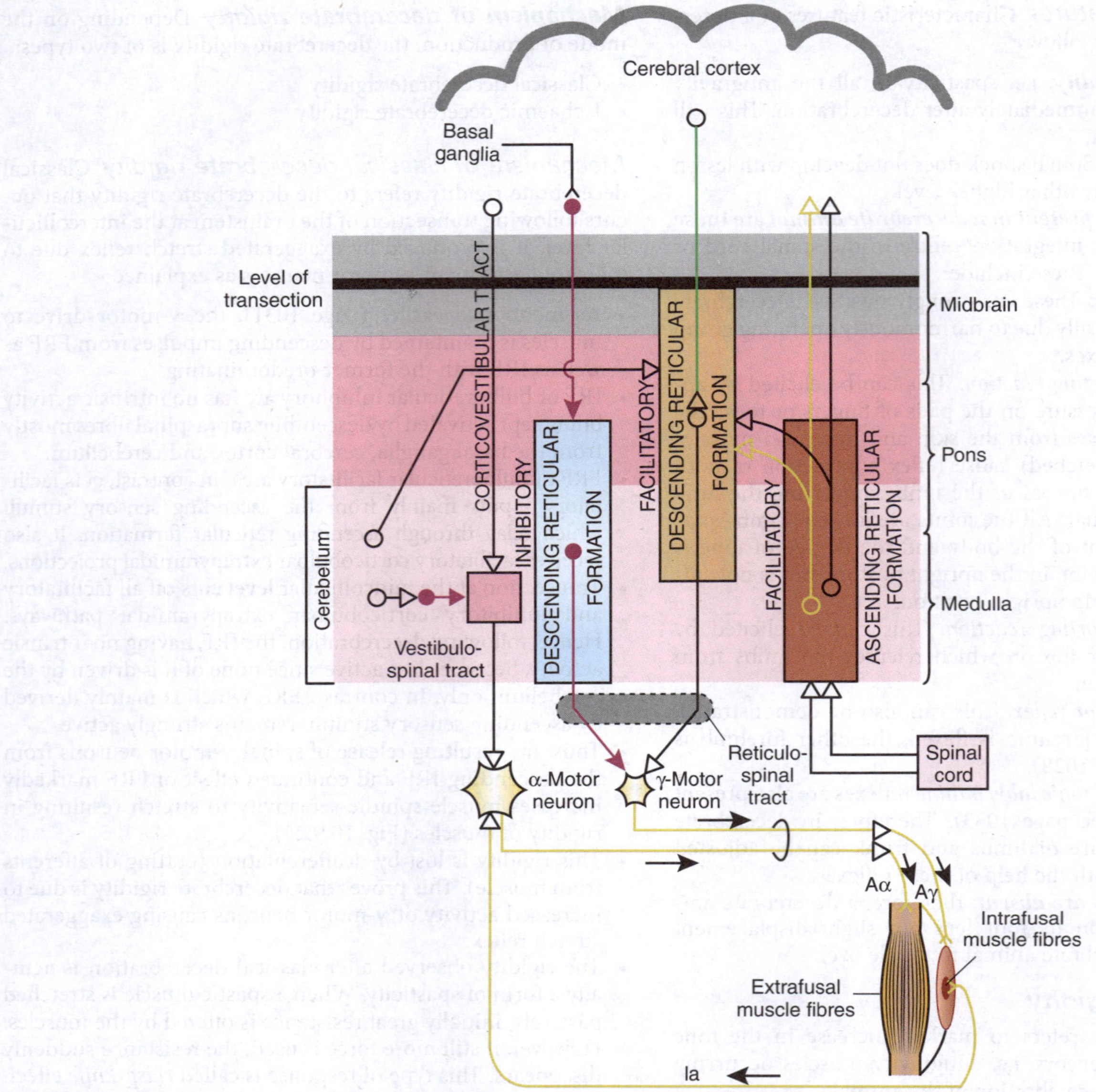

Fig. 10.9.25 Supraspinal control of stretch reflex. Note the pathway cut in the transaction at midcollicular level producing decerebrate rigidity.

- This rigidity is not lost by deafferentation (cutting off afferents from muscles). This proves that ischaemic decerebrate rigidity is not due to increased γ-motor neuron activity but is due to increased α-motor neuron activity.

Classical versus ischaemic decerebrate rigidity. Differences between classical and ischaemic decerebrate rigidity are summarized in Table 10.9.3.

Role of Midbrain: Mesencephalic Animal or High Decerebrate Animal

Mesencephalic or high decerebrate animal is one in whom the brainstem is transected at the rostral border of the midbrain.

Characteristic features of a mesencephalic animal are as follows:

1. ***Decerebrate rigidity***, similar to that of a bulbospinal animal, is present but it disappears when the limb is performing a reflex activity.
2. ***No spinal shock*** is present, similar to a bulbospinal animal.
3. ***Not only can the animal stand***, but also typical quadrupedal walking movements can be reflexly performed.
4. ***Righting reflexes*** having integration centre in the midbrain are present. These include:
   - Labyrinthine righting reflex
   - Neck righting reflex
   - Body-on-head righting reflex
   - Body-on-body righting reflex

   For details of these reflexes, see page 1034. The chief advance in postural regulation in a mesencephalic animal over a bulbospinal animal lies in the presence of righting reflexes. By means of the righting reflexes, the midbrain animal can bring its head the right way up and get the body into the erect position under all circumstances.
5. ***Pupillary light reflexes*** having an integration centre in the midbrain are present (for details, see page 1132).
6. ***Nystagmus***, the reflex response to rotational acceleration, can be elicited (see page 1044).

Table 10.9.3 Differences between classical and ischaemic decerebrate rigidity

Classical decerebrate rigidity	Ischaemic decerebrate rigidity
1. *Produced by* transection of brainstem between superior and inferior colliculi	Ligating both the common carotid arteries and the basilar artery at the junction of pons and medulla
2. *Rigidity observed* is type of spasticity which exhibits clasp-knife effect	Rigidity produced is due to marked muscle tone which does not exhibit clasp-knife effect
3. *Rigidity is mainly due to* increased activity of γ-motor neurons, hence also called γ-rigidity	Increased α-motor neuron activity, hence also called α-rigidity
4. *Deafferentation, i.e. cutting off posterior nerve root,* abolishes rigidity, proving that it is reflex in origin	Does not abolish rigidity, indicating that hypertonia is induced directly and not reflexly
5. *Local injection of procaine into nerve trunk* reduces spasticity	Does not reduce rigidity
6. *Systemic administration of chlorpromazine* reduces spasticity	Has no effect on rigidity
7. Removal of anterior lobe of cerebellum increases rigidity	Has no effect

Role of Cerebellum

Spinocerebellum regulates the postural reflexes by modifying muscle tone. It facilitates the γ-motor neurons in the spinal cord via cerebello-vestibulo-spinal and cerebello-reticulo-spinal tracts. The γ-motor neurons reflexly modify the activity of α-motor neurons and thus regulate the muscle tone. Thus, the cerebellum forms an important site of linkage of α–γ systems responsible for muscle tone (for details, see page 910).

Applied Aspects

Unilateral cerebellar disease in humans causes:

1. ***Atonia or hypotonia*** occurs in the skeletal muscles of the same side.
2. ***Attitude changes*** include:
   - Rotation of the face towards the opposite side
   - Lowering of the shoulder on the affected side
   - Outward rotation and abduction of the leg on the involved side
   - Trunk bent with concavity towards the affected side (this is because the weight of the body is thrown on the unaffected leg)
3. ***Deviation movement:*** Arm held straight out in front of the body deviates laterally when the eyes are closed.
4. ***Deep or tendon reflexes*** become weak and pendular.

Role of Basal Ganglia: Decorticate Animal

Decorticate animal is one in whom the whole cerebral cortex is removed but the basal ganglia and brainstem are left intact.

Postural characteristics of a decorticate animal are as follows:

Moderate rigidity is present due to loss of the cortical area that inhibits spinal γ-motor neuron discharge via reticular formation. It is seen only when the animal is at rest. It commonly occurs on the hemiplegic side after haemorrhage or thrombosis in the internal capsule.

Decorticate animal does not have such intense hypertonia as a decerebrate preparation. This is because the basal ganglia that are intact in a decorticate animal activate the descending IRF and thereby prevent hypertonia.

Typical posture in a decorticate human consists of full extension of legs, arms lying across the chest, with semiflexion at the elbow, slight pronation of the forearm and flexion of the wrist and fingers (Fig. 10.9.26).

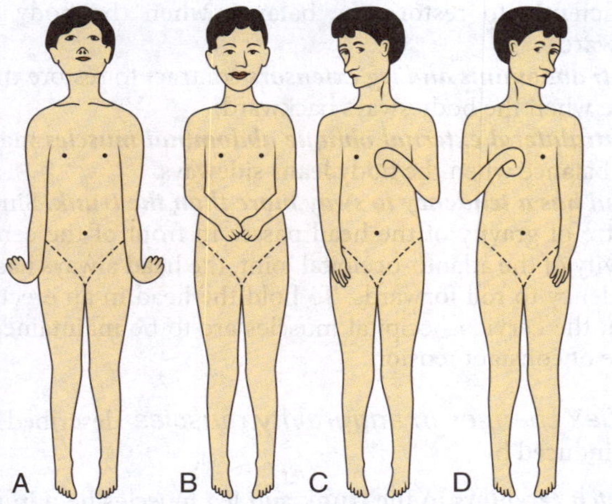

Fig. 10.9.26 Decerebrate (**A**) and decorticate (**B–D**) rigidity in humans.

Postural reflexes: In a decorticate human or animal, the following reflexes can be elicited:

- Typical neck reflexes (page 1034)
- Righting reflexes (page 1034)
- Postural reflexes which are seriously disrupted by decortication are as follows:
  - Hopping reactions
  - Placing reactions

Important Note

It is easier to maintain a decorticate animal than a midbrain animal because temperature regulation and integration of visceral homeostatic mechanism are present in the hypothalamus.

MECHANISM OF STANDING IN HUMANS

As mentioned earlier, a tall human has to stand over a narrow base of feet; therefore, maintenance of an erect posture is more difficult than in the quadruped animals. Mechanisms that play an important role in erect standing posture are given next.

Reflex adjustment in muscle tone of antigravity muscles undoubtedly plays the most important role in making the humans stand erect. From this statement, it may be presumed that a continued contraction of most of the trunk and leg muscles keeps the posture upright. However, electromyographic studies have revealed very little muscle activity in a person standing quietly in upright position.

Configuration of hip and knee joints is such that they are kept extended by the gravity itself. However, a little activity of the antigravity muscles is required to maintain the very precarious balance. This explains the little muscle activity revealed by electromyographic studies.

The effect of gravity has to be opposed by reflex contraction of some of the antigravity muscles all the time; otherwise, a standing human may fall in any direction (forwards, backwards or sideways). The different antigravity muscles which oppose the fall under various circumstances are as follows:

Extensors of the trunk and flexors of the legs contract sufficiently to restore the balance when the body sways forward.
Recti abdominis and leg extensors contract to restore the balance when the body sways backward.
Contralateral external oblique abdominal muscles maintain the balance when the body leans sideways.
Head has a tendency to sway more than the trunk. Since the centre of gravity of the head passes in front of the centre of gravity of the atlanto-occipital joint, the head always has got a tendency to roll forwards. To hold the head in an erect position, the cervico-occipital muscles are to be maintained in a state of constant tension.

Reflex changes in antigravity muscles described above are induced by:

Stretch receptors in the trunk and leg muscles help in maintaining the erect position of the head.
Visual afferents also play an important role in reflex maintenance of upright posture in humans. This is why, when the eyes are closed, the upright posture is less steady and there occurs more swaying (bending) of the trunk.
Vestibular afferents help in maintaining the erect position of the head.

VESTIBULAR APPARATUS AND EQUILIBRIUM

FUNCTIONAL ANATOMY

The internal ear or labyrinth is situated in the petrous part of the temporal bone. It consists of bony labyrinth and membranous labyrinth (Fig. 10.9.27).

Bony labyrinth consists of three parts – vestibule, semicircular canals and cochlea.
Membranous labyrinth is lodged within the bony labyrinth. It is filled with endolymph, which resembles intracellular fluid, and is surrounded by perilymph, which resembles extracellular fluid in its composition. It consists of:

- *Utricle and saccule*, which are lodged in the bony vestibule, and are collectively called *otolith organs*
- *Three semicircular ducts*, which lie within the body of semicircular canals
- *Duct of the cochlea*, which lies within the bony cochlea

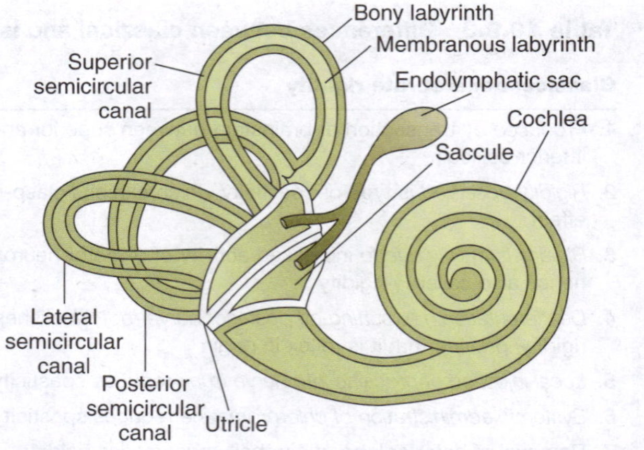

Fig. 10.9.27 Vestibular apparatus: semicircular canals and otolith organs.

Vestibular Apparatus

The semicircular canals, and the utricle and saccule collectively form the vestibular apparatus. The vestibular apparatus plays important role in maintaining posture and equilibrium.

Semicircular canals The three semicircular canals are arranged at right angles to each other, so that all the three planes are represented as (Fig. 10.9.28):

Anterior semicircular canal is vertical and placed at right angles to the long axis of the petrous bone. Thus, it lies in a plane that points forward and outward at about 45° from the sagittal plane.
Posterior semicircular canal is also vertical but is placed parallel to the long axis of the petrous bone. Thus, it lies in a plane that points backward and outward at about 45° from the sagittal plane.
Lateral semicircular canal is set in a horizontal position making an angle of about 30° with the horizontal plane.

> **Important Note**
>
> It is important to note that:
>
> - The right anterior and left posterior canals lie in one plane, whereas the left anterior and right posterior canals lie in the other plane.
> - One end of each semicircular canal is dilated and is called *ampulla*. The ampulla contains the receptor organ known as *crista ampullaris*.
> - The semicircular canals open into the utricle by means of five orifices. The ampullary end of each canal and the narrow end of the horizontal canal open independently, whereas narrow ends of anterior and posterior canals open jointly by a common orifice.

Otolith organ Otolith organ refers to the combined two vestibular sacs called the utricle and saccule.

Utricle is the larger of the two vestibular sacs in which open the three semicircular canals. It is indirectly connected to the saccule and ductus endolymphaticus by the *ductus utriculosaccularis*. The *ductus endolymphaticus*, after being joined by the ductus utriculosaccularis, passes on to end in a small bag-like structure called *endolymphatic sac* (Fig. 10.9.27).
Saccule is a globular sac that is connected to the utricle indirectly through the ductus utriculosaccularis, and cochlea via the *ductus reunion* (Fig. 10.9.27).

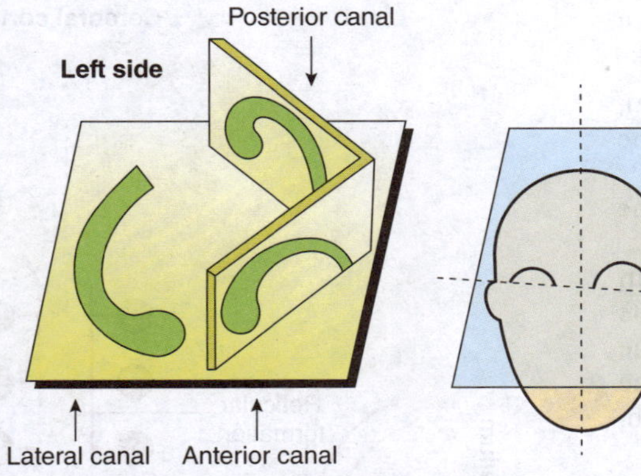

Fig. 10.9.28 Position of semicircular canals when head is tilted forward at 30°.

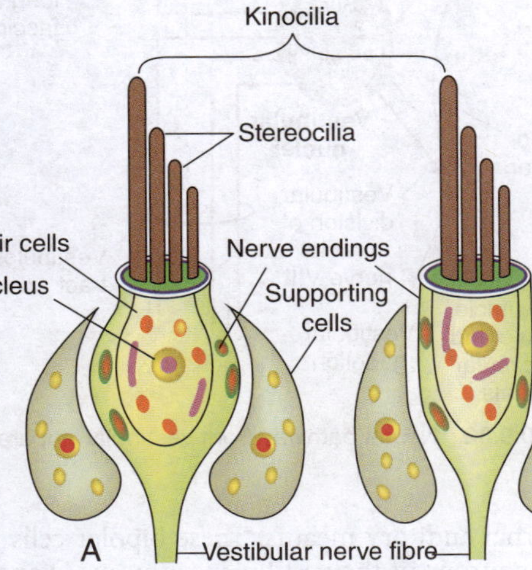

Fig. 10.9.29 Structure of crista ampullaris.

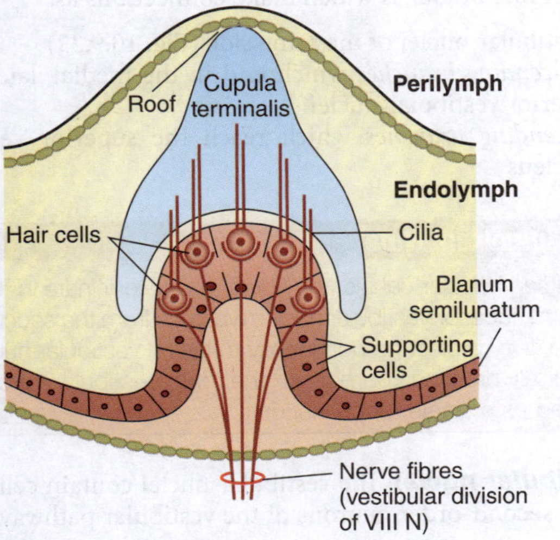

Fig. 10.9.30 Structure of hair cells: **A**, type I; and **B**, type II.

VESTIBULAR RECEPTORS

The receptor cells of the vestibular system are called hair cells, which are slowly adapting mechanoreceptors.

- The hair cells of the semicircular canals are located in a mass of tissue within the ampulla called *crista ampullaris*.

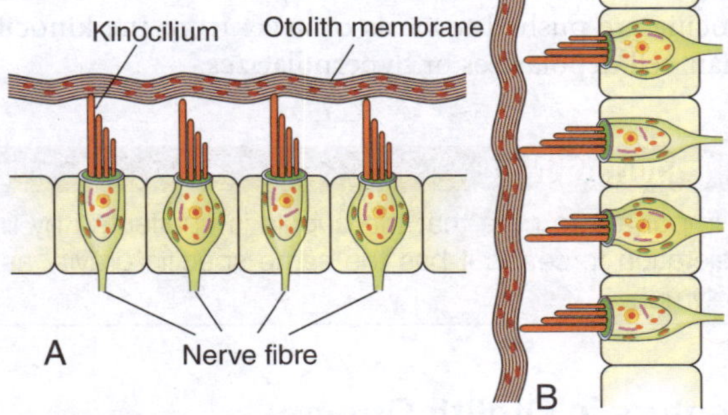

Fig. 10.9.31 Structure of macula of: **A**, utricle (horizontally placed); and **B**, saccule (vertically placed).

- The hair cells of the utricle and saccule are located in a mass of tissue called the *macula*.

Hair cells (Fig. 10.9.31) The vestibular hair cells are of two types:

Type I hair cells are flask shaped. These make synaptic contacts with afferent nerve fibres only (Fig. 10.9.29A).

Type II hair cells are cylindrical in shape and make synaptic contacts with both afferent and efferent nerve fibres (Fig. 10.9.29B).

Cilia of hair cells: The apex of each hair cell has a cuticular plate from which arise about 40–60 cilia. These cilia are called *stereocilia*, which are motile.

A large nonmotile cilium located at one end of the cell is called *kinocilium*.

Activity of hair cells Hair cells are polarized cells. The membrane potential of hair cells is about −60 mV. When the stereocilia are bent towards the kinocilium, the cell depolarizes and membrane potential is decreased to about −50 mV. When the stereocilia are bent away from the kinocilium, the cell hyperpolarizes. The changes in the activity of hair cells are conveyed to the central nervous system by afferent fibres which form the vestibular part of cranial nerve VIII. The mechanoelectrical transduction in vestibular hair cells is same as that occurring in auditory hair cells (see page 1143).

Receptors in Semicircular Canals

The receptors, i.e. the hair cells of the semicircular canals, are located on a raised mass of tissue in the ampulla, called the *crista ampullaris*.

Structure of crista ampullaris The crista ampullaris is a ridge-like area having the following structures (Fig. 10.9.30):

Neuroepithelium is formed by the hair cells (described above), which are innervated by the primary afferent fibres of the vestibular nerve.
Secretory epithelial cells surround the hair cells and form the so-called planum semilunatum around them.
Cupula is a dome-shaped large mass of gelatinous material in which are embedded the cilia arising from the hair cells. At its free end, the cupula is in loose contact with the wall of the ampulla. As a result, it forms a compliant seal that closes the lumen of the canal, preventing free circulation of endolymph.

Stimulation of receptors in semicircular canals The movements produced in the endolymph by the angular movements of the head push the cupula backwards, causing the cilia of hair cells to bend. Depending on whether the stereocilia are pushed towards or away from the kinocilium, the hair cell depolarizes or hyperpolarizes.

Important Note

It is important to note that the cupula is unaffected by linear acceleration force, as it has the same specific gravity as the endolymph.

Receptors in Otolith Organs

The receptors (hair cells) of the otolith organs (utricle and saccule) are located in a raised mass of tissue called macula.

Structure of macula The macula consists of (Fig. 10.9.31):

Neuroepithelium of the macula like that of the crista ampullaris is formed by hair cells (both type I and II).
Supporting cells are present around the hair cells.
Otolith membrane: It is a flat gelatinous membrane covering the hair cells. This contains crystals of calcium carbonate called *otoliths or otoconia* which increase its specific gravity as compared with endolymph. The cilia of hair cells project in the gelatinous membrane.

Stimulation of receptors in otolith organs. The movements produced in the otolith membrane by linear acceleration of the head cause the cilia of hair cells to bend. This leads to excitation of vestibular afferents supplying these cells. *Orientation of the macula* is (Fig. 10.9.31):

Macula of the utricle is directed horizontally so its cilia are in a vertical plane, which are stimulated by horizontally directed linear acceleration, e.g. moving in a car.
Macula of the saccule is directed vertically, so its cilia are in a horizontal plane and are stimulated by vertically directed linear acceleration, e.g. moving in a lift.

VESTIBULAR PATHWAYS

Receptors are the hair cells located in the crista ampullaris of the semicircular canal and maculae of the utricle and saccule.

First-order neurons The afferent fibres carrying impulses from the hair cells are dendrites of the bipolar cells, having their cell bodies in the vestibular or Scarpa's ganglion situated

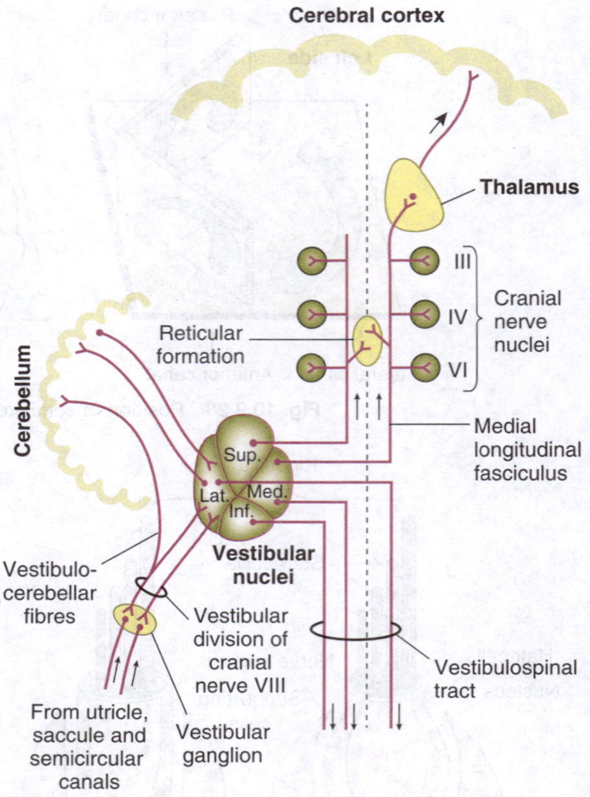

Fig. 10.9.32 Neural pathway from vestibular apparatus.

in the internal auditory meatus. These bipolar cells form the first-order neurons of the vestibular pathway. Axons of these cells form the vestibular division of the vestibulocochlear (VIII) nerve which enters the medulla ventral to the inferior cerebellar peduncle. These axons divide into ascending and descending branches which make connections as:

- Vestibular nuclei of the same side (Fig. 10.9.32)
- *Descending branches* which end in the medial, lateral and inferior vestibular nuclei
- *Ascending branches* which reach the superior vestibular nucleus

Important Note

From semicircular canals, the fibres mainly terminate in the medial and superior vestibular nuclei, whereas from the saccule and utricle, they project predominantly to lateral vestibular nuclei.

For all practical purposes, the four vestibular nuclei are treated as a single functional unit.

Vestibular nuclei The vestibular nuclei contain cell bodies of the second-order neurons of the vestibular pathway.

Afferent connections In addition to the main afferents from the vestibular apparatus, the vestibular nuclei also receive inhibitory fibres from the cerebrum and cerebellum (Fig. 10.9.32).

Efferent connections Efferents from vestibular nuclei are as follows:

Vestibulospinal tracts (anterior and lateral) end directly and also via short interneurons around the ventral horn cells.

The inputs from the vestibular nuclei are *excitatory to antigravity* α-motor neurons.

Vestibulo-ocular tract: These are the fibres which ascend through the *medial longitudinal fasciculus* and terminate in the nuclei of cranial nerves III, IV and VI. These fibres are concerned with movements of eyeballs in relation to the position of the head.

Vestibulocerebellar fibres pass through the inferior cerebellar peduncle and terminate in the flocculonodular lobe and fastigial nuclei in the cerebellum of both sides.

Vestibuloreticular spinal tract: Some fibres from the vestibular nuclei reach the reticular formation of the brainstem, ultimately forming the vestibulo-reticulo-spinal tract.

Vestibulo-rubro-spinal tract: Some fibres from the vestibular nuclei reach the red nucleus forming the vestibulo-rubro-spinal tract.

Vestibulo-thalamo-cortical fibres: Some fibres from the vestibular nuclei pass via the medial lemniscus to the opposite thalamus and thence to the opposite temporal lobe.

MECHANISM OF FUNCTIONING OF VESTIBULAR APPARATUS

A. Mechanism of Functioning of Semicircular Canals

Salient features of functioning of semicircular canals

Salient features of functioning of semicircular canals are as follows:

Receptors of semicircular canals are stimulated by rotatory movements or *angular acceleration* of the head.

Semicircular canals are oriented in three different planes, so movement of the head in any direction generates a unique pattern of activity within the semicircular canals. The three axes of the semicircular canals are those activated while:

- Nodding the head up and down (as in signifying yes). This movement occurs along the transverse axis.
- Shaking the head from side to side (as in signifying no). This movement occurs along the vertical axis.
- Tilting the head so that the ear touches the shoulders. This movement occurs along the anteroposterior axis.

Receptors of horizontal canals are stimulated during rotation of the head in the vertical axis, whereas receptors of vertical canals are stimulated during rotation of the head in the anteroposterior or transverse axis. However, the mechanism of stimulation of receptors is same in all the canals.

Receptors of semicircular canals are stimulated only at the beginning and at the stoppage of rotatory movements. During continued rotation at a constant speed, these receptors are not stimulated; rather, they are adapted as explained.

Mechanism of stimulation and adaptation of receptors of semicircular canals Mechanism of stimulation and adaptation of receptors of semicircular canals is explained in the subsequent text during rotation of the head in the vertical axis.

1. At the beginning of movement of head

Movements to the right (i.e. clockwise rotation along the vertical axis) stimulate the hair cells in the right horizontal canal and inhibit these in the left horizontal canal. As shown in Fig. 10.9.33, when the head begins to move, the horizontal canals move in the clockwise direction but the endolymph within the semicircular canals lags behind because of inertia. This phenomenon causes relative displacement of endolymph in the direction opposite to that of the rotation of the head. That is, the endolymph is pushed in the anticlockwise direction (Fig. 10.9.33B).

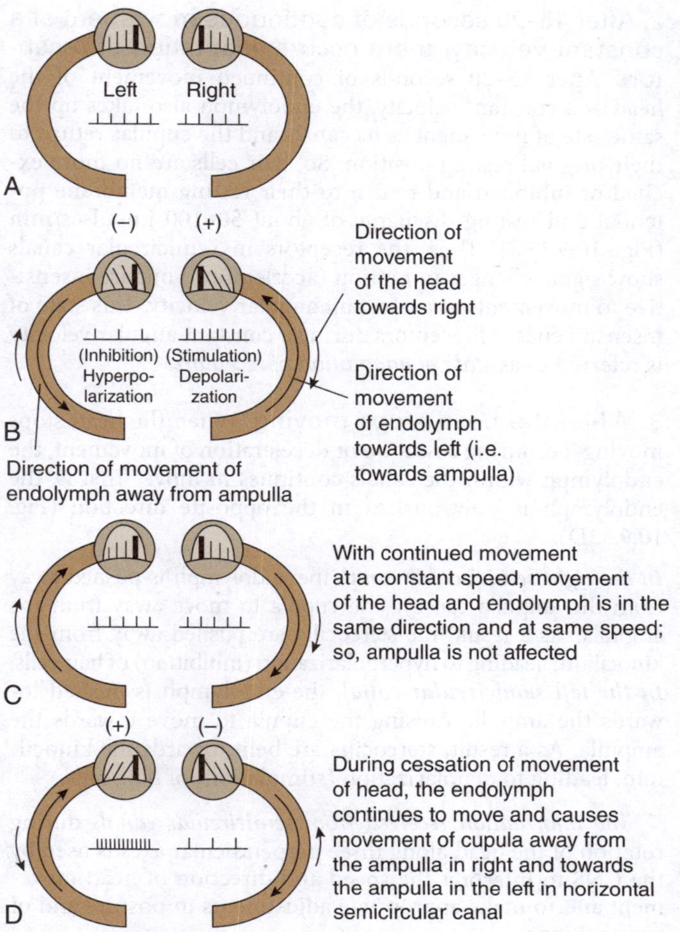

Fig. 10.9.33 Mechanism of stimulation of receptors in horizontal (lateral) semicircular canal during rotation of head towards the right: **A**, resting position; **B**, when head begins to rotate to the right; **C**, after 15–20 seconds of continued movement of head at a constant speed; and **D**, when the head stops moving.

In the right semicircular canal, the endolymph is pushed towards the ampulla causing the cupula to move towards the ampulla. As a result, the stereocilia are pushed towards the kinocilium, leading to depolarization (stimulation) of hair cells.

In the left semicircular canal, the endolymph is pushed away from the ampulla causing the cupula to move away from the ampulla. As a result, the stereocilia are pushed away from the kinocilium, leading to hyperpolarization (inhibition) of hair cells. This combination of excitation of one ampulla and inhibition of the ampulla from the other canal forms the basis of the direction of movement. At the beginning of movement, frequency of discharge from excited hair cells may increase to a frequency of 100–500 impulses/min from a resting discharge of 50–100 impulses/min.

Movements to the left (i.e. counterclockwise movements), on the other hand, stimulate the hair cells in the left horizontal semicircular canal and inhibit those in the right horizontal canal by the same mechanism as explained above.

2. After 15–20 seconds of continuous movement at a constant velocity, there occurs adaptation of receptors After 15–20 seconds of continued movement of the head at a constant velocity, the endolymph also takes up the same rate of movement as its canals and the cupulas return to their original resting position. So, hair cells are no more excited or inhibited and return to their resting membrane potential and resting discharge of about 50–100 impulses/min (Fig. 10.9.33C). Thus, the receptors in semicircular canals show signal changes in motion (acceleration) but are insensitive to movements at a constant angular velocity. This state of insensitiveness of receptors during a constant angular velocity is referred to as *state of adaptation of receptors*.

3. When the head stops moving When the head stops moving, i.e. during cessation or deceleration of movement, the endolymph within the canals continues to move. That is, the endolymph is now pushed in the opposite direction (Fig. 10.9.33D):

In the right semicircular canal, the endolymph is pushed away from the ampulla causing the cupula to move away from the ampulla. As a result, the stereocilia are pushed away from the kinocilium, leading to hyperpolarization (inhibition) of hair cells.
In the left semicircular canal, the endolymph is pushed towards the ampulla causing the cupula to move towards the ampulla. As a result, stereocilia are bent towards the kinocilium, leading to depolarization (stimulation) of hair cells.

The information received from semicircular canals during rotation of the head along three perpendicular axes is used by the CNS to interpret the speed and direction of head movement and to make appropriate adjustments in posture and of eye positions.

B. Mechanism of Functioning of Utricle and Saccule

General features of functioning of the utricle and saccule are as follows:

- These provide information about linear acceleration and change in head position relative to the force of gravity.
- *Receptors* (hair cells) present in the maculae of the utricle and saccule act as stretch receptors, the effective stimulus being the pull of gravity on the otolith membrane. These receptors discharge tonically even in the absence of head movement, because of pull of gravity on the otolith. So, these receptors show little adaptation (of receptors of semicircular canals).
- During linear acceleration of the head, the otolith membrane having more specific gravity lags behind due to inertia. This causes cilia of hair cells embedded in the otolith membrane to bend. This leads to excitation of vestibular afferents supplying these cells.

Functioning of utricle As mentioned earlier, the macula of the utricle is directed horizontally and so its cilia are in the vertical plane (Fig. 10.9.31). These vertically oriented cilia are stimulated by horizontally directed linear acceleration, e.g. moving in a car. These hair cells are also stimulated during dorsiflexion or ventroflexion of the head, i.e. by nodding the head up and down (as in signifying yes).

Functioning of saccule As mentioned earlier, the macula of the saccule is directed vertically and so its cilia are in the horizontal plane (Fig. 10.9.31). These horizontally oriented cilia are stimulated by vertically directed linear acceleration, e.g. moving in a lift up or down. These hair cells are also stimulated when the head is tilted sideways, e.g. if the head is tilted laterally to the right, the otolith membrane of the macula of the right saccule hangs downwards and pulls on its macula which is maximally stimulated, and the otolith membrane of the left saccule points upwards and rests on the macula, this being the position of minimal stimulation of the nerve endings.

Vestibular Reflexes

1. Vestibulo-Ocular Reflex (VOR)

The VOR maintains visual fixation during movements of the head by producing reflex nystagmus and postrotatory nystagmus as described.

Nystagmus For example, when the head is rotated to the left, the eyes move slowly towards the right in order to keep the image on the fovea. When the eyes have rotated as far as they can, they are rapidly returned to the centre of the socket. These reflex movements of the eyes are called nystagmus. Thus, nystagmus has two components of the movements:

Slow components, i.e. slow movement of the eyes to maintain visual fixation is initiated by receptors in the semicircular canals. When the head rotates to the left, receptors in the left horizontal canal are stimulated. Their axons activate reflex movements of the eyes towards the right through the impulses reaching the nuclei of cranial nerves III, IV and VI.
Quick component: When slow movement of the eyeballs is limited, the eyeballs move to a new fixation point in the direction of rotation of the head. This movement to a new fixation point occurs with a jerk. So, it is called the quick component. The quick component of nystagmus is due to impulses from the vestibular nuclei to the ocular muscle.

Postrotatory nystagmus occurs after the body has been rotated and the movement ceases. This is due to movement of the cupula in the opposite direction caused by the endolymph when rotation is stopped. Thus, the postrotatory nystagmus rotates in a direction opposite to the original nystagmus and continues until the cupula returns to its resting position. It can be demonstrated by Barany chair.

Applied Aspects

Nystagmus present in the resting state is a sign of pathology. There are two types of nystagmus:

(i) Congenital nystagmus, which is seen at birth
(ii) Acquired nystagmus, which occurs in later life. It is seen in various clinical conditions like:
- Fracture of the temporal bone affecting semicircular canals
- Damage to the flocculonodular lobe of the cerebellum or to the fastigial nucleus
- Also associated with multiple sclerosis, head injury, brain tumours and during stroke

Treatment: For acquired nystagmus, the best treatment is to treat the underlying cause.

- *Surgery:* Some cases of acquired nystagmus are successfully treated by rectus muscle surgery.
- *Botox:* For short term, nystagmus can be corrected by injection of Botox (botulinum toxin) to paralyse the ocular muscles.

2. Otolith Reflexes

Otolith organs initiate a reflex that prevents leg injuries when an individual walks downstairs or jumps from a platform. When making such a descent, the muscles of the leg begin to contract before the feet reach the ground to cushion the force of impact.

- The otolith receptors responsible for this reflex are stimulated by the linear acceleration of the head that occurs during descent.
- Individuals lacking otolith reflexes are prone to leg injuries because of the large contact force that occurs during descent (e.g. stepping off a bus).

FUNCTIONS OF VESTIBULAR APPARATUS

1. Role in maintenance of equilibrium The otolith organs detect change in position of the head and help in maintenance of equilibrium under static condition.

- The otolith organs also detect linear acceleration of the head and help in maintenance of equilibrium during such movements.
- Semicircular canals detect angular acceleration and help in maintaining equilibrium during dynamic phase. They also have a predictive function.
- When the person is in dynamic state, they predict ahead of time that the person is likely to fall off balance and help the nervous system to do adjustments to prevent a fall.

2. Role in maintenance of posture The vestibular apparatus plays an important role in maintenance of posture through vestibular reflexes, which include:

- Vestibular placing reaction
- Righting reflexes
- VOR
- Vestibulo-otolith reflex

MAINTENANCE OF EQUILIBRIUM

Equilibrium refers to maintenance of line of gravity constant at rest and during movement by adjusting the tone of different muscles, whereas the term posture signifies an unconscious adjustment of tone of different muscles so as to maintain balance during rest as well as during movements.

Role of Various Parts of Neural System in Maintaining Equilibrium

1. Role of vestibular apparatus Role of the vestibular apparatus is as described above.

2. Role of cerebellum Role of the cerebellum is as follows:

Uvula of the cerebellum gets impulses from the macula of the utricle and saccule and helps in maintaining equilibrium under static conditions.

Flocculonodular lobe of the cerebellum gets impulses from the semicircular canals and helps in maintaining equilibrium during rapid changes in direction of motion.

3. Role of brainstem Main role is played by four pairs of vestibular nuclei present in the brainstem:

Superior vestibular nuclei receive signals from semicircular canals and send impulses to:

- *Medial longitudinal fasciculus* to cause corrective movements of eyes
- *Medial vestibular tract* to cause appropriate movements of the neck and head

Medial vestibular nuclei receive signals from semicircular canals and send signals to:

- *Medial longitudinal fasciculus* to cause corrective movements of eyes
- *Vestibulospinal tract* to cause appropriate movements of the head and neck

Lateral vestibular nuclei receive signals from otolith organs and in turn send signals through the lateral vestibulospinal tract to the spinal cord for controlling body movements.

Inferior vestibular nuclei receive signals from semicircular canals and utricle and in turn send signals to:

- Cerebellum
- Reticular formation of the brainstem

4. Role of other factors in maintenance of equilibrium *Neck proprioceptors* transmit information about orientation of the head with respect to the body to vestibular and reticular nuclei of the brainstem and cerebellum.

Neck reflexes must function opposite to vestibular reflexes to maintain equilibrium of the entire body. When the vestibular apparatus is destroyed, the bending of the head produces muscular reflexes (called neck reflexes) in the forelimbs.

Body exteroceptors and proprioceptors transmit information from other parts of the body besides the neck and play an important role in maintenance of equilibrium, for example, pressure from the foot pad informing whether weight is more forward or backward on the feet. This information is useful for maintenance of equilibrium.

Visual receptors also play an important role in maintenance of equilibrium. It has been noted that after complete destruction of the vestibular apparatus and loss of proprioceptive information, a person can still use the visual mechanism effectively to maintain balance. But in such cases, if the eyes are closed or the person is moving rapidly, balance is lost.

Applied Aspects

The important applied aspects in relation to the vestibular apparatus which need special emphasis are as follows:

- Vestibular dysfunctions
- Experimental stimulation of the semicircular canal

A. Vestibular Dysfunctions

1. Motion Sickness

Motion sickness is a symptom complex occurring due to excessive and repeated stimulation of the vestibular apparatus while travelling in an automobile, ship, aircraft or spacecraft. The psychological factors, like anxiety about the unfamiliar mode of travel, may be additional factors in causation of motion sickness.

The disease occurring during travelling by a ship is referred to as *sea sickness*.

Characteristic features of motion sickness are as follows:

- Unpleasant sensation of rotation accompanied by nausea, vomiting, sweating, pallor, salivation, headache, disorientation and even diarrhoea. Most of the symptoms and signs are the effects of vestibular stimulation on the medullary autonomic centres.

Prevention: Motion sickness can be prevented by taking antiemetic drugs such as *Avomine* and by avoiding greasy and bulky food before travelling.

- Space motion sickness is usually experienced by the astronauts when they are first exposed to microgravity environment. The symptoms of nausea, vomiting and dizziness experienced usually wear off after a few days, and may occur in reentry into the gravity force. These symptoms occur due to mismatched neural signal inputs by the vestibular apparatus and other gravity sensors.

2. Benign Paroxysmal Positional Vertigo (BPPV)

It is an important common vestibular disorder that is characterized by episodes of vertigo associated with turning of the head in a particular position. This occurs due to separation of otoconia from the otolith membrane, which get lodged into the cupula or semicircular canal.

Treatment: Usually symptoms of BPPV disappear after a few weeks. Canalith repositioning or Epley manoeuvre (a simple slow manoeuvre) is advised to maintain position of the head so that otoconia move from the semicircular canal back into the vestibule (utricle).

3. Ménière Disease

Ménière disease is also called endolymphatic hydrops.

Causes: It is caused by overdistension of the membranous labyrinth, probably due to oversecretion. Other causes include:

- Ischaemia and vasospasm causing decreased blood supply to the labyrinth
- Emotional factors, i.e. sympathetic overactivity

Characteristic features: Ménière disease originates in the labyrinth and typically presents as a triad consisting of:

- Fluctuating deafness (hearing loss) of sensorineural (SN) type
- Tinnitus which may be very troublesome
- Episodic attacks of rotatory vertigo

The disease is usually unilateral to start with and the common age of onset is 35–50 years and comes in attacks. The patient usually has nausea, vomiting and fullness of the ear in addition to the above-listed triad.

Diagnosis: Electrocochleography (ECOG) is gold standard for diagnosis of Ménière disease.

Treatment: The symptoms of Ménière disease can be controlled by reducing fluid retention by dietary changes like low-salt/salt-free diet.

Medical treatment includes:

- Vestibular suppressants such as meclizine (antihistaminic drug; it acts by decreasing excitability of the labyrinth, and also blocks conduction in the middle ear–vestibular–cerebellar pathway)
- Diuretics
- Chemical labyrinthectomy by injecting gentamicin

Surgical treatment includes:

Endolymphatic sac compression

Sacculotomy (i.e. through the footplate of the stapes, the saccule is punctured with a needle)

Lermoyez syndrome is a variant of Ménière disease. There is sensorineural hearing loss (SNHL) and tinnitus followed by attacks of vertigo, i.e. reversal of Ménière triad.

- In patients with frequent attacks, the implantation of a small tube or shunt into the abnormally swollen endolymphatic sac is done.

4. Labyrinthectomy: Bilateral and Unilateral

Bilateral labyrinthectomy, i.e. removal of the labyrinthine apparatus on both sides, is characterized by:

- *Equilibrium* is maintained by visual sensation. The individual cannot right himself/herself when blindfolded.
- *Postural reflexes* are severely affected.
- *Muscle tone* is decreased but there is no permanent loss.
- *Hearing* loss is also present.

Unilateral labyrinthectomy, i.e. removal of the labyrinthine apparatus on one side, is characterized by the following immediate and permanent effects:

- ***Immediate effects*** occurring due to unopposed action of an intact labyrinth are as follows:
  - *Oblique deviation of the eyeballs*, i.e. one eyeball is rolled upwards and outwards and the other downwards and inwards
  - *Nystagmus*
  - *Rotation and lateral flexion of the head*, so that the occiput is turned to the side of lesion
  - *Flexion of limbs* on the side of lesion and extension of limbs on the opposite side
- ***Permanent effects*** are as follows:
  - Nystagmus occurs.
  - Reciprocal changes in the tone and head rotation persist.
  - Rotation of the trunk decreases.

B. Experimental Stimulation of Semicircular Canals

The semicircular canals can be stimulated by two methods:

- Rotational movement by Barany chair
- Caloric stimulation

1. Stimulation by Rotational Movement Using Barany Chair

Method: The subject is made to sit in the chair with the head tilted forward at 30°. The chair is rotated at 30 rpm for 20 seconds.

Effects: During rotation with eyes open, *nystagmus* occurs continuously throughout the period of rotation. *After rotation* in Barany chair for 20 seconds at 30 rpm, the following effects are noted:

- *Postrotatory nystagmus* occurs for about 30 seconds.
- *Dizziness*, i.e. feeling of unsteadiness, occurs immediately after stoppage of rotation. It is associated with feeling of rotation in the opposite direction.
- *Vertigo*, i.e. feeling of rotation even after stoppage of rotation, occurs.
- *Nausea and vomiting* may occur after rotation for a longer period.

2. Caloric Stimulation

The semicircular canals can be stimulated by introducing hot (40°C) or cold (30°C) water into the external auditory meatus.

Mechanism: The transmission of change in temperature into the labyrinth alters the specific gravity of the endolymph.

As a result, the cupula is set into motion and the hair cells are stimulated.

Effects: Caloric stimulation produces the same effects as rotational movement, i.e. there occur:

- Vertigo
- Dizziness
- Nystagmus

If cold water is poured into the right ear, the patient develops left jerk nystagmus (rapid phase towards the left), whereas the reverse happens with warm water. It can be remembered by the mnemonic 'COWS' (cold–opposite–warm–same).

Significance Caloric stimulation is used as a clinical test for diagnostic purpose.

While irrigating the ear canal for treatment of ear infections, it must be ensured that fluid used is at the body temperature level; otherwise, the annoying symptom of caloric stimulation will occur.

Self-Assessment

1. Discuss the CNS levels which control the body movements.
2. Discuss the role of stretch reflex in maintenance of muscle tone.
3. Classify the various physiological and pathological reflexes and their significance.
4. Describe briefly the following:
   - Vestibular apparatus and its significance
   - Mechanism of standing in humans
5. Write notes on the following:
   - Decerebrate rigidity
   - Tonic neck reflex
   - Inverse stretch reflex
   - Vestibular function tests
   - Withdrawal reflex response

Clinical Cases

Case 1

A 55-year-old hypertensive patient had stroke and was referred to the emergency department. Examination revealed the following signs:

Patient in a conscious state
Muscles of lower limbs stiff
No muscle wasting
Patient unable to sit/stand
Deep tendon reflexes slow

Q1. What is this condition known as?
Q2. What is the cause for stiffness of muscles?
Q3. What is the state of ventral horn cells in this condition?

Case 2

A 60-year-old hypertensive lady suddenly became unconscious; on recovery, the signs and symptoms noticed are as follows:

The patient is unable to move her right leg.
The superficial reflexes are normal.
Ankle jerk shows clonus.
There is no muscle wasting.

Q1. What is the cause for ankle clonus?
Q2. Which type of ventral horn neurons of the spinal cord is involved?

Case 3

A 66-year-old female presented in the neurology department with the face turned towards the right side, and the shoulder of the left side bending lower as compared with that of the right.

On examination, there was outward rotation of the left leg trunk bent towards the left side. When she was asked to hold the upper limbs straight in front of her body with closed eyes, her arms deviated laterally. The deep tendon reflexes were delayed and weak and pendular.

Q1. In which disease do above-mentioned signs and symptoms develop?
Q2. Which is the site of lesion and of which side?
Q3. Why do the arms move laterally with closed eyes?

Case 4

In a 2-year-old male child, the mother noticed quick eyeball movements for which she consulted the paediatrician and the case was referred to an ophthalmologist. Examination and history revealed that side-to-side movements of both eyes were occurring for the last 1 week and were not controlled. There was no history of trauma during childbirth and afterwards. The child was born by normal vaginal delivery.

Q1. What is this condition called?
Q2. What are components of this condition?
Q3. What are the causes?

Case 5

A 25-year-old female experienced giddiness, nausea, vomiting and severe headache while travelling by road to a hill station.

Q1. What is the diagnosis?
Q2. What is the cause for signs and symptoms?
Q3. How can these signs and symptoms be prevented?

Case 6

A 30-year-old male visited the ENT department with complaints of frequent episodes of vertigo while turning the head to the right side to see the back while starting his bike.

Q1. What is this condition called?
Q2. What is the cause for this phenomenon?
Q3. Which manoeuvre is advised to avoid such symptoms?

Case 7

A 54-year-old male presented in the ENT department with complaints of decrease in hearing ability, ringing sensations in the ears and giddiness especially during rotation movements and a feeling of ear fullness.

Q1. What is the probable diagnosis?
Q2. Which test should be done to confirm the diagnosis?
Q3. What treatment is recommended to treat the symptoms?

10.10 Limbic System and Physiology of Emotional, Behavioural and Motivational Mechanisms

CHAPTER OUTLINE

LIMBIC SYSTEM

PHYSIOLOGICAL ANATOMY

Components of Limbic System

The term limbic has been derived from the word 'limbus' which means a ring. Thus, the term limbic system is applied for those parts of the cortex (limbic cortex or limbic lobe) and subcortical structures that form a ring around the brainstem. Previously, this area was called rhinencephalon because of its relation to olfaction. It is now known to play, apart from olfaction, a role in functions like behavioural activity, emotions, motivational drives, memory and regulation of viscera, and so it is also referred to as 'visceral brain'. Components of the limbic system are as follows (Fig. 10.10.1):

Limbic cortex or the so-called limbic lobe surrounds the subcortical structures of the limbic system. Phylogenetically, limbic cortex is an older part of the cerebral cortex (allocortex) having primitive histological structures, i.e. only three layers (page 938). Rest of the cerebral cortex is greatly developed (neocortex) and in most areas has six layers (page 939).

Limbic cortex is composed of (Figs 10.10.1 and 10.10.2):

- Orbitofrontal cortex
- Subcallosal gyrus
- Cingulate gyrus
- Parahippocampal gyrus
- Uncus

Subcortical structures included in the limbic system are as follows:

- Hypothalamus
- Septum
- Paraolfactory area
- Anterior nuclei of the thalamus
- Amygdala
- Portions of basal ganglia
- Hippocampus

Connections

Bundles of axons connecting the various components of limbic system are as follows (Fig. 10.10.3):

- Fornix (see page 929)
- Mammillothalamic tract (see page 930)
- Stria terminalis (see page 929)
- Stria medullaris thalami
- Medial forebrain bundle (see page 928)

Papez circuit refers to a closed circuit formed by connections between the cingulate gyrus (located in the prefrontal lobe), hippocampus, mammillary bodies and anterior nucleus of the thalamus (Fig. 10.10.4). This circuit is responsible for resting EEG (page 1049) and for those emotions and aspects of behaviour that are related to preservation of the individual and species. ***Efferent projection of the limbic system*** is shown in Fig. 10.10.5.

Characteristic features of limbic system connections are as follows:

Limbic system *has very little connection with the neocortex.* Because of this, emotional and instinctual behaviour is not under

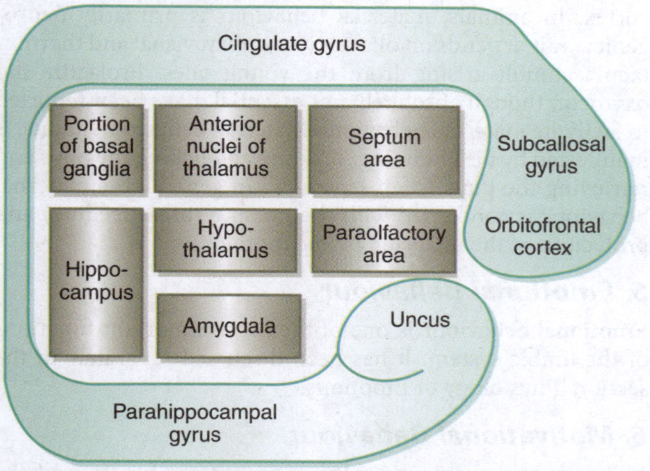

Fig. 10.10.1 Diagrammatic representation of the structures forming limbic system.

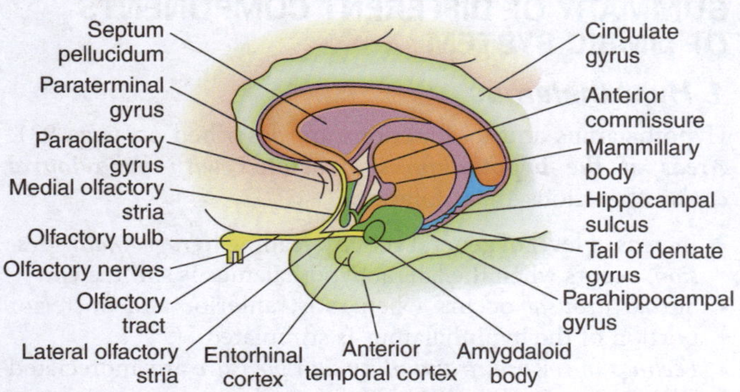

Fig. 10.10.2 Medial surface of right cerebral hemisphere showing limbic cortex (limbic lobe) and other components of limbic system.

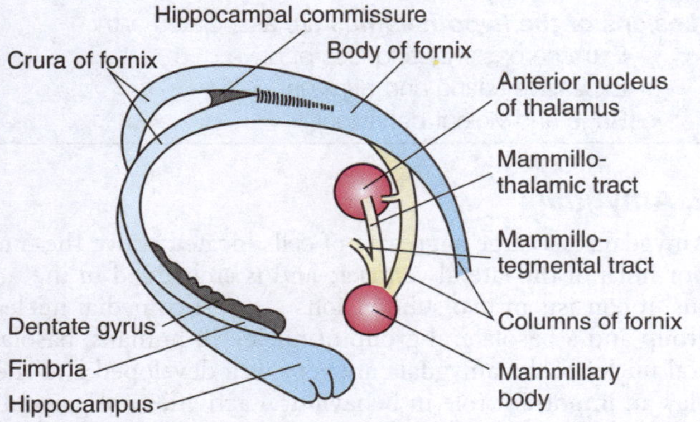

Fig. 10.10.3 The fornix and related pathways of the limbic system.

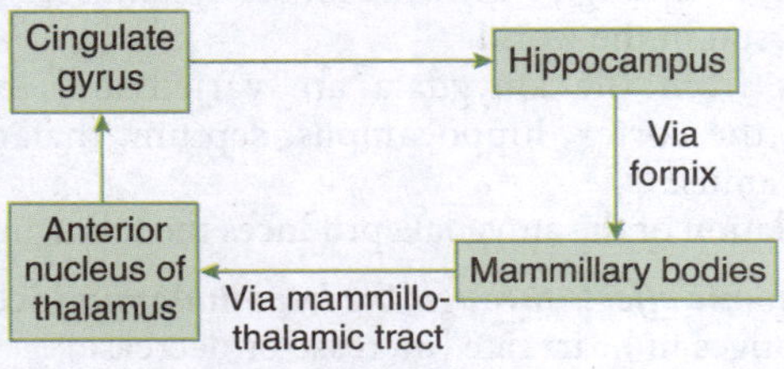

Fig. 10.10.4 The Papez circuit.

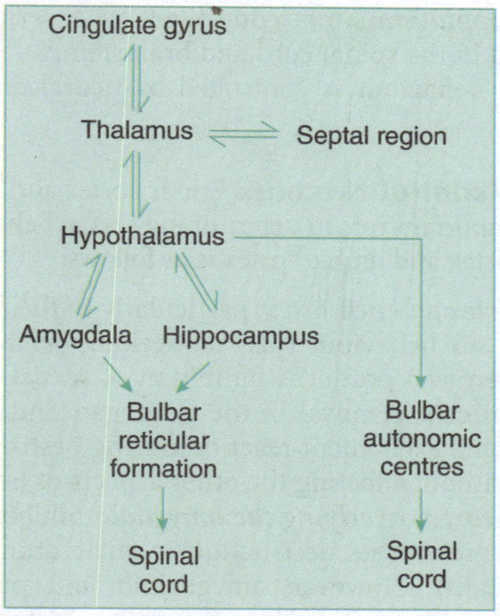

Fig. 10.10.5 Efferent projection of limbic system.

voluntary control, especially in lower animals. Thus, from a functional point of view, neocortical activity does modify emotional behaviour but it cannot be turned on and off at will.

Prolonged afterdischarge is shown by the anatomic closed circuit of the limbic system following a sensory experience. Therefore, the emotional responses are usually prolonged, i.e. continue long after the end of the stimuli that produce them.

FUNCTIONS OF LIMBIC SYSTEM

Most of the functions of the limbic system are intimately related to the functions of the hypothalamus which have been described in Chapter 10.3, page 931. These include those given next.

1. Autonomic Functions

Stimulation of many parts of the limbic system, especially that of the amygdala, produces autonomic responses such as changes in cardiovascular, respiratory and gastrointestinal systems through the hypothalamus. Such changes are also observed during emotional states. Autonomic functions of the hypothalamus are described on page 931.

2. Regulation of Feeding Behaviour

Limbic system regulates feeding behaviour mainly through the hypothalamus and amygdala.

Hypothalamus Hypothalamus regulates food intake through the *feeding centre* and *satiety centre* (for details, see page 932).

Amygdala Stimulation of the amygdala produces movements associated with eating (chewing, swallowing and licking). On the other hand, lesions of the amygdala produce moderate hyperphagia (overeating). There may be indiscriminate ingestion of edible or nonedible materials.

3. Regulation of Sexual Behaviour and Reproduction

The sexual activity comprises two components.

Sexual behaviour The basic sex drive (urge to copulate) is an instinctual behaviour like food intake. It is the function of the limbic system and hypothalamus which in turn are influenced by gonadal hormones and cerebral cortex.

Act of copulation: It is controlled by a series of reflexes integrated in the spinal cord and brainstem.

Sexual behaviour is controlled by neural and endocrinal factors.

i. Neural control Neocortex, limbic cortex and hypothalamus play an important role in determining sexual behaviour. Role of the neocortex and limbic cortex is as follows:

Limbic cortex and neocortex, particularly in the frontal region, stimulate sex behaviour (partner-seeking behaviour). Therefore, its removal produces inhibition of sexual behaviour. In female animals, removal of the neocortex and limbic cortex abolishes the excitement reaction during oestrous cycle (heat period) without affecting the other aspects of heat.

Piriform cortex overlying the amygdala inhibits sex drive in males. Therefore, its destruction in male animals produces hypersexuality. However, amygdaloid and periamygdaloid lesions do not produce hypersexuality in female animals. In human males, also bilateral lesions of this area produce hypersexuality (*Klüver–Bucy syndrome*) (see page 1051).

Role of hypothalamus Anterior hypothalamus and median forebrain bundle stimulation elicits sex behaviour in males as well as in females. A decorticate female animal will have regular oestrous cycle provided the hypothalamus is intact. Lesions of the anterior hypothalamus abolish oestrous cycle in female animals and sexual interest in male animals (for further details, see page 933).

Role of encephalization In humans, sex behaviour is largely encephalized, i.e. the perception that sexual act produces pleasure is a big cause of sex behaviour. Therefore, menopausal women (akin to castrated female animals) continue to have sex behaviour. Furthermore, sex behaviour is strongly influenced, in humans, by social customs, rules and social taboos.

ii. Endocrinal control involves:

Role of gonadal hormones

In males, testosterone stimulates sex drive. Castration (removal of testes) is associated with a marked decrease in sex drive, which can be restored by injection of testosterone. Surprisingly, administration of oestrogen also produces a stimulation of sex drive and sex behaviour.

In female animals, plasma oestrogen levels are raised during oestrous period. In human females, sexual activity persists throughout the menstrual cycle, which is slightly increased during the time of ovulation. Castration in female animals (removal of ovaries) causes decline and eventual abolishment of sex drive.

Role of pheromones Pheromones are chemicals which by their smell act as sex attractants in animals. It has been observed that in monkeys, sexual drive is greater in the male when exposed to a female at the time of ovulation than when exposed to a female at other time of ovarian cycle. Certain fatty acids present in the vaginal secretions during ovulation are supposed to attract the male monkey by their smell.

The role of pheromones in human sexuality is, however, uncertain.

4. Maternal Behaviour

Maternal behaviour, as demonstrated in rats, is the function of the cingulate gyrus and retrosplenial portion of the limbic cortex. In animals, maternal behaviour is primarily neurogenic, i.e. it depends on olfactory, auditory, visual and thermotactile stimuli arising from the young ones. Prolactin and oxytocin, though absolutely not essential, have been reported to facilitate maternal behaviour. Maternal behaviour, in rats, is manifested by nest building, suckling and licking the pups and retrieving the pups when separated. In general, the maternal behaviour is concerned with the nursing (breastfeeding) and protection of the offspring by the mother.

5. Emotional Behaviour

Emotional behaviour is one of the most important functions of the limbic system. It has been discussed separately in the section 'Physiology of Emotions'.

6. Motivational Behaviour

Motivational behaviour is also an important function of the limbic system and has been discussed separately in the section 'Physiology of Motivation'.

SUMMARY OF DIFFERENT COMPONENTS OF LIMBIC SYSTEM

1. Hypothalamus

Hypothalamus and its functions are described on page 931.
Areas of the hypothalamus associated with behavioural control functions are as follows:

- Increased level of general activity, leading to *rage and aggression*, occurs when the lateral hypothalamus is stimulated.
- *Sexual arousal* occurs when most anterior and posterior portion of the hypothalamus is stimulated.
- *Feelings of reward, tranquillity and pleasure* are appreciated when the reward centre is stimulated.
- *Fearing, feeling of punishment and aversion* are felt when the punishment centre is stimulated.

Applied Aspects

Lesions of the hypothalamus are associated with:
- Extreme passivity and loss of drive
- Excessive eating and drinking
- Rage and violent behaviour

2. Amygdala

Amygdala is a large aggregate of cells located above the inferior horn of the lateral ventricle and is embedded in the uncus. It consists of two subdivisions – a corticomedial nuclear group and a basolateral group of nuclei. In humans, basolateral nuclei of the amygdala are very well developed and they play an important role in behavioural activities not generally associated with olfactory stimuli.

Afferents to the amygdala come from all portions of the limbic cortex as well as from the neocortex and, therefore, it is called the 'window' through which the limbic system sees the place of the person in the world.

Efferents from the amygdala are varied and extensive, reaching the cortex, hippocampus, septum, thalamus and hypothalamus.

Stimulation of the amygdala produces the following effects:

1. ***Autonomic effects through the hypothalamus*** include:
   - Changes in heart rate (increase or decrease)

- Changes in blood pressure (increase or decrease)
- Changes in gastrointestinal secretion and motility
- Defaecation and micturition
- Pupillary dilatation
- Piloerection
- Secretion of anterior pituitary hormones

2. ***Involuntary movements*** which can be elicited are as follows:
   - Tonic movements such as raising of the head or bending of the body
   - Clonic rhythmic movements
   - Circling movements
   - Clonus
   - Movements associated with olfaction and eating (chewing, swallowing, etc.)
3. ***Behavioural effects*** are as follows:
   - Reaction of reward and punishment (rage and escape)
   - Sexual activities including erection, copulatory movements, ovulation, uterine activity and premature labour

Applied Aspects

Bilateral destruction of the temporal pole is associated with destruction of the amygdala which leads to *Klüver–Bucy syndrome* characterized by:

- Extreme orality, i.e. excessive tendency to examine objects orally
- Loss of fear
- Decreased aggressiveness
- Tameness
- Changes in eating behaviour
- Psychic blindness
- Excessive sexual drive

3. Hippocampus

Hippocampus is formed due to projection of the hippocampal sulcus into the floor of the inferior horn of the lateral ventricle.

Connections: Hippocampus has many indirect connections to many portions of the cerebral cortex.

Stimulation of the hippocampus can evoke rage, passivity and excessive sexual drive. It is also hyperexcitable, and weak stimuli can produce epileptic seizures.

Functions of the hippocampus are as follows:

- Like the amygdala, it is an additional channel through which incoming signals can lead to an appropriate behavioural pattern.
- It is suggested that the hippocampus also provides the signal for memory consolidation, e.g. the transformation from short-term to long-term memories of verbal and symbolic type.

Applied Aspects

Lesions of the hippocampus lead to *anterograde amnesia*, i.e. a profound inability to form new memories based on any type of verbal symbolism (language).

4. Limbic Cortex

Limbic cortex acts as an association area for control of behaviour:

Anterior temporal cortex has gustatory and olfactory association.

Parahippocampal gyrus has complex auditory association, and complex thought association derived from Wernicke's area of the posterior temporal lobe.

Posterior cingulate cortex has sensory motor association.

Applied Aspects

Lesions of different parts of the limbic cortex produce certain symptoms that suggest their functions, e.g.:

- *Bilateral destruction of the anterior temporal cortex* leads to Klüver–Bucy syndrome as described above.
- *Bilateral lesions in the posterior orbitofrontal cortex* lead to insomnia and restlessness.
- *Bilateral destruction of anterior cingulate and subcallosal gyri* evokes an extreme rage reaction.

PHYSIOLOGY OF EMOTIONS

COMPONENTS OF EMOTIONS

Emotions refer to an aroused state involving intense feeling, autonomic activation and related behaviour which accompany many of our conscious experiences. They have two major components – mental and physical. The components of emotions are explained in the subsequent text by considering the example of response of an individual to sudden very loud noise.

I. Mental or Sensory Component

Mental or sensory component of emotions comprises cognition, affect and conation.

Cognition It refers to a phenomenon by which one becomes aware (sees) and recognizes a situation, for example, when an individual hears a sudden very loud noise, and from his/her experience recognizes it to be bomb blast. This is called cognition. Thus, mere seeing but not recognizing is not cognition.

Affect It is a German word which means development of a feeling. In the above-stated example, the person after cognizing the loud sound as bomb blast is frightened; this feeling of frightening is called affect.

Conation It is the force that directs or urges to take some action. For example, the desire to run away from the site of loud noise after getting frightened is conation.

II. Physical or Expressive or Peripheral Component

Physical or expressive Physical or expressive or peripheral component of the emotions is the motor side of emotional behaviour. It consists of two subcomponents – somatic and autonomic:

Somatic part of the physical component of emotions basically comprises changes in the skeletal muscles. The accomplishment of the act of running away from the site of noise in the above-stated example constitutes the somatic part of the physical component.

Autonomic part of the physical component of emotions involves the coordinated activity of the sympathetic and parasympathetic nervous system. For example, occurrence of tachycardia, raised blood pressure and increased respiration rate after getting frightened from the sudden loud noise constitute the autonomic part of the physical component.

Sympathetic expression: Fear (as in the above-stated example) is associated with sympathetic expression which is characterized by an increase in heart rate, increase in respiration rate, cutaneous vasoconstriction, sweating (cold sweat), piloerection, pupillary dilatation and dryness of the mouth.
Parasympathetic expression is noticed during grief or pleasure.

Important Note

In many instances, the somatic part of the physical component of emotions may be absent. For example, after getting insulted and provoked, one may beat the insulter (somatic part present). In contrast, the other individual may feel enraged and develop high blood pressure plus tachycardia but restrains himself/herself and does not show any somatic side of expression (indeed, this is common in civilized societies).

Functions Served by Peripheral Component of Emotions

Preparatory function, i.e. the body is prepared for action. It involves:

- *General arousal*, which prepares the organism as a whole for action
- *Specific arousal*, which prepares the organism for a particular behaviour. For example, *sexual arousal* involves:
  - General arousal in the form of tachycardia that prepares for physical exertion
  - Specific arousal in the form of tumescence

THEORIES OF GENESIS OF EMOTIONS

Physical changes are secondary to emotional feelings or vice versa has been the matter of debate. The theories given in the subsequent text have been put forward from time to time in this regard; the genesis of emotions as explained by Arnold is as given next.

Arnold's theory According to this theory of genesis of emotions (Fig. 10.10.6):

- By *cognition*, one becomes aware and recognizes a situation.
- By *unconscious evaluation*, the situation is judged as to be harmful or beneficial.
- *Affect* is conscious reflection of unconscious appraisal. A feeling is thus generated consciously in response to unconscious evaluation of a situation. Such a feeling may be in the form of fear, joy, grief or rage.

Thus, according to Arnold's theory, emotions have their own logic and the peripheral component of emotions results from unconscious evaluation of situation as potentially harmful or harmless. Therefore, in response to a particular situation, different individuals react differently, e.g. in response to a bomb blast by terrorist attacks:

- Some will be frightened.
- Proterrosist persons will have a feeling of joy.
- Antiterrorists will develop a feeling of rage and so on.
- Furthermore, Arnold pointed out that autonomic responses are not an essential component of emotions.

The James–Lange theory of emotion suggests that emotions occur as a result of physiological reaction.

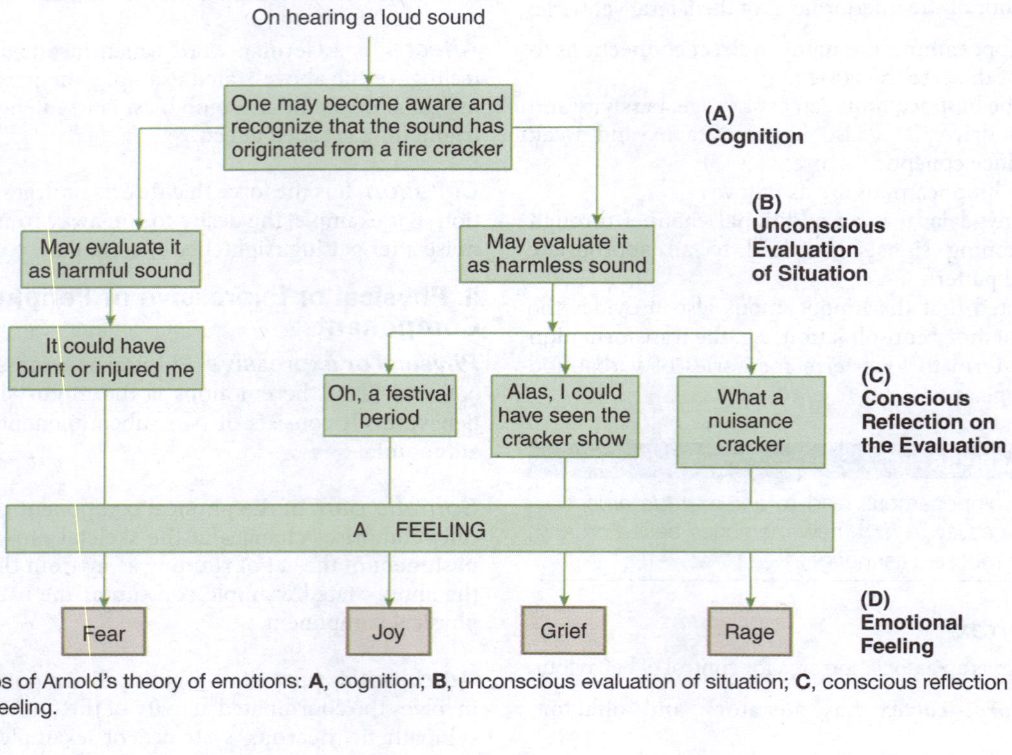

Fig. 10.10.6 Steps of Arnold's theory of emotions: **A**, cognition; **B**, unconscious evaluation of situation; **C**, conscious reflection on the evaluation; and **D**, emotional feeling.

EMOTIONAL BEHAVIOUR

Different emotions produce different sets of behaviour. Physiological basis of most emotional behaviours has been studied extensively in animals and little bit in humans. Behaviour is considered an expression of emotions. Some of the emotional behaviours are as follows:

- Rage, fear and placidity (see page 933)
- Sexual behaviour (see page 933)
- Feeling of reward and punishment (see page 1054)

NEURAL SUBSTRATE OF EMOTIONS

1. Role of Central Nervous System

i. Role of cerebral cortex Cerebral cortex, especially the frontal, cingulate and parahippocampal cortices, plays an important role in *affective component* of *emotions*:

- Detailed processing of conscious experience of emotional feeling occurs in the cerebral cortex.
- Cortical mechanisms also provide the means by which memory and imagination too can evoke emotional feeling.
- Cortex also provides the mechanisms that direct the motor responses to the external event during emotional behaviour, e.g. to approach or avoid a situation.
- Cortical mechanisms also provide the means which account for the modulation, direction, understanding or even inhibition of emotional behaviour. For example, once we know that an explosive sound came from only a fire cracker, the fear subsides by cortical suppression of reflex emotional responses.

Applied Aspects

Lesions of the cerebral cortex concerned with emotions are associated with emotional disturbances as:

Lesions of the orbitofrontal cortex reduce the normal aggressiveness and emotional responsiveness.

Lesions of the ventromedial frontal cortex have normal autonomic response mechanism, i.e. patients show normal galvanic skin responses (sweating measured electrically) to *startle* stimuli, such as unexpected loud noises or bright lights. However, when they are shown emotionally disturbing pictures, they fail to show the expected autonomic response to these emotionally charged stimuli.

Lesions of the anterior cingulate cortex reduce the emotional response to chronic intractable pain. Such patients experience pain as a sensation and exhibit appropriate autonomic reactions, but the sensation is not perceived as intensely unpleasant.

Lesion of the prefrontal cortex leads to:

- *Frontal abulic syndrome* – occurs due to prefrontal cortex lesion, characterized by loss of initiative, creativity and curiosity, emotional baldness and apathy
- *Frontal disinhibition syndrome* – characterized by severe impairment in judgement and person being socially disinhibited

ii. Role of hypothalamus Hypothalamus and other components of the limbic system are intimately concerned with physiology of emotions. Functions of all these components have been described on page 1054. However, their role as neural substrates of emotions is described in the subsequent text even at the cost of repetition.

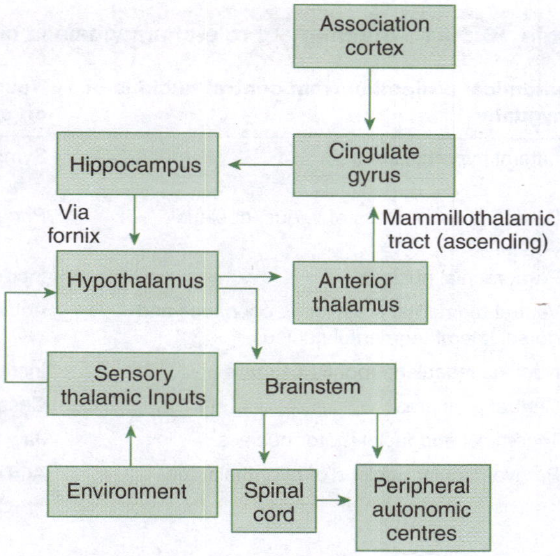

Fig. 10.10.7 The Papez model of emotions.

Hypothalamus has been considered the main seat of emotions. Papez suggested a model of emotional expression and experience on the basis of clinical and to some extent anatomical facts (Fig. 10.10.7).

- *Sensory input* from environment passes through the thalamus to the hypothalamus.
- *Ascending output from the hypothalamus* passes on through the mammillothalamic tract to the anterior thalamus and on to the cingulate cortex.
- *Output from the cingulate cortex* interacts with the sensory cortical signals in the association cortex.
- Thus, the sensory information from the cortex, particularly that from the frontal lobe, is lent an emotional flavour and reaches the hippocampus.
- *Hippocampus* projects onto the hypothalamus through the fornix and thus completes the so-called Papez circuit (Fig. 10.10.4).
- *Descending projections from the hypothalamus* pass through the brainstem down to the spinal cord and out into the peripheral autonomic nervous system. The output of the peripheral autonomic nervous system produces the manifestation of emotional expressions.
- *Areas of the hypothalamus concerned with various emotional behaviour* are given on page 933.

iii. Role of amygdala Salient anatomical and functional features of the amygdala are described on page 1050. As far as emotions are concerned, the amygdala coordinates the affective component of emotions (function of the cerebral cortex) with the autonomic response to emotions (function of the hypothalamus).

Affective component of the emotions is influenced by the amygdala through the *ventral amygdalofugal pathway* that projects from the central nucleus of the amygdala to the brainstem, the dorsal medial nucleus of the thalamus and the association areas of the cortex, especially the rostral cingulate gyrus of the cortex and the orbitofrontal cortex.

Table 10.10.1 Summary of role of amygdala in emotions

Anatomical projection from central nucleus of amygdale	Neuroendocrinal response on stimulation	Peripheral signs of emotions
1. Lateral hypothalamus	Sympathetic stimulation	Increased heart rate, increased blood pressure and pupillary dilatation
2. Dorsal motor nucleus of vagus, nucleus ambiguus	Parasympathetic stimulation	Bradycardia, urination, defaecation
3. Parabrachial nucleus	Increased respiration	Panting, respiratory distress
4. Ventral tegmental area, locus coeruleus and dorsal lateral tegmental nucleus	Activation of catecholamines	Behavioural and electroencephalographic arousal
5. Nucleus reticularis, pontis caudalis	Increased reflexes	Increased startle
6. Central grey area	Cessation of behaviour	Social interaction
7. Trigeminal and facial motor nucleus	Jaw movements and mouth opening	Facial expression of fear
8. Paraventricular nucleus of hypothalamus	ACTH release	Corticosteroid release (stress response)

Peripheral component of emotions is influenced by the amygdala through the *stria terminalis* that projects from the central nucleus of the amygdala to:

- *Hypothalamus*, which mediates neuroendocrinal response to fearful and stressful stimuli
- *Nucleus accumbens* that controls the body language in emotional states

Summary of role of amygdala in emotions: Various anatomical projections from the central nucleus of the amygdala, neuroendocrinal response and the peripheral signs of emotions produced are summarized in Table 10.10.1.

Concepts of extended Papez circuit: Recently, a concept of extended Papez circuit has been described in which the focus has been shifted to the main role of the amygdala in emotions (Fig. 10.10.8). The Papez circuit of emotions, described by James Papez in 1937, points out that the circuit is completed by projection of the hippocampus to the hypothalamus through the fornix (Fig. 10.10.7).

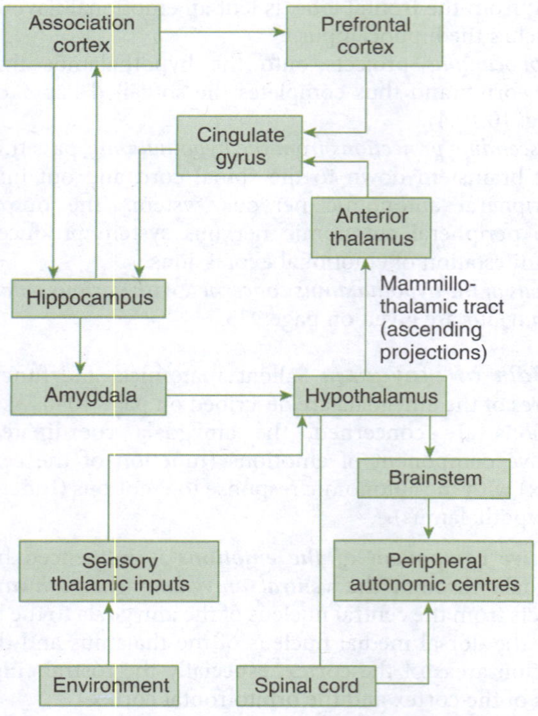

Fig. 10.10.8 The extended Papez circuit of emotions.

2. Role of Peripheral Nervous System

Autonomic as well as somatic motor peripheral nervous system is involved in the peripheral expression of the emotions.

i. Autonomic nervous system is the chief mediator of the emotional output. There is some degree of specificity in the pattern of autonomic expressions depending on the type of emotion in question and also whether the autonomic response is primary, i.e. independently determined, or secondary to the somatomotor behaviour. Cannon described the emotional response to an emergency or involving diffuse sympathetic activation and outpouring into the blood of excitatory substances, i.e. the catecholamines.

ii. Somatic motor nervous system is involved in the somatic part of the physical component of emotions, which basically comprises changes in skeletal muscles.

PHYSIOLOGY OF MOTIVATION

Motivation is that component of behaviour which is responsible for accomplishing a particular task.

NEURAL MECHANISM OF MOTIVATION

Neural mechanisms involved in motivation are based on the concept of reward and punishment. It has been elucidated by the effects of self-stimulation of the brain.

CONCEPT OF REWARD AND PUNISHMENT

Almost anything that we do is related in some way to reward and punishment. If we do something that is rewarding, we continue to do it. If we do something that is punishing, we cease to do it.

Reward and punishment centre It appears that conditions which result in stimulation of the reward centre produce motive to do a job. For details about *reward and punishment* centres, see page 933.

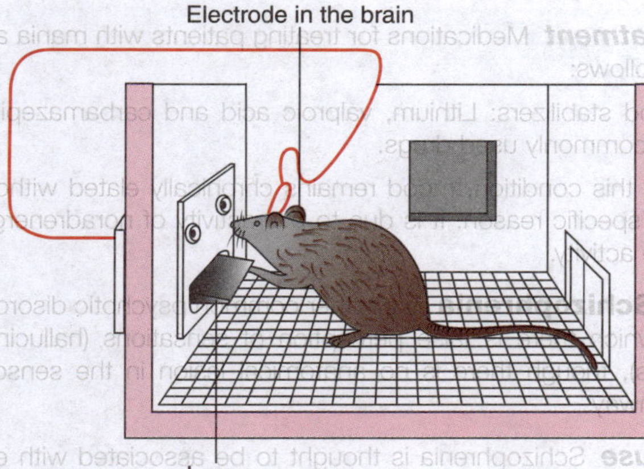

Fig. 10.10.9 Experimental set-up to demonstrate reward and punishment centres by self-stimulation.

Experiment to demonstrate activity of reward and punishment centres: This experiment demonstrates that the animal itself regulates the stimulation of reward and punishment centres (self-stimulation). The *Hess technique* of experiment is as follows: a rat is placed in a cage having a bar (lever) that can be pressed by the rat. The electrical connections are made in such a way that on pressing the bar, a stimulus may be applied to the brain of the rat through an electrode (Fig. 10.10.9). The following observations are made:

- *When no stimulus is applied* to the brain on pressing the bar, the animal presses it occasionally (at random).
- *When stimulation is applied to the reward centre* (located along the course of the medial forebrain bundle, especially in the lateral and ventromedial nucleus of the hypothalamus) on pressing the bar, the animal presses the bar repeatedly at a rate much above the rate of random pressing. It has been reported that stimulation of the reward centre produces a *pleasure sensation* (feeling of complete relaxation).
- Furthermore, it has been observed that even if a painful barricade is placed between the rat and the bar (lever), the rat ignores the pain to cross the barrier to press the bar. This means that the rat must have developed a strong motive to derive pleasure sensation.
- Instead of a painful barrier, if a complicated maze is made between the rat and the bar (lever), the rat learns to cross the maze. This means that development of a motive is a strong factor for learning. From this, it can be concluded that if there is no motive to do a job, people will neither do the job nor learn to do the job.
    - It has been observed that self-stimulation increases when the animal is deprived of food and decreased by castration (restarted by the administration of sex hormones).
    - When stimulation is applied to the punishment centre (located in the medial hypothalamus, periventricular zone) on pressing the bar, the animal avoids further stimulation of this area. The pressing rate of the bar is decreased much below the rate of random pressing. It has been reported that electrical stimulation of the punishment centre leads to pain, fear, defence, escape reactions and the other elements of punishment.

ROLE OF NEUROTRANSMITTERS

Neurotransmitters (NTs) involved in the pathway that stimulate the *reward centre* are as follows:

- Catecholamines (norepinephrine and dopamine [DA])
- Morphine
- Enkephalin

Drugs that increase stimulation of the reward centre are those which increase synaptic activity in the catecholamine pathway, e.g.:

- *Amphetamine* causes increased release of DA.
- *Nicotine and alcohol* increase the amount of DA.
- *Cocaine* inhibits the reuptake of DA and norepinephrine.

Applied Aspects

Addiction: Tobacco, alcohol, cannabis, opiates, LSD, cocaine and amphetamine are well known to produce addiction. These drugs act by increasing dopaminergic activity in the reward centre. Thus, a strong motive develops to use them again and again.

Learning: Catecholamines and enkephalins are also involved in pathways responsible for learning. Therefore, it seems that reward and punishment constitute the incentives for learning.

Drugs that decrease stimulation of the reward centre are those which lower synaptic activity in the catecholamine pathway, e.g. chlorpromazine hydrochloride (Largactil).

MONOAMINERGIC NEURONAL TRACTS AND PHYSIOLOGICAL BASIS OF PSYCHOTIC DISORDERS

MONOAMINERGIC NEURONAL TRACTS

Apart from sensory and motor tracts, the CNS also has a third kind of tract called monoaminergic tracts (because they secrete monoamines like noradrenaline [NA], DA, serotonin [5-HT] as NTs). Nevertheless, there are many neuronal tracts (NTs) and some of them are opioid peptides instead of monoamines. Therefore, the term monoaminergic neurons is less popular nowadays. In fact, the tracts are better known by the name of NT, e.g. noradrenergic tracts, dopaminergic tracts and serotonergic tracts.

Adrenergic Tracts

Fibres of adrenergic tracts arise chiefly from *locus coeruleus* and *lateral tegmentum* of the midbrain, and spread extensively to terminate in many parts of CNS, including the cerebral cortex, limbic system, cerebellum and spinal cord.

Function of noradrenergic fibres can typically be explained by describing the deficits seen in individuals with deficiency of NA in these fibres, which include:

- Abnormal mood (i.e. mood is down, and depression develops)
- Increase in hunger and appetite
- Increased sleep

Dopaminergic Tracts

Two major dopaminergic pathways that arise from the midbrain are as follows:

Nigrostriatal, from the substantia nigra of the midbrain to the corpus striatum

Mesolimbic, from the mesencephalon to the nucleus accumbens which is situated little cranial to the corpus striatum

Functions of dopaminergic pathways are understood from the abnormalities of these tracts:

- Damage of the nigrostriatal pathway or dopaminergic receptor deficiency causes *parkinsonism* (for details, see page 918).
- Excessive dopaminergic activity in mesolimbic fibres leads to schizophrenia.

Applied Aspects

Physiological Basis of Psychotic Disorders

1. Depression

In a normal person, the mood usually swings, i.e. with bad news (e.g. failure in examination), the mood is down, and with good news (e.g. distinction in examination), the mood is elated. However, when mood chronically remains down without any specific reason, then the condition is called depression.

Signs and Symptoms are as follows:

- Chronic depression of mood
- Lack of interest
- Suicidal tendency
- Excessive sleep and overeating

Causes The physiological basis of this disorder is decreased activity of either noradrenergic or serotoninergic fibres. Serotonin is the main NT that allows communication with different brain regions involved in processing the emotions.

Observations suggested that patients with depression have less number of receptors on the hippocampus.

- Researchers have also documented that some persons with depression have high levels of increased amount of cortisol (stress hormone) and cortisol has a toxic effect on the hippocampus.

The defect may be at the receptor level or there is deficiency of NTs (NA or serotonin).

Treatment Drugs that increase the excitatory effects of NA are effective in treating depression; these include monoamine oxidase (MAO) inhibitors, tricyclic antidepressants and drugs that enhance the action of serotonin. Manic-depressive conditions (bipolar disorder) can be effectively treated by lithium compounds that diminish the actions of NA and serotonin.

2. Mania Syndrome are:

Mania syndrome is a state of abnormal elevated period of great excitement/euphoria, delusions and overactivity.

Signs and Symptoms are as follows:

- Patient usually disconnected and has very fast thoughts
- Inappropriate elation or euphoria, irritability and social behaviour
- Increased sexual desires
- High volume and speed of talking
- Markedly increased energy

Treatment Medications for treating patients with mania are as follows:

Mood stabilizers: Lithium, valproic acid and carbamazepine are commonly used drugs.

In this condition, mood remains chronically elated without any specific reason. It is due to overactivity of noradrenergic fibre activity.

3. Schizophrenia is another common psychotic disorder in which there is false perception of sensations (hallucinations), though there is no anatomical lesion in the sensory pathway.

Cause Schizophrenia is thought to be associated with excessive activity of the dopaminergic mesolimbic pathway (mainly due to overactivity of D_2 receptors). Evidence supporting this theory derives from the fact that schizophrenic symptoms are reduced by drugs such as chlorpromazine and haloperidol that diminish DA release at axon terminals (drugs that block D_2 receptors). Recently developed antipsychotic agents are effective, but they bind to D_2 receptors to a limited degree; however, they bind effectively to D_4 receptors. This effect leads to a possibility that schizophrenia is associated with D_4 receptor abnormality.

Characteristic Features of schizophrenia are as follows:

- *Hallucinations*, auditory as well as visual
- *Delusions* of grandeur, intense fear or paranoia
- *Withdrawal from the society* (i.e. the patient prefers extreme isolation, avoids company with persons and has no interest in the surroundings)

Treatment The drugs which decrease the DA concentration in the central nervous system are used. But the main drawback of these drugs is that they cause deficiency of DA, which precipitates parkinsonism. Agranulocytosis is a potential side effect of most of the antipsychotic drugs. However, certain drugs that do not cause agranulocytosis but effectively reduce the symptoms of schizophrenia are as follows:

- Risperidone
- Aripiprazole
- Olanzapine
- Paliperidone

Self-Assessment

1. Discuss the components and functions of limbic system.
2. Discuss the physiological aspects of genesis of emotions.
3. Discuss the physiology of motivation.
4. Describe about the following:
   - Monoaminergic neuronal tracts
   - Klüver–Bucy syndrome
5. Write notes on the following:
   - Papez circuit
   - Addiction
   - Depression

Clinical Cases

Case 1

A 45-year-old male had a head injury in a road accident and was in coma state for 6 months and recovered, but developed abnormal behaviour in terms of:

Excessive tendency to examine the things orally
Becoming a very quiet person in spite of having a very aggressive behaviour before the accident
Change in eating behaviour (excessive heating)
Excessive sexual drive

Q1. What is the probable diagnosis?
Q2. Lesion of which part of the brain causes this condition?

Case 2

A 35-year-old orthopaedic surgeon addicted to smoking for more than 10 years cannot do surgery without.

Q1. What is the mechanism of addiction?
Q2. What are the effects of addiction?
Q3. Which part of the brain is most affected?
Q4. What is the role of neurotransmitters in addiction?

Case 3

An 18-year-old boy did not crack the NEET examination and tried suicide; after that, he has lack of interest in studies, his sleep pattern has changed (all the times he is sleepy) and he does not interact with friends and family members.

Q1. What is the probable diagnosis?
Q2. Which neurotransmitter is responsible for above-mentioned signs and symptoms?
Q3. What should be the treatment plan in such type of cases?

Case 4

A 25-year-old male was brought to the psychiatry department for his abnormal behaviour with complaints like having hallucinations, having feeling of extreme fear, remaining isolated, not mixing with family members, not actively participating in family activities such as wedding ceremonies or birthday parties, and at times speaking very loudly.

Q1. What is the probable diagnosis?
Q2. What is the pathophysiology of this condition?
Q3. What is the treatment plan for this condition?

10.11 Reticular Formation, Electrical Activity of the Brain, and Alert Behaviour and Sleep

CHAPTER OUTLINE

RETICULAR FORMATION AND RETICULAR ACTIVATING SYSTEM

Reticular formation (RF) refers to the complex network of neurons and nerve fibres which occupy the midventral portion of the brainstem around the central cavity and is exclusive of the specific nuclei and tracts. In other words, it is formed by neurons and processes left over after all well-defined named nuclei and pathways have been accounted for. Phylogenetically, it represents the old reticular core of the brain. The brainstem RF comprises the medullary RF, pontine RF and midbrain RF. Structurally, brainstem RF consists of:

- Neuronal aggregates
- Afferent connections] Reticular pathway
- Efferent connections]

NEURONAL AGGREGATES OF RF

Reticular Nuclei

A number of reticular nuclei have been described. The limits of such nuclei are ill-defined (and often controversial), and their functional significance is often obscure. These can be divided into three longitudinal columns (in each half of the brainstem):

Nuclei of the median column lie next to the middle line and are called *nuclei of raphe*, e.g. raphe nuclei in the midbrain.

Nuclei of the medial column lie laterally to the nuclei of the median column. These are made of large cells and so also called *magnocellular nuclei*, e.g. nucleus gigantomedullaris in the medulla and pontine tegmental nuclei.

Nuclei of the lateral column lie laterally to the nuclei of the medial column. These are made of small neurons and so also called *parvocellular nuclei*. Examples of such nuclei are central nucleus of the medulla and central nucleus of the pons.

Functional Neuronal Aggregates

Functional neuronal aggregates, though not anatomical entities, have been described to have fairly well-defined physiological functions. These include:

- Cardiac centres
- Respiratory centres
- Vasomotor centres
- Salivatory centres
- Chemoreceptor neurons

RETICULAR PATHWAYS

Connections of RF are as follows:

- Afferent connections
- Efferent connections, which include:
  - Descending projections
  - Ascending projections

The afferent and efferent connections of the RF form several pathways. Some of the major pathways are as follows:

- Cortico-reticulospinal pathways
- Cortico-reticulocerebellar and cortico-reticulo-basal ganglia connections
- Visceral control pathways
- Reticular activating system (RAS)

1. Cortico-Reticulospinal Pathways

Afferents of this pathway to neurons of RF come from the motor and other areas of the cerebral cortex.

Areas of RF which receive impulses from the cerebral cortex are as follows:

- Bulboreticular inhibitory area located in the lower part of the medulla (see page 893)
- Bulboreticular facilitatory area located in the pons (see page 893)

2. Cortico-Reticulocerebellar and Cortico-Reticulo-Basal Ganglia Connections

Some afferents from the cerebral cortex, after relaying in RF, project to the cerebellum and basal ganglia. The influence of the cerebellum and basal ganglia on the motor function has been described in Chapter 10.9; see page 1025.

3. Visceral Control Pathways

Certain centres in the RF regulate respiration, heart rate and blood pressure. These effects are mediated through connections between the RF and the autonomic centres in the brainstem and spinal cord, but the pathways concerned are not well defined.

4. Reticular Activating System (RAS)

RAS, also known as ascending reticular activating system (ARAS), is a complex polysynaptic pathway that projects diffusely from the brainstem RF to the cerebral cortex.

Collaterals to RAS funnel from the following sources (Fig. 10.11.1):

- Long, ascending sensory pathways such as spinothalamic tracts are the important sources of collaterals to RAS. The fibres of the tracts, which convey slow pain, send the richest collateral connections to the RAS.
- In addition to long ascending sensory tracts, collateral to the RAS also funnel from the trigeminal, auditory, visual and olfactory pathway systems.

Efferent projections from RAS are as follows:

- Majority of RAS fibres end in nonspecific thalamic nuclei (intralaminar and midline nuclei), and from there are projected diffusely and nonspecifically to the whole neocortex (Fig. 10.11.1).
- Another part of RAS bypasses the thalamus to project diffusely to the cortex.

The RAS fibres occupy the core portion of the brainstem (Fig. 10.11.1), whereas the specific fibres occupy the lateral parts of the brainstem.

Stimulation of RAS: The RAS is stimulated by impulses funnelled into it through the collateral described above. Thus, the RAS is a *nonspecific system* which can be excited by

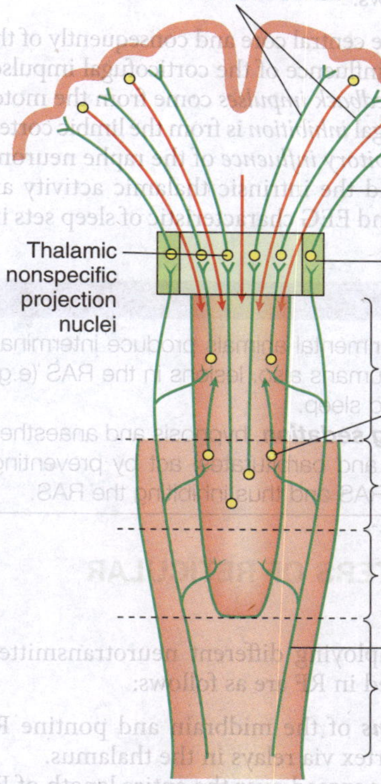

Fig. 10.11.1 Diagrammatic depiction of reticular activating system (RAS) vis-à-vis specific sensory projections.

any sensation. In contrast, the classic sensory pathways are specific in that the fibres in them are activated by only one type of sensory stimulation.

Functions of RAS are as follows:

- RAS sends a strong facilitatory drive to the central neurons, raising their background excitability and increasing their responsiveness to specific stimuli. Thus, when RAS is stimulated, there is wakefulness and alertness of the subject and the subject becomes fully conscious. This alertness is necessary even for proper sense perception. Thus, only an alert subject can correctly sense a touch sensation. Conversely, when the RAS is inhibited, the subject is asleep.
- Besides increasing the general background of excitation, RAS is also responsible for selective attention and, in corollary, the sensory inattention. The selective attention and inattention are due to (i) filtering of stimuli by the noradrenergic neurons of the central reticular core through centrifugal sensory central pathways and (ii) habituation of the reticular neurons.
- The thalamic reticular neurons are capable of intrinsic, spontaneous activity at their own rate of 8–13 impulses/s. In the absence of a bombarding drive from the RAS, these neurons pace the postsynaptic potential of the cortex and thus contribute to the alpha rhythm of the electroencephalogram (EEG). On the other hand, when the influence of facilitatory drive from RAS is strong, low intrinsic rate of thalamic reticular neurons is overwhelmed and there is an overall increase in excitability, marked by the beta rhythm of the EEG.

Control of RAS activity in addition to stimulation by sensory collaterals is as follows:

- The neural activity of the central core and consequently of the RAS is under feedback influence of the corticofugal impulses to the RF. *Facilitatory feedback impulses* come from the motor cortex, whereas centrifugal *inhibition* is from the limbic cortex.
- Under the specific *inhibitory influence* of the raphe neurons, both the RAS drive and the intrinsic thalamic activity are considerably reduced and EEG characteristic of sleep sets in.

Applied Aspects

Lesions of RAS in experimental animals produce interminable sleep and coma. In humans also, lesions in the RAS (e.g. tumours) cause prolonged sleep.

Many agents producing sedation, hypnosis and anaesthesia (e.g. benzodiazepine and barbiturates) act by preventing synaptic transmission in RAS and thus inhibiting the RAS.

NEUROTRANSMITTERS OF RETICULAR FORMATION

Some of the systems employing different neurotransmitters which have been identified in RF are as follows:

Large cholinergic neurons of the midbrain and pontine RF project to the cerebral cortex via relays in the thalamus.

Small adrenergic neurons spread over the entire length of RF and also project extensively to the cerebral cortex via relays in the intralaminar nuclei of the thalamus.

Noradrenergic neurons from several areas of the RF project to the cerebellum.

Dopaminergic neurons of midbrain RF and substantia nigra project to several basal ganglia.

Serotonergic neurons of the raphe nuclei in the lower pontine and medullary RF project to the thalamus and cerebral cortex besides projecting to the hypothalamus and limbic structures.

Serotonergic neurons in the raphe nuclei of medullary RF also project to the substantia gelatinosa of the spinal cord where they control transmission of pain impulses.

In the serotonergic system, a neuroactive peptide usually coexists in the same neuron. Serotonergic neurons, having different peptides accompanying them, may project to different cells, or different combinations of transmitters may control the activity of the same cell differently. One of the substances may act as a transmitter, and the other as a modulator.

The possibilities for different ways in which combinations of neurotransmitters may exert their effect are virtually endless.

FUNCTIONS OF RETICULAR FORMATION

1. Sleep–wakefulness The RAS of RF is the neural substrate of the consciousness and sleep–waking cycle (for details, see page 1068).

2. Selective attention and sensory inattention The RF is also responsible for selective attention and sensory inattention, through the corticofugal control of sensory input and due to habituation.

3. Conditioning and learning RF is an integral part of the neural substrate for conditioning and learning (for details, see page 1083).

4. Control of muscle tone and regulation of postural reflex changes RF modulates the tone of extensor (antigravity) muscles. The pontine (medial) reticulospinal tract has an excitatory influence and the medullary (lateral) reticulospinal tract has an inhibitory influence on extensor muscle tone (for details, see page 1025).

5. Autonomic functions The visceral regulating centres are an integral part of the RF. The influence of higher neurons over the viscera and autonomic functions are mediated through the visceral centres in RF.

6. Modulation of pain Serotonergic neurons of the modulatory raphe nuclei form a part of the endogenous pain relief system. By affecting the transmission of pain impulses through the substantia gelatinosa of the spinal cord, these neurons modulate the perception of pain (for details, see page 1005).

7. Control of neuroendocrine system The RF projections play a role in the control of neuroendocrine systems in the hypothalamus.

ELECTRICAL ACTIVITY OF THE BRAIN

EVOKED CORTICAL POTENTIALS

Evoked potential refers to surface electrical activity recorded from the surface of the scalp in response to a specific and adequate stimulus – auditory, visual or somatosensory. Stimulation by a specific adequate stimulus produces two types of electrical activity in the cerebral cortex known as primary evoked potential and diffuse secondary response. It is important to note that the evoked potential recorded is barely discernible amidst the backdrop of EEG waves (the noise). In order to identify the evoked potential, the technique of averaging is used in order to enhance the signal-to-noise ratio.

Primary evoked potential: This is the initial, brief (lasting for few milliseconds) and localized response over the specific sensory cortex. For example, in the foot area of the postcentral gyrus, if an electrical shock is administered over the foot or over the occipital lobe after photopic stimulation, the primary evoked potential is characterized by (Fig. 10.11.2):

- There is latency of about 5–12 milliseconds (average 10 milliseconds).
- First, there appears a surface-positive wave which is followed by a small negative wave.

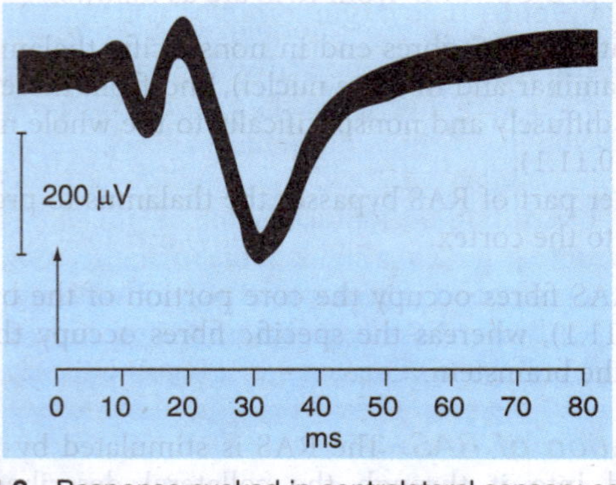

Fig. 10.11.2 Response evoked in contralateral sensory cortex by stimulation of sciatic nerve in a cat. The upward deflection is surface negative.

- The primary evoked potential is highly specific in its location and can be observed only where the pathway from a particular sensory organ ends, i.e. it is produced by conduction of sensory signals through the specific sensory pathways.

Secondary diffuse response is characterized by:

- There is latency of about 20–80 milliseconds (average 50 milliseconds), i.e. it appears at about 50 milliseconds of sensory stimulus.
- Positive–negative wave sequence of the secondary diffuse response is frequently larger and more prolonged than the positive–negative wave sequence of primary evoked potential.
- The surface-positive diffuse secondary response, unlike the primary, is not highly localized. It can be recorded at the same time from most of the cerebral cortex. It is due to spread of impulses through the RAS to the cerebral cortex.

Types of Evoked Potentials

Depending on the type of stimulus, the evoked potential can be:

- Visual evoked potential (VEP)
- Brainstem auditory evoked potential (BAEP)
- Somatosensory evoked potential (SEP)

Depending on the latency of response, evoked potential can be classified into:

- Stimulus-related potentials (short, mid and long latency)
- Event-related or endogenous potentials

Stimulus-Related Potentials

Stimulus-related potential refers to a series of waves that relates to the sensory modality. For example, the auditory stimulus-related response has been divided into three sequential time periods:

- Early latency response (ELR)
- Mid-latency response (MLR)
- Long latency response (LLR)

1. ELR to an auditory stimulus is characterized by a latency of <10 milliseconds and is named 'BAEP'.

Waves of ELR: ELR consists of a series of waves named I–VII (Fig. 10.11.3).

Wave I represents the volume-conducted electrical activity from the auditory nerve.

Wave II represents the volume-conducted electrical activity from the pons.

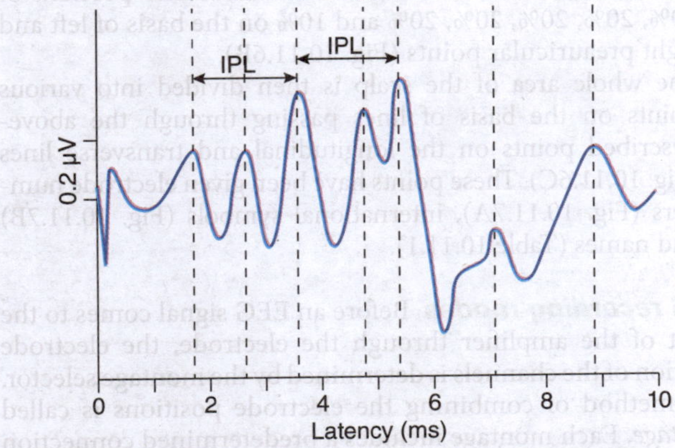

Fig. 10.11.3 Early latency response to an auditory stimulus of 60 dB at 10/s (brainstem auditory evoked potential).

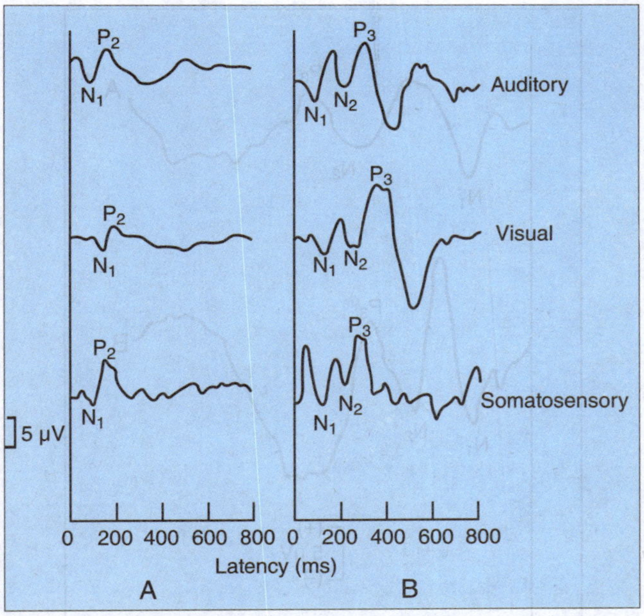

Fig. 10.11.4 Stimulus-related **(A)** and event-related **(B)** long latency potential evoked by auditory, visual and somatosensory stimuli.

Wave III represents the volume-conducted electrical activity from the midbrain.

Interpeak latency (IPL) indirectly reflects the neural conduction in the corresponding segment of the central auditory pathway as:

I–III IPL, i.e. IPL between waves I and III, is a measure of conduction in the more caudal segment of the brainstem auditory pathway, i.e. the auditory nerve and pontomedullary portion.

III–V IPL is a measure of conduction in the more rostral (pontine and midbrain) portions of the pathway.

2. MLR to an auditory stimulus is characterized by a latency of 10–50 milliseconds. It is considered to represent the electrical activity arising in the thalamocortical radiations, the primary auditory cortex and the early association cortex.

3. LLR to an auditory stimulus is characterized by a latency of more than 50 milliseconds. The neural generators of LLR are unknown. It is a negative–positive complex comprising (Fig. 10.11.4):

- A large negative wave (N_1)
- A large positive wave (P_2)

The visual and somatosensory stimuli too elicit a similar response (Fig. 10.11.4). All these responses are stimulus evoked and reflect the functional integrity of the sensory pathways in the CNS. Unlike the event-related potentials (ERPs, discussed in the subsequent text), they are largely independent of the subject's attention or level of arousal.

Event-Related Potentials

ERPs are dependent on the subject's attention or level of arousal (cf. stimulus-related potential, as described above). They are elicited only when the subject is required to distinguish one stimulus (the target) from the other (the nontargets). The ERPs primarily depend on the setting in which the target stimulus occurs and are relatively independent of the physical characteristics of that stimulus. Thus, ERPs are related to the

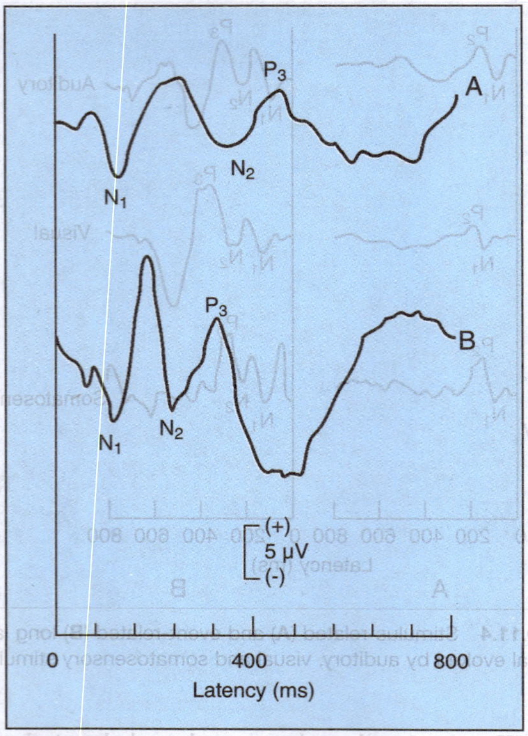

Fig. 10.11.5 Event-related potential (ERP) in a patient with dementia (**A**) shows prolonged latency and reduced amplitude of P_3 component as compared with in a normal subject (**B**).

cognitive events associated with the distinction of target from nontarget stimuli. LLR in ERPs is also a negative–positive complex comprising (Fig. 10.11.4):

- A negative wave (N_2)
- A positive wave (P_3)

Clinical Uses of Evoked Potentials

Stimulus-related evoked potentials reflect the functional integrity of the sensory pathways from the receptor to the cortex. Therefore, any delay in conduction as depicted by delayed peak or IPLs would be of diagnostic value. The lesions interrupting the conduction pathways can be inflammations, demyelinating disorders, degenerative lesions and tumours. For example, in patients with optic neuritis due to multiple sclerosis (a demyelinating disorder), the abnormal VEP is diagnostic.

Event-related evoked potentials are related to cognitive behaviour. Therefore, considerable interest has developed in the possible clinical use of these potentials in the evaluation of patients who suffer from disorders of cognition. The use of ERPs in the clinical assessment of dementia and delirium is fairly well established by now. *Dementia* refers to an abnormal deterioration of intellect affecting several areas of cognitive functions, such as abstraction, orientation, judgement and memory more than 50%. Cases of dementia are due to age-related, senile dementia of Alzheimer type. ERPs in patients with dementia are characterized by prolonged latency and reduced amplitude of P_3 component (Fig. 10.11.5).

ELECTROENCEPHALOGRAM

The term EEG (introduced by the German psychiatrist Hans Berger) refers to record of spontaneous electrical activity of the brain taken from the surface of the scalp (cf. evoked potential which is the surface electrical activity recorded in response to a specific and adequate stimulus). The spontaneous electrical activity of the brain is due largely to graded or summated post-synaptic potentials in the many hundreds or thousands of brain neurons that underlie the recording electrode at the surface of the scalp. The electrical activity of the brain can also be recorded from the pial surface of the brain cortex after opening the skull (e.g. during brain surgery). The term *electrocorticogram* (ECoG) is used to denote such a record.

Electroencephalography

Electroencephalography refers to the technique of EEG recording.

Bipolar Versus Unipolar Electroencephalogram

Bipolar EEG is the record of potential variations between a pair of scalp (cortex) electrodes.

Unipolar EEG is the record of potential variation between an active scalp (cortical) electrode and a theoretically indifferent electrode placed on some part of the body (distant from the cortex such as earlobe).

Thus, the electroencephalography basically involves record of potential difference between a pair of scalp electrodes (bipolar electroencephalography) or between an active scalp electrode and an indifferent electrode (unipolar electroencephalography). The electrodes are connected to a cathode ray oscilloscope (CRO) via a suitable amplifier. The modern EEG machine has 8–16 channels, which can simultaneously record electrical activity from areas of many scalp electrodes.

Location of electrodes Different techniques such as Illinois, Montreal, AIRD and Cahn methods have been described to determine the electrode attaching positions. The most popular method is the *International 10–20 system (Montreal method)* recommended by the International Federation of Societies for Electroencephalography and Clinical Neurophysiology. This system is based on measurement from four standard points on the head – the nasion, the union and the left and right preauricular points. This system is named '10–20 system', because electrodes are spaced either 10% or 20% of the total distance between a given pair of skull landmarks as (Fig. 10.11.6):

- The longitudinal line of the head is divided into portions of 10%, 20%, 20%, 20%, 20% and 10% on the basis of nasions and inions (Fig. 10.11.6A).
- The transverse line of the head is divided into portions of 10%, 20%, 20%, 20%, 20% and 10% on the basis of left and right preauricular points (Fig. 10.11.6B).
- The whole area of the scalp is then divided into various points on the basis of lines passing through the above-described points on the longitudinal and transverse lines (Fig. 10.11.6C). These points have been given electrode numbers (Fig. 10.11.7A), international symbols (Fig. 10.11.7B) and names (Table 10.11.1).

EEG recording modes Before an EEG signal comes to the input of the amplifier through the electrode, the electrode position of the channels is determined by the montage selector. The method of combining the electrode positions is called *montage*. Each montage includes a predetermined connection format. The predetermined combinations of electrode

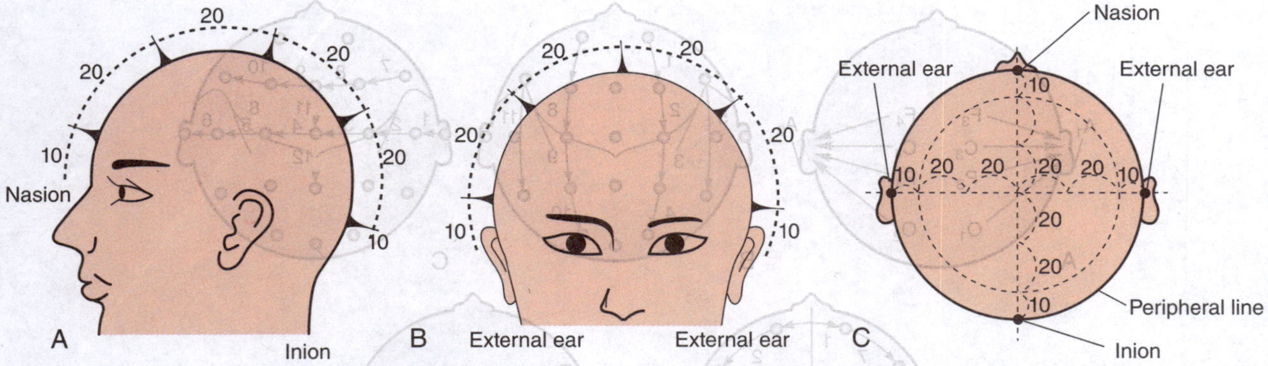

Fig. 10.11.6 Reference points in International '10–20 system' of electrode position for EEG recording: **A**, divisions of longitudinal nasion–inion line; **B**, transverse left and right earline; and **C**, various points on the scalp on the basis of lines passing through. EEG, electroencephalogram.

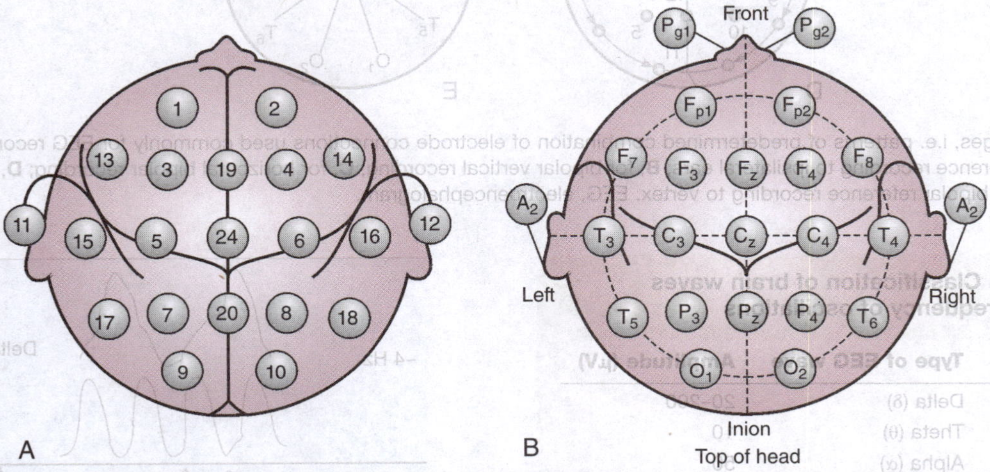

Fig. 10.11.7 Numbers (**A**) and symbols (**B**) for different electrode positions for EEG recording on the scalp. EEG, electroencephalogram.

Table 10.11.1 Name, number and position of electrodes on the scalp for recording electroencephalogram

Electrode number			International symbol			Name
Left	**Right**	**Midline**	**Left**	**Right**	**Midline**	
1	2	–	FP_1	FP_2	–	Frontal pole
3	4	–	F_3	F_4	–	Frontal
5	6	–	C_3	C_4	–	Centre
7	8	–	P_3	P_4	–	Parietal
9	10	–	O_1	O_2	–	Occipital
13	14	–	F_7	F_8	–	Anterior temporal
15	16	–	T_3	T_4	–	Middle temporal
17	18	–	T_5	T_6	–	Posterior temporal
–	–	19	–	–	F_Z	Midline frontal
–	–	24	–	–	C_Z	Midline central
–	–	20	–	–	P_Z	Midline parietal
11	12	–	A_1	A_2	–	Auricular

connections are called patterns. EEGs used in hospitals and other medical facilities are usually operated with montages having the following patterns (Fig. 10.11.8):

- Pattern for monopolar reference recording to ipsilateral ears (Fig. 10.11.8A)
- Pattern for vertical bipolar recording or parasagittal chains (Fig. 10.11.8B)
- Pattern for horizontal bipolar recording (Fig. 10.11.8C)
- Pattern for crown bipolar recording (Fig. 10.11.8D)
- Pattern for bipolar reference recording to vertex (Fig. 10.11.8E)

Normal Electroencephalogram

The EEG consists of waves which are oscillations in the electrical potential of the brain having the following characteristics:

- The oscillations differ in the frequency and amplitude at different points on the scalp and during different stages of mental alertness.
- *Frequencies* of brain waves range from 1 to more than 50 cycles/s.
- *Amplitude* of brain waves may vary from 50 to 200 μV.
- Much of the time, brain waves are *irregular* and no general pattern is obtained. At other times, distinct patterns do appear.
- Different waves recorded in a normal person, depending on their frequency, are classified as alpha, beta, theta and delta waves (Table 10.11.2; Fig. 10.11.9).

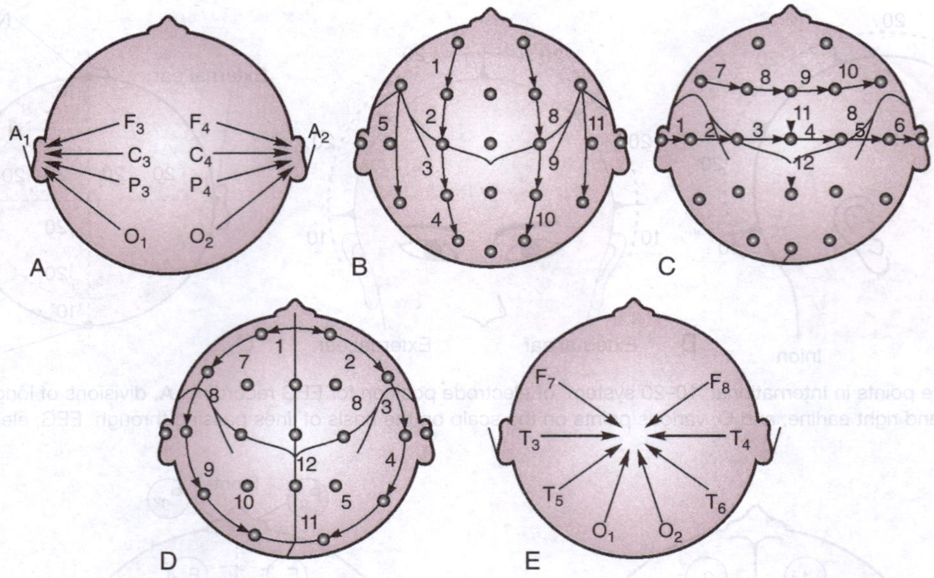

Fig. 10.11.8 Montages, i.e. patterns of predetermined combination of electrode connections used commonly for EEG recording in hospitals: **A**, for monopolar reference recording to ipsilateral ears; **B**, for bipolar vertical recording; **C**, for horizontal bipolar recording; **D**, for crown bipolar recording; and **E**, for bipolar reference recording to vertex. EEG, electroencephalogram.

Table 10.11.2 Classification of brain waves depending on frequency of oscillations

Frequency (Hz)	Type of EEG wave	Amplitude (μV)
1–4	Delta (δ)	20–200
4–7	Theta (θ)	10
8–13	Alpha (α)	50
14–30	Beta (β)	5–10

EEG, electroencephalogram.

Waves of EEG (Fig. 10.11.9)

Different types of EEG waves recorded are given next.

Alpha waves These are the most prominent component of EEG obtained from adult humans who are awake but quiet and at rest with the eyes closed. Alpha waves are said to result from spontaneous activity of nonspecific thalamocortical system.

Characteristic features of alpha waves are as follows:

Frequency of alpha waves varies from 8 to 13 Hz. The mean peak frequency in a large number of normal adults is 4.2 Hz.

Amplitude of these waves slowly waxes and wanes, but the average amplitude is about 50 μV.

Location: Alpha waves are most marked in the parieto-occipital area of the scalp, though these are observed sometimes from other locations as well.

Alpha waves *disappear* during sleep.

Causes of decreased frequency of alpha waves are as follows:

- Old age, due to decreased cerebral perfusion leading to decreased cerebral metabolism
- Low blood glucose level
- Low body temperature
- Low levels of adrenal glucocorticoids
- High arterial partial pressure of CO_2
- Sleep

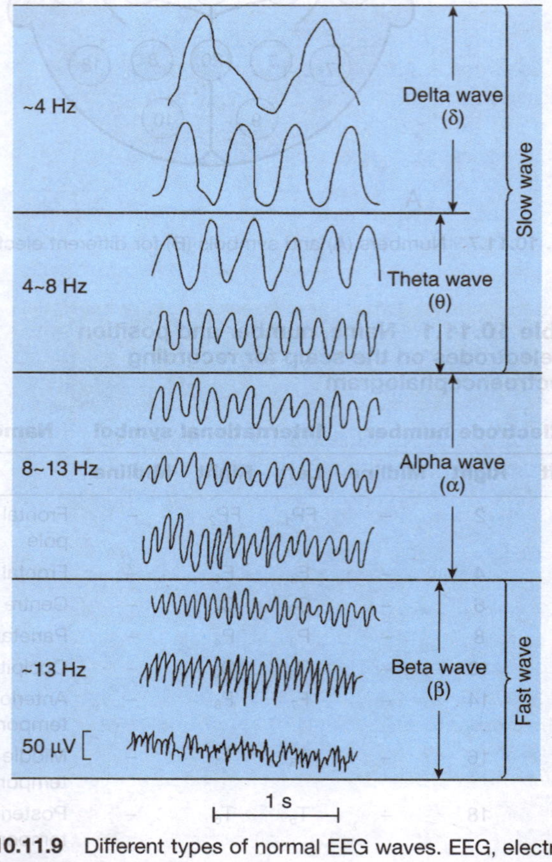

Fig. 10.11.9 Different types of normal EEG waves. EEG, electroencephalogram.

- Frequency and magnitude of alpha rhythms also reduced in encephalopathies (metabolic, toxic or due to hyponatraemia and vitamin B_{12} deficiency)
- Acute intoxification with alcohol, drugs like amphetamine, barbiturates, phenytoin and antipsychotic drugs

Causes of increased frequency of alpha waves are as follows:

- High blood glucose level
- Rise in body temperature
- Low arterial pCO_2 (forced overbreathing to decrease pCO_2 is sometimes used clinically to elicit latent EEG abnormalities)
- High levels of adrenal glucocorticoids
- Alerting states

Alpha block Alpha block or alpha attenuation refers to a phenomenon in which the alpha waves attenuate and are replaced by the fast, irregular waves of low amplitude. It occurs when:

- The persons open their eyes.
- The individual engages in conscious mental activity such as doing mathematical calculations.
- Any form of stimulation is applied (Fig. 10.11.10).

The term *aroused* or *alerting response* is also used to denote an alpha block, since it is correlated with arousal or alerting response.

The term desynchronization has also been suggested for alpha block, because it represents breaking up of the obviously synchronized neural activity necessary to produce regular alpha waves. However, the term desynchronization is misleading as the fast EEG activity seen in alert states is also synchronized, but at a higher rate.

Beta waves Beta waves are seen under the following conditions:

- Tension and CNS activation lead to the appearance of beta waves.
- Arousal response (or alpha block) also leads to the appearance of beta waves.
- Infants have fast beta-like activity in EEG and occipital rhythm is slow, 0.5–2/s patterns.
- Barbiturates induce beta activity typically at a frequency of 18–24 Hz.

Characteristics of beta waves of EEG are as follows:

Frequency of beta waves is usually between 14 and 30 cycles/s.
Amplitude (voltage) of beta waves (5–10 μV) is much lower than that of alpha waves (50 μV).
Location: They are frequently recorded from the parietal and frontal regions.

Theta waves Theta (θ) waves usually do not occur in normal waking individuals (except in newborn infants). Theta component persists in adult life in 10%–15% of normal subjects.

Usually theta waves are seen under the following conditions:

- Emotional stress in adults, particularly during disappointment and frustration, leads to the appearance of theta waves.
- Many brain disorders also lead to the appearance of theta waves.
- Theta component of EEG often accentuates during crying in children.

Characteristic features of theta waves are as follows:

Frequency is between 4 and 7 Hz.
Amplitude (10 μV) is slightly larger than that of beta waves.
Location: They are recorded from the temporal and parietal region in children.

Delta waves do not occur in normal waking individuals. They *can be produced* by overbreathing.

They *occur strictly* in the cortex independent of activities in lower regions of the brain; therefore, they occur in sleep when the cortex is released from the activating influence of lower centres.

These are seen in the following conditions:

- Deep sleep (stages III and IV of non–rapid eye movement [NREM] sleep)
- Infancy
- Serious brain damage

Characteristic features (Fig. 10.11.9) are as follows:

Frequency is less than 4 Hz.
Amplitude is very high (20–200 μV).

Neurophysiological Basis of EEG

The neurophysiological basis of EEG has not been fully elucidated. Some of the important points in this regard are given next.

Cortical grey matter along with its thalamic connection plays an important role in the EEG. Largely, the activity recorded in the EEG is that of rhythmically discharging cell bodies in the most superficial layers of cortical grey matter. Thalamus discharge synchronizes this activity.

Current flow in the fluctuating dipoles formed by the cell bodies and dendrites of the cortical cells accounts for the potential changes recorded as EEG. The dendrites are the sites of nonpropagated hypopolarizing and hyperpolarizing local potential changes. The cell–dendrite relationship is, therefore, that of a constantly shifting dipole. Hence, they become sites of current sink. The dense dendritic tree is present in a particular (vertical) orientation and this results in the brainwave patterns (Fig. 10.11.11). In general, when the sum of the dendritic activity is positive relative to the cell, the cell is hyperpolarized and less excitable, and when it is negative, the cell is depolarized and hyperexcitable. Thus, the EEG is due to graded potentials which are summated postsynaptic potentials in the brain neurons (Fig. 10.11.11).

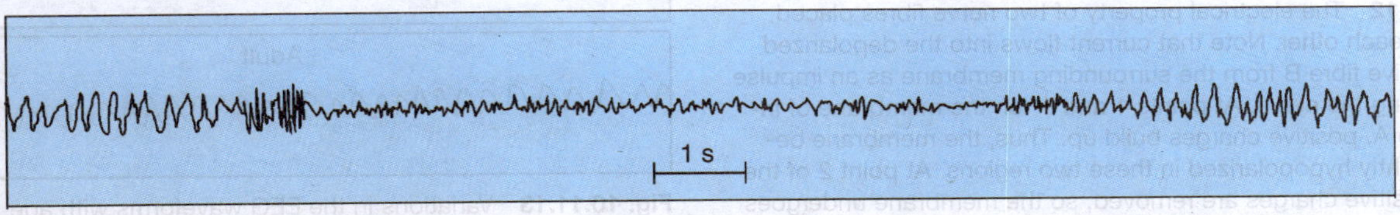

Fig. 10.11.10 Electroencephalography depicting alpha block produced by olfactory stimulus in a rabbit.

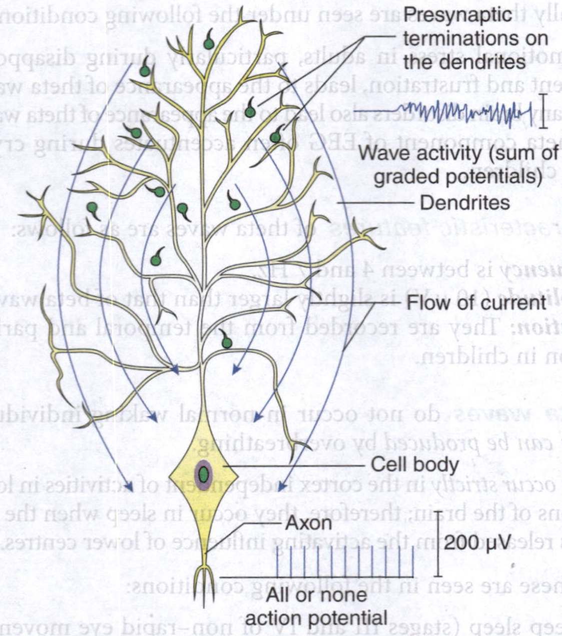

Fig. 10.11.11 Electrical activity recorded from vertically oriented dendritic tree of pyramidal cells in the cerebral cortex compared with that recorded from an axon.

Synchronizing mechanisms: Synchronizing activity of neighbouring cells and rhythmic discharge from the thalamus are responsible for the synchronizing mechanism.

1. ***Synchronizing activity of neighbouring cells*** is due to:
   - The effect of parallel neural processes on each other in a volume conductor (Fig. 10.11.12)
   - The interconnection of neurons by the inhibitory pathway
2. ***Rhythmic discharge from the thalamus*** also responsible for synchronization of EEG waves is evident from the following observations:
   - Stimulation of certain thalamic nuclei of the frequency of about 8 cycles/s produces on EEG record with similar frequency in greater part of the ipsilateral cerebral cortex. The amplitude of the waves also waxes and wanes, i.e. alpha rhythms are produced.
   - Large lesions of the thalamus produce disturbances in the synchronized activity of the EEG on the side of lesion.

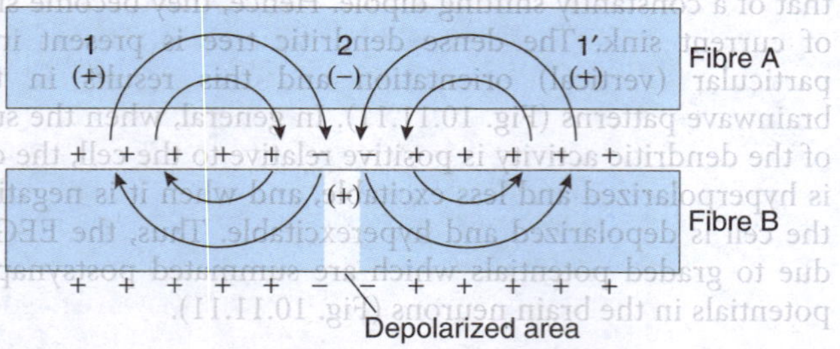

Fig. 10.11.12 The electrical property of two nerve fibres placed parallel to each other. Note that current flows into the depolarized area of active fibre B from the surrounding membrane as an impulse passes along the nerve. At points 1 and 1′ on the membrane of inactive fibre A, positive charges build up. Thus, the membrane becomes slightly hypopolarized in these two regions. At point 2 of the fibre A, positive charges are removed, so the membrane undergoes a slight depolarization at this point.

Desynchronizing mechanisms Desynchronization, as mentioned earlier in the section 'Alpha Block', refers to replacement of a rhythmic EEG pattern with irregular low-voltage activity (arousal reaction). It occurs due to sensory stimulation of the RAS as is evident from the following observations:

- Stimulation of specific sensory system up to the midbrain only (up to where RF is present) produces desynchronization, and the stimulation of these systems above the midbrain does not produce desynchronization.
- Large lesions of the midbrain that interrupt the medial lemnisci and other ascending specific sensory systems fail to prevent the desynchronization produced by specific sensory stimulation below the midbrain level.
- High-frequency stimulation of RF in the midbrain like that of nonspecific projection nuclei of the thalamus produces desynchronization and arousal in sleeping animals.
- Lesions in the midbrain tegmentum that disrupt the RAS without damaging the specific systems are associated with a synchronized EEG pattern that is unaffected by sensory stimulation.

Variations in the EEG wave formation with age EEG wave formation in humans at rest varies with age as (Fig. 10.11.13):

In infants (up to 1 year of age), the occipital rhythm is slow (0.5–2 Hz) than that of adults (8–13 Hz).

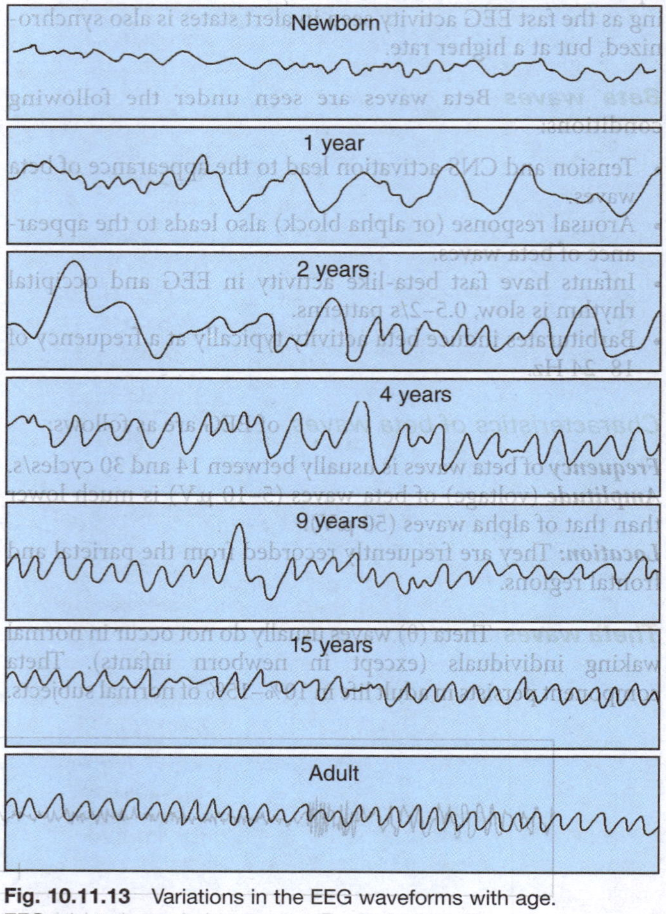

Fig. 10.11.13 Variations in the EEG waveforms with age. EEG, electroencephalogram.

In children, the occipital rhythm speeds up and the adult alpha pattern gradually appears during adolescence.

- In children 4 years of age, theta and alpha waves of 7–8 Hz appear.
- In 9-year-old children, an alpha wave of about 10 Hz appears in the occipital region.
- After 15 years of age, the EEG waveforms become almost the same as those of adults.

In adults (between 15 and 60 years), the EEG waveforms and the typical adult alpha pattern are seen. However, even during these ages, the slow waves decrease as the age rises and the fast waves increase in those *older than 60 years*; the slow waves increase again as the age increases.

Applied Aspects

Abnormal EEG Waveforms

1. Epilepsy

Epilepsy is a syndrome in which there are recurring seizures due to damage to the brain.

Electroencephalographic inspection is indispensable to the diagnosis of epilepsy. Epileptic seizure represents highly synchronized but abnormal neuronal activity. The waveforms of epilepsy (Fig. 10.11.14) include idiopathic abnormal waves such as a spike, sharp wave and spike-and-slow-wave complexes. Between these abnormal waves, an irregular slow wave appears and the background waveform is disturbed. An abnormal wave sometimes appears isolated in the limited part or continues all over the waveform. The generating condition and form are different case by case. A general spike-and-slow-wave complex of 3 Hz appears in the case of absence seizures (characteristic features of tyknoleptic petit mal). Autonomic nerve fit is characterized by a positive spike of 14 or 6 Hz. Nod spasm is characterized by seriously abnormal rhythm and is called a wasting syndrome and seen in babies. Serious fit is usually accompanied by a spasm and consciousness is lost. The EEG waveform shows continuous spikes or sharp waves.

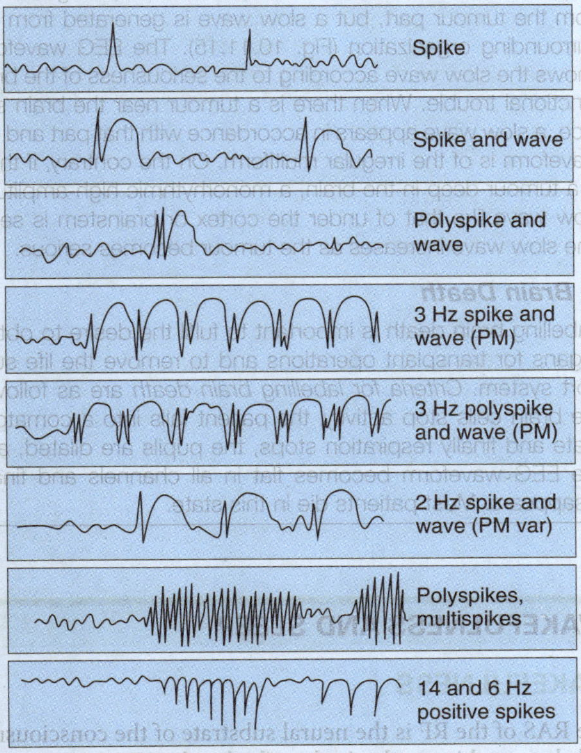

Fig. 10.11.14 EEG waveform of epilepsy. EEG, electroencephalogram; PM, petit mal.

Epileptic seizures are of two types – partial and generalized.

(i) ***Partial seizures*** usually occur due to involvement of a small group of neurons due to causes like head injury, infection, tumour or stroke. The partial seizures are further of two subtypes – simple and complex.
  - *Simple partial seizure:* In this type, there is no loss of consciousness. The typical seizure is characterized by localized jerky movements in one hand progressing to clonic movements of the entire arm, lasting for about 60–90 seconds.
    - The seizure is always preceded by typical aura comprising abnormal sensations. The time period for normal neurological activity to return back after the seizure is called the postictal period.
  - *Complex partial seizure* is not associated with altered consciousness.

(ii) ***Generalized seizures:*** In this type, there is simultaneous widespread electrical activity in both the cerebral hemispheres. Generalized seizures are also of further two subtypes – convulsive and nonconvulsive – depending on tonic and clonic movements.
  - *Tonic–clonic seizure*, formerly called *grand mal epilepsy* or convulsive generalized seizure, is characterized by tonic phase (in which there is sudden onset of contractions of the limb muscles for about 30 seconds) followed by clonic phase (alternating contraction and relaxation of limb muscles causing jerky movements) lasting for 1–2 minutes. EEG changes during tonic phase show fast activity and slow-wave activity (each slow wave preceded by spike) occurs during clonic phase.
  - *Absence seizure*, formerly called *petit mal epilepsy*, is a nonconvulsive generalized seizure, characterized by momentary loss of consciousness only. There is no typical aura and postictic period. EEG changes show doublets (3/s), each comprising a typical spike-and-wave pattern lasting for 10 seconds. This pattern of EEG occurs due to activation of low-threshold T-type Ca^{2+} channels of thalamic neurons.

Pathophysiology: Epilepsy occurs due to release of glutamate from astrocytes. The current view suggests that there is structural basis for increase in excitability due to reorganization of astrocytes along with sprouting of dendrites and new synapse formation.

Genetic mutation: Mutation of certain ion channels has been associated with idiopathic epilepsy which occurs in different forms:

- *Childhood absence epilepsy (CAE)* is associated with mutation of a subunit gene (responsible for GABA receptors called GABA B_3).
- *Inherited form* of generalized epilepsy with fever (febrile seizures) is associated with mutation of sodium channel subunit gene called SCNIA and SCNIB mutations.

Treatment: The basis of therapeutic measures for epilepsy is to reduce excitability, by enhancement of inhibitory neuronal transmission (increased release of GABA).

The anticonvulsant drugs include:

- Gabapentin acts by decreasing Ca^{2+} influx into the cells and reduces glutamate release.

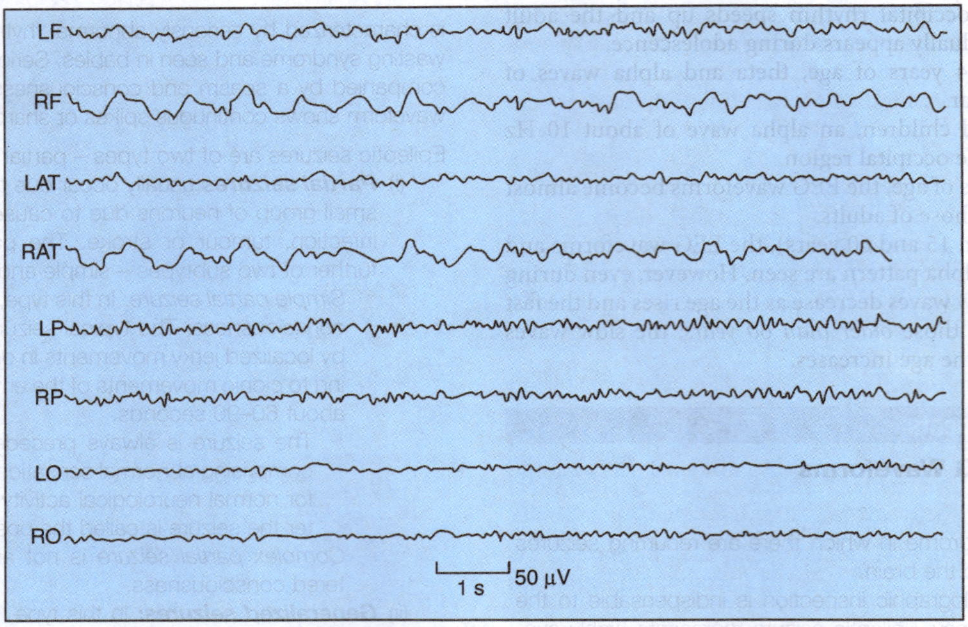

Fig. 10.11.15 EEG waveform of brain tumour. EEG, electroencephalogram.

- Topiramate blocks voltage-gated Na^+ channels associated with glutamate receptors resulting in potentiation of inhibitory effect of GABA.
- Ethosuximide reduces low-threshold T-type Ca^{2+} currents in thalamic neurons, therefore effectively used for treatment of absence seizures.
- Phenytoin and valproate act on voltage-gated Na^+ channels to reduce glutamate release, thus block firing of neurons.

Surgery: The seizures associated with the temporal lobe are treated by surgical treatment.

Vagal nerve stimulation is effective in partial seizures.

Activation Activation is made to detect latent epilepsy, which cannot be detected by ordinary EEG recording. A flash stimulus, hyperventilation, sleep or drug administration is used to induce an epileptic attack.

2. Consciousness Dysfunction

A slow wave appears in the case of consciousness dysfunction according to the degree of seriousness. In the serious case, a general slow wave or delta wave prevails in the EEG waveform. In the more serious cases, the waveform becomes flat or sometimes disappears. However, there are many exceptions. Disturbances of consciousness include coma, syncope and stupor.

(i) ***Coma:*** Coma refers to a permanent state of sleep which is characterized by a loss of consciousness from which arousal cannot be elicited. It is produced by lesions blocking the connection between the ascending RAS and the thalamus.

- O_2 consumption of the brain is reduced in coma. This is in marked contrast to normal sleep, in which there is no change in brain O_2 consumption from the waking state.
- During state of coma, stimulation of sensory pathways can cause a momentary desynchronization of the EEG but does not produce any behavioural changes.

(ii) ***Syncope*** (fainting) refers to a transient pathological loss of consciousness.

(iii) ***Stupor*** is the more persistent loss of consciousness, from which arousal can be obtained.

3. Organic Brain Dysfunction

An abnormal wave appears when brain functional trouble occurs due to cerebral tumour, brain–blood vessel trouble (bleeding, clogging, artery/vein leakage, hardened brain artery, etc.) or brain injury caused by an external wound of the head. For example, in the case of brain tumour, no waveform is generated from the tumour part, but a slow wave is generated from the surrounding organization (Fig. 10.11.15). The EEG waveform shows the slow wave according to the seriousness of the brain functional trouble. When there is a tumour near the brain surface, a slow wave appears in accordance with that part and the waveform is of the irregular multiform. On the contrary, if there is a tumour deep in the brain, a monorhythmic high-amplitude slow wave like that of under the cortex or brainstem is seen. The slow wave increases as the tumour becomes serious.

4. Brain Death

Labelling brain death is important to fulfil the desire to obtain organs for transplant operations and to remove the life support system. *Criteria for labelling brain death* are as follows: the brain cells stop activity, the patient falls into a comatose state and finally respiration stops, the pupils are dilated, and the EEG waveform becomes flat in all channels and finally disappears. Most patients die in this state.

WAKEFULNESS AND SLEEP

WAKEFULNESS

The RAS of the RF is the neural substrate of the consciousness and sleep–waking cycle. As described earlier, RAS is a complex polysynaptic pathway that projects diffusely from the brainstem RF to the cerebral cortex, both directly and via the thalamus (for details, see page 927). The RAS is stimulated by impulses funnelling into it through the collaterals from the specific sensory pathways. The RAS, in turn, sends a strong facilitatory drive to the cerebral cortex, raising the background excitability and increasing the responsiveness of central neurons to specific stimuli. According to Dr Magoun, an American brain physiologist, projection of nonspecific stimuli by RAS to the cortex is responsible for wakefulness and alertness of the subject and the subject becomes fully conscious. When such impulse projection becomes less frequent, it is called sleep. When the pulse activity stops, it is called a dead sleep.

Neural Substrate for Wakefulness

In addition to the projections from the RAS, the wakefulness and consciousness are maintained by a continuous sensory input to the cortex from the visceral as well as somatic systems via the nonspecific thalamic system, subthalamus, hypothalamus and basal forebrain. This is proved by *cerveau isolé* (transections separating the cerebrum from the brainstem and spinal cord) which produces a sleep-like state with cortical slow waves. The neural substrates of wakefulness-generating systems are described briefly.

1. Reticular activating system RAS, as discussed above, is mainly responsible for the tonic maintenance of the cortical activation and behavioural arousal of the wakefulness. The cortical activation and behavioural arousal are controlled by two different mechanisms:

- Cortical activations without behavioural arousal are produced by the central tegmentum of the midbrain.
- Behavioural arousal without cortical activation is produced by the ventral tegmentum of the midbrain.

2. Thalamus The nonspecific thalamic system formed by the ventromedial, intralaminar and midline nuclei is involved in the activation of the entire cerebral cortex. These nuclei get tonic drive from the RF, and, in turn, project diffusely to the cerebral cortex.

3. Hypothalamus and subthalamus The ascending impulses from midbrain RF also relay to the cerebral cortex through the posterior hypothalamus and subthalamus. In addition, the posterior hypothalamus also acts as the waking centre, as its stimulation causes wakefulness. Conversely, lesions of the posterior hypothalamus result in coma.

4. Basal forebrain It comprises the nucleus basalis of Meynert (substantia innominata), nuclei of the diagonal band and septum. The basal forebrain receives impulses from the RF, and, in turn, project to the cerebral cortex and is responsible for cortical activation of wakefulness.

Chemical Mediators of Wakefulness

Chemical mediators of wakefulness include:

- Neurotransmitters
- CSF-borne peptides
- Blood-borne peptides

Neurotransmitters

1. Catecholamines Norepinephrine neurons of the locus coeruleus and brainstem, which project diffusely to the forebrain, including the cortex, play an integral role in the cortical activating system. This fact is corroborated by the following observations:

***L*-DOPA** (a precursor of catecholamine) has been reported to cause improvement in comatose states due to cerebral lesions.

Reserpine, a drug which depletes catecholamines in nerve terminals, induces drowsiness.

Amphetamine, a sympathomimetic amine, produces intense arousal and cortical activation.

Cocaine also produces increased arousal and alertness. It acts by blocking reuptake of norepinephrine at the nerve terminals.

2. Acetylcholine Cholinergic neurons, which contribute to wakefulness and cortical activation, can be divided into two major groups:

i. ***Neurons located in the caudal mesencephalic oral pontine RF:*** These project forward into the forebrain, particularly into the medial intralaminar thalamic nuclei, and also into the lateral hypothalamus and the frontal cortex.
ii. ***Neurons located within the basal forebrain*** consist of substantia innominata or the nucleus basalis of Meynert, nuclei of diagonal band and septum. These project to the entire cerebral cortex in a widespread manner.

Important Note

Role of cholinergic neurons in wakefulness is also corroborated by the following observations:

- *Cholinergic agonists and anticholinesterases* (e.g. neostigmine) promote cortical activation and wakefulness.
- *Acetylcholine (ACh) antagonist* like atropine produces a decrease in vigilance due to loss of cortical activation.
- *Alzheimer disease*, which is associated with loss of cholinergic innervation of the cerebral cortex and degeneration of cholinergic neurons of the basal forebrain, in addition to dementia, is also characterized by sleep disturbances.

3. Histamine The histamine-containing neurons are located in the posterior hypothalamus. These account for:

- Arousing effect produced by intraventricular administration of histamine
- Sedative effect produced by antihistaminic drugs

4. Glutamate It is an excitatory neurotransmitter released from the cerebral cortex in highest quantities during cortical activation of spontaneous waking or that induced by stimulation of the midbrain RF.

CSF-Borne Peptides

It has been presumed that wakefulness-promoting factors (probably peptides) are present in CSF, since CSF taken from a waking donor animal is reported to produce wakefulness and cortical activation in the recipient animal. Some of the CSF-borne peptides, which have been known to produce wakefulness, include:

- Substance P
- Hypothalamic releasing factors
- Vasoactive intestinal peptide (VIP)

Blood-Borne Peptides

Blood-borne peptides that act as wakefulness-promoting factors are as follows:

Epinephrine and histamine: These do not cross the blood–brain barrier but act on the circumventricular organs that lie outside the blood–brain barrier and mediate cortical arousal.

Glucocorticoids: These readily cross the blood–brain barrier and act directly on the neurons to enhance arousal in stress.

SLEEP

Sleep refers to a state of unconsciousness from which the individual can be aroused by sensory or other stimuli. When asleep, an individual is not aware of the environment and is unable to perform activities that require consciousness. During sleep, the stimulus pulse transfer becomes less frequent between the RF and the cerebral cortex.

Factors Affecting Sleep

Sleep time remains fairly stable from day to day even under widely varying conditions, and is only modestly affected by variations in activity and sensory stimulation. However, the factors which minimize sensory stimulation and favour the onset of natural sleep are as follows:

- Darkened room
- Comfortable surrounding temperature
- Silence
- Physical and mental relaxation
- Satiation of a basic urge such as hunger or sex
- Low-frequency stimulation, such as by patting, rocking in a cradle or sitting in a moving vehicle

The above-described factors have only a modest effect, if any. The only behavioural factor that reliably and substantially increases sleep is prior sleeplessness. On the other hand, anxiety and emotional stimuli by release of epinephrine cause activation of RAS and make sleep more difficult.

Types and Stages of Sleep

Sleep is of two types – NREM sleep and rapid eye movement (REM) sleep, which alternate in a sleep cycle. The presence of sleep can be assessed by behavioural analysis and more accurately by electrical records of physiological activities during sleep.

Behaviourally, sleep is defined by four criteria:

- Reduced motor activity
- Decreased response to stimulation
- Stereotypic postures (in humans, e.g. lying down with eyes closed)
- Relatively easy reversibility (distinguishing it from coma and hibernation)

Polysomnography refers to electrical records of physiological indicators of sleep, which include:

- *Electroencephalography* (EEG) that measures the collective activity of cortical neurons. EEG changes of sleep are described in detail.
- *Electromyography* (EMG), which monitors the muscle activity. The motor unit potential shows a gradual diminution as sleep approaches.
- *Electro-oculography* (EOG) that monitors the eye movements. EOG shows slow eye movements (SEMs) as sleep approaches. These generally disappear within several minutes of the EEG changes. REMs are recorded during REM sleep.

Non-REM Sleep

NREM sleep is also known as *slow-wave sleep* (SWS), because in this type of sleep, brain waves are very slow.

In normal adults, sleep mostly begins with NREM sleep. It is a rest type of sleep which a person experiences during the first hour of sleep after having been awake for many hours. The NREM sleep alternates with REM sleep during the sleep cycle.

The NREM sleep is discussed under the following headings:

- Stages and EEG patterns of NREM sleep
- Physiological changes during NREM sleep
- Behavioural changes during NREM sleep
- Intellectual changes during NREM sleep

Stages and EEG Stages and EEG patterns of non-REM sleep are given next.

Stage of wakefulness As described above, the state of wakefulness and consciousness results due to stimulatory impulses from RAS to the cerebral cortex.

EEG pattern during wakefulness is characterized by asynchronous and low-amplitude brain waves called beta waves (Fig. 10.11.16A).

State of quiet, wakeful rest with eyes closed State of quiet, wakeful rest with eyes closed is the period in between the stage of wakefulness and stage of sleep.

EEG pattern during quiet wakeful resting stage, as described earlier (page 1064), is characterized by alpha waves, which are highly synchronized, large waves having a frequency of 8–13 cycles/s (Fig. 10.11.16B).

State of non-REM sleep When an individual from the state of quiet rest with eyes closed enters the state of NREM sleep, the consciousness is reduced. The NREM sleep, also known as SWS, progresses in an orderly way from light to deep sleep in four stages:

Stage 1 of NREM sleep (stage of very light sleep): EEG pattern in this stage is characterized by low-amplitude mixed-frequency activity (Fig. 10.11.16C). There is still considerable sensitivity to sensory stimuli. However, the mild-to-moderate stimuli are often unable to produce a full arousal; instead, they produce a sharp electronegative wave at the vertex called *vertex sharp wave* or *V-wave*.

Stage 2 of NREM sleep, also called stage of light sleep, is characterized by appearance of sleep spindles. These are bursts of alpha-like 10- to 14-Hz, 50-μV waves which periodically interrupt the alpha rhythm (Fig. 10.11.16D).

- Auditory stimuli during this phase readily evoke the K-complexes in the EEG. They also occur spontaneously during this stage. The K-complex consists of one or two high-voltage waves followed by a brief 14-Hz activity (Fig. 10.11.16D).

Stage 3 of NREM sleep or stage of moderate deep sleep is characterized by an EEG that displays high-amplitude slow (0.5–2 Hz) waves (Fig. 10.11.16E).

Stage 4 of NREM sleep or stage of deep sleep produces an EEG pattern characterized by dome-like, very slow, large waves called *delta waves* (Fig. 10.11.16F). Thus, the characteristics of

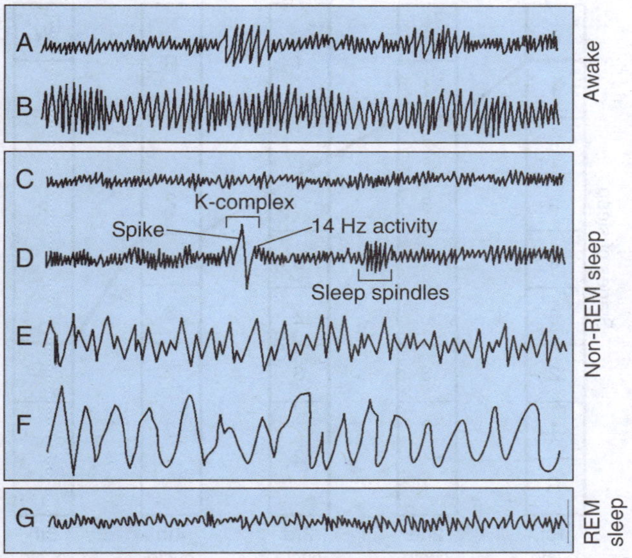

Fig. 10.11.16 EEG patterns of wakefulness and different stages of sleep: **A**, during wakefulness; **B**, during quiet wakeful resting; **C**, during stage 1 of non-REM sleep; **D**, during stage 2 of non-REM sleep; **E**, during stage 3 of non-REM sleep; **F**, during stage 4 of non-REM sleep; **G**, during stage of REM sleep. EEG, electroencephalogram; REM, rapid eye movement.

deep sleep are a pattern of rhythmic slow waves, indicating marked *synchronization*.

Physiological changes during non-REM sleep are as follows:

- Muscle tone decreases progressively.
- Heart rate and blood pressure are decreased.
- Respiration rate is also decreased.
- Eyes begin slow, rolling movement until they finally stop in stage 4 (deep sleep) with eyes turned upwards.
- Body metabolism is lowered.
- Pituitary shows pulsatile release of growth hormones and gonadotropin.

Behavioural changes during non-REM sleep: Behaviourally, the NREM sleep is characterized by:

- Progressive reduction in consciousness occurs.
- An increasing resistance to being awakened occurs; it is more difficult to wake up a person from stages 3 and 4 than from stages 1 and 2 of NREM sleep.
- It is more difficult to wake up a young person than the elderly from sleep, because the elderly person spends very little time in stages 3 and 4 of NREM stage.
- When awakened, the person does not report dreaming.
- Response to visual stimuli is present in <15% of the time during stages 1 and 2.
- Auditory reaction times become longer as stage 1 sleep approaches. At the sleep onset, the auditory response is absent.
- There is some response to meaningful stimuli even in sleep, which indicates that sensory processing continues at some level after the onset of sleep. This is apparent from the *discriminate responses* during sleep to meaningful versus non-meaningful stimuli. Examples of discriminate responses are as follows:
  - There is a lower arousal threshold for one's own name than for someone else's name.
  - A sleeping mother is more likely to hear her own baby's cry than the cry of an unrelated infant.
  - A captain wakes up to the cry of 'iceberg' in the midst of the din and bustle of a ship.

Intellectual functions during non-REM sleep During NREM sleep, thoughts become illogical and incoherent towards the onset of sleep.

Retrograde amnesia occurs during transition from wakefulness to sleep. This is because sleep inactivates the consolidation of short-term into long-term memory. Examples of retrograde amnesia include:

- Inability to grasp the instant of sleep onset in memory
- Not remembering the ringing of alarm clock
- Morning amnesia for coherent sleep talking
- Poor recall of midnight dreams

Memory for the few minutes before sleep is lost, if sleep persists for approximately 10 minutes. Patients suffering from syndromes of excessive sleepiness may experience similar memory problems in the daytime if sleep becomes intrusive.

REM Sleep

REM sleep is also called 'fast-wave (desynchronized) sleep', or 'paradoxical sleep' or 'dream sleep' or 'deepest sleep' (as explained below). In adults, the REM sleep follows NREM sleep, whereas their entry into sleep occurs via REM sleep.

EEG pattern of REM sleep During REM sleep, EEG is characterized by a high-frequency and low-amplitude pattern (β rhythm), i.e. some desynchronized pattern that is seen in the waking state (Fig. 10.11.16G). Hence, REM sleep is also called 'fast-wave sleep' or 'desynchronized sleep'. However, the individual clearly is unresponsive to environment stimuli, and thus is asleep. Furthermore, it is usually more difficult to awaken in REM sleep than in NREM sleep. Because of the EEG pattern of wakefulness, the REM is also called 'paradoxical sleep'.

In cats, REM sleep is also associated with ponto-geniculo-occipital (PGO) waves. The PGO waves are not detectable in humans by scalp EEG, but are recordable by depth EEG recordings. These waves originate in the pons and pass rapidly to the lateral geniculate body and then to the cerebral cortex and hence the name PGO. These waves activate the reticular inhibiting area in the medulla producing hypotonia.

Behavioural changes during REM sleep are as follows:

- *Arousal:* As mentioned above, it is difficult to arouse an individual from REM sleep as it is from deep sleep.
- However, when awakened from REM sleep, the individual is immediately alert and aware of the environment. *Dreaming* occurs during REM sleep, so it is also called 'dream sleep'. There is vivid dream recall from approximately 80% of arousals from REM sleep.

Physiological changes during REM sleep are as follows:

REMs are the hallmark of this state of sleep and that is why the name REM sleep. REMs (saccadic eye movements) are bursts of small jerky movements that bring the eye from one fixation point to another to allow a sweeping of visual images of dreams.

Heart rate and respiration rate become irregular.

Muscle tone is reduced due to inhibition of spinal motor neurons via brainstem mechanisms. Snoring during sleep results from partial obstruction of airways caused by a relaxed tongue (due to muscular atonia) in supine position.

Twitching of limb musculature occurs occasionally. Because muscle tone is reduced tremendously during REM sleep, frequency and intensity of muscle twitching does not produce injuries or awaken the individual.

Middle ear muscles are also active during REM sleep.

Penile erection in males and engorgement of clitoris in females may occur during REM sleep.

Impaired thermoregulation: Sweating or shivering during sleep in response to ambient temperature occurs in NREM sleep and ceases in REM sleep.

Teeth grinding (bruxism) may be seen in children.

Sleep Cycle

In a normal adult, the average sleep period of about 7–8 hours is divided into approximately five cycles during which NREM sleep and REM sleep alternate with each other. There is an orderly progression of sleep states and stages during a typical sleep cycle as described in the subsequent text (Fig. 10.11.17).

- *Sleep onset* in normal adults usually occurs with NREM sleep.
- *Stage 1 (very light sleep)* of NREM sleep is initiated after a state of drowsiness as soon as an individual falls asleep.
- *Stage 2 (light sleep), stage 3 (moderate deep sleep)* and stage 4 (deep sleep) of NREM sleep are then reached progressively during the next hour or so. After approximately 15 minutes of deep sleep, the depth of sleep starts to decrease progressively from stage 4 to 1.
- *State of REM sleep* is then reached (after about 90 minutes of NREM sleep during the first sleep cycle). After the end of REM sleep (5 minutes), the first cycle is completed and is followed by the next sleep cycles (about five cycles during normal sleep of about 7 hours).
- Transition from sleep to the awake state occurs either at the end of REM sleep or at the end of the second stage of NREM sleep of the last sleep cycle.

Duration of sleep cycles and sleep stages

The average duration of each sleep cycle is about 90 minutes (range 70–120 minutes). Duration of different sleep stages is different in different cycles as (Fig. 10.11.18):

- Duration of NREM sleep, which is about 85 minutes (out of total 90 minutes) in the first cycle, decreases progressively in the subsequent sleep cycles.
- About 25% of the entire sleep period is passed in REM sleep.
- Duration of REM sleep, which is about 5 minutes (out of total 90 minutes) in the first cycle, increases progressively in the next cycle.

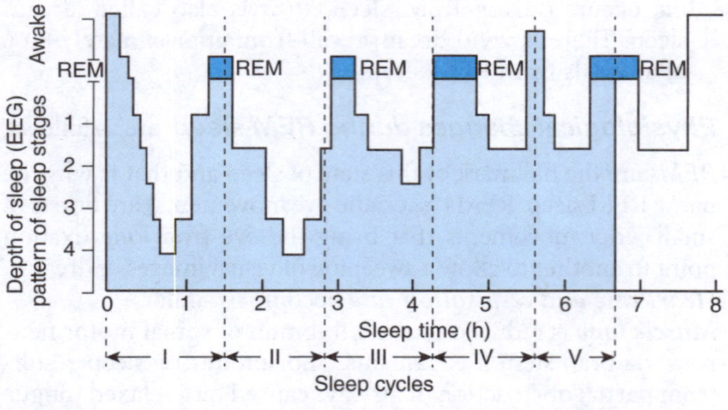

Fig. 10.11.17 Typical sleep cycles in an adult individual.

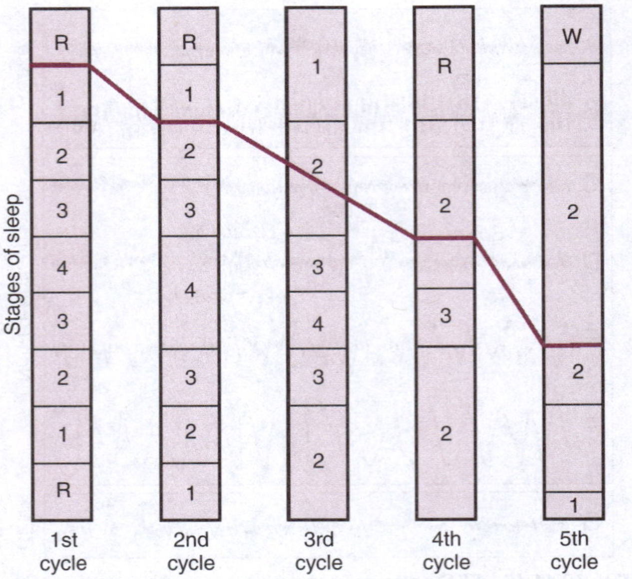

Fig. 10.11.18 Duration of different stages of non-REM sleep and REM sleep. Note that all the five sleep cycles have been shown of equal duration just for comparative depiction of duration in percentage of different stages. However, in reality, the cycle varies in duration. R, REM sleep; REM, rapid eye movement; W, wake.

- Duration of deeper stages (3 and 4) of NREM sleep is maximum during the first cycle and then decreases progressively and may even disappear altogether from the later cycles.
- Duration of the second stage of NREM sleep increases progressively from the first cycle onwards and may even occupy most of the NREM portion of later cycles. About 50% of the entire sleep period is spent in the second stage of NREM sleep.
- As morning approaches, the individual may be periodically awakened during later sleep cycles.
- The approximate duration (%) of different stages of sleep during the first cycle and during the entire sleep is given in Table 10.11.3.

Variations in sleep cycles

Variations in sleep cycle, from the typical adult pattern depicted in Figs 10.11.17 and 10.11.18, occur under certain circumstances. In adults, onset of sleep with REM sleep occurs under special circumstances such as in jetlag, chronic sleep deprivation, narcolepsy, acute withdrawal of REM-suppressing drugs and endogenous depressions.

Table 10.11.3 Approximate duration of different stages of sleep in first sleep cycle and during entire sleep

Stage of sleep	First cycle (%)	Entire sleep (%)
Non-REM sleep		
Stage 1	5	4
Stage 2	20	50
Stage 3	30	6
Stage 4	40	15
REM sleep	5	25

REM, rapid eye movement.

Variations in total sleep duration Average sleep time per day differs according to the age:

- During infancy: 16 hours
- During childhood: 10 hours
- During adulthood: 7–8 hours
- During old age: <8 hours

Variation in time period of different stages of sleep occurs due to the following:

Effects of age on sleep cycle are as follows:

- Prematurely born infants spend about 80% of their sleep time in REM sleep.
- Full-term infants spend only 50% of their sleep time in REM sleep.
- The total time spent in REM sleep is reduced to about 1.5–2 hours by puberty and remains unchanged thereafter.
- From the above, it is clear that the reduction in sleep time from 16 hours in infants (8 hours REM and 8 hours NREM sleep) to 10 hours during childhood (2 hours REM and 8 hours NREM sleep) occurs almost entirely by a reduction of the amount of time spent in REM sleep (Fig. 10.11.19).
- In adulthood, reduction in total sleep time to 8 hours (2 hours REM and 6 hours NREM sleep) from 10 hours in childhood is by a reduction in the time spent in deep stages of NREM sleep (Fig. 10.11.19).
- *In old age*, there is very high variability in the type and duration of sleep. By the age of 60 years, SWS may no longer be present, particularly in men. Women appear to maintain SWS later in life than men. REM sleep as a percentage of total sleep is maintained well in healthy old age.

Effects of prior sleep deprivation are as follows:

- *Following differentially deprived of REM or SWS*, a preferential rebound of that stage of sleep will occur when natural sleep is resumed.
- *Following a total sleep loss of one or more nights*, SWS tends to be recovered first. REM sleep tends to recover only after the recuperation of SWS.

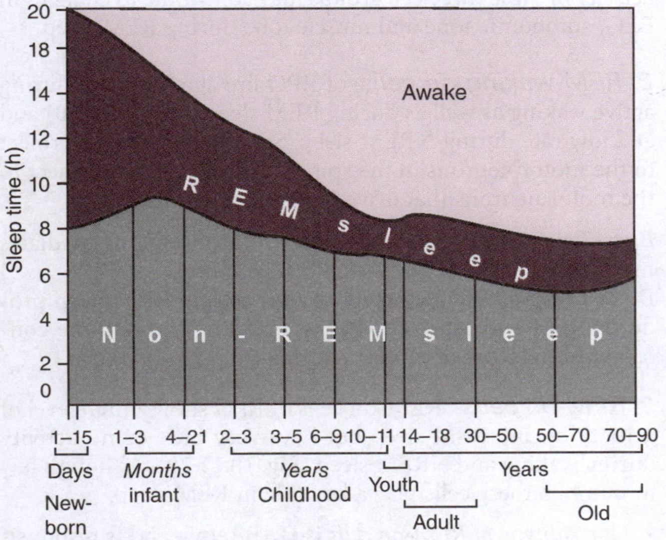

Fig. 10.11.19 Variation of total period of wakefulness, non-REM sleep and REM sleep with age. REM, rapid eye movement.

- *Recovery sleep*, whether following differential or total sleep loss, is usually deeper than basal sleep, i.e. it has a higher arousal threshold throughout NREM and REM sleep.

Effect of temperature Sleep in general and REM sleep in particular are disrupted by extremes of temperature.

Effect of circadian rhythms The distribution of sleep stages is affected by the time of the day/night at which sleep occurs first. Since REM sleep peaks in the morning hours, if sleep onset is delayed until morning, REM sleep will tend to predominate and may even occur at the onset of sleep.

Effects of drugs are as follows:

- *Benzodiazepines* (such as diazepam) reduce NREM sleep (SWS).
- *Barbiturates, tricyclic antidepressants and monoamine oxidase* inhibitors (MAOIs) reduce REM sleep.
- *Alcohol* intake immediately before sleep produces REM suppression early in the night.

Genesis of Sleep

The sleep state does not result from the passive withdrawal of arousal due to fatigue of RAS as thought earlier. Now, it is established that the sleep is produced by an active process which is different for NREM sleep and REM sleep.

Genesis of non-REM Sleep

The NREM sleep is generated by interaction of neurons, which are grouped as:

- Diencephalic sleep zone
- Medullary synchronizing zone
- Basal forebrain sleep zone

Diencephalic sleep zone lies in the hypothalamus and the nearby intralaminar and anterior thalamic nuclei. *A sleep facilitatory centre* is considered to be located in the anterior hypothalamus, as its stimulation causes sleep. The posterior hypothalamus acts as a *waking centre*, as its stimulation causes wakefulness. *The diencephalic sleep zone must be stimulated at a low frequency (about 8 Hz) to produce sleep.*

Medullary synchronizing zone is in the RF of the medulla oblongata at the level of the *nucleus of the tractus solitarius* (NTS). Like diencephalic sleep zone, this zone also produces sleep when stimulated at a *low frequency*.

Basal forebrain sleep zone includes the *preoptic area and the diagonal band of Broca*. Unlike the other two zones, stimulation of this zone at low, as well as high, frequency produces sleep.

Activity of non-REM on cells The NREM on cells is due to GABAergic inhibitory neurons that mediate sleep-inducing action of the above-described sleep zones. These cells are thought to produce sleep by inhibiting the histaminergic cells in the posterior hypothalamus as well as cells of the nucleus reticularis pontis oralis (RPO) in the midbrain that mediate arousal. They are maximally active in NREM sleep and inactive during waking and REM sleep (Fig. 10.11.20). Many NREM on cells are activated by heat and thus may mediate the *sleep-inducing effects of elevated temperature.*

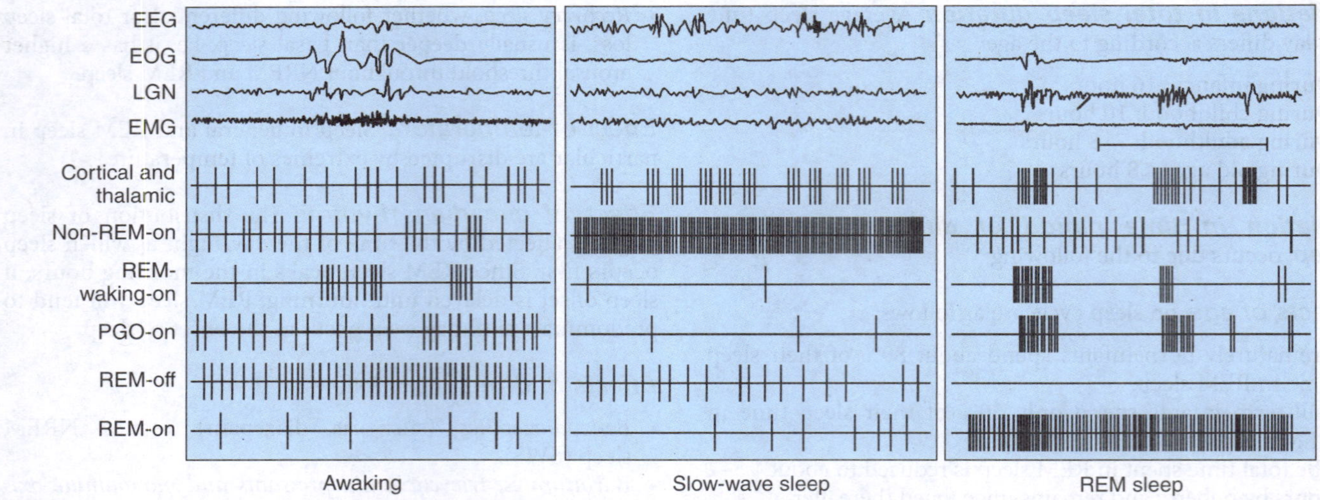

Fig. 10.11.20 The pattern of activity of key cell groups during waking and slow-wave and REM sleep. Each vertical line represents an action potential. EEG, electroencephalogram; EMG, electromyography of dorsal neck cell; EOG, electro-oculogram depicting eye movement; LGN, recording from lateral geniculate nucleus showing ponto-geniculo-occipital (PGO) spike activity during REM sleep; REM, rapid eye movement.

Mechanism of production of sleep spindles and slow waves of non-REM sleep The NREM sleep is characterized by EEG spindles and slow waves that are produced by synchronized postsynaptic potentials in the cortical neurons. These synchronized synaptic potentials are generated by the rhythmic firing of thalamic relay neurons that project to the cortex (Fig. 10.11.20). The rhythmic firing of relay neurons is a result of action of GABAergic inhibitory neurons in the nucleus reticularis that forms a shell around the thalamus.

Genesis of REM sleep

REM sleep is generated by the interaction of neurons in the caudal midbrain and pons with the neurons in the medulla and forebrain.

REM sleep as described earlier is characterized by:

- Blockage of EEG spindles and slow waves
- Occurrence of PGO waves
- Muscle atonia
- Phasic motor action

Genesis of the above components of REM sleep is discussed.

Role of cholinergic neurons of midbrain and the adjacent dorsal pons These cells form an important component of the midbrain arousal system and are maximally active during waking and REM sleep. Their activity contributes to the blocking of the slow waves of EEG ACh, and other transmitters released by these cells depolarize the GABAergic inhibitory neurons in the reticularis nucleus. This depolarization prevents the hyperpolarization that activates the low-threshold Ca^{2+} channels, which in turn initiate the rhythmic firing of the reticular neurons. In the absence of rhythmic firing of the reticular neurons, the thalamocortical relay cells fire only asynchronously, and this asynchronous activity results in the low-voltage EEG, characteristic of waking and REM sleep.

Role of nucleus reticularis pontis oralis The nucleus RPO forms another important neuronal machinery for genesis of REM sleep. Three classes of neurons in the RPO of particular interest are as follows:

1. Cholinergic PGO-on cells: The discharge of these neurons produces the so-called PGO spikes that are characteristic of REM sleep (Fig. 10.11.20). The term PGO spikes comes from the fact that they originate in the lateral pontine tegmentum and pass rapidly to the lateral geniculate body and thence to the occipital cortex.

Regulation of PGO-on cells: The PGO-on cells are regulated by serotonergic REM-off cells (Fig. 10.11.20) in the raphe nuclei of the brainstem, noradrenergic neurons in the locus coeruleus and histaminergic neurons in the posterior hypothalamus. All these neurons contribute to wakefulness and block the activity of PGO-on cells during waking. However, in the transition from NREM to REM sleep, all these neurons remain silent and allow the PGO-on cells to begin discharging in bursts generating PGO spikes. It appears that cessation of activity in these three cell groups may contribute to changes in EEG, autonomic tone and muscle tone during REM sleep.

2. REM-waking-on cells of RPO fire at a high rate during active waking as well as during REM sleep (Fig. 10.11.20) and at a low rate during NREM sleep. Some of these cells project to the motor neurons in the spinal cord, and others project to the motor neurons that drive the extraocular muscles.

Burst firing of REM-waking-on cells during waking mediates movements of the head, neck, limbs and eyes.
Burst firing of REM-waking-on cells during REM sleep produces REM and muscle twitches, breaking through the concurrent inhibition of motor neurons.

3. REM-on cells: REM-on cells of RPO show a high level of activity during REM sleep but have very little or no activity during waking and NREM sleep (Fig. 10.11.20). Although few in number, these cells play a key role in REM sleep.

- *One subtype of REM-on cells* is GABAergic and is responsible for inhibition of activity in serotonergic and noradrenergic cells during REM sleep.

- *Another subtype of REM-on cells* is possibly glutamatergic and is responsible for loss of muscle tone in REM sleep.

Important Note

Important points to be noted:
- *Reserpine*, a drug which depletes serotonin and catecholamines, blocks SWS and some aspects of REM sleep but increases PGO spike activity.
- *Barbiturates* decrease the amount of REM sleep.

Chemical Mediators of Sleep

Neurotransmitters employed by neurons forming the neural substrate of sleep as discussed above include:
- Serotonin
- ACh
- Noradrenaline

Endogenous sleep-producing substance (S/S): For nearly a century, sleep researchers have searched for substances that might be responsible for induction of sleep. However, no endogenous substance is yet widely accepted as causing sleep. The substances that have been identified by experiments on sleep-deprived animals as S/S are as follows:
- *Muramyl dipeptide* (MDP), a chemical related to substances found in bacterial cell walls
- *Interleukin-1* (IL-1), a cytokine that may mediate the effects of MDPs as well as immune response
- *Adenosine*
- *Delta sleep-inducing peptide* (DSIP), a substance isolated from the blood of sleeping rabbits
- *Prostaglandin* D_2
- *Arginine vasotocin (AVT)*

Physiological Significance of Sleep

Sleep is an indispensable phenomenon. Its physiological significance is highlighted.

1. ***Sleep may serve as a period of body's rest and metabolic restoration*** as evidenced by the following physiological changes during NREM sleep:
   - Pulsatile release of growth hormone and gonadotropins from the pituitary
   - Decrease in blood pressure, heart rate and respiration
2. ***Sleep is necessary for certain forms of learning.*** In experimental animals, learning sessions do not improve performance until a period of SWS or SWS plus REM sleep has occurred. However, it is not known why sleep is necessary, and there is as yet no clinical correlate to this experimental observation.
3. ***REM sleep is necessary for mental well-being.*** The correlation between dreaming and REM sleep indicates that the brain is highly active at this time. This may allow for the expression, through dreams, of concern in the subconscious and for long-term chemical and structural changes that the brain must undergo to make learning and memory possible.
4. ***REM sleep plays an important role in homeostatic mechanism.*** It is evident from the observation that when the experimental animals are completely deprived of REM sleep for long periods, they lose weight in spite of increased caloric intake and finally die.

Sleep–Wake Cycle and Factors Affecting Sleep

Sleep and wakefulness, like many of the body's regulatory mechanisms, have a circadian rhythm of about 24 hours. A newborn infant has many cycles of sleep and wakefulness in 24 hours, but after the age of 2 years, a single sleep–wake cycle is established. In a normal adult, the sleep–wake cycle consists of 7–8 hours of sleep and 16–17 hours of wakefulness.

Control of Sleep–Wake Cycle

Sleep–wake cycle, like other circadian rhythms, is endogenous. The biological clock controlling the circadian rhythms is the *suprachiasmatic nucleus* of the anterior hypothalamus. The circadian rhythms are endogenous and can persist without environmental cues; however, under normal circumstances, the rhythms are modulated by external timing cues called *zeitgebers* (time givers) that adapt the rhythm to the environment. Sunlight is a powerful timing cue. Light entrains this rhythm by means of the *retinohypothalamic tract*. Although the suprachiasmatic nucleus regulates the timing of sleep, it is not responsible for sleep itself.

Neurochemical mechanisms Transition between sleep and wakefulness manifests as circadian rhythm. The RAS of the brainstem is composed of a group of neurons (locus coeruleus and raphe nuclei) that releases norepinephrine, serotonin or ACh. When the activity of these neurons increases, there is decreased activity of ACh-containing neurons of the pontine RF. This pattern of neuronal activity is responsible for the awake state, whereas reverse of this pattern is responsible for REM sleep.

NREM sleep occurs when there is greater even balance (i.e. increase in GABA and decrease in histamine) that promotes NREM sleep via deactivation of the thalamocortical neurons (Fig. 10.11.21). Posterior hypothalamic neurons produce orexin that is considered to be an important factor for switching between sleep and awake state.

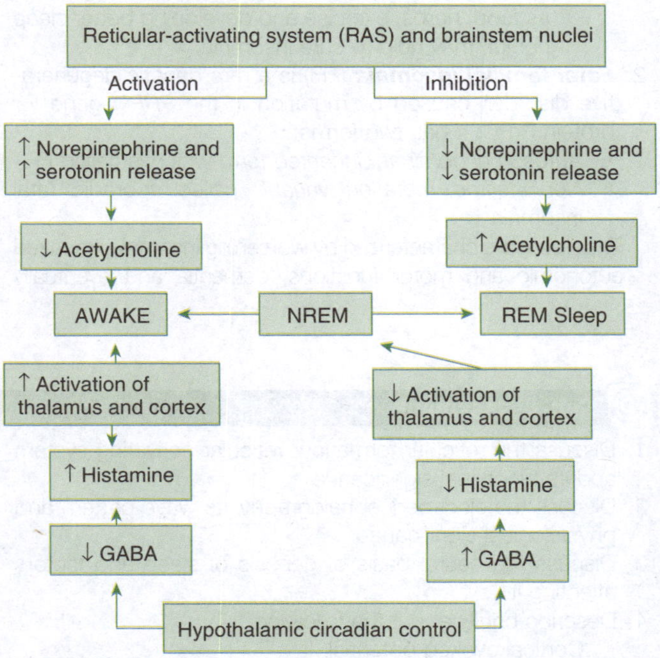

Fig. 10.11.21 Alternating activity of brainstem and hypothalamic neurons influencing sleep and wake cycle.

Applied Aspects

Sleep Disorders

1. ***Insomnia*** refers to an inability to have sufficient or restful sleep despite an adequate opportunity for sleep. It is a subjective problem that occurs at one time or another in almost all adults.

   Types of insomnia: There are two types of insomnia:

   Primary insomnia: It means that a person is having sleep problems which are not directly associated with any another health condition.

   Secondary insomnia: It means that a person is having sleep problems due to other associated health problems like asthma, depression and arthritis or due to intake of certain drugs.

   Causes of insomnia include:
   - Significant life stress
   - Illness
   - Emotional discomfort
   - Environmental factors such as noise, light and extreme variations in temperature
   - Medications used as a part of treatment of other diseases – hypertension, asthma, etc.
   - Interference with normal sleep schedule (jet lag)
   - Pain

   Signs and symptoms include:
   - Sleepiness during the daytime
   - General fatigue/tiredness
   - Irritability
   - Inability to concentrate and memory disturbances

   Treatment: Insomnia can be relieved temporarily by sleeping pills, especially benzodiazepines. Prolonged use of these drugs can be habit-forming and can compromise daytime performance.
   - Melatonin – might be helpful to regulate sleep–wake cycle
   - Magnesium – also plays a key role with sleep
   - *Sleeping habits and natural insomnia remedies*, such as food, herbs, exercise and developing better sleep habits, may help to cure insomnia.

2. ***Fatal familial insomnia*** (FFI) is a rare genetic degenerative disorder, caused by mutation in the *PRPN* gene for protein PrPC. It has two forms:
   - *Autosomal dominant inherited form* which is called FFI
   - *Noninherited mutation variant*, called sporadic fatal insomnia

   The disease is characterized by worsening insomnia, impaired autonomic and motor functions, dementia and eventually death. It is a progressive disease that occurs in both an inherited and a sporadic form.

3. ***Narcolepsy*** refers to an irresistible urge to sleep. As mentioned in the section 'Sleep Cycle', in adults, the sleep onset occurs with NREM sleep, which is followed by REM sleep. However, in narcolepsy, REM sleep is entered directly from the waking states.

   Causes: The main cause of narcolepsy is deficiency or lack of hypocretin (neurochemical), also known as orexin, which regulates sleep.

   Signs and symptoms: Narcolepsy may manifest as:

   Episodes of sudden sleep: The individuals go to sleep while performing daytime tasks.

   Cataplexy: In some narcoleptics, the profound reduction in muscle tone characteristic of REM sleep can occur without loss of consciousness. During such an attack, called cataplexy, the individual suddenly becomes paralysed, falls to the ground and is unable to move.

   Dream-like state during wakefulness is another mode of manifestation of narcolepsy. Narcoleptics describe it as a hallucination.

4. ***Some sleep disorders associated with NREM sleep (SWS)***, or, more specifically, occurring during arousal from SWS, are as follows:

   Sleepwalking (somnambulism): Episodes of sleepwalking are more common in children than in adults and occur predominantly in males. These episodes may last for several minutes. Such individuals walk with their eyes open and avoid obstacles, but when awakened, they cannot recall the episode.

   Bed-wetting (nocturnal enuresis), i.e. involuntary voiding of urine, occurs in some children during SWS.

   Nightmares (pavor nocturnus or episodes of night terror): During a nightmare that occurs in SWS, the individual wakes up screaming and appears terrified. However, no reason for acute anxiety is recalled. By contrast, terrifying dreams that occur during REM sleep are graphically remembered.

5. ***REM behaviour disorder:*** It is a newly recognized condition in which REM sleep is not associated with inhibition of muscle tone. Consequently, such persons act out their dreams, i.e. they thrash about and may even jump out of bed, ready to do battle with imagined aggression. The generalized or localized muscle contraction associated with vivid visual imagery, i.e. the motor response to some of the dream events, is referred to as *hypnic myoclonia*.

Self-Assessment

1. Discuss the reticular formation, reticular activating system and its functional significance.
2. Discuss the electroencephalography, its wave pattern and physiological significance.
3. Discuss the neural basis of genesis of sleep and factors affecting it.
4. Describe briefly about the following:
   - Cortical evoked potential
   - EEG changes during REM and non-REM sleep
5. Write notes on the following:
   - Alpha block
   - Wakefulness
   - Sleep cycle
   - Narcolepsy

Clinical Cases

Case 1

A 50-year-old female was presented by a family member in the emergency department with loss of consciousness and sudden jerky body movements. On regaining consciousness, the patient's history revealed that while she was sitting in her lawn on the chair and taking morning coffee, suddenly she felt light-headedness and then she could not remember.

According to the family member, her eyes were rolled upwards on one side; the family member helped her to lie down on the bed, and then the jerky types of movements started.

On the physical examination, no abnormal finding was noticed, and the vital and biochemical findings were within the normal range. The probable diagnosis made was a case of epilepsy and the patient was advised EEG.

Q1. What changes in EEG are expected in this case?
Q2. What are the types of epilepsy?
Q3. What is the pathophysiology of epilepsy?
Q4. What is the treatment plan for epilepsy?

Case 2

A 35-year-old female met with an accident and was on life support system in ICU for the last 5 months. The family members had a desire for her organ donation to needy patients.

Q1. To remove life support system and to label the patient brain dead, what criteria should be followed?

Case 3

An 18-year-old boy had a fall from his roof and was brought to the emergency in an unconscious state. There was no sign of internal or external injury and blood loss. On examination, he did not respond to sensory stimulation. The attending physician declared that the patient was in coma.

Q1. What are the EEG findings suggestive of coma?
Q2. Which part of the brain lesion causes this state?
Q3. How is coma state different from deep sleep?

Case 4

A 21-year-old male medical student complains of inability to sleep well for the last 1 year in the night and feeling lot of tiredness in the daytime and does not feel alert and cannot concentrate on studies.

Q1. What is this condition called?
Q2. What are the types of this condition?
Q3. Is any family history related to this condition?
Q4. What is the treatment basis?

10.12 Some Higher Functions of Nervous System

CHAPTER OUTLINE

LANGUAGE AND SPEECH

NEUROPHYSIOLOGY OF LANGUAGE AND SPEECH

Communication through language is a unique faculty, which places the humans much above the animals. Language refers to that faculty of nervous system which enables the humans to understand the spoken and printed words, and to express ideas in the form of speech and writing. There are two aspects of communications – language input (the sensory aspect) and language output (the motor aspect). Sensory aspect of language includes the visual, auditory and proprioceptive impulses, whereas the motor aspect includes the mechanisms concerned with expression of spoken (sound) language and written language.

Components of Sound-Based Language

Before understanding neurophysiology of language, it will be worthwhile to become familiar with the different components of sound-based language which include phonemes, morphemes, syntax, lexicon, semantic, prosody and discourse. These components are applicable not only to sound-based but also to sign languages. For example, a morpheme in sign language would be the smallest meaningful movement.

Phonemes refer to the fundamental sounds in a language whose linking together in a particular order forms morphemes.
Morphemes, a combination of phonemes, are the smallest meaningful units of words. Morpheme may be a word itself or some morphemes may combine to form a word.
Words are made of syllables which include consonants and vowels. Use of syllables is a unique characteristic of human language.
Lexicon refers to collection of all words in a given language.
Syntax refers to linking together of different words by the use of verbs and appropriate choice of verb tenses, i.e. making a sentence (called rules of grammar in popular usage). Children develop syntax independent of formal training, which suggests that there is an innate basis for the development of human language.
Semantic refers to understanding the meaning of lexicons and syntaxes.
Discourse refers to linking together of sentences in such a way that they constitute a meaningful narrative.
Prosody refers to rise and fall of the pitch of the voice in speaking that can modify the literal meaning of words and sentences.

Wernicke's Theory of Language

To explain the mechanism of speech, Wernicke put forward a theory of language production in the brain (a neurological model of language), which was later revived by Gestiwind. This theory was formulated on the basis of defects in language observed in patients with lesions of different parts of the cortex. According to this theory, utterance arises in Wernicke's area and is passed on to Broca's area via the arcuate fasciculus. After the sentence is formulated in Broca's area, it is transferred to the motor cortex where the articulation is programmed by activation of appropriate muscles in the mouth and face, etc. The essentials of this theory have survived more than 100 years. However, modifications have been made in it regarding the areas in which lesions produce the distinct varieties of aphasia.

Development of Speech

Development of speech involves coordinated activity of three important areas of the cerebral cortex, namely Wernicke's area, Broca's area and motor areas of the categorical (dominant) hemisphere.

Development of speech in a child occurs in two stages.

First stage In this stage, there occurs an association of certain words with visual, tactile, auditory and other sensations, aroused by objects in the external world, which is stored in the memory.

Second stage This stage of development of speech involves establishment of new neuronal circuits. When a definite meaning has been attached to certain words, pathway between the auditory area (area 41) and the motor area for the muscles of articulation which helps in speech (area 44) is established. And the child attempts to formulate and pronounce the words, which are learnt.

Mechanism of Speech and Speech Centres

Speech is of two types – spoken and written.

Spoken speech involves both understanding of spoken words and expressing ideas in the form of spoken words.

Written speech also involves both understanding of written words and expression of ideas in the form of written words.

Mechanism of speech involves coordinated activities of the central speech apparatus and peripheral speech apparatus. The central speech apparatus consists of cortical and subcortical centres. The peripheral speech apparatus includes the larynx or sound box, pharynx, mouth, nasal cavities, tongue and lips. All the structures of the peripheral speech apparatus work in coordination with the respiratory system, under the influence of motor impulses from the respective motor areas of the cerebral cortex.

Mechanism of speech and the centres concerned with can be described separately for:

- Understanding of speech
- Expression of speech

Understanding of Speech (Sensory Aspects of Communication)

Different mechanisms are involved in the understanding of a spoken speech and written speech.

Understanding of spoken speech Understanding of the spoken words is accomplished by the following activities:

1. Hearing of the spoken words requires an intact auditory pathway from the ears to the primary auditory areas.

Primary auditory areas, also called auditory sensory areas, include the Brodmann areas 41 and 42 and form the centre for hearing.

- *Location:* Primary auditory areas are located in the middle of the superior temporal gyrus on the upper margin and on its deep or insular aspect (Fig. 10.12.1).

Connections: *Afferents* are received from the medial geniculate body (via auditory radiations) and pulvinar of the thalamus.

Efferents are sent to the medial geniculate body, superior colliculus and pulvinar.

Functions: This area perceives the nerve impulses as sound, i.e. auditory information such as loudness, pitch, source and direction of sound.

2. Recognition and understanding of the spoken words is carried by *auditory association areas* (21 and 20) located in the middle and inferior temporal gyrus, respectively

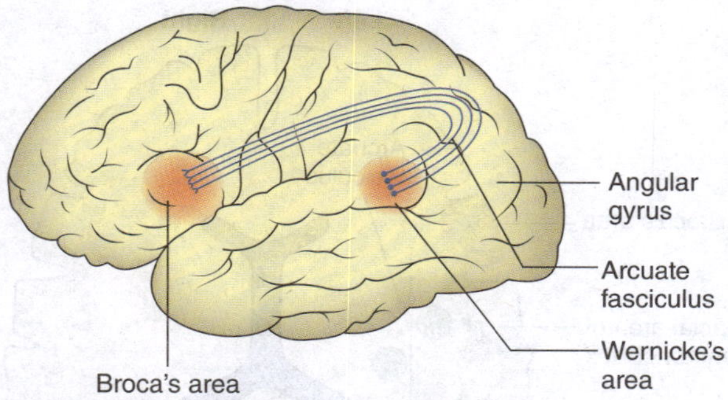

Fig. 10.12.1 Lateral surface of left (categorical) hemisphere showing location of primary areas of language.

(Fig. 10.12.1). These areas receive impulses from the primary area and are concerned with interpretation and integration of auditory impulses.

3. Interpretation and comprehension of the speech ideas: This involves the activities of *Wernicke's area.*

Wernicke's area (area 22) is a *sensory* speech centre, located in the posterior part of the superior temporal gyrus, behind the areas 41 and 42 (Fig. 10.12.1) in the categorical hemisphere, i.e. dominant hemisphere.

Functions of this area are as follows:

- Interpretation of the meaning of what is heard
- Comprehension of the spoken language and the formation of idea that are to be articulated in speech

Understanding of written speech Understanding of the written speech is accomplished by the following activities (Fig. 10.12.2):

1. Perception of written words requires an intact visual pathway from the eyes to the primary visual cortex.

Primary visual cortex, also called striate area (area 17), or the centre of vision lies on the medial surface of the occipital lobe in and near the calcarine sulcus occupying parts of the lingual gyrus and cuneus. It also extends to the superolateral surface of the occipital pole limited by the lunate sulcus.

Afferents to area 17 are fibres of the optic radiations, which bring impulses from parts of both retinae, and these parts are represented within the area in a specific orderly manner.

Functions: Primary visual cortex is concerned with perception of visual impulses.

2. Interpretation of written speech is by visual association areas.

Visual association areas (area 18 and 19), located in the walls and in front of the lunate sulcus, are concerned with the interpretation of written words. These areas are involved in the recognition and identification of the written words in the light of past experience.

3. Generation of thoughts/ideas in response to written speech:

Dejerine's area (area 38), located in the angular gyrus behind the Wernicke's area in the dominant hemisphere, is involved in the activity of generation of thoughts/ideas in response to

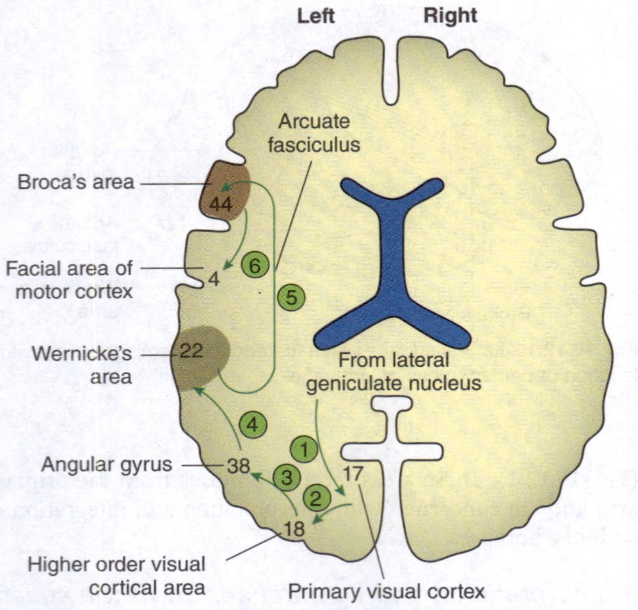

Fig. 10.12.2 Neural pathway in brain involved in the understanding and expression of written speech.

the written speech. This area is also called *visual speech centre* and along with the Wernicke's areas (auditory speech centre) forms the so-called sensory speech centre.

Expression of Speech (Motor Aspect of Communication)

Expression of speech in response to both spoken speech and written speech can be in the form of spoken speech or written speech or both. It involves the activities of *motor speech centres*, which include Broca's area (area 44) and Exner's area.

1. Expression in the form of spoken speech Expression in the form of spoken speech involves the activities of the motor speech (Broca's area) area.

Broca's area or motor speech area (area 44) is a special area of the premotor cortex situated in the inferior frontal gyrus.

Functions: This area, especially in the dominant hemisphere (left hemisphere in a right-handed person), processes the information received from the sensory speech centres (Wernicke's area and Dejerine's area) into a detailed and coordinated pattern for vocalization, which is then projected to the motor cortex for implementation. Thus, Broca's area is concerned with the movements of those structures which are responsible for the production of voice and articulation of speech, i.e. it causes activation of vocal cords simultaneously with movements of the mouth and tongue during speech; lesions of this area cause motor aphasia.

Important Note

- In adulthood, if a person learns a second language by fMRI, it is observed that a separate area lying adjacent to the Broca's area is involved for this action.
- Another observation revealed that if a person learns a second language in early life, then only single area is involved for both languages.

2. Expression in the form of written speech Expression in the form of written speech is the function of Exner's area (Fig. 10.12.2).

Exner's area (motor writing centre) is situated in the middle frontal gyrus in the categorical (dominant) hemisphere in the premotor cortex. It processes the information received from Broca's area into a detailed and coordinated pattern, and then along with the motor cortex (area 4) initiates the appropriate muscle movements of the hand and fingers to produce written speech.

Concept of Dominant Hemisphere for Language

In the human cerebral cortex, the interpretive functions of Wernicke's area, the angular gyrus and the frontal motor speech areas (i.e. the ability to understand or express oneself by spoken or written speech) are more highly developed in one hemisphere called the *dominant hemisphere*. How one hemisphere comes to be dominant is not yet understood. It is important to note that:

- In approximately 95% of all individuals, the left hemisphere is dominant regardless of handedness.
- Since the motor area concerned with the hand movements is closely associated with the centre for speech, this explains the right-handedness in more than 90% of the individuals.
- Right hemisphere dominance is seen in only 15% of left-handers.
- About 70% of left-handers also have left hemisphere dominance.
- The area in the nondominant hemisphere that corresponds to Wernicke's area is also involved in language function. It is responsible for understanding the emotional content or intonation of spoken language. It also serves equally important functions of understanding and interpreting nonverbal, visual or auditory experiences such as recognition of visual patterns or faces and interpretation of music.

Concept of Categorical and Representational Hemispheres

Presently, it is believed that the left hemisphere is not really dominant over the right hemisphere. In fact, the two halves of the brain have independent capabilities of consciousness, memory storage and control of motor activities and speech. The corpus callosum and anterior commissure connect the two halves of the brain. By these connections, information stored in one hemisphere is made available to the other hemisphere and then the activities of two hemispheres are coordinated.

As summarized in the subsequent text, some specialized higher functions are allowed to each hemisphere. Therefore, the terms 'dominant' and 'nondominant' have been replaced by *categorical* and *representational* hemisphere, respectively.

Functions allotted to left hemisphere in right-handed person Functions allotted to the left hemisphere in a right-handed person are as follows:

- Right-hand control
- Spoken language
- Written language
- Mathematical skills
- Scientific skills
- Reasoning

Functions allotted to right hemisphere in a right-handed person Functions allotted to the right hemisphere in a right-handed person are as follows:

- Left-hand control
- Music awareness
- Three-dimensional awareness
- Art awareness
- Insight
- Imagination

Applied Aspects

Speech Disorders

1. Dysarthria

Dysarthria is a disorder of speech in which articulation of words is impaired, but the comprehension of spoken and written speech is not affected. It may be due to paresis, or incoordination of the muscles involved in the production of speech as seen in lesions of the pyramidal tract, cranial nerves, cerebellum or basal ganglia.

2. Aphasia

Aphasia refers to inability to understand spoken or written speech or inability in expressing the spoken or written speech in the absence of mental confusion or motor deficit. Depending on the site of lesion, the aphasia may be:

- Sensory aphasia
- Motor aphasia
- Global aphasia

Sensory Aphasia Sensory or receptive aphasia is also known as Wernicke's aphasia.

Site of lesion is the Wernicke's area.

Characteristic features of sensory aphasia are as follows:

1. ***Difficulty in understanding the meaning of speech:*** In this condition, the affected individuals are capable of hearing or identifying written or spoken words, but they do not comprehend the meaning of the words.
2. ***Motor speech*** is intact, and the patients talk very fluently (or rather excessively); that is why, it is also called *fluent aphasia*. However, the speech does not make much sense and is often associated with:
   - *Anomia:* It refers to the inability to find an appropriate word to express a thought.
   - *Neologism:* It refers to using or creating new words or new meanings for established words.
   - *Paraphasias:* It refers to production of unintended words or phrases during effort to speak.
   - *Conduction aphasia:* It is another form of fluent aphasia. In this condition, the patient can speak well and has good auditory comprehension, but cannot put words together. Earlier it was thought to be due to lesion of the arcuate fasciculus (which connects the Wernicke's area to the Broca's area), but the latest view is that lesion occurs near the auditory cortex in the perisylvian fissure.
3. *Impairment in reading and writing:* Since the patient cannot comprehend the written words (*word blindness*), he/she is unable to read aloud or copy print into writing.

Motor Aphasia is also known as Broca's aphasia.

Site of lesion is the Broca's motor speech area (area 44) in the frontal lobe.

Characteristic features of Broca's aphasia are as follows:

1. ***Comprehension of written or spoken*** speech is good.
2. ***Difficulty in speaking:*** The affected individual is able to formulate verbal language in his/her mind but cannot vocalize the response. The defect is not in the control of musculature needed for speech but rather in the elaboration of the complex patterns of neural and muscle activation, i.e. *effect* which defines the motor aspect of language.
3. ***Speech is nonfluent***, i.e. the patient utters only a few words with great difficulty. Because of this, motor aphasia is also known as *nonfluent aphasia* or *expressive aphasia*.
4. ***Inability to write*** (*agraphia*) is present.

Global Aphasia refers to total inability to use language communication.

Site of lesion: This condition is produced as a result of loss of both Wernicke's and Broca's areas. In this situation, speech becomes scanty and fluent. In case of deaf subjects, if a lesion occurs in the categorical hemisphere, then these individuals are unable to communicate in sign language.

Anomic aphasia: There is deficit in naming. In this condition, lesion usually involves middle and inferior temporal gyri. It is the most common language disturbance that usually occurs in Alzheimer disease, head injury and metabolic encephalitis.

Cause of Aphasia are mostly produced by thrombosis or embolism of a blood vessel in the dominant hemisphere. They are commonly associated with right-sided motor and sensory deficit but may also occur independently, when the lesion is restricted to cortical association area.

LEARNING AND MEMORY

LEARNING

Learning and memory are closely related. Learning is impossible without memory and memory has no meaning without learning. In fact, learning and memory are two sides of a coin. Learning refers to a neural mechanism by which the individual changes his/her behaviour on the basis of past experience. Two patterns of learning are given next.

Incidental Learning

Incidental learning is in which the behavioural changes are not immediately apparent. The individuals acquire information about the world while attending incidentally to sensory inputs, and thereby develop the potential to behave differently.

Reflex Learning

Reflex learning is in which the learning is associated with an immediate behavioural change. The two broad classes of reflex learning are as follows:

- Nonassociative learning
- Associative learning

A. Nonassociative Learning

In nonassociative learning, the subject learns about the properties of a single stimulus. It results when an animal or person is repeatedly exposed to a single type of stimulus. Two forms of nonassociative learning are common in everyday life – habituation and sensitization.

Habituation Habituation refers to decrease in response to a benign (neutral type) stimulus, when the stimulus is presented repeatedly. When the stimulus is applied for the first time, it is novel and evokes a reaction. This response is called *orientation reflex* or 'what is it' response. However, due to habituation, lesser and lesser response is evoked on repeated stimulation. Eventually, the subject totally ignores the stimulus and thus gets habituated to it. The response presumably diminishes because the individual learns that the stimulus is not important. For example, when a new clock is presented to a subject, at first, the ticking noise may be annoying and may cause some difficulty in sleeping. However, after several nights, the clock is no longer noticed.

It is important to note that presentation of another, usually noxious stimulus results in recovery of the habituated response, i.e. *dishabituation*. Dishabituation is a major criterion to demonstrate that habituation has indeed occurred.

Cellular basis of habituation has been studied in lower animals like snail (*Aplysia*). Habituation of the gill withdrawal reflex occurs when the siphon of the snail is touched repeatedly, and the snail does not withdraw its gill anymore. Habituation is associated with a decrease in neurotransmitter released at the synapses, which in turn is due to the inactivation of Ca^{2+} influx at the axon endings (Fig. 10.12.3). However, the mechanism of inactivation of Ca^{2+} channels is not known.

Sensitization Sensitization is opposite to habituation. In it, repeated application of a distinctly pleasant or unpleasant (strong) stimulus produces greater and greater response. For example, an animal responds more vigorously to a mild tactile stimulus, after it has received a painful pinch. Similarly, a spanking can lead to a greater likelihood that a child will obey

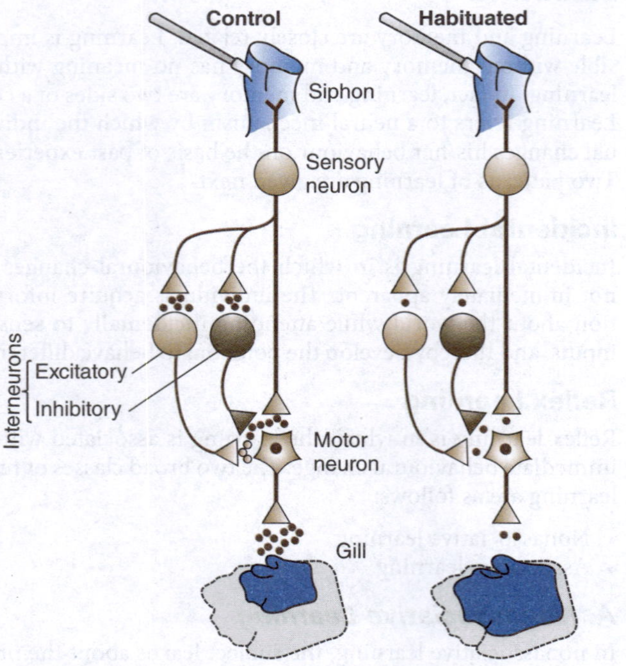

Fig. 10.12.3 Cellular mechanism of habituation as studied in the gill withdrawal reflex of marine snail (*Aplysia*) (presynaptic inhibition).

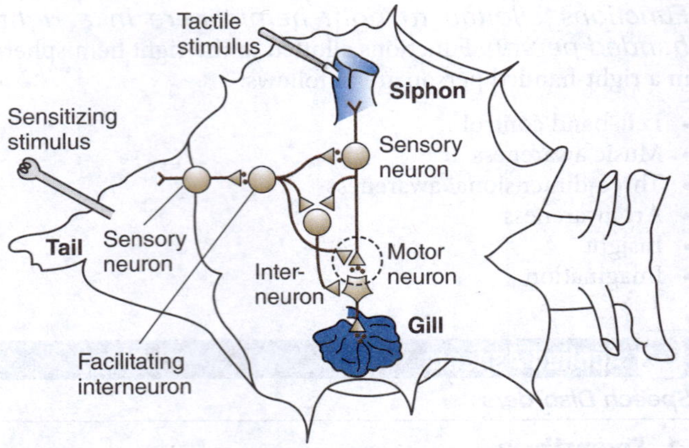

Fig. 10.12.4 Cellular mechanism of short-term sensitization as studied in the gill withdrawal reflex (presynaptic facilitation).

a parent's admonition. Thus, in sensitization, learning occurs in a direction opposite to that seen in habituation, presumably so that the behaviour becomes directed towards escape from the stimulus. Moreover, a sensitizing stimulus can override the effects of habituation, i.e. can cause dishabituation (as described above).

Cellular mechanism of sensitization has also been studied in lower animals like *Aplysia* (snail). After a painful stimulus is applied to the tail repeatedly, the snail subsequently withdraws its gill much more vigorously in response to an innocuous touch on the siphon. The sensitization is associated with increased release of neurotransmitters from the axonal endings of the sensory neuron. This result due to presynaptic facilitation of synaptic transmission is brought about by a third neuron called the facilitatory neuron (Fig. 10.12.4). The transmitter released by the presynaptic interneuron is serotonin (5-HT). Here, it binds to two serotonin receptors on the sensory nerve terminals (Fig. 10.12.5). One engages a G protein (G_s), which increases the activity of adenylyl cyclase. The adenylyl cyclase converts adenosine triphosphate (ATP) to cyclic adenosine monophosphate (cAMP), thereby increasing the level of cAMP in the terminal of sensory neuron. The cAMP activates the cAMP-dependent protein kinase A (PKA) by attaching to its inhibitory regulatory subunit, thus releasing its active catalytic subunit. The catalytic subunit of PKA acts along three biochemical pathways to cause increased release of neurotransmitter at axonal nerve ending of sensory neurons.

- In *pathway 1*, the catalytic subunit phosphorylates K^+ channels, thereby decreasing the K^+ current. This prolongs the action potential and increases the influx of Ca^{2+}, thus augmenting transmitter release.
- In *pathway 2*, vesicles containing transmitter are mobilized to the releasable transmitter pore at the active zone and the efficiency of exocytotic release machinery is also enhanced.
- In *pathway 3*, L-type Ca^{2+} channels are opened. Serotonin acting through a second receptor engages the G protein (Go) that activates a phospholipase C (PLC), which in turn stimulates intramembranous diacylglycerol to activate protein kinase C (PKC).

As shown in Fig. 10.12.5, the pathways 2–2a and 3–3a involve in the joint action of PKA and PKC.

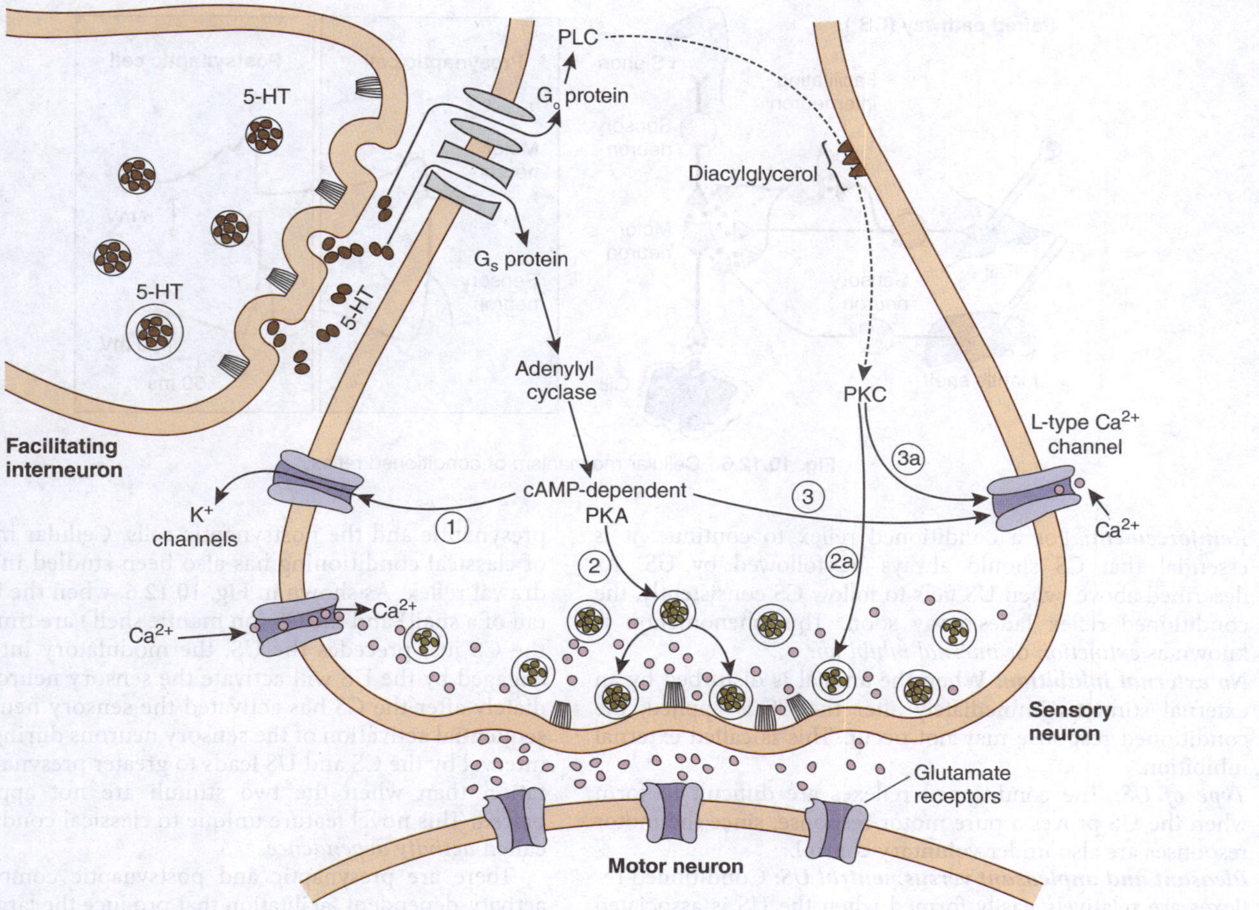

Fig. 10.12.5 Pathways involved in increased release of neurotransmitter (responsible for sensitization).

B. Associative Learning

In associative learning, the subject learns about the relationship between two stimuli or between a stimulus and behaviour. Two forms of associative learning have been distinguished based on the experimental procedures used to establish the learning:

- Classical conditioning
- Operant conditioning

Classical conditioning Classical conditioning involves learning a relationship between two stimuli. It is also termed Pavlovian conditioning, conditioned reflex type I, respondent conditioning or type S conditioning.

Characteristic features of a classical conditioned reflex are as follows:

- A conditioned reflex is a reflex response to a stimulus that previously elicited little or no response, *acquired by repeatedly pairing the stimulus with another stimulus* that normally does produce the response. Thus, in classical conditioning, a temporal association is made between a neutral conditioned stimulus (CS) and an unconditioned stimulus (US) that elicits an unlearned response. It is *peculiar to the individual* and refers to the fact that certain conditions must be present if this class of response is to develop. It depends for its appearance on the *formation of new functional connections in CNS*.
- *Reinforcement*, i.e. a process of following a CS with the basic US, is must for retaining a conditioned reflex; otherwise, it will be *extinct*.

Pavlov's experiment to demonstrate classical conditioned reflex is as follows:

- When food, i.e. a US, is presented to a hungry dog, it produces salivation (an unconditioned response).
- If a bell is rung (CS) just before the food (US) is presented, the dog learns to associate the bell (CS) with the food (US).
- Eventually, ringing the bell (CS) alone causes salivation.
- Of course, if the food fails to appear consistently when the bell is rung, the conditioned response fades away, a process called *extinction* or *internal inhibition*. Thus, a conditioned reflex needs to be reinforced frequently; otherwise, it dies out.

Prerequisites for development of conditioned reflex

Alertness and good health: The animal must be alert and in good health.

Timing of CS and US stimuli is critical in classical conditioning. The CS must precede the US, often within an interval of about 0.5 second. If the CS follows US, no conditioned response is developed.

Duration of CS: The CS must be allowed to continue to act so as to overlap the US. Almost any stimulus, if suitably employed, may become the CS.

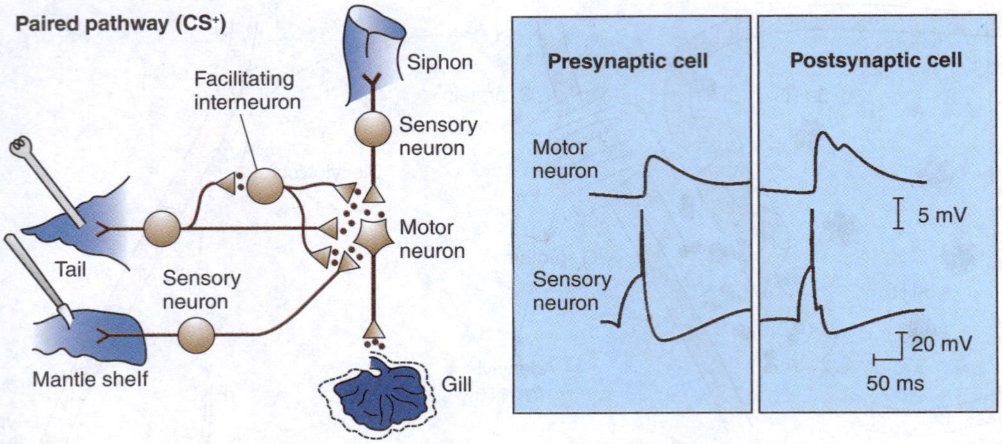

Fig. 10.12.6 Cellular mechanism of conditioned reflex.

Reinforcement: For a conditioned reflex to continue, it is essential that CS should always be followed by US. As described above, when US fails to follow CS consistently, the conditioned reflex fades away soon. This phenomenon is known as *extinction* or *internal inhibition*.

No external inhibition: When the animal is disturbed by an external stimulus immediately after the CS is applied, the conditioned response may not occur. This is called external inhibition.

Type of US: The conditioned reflexes are difficult to form when the US proves a pure motor response, since the motor responses are also under voluntary control.

Pleasant and unpleasant versus neutral US: Conditioned reflexes are relatively easily formed when the US is associated with a pleasant or unpleasant effect than when associated with a neutral effect. For example, stimulation of the brain reward system is a powerful US; this is called pleasant or *positive reinforcement*. Similarly, stimulation of the avoiding system or a painful shock to the skin is also a powerful US, and this is called an unpleasant or *negative reinforcement*.

Physiological basis of conditioned reflexes

Physiologically, the occurrence of conditioned reflex is explained by the formation of a new functional connection in the nervous system. For example, in Pavlov's classical experiments, salivation in response to ringing of a bell indicates that a functional connection has developed between the auditory pathways and the autonomic centres controlling salivation.

Site of formation of functional connections can be intracortical as well as subcortical.

Evidences in favour of the intracortical level are as follows:

- In decorticate animals, the conditioned reflexes can be built up with great difficulty.
- Presence of the sensory cortex is must to understand a complex sensory CS.

Evidence in favour of the subcortical level: Nondiscriminative conditioned reflexes to simple sensory stimuli can be formed in the absence of a whole neocortex. This indicates that the new functional connections can also be formed at the subcortical level.

Cellular mechanism of conditioned reflex

Classical conditioning involves presynaptic facilitation of synaptic transmission that is dependent on activity in both the presynaptic and the postsynaptic cells. Cellular mechanism of classical conditioning has also been studied in gill withdrawal reflex. As shown in Fig. 10.12.6, when the US (to the tail of a snail) and the CS (on mantle shelf) are timed so that the CS just precedes the US, the modulatory interneurons engaged by the US will activate the sensory neurons immediately after the CS has activated the sensory neurons. This sequential activation of the sensory neurons during a critical interval by the CS and US leads to greater presynaptic facilitation than when the two stimuli are not appropriately paired. This novel feature unique to classical conditioning is called *activity dependence.*

There are presynaptic and postsynaptic components to activity-dependent facilitation that produce the large increase in transmitter release that occurs with classical conditioning. Furthermore, it is important to note that classical conditioning requires the activation of *N*-methyl-D-aspartate (NMDA) receptors for glutamate present on the motor cell, as opposed to the non-NMDA receptors that are activated during sensitization.

Presynaptic components include:

- Activation of adenylyl cyclase by Ca^{2+} influx, representing the CS
- Activation of serotonergic receptors coupled to adenylyl cyclase, representing the US

Postsynaptic component includes:

- A retrograde signal indicating that the postsynaptic cell has been adequately activated by US

Operant conditioning

Operant conditioning is also termed instrumental conditioning, type II conditioning, type R conditioning or trial-and-error conditioning. It involves associating a specific behaviour with a reinforcement event. In it, the organism's behaviour is instrumental in conditioning. Therefore, the organism learns which of its actions are responsible for the occurrence of reinforcement event. *Operant conditioning* is of two types:

Reward conditioning: In it, a naturally occurring response is strengthened by positive reinforcement (reward).

Aversive conditioning: In it, a naturally occurring (innate) response is weakened by a negative reinforcement (punishment).

Experiment to demonstrate operant conditioning

A hungry animal (e.g. rat) is placed in a cage with a lever (bars) protruding in the cage. Because of naturally occurring (innate) response, the rat will randomly press the lever.

- If pressing of the lever is not associated with any event, the pressing of the lever will be at a random rate.
- If pressing the lever is associated with a positive reinforcement, i.e. reward (e.g. food), the rate of pressing the lever will be much more than the random rate (*reward conditioning*).
- If pressing of the lever is associated with a negative reinforcement, i.e. punishment (e.g. electric shock), the lever-pressing rate will be much less than the random rate (*aversive conditioning*).

Neural mechanism of operant conditioning Operant and classical conditioning involve different kinds of association – classical conditioning involves learning an association between two stimuli, whereas operant conditioning involves learning the association between a behaviour and a reward; one might suppose the two forms of learning are mediated by different neural mechanisms. However, the laws of operant and classical conditioning are quite similar, suggesting that the two forms of learning may use the same neural mechanisms.

MEMORY

As mentioned earlier, memory and learning are closely related to each other. Memory refers to the acquisition, storage and retrieval of sensory information, whereas learning is the change in behaviour based on the sensory information stored in the brain. The brain has different sites and mechanisms for handling different types of information.

Memory can be classified in two ways.

I. Physiologically, on the basis of how information is stored and recalled The memory can be classified as implicit memory and explicit memory.

Implicit memory, also called nondeclarative or reflexive memory, refers to information about how to perform something. It is not associated with awareness and does not involve processing in the hippocampus in most instances.

Explicit memory, also termed declarative or recognition memory, refers to factual knowledge of people, places and things and what these facts mean. It is associated with consciousness or at least awareness, and is dependent for its retention on the hippocampus and other parts of the medial temporal lobes of the brain.

II. Depending on permanency of storage Depending on permanency of storage, memory is short-term, intermediate long-term and long-term memory.

1. ***Short-term memory***, also termed *primary memory*, lasts for seconds to hours. Example of short-term memory includes memory of a new telephone number after calling the operator or after looking into directory. Most of the times, such a telephone number is forgotten after few minutes.
2. ***Intermediate long-term memory*** (or secondary memory) lasts for days to weeks but is eventually lost.
3. ***Long-term memory*** (or tertiary memory), once stored, can be recalled years later or for a lifetime.

Implicit Memory

Implicit memory, also termed *reflexive* or *nondeclarative memory*, refers to information about how to perform something. Unlike explicit memory, it does not depend directly on conscious processes nor does recall require a conscious search of memory. This type of memory builds up slowly, through repetition over many trials, and is expressed primarily in performance, not in words. Examples of implicit memory include motor skills, habits, behavioural reflexes and the learning of certain types of procedures and rules, which, once acquired, become unconscious and automatic. It also includes priming in which recall of words and objects is improved by prior exposure to them. An example is improved recall of a word by a subject with amnesia when presented with first few letters of it. Most forms of implicit memory are acquired through different forms of reflexive learning which comprise:

1. ***Nonassociative learning*** that includes:
   - Habituation
   - Sensitization
2. ***Associative learning*** that includes:
   - Classical conditioning
   - Operant conditioning

Different forms of reflexive learning, which comprise implicit memory, have been described above (page 1081). These involve different brain regions:

- Memory acquired through *fear conditioning*, which has an emotional component, is thought to involve the *amygdala*.
- Memory acquired through *operant conditioning* requires the *striatum* and *cerebellum*.
- Memory acquired through classical conditioning, sensitization and habituation involves changes in the sensory and motor systems involved in the learning.

Explicit Memory

Explicit memory, also termed *declarative* or *recognition memory*, refers to factual knowledge of people, places and things, and what these facts mean. This is recalled by a deliberate conscious effort. Explicit memory is highly flexible and involves the association of multiple bits and pieces of information. In contrast, implicit memory is more rigid and tightly connected to the original stimulus conditions under which the learning occurred.

Explicit memory can be further classified as:

- *Semantic memory* (a memory of facts)
- *Episodic memory* (a memory of events and personal experience)

Semantic (factual) memory The semantic memory is that form of long-term explicit memory that embraces knowledge of objects, facts and concepts as well as words and their meaning. It includes the naming of objects, the definition of spoken words and verbal fluency. *Semantic memory* is stored in a distributed fashion in different association cortices. For example, the word alarm clock immediately brings its features in our mind from our past experience (stored memory) as follows:

Visual memory reminds us about its shape, needles depicting hours, minutes, seconds and markings for 1–12 o'clock hours, etc.

Auditory memory reminds us about its sound (ringing of alarm).

Somatosensory memory reminds us that it is made of a plastic or metallic box, having a smooth, transparent glass. The visual, auditory and somatosensory memory which reminds us about different attributes is stored in different areas of the neocortex. Whenever the information about the features of an alarm clock has to be recalled, the recall is built up from distinct bits of information, each of which is stored in specialized (dedicated) memory stores of the neocortex. Thus, there is no general semantic memory store, i.e. semantic knowledge is not stored in a single region.

Applied Aspects

Damage to a specific cortical area leads to loss of specific information, and therefore a fragmentation of knowledge as exemplified:

Associative visual agnosia results from damage to the posterior parietal cortex. In it, the patient cannot name objects but can identify them by selecting the correct drawing and can faithfully reproduce detailed drawings of the object.

Appreciative visual agnosia occurs in damage to occipital lobes and surrounding region. In it, patients are unable to draw objects but they can name them if appropriate perceptual cues are available.

Episodic (autobiographical) memory Episodic memory refers to memory of events and personal experiences. For example, we use episodic memory when we recall that last Sunday, I visited my friend's house in Kailash Colony of New Delhi.

Episodic memory is stored in association areas of prefrontal cortex These prefrontal areas work with other areas of the neocortex to allow recollection of when and where a past event occurred. Therefore, a particularly striking symptom in patients with frontal lobe damage is *source amnesia*, i.e. tendency to forget how information was acquired. Since the ability to associate a piece of information with the time and place it was acquired is at the core of how accurately we remember the individual episodes of our lives, a deficit in source information interferes dramatically with the accuracy of recall of episodic knowledge.

Mechanism (Physiological and Cellular or Molecular Basis) of Memory

Studies of memory retention and disruption of memory have revealed that both explicit and implicit memories are stored in stages by different mechanisms. Input to the brain is processed into *short-term memory* before it is transformed through one or more stages (intermediate long-term memory) into more permanent long-term storage.

Mechanism of Implicit Memory

As mentioned earlier, most forms of implicit memory are acquired through different forms of reflexive learning (habituation and sensitization) and associative learning (classical and operant conditioning). Short-term storage of implicit memory for these simple forms of learning results from *changes in the effectiveness of synaptic transmission*:

***Habituation** involves an activity-dependent presynaptic depression of synaptic transmission*, resulting from the decrease in neurotransmitter released at the synapses.

- Cellular basis of habituation is described on page 1082.

***Sensitization** involves presynaptic facilitation of synaptic transmission*, which is associated with increased release of neurotransmitters from the axonal ending of the sensory neuron.

- Cellular mechanism *of sensitization* is described on page 1082.

***Classical conditioning** involves presynaptic facilitation of synaptic transmission that is dependent on activity in both the presynaptic and the postsynaptic cells.*

- *Physiological basis and cellular mechanism of classical conditioning* are described on page 1084.

Mechanism of long-term storage of implicit memory

The process by which transient short-term memory is converted into a stable long-term memory is called consolidation. *Consolidation of long-term implicit memory* for simple forms of learning involves three processes:

- Gene expression
- New protein synthesis
- Growth (or pruning) of synaptic connections

Molecular biological analysis of long-term storage of implicit memory reveals that it involves the cyclic AMP-protein kinase A (cAMP–PKA) mitogen-activated protein kinase (MAPK)–cyclic-AMP response element-binding proteins (CREB) pathway.

Mechanism of Explicit Memory

Both semantic and episodic types of explicit memory are the result of at least four related but distinct types of processing – encoding, consolidation, storage and retrieval.

Mechanism of short-term explicit memory Encoding refers to the process by which newly learned information is attended to and processed when first encountered. The extent and nature of this encoding are critically important for determining how well the learned material will be remembered at later times. For a memory to persist and be well remembered, the incoming information must be encoded thoroughly and deeply.

Neural substrate for encoding of explicit memory As mentioned earlier, the explicit memory is associated with consciousness (or at least awareness) and is dependent for its retention on the *hippocampus* and other parts of *medial temporal lobes* of the brain.

Studies with human patients and with experimental animals suggest that knowledge stored as explicit memory is processed as (Fig. 10.12.7):

- Sensory information is first acquired through processing in one or more of the three polymodal association cortices (the *prefrontal*, *limbic* and *parietal–occipital–temporal cortices*) that synthesize visual, auditory and somatic information. Together, these pathways are called perforant pathway.
- From polymodal association cortices, the information is conveyed in series to the *parahippocampal* and *perirhinal cortices*, then the *entorhinal cortex*, the dentate gyrus, the hippocampus, the subiculum and finally back to the entorhinal cortex.
- From the entorhinal cortex, the information is sent back to parahippocampal and perirhinal cortices and finally back to polymodal association areas of the neocortex.
- Role of the hippocampus in learning and memory:
  - Hippocampus is a part of hippocampal formation which includes subiculum, hippocampus and dentate gyrus. Hippocampus, also called cornu ammonis (CA), is basically divided into four regions as CA_1, CA_2, CA_3 and

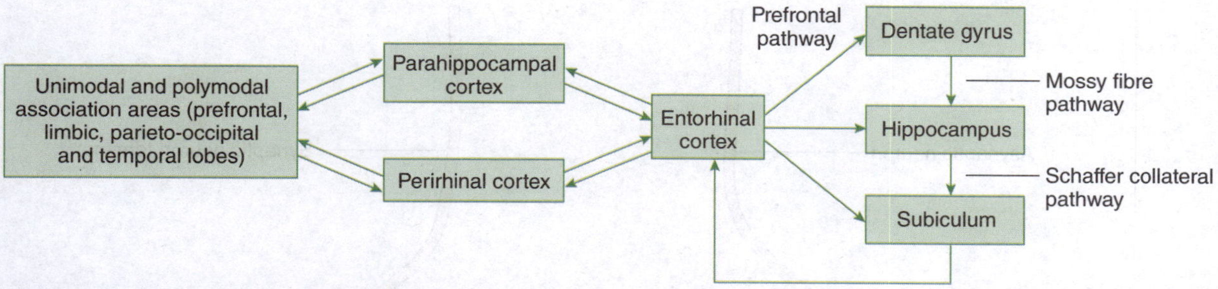

Fig. 10.12.7 Neural substrate for encoding of explicit memory (the input and output pathways of the hippocampal formation).

CA_4. The major function of the hippocampus is in conversion of short-term memory into long-term memory.

Applied Aspects

The CA_1–subiculum interface region is referred to as *Sommer sector* in pathological conditions, because lesion of this region leads to memory loss and the affected person suffers difficulty in converting short-term memory to long-term memory (anterograde amnesia).

Physiological processes in the neural substrate associated with storage of short-term explicit memory (*hippocampus*) are as follows:

- *Continuous neural activity* is present in reverberating circuits.
- *Activation of synapses* occurs on presynaptic terminals that typically result in prolonged facilitation, i.e. long-term potentiation (LTP), or prolonged inhibition, i.e. long-term depression (LTD).
- *Accumulation of calcium* in axon terminals may eventually lead to enhanced synaptic output from the terminal.

Long-term potentiation The LTP involves protein synthesis and growth of presynaptic and postsynaptic neurons and their connections. It is a rapidly developing postsynaptic potential that occurs in response to repeated stimulation of presynaptic neuron. It lasts for a prolonged period (for days).

Mechanisms: There are different mechanisms for development of LTP. Though LTP develops in different parts of the nervous system, it has been studied in great detail in the hippocampus, specifically for connections of pyramidal cells of cortical area 3 region and of CA_1 region via collaterals called Schaffer collaterals. The underlying mechanisms depend on changes in the following types of receptors:

NMDA receptors, which are Na^+-dependent receptors

α-Amino-3-hydroxy-5-methylisoxizal-4-propionic acid (AMPA) receptors or Na^+-independent receptors

The sequence of events is as follows (Fig. 10.12.8):

- At resting membrane potential, glutamate releases from the presynaptic neuron.
- Glutamate binds to NMDA receptors as well as to non-NMDA or AMPA receptors.
- LTP initiated by NMDA receptors increases intracellular Ca^{2+}, either in presynaptic or in postsynaptic neurons, whereas in activation of AMPA receptors, there is increased Na^+ and K^+ flow (because of the presence of Mg^{2+} on NMDA receptors that blocks their flow through these receptors).
- However, depolarization triggered by the activation of AMPA receptors relieves the Mg^{2+} blocked in the NMDA receptors and Ca^{2+} enters the postsynaptic neurons.
- The increase in cytoplasmic Ca^{2+} activates Ca^{2+}/calmodulin kinase, PKC and tyrosine kinase, which together induce LTP.
- The Ca^{2+}/calmodulin kinase II phosphorylates the AMPA receptors, increasing their conductance and causing movement of more AMPA receptors to the synaptic membrane from the cytosolic storage site.
- As there is an initiation of LTP, nitric oxide releases by the postsynaptic neuron that passes retrogradely to the presynaptic neuron and causes long-term quantitative increase in the release of glutamate.

In the hippocampus, LTP occurs in mossy fibres that connect granule cells in the dentate cortex. LTP is induced due to increase in Ca^{2+} in the presynaptic neuron rather than in the postsynaptic neuron in response to tetanic stimulation and is independent of NMDA receptors. The increased influx of Ca^{2+} in presynaptic neuron activates Ca^{2+}/calmodulin-dependent adenylyl cyclase that increases cAMP.

Long-term depression LTD is just opposite to LTP. It is characterized by a decrease in synaptic strength, due to slower stimulation of presynaptic neurons, and is associated with lesser rise in the intracellular Ca^{2+}. LTD was first noticed in the hippocampus, but subsequently, it was observed in many other regions of CNS also. It is also observed in same fibres in which LTP is present.

Mechanism of intermediate long-term memory

Intermediate long-term memory can result from temporary chemical or physical changes in either the presynaptic or the postsynaptic membrane that can persist for a few minutes to several weeks. The newly stored sensory information is still labile during this stage, which is converted into long-term memory after the process of consolidation is complete.

Physiological process in the neural substrate associated with intermediate long-term memory is that of synaptic facilitation and has been studied in the snail *Aplysia*. As shown in Figs 10.12.4 and 10.12.5, stimulation of a facilitator terminal at the same time as activation of another sensory input causes serotonin to be released at synaptic sites on the sensory terminal. Stimulation of serotonin receptors activates adenylyl cyclase in the main sensory terminal, resulting in formation of cAMP, which causes the release of a protein kinase and leads to phosphorylation of protein that blocks potassium channels in the sensory terminal, resulting in increased neurotransmitter release from the sensory terminal, thereby facilitating transmission at this synapse.

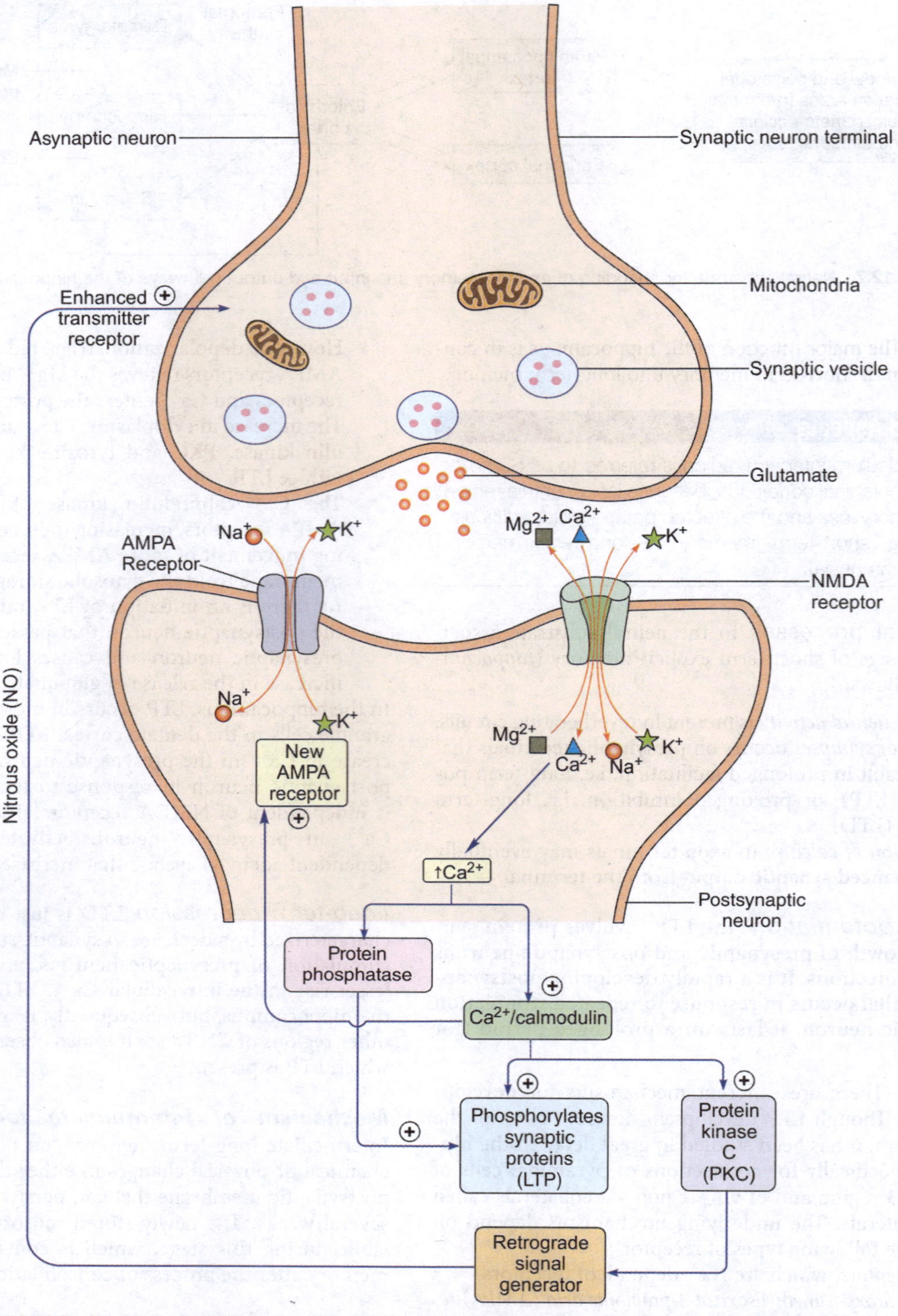

Fig. 10.12.8 Production of LTP in Schaffer collaterals in the hippocampus. LTP, long-term potentiation.

Mechanism of long-term memory For memories to be converted to long-term memories, they must be consolidated.

Consolidation of memory: Consolidation refers to those processes that alter the newly stored and still labile information so as to make it more stable for long-term storage. In general, 5–10 minutes is required for minimal consolidation, whereas 1 or more hours may be needed for strong consolidation. If this time is not allowed for the consolidation to occur, the data in short-term memory are completely forgotten. This is seen in patients with concussion injury and after electroconvulsive therapy (ECT) who are unable to recall the events immediately preceding the concussion or convulsion. This phenomenon is called *retrograde amnesia*. A similar retrograde amnesia occurs before the onset of sleep. This is the reason one is unable to remember the precise time of one's own sleep onset.

Rehearsal mechanism is thought to represent the consolidation process. Rehearsal of the same information again and again in the mind potentiates the transfer from short-term to long-term memory. Over time, the important features of sensory experience become progressively more fixed in memory stores. Also during consolidation, memories are codified into different classes of information. For example, new and old experiences related to a topic are compared for similarities and differences, and it is the later information that is stored.

Process of consolidation involves the expression of genes and synthesis of new proteins, giving rise to structural changes that store memory stably over time. The structural changes include:

- An increase in the number of synaptic vesicle release sites
- An increase in the number of available synaptic vesicles
- An increase in the number of synaptic terminals
- Changes in the shape or number of postsynaptic spines

Storage of memory refers to the mechanism and sites by which memory is retained over time. One of the remarkable features about long-term storage is that it seems to have an almost unlimited capacity. In contrast, short-term working memory is very limited.

Neural substrate for long-term storage memory The encoding process for short-term explicit memory involves the hippocampus, whereas long-term memories are stored in the various parts of the neocortex. Apparently, the various parts of the memories – visual, olfactory, auditory, etc. – are located in the cortical regions concerned with these functions, and the pieces are tied together by long-term changes in the strength of transmission at relevant synaptic junctions, so that all the components are brought to consciousness when the memory is recalled.

Retrieval of Memory

Retrieval refers to those processes that permit the recall and use of stored information. It involves bringing different kinds of information together that are stored separately in different storage sites. Retrieval of memory is much like perception; it is a constructive process and therefore subject to distortion, much as perception is subject to illusions.

Retrieval of information is most effective when it occurs in the same context in which the information was acquired and in the presence of same cues (retrieval cues) that were available to the subject during learning. However, once established, long-term memories can be recalled or accessed by a large number of different associations. For example, the memory of a vivid scene can be evoked not only by a similar scene but also by a sound or smell associated with the scene. Thus, there must be multiple routes or keys to each stored memory.

Working memory Both the initial encoding and the ultimate recall of explicit memory (and perhaps some forms of implicit memory as well) are thought to require recruitment of stored information into a special short-term memory store called *working memory*. Working memory has three component systems:

- Attentional control system
- Rehearsal systems that include:
  - Articulatory loop
  - Visuospatial sketch pad

Attentional control system or (central executive) actively focuses perception on specific events in the environment. It is located in the prefrontal cortex and has a very limited capacity (less than a dozen items). It regulates the information flow to two rehearsal systems that are thought to maintain memory for temporary use.

Rehearsal systems include the articulatory loop and the visuospatial sketch pad.

Articulatory loop is a storage system with a rapidly decaying memory trace where memory for words and numbers can be maintained by subvocal speech. It is this system that allows one to hold information in mind, through repetition, i.e. a new telephone number as one prepares to dial it.

Visuospatial sketch pad represents both the visual properties and the spatial location of the object to be remembered. This system allows one to store the image of the face of a person one meets at a dinner party.

The two rehearsal memory systems are thought to be located in different parts of the posterior association cortices. The information processed in either of these systems has the possibility of entering long-term memory.

Important Note

Hebb's rule: According to Hebb's rule, if one neuron excites another neuron repeatedly and persistently, then the synapse between those two neurons gets strengthened. This is seen as conversion of short-term memory into long-term memory in the hippocampus. That is why it is always suggested that for better academic performance, revision is the key to success.

Other brain areas involved in learning and memory:

- *Mammillary bodies* form a part of Papez circuit concerned with learning and memory. Lesion of mammillary body causes Wernicke–Korsakoff syndrome (see page 935).
- *Anterior nucleus of thalamus:* Lesion of this region causes loss of recent memory.
- *Basal forebrain:* Nucleus basalis of Meynert projects cholinergic fibres to the hippocampus; therefore, loss of these fibres causes Alzheimer disease.
- *Amygdala* is concerned with emotionally related memories.

INTERHEMISPHERIC TRANSFER OF LEARNING AND MEMORY

Much information is transferred between the two hemispheres through the corpus callosum, although some is transmitted through other commissures (e.g. the anterior commissure or hippocampal commissure).

Experiment to demonstrate importance of the corpus callosum for interhemispheric transfer of information is as follows (Fig. 10.12.9):

- An experimental animal (cat or monkey), with an intact optic chiasma and corpus callosum, and the left eye closed, is conditioned to a visual discrimination task (Fig. 10.12.9A_1).
- When the animal is asked to perform the same task with the left eye open and the right eye closed, the task can still be performed (Fig. 10.12.9A_2) indicating that both hemispheres have learned the task. Conclusion is that interocular transfer

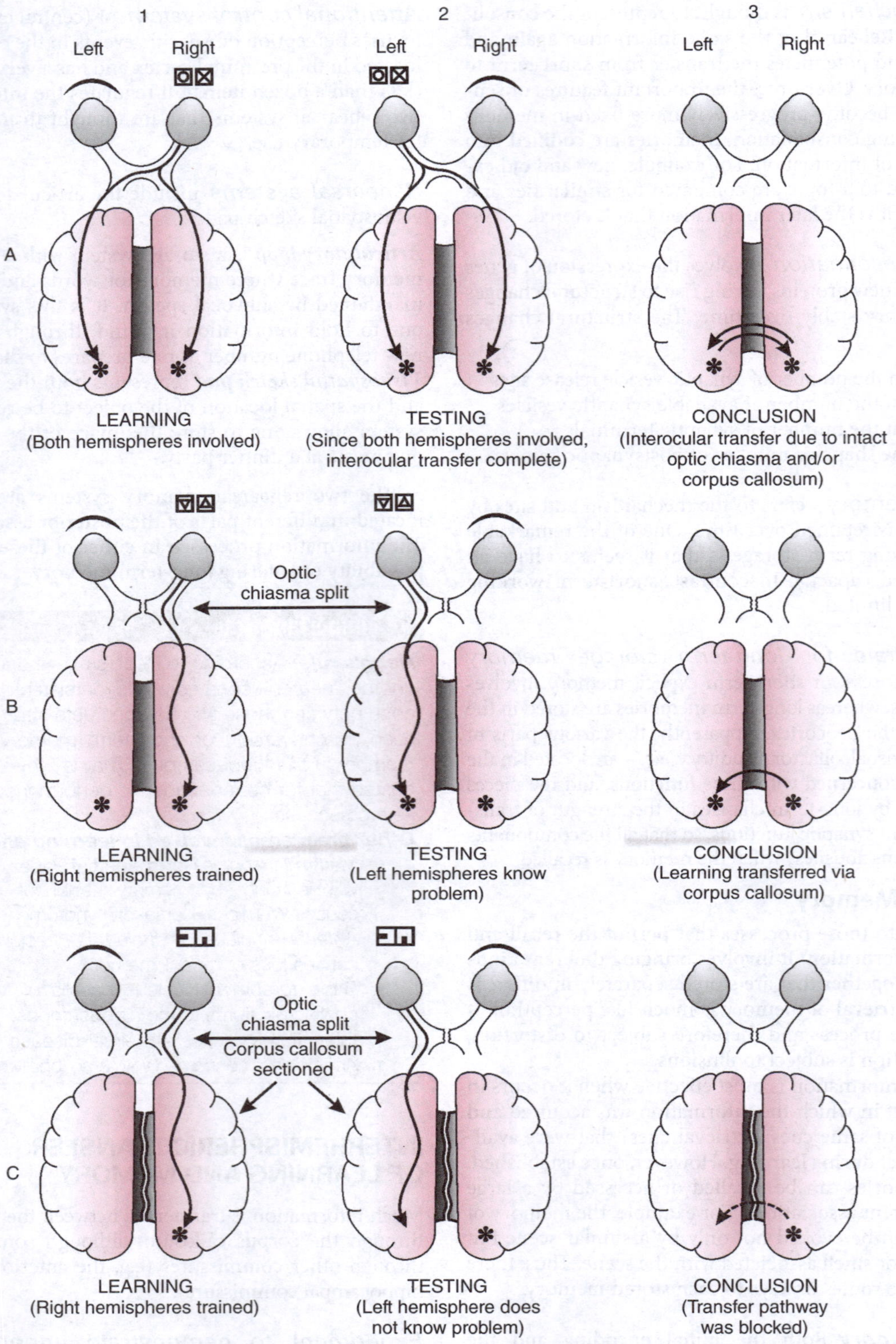

Fig. 10.12.9 Experiment to demonstrate importance of corpus callosum for interhemispheric transfer of learning and memory (for details, see text).

has occurred due to either intact optic chiasma or corpus callosum (Fig. 10.12.9A_3).

- When the optic chiasma is transected before the animal is trained (Fig. 10.12.9B_1), the result is the same (Fig. 10.12.9B_2), concluding that learning is transferred via the corpus callosum (Fig. 10.12.9B_3).
- When both the optic chiasma and the corpus callosum are cut before training (Fig. 10.12.9C_1), information is not transferred (Fig. 10.12.9C_2), and each hemisphere must learn the task independently. This confirms the fact that the learning is transferred via corpus callosum (Fig. 10.12.9C_3).

Similar results about failure of intercortical transfer of learning and memory are also seen in human patients, who have had a surgical transection of the corpus callosum to prevent inter-hemispheric spread of epilepsy. Studies in subjects indicate that the transfer of visual memory occurs in the posterior part of the corpus callosum, whereas transfer of auditory and somaesthetic memory occurs in the anterior part of the corpus callosum.

Furthermore, functional capabilities of the two hemispheres when compared by exploring the performance of individuals with a transected corpus callosum have yielded the following results:

- Right hemisphere specializes in spatial task, facial expression, body language and speech into notion.
- Patients with a transected corpus callosum lack coordination. For example, when they are dressing, one hand may button a shirt while the other tries to unbutton it.
- From this experiment, it can be concluded that the two hemispheres can operate quite independently when they are no longer interconnected.

Applied Aspects

- Drugs facilitating memory
- Amnesia
- Alzheimer disease and senile dementia
- Confabulation
- Strangeness and familiarity

Drugs Facilitating Memory

Learning and memory are reported to improve in animals when a variety of CNS stimulants are administered immediately, before or after the learning sessions.

Common CNS stimulants that facilitate learning and memory are caffeine, amphetamine, physostigmine, nicotine, pemoline, strychnine and pentylenetetrazol.

Mechanism of action: CNS stimulants act probably by facilitating consolidation of memory. For example, physostigmine acts by inhibiting acetylcholinesterase and, hence, preventing breakdown of acetylcholine, whereas nicotine stimulates cholinergic receptors.

Amnesia

Amnesia refers to loss of memory. It is of two types – antegrade amnesia and retrograde amnesia.

Antegrade amnesia refers to inability of an individual to establish new long-term memories of those types of information that form the basis of intelligence. This usually occurs in lesions involving the hippocampus.

Retrograde amnesia refers to inability of an individual to recall past memories. Amnesia is much greater for events of recent past than those of remote past. Memories of distant past are rehearsed so many times that the memory traces are deeply engrained and elements of these memories are stored in the widespread areas of the brain. Retrograde amnesia occurs in lesions involving the temporal lobe (*temporal lobe syndrome*).

Alzheimer Disease and Senile Dementia

Senile Dementia

Senile dementia refers to a clinical syndrome in elderly people that is characterized by progressive impairment of memory and cognitive capacities. There are a number of diseases that are manifested by dementia in mid and late life.

Common causes of dementia in the elderly are as follows:

- Alzheimer disease
- Cerebrovascular disease
- Lewy body dementia
- Parkinsonism
- Prion diseases

Alzheimer Disease

Alzheimer disease is the most common cause of dementia in the elderly persons.

Pathophysiology: Both genetic and environmental factors may be responsible for the aetiology of the disease. Alzheimer disease is a prototypical neurodegenerative disease. It is characterized by a series of abnormalities in the brain that selectively affect neurons in specific regions, particularly in the neocortex, entorhinal area, hippocampus, amygdala, nucleus basalis, anterior thalamus, locus coeruleus and raphe complex. There is a severe loss of cholinergic neurosis in the affected areas. The major cholinergic pathways involved in Alzheimer disease are shown in Fig. 10.12.10.

- Familial form of disease is seen in early onset disease, and is caused by mutation in the presenilin-1 (PS-1) gene, presenilin-2 (PS-2), beta-amyloid precursor protein (APP) and apolipoprotein E (APO-E). PS-1 gene is located on chromosome 14 and encodes protein S182. Mutation in PS-1 gene is the most common cause of early onset Alzheimer disease.
- PS-2 gene is located on chromosome 1 and encodes protein STM 2.
- APO-E gene is located on chromosome 19 and involved in cholesterol transport. APOE4 is an important biological marker associated with risks of Alzheimer disease.
- APP gene is located on chromosome 21. Mutation in this gene is responsible for overproduction of PS-1 and PS-2. It is transmitted as an autosomal dominance. Each mutation leads to overproduction of β-amyloid protein. Recently, it is found that mutation of α_2-macroglobulin gene is associated with late-onset disease.

Alzheimer disease is associated with cytoskeletal abnormalities in the affected nerve cells, the most important being accumulation of neurofibrillary tangles in the neuronal cytoplasm made up of hyperphosphorylated *tau* protein that binds to microtubules. Amyloid plaque (fibrillar peptides) deposits surrounded by altered nerve fibres and glial cells are one of the hallmarks of Alzheimer disease.

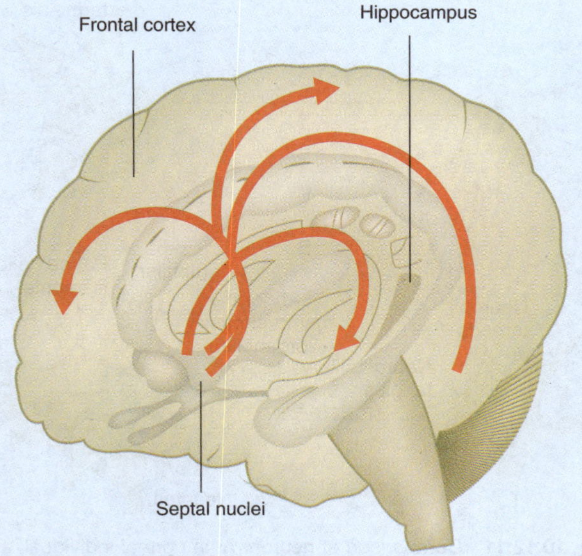

Fig. 10.12.10 Major cholinergic pathways involved in Alzheimer disease.

Important Note

The β-amyloid plaques are the products of APP, a normal transmembrane protein that projects into the extracellular fluid from nerve cells. This protein is hydrolysed at three sites by α-, β- and γ-secretase. The polypeptides formed after hydrolysation by γ-secretase are toxic. These polypeptides get aggregated and stick on to AMPA receptors and Ca^{2+} channels and thus prevent Ca^{2+} influx, and also induce inflammatory reaction and formation of intracellular tangles (Fig. 10.12.11).

Characteristic features of Alzheimer disease are as follows:

- Loss of recent memory occurs in an otherwise alert individual.
- Impairment occurs in other areas of cognition such as language, problem solving, judgement, calculation, attention and perception.
- Psychiatric symptoms begin to appear as the disease progresses.
- Extrapyramidal and akinetic hypertonic symptoms also appear in later stages.
- There may occur loss of spatial orientation.
- Finally, the patient has to lead a vegetative life without memory, without thinking power, speechless, with inability to understand anything, and with *apraxia* (inability to perform voluntary movements) and *agnosia* (inability to recognize objects in spite of intact sensory modality).

Treatment: There is no effective treatment for Alzheimer disease; as yet, *physostigmine*, which inhibits cholinesterase, causes some improvement. Presently, focus is on treating associated symptoms such as depression, agitation, sleep disorders, hallucinations and delusions.

- *Memantine* is a NMDA receptor antagonist that prevents glutamate-induced excitability in the brain and is useful for treating patients with moderate to severe Alzheimer.
- *Lipid-lowering statins* like rosiglitazone are effective if used prior to the onset of disease.
- *Secretase inhibitors* are useful.

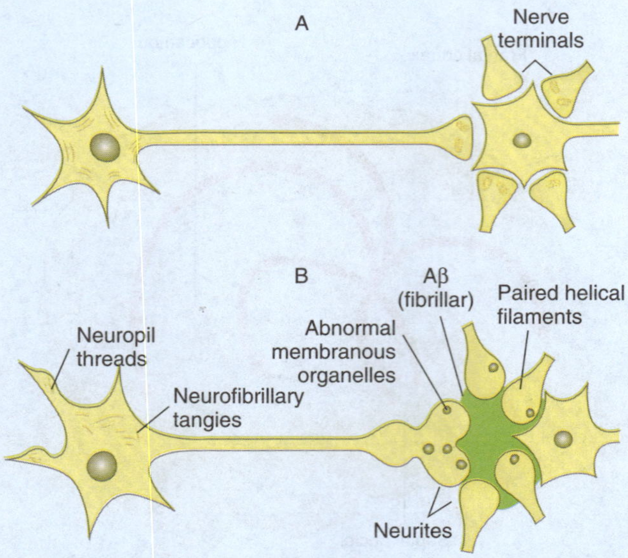

Fig. 10.12.11 Comparison of neuron: **A**, in normal individual; and **B**, with abnormalities associated with Alzheimer disease.

- *R-flurbiprofen* is useful in blocking the production of β-amyloid protein.
- *Vaccines* that allow the body's immune system to produce antibodies against these proteins are under trial.

In a prospective study, it is mentioned that if a person is doing frequent effortful mental activities like solving crossword and puzzles, the onset of cognitive dementia slows down. Explanation is based on the fact that the hippocampus and its connections have plasticity.

Confabulation

Confabulation occurs in patients with lesion of the ventromedial part of the frontal lobe. In this condition, individuals perform poorly on memory tests but describe the events spontaneously which have not occurred (called honest lying, see page 935).

Strangeness and Familiarity

Normally, the sense of familiarity helps the normal individuals to adjust according to the surrounding environment. In strange surroundings, the person becomes alert and more vigilant, and in familiar surroundings, the vigilance is relaxed.

It is observed that on stimulation of some parts of the temporal lobe in humans, there is change in the interpretation of surroundings (i.e. the person feels strange in familiar surroundings and there is an inappropriate feeling of familiarity in new surroundings). This condition is clinically known as *déjà vu phenomenon* from a French word meaning 'already seen'. Sometimes, this phenomenon occurs in normal individuals, but in a patient suffering with temporal epilepsy, this occurs as an aura.

HIGHER INTELLECTUAL FUNCTIONS OF THE PREFRONTAL ASSOCIATION CORTEX

Prefrontal cortex refers to the portion of frontal lobes in front of the motor cortex. This area, like other association areas, is better developed in humans than in any other species. The function of the prefrontal cortex is complex and multifactorial, and is typically explained by describing the deficits seen in individuals in whom the prefrontal lobotomy has been performed for tumour of this region. The functions thought to be performed by the prefrontal cortex are given next.

1. ROLE IN THOUGHT PROCESS

Prefrontal cortex gathers information from widespread area of the brain to develop solutions to problems, whether they require motor or nonmotor responses. Without this function, thoughts lose their logical progression, and the individual loses the ability to focus attention and is easily distracted in the sequence of thoughts. Hence, any activity involving a number of steps in sequence cannot be performed properly. In other words, there occurs *inability to progress towards goals* or *to carry through sequential thoughts*.

2. SITE OF WORKING MEMORY AND INTELLECTUAL FUNCTIONS

Prefrontal cortex is considered the site of 'working memory'. Working memory refers to the ability to hold and sort bits of information to be used in problem-solving function. By combining these stored bits of information, an individual can prognosticate, plan for the future, delay a response while further information is gathered, consider the consequences of actions before they are performed, correlate information from many different sources and control actions in accordance with societal or moral laws. All of these are considered as *intellectual functions* of the highest order and seem to be definitive for the human experience.

The patients with lesions of the prefrontal cortex have great difficulty in abstract thinking, e.g. planning for future or considering the consequences of a particular motor activity beforehand. The patient cannot act within the norm of social or moral behaviour.

3. ROLE IN EPISODIC MEMORY

Patients with prefrontal lesions show a difficulty in remembering the temporal sequence of events, i.e. they cannot remember how long ago they saved an event or picture card (episodic memory, i.e. a memory for events and personal experience).

Self-Assessment

1. Discuss the mechanism of development of speech.
2. Discuss the neurophysiology of learning and its retrieval.
3. Discuss the types of memory and neural substrate for storage.
4. Describe the following:
   - Concept of categorical and representational hemispheres
   - Classical conditioned reflex and its physiology
5. Write notes on the following:
   - Long-term potentiation
   - Strangeness and familiarity
   - Senile dementia
   - Retrograde amnesia

Clinical Cases

Case 1

A 45-year-old female was operated for left meningioma through middle temporal gyrus approach. Now, she has difficulty in speaking, the speech is nonfluent, and she can understand but cannot write.

Q1. What is the probable diagnosis?
Q2. What are the types of this condition?
Q3. What is the site of lesion?
Q4. What is the other name for this condition?

Case 2

A 46-year-old male suffered from a head injury in an accident and was in coma state for few months; after recovery, he lost memory about all incidences which occurred before the injury and also had difficulty in recognizing the persons.

Q1. What is this condition known as?
Q2. Which is the site of lesion?

Case 3

An 85-year-old lady has difficulty in remembering the recent incidences, even what she has eaten in the morning; her past memory is very sharp; doctors diagnosed this condition as age-related dementia (Alzheimer disease).

Q1. What is the pathophysiology of this condition?
Q2. Which neurons are affected mainly and of which part of the brain?
Q3. What are the characteristic features of this disease?
Q4. What is the treatment for this condition?

SPECIAL SENSES SECTION 11

SECTION OUTLINE

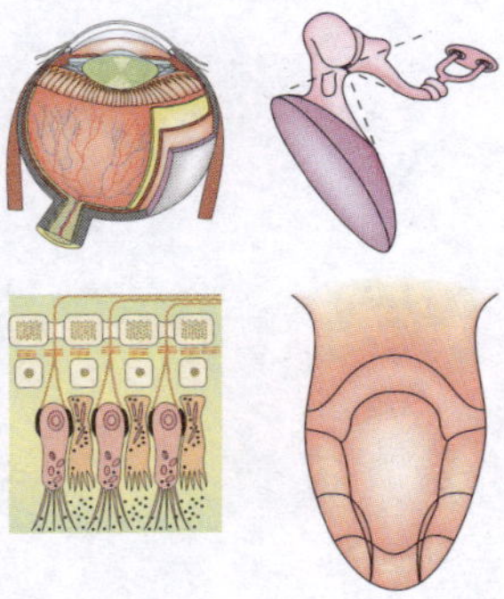

INTRODUCTION

As we have studied, the sensory division of the human nervous system is concerned with collection of the information about the outside world and the changes occurring within the body itself. The term *sensation* refers to the conscious perception of sensory information reaching the brain. The sensations have been broadly divided into general and special sensations.

General sensations These, depending on their point of origin, can be classified into three main groups:

- *Exteroceptive sensations*, i.e. those arising from the skin, e.g. touch and temperature sensation
- *Visceral sensations*, i.e. those arising from the viscera
- *Proprioceptive and kinaesthetic sensations*, i.e. those arising from the muscles, tendons and joints

Special sensations There are a few organs in the body which collect information of special significance to us from the external environment and are, therefore, called the organs of special senses. These organs of special senses have developed in the heads of animals, along with corresponding neural systems in the brain, during the involutionary process of encephalization. These special sensory systems include:

- *The sense of vision*, which allows the animal to detect and analyse light
- *The sense of hearing*, which makes possible the detection and analysis of sound
- *The chemical senses of taste and smell*, which are responsible for appreciation of chemical signals in the environment

GENERAL VERSUS SPECIAL SENSATIONS

Location of receptors: Receptors for general sensations are located throughout the body, e.g. touch, pain, pressure and temperature sensations, whereas the receptors for special senses are located at one place in the head near the nervous system, e.g. receptors for vision, hearing, taste and smell.

Response of receptors: The receptors for general sensations get easily stimulated by different stimuli; however, they respond maximally to an adequate stimulus. Furthermore, the receptor response is nonspecific to different stimuli. In contrast, the receptors for special senses are specialized and respond only to one type of stimulus. Furthermore, the receptor response is more complex and makes coordination within the CNS.

This section is devoted to special sensations, whereas the general sensations have been discussed in Chapter 10.8; see page 989 on the somatosensory system.

11.1 Sense of Vision

CHAPTER OUTLINE

INTRODUCTION AND FUNCTIONAL ANATOMY

INTRODUCTION

Sense of vision, the choicest gift from the Almighty to the humans and other animals, is a complex function of the two eyes and their central connections. The eyeballs are able to perform their function with the help of the following physiological activities:

- Maintenance of clear media of the eye
- Maintenance of normal intraocular pressure (IOP)
- The image-forming mechanism
- Physiology of vision
- Physiology of binocular vision
- Physiology of the pupil
- Physiology of ocular motility

Before discussing the details of the above-mentioned physiological considerations, it will be worthwhile to be conversant with the broad outlines of functional anatomy of the eyeball and related structures.

FUNCTIONAL ANATOMY

There are two eyeballs, each being suspended by *extraocular muscles* and fascial sheaths in a quadrilateral pyramid-shaped bony cavity called *orbit*. Each eye is protected anteriorly by two shutters called the *eyelids*. The anterior part of the sclera and posterior surface of the eyelids are lined by a thin membrane called *conjunctiva*. For smooth functioning, the cornea and conjunctiva are to be kept moist by tears, which are produced by the lacrimal gland and drained by lacrimal passages, which together form the *lacrimal apparatus*. The eyelids, the eyebrows, the conjunctiva and the lacrimal apparatus are collectively known as the *appendages of the eye*. A brief account of anatomy of the eyeball and its related structures is given.

Eyeball

Each eyeball (Fig. 11.1.1) is a cystic structure kept distended by the pressure inside it. Although generally referred to as a globe, the eyeball is not a sphere but an oblate spheroid.

Dimensions of an Adult Eyeball

Anteroposterior diameter	: 24 mm
Horizontal (transverse) diameter	: 23.5 mm
Vertical diameter	: 23 mm
Circumference	: 75 mm
Volume	: 6.5 mL
Weight	: 7 g

Coats of the Eyeball

The eyeball comprises three coats – outer (fibrous coat), middle (vascular coat) and inner (nervous coat).

1. Outer fibrous coat The fibrous coat (Fig. 11.1.1) is a dense strong wall which protects the intraocular contents. Anterior one-sixth of this fibrous coat is transparent and is called cornea. The posterior five-sixth opaque part is called sclera. Junction of the cornea and the sclera is called limbus.

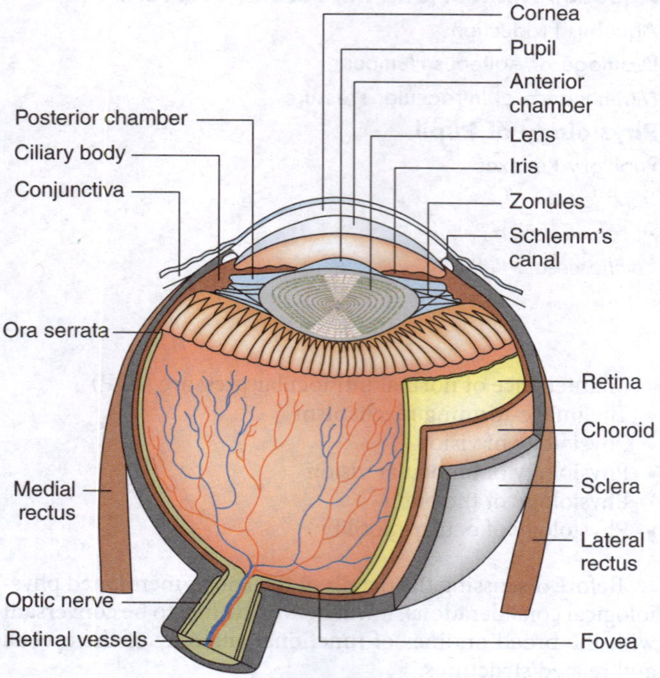

Fig. 11.1.1 Gross anatomy of eyeball.

Cornea The cornea is a transparent, avascular, watch glass–like structure with a smooth shining surface. The average diameter of the cornea is 11–12 mm. Its thickness in the central part is 0.52 mm and in the peripheral part 0.67 mm.

Sclera The sclera is a strong, opaque, white fibrous layer. It is a relatively avascular structure about 1 mm in thickness. It is pierced by nerves and vessels entering the eyeball. Histologically, the sclera consists of three layers – episcleral tissue, sclera proper and lamina fusca.

2. Middle vascular coat The middle vascular coat (Fig. 11.1.1), also known as uveal tract, from anterior to posterior, can be divided into three parts – iris, ciliary body and choroid. The blood supply of the uveal tract is derived from the short posterior ciliary arteries, long posterior ciliary arteries and anterior ciliary arteries.

Iris Iris is a coloured, circular diaphragm with a central aperture of 3–4 mm size known as pupil. The pupil regulates the light reaching the retina. It constricts and dilates by the contraction of sphincter pupillae and dilator pupillae muscles of the iris, respectively. The sphincter pupillae is supplied by the parasympathetic nerves, whereas the dilator pupillae is supplied by the sympathetic nerves.

Ciliary body The ciliary body is the middle part of the uveal tract. In cut section, it is triangular in shape with the base forwards. Anteriorly, the iris is attached to about the middle of the base of the ciliary body. Posteriorly, the ciliary body becomes continuous with the choroid. The ciliary body can be divided into two parts – anterior known as pars plicata and posterior known as pars plana.

The ciliary body contains a nonstriated muscle called the ciliary muscle which is supplied by parasympathetic fibres and takes part in the process of accommodation of the eye.

There are about 70–80 finger-like projections from the pars plicata part of the ciliary body. These are called *ciliary processes* and are the site of aqueous humour production – a watery fluid which maintains the IOP of the eyeball.

Choroid Choroid is a dark brown highly vascular layer situated in between the sclera and the retina. It supplies nutrition to the outer layers of the retina. The inflammations of the choroid invariably involve the underlying retina.

3. Inner nervous coat (retina) Retina, the innermost tunic of the eyeball, is a thin, delicate, transparent membrane. It is the most highly developed tissue of the eye. It is concerned with the visual functions (details on page 1107).

Interior of the Eyeball

Interior of the eyeball consists of anterior and posterior chambers containing the aqueous humour, the lens and the vitreous.

Anterior chamber is the space bounded anteriorly by the back of the cornea and posteriorly by the anterior surface of the iris. ***Posterior chamber*** is the space between the front of the crystalline lens and the back of the iris. Through the pupil, anterior and posterior chambers communicate with each other. *Aqueous humour* is a watery fluid present in the anterior and posterior chambers of the eyeball.

Crystalline Lens

The lens is a transparent, biconvex, crystalline structure placed between the iris and the vitreous. It is suspended from the ciliary body by the suspensory ligaments or zonules of Zinn. Refractive power of the lens is about 15–16 D. Lens is elastic in nature and its power changes with accommodation. Elasticity of the lens gradually decreases with the age. It is an avascular structure and derives its nutrition from the aqueous humour.

Vitreous Humour

Vitreous humour is an inert, transparent, jelly-like structure that fills the posterior four-fifths of the cavity of the eyeball. It serves the optical function. It consists of 90% water, some salts and mucoproteins.

Extraocular Muscles, Appendages of Eye and Orbit

Extraocular muscles A set of six extraocular muscles (four recti and two obliques) controls the movements of each eye (see page 1128).

Appendages of the Eye include:

Eyebrows The two eyebrows are arched structures placed horizontally over the superciliary ridge of the frontal bone, separated from each other by a smooth hairless prominent area known as glabella. The surface of the eyebrows is covered by hair which project obliquely from the skin and form an important part of the eyebrows. They protect the eyeball from sweat, dust and other foreign bodies.

Eyelids The eyelids are mobile tissue curtains placed in front of the eyeballs. These act as shutters protecting the eyes from injuries and excessive light. These also perform an important function of spreading the tear film over the cornea and conjunctiva.

Eyelashes are short curved hair present on the lid margins (free edges of the eyelids).

Conjunctiva The conjunctiva is a translucent mucous membrane which lines the posterior surface of the eyelids and anterior aspect of the eyeball up to the limbus. It consists of the following parts:

1. *Palpebral conjunctiva* lines the posterior surface of the eyelids.
2. *Bulbar conjunctiva* covers the anterior part of the eyeball up to the limbus.
3. *Fornices:* Superior and inferior conjunctival fornices are the cul-de-sac formed at the junction of the bulbar conjunctiva with the palpebral conjunctiva.
4. *Plica semilunaris* is a pinkish crescentic fold of the conjunctiva present in the medial canthus.

Orbit The bony orbits are quadrangular truncated pyramids situated between the anterior cranial fossa above and the maxillary sinuses below. Seven bones take part in its formation. It has four walls (medial, lateral, superior and inferior), a base and an apex.

MAINTENANCE OF CLEAR REFRACTIVE MEDIA OF THE EYE

The main prerequisite for visual function is the maintenance of clear refractive media of the eye. The major factor responsible for transparency of the ocular media is their avascularity. The structures forming refractive media of the eye from anterior to posterior are as follows:

- Tear film
- Cornea
- Aqueous humour (see page 1130)
- Crystalline lens
- Vitreous humour

PHYSIOLOGY OF TEARS

Lacrimal Apparatus

The lacrimal apparatus (Fig. 11.1.2) comprises the structures concerned with the formation (main lacrimal gland and accessory lacrimal glands) and drainage (lacrimal passages – puncta, canaliculi, lacrimal sac and nasolacrimal duct) of tears.

Tear Film and its Functions

Tear film Tear film refers to the fluid covering the cornea and conjunctiva. Tears are composed of 98% water and 1.5% sodium chloride (which gives the tears their salty flavour). They also contain antibacterial substances like lysozyme, betalysin and lactoferrin. Anatomically, the precorneal tear film has been described to consist of three layers, which from posterior to anterior (Fig. 11.1.3) are as follows:

1. ***Mucous layer:*** It consists of mucus secreted by conjunctival goblet cells.
2. ***Aqueous layer:*** It is formed by tears secreted by the main and accessory lacrimal glands.
3. ***Lipid layer:*** This, outermost layer, is formed by secretions of meibomian, and Zeis and Moll's glands.

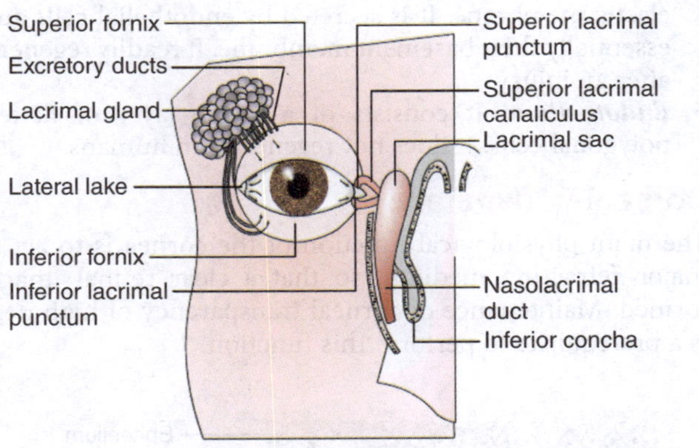

Fig. 11.1.2 The lacrimal apparatus.

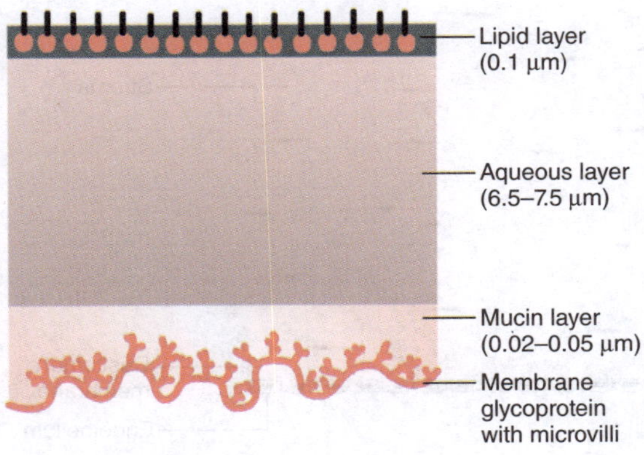

Fig. 11.1.3 Structure of tear film.

Functions of the tear film

1. It keeps the cornea and conjunctiva moist.
2. It provides oxygen to the corneal epithelium.
3. It washes away debris and noxious irritants.
4. It prevents infection due to presence of antibacterial substances.
5. It facilitates movements of the lids over the globe.

PHYSIOLOGY OF CORNEA

Cornea forms the main refracting medium of the eye. It is a transparent watch glass–like structure, the anterior surface of which is bathed with tears, and the endothelial surface is bathed in aqueous humour.

Histological Structure

Histologically, the cornea consists of the following five layers (Fig. 11.1.4):

1. ***Epithelium:*** It is of stratified squamous type and consists of five to six layers of cells.
2. ***Bowman's membrane:*** It is an acellular structure which consists of condensed collagen fibrils. Once damaged, it does not regenerate and leaves behind a faint corneal scar.
3. ***Stroma (substantia propria):*** It forms 90% of corneal thickness. It mainly consists of collagen fibrils arranged in sets of regular lamellae, lying parallel to the surface. The corneal lamellae are embedded in the ground substance. The ground substance consists of acid mucopolysaccharides, chondroitin sulphate (types A and C) and keratin sulphate. Scattered between the lamellae are the corneal corpuscles (keratocytes) and a few wandering leucocytes and macrophages.
4. ***Descemet's membrane:*** It is a thin but strong homogeneous elastic membrane. It is secreted by endothelial cells and is essentially their basement membrane. It readily regenerates after an injury.
5. ***Endothelium:*** It consists of a single layer of flattened polygonal cells. It does not regenerate in humans.

Corneal Transparency

The main physiological function of the cornea is to act as a major refracting medium, so that a clear retinal image is formed. Maintenance of corneal transparency of high degree is a prerequisite to perform this function.

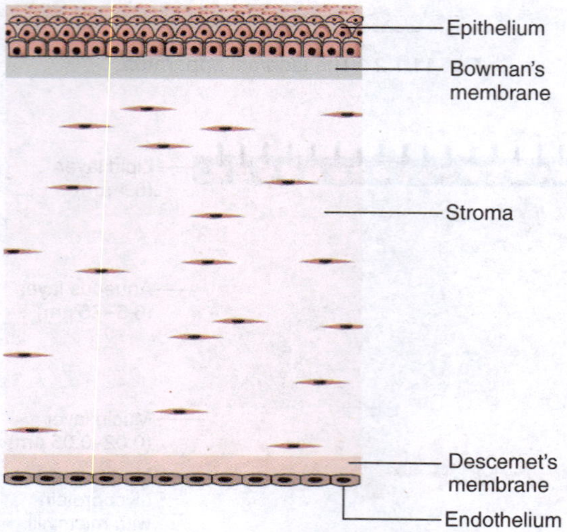

Fig. 11.1.4 Microscopic structure of cornea.

Factors responsible for corneal transparency Factors responsible for corneal transparency are as follows:

1. Anatomical factors contributing to corneal transparency are as follows:

- Avascularity of the cornea
- Absence of pigment in the cornea
- Demyelinated nerve supply
- Regular arrangement, nonkeratinization and homogenicity of refractive index of corneal epithelium
- A peculiar regular arrangement of the stromal lamellae (lattice theory)
- Paucity of cells in the stroma
- Regular arrangement of endothelial cells

2. Relative dehydration of stroma: The normal cornea maintains itself in a state of relative dehydration which is essential for the corneal transparency. The water content of the normal cornea is approximately 80%. It is kept constant by a balance of factors which draw water in the cornea and the factors which prevent the flow of water in the cornea.

Factors maintaining relative corneal dehydration are as follows:

- *Stromal swelling pressure* is the pressure (60 mm Hg) exerted by the glycosaminoglycans (GAGs).
- Barrier function of the epithelium is largely impermeable to water.
- Endothelial active pump system pumps fluid and electrolytes from the stroma to the aqueous. It includes Na^+–K^+-ATPase pump system.
- Special intercellular junctions in the endothelium also act to some extent as a barrier for the fluid.
- IOP should be optimum to control fluid transport in the cornea.

Source of Nutrition

Peripheral cornea receives its nutrients via the bloodstream of the perilimbal plexus.

Central cornea is avascular and nutrients enter by either simple diffusion or active transport through aqueous humour. Oxygen is derived directly from air through the tear film. It is an active process undertaken by the epithelium.

Applied Aspect

Cornea is an avascular structure; therefore, corneal grafts are very well taken up in cases like blindness due to corneal opacities.

Metabolism

Cornea requires energy to maintain its deturgescence and also for epithelial cell renewal.

Energy in the form of ATP is provided by the metabolism of glucose. The most actively metabolizing layers of the cornea are epithelium and endothelium, the former being 10 times thicker than the latter and requiring a proportionately large supply of metabolic substrate. About 65% of corneal metabolism occurs via glycolysis and the remainder by way of Krebs cycle and hexose monophosphate (HMP) shunt.

PHYSIOLOGY OF CRYSTALLINE LENS

Structure of Lens

The lens is a transparent, biconvex, crystalline structure. Its diameter is 9–10 mm and thickness varies with age from

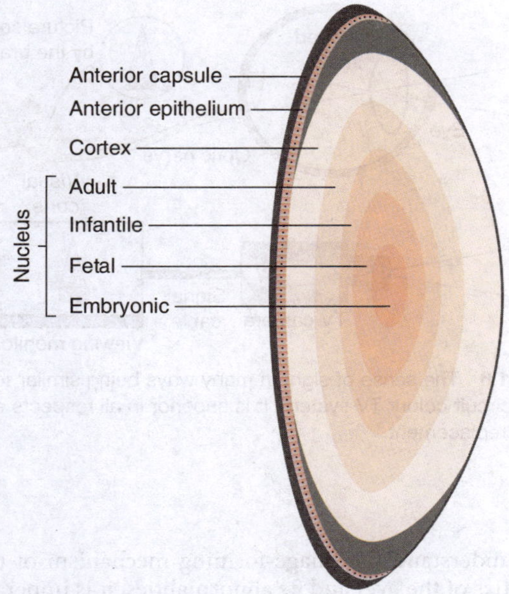

Fig. 11.1.5 Structure of crystalline lens.

3.5 mm (at birth) to 5 mm (at extreme of age). It consists of the layers given next (Fig. 11.1.5).

1. Lens capsule It is a thin, transparent, hyaline membrane surrounding the lens.

2. Anterior epithelium It is a single layer of cuboidal cells which lies deep to the anterior capsule. In the equatorial region, these cells become columnar, which are actively dividing and elongating to form new lens fibres throughout the life.

3. Lens fibres These form the main bulk of the lens and are arranged compactly as nucleus and cortex of the lens.

Nucleus is the central part containing the oldest fibres. It consists of different zones - embryonic nucleus, fetal nucleus, infantile nucleus and adult nucleus.
Cortex is the peripheral part which comprises the youngest fibres.

4. Suspensory ligaments of lens (zonules of Zinn) These consist essentially of a series of fibres by which the lens is suspended from the ciliary body.

Lens Transparency

Factors that play a significant role in maintaining outstanding clarity and transparency of the lens are as follows:

- Avascularity
- Tightly packed nature of lens cells
- The arrangement of lens protein
- Semipermeable character of lens capsule
- Same index of refraction in all parts of the lens
- Pump mechanism of lens fibre membranes that regulates the electrolyte and water balance in the lens, maintaining relative dehydration
- Auto-oxidation and high concentration of reduced glutathione in the lens that maintains the lens proteins in a reduced state and ensures the integrity of the cell membrane pump

Metabolism

Lens requires a continuous supply of energy (ATP) for active transport of ions and amino acids, maintenance of lens dehydration and a continuous protein and GSH synthesis. Most of the energy produced is utilized in the epithelium which is the major site of all active transport processes. Only about 10%–20% of the ATP generated is used for protein synthesis.

Source of Nutrient Supply

The crystalline lens, being an avascular structure, is dependent for its metabolism on chemical exchanges with the aqueous humour.

Pathways of Glucose Metabolism

Glucose is very essential for the normal working of the lens. Metabolic activity of the lens is largely limited to the epithelium and cortex, whereas the nucleus is relatively inert. In the lens, 80% of glucose is metabolized anaerobically by the glycolytic pathway, 15% by pentose HMP shunt and a small proportion via oxidative Krebs citric acid cycle. Sorbitol pathway is relatively inconsequential in the normal lens; however, it is extremely important in the production of cataract in diabetic and galactosaemic patients.

Applied Aspects

Cataract Any opacity in the lens or its capsule is called cataract.

Pathogenesis Three basic mechanisms which cause cataract are as follows:

- Damage to the lens capsule that changes its membranous properties
- Change in the lens fibre protein synthesis
- Increased lens hydration

Mechanism of loss of transparency: It is basically different in nuclear and cortical senile cataracts.

1. **Cortical senile cataract:** Its main biochemical features are decreased levels of total proteins, amino acids and potassium associated with increased concentration of sodium and marked hydration of the lens, followed by coagulation of proteins. The probable course of events leading to senile opacification of the cortex may be as shown in the following flowchart:

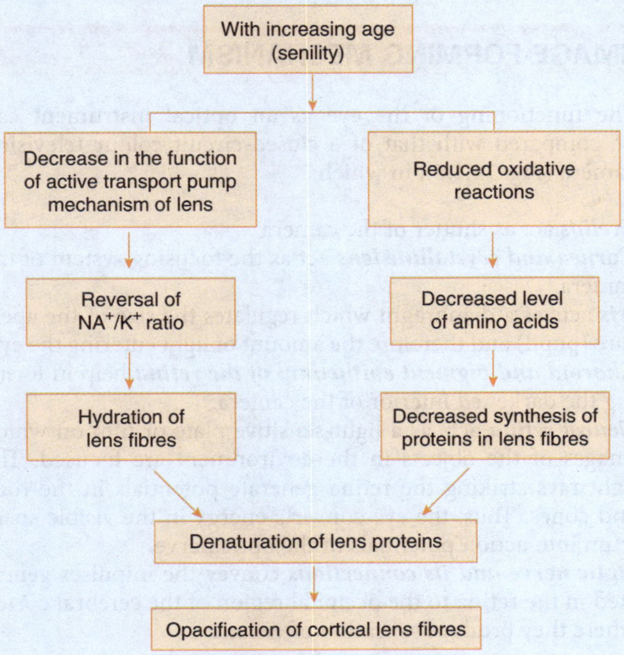

2. **Nuclear senile cataract:** In it, the usual degenerative change is intensification of the age-related nuclear sclerosis associated with dehydration and compaction of the nucleus resulting in a hard cataract. It is accompanied by a significant increase in water-insoluble proteins. However, the total protein content and distribution of cations remain normal. There may or may not be associated deposition of pigment urochrome and/or melanin derived from the amino acids in the lens.

PHYSIOLOGY OF VITREOUS HUMOUR

Vitreous humour is an inert, transparent, colourless, jelly-like structure that fills the posterior four-fifth of the cavity of the eyeball and is about 4 mL in volume.

Structure

The normal youthful vitreous gel is composed of a network of randomly oriented collagen fibrils interspersed with numerous spheroidal macromolecules of hyaluronic acid. The collapse of this structure with age or otherwise leads to conversion of gel into solution. The vitreous body can be divided into two parts – *cortex* (peripheral part) and *nucleus* (the main vitreous body).

Biochemical composition The vitreous body is composed of three major structural components – water, collagen-like fibres and hyaluronic acid, GAGs and a few other minor components.

Metabolic activities Cortical vitreous, though representing only 2% of the total vitreous volume, is the metabolic centre of the vitreous body. Hyalocytes present mainly in this part of the vitreous are involved in the production of hyaluronic acid.

Functions The vitreous gel mainly serves the *optical function*. In addition, it mechanically stabilizes the shape and volume of globe, and is a pathway for nutrients to reach the lens and retina.

IMAGE-FORMING MECHANISM

The functioning of the eye as an optical instrument can be compared with that of a closed-circuit colour television camera (Fig. 11.1.6), in which:

Eyelids act as shutter of the camera.
Cornea and crystalline lens act as the focusing system of the camera.
Iris acts as a diaphragm which regulates the size of the aperture (pupil) and therefore the amount of light entering the eye.
Choroid and pigment epithelium of the retina help in forming the darkened interior of the camera.
Neural retina acts as a light-sensitive plate or film on which images of the objects in the environment are focused. The light rays striking the retina generate potentials in the rods and cones. Thus, the eye converts energy in the visible spectrum into action potentials in the optic nerve.
Optic nerve and its connections convey the impulses generated in the retina to the occipital region of the cerebral cortex where they produce sensation of vision.

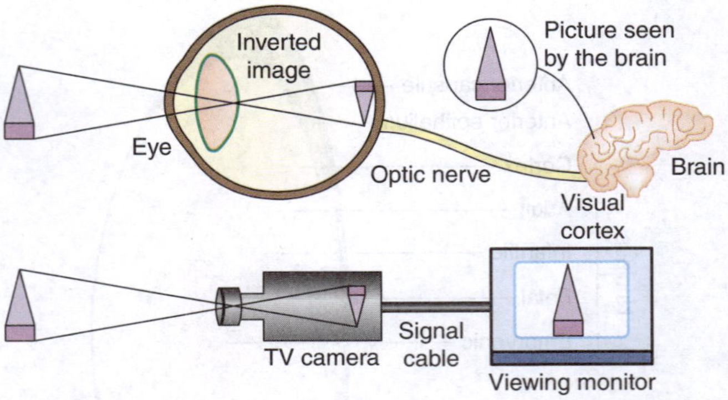

Fig. 11.1.6 The sense of sight in many ways being similar to a closed-circuit colour TV system. It is superior in all respects except ease of replacement.

To understand the image-forming mechanism of the eye (i.e. optics of the eye) and its abnormalities, it is imperative to have some knowledge about the light and geometrical optics.

OPTICS OF THE EYE

As an optical instrument, the eye can be compared with a camera with the retina acting as a unique kind of 'film'. The focusing system of the eye is composed of several refracting structures; these include (the numbers in parentheses are their refractive indices): (i) cornea (1.37), (ii) aqueous humour (1.33), (iii) crystalline lens (1.42) and (iv) vitreous humour (1.33). These constitute a homocentric system of lenses, which when combined in action form a very strong refracting system of a short focal length. The total dioptric power of the eye is about +60 D out of which about +44 D is contributed by cornea and +16 D by the crystalline lens.

Cardinal Points of the Eye

Listing and Gauss, while studying refraction by lens combinations, concluded that for a homocentric lens system, there exist three pairs of cardinal points, which are two principal foci, two principal points and two nodal points, all situated on the principal axis of the system. Therefore, the eye, forming a homocentric complex lens system, when analysed optically according to Gauss' concept can be resolved into six cardinal points (schematic eye). The cardinal data of the ***schematic eye*** are as follows (Fig. 11.1.7A):

- Total dioptric power is +58 D, of which the cornea contributes +43 D and the lens +15 D.
- The principal foci F_1 and F_2 lie 15.7 mm in front of and 24.4 mm behind the cornea, respectively.
- The principal points P_1 and P_2 lie in the anterior chamber 1.35 and 1.60 mm behind the anterior surface of the cornea, respectively.
- The nodal points N_1 and N_2 lie in the posterior part of the lens 7.08 and 7.33 mm behind the anterior surface of the cornea, respectively.

Reduced Eye

Listing's reduced eye: The optics of the eye otherwise is very complex. However, for understanding, Listing has simplified the data by choosing single principal point and single nodal

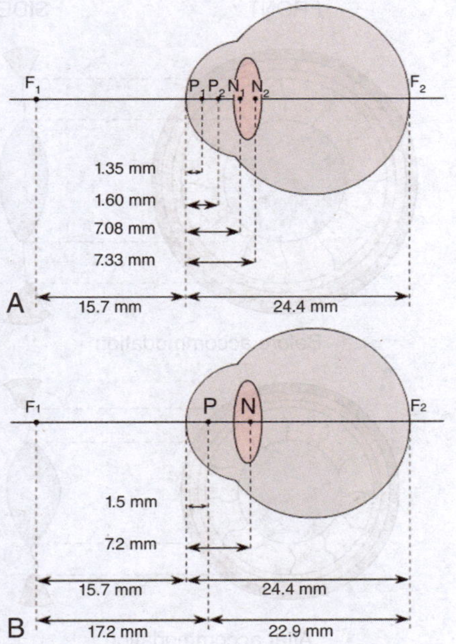

Fig. 11.1.7 Cardinal points of: **A**, schematic eye; and **B**, Listing's reduced eye.

point lying midway between two principal points and two nodal points, respectively. This is called Listing's reduced eye. The simplified data of this eye (Fig. 11.1.7B) are as follows:

- Total dioptric power is +60 D.
- The principal point (P) lies 1.5 mm behind the anterior surface of the cornea.
- The nodal point (N) is situated 7.2 mm behind the anterior surface of the cornea.
- The anterior focal point is 15.7 mm in front of the anterior surface of the cornea.
- The posterior focal point (on the retina) is 24.4 mm behind the anterior surface of the cornea.
- The anterior focal length is 17.2 mm (15.7 + 1.5) and the posterior focal length is 22.9 mm (24.4 − 1.5).

Axes of the Eye

The eye has three principal axes (Fig. 11.1.8):

Optical axis is the line passing through the centre of the cornea (P) and centre of the lens (N), and meets the retina (R) on the nasal side of the fovea.

Visual axis is the line joining the fixation point (O), nodal point (N) and fovea (F).

Fixation axis is the line joining the fixation point (O) and the centre of rotation (C).

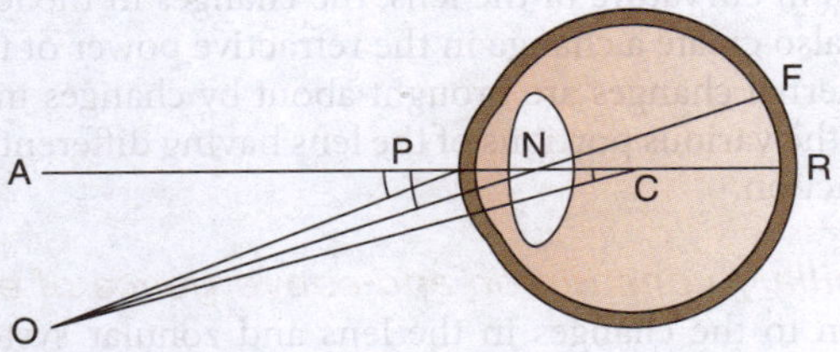

Fig. 11.1.8 Axes of the eye. AR, optical axis; OC, fixation axis; OF, visual axis.

ACCOMMODATION

Definition of Accommodation and Related Terms

Accommodation

As we know, in an emmetropic eye, parallel rays of light coming from infinity are brought to focus on the retina, with accommodation at rest. Our eyes have been provided with a unique mechanism by which we can focus even the diverging rays coming from a near object on the retina in a bid to see clearly (Fig. 11.1.9). This mechanism is called accommodation. In it, there occurs increase in the power of the crystalline lens.

Far point, Near Point, Range and Amplitude of Accommodation

The nearest point at which small objects can be seen clearly is called near point or *punctum proximum* and the distant (farthest) point is called far point or *punctum remotum*. The distance between the near point and the far point is called *range of accommodation*. The difference between the dioptric power needed to focus at near point (*P*) and that needed to focus at far point (*R*) is called *amplitude of accommodation* (*A*). Thus, $A = P - R$.

Far point and near point of the eye vary with the static refraction of the eye. In a hypermetropic eye, far point is virtual and lies behind the eye, whereas in a myopic eye, it is real and lies in front of the eye (Fig. 11.1.10). In an emmetropic eye, far point is at infinity and near point varies with age, being about 7 cm at age of 10 years, 25 cm at the age of 40 years and 33 cm at the age of 45 years. Thus, the amount that the eye can alter its refraction is greatest in childhood and slowly decreases until it is lost in middle age.

Mechanism of Accommodation

As we know, accommodation is a process by which one can focus the objects at different distances in a bid to have a clear vision. Its mechanism varies from species to species. Just for an interest, examples of a few species are as follows:

- Some fishes retract their lenses to focus on distant objects.
- Snakes and frogs have a mechanism to move the lens forward for near vision.
- Horses, by moving their heads, tilt the retina so that different regions lie at appropriate distances behind the lens. In humans, the process of accommodation is achieved by a change in the shape of the lens.

Theories of Mechanism of Accommodation in Humans

Relaxation theory This theory was first proposed by Thomas Young and elaborated by Helmholtz in 1885, by whose name it is known generally. The importance given to the lens

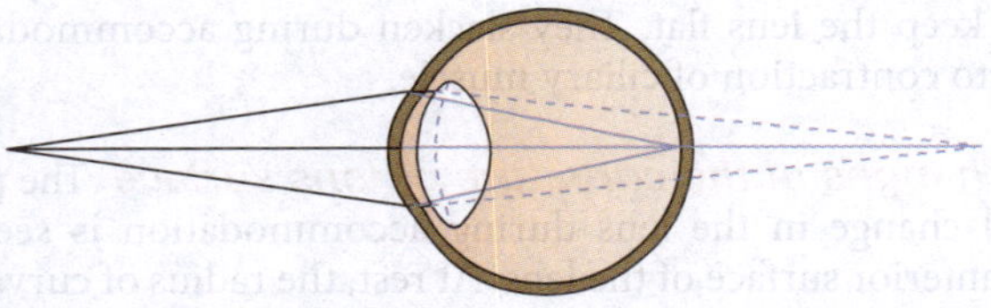

Fig. 11.1.9 Effect of accommodation on divergent rays entering the eye.

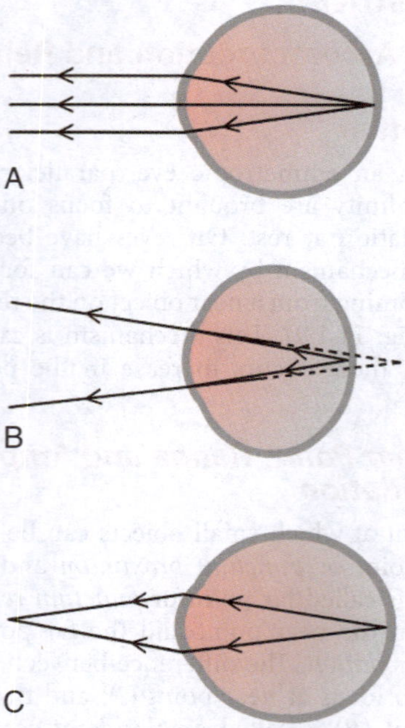

Fig. 11.1.10 Far point in: **A**, emmetropic eye; **B**, hypermetropic eye; and **C**, myopic eye.

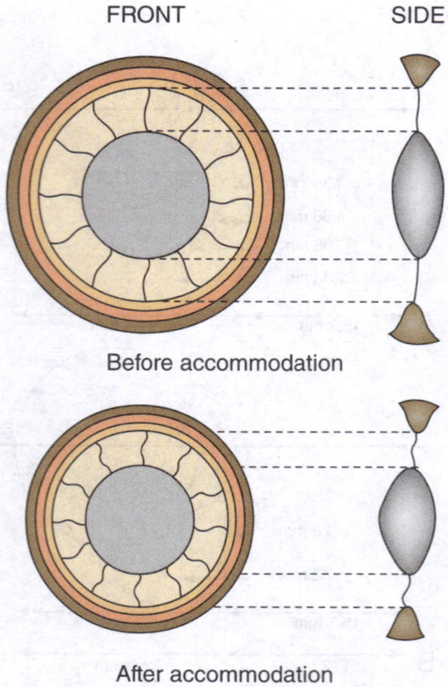

Fig. 11.1.11 Changes in the ciliary body ring zonules and shape of lens during accommodation.

capsule was emphasized by Fincham in 1937. The main points of the relaxation theory are as follows:

- When the eye is at rest (unaccommodated), the malleable substance of the young lens is compressed in its capsule (which is an elastic structure) by tension of the zonules. The surfaces of the compressed lens are less curved and these change the dioptric power in the lens.
- Zonules are kept under tension by a pull executed on them by the elastic choroid (Helmholtz original assumption). However, recently, it is being assumed by many workers that the zonules are kept under tension by the relaxation of fibres of the ciliary muscle.
- Contraction of the ciliary muscle causes the ciliary ring to shorten and move forward the equator of the lens. It also pulls the choroid forward. As a result, the zonules are relaxed *(basic mechanism of relaxation theory)*, the tension on the capsule is relieved and the lens attains a more spherical shape. As the refractive index of the lens (1.39) is more than the refractive index of the aqueous and vitreous, an increase in convexity of the lens increases its dioptric power and thus allows the near objects to be focused clearly on the retina.

Ocular Changes in Accommodation

The changes which take place in the eye during accommodation can be summarized as given next.

1. Slackening of the zonules Zonules are normally tense and keep the lens flat. They slacken during accommodation due to contraction of ciliary muscle.

2. Changes in the curvature of lens surface The principal change in the lens during accommodation is seen in the anterior surface of the lens. At rest, the radius of curvature of the anterior surface of the lens is 11 mm and that of the posterior surface is 6 mm. In accommodation, the curvature of the posterior surface remains almost the same, but the anterior surface changes, so that in strong accommodation, its radius of curvature becomes about 6 mm in the periphery and 3 mm in the central part which bulges more. The central part of the anterior surface bulges more because the anterior capsule is thinner here (Fig. 11.1.11) as compared with the peripheral part. The posterior capsule is the thinnest region and so the posterior surface has a greater curvature even in the unaccommodated lens.

3. Anterior pole Anterior pole of the lens moves forward carrying the iris with it, resulting in shallowing of the anterior chamber in the centre.

4. Axial thickness Axial thickness of the lens is increased owing to forward movement of the anterior pole (posterior pole remaining fixed).

5. Changes in the tension of lens capsule Changes in the tension of lens capsule have also been studied. During accommodation, the anterior capsule becomes slack.

6. Lens sinks down Because the accommodated lens is held less firmly by its zonular attachment, it is influenced by the force of gravity and tends to sink within the globe.

7. Changes within the lens substance In addition to the changes in curvature of the lens, the changes in the lens substance also create a change in the refractive power of the lens. The internal changes are brought about by changes in curvature of the various portions of the lens having different indices of refraction.

8. Pupillary constriction and convergence of eyes In addition to the changes in the lens and zonular system, the pupil constricts and the eyes converge, almost simultaneously. These changes occur in a bid to achieve clear vision for near objects. The pupillary constriction is a synkinesis and not a true reflex, for it does not depend on either accommodation or convergence alone for its appearance.

9. Choroid The choroid is stretched forward by the ciliary muscle contraction.

10. Ora serrata The ora serrata moves forward about 0.05 mm with each dioptre of accommodation.

Optical Aberrations of the Eye

The eye, in common with many optical systems in practical use, is by no means optically perfect; the lapses from perfection are called aberrations. Fortunately, the eyes possess those defects to so small a degree that, for functional purposes, their presence is immaterial. It has been said that despite imperfections, the overall performance of the eye is little short of astonishing. Physiological optical defects in a normal eye include those given next.

1. Diffraction of light Diffraction is bending of light caused by the edge of an aperture or the rim of a lens. Even a perfect lens, free from aberrations, will not focus light to a point due to diffraction. The actual pattern of a diffracted image point produced by a lens with a circular aperture or pupil is a series of concentric bright and dark rings (Fig. 11.1.12). At the centre of the pattern is a bright spot known as the Airy disc after Sir George Airy who was the first to report it.

2. Spherical aberrations Spherical aberrations occur owing to the fact that spherical lens refracts peripheral rays more strongly than paraxial rays which in the case of a convex lens brings the more peripheral rays to focus closer to the lens (Fig. 11.1.13).

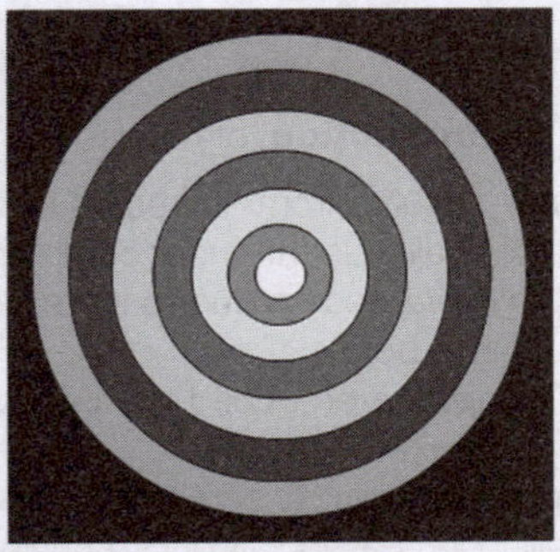

Fig. 11.1.12 The diffraction of light. Light brought to a focus does not come to a point, but gives rise to blurred disc of light surrounded by several dark and light bands (the Airy disc).

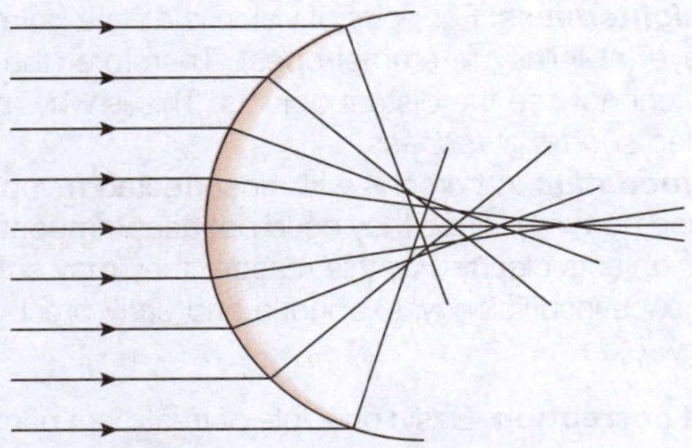

Fig. 11.1.13 Spherical aberration.

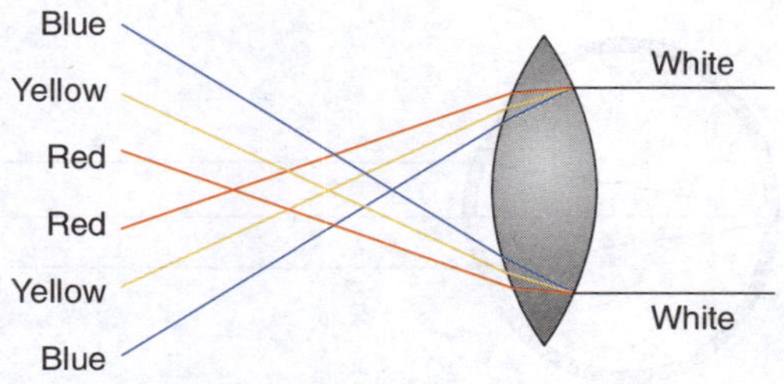

Fig. 11.1.14 Chromatic aberration.

The factors which contribute in diminishing the spherical aberrations of a human eye are as follows:

- Peculiar curvature of the cornea, i.e. flatter periphery than the centre
- Peculiar structure of the crystalline lens in which the central portions have a greater density and are arranged in layers of greater curvature than the peripheral portion
- Blocking the peripheral rays to enter the eye by the iris and thus in ordinary circumstances refraction of only paraxial rays of light taking place

3. Chromatic aberrations Chromatic aberrations result owing to the fact that the index of refraction of any transparent medium varies with the wavelength of incident light. In a human eye, which optically acts as a convex lens, blue light is focused slightly in front of the red (Fig. 11.1.14). In other words, the emmetropic eye is, in fact, slightly hypermetropic for red rays and myopic for blue and green rays. This fact forms the basis of bichrome test used in subjective refraction.

Applied Aspects

Common Defects of the Image-Forming Mechanism

Emmetropia

Emmetropia (optically normal eye) can be defined as a state of refraction when the parallel rays of light coming from infinity are focused at the sensitive layer of the retina with the accommodation being at rest (Fig. 11.1.15).

Ametropia

Ametropia, a condition of refractive error is defined as a state of refraction when the parallel rays of light coming from infinity (with accommodation at rest) are focused either in front or behind the sensitive layer of the retina, in one or both the meridia. It includes myopia, hypermetropia and astigmatism.

Hypermetropia. Hypermetropia, hyperopia or long-sightedness is the refractive state of the eye in which the parallel rays of light

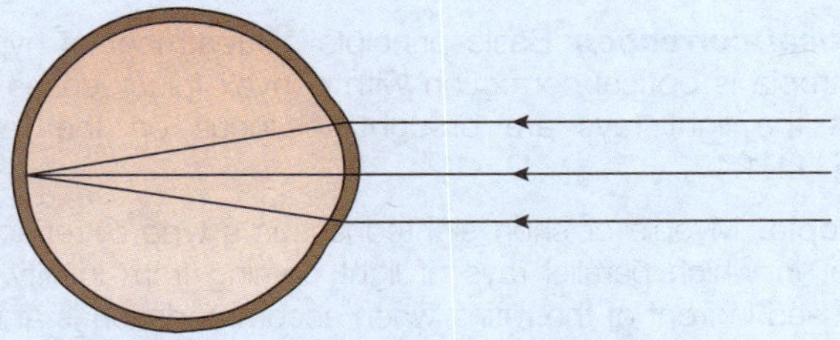

Fig. 11.1.15 Refraction in an emmetropic eye.

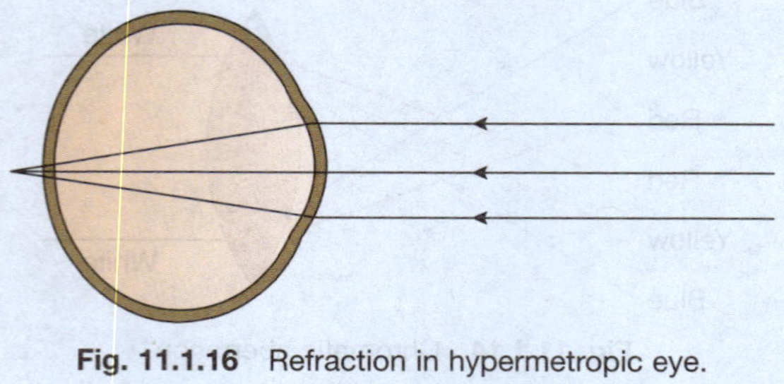

Fig. 11.1.16 Refraction in hypermetropic eye.

coming from infinity are focused behind the retina with accommodation being at rest (Fig. 11.1.16).

Mechanism of production Aetiologically, hypermetropia may be axial, curvatural, index, positional and due to absence of the lens.

1. *Axial hypermetropia* is by far the most common form. In this condition, there is an axial shortening of the eyeball. About 1 mm shortening of the anteroposterior diameter of the eye results in 3 D of hypermetropia.
2. *Curvatural hypermetropia* is the condition in which the curvature of the cornea, lens or both is flatter than the normal. About 1 mm increase in radius of curvature results in 6 D of hypermetropia.
3. *Index hypermetropia* occurs due to change in refractive index of the lens in old age. It may also occur in diabetic patients under treatment.
4. *Positional hypermetropia* results from posteriorly placed crystalline lens.
5. *Absence of crystalline lens* either congenitally or acquired (following surgical removal or posterior dislocation) leads to aphakia – a condition of high hypermetropia.

Characteristic features are as follows:

Far-sightedness: Persons with mild to moderate hypermetropia, in their young age, can see the distant objects clearly using their accommodation. This is why hypermetropia is also called far-sightedness or long-sightedness.

Near point of vision moves further away and the patient may have sometimes problem in near vision, when most of the accommodation is used for correcting for vision. Because of this, hypermetropia requires presbyopic correction at a younger age.

Asthenopic symptoms: Due to sustained accommodation (i.e. prolonged muscular effort), individuals may develop mild headache, eye ache, feeling of tiredness and discomfort in reading. All these symptoms are collectively called asthenopic symptoms.

Accommodative convergent squint may develop in children with moderate to high hypermetropia (usually by the age of 2–3 years) due to excessive use of accommodation.

Optical correction Basic principle of treatment of hypermetropia is optical correction with convex (plus) lenses, so that the light rays are brought to focus on the retina (Fig. 11.1.17).

Myopia. Myopia or short-sightedness is a type of refractive error in which parallel rays of light coming from infinity are focused in front of the retina when accommodation is at rest (Fig. 11.1.18).

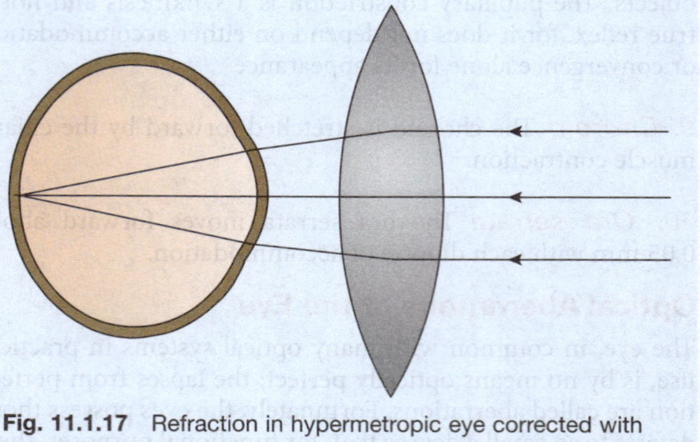

Fig. 11.1.17 Refraction in hypermetropic eye corrected with convex lens.

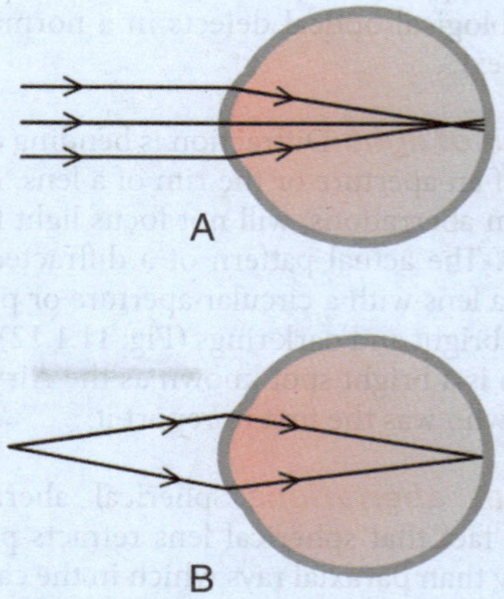

Fig. 11.1.18 Optics of myopia: **A**, parallel rays are focused in front of retina; and **B**, divergent rays from an object situated at a far point of the eye are focused at the retina.

Mechanisms of production of myopia are the following:

1. ***Axial myopia*** results from increase in anteroposterior length of the eyeball. It is the most common form.
2. ***Curvatural myopia*** occurs due to increased curvature of the cornea, lens or both.
3. ***Positional myopia*** is produced by anterior placement of the crystalline lens in the eye.
4. ***Index myopia*** results from increase in the refractive index of the crystalline lens associated with nuclear sclerosis.
5. ***Myopia due to excessive accommodation*** occurs in patients with spasm of accommodation.

Characteristic features are as follows:

Short-sightedness: Far point of vision is a finite point in front of the eye (at infinity in emmetropes). Therefore, the myopic persons cannot see the distant objects. This is why myopia is also called *short-sightedness*.

Accommodation in persons with uncorrected myopia is not developed normally, since they need not accommodate to see the near objects clearly. For this reason, they may suffer from convergence insufficiency, exophoria and early presbyopia as they grow older.

Optical correction Basic principle of treatment of myopia is optical correction with concave (minus) lenses, so that the

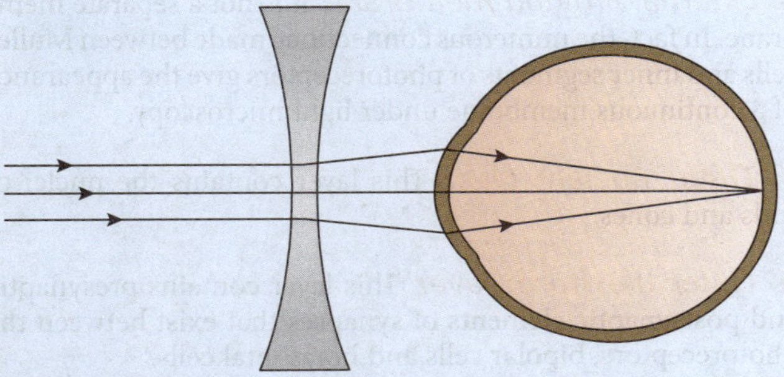

Fig. 11.1.19 Refraction in a myopic eye corrected by concave lens.

clear image is formed on the retina (Fig. 11.1.19). A myopic patient may not need glasses for near vision in old age, because his/her near point may be at a reading distance (which recedes back in emmetropic presbyopes).

Astigmatism. Astigmatism is a type of refractive error in which the refraction varies in the different meridia. Consequently, the rays of light entering the eye cannot converge to a point focus but form focal lines. Broadly, there are two types of astigmatism – regular and irregular.

Regular astigmatism The astigmatism is regular when the refractive power changes uniformly from one meridian to another (i.e. there are two principal meridia).

Irregular astigmatism It is characterized by an irregular change of refractive power in different meridia. There are multiple meridia which admit no geometrical analysis.

Presbyopia

Presbyopia (eyesight of old age) is not an error of refraction but a condition of physiological insufficiency of accommodation, leading to failing vision for near. To understand the condition of presbyopia, a working knowledge about accommodation is mandatory (see page 1103).

Since we usually keep the book at about 25 cm, we can read comfortably up to the age of 40 years. After the age of 40 years, the near point of accommodation recedes beyond the normal reading or working range. This condition of failing near vision due to age-related decrease in the amplitude of accommodation or increase in punctum proximum is called presbyopia.

Pathophysiology of presbyopia. Decrease in the accommodative power of the crystalline lens with increasing age, leading to presbyopia, occurs due to: (i) decrease in the elasticity and plasticity of the crystalline lens (which results from age-related sclerosis) and (ii) age-related decrease in the power of ciliary muscles.

Symptoms. Symptoms of presbyopia are as follows:

- Difficulty in near vision (to start with in the evening and in dim light and later even in good light) occurs.
- Asthenopic symptoms due to fatigue of the ciliary muscle are also complained after reading or doing any near work.

Treatment. The treatment of presbyopia is the prescription of appropriate convex glasses for near work.

PHYSIOLOGY OF VISION

Physiology of vision is a complex phenomenon which is still poorly understood.

The main mechanisms concerned with vision

Initiation of vision (phototransduction) is a function of photoreceptors (rods and cones).

Processing and transmission of visual sensation is a function of the image processing cells of the retina and visual pathway.

Visual perceptions are a function of the visual cortex and related areas of the cerebral cortex. They are based on the activities of serial processing stations in the visual pathway and parallel processing pathways. The visual perceptions are the functional elements of the vision, i.e. the sensations which result from stimulation of the retina with light. These are of four kinds, namely the light sense, the form sense, the contrast sense and the colour sense. Furthermore, different cortical areas make different contributions to the processing of motion, depth, form and colour.

For the purpose of understanding, the description of physiology of vision can be organized as:

- Retina, photoreceptors and visual pigment
- Phototransduction
- Processing and transmission of visual impulse in the retina
- Processing and transmission of visual impulse in the visual pathway
- Processing and analysis of visual impulse in the visual cortex
- Concept of serial and parallel processing of visual information

RETINA, PHOTORECEPTORS AND VISUAL PIGMENTS

Before embarking on the complex physiological processes concerning initiation and transmission of visual sensation, a brief description of the retina, photoreceptors and visual pigments will be useful.

Retina

Gross Anatomy

Retina, the innermost tunic of the eyeball, is a thin, transparent membrane. It is concerned with the visual functions. Grossly, the retina exhibits three distinct areas – optic disc, macula lutea and peripheral retina (Fig. 11.1.20).

Optic disc It is a well-defined, circular, pink-coloured disc of 1.5 mm diameter. It has only nerve fibre layer, so it does not excite any visual response. It produces a *blind spot* in the field of vision.

Macula lutea (yellow spot) It is a comparatively dark area situated at the posterior pole temporal to the optic disc. Its central depressed area 1.5 mm in diameter is called *fovea centralis*, which is the most sensitive part of the retina. Visual acuity is maximum in this part of the retina.

Ora serrata It is the anterior serrated margin where the retina ends.

Microscopic Structure

Retina consists of 10 layers, which from outside to inwards are given next (Fig. 11.1.21).

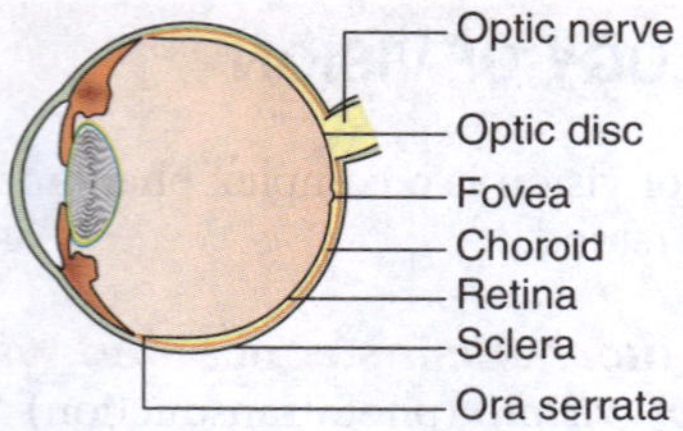

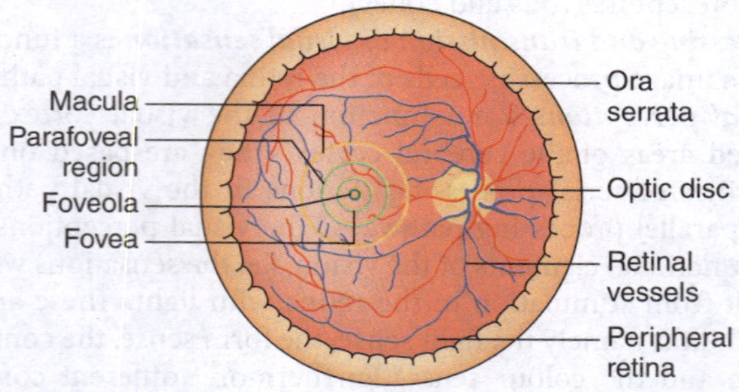

Fig. 11.1.20 Gross anatomy of retina.

1. Layer of pigment epithelium It is a single layer of hexagonal cells containing melanin pigments. It serves the following *functions*:

- Absorbs stray light, and thereby reduces light scatter
- Phagocytoses the ends of the outer segments of rods which are continuously shed
- Reconverts the metabolized photopigment into a form that can be reused after it is transported back to photoreceptor
- Acts as a tight junction between the cells that forms the outer blood–retinal barrier

2. Layer of rods and cones It consists of the outer segments of the photoreceptors (rods and cones). Photoreceptors are the end organs of vision.

3. External limiting membrane It is not a separate membrane. In fact, the numerous connections made between Muller cells and inner segments of photoreceptors give the appearance of a continuous membrane under light microscopy.

4. Outer nuclear layer This layer contains the nuclei of rods and cones.

5. Outer plexiform layer This layer contains presynaptic and postsynaptic elements of synapses that exist between the photoreceptors, bipolar cells and horizontal cells.

6. Inner nuclear layer It contains the cell bodies and nuclei of bipolar cells, amacrine cells and horizontal cells.

7. Inner plexiform layer It is the layer of synapse between bipolar cells, ganglion cells and amacrine cells.

8. Ganglion cell layer It consists of ganglion cells, which are the output cells of the retina. They transmit visual information to the brain.

9. Nerve fibre layer It consists of the axons of ganglion cells which pass through the lamina cribrosa to form the optic nerve. These fibres remain unmyelinated in the retina, but become myelinated in the optic nerve.

10. Inner limiting membrane It is formed by projections of the Muller's cells and separates the retina from the vitreous.

Structural characteristics of fovea centralis Foveal region has the highest visual resolution because of the following structural characteristics:

- Rods are absent and cone density is maximum.
- Foveal cones have unusually long and thin outer segments. This shape allows a high packing density.

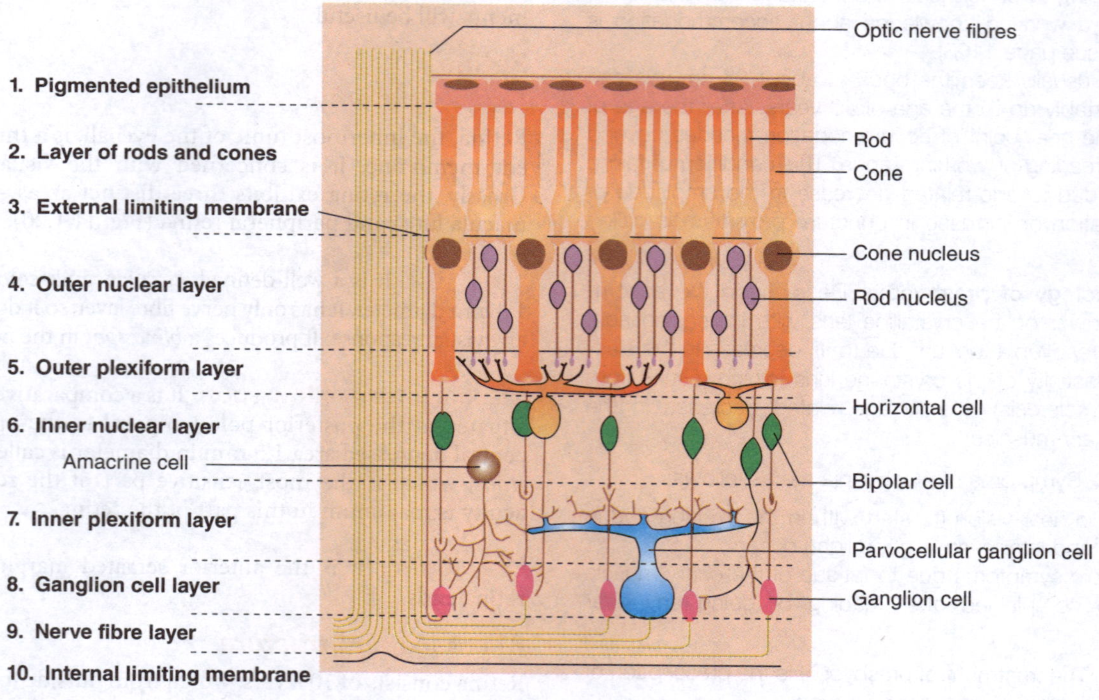

Fig. 11.1.21 Microscopic structure of retina.

- All other inner layers of the retina are pushed aside in this area. This arrangement allows light to reach the cones without having to pass through the inner layers of the retina, and thereby reduces distortion of the image.
- The most central part of the fovea (foveola) is devoid of even capillaries, whereas the rest of the fovea contains fine capillaries but no large vessels which encircle this area.
- There is no convergence of efferents of the foveal cones. Each foveal cone relays to single ganglion cell. Hence, there is disproportionate large representation of the fovea in the visual cortex.

Applied Aspects

Age-related macular degeneration (ARMD) occurs due to blood vessel growth over the macula leading to loss of central vision. This disease is more common in females.

Types: ARMD is of two types—dry ARMD and wet ARMD.

- In dry ARMD, there occurs slow damage of cones resulting in loss of central vision.
- In wet ARMD, the increased activity of vascular endothelial growth factor (VEGF) promotes proliferation of fragile blood vessels under the macula resulting in leakage of blood/fluid.

Retinal detachment (RD) is an emergency condition in which the neural layer of the retina gets separated from the pigment layer.

Causes: There are many causes of RD, but the most common causes are ageing or an eye injury.

Types: Three types of RD are as follows:

Rhegmatogenous
Tractional
Exudative

Signs and symptoms include:

Sudden loss of vision
Small dark spots or linear lines that float across the vision (floaters)
Flashes of light and dark shadows in the field of vision

Treatment of RD depends on the type and extent. It includes:

Laser surgery and freezing treatment (cryopexy) if there is a small hole or tear in the retina
If a large part of the retina is detached from the back of the eye, retina surgery is required to move the retina back into its place.

Photoreceptors

Density and Distribution of Photoreceptors

- Rods and cones *(photoreceptors)* are the end organs of vision which transform light energy into visual (nerve) impulse.
- Rods contain a photosensitive substance, visual purple *(rhodopsin)*, and subserve the peripheral vision and vision of low illumination (scotopic vision).
- Cones also contain a photosensitive substance and are primarily responsible for highly discriminatory central vision (photopic vision) and colour vision.
- There are about 120 million rods and 6.5 million cones.
- The highest density of cones is at the fovea with an average of 199,000 cones/mm^2. The number of cones falls off rapidly outside the fovea.
- Rods are absent at the fovea in an area of 0.35 mm (rod-free zone) which corresponds to 1.25° of the visual field, but are present in a large number (160,000/mm^2) in a ring-shaped zone 5–6 mm from the fovea.

Structure of Photoreceptor

Each *photoreceptor* consists of a cell body and nucleus (which lie in the outer nuclear layer), a cell process that extends into outer plexiform layer and inner and outer segments (which form the layer of rods and cones) (Fig. 11.1.22). The long axis of the photoreceptor is oriented perpendicular to the retinal surface.

Rod cell Each rod is about 40–60 μm long and consists of the following:

Outer segment of the rod is cylindrical, highly refractile and transversely striated, and contains visual purple. It is composed of numerous lipid protein lamellar discs stacked one on top of the other and surrounded by a cell membrane.

Inner segment of the rod is thicker than the outer segment. It consists of two regions – ellipsoid and myoid. *An outer rod fibre* arises from the inner end of the rod, which passes through the external limiting membrane and swells into a densely staining nucleus – the rod granule (lies in the outer nuclear layer), and then terminates as *inner rod fibre* (lies in the outer molecular layer) which at its end has got an end bulb called the rod spherule that is in contact with the cone foot.

Cone cell Each cone cell is 40–80 μm long. It is longest at the fovea (80 μm) and shortest at the periphery (40 μm).

Cone outer segment is conical in shape, much shorter than that of the rod, and contains the iodopsin. The lamellar discs, which are narrower than those of the rods, are, in fact, infoldings of plasma membrane. There are about 1000–1200 discs/cone.

Cone inner segment and cilium are similar to the rod structures; however, the cone ellipsoid is very plump and contains a large number of mitochondria.

Unlike the rod, the inner segment of the cone becomes directly continuous with its nucleus and lies in the outer nuclear layer. A stout cone inner fibre runs from the nucleus which at the end is provided with lateral processes called *cone foot* or *cone pedicle* (lies in the outer plexiform layer).

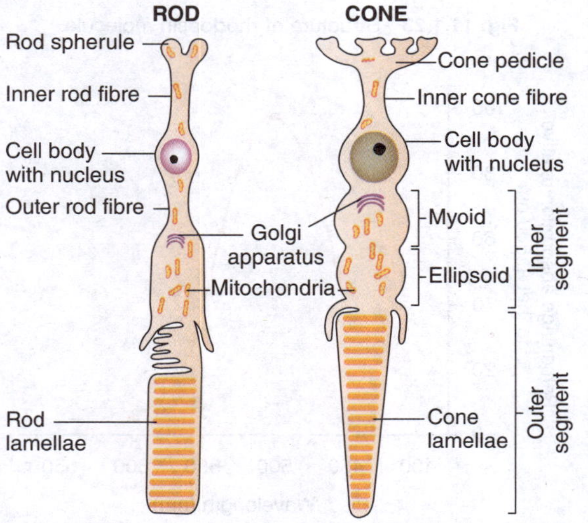

Fig. 11.1.22 Microscopic structure of rod and cone cells.

Visual Pigments

The visual pigments are those substances which have the property of absorbing light. These include *rhodopsin* and cone pigments.

Rhodopsin (Visual Purple)

Rhodopsin is the photosensitive visual pigment present in the discs of the rod outer segments. It consists of a protein opsin (called scotopsin) and a carotenoid called retinal (the aldehyde of vitamin A).

Human rhodopsin has a molecular weight of 40,000. It is one of the many serpentine receptors coupled to G-proteins. Its structure is shown in Fig. 11.1.23.

The absorption spectrum of rhodopsin as shown in Fig. 11.1.24 depicts that its peak sensitivity to light lies within the narrow limits of 493–505 nm. It absorbs primarily yellow wavelength of light, transmitting violet and red to appear purple by transmitted light; it is therefore also called visual purple.

Cone Pigments

The visual pigments present in the cones have not been so intensively studied as the rhodopsin. There are three kinds of cones in primates. Cone pigments are somewhat different from the rhodopsin, in that they respond to specific wavelength of light, giving rise to colour vision. These differences are present in the opsin portion of the molecule, whereas the chromophore 11-*cis*-retinal remains the same. The peak absorbance wavelength of the 'blue'-, 'green'- and 'red'-sensitive cones lies at about 435, 535 and 580 nm, respectively.

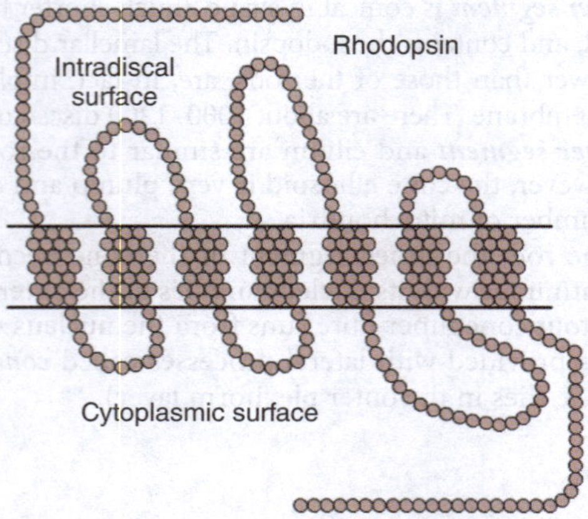

Fig. 11.1.23 Structure of rhodopsin molecule.

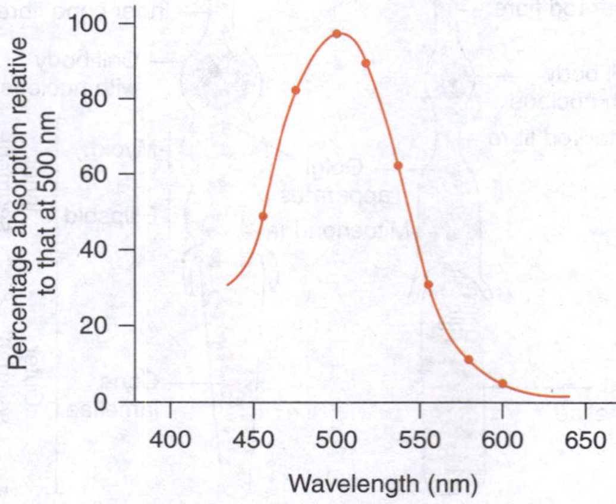

Fig. 11.1.24 Absorption spectrum of rhodopsin.

Light-induced changes Light falling on the retina is absorbed by the visual pigments and initiates *photochemical changes* which in turn trigger a sequence of events that cause phototransduction. The photochemical changes occurring in the rods and cones are similar, but they have been studied in detail in the rods and can be described under three headings:

- Rhodopsin bleaching
- Rhodopsin regeneration
- Visual cycle

Rhodopsin bleaching As mentioned earlier, the rhodopsin consists of a protein called *opsin* and a carotenoid called retinene (vitamin A aldehyde or 11-*cis*-retinal). The light absorbed by the rhodopsin converts its *11-cis-retinal* into *all-trans-retinal*. This light-induced isomerization of 11-*cis*-retinal into all-*trans*-retinal occurs through formation of many intermediates which exist for a transient period (Fig. 11.1.25). One of the intermediate compounds (*metarhodopsin II*, also called activated rhodopsin) of the above-mentioned isomerization chain reaction acts as an enzyme to activate many molecules of transducin. The activated transducin triggers the phototransduction.

The all-*trans*-retinal (produced from light-induced isomerization of 11-*cis*-retinal) can no longer remain in combination with the opsin and thus there occurs separation of opsin and all-*trans*-retinal. This process of separation is called *photodecomposition* and the rhodopsin is said to be bleached by the action of light.

Rhodopsin regeneration The all-*trans*-retinal separated from the opsin (as above) subsequently enters the chromophore pool existing in the photoreceptor outer segment and

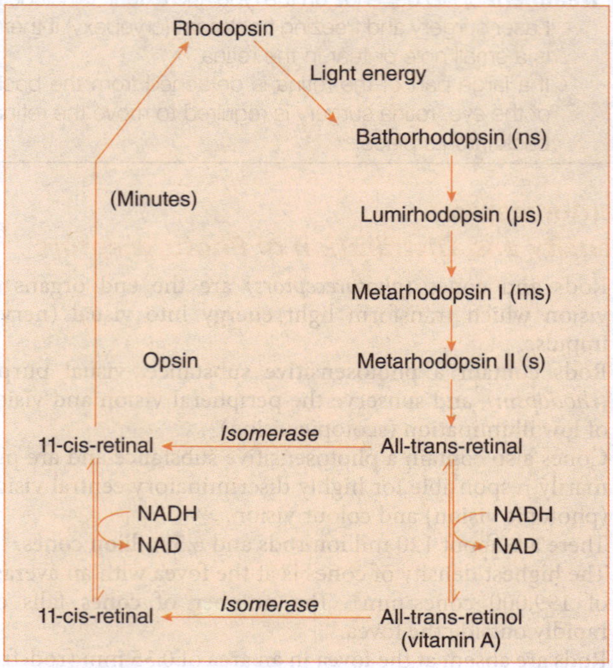

Fig. 11.1.25 Light-induced changes in rhodopsin.

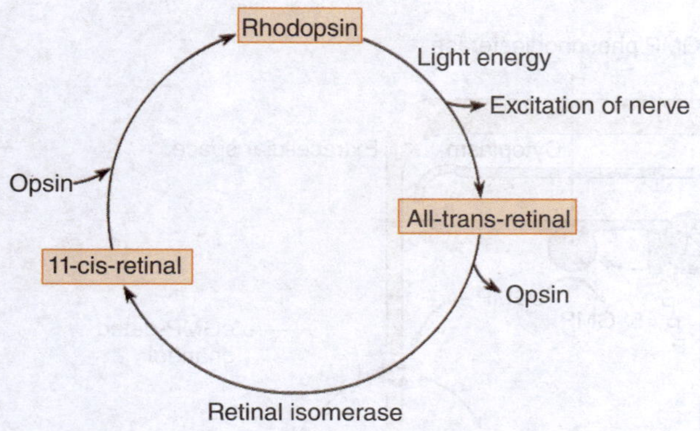

Fig. 11.1.26 Visual cycle.

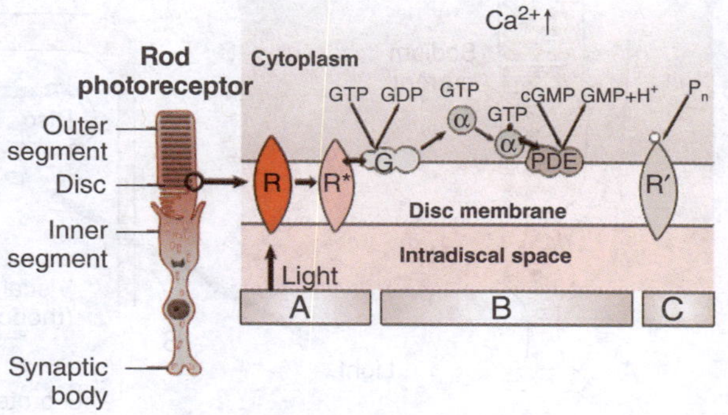

Fig. 11.1.27 The scheme for reaction triggered by rhodopsin bleaching which affects cyclic GMP in the photoreceptors: **A**, light-induced conversion of rhodopsin to its active form; **B**, activation of G-protein (G) and activation of cGMP phosphodiesterase (PDE) protein; and **C**, phosphorylation of photolysed rhodopsin.

the retinal pigment epithelial cells (for this, close approximation of RPE and photoreceptor is must). The all-*trans*-retinal may be further reduced to retinol by alcohol dehydrogenase, and then esterified to re-enter the systemic circulation.

The first stage in the reformation of rhodopsin, as shown in Fig. 11.1.25, is isomerization of all-*trans*-retinal back to 11-*cis*-retinal. The process is catalysed by the enzyme *retinal isomerase*. Energy for the regeneration process is supplied by the overall metabolic pool of the photoreceptor outer segment. The 11-*cis*-retinal in the outer segments of photoreceptors reunites with the opsin to form rhodopsin. This whole process is called regeneration of the rhodopsin. Thus, the bleaching of the retinal photopigments occurs under the influence of light, whereas the regeneration process is independent of light, proceeding equally well in light or darkness. The amount of rhodopsin in the rods, therefore, varies inversely with the incident light.

Visual cycle In the retina of living animals, under constant light stimulation, a steady state must exist under which the rate at which the photochemicals are bleached is equal to the rate at which they are regenerated. This equilibrium between the photodecomposition and the regeneration of visual pigments is referred to as *visual cycle* (Fig. 11.1.26).

PHOTOTRANSDUCTION

Phototransduction refers to conversion of light energy into nerve impulse. It involves a cascade of biochemical reactions in the steps given next (Fig. 11.1.27).

Activation of rhodopsin As described above, following exposure to light, the rhodopsin undergoes a series of spontaneous transformation, leading to formation of an active form of rhodopsin, the *metarhodopsin II*.

Activation of transducin The activated rhodopsin acts as an enzyme to activate many molecules of transducin (G-protein), which initiates the cascade of cellular responses by catalysing the exchange of GDP bound to transducin α-subunit for GTP. Then, transducin gets replaced by GTP and the α-subunit separates.

Conversion of cGMP to GMP The α-subunit activates the many molecules of the enzyme phosphodiesterase (PDE) which catalyses conversion of cGMP to GMP leading to reduction in the concentration of cGMP within the photoreceptor.

Production of receptor potential Reduction in the cGMP is responsible for producing receptor potential as explained next (Fig. 11.1.28).

- In dark, the Na^+ channels present in the cell membrane of the outer segment of photoreceptor are kept open by cGMP. So, a net influx of Na^+ results in a continuous current called *dark current*. The dark current causes the receptor cell to be maintained in a constant state of depolarization (the resting potential is about −40 mV). The intracellular Na^+ concentration is kept at a steady-state level by sodium pump (Na^+–K^+-ATPase) located in the inner segment.
- When light strikes the photoreceptor, the amount of cyclic GMP in the photoreceptor is reduced (as discussed above), so some of the Na^+ channels (which were kept open by cyclic GMP in dark) are closed, and the result is a hyperpolarizing receptor potential. Thus, the photoreceptor potential is different from the receptor potentials in almost all other sensory receptors in that the excitation of photoreceptor causes increased negativity of the membrane potential (hyperpolarization), rather than decreased negativity (depolarization) which is the characteristic of all other receptors. Normally, in dark, the electronegativity inside the rod membrane is about −40 mV and after excitation it approaches about −70 to −80 mV. Furthermore, the eye is unique in that the receptor potential of the photoreceptors is local graded potential, i.e. it does not propagate and does not follow the 'all-or-none law'.

The sequence of events in photoreceptors by which incident light leads to production of a nerve impulse (*phototransduction*) is summarized in Fig. 11.1.29.

Cone Versus Rod Receptor Potential

The cone receptor potential has a sharp onset and offset, whereas the rod receptor potential has a sharp onset and slow offset. The curve relating the amplitude of receptor potentials to the stimulus intensity has similar shapes in rods and cones, but the rods are much more sensitive. Therefore, rod responses are proportionate to stimulus intensity at levels of illumination that are below the threshold for cones. On the other hand, cone responses are proportionate to stimulus intensity at high levels of illumination when the rod responses

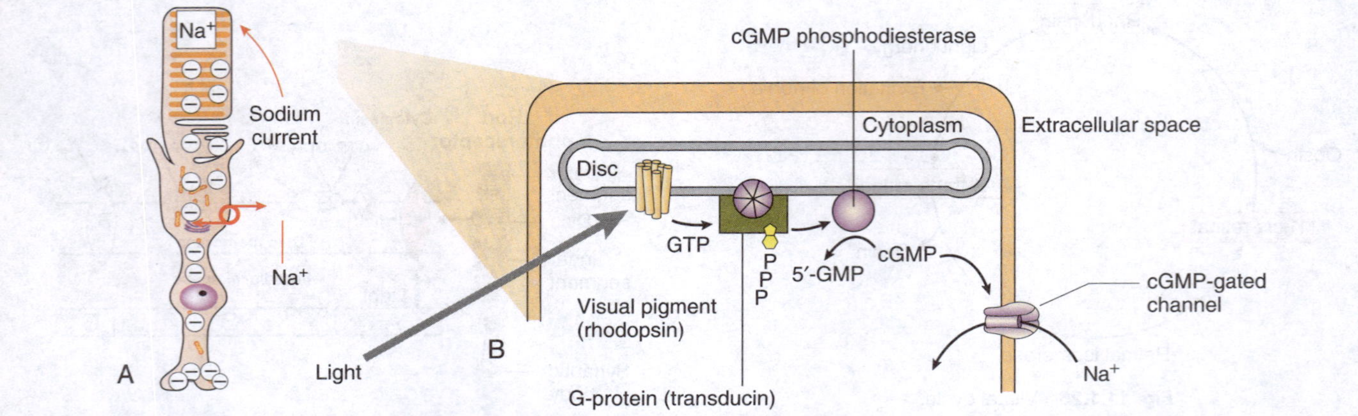

Fig. 11.1.28 Potential changes in a photoreceptor: **A**, in dark, Na^+ channels are opened by the cGMP and due to Na^+ influx, dark current results and membrane is kept depolarized (at resting membrane potential of −40 mV); and **B**, when light falls on the retina, the activated rhodopsin reduces intracellular levels of cGMP and consequently the Na^+ channels are blocked. This results in hyperpolarization (photoreceptor potential).

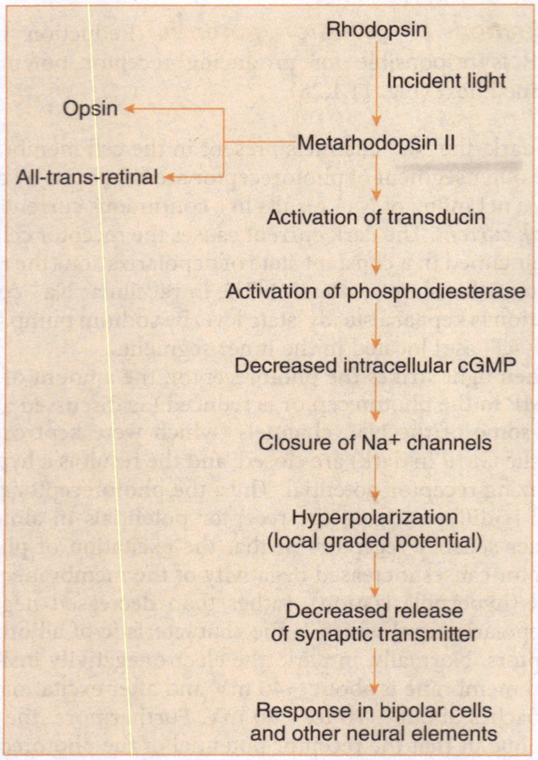

Fig. 11.1.29 Sequence of events involved in phototransduction process in the photoreceptors.

are maximal and cannot change. That is why cones generate good response to change in light intensity above background but do not represent absolute illumination well, whereas rods detect absolute illumination.

PROCESSING AND TRANSMISSION OF THE VISUAL IMPULSE IN RETINA

The receptor potential generated in the photoreceptors is transmitted by *electrotonic conduction* (i.e. direct flow of electric current, not action potential to other cells of the retina, i.e. horizontal cells, amacrine cells and ganglion cells). However, the ganglion cells transmit the visual signals by means of action potential to the neurons of the lateral geniculate body (LGB) and then later to the primary visual cortex.

Role of different cells in the processing of retinal image can be discussed in terms of the following concepts which have been evolved in physiology of vision:

- Concept of receptive field
- Concept of serial processing of the image (see page 1119)
- Concept of parallel processing pathway (see page 1118)

Concept of Receptive Field

The concept of receptive field has been evolved to explain the processing of visual signal. In general sense, the receptive field is defined as the influence area of a sensory neuron. It is circular in configuration.

Receptive field of individual photoreceptor is small and circular. Light falling in the receptive field hyperpolarizes the cell (as described above). In the dark, i.e. when the photoreceptor is depolarized, a neurotransmitter (glutamate) is released from its terminal. When hyperpolarized, the photoreceptor will therefore release less neurotransmitter.

Horizontal cells have a very large receptive field in comparison to the photoreceptor cell. A horizontal cell transmits signals horizontally in the outer plexiform layer from rods and cones to the bipolar cells. Their main function is to *enhance the visual contrast by causing lateral inhibition, i.e.* they play a role in processing of *spatial information* (Fig. 11.1.30).

Bipolar cells: There are two types of bipolar cells; one type of cells (which are inhibited by glutamate) is depolarized, whereas the other (which are excited by glutamate) is hyperpolarized when the photoreceptors are excited (Figs 11.1.30 and 11.1.31). Thus, the two different types of bipolar cells provide opposing excitatory and inhibitory signals in the visual pathway.

- *Receptive field* of the bipolar cell is also circular in configuration *but* has *got centre-surround antagonism*. As shown in Fig. 11.1.31 in case of centre-depolarizing cells (also called 'on cell'), the light striking the centre of receptive field activates and the light striking the surround' inhibits bipolar cell output. The reverse occurs in the centre-hyperpolarizing cell (also called 'off cell'), i.e. the

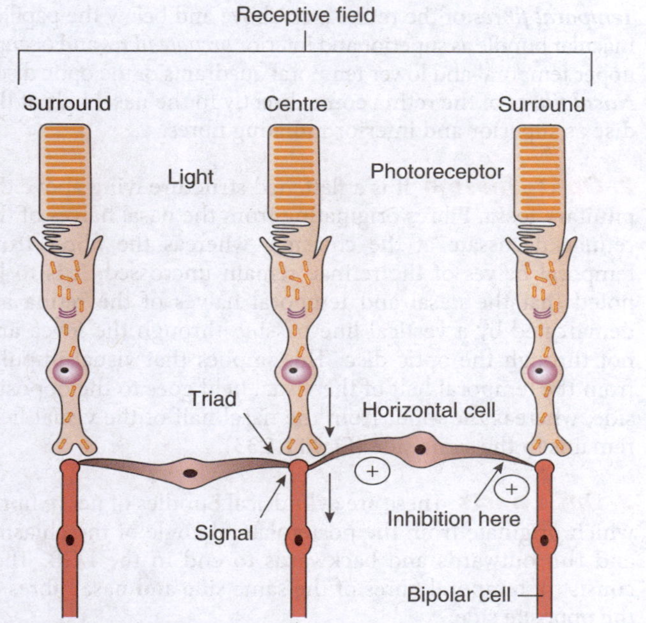

Fig. 11.1.30 Horizontal cells showing phenomenon of lateral inhibition in the surround receptive plexiform layer. The central photoreceptor has been stimulated with light and inner portion of the cell membrane becomes more negative. The signal is transmitted upward to bipolar cell and horizontally to horizontal cells. This horizontal transmission results in inhibition of receptor bipolar synapse of neighbouring photoreceptor element. The stimulated bipolar cell may be hyperpolarized or depolarized.

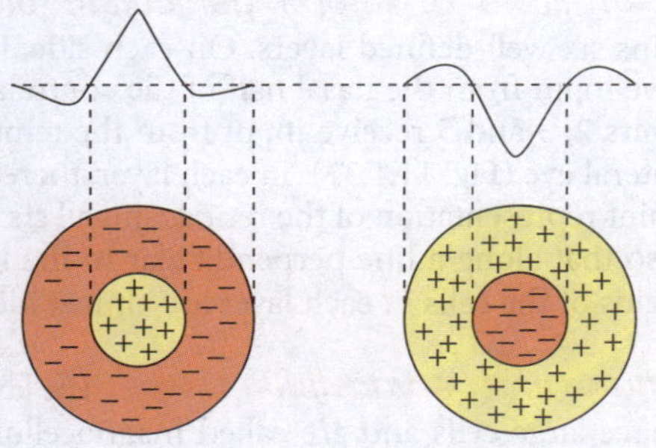

Fig. 11.1.31 The centre-surround response to light in 'on' or centre-depolarizing bipolar cell (left) and 'off' or centre-hyperpolarizing bipolar cell (right). Plus (+) signs indicate region giving depolarizing response and minus (−) signs a hyperpolarizing one.

light striking the 'centre' is inhibitory and the light striking the 'surround' is excitatory to bipolar cell output. The size of the centre of the bipolar cell receptive field is determined by the reach of its dendrites and that of the much larger 'surround' is determined by the spread of interconnected horizontal cells.

- The importance of the above-described reciprocal relationship between the depolarizing and hyperpolarizing bipolar cells is that it provides a second mechanism for lateral inhibition *(spatial information processing)* in addition to horizontal cell mechanism. Furthermore, this reciprocal relationship allows half of the bipolar cells to transmit positive signals and the other half to transmit negative signals; both of these have a useful role in transmitting visual information to the brain.

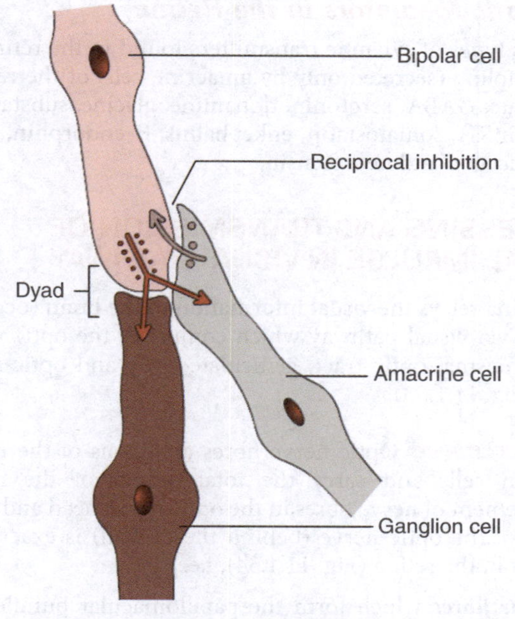

Fig. 11.1.32 Bipolar–amacrine ganglion cell interaction.

Amacrine cells: Amacrine cells receive information at the synapse of bipolar cell axon with ganglion cell dendrite (Fig. 11.1.32) and use this information for *temporal processing*. Furthermore, these cells receive input from different combinations of on-centre and off-centre bipolar cells. Therefore, the *receptive fields of amacrine cells* are mixture of on-centre and off-centre regions. Many different types of amacrine cells utilize at least eight different neurotransmitters. Thus, the contributions of amacrine cells to visual processing are complex.

Ganglion cells: The electrical response of bipolar cells (local graded potential) after modification by the amacrine cells is transmitted to the ganglion cells which in turn transmit their signals by means of action potentials to the brain.

Receptive field of ganglion cells like that of bipolar cells has got a centre-surround antagonism. Furthermore, like bipolar cells, the ganglion cells are also of two types in terms of their centre response – *'on-centre' cells* that increase their discharge and *'off-centre'* cells that decrease their discharge on illumination of the centre of their receptive fields.

Another group of ganglion cells in the retina contains the pigment melanopsin, functioning independently of rods and cones of the retina. These ganglion cells get depolarized in response to light.

Important Note

Melanopsin-containing ganglion cells project to suprachiasmatic nucleus of the hypothalamus and mediate circadian rhythm. These cells also project to Edinger–Westphal nucleus and have a role in pupillary reflex.

Concept of Parallel Processing Pathway

See page 1118.

Concept of Serial Processing of Image in Retina

See page 1119.

Synaptic Mediators in the Retina

Various types of synaptic transmitters found in the retina are acetylcholine (secreted only by amacrine cells of the retina), glutamate, GABA, serotonin, dopamine, glycine, substance P, TRH, GnRH, somatostatin, enkephalins, β-endorphin, CCK, VIP, glucagon and neurotensin.

PROCESSING AND TRANSMISSION OF VISUAL IMPULSE IN VISUAL PATHWAY

The retina relays the visual information to the brain (occipital cortex) via visual pathway which comprises the optic nerve, optic chiasma, optic tract, geniculate body and optic radiations (Fig. 11.1.33).

1. Optic nerve Optic nerve fibres are axons of the retinal ganglion cells and carry the total output of the retina. Arrangement of nerve fibres in the optic nerve head and distal region of the optic nerve (behind the eyeball) is exactly the same as in the retina (Fig. 11.1.34), i.e.:

Macular fibres which form the papillomacular bundle pass straight in the temporal part of the optic disc.

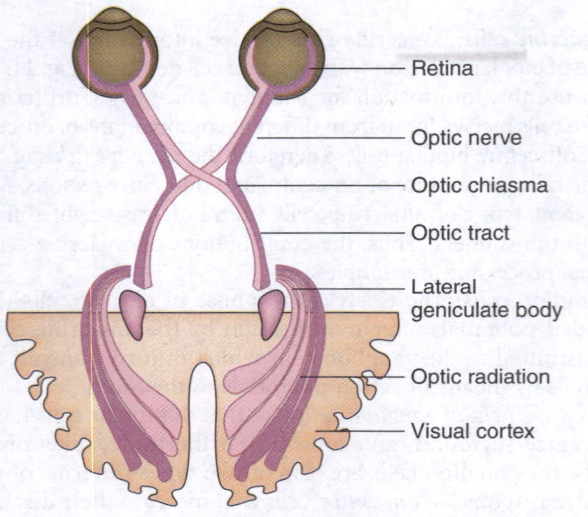

Fig. 11.1.33 Components of visual pathway.

Temporal fibres of the retina arch above and below the papillomacular bundle as superior and inferior *arcuate fibres* and occupy upper temporal and lower temporal quadrants of the optic disc.

Nasal fibres of the retina come directly to the nasal half of the disc as superior and inferior radiating fibres.

2. Optic chiasma It is a flattened structure lying above the pituitary fossa. Fibres originating from the nasal halves of the retinae decussate at the chiasma, whereas the fibres from temporal halves of the retinae remain uncrossed. It is to be noted that the nasal and temporal halves of the retina are demarcated by a vertical line passing through the fovea and not through the optic disc. This implies that visual impulse from the temporal half of the visual field goes to the opposite side, whereas the input from the nasal half of the visual field remains in the same side (Fig. 11.1.33).

3. Optic tracts These are cylindrical bundles of nerve fibres which originate from the posterolateral angle of the chiasma and run outwards and backwards to end in the LGB. They consist of temporal fibres of the same side and nasal fibres of the opposite side.

4. Lateral geniculate bodies These are oval structures situated at the posterior termination of the optic tracts.

Retinotopic projection The optic tract fibres, which are axons of retinal ganglion cells, project a detailed spatial representation of the retina on the LGB, with precise point-to-point localization.

Lamellar structure of lateral geniculate body Each LGB contains six well-defined layers. On each side, layers 1, 4 and 6 receive input from the nasal half of the contralateral eye, whereas layers 2, 3 and 5 receive input from the temporal half of the ipsilateral eye (Fig. 11.1.35). In each layer, there is precise point-to-point representation of the retina, and all six layers are in register so that along a line perpendicular to the layers, the receptive fields of the cells in each layer are almost identical.

Magnocellular and parvocellular layers The layers 1 and 2 of LGB have large cells and are called magnocellular layers, whereas layers 3–6 have small cells and are called parvocellular

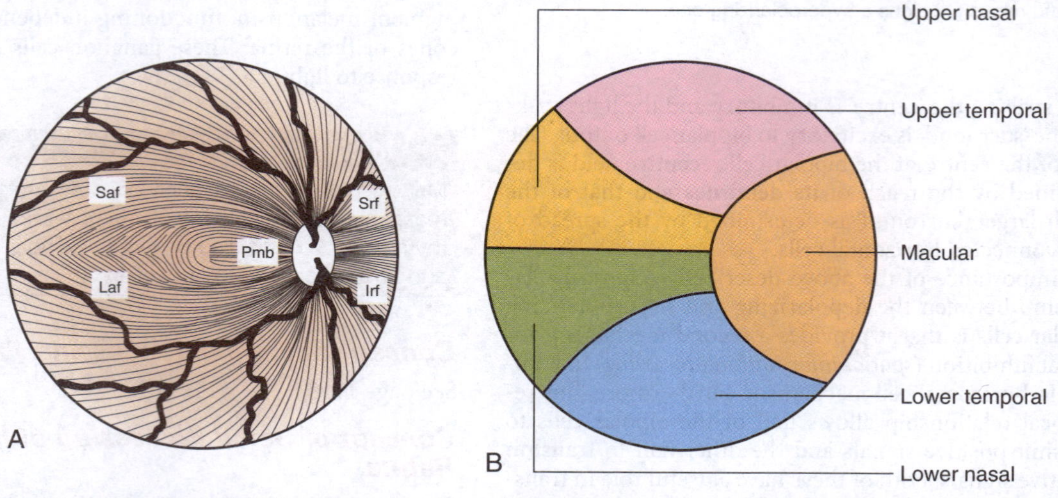

Fig. 11.1.34 Arrangement of nerve fibres: **A**, in the retina, optic disc and distal part of optic nerve; and **B**, in proximal region of optic nerve.

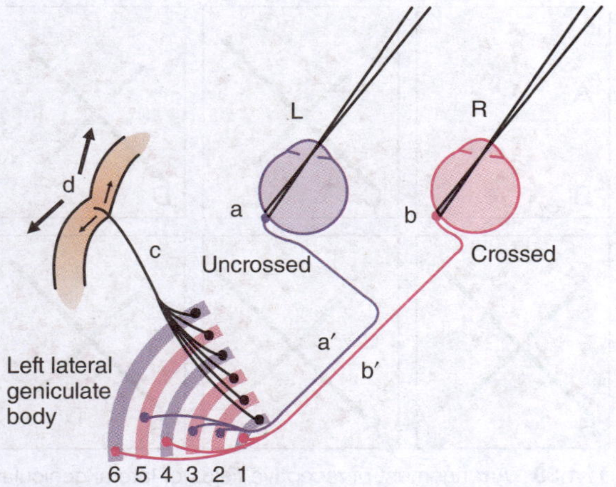

Fig. 11.1.35 Arrangement of termination of axons of ganglion cells (second-order neurons) of two eyes in the lateral geniculate body (LGB) (for explanation, see text).

layers. The inputs to the magnocellular layer come from the M ganglion cells of retinae, whereas inputs to the parvocellular layer come from the P ganglion cells of retinae.

Functions of LGB Two principal functions served by LGB are as follows:

1. ***Relay station:*** LGB serves as a relay station to relay the visual information from the ganglion cells to the visual cortex via parvocellular and magnocellular pathways, which travel through optic radiations to the visual cortex. The relay function is very accurate, so much so that there is exact point-to-point transmission with a high degree of spatial fidelity all the way from the retina to the visual cortex. The signals from the two eyes are kept apart in LGB.
2. ***Visual perception and to 'gate' the transmission of signals,*** i.e. to control how much of the signals be allowed to pass to the cortex: It is worth noting that only 10%–20% of the input to the LGB comes from the retina. The major inputs (80%–90%) come as corticofugal fibres from the primary visual cortex and other brain regions. The feedback pathway from the visual cortex has been shown to be involved in the visual processing related to the perception of orientation and motion. These inputs also control the flow of visual information from the retina to the cortex.

5. Optic radiations The optic radiations are composed of axons of the lateral geniculate relay cells which project to the visual cortex on the same side. The optic radiations maintain a *retinotopic organization* in their passage to the visual cortex.

PROCESSING AND ANALYSIS OF VISUAL IMPULSE IN THE VISUAL CORTEX

Retinotopic Organization

Just as the ganglion cell axons project a detailed spatial representation of the retina on the LGB, the LGB projects a similar point-to-point representation on the visual cortex. The visual cortex is, therefore, also called the *cortical retina,* since a true copy of the retinal image is formed here. It is only in the visual cortex that impulses originating from corresponding points of two retinae meet. Thus, the right visual cortex is concerned with the perception of objects situated to the left of the vertical median line in the visual fields, and the left visual cortex with the objects situated to the right.

Functional Anatomy and Organization of the Visual Cortex

Classical nomenclature Classically, the visual cortex has been divided into:

- Primary visual cortex or striate cortex (area 17)
- Peristriate cortex or visual association area (area 18)
- Parastriate cortex or visual association area (area 19)

1. ***Primary visual cortex,*** also called striate cortex or area 17, lies in the medial surface of the occipital lobe in and near the calcarine sulcus occupying parts of the lingual sulcus and coneum. Retina is represented in the primary visual cortex as (Fig. 11.1.36):
   Peripheral part in the anterior part of area 17, upper quadrants project on the upper wall of the calcarine sulcus and lower quadrants on the lower walls of the sulcus.
   Macular part projects mainly to the posterior part of area 17 and anteriorly to a thin strip along the calcarine sulcus. The macular area occupies nearly one-third of area 17.
2. ***Peristriate cortex*** or visual association area 18 lies in the walls of the lunate sulcus.
3. ***Parastriate cortex*** or visual association area 19 lies in the cortex in front of the lunate sulcus.

Modified nomenclature of visual areas It is now believed that some other parts of the brain are also involved in visual processing and so a modified nomenclature recognizing five visual areas has been described as:

V1 (visual area 1): It mainly includes the primary visual cortex or Brodmann's area 17.
V_2 (visual area 2): It occupies the greater part of Brodmann's area 18, but not the whole of it.
V_3 (visual area 3): It occupies a narrow strip over the anterior part of area 18.
V_4 (visual area 4): It occupies the area 19.
V_5 (visual area 5) or middle temporal (MT) area: It is located at the posterior end of the superior temporal gyrus.

Histological Layers of Primary Visual Cortex

Primary visual cortex, like other portions of the cerebral cortex, has six distinct layers (Fig. 11.1.37). Layers I, II and III are

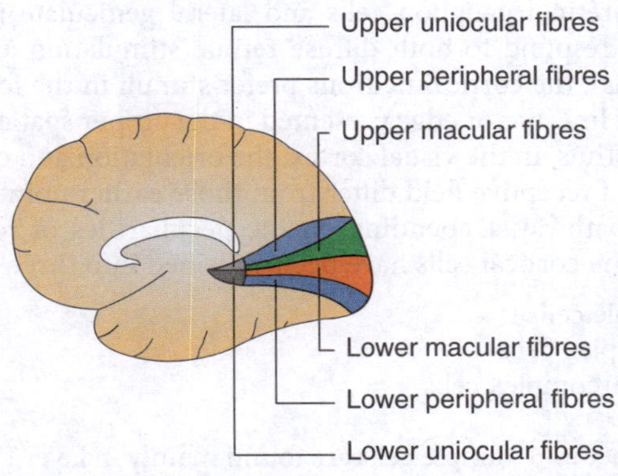

Fig. 11.1.36 Arrangement of termination of retinal fibres in visual cortex.

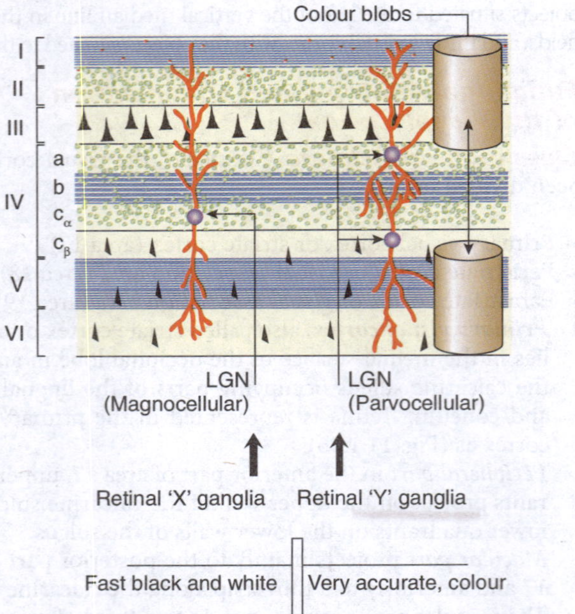

Fig. 11.1.37 Layers of visual cortex.

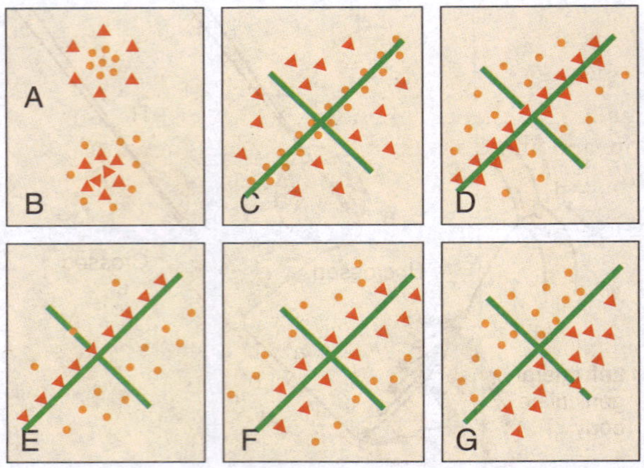

Fig. 11.1.38 Arrangement of receptive fields of lateral geniculate body and primary visual cortex: **A**, 'on-centre' geniculate receptive field; **B**, 'off-centre' geniculate receptive field; and **C–G**, arrangement of receptive field of simple cell. Dots represent areas that give excitatory responses (on response) and triangles represent areas that give inhibitory responses (off response). Receptive field axes are shown by continuous lines through field centres.

thin and contain pyramidal cells. Layer IV is the thickest and contains stellate cells. Layer IV may be further subdivided into layers a, b, cα and cβ; layers IV a and b contain the white stripe of Gennari. Layers V and VI are again relatively thin.

Physiological Considerations of Visual Cortex

The present information available on physiology of the visual cortex is just a tip of the iceberg. Much credit goes to Hubel and Wiessel for the present-day knowledge. Some of the aspects of physiology of the visual cortex which have been delineated, though incompletely, can be discussed under the following headings:

- Concept of receptive field of striate cortex
- Columnar organization of striate cortex
- Serial versus parallel analysis of visual image
- Role of extrastriate cortex in visual functions
- Psychophysiological aspects of visual functions

Concept of Receptive Field of Striate Cortex

Unlike retinal ganglion cells and lateral geniculate neurons (which respond to both diffuse retinal stimulation and spot stimulus), the cortical neurons prefer stimuli in the form of a straight line, bar or edge presented in the proper spatial orientation. Thus, in the visual cortex, the orientation and configuration of receptive field differ from those earlier points in the visual pathway. Depending on the peculiarities of receptive fields, the cortical cells have been classified into three types:

- Simple cells
- Complex cells
- Hypercomplex cells

Simple cells Simple cells are found mainly in layer IV of the primary visual cortex (area 17) and form the first relay station within the visual cortex. These respond to bars of light, lines or edges, but only when they have a particular orientation. The orientation of a stimulus that is most effective in evoking a response is called the *receptive field axis orientation*. The receptive field of simple cells can be mapped with small spots of light into *on-areas* and *off-areas*, which, like those of cells in the LGB, are mutually antagonistic. However, unlike lateral geniculate neurons, the receptive fields of simple cells are arranged in parallel bands of 'on' and 'off' regions, rather than concentric centre-surround arrangement of the geniculate body (Fig. 11.1.38A and B). Receptive fields of simple cells often have a central band that is either an 'on-region' or an 'off-region', with parallel flanking region on two sides that are opposite (Fig. 11.1.38C–G).

Thus, the simple cell receptive fields play an important role not only in the detection of lines and borders in the different areas of retinal image but also in the detection of the orientation of each line or border – that is whether it is vertical or horizontal, or lies at some degree of inclination. It is assumed that for each such orientation of a line, a specific neuronal simple cell is stimulated.

Complex cells These cells are found in the cortical layers above and below layer IV of areas 17, 18 and 19 of the visual cortex, and only rarely in layer IV itself. They resemble simple cells in requiring a preferred orientation of a linear stimulus but are less dependent on the location of a stimulus in the visual field than the simple cells. They often respond maximally when a linear stimulus is moved laterally without a change in its orientation. Unlike simple cells, it is not possible to map out distinct antagonistic 'on' and 'off' regions in the receptive fields of complex cells. Complex cells often receive input from both eyes and are thus called binocular. The receptive fields of a given binocular complex cell are on corresponding parts of the two retinae and have identical receptive field properties.

Four types of complex cell receptive fields are described according to their preferred stimulus:

- Activated by a slit-nonuniform field
- Activated by a slit-uniform field
- Activated by an edge
- Activated by a dark bar

Thus, the complex cell receptive fields play an important role in the detection of lines, bars and edges, but especially so when they are moving. In other words, by means of simple and complex cells, the person perceives the features, orientation and movements of the objects. Therefore, simple and complex cells together are known as 'feature detectors'.

Hypercomplex cells These are found in cortical layers II and III of the areas 17, 18 and 19. These cells retain all the properties of complex cells but also have the added feature of requiring the line stimulus to be of a specific length. The stimuli to which they respond vary greatly, as does their complexity.

Four types of 'lower' hypercomplex cells and two categories of 'higher' hypercomplex cells were described by Hubel and Wiesel. Dreher has classified hypercomplex cells into two types – I and II.

Thus, the hypercomplex cells play a role in the detection of lines of specific length, angles or other shapes.

Columnar Organization of the Striate Cortex (Fig. 11.1.39)

The primary visual cortex is organized into vertically oriented functional modules called the *hypercolumns*, each of which processes visual information from a specific region of the visual field. The term hypercolumn refers to a set of columns responsive to lines of all orientation from a particular region in space. These vertically oriented columnar units are linked with one another by means of horizontal connections that link cells within a layer. Each hypercolumn includes sets of three types of vertical columns, which are as follows (Fig. 11.1.39):

- Orientation columns
- Ocular dominance columns
- Colour blobs

Orientation columns Like the somatic sensory cortex, the primary visual cortex is organized into narrow columns of cells, running from the pial surface to the white matter. Thus, the orientation column is the unit of organization in the visual cortex which can be defined as *vertical grouping of cells with identical orientation specificity*. The visual cortex is thus organized into several million vertical columns of neuronal cells, each being about 30–100 μm wide and 2 mm deep.

It has been observed that the orientation preferences of neighbouring columns differ in a systematic way; as one moves from column to column across the cortex, there are sequential changes in orientation preference of 5–10° (Fig. 11.1.40). Thus, it is possible to speculate that for each ganglion cell receptive field in the visual field, there is a collection of columns in a small area of the visual cortex representing the possible preferred orientation at small intervals throughout the full 360°.

Ocular dominance columns Ocular dominance columns refer to an independent system of columns which exist in the visual cortex with respect to the binocular input to cortical cells. As discussed earlier, the simple cells in layer IV of the striate cortex receive input from one eye only, whereas most complex and hypercomplex cells in layers above and below the layer IV receive input from both eyes. Although most cortical neurons are binocularly activated, there remains a strong monocular dominance. Neurons with receptive fields dominated by one eye are grouped alternately into left eye and right eye columns that are 0.25–0.5 mm in width (Fig. 11.1.41).

Thus, a group of binocular complex and hypercomplex cells in layers II, III, V and VI that receive a stronger input from one of the two eyes, along with the cells in layer IV that receive input from the same eye, is called an ocular dominance column.

The reason for the existence of rigorously ordered, complex binocular input to some complex cells is unknown but may have something to do with *binocular stereoscopic vision*.

Colour blobs Interspersed among the primary visual columns are special column-like areas called *colour blobs* (Fig. 11.1.39). These receive lateral signals from the adjacent

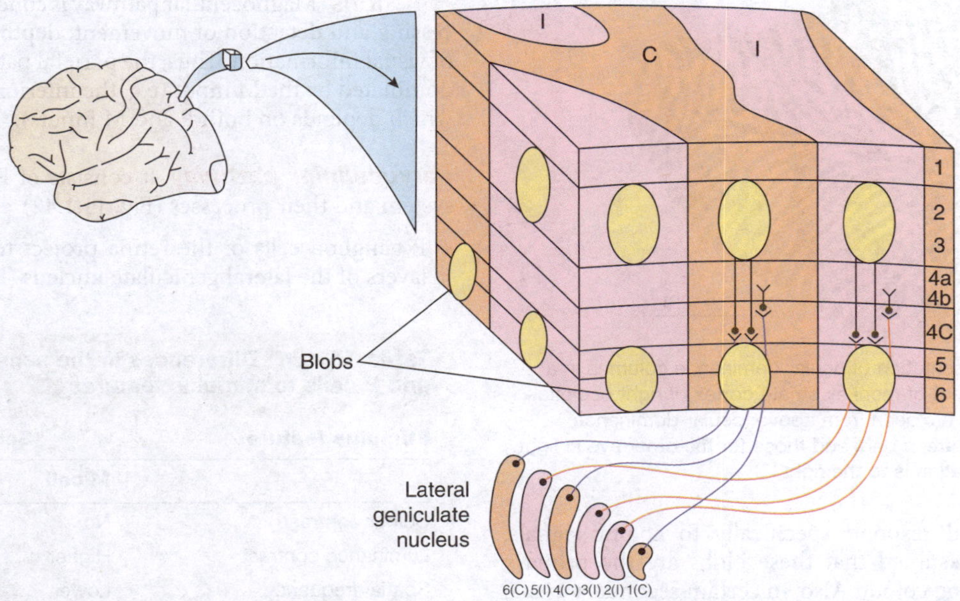

Fig. 11.1.39 Organization of the orientation columns, ocular dominance columns and blobs in the primary visual cortex. C, contralateral inputs; I, ipsilateral inputs.

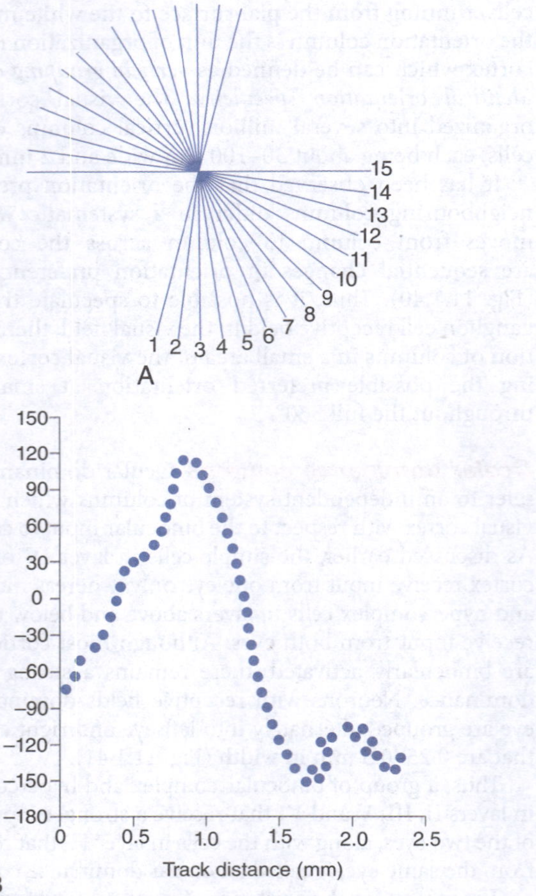

Fig. 11.1.40 **A**, Orientation preferences of 15 neurons encountered as a microelectrode penetrated the visual cortex obliquely. The preferred orientation changed steadily in a counterclockwise direction. **B**, Results of a similar experiment plotted against distance the electrode travelled. In this case, there were a number of reversals in direction of rotation.

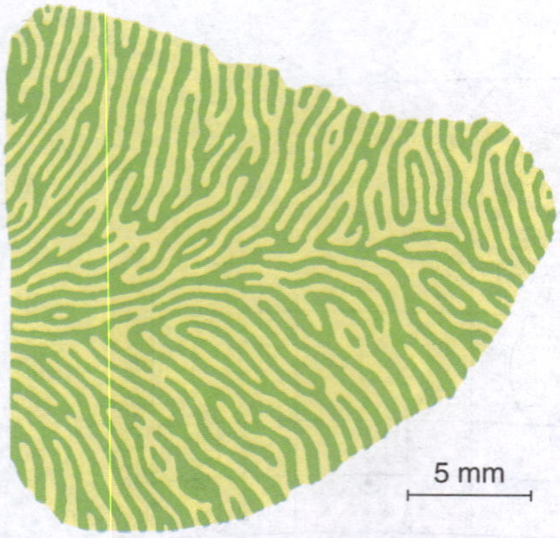

Fig. 11.1.41 Representation of ocular dominance columns in a relatively large segment of monkey striate cortex of right occipital lobe. View is of layer IVc seen from above; ocular dominance columns for one eye are in dark and those for the other eye in light. The foveal representation is to the right.

visual column and respond specifically to colour signals. Therefore, it is presumed that these blobs are the primary areas for deciphering colour. Also, in certain secondary visual areas, additional colour blobs are found, which presumably perform still higher levels of colour deciphering.

Applied Aspects

- *Anton syndrome* is a cortical blindness in which an individual is usually unaware about the blindness. In this condition, the pupillary light reflex remains intact. The common cause is bilateral infarction due to occlusion/spasm of the distal posterior cerebral artery.
- *Prosopagnosia* is the inability to recognize familiar faces, usually seen in lesion of the anterior and inferior temporal cortex.

Concept of Serial and Parallel Processing of Visual Information

It is now clear that visual image is deciphered and analysed in both parallel and serial fashions.

Parallel Processing Pathways

Two kinds of cells can be distinguished in the visual pathway starting from the ganglion cells of the retina including neurons of the LGB, striate cortex and extrastriate cortex. These are large cells (magno or M cells) and small cells (parvo or P cells). There are striking differences between the sensitivity of M and P cells to stimulus features (Table 11.1.1).

The visual pathway is now being considered to be made of two lanes – one made of the large cells is called magnocellular pathway, and the other of small cells is called parvocellular pathway. These can be compared with two lanes of a road. The M pathway and P pathway are involved in the *parallel processing* of the image, i.e. analysis of different features of the image.

Magnocellular pathway It is formed by the M cells and their processes (Fig. 11.1.42). M ganglion cells of the retina project to the magnocellular layers of the lateral geniculate nucleus (layers 1 and 2). The magnocellular projections from the LG nucleus project to the striate cortex first to layer IVc and then to layer IV_b. Cells in layer IV_b project directly to the MT area and also the thick stripes in area V, from which cells also project to MT. From MT, the M pathway extends to the posterior parietal cortex as dorsal cortical pathway.

Functions Magnocellular pathway is concerned with the processing and detection of movement, depth and flicker feature of visual information. Thus, the parietal pathway appears to be dominated by the M input (e.g. the inferior temporal pathway which depends on both P and M inputs).

Parvocellular pathway It consists of P cells of the visual system and their processes (Fig. 11.1.42):

- P ganglion cells of the retina project to the parvocellular layers of the lateral geniculate nucleus (layers 3–6).

Table 11.1.1 Differences in the sensitivity of M and P cells to stimulus features

Stimulus feature	Sensitivity	
	M cell	P cell
Colour contrast	No	Yes
Luminance contrast	Higher	Lower
Spatial frequency	Lower	Higher
Temporal frequency	Higher	Lower

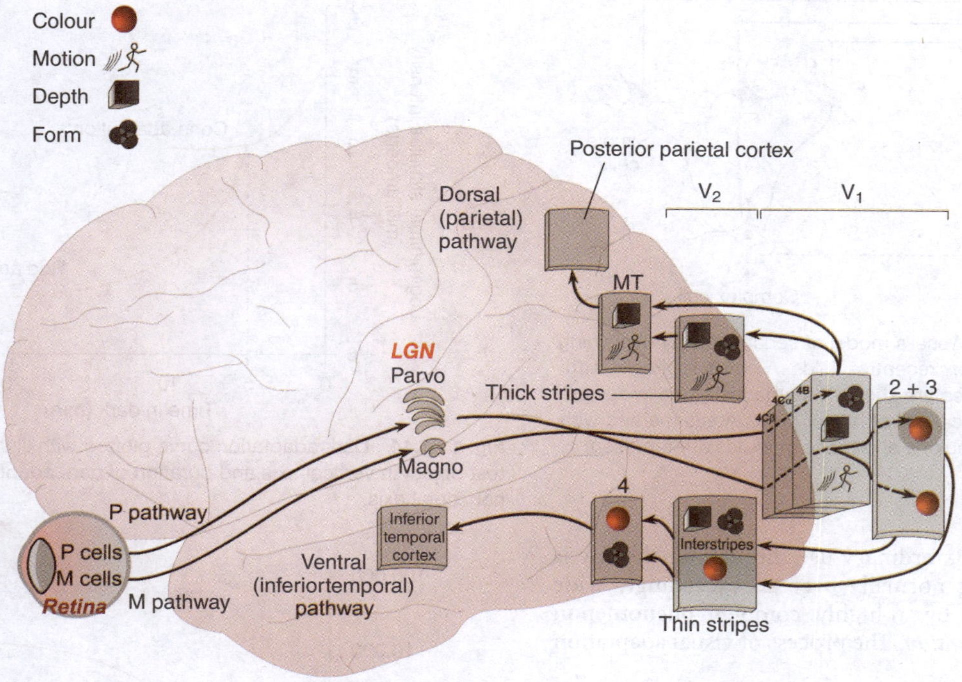

Fig. 11.1.42 The magnocellular (M) and parvocellular pathway (P) from retina project through lateral geniculate body (LGB) to V_1. Separate pathways to temporal and parietal cortices course through the extrastriate cortex beginning in V_2.

- Parvocellular projections from the LG nucleus project to the layer IVcα of the striate cortex, from which cells project to the blobs and interblobs of V_1.
- The blobs send a strong projection to the thin stripes in V, whereas interblobs send strong projection to the interstripes in V_2.
- The thin stripe and interstripe area of V project to discrete subregions of V_4, from which the cells project to the inferior temporal cortex as *ventral cortical pathway*.

Function The parvocellular pathway is concerned with colour vision, texture, shape and fine details.

Concept of Serial Processing of Visual Information

The successive cells in the visual pathway starting from the photoreceptors to the cells of LGB are involved in an increasingly complex analysis of an image. This is called sequential or serial processing of visual information.

Serial processing in the retina In a sense, the processing of visual information in the retina involves the formation of three images:

First image is formed by the action of light on the photoreceptor. Photoreceptors break up the image into small spots of light or darkness (much like a scanner that breaks down a picture into small pixels).
Second image: The first image is converted into the second image by bipolar cells. In the formation of the second image, the signal is altered by horizontal cells which cause *spatial summation* by lateral inhibition.
Third image: The second image is converted into the third image by the ganglion cells. In the formation of the third image, the signal is altered by amacrine cells which cause *temporal summation*. Thus, image processing in ganglion cells results in the sharpening of the image contrast. The image is thus analysed mostly in terms of contours of the light–darkness boundaries and areas of uniform light or darkness elicit very little neural response. Thus, the image processing system in ganglion cells yields a high-contrast line diagram of the original image. There is a little change in the impulse pattern in the LGBs, so the third image reaches the occipital cortex.

Serial analysis of visual image in the visual cortex A hierarchical model for cell interconnections has been suggested in the visual cortex. The sequence from simple to complex and to hypercomplex forms a system of serial analysis with more and more details being deciphered. A complex cell is thought of as receiving input from several simple cells of the same orientation whose receptive fields are overlapping to produce the complex cell receptive field (Fig. 11.1.43). Since the complex cells are binocular and simple cells are mainly monocular, this adds support to the idea that complex cells are at a more advanced stage of processing.

VISUAL PERCEPTION

It is a complex integration of light sense, form sense, sense of contrast and colour sense. The receptive field organization of the retina and cortex are used to encode this information about a visual image.

Light Sense

It is awareness of the light. The minimum brightness required to evoke a sensation of light is called the *light minimum*. It should be measured when the eye is dark adapted for at least 20–30 minutes.

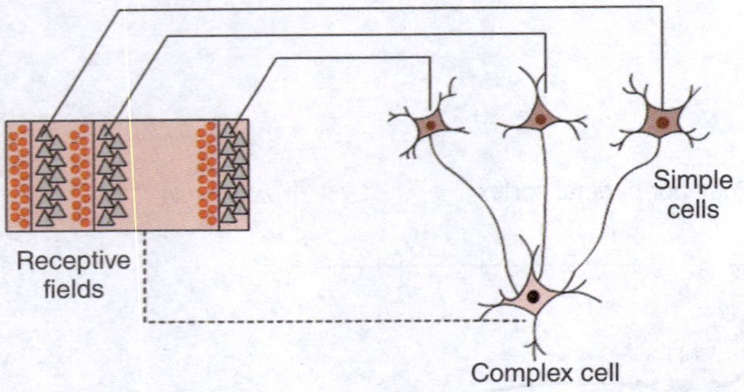

Fig. 11.1.43 Hubel and Wesel's model of serial pathway explaining the organization of complex receptive fields. A number of cells with simple fields, of which three are shown schematically, are imagined to project to a single cortical cell of higher order. Areas marked with represent the excitatory regions and those marked with represent the inhibitory region.

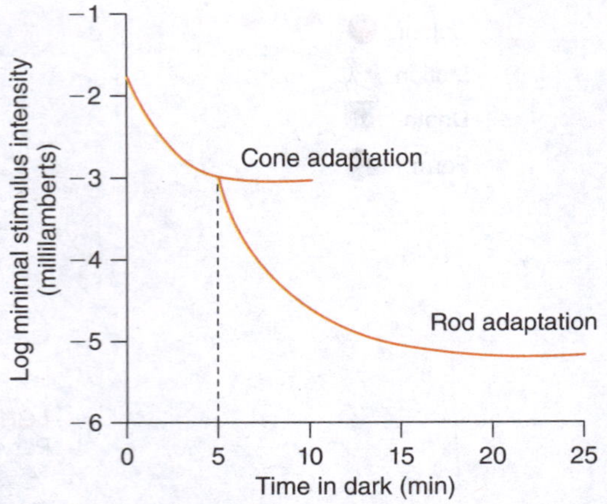

Fig. 11.1.44 Dark adaptation curve plotted with illumination of test object in vertical axis and duration of dark adaptation along the horizontal axis.

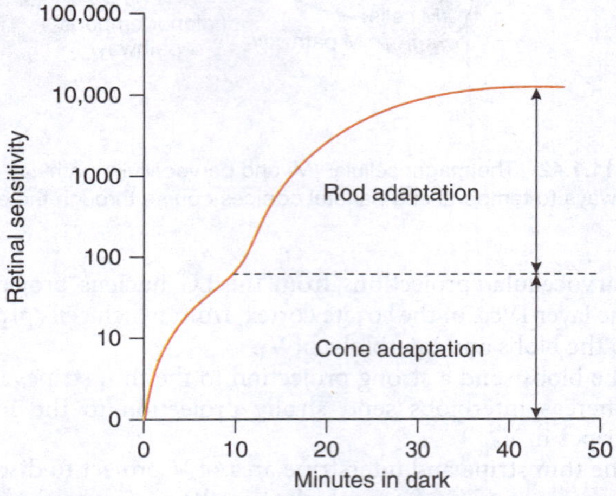

Fig. 11.1.45 Dark adaptation curve plotted with retinal sensitivity along the vertical axis and duration of dark adaptation along the horizontal axis.

The human eye in its ordinary use throughout the day is capable of functioning normally over an exceedingly wide range of illumination by a highly complex phenomenon termed the *visual adaptation*. The process of visual adaptation primarily involves:

- *Dark adaptation* (adjustment in dim illumination)
- *Light adaptation* (adjustment to bright illumination)

Dark Adaptation

It is the ability of the eye to adapt itself to decreasing illumination. When one goes from bright sunshine into a dimly lit room, one cannot perceive the objects in the room until some time has elapsed. During this period, the eye is adapting to low illumination. The time taken to see in dim illumination is called *dark adaptation time*. The rods are much more sensitive to low illumination than cones. Therefore, rods are used more in dim light *(scotopic vision)* and cones in bright light *(photopic vision)*.

Dark adaptation curve Dark adaptation curve plotted with illumination of test object along the vertical axis and duration of dark adaptation along the horizontal axis shows that visual threshold falls progressively in the darkened room for about half an hour until a relative constant value is reached (Fig. 11.1.44). The dark adaptation curve plotted with retinal sensitivity along the vertical axis and duration of dark adaptation along the horizontal axis (Fig. 11.1.45) shows that the sensitivity of the retina is very low on first entering the darkness, but within 1 minute, the sensitivity has increased 10-fold, that is, the retina can respond to light of one-tenth the previously required intensity. At the end of 20 minutes, the sensitivity has increased about 6000-fold, and at the end of 40 minutes, it has increased about 25,000-fold.

It can be seen that the decrease in threshold of the retina (Fig. 11.1.44), i.e. increase in sensitivity of the retina (Fig. 11.1.45), proceeds in two steps: (i) the first is rapid, of short duration and small in extent; and (ii) the second is slow, more prolonged and larger. This indicates that two processes are at work, each having different characteristics, and that the break in the curve is the point at which one process is about to finish and the second one is just commencing. The analyses have revealed that the first plateau of the curve represents cone threshold (reached in about 5 minutes) and the second plateau represents rod threshold (reached after about 30 minutes). The inflection of the dark adaptation curve where the rod limb begins is called the cone–rod break or alpha point, and it usually occurs after 7–10 minutes of adaptation. The final rod phase of adaptation does not begin until 93% of rhodopsin has already regenerated.

Mechanism of dark adaptation Mechanism of dark adaptation involves:

1. ***Visual pigment mechanism:*** Dark adaptation primarily involves a reversal of the mechanism of light adaptation, i.e. regeneration of visual pigments (rhodopsin and cone pigments, see page 1110).
2. ***Change in pupillary size:*** The pupil dilates and can cause adaptation of approximately 30-fold because of changes in the amount of light allowed through the pupil.
3. ***Neural mechanism:*** The mechanism of neural adaptation involves neurons of the visual chain in the retina itself. The neurobiological adaptation is based on feedback inhibition and the mechanism of adaptation that lies within the neuron itself.

Important Note

The persons who require maximum visual sensitivity in dim light, e.g. aircraft pilots, radiologists and drivers, are advised to use red goggles before entering in the dark to avoid 20- to 30-minute time required for dark adaptation.

Applied Aspects

Dark Adaptation and Vitamin A Deficiency

Severe deficiency of vitamin A elevates the threshold for dark adaptation curve due to depletion of photosensitive pigment. *Nyctalopia*, i.e. night blindness, is another important feature of vitamin A deficiency. Other causes of nyctalopia are retinitis pigmentosa and congenital night blindness.

Vitamin A deficiency is termed xerophthalmia (dry eye). The manifestations of xerophthalmia are as follows:

- *Conjunctival xerosis:* In this condition, the conjunctiva becomes muddy and wrinkled.
- *Bitot's spots* are triangular pearly white spots on the bulbar conjunctiva which appear on either side of the cornea.
- *Corneal xerosis* is characterized by loss of corneal lustre and punctate keratopathy.
- *Keratomalacia:* In this condition, corneal stroma is involved resulting in corneal ulcerations.

Treatment: Early stage of xerophthalmia is treated by administration of 200,000 IU of retinal palmitate orally on 2 successive days.

Prevention: For prevention, a single dose of 200,000 IU of vitamin A is administered orally every 6 months up to 1–6 years of age (preschool children).

Light Adaptation

When one passes suddenly from a dim to a brightly lighted environment, the light seems intensely and even uncomfortably bright until the eyes adapt to the increased illumination and the visual threshold rises. The process by means of which the retina adapts itself to bright light is called *light adaptation*. Unlike dark adaptation, the process of light adaptation is very quick and occurs over a period of 5 minutes. Strictly speaking, light adaptation is merely the disappearance of dark adaptation.

Mechanism of light adaptation It involves the following processes:

1. ***Neural adjustment*** of sensitivity which takes place rapidly is more important and is responsible for the *transient effect* seen in the light adaptation curve (Fig. 11.1.46B and C).
2. ***Visual pigment mechanism*** involves reduction of quantity of rhodopsin and cone pigment because of their bleaching in light (see page 1110) and is responsible for the *photochemical effect* in the light adaptation curve (Fig. 11.1.46D).
3. ***Pupillary mechanism:*** The pupil constricts in bright light and decreases the amount of light entering the eye.

Form Sense

It is the ability to discriminate between the shapes of the objects. Cones play a major role in this faculty. Therefore, form sense is most acute at the fovea, where there are maximum number of cones, and decreases very rapidly towards the periphery (Fig. 11.1.47). Visual acuity recorded by Snellen's test chart is a measure of the form sense.

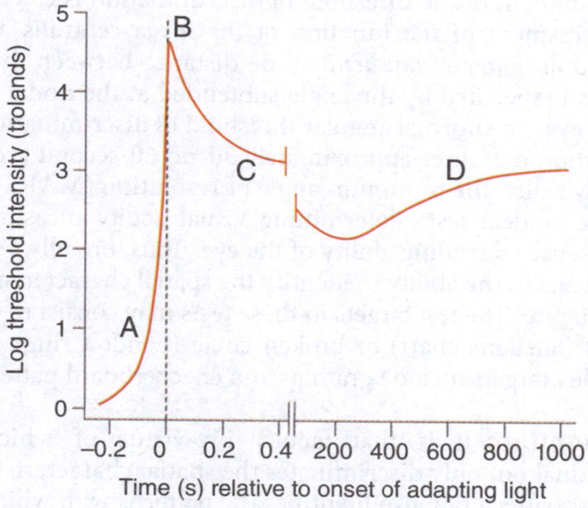

Fig. 11.1.46 Time course of light adaptation measured by an increment threshold technique: **A**, anticipatory effect; **B** and **C**, transient effect; and **D**, photochemical effect.

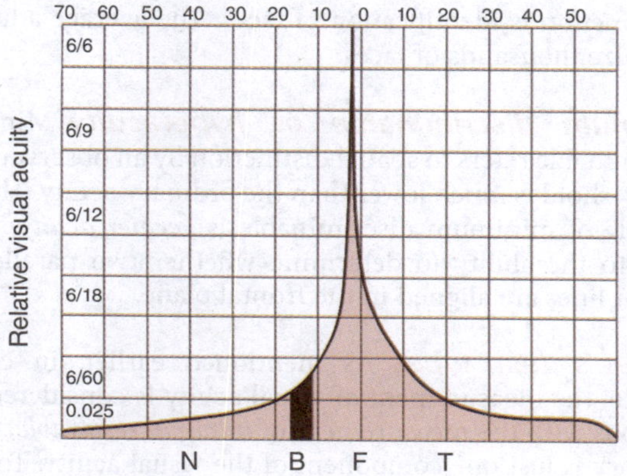

Fig. 11.1.47 Visual acuity (form sense) in relation to the regions of the retina. B, blind spot; F, foveal region; N, nasal retina; T, temporal retina.

Components of Visual Acuity

In clinical practice, measurement of the threshold of discrimination of two spatially separated targets (a function of the fovea centralis) is termed visual acuity. However, in theory, visual acuity is a highly complex function that consists of the components given next.

Minimum visible The ability to determine whether an object is present in an otherwise empty visual field is termed *visibility* or *detection*. This kind of task is referred to as the *minimum visible* or *minimum detectable function*. The limit of visibility reflects the absolute threshold of vision. The minimum visible spatial threshold level will depend on the specification of stimulus such as size, shape and illumination.

Resolution (ordinary visual acuity) Discrimination of two spatially separated targets is termed resolution. The minimum separation between the two points, which can be discriminated as two, is known as *minimum resolvable*.

Measurement of the threshold of discrimination is essentially an assessment of the function of the fovea centralis and is termed *ordinary visual acuity*. The distance between the two targets is specified by the angle subtended at the nodal point of the eye. The normal angular threshold of discrimination for resolution measures approximately 30- to 60-second arc; it is usually called the minimum angle of resolution (MAR).

The clinical tests determining visual acuity measure the form sense or reading ability of the eye. Thus, broadly, resolution refers to the ability to identify the spatial characteristics of a test figure. The test targets in these tests may consist of either letters (Snellen's chart) or broken circle (Landolt ring). More complex targets include gratings and checkerboard patterns.

Recognition It is that faculty by virtue of which an individual not only discriminates the spatial characteristics of the test pattern but also identifies the patterns with which he/she has had some experience. Recognition is thus a task involving cognitive components in addition to spatial resolution. For recognition, the individual should be familiar with the set of test figures employed in addition to being able to resolve them. The most common example of recognition phenomenon is identification of faces. The average adult can recognize thousands of faces.

Minimum discriminable or hyperacuity Minimum discriminable refers to spatial distinction by an observer when the threshold is much lower than the ordinary acuity. The best example of minimum discriminable is *vernier acuity*, which refers to the ability to determine whether two parallel and straight lines are aligned in the frontal plane.

Snellen's test types As mentioned earlier, in clinical practice, the measurement of visual acuity is considered synonymous with the measurement of *minimal resolvable*, which in theory is just one component of the visual acuity. To measure the minimal resolvable, Snellen constructed certain test types, which are now routinely used to test the distant central visual acuity.

The fact that two distant points can be visible as separate only when they subtend an angle of 1 minute at the nodal point of the eye forms the basis of Snellen's test types. It consists of a series of black capital letters on a white board, arranged in lines, each progressively diminishing in size. The lines comprising the letter have such a breadth that they will subtend an angle of 1 minute at the nodal point. Each letter of the chart is so designed that it fits in a square, the sides of which are five times the breadth of the constituent lines. Thus, at the given distance, each letter subtends an angle of 5 minutes at the nodal point of the eye (Fig. 11.1.48). The letter of the top line of Snellen's chart (Fig. 11.1.49) should be read clearly at a distance of 60 m. Similarly, the letters in the subsequent lines should be read from a distance of 36, 24, 18, 12, 9, 6, 5 and 4 m.

Critical flicker fusion frequency When intermittent light stimuli are presented to the eye, a sensation of 'flicker' is evoked. As the frequency of presentation of the stimuli is increased, a point is reached at which flicker sensation fuses to form the sensation of continuous stimulation. This frequency is known as the critical flicker fusion (CFF) frequency. The CFF frequency serves as a measure of the temporal resolving power of the visual system under the particular condition of stimulation. Motion pictures move because the frames are presented at a rate above the CFF, and movies begin to flicker when the projector slows down.

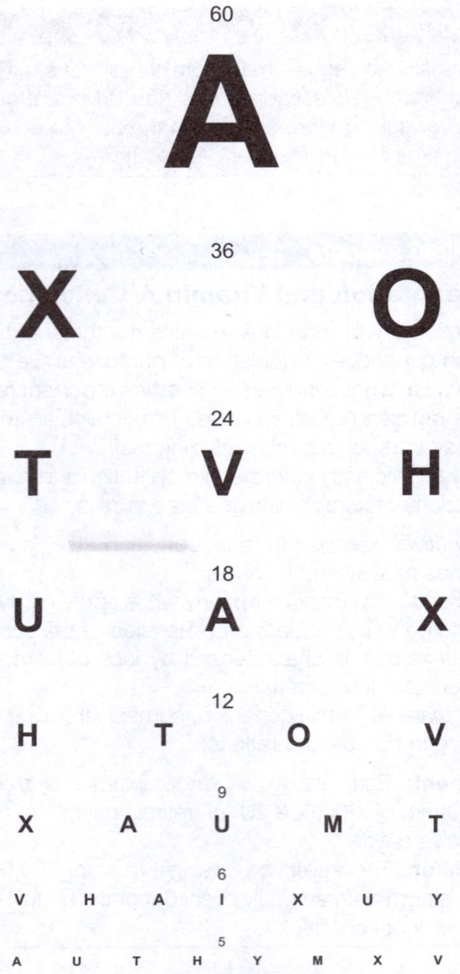

Fig. 11.1.48 Snellen's test types.

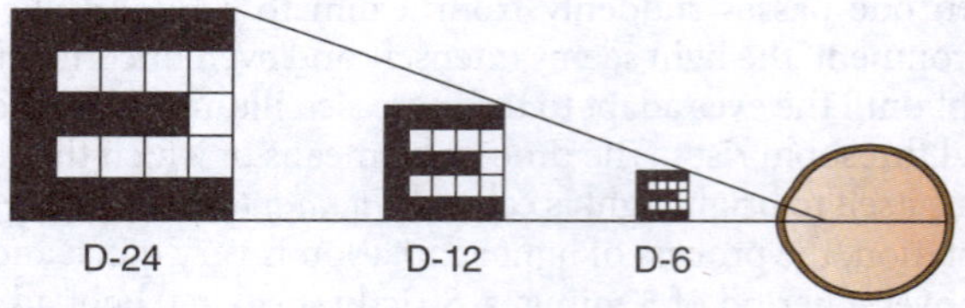

Fig. 11.1.49 Principle of Snellen's test type.

Colour Sense

Colour sense is the ability of the eye to discriminate between colours excited by light of different wavelengths. Some broad facts about colour vision are as follows:

- Colour vision is a function of cones and thus better appreciated in photopic vision.
- The sensation of colour is subjective. Individuals are taught names for their colour sensations and subsequently use these names whenever the same sensation is obtained.
- There are three different types of cones, i.e. red sensitive, green sensitive and blue sensitive, which combinedly perform the function of colour vision.

- All colours are a result of admixture in different proportion of three primary colours – red (723–647 nm), green (575–492 nm) and blue (492–450 nm).
- Colours have three attributes – hue, intensity and saturation.
- For any colour, there is a complementary colour that, when properly mixed with it, produces a sensation of white.
- The colour perceived depends in part on the colour of other objects in the visual field. Thus, for example, a red object is seen red if the field is illuminated with green or blue light but as pale pink or white if the field is illuminated with red light.
- A normal person can see all wavelengths between violet and red. If the wavelength is shorter than that of violet, the light becomes ultraviolet (UV) and is beyond visibility. If the wavelength is greater than 750 nm, the light is infrared and is again beyond visibility. Human beings could have seen even UV light as blue cones retain some sensitivity at around 10 nm, but crystalline lens blocks all UV rays. Consequently, after cataract operation, one can see the UV rays to some extent.
- In dim light, all the colours are seen as grey; this is called Purkinje shift phenomenon.

Mechanism (Neurophysiology) of Colour Vision

Theories of colour vision The process of colour analysis begins in the retina and is not entirely a function of the brain. Many theories have been put forward to explain the colour perception, but two have been particularly influential.

1. Trichromatic theory The trichromacy of colour vision was originally suggested by Young and subsequently modified by Helmholtz. Hence, it is called Young–Helmholtz theory. It postulates the existence of three kinds of cones, each containing a different photopigment and maximally sensitive to one of three primary colours, i.e. red, green and blue. The sensation of any given colour is determined by the relative frequency of the impulse from each of the three cone systems. In other words, a given colour consists of admixture of the three primary colours in different proportions. The correctness of the Young–Helmholtz trichromacy theory of colour vision has now been demonstrated by the identification and chemical characterization of each of the three pigments by recombinant DNA technique, each having different absorption spectrum as (Fig. 11.1.50):

Red-sensitive cone pigment, also known as *erythrolabe or* long wavelength-sensitive (LWS) cone pigment, absorbs maximally in a yellow portion with a peak at 565 nm. But its spectrum extends far enough into the long wavelength to sense red.
Green-sensitive cone pigment, also known as *chlorolabe* or medium wavelength-sensitive (MWS) cone pigment, absorbs maximally in the green portion with a peak at 535 nm.
Blue-sensitive cone pigment, also known as *cyanolabe or* short wavelength-sensitive (SWS) cone pigment, absorbs maximally in the blue-violet portion of the spectrum with a peak at 440 nm.

Thus, the Young–Helmholtz theory concludes that blue, green and red are primary colours, but the cones with their maximal sensitivity in the yellow portion of the spectrum are light at a lower threshold than green.

It has been studied that the gene for human rhodopsin is located on chromosome 3, and the gene for the blue-sensitive cone is located on chromosome 7. The genes for the red- and

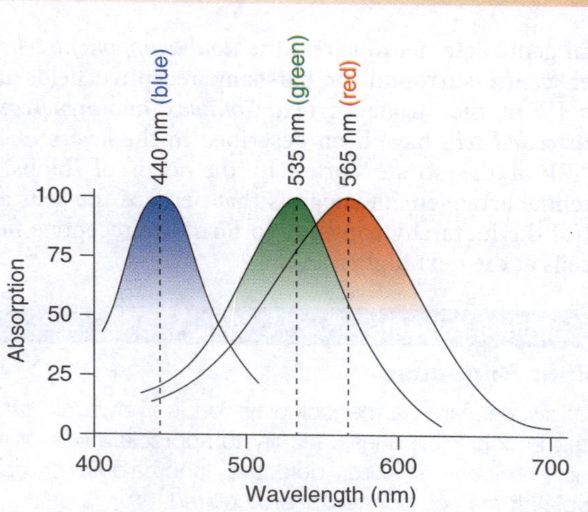

Fig. 11.1.50 Absorption spectrum of three cone pigments.

green-sensitive cones are arranged in tandem array on the q arm of the X chromosomes.

2. Opponent colour theory The opponent colour theory of Herring points out that some colours appear to be 'mutually exclusive'. There is no such colour as 'reddish green', and such phenomenon can be difficult to explain on the basis of trichromatic theory alone. In fact, it seems that both theories are useful in that:

- The colour vision is trichromatic at the level of photoreceptors.
- Colour opponency occurs at ganglion cell onwards.

According to opponent colour theory, there are two main types of colour-opponent ganglion cells:

a. ***Red-green opponent colour cells*** use signals from red and green cones to detect red/green contrast within their receptive field.
b. ***Blue-yellow opponent colour cells obtain a yellow signal*** from the summed output of red and green cones, which is contrasted with the output from blue cones within the receptive field.

Analysis of Colour Signals in the Visual Cortex

Colour information from the parvocellular portion of the LGB is relayed to the layer IVc of the *striate cortex* (area 17). From there, the information passes to the blobs in layers II and III. The neurons in the *blobs* lack orientation specificity but respond to colours. Like the ganglion cells and LGB cells, they are *centre-surround cells*. Many are *double-opponent cells*, which, for example, are stimulated by green centre and inhibited by green surround and are inhibited by red centre and stimulated by red surround. From the blobs, colour information is relayed to thin strips in the visual association area and from there to a *specialized area concerned* with colour, which in humans is in the lingual and fusiform gyri of the occipital lobe.

Hierarchy of colour-coded cells The phenomenon of hierarchy of colour-coded cells suggests a system of *serial analysis* of colour sense. The colour-coded cells have been reported to be arranged in a hierarchical manner as follows: the *opponent colour cells* being located in ganglion cells and lateral geniculate neurons and the *double opponent cells* with either 'centre-surround' or bar-flank receptive fields in the layer IV of the striate cortex. *Complex and hypercomplex colour-coded cells* have been described in the layers II, III, V and VI of the striate cortex in the form of 'blobs'. This sequential arrangement suggests that perhaps the cells at one level of the hierarchy converge to form the receptive field of the cells at the next higher level.

Applied Aspects

Colour Blindness

An individual with normal colour vision is known as *'trichromate'*. In colour blindness, faculty to appreciate one or more primary colours is either defective (anomalous) or absent (anopia). It may be congenital or acquired.

1. Congenital Colour Blindness

It is an inherited condition affecting males more (3%–4%) than females (0.4%). It may be of the following types:

- Dyschromatopsia
- Achromatopsia

I. Dyschromatopsia. Dyschromatopsia literally means colour confusion due to deficiency of the mechanism to perceive colours. It can be classified into:

- Anomalous trichromatism
- Dichromatism

a. ***Anomalous trichromatism:*** Here the mechanism to appreciate all the three primary colours is present but is defective for one or two of them. It may be of the following types:
   - *Protanomalous*, i.e. defective red colour appreciation
   - *Deuteranomalous*, i.e. defective green colour appreciation
   - *Tritanomalous*, i.e. defective blue colour appreciation

b. ***Dichromatism:*** In this condition, faculty to perceive one of the three primary colours is completely absent. Such individuals are called dichromates and may have one of the following types of defects:
   - *Protanopia*, i.e. complete red colour defect
   - *Deuteranopia*, i.e. complete defect for green colour
   - *Tritanopia*, i.e. absence of blue colour appreciation

Red-green deficiency (protanomalous, protanopia, deuteranomalous and deuteranopia) is more common. Such a defect is a source of danger in certain occupations such as drivers, sailors and traffic police.

Blue deficiency (tritanomalous and tritanopia) is comparatively rare.

II. Achromatopsia. It is an extremely rare condition presenting as cone monochromatism or rod monochromatism.

Cone monochromatism is characterized by the presence of only one primary colour and thus the persons are truly colour blind. Such patients usually have a visual acuity of 6/12 or better.

Rod monochromatism may be complete or incomplete. It is inherited as an autosomal recessive trait. It is characterized by:

- Total colour blindness
- Day blindness (visual acuity is about 6/60)

It may follow damage to the macula or optic nerve. Usually, it is associated with a central scotoma or decreased visual acuity. It may manifest as:

- *Blue-yellow impairment*
- *Red-green deficiency*

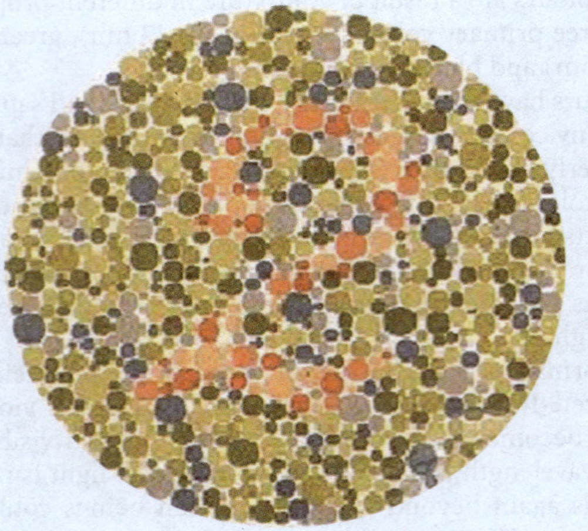

Fig. 11.1.51 Ishihara chart.

- *Acquired blue colour defect* (blue blindness) (it may occur in old age due to increased sclerosis of the crystalline lens; it is owing to the physical absorption of the blue rays by increased amber-coloured pigment in the nucleus)

Tests for Colour Vision Commonly employed colour vision tests are given next.

1. Pseudoisochromatic chart test. It is the most commonly employed test using Ishihara's plates. In this, there are patterns of coloured and grey dots which reveal one pattern to the normal individuals and another to the colour deficients. It is a quick method of screening colour blinds from the normal (Fig. 11.1.51).

Another test based on the same principle is *Hardy–Rand–Rittler plate test*.

2. The lantern test. In this test, the subject has to name the various colours shown to him/her by a lantern and the judgement is made by the mistake he/she makes. *Eldridge-Green lantern* is the most popular.

3. Farnsworth–Munsell 100 hue test. It is a spectroscopic test in which a subject has to arrange the coloured chips in ascending order. The colour vision is judged by the error score, i.e. greater the score, poorer is the colour vision.

4. City University colour vision test. It is also a spectroscopic test in which a central coloured plate is to be matched to its closest hue from four surrounding colour plates.

5. Nagel anomaloscope test. In this test, the observer is asked to mix red and green colours in such a proportion that the mixture should match the given yellow-coloured disc. The judgement about the defect is made from the relative amounts of red and green colours and the brightness setting used by the observer.

6. Holmgren wool test. In this, the subject is asked to make a series of colour matches from a selection of skeins of coloured wools.

Contrast Sensitivity

Contrast sensitivity is the ability to perceive slight changes in luminance between regions which are not separated by definite borders and is just as important as the ability to perceive sharp outlines of relatively small objects. It is only the latter ability which is tested by means of the Snellen's test types. In many diseases, loss of contrast sensitivity is more important and disturbing to the patient than the loss of visual acuity.

Encoding of Contrast

Contrast is encoded when one ganglion cell is stimulated and its neighbour is inhibited.

At the border between light and dark areas of image, the neighbouring cells respond in opposite way, i.e.:

- *In the lighted portion* of the border between light and dark, the centre of the receptive field is illuminated, whereas its surround is not. Therefore, the on-centre ganglion cell activity is increased.
- *In the darkened portion*, the surround of the receptive field is illuminated, whereas its centre is not. Therefore, the on-centre ganglion cell activity is decreased.

When both the centre and the surround of the receptive field are totally in the illuminated or darkened portion of the image, no change in ganglion cell activity occurs.

ELECTROPHYSIOLOGICAL TESTS

The electrophysiological tests allow objective evaluation of the retinal functions. These include electroretinography (ERG), electro-oculography (EOG) and visual evoked response (VER).

Electroretinography ERG is the record of changes in the resting potential of the eye induced by a flash of light. It is measured in a dark-adapted eye with the active electrode (fitted on contact lens) placed on the cornea and the reference electrode attached on the forehead.

Normal record of ERG consists of the following waves (Fig. 11.1.52):

a-Wave: It is a negative wave possibly arising from the rods and cones.
b-Wave: It is a large positive wave which is generated by Muller cells, but represents the activity of the bipolar cells.
c-Wave: It is also a positive wave representing metabolic activity of pigment epithelium.

Both scotopic and photopic responses can be elicited in ERG. Foveal ERG can provide information about the macula.

Uses: ERG is very useful in detecting functional abnormalities of the outer retina (up to bipolar cell layer), much before the ophthalmoscopic signs appear. However, ERG is normal in diseases involving ganglion cells and the higher visual pathway, such as optic atrophy.

Electro-oculography EOG is based on the measurement of resting potential of the eye which exists between the cornea (+ve) and the back of the eye (−ve).

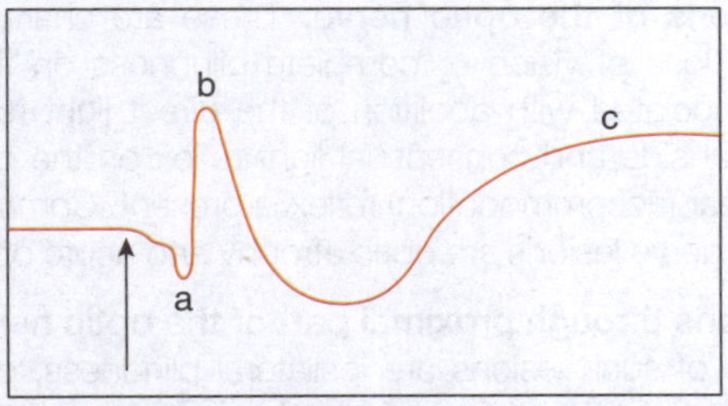

Fig. 11.1.52 Components of normal electroretinogram (ERG).

Normally, the resting potential of the eye decreases during dark adaptation and reaches its peak in light adaptation.

Interpretation of results: Results of EOG are interpreted by finding out the Arden ratio as:

$$\text{Arden ratio} = \frac{\text{Maximum height of light peak}}{\text{Minimum height of dark peak}} \times 100$$

- *Normal curve* values are 185 or greater.
- *Subnormal curve* values are less than 150.
- *Flat curve* values are less than 125.

Uses: Since the EOG reflects the presynaptic function of the retina, any disease that interferes with the functional interplay between the retinal pigment epithelium and the photoreceptors will produce an abnormal or absent light rise in the EOG. Thus, EOG is affected in diseases such as retinitis pigmentosa, vitamin A deficiency, retinal detachment and toxic retinopathies. Hence, EOG serves as a test that is supplementary and complementary to ERG and in certain states is more sensitive than the ERG.

Visual evoked response As we know when light falls on the retina, a series of nerve impulses are generated and passed on to the visual cortex via the visual pathway. The changes produced in the visual cortex by these impulses can be recorded by electroencephalography (EEG). Thus, VER is nothing but the EEG recorded at the *occipital lobe. VER* is the *only clinically objective technique available to assess the functional state of the visual system beyond the retinal ganglion cells*. Since there is disproportionately large projection of the macular area in the occipital cortex, the VER represents the macula-dominated response. VER is of two types depending on the techniques used:

1. ***Flash VER:*** It is recorded by using an intense flash stimulation. It merely indicates that light has been perceived by the visual cortex. It is not affected by the opacities in the lens and cornea.
2. ***Pattern reversal VER:*** It is recorded using some patterned stimulus, as in the checkerboard. In it, the pattern of the stimulus is changed (e.g. black squares go white and white become black) but the overall illumination remains the same. The pattern reversal VER depends on form sense and thus may give a rough estimate of the visual acuity.

FIELD OF VISION AND BINOCULAR VISION

FIELD OF VISION

The visual field is a three-dimensional area that can be seen around an object of fixation. The extent of a normal visual field with a 5-mm white colour object is superiorly 60°, inferiorly 70°, nasally 60° and temporally 90° (Fig. 11.1.53). The field for blue and yellow is roughly 10° less and that for red and green colour is about 20° less than that for white. Perimetry with a red-coloured object is particularly useful in the diagnosis of bitemporal hemianopia due to chiasmal compression and in the central scotoma of retrobulbar neuritis.

Perimetry: It is the procedure for estimating extent of the visual fields. It is of the following two types:

1. ***Kinetic perimetry:*** In this, the stimulus of known luminance is moved from the periphery towards the centre to establish isopters.

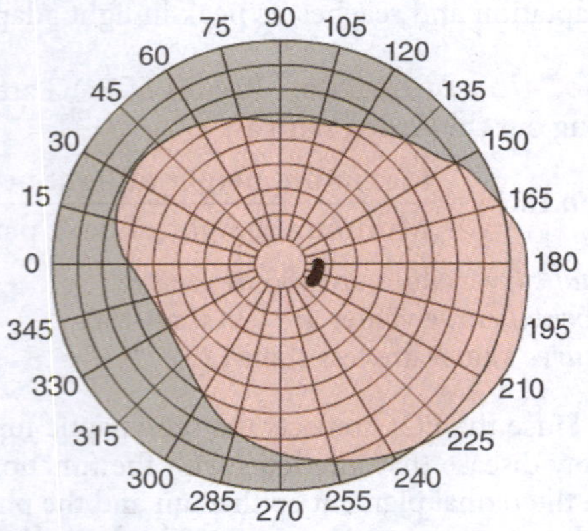

Fig. 11.1.53 Extent of normal visual field.

2. ***Static perimetry:*** This involves presenting a stimulus at a predetermined position for a preset duration with varying luminance.

Methods of Estimating the Visual Fields

A. Peripheral field charting Peripheral field charting is done by:

- Confrontation method
- Perimetry: Lister's, Goldmann's and automated

B. Central field charting is done by:

- Campimetry or scotometry
- Goldmann's perimetry
- Automated field analysis

1. Confrontation method: This is a rough but rapid and extremely simple method of estimating the peripheral visual field. Assuming the examiner's fields to be within the normal range, they are compared with the patient's visual fields.

2. Lister's perimeter: It has a metallic semicircular arc, graded in degrees, with a white dot for fixation in the centre. The arc can be rotated in different meridia. With the help of this perimeter, extent of peripheral field is charted (Fig. 11.1.54).

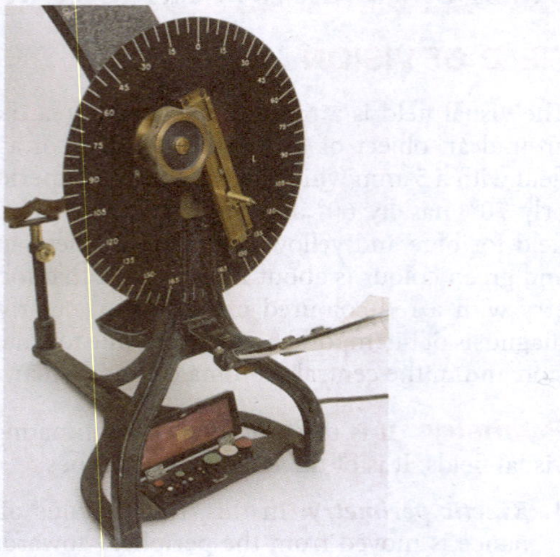

Fig. 11.1.54 Perimeter.

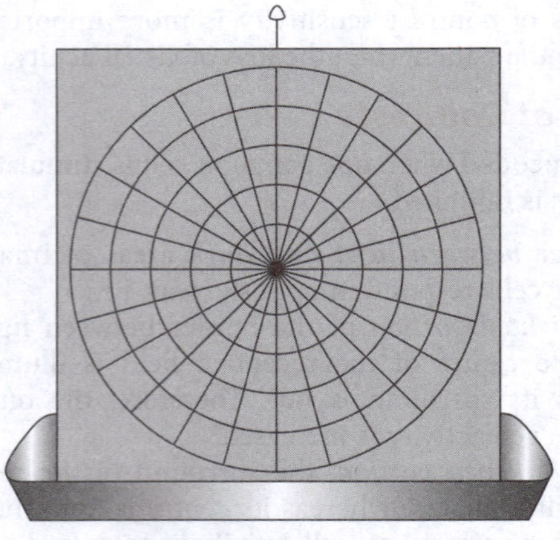

Fig. 11.1.55 Bjerrum's screen.

3. Campimetry (scotometry) is done to evaluate the central and paracentral areas (30°) of the visual field. The Bjerrum's screen is used and can be of size 1 or 2 m^2 (Fig. 11.1.55). Initially, the *blind spot* physiological scotoma is charted, which is normally located about 15° temporal to the fixation point. Dimensions of blind spots are horizontally 7–8° and vertically 10–11°. *Central/paracentral scotomas* can be found in optic neuritis and open-angle glaucoma.

4 Goldmann's perimeter: It consists of a hemispherical dome. Its main advantage over the tangent screen is that the test conditions and the intensity of the target are always the same. It permits greater reproducibility.

5. Automated perimeters are computer assisted and test visual fields by a static method. They automatically test supra-threshold and threshold stimuli and quantify depth of field defect.

Applied Aspects

Common Causes of Defects in the Field of Vision

The most common causes of field defects are given next.

I. Glaucomatous Field Defects

A typical pattern of field defects is seen in patients with chronic glaucomas.

II. Field Defects in Lesions of the Optic Disc and Optic Nerve

Central and paracentral scotomas can be found in patients with papillitis (inflammation of the optic disc) and optic neuritis.

III. Field Defects in Lesions of Visual Pathway

Salient features and important causes of lesions of the visual pathway at different levels (Fig. 11.1.56) are given next.

1. Lesions of the optic nerve. These are characterized by marked loss of vision or complete blindness on the affected side associated with abolition of the direct light reflex on the ipsilateral side and consensual light reflex on the contralateral side. Near (accommodation) reflex is present. *Common causes* of optic nerve lesions are optic atrophy and acute optic neuritis.

2. Lesions through proximal part of the optic nerve. Salient features of such lesions are ipsilateral blindness, contralateral hemianopia and abolition of direct light reflex on the affected

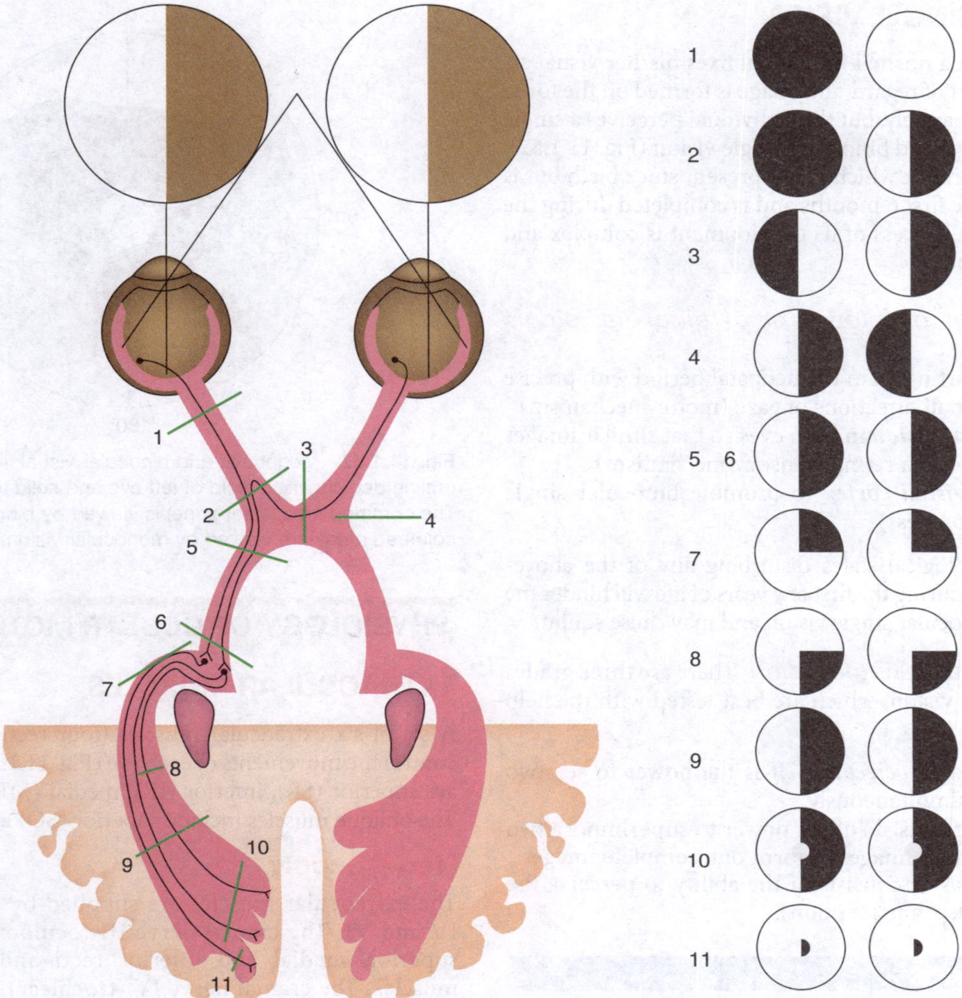

Fig. 11.1.56 Lesions of the visual pathways at the level of: 1, optic nerve; 2, proximal part of optic nerve; 3, central chiasma; 4, lateral chiasma (both sides); 5, optic tract; 6, geniculate body; 7, part of optic radiations in temporal lobe; 8, part of optic radiations in parietal lobe; 9, optic radiations; 10, visual cortex sparing the macula; and 11, visual cortex, only macula.

side and consensual on the contralateral side. Near reflex is intact.

3. Sagittal (central) lesions of the chiasma. These are characterized by bitemporal hemianopia and bitemporal hemianopic paralysis of pupillary reflexes. These usually lead to partial descending optic atrophy.

Common causes of central chiasmal lesion are suprasellar aneurysms and tumours of the pituitary gland.

4. Lateral chiasmal lesions. Salient features of such lesions are binasal hemianopia associated with binasal hemianopic paralysis of the pupillary reflexes. These usually lead to partial descending optic atrophy. *Common causes* of such lesions are distension of the third ventricle causing pressure on each side of the chiasma.

5. Lesions of optic tract. These are characterized by incongruous homonymous hemianopia associated with contralateral hemianopic pupillary reaction (Wernicke's reaction).

6. Lesions of lateral geniculate body. These produce homonymous hemianopia with sparing of pupillary reflexes, and may end in partial optic atrophy.

7. Lesions of optic radiations. Their features vary depending on the site of lesion. Involvement of total optic radiations produces complete homonymous hemianopia (sometimes sparing the macula). Inferior quadrantic hemianopia (*pie on the floor*) occurs in lesions of the parietal lobe (containing superior fibres of optic radiations). Superior quadrantic hemianopia (*pie in the sky*) may occur following lesions of the temporal lobe (containing inferior fibres of optic radiations). Pupillary reactions are normal as the fibres of the light reflex leave the optic tracts to synapse in the superior colliculi.

Common lesions of the optic radiations include vascular occlusions.

8. Lesions of the visual cortex. Congruous homonymous hemianopia (usually sparing the macula) is a feature of occlusion of the posterior cerebral artery supplying the anterior part of the occipital cortex. Congruous homonymous macular defect occurs in lesions of the tip of the occipital cortex following a head injury or gunshot injuries. Pupillary light reflexes are normal and optic atrophy does not occur following visual cortex lesions.

BINOCULAR SINGLE VISION

Definition When a normal individual fixes his/her visual attention on an object of regard, the image is formed on the fovea of both the eyes separately, but the individual perceives a single image. This state is called binocular single vision (Fig. 11.1.57). It is a conditioned reflex which is not present since birth but is acquired during the first 6 months and is completed during the first few years. The process of its development is complex and partially understood.

Prerequisites for development of binocular single vision

1. ***Straight eyes*** starting from the neonatal period with precise coordination for all directions of gaze (motor mechanism)
2. ***Reasonably clear vision*** in both eyes so that similar images are presented to each retina (sensory mechanism)
3. ***Ability of the visual cortex*** to promote binocular single vision (mental process)

Therefore, pathological states disturbing any of the above-stated mechanisms during the first few years of life will hinder the development of binocular single vision and may cause squint.

Grades of binocular single vision There are three grades of binocular single vision, which are best tested with the help of a synoptophore:

Grade I: *Simultaneous perception.* It is the power to see two dissimilar objects simultaneously.
Grade II: *Fusion.* It consists of the power to superimpose two incomplete but similar images to form one complete image.
Grade III: *Stereopsis.* It consists of the ability to perceive the third dimension (depth perception).

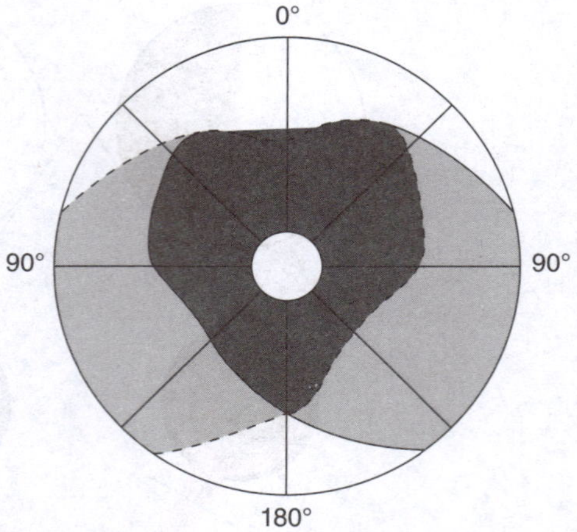

Fig. 11.1.57 Monocular and binocular visual fields. The dashed outline depicts visual field of left eye and solid line that of right eye. The common area (clear zone) is viewed by binocular vision and coloured areas are viewed by monocular vision.

Applied Aspects

Anomalies of Binocular Vision

Anomalies of binocular vision include suppression, amblyopia and diplopia.

1. Suppression

It is a temporary active cortical inhibition of the image of an object formed on the retina of the squinting eye. This phenomenon occurs only during binocular vision (with both eyes open). However, when the fixating eye is covered, the squinting eye fixes (i.e. suppression disappears).

2. Amblyopia

It is an impairment of vision in the absence of any organic disease of ocular media and visual pathway. Types of functional amblyopia are as follows:

- Anisometropic amblyopia which usually occurs when the difference in refractive error of the two eyes is more than 2.5 D
- Stimulus deprivation amblyopia (amblyopia ex anopsia) which may occur in children with cataract, corneal opacity and severe ptosis
- Strabismic amblyopia which results from prolonged uniocular suppression

3. Diplopia

Diplopia occurs due to formation of image on dissimilar points of the two retinae. It is the main symptom of paralysis of extraocular muscles.

PHYSIOLOGY OF OCULAR MOTILITY

EXTRAOCULAR MUSCLES

A set of six extraocular muscles (four recti and two obliques) control the movements of each eye (Fig. 11.1.58). Rectus muscles are superior (SR), inferior (IR), medial (MR) and lateral (LR). The oblique muscles include superior (SO) and inferior (IO).

Nerve Supply

The extraocular muscles are supplied by cranial nerves III, IV and VI. The cranial nerve III (oculomotor) supplies the superior, medial and inferior recti and inferior oblique muscles. The cranial nerve IV (trochlear) supplies the superior oblique and the nerve VI (abducent) supplies the lateral rectus muscle.

Actions The extraocular muscles rotate the eyeball around vertical, horizontal and anteroposterior axes. Medial and lateral rectus muscles are almost parallel to the optic axis of the eyeball; so they have got only the main action. In contrast, superior and inferior rectus muscles make an angle of 23° and reflected tendons of the superior and inferior oblique muscles of 51° with the optical axis in the primary position; so they have subsidiary actions in addition to the main action. Actions of each muscle (Fig. 11.1.59) are shown in Table 11.1.2.

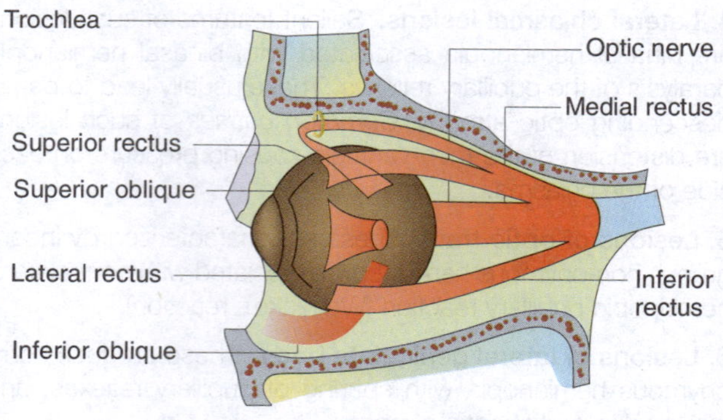

Fig. 11.1.58 Extraocular muscles.

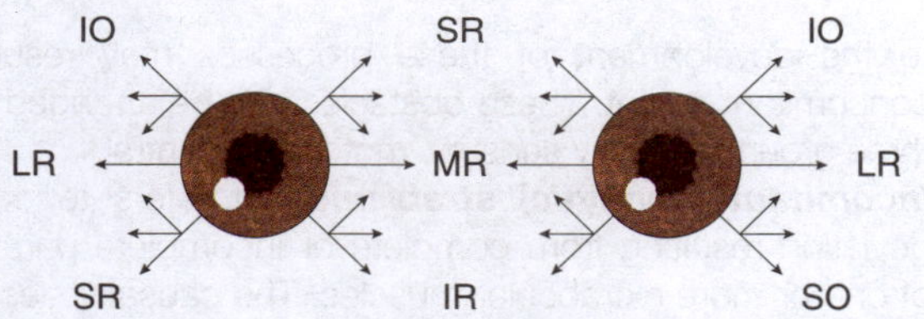

Fig. 11.1.59 Action of extraocular muscles. IO, inferior oblique; IR, inferior rectus; LR, lateral rectus; MR, medial rectus; SO, superior oblique; SR, superior oblique.

Table 11.1.2 Actions of extraocular muscles

Muscle	Primary action	Secondary action	Tertiary action
MR	Adduction	–	–
LR	Abduction	–	–
SR	Elevation	Intorsion	Adduction
IR	Depression	Extorsion	Adduction
SO	Intorsion	Depression	Abduction
IO	Extorsion	Elevation	Abduction

IO, inferior oblique; IR, inferior rectus; LR, lateral rectus; MR, medial rectus; SO, superior oblique; SR, superior rectus.

OCULAR MOVEMENTS

Types of Ocular Movements

A. Uniocular movements are called 'ductions' and include:

1. *Adduction:* It is an inward movement (medial rotation) along the vertical axis.
2. *Abduction:* It is an outward movement (lateral rotation) along the vertical axis.
3. *Supraduction:* It is an upward movement (elevation) along the horizontal axis.
4. *Infraduction:* It is a downward movement (depression) along the horizontal axis.
5. *Incycloduction* (intorsion): It is a rotatory movement along the anteroposterior axis in which the superior pole of the cornea (12-o'clock point) moves medially.
6. *Excycloduction* (extorsion): It is a rotatory movement along the anteroposterior axis in which the superior pole of the cornea (12-o'clock point) moves laterally.

B. Binocular movements: These are of two types – versions and vergences.

a. Versions, also known as conjugate movements, are synchronous (simultaneous) symmetric movements of both eyes in the same direction. These include:

1. ***Dextroversion:*** It is the movement of both eyes to the right. It results due to simultaneous contraction of the right lateral rectus and left medial rectus.
2. ***Levoversion:*** It refers to movement of both eyes to the left. It is produced by simultaneous contraction of the left lateral rectus and right medial rectus.
3. ***Supraversion:*** It is an upward movement of both eyes in primary position. It results due to simultaneous contraction of the bilateral superior recti and inferior obliques.
4. ***Infraversion:*** It is a downward movement of both eyes in primary position. It results due to simultaneous contraction of the bilateral inferior recti and superior obliques.
5. ***Dextrocycloversion:*** It is a rotational movement around the anteroposterior axis, in which the superior pole of the cornea of both the eyes tilts towards the right.
6. ***Levocycloversion:*** It is just the reverse of dextrocycloversion. In it, the superior pole of the cornea of both the eyes tilts towards the left.

b. Vergences, also called disjugate movements, are synchronous and symmetric movements of both eyes in opposite directions, e.g.:

1. ***Convergence:*** It is a simultaneous inward movement of both eyes which results from contraction of the medial recti.
2. ***Divergence:*** It is a simultaneous outward movement of both eyes produced by contraction of the lateral recti.

SUPRANUCLEAR CONTROL OF EYE MOVEMENTS

There exists a highly accurate, still not fully elucidated, supranuclear control of eye movements which keeps the two eyes yoked together so that the image of the object of interest is simultaneously held on both foveae despite movement of the perceived object or the observer's head and/or body.

The following supranuclear eye movement systems have been recognized:

1. Saccadic system
2. Smooth pursuit system
3. Vergence system
4. Vestibular system
5. Optokinetic system
6. Position maintenance system

All these systems perform specific functions and each one is controlled by a different neural system but share the same final common path – the motor neurons that supply the extraocular muscles.

1. Saccadic system Saccades are sudden, jerky conjugate eye movements that occur as the gaze shifts from one object to another. Thus, they are performed to bring the image of an object quickly on the fovea. Though normally voluntary, saccades may be involuntary, aroused by peripheral, visual or auditory stimuli.

2. Smooth pursuit eye movement system Smooth pursuit movements are tracking movements of the eye as they follow moving objects. These occur voluntarily when the eyes track moving objects but take place involuntarily if a repetitive visual pattern is displayed continuously. When velocity of the moving object is more, the smooth pursuit movement is replaced by *small saccades (catch-up saccades)*.

3. Vergence movement system Vergence movements allow focusing of an object which moves away from or towards the observer or when visual fixation shifts from one object to another at a different distance. They are very slow (about 20°/s) disjugate movements. They have a latency of about 160 milliseconds.

4. Vestibular eye movement system Vestibular movements are usually effective in compensating for the effects of head movements in disturbing visual fixation. These movements operate through the vestibular system (see page 1044).

Most rotations of the head do not involve angular rotations as fast as 300°/s and the vestibular system can compensate for these. However, when the body is rotated at great speeds around a vertical axis (e.g. a skater performing a spin), eye movements show the so-called oculovestibular nystagmus, with a slow motion of the eyes in the opposite direction to that of rotation – this is initiated by the vestibular mechanism – followed by a quick jerky binocular 'return' movement in the direction of rotation. This sequence is repeated as long as the angular acceleration lasts. It is likely that the fast component of nystagmus is mediated by mechanisms similar to those responsible for saccades.

5. Optokinetic system This system helps to hold the images of the seen world steady on the retinae during sustained head rotation. This system becomes operative when the vestibular reflex gets fatigued after 30 seconds. The optokinetic response is evoked by rotation of the visual field before the eyes. It consists of a movement following the moving scene, succeeded by a rapid saccade in the opposite direction. In fact, the transient head rotation stimulates both the vestibulo-ocular reflex with a latency of only 10 milliseconds and the optokinetic reflex with a latency of 70 milliseconds. However, during sustained rotation with eyes open, the vestibulo-ocular reflex ceases, whereas the optokinetic system maintains a steady discharge from the vestibular nuclei to sustain the compensatory optokinetic nystagmus.

6. Position maintenance system This system helps to maintain a specific gaze position by means of rapid micromovements called *flicks* and slow micromovements called *drifts*. This system coordinates with other systems. ***Neural pathway*** for this system is believed to be the same as for saccades and smooth pursuits.

Applied Aspects

Strabismus and Nystagmus

Strabismus

Definition. Normally, visual axes of the two eyes are parallel to each other in the 'primary position of gaze' and this alignment is maintained in all positions.

A misalignment of the visual axes of the two eyes is called squint or strabismus.

Manifest squint (heterotopia)

It is of two types:

- Concomitant strabismus
- Incomitant strabismus

1. ***Concomitant (nonparalytic) strabismus:*** It is a type of manifest squint in which the amount of deviation in the squinting eye remains constant (unaltered) in all the directions of gaze, and there is no associated limitation of ocular movements.

   Aetiology of concomitant strabismus is not clearly defined. The causative factors differ in individual cases. As we know, the binocular vision and coordination of ocular movements are not present since birth but are acquired in the early childhood. The process starts by the age of 3–6 months and is completed up to 5–6 years. Therefore, any obstacle to the development of these processes may result in concomitant squint. These obstacles can be arranged into three groups, namely sensory, motor and central.
2. ***Incomitant (paralytic) strabismus:*** It refers to ocular deviation resulting from complete or incomplete paralysis of one or more extraocular muscles. The causative lesions may be neurogenic, myogenic or at the level of neuromuscular junction.

Nystagmus

It is defined as regular and rhythmic to-and-fro involuntary oscillatory movements of the eyes.

Aetiology. It occurs due to disturbance of the factors responsible for maintaining normal ocular posture. These include disorders of the sensory visual pathway, vestibular apparatus, semicircular canals, midbrain and cerebellum.

Features of nystagmus. It may be characterized by any of the following features:

1. It may be *pendular or jerk nystagmus*. In pendular nystagmus, movements are of equal velocity in each direction. It may be horizontal, vertical or rotatory. In jerk nystagmus, the movements have a slow component in one direction and a fast component in the other direction. The direction of jerk nystagmus is defined by direction of the fast component (phase). It may be right, left, up, down or rotatory.
2. Nystagmus movements may be *rapid or slow*.
3. The movements may be *fine or coarse*.
4. Nystagmus may be *latent or manifest*.
   For details, see page 1044.

AQUEOUS HUMOUR AND INTRAOCULAR PRESSURE

AQUEOUS PRODUCTION

The aqueous humour is a clear watery fluid filling the anterior chamber (0.25 mL) and posterior chamber (0.06 mL) of the eyeball. In addition to its role in maintaining a proper IOP, it also plays an important metabolic role by providing substrates and removing metabolites from the avascular cornea and the lens. Constituents of normal aqueous humour are water (99.9%), proteins (0.04%) and others including (in millimoles per kilogram) Na^+ (144), K^+ (4.5), Cl^- (110), glucose (6.0), lactic acid (7.4), amino acids (5) and inositol (0.1).

Aqueous humour is derived from plasma within the capillary network of ciliary processes. The normal aqueous production rate is 2.3 mL/min. The three mechanisms – *diffusion, ultrafiltration and secretion* (active transport) – play a part in its production at different levels. The steps involved in the process of production are as follows:

1. First of all, by *ultrafiltration*, most of the plasma substances pass out from the capillary wall, loose connective tissue and pigment epithelium of the ciliary processes. Thus, the plasma filtrate accumulates behind the nonpigmented epithelium of ciliary processes.
2. The tight junctions between the cells of the nonpigmented epithelium create part of blood–aqueous barrier. Certain substances are actively transported *(secreted)* across this barrier into the posterior chamber. The active transport is brought about by Na^+–K^+-activated ATPase pump and

carbonic anhydrase enzyme system. Substances that are actively transported include sodium, chlorine, potassium, ascorbic acid, amino acids and bicarbonates.

Active transport of these substances across the nonpigmented ciliary epithelium results in an osmotic gradient leading to the movement of other plasma constituents into the posterior chamber by ultrafiltration and *diffusion*. Sodium is primarily responsible for movement of water into the posterior chamber.

Control of aqueous formation: The diurnal variation in IOP certainly indicates that some endogenous factors do influence the aqueous formation. The exact role of such factors is yet to be clearly understood. Vasopressin and adenylyl cyclase have been described to affect aqueous formation by influencing active transport of sodium.

Ultrafiltration and diffusion, the passive mechanisms of aqueous formation, are dependent on the level of blood pressure in the ciliary capillaries, the plasma osmotic pressure and the level of IOP.

DRAINAGE OF AQUEOUS HUMOUR

Aqueous humour flows from the posterior chamber into the anterior chamber through the pupil against slight physiological resistance. From the anterior chamber, the aqueous is drained out by two routes:

- Trabecular (conventional outflow)
- Uveoscleral (unconventional) outflow

A. Trabecular (Conventional) Outflow

It is the main outlet for aqueous from the anterior chamber. Approximately, 90% of the total aqueous is drained out via this route. The aqueous outflow system includes the trabecular meshwork, Schlemm's canal, collector channels, aqueous veins and episcleral veins (Fig. 11.1.60).

1. Trabecular meshwork It is a sieve-like structure through which aqueous humour leaves the eye. It consists of three portions:

- *Uveal meshwork*
- *Corneoscleral meshwork*
- *Juxtacanalicular (endothelial) meshwork*

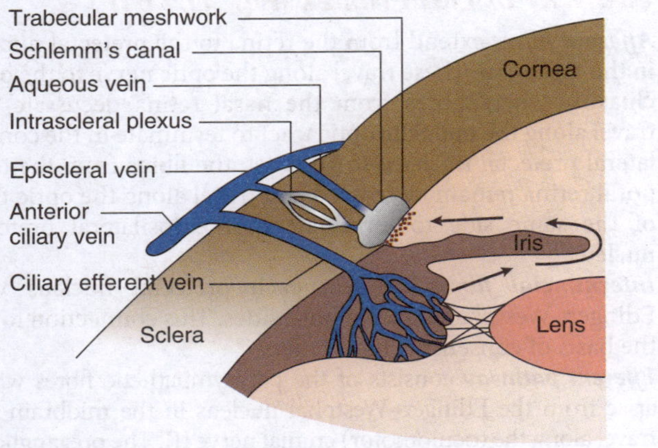

Fig. 11.1.60 The aqueous outflow system.

2. Schlemm's canal This is an endothelial-lined oval channel present circumferentially in the scleral sulcus. The endothelial cells of its inner wall are irregular spindle-shaped and contain giant vacuoles. The outer wall of the canal is lined by smooth flat cells and contains the openings of collector channels.

Free flow of aqueous occurs from the trabecular meshwork up to the inner wall of Schlemm's canal which appears to provide some resistance to outflow.

Mechanism of aqueous transport across inner wall of Schlemm's canal: It is partially understood. *Vacuolation theory* is the most accepted view. According to it, transcellular spaces exist in the endothelial cells forming the inner wall of Schlemm's canal. These open as a system of vacuoles and pores, primarily in response to pressure, and transport the aqueous from juxtacanalicular connective tissue to Schlemm's canal.

3. Collector channels These, also called intrascleral aqueous vessels, are about 25–35 in number and leave the Schlemm's canal at oblique angles to terminate into episcleral veins in a laminated fashion. These intrascleral aqueous vessels can be divided into two systems (Fig. 11.1.60). The larger vessels *(aqueous veins)* run a short intrascleral course and terminate directly into episcleral veins (*direct system*). Many smaller collector channels form an intrascleral plexus before eventually going into episcleral veins (*indirect system*).

From Schlemm's canal, the aqueous is transported via external collector channels into the episcleral veins by direct and indirect systems. A pressure gradient between IOP and intrascleral venous pressure (about 10 mm Hg) is responsible for unidirectional flow of aqueous.

B. Uveoscleral (Unconventional) Outflow

It is responsible for about 10% of the total aqueous outflow. Aqueous passes across the ciliary body into the suprachoroidal space and is drained by the venous circulation in the ciliary body, choroid and sclera.

The drainage of aqueous humour is summarized in the flowchart.

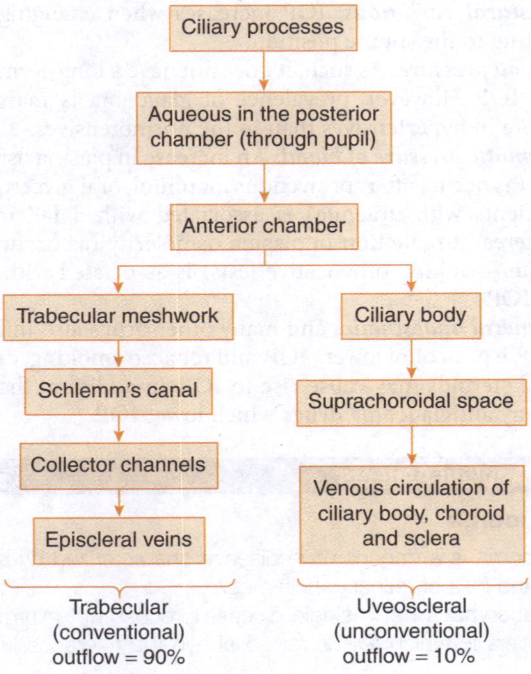

MAINTENANCE OF INTRAOCULAR PRESSURE

The IOP refers to the pressure exerted by intraocular fluids on the coats of the eyeball. The normal IOP varies between 10 and 21 mm Hg (mean 16 ± 2.5 mm Hg). The normal level of IOP is essentially maintained by a dynamic equilibrium between the formation and the outflow of the aqueous humour. Various factors influencing IOP can be grouped as given next.

A. Local factors include:

1. ***Rate of aqueous formation*** influences IOP levels. The aqueous formation in turn depends on many factors such as permeability of ciliary capillaries and osmotic pressure of the blood.
2. ***Resistance to aqueous outflow (drainage):*** From the clinical point of view, this is the most important factor. Most of the resistance to aqueous outflow is at the level of the trabecular meshwork.
3. ***Increased episcleral venous pressure*** may result in rise of IOP. The Valsalva manoeuvre causes temporary increase in episcleral venous pressure and rise in IOP.
4. ***Dilatation of the pupil*** in patients with a narrow anterior chamber angle may cause rise of IOP owing to a relative obstruction of the aqueous drainage by the iris.

B. General factors General factors include:

1. ***Heredity:*** It influences IOP, possibly by multifactorial modes.
2. ***Age:*** The mean IOP increases after the age of 40 years, possibly due to reduced facility of aqueous outflow.
3. ***Sex:*** IOP is equal between the sexes in ages 20–40 years. In older age groups, increase in mean IOP with age is greater in females.
4. ***Diurnal variation of IOP:*** Usually, there is a tendency of higher IOP in the morning and lower in the evening. This has been related to diurnal variation in the levels of plasma cortisol. Normal eyes have a smaller fluctuation (<5 mm Hg) than glaucomatous eyes (>8 mm Hg).
5. ***Postural variations:*** IOP increases when changing from sitting to the supine position.
6. ***Blood pressure:*** As such, it does not have a long-term effect on IOP. However, prevalence of glaucoma is marginally more in hypertensives than in the normotensives.
7. ***Osmotic pressure of blood:*** An increase in plasma osmolarity (as occurs after intravenous mannitol, oral glycerol or in patients with uraemia) is associated with a fall in IOP, whereas a reduction in plasma osmolarity (as occurs with water-drinking provocative tests) is associated with a rise in IOP.
8. ***General anaesthetics*** and many other drugs also influence IOP, e.g. alcohol lowers IOP, and tobacco smoking, caffeine and steroids may cause rise in IOP. In addition, there are many antiglaucoma drugs which lower IOP.

Applied Aspects

Glaucoma

Glaucoma is a degenerative disease characterized by raised IOP and loss of retinal ganglion cells.

Glaucoma is not a single disease process but a group of disorders in which IOP is raised above the tolerance limit of the affected eye, resulting in a damage to the optic nerve head and irreversible visual field defects.

This definition is not so simple as it apparently looks, since it is impossible to know the tolerance limit of the individual eye. Consequently, the term *ocular hypertension* is used for cases having constantly raised IOP without any associated glaucomatous damage (normal 10–20 mm Hg). Conversely, the term *normal-* or *low-tension glaucoma (NTG/LTG)* is suggested for the typical cupping of the disc and/or visual field defects associated with a normal or low IOP.

Types of Glaucomas

1. ***Congenital and developmental glaucomas*** occur due to developmental anomalies of the angle of the anterior chamber.
2. ***Primary glaucomas*** occur without any obvious systemic or ocular cause, usually after the age of 40 years. These are of two types:
   - *Primary open-angle glaucoma*, which occurs due to sclerosis of the trabecular meshwork
   - *Primary angle-closure glaucoma*, which occurs due to closure of the angle of the anterior chamber
3. ***Secondary glaucomas*** are characterized by rise in IOP, secondary to some other ocular disease, e.g. phacomorphic glaucoma associated with swollen cataractous lens.

Treatment The main aim of treatment is to normalize the raised IOP. The drugs which lower the IOP are as follows:

- *Carbonic anhydrase inhibitors* decrease the production of aqueous humour.
- *Prostaglandins* increase the outflow of the aqueous.
- *Cholinergic agonists* increase the aqueous outflow by ciliary muscle contraction.

PHYSIOLOGY OF PUPIL

PUPILLARY REFLEXES

Light Reflex

When light is shone in one eye, both the pupils constrict. Constriction of the pupil to which light is shone is called *direct light reflex* and that of the other pupil is called *consensual (indirect) light reflex*. Light reflex is initiated by rods and cones.

Pathway of Light Reflex (Fig. 11.1.61)

Afferent fibres extend from the retina to the pretectal nucleus in the midbrain. These travel along the optic nerve to the optic chiasma where fibres from the nasal retina decussate and travel along the opposite optic tract to terminate in the contralateral pretectal nucleus. In contrast, the fibres from the temporal retina remain uncrossed and travel along the optic tract of the same side to terminate in the ipsilateral pretectal nucleus.

Internuncial fibres connect each pretectal nucleus with Edinger–Westphal nuclei of both sides. This connection forms the basis of consensual light reflex.

Efferent pathway consists of the parasympathetic fibres which arise from the Edinger–Westphal nucleus in the midbrain and travel along the (oculomotor) cranial nerve III. The preganglionic fibres enter the inferior division of the cranial nerve III and

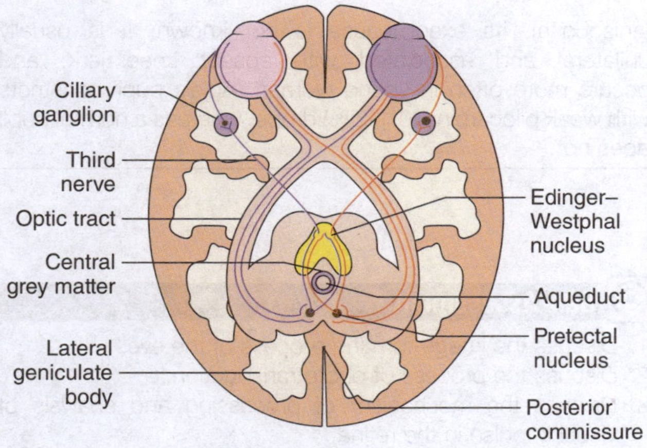

Fig. 11.1.61 Pathway of the light reflex.

via the nerve to the inferior oblique reach the ciliary ganglion to relay. Postganglionic fibres travel along the short ciliary nerves to innervate the sphincter pupillae.

Functions of light reflex:

- Pupillary constriction associated with light reflex prevents excessive bleaching of the visual pigment by reducing the amount of light entering the eye.
- Light reflex helps in light and dark adaptation; thus, it plays a role in maximizing visual acuity at different light levels.

Accommodation Reflex

During accommodation, when eyes are focused from a distant to a near object to achieve clear vision, three reactions occur, i.e.:

- Changes in the radius of curvature of the lens (more convex) by contraction of ciliary muscles
- Pupillary constriction (meiosis) by contraction of sphincter pupillae
- Convergence of eyes due to contraction of medial recti of eyeballs

Near Reflex

Near reflex occurs on looking at a near object. It consists of two components: (i) convergence reflex, i.e. contraction of the pupil on convergence; and (ii) accommodation reflex, i.e. contraction of the pupil associated with accommodation.

Pathway of convergence reflex (Fig. 11.1.62) Its afferent pathway is still not elucidated. It is assumed that the afferents from the medial recti travel centrally via the third nerve to the mesencephalic nucleus of the cranial nerve V, to a presumptive convergence centre in the tectal or pretectal region. From this, the impulse is relayed to the Edinger–Westphal nucleus and the subsequent efferent pathway of near reflex is along the third nerve. The efferent fibres relay in the accessory ganglion before reaching the sphincter pupillae.

Pathway of accommodation reflex (Fig. 11.1.62) The afferent impulses extend from the retina to the parastriate cortex via the optic nerve, chiasma, optic tract, LGB, optic radiations and striate cortex. From the parastriate cortex, the impulses are relayed to the Edinger–Westphal nucleus of both sides via the occipitomesencephalic tract and the pontine

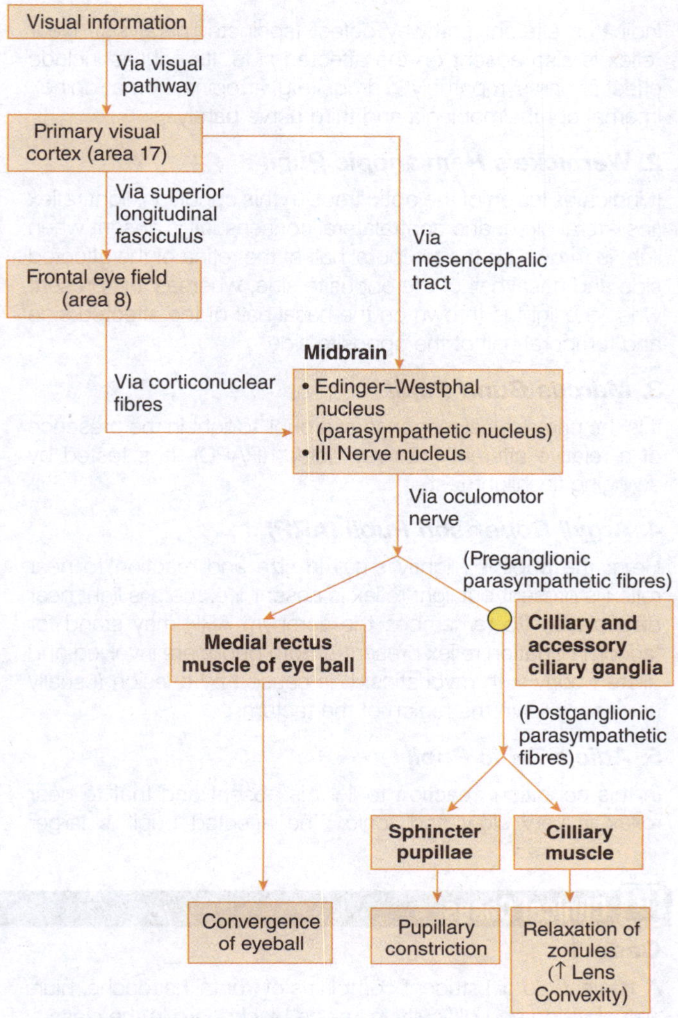

Fig. 11.1.62 Pathway of the accommodation reflex.

centre. From the Edinger–Westphal nucleus, the efferent impulses travel along the third nerve and reach the sphincter pupillae and ciliary muscle after relaying in the accessory and ciliary ganglia.

For convergence reaction, impulses from the visual cortex reach the frontal eye field (area 8) through association fasciculus (superior longitudinal fasciculus). From the frontal eye field, the corticonuclear fibres project to the third nerve nuclei of both sides and through oculomotor nerves supply the medial recti of the eyeballs.

Psychosensory Reflex

It refers to dilatation of the pupil in response to sensory and psychic stimuli. It is very complex and its mechanism is still not elucidated.

Applied Aspects

Abnormalities of Pupillary Reactions

1. Efferent Pathway Defect

Absence of both direct and consensual light reflexes on the affected side (say right eye) and presence of both direct and consensual light reflexes on the normal side (i.e. left eye) indicates efferent pathway defect (sphincter paralysis). Near reflex is also absent on the affected side. Its causes include effect of parasympatholytic drugs (e.g. atropine, homatropine), internal ophthalmoplegia and third nerve paralysis.

2. Wernicke's Hemianopic Pupil

It indicates lesion of the optic tract. In this condition, light reflex (ipsilateral direct and contralateral consensual) is absent when light is thrown on the temporal half of the retina of the affected side and nasal half of the opposite side, whereas it is present when the light is thrown on the nasal half of the affected side and temporal half of the opposite side.

3. Marcus Gunn Pupil

It is the paradoxical response of a pupil to light in the presence of a relative afferent pathway defect (RAPD). It is tested by swinging flashlight test.

4. Argyll Robertson Pupil (ARP)

Here, the pupil is slightly small in size and reaction to near reflex is present but light reflex is absent, i.e. there is light near dissociation (to remember, the acronym ARP may stand for 'accommodation reflex present'). Both pupils are involved and dilate poorly with mydriatics. It is caused by a lesion (usually neurosyphilis) in the region of the tectum.

5. Adie's Tonic Pupil

In this condition, reaction to light is absent and that to near reflex is very slow and tonic. The affected pupil is larger (anisocoria). Its exact cause is not known. It is usually unilateral and associated with absent knee jerk, and occurs more often in young women. Adie's pupil constricts with weak pilocarpine (0.125%) drops, whereas a normal pupil does not.

Self-Assessment

1. Discuss the image-forming process of the eye.
2. Discuss the process of phototransduction.
3. Discuss the mechanism of processing and analysis of visual impulse in the retina.
4. Describe the following:
   - Concept of serial and parallel processing of visual information
   - Formation, drainage and significance of aqueous humour
5. Write notes on the following:
   - Supranuclear control of ocular motility
   - Pupillary reflex
   - Accommodation
   - Visual pigments
   - Colour sense
   - Ocular dominance columns
   - Visual evoked potential
   - Concept of binocular single vision

Clinical Cases

Case 1

A 10-year-old girl student complains of frontal headache, blurring of vision and difficulty in seeing blackboard in the class.

Q1. The student is suffering from which refractive error?
Q2. What are the tests to be carried out to confirm the refractive error?
Q3. How should this error be corrected?

Case 2

A 55-year-old female visited eye OPD with complaints of headache, and inability to read small letters of the newspaper and perform fine needle work.

Q1. What is the reason for these symptoms?
Q2. What is the pathophysiology of this condition?
Q3. What is the corrective measure?

Case 3

A 7-year-old male child was referred to the eye department for complaints of difficulty in seeing in the night.

The eye examination observations showed muddy wrinkled conjunctiva with white patchy spots on the bulbar conjunctiva.

Q1. What is the probable diagnosis?
Q2. What is the main cause of this condition?
Q3. What is the pathophysiology of difficulty in seeing during night?

Case 4

A 60-year-old male presented with complaints of blurring of vision, change in the number of his glasses every 2–3 months and feeling difficulty in driving also. The ophthalmologist examined him thoroughly and the patient was diagnosed to be a case of senile cataract.

Q1. What is the pathophysiology of this condition?
Q2. What is the treatment?

Case 5

A 25-year-old male was selected for driver post; before joining, he underwent medical examination. Observations during eye examination were as follows:

Visual acuity: 6/36
Intraocular pressure: Within normal range
Colour vision test: Unable to appreciate red colour

Q1. He is suffering from which type of colour vision defect?
Q2. What is the pathophysiology of colour vision defects?

Case 6

A 64-year-old female presented with a history of redness, pain and diminishing of vision in the left eye for 3 days.

Signs and symptoms revealed coloured haloes around the white light.

Examination and test findings showed raised intraocular pressure, and the patient was advised further tests – visual field charting and fundus examination.

Q1. What is the probable diagnosis?
Q2. What changes are expected in fundus examination in this case?
Q3. What is the visual field pattern in this case?

Case 7

A 35-year-old male presented with severe headache and loss of vision, and was suspected to be a case of glaucoma and investigated.

Intraocular pressure was within normal range.
Visual field analysis showed bitemporal hemianopia.
There were no obvious fundus findings.

Q1. What is the site of lesion in this case?
Q2. What is the common cause for this condition?
Q3. What is the reason for severe headache and vomiting in this case?

Case 8

A 20-year-old girl presented with double vision and blurring of vision and she had inability to position the eye when looking towards the right side.

Thorough eye examination concluded this to be a case of ophthalmoplegia due to sixth nerve palsy.

Q1. What is position of eyeballs when looking towards the right side?
Q2. What is the cause for double vision?

11.2 Sense of Hearing

CHAPTER OUTLINE

FUNCTIONAL ANATOMY

EAR

The mechanism of hearing is closely associated with the mechanism of equilibrium; therefore, the inner ear acts as an organ of hearing and equilibrium. For hearing, the sound waves have to pass through the three subdivisions of the ear, which are as follows (Fig. 11.2.1):

- External ear
- Middle ear
- Internal ear

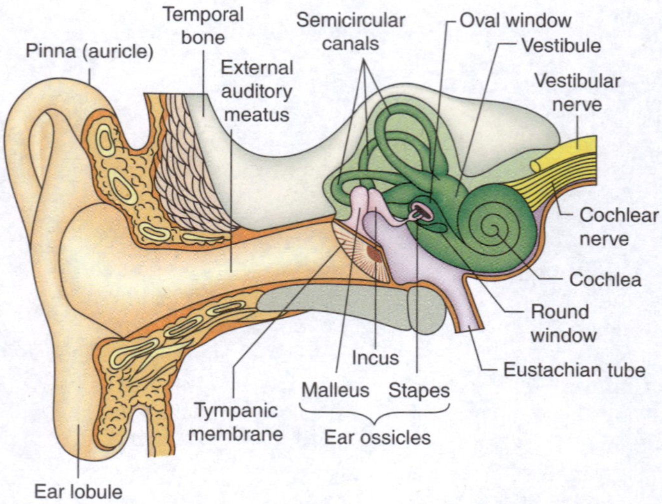

Fig. 11.2.1 Structure of three subdivisions of the ear.

External Ear

The external ear consists of the pinna (auricle) and the external auditory meatus.

Pinna or auricle consists of a single convoluted plate of elastic cartilage covered by skin which is tightly attached to the underlying perichondrium.

Functions: The pinna collects and reflects the sound waves into the external auditory canal.

- In lower animals, the pinna is more important, in whom it can be moved by muscular action in the direction of sound source.
- In humans, the pinna is not moveable, but its peculiar shape aids in *discerning* the source of sound (e.g. in front of vs. behind the head).

External auditory meatus extends from the pinna to the tympanic membrane. It consists of two distinct portions – external one-third, cartilaginous portion and internal two-third,

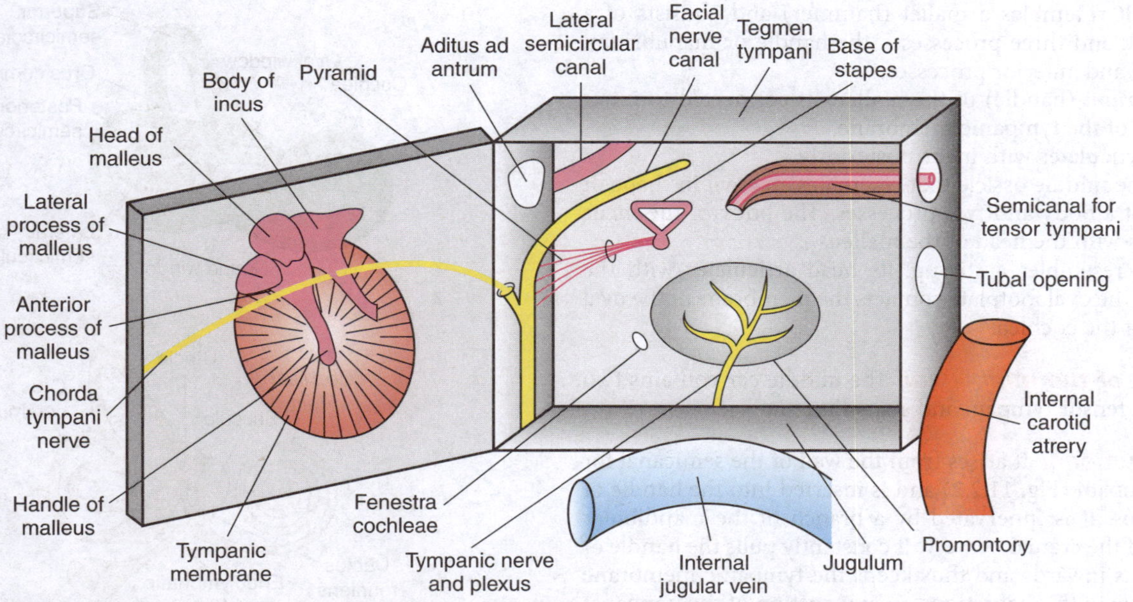

Fig. 11.2.2 Schematic diagram of the six-sided tympanic cavity (middle ear) with the lateral wall open to depict the features on various boundaries.

bony portions. It is lined with skin, which in the cartilaginous part secretes wax (from the ceruminous glands) and oil (from the sebaceous glands).

Middle Ear

Walls of middle ear The middle ear or the tympanic cavity is a six-sided air-filled rectangular space in the petrous part of temporal bone with a roof, a floor, and an anterior, a posterior, a medial and a lateral wall (Fig. 11.2.2).

Lateral wall is formed by tympanic membrane which shuts the medial end of the external auditory meatus. The tympanic membrane is a cave-shaped structure with concavity directed towards the external auditory meatus. Point of maximum convexity is called umbo. It consists of connective tissue covered with skin on the outside and mucous membrane on the inside.

Anterior wall contains two canals – upper one lodges tensor tympani muscle and lower one lodges the Eustachian tube (Fig. 11.2.2).

Eustachian tube or the pharyngotympanic tube connects the middle ear cavity with the pharynx. Air can pass through this tube into the middle ear. Therefore, it serves the function of equalization of pressure on two sides of the tympanic membrane. When its pharyngeal opening is blocked, e.g. in common cold, the air cannot pass into the tympanic cavity. The air present in the middle ear gets absorbed by the mucous membrane and the tympanic membrane is retracted inwards. As a result, the vibrations of the tympanic membrane get decreased or abolished, causing discomfort and loss of hearing.

Posterior wall of the middle ear communicates with air cavities in the mastoid process.

Medial wall (labyrinthine wall): It contains two windows (Fig. 11.2.2):

Oval window (fenestra vestibuli) is present above, in which footplate (face plate or stapes) is attached. It leads to the vestibule of the internal ear and transmits the sound vibrations of the ossicles to the perilymph of scala vestibuli.

Round window (fenestra cochlea) is present in the lower part, and is closed by a thin membrane called *secondary tympanic membrane*. It accommodates the pressure waves transmitted to the perilymph of the scala tympani.

Roof: It is formed by a thin bone called the tegmen tympani of the petrous temporal bone and separates the middle ear from the middle cranial fossa.

Floor: It is formed by a convex plate of bone which separates the middle ear from the jugular fossa which lodges the superior bulb of the internal jugular vein.

Ear ossicles The three ear ossicles (auditory ossicles) include malleus, incus and stapes. They are attached to each other by ligaments and form a chain (Fig. 11.2.3).

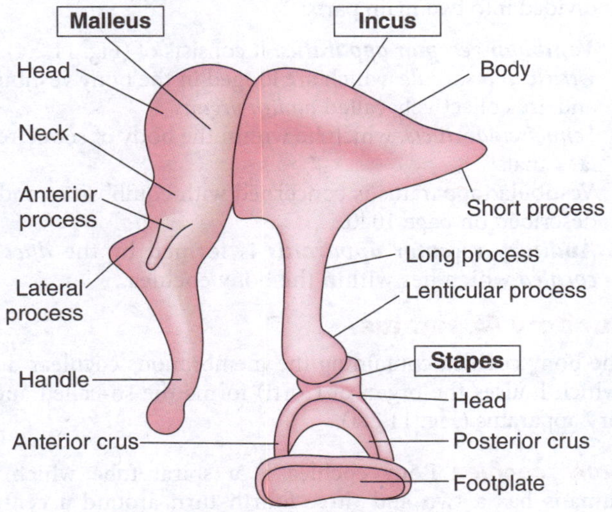

Fig. 11.2.3 Ear ossicles and their parts.

Malleus: It resembles a mallet (hammer) and consists of a head, neck and three processes – the handle or manubrium, the lateral and anterior processes.

Manubrium (handle) of the malleus is connected to inner surface of the tympanic membrane.

Head articulates with incus posteriorly.

Incus is the middle ossicle that resembles an anvil in shape. It consists of a body and two processes. The body of the incus articulates with the head of the malleus.

Stapes: It resembles a stirrup. Its head articulates with the incus and the oval footplate contacts the membrane of the oval window of the cochlea.

Muscles of the middle ear The middle ear contains two muscles – tensor tympani and stapedius.

Tensor tympani It arises from the wall of the semicanal for tensor tympani (Fig. 11.2.2) and is inserted into the handle of the malleus. It is innervated by a branch of the mandibular division of the cranial nerve V. It constantly pulls the handle of the malleus inwards and thus keeps the tympanic membrane tensed. Due to this, vibrations on any portion of the tympanic membrane are transmitted to the malleus.

Stapedius It arises from the posterior wall of the middle ear and is inserted on the neck of the stapes. It is innervated by a branch from the facial nerve and on contraction it pulls the footplate of the stapes out from the oval window.

Function Both muscles of the middle ear act simultaneously and reflexly in response to loud sound and attenuate the sound (see also page 1143).

Internal Ear

The internal ear or labyrinth is situated in the petrous part of the temporal bone. It consists of bony labyrinth and membranous labyrinth (Fig. 11.2.4).

Bony labyrinth consists of three parts – vestibule, semicircular canals and the cochlea.

Membranous labyrinth is lodged within the bony labyrinth. It is filled with endolymph (which resembles intracellular fluid [ICF]) and is surrounded by perilymph (which resembles extracellular fluid [ECF] in its composition). The inner ear can be divided into two main parts:

1. ***Vestibular receptor apparatus:*** It consists of (Fig. 11.2.4):
   Utricle and saccule, which are lodged in the bony vestibule, and are collectively called *otolith organs*
   Semicircular ducts, which lie within the body of semicircular canals
   Vestibular apparatus is concerned with equilibrium and is described on page 1040.
2. ***Auditory receptor apparatus*** is formed by the *duct of cochlea* which lies within the bony cochlea.

Auditory Apparatus

The bony cochlea containing the membranous cochlear duct (which houses the organ of Corti) forms the so-called auditory apparatus (Fig. 11.2.4).

Bony cochlea Bony cochlea is a spiral tube which in humans has a two and three-fourth turn around a central bone called the *modiolus*.

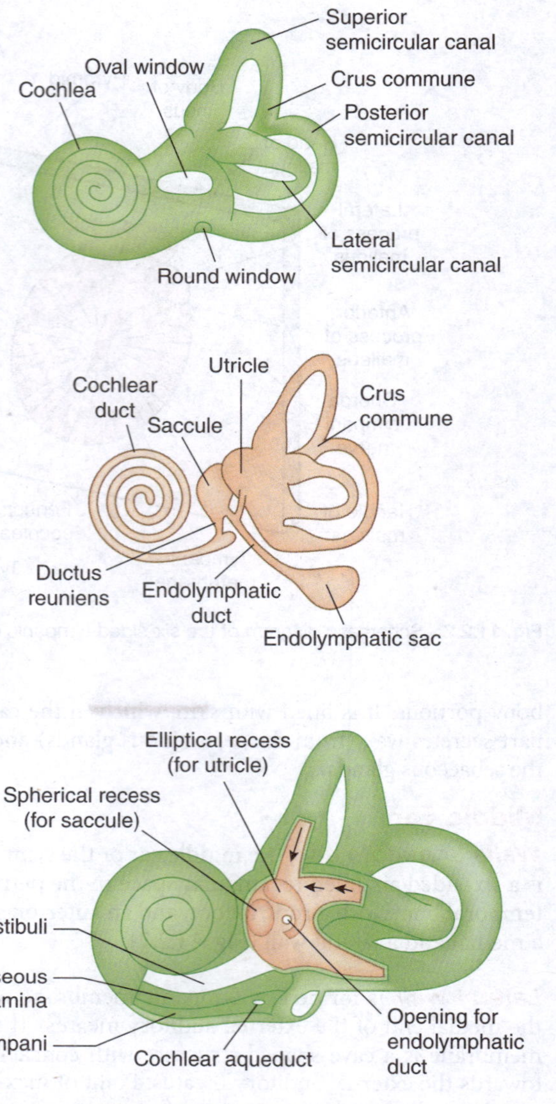

Fig. 11.2.4 Structure of inner ear: **A**, left bony labyrinth; **B**, left membranous labyrinth; and **C**, cut section of bony labyrinth.

The base of the modiolus is directed towards the internal acoustic meatus and transmits vessels and nerves to the cochlea. Around the modiolus and winding spirally like the thread of a screw is a thin plate of bone called *osseous spiral lamina*. It divides the bony cochlea incompletely and gives attachment to the basilar membrane. Two membranes (basilar membrane and Reissner membrane) divide the bony cochlea into three compartments (Fig. 11.2.5):

- Scala vestibuli
- Scala media (membranous cochlear duct)
- Scala tympani

Scala vestibuli and scala tympani Scala vestibuli and scala tympani are filled with perilymph and communicate with each other at the apex of the cochlea through an opening called *helicotrema*.

Scala vestibuli is separated from the scala media by *Reissner membrane* and is closed by the footplate of the stapes which separates it from the air-filled middle ear (Figs 11.2.5 and 11.2.6).

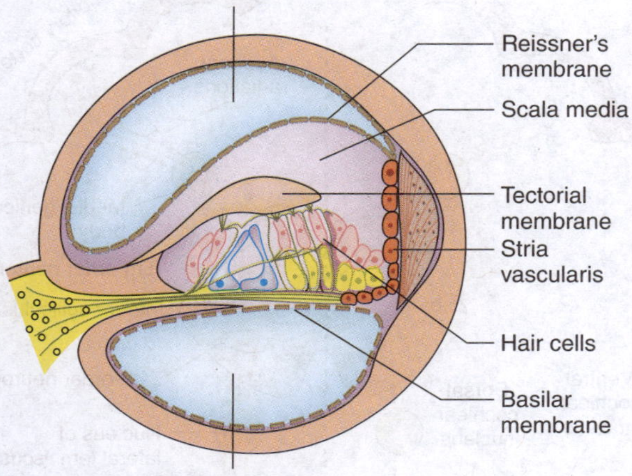

Fig. 11.2.5 Vertical section through cochlea showing scala vestibuli, scala media (cochlear duct) and scala tympani. Note the location of organ of Corti over the basilar membrane in the cavity of cochlear duct.

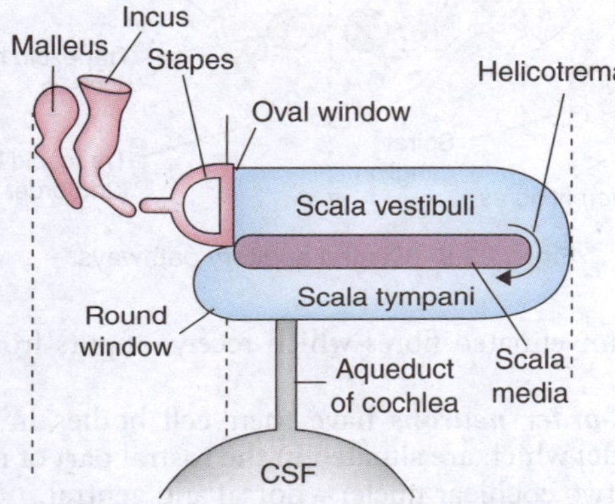

Fig. 11.2.6 Diagrammatic depiction of arrangement of perilymphatic system, three compartments of cochlea (scala vestibuli, scala media and scala tympani) and ear ossicles of the middle ear. Note that the CSF passes into scala tympani through aqueduct of cochlea.

Scala tympani is separated from the scala media by the *basilar membrane* and is closed by the *secondary tympanic membrane*. It is also connected with the subarachnoid space through the aqueduct of the cochlea (Figs 11.2.5 and 11.2.6).

Scala media or cochlear duct or membranous cochlea appears triangular on cross-section. Its three walls are formed by (Fig. 11.2.5):

Basilar membrane, which is attached medially to the osseous spiral lamina and laterally to the fibrous spiral ligament (which lines the bony cochlea), forms the inferior wall of the cochlear duct. The basilar membrane supports the *organ of Corti*.

Reissner membrane, which is attached medially to the wall of the limbus and laterally to the upper margin of the stria vascularis, forms the superior wall of the cochlear duct.

Stria vascularis forms the lateral wall of the cochlear duct. It consists of vascular epithelium and is concerned with secretion of *endolymph*.

Perilymph and endolymph

Perilymph is the fluid present in the scala tympani and scala vestibuli compartments of the cochlea. Its composition is similar to that of ECF in that it is high in Na^+ and low in K^+.

Endolymph is the fluid present within the scala media or the membranous cochlea. Its composition is similar to that of ICF in that it is high in K^+ and low in Na^+. It is secreted by the stria vascularis which forms the lateral wall of scala media.

Organ of Corti

The organ of Corti, the sense organ of hearing, is situated on the top of the basilar membrane in the scala media (Fig. 11.2.5). It contains the auditory receptors or the peripheral receptors of sense of hearing. Important components of the organ of Corti are given next (Fig. 11.2.7).

1. Rods of corti These are two projections (inner and outer rods) from the basilar membrane into the scala media. In between the two rods is the *tunnel of Corti* which contains a fluid called cortilymph. The exact function of the rods and cortilymph is not known.

2. Hair cells Hair cells are receptor cells that transduce sound energy into electrical energy. Two groups of hair cells lie on the basilar membrane (Fig. 11.2.7).

Inner hair cells: These form a single row of cells internal (i.e. medial) to the inner rod. These are about 3500 in number. These cells are probably more important in the transmission of auditory impulses. These are responsible for fine auditory transmission.

Outer hair cells: These are about 20,000 in number and are arranged in three or four layers external (i.e. lateral) to the outer rod. These are responsible for *detecting the presence of sound*. They mainly receive efferent innervation from the olivary complex and are concerned with modulating the function of inner hair cells.

Structure of a hair cell: The inner hair cells are flask-shaped, whereas the outer hair cells are cylindrical. On the upper surface of the hair cells are present tiny cilia (*stereocilia*) which protrude into the overlying tectorial membrane.

3. Supporting cells Supporting cells of the following types are known (Fig. 11.2.7):

- Inner phalangeal cells support the inner hair cells.
- Deiters cells (outer phalangeal cells) are situated between the outer hair cells and provide support to the latter.
- Hensen cells lie outside the Deiters cells.
- Claudius cells lie outside the Hensen cells.

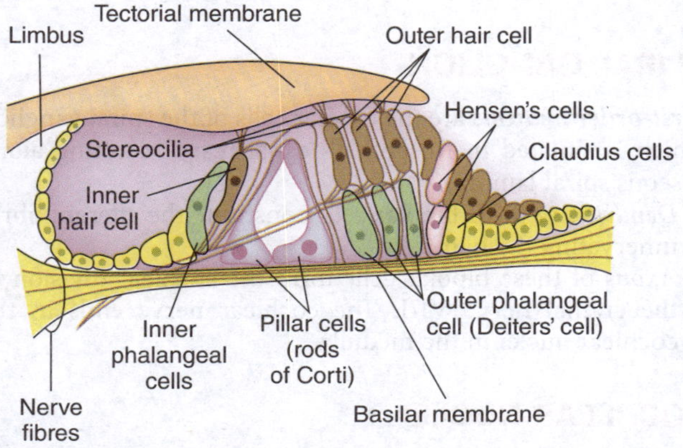

Fig. 11.2.7 Structure of organ of Corti. Note the connections between tectorial membrane and cilia of hair cells.

4. Tectorial membrane It consists of gelatinous matrix with delicate fibres. It is a thin but stiff membrane made of glycoprotein material. This membrane is attached to the upper surface of the spiral lamina, and its free edge extends just beyond the outermost neuroepithelial cells.

The shearing force between the hair cells and the tectorial membrane produces the stimulus to hair cells.

Nerve supply of hair cells consists of:

Afferent fibres supplying the hair cells constitute the cochlear division of the cranial nerve VIII. Cell bodies of these fibres are located in the spiral ganglion.

Inner hair cells receive 90%–95% of the afferent fibres and so are more important in the transmission of auditory impulses.

Outer hair cells receive only 5%–10% of the afferent fibres.

Important Note

There are about 30,000 fibres in each auditory nerve, so there is no net convergence of receptors on the first-order neurons. Most of the afferent fibres, however, supply more than one hair cell and, conversely, most of hair cells are supplied by more than one fibre.

Efferent fibres to the hair cells come from both the ipsilateral and the contralateral sides via the olivocochlear bundle. Their cell bodies are situated in the superior olivary complex. These fibres descend to join the cranial nerve VIII. Outer hair cells receive most of the efferent fibres, whereas inner hair cells receive only a few efferent fibres. The efferent fibres are cholinergic and cause inhibition of afferent fibres by liberating a hyperpolarizing mediator which is probably acetylcholine (ACh). Thus, the outer hair cells are mainly concerned with modulation of the function of inner hair cells.

AUDITORY PATHWAYS

Auditory pathways comprise the following relay stations (Fig. 11.2.8):

- Spiral ganglion
- Superior olivary nucleus complex, trapezoid nucleus and nucleus of the lateral lemniscus
- Inferior colliculus
- Medial geniculate body
- Auditory cortex

SPIRAL GANGLION

First-order neurons are the bipolar cells of the spiral ganglion which is situated in Rosenthal's canal (canal running along osseous spiral lamina).

Dendrites of these bipolar cells constitute the afferent fibres innervating the hair cells.

Axons of these bipolar cells form the cochlear division of the cranial nerve VIII. The cochlear nerve ends in the cochlear nuclei in the medulla.

COCHLEAR NUCLEI

Ninety-five per cent of the fibres in the cochlear nuclei are myelinated that receive inputs from inner hair cells and only

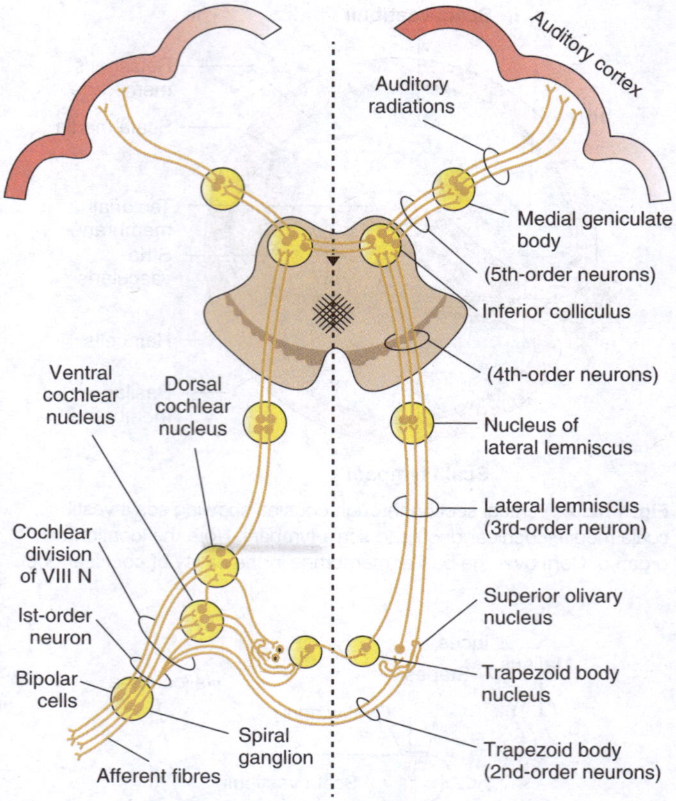

Fig. 11.2.8 Central auditory pathways.

5% are unmyelinated fibres which receive inputs from outer hair cells.

Second-order neurons have their cell bodies in the cochlear nuclei which are situated in the rostral part of medulla. There are two cochlear nuclei – dorsal and ventral.

The axons of second-order neurons from cochlear nuclei pass medially in the dorsal part of the pons. Most of them cross to the opposite side, but some remain uncrossed.

- The crossing fibres of two sides form a conspicuous mass of fibres called the *trapezoid body*.
- Some crossing fibres run separately in the dorsal part of the pons and do not form part of the trapezoid body.

SUPERIOR OLIVARY NUCLEUS COMPLEX, TRAPEZOID NUCLEUS AND NUCLEUS OF LATERAL LEMNISCUS

Third-order neurons have their cell bodies mainly in the superior olivary complex (made up of a number of nuclei) and also in the trapezoid nucleus and nucleus of the lateral lemniscus.

Superior olivary nuclear complex receives the large majority of lateral lemniscus fibres from the cochlear nuclei. Axons arising from the superior olivary complex form an important ascending bundle called the *lateral lemniscus*. Superior olivary nucleus receives information from both the ears (bilateral). It also sends efferents to the outer hairs cells in the form of olivocochlear bundle that modulates the sensitivity of these hair cells and blocks background noise.

Trapezoid nucleus: Some cochlear fibres that do not relay in the superior olivary nucleus join the lateral lemniscus after relaying in the scattered groups of cells lying within the trapezoid body (which constitute the *trapezoid nucleus*).

Nucleus of the lateral lemniscus refers to the collection of cells that lie within the lemniscus itself. Some cochlear fibres relay in these cells.

The fibres of the *lateral lemniscus* ascend to the midbrain and terminate in the inferior colliculus.

INFERIOR COLLICULUS

Fourth-order neurons have their cell bodies in the inferior colliculus where the fibres of the lateral lemniscus terminate. Fibres arising in the inferior colliculus enter the inferior brachium to reach the medial geniculate body.

MEDIAL GENICULATE BODY

Fifth-order neurons have their cell bodies in the medial geniculate body where most of the fibres arising in the inferior colliculus terminate. Some fibres from the lateral lemniscus reach this body without relay in the inferior colliculus. Fibres arising in the medial geniculate body form the acoustic radiation which ends in the acoustic area of the cerebral cortex.

AUDITORY CORTEX

Major areas constituting the auditory cortex present in the temporal lobe are as follows:

- Primary auditory cortex (areas 41 and 42)
- Auditory association areas (areas 22, 21 and 20) (for details, see page 946)

PHYSIOLOGY OF HEARING

Hearing, i.e. detection of sound waves, may serve to warn of impending danger or localize friends. But most importantly, audition allows social communication. Physiology of audition can be discussed under the following headings:

- Stimuli or sound waves
- Conduction of sound waves
- Transduction of sound waves
- Neural transmission of signals
- Encoding of signals

STIMULI OR SOUND WAVES

Definition

Stimuli for the receptors of hearing are sound waves. Sound is a form of energy produced by a vibrating object. A sound wave consists of alternating phases of compression and rarefaction of molecules of the medium (air, liquid or solid) in which it travels.

Physical Properties of Sound

Physical properties of sound and certain terms which are frequently used in audiology and acoustics are as follows (Fig. 11.2.9):

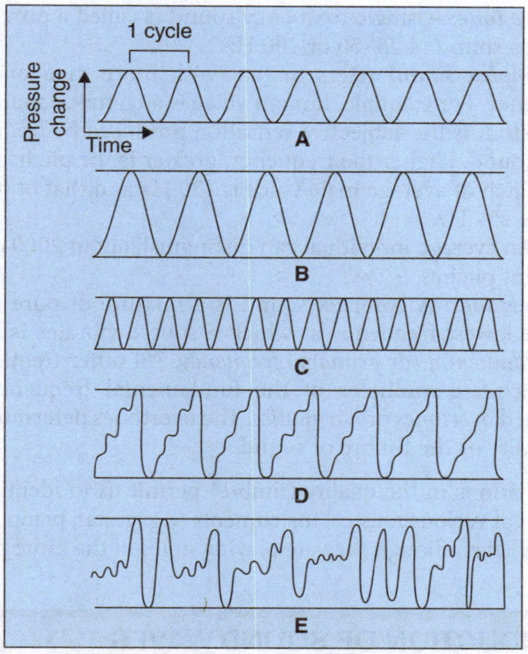

Fig. 11.2.9 Characteristics of sound wave: **A**, pure tones; **B**, increase in amplitude (intensity) of sound wave, and thus the sound is louder; **C**, increase in frequency (pitch); **D**, complex waveform due to mixture of pure tones and overtones, determines the quality of sound (timbre); and **E**, aperiodic irregular waveform (noise).

1. ***Speed of sound:*** Speed or velocity of the sound waves is different in different media:
   In the air, at 0°C, at sea level, sound travels at a rate of approximately 330 m/s (1100 feet/s), whereas at 20°C, it travels at a rate of 349 m/s (1150 feet/s).
   In the water, at 20°C, sound travels at a much faster speed of 1450–1500 m/s. The speed is faster in salt water as compared with that in fresh water. Furthermore, the speed of sound in water slightly increases with temperature and altitude.
2. ***Frequency of sound*** refers to the number of waves per second.
   - The *unit* of frequency is hertz.
   - Range of human hearing is approximately 20–20,000 Hz.
   - Range of average speaking voice is approximately 2000–5000 Hz.
3. ***Amplitude (intensity) of sound*** is the strength which determines its loudness. The intensity of sound is measured in terms of maximum pressure change at the tympanic membrane which is more commonly expressed as *sound pressure level* (SPL). The unit of SPL is decibel (dB), which is expressed as:

$$\text{dB} = 20\log\frac{P_S}{P_R}$$

   where P_S is the pressure of the stimulus sound and P_R is the pressure of the reference sound.
   Reference (standard) pressure is 0.0002 dyne/cm^2. It is defined as a sound pressure that is just detectable, i.e. auditory *threshold*.
   Thus, sound intensities are measured on a ratio scale using a subjective intensity (i.e. the threshold), rather than an arbitrary intensity, as a base.
   At a distance of 1 m, intensity of some common sounds is as follows:
   - Whisper : 30 dB
   - Normal conversation : 60 dB
   - Rock music : 90 dB
   - Discomfort of the ear is produced by sounds of : 120 dB
   - Pain in the ear is produced by sound of above (10^7 times threshold) : 140 dB

4. ***Pure tone:*** A single frequency sound is called a pure tone, e.g. a sound of 25–50 or 100 Hz.
5. ***Complex sound*** refers to that with more than one frequency. For example, human voice is a complex sound.
6. ***Pitch:*** It is the subjective sensation produced by frequency of sound. Higher the frequency, greater is the pitch.
   - Pitch of average male voice is 120 Hz and that of female is 250 Hz.
   - An average individual can distinguish about 2000 different pitches.
7. ***Overtones:*** A complex sound is a mixture of pure tones. The lowest frequency at which a source vibrates is called *fundamental (or primary) frequency*. All other frequencies which are multiples of the fundamental frequency are called *overtones* or *harmonics*. The overtones determine the quality or the timbre of sound.

Variations in the quality (timbre) permit us to identify the sounds of various musical instruments (e.g. guitar, piano, *tabla*, *sarangi*) even though they are playing notes of the same pitch.

CONDUCTION OF SOUND WAVES

ROLE OF EXTERNAL EAR

the External ear captures the sound waves.

Pinna collects and reflects the sound waves into the external auditory meatus. Its peculiar shape, in humans, aids in discerning the source of sound (e.g. in front vs. behind the head).
External auditory meatus conducts the sound waves to the tympanic membrane. Its S-shaped course:
- Helps in amplifying the sound waves
- Prevents mechanical injury to the tympanic membrane
- Helps in maintaining favourable temperature and humidity for normal functioning of the tympanic membrane

ROLE OF MIDDLE EAR

Conduction of sound stimulus by tympanic membrane to ear ossicles The sound waves that pass through the pinna and external auditory meatus strike the tympanic membrane. The presence of air at atmospheric pressure on both sides of the membrane enables it to vibrate. Eustachian tube does the function of equalization of pressure on two sides of the tympanic membrane. The vibrating tympanic membrane causes the ear ossicles to vibrate. Thus, the tympanic membrane acts as:

Pressure receiver, i.e. it is extremely sensitive to pressure changes produced by sound waves.
Resonator, i.e. it starts vibrating with pressure changes produced by sound waves.
Critically dampens, i.e. the vibrations of the tympanic membrane cease immediately after the end of sound.

Conduction of sound waves mechanically from middle ear to inner ear Various mechanisms which play a role during conduction of sound waves mechanically from the middle ear to the inner ear are as follows:

- Impedance matching mechanism
- Phase differential between oval and round windows
- Natural resonance of the external ear and middle ear
- Attenuation reflex

Impedance Matching Mechanism

The air-filled middle ear conducts sound waves mechanically to the fluid-filled internal ear through the ossicular system. Effective transfer of sound energy from an air to a fluid medium is difficult because most of the sound is reflected as a result of the different mechanical properties of the two media, i.e. *impedance mismatching*. This fact can be appreciated by the observation that a person under water cannot hear any sound made in the air. This happens because 99.9% of the sound energy is reflected away from the surface of water because of the impedance offered by it. Exactly a similar situation exists in the ear when the air-filled middle ear has to conduct the sound to the fluid-filled inner ear. Nature has compensated for it by providing impedance matching mechanism to the middle ear.

- The middle ear functions as an impedance matching device, primarily by amplifying the sound pressure. It is accomplished by the following three mechanisms (Fig. 11.2.10):
  1. ***Lever action of ossicles:*** The handle of the malleus is 1.3 times longer than the long process of the incus; this provides a mechanical leverage advantage, due to which the middle ear ossicles increase the force of movement by 1.3 times.
  2. ***Hydraulic action of the tympanic membrane*** is exerted because the effective vibratory area of the tympanic membrane (about 55 mm^2) is much greater than the stapes oval window surface area (about 3.2 mm^2). This size difference means that the force produced by the sound is concentrated over a smaller area, thus amplifying the pressure exerted on the oval window (17-fold).
  3. ***Curved membrane effect:*** Movements of the tympanic membrane are more at the periphery than at the centre where the malleus handle is attached. This too provides some leverage.

Thus, the above-mentioned three mechanisms together increase the sound pressure 22-fold (i.e. 17 × 1.3). In this way, the impedance mismatching between the air-filled middle ear and the fluid-filled inner ear is mostly compensated. Therefore, when the tympanic membrane and the ossicles are removed, and the sound waves strike the oval window directly, even very loud sounds are heard as whispers.

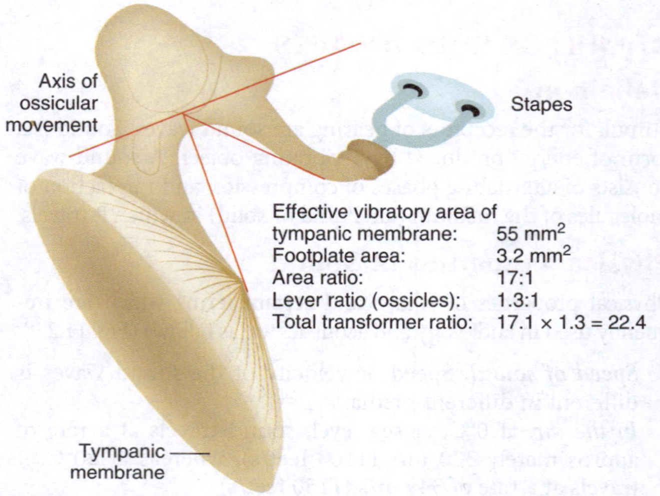

Fig. 11.2.10 Amplification of sound pressure by the combined hydraulic effect of tympanic membrane and leverage effect of ear ossicles.

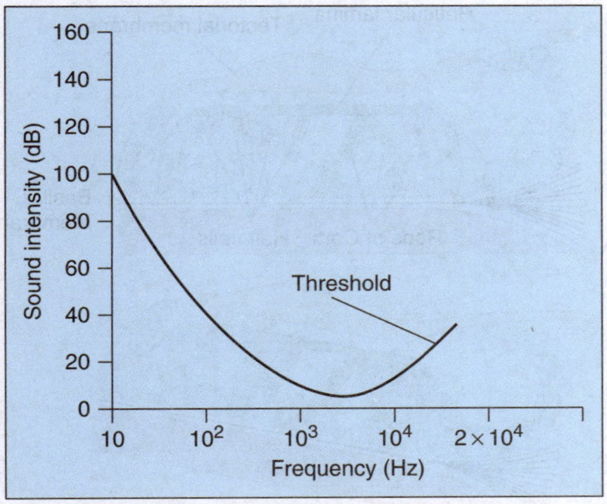

Fig. 11.2.11 Minimum audibility curve.

Minimum audibility curve: It is important to note that:

- Amplification of sound intensity is greatest between 1000 and 3000 Hz.
- Sounds below 16 Hz or above 20,000 Hz are not amplified at all.
- Because of the above, the human ear can perceive pitch of sound between 16 and 20,000 Hz, but maximum sensitivity is between 1000 and 3000 Hz. This effect is the basis of so-called minimum audibility curve (Fig. 11.2.11).

Phase Differential between Oval and Round Windows

Sound waves striking the tympanic membrane do not reach the oval and round windows simultaneously. There is a preferential pathway to the oval window because of the ossicular chain. Thus, when the oval window is receiving wave of compression, the round window is at the phase rarefaction. If the sound waves were to strike both the windows simultaneously, they would cancel each other's effect with no movement of perilymph and no hearing. This acoustic separation of windows is achieved by the presence of an intact tympanic membrane and a cushion of air in the middle ear around the round window.

Natural Resonance of External and Middle Ear

The external ear and middle ear due to the inherent anatomic and physiological properties allow certain frequencies of sound to pass more easily to the inner ear. The natural resonance of different structures is as follows:

- External auditory canal 3000 Hz
- Tympanic membrane 800–1600 Hz
- Middle ear 800 Hz
- Ossicular chain 500–2000 Hz

Thus (from the above), the greatest sensitivity of the sound transmission is between 500 and 3000 Hz, and these are the frequencies most important to humans in day-to-day conversation.

Attenuation Reflex

Attenuation reflex, also called tympanic reflex or acoustic reflex, is a preventive reflex which reduces sound pressure amplitude by affecting the mobility and transmission properties of the auditory ossicles.

- *Stimulus* for this reflex is loud sound.
- *Latent period* is 40–80 milliseconds.
- *Reflex activity:* The two muscles of the middle ear (tensor tympani and stapedius) contract reflexively in response to intense sound.

Contraction of tensor tympani muscle pulls the malleus inwards, whereas contraction of the stapedius muscle pulls the stapes outward. These two opposing forces make the ossicular system very rigid and therefore it fails to vibrate with the sound waves. Thus, sound is not allowed to enter the inner ear (i.e. is attenuated or intensity is reduced by 30–40 dB).

Advantages of attenuation reflex are as follows:

- It prevents occurrence of damage to the cochlea from the intense sounds like that of loud music and of jet aircraft.
- It attenuates and masks all the low-frequency environmental sounds and allows the person to concentrate on the sound above 1000 Hz, where most of the prominent information in voice communication is transmitted.
- It occurs just prior to vocalization and chewing, which suggests that the middle ear muscles may act to reduce the intensity of the sounds produced by these activities.

Important Note

Because the latent period of attenuation reflex is 40–80 milliseconds, sudden, brief, extremely loud sound such as due to bomb explosion or gun shot is likely to cause deafness due to damage to the cochlea.

TRANSDUCTION OF SOUND WAVES

Transduction of mechanical sound wave into electrical signal occurs in the organ of Corti of the inner ear (revise structure of the inner ear and organ of Corti given on page 1139). Steps involved in the process of transduction are given next.

VIBRATION OF BASILAR MEMBRANE

Sound waves from the middle ear are passed on to the inner ear through the oval window by in-and-out motion of the stapes (Fig. 11.2.12):

- Sound waves entering the inner ear from the oval window spread along the scala vestibuli as a travelling wave.
- Most of the sound energy is transferred directly from the scala vestibuli to the scala tympani. Very little of the sound wave ever reaches the helicotrema at the apex of the cochlea.
- As the sound energy passes from the scala vestibuli to the scala tympani, it causes the basilar membrane to vibrate. It is important to note that the part of the cochlea where height of pressure wave reaches its maximum varies with the frequency of sound (travelling wave theory of von Békésy) (see page 1147).

STIMULATION OF THE HAIR CELLS

The up-and-down movements of the basilar membrane in turn cause the organ of Corti to vibrate up and down. The tops

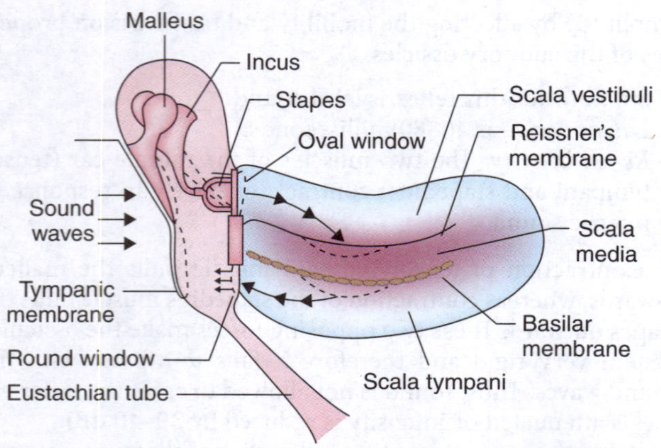

Fig. 11.2.12 Diagrammatic depiction of the mechanism of vibrations of basilar membrane produced by in-and-out motion of stapes (for details, see text).

of the hair cells in the organ of Corti are held rigid by the reticular lamina and the hair of the outer hair cells are embedded in the tectorial membrane (Fig. 11.2.13). Because the tectorial and basilar membranes are attached at different points on the limbus (Fig. 11.2.13A), they slide past each other as they vibrate up and down.

Owing to the shear forces set up by the relative displacement of the basilar membrane and the tectorial membrane, the stereocilia of hair cells bend back and forth as:

- When the organ of Corti moves up, the tectorial membrane slides forward relative to the basilar membrane, bending the stereocilia away from the limbus (Fig. 11.2.13B).
- When the organ of Corti moves down, the tectorial membrane slides backwards relative to the basilar membrane and bends the stereocilia towards the limbus (Fig. 11.2.13C).
  The bending of stereocilia stimulates (excites) the hair cells.
- *Depolarization occurs* when the stereocilia bend away from the limbus.
- *Hyperpolarization* occurs when the stereocilia bend towards the limbus.

Membrane Potential Changes in the Hair Cells

The bending of the stereocilia produces a change in the membrane potential of the hair cells proportionate to the degree of displacement (generator potential). The electrical activity of the inner ear can be considered as follows:

- Resting condition
- During stimulation of the ear

Potentials Recorded from the Ear Under Resting Condition

Under resting condition (when the ear is not stimulated with sound), two different potentials are recorded:

- Endocochlear potential
- Resting potential of the hair cells

Endocochlear potential The endolymph contains a high concentration of K^+ (135 mEq/L) and is electrically positive in comparison to perilymph. The +80 mV electrical potential which exists between endolymph of the scala media and perilymph of the scala vestibuli and scala tympani is called *endolymphatic* or *endocochlear potential. Source* of endolymphatic potential is the stria vascularis which covers the lateral wall of the scala media. The characteristic features of the cells of the stria vascularis which contribute to high K^+ concentration of endolymph are as follows:

- High concentration of Na^+–K^+-ATPase
- Presence of a unique electrogenic K^+ pump

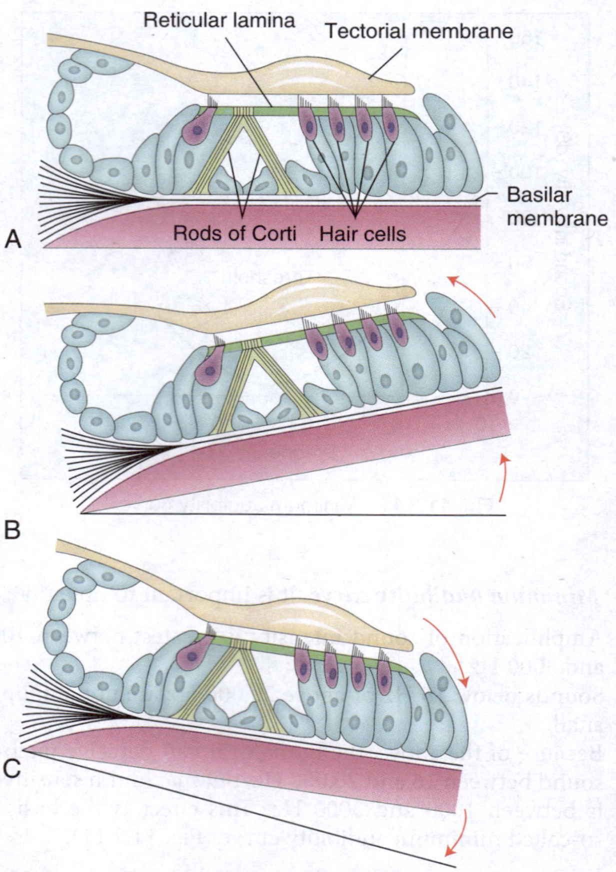

Fig. 11.2.13 Demonstration of bending of stereocilia with movement of organ of Corti: **A**, the tectorial membrane and basilar membrane are attached to limbus at different points; **B**, upward movement of organ of Corti causes bending of cilia away from limbus; and **C**, downward movement of organ of Corti causes cilia to bend towards limbus.

Resting potential of the hair cells Each hair cell has a negative resting membrane potential. Therefore, ICF is at a potential of −70 mV with respect to perilymph of the scala tympani. At the upper end of hair cell, the potential difference between ICF and endolymph is, therefore, −150 mV (−70 − [+80]). However, there is not much difference between K^+ concentration of endolymph and ICF. The large negative potential and lack of a K^+ concentration difference between the inside and the outside of the hair cells make these cells very sensitive. Therefore, slightest movement of the hair stimulates the cells.

Potentials Recorded from the Ear on Stimulation

When the ear is stimulated by sound, two types of potentials can be recorded:

- Cochlear microphonic potential
- Action potential in the auditory nerve

Cochlear microphonic potential When stimulated by the sound wave, the changes in membrane potential of the hair cells result from changes in cation conductance at their apical ends. The gating of K^+ channels is controlled by bending of stereocilia as:

- When the stereocilia bend away from the limbus, they cause K^+ channels to open; K^+ then flows into the cell and the *hair cell depolarizes*.
- When the stereocilia bend towards the limbus, they cause K^+ channels to close and the *hair cell hyperpolarizes*.

The sum of receptor potentials of a number of hair cells when recorded extracellularly is called *cochlear microphonic potential*. It is an oscillatory event that can be recorded by placing one electrode in the scala media and other electrode in the scala tympani.

Cochlear microphonic potentials are similar to generator potential, because:

- These have no latency or refractory period.
- These do not obey all-or-none law.
- These are resistant to ischaemia and anaesthesia.

Relationship between intensity of sound and cochlear microphonic potential: The cochlear microphonic potentials recorded have the same form and polarity as those of the acoustic stimulus. The excitatory phase of cochlear microphonic potential (i.e. increasing negativity in the scala media) is associated with a current flow outwards across the membrane of the nerve fibres (Fig. 11.2.14). As shown in Fig. 11.2.14, the base of the cochlea responds to all frequencies of sound, whereas the apex responds to only low frequencies of sound.

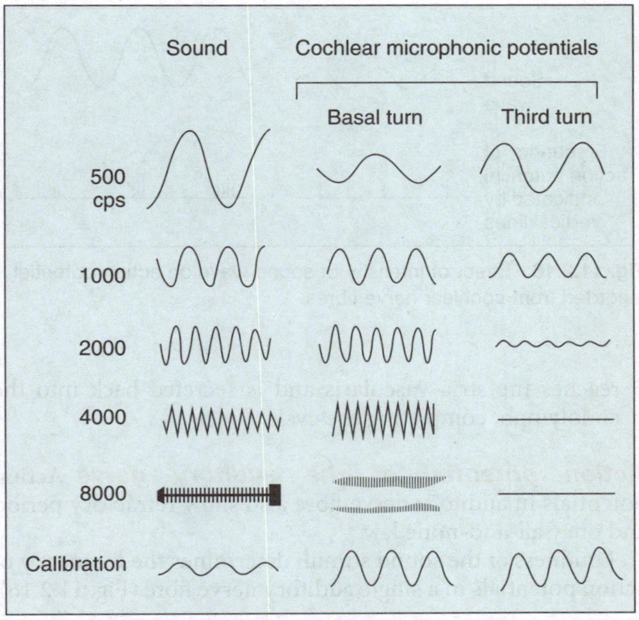

Fig. 11.2.14 Relationship between the intensity (loudness) of sound and cochlear microphonic potentials recorded through basal turn and third turn of cochlea.

Important Note

When the organ of Corti is damaged by prolonged exposure to a loud tone, the cochlear microphonic potential produced by this particular band of frequency is abolished.

Genesis of action potential in afferent nerve fibres

The stereocilium of hair cells of the organ of Corti is linked to the site of neighbouring hair cell by a very fine process called tip link. The arrangement is such that tip link ties the tip of stereocilium to the side of its higher neighbouring stereocilium (Fig. 11.2.15). At the junction, mechanosensitive cation channels are present at the higher process. The events of genesis of action potential are as follows:

- When shorter stereocilia are pushed towards the higher neighbouring ones, the channels get open up and K^+ and Ca^{2+} influx causes depolarization.
- The molecular motors (myosin based) present in the higher neighbouring process next move the channel towards the base, thereby releasing tension in the tip link. This causes closure of the mechanosensitive cation channel and permits restoration of the resting state.
- The depolarization of hair cells causes release of neurotransmitter (glutamate), which initiates depolarization of neighbouring afferent neurons and causes generation of action potential.
- The K^+ that enters the hair cells through mechanosensitive channels is recycled (Fig. 11.2.15). It enters through tight junctions into the neighbouring supporting cells and

Fig. 11.2.15 Schematic representation of the role of tip links in the responses of hair cells.

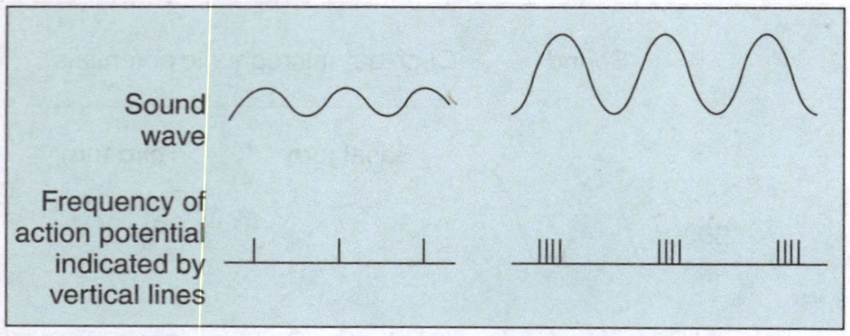

Fig. 11.2.16 Effect of intensity of sound wave on action potential recorded from cochlear nerve fibres.

reaches the stria vascularis and is secreted back into the endolymph, completing the cycle.

Action potential of the auditory nerve Action potentials in auditory nerve fibre also show refractory period and obey all-and-none law.

Loudness of the sound stimuli determines the frequency of action potentials in a single auditory nerve fibre (Fig. 11.2.16):

At low sound intensities, each axon discharges to sounds of only one frequency called the characteristic frequency, which varies from axon to axon depending on the part of the cochlea from where the fibre originates.
At higher sound intensities, the individual axon responds to an increasingly wide range of sound frequencies.
Refractory period of auditory nerve fibre is 1 millisecond. Therefore, maximum rate of discharge through fibre can be only 1000 impulses/s. At a very low frequency (20–200 cycles/s), there is a synchronization between the sound frequency and the rate of discharge.

NEURAL TRANSMISSION OF SIGNALS

The electrical signals which emanate from transduction of the sound waves in the hair cells are transmitted through a complex auditory pathway which consists of the following relay stations (Fig. 11.2.8):

- Spiral ganglion
- Cochlear nuclei
- Superior olivary nuclear complex, trapezoid nucleus and nucleus of the lateral lemniscus
- Inferior colliculus
- Medial geniculate body
- Auditory cortex

Revise anatomical details of the auditory pathway before proceeding further (see page 1140).

SALIENT FEATURES OF AUDITORY PATHWAY

Some salient features of the auditory pathway which need special emphasis are given next.

1. Bilateral representation From the medulla onwards, each ear is bilaterally represented in the auditory pathway with only slight preponderance in the contralateral pathway. Because of the bilateral representation, lesion beyond the medulla has slight effect on the auditory acuity.

2. Descending pathway There is not only an ascending auditory pathway but also a significant descending pathway forming feed-forward and feed-backward loops.

3. Role in brainstem and spiral acoustic reflexes Auditory pathway is also involved in the brainstem and spiral acoustic reflexes and brainstem mechanism for auditory visual reflexes. The integration of visual and auditory information occurs due to interconnection of the superior and inferior colliculi.

4. Role in general arousal The auditory pathways in the brainstem give collaterals to the reticular formation and the cerebellum and thus play a role in general arousal.

5. Spatial organization The different parts of the organ of Corti respond to tones of different frequencies from basilar to apical part of the cochlea. Neurons receiving fibres from different parts of the spiral ganglion are arranged in a definite sequence in the cochlear nuclei. The tonotopic organization which is prominent in cochlear nuclei is maintained in the superior olivary nucleus, inferior colliculus, medial geniculate body and auditory cortex. This *tonotopic organization* resembles the retinotopic organization of the visual pathway and somatotopic organization of the somatosensory system.

6. Features of auditory cortex The auditory cortex exhibits the following characteristic features:

i. *Tonotopic organization*, as described above
ii. *Column organization*

In addition to the tonotopic organization, the auditory cortex also exhibits feature extractions. For example, some neurons are selected for the direction of frequency modulation. Neurons in the primary auditory cortex form the so-called isofrequency, summation and suppression columns.

Isofrequency columns: Neurons arranged in these columns have the same characteristic frequency.
Summation columns: Neurons in these columns are more responsive to binaural than to monaural input.
Suppression columns: Neurons in these columns are less responsive to binaural than to monaural stimulation and accordingly the response to one ear is dominant.

7. Features of other cortical areas concerned with audition

i. ***Hemispheric specialization:*** Although the auditory area looks very much the same on the two sides of the brain, there is marked hemispherical specialization. For example, Brodmann area 22 is concerned with the processing of auditory signals related to speech. During language processing, it is much more active on the left side than on the right side. Area 22 on the right side is more concerned with melody, pitch and sound intensities.
ii. ***Plasticity of auditory pathways:*** There exists a great plasticity in the auditory pathways, i.e. they are modified by experience. Examples of auditory plasticity in humans include the following observations:
   - In individuals who become deaf before language skills are fully developed, viewing sign language activates auditory association areas.
   - Conversely, individuals who become blind early in life are demonstrably better at localizing sound than individuals with normal eyesight.

- In right-handed individuals, planum temporale, i.e. a portion of the posterior superior temporal gyrus involved in language-related auditory process, is larger in the left cerebral hemisphere than in the right.
- Musicians have an increase in the size of auditory area activated by musical tones. They also have a larger cerebellum than nonmusicians, presumably because of learned precise finger movements.

NEURAL PROCESSING OF AUDITORY INFORMATION

Neural processing of auditory information involves:

- Encoding of frequency (pitch determination)
- Encoding of intensity (determination of loudness)
- Feature detection
- Localization of sound in space

ENCODING OF SOUND FREQUENCY

The human auditory mechanism has a remarkable power to discriminate between the sounds in the range 60–20,000 Hz. Cochlear nerve fibres encode frequency of sound stimulus. *Duplex theory*, which includes both place theory and frequency theory, is required to explain the frequency coding of sound.

Place theory or Békésy travelling wave theory This theory can explain the discrimination between sound frequencies above 2000 Hz and up to 20,000 Hz. Salient features of this theory are given next.

Basilar membrane is a mechanical analyser of source frequency. The basic pattern of movement of the basilar membrane is that of a travelling wave (Fig. 11.2.17). The high-frequency sound waves produce waves of maximum height near the oval window, whereas low-frequency sounds produce waves of maximum height near the helicotrema (Fig. 11.2.17). Correspondingly, the basilar membrane near the oval window vibrates in response to high-frequency sounds. This aspect of the basilar membrane gives it the name '*frequency analyser*'.

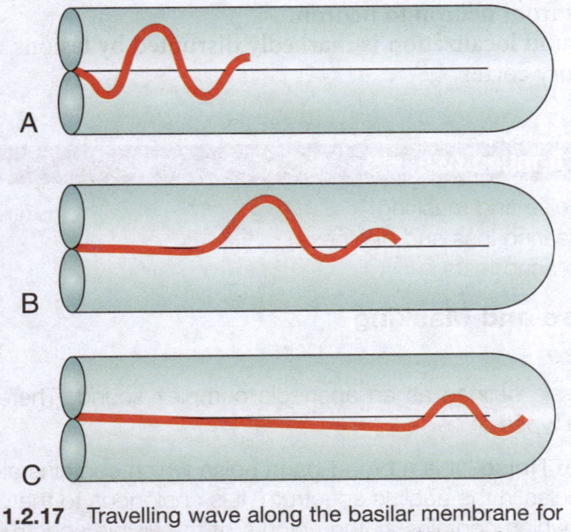

Fig. 11.2.17 Travelling wave along the basilar membrane for **(A)** high-frequency, **(B)** medium-frequency and **(C)** low-frequency sounds.

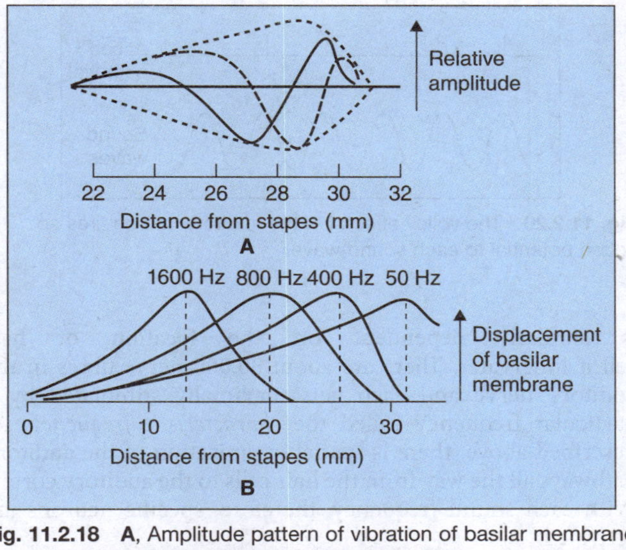

Fig. 11.2.18 A, Amplitude pattern of vibration of basilar membrane for a medium-frequency sound wave; and **B**, displacement of the basilar membrane by the waves generated by stapes vibrations of frequencies shown at the top of each curve.

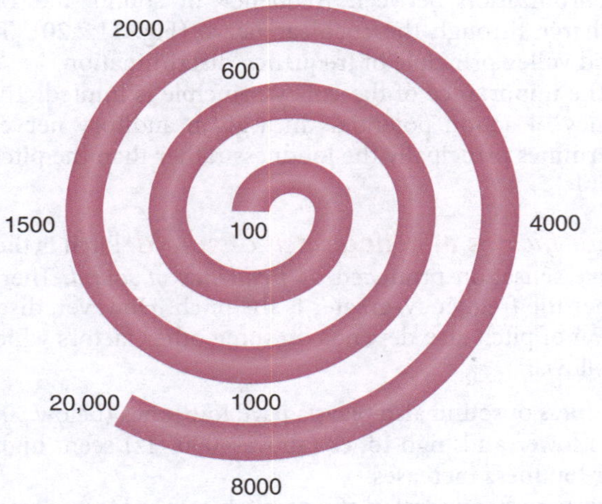

Fig. 11.2.19 Frequency localization in the cochlea. Higher frequencies are localized in the basal turn and then progressively decrease towards the apex.

As the distance of the basilar membrane from the oval window increases, there is gradual decrease in the frequency of sounds to which the membrane responds. Near the helicotrema, the basilar membrane responds to very low-frequency sound (Fig. 11.2.18). This differential response to different frequencies of sound is possible because of a systematic variation in the mechanical properties along the basilar membrane. The basilar membrane is the narrowest and stiffest at the base of the cochlea (near the oval and round windows) and the widest and most compliant at the apex of the cochlea (near the helicotrema).

Thus, as per the travelling wave theory of von Békésy, the higher frequencies are represented in the basal turn of the cochlea and the progressively lower ones towards the apex (Fig. 11.2.19).

Different hair cells respond to different frequencies of sound depending on their location on the basilar membrane. The auditory nerve fibre activated by a particular sound frequency

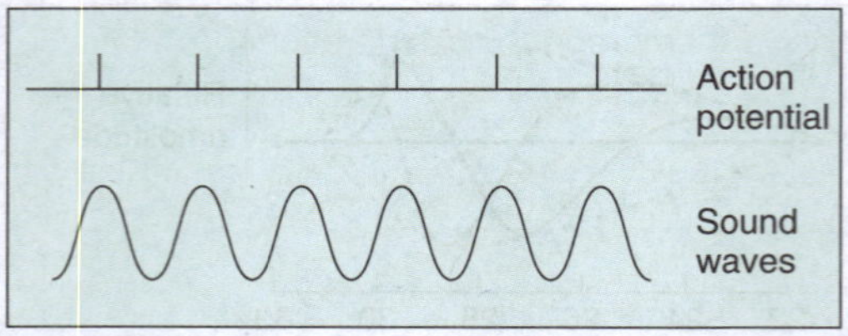

Fig. 11.2.20 The volley effect, i.e. the auditory neuron fires an action potential to each sound wave.

is similarly dependent on the location of hair cell it innervates. There are about 30,000 nerve fibres in the auditory nerve and each gets maximally stimulated by a particular frequency called the *characteristic frequency*. As described above, there is spatial organization of the auditory pathways all the way from the hair cells to the auditory cortex. With each sound frequency, therefore, specific neurons are activated.

Frequency theory Frequency theory or *volley principle* accounts for the coding of low frequencies of sound up to 2000 Hz. For very low frequencies of sound, there is a synchronization between frequency of sound and rate of discharge through the cochlear nerve (Fig. 11.2.20). This is called volley principle of frequency discrimination.

The importance of the volley principle is limited. The frequency of action potentials in a given auditory nerve fibre determines principally the loudness rather than the pitch of a sound.

Other factors affecting pitch of sound Pitch is the subjective sensation produced by *frequency of sound*. Therefore, higher the frequency, greater is the pitch. However, discrimination of pitch also depends on some other factors which are as follows:

Loudness of sound also plays a part; low tones (below 500 Hz) seem lower and high tones (above 4000 Hz) seem higher as their loudness increases.

Duration of sound also affects pitch to a minor degree. The pitch of a tone cannot be perceived unless it lasts for more than 0.01 second and with durations between 0.01 and 0.1 second, pitch rises as duration increases.

ENCODING OF INTENSITY

Encoding of sound intensity (loudness) occurs at the level of cochlear nerve fibres by the following mechanisms:

Increase in frequency of firing of an auditory nerve fibre: With the increase in intensity (loudness) of sound wave, the amplitude of vibration of the basilar membrane increases, which in turn increases the frequency of firing in an auditory nerve fibre.

Increase in number of nerve fibre stimulation: As amplitude of vibration increases, a larger portion of the basilar membrane is vibrated and thus more and more hair cells are stimulated. This increases the number of auditory nerve fibres which are activated.

Stimulation of inner hair cells: Certain hair cells (inner hair cells) are not stimulated unless the sound is very loud. Stimulation of these cells, therefore, apprises the nervous system that intensity of sound is high.

FEATURE DETECTION

Higher auditory centres respond to particular features of sound stimuli. For example, cortical neurons may respond specifically to a shift from high- to low-frequency notes, which is why lesions of the auditory cortex may not impair the ability to discriminate frequency. Instead, lesions of the auditory cortex cause a loss of ability to recognize a patterned sequence of sounds.

LOCATION OF SOUND IN SPACE

A human can distinguish sounds originating from sources separated by as little as 1°. Binaural receptive fields (which are a feature of most auditory neurons above the level of cochlear nuclei) contribute to sound localization. In other words, relay nuclei in the brainstem (especially the superior olivary nuclei complex) mediate localization of sound sources. The auditory system uses the following clues to judge the origin of sound:

Time lag between the entry of sound in two ears: For example, if the sound originates from the right side of a person, it reaches the right ear earlier than the left ear. The interaural time difference is a more important clue. The detectable time difference is of 20 microseconds, especially for relatively low-frequency sounds (below 3000 Hz). The medial superior olivary nuclei include many neurons responsive to low-frequency inputs.

Differences in the intensity that reaches the two ears: Interaural intensity clues are the most important for high-frequency stimuli (above 3000 Hz), because the head absorbs shorter-wavelength sounds better than long-wavelength sounds. The *lateral superior olivary* nuclei are most sensitive to high-frequency stimuli and thus differences in the sound intensity that reaches the two ears to provide information about the source of sound.

Quality of sound: The sound coming directly in front of an individual differs in quality than that coming from behind, because the pinna is directed slightly forward. Therefore, quality of sound waves changes after reflection from the pinnal surface; it moves up and down. Change in quality of the sound wave is an important factor in localizing the sound in vertical plane.

Neurons in the auditory cortex that receive input from both ears respond maximally or minimally when the time of arrival of a stimulus at one ear is delayed by a fixed period relative to the time of arrival at the other ear. This fixed period varies from neuron to neuron.

Sound localization is markedly disrupted by lesions of the auditory cortex.

Applied Aspects

- Noise and masking
- Hearing loss and deafness
- Hearing tests

Noise and Masking

Noise

Noise is defined as an aperiodic complex sound. There are three types of noise.

White Noise. It is a broad-band noise which contains all frequencies in the audible spectrum. It is analogous to the white light which contains all the colours of the visible spectrum. It is used for masking.

Narrow-Band Noise. It is a white noise, out of which certain frequencies above and below the given noise have been filtered out. Thus, its frequency range is smaller than that of the broad-band white noise. It is used to mask the tested frequency in pure-tone audiometry.

Speech Noise. It is a noise having all frequencies in the speech range (300–3000 Hz). All other frequencies are filtered out.

Masking

Masking refers to a phenomenon in which the presence of one type of sound decreases the ability of the ear to hear another type of sound. In other words, masking represents the inability of the auditory mechanism to separate the simultaneous stimulation into separate components. Masking is more effective for sounds with similar frequencies than for sounds with widely different frequencies. Low-frequency tones mask high-frequency tones more easily than the reverse. Example of masking observed is the difficulty in conversation in noisy surroundings.

Clinical Applications of masking:
In clinical audiometry, one ear is kept busy by a sound while the other is being tested. Masking of the nontest ear is essential in all bone conduction (BC) tests.

Hearing Loss, Deafness and Tinnitus

Hearing loss refers to impairment of hearing and its severity may vary from mild to profound.

Deafness is labelled when there is little or no hearing at all.

Degree of hearing loss: WHO (1980) recommended the classification given in Table 11.2.1 on the basis of pure-tone audiogram taking the average of the thresholds of hearing for frequencies of 500, 1000 and 2000 Hz.

Types of hearing loss: Hearing loss can be of three types:

- Conductive hearing loss
- Sensorineural (SN) hearing loss
- Mixed hearing loss

1. Conductive Hearing Loss

Any disease process which interferes with the conduction of sound from the external ear to the cochlea causes conductive hearing loss.

Causes. The causes of conduction hearing loss may lie in the:

- *External ear:* Any obstruction in the ear canal, e.g. by wax (cerumen), tumours, atresia and otitis externa, i.e. inflammation of the external ear (swimmer's ear)
- *Tympanic membrane,* e.g. perforation
- *Middle ear cavity*, e.g. fluid in the middle ear (as in otitis media)
- *Ear ossicles,* e.g. disruption of ear ossicles and fixation of ear ossicles (otosclerosis)
- *Eustachian tube* obstruction as in retracted tympanic membrane

Characteristic Features Characteristically, hearing loss is partial and never complete because skull bones themselves conduct sound to the cochlea (BC) and the basilar membrane can be set into vibrations.

- Hearing loss is fairly uniform throughout the frequency wave.
- Speech discrimination is good.

Hearing tests: See Table 11.2.2.

Management: Treatment of the cause is done.

2. Sensorineural Hearing Loss

SN hearing loss results from lesions of the cochlea (*sensory type*) or cranial nerve VIII and its central connections (neural type). It can be congenital or acquired.

Congenital SN hearing loss is present at birth. It may be due to anomalies of the inner ear or damage to the hearing apparatus by prenatal or perinatal factors.

Acquired SN hearing loss appears later in life. Cause may be genetic (delayed onset) or nongenetic.

Genetic causes of hearing loss include:

- Mutation of gene GJB_2 for connexin-26 protein. This defect prevents K^+ recycling through the sustentacular cells.
- Mutations in myosin like myosin VIIa (associated with actin in hair cell processes), myosin-1β (part of molecular motor that adjusts tension on tip links) and myosin VI (involved in formation of cilia) lead to hearing loss.
- Mutation of α-tectin: α-Tectin is one of the major proteins present in the tectorial membrane.
- Pendred syndrome – associated with deafness and goitre – is caused by mutation of multifactorial anion exchanger gene SLC26A4.
- Long QT syndrome in which a type of K^+ channel protein ($KVLQT_1$) is mutated. In a normal individual, K^+ channel is responsible for maintaining high K^+ concentration in endolymph and normal QT interval (see page 265).
- Bartter syndrome: Mutation of bartin, a membrane protein, causes deafness and renal manifestations (see page 492).

Causes of nongenetic acquired SN deafness:

- *Infection* of the labyrinth (viral, bacterial or spirochaetal)
- *Acoustic trauma*, i.e. injury to the labyrinth or the eighth nerve
- *Noise trauma or noise*-induced hearing loss (NIHL) that occurs due to prolonged exposure to industrial noise or in leisure activity and causes high-frequency hearing loss (the hair cells are damaged by excessive noise; the outer hair cells are more vulnerable than the inner cells)
- *Ototoxicity* (certain drugs cause damage to the inner ear, e.g. streptomycin, neomycin, quinine and chloroquine; these drugs especially cause damage to the outer hair cells or stria vascularis)
- *Neoplasms*, e.g. acoustic neuroma
- *Systemic disorders*, e.g. diabetes mellitus and hypertension

Table 11.2.1 WHO classification of hearing loss

Degree of hearing loss	Hearing threshold in better ear (average of 500, 1000 and 2000 Hz) (dB)
0: Not significant	0–25
1: Mild	26–40
2: Moderate	41–55
3: Moderately severe	56–70
4: Severe	71–91
5: Profound	>91
6: Total	

- *Presbycusis* that refers to gradual hearing loss associated with ageing, and occurs due to gradual loss of hair cells and neurons

Characteristic Features. Characteristic features are as follows:

- Usually loss of hearing is complete.
- Speech discrimination is poor.
- Hearing loss may exceed 60 dB.

Hearing tests: See Table 11.2.2.

Management. Management includes:

- *Treatment of the cause* when possible
- *Hearing aids* for rehabilitation
- *Cochlear implants* – the devices which consist of:
  - Microphone that picks up environmental sound
  - Speech processor that selects and arranges these sounds
  - Transmitter and receiver/stimulator that converts those sounds into electrical impulses
  - Electron array that sends impulses to the auditory nerve

Advantage: In a deaf person, though cochlear implants cannot restore normal hearing, they can promote useful representation of environment sound.

In adult-onset deafness, the person can learn to associate signals with sound that he/she remembers.

With the help of a cochlear implant with intensive therapy, a deaf child can acquire language and speech skill.

Stem cell: With the help of stem cells, hair cells can be developed.

3. Mixed Hearing Loss

Both conductive and SN hearing loss are present in the same ear and are characterized by:

- Air–bone gap indicating conductive hearing loss
- Impairment of BC indicating SN hearing loss

Tinnitus. Tinnitus refers to ringing sensation in the ear. It is caused by irritative stimulation of either the inner ear or the vestibulocochlear nerve.

Hearing Aids. Hearing aids are sound amplifying devices designed to help the people suffering with hearing loss.

Types: The hearing aids are categorized into five types:

In the ear (ITE)
Behind the ear (BTE)
Receiver in the ear (RITE)
In the canal (ITC)
Contralateral routing signals (CROS)/bicontralateral routing sounds (BiCROS)

Mechanism of action: Hearing aids work by amplifying sound through three-part system:

Microphone receives sound and converts it into digital signal.
Amplifier increases the strength of digital signals.
Speaker produces the amplified sound into the ear.

Cochlear implants: A cochlear implant is a small electronic device that provides a sense of sound into the ear to the people who are deaf or hard of hearing. It is basically an electrode which by surgical procedure is implanted in the cochlea. Its processor is placed behind the ear between the muscle and the bone.

Mechanism of action: A cochlear implant directly stimulates the auditory nerve bypassing the damaged part of the auditory apparatus. The signals generated by the implant are transmitted through the nerve to the brain that recognize the signals as sound.

Hearing Tests

A. Clinical Tests of Hearing

1. Finger Friction Test. It is a rough and quick method for screening. In it, the thumb and index finger are rubbed near the ear and the patient is asked to appreciate with the eyes closed.

2. Watch Test. A clicking watch is brought close to the ear and the distance at which it is heard is noted.

3. Human Speech Voice Test. Normally, a conversational voice (60 dB) and whisper should be heard at 6 m with the eyes closed (to avoid lip reading) in a quiet room. The commonly used *spondees* (phonetically balanced words) are black-night, football, daydream or numbers with letters such as X3B, 2AZ and MOD. The distance at which the conversational voice is heard is measured.

4. Tuning Fork Tests. These tests are performed with tuning forks of different frequencies (commonly used are 256 and 512 Hz). These are quite useful in distinguishing conductive deafness from SN deafness. Commonly used tests are as follows:

i. ***Rinne test:*** In this test, air conduction (AC) of the ear is compared with BC. Base of a vibrating tuning fork is placed on the mastoid bone (Fig. 11.2.21A), and when the patient stops hearing, it is brought beside the meatus (Fig. 11.2.21B). If he/she still hears, AC is more than BC and Rinne test is positive.
   - In normal subjects, Rinne test is positive.
   - In conductive deafness, Rinne test is negative.
   - In partial nerve deafness, Rinne test is positive.
   - In complete nerve deafness, both bone-conducted and air-conducted sounds are not perceived.

ii. ***Weber test:*** In this test, base of the vibrating tuning fork is placed in the middle of the forehead (Fig. 11.2.21C) or vertex and the patient is asked in which ear the sound is heard better.
   - *Normally*, the sound is heard equally in both ears.
   - In *conductive hearing loss*, the sound is lateralized (better heard) towards the affected ear. This is because the masking effect of environmental noise is absent in the affected ear.

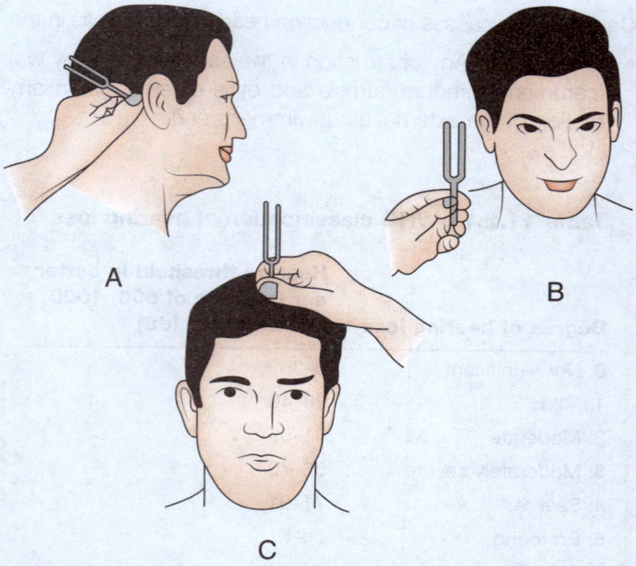

Fig. 11.2.21 Tuning fork test: **A**, test for bone conduction; **B**, test for air conduction; and **C**, Weber test.

- In *SN hearing loss*, the sound is lateralized towards the better ear, because the sound is reaching the normal cochlea through bone.

iii. ***Absolute bone conduction (ABC) test:*** In this test, the patient's BC is compared with that of the examiner (presuming that the examiner has normal hearing). External auditory meatus of both the examiner and the patient should be occluded (by pressing the tragus inwards), to prevent the ambience noise entering through AC route.
   - Normally, and in conduction deafness, both the examiner and the patient hear the fork for the same duration of time.
   - In SN deafness, the patient hears the fork for a shorter duration.

iv. ***Schwabach test:*** It is similar to the ABC test except that the external auditory meatus is not occluded in this test.
   - *Normally*, both the examiner and the subject hear the sound equally well.
   - In *conductive deafness*, the patient hears the fork for a longer period than the examiner (because there is no masking effect of environmental noise).
   - In *SN deafness*, the examiner hears the fork for a longer duration than the patient.

Table 11.2.2 summarizes the interpretation of tuning fork tests.

B. Audiometric Tests

Audiometer is the device used to perform audiometry. Audiometry refers to measurement of auditory acuity (sharpness of hearing) using the audiometer. An audiometer consists of the following main parts:

- Electronic oscillator: It can generate pure tones of frequencies ranging from low to high.
- Intensity dial: It helps to adjust the threshold intensity of hearing for each tone.
- Headphone: It helps to deliver the pure tones of various frequencies to each ear separately.

Types of audiometric tests performed in clinical practice are as follows:

- Pure-tone audiometry
- Békésy audiometry
- Impedance audiometry

1. Pure-Tone Audiometry. It is performed in a soundproof room. Each ear is tested separately. Usually AC thresholds are measured for tones of 125, 250, 500, 1000, 2000, 4000 and 8000 Hz, and BC thresholds for 250, 500, 1000, 2000 and 4000 Hz. The results are interpreted as:

- Audiometer is so calibrated that the hearing of a normal person, for both AC and BC, is at 0 dB and there is no A–B gap, whereas tuning fork tests normally show AC > BC.
- The amount of intensity that has to be raised above the normal level is a measure of the degree of hearing loss at that frequency. It is charted in the form of a graph called *audiogram* (Fig. 11.2.22).
- Threshold of BC is a measure of cochlear function.
- Difference in the thresholds of AC and BC (A–B gap) is a measure of degree of conductive deafness.

2. Speech Audiometry. In this test, the patient's ability to hear and understand speech is measured. In it, a set of spondee words (two-syllable words with equal stress on each, e.g. baseball, sunlight and daydream) with variable intensity is delivered to each ear. The following two parameters are measured:

- Speech reception threshold (SRT)
- Discrimination score (DS)

3. Békésy Audiometry. It is a self-recording audiometry in which various pure-tone frequencies automatically move from low to high.

4. Impedance Audiometry. It is an objective test, which is particularly useful in children. It consists of two tests:

- Tympanometry
- Acoustic reflex measurements

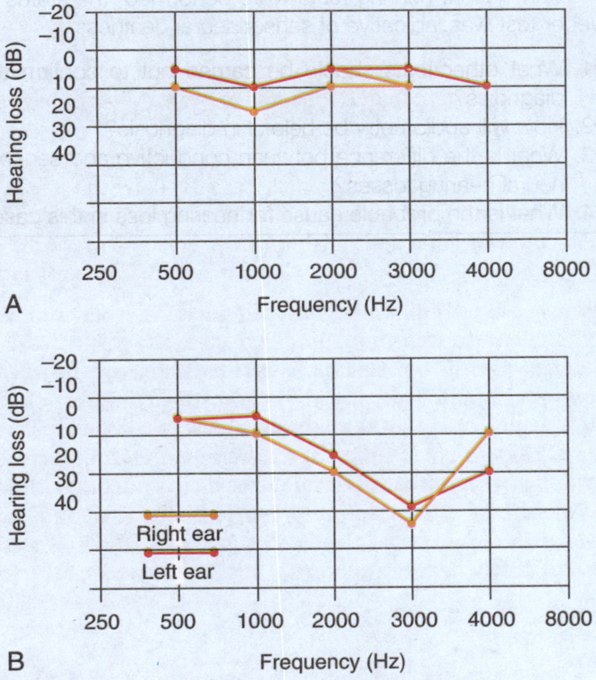

Fig. 11.2.22 Audiogram showing: **A**, normal hearing; and **B**, loss of 20 dB hearing for 3000 Hz frequency in both ears.

Table 11.2.2 Tuning fork tests and their interpretation

Test	Normal	Conductive hearing loss	Sensorineural hearing loss
Rinne test	AC > BC Rinne +ve	BC > AC Rinne −ve	AC > BC in partial deafness
Weber test	Not lateralized	Lateralized towards affected ear	Lateralized towards healthy ear
Absolute bone conduction test	Same as examiner's	Same as examiner's	Reduced
Schwabach test	Equal	Better conduction in patient	Better conduction in examiner

AC, air conduction; BC, bone conduction.

C. Special Tests for Hearing

Certain special tests have been devised to elucidate different aspects of hearing loss. Some of these tests include:

- Recruitment
- Short increment sensitivity index (SISI)
- Threshold tone decay test
- Evoked response audiometry which includes:
  Electrocochleography (ECoG) is the technique of recording electrical potentials generated in the internal ear. The potentials recorded are called *cochlear microphonics* (see page 1148).
- Auditory brainstem responses (see page 1061):
  - Otoacoustic emissions were first demonstrated experimentally by David Kamp, hence called Kamp waves; they are related to the amplification activity of the cochlea and are mainly generated by the outer hair cells of the organ of Corti. Otoacoustic emission testing is a simple, noninvasive test for finding hearing defects especially in newborn babies and small children.

Self-Assessment

1. Discuss the role of middle ear in conduction of sound information.
2. Discuss the process of sound transduction.
3. Discuss neural processing of audition.
4. Describe briefly the following:
   - Cochlear microphonics
   - Features of cortical areas concerned with audition
5. Write notes on the following:
   - Attenuation reflex
   - Impedance matching mechanism
   - Travelling wave theory
   - Pure-tone audiometry
   - Noise

Clinical Cases

Case 1

A 55-year-old male was referred to the ENT department because of the following complaints:

Problem following conversation when three to four persons were conversing

Inability to hear in noise

Feeling of fullness in the ears, dizziness and ringing sensations in the ears

Personal history revealed that the patient was diabetic and hypertensive for the last 1 month and was taking antibiotic streptomycin for infection.

On examination, hearing tests were performed; the status of Weber test was indicative of sensorineural deafness.

Q1. What other tests should be carried out to confirm the diagnosis?

Q2. How will audiometry be helpful in diagnosis?

Q3. What is the difference between conductive and sensorineural hearing losses?

Q4. What is the probable cause for hearing loss in this case?

Case 2

A 3-month-old baby girl was referred to the ENT department for not responding to sounds. The history revealed that at the time of birth, the baby remained admitted in NICU for about 1 month due to some infection. The case was labelled congenital deafness.

Q1. What are the causes of congenital deafness?

Q2. What is the best test for diagnosis of congenital deafness?

Q3. What are the risk factors for congenital deafness?

Q4. What are the effects of congenital deafness in later life?

11.3 Chemical Senses: Smell and Taste

CHAPTER OUTLINE

SENSE OF SMELL

The sense of smell or olfaction is well developed in animals like dogs and rabbits to give warning of the environmental dangers. Such animals are called *macrosomatics*. In humans, apes and monkeys (primates), the sense of smell is comparatively less developed, but still it is important for pleasure and for enjoying the taste of food. Therefore, the humans and primates are called *microsomatics*.

SITE OF OLFACTION

The olfactory stimuli are detected by specialized receptors located on the free nerve endings of the olfactory nerves which are located in the:

- Olfactory mucosa of the nose in human beings
- Vomeronasal organ in reptiles and certain mammals

Olfactory Mucosa

In humans, the olfactory mucosa is confined to upper one-third of the nasal cavity. It includes the roof of the nasal cavity and the adjoining areas on the medial wall (septum) and superior nasal concha on the lateral wall (Fig. 11.3.1). The olfactory neuroepithelium is a patch of thin and dull yellow mucosa about 2.5 cm^2 in area. A mucous layer covers the entire epithelium.

Histological Structure

Histologically, the olfactory mucosa consists of three types of cells (Fig. 11.3.2):

1. *Receptor cells:* About 10–20 million receptor cells are present in the olfactory mucosa. These cells are bipolar neurons which lie between the supporting (sustentacular) cells. The dendrites of the receptor cells terminate in a knob from which 6–12 fine cilia project and form a dense mat into the mucous layer of the olfactory mucosa. Their axons are fine unmyelinated fibres which form the olfactory nerves.

Characteristic features of olfactory receptor cells which differentiate them from other sensory neurons are as follows:
- These are the only sensory neurons whose cell bodies are closest to the external environment.
- These cells have a short life span of about 60 days and get replaced by proliferation of basal cells. This natural turnover is a unique feature of these sensory neurons.

2. *Supporting cells,* also known as sustentacular cells, are columnar in shape. Microvilli extend from the surface of these cells into the mucous layer covering the olfactory mucosa. These cells secrete mucus.

The *Bowman's glands* lying just under the basement membrane also secrete mucus.

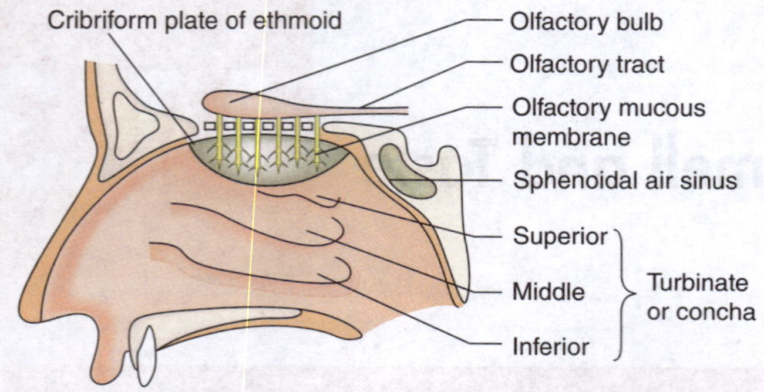

Fig. 11.3.1 Location of olfactory mucosa.

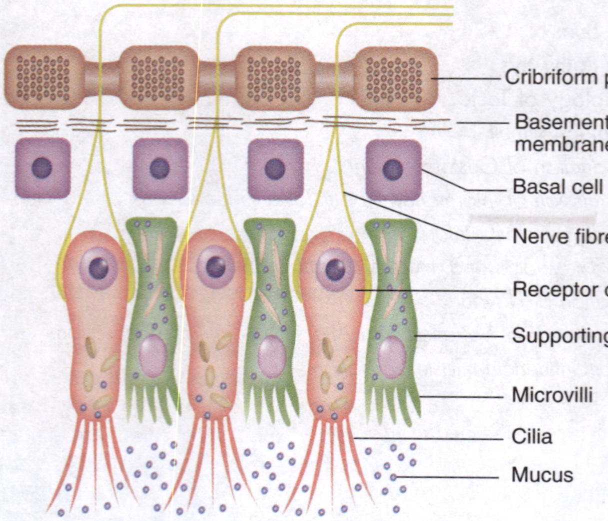

Fig. 11.3.2 Histological features of olfactory mucosa.

3. Basal cells are stem cells from which new receptor cells are formed. As mentioned above, there is a continuous replacement of receptor cells by mitosis of basal cells.

Distinguishing features of olfactory mucosa from the surrounding respiratory mucosa of the nasal cavity are as follows:
- Presence of receptor cells
- Presence of Bowman's glands
- Absence of rhythmic ciliary beating (which is a characteristic feature of respiratory mucosa)
- Presence of a distinctive yellow-brown pigment

Nerve Supply of Olfactory Mucosa

Special sensory nerves innervating the olfactory mucosa are 15–20 bundles of olfactory nerve fibres (cranial nerve I) which convey sense of smell.

General sensory nerves supplying the olfactory mucosa are branches of the trigeminal nerve (cranial nerve V). The irritative character of some odorants results from stimulation of free nerve endings of the trigeminal nerve. Therefore, vapours of ammonia are never used to test the sense of smell as they stimulate fibres of the trigeminal nerve and cause irritation in the nose rather than stimulating the olfactory receptors.

Vomeronasal Organ (Jacobson's Organ)

It is a pouch-like structure found along the nasal septum in the nose of some animals (rodents and various other animals). Receptors present in the vomeronasal organ are concerned with perception of odour that emanates from the *pheromones* and foodstuffs and are thus related to food and sex behaviour of the animals. Nerve fibres emerging from the vomeronasal organ project to the *accessory olfactory bulb* and from those primarily to areas in the amygdala and hypothalamus that are concerned with reproduction and eating behaviour.

Vomeronasal organ is not well developed in humans, but there is an anatomically separate and biochemically unique area of olfactory mucous membrane in a pit in the anterior third of the nasal septum which appears to be a homologous structure.

Pheromones These are hormone-like substances which emit specific odour and produce hormonal, behavioural or other physiological changes in another animal of the same species. Usually a pheromone is secreted by an animal during mating season only. The smell of pheromones often is the cause of sex, which an animal follows to find out its mating partner which may be waiting at a distance. It is being assumed that pheromone also exists in humans and that there is close relationship between smell and sexual function.

OLFACTORY PATHWAYS

Olfactory pathways comprise those given next.

1. Olfactory nerves There are about 15–20 olfactory nerve filaments which consist of the axons of the bipolar olfactory neurons which pierce the cribriform plate to reach the olfactory bulb.

2. Olfactory bulb Olfactory bulb (Fig. 11.3.3) is an oval flattened strip of grey matter lying on the cribriform plate which receives the olfactory nerve filaments. There is a point-to-point representation of olfactory mucosa in the olfactory bulb. The upper part of the mucosa is represented in the anterior part of the bulb, whereas the lower part is represented posteriorly. The olfactory bulb contains three types of cells – mitral cells, tufted cells and interneurons (granule cells and periglomerular cells). The mitral and tufted cells constitute second-order neurons.

Dendrites of mitral and tufted cells branch and form synapses with the axon terminals of olfactory neurons (first-order neurons) to constitute globular masses called olfactory glomeruli. Olfactory axons converge extensively onto mitral cell dendrites; as many as axons from 1000 olfactory neurons synapse on the dendrites of a single mitral cell.

Granule and periglomerular cells are inhibitory neurons. They form dendrodendritic reciprocal synapses with the dendrites of the mitral cells. The periglomerular cells also participate in the formation of olfactory glomeruli.

Axons of the mitral and tufted cells leave the olfactory bulb and run in the olfactory tract.

3. Olfactory tract It lies in the olfactory sulcus on the orbital surface of the frontal lobe and proceeds backwards from each olfactory bulb to the region of anterior perforated substance on the base of the brain where it divides into lateral, intermediate and medial olfactory striae (Fig. 11.3.4). *Olfactory trigone* refers to the flattened part of the olfactory tract, near the anterior perforated substance before it divides into the striae.

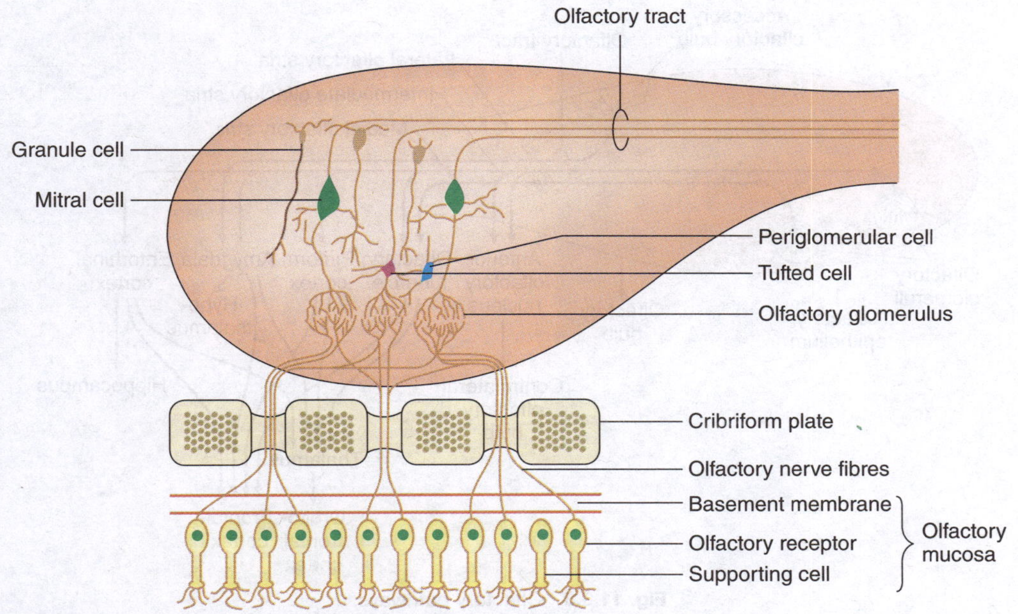

Fig. 11.3.3 Diagrammatic depiction of the synapses between axons of olfactory neurons (first-order neurons) with the dendrites of mitral and tufted cells (second-order neurons) to form the olfactory glomeruli which lie in the olfactory bulb. The inhibitory neurons present in the olfactory bulb are granule cells and periglomerular cells.

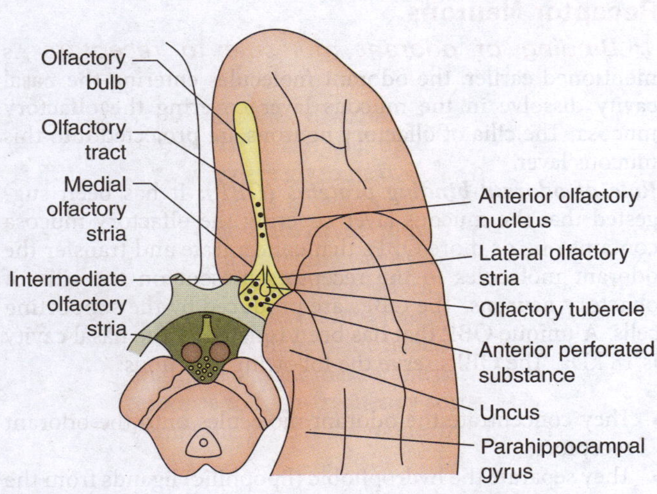

Fig. 11.3.4 Olfactory bulb and olfactory tract.

Anterior olfactory nucleus: It is made up of scattered neurons within the olfactory tract. Neurons in this structure receive synaptic connections from neurons of the olfactory bulb and send axons through the anterior commissure to excite inhibitory neurons on the contralateral olfactory bulb (Fig. 11.3.5).

Olfactory striae: Three striae are derived from each olfactory tract (Fig. 11.3.5):

Lateral olfactory stria: Axons of the lateral olfactory stria synapse in the primary olfactory receiving area which includes the *prepiriform cortex* (and in many animals the piriform lobe).
Medial olfactory stria includes projections to the *amygdaloid nucleus*, as well as to part of the cortex of the basal forebrain.
Intermediate olfactory stria terminates in the *olfactory tubercle*, an area of the cortex rostral to the anterior perforated substance.

4. ***Olfactory cortex*** It includes the anterior olfactory nucleus, prepiriform cortex, olfactory tubercle and amygdala. All these are parts of the limbic system.

PHYSIOLOGY OF OLFACTION

Odoriferous Stimuli

The odoriferous (smell-producing molecules) stimuli enter the nasal cavity while breathing. During quiet breathing, the air passes through the lower parts of the nasal cavity. Through eddy currents, however, some air does reach the olfactory epithelium. The amount of air reaching the olfactory mucosa can be increased by sniffing which causes turbulence in the airflow in the nasal cavity. Sniffing is an act of deep breathing (semireflex response) which occurs when a new odour is encountered. The odorant molecules must dissolve in the mucous layer (lining the olfactory mucosa) before they can come in contact with olfactory receptors.

Characteristic features of odorant molecules To be effective, an odorant molecule must be:

Volatile, because the olfactory receptors respond to chemicals transported by the air into the nose
Water soluble (to some extent), to penetrate the watery mucous layer (lining the nasal epithelium) to reach the receptor cell membrane
Lipid soluble (to some degree), to penetrate the cell membranes of the olfactory receptor cells to stimulate those cells

Types of odorant stimuli There seem to be more than 50 *primary smell sensations* (in contrast to 3 primary sensations of colour and 4 primary sensations of taste). Although the olfactory capability of humans is somewhat limited, compared with that of macrosomatic animals, humans are able to perceive more than 10,000 different odorous molecules.

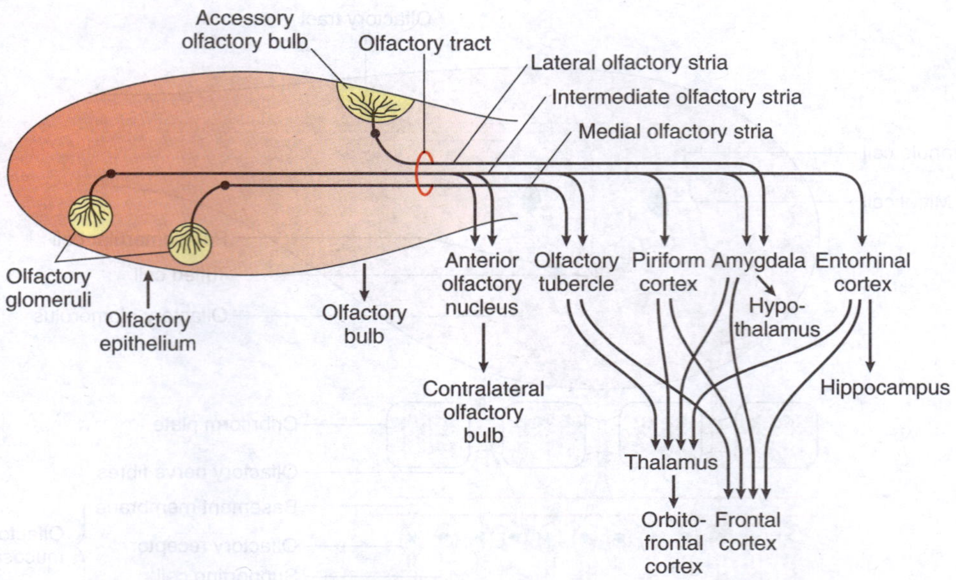

Fig. 11.3.5 Olfactory pathways.

Common odours encountered are named as:

- *Aromatic or resinous odours*, e.g. camphor, lavender and cloves
- *Fragrant odours*, e.g. perfumes and flowers
- *Ethereal odours*, e.g. ether and chloroform
- *Garlic odours*, e.g. garlic, onion and sulphur compounds
- *Burning odours*, tobacco and burning of feathers, meat and bones
- *Nauseating odours*, e.g. excreta and decomposed meat and vegetables
- *Goat odours*, e.g. sweat and ripe cheese
- *Repulsive odours*, e.g. odour of the bed bug
- *Musky odours*, e.g. musk

Olfactory Receptors

The cilia of the olfactory neurons are specialized for odour detection. They have specific receptors for odorants as well as the transduction machinery needed to amplify sensory signals and generate action potentials in the neuron's axon. Some important points about olfactory receptors:

- A large family of odorant receptors permits discrimination of a wide variety of odorants.
- A large multigene family (approximately 500) appears to code for as many as 1000 different types of odorant receptors.

The odorant receptors are G-protein-coupled receptors (GTcRs) belonging to a large superfamily of structurally related receptor proteins that transduce signals by interactions with G-proteins.

Important Note

In 2004, Nobel Prize in Physiology and Medicine was awarded to Linda Buck and Richard Avel for discovery of odorant receptors and organization of the olfactory system.

Steps in Transduction in the Olfactory Receptor Neurons

1. Binding of odorant molecule to receptors As mentioned earlier, the odorant molecules entering the nasal cavity dissolve in the mucous layer covering the olfactory mucosa. The cilia of olfactory neurons are projected into this mucous layer.

Role of odorant-binding proteins (OBP): It has been suggested that the mucous layer covering the olfactory mucosa contains one or more OBPs that concentrate and transfer the odorant molecules to the receptors present on the cilia of olfactory neurons. The OBPs are produced by the supporting cells. A unique OBP that has been isolated in the nasal cavity is 18 kDa. The OBPs serve the following functions:

- They concentrate the odorant molecules onto the odorant receptors.
- They separate the hydrophobic (lipophilic) ligands from the air and transfer them to an aqueous phase.
- They may help in odour clearance by sequestering odorous molecules from the sites of recognition.

2. Activation of receptor The interaction of an odorant with its receptor induces an interaction between the receptor and a heterotrimeric G-protein. This interaction causes dissociation of α-, β- and γ-subunits of G-protein. The α-subunit then stimulates adenylyl cyclase to produce cAMP.

3. Depolarization receptor potential The increased intracellular cAMP opens cyclic nucleotide-gated (CNG) cation channels, leading to cation influx (Ca^{2+} and Na^{+}) and a change in membrane potential in the cilium membrane, i.e. produces a depolarizing receptor potential (Fig. 11.3.6).

4. Action potentials The receptor potential depolarizes the initial segment of the axon to threshold leading to the generation of action potentials in the sensory axon and the *transmission of signal to the olfactory bulb.*

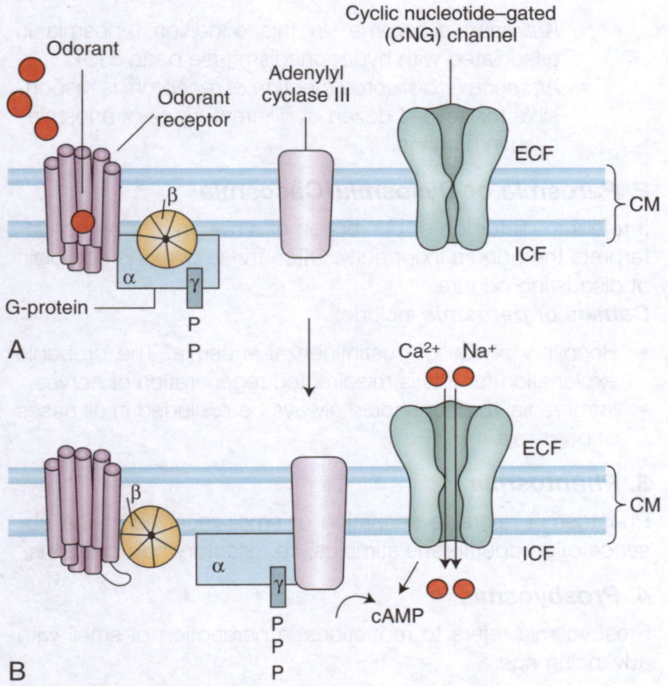

Fig. 11.3.6 Transduction of olfactory signals: **A**, receptor activation; and **B**, depolarization.

Important Note

A specific olfactory receptor does not respond to a particular compound or category of compounds. Instead, an individual receptor responds to many odours. Furthermore, no two receptor cells have identical responses to a series of stimuli. Sensory perception, therefore, is based on the pattern of receptors activated by the stimulus.

Processing of Olfactory Sensation in the Olfactory Bulb

Odorant information is encoded spatially in the olfactory bulb. In the olfactory glomeruli, there is lateral inhibition mediated by periglomerular cells and granule cells (Fig. 11.3.3). Another potential source of signal refinement, or adjustment, is the multiple inputs to the olfactory bulb from the olfactory areas of the cortex as well as the basal forebrain and midbrain. Thus, sensory information is extensively processed, and perhaps refined, in the olfactory bulb before it is sent to the olfactory cortex.

In the olfactory bulb, mitral cells and tufted cells are excitatory cells; on activation, these cells release excitatory neurotransmitter glutamate, whereas periglomerular and granule cells are inhibitory cells, and release GABA on activation. Thus, they play an important role in processing olfactory sensation.

Transmission of Odorant Information to the Olfactory Cortex and Neocortex

- From the olfactory bulb, the odorant information is first transmitted to the *olfactory cortex* which includes piriform cortex, parts of amygdala, the olfactory tubercle and parts of entorhinal cortex.
- From the olfactory cortex, information is relayed to the frontal cortex (directly) and orbitofrontal cortex (via the thalamus) (Fig. 11.3.5).

Important Notes

- The olfactory pathway is the only sensory system that does not have an obligatory synaptic relay in the thalamus. The olfactory tracts project directly to the olfactory cortex, whereas all other sensations are first processed in the thalamus before projection to the cerebral cortex. This may reflect the phylogenetic primitiveness of the olfactory system. Furthermore, because of this, olfactory stimuli have an unusually direct and widespread effect on emotions, motivation and certain kind of memory.
- Traditionally, olfactory sense bypasses the thalamus.

However, olfactory information does reach the mediodorsal nucleus of the thalamus, and it is then transmitted to the prefrontal and orbitofrontal cortex (neocortex). This pathway is concerned with conscious discrimination of odours.

Role played by different regions of the cerebral cortex involved in processing of olfactory information is summarized as:

- *Piriform cortex* is activated by sniffing in humans.
- *Amygdala* and hypothalamus are probably involved with the emotional and motivational responses to olfactory stimuli as well as many of the behavioural and physiological effects of odour. In animals, effects of pheromones are also thought to be mediated by signals from the main and accessory olfactory bulbs to the amygdala and hypothalamus.
- *Entorhinal cortex* is concerned with olfactory memories.
- *Neocortex (orbitofrontal and frontal cortex)* is thought to be concerned with conscious discrimination of odours. People with lesions of the orbitofrontal cortex are unable to discriminate odours.

Factors Influencing Olfactory Function

1. Threshold of olfactory receptors The threshold of olfactory receptors varies from substance to substance. For example, methyl mercaptan, a substance which gives garlic its characteristic odour, has an extremely low threshold. It can be smelled at a concentration of less than 500 mg/L of air (Table 11.3.1).

2. Intensity/concentration of the odour Like taste receptors, the intensity discrimination of any odour by olfactory

Table 11.3.1 Threshold concentrations of some odoriferous substances

Substance	Concentration (mg/L of air)
Ethyl ether	5.83
Chloroform	3.30
Pyridine	0.03
Oil of peppermint	0.02
Iodoform	0.02
Butyric acid	0.009
Propyl mercaptan	0.006
Artificial musk	0.00004
Methyl mercaptan	0.0000004

receptors is poor. The concentration of an odoriferous substance must be changed by about 30% before a difference can be detected.

- Solubility of the odorant: Relatively high water and lipid solubility is the characteristic of substances with strong odours.

3. Structural configuration of odorant Odoriferous molecules are generally small and contain 3–20 carbon atoms. It is important to note that molecules with the same number of carbon atoms but different structural configurations have different odours.

4. Adaptation Olfactory sensation adapts very rapidly with continued exposure to an odour. When one is continuously exposed to even the most disagreeable odour, perception of the odour decreases and eventually ceases. However, a brief exposure to fresh air allows one to smell the unpleasant odour again. Unlike adaptation of touch receptors, the adaptation of olfactory receptors may not be always functionally useful.

Physiological mechanisms responsible for olfactory adaptation are the following:

Inactivation or desensitization of the receptor due to phosphorylation of the receptor by a protein kinase may occur following interaction of an odorant receptor with its ligand.

Adjustment in the sensitivity of CNG ion channels to cAMP with different concentrations of odorant seems to be another physiological mechanism responsible for adaptation of olfactory neurons (when CNG A4 is knocked out, adaptation is slowed). This effect is conceptually analogous to light adaptation in the visual system, in which light sensitivity is adjusted to match the intensity of light in the environment.

Important Note

Sense of olfaction is more acute in females than in males.

- It is more acute at the time of ovulation.

Applied Aspects

Abnormalities of Olfaction

1. Anosmia and Hyposmia or Microsmia

Anosmia is total loss of sense of smell, whereas hyposmia refers to diminished olfactory sensitivity.

Causes of anosmia or hyposmia *are as follows:*

Injuries to olfactory nerves or olfactory bulb in fractures of anterior cranial fossa cause anosmia or hyposmia

Intracranial lesions like abscess, tumour or meningitis which may cause pressure on the olfactory tracts may also cause anosmia or hyposmia

Nasal obstruction due to nasal polyp, enlarged turbinates or marked oedema of nasal mucosa in allergic or vasomotor stimuli

- *Atrophic rhinitis*, a degenerative disease of nasal mucosa, also causes anosmia.
- *Old age:* Olfactory thresholds increase with advancing age, and more than 25% of humans older than 80 years have an impaired ability to identify smells.
- *Kallmann syndrome:* In this condition, anosmia is associated with hypogonadism (see page 815).
- *Absence or disrupted function of receptors* is responsible for several dozen of different types of anosmias seen in humans.

2. Parosmia or Dysosmia/Cacosmia

It refers to distortion or perversion of smell. In it, a person interprets the odours incorrectly. Often these persons complain of disgusting odours.

Causes of parosmia include:

- Recovery phase of postinfluenzal anosmia. The probable explanation for this is misdirected regeneration of nerves.
- Intracranial tumour should always be excluded in all cases of parosmia.

3. Phantosmia

Phantosmia refers to sensation of smell received in the absence of an odoriferous stimulus, i.e. olfactory hallucinations.

4. Presbyosmia

Presbyosmia refers to reductions in perception of smell with advancing age.

5. Drugs

Drugs causing deterioration of sense of olfaction are amoxicillin, doxycycline, captopril, erythromycin and intranasal sprays containing zinc.

CNS disorders accompanied by olfactory impairment are as follows:

- Parkinson disease (see page 918)
- Alzheimer disease (see page 1091)
- Huntington disease (see page 921)
- Down syndrome (see page 46)
- Multiple sclerosis (see page 897)
- Narcolepsy (see page 1076)

Measurement of Sense of Smell

1. Qualitative Testing

Qualitatively, sense of smell can be tested by asking the patient to smell common odours such as onion, peppermint, rose, garlic or cloves from each side of the nose separately, with the eyes closed.

2. Olfactometry

Olfactometry is the method of quantitative estimation of sense of smell with the help of an instrument called olfactometer. *Olfactometer* consists of two glass tubes – outer and inner sliding one over the other. The inner tube is graduated. The inner surface of the outer tube contains the smelling substance. The curved end of the inner tube is introduced into the nostril and the subject is asked to breathe quietly. The distal end of the outer tube is closed and withdrawn gradually. The highest figure is noted as soon as the odour is perceived first of all. This reading gives the subject's threshold for smell in terms of olfactories.

3. Electro-Olfactogram

Electro-olfactogram is available but not widely used.

4. 40-Item University of Pennsylvania Smell Identification Test

The 40-Item University of Pennsylvania Smell Identification Test (UPSIT) is the most widely used test for smell testing.

SENSE OF TASTE

Sense of taste (gustation) is a chemical sense that is stimulated by food and drink. It contributes considerably to the quality of life and is an important stimulant for digestion. Taste must be distinguished from flavour, which includes the olfactory, tactile and thermal attributes of food in addition to taste.

SITE OF TASTE

The taste (gustatory) stimuli are detected by specialized chemoreceptors called taste receptors or taste cells. The taste receptors are clustered in the taste buds located on the tongue, palate, pharynx, epiglottis and upper third of the oesophagus.

Tongue, the main site of taste detection, contains numerous taste buds on its dorsal surface. The mucous membrane of the dorsal surface of the tongue exhibits numerous papillae, which increase the surface area of the mucosa available for taste receptors. The taste buds are located in the walls of these papillae.

Papillae

Papillae, present on the tongue, are of four types (Fig. 11.3.7).

1. Circumvallate papillae These are large (2–4 mm in diameter) papillae, about 10–12 in number, forming a single row in front of the sulcus terminalis. Sulcus terminalis is a V-shaped groove (with the apex posteriorly), which separates the anterior two-thirds of the dorsum of the tongue from the posterior one-third. Each circumvallate papilla is surrounded by a groove. About 200 taste buds are located along the sides of each circumvallate papilla.

2. Fungiform papillae These are bright red, flat dot-like structures (each of about 1 mm in diameter) located in the anterior two-thirds of the tongue along the edges, dorsum and tip. There are 8–10 taste buds on each papilla.

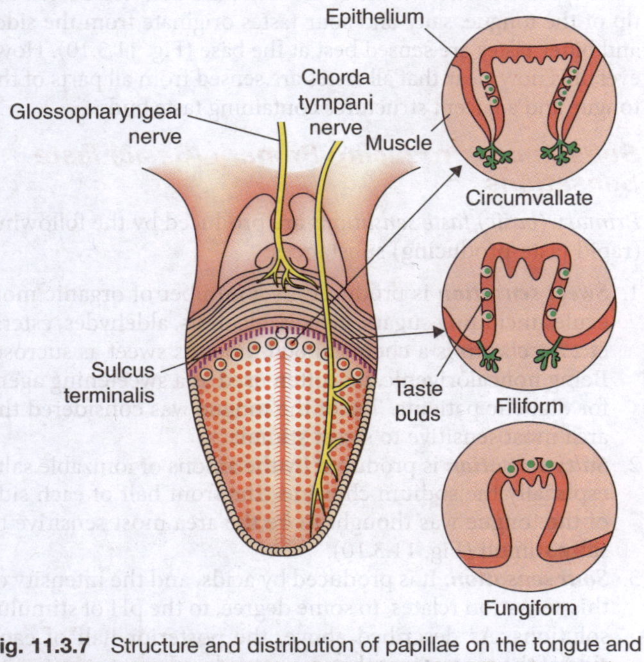

Fig. 11.3.7 Structure and distribution of papillae on the tongue and arrangement of taste buds in the three types of papillae. Innervation by the cranial nerves is also indicated.

3. Foliate papillae These are transverse mucosal folds, found on the posterolateral surfaces of the tongue anterior to the circumvallate papillae. Each foliate papilla has numerous taste buds.

4. Filiform papillae These are small conical projections, covering the entire remaining surface of the dorsum of the anterior two-thirds of the tongue, giving it a velvety appearance. They are arranged in rows parallel to the sulcus terminalis. They are not gustatory structures, i.e. *do not contain taste buds*. However, they may play a role in breaking up food particles and are also called *mechanical papillae* in contrast to the other three forms which are called gustatory papillae.

Taste Buds

Distribution The taste buds are concerned with the sensation of taste. As mentioned above, taste buds are located on the tongue papillae, hard and soft palate, epiglottis, pharynx and upper third of the oesophagus.

Structure Each taste bud is barrel shaped. It consists of a cluster of cells with a small opening (taste pore) in the surface that allows substances to reach the interior of the taste bud. Each taste bud measures about 50–70 μm in diameter and consists of the following cells (Fig. 11.3.8):

1. ***Receptor cells:*** Each taste bud has about 100 receptor cells (modified epithelial cells). These are of further three types – dark cells, light cells and intermediate cells which respond to taste stimuli or tastants.
   The characteristic features are as follows:
   - The receptor cells are elongate and bipolar shaped, and extend from the epithelial opening of the taste bud to its base.
   - The taste cells have a short life (about 10 days) and are continuously replaced by new taste cells differentiating them from the basal cells.
   - Through the taste pore, microvilli (cilia) of all the taste cells protrude into the oral cavity and come in contact with the saliva.
   - The taste cells are innervated by sensory neurons (primary gustatory afferent fibres) at their basal pole. Although taste cells are non-neuronal epithelial cells, the contacts between these cells and sensory cells have morphological characteristics of chemical synapses.

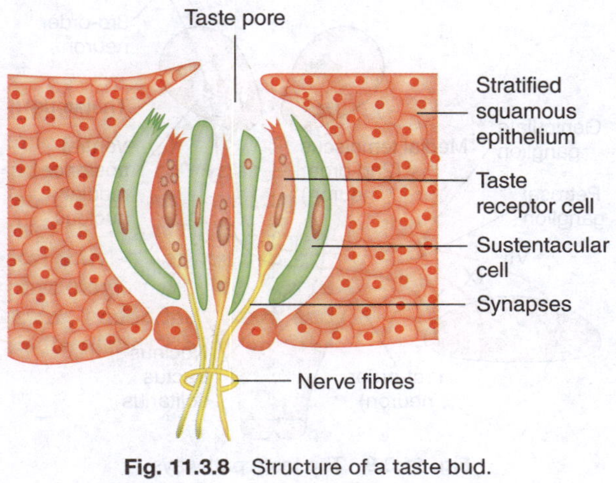

Fig. 11.3.8 Structure of a taste bud.

Each taste nerve fibre innervates taste cells in several taste buds and conversely, each taste bud is innervated by approximately 50 nerve fibres.

2. ***Basal replacement cells:*** These are small round cells present at the bottom of the taste bud (Fig. 11.3.8). They are thought to be stem cells which are continuously being differentiated into taste cells.
3. ***Supporting cells:*** In addition to taste cells and basal cells, the taste buds contain supporting or sustentacular cells.

Innervation The special sensory nerve fibres innervating the taste cells come from the branches of the facial, glossopharyngeal and vagus nerves (cranial nerves VII, IX and X, respectively). Further details of taste nerve fibres are described in the section 'Taste Pathways'. The tactile and temperature receptors of the mouth, tongue and pharynx are innervated by the trigeminal nerve (cranial nerve V).

TASTE PATHWAYS

The taste pathways consist of three orders of neurons (Fig. 11.3.9).

First-order neurons The cell bodies of the first-order neurons innervating the taste cells in taste buds are located in different ganglia of the cranial nerves VII, IX and X as:

From the taste buds located on anterior two-thirds of the tongue, the taste fibres run in the lingual nerve which branches from the chorda tympani nerve which is a branch of the facial nerve. The cell bodies are located in the geniculate ganglion.

From the taste buds located on the posterior one-third of the tongue, the taste fibres run in the glossopharyngeal nerve. The cell bodies lie in the *superior and inferior ganglia* of this nerve.

From the taste buds located on the pharyngeal aspect of the tongue, epiglottis, and hard and soft palate, the taste fibres run in the vagus nerve. The cell bodies are located in the superior and inferior ganglia of the vagus nerve.

Termination of first-order neurons: Ultimately all the taste fibres, travelling in different cranial nerves, join the tractus solitarius to terminate in the nucleus of tractus solitarius (NTS) (Fig. 11.3.9).

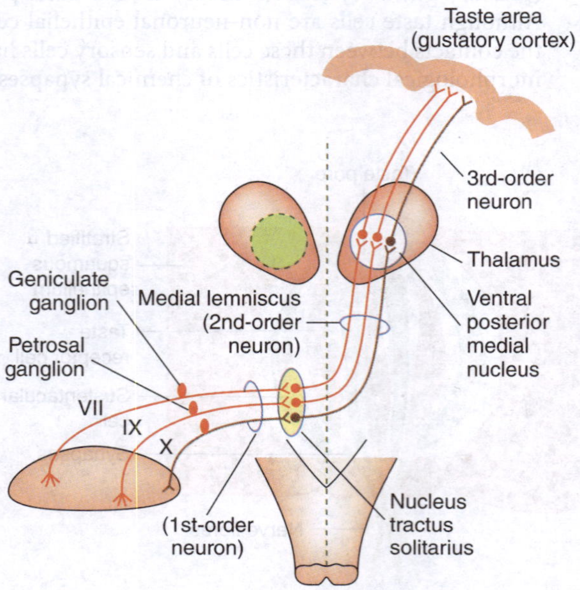

Fig. 11.3.9 The taste pathways.

Second-order neurons The cell bodies of second-order neurons of taste pathways are located in the *NTS* in the medulla. Axons of the second-order neurons cross the midline to join the medial lemniscus and terminate with the cranial nerve V fibres (carrying pain, touch and temperature fibres) in the ventral posterior medial nucleus of the thalamus.

Third-order neurons The cell bodies of third-order neurons are located in the *ventral posterior medial nucleus of the thalamus*. Axons of third-order neurons proceed to terminate in the inferior part of the postcentral gyrus, i.e. the part of sensory cortex called taste cortex (anterior insula and frontal operculum) (Fig. 11.3.9).

PHYSIOLOGY OF TASTE

Gustatory Stimuli

Types of Stimuli and Most Sensitive Areas of Tongue

As mentioned earlier, the taste buds containing taste receptors are concerned with perception of sensation of taste. In humans, the taste buds are located in the three types of gustatory papillae (Fig. 11.3.7). There are about 10,000 taste buds, which after the age of 45 years start decreasing in number, resulting in blunting of taste sensations in old age.

Conventionally, four basic types of taste sensations have been described – *sweet, salt, sour* and *bitter*. Recently, a fifth stimulus type called *umami* has also been considered in the list of basic tastes. All other taste sensations (hundreds in humans) are assumed to result from various combinations of these five primary (basic) taste sensations. In addition to the above, associated sensations of olfaction, heat, cold and texture contribute to different flavours. Earlier, it was believed that there are special areas on the surface of the tongue for each of the four conventional basic types of tastes, i.e. the sweet tastes are detected best at the tip of the tongue, salty and sour tastes originate from the sides and bitter tastes are sensed best at the base (Fig. 11.3.10). However, it is now clear that all tastes are sensed from all parts of the tongue and adjacent structures containing taste buds.

Substances Producing Primary (Basic) Taste Sensations

Primary (basic) taste sensations are produced by the following (rapid taste-producing) substances:

1. ***Sweet sensation*** is produced by a number of organic molecules including sugars, glycols, alcohols, aldehydes, esters, etc. Saccharin is a chemical 600 times as sweet as sucrose. Being noncalorigenic, it is often used as a sweetening agent for diabetic patients. Tip of the tongue was considered the area most sensitive to sweet stimuli.
2. ***Salty sensation*** is produced by the anions of ionizable salts especially the sodium chloride. The front half of each side of the tongue was thought to be the area most sensitive to salty stimuli (Fig. 11.3.10).
3. ***Sour sensation:*** It is produced by acids, and the intensity of this sensation relates, to some degree, to the pH of stimulus solutions. As described above, the posterior half of each side of the tongue was the area considered most sensitive to sour stimuli (Fig. 11.3.10).

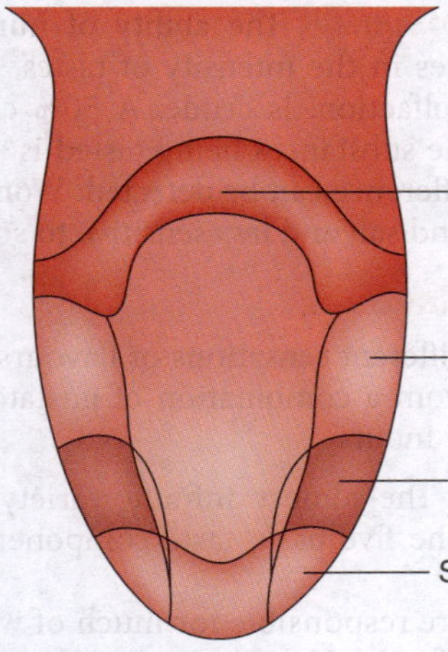

Fig. 11.3.10 Distribution of four primary taste sensations (according to old view).

4. ***Bitter sensation*** is produced by alkaloids such as quinine, caffeine, nicotine and strychnine. Many alkaloids are harmful when swallowed. Perhaps, the highly bitter taste has been given by the nature to these substances to prevent their ingestion by humans and animals.
5. ***Umami sensation:*** It has been recently added to the four basic taste sensations. It is produced by glutamate, particularly by monosodium glutamate used extensively in Asian cooking. This taste is pleasant and sweet but differs from the standard sweet taste.

Transduction of Gustatory Stimuli

Transduction of gustatory stimuli into electrical signals is initiated at the level of receptors. The taste receptors are chemoreceptors which are stimulated by substances dissolved in the mouth by saliva. The dissolved substances act on the microvilli of taste receptors exposed in the taste pore of taste buds. This interaction typically depolarizes the cell either directly or via the action of second messengers. This causes the development of *receptor potential* in the receptor cell which in turn generates action potential in the sensory nerves. The receptors for different taste modalities have been divided into two major types – ligand-gated channels (ionotropic) and GTcRs (or metabotropic). In human beings, GPCR$_s$ are taste receptor types, i.e. T_1R_1, T_1R_2, T_1R_3, T_2R and mGLuR4. G protein present in taste receptors is gustducin.

The mechanisms involved in the transduction of five types of basic taste stimuli into electrical signals are different. These are described briefly (Fig. 11.3.11):

1. ***Sweet tastants*** are known to depolarize the taste receptors of family T_1R_2 and T_1R_3 by two different mechanisms:
   i. ***By activating adenylate cyclase:*** Some sweet receptors couple to a G protein that interacts with adenylyl cyclase, causing an increase in cAMP that leads to the closing of K^+-selective channels. Since these channels are normally open at the resting membrane potential, their closure leads to depolarization of the taste cells (Fig. 11.3.11A).
   ii. ***By stimulating inositol triphosphate (IP_3) production:*** Some sweet tastants are also thought to bind to receptors that couple to gustducin or a G protein that stimulates IP_3 production. The increase in IP_3 is likely to cause the release of Ca^{2+} from intracellular stores.

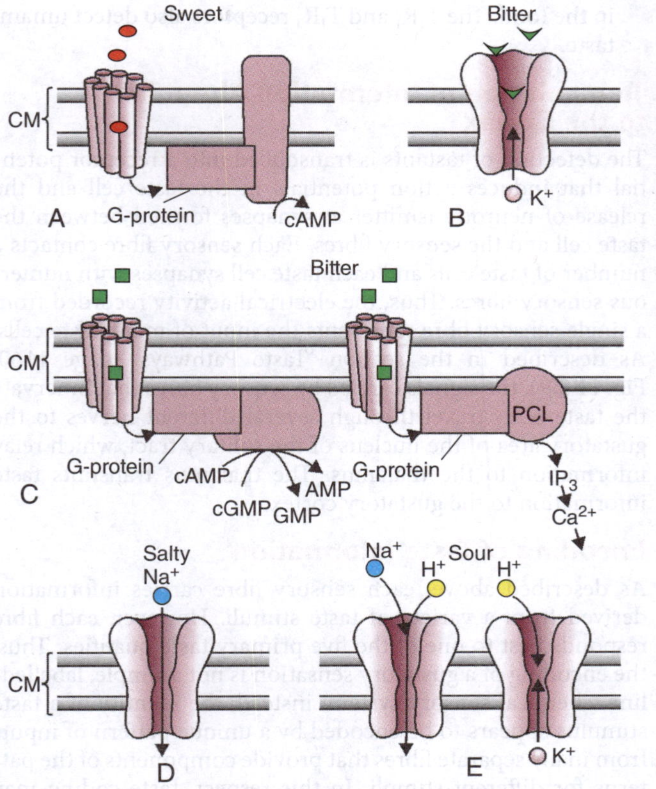

Fig. 11.3.11 Transduction of basic taste stimuli (tastants) into electrical signals by different mechanisms: **A**, sweet tastants; **B** and **C**, bitter tastants; **D**, salty tastants; and **E**, sour tastants (for details, see text).

2. ***Bitter tastants*** are known to depolarize the taste receptors of GPCR$_s$ TR_2 family by three different mechanisms (Fig. 11.3.11B and C).
   i. ***By stimulating IP_3 production:*** Some bitter tastants are thought to bind to receptors that couple to G protein which stimulates IP_3 production. IP_3 increases intracellular Ca^{2+} level, which leads to release of synaptic transmitter and the activation of the gustatory nerve fibre.
   ii. ***By lowering intracellular levels of cAMP and cGMP:*** Receptors for some bitter tastants may be coupled to the taste cell–specific G protein gustducin. The G protein gustducin activates a phosphodiesterase that may reduce intracellular levels of both cAMP and cGMP.
   iii. ***By blocking apical K^+ channel:*** At least one bitter stimulus, the quinine may depolarize the taste cells by blocking apical K^+ channels.
3. ***Salty tastants*** depolarize taste cells by activating an amiloride-sensitive Na^+ channel (ENaC) (Fig. 11.3.11D). No specific Na^+ receptor has been identified.
4. ***Sour tastants*** depolarize the taste cells by permeation or blockade of apical ion channels by proteins. As shown in Fig. 11.3.11E, sour taste can result either from the passage of H^+ through amiloride-sensitive Na^+ channels or from the blockade of K^+ channels, which are normally open at resting membrane potential.
5. ***Umami taste*** is transduced by a specific type of truncated metabotropic glutamate receptor (mGluR4), and the agonists are purine 5-ribonucleotides such as AMP and GMP

in the food. The T_1R_1 and T_1R_3 receptors also detect umami taste.

Transmission of Information About Taste to the Cortex

The detection of tastants is transduced into a receptor potential that induces action potentials in the taste cell and the release of neurotransmitter at synapses formed between the taste cell and the sensory fibres. Each sensory fibre contacts a number of taste cells and each taste cell synapses with numerous sensory fibres. Thus, the electrical activity recorded from a single sensory fibre represents the input of many taste cells. As described in the section 'Taste Pathways' (page 1160, Fig. 11.3.9), the signals carried by sensory fibres that innervate the taste buds travel through several different nerves to the gustatory area of the nucleus of the solitary tract, which relay information to the thalamus. The thalamus transmits taste information to the gustatory cortex.

Encoding of Taste Information

As described above, each sensory fibre carries information derived from a variety of taste stimuli. However, each fibre responds best to one of the five primary taste qualities. Thus, the encoding of a gustatory sensation is not a simple, labelled-line, chemical sensory system; instead, the identity of a taste stimulus appears to be encoded by a unique pattern of inputs from many separate fibres that provide components of the patterns for different stimuli. In this respect, taste coding may resemble sensory information coding in other systems, including the visual and auditory systems, in which late steps in the processing of information involve a comparison of the activity of different cells that respond preferentially, but not exclusively, to certain features of sensory stimuli.

Taste Thresholds and Intensity Discriminations

Taste threshold Taste threshold refers to the minimum concentration at which a substance can be perceived. To be recognized as salty, a substance need only be 0.01 M, whereas for quinine to be perceived as bitter, its concentration need only be 0.000008 M. This correlates with the notion that bitter serves a protective function against dangerous alkaloids; thus, its intensity is high. The threshold concentrations of some substances to which the taste buds respond are shown in Table 11.3.2.

Table 11.3.2 Threshold concentrations of some taste-producing substances

Substance	Taste	Threshold concentration (μmol/L)
Hydrochloric acid	Sour	100
Sodium chloride	Salt	2000
Strychnine hydrochloride	Bitter	1.6
Quinine	Bitter	8
Glucose	Sweet	80,000
Sucrose	Sweet	10,000
Saccharine	Sweet	23

Intensity discrimination The ability of humans to discriminate differences in the intensity of tastes, like intensity discrimination in olfaction, is crude. A 50% change in the concentration of the substances being tasted is necessary before an intensity difference can be detected. Women are more sensitive to sweet and salt and less sensitive to sour.

Sensation of Flavours

The multitude of different sensations of flavours that one experiences results from a combination of gustatory, olfactory and somatosensory inputs.

Gustatory inputs: The almost infinite variety of tastes is synthesized from the five basic taste components described earlier.

Olfactory inputs are responsible for much of what we think as the flavour of foods. Volatile molecules released from foods or beverages in the mouth are pumped into the back of the nasal cavity (retronasally) by the tongue, cheek and throat movements that accompany chewing and swallowing. Although the olfactory epithelium of the nose clearly makes a major contribution to sensations of taste, we experience taste as being in the mouth, not in the nose. It is thought that the somatosensory system is involved in this localization and that the coincidence between somatosensory stimulation of the tongue and retronasal passage of odorants into the nose causes the odorants to be perceived as flavours in the mouth.

Somatosensory input frequently contributes to the sensation of flavour. This component includes the texture (consistency) and temperature of foods as well as pain sensations evoked by spicy and minty foods and by carbonation.

Phenomenon of Variation and After-Effects in Taste Sensations

It has been reported that taste sensations exhibit after-reactions and contrast phenomena. These are similar in some way to visual after-images and contrasts. Some of these occur due to chemical tricks, whereas others are considered to be the result of a true *central phenomenon*.

Factors Influencing Taste Sensation

1. Area of stimulation The perception of sense of taste is directly proportional to the area of taste buds stimulated. Therefore, stimulation of a small area of the tongue by one drop of solution produces a weaker sensation than the same solution by the whole mouth.

2. Temperature of the tastant An optimal response to taste-producing substances is obtained when their temperature is between 30°C and 40°C.

3. Age of the person After the age of 45 years, the number of taste buds starts decreasing resulting in the blunting of sensation of taste.

4. Sex In general, women are more sensitive to sweet and salt and less sensitive to sour.

5. Adaptation Taste sensation adapts rapidly when a taste-producing substance is kept for a long time in one place in the mouth. The adaptation is peripheral. Further adaptation to

one acid produces adaptation to other acids, because H^+ is the stimulus in all cases.

6. Interaction between taste-producing substances Interaction between taste-producing substances also affects taste sensation. For example, the reduction of sour taste of fruits by sucrose is a well-known phenomenon.

7. Effect of taste-modifying proteins A taste-modifier protein, *miraculin*, has been discovered in a West African plant. When applied to the tongue, this protein makes acids taste sweet.

8. Abnormalities of taste sensations Abnormalities of taste sensations obviously affect the various taste sensations.

Applied Aspects

Abnormalities of Taste Sensations

1. Ageusia

Ageusia refers to absence of taste sensation.

Causes of ageusia are as follows:

- *Lesions of the mandibular* division of the trigeminal nerve (through lingual branch of which the chorda tympani nerve reaches the tongue) cause loss of taste sensations in the anterior two-thirds of the tongue.
- *Lesions of the facial nerve* also lead to loss of taste sensations in the anterior two-thirds of the tongue.
- *Lesions of the glossopharyngeal nerve* are associated with absence of taste sensations from the posterior one-third of the tongue.
- *Drugs* like cisplatin, captopril and penicillamine, which contain sulphydryl groups, cause temporary loss of taste sensation. The reason for this effect of sulphydryl compounds is not known.
- *Familial dysautonomia:* It is a congenital widespread sensory disorder characterized by absence of taste sensations associated with other abnormalities such as postural hypotension, lacrimation, hyporeflexia and insensitivity to temperature and noxious stimuli.

2. Hypogeusia

Hypogeusia refers to diminished taste sensitivity. In it, the taste sensations are not completely lost but there occurs an increase in the threshold for different taste sensations. Many different conditions that can produce hypogeusia are deficiency of vitamin B_3 or zinc, tobacco chewing and ageing.

3. Dysgeusia

Dysgeusia refers to disturbed sense of taste in which foul, salty and metallic taste persists in the mouth. Dyspepsia is sometimes associated with burning mouth syndrome.

It is a feature of temporal lobe syndrome, particularly when the anterior region of the temporal lobe is affected. The patient usually experiences paroxysmal hallucinations of taste and smell, which are usually unpleasant.

Burning mouth syndrome is a condition in which a person perceives burning pain sensation even when the mucosa of the mouth is normal.

Causes: The underlying pathophysiology is not well understood, but certain factors that can cause this condition are as follows:

Oral habits like tooth grinding/jaw clinching
Endocrinal disorders like diabetes and hypothyroidism
Allergy to dental materials (metals) and certain food products
Nutritional deficiency like deficiency of vitamin D, low levels of vitamin B, iron and zinc
Infection of the mouth (fungal)
Acid reflux

Treatment: To relieve the symptoms, magic mouthwash is commonly recommended, which consists of viscous lidocaine, diphenhydramine, topical steroids, antifungal medication and antibiotic.

4. Selective Taste Blindness

Selective taste blindness is an inherited autosomal recessive trait characterized by markedly elevated threshold for phenylthiocarbamide (PTC, a chemical substance with very bitter taste). Such individuals are called *nontasters for PTC*. The defect is highly selective since there is no taste blindness to other substances producing bitter taste and to the substances producing salty, sour or sweet tastes. Probably, there is a particular receptor protein, which is not synthesized in these individuals.

5. Hypersensitivity to Taste

Individuals with hypersensitivity to taste, particularly to bitter taste, are called supertasters. The exact reason is not known; it may be due to an increased number of fungiform papillae.

6. Taste Disturbances

Taste disturbances also occur in conditions in which levels of norepinephrine and serotonin are altered (e.g. during anxiety and depression) because these substances act as neuromodulators, thus contributing towards altered taste threshold.

Important Notes

- In pregnant women, especially during the first trimester, disliking for bitter taste increases. This ensures that women avoid poisons during fetal development.
- During second and third trimesters, increased liking for salty taste ensures adequate supply of electrolytes.

Self-Assessment

1. Discuss the physiology of olfaction.
2. Discuss the physiology of taste sensation.
3. Describe the following:
   - Sensation of flavour
   - Olfactory receptors
4. Write notes on the following:
   - Pheromones
   - Odorant binding proteins
   - Vomeronasal organ
   - Umami sensation
   - Selective taste blindness

Clinical Cases

Case 1

A 56-year-old diabetic patient was treated for chronic sinusitis and upper respiratory tract infection due to COVID-19 and recovered after the treatment. Presently, he complains of reduced ability of smelling different odorants.

Q1. What is this condition known as?
Q2. What is the transmission pathway?
Q3. What is the site of lesion in this case?

Case 2

A 60-year-old male suffering from cancer is undergoing chemotherapy followed by radiotherapy; now, he complains of foul, salty and metallic taste persisting all the time in the mouth and sometimes a burning pain sensation in the mouth.

Q1. What is this condition?
Q2. What is the name given to burning pain in the mouth in this condition?
Q3. What are the other causes for this condition?

PART III

SPECIALIZED INTEGRATIVE PHYSIOLOGY

PART OUTLINE

SPECIALIZED INTEGRATIVE PHYSIOLOGY

SECTION 12

SECTION OUTLINE

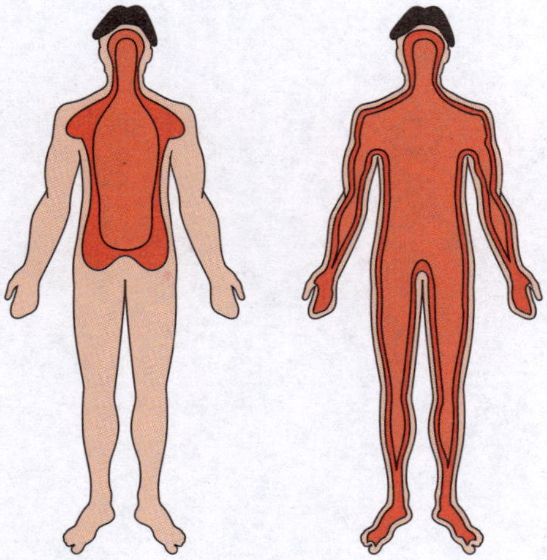

INTRODUCTION

This section includes chapters on miscellaneous topics and not on different physiological aspects related to each other as is in the case of systemic physiology. In systemic physiology, each section, say, for example, the section '*Respiratory System*' (see page 377), includes various chapters dealing with the different aspects of respiration. The only similarity between the various physiological aspects discussed in different chapters of this section is that each involves an integrated role of two or more than two systems to perform a highly specialized physiological activity. For instance, the chapter '*Physiology of Exercise and Sports*' includes integrated role of physiological activities related to the skeletal muscle system, respiratory system, cardiovascular system, endocrine system and nervous system. Similarly, the chapter '*Physiology of Body Temperature Regulation*' highlights the nicely integrated role of the cardiovascular system, respiratory system, skin and nervous system to perform the highly specialized task of regulating the body temperature. In other words, this section is perfect demonstration of unity in diversity. Various diverse aspects of physiology discussed in this section are enumerated above.

12.1

Physiology of Exercise and Sports

CHAPTER OUTLINE

INTRODUCTION

Physiology of exercise has generated significant interest and has gained importance because of:

- The current concern with physical conditioning and improvement in performance of athletes, sports persons, military and paramilitary personnel all over the world
- Role of exercise in prevention of cardiovascular diseases and physical fitness of population groups
- Role of exercise (stress tests) in evaluation of the cardiovascular and respiratory systems
- Role of exercise in rehabilitation of the cardiac invalids

EXERCISE: TYPES AND GRADING

Exercise, to be more precise, muscular exercise, is a period of enhanced energy expenditure by skeletal muscles, which is met by many complex adjustments of metabolism, respiration, circulation and temperature regulation.

Types of Exercise

Exercise may be dynamic or isotonic and static or isometric.

Dynamic exercise involves isotonic muscle contractions. External work is involved in this type of exercise.

Static exercise involves isometric muscle contractions.

Quite a few changes in exercise depend on whether the exercise is predominantly isotonic or isometric. The differences in the two forms of exercise originate because isotonic exercise is associated with a fall in peripheral resistance, whereas isometric exercise is associated with a rise in peripheral resistance. The differences in the responses to two types of exercise will be summarized later.

Grading of Exercise

WHO (1978) has classified muscular exercise into four grades depending on the heart rate and oxygen consumption. Oxygen consumption can be expressed as litres per minute or as relative load index (RLI), i.e. percentage of maximum O_2 utilization. The oxygen utilization can also be expressed as metabolic energy expenditure (MET) test. One MET is equivalent to

Table 12.1.1 Grades of exercise

Grade level		Heart rate (beats/min)	O_2 consumption (L/min)	Relative load index (RLI) (percentage of maximum O_2 consumption)	METs
I	Light (mild)	<100	0.4–0.8	<25	<3
II	Moderate	100–125	0.8–1.6	25–50	3.1–4.5
III	Heavy	125–150	1.6–2.4	51–75	4.6–7
IV	Severe	>150	>2.4	>75	>7

MET, metabolic energy expenditure.

resting O_2 uptake of 250 mL/min for an average adult man and 200 mL/min for an average woman. Thus, exercise of two METs requires twice the resting metabolism and twice the amount of O_2 per minute and so on. The four grades of exercise are shown in Table 12.1.1.

Important Note

The figures shown in Table 12.1.1 are true for cold climates. In tropical countries like India, the environmental heat further increases the stress and even in moderate exercise, heart rate increases like in heavy exercise.

MUSCLES IN EXERCISE

Muscle Strength, Power and Endurance

For details, see page 101.

Muscle Metabolic Systems in Exercise

For details, see page 105.

ADJUSTMENTS TO EXERCISE

Adjustments to physical (muscular) exercise depend on the type of exercise, grade of exercise, cardiac reserve (i.e. efficiency of the heart), muscle power, training, motivation and the state of nutrition.

Response to exercise: The term 'response to exercise' is used to describe short-term adjustments to a bout of acute exercise, which differ in both quantity and quality in trained and untrained individuals.

Effects of training: The term 'effect of training' is used to describe long-term adjustments (adaptations) to chronic exercise.

RESPONSES TO EXERCISE

Exercise, basically, is a period of enhanced energy expenditure. The energy for muscular exercise is provided by the increased fuel consumption, which is reflected as *greater O_2 consumption and CO_2 production*. The increased O_2 delivery to the tissues and removal of CO_2 from the tissues is achieved by:

- Cardiovascular responses to exercise
- Respiratory responses to exercise
- Changes at tissue levels during exercise

In addition, endocrine responses to exercise occur and play a regulatory role by regulating the water loss and availability of fuel during exercise.

A. OXYGEN CONSUMPTION DURING EXERCISE

Oxygen Consumption

Oxygen consumption during exercise: The energy for muscular work during exercise is provided by increased fuel consumption, which is reflected in greater O_2 consumption and CO_2 production.

Oxygen consumption (VO_2) during rest is about 250 mL/min, which increases linearly with severity of exercise up to a certain limit, beyond which a plateau is reached (Fig. 12.1.1).

Maximal oxygen consumption (VO_2 max) is the term used to define the level of oxygen consumption beyond which no further increase in O_2 consumption occurs with further increase in the severity of exercise.

- Thus, VO_2 max refers to the maximum amount of oxygen that can be consumed by a person while performing severe exercise (irrespective of the demand).
- Average VO_2 max in an adult is 3 L/min and in a trained athlete, it may be as high as 5 L/min.
- VO_2 max is probably the best physiological indicator of a person's capacity to continue severe work, i.e. it determines the maximum *aerobic work capacity*.
- VO_2 max represents the highest attainable rate of aerobic metabolism during performance of rhythmic muscular work that exhausts the subject within 5–10 minutes.
- VO_2 max increases during childhood and reaches a peak during early adulthood; after that, a gradual and steady decline takes place with the increasing age.
- VO_2 max of a normal individual is limited by the degree to which cardiac output can increase and not by the ventilatory capacity or oxygen diffusion capacity of the lungs. The ability of the active tissues to extract O_2 delivered by

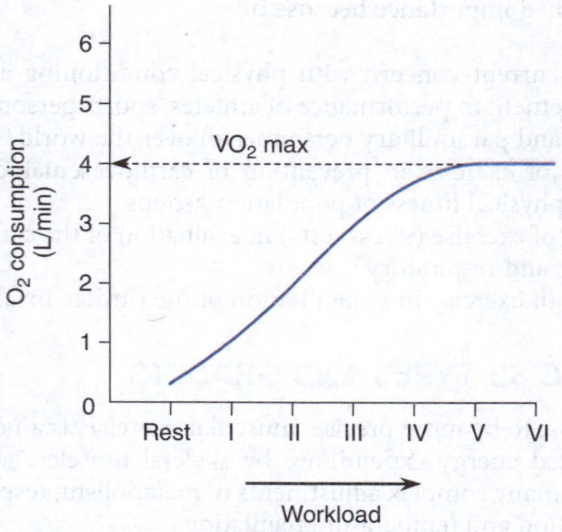

Fig. 12.1.1 Oxygen consumption during exercise.

circulation or peripheral factors (muscle mass) may be the other possible limiting factors for VO_2 max.

Oxygen Deficit and O_2 Debt

The period of muscular exercise can be divided into three phases (Fig. 12.1.2).

1. Adaptation phase Adaptation phase refers to the beginning of muscular exercise (first 2–4 minutes) during which oxygen consumption increases linearly and reaches the maximal O_2 consumption (VO_2 max). The VO_2 max at this stage is much less than the oxygen demand; thus, an *oxygen deficit* is established at the beginning of exercise which continues throughout the period of exercise. So, the energy requirement over and above the limits of O_2 consumption is met with by the anaerobic pathway.

2. Steady phase Steady phase of exercise is characterized by a maximum O_2 consumption (VO_2 max) throughout, i.e. a plateau phase of O_2 consumption and work done relationship. During this phase also, as mentioned above, the excess energy requirement is met with by the anaerobic pathway, i.e. by breakdown of creatine phosphate and muscle glycogen. As a result of anaerobic release of energy in the muscles, the blood levels of lactic acid begin to rise steeply when the oxygen consumption exceeds 2 L/min (Fig. 12.1.3). In the blood, lactic acid is buffered by the bicarbonate buffer as:

$$H^+ + HCO_3^- \Leftrightarrow H_2CO_3 \Leftrightarrow CO_2 + H_2O$$

The extra CO_2 so evolved is removed by hyperventilation. Since CO_2 evolved is more than O_2 consumed, the respiratory quotient (CO_2 evolved/O_2 consumed) may reach 1.5–2 during severe exercise.

The anaerobic mechanism of energy release permits an individual to utilize energy far in excess of the capacity for oxidative metabolism. The amount of energy that a person may draw from the anaerobic metabolism in the muscle is limited by his/her tolerance for metabolic acidosis produced by the lactic acid. Trained athletes have a greater tolerance for lactoacidosis than untrained individuals. Furthermore, trained athletes produce smaller amounts of lactic acid for a given amount of submaximal work than an untrained individual.

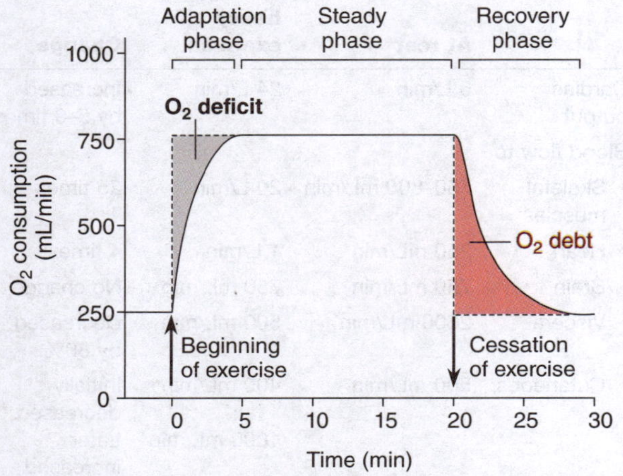

Fig. 12.1.2 Oxygen deficit and oxygen debt.

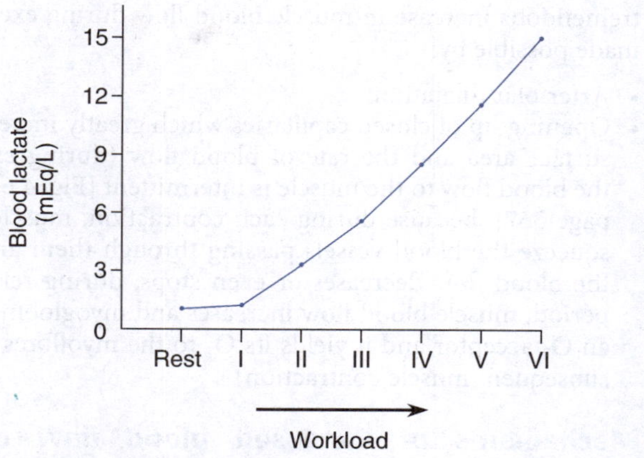

Fig. 12.1.3 The relationship between blood lactate and severity of exercise.

3. Recovery phase Recovery phase refers to the period after cessation of exercise during which extra amount of O_2 is consumed. The amount of extra O_2 consumed during recovery phase is called O_2 debt and is proportionate to the extent to which energy demands during exercise exceeded the capacity of aerobic synthesis of energy store, i.e. the extent to which *oxygen deficit* occurred during exercise. In other words, the O_2 deficit that occurs during exercise is repaid during the recovery phase, in the form of O_2 debt. The extra amount of O_2 consumed during recovery phase (O_2 debt) is used:

- To remove the excess lactate collected due to anaerobic glucose breakdown
- To replenish the ATP and phosphorylcreatine store
- To replace the small amount of O_2 that has come from myoglobin
- To resupply dissolved O_2 in tissue fluids and blood

During recovery phase, the respiratory quotient falls to low values since CO_2 is retained to form HCO_3^- and lactate is mobilized by the Cori's cycle.

B. CARDIOVASCULAR RESPONSES TO EXERCISE

To meet the increased energy demand of muscles during exercise, the primary cardiovascular response is in the form of:

- Increase in the skeletal muscle blood flow
- Redistribution of blood flow in the body
- Increase in the cardiac output
- Blood pressure changes
- Changes in blood volume

I. Skeletal Muscle Blood Flow

At rest, the blood flow to the skeletal muscle is about 2–4 mL/100 g/min of muscle tissue. Since the whole-body skeletal muscles weigh about 30 kg in adults, the total blood flow to the body muscles is about 750–800 mL/min which is about one-sixth of the cardiac output at rest. At rest, about 20%–25% of muscle capillaries have flowing blood.

During exercise: During strenuous exercise, muscle blood flow can increase up to 20 times, i.e. about 50–80 mL/100 g/min muscle tissue or greater than 20 L/min to the whole-body skeletal muscle mass. This is called *exercise hyperaemia*. This tremendous increase in muscle blood flow during exercise is made possible by:

- Arteriolar dilatation
- Opening up of closed capillaries which greatly increase the surface area and the rate of blood flow (during exercise, the blood flow to the muscle is intermittent [Fig. 4.6.13, see page 357], because during each contraction, muscle fibres squeeze the blood vessels passing through them and thus the blood flow decreases or even stops; during relaxation period, muscle blood flow increases and myoglobin acts as an O_2 acceptor and it yields its O_2 to the myofibres during subsequent muscle contraction)

Mechanisms of increased blood flow during exercise

1. Local metabolic control mechanism Local metabolic control mechanism is chiefly responsible for the tremendous increase in skeletal muscle blood flow during exercise (exercise hyperaemia) (see page 358). The muscle contraction increases the metabolic rate of tissue, which in turn reduces oxygen concentration in the muscle. The *decreased tissue pO_2* leads to vasodilation. In addition, in the exercising skeletal muscles, there occurs accumulation of carbon dioxide, lactic acid, potassium ions and hydrogen ions, and a rise in temperature. Each of these factors acts as a vasodilator. All these factors lead to dilatation of arterioles and precapillary sphincters, and a 10- to 100-fold increase in the number of open capillaries in the skeletal muscle. The accumulated metabolites also maintain some increase in blood flow during recovery from the exercise.

The regulation of blood flow by local metabolic factors is a self-adjusting mechanism as explained. Vasodilatation increases blood flow, which brings in more oxygen and nutrients, and washes away the accumulated metabolites. When the demand is no longer heavy, the enhanced blood flow tends to reverse the changes which initiated vasodilatation.

2. Neural control mechanism Vessels of the skeletal muscles are supplied by both sympathetic vasoconstrictor and sympathetic vasodilator fibres.

Sympathetic vasoconstrictor control: Most of the basal tone of the resistance vessels of skeletal muscle is myogenic with very little contribution by noradrenergic sympathetic nerve fibres. Thus, it is obvious that exercise hyperaemia is independent of sympathetic discharge and is mainly due to metabolic factors as described above.

Sympathetic vasodilator (cholinergic) fibres are unique to skeletal muscles. Previously, it was thought that these fibres are stimulated due to sympathetic overactivity in exercise and increase the blood flow to the muscles. However, now it has been established that the sympathetic vasodilator fibres dilate only the arterioles and not the precapillary sphincters and so do not increase the blood flow to muscles either during or before exercise (see page 358).

3. Humoral control mechanism The skeletal blood vessels contain both α-adrenergic and β-adrenergic receptors. During strenuous exercise, norepinephrine and epinephrine are released into the systemic circulation from the adrenal medulla which tend to produce vasoconstriction and vasodilatation by acting on α- and β-receptors, respectively. These two factors counter each other and hence may not contribute significantly to the increased skeletal blood flow during exercise. However, some authors do believe that adrenaline through the β-receptor-mediated vasodilation may contribute to increase in muscle blood flow before, during and after the exercise.

Blood flow through nonexercising muscles Blood flow through nonexercising muscles is also reported to increase during exercise. This may be because of the fact that sympathoadrenal discharge may not distinguish between the blood vessels of exercising and nonexercising muscles. However, blood flow in exercising muscles is increased more than in the nonexercising muscles because of the effect of local metabolic factors and intrinsic nerves.

II. Redistribution of Blood Flow

As mentioned earlier, the tremendous increase in skeletal muscle blood flow is possible due to increased cardiac output (discussed later in detail) and redistribution of cardiac output in the manner given next (Table 12.1.2).

Coronary blood flow Coronary blood flow at rest is about 250 mL/min (about 70 mL/100 g tissue/min) with 70%–80% coefficient of O_2 utilization. During exercise, coronary blood flow is increased by four to five times with 100% O_2 utilization. This occurs due to:

Increased coronary blood flow due to sympathetic stimulation by the following mechanisms:

- Increased activity of the heart
- Increased cardiac output ($\geq$5-fold)
- Increase in mean arterial pressure

Coronary vasodilatation produced by:

- Catecholamine
- Hypoxia
- Fall in blood pH
- ATP and ADP

Visceral blood flow Visceral blood flow is temporarily curtailed in coordination with increase in muscle blood flow. It is brought about by the increased sympathoadrenal

Table 12.1.2 Redistribution of blood flow during exercise

	At rest	During heavy exercise	Change
Cardiac output	5 L/min	24 L/min	Increased by 5–6 times
Blood flow to			
• Skeletal muscles	750–800 mL/min	20 L/min	25 times
• Heart	250 mL/min	1 L/min	4 times
• Brain	750 mL/min	750 mL/min	No change
• Visceral	2600 mL/min	500 mL/min	Decreased by 80%
• Cutaneous	500 mL/min	400 mL/min	Initially decreased
		1000 mL/min	Later increased

discharge. Renal and splanchnic vessels have only sympathetic noradrenergic vasoconstrictor fibres and they respond to adrenaline with vasoconstriction because they are furnished with α-adrenergic receptors.

Splanchnic blood flow Splanchnic blood flow is decreased by 80% in severe exercise.

Renal blood flow Renal blood flow is also decreased by 50%–80% in severe exercise. Prolonged, heavy exercise may produce a condition known as *athletic pseudonephritis*, which is characterized by increase in proteins, haematuria, cells and other abnormal substances in urine. It occurs because:

- Decreased renal blood flow produces glomerular capillary hypoxia and increases permeability to large molecules.
- Increase in urine proteins occurs in exercise.

Important Note

Athletic pseudonephritis is a transient condition that settles completely within 3–4 days of rest.

Cutaneous blood flow Cutaneous blood flow at rest is about 500 mL/min.

- *Decrease* in cutaneous blood flow occurs initially in the beginning of exercise due to reflex vasoconstriction.
- *Increase* in cutaneous blood flow is noted in sustained exercise when body temperature rises to dissipate the heat generated during exercise, as the blood flow through the skin is controlled predominantly by the requirements of temperature regulation.

Cerebral blood flow Cerebral blood flow at rest is about 750 mL/min and remains unchanged during any grade of muscular exercise. This is because the blood flow through the brain is governed primarily by local metabolites.

Adipose tissue blood flow Adipose tissue blood flow is increased by four times during exercise. This helps to deliver fatty acids mobilized from triglyceride stores to the working muscles.

III. Increase in Cardiac Output

Normal cardiac output is about 5–6 L/min. During exercise, the cardiac output is increased depending on the severity of exercise. In maximum exercise, it may increase by five to six times. Maximal cardiac output is greater in conditioned athletes than in unconditioned individuals (e.g. 30–35 L/min in Olympic-class runners compared with 15 L/min in unconditioned adults). Since cardiac output is the product of heart rate and stroke volume, an increase in both contributes to the increase in cardiac output during exercise (Fig. 12.1.4).

Increase in heart rate Heart rate increases linearly with the severity of exercise (Fig. 12.1.4) up to a maximum, which is determined by the subject's age. The *maximum heart rate* (HR max) is approximately equal to 210 − (0.65 × age [in years]), and is *unaffected by conditioning*. Increase in the heart rate causes palpitation that everyone has personally experienced during exercise. The increase in heart rate occurs as soon as exercise begins or may be seen even before the exercise begins (anticipatory tachycardia).

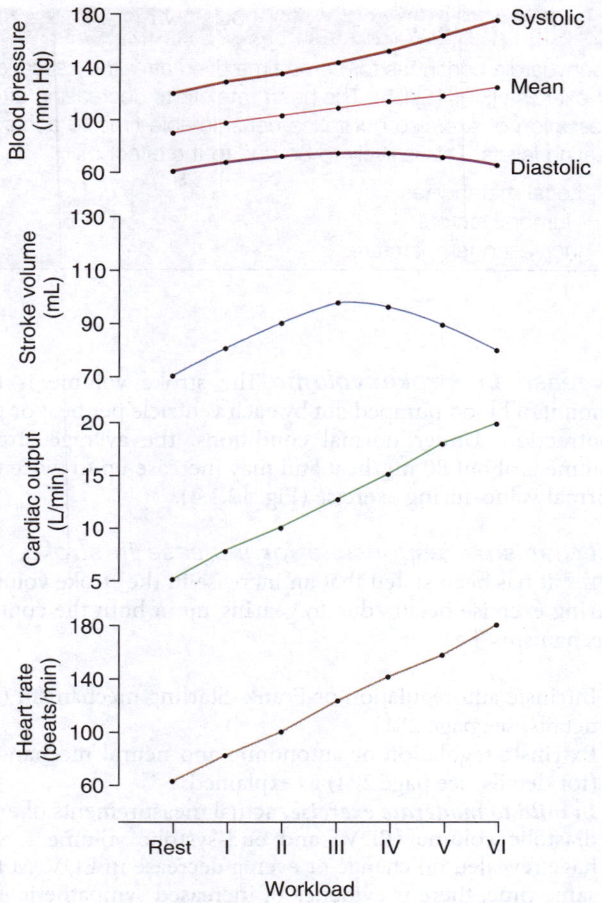

Fig. 12.1.4 Effect of severity of muscular exercise on cardiovascular functions.

Factors contributing to tachycardia Factors contributing to tachycardia during exercise are as follows:

Increased sympathetic discharge which originates centrally, probably from the subthalamic movement centre whenever there is an increase in motor activity, is responsible for tachycardia. Even the thought of exercise stimulates the hypothalamic defence area, bringing about intense sympathetic discharge and causing anticipatory tachycardia.

Peripheral reflexes originating from the exercising muscles (muscle spindles, muscle–tendon receptors and organ of Corti) and joints are responsible for the increase in heart rate which occurs as soon as exercise begins.

Local metabolic factors possibly contribute to the sustained increase in heart rate during prolonged exercise. Muscle tissue has free nerve endings that are stimulated by lactic acid, potassium ions and other metabolites, which collect in exercising muscles.

Humoral factors such as release of adrenaline and noradrenaline and possibly thyroid hormones during exercise also contribute to increase in heart rate during sustained exercise.

Intrinsic factor which increases the heart rate during exercise is the stimulation of SA node in the right atrium due to increased venous return. This is known as *Bainbridge reflex*.

Increased temperature in the myocardium due to increased activity of the heart during exercise may directly increase the rhythmicity of the pacemaker.

> **Important Note**
>
> Tachycardia continues for some time even after the cessation of exercise (Fig. 12.1.5). The heart rate starts decreasing after cessation of exercise but takes considerable time to achieve resting levels. This is likely to be due to the effect of:
>
> - Local metabolites
> - Humoral factors
> - Increased temperature

Increase in stroke volume The stroke volume is the amount of blood pumped out by each ventricle per beat or per contraction. Under normal conditions, the average stroke volume is about 80 mL/beat and may increase up to twice the normal value during exercise (Fig. 12.1.4).

Mechanisms responsible for increase in stroke volume It has been stated that an increase in the stroke volume during exercise occurs due to gearing up of both the control mechanisms, i.e.:

- Intrinsic autoregulation or Frank–Starling mechanism (for details, see page 281)
- Extrinsic regulation or autonomic and neural mechanism (for details, see page 284) as explained:
  In mild to moderate exercise, actual measurements of end-diastolic volume (EDV) and end-systolic volume (ESV) have revealed no change or even a decrease in EDV. At the same time, there is evidence of increased sympathetic discharge to the heart in the form of increased heart rate. It has been explained that *increased venous return* produced by skeletal vasodilatation, muscle pump action and increased respiration (thoracic pump) is tackled by *improved pumping of the heart* due to sympathetic activity and so the Frank–Starling mechanism does not operate. Therefore, it can be concluded that during mild to moderate exercise, the pumping ability of the heart is enhanced mainly by greater sympathetic discharge.
  In severe exercise, when venous return is large enough to raise the EDV, Frank–Starling mechanism also comes into play over and above the increased sympathetic discharge and thus results in very high cardiac output.

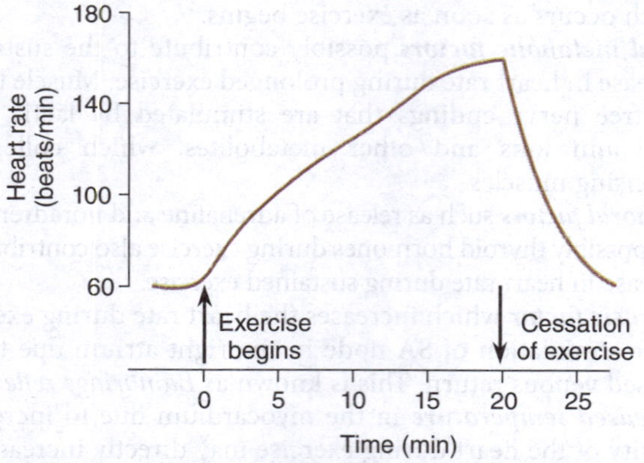

Fig. 12.1.5 Heart rate response to moderate exercise.

> **Important Notes**
>
> It is important to note that:
>
> - ***Starling's law of the heart*** does not allow further increase in stroke volume once the heart rate increases to 120/min.
> - ***Endurance training increases stroke volume*** of the heart by increasing the ventricular EDV. Thus, conditioned athletes can maintain any level of cardiac output at a lower heart rate than nonconditioned individuals.

IV. Blood Pressure Changes During Exercise (Figs 12.1.4 and 12.1.6)

In Systemic Circulation

Systolic blood pressure is always raised by exercise, since it depends on the cardiac output which is increased in exercise. The blood pressure remains elevated during exercise and is not reflexly corrected by baroreceptor reflex. This has been explained by the fact that the neurons descending from the hypothalamic defence centre inhibit the baroreceptor afferents.

Diastolic blood pressure which primarily depends on the peripheral resistance may mildly increase or decrease or remain unchanged depending on the change in total peripheral resistance. Mostly, the vasodilatation in the skeletal muscles balances the vasoconstriction in other tissues, so the diastolic blood pressure is usually not changed much.

Mean blood pressure is usually increased. It helps to increase the skeletal muscle blood flow by providing greater pressure head in the face of dilated resistance vessels.

In Pulmonary Circulation

Pressure in the pulmonary artery does not rise much during exercise due to intrathoracic location of blood vessels which provide low resistance to blood flow, and due to marked increase in the number of open capillaries in lungs during exercise.

Systolic blood pressure in pulmonary artery may rise during heavy exercise to 25–30 from 15–20 mm Hg at rest.

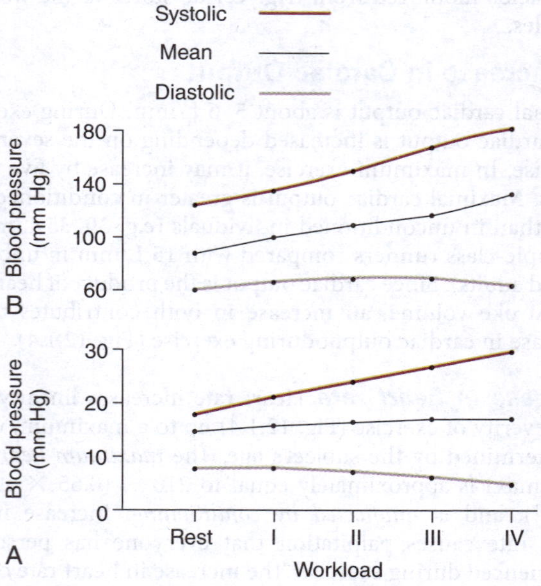

Fig. 12.1.6 Blood pressure response to exercise: **A**, pulmonary; and **B**, systemic.

Diastolic blood pressure may rise from 5–8 mm Hg at rest to 8–10 mm Hg.

Mean blood pressure may reach 15 from 8–12 mm Hg at rest.

V. Changes in Blood Volume During Exercise

Blood volume during exercise is decreased by 15% resulting in haemoconcentration. Blood volume is decreased due to more plasma loss at the capillary level due to the following reasons:

- Increased hydrostatic pressure in capillaries
- Increased tissue fluid osmotic pressure due to accumulation of osmotically active metabolites in tissue spaces such as potassium, phosphate and lactic acid

Advantages include:

Oxygen-carrying capacity of blood is increased because of increased concentration of red blood cells.

Buffering capacity of blood is increased due to increased concentration of plasma proteins.

Disadvantages are as follows:

Blood flow decreases due to increased viscosity of blood.

WBC count increases due to washing out of WBCs from storage places and bone marrow.

Summary of Cardiovascular Responses to Exercise

The cardiovascular responses to exercise are summarized in Fig. 12.1.7.

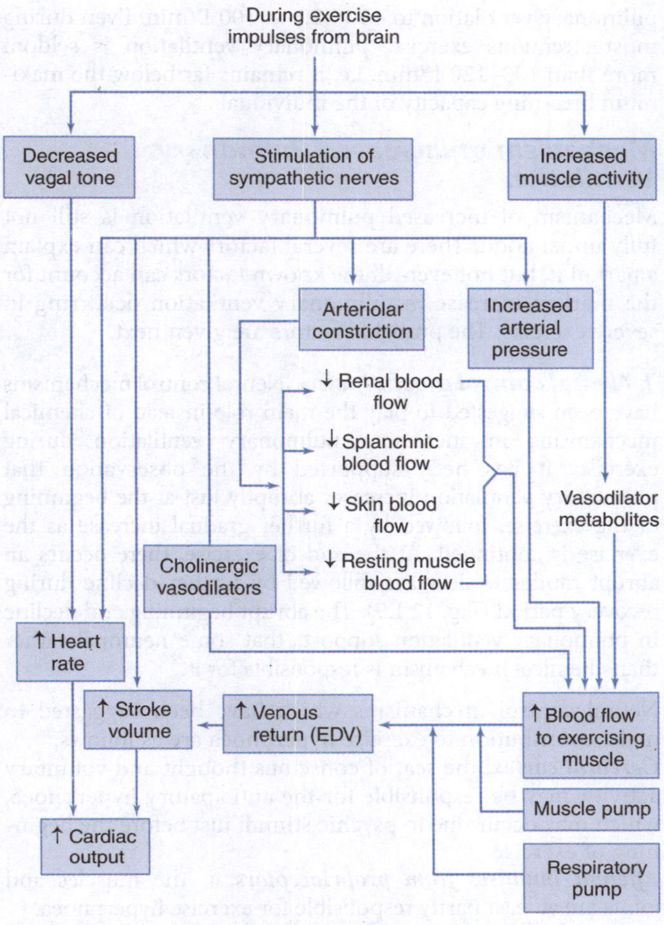

Fig. 12.1.7 Summary of cardiovascular responses to exercise.

C. RESPIRATORY RESPONSES TO EXERCISE

Exercise is the most frequently faced stress by the respiratory system in day-to-day life. During heavy exercise, up to 25-fold increase in O_2 consumption and CO_2 production may occur. The O_2 consumption does not decrease with training at any workload (i.e. training does not improve the body's efficiency unless muscle coordination is improved by practice). The respiratory system meets this metabolic demand so well that alveolar and arterial pO_2 and pCO_2 are practically maintained normal even during the most strenuous exercise. This is made possible by the following respiratory responses to exercise.

I. Increase in Pulmonary Ventilation

The pulmonary ventilation increases linearly with the increase in intensity of exercise (O_2 consumption) until the anaerobic threshold is reached (Fig. 12.1.8). Anaerobic threshold is defined as the level of activity (exercise) that produces an elevation of blood lactate levels, which results from a shift from aerobic to anaerobic metabolism. The anaerobic threshold occurs at a higher level of activity in conditioned athletes than in unconditioned individuals. The anaerobic threshold occurs at approximately 60% of the maximal exercise level, regardless of the level of physical fitness (Fig. 12.1.8). Above the anaerobic threshold, the pulmonary ventilation increases out of proportion to the increase in O_2 consumption because lactic acid that is generated imposes an additional respiratory drive. During this period, the arterial pCO_2 may drop significantly, because excretion of CO_2 exceeds production (Fig. 12.1.8).

Pulmonary ventilation increases because of increase in depth as well as rate of respiration. As the severity of exercise is gradually increased, the depth of breathing (tidal volume) rapidly increases to an optimum value, beyond which ventilation is chiefly increased by increase in the rate of respiration. During quiet breathing at rest, the respiratory rate is about 12–14/min and the tidal volume is about 0.5 L and hence the pulmonary ventilation is about 12 × 0.5 to 14 × 0.5 = 6–7 L/min. During heavy exercise, the rate of respiration may increase to 40/min and the tidal volume to 2.5 L, increasing

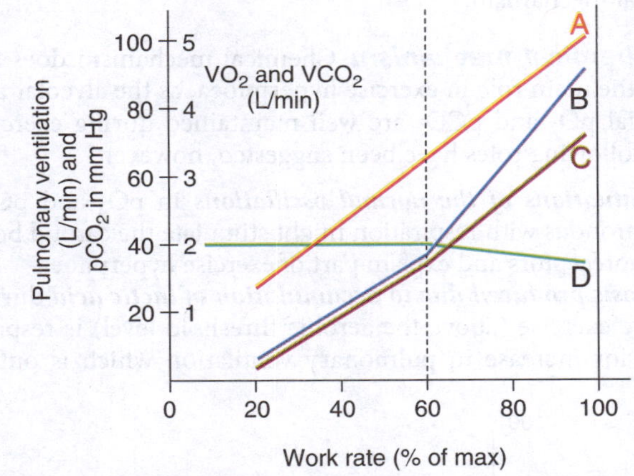

Fig. 12.1.8 The effect of exercise on respiratory parameters of gas exchange: **A**, pulmonary ventilation; **B**, CO_2 excretion in expired air (VCO_2); **C**, oxygen consumption (VO_2); and **D**, arterial pCO_2. The dashed line indicates onset of anaerobic threshold.

pulmonary ventilation to 40 × 2.5 = 100 L/min. Even during most strenuous exercise, pulmonary ventilation is seldom more than 100–120 L/min, i.e. it remains far below the maximum breathing capacity of the individual.

Mechanism of Increased Pulmonary Ventilation

Mechanism of increased pulmonary ventilation is still not fully understood. There are several factors which can explain a part of it, but not even all the known factors can account for the marked increase in pulmonary ventilation occurring in severe exercise. The probable factors are given next.

1. Neural control mechanisms Neural control mechanisms have been suggested to play the main role instead of chemical mechanisms in increasing pulmonary ventilation during exercise. It has been supported by the observation that pulmonary ventilation increases abruptly just at the beginning of the exercise, followed by a further gradual increase as the exercise is continued. At the end of exercise, there occurs an abrupt moderate decrease followed by further decline during recovery period (Fig. 12.1.9). The abrupt beginning and decline in pulmonary ventilation supports that some neuronal rather than chemical mechanism is responsible for it.

Neural control mechanisms which have been suggested to make contribution to exercise hyperpnoea are as follows:
Cerebral cortex, the seat of conscious thought and voluntary activity, may be responsible for the anticipatory hyperpnoea, which may occur due to psychic stimuli just before the beginning of exercise.
Afferent impulses from proprioceptors in the muscles and joints are at least partly responsible for exercise hyperpnoea.
Increase in body temperature during sustained exercise may also make some contribution to exercise hyperpnoea through neural mechanism.

2. Chemical mechanism Chemical mechanism does not play the main role in exercise hyperpnoea, as the alveolar and arterial pO_2 and pCO_2 are well maintained during exercise. The following roles have been suggested, however:

Accentuations of the normal oscillations in pO_2 and pCO_2 synchronous with respiration might stimulate the carotid body chemoreceptors and explain part of exercise hyperpnoea.
Acidosis produced due to accumulation of lactic acid during severe exercise (above the aerobic threshold level) is responsible for increase in pulmonary ventilation which is out of proportion to the O_2 consumption. During this period, arterial pCO_2 may drop significantly.

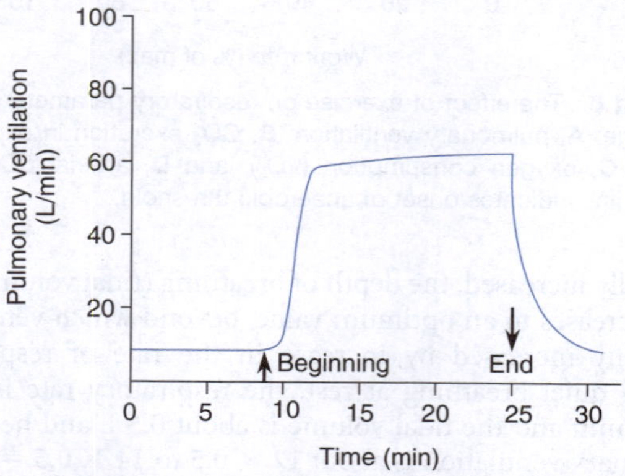

Fig. 12.1.9 Ventilatory response to mild exercise showing abrupt change at beginning and at the end of exercise.

3. Humoral mechanisms Humoral mechanisms are not reported to play any role in exercise hyperpnoea.

II. Increase in Oxygen Uptake in the Lungs

The oxygen uptake by blood in the lungs increases from 250 mL/min at rest to about 4 L/min during heavy exercise. This is made possible by the changes given next.

1. Increased pulmonary perfusion This happens due to increase in cardiac output from 5 L/min at rest to about 30 L/min during heavy exercise. This applies as much to the right ventricle as to the left. Thus, during exercise, about six times more blood passes through the lungs per minute and so more O_2 per minute is carried by the blood from the lungs.

2. Increased alveolar capillary pO_2 gradient During exercise, because of greater extraction of O_2 by the muscles, the O_2 content of the mixed venous blood reaching the lungs may be as low as 3 mL/100 mL of blood (compared with 14–15 mL% at rest). Thus, the alveolar capillary pO_2 gradient is increased due to marked desaturation of the venous blood and so more O_2 is taken up by the blood in the lungs.

3. Increased pulmonary diffusion capacity About sixfold increase in pulmonary blood flow due to increased cardiac output during exercise is not accompanied by rise in the pressure in the pulmonary capillaries. This is made possible by the opening of several pulmonary capillaries which are closed at rest. As a result, the alveoli are better perfused with blood. The larger number of opened-up capillaries increases the surface area available for diffusion. In this way, there occurs threefold increase in the diffusion capacity of the lungs from 21 mL/min/mm Hg at rest to about 65 mL/min/mm Hg during exercise.

D. CHANGES AT THE TISSUE LEVEL

The cardiovascular and respiratory changes described above supply large amounts of O_2 from the alveolar air to the blood and remove equally huge amounts of CO_2 from the blood to the alveoli and ultimately to the atmosphere. The changes at the tissue level which facilitate transfer of large amount of O_2 from the blood to the exercising muscles and that of CO_2 from the tissues to the blood are given next.

Blood flow Blood flow to the skeletal muscles is increased from 2 to 4 mL/min/100 g of muscles during strenuous exercise. Increased blood flow brings more O_2 to the tissue per minute. *Capillary bed* of the contracting muscles is dilated and many previously closed capillaries are open. Because of these changes, the mean distance from the blood to the tissue cells is greatly decreased; this facilitates movement of O_2 from the blood to the cells.

Gradient of pO_2 Gradient of pO_2 between capillary blood and tissue fluid is increased. This happens because during exercise, contracting muscles extract more O_2 from tissue fluid. Due to increased gradient of pO_2 between capillaries and tissue fluid, more O_2 is removed from the capillary blood into the tissue fluid.

O_2–Hb dissociation curve O_2–Hb dissociation curve shifts to the right due to accumulation of CO_2, rise in temperature and rise in red blood cell 2,3-DPG. This results in a threefold increase in O_2 extraction from each unit of blood. Since there is associated (about 30-fold) increase in muscle blood flow (as mentioned above), a net increase of about 100-fold in metabolic rate of muscle is possible during exercise.

E. ENDOCRINAL RESPONSES TO EXERCISE

Endocrines play an important role in adjustment to exercise. However, it has still not been fully elucidated. The hormones that are increased during exercise along with the role played by them are given next.

1. Antidiuretic hormone Antidiuretic hormone (ADH) secretion is markedly increased during exercise. It helps to maintain fluid balance by reducing urine flow so that enough fluid is available for excessive sweating required to dissipate heat.

2. Adrenocorticotropic hormone Adrenocorticotropic hormone (ACTH) is released during endurance events and probably helps by mobilizing fats for providing energy directly as well as by stimulating glucocorticoid secretion.

3. Endorphin Endorphin secretion is significantly increased during exercise. They improve tolerance to discomfort associated with exercise by relieving pain. They also relieve mental stress and induce a feeling of well-being.

4. Cortisol Cortisol secreted during exercise is helpful in reducing exercising stress. It also mobilizes proteins and fats. Fatty acids are particularly useful as fuel during exercise. Consequently, carbohydrates are spared to be used by the brain.

5. Aldosterone Aldosterone secreted during exercise reduces urinary loss of water and sodium like ADH. This helps to maintain fluid balance in the presence of excessive sweating during exercise.

6. Adrenaline and noradrenaline Adrenaline and noradrenaline secretion is increased significantly in intense exercise. These hormones mobilize fatty acids and glucose and thus improve the availability of fuel.

7. Insulin Insulin secretion is decreased during exercise. However, due to training tissue, sensitivity to insulin improves at rest and decreases during exercise. The improved sensitivity at rest accounts for the improvement in glucose tolerance test seen as a result of regular exercise. Because of this effect, exercise is considered one of the most useful components for the treatment of diabetes.

8. Glucagon Prolonged exercise stimulates secretion of glucagon. It mobilizes glucose from glycogen and fatty acids from the adipose tissue, and thereby improves fuel availability during prolonged exercise.

EFFECTS OF TRAINING

Training to the body tissues is provided by different sets of exercise regimes. Endurance training (aerobic) produces different effects in the skeletal muscles than weight training. Training effects are specific for the particular muscle groups involved. Only aerobic exercises produce cardiovascular conditioning.

Usefulness of training to the body systems is highlighted:

- Training is most essential for the performance by athletes and sports persons, and it forms the main aspect of sports physiology.
- Training by regular physical exercise is likely to slow the ageing process, and helps to prevent several degenerative and metabolic diseases and thereby makes life healthier and longer.
- One of the clear-cut benefits of exercise regime is psychological; patients who exercise regularly 'feel better'. Such effects may also be attributed to release of endorphins during exercise. Endorphins are reported to relieve mental stress and induce a sense of well-being, and even euphoria.
- Regular exercise is one of the most useful components of treatment of diabetes because it reduces insulin requirement by virtue of improvement in glucose tolerance.
- There is some evidence that regular exercise decreases the incidence and severity of myocardial infarctions, although there continues to be debate on this point.

Effects of training on the body tissues can be described as:

- Effects of training on the cardiovascular system
- Effects of training on the respiratory system
- Effects of training on skeletal muscles
- Psychological effects of training

I. EFFECTS OF TRAINING ON CARDIOVASCULAR SYSTEM

Athletic training by regular exercise has a favourable influence on cardiovascular functions. Only aerobic exercises produce cardiovascular conditioning. *Optimal cardiovascular conditioning* requires attaining a heart rate of 60%–70% of the maximum for 20–30 minutes, three to four times a week for at least 3 months. Athletic training produces the effects given next on the cardiovascular system.

1. Low resting heart rate Athletic training by some unknown mechanism increases the vagal tone. Consequently, trained athletes have a low resting heart (50–60/min). This is useful during exercise because it increases the range through which the heart rate can increase without any change in the maximal heart rate. The maximal heart rate (HR max) is approximately equal to 210 − (0.65 × age [in years]), and is unaffected by conditioning.

2. Higher resting stroke volume The aerobic athletic training leads to cardiac hypertrophy and increase in EDV which increase the resting stroke volume to about 105 mL compared with about 75 mL in an untrained individual.

3. Much larger cardiac output during exercise Because of the low resting heart rate and higher resting stroke volume, a trained athlete can achieve much larger cardiac output during exercise than an untrained individual as illustrated in Table 12.1.3 by arbitrary but plausible figures. An Olympic-class runner can achieve a maximal cardiac output of about 30–35 L/min compared with only 15 L/min in unconditioned adults.

Table 12.1.3 Effect of aerobic training on cardiovascular functions

	At rest		During maximal exercise	
	Untrained individual	Trained athlete	Untrained individual	Trained athlete
Heart rate (beats/min)	72	50	180	180
Stroke volume (mL/beat)	75	100	100	160
Cardiac output (L/min)	5	5	18	29

II. EFFECTS OF TRAINING ON RESPIRATORY SYSTEM

1. Increase in Maximal Oxygen Consumption

The O2 consumption does not decrease with training at any workload, i.e. training does not improve the body's efficiency unless muscle coordination is improved by practice.

Maximal O_2 consumption (VO_2 max) increases by 5%–20% by conditioning (athletic training) because of:

- Increase in cardiac output
- Increase in arteriovenous O_2 difference

Values of VO_2 max (arbitrary but plausible) are as follows:

- Average untrained male: 3600 mL/min
- Average trained male: 4000 mL/min
- Male marathon runner: 5100 mL/min

Of course, the maximum oxygen consumption increases during training, but high values in marathon runners may be partly genetically determined by factors such as large lung capacity in relation to body size and strength of respiratory muscles.

2. Increase in Maximal Minute Ventilation

Endurance (aerobic) training increases maximal minute ventilation that is achieved during exercise but does not improve the maximum voluntary ventilation.

- Specific respiratory muscle training allows one to increase the duration and intensity of exercise.

3. Increase in Pulmonary Oxygen-Diffusing Capacity

The oxygen-diffusing capacity is the rate at which O_2 diffuses from the alveoli into the blood per millimetre of mercury oxygen pressure. During exercise, diffusing capacity increases in a nonathlete from a resting value of 23 to 48 mL/min/mm Hg. Athletic training allows more increase in diffusion capacity of the lungs for oxygen because by training, the pulmonary capillary density increases.

4. No effect on Vital Capacity

There is no consistent effect of training on vital capacity or other measures of pulmonary function. It implies that, in a healthy individual, pulmonary function is usually not a limiting factor in determining the maximum intensity of exercise that one can undertake.

III. EFFECTS OF TRAINING ON SKELETAL MUSCLES

Regular muscular exercise may lead to the changes given next in the muscles.

Increased Muscle Strength

Increased muscle strength due to training results from:

Increase in muscle mass which is entirely the result of an increase in the size of muscle fibres (*hypertrophy*) and not due to increase in the number of muscle fibres (hyperplasia). Furthermore, it is observed that increase in muscle strength is out of proportion to the increase in muscle mass. Other factors which contribute to increase in muscle strength are as follows:

More effective and efficient deployment of motor units

Increase in the production of contractile proteins such as actin and myosin which is mediated by somatomedins (the increased amount of contractile proteins increases the cross-bridges available for generating force during muscle contraction)

Changes in the Muscle Fibres

Changes in the muscle fibres that enhance the capacity of the muscles to extract more O_2 and improve the ability of the muscle fibres to provide energy during prolonged exercise are as follows:

- Increase in the capillary network which is demonstrated as significant increase in the capillary to muscle fibre ratio on muscle biopsy
- Increase in the number of mitochondria in muscle fibres
- Increase in the mitochondrial enzymes involved during oxidative metabolism
- Increase in the muscle glycogen stores
- Increase in the stored triglycerides

Fast- and Slow-Twitch Muscle Fibres and Different Types of Exercise

Fast-twitch muscle fibres generate a great amount of power in a short period of time, such as during a sprint. In other words, the fast-twitch fibres give a person the ability to rapidly and forcefully contract his/her muscles. Fast-twitch fibres are able to generate more power because:

- They are about twice as large in diameter as slow-twitch fibres.
- The enzymes that release energy from the phosphagen and glycogen lactic acid energy systems are two- to threefold as active in the fast-twitch fibres.

Slow-twitch fibres are used in endurance exercise, i.e. prolonged lower leg muscle activity, such as marathons. The difference in the activities of fast-twitch and slow-twitch muscle fibres is because of the differences given next between the two types of muscle fibres. Slow-twitch fibres use more for endurance exercise while employing the anaerobic system of energy because in comparison to fast-twitch fibres, they contain:

- Higher number of mitochondria
- More myoglobin, which is a haemoglobin-like substance that combines with oxygen in muscle
- More capillary density

Training results in metabolic drift of both fast- and slow-twitch fibres towards the mitochondrial characteristics of slow muscle fibres, which are better suited for endurance events.

IV. PSYCHOLOGICAL EFFECTS OF TRAINING

Regular training improves the psychology of the individual and thus the psychic stimuli to vasomotor centre and respiratory centres are reduced. Consequently, during exercise, there occurs:

- Less increase in sympathetic activity
- Less decrease in parasympathetic activity

V. METABOLIC EFFECTS OF TRAINING

Metabolic adjustments during exercise are the result of increase in energy stores and mitochondrial changes in the muscles described above. Due to these changes, the ability of the muscle to extract oxygen improves and there is shift towards aerobic metabolism, which is more efficient than anaerobic metabolism. Consequently, there is less accumulation of lactic acid and smaller fall in the pH of the body fluids. These changes facilitate mobilization of fatty acids from tissue stores into the blood. Shift in metabolism towards more utilization of fats is a very useful adaptation because fat stores are virtually unlimited compared with the extremely meagre glycogen store. So, fat utilization spares glycogen. As physical performance is a direct function of glycogen stores, endurance of the individual increases.

Summary of Effects of Training

In nutshell, physical training decreases the O_2 deficit and thus increases the physical performance or fitness, which is inversely related to O_2 deficit. In summary, the physical training decreases O_2 deficit by the following effects:

1. ***Increasing maximal O_2 consumption (VO_2 max)*** because of:

Greater increase in cardiac output due to:
- Low resting heart rate
- High resting stroke volume

Increase in arteriovenous O_2 difference

2. *Increasing oxygen availability* by:
   - Increasing pulmonary diffusion

3. *Enhancing the capacity of the muscles to extract more O_2* due to:
   - Increase in capillary network in the muscle
   - Increase in the number of mitochondria in muscle fibres
   - Increase in the mitochondrial enzymes

4. *Increasing the strength of muscles* by hypertrophy

5. *Increasing the endurance of muscles* by:
   - Metabolic changes leading to more utilization of fats as energy store
   - Sparing of glycogen (physical performance is a direct function of glycogen stores)

6. *Psychological improvement makes it possible to perform better during exercise* with:
   - Less increase in sympathetic activity
   - Less decrease in parasympathetic activity

All the aforementioned factors help in decreasing the dependence on anaerobic mechanism.

Self-Assessment

1. Discuss the oxygen consumption during exercise.
2. Discuss the cardiovascular and respiratory responses to exercise.
3. Discuss the effect of training on exercise response.
4. Describe briefly the following:
   - Phases of oxygen debt
   - Role of catecholamine during exercise

12.2 Environmental Physiology

CHAPTER OUTLINE

HIGH-ALTITUDE PHYSIOLOGY

INTRODUCTION

Atmosphere refers to the medium in which aerospace physiology occurs. This is divided into the following major zones:

- *Troposphere* extends from sea level to about 18 km (58,000 feet).
- *Stratosphere* extends from 18 to 50 km. The so-called *ozone layer* is found between 12 and 44 km.
- *Mesosphere* extends from 50 to 85 km.
- *Thermosphere* extends from 85 to 700 km.
- *Exosphere* extends beyond 700 km and is called true outer space.

Critical altitudes which are important from the physiological point of view are as follows:

- *At 10,000 feet altitude*, usually no symptoms or some degree of hypoxia may be present, but the body can easily acclimatize to the lack of oxygen. Therefore, *high altitude* is classically defined as an altitude in excess of 10,000 feet (3 km).
- *An altitude of 18,000 feet* is the highest altitude at which permanent inhabitation is possible.
- *Above 20,000 feet altitude*, hypoxia can endanger life, unless O_2 is added to the inhaled air.
- *At an altitude of about 35,000 feet*, modern aircraft commonly fly. The use of pressurized cabins in these aircraft helps to provide an environment similar to that at sea level.
- *Above 40,000 feet altitude*, the ozone layer starts.

Composition of air and effect of altitude on it: Composition of air (Table 12.2.1) does not change with altitude, i.e. composition of atmosphere (percentage of gases) remains constant from sea level to about 30,000 feet.

Barometric pressure and partial pressure of gases: Barometric pressure at sea level is 760 mm Hg and it falls progressively with the increasing height (Table 12.2.2). With decrease in total pressure of air at increasing altitude, partial pressure of gases will change as:

According to Dalton's law, the total pressure of air (*P*) is equal to the sum of partial pressures of the gases contained, i.e. $P = pO_2 + pCO_2 + pN_2 + pH_2O$.

pH_2O in alveolar air at sea level is 47 mm Hg (Table 12.2.2). It is entirely determined by the body temperature and does not change with altitude. As the body can regulate and maintain the temperature at 37°C, pH_2O remains constant at 47 mm Hg.

pCO_2 in alveolar air at sea level is 40 mm Hg (Table 12.2.2) and depends on the metabolic production of the body. As the metabolic production of CO_2 does not alter with increasing altitude, the alveolar pCO_2 does not change with altitude until the breathing is affected by the effect of hypoxia.

pO_2 and pN_2 in alveolar air at sea level are 104 and 569 mm Hg, respectively. With increasing altitude, there is decrease in total pressure of air. So, the pO_2 and pN_2 levels will decrease proportionately (as the pH_2O and pCO_2 remain unchanged).

Values of pO_2 in alveolar air and atmospheric air at different altitudes are shown in Table 12.2.2.

Changes in the body at high altitude are produced mainly by hypoxic *hypoxia* produced by falling pO_2. *Other factors* which produce changes in the body at high altitude are effects of expansion of gases, fall in atmospheric temperature, light rays and gravity.

HYPOXIA AT HIGH ALTITUDE

The effects of hypoxic hypoxia produced by decreasing pO_2 at high altitude depend on:

- The level of altitude
- Rate at which hypoxia develops, i.e. hypoxia occurs due to rapid ascent (acute hypoxia) or slow ascent (subacute hypoxia)

Table 12.2.1 Concentration and partial pressure of gases in atmospheric air and alveolar air

Gas	Atmospheric air: Concentration (%)	Atmospheric air: Partial pressure (mm Hg)	Alveolar air: Concentration (%)	Alveolar air: Partial pressure (mm Hg)
Nitrogen	78.62	597.0	74.9	569
Oxygen	20.84	159.0	13.6	104
Carbon dioxide	0.04	0.3	5.3	40
Water vapour	0.50	3.7	6.2	47
Total	**100**	**760.0**	**100**	**760**

Table 12.2.2 Barometric pressure, pO_2 and common effects at different altitudes

Level of altitude (feet [km])	Barometric pressure (mm Hg)	Atmospheric air pO_2 (mm Hg)	Alveolar air pO_2 (mm Hg)	Alveolar air pCO_2 (mm Hg)	Percentage oxygen saturation of haemoglobin	Common effects	Stage of hypoxia
0 (sea level)	760	159	104	40	100	Nil	–
5000 (1.5)	630	130	80	40	95	No effects	
10,000 (3)	520	110	60	40	90	Usually no symptoms except at night, there may be some reduction in visual capacity	**Stage of indifference** • The rapid ascent up to *10,000 feet is* safe zone of ascent • Classically, high altitude is in excess of 10,000 feet • No hypoxia up to pO_2 60 mm Hg
15,000 (4.5)	480	90	50	36	80	Effects of hypoxia in the form of CVS and respiratory system symptoms	**Stage of reaction** • At altitude 10,000–15,000 feet • Moderate hypoxic symptoms due to pO_2 40–60 mm Hg
18,000 (5.5)	400	80	40	30	70	Above-mentioned effects of hypoxia plus hypoxic symptoms due to involvement of CNS	**Stage of disturbance** • At altitude 15,000–20,000 feet • Severe hypoxia due to pO_2 30–40 mm Hg • Needs to be treated with O_2 therapy
20,000 (6)	350	70	<40	<30	<70	Hypoxic symptoms due to CNS involvement aggravate; unconsciousness occurs when Hb saturation falls below 60%	
30,000 (9)	226	47	21	24	20	Severe hypoxic symptoms even with oxygen therapy	**Critical stage** • Survival is not possible without O_2 therapy above 20,000 feet altitude called *critical* survival altitude
40,000 (12)	140	30	12	24	15		

- Duration of exposure to hypoxia, i.e. whether short-term stay or long-term stay (chronic hypoxia)

Barometric Pressure and pO_2 at Different Altitudes and its Effect on the Body

The barometric pressure, partial pressure of oxygen (pO_2) and common effects at different altitudes are given in Table 12.2.2.

Stages of Hypoxic Hypoxia

In a classical mould, four stages of hypoxic hypoxia depending on the value of pO_2 are described (Table 12.2.2):

1. ***Stage of indifference*** is usually characterized by no symptoms of hypoxia as pO_2 remains above 60 mm Hg. This occurs up to an altitude of 10,000 feet.
2. ***Stage of reaction*** starts above 10,000 feet altitude and is characterized by development of moderate hypoxia up to 15,000 feet altitude at pO_2 levels of 40–60 mm Hg. Hypoxic symptoms include:
   - *Cardiovascular involvement* in the form of tachycardia and hypertension
   - *Respiratory symptoms* in the form of increased pulmonary ventilation
   - *Early CNS involvement* in the form of impaired judgement, feeling of overconfidence, talkativeness, reduction in visual acuity, emotional outburst of laughing or crying, etc.
3. ***Stage of disturbance*** occurs when pO_2 values fall between 30 and 40 mm Hg, usually between 15,000 and 20,000 feet altitude. It is characterized by development of severe hypoxia. In addition to the symptoms described above, the CNS involvement is aggravated.
4. ***Critical stage*** occurs above 20,000 feet altitude and survival is not possible without O_2 therapy.

Clinical Types of Hypoxic Hypoxia at High Altitude

Clinically, three types of hypoxia occurring at high altitude are described:

1. Fulminating hypoxia
2. Acute hypoxia
3. Chronic hypoxia (for details, see page 451)

Applied Aspects

Clinical Syndromes Caused by High Altitude

The three specific entities (clinical syndromes) which need to be discussed in relation to the effects of low pO_2 at high altitude are as follows:

- High-altitude pulmonary oedema (HAPO)
- Acute mountain sickness
- Chronic mountain sickness

High-Altitude Pulmonary Oedema

HAPO usually occurs as an effect of rapid ascent at high altitude (above 10,000 feet).

Individuals who develop HAPO: It is seen in the following individuals:

- About 75%–80% of individuals who engage in heavy physical work during the first 3–4 days after rapid ascent to high altitude develop HAPO.
- Individuals who are acclimatized to high altitude, stay for more than 2 weeks at sea level and then rapidly reascend at high altitude develop HAPO.

Mechanism of development of HAPO: Since HAPO does not develop in individuals who ascend slowly at high altitude and avoid physical exertion for the first few days, the mechanism of development of HAPO may probably be the following: Sympathetic activity increased by physical work is over and above the sympathetic stimulation caused by hypoxia (due to low pO_2) and cold (as the temperature falls by 2°C for every 1000 feet increase in altitude). The resultant marked increase in sympathetic activity produces vasoconstriction leading to increase in pulmonary capillary hydrostatic pressure. Normally, pulmonary capillary hydrostatic pressure, which is less than 10 mm Hg, and osmotic pressure of 25 mm Hg keep the alveoli dry. Thus, increased pulmonary capillary hydrostatic pressure drives the fluid out of the pulmonary capillaries producing pulmonary oedema. When the hypoxia is very severe, even generalized oedema may develop by a similar mechanism.

Characteristics of HAPO include:

- It responds to rest and O_2 therapy because it occurs due to aggravation of hypoxia and not due to cardiovascular or lung disease.
- It is associated with increased pulmonary artery pressure; it also responds to calcium channel blockers such as nifedipine, which lowers the pulmonary artery pressure.

Signs and symptoms are fatigue, tightness of chest, dyspnoea, cough on exertion and cyanosis.

Diagnosis is mainly based on X-ray chest showing patchy alveolar infiltration with a normal-sized heart.

Treatment includes rest and oxygen therapy.

Acute Mountain Sickness

Individuals who ascend to high altitudes gradually do not develop severe effects of hypoxia because the body gets some time to adjust to it.

Acute mountain sickness refers to the symptom complex which occurs in an individual residing at sea level who ascends to a high altitude over a period of 1–2 days for the first time. The symptoms develop between 8 and 24 hours after arrival at high altitude, and last for 4–8 days.

Characteristic features of acute mountain sickness are headache, nausea, vomiting, irritability, insomnia and breathlessness.

Cause of acute mountain sickness is not definitely known, but it appears to be associated with cerebral oedema or alkalosis.

Mechanism of cerebral oedema: The low pO_2 at high altitude causes arteriolar dilation which is normally compensated by cerebral autoregulation. However, once the limit of the cerebral circulation autoregulatory mechanism is reached, there occurs an increase in capillary pressure that favours increased transudation of fluid into brain tissue.

Treatment: The symptoms of acute mountain sickness can be reduced by:

Decreasing cerebral oedema by administration of large doses of glucocorticoids

Decreasing alkalosis by administration of acetazolamide (acetazolamide decreases H^+ excretion through kidneys by inhibiting the enzyme carbonic anhydrase)

Chronic Mountain Sickness

Chronic mountain sickness *(Monge disease)* occurs in some long-term residents of high altitude who develop extreme polycythaemia, cyanosis, malaise, fatigue and exercise intolerance. These individuals must be removed to a lower altitude to prevent rapid development of fatal pulmonary oedema.

Physiological Compensatory Responses to High-Altitude Hypoxia

Two types of physiological compensatory responses known to occur in individuals exposed to high-altitude hypoxia are accommodation and acclimatization.

Accommodation refers to immediate reflex adjustments of the respiratory and cardiovascular systems to hypoxia (for details, see page 453).

Acclimatization refers to changes in the body tissues in response to long-term exposure to hypoxia, such as when a person living at sea level goes and stays at high altitude for a long time (for details, see page 453).

OTHER EFFECTS OF HIGH ALTITUDE

Factors other than hypoxia which produce changes in the body at high altitude are as follows:

- Effects of expansion of gases
- Effects of fall in atmospheric temperature
- Effects of light rays

Effects of expansion of gases According to Boyle's law of gases, the pressure (P) of a given mass of gas is inversely proportional to its volume (V), i.e. $p \propto 1/V$.

Therefore, at high altitude, barometric pressure and partial pressure of a gas are decreased, and its volume is increased. For example, if at sea level, with atmospheric pressure of 760 mm Hg, the volume of a given gas is 1 L:

- *At an altitude of 18,000 feet* where atmospheric pressure is about 400 mm Hg, the volume of gas increases to about *2 L*.
- *At an altitude of 30,000 feet* where atmospheric pressure is about 225 mm Hg, the volume of the gas increases to about *3 L*.

Rapid decompression Rapid decompression refers to a situation in which the body is suddenly exposed to low atmospheric pressure. Such a situation may be encountered when the cabin pressure failure accidentally occurs in an aircraft flying at high altitude. Immediately, all the body gases expand as expected as per Boyle's law of gases.

Effects of expansion of gases in the body are as follows:

In the gastrointestinal tract, the expansion of gases may cause painful distension of the stomach and intestines. This effect can be reduced by supporting the abdomen by a belt or by evacuation of gases while ascending rapidly.

In the lungs, the expansion of gases may sometimes destroy the alveoli.

In the paranasal sinuses, the expansion of gases may cause tissue damage.

Decompression sickness may occur in an aviator if he/she is exposed to an ambient altitude in excess of about 22,000 feet (below this altitude, decompression sickness is almost nonexistent). This may happen as a corollary to rapid decompression.

Effects of Fall in Atmospheric Temperature

The atmospheric temperature falls by 2°C for every 1000 feet increase in altitude above sea level. Therefore, at different altitudes, the atmospheric temperature changes as follows:

- At an altitude of 10,000 feet, it is about 0°C.
- At an altitude of 20,000 feet, it is about −22°C.
- At an altitude of 40,000 feet, it is about −44°C.

Effects of low temperature on the human body depend not only on the atmospheric temperature but also on the wind velocity and humidity. The high wind velocity, as well as high humidity, makes the cold more severe. For example, an atmospheric temperature of 0°C, if accompanied by a wind velocity of 70 km/h, is equivalent to a temperature of −20°C when the air is still. Due to this, one feels colder while riding a motorcycle as compared with while walking, or standing still.

In general, the effects of low temperature on the body can be described as:

- Effects of acute cold exposure (see page 1206)
- Effects of long-term cold exposure (see page 1206)

Effects of Light Rays

At high altitude, atmosphere filters less of ultraviolet (UV) radiations; with every 1000 m increase in altitude, UV level increases by 10%–20%. UV rays at high altitude also cause many hazardous effects such as skin irritation; exposure to UV radiations is a major risk factor for skin cancer.

PHYSIOLOGY OF HIGH ATMOSPHERIC PRESSURE

INTRODUCTION

Atmospheric pressure of 760 mm Hg at sea level is considered 1 atm pressure.

Pressure increases by 1 atm for a depth of every 10 m (33 feet) as one descends under water. Thus, a person under sea at a depth of 10 m (33 feet) is exposed to a pressure of 2 atm, 1 atm due to the air above the sea level and another 1 atm due to 10 m column of water. As the depth under water increases, the pressure also increases proportionately (Table 12.2.3).

Decrease in volume of gases occurs due to compression as the pressure increases under water. According to Boyle's law, the volume to which a given quantity of gas is compressed is inversely proportional to the pressure. Therefore, 1 L of volume of air at sea level with 1 atm pressure compresses to 0.5 L volume at a depth of 10 m under water, where pressure is 2 atm. With further increase in the pressure, the volume decreases proportionately (Table 12.2.3).

High atmospheric pressure is met under the following conditions:

- Deep sea diving
- Going under the sea in submarines
- Caisson workers, i.e. the persons who dig underwater tunnels work in a chamber (caisson chamber) in which atmospheric pressure is high to prevent entry of water

Physiological problems associated with life under high pressure may be classified as:

- Physiological problems at depth (due to compression effect of high atmospheric pressure)

Table 12.2.3 Effect of sea depth on pressure and volume of gas

Depth (m [feet])	Pressure (atm)	Volume (L)
Sea level	1	1
10 (33)	2	1/2 (0.5)
20 (66)	3	1/3 (0.33)
30 (100)	4	1/4 (0.25)
40 (133)	5	1/5 (0.2)
50 (166)	6	1/6 (0.167)
60 (200)	7	1/7 (0.143)
90 (300)	10	1/10 (0.1)
120 (400)	13	1/13 (0.077)
150 (500)	16	1/16 (0.062)

- Physiological problems of ascent (due to decompression phenomenon)

PHYSIOLOGICAL PROBLEMS: UNDER DEPTH

If appropriate preventive measures are not taken, then the individuals working at depth under water will face the physiological problems given next.

Physiological problems due to mechanical effects of high atmospheric pressure At a depth of more than 30 m (100 feet), due to the mechanical effects of increased atmospheric pressure, there may occur:

- Caving in of the chest
- Damage to the face
- Squeezing of air in the paranasal sinuses and middle ear

Physiological problems due to effect of high pressure on respiratory gases Air under high atmospheric pressure is breathed under water. At high atmospheric pressure, the partial pressure of oxygen (pO_2), nitrogen (pN_2) and carbon dioxide (pCO_2) also increases, producing the physiological problems given next.

Applied Aspects

1. Effects of Increased pO_2 (Oxygen Toxicity)

Oxygen toxicity may be acute or chronic.

Acute oxygen toxicity occurs on exposure to 4 atm pressure of oxygen (pO_2 in lungs is approx 3000 mm Hg).

- Acute oxygen poisoning is typically characterized by nervous system complications as the *brain tissue is especially susceptible to acute oxygen poisoning*.
- *Mechanism of damage to the nervous system* is as described. At 4 atm pressure, the amount of oxygen dissolved is markedly increased to 9 mL/100 mL compared with about 2 mL at 1 atm. This raises the tissue pO_2 level. At high tissue pO_2, the molecular oxygen is converted into active oxygen, i.e. superoxide anion (O_2^-) which is a free radical. The oxygen free radicals oxidize the polyunsaturated fatty acids of the cell membranes as well as the cellular enzymes, thus damaging the cellular metabolic system severely. Nervous tissues, because of their high lipid content, are especially susceptible to damage by oxygen free radicals producing nervous complications.
- *Nervous complications of acute oxygen poisoning* include disorientation, dizziness, convulsions and even coma.

Chronic oxygen toxicity occurs due to prolonged exposure (8–24 hours) to oxygen at 1 or 1.5 atm pressure. Chronic oxygen poisoning causes the following bronchopulmonary problems:

Irritation of airways in the form of nasal congestion, sore throat, substernal discomfort, sneezing, coughing and bronchoconstriction may occur after 8 hours of exposure.

Pulmonary oedema and atelectasis begin to develop after 12 hours of exposure.

Bronchopneumonia may be initiated when exposure is continued for more than 24 hours. It is initiated because of inhibition of ability of lung macrophages to kill bacteria, and decreased production of surfactant.

2. Effects of Increased pN_2 (Nitrogen Narcosis)

The partial pressure of nitrogen (pN_2) rises in the blood when an individual is made to breathe compressed air for an hour or more at high atmospheric pressure, deep underwater. Due to increased pN_2, the nitrogen dissolves *gradually* into the body fluids and more easily into fats. The cell membrane of neurons contains high lipid content, so more nitrogen is dissolved in the neurons of the brain. The nitrogen dissolved in the cell membranes of neurons alters the ionic conductance through the membrane, and finally decreases the neuronal excitability, producing nitrogen toxicity known as nitrogen narcosis.

Nitrogen narcosis is characterized by:

- *At a depth of about 120 feet* (4–5 atm pressure), there occurs euphoric symptoms. The individual becomes jovial and carefree. These are followed by impairment of mental functions and intelligence.
- *At a depth of 150–200 feet* (about 6–7 atm pressure), the individual becomes drowsy and has poor muscular coordination.
- *At a depth of 200–250 feet* (7–8 atm pressure), the individual becomes extremely fatigued, weak and in stupor.
- *Beyond a depth of 250 feet* (above 8 atm pressure), there occurs deep narcosis and the individual becomes unconscious and insensitive to stimuli (anaesthetized) and ultimately may even die.

Important Note

It is important to note that very short-lasting dives do not result in nitrogen narcosis, no matter how deep. This is because the nitrogen takes time to get dissolved.

3. Effects of Carbon Dioxide Build-up

Carbon dioxide build-up occurs when the individual rebreathes the CO_2 which he/she produces. This happens in the absence of an apparatus which absorbs CO_2 or releases expired CO_2 into the atmosphere. With the passage of time, pCO_2 in the body fluids may build up to reach toxic levels. The maximum tolerated CO_2 build-up is up to an alveolar pCO_2 of 80 mm Hg, beyond which respiratory acidosis and carbon dioxide narcosis may occur.

Physiological Problems of Ascent

The two physiological problems which occur when an individual ascends back to sea level after sufficient exposure to high atmospheric pressure in the deep sea are as follows:

- Decompression sickness
- Air embolism

1. Decompression Sickness

Decompression sickness is also known as caisson disease, dysbarism, compressed air sickness, the bends and divers' palsy.

Causes of Decompression Sickness

As discussed earlier, under high atmospheric pressure (deep in the sea), the nitrogen present in the breathed air is dissolved in the body fluids and fats in considerably increased amounts. When the individual ascends rapidly to sea level after sufficient exposure to high atmospheric pressure deep underwater, nitrogen is decompressed and escapes from the tissues at a faster rate. Being gas, it forms bubbles while escaping rapidly from the tissues. The gas bubbles block the blood vessels producing tissue ischaemia, and, sometimes, result in tissue death. The symptoms produced by escaping gas bubbles constitute *decompression sickness*.

Symptoms of Decompression Sickness

Symptoms of decompression sickness are caused by the escape of nitrogen bubbles from the various tissues and are as follows:

Pain in joints and muscles of the legs or arms is the most frequently occurring symptom. The joint pain accounts for the term '*bends*' that is often used to describe decompression sickness. Pain is produced due to the escape of nitrogen bubbles from the myelin sheath of sensory nerves supplying the joints and muscles.

Sensation of numbness, tingling or pricking (paraesthesia) and itching may also be produced due to the escape of bubbles from the myelin sheath of sensory nerves.

The chokes may also occur in patients with decompression sickness. They refer to serious shortness of breath, which is often followed by severe pulmonary oedema, and, occasionally, even death. This is caused by a massive number of microbubbles plugging the capillaries of the lungs.

Paralysis of muscles may occur temporarily due to escaping nitrogen bubbles from the myelin sheath of motor nerves. This is called *divers' palsy* (one of the names of this disease).

Coronary ischaemia or myocardial infarction may occur due to blockage of coronary capillaries by the nitrogen bubbles.

Neurological symptoms like dizziness, paralysis of muscles, or collapse and unconsciousness may occur due to blockage of blood vessels of the brain and spinal cord.

Treatment of Decompression Disease

Treatment of decompression disease includes:

- *Tank decompression* is used for treatment of decompression disease. The diver, i.e. the affected individual, is placed in a pressurized tank and recompression is done, first to dissolve the N_2 bubbles, and then the pressure is lowered gradually back to normal atmospheric pressure. In this way, a slow decompression is performed so that the body can get rid of N_2 without producing any harmful effects.

2. Air Embolism

Air embolism is another physiological problem which may occur during rapid ascent from a depth below the sea level.

Cause of Air Embolism

Air embolism, i.e. entry of air into the blood circulation, occurs following a rupture of pulmonary capillaries, arteries and veins caused by sudden expansion of gases in the lungs due to a sudden fall in the atmospheric pressure (*explosive decompression*). Such a situation may typically occur in deep sea divers or caisson workers who breathe oxygen–helium mixture at high pressure. A similar situation may also occur in rockets (i.e. spacecraft in which high pressure is maintained according to height of ascent). Due to accidental leakage in a pressurized cabin, sudden reduction in pressure occurs, causing expansion of gases in the lungs.

Manifestations of air embolism include chest pain, tachypnoea, systemic hypotension and hypoxaemia. In severe cases, air emboli may travel to the systemic circulation, block the blood flow to some vital organs and may even result in death.

Prevention of Physiological Problems Occurring at Depth and on Ascent.

We have studied that without appropriate preventive measures, physiological problems occur at depth (oxygen toxicity and nitrogen narcosis) and on ascent (decompression disease and air embolism). So, professional sea divers and caisson workers must adopt some preventive measures to avoid occurrence of these problems.

Measures for Short-Duration Dive Up to 20 m

A short-duration dive up to 20 m is made safe by adopting a simple and safe strategy in which the divers take a few rapid and deep breaths before diving which washes off carbon dioxide; nitrogen does not get enough time to dissolve and oxygen toxicity cannot occur as the diver holds the breath. Traditionally, pearls and sponge divers have been adopting this strategy.

Measures for Deeper and Longer Dives

Deeper and longer dives can be made safer by adopting the preventive measures given next.

1. Use of Breathing Apparatus. Use of breathing apparatus which delivers gas to breathe and either absorbs carbon dioxide (closed-circuit apparatus) or releases carbon dioxide as bubbles into the surroundings (open-circuit apparatus) helps in making deeper and longer dives safer. An example of such an apparatus is self-contained underwater breathing apparatus (SCUBA) diving gear.

SCUBA diving: SCUBA is a compact arrangement for breathing which the diver can carry with him/her under water. In this apparatus, the air is compressed so that more air is carried in less volume and also the gas amounts to a substantial quantity even when the ambient pressure is high. The cylinder of compressed air is connected via a mask and tube for breathing through a valve. The valve ensures that whenever the diver makes an inspiratory effort, an appropriate quantity of compressed air is delivered and the expired air is released into the water (outside the apparatus). The amount of gas in SCUBA required for a deeper dive is more than that for a less deep dive.

2. Use of Breathing Mixture Containing Helium and Oxygen at Low Concentration. Use of a breathing mixture containing helium and oxygen at low concentration is less harmful than breathing natural air because:

Low oxygen concentration prevents occurrence of oxygen toxicity.

Helium when replaced with nitrogen provides the following advantages:

- Because of its smaller molecules and lower density than nitrogen, it is easier to breathe, it diffuses faster and it is easier to eliminate its bubbles from the body.
- The amount of helium trapped in the body under high atmospheric pressure is much less than that of nitrogen because its solubility in the body fluids is less than half that of nitrogen.
- Being less toxic than nitrogen, its narcotic effect is only one-fifth that of nitrogen.

3. Slow Ascent or use of Decompression Tank. Slow ascent with short stay at regular intervals, i.e. slow and stepwise ascent, ensures that only a small amount of bubbles is formed at a time. These bubbles are eliminated before further ascent. In this way, decompression sickness can be prevented effectively.

Decompression tank is based on the principle of slow ascent. After a rapid ascent, the individual is placed in a pressurized tank whose pressure is lowered gradually to normal atmospheric pressure. Usually, no decompression is required after a 30-m dive for less than 30 minutes. Decompression for a period of 3 hours is required for a 60-minute dive at a depth of 60 m, and for a 20-minute dive at a depth of 100 m.

Self-Assessment

1. Discuss the clinical effects of hypoxia at high altitude.
2. Describe the following:
   - Physiological problems faced under depth
   - Pathophysiology of decompression sickness
3. Write notes on the following:
   - SCUBA diving
   - Air embolism
   - Acute mountain sickness

Clinical Cases

Case 1

A labourer from a village in Uttar Pradesh was appointed by a construction company at high altitude. He started hard work of digging immediately after reaching. He felt tired and after 2 hours, he developed dry cough, breathlessness and feeling of tightness of the chest and was shifted to the emergency. On the basis of history, onset and signs and symptoms, the probable diagnosis made was high-altitude pulmonary oedema.

Q1. What investigative tests should be done to confirm the diagnosis?
Q2. What is the pathophysiology of this condition?
Q3. What is the immediate treatment?
Q4. How can this condition be prevented?

Case 2

During Armed Forces training, a trainee was doing diving practice. About 2 hours after finishing the practice, he developed dizziness, pain in the left knee, blurring of vision and shortness of breath.

Q1. What is this condition called?
Q2. What is the pathophysiology of this condition?
Q3. What is the immediate treatment?
Q4. What are the preventive measures for this condition?

12.3 Physiology of Acid–Base Balance

CHAPTER OUTLINE

GENERAL CONSIDERATIONS

ACIDS AND BASES

Acids and bases: Acid refers to a substance that acts as proton (H^+) donor, whereas base refers to a substance that accepts proton (H^+). Examples of a few acids and their corresponding bases are:

Acid	*Base*
HCl	$H^+ + Cl^-$
H_2CO_3	$H^+ + HCO_3^-$

Alkalies refer to metallic hydroxides, e.g. NaOH and KOH. These compounds do not directly satisfy the criteria of bases. However, they dissociate to form metallic ion and OH^- which being the base accepts H^+ ions. Therefore, for all practical purposes, alkalies are considered bases.

Strong acids and bases: Acid or base having a strong tendency to dissociate into ions is called strong acid or strong base, and the acid or base having a weak tendency to dissociate into ions is called weak acid or weak base. In general, a strong acid has a weak base, whereas a weak acid has a strong base. For example, strong acid HCl has weak base Cl^-, and weak acid HCN has a strong base CN^-.

Ampholytes refer to the substances that can act as both acids and bases. Water is the best example of an ampholyte.

CONCEPT OF pH AND H^+ CONCENTRATION

H^+ ion concentration: The acidic or basic nature of a solution is measured by H^+ ion concentration. Since the concentration of H^+ ions in biological fluids is exceedingly low, the conventional units such as milliequivalent per litre or moles per litre are not commonly used to express H^+ ion concentration. For example, the normal Na^+ concentration of arterial plasma is about 140 mEq/L, whereas H^+ ion concentration is 0.00004 mEq/L.

pH is the term suggested to express H^+ ion concentration. It is defined as the negative logarithm of H^+ concentration.

$$pH = -\log\left[H^+\right]$$

It is important to note that pH and $[H^+]$ are inversely related. For example, pH of plasma with an H^+ ion concentration of 0.00004 mEq/L is 7.4, whereas pH of HCl with an H^+ ion concentration of 150 mEq/L is 0.8.

Neutral pH, acidic pH and alkaline pH: Pure water has an equal concentration of H^+ and OH^- ions, i.e. 10^{-7} M each. Thus, pure water has pH of 7 which is neutral. Therefore, solutions with pH less than 7 are considered acidic and those with pH more than 7 are considered alkaline.

H^+ CONCENTRATION AND pH OF BIOLOGICAL FLUIDS

The H^+ concentration and pH of some biological fluids are depicted in Table 12.3.1.

MAINTENANCE OF BLOOD pH

GENERAL CONSIDERATIONS

Blood and Plasma pH

- The term blood pH always refers to plasma pH.
- Normal plasma pH is 7.4 (H^+ concentration ~40 nEq/L), which is higher than the intracellular pH of the erythrocyte (7.2).
- Plasma pH compatible with life varies from 7.7 to 6.9 (H^+ concentration is 20–120 nEq/L).

Table 12.3.1 H^+ concentration and pH of biological fluids

Fluid	H^+ concentration nEq/L	mol/L	pH
1. Pure water	100	1×10^{-7}	7.0
2. Blood			
• Normal mean	40	3.98×10^{-8}	7.4
• Normal range	44–36	4.36×10^{-8} to 3.6×10^{-7}	7.36–7.44
• Acidosis (severe)	126	1.26×10^{-7}	6.9
• Alkalosis (severe)	20	2.00×10^{-8}	7.7
3. Cerebrospinal fluid (CSF) (normal range)	44–36	4.36×10^{-8} to 3.6×10^{-7}	7.36–7.44
4. Gastric juice (pure)	100,000,000	1×10^{-1}	1.0
5. Pancreatic juice	10	1×10^{-8}	8.0
6. Urine			
• Normal average	1000	1×10^{-6}	6.0
• Maximum acidity	31,600	3.16×10^{-5}	4.5
• Maximum alkalinity	10	1×10^{-8}	6.0
7. Intracellular fluid (ICF)	158	1.58×10^{-7}	6.8

- At rest, normal pH of mixed venous blood is 7.38 compared with 7.41 of arterial blood, because of uptake of CO_2 by blood as it perfuses the tissues.
- Normally, the pH of extracellular fluid (ECF) is maintained between a narrow range of 7.35 and 7.45.

Dietary and Metabolic Production of Acids and Bases

The daily consumed diet contains many acids and alkalies. The diet rich in animal proteins results in acid production, whereas the vegetarian diet has an alkalizing effect on the body. In addition, cellular metabolism produces a number of acidic and alkaline substances that have an impact on the body pH. Finally, alkalies are normally lost in the faeces. As a net result, the dietary and metabolic products add some acid to the body fluids, which need to be excreted daily at an equivalent rate so that acid–base balance can be maintained. If acid addition exceeds excretion, acidosis results, and, conversely, if acid excretion exceeds addition, alkalosis results.

Acid production by the body The metabolic activities of the body are accompanied by production of two types of acids.

1. Volatile acids CO_2 is the volatile acid produced from the aerobic metabolism of cells. It is also a major end product in oxidation of carbohydrates, fats and amino acids. CO_2 accounts for greater than 12,000 mEq/L of H^+ per day. It is considered acid, because CO_2 combines with H_2O (by a reaction catalysed by carbonic anhydrase [CA]) to form weak acid H_2CO_3, which dissociates into H^+ and HCO_3 by the following reaction:

$$CO_2 + H_2O \xrightleftharpoons{CA} H_2CO_3 \rightleftharpoons H^+ + HCO_3^-$$

It is called volatile, because it is a gas, and under normal circumstances, almost all the CO_2 is excreted by lungs.

2. Nonvolatile acids Nonvolatile acids, also called fixed acids, contribute about 50–100 mEq H^+ per day, depending on the diet. *These include:*

- *Sulphuric acid*, a product of sulphur-containing amino acids such as cysteine and methionine
- *Phosphoric acid*, a product of phospholipid metabolism
- *Hydrochloric acid*, a product of amino acids such as lysine, arginine and histidine
- *Organic acids* are other fixed acids that may be overproduced in disease:
  - *Lactic acid* produced in conditions of severe exercise, hypovolaemia and circulatory shock
  - *Acetic acid* and *β-hydroxybutyric acid* produced in conditions of starvation and uncontrolled diabetes mellitus
  - *Uric acid* produced in metabolism of nucleoproteins

Production of bases by the body In normal circumstances, a negligible amount of bases is formed in the body.

- *HCO⁻* produced by the metabolism of organic anions (e.g. citrate) offsets nonvolatile acid production to some degree.
- *Ammonia* produced in the amino acid metabolism is converted to urea; hence, its contribution as a base in the body is insignificant.

DEFENCES AGAINST CHANGES IN H^+ CONCENTRATION

There are three lines of defence to regulate the body's acid–base balance and maintain the blood pH (around 7.4):

I. ***Buffer systems of body fluid:*** These:
  - Form the first line of defence
  - Act instantaneously in ECF
  - Immediately combine with H^+ to prevent changes in H^+ concentration and form a temporary measure to control changes in H^+ concentration

II. ***Respiratory mechanism*** to regulate acid–base balance:
  - Forms the second line of defence
  - Acts within a few minutes
  - Acts via the respiratory centre to regulate removal of CO_2 (and therefore H_2CO_3)
  - Forms a short-term measure to regulate changes in H^+ concentration

III. ***Renal mechanism*** to regulate acid–base balance:
  - Forms the third line of defence
  - Takes days or weeks
  - Is slow, but is the most powerful and effective in regulating pH
  - Acts by reabsorbing filtered HCO_3, generating new HCO_3^- and excreting H^+ as titrable acid and ammonium ion
  - Thus, provides a permanent solution to acid–base balance

I. BUFFER SYSTEM: PRIMARY DEFENCE

A buffer is a solution, consisting of a weak acid and its salt with a strong base, which prevents a change in pH when H^+ ions are added to or removed from a solution. Buffers are most effective within 1.0 pH unit of the pK of the buffer (i.e. in the linear portion of the titration curve). Buffering capacity is dependent on the absolute concentration of salt and acid. It must be borne in mind that a buffer cannot remove H^+ ions from the body. It temporarily acts as a shock absorbent to reduce the free H^+ ions. The H^+ have to be ultimately eliminated by the renal mechanism.

When acid is added to a buffer solution, its H^+ ion concentration is increased and the reaction is forced towards right leading to increase in undissociated molecules; therefore, increase in H^+ concentration is less.
When base is added to buffer, reaction shifts towards left; more H^+ ions are released from the buffer to combine with base, thereby limiting the decrease in H^+ concentration.

Henderson–Hasselbalch equation which is used to calculate the pH in a buffer system can be derived as follows: the general equation for a buffer is

$$HA \rightleftharpoons H^+ + A^-$$

A^- represents any anion from a buffer (i.e. H^+ acceptor) and HA the undissociated acid from a buffer (i.e. H^+ donator). By the law of mass action, at equilibrium:

$$K = \frac{[H^+][A^-]}{[HA]} \quad (1)$$

where K is the dissociation constant of the acid HA.

The equation to represent free H^+ ion in a solution can be rewritten as:

$$[H^+] = K = \frac{HA}{[A^-]}$$

$$\text{We know that pH} = \log\frac{1}{[H^+]} \quad (2)$$

By taking the reciprocals and logarithms (for log, multiplication becomes addition):

$$\log\frac{1}{[H^+]} = \log\frac{1}{K} + \log\frac{[A^-]}{[HA]} \quad (3)$$

$$\text{As } \log\frac{1}{K} = pK$$

Equation (3) may be rewritten as:

$$pH = pK + \log\frac{[A]}{[HA]}$$

From this equation, it is evident that buffering capacity of a buffer system is greatest when amount of anions [A] and undissociated acid [HA] is same, i.e.:

$$\frac{[A^-]}{[HA]} = 1, \text{ or } \log\frac{[A^-]}{[HA]}$$

Thus, pH = pK. Therefore, most effective buffers in the body are those with pK close to the pH in which they operate.

Isohydric principle states that when there is a change in H^+ concentration in the ECF, balance of all the buffer systems changes at the same time. According to this principle, all buffers in a common solution are in equilibrium with the same H^+ concentration, i.e.:

$$[H^+] = K_1 \times \frac{HA_1}{A_1} = K_2 \times \frac{HA_2}{A_2} = K_3 \times \frac{HA_3}{A_3}$$

where:

- K_1, K_2 and K_3 are dissociation constants of the three acids.
- HA_1, HA_2 and HA_3 are undissociated acids.
- A_1, A_2 and A_3 are the concentrations of free negative anions.

Classification of the buffer systems Buffer systems in the body can be classified by different methods.

A. Bicarbonate versus nonbicarbonate buffers Bicarbonate versus nonbicarbonate buffers include:

1. *Bicarbonate buffer* forms 53% of the buffering in the whole body. Out of it:
   - Plasma HCO_3^- contributes 35%.
   - Erythrocyte HCO_3^- contributes 18%.
2. *Nonbicarbonate buffers* form remaining 47% of the buffering in the whole body, with a contribution from:
   - Haemoglobin and oxyhaemoglobin 35%
   - Plasma proteins 7%
   - Organic phosphate 3%
   - Inorganic phosphate 2%

B. Extracellular versus intracellular buffers Extracellular versus intracellular buffers are as follows:

1. *Bicarbonate* (HCO_3^-) is the major extracellular buffer, which is produced from CO_2 and H_2O.
   - The pK of the CO_2/HCO_3^- buffer pair is 6%.
2. *Phosphate* is a minor extracellular buffer.
   - The pK of H_2PO^-/HPO^{2-} buffer pair is 68%.
   - Phosphate is most important as urinary buffer; excretion of H^+ as $H_2PO_4^-$ is called titrable acid.
3. *Plasma proteins* form the nonbicarbonate buffer in the blood and are responsible for 7% of the total buffering of blood.
4. *Haemoglobin*, though found intracellularly, is more conventionally regarded as part of the extracellular system (as described later).

C. Intracellular buffers Intracellular buffers include:

1. *Organic phosphates* include AMP, ADP, ATP and 2,3-diphosphoglycerate (2,3-DPG).
2. *Proteins* of the skeletal muscle form 6 mEq/L.
3. *HCO_3^-* present in intracellular fluid (ICF) of skeletal and cardiac muscles constitutes 12 mEq/L.
4. *Haemoglobin* is an intracellular buffer but is considered an extracellular buffer as mentioned above.

Major Buffer Systems of the Body

The major buffer systems involved in the maintenance of body pH are as follows:

- Bicarbonate buffer
- Phosphate buffer
- Protein buffer

1. Bicarbonate Buffer System

The carbonic acid–sodium bicarbonate (H_2CO_3–$NaHCO_3$) is the most predominant buffer system of the ECF and particularly the plasma H_2CO_3 in the body is formed by CO_2 and H_2O:

$$CO_2 + H_2O \xrightarrow{\text{carbonic anhydrase}} H_2CO_3$$

This reaction is catalysed by the enzyme CA, which is present in the RBCs, walls of the lungs, alveoli and epithelial cells of renal tubules.

Dynamics of bicarbonate buffer system Carbonic acid dissociates into hydrogen and bicarbonate ions:

$$H_2CO_3 \rightleftharpoons H^+ + HCO_3^-$$

According to Henderson–Hasselbalch equation for this system:

$$pH = pK + \log\frac{[HCO_3^-]}{[H_2CO_3]} \quad (4)$$

The p*K* for the system in an ideal solution is low (about 3), and the amount of H_2CO_3 is small and hard to measure accurately. However, in the body, H_2CO_3 is in equilibrium with CO_2, i.e.:

$$H_2CO_3 \rightleftharpoons CO_2 + H_2O$$

If the p*K* is changed to pK_1 and CO_2 is substituted for H_2CO_3, the pK_1 is 6.1:

$$pH = 6.10 + \log\frac{[HCO_3^-]}{[CO_2]} \quad (5)$$

Since the amount of dissolved CO_2 is proportionate to the partial pressure of CO_2 and the solubility coefficient of CO_2 in millimole per litre per millimetre of mercury is 0.0301, the clinically relevant form of this equation is as follows:

$$pH = 6.10 + \log\frac{[HCO_3^-]}{[0.0301\ pCO_2]} \quad (6)$$

$[HCO_3^-]$ cannot be measured directly but can be calculated from the values of pH and pCO_2 which can be measured with suitable accuracy using pH and pCO_2 glass electrodes.

Blood pH and the ratio of HCO_3^- to H_2CO_3: The pH of arterial plasma with normal CO_2 tension (pCO_2) of 40 mm Hg and normal HCO_3^- concentration of 24 mmol/L can be calculated from Equation (6) as follows:

$$\begin{aligned} pH &= 6.10 + \log\frac{24\ \text{mmol/L}}{0.301 \times 40\ \text{mm Hg}} \\ &= 6.10 + \log\frac{24}{1.2} \\ &= 6.1 + \log 20 \\ &= 6.1 + 1.3 \\ &= 7.4 \end{aligned}$$

The pK_1 of this system (6.1) is still low, relative to the pH of the blood (7.4), but the system is one of the most effective buffer systems in the body because the amount of dissolved CO_2 is controlled by respiration, and plasma concentration of HCO_3 is regulated by the kidney. Therefore, pH of ECF can be precisely controlled.

Actions of bicarbonate buffer system Actions of bicarbonate buffer system are as follows:

1. Effective buffering of H^+: It is evident that at a blood pH 7.4, the ratio of bicarbonate to carbonic acid is 20%. Thus, the bicarbonate concentration is much higher (20 times) than that of carbonic acid in the blood. This is referred to as alkali reserve and is responsible for effective buffering of H^+.

Addition of strong acid, e.g. HCl, is followed by buffering of H^+ by the following reaction:

$$\uparrow H^+ + HCO_3^- \rightarrow \text{More } H_2CO_3 \rightarrow CO_2 + H_2O$$
$$\downarrow$$
$$\text{Elimination of } CO_2 \leftarrow \uparrow \text{Respiration}$$

2. Effective buffering of base: On addition, the strong base (e.g. NaOH) is converted into a weak base ($NaHCO_3$), as shown:

$$NaOH + H_2CO_3 \rightarrow NaHCO_3 + H_2O \rightarrow Na^+ + HCO_3^-$$

- As a consequence, the concentration of H_2CO_3 decreases and that of HCO_3 increases. Therefore, more CO_2 combines with H_2O to form new carbonic acid.

$$H_2O + CO_2 \rightleftharpoons H_2CO_3$$

- Decrease in CO_2 (as above) inhibits the respiration, leading to correction of CO_2 deficiency.
- Increase in HCO_3^- is corrected by increased renal excretion of HCO_3^-.

2. Phosphate Buffer System

Inorganic orthophosphate buffer system Inorganic orthophosphate buffer system is formed by sodium dihydrogen phosphate and disodium hydrogen phosphate ($NaH_2PO_4 \sim Na_2HPO_4$), which exist at a plasma pH of 7.4 in a concentration ratio of 1:4.

Sites of operation of NaH_2PO_4–Na_2HPO_4 buffer

1. ***In ECF (plasma and interstitial fluid)***, the $HPO_4^{2-}/H_2PO_4^-$ buffer exists in small concentration (0.66 mmol/L) and thus contributes little to the buffering capacity of plasma. However, it is important to note that this buffer pair with a p*K* of 6.8 would be a more effective buffer than HCO_3^-/CO_2 system (p*K* = 6.1) if it were present in an appreciable concentration.
2. ***In ICF***, the $HPO_4^{2-}/H_2PO_4^-$ forms an important buffer pair because:
   - Its concentration in ICF is high (6 mmol/L).
   - Its p*K* (6.8) is much closer to pH of ICF (6.9).
3. ***In renal tubules***, the $HPO_4^{2-}/H_2PO_4^-$ forms an effective extracellular buffer because:
   - Phosphate becomes greatly concentrated in the tubular fluid due to reabsorption of H_2O.
   - pH of tubular fluid and urine is more acidic than the pH of ECF, i.e. is close to p*K* of phosphate buffer. The $HPO_4^{2-}/H_2PO_4^-$ system is a major elimination route for H^+ via the urine (see page 516).

Mechanism of action of $HPO_4^{2-}/H_2PO_4^-$ This nonbicarbonate buffer system can buffer both noncarbonic and carbonic acid.

- It equilibrates as:

$$H_2PO_4^- \rightleftharpoons H^+ + HPO_4^{2-}$$

- *On addition of strong acid*, e.g. HCl, it forms a weak acid:

$$HCl + Na_2HPO_4 \rightleftharpoons \underset{\text{(weak acid)}}{NaH_2PO_4} + NaCl$$

- *On addition of strong base*, e.g. NaOH, it forms a weak base:

$$NaOH + NaH_2PO_4 \rightleftharpoons \underset{\text{(weak base)}}{Na_2HPO_4} + H_2O$$

Organic phosphate buffer system Organic phosphates (such as AMP, ADP, ATP and 2,3-DPG) exist in quantitatively significant amount in ICF (8.4 mmol/L), giving this compartment the capacity to effectively buffer both noncarbonic and carbonic acids, as well as alkali.

3. Protein Buffer System

The protein buffer system of the blood is constituted by the plasma proteins and haemoglobin combinedly. The buffering capacity of proteins is dependent on the *pK* of ionizable groups of amino acids. The *imidazole group of histidine* (*pK* 6.7) is the most effective contributor of protein buffers.

Plasma protein buffer system Plasma protein buffer system accounts for 15% of the buffering capacity of the whole blood. Plasma proteins are effective buffers because both their free carboxyl and free amino groups dissociate:

$$RCOOH \rightleftharpoons RCOO^- + H^+;$$

$$pH = pK_1\ RCOOH + \log\frac{[RCOO^-]}{[RCOOH]}$$

$$RNH_3^+ \rightleftharpoons RNH_2^+ + H^+;$$

$$pH = pK_1\ RNH_3 + \log\frac{RNH_2^+}{RNH_3}$$

Because of their amphoteric nature, plasma proteins can combine with acids and bases as:

In acidic pH, the NH_2 group of the proteins acts as a base and accepts protons and is converted to NH_3.
In alkaline pH, the –COOH group of the proteins acts as an acid and can donate a proton and thus becomes COO^-.
At normal pH of blood, proteins act as acids and combine with cations (mainly sodium).

Haemoglobin buffer system Haemoglobin buffer system (Hb/HHb and $HbO_2^-/HHbO_2$) accounts for 35% of the total buffering capacity of the whole blood. It mainly buffers the fixed acids, besides being involved in the transport of gases (O_2 and CO_2).

Haemoglobin – intracellular versus extracellular buffer concept: Haemoglobin, though found intracellularly, is more conventionally regarded as part of the extracellular buffer system because:

- Haemoglobin is confined to the erythrocytes which are a cellular component of ECF.
- Haemoglobin is readily available for the buffering of extracellular acids.
- Haemoglobin is the primary noncarbonated buffer of the body.

Buffering system in haemoglobin is provided by dissociation of imidazole group of histidine residues:

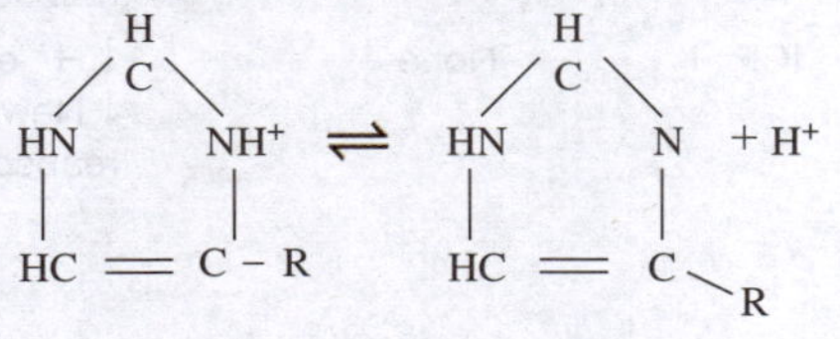

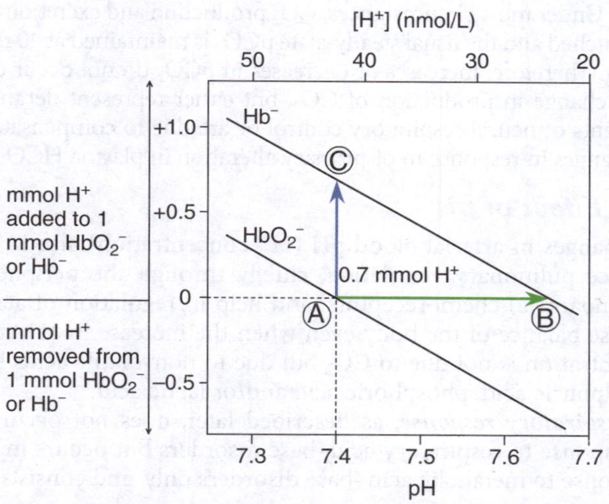

Fig. 12.3.1 Titration curves for oxyhaemoglobin and deoxyhaemoglobin (for explanation, see text).

Hb is a major buffer in blood; although between pH 7 and 7.7, it contributes relatively less to buffering capacity. This is because:

- Haemoglobin molecules are present in large amounts. One litre of whole blood contains about 150 g (2.3 mmol) of haemoglobin.
- Haemoglobin molecule contains 38 histidine residues.

Deoxyhaemoglobin (Hb) is a better buffer than oxyhaemoglobin (HbO_2), because the imidazole groups of Hb dissociate less than those of HbO_2, making Hb a weaker acid.

Titration curves for Hb and HbO_2 (Fig. 12.3.1) illustrating the importance of haemoglobin as a buffer indicate that:

- The complete deoxygenation of 1 mmol of HbO_2 to liberate 1 mmol of O_2 results in the neutralization of 0.7 mmol of H^+ without a change in pH (arrow AC in Fig. 12.3.1). Such a reaction is called *isohydric buffering*.
- When the oxyhaemoglobin (HbO_2) at pH 7.4 is completely reduced to deoxyhaemoglobin (Hb), there occurs an increase in pH (arrow AB in Fig. 12.3.1).

II. RESPIRATORY MECHANISM FOR pH REGULATION

Second line of defence against acid–base disorders is formed by the respiratory mechanism, which provides a short-term but rapid control. It acts via the respiratory centre, located in the medulla to regulate removal of CO_2 and, therefore, carbonic acid (H_2CO_3) concentration in the blood.

Role of Respiratory Centres

Respiratory centres are influenced by both CO_2 and H^+ concentrations – through central and peripheral chemoreceptors.

1. Effect of CO_2

CO_2 influences the respiratory centre through peripheral as well as central chemoreceptors. It is a highly diffusible gas and can easily cross the blood–brain–CSF barriers and influence the medullary central chemoreceptors. In contrast, H^+ cannot cross these barriers easily. Therefore, central chemoreceptors are most sensitive to changes in arterial pCO_2 and less so to changes in H^+ concentration.

Under most circumstances, CO_2 production and excretion are matched and the usual steady-state pCO_2 is maintained at 40 mm Hg. Therefore, increases or decreases in pCO_2 do not occur due to change in production of CO_2, but either represent derangements of neural respiratory control or are due to compensatory changes in response to or primary alteration in plasma HCO_3^-.

2. Effect of pH

Changes in arterial blood pH (H^+ concentration) also influence pulmonary ventilation, chiefly through the peripheral (sinoaortic) chemoreceptors, and help in regulation of acid–base balance of the body even when the increase in H^+ concentration is not due to CO_2 but due to nonvolatile acids like sulphuric acid, phosphoric acid and/or lactic acid.

Respiratory response, as described later, does not occur in response to respiratory acid–base disorders but occurs in response to metabolic acid–base disorders only, and consists of:

1. *Hyperventilation:* It occurs in response to metabolic acidosis and results in lowering of pCO_2 to match the decreased HCO_3^-.
2. *Hypoventilation* occurs in response to metabolic alkalosis and results in raising the pCO_2 to match the increased HCO_3^-.

III. RENAL MECHANISM FOR pH REGULATION

The kidneys regulate pH through three main processes:

- 'Reabsorption' of filtered HCO_3^-
- 'Generation' of new HCO_3^-
- H^+ excretion in the form of titrable acid and NH_4^+ (for details, see description of acidification of urine [page 516])

Applied Aspects

Acid–Base Disorders

Acidosis refers to decline in blood pH, whereas *alkalosis* refers to rise in blood pH. As described above, our body has been provided with an efficient system for the maintenance of acid–base equilibrium with a result that the pH of blood is almost constant (7.4). The blood pH compatible to life is 6.8–7.8, beyond which life cannot exist.

Acid–base disorders can be classified into two groups:

I. *The simple acid–base disorders* include:
- Metabolic acidosis
- Metabolic alkalosis
- Respiratory acidosis
- Respiratory alkalosis

II. *Mixed acid–base disorders* include:
- Metabolic acidosis and respiratory acidosis
- Metabolic acidosis and respiratory alkalosis
- Metabolic alkalosis and respiratory alkalosis
- Metabolic alkalosis and respiratory acidosis

Simple Acid–Base Disorders

The physiological aspects of single acid–base disorders are summarized in Table 12.3.2 and described next.

Metabolic Acidosis

Physiological Disturbance. Physiological disturbance that produces metabolic acidosis is either increased net nonvolatile acid load or loss of base (HCO_3^-).

Primary Disturbance. Primary disturbance in metabolic acidosis is *decreased plasma [HCO_3^-]* (which has been either used to buffer the extra fixed acid or lost from the body) producing a *low plasma pH*.

Causes. Causes of metabolic acidosis include:

1. *Addition of nonvolatile acids* to the body can occur in:
   - Diabetic ketoacidosis causing accumulation of acetoacetic acid and β-OH-butyric acid
   - Lactic acidosis in hypoxia
   - Methanol/formaldehyde intoxication which produces formic acid
2. *Loss of nonvolatile alkali* from the body occurs in:
   - Diarrhoea (GIT loss of HCO_3^-)
   - Type 2 renal tubular acidosis (renal loss of HCO_3^-)
3. *Failure of the kidney to excrete sufficient net acid to replenish HCO_3^- used to titrate the net daily acid load*, as may occur in:
   - Chronic renal failure (failure to excrete H^+ as titrable acid and NH_4)

Table 12.3.2 Summary of characteristics of simple acid–base disorders

		Arterial plasma (approximate values)			Defence mechanism		
Disorder	**Primary disturbance**	**pH (normal 7.4)**	**HCO_3^- (mEq/L) (normal 24)**	**pCO_2 (mm Hg) (normal 40)**	**Buffering**	**Respiratory compensation**	**Renal compensation**
Metabolic acidosis	↓ Plasma HCO_3^-	↓ (7.28)	↓ (18)	→ (40)	ECF and ICF	Hyperventilation (↓ pCO_2)	↑ H^+ excretion ↑ New HCO_3^- reabsorption
Metabolic alkalosis	↑ Plasma HCO_3^-	↑ (7.5)	↑ (30)	→ (40)	ECF and ICF	Hypoventilation (↑ pCO_2)	↓ H^+ excretion ↓ New HCO_3^- reabsorption
Respiratory acidosis	↑ pCO_2	↓ (7.34)	↑ (25)	↑ (48)	ICF	None	↑ H^+ excretion ↑ New HCO_3^- reabsorption
Respiratory alkalosis	↓ pCO_2	↑ (7.53)	↓ (22)	↓ (27)	ICF	None	↓ H^+ excretion ↓ New HCO_3^- reabsorption

↑, increased; ↓, decreased; →, normal; ECF, extracellular fluid; ICF, intracellular fluid.

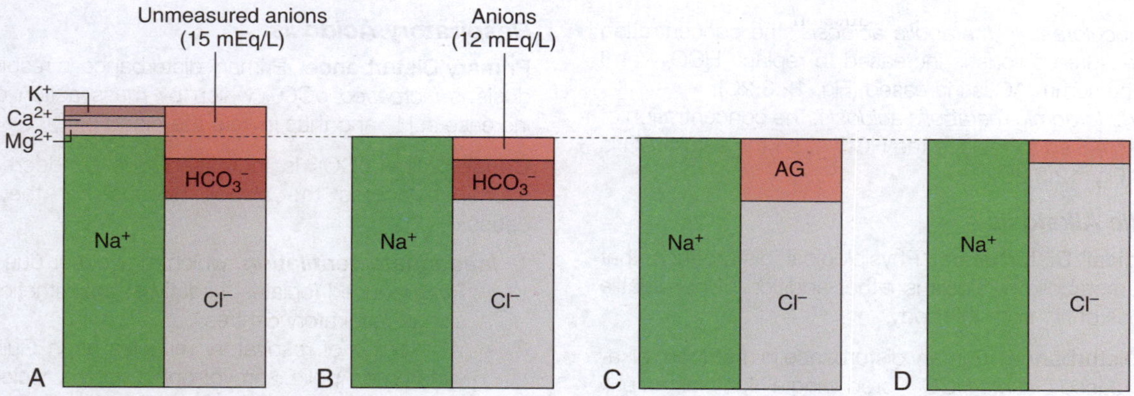

Fig. 12.3.2 Concept of anion gap: **A**, normal ionogram showing the major cations (Na^+) and the minor cations (K^+, Ca^{2+} and Mg^{2+}), the major anions are HCO_3^- and Cl^- and the unmeasured anion constitute the anion gap; **B**, simplified ionogram showing Na^+ as the only cation and making the anion column fall as the Na^+ column; **C**, ionogram depicting increased anion gap in normochloraemic metabolic acidosis; and **D**, ionogram depicting normal anion gap but increased [Cl^-] in hyperchloraemic metabolic acidosis.

- Type I distal renal tubular acidosis (failure to excrete titrable acid and NH_4)

Uncompensated Metabolic Acidosis. Uncompensated metabolic acidosis characterized by a low plasma pH and low plasma HCO_3^- is expressed as:

$$\downarrow \text{pH} = pK + \log \frac{HCO_3^- \downarrow}{pCO_2}$$

Compensatory Mechanisms. When metabolic acidosis is produced by nonrenal factors, the respiratory and renal compensatory mechanisms tend to minimize the change in pH of blood. In renal failure, only respiratory compensation is possible.

1. ***Respiratory compensation:*** Increased (H^+) stimulates the respiratory centre through peripheral chemoreceptors and produces *hyperventilation* (Kussmaul *breathing*) which in turn decreases the arterial pCO_2 value and minimizes the degree of acidosis. Respiratory compensatory mechanism is prompt but short term.
   Compensated metabolic acidosis characterized by near-normal pH with ↓ pCO_2 to compensate the ↓ HCO_3^- is expressed as:
   $$\text{pH} = pK + \log \frac{HCO_3^- \downarrow}{pCO_2 \downarrow}$$
2. ***Renal compensation*** is slow, but an effective mechanism to control metabolic acidosis. It consists of:
   - *Increased excretion of fixed H^+* as titrable acid and NH_4
   - *Increased reabsorption of 'new HCO_3^-'*, which replenishes the HCO_3^- used in buffering the added fixed H^+
   - *An adaptive increase in NH_3* synthesis in chronic metabolic acidosis that helps in the excretion of excess H^+

Hyperchloraemic Versus Normochloraemic Metabolic Acidosis

Normochloraemic metabolic acidosis is characterized by decreased plasma HCO_3^- and low plasma pH with normal serum Cl^- levels. As described above, the metabolic acidosis caused by conditions adding nonvolatile acid to the body or due to renal failure to excrete H^+ is normochloraemic type of metabolic acidosis.

Hyperchloraemic metabolic acidosis is characterized by decreased plasma HCO_3^- and low plasma pH with an increase in plasma Cl^-.

This type of metabolic acidosis occurs in:

- *Diarrhoea*, in which HCO_3^- is lost from the gut in exchange of Cl^-
- *Type 2 renal tubular acidosis*, in which failure to reabsorb HCO_3^- by the kidneys is accompanied by excessive reabsorption of Cl^-

Anion gap concept

Anion gap (AG) helps to differentiate hyperchloraemic metabolic acidosis from normochloraemic metabolic acidosis.

According to law of electroneutrality, the total concentration of cations and that of anions in serum are equal. Routine serum electrolyte determinations measure essentially all cations but only a fraction of the anions. This apparent disparity between the total cation concentration and the total anion concentration is termed the AG (Fig. 12.3.2). It is a virtual measurement and does not represent any specific ionic constituent as shown (Fig. 12.3.2A):

$$\left[Na^+ + K^+ + Ca^+ + Mg^+\right] = \left[HCO_3^- + Cl^- + \text{unmeasured anions}\right](AG)$$

$$\text{Therefore, } AG = \left[Na^+ + K^+ + Ca^+ + Mg^+\right] - \left[HCO_3^- + Cl^-\right]$$

Often the AG is calculated with Na^+ as the major cation, as K^+, Ca^{2+} and Mg^{2+} have a relatively minor quantitative contribution. The equation then becomes (Fig. 12.3.2B):

$$\begin{aligned} AG &= \left[Na^+\right] - \left[HCO_3^- + Cl^-\right] \\ &= [142 \text{ mEq/L}] - [25 \text{ mEq/L} + 105 \text{ mEq/L}] \\ &= 142 \text{ mEq/L} - 130 \text{ mEq/L} \\ &= 12 \text{ mEq/L} \end{aligned}$$

The AG, which has a normal value of 12 ± 4 mEq/L, reflects the concentration of those anions which are actually present but are not determined routinely (i.e. other than HCO_3^- and Cl^-) and include polyanionic plasma proteins (primarily albumin), inorganic phosphates, sulphate and ions of organic acids.

AG in metabolic acidosis: As mentioned above, in metabolic acidosis, the serum HCO_3^- decreases, since it is utilized in buffering the fixed acid. For electroneutrality, the concentration of another anion must increase to replace HCO_3^-. That anion can be Cl^- or the unmeasured anions (which constitute AG).

In normochloraemic metabolic acidosis, the concentration of unmeasured anions is increased to replace HCO_3^- and hence the serum AG is increased (Fig. 12.3.2C).
In hyperchloraemic metabolic acidosis, the concentration of Cl^- is increased to replace the HCO_3^-, so the serum AG is normal (Fig. 12.3.2D).

Metabolic Alkalosis

Physiological Disturbance. Physiological disturbance that produces metabolic alkalosis is either addition of nonvolatile alkali or loss of H^+ from the body.

Primary Disturbance. Primary disturbance in metabolic alkalosis is *increased plasma* HCO_3^- producing a high plasma pH.

Causes. Causes of metabolic alkalosis include:

1. *Addition of nonvolatile alkali* to the body, e.g. in:
   - Ingestion of antacids
2. *Volume contraction alkalosis* may occur with:
   - Haemorrhage
   - Loop or thiazide diuretics
3. *Loss of H^+ from the body* (a common cause) may occur in:
   - Vomiting (H^+ is lost from the stomach)
   - Hyperaldosteronism (increased H^+ secretion by distal tubule)

Uncompensated Metabolic Alkalosis Uncompensated metabolic alkalosis, characterized by a high plasma pH and high plasma HCO_3^-, is expressed as:

$$\uparrow \text{pH} = pK + \log \frac{HCO_3^- \uparrow}{pCO_2}$$

Compensatory Mechanisms

1. ***Respiratory compensation:*** Increased pH (or decreased H^+) inhibits the respiratory centre through peripheral chemoreceptors and produces *hypoventilation* which in turn elevates pCO_2 and thus normalizes plasma pH.
2. ***Compensated metabolic alkalosis*** characterized by near-normal pH with ↑ pCO_2 to compensate the ↑ HCO_3^- is expressed as:

$$\text{pH} = pK + \log \frac{HCO_3^- \uparrow}{pCO_2 \uparrow}$$

Important Note

It is important to note that the magnitude of respiratory compensation is limited by the fact that hypoventilation results in decreased arterial pO_2 which stimulates the respiratory centres via peripheral chemoreceptors.

3. ***Renal compensation*** for metabolic alkalosis consists of:
   - *Decreased H^+ secretion* by the renal tubules
   - *Increased HCO_3^- excretion*, as the filtered load of HCO_3^- exceeds the ability of renal tubule to reabsorb it (the urinary loss of HCO_3^- decreases the plasma level of HCO_3^-, thereby restoring the pH of blood to near normal)

Important Note

It is important to note that if metabolic alkalosis is accompanied by ECF volume contraction (e.g. following persistent vomiting), the resultant hypovolaemia becomes a strong stimulus for Na^+ reabsorption by increased H^+ secretion (because of Na^+/H^+ antiport system) and thus HCO_3^- reabsorption increases, worsening the metabolic alkalosis.

Respiratory Acidosis

Primary Disturbance. Primary disturbance in respiratory acidosis is *increased pCO_2*, which by mass action causes an increase in H^+ and thus lowers the blood pH.

Causes. The pCO_2 is increased due to decreased gas exchange across the alveoli because of the following causes:

1. ***Inadequate ventilation***, which may occur due to:
   - Drug-induced (opiates, sedatives, anaesthetics) depression of respiratory centres
   - Weakening of respiratory muscles as in Guillain–Barré syndrome, polio, amyotrophic lateral sclerosis and multiple sclerosis
   - Airway obstruction
2. ***Impaired gas diffusion***, which may occur in cardiovascular diseases or lung diseases (e.g. adult respiratory distress syndrome, chronic obstructive pulmonary disease)

Uncompensated respiratory acidosis. Uncompensated respiratory acidosis, characterized by low plasma pH and high pCO_2, is expressed as:

$$\downarrow \text{pH} = pK + \log \frac{HCO_3^-}{pCO_2 \uparrow}$$

Compensatory Mechanism

Important Note

There is no respiratory compensation for respiratory acidosis.

Buffering in respiratory acidosis, in contrast to that in metabolic acidosis, occurs almost entirely in the intracellular compartment.

Renal compensation: Increased pCO_2 supplies more H^+ to renal tubule cells for secretion which leads to:

- Excretion of H^+ as titrable acid and NH_3 is increased.
- Reabsorption of new HCO_3^- is increased.
- The resulting increase in serum HCO_3^- helps to normalize the pH. Thus, acidosis is mostly but not completely compensated by the renal mechanism.

Acute Versus Chronic Respiratory Acidosis. As the renal compensatory response takes several days to develop, the respiratory acidosis can be divided into acute and chronic phases.

1. *Acute respiratory acidosis* is labelled when not enough time has elapsed and the renal compensation has not yet occurred. During this phase, the body relies on intracellular buffering to minimize the change in pH. Because of intracellular buffering, plasma HCO_3^- increases by 1 mEq/L for every 10 mm rise in pCO_2 during this period.
2. *Chronic respiratory acidosis* is labelled when renal compensation occurs. During this phase, plasma HCO_3^- increases by 3.5 mEq/L for every 10 mm rise in pCO_2.
3. *Compensated respiratory acidosis* characterized by near-normal pH with increased plasma HCO_3^- to compensate the increased pCO_2 is expressed as:

$$\text{pH} = pK + \log \frac{HCO_3^- \uparrow}{pCO_2 \uparrow}$$

Respiratory Alkalosis

Primary Disturbance. Primary disturbance in respiratory alkalosis is decreased pCO_2 associated with low (H^+) and, thus, an elevated plasma pH.

Causes. The pCO_2 is decreased due to increased gas exchange in the lungs because of increased ventilation as seen in the following conditions:

Pneumonia and pulmonary embolus (ventilation rate is increased secondary to hypoxaemia)
High altitude (ventilation rate is increased secondary to hypoxaemia)
Psychogenic hyperventilation that may occur as a response to anxiety or fear
Salicylate intoxication (hyperventilation occurs due to direct stimulation of medullary respiratory centres)

Uncompensated Respiratory Alkalosis. Uncompensated respiratory alkalosis, characterized by high plasma pH and low pCO_2, is expressed as:

$$\uparrow pH = pK + \log \frac{HCO_3^-}{pCO_2 \downarrow}$$

Compensatory Mechanisms

Important Note

There is no respiratory compensation for respiratory alkalosis.

Buffering in respiratory alkalosis, in contrast to that in metabolic alkalosis, occurs almost entirely in the intracellular compartment.

Renal compensation: Decreased pCO_2 causes a deficit of H^+ in the renal cells for secretion which leads to:

- Decreased excretion of H^+ as titrable acid and NH_4^+
- Decreased reabsorption of new HCO_3^-
- Decreased reabsorption of the filtered HCO_3^-

The resulting decrease in serum HCO_3^- helps to normalize the pH. In this way, alkalosis is mostly but not completely compensated by the renal mechanism.

Acute Versus Chronic Respiratory Alkalosis. As the renal compensatory response takes several days to develop, the respiratory alkalosis can be divided into acute and chronic phases:

1. ***Acute respiratory alkalosis*** is labelled when not enough time has elapsed and renal compensation has not yet occurred. During this phase, the body relies on intracellular buffering to minimize the change in pH. Because of intracellular buffering, plasma HCO_3^- decreases by 2 mEq/L for every 10 mm Hg fall in pCO_2.
2. ***Chronic respiratory alkalosis*** is labelled when renal compensation occurs. During this phase, plasma HCO_3^- decreases by 5 mEq/L for every 10 mm Hg reduction in pCO_2 by the renal compensatory mechanism as described above.

Compensated Respiratory Alkalosis. Compensated respiratory alkalosis, characterized by near-normal pH with decreased plasma HCO_3^- to compensate the decreased pCO_2, is expressed as:

$$pH = pK + \log \frac{HCO_3^- \downarrow}{pCO_2 \downarrow}$$

Table 12.3.3 Predicted physiological responses in simple acid–base disorders

Acid–base disorder	Primary disturbance	Predicted compensatory response
Metabolic acidosis	↓ $[HCO_3^-]$	↓ pCO_2 by 1.30 mm Hg/mEq/L decrease in HCO_3^-
Metabolic alkalosis	↑ $[HCO_3^-]$	↑ pCO_2 by 0.7 mm Hg/mEq/L increase in HCO_3
Respiratory acidosis		
• Acute	↑ pCO_2	↑ $[HCO_3^-]$ by 0.1 mEq/L/mm Hg increase in pCO_2
• Chronic	↑ pCO_2	↑ $[HCO_3^-]$ by 0.4 mEq/L/mm Hg increase in pCO_2
Respiratory alkalosis		
• Acute	↓ pCO_2	↓ $[HCO_3^-]$ by 0.2 mEq/L/mm Hg decrease in pCO_2
• Chronic	↓ pCO_2	↓ $[HCO_3^-]$ by 0.4 mEq/L/mm Hg decrease in pCO_2

Summary of characteristics of simple acid–base disorders

Various characteristics of simple acid–base disorders are summarized in Table 12.3.2.

Predicted Physiological Responses to Simple Acid–Base Disorders

As described above, the primary respiratory disturbances (primary change in pCO_2) involve secondary metabolic responses (secondary change in HCO_3^-) and primary metabolic disturbances elicit predictable respiratory responses. Predicted physiological compensation in various acid–base disturbances is summarized in Table 12.3.3.

ANALYSIS AND CLINICAL EVALUATION OF ACID–BASE DISORDERS

THREE-STEP APPROACH FOR ANALYSIS OF ACID–BASE DISORDERS

Three-step approach for analysis of acid–base disorders is summarized in Fig. 12.3.3. It consists of the following three steps:

- ***Step I:*** Estimate pH to know acidosis ($pH < 7.4$) or alkalosis ($pH > 7.4$).
- ***Step II:*** Detect primary disturbance to know whether the disorder is metabolic (primary disturbance of HCO_3^-) or respiratory (primary disturbance of pCO_2).
- ***Step III:*** Analysis of compensatory response can be done from the values of plasma HCO_3^- and pCO_2.

Determination of Anion Gap

As described above (page 1193), the determination of anion gaps is useful in differential diagnosis of metabolic acidosis. The anion gap is increased in metabolic acidosis due to ketoacidosis, lactic acidosis and other forms of acidosis in which organic anions are increased. It is not increased in hyperchloraemic acidosis.

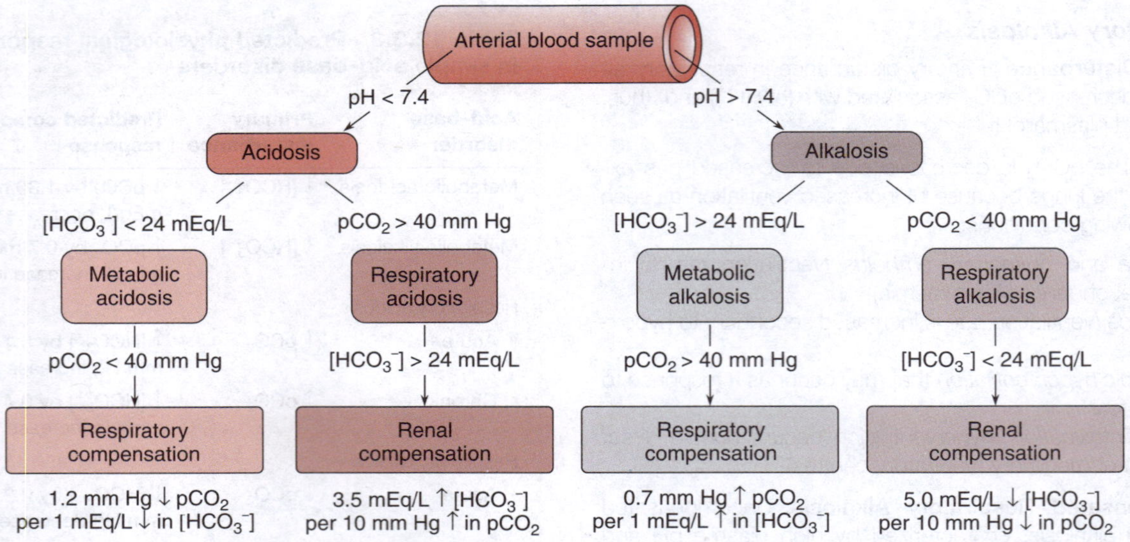

Fig. 12.3.3 Algorithm of three-step approach for analysis of acid–base disorder.

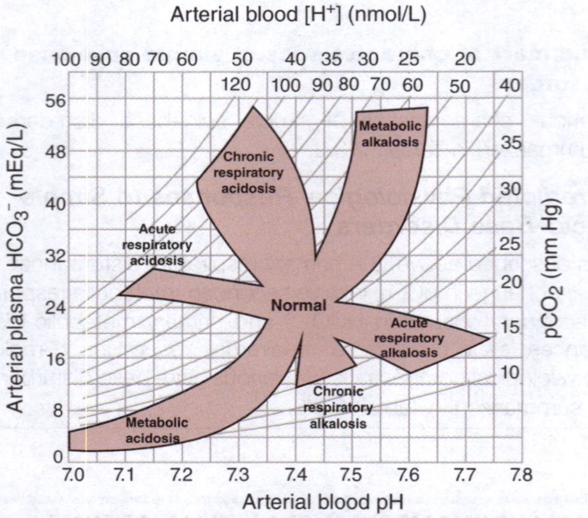

Fig. 12.3.4 Acid–base nomogram (for explanation, see text).

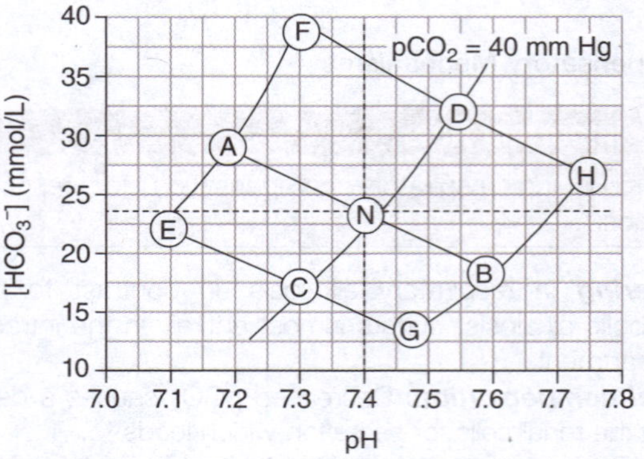

Fig. 12.3.5 Interpretation of acid–base abnormalities using the pH–[HCO_3^-] diagram (Davenport diagram; for explanation, see text). Acid–base nomogram (for explanation, see text).

GRAPHIC ANALYSIS OF CHANGES IN pH, PCO_2 AND HCO_3^-

Acid–base nomogram Acid–base nomogram (Fig. 12.3.4) is the graphical display of changes in pCO_2 (curved lines in Fig. 12.3.4), plasma HCO_3^- and pH of arterial blood in respiratory and metabolic acid–base disorders. This nomogram is useful in predicting compensatory responses to simple acid–base disorder. Although the shaded areas of nomogram show the 95% confidence limits for normal compensation in simple disturbances, finding acid–base values within the shaded area does not necessarily rule out a mixed disturbance. Note that the shifts in HCO_3^- and pH as acute respiratory acidosis and alkalosis are compensated producing their chronic counterparts.

Davenport diagram: Graphic display of true plasma pH, HCO_3^- and pCO_2 in metabolic acidosis and alkalosis Fig. 12.3.5 is the typical graphical display of true plasma pH, HCO_3^- and pCO_2 in uncompensated and compensated metabolic acidosis and metabolic alkalosis. It shows the relationship between pH and HCO_3^- at a constant pCO_2, and hence is also called *pCO_2 isobar*. Thus, acid–base imbalances are determined graphically, with reference to the intercept of pCO_2 isobar of 40 mm Hg (line CND, Fig. 12.3.5) and the normal buffer line (line ANB, Fig. 12.3.5). The intercept of these two curves marks the point of normality (N) which is associated with a pH of 7.4 (the abscissa) and a [HCO_3^-] of 24 mmol/L (the ordinate). Thus, the point N is the triple intercept that defines the pH, [HCO_3^-] and pCO_2 of true arterial plasma of a normal individual.

Interpretation of acid–base abnormalities using Davenport diagram (pH, HCO_3^- diagram) is made as:

- *Point A* represents uncompensated respiratory acidosis.
- *Point B* represents uncompensated respiratory alkalosis.
- *Point C* represents uncompensated metabolic acidosis.
- *Point D* represents uncompensated metabolic alkalosis.
- *Point E* represents respiratory acidosis + metabolic acidosis.
- *Point F* represents respiratory acidosis + metabolic alkalosis.
- *Point G* represents respiratory alkalosis + metabolic acidosis.
- *Point H* represents respiratory alkalosis + metabolic alkalosis.

Siggaard-Andersen curve nomogram Siggaard-Andersen (SA) curve nomogram (Fig. 12.3.6) has pCO_2 plotted on a log

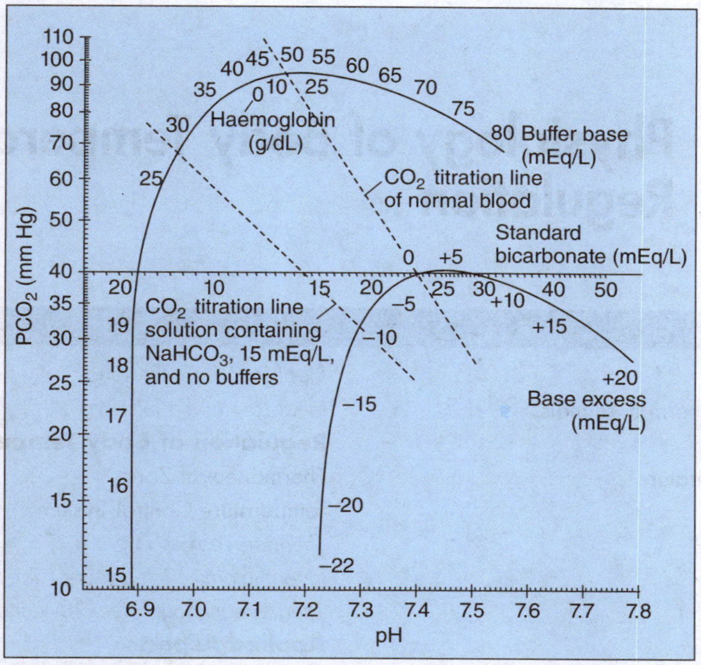

Fig. 12.3.6 Siggaard-Andersen curve nomogram to plot the acid–base characteristics of arterial blood.

scale on the vertical axis and pH on the horizontal. This nomogram is helpful in clinical situations to plot the acid–base, a characteristic of arterial blood.

Protocol for using a nomogram Arterial capillary blood is drawn anaerobically and pH is measured. pH of the same blood after equilibration with each of two gas mixtures containing known amounts of CO_2 is determined.

- pH values at known pCO_2 levels are plotted and connected to provide CO_2 titration line from blood sample.
- pH of the blood sample before equilibration is plotted on this line and actual pCO_2 of sample read off the vertical line.

The following values can be determined:

- Standard HCO_3^- content of sample, i.e. measure of the alkali reserve of the blood
- Buffer base (normal value 48 mEq/L)
- Base excess that is represented by the point at which CO_2 calibration line intersects the lower curved scale on the nomogram (it is positive in alkalosis and negative in acidosis)

Self-Assessment

1. Discuss the mechanism of pH regulation.
2. Discuss the role of body buffer system in maintenance of pH.
3. Describe the following:
   - Anion gap and its determination
   - Acid–base nomogram and its significance
4. Write notes on the following:
   - Siggaard-Andersen curve nomogram
   - Henderson–Hasselbalch equation
   - Metabolic acidosis
   - Respiratory alkalosis
   - Extracellular versus intracellular buffers

Clinical Cases

Case 1

A 58-year-old male presented to the emergency department in a confused state with severe headache and jerky movements of the limbs.

History revealed that the patient was a chronic smoker and was a diagnosed case of COPD.

Examination showed central cyanosis.

Serum electrolytes showed raised HCO_3^- and hypokalaemia. X-ray chest showed emphysema and fibrosis.

Q1. On the basis of signs and symptoms and investigations, what is the diagnosis?

Q2. What are the compensatory mechanisms to improve the situation?

Q3. What are the other causes of this condition?

Q4. What is the treatment plan?

Q5. What are the complications if not treated timely?

Case 2

A 20-year-old male student suffering from acute diarrhoea and vomiting due to food poisoning was brought to the emergency department in a state of dizziness with breathlessness and muscle twitching.

Examination and investigations showed numbness and tingling sensations, and respiratory rate 30/min; serum electrolyte analysis indicated raised bicarbonates, blood pH >7.4 and urine pH 5.0.

Q1. On the basis of above-mentioned signs and symptoms and investigation findings, the patient is suffering from which acid–base disorder?

Q2. Why is the urine pH <6.0 in this case?

Q3. What are the compensatory mechanisms that come into action for improvement?

Q4. What should be the treatment plan in this case?

12.4 Physiology of Body Temperature Regulation

CHAPTER OUTLINE

BODY TEMPERATURE

HOMEOTHERMIC VERSUS POIKILOTHERMIC ANIMALS

Homeothermic animals, also called warm-blooded animals, are able to maintain their body temperature within a normal narrow range in spite of wide variations in the environmental temperature. Birds and mammals, including humans, belong to this category.

Poikilothermic animals, also called cold-blooded animals, do not have an efficient temperature-regulating system; therefore, their body temperature fluctuates with the fluctuations in the environmental temperature. The reptiles, amphibians and fishes belong to this category.

NORMAL BODY TEMPERATURE

There is a slight variation in normal temperature in different parts of the body:

Oral temperature, when measured with the help of a clinical thermometer, varies from 36.0°C to 37.5°C (97.5–99°F) with an average of 37°C (98.6°F). It is affected by hot and cold drinks and food, smoking, chewing gums and mouth breathing.

Axillary temperature is slightly lower (about 0.5°C) than the oral temperature.

Rectal and oesophageal temperatures are slightly higher (about 0.5°C) than the oral temperature.

Superficial skin or surface temperature varies to some extent with the environmental temperature (see 'shell temperature').

Extremities are generally cooler than the rest of the body.

Scrotal temperature is carefully regulated at 32°C (89.6°F).

Concept of core versus shell temperature: The body is hypothetically divided into core and shell (Fig. 12.4.1).

Shell temperature, i.e. temperature of the limbs and the surface layer of the trunk, i.e. skin and underlying structure, exhibits variations of the temperature with the change in external temperature.

In cold weather, the temperature of the shell may be several degrees lower than the core temperature (Fig. 12.4.1A). This decreases the loss of body heat to the environment by conductional radiation. In hot environment, the shell temperature approaches the core temperature (Fig. 12.4.1B), and this helps in heat loss by conduction and radiation.

Core temperature, i.e. temperature of deeper body structures (e.g. temperature of intra-abdominal, intrathoracic and intracranial structures), is maintained strictly constant. It has been widely assumed to be an accurate index of the temperature of blood to which hypothalamic thermoregulatory receptors are exposed. The core temperature is always slightly more than the oral temperature (about 37.8°C or 100°F). Rectal, vaginal and oesophageal temperatures represent the core temperature. Oesophageal temperature taken at the heart level is a good index of rapid changes of cardiac and aortic blood temperature. In contrast, rectal temperature gives a poor reflection of rapid changes of blood temperature and may be misleading.

Lower versus upper lethal core temperature: As shown in Fig. 12.4.2, the *lower lethal core temperature* is about 26°C, at which cardiac arrhythmias occur and lead to death due to cardiac failure. *Upper lethal core temperature* is 43.5°C, which leads to death due to heat stroke. A core temperature of 41°C for prolonged periods produces irreversible brain damage.

FACTORS AFFECTING BODY TEMPERATURE

I. Physiological Variations

1. Diurnal variation Body temperature is *highest* in the evening (after day's labour – between 5 and 7 p.m.) and *lowest* in early hours of morning (after night's rest between 2 and

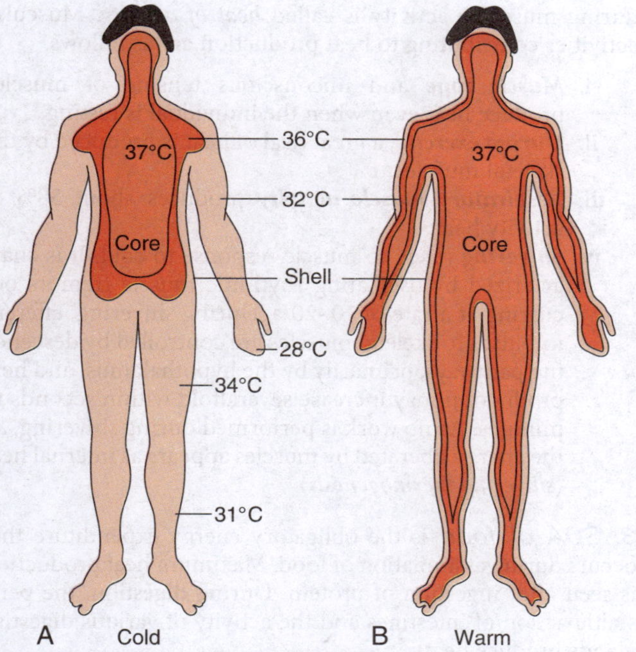

Fig. 12.4.1 Concept of body core and shell temperature. Dark areas represent body core and superficial light areas represent body shell.

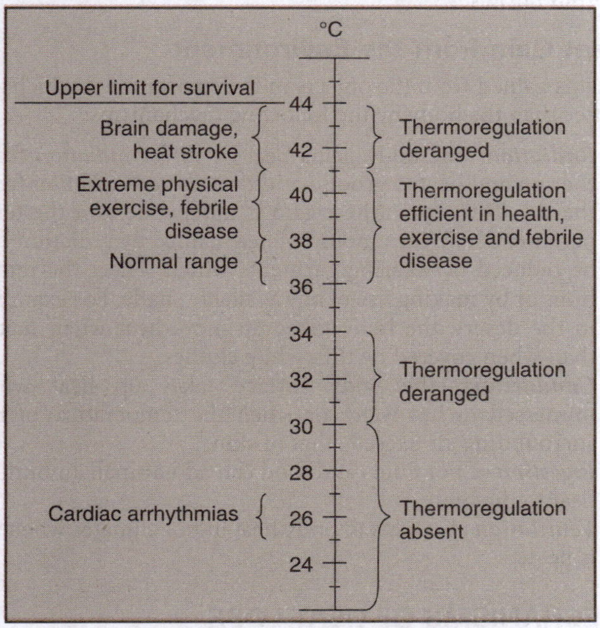

Fig. 12.4.2 Effects of alteration of body temperature.

4 a.m.). Difference between the two values may be 1°C. In the night workers, the rhythm is reversed. This diurnal variation is related to exercise and specific dynamic action (SDA) of food. Fasting and absolute bed rest abolish this variation.

2. Age *Infants* have imperfect regulation of temperature. Hence, range of variation is wider. A fit of crying may raise and a cold bath may lower the body temperature.

In old age, the body temperature tends to be subnormal due to decreased activity and decreased basal metabolic rate (BMR). In addition, due to compromised circulatory system, older individuals cannot tolerate extremes of environmental temperature.

3. Sex *Females* have a slightly low body temperature due to relatively low BMR and thick layer of subcutaneous fat (nonconductor). Furthermore, due to thermogenic effect of progesterone, the body temperature is higher in *postovulatory phase* of menstrual cycle than in the preovulatory phase.

4. Size Heat production and heat loss depend on the ratio of mass to body surface area. In a mouse, heat production is 450 kcal/kg body weight/24 h, whereas in a horse, it is only 14.5 kcal/kg body weight/24 h.

5. Food Protein food, due to high SDA, may raise body temperature. The act of ingestion of food may also raise body temperature.

6. Exercise increases temperature Only 25% of muscular energy is converted into mechanical work; the rest comes out as heat. Inability of heat-dissipating mechanisms to handle the greatly increased amount of heat produced increases body temperature. Furthermore, there occurs resetting of the thermostat at a higher body temperature.

7. Atmospheric conditions Temperature, humidity and movement of air are directly concerned with the amount of heat loss from the surface and thus affect body temperature.

8. Sleep Because of muscular inactivity, sleep results in a slight fall of body temperature.

9. Emotions Body temperature may rise due to emotional disturbances. The rise of temperature may be as high as 2°C.

10. Posture, piloerection and clothing Posture, piloerection and clothing are also important factors that affect the body temperature. All animals and even humans may conserve heat or may prevent heat loss by curling up during exposure to cold.

II. Pathological Variations

1. Hyperthermia or fever Hyperthermia or fever refers to the pathologically raised body temperature. Common causes of fever are as follows:

- *Pyrogens* are the toxic substances which raise the body temperature by affecting the hypothalamus. They are released during infections (bacterial, viral, parasitic, etc.).
- *In hyperthyroidism*, body temperature is raised due to increased BMR.
- *Lesions of the brain* and diabetes insipidus may be associated with raised temperature.

2. Hypothermia Hypothermia refers to lowered body temperature (below normal) due to some pathological causes, such as:

- Hypothyroidism
- Hypopituitarism
- Lesions in the hypothalamus
- Haemorrhage in certain parts of the brain, particularly pons

HEAT BALANCE

Heat balance refers to the balance between the mechanisms of net heat gains by the body and mechanisms of heat losses from the body (Fig. 12.4.3). The heat balance in the body is maintained by adjusting the heat production in accordance with heat loss and vice versa. In turn, the heat balance maintains the body temperature at a constant level.

MECHANISMS OF HEAT GAIN

The main mechanisms responsible for heat gain by the body are as follows:

- Heat production in the body
- Heat gain from the environment

Heat Production or Thermogenesis

Thermogenesis refers to heat production in the body by various physiological/metabolic processes which include:

1. Basal metabolic activity: The main mechanism responsible for heat production in the body is physiological oxidation of food materials, i.e. combustion of carbohydrates, proteins and fats; 1 g of each yields about 4, 4 and 9 cal, respectively. This is called *heat of metabolism*. Of all the organs, the liver contributes the highest amount of heat of metabolism. Heat produced by the liver and heart is relatively constant.

2. Muscular activity: Though heat produced by skeletal muscles is variable and depends on the physiological activity, skeletal muscles are a major source of heat. The heat produced during muscular activity is called *heat of activity*. Muscular activities contributing to heat production are as follows:

i. ***Muscle tone*** and unconscious tensing of muscles produce heat even when the individual is resting.
ii. ***During exercise***, a great deal of heat is produced by the skeletal muscles.
iii. ***Respiratory muscle activity*** produces about 38% of activity heat.
iv. ***Shivering*** refers to muscle response to cold. It is characterized by oscillating rhythmic muscle tremors occurring at a rate of 10–20/s. During shivering, efferent impulses to skeletal muscles are controlled by descending pathways, primarily by the hypothalamus, and heat production may increase severalfold within seconds to minutes. As no work is performed during shivering, all the energy liberated by muscles appears as internal heat (*shivering thermogenesis*).

3. SDA of food is the obligatory energy expenditure that occurs during assimilation of food. Maximum heat production is seen after ingestion of protein. During digestion, the peristaltic action of intestines and the activity of various digestive glands produce heat.

4. Nonshivering thermogenesis refers to heat production due to increase in the metabolic rate resulting from the increased secretion of epinephrine and to a certain extent thyroid hormone.

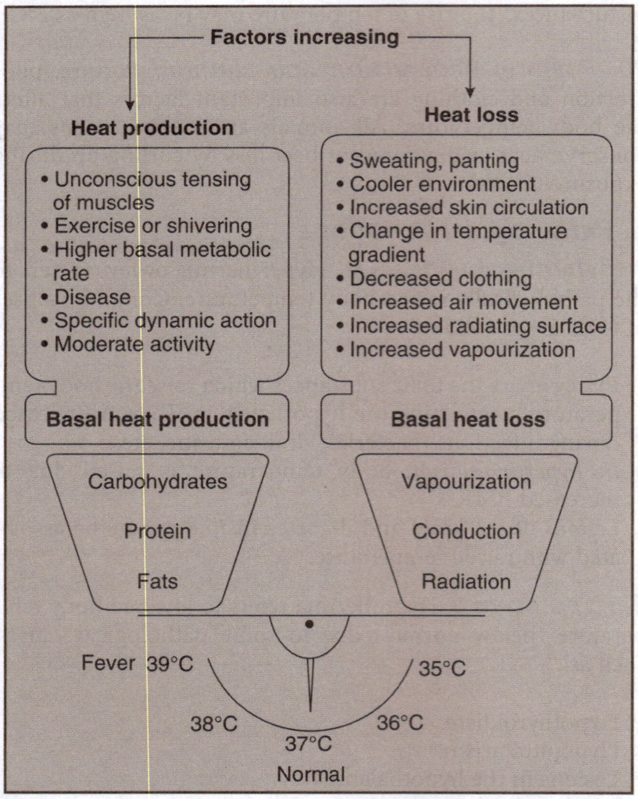

Fig. 12.4.3 Balance between factors contributing to heat gain and heat loss from the body.

Heat Gain from the Environment

Heat is gained from the objects in the environment which are hotter than the body by the following mechanisms:

1. ***Radiation:*** The body gains heat by *direct radiation* from the sun and heated ground and by *reflected radiation* from the sky. This type of heat gain is independent of the temperature of air. The amount of heat gained by radiation can be reduced by wearing garments which reflect the radiations or by making use of any available shade. For example, in the desert, the body takes up more heat when naked than when covered by thin white clothes.
2. ***Conduction:*** The body surface takes up heat when immersed in hot water or when the temperature of the surrounding air exceeds that of skin.
3. ***Ingestion*** of hot fluids and food can add a small amount of heat to the body.
4. ***Ventilation*** also adds to body heat in hot climates when air is heated.

MECHANISMS OF HEAT LOSS

Heat is lost from the body by the following routes:

- Heat loss from the skin
- Heat loss from the lungs
- Heat loss in the excreta

I. Heat Loss from the Skin

Mechanisms of heat loss from the skin surface include (Table 12.4.1):

1. Radiation refers to transfer of heat from an object to another object with which it is not in contact. The magnitude of heat loss by radiation depends on the size of the body surface and the average temperature difference between the skin and the

Table 12.4.1 Mechanisms of heat loss from the body

Mechanism	Amount of heat loss (cal)		Percentage	
Radiation	1500		50	70
Conduction and convection	600		20	
Evaporation of water from:				
• Skin	690	1000	20	27
• Lungs	210		7	
Warming inspired air	60		2	
Excreta (urine and faeces)	30		1	
Total	3000		100	

surrounding objects. About 50% of the total heat loss from the body occurs by radiation. The colour of clothing may play a part but the colour of the human skin has no effect on the radiation.

2. Conduction refers to heat exchange between objects at different temperatures that are in contact with one another. The amount of heat transferred by conduction is proportionate to the temperature difference between the two objects.

3. Convection refers to the movement of molecules of a gas or liquid at one temperature to another location that is at a different temperature. Thus, the heat loss through this process depends on the temperature of the surrounding atmosphere. When the temperature of the surrounding atmosphere is low, heat is lost from the skin to the surrounding air. The molecules of air gradually get warmed and move away from the skin. Another layer of the cooler air takes its place. Thus, heat loss through convection depends on the relative density and temperature of air and wind velocity.

Important Note

About 20% of heat is lost from the body by conduction and convection.

4. Evaporation: About 27% of the heat is lost by evaporation from the skin, mucous membranes and respiratory passages. Vaporization of 1 g (approximately 1 mL) of water resumes about 0.6 kcal of heat. Evaporation from the skin accounts for loss of only 600 cal (20%) per day which occurs in two forms:

i. ***Insensible water loss (perspiration):*** Perspiration occurs due to continuous diffusion of fluid through the epidermis (in absence of sweating). It occurs over the entire body surface at a uniform rate and is largely independent of environmental conditions. Perspiration amounts to about 60 mL/day and is equivalent to heat loss by evaporation of approximately 400 kcal/day. But this heat loss is not under control and, therefore, cannot be changed as required.

ii. ***Evaporation of sweat:*** The eccrine sweat glands play a very important role in thermoregulation of the body. *Thermal sweating* from the eccrine sweat glands increases when the external or internal body temperature rises (details are given). Sweat is vaporized from the skin, which decreases its temperature. Evaporation decreases to a great extent if the humidity of the atmosphere is high, and thus body temperature regulation becomes seriously affected.

Factors Affecting Cutaneous Heat Loss

1. Gradient between the temperature of the skin and the environmental temperature is the most important factor determining the cutaneous heat loss, especially by the radiation, conduction and convection mechanisms. The temperature of the skin that depends on the amount of heat reaching the surface from the deeper tissues can be varied by changing the blood flow to the skin depending on the requirement. This is accomplished by the radiator system of the body.

Radiator system of the body is formed by the cutaneous circulation. Blood vessels penetrate fatty subcutaneous insulator tissue and are distributed profusely beneath the skin. There is a venous plexus underneath the skin, which is supplied by inflow of blood from the skin capillaries. In exposed areas of the body, such as hands, feet and ears, there is arteriovenous anastomosis (blood is supplied to the plexus directly from the small arteries). The rate of blood flow through venous plexus can be varied as:

When the cutaneous blood vessels are dilated, the blood flow to the venous plexus can be increased up to 30% of the total cardiac output. As the warm blood fills the subcutaneous venous plexus, the skin temperature approaches the deep tissue temperature. It promotes heat loss.

When the cutaneous blood vessels are constricted, e.g. on exposure to extreme cold, the rate of blood flow to the venous plexus can be reduced to as low as 2%–3% of cardiac output. Consequently, the skin temperature, especially of the hands and feet, becomes much lower than the deep tissue temperature (Fig. 12.4.4). In this way, heat loss is minimized by decrease in the temperature gradient between the skin and the environment.

Changing flow of blood through the skin is thus the effective mechanism of controlling heat loss. The skin therefore forms an effective radiator system.

2. Insulator system: The subcutaneous fat acts as the heat insulator for the body. Fat conducts heat only one-third as readily as other tissues. This insulation is important in maintaining the core temperature even though the skin temperature varies with that of the surroundings. Women

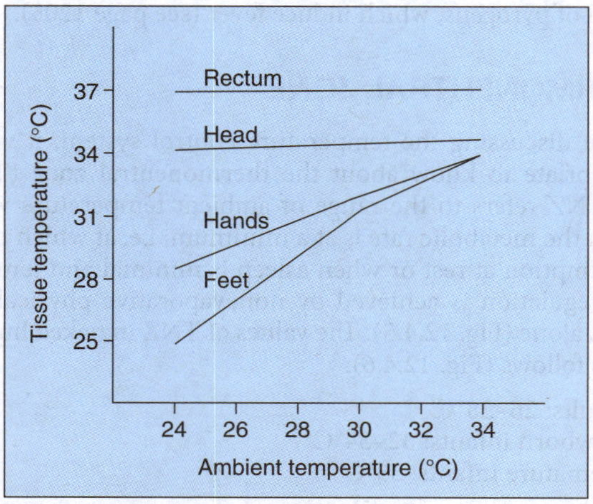

Fig. 12.4.4 Effect of exposure of naked individuals to low ambient temperature on different parts of the body.

have a thicker layer of subcutaneous fat than men; this is partly the reason why in winter, males feel more cold than the females. This is in spite of the fact that males produce more heat because of higher BMR.

3. Piloerector muscle contracts in response to cold and causes erection of the hair. The layer of air entrapped between the hair acts as an insulator and thus reduces the cutaneous heat loss.

4. Clothing: Woollen clothes offer better protection against cold than cotton clothes, because of a larger amount of air entrapped in the former. In animals, the fur and feathers serve the same purpose more effectively.

II. Heat Loss from the Lungs

Heat loss from the lungs occurs by three processes:

1. Evaporation of water in expired air causes heat loss. On an average, the water loss from the lungs is approximately 300 mL/day equivalent to heat loss of 200 kcal. It is the main mechanism through which heat is lost in dogs and sheep.

2. Warming inspired air to the body temperature accounts for 2% of heat loss in humans.

3. Panting: Some mammals lose heat by panting. Panting refers to rapid shallow breathing which greatly increases the amount of water to be evaporated in the mouth and respiratory passages and thereby results in the heat loss.

III. Heat Loss in the Excreta

About 1% of the total body heat loss occurs in the excreta (urine and faeces).

REGULATION OF BODY TEMPERATURE

Like other homeothermic animals, humans have been provided with a *temperature control system* which maintains the internal (core) body temperature constant within the range of ±1°F of the normal temperature. Normal body temperature is the 'set point' in the system of temperature regulation. In humans, the set point of the temperature control system is approximately 98.6°F (37°C), although it normally varies somewhat diurnally, decreasing to a minimum during sleep. The set point can be altered by pathological status, for example, by the action of pyrogens, which induce fever (see page 1205).

THERMONEUTRAL ZONE

Before discussing the temperature control system, it will be appropriate to know about the thermoneutral zone (TNZ). The TNZ refers to the range of ambient temperature within which the metabolic rate is at a minimum, i.e. at which the O_2 consumption at rest or when asleep is minimal and temperature regulation is achieved by nonevaporative physical processes alone (Fig. 12.4.5). The values of TNZ in naked humans are as follows (Fig. 12.4.6):

- Adults: 26–28°C
- Newborn infants: 32–34°C
- Premature infants: 35°C

Certain other terms which need mention are given next.

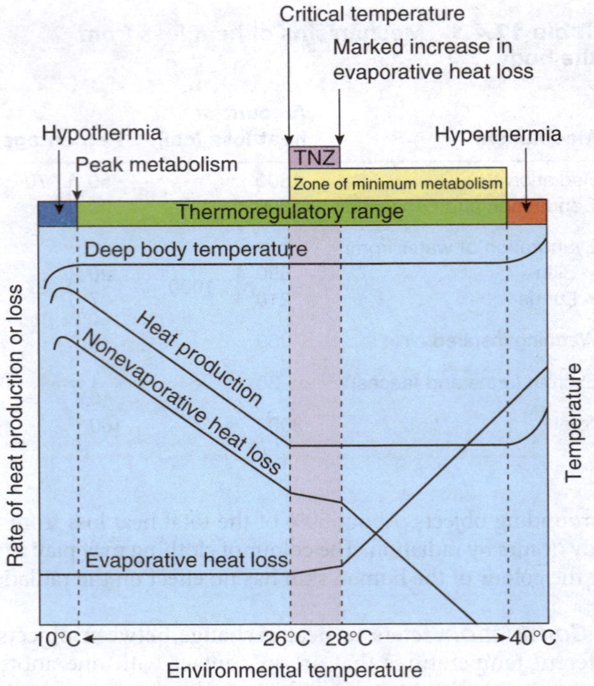

Fig. 12.4.5 Thermoneutral zone and rate of heat production and heat loss in relation to environmental temperature.

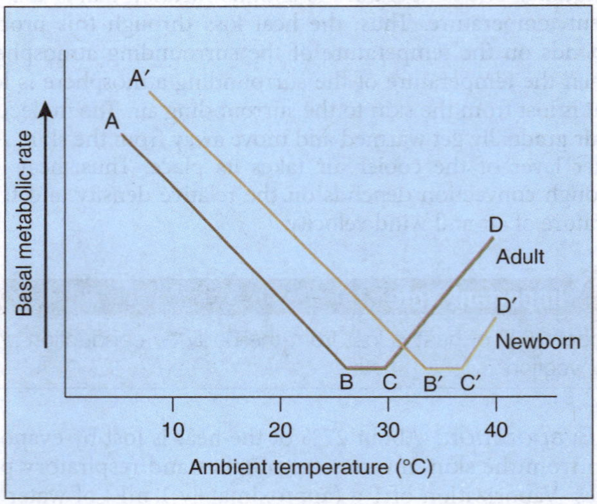

Fig. 12.4.6 Thermoneutral zone of the newborn (B′–C′) compared with that of an adult human (B–C).

Critical temperature It is the lower limit of TNZ. Below it, the metabolic heat production of a resting thermoregulating animal increases to maintain thermal balance (Fig. 12.4.5).

Preferred ambient temperature Preferred ambient temperature (PAT) is the range of ambient temperature associated with thermal comfort. It is not the same as TNZ. It is important to note that:

- When humidity is high, the PAT would be lower than the TNZ.
- When air movement is brisk, the PAT would be higher than the TNZ.

Thermal comfort Thermal comfort is maximum when the skin temperature is about 33°C and also depends on:

- Level of humidity
- Amount of air movement
- Level of body activity
- Amount of clothing

TEMPERATURE CONTROL SYSTEM

The temperature control system comprises the hypothalamus with integrated autonomic, endocrine and skeletomotor responses. The components of the temperature control system are as follows:

- Thermoreceptors
- Hypothalamus, the thermostat and integrator of temperature control system
- The thermoregulatory effector mechanisms

Thermoreceptors

Thermoreceptors or temperature receptors which give information about the body temperature to the temperature control centre in the hypothalamus are of two types – peripheral thermoreceptors and central thermoreceptors.

1. Peripheral thermoreceptors are present throughout the body in the skin and mucous membrane (and probably other organs such as muscle and viscera).

Cutaneous thermoreceptors sense the ambient temperature; 90% of them are cold receptors.

Deep receptors, present in the viscera, sense the core temperature unlike cutaneous receptors that sense the surface temperature. However, like cutaneous receptors, the deep receptors also mainly detect cold than warmth. Probably, both the cutaneous and deep receptors are concerned with preventing hypothermia.

2. Central thermoreceptors are mainly present in the hypothalamus. The hypothalamic receptors are probably neurons whose firing rate is highly dependent on local temperature, which in turn is importantly affected by the temperature of blood.

Hypothalamus: Integrator of Temperature Control System

The integrator and many controlling elements for temperature regulation appear to be located in the hypothalamus. The system acts as a *servomechanism* (a control system that uses negative feedback to operate another system) with a *set point* at normal body temperature (98.6°F or 37°C). The hypothalamic neurons involved in temperature regulation can be divided into three types, depending on the function subserved by them:

- Sensing neurons or feedback detectors
- Heat loss centre or antirise centre
- Heat production and conservation centre or antidrop centre

Sensing neurons or feedback detectors These neurons, located in the anterior hypothalamus, collect information about temperature from both the central and peripheral thermoreceptors.

Two types of neurons have been identified in this area:

- *Warm-sensitive neurons,* which respond to information from warmth receptors
- *Cold-sensitive neurons,* which respond to cold receptors

The central and peripheral thermoreceptors rarely provide identical information about body temperature. In dealing with the body temperature, therefore, the hypothalamus calculates an integrated temperature from the feedback received.

Heat loss centre (antirise centre) is composed of neurons in the preoptic region and anterior or rostral hypothalamus. It organizes the heat loss responses as illustrated:

Electrical stimulation of this area produces heat loss by cutaneous vasodilatation, sweating and panting, and decreases heat production by inhibiting shivering.

Applied Aspects

Lesions of heat loss centre, conversely, prevent sweating and cutaneous vasodilatation and they cause hyperthermia (neurogenic fever) when the individual is placed in a warm environment.

Heat production and conservation centre (antidrop centre) is formed by the neurons in the area of *posterior or caudal hypothalamus* which is dorsolateral to the mammillary body. These neurons organize the heat production and conservation responses as illustrated:

Stimulation of this area conserves heat by cutaneous vasoconstriction and activates heat production by evoking shivering and increasing the metabolic rate through the release of thyroid-stimulating hormone (TSH).

Applied Aspects

Lesions in this area interfere with heat production and conservation, and they can cause *hypothermia* when the subject is in cold environment.

Thermoregulatory Effector Mechanisms

As described above, the effector mechanisms of thermoregulation are integrated by a thermostat located in the hypothalamus, and the *hypothalamic thermostat* has a set point which is normally at 98.6°F (37°C). Error signals that represent a deviation from the set point, due to either raised or lowered body temperature, evoke responses that tend to restore body temperature towards the set point. These responses are mediated by autonomic, somatic and endocrine systems. The thermoregulatory effector mechanisms activated by the hypothalamus can be grouped as:

A. Mechanisms activated by heat are as follows:

I. Mechanisms increasing heat loss:

1. Cutaneous vasodilatation
2. Sweating
3. Increased respiration/panting

II. Mechanisms decreasing heat production are as follows:

1. Anorexia
2. Behavioural responses

B. Mechanisms activated by cold are as follows:

I. Mechanisms conserving heat:

1. Cutaneous vasoconstriction
2. Piloerection
3. Behavioural mechanisms

II. Mechanisms increasing heat production:

1. Shivering
2. Thermogenic chemical (nonshivering) thermogenesis
3. Behavioural responses

A. Mechanisms Activated by Heat

I. Mechanisms increasing heat loss Mechanisms increasing heat loss include those given next.

1. Cutaneous vasodilatation As described on page 1200, the cutaneous vessels form the radiator system of the body. Cutaneous vasodilatation occurring on exposure to heat stresses increases cutaneous blood flow from 4–5 mL/100 g skin weight/min to as high as 150 mL/100 g of skin weight/min. By this, warm blood from the deeper tissues is brought to the surface, and heat loss by conduction, radiation and convection is facilitated as described above.

Mechanisms of cutaneous vasodilatation: Cutaneous vasodilatation is produced through a local effect, spinal reflex as well as the hypothalamus.

i. *Local effect:* Body kinins released from the secretory activity of sweat glands cause local vasodilatation.
ii. *Spinal reflex* evoked by peripheral thermoreceptors produces localized vasodilatation.
iii. *Hypothalamus-controlled vasodilatation:* Impulses from the heat loss centre of the hypothalamus produce inhibition of the sympathetic discharge to cutaneous vessels causing vasodilatation and accumulation of blood in subpapillary venous plexus. The effect of sympathetic inhibition is particularly prominent in the hands, feet and ear lobules, where A-V anastomoses present in the skin are normally kept closed by the strong sympathetic discharge.

2. Sweating As mentioned earlier, the evaporation of sweat is the most important mechanism of heat loss, especially when a person is exposed to the environmental temperature greater than the body temperature.

Sweat glands: There are two types of sweat glands – eccrine and apocrine.

Eccrine sweat glands are distributed all over the body. Their ducts open on the surface of the skin independent of hair follicles. These glands play the main role in thermoregulation of the body.

Apocrine glands are found in the skin of the axilla, pubic, circumareolar and circumanal areas. Their ducts open into a hair follicle above the opening of sebaceous glands. These glands do not have any thermoregulatory function.

Mechanism of heat-induced sweating: When the environmental temperature rises above the *thermal comfort level* (about 33°C), sweating is induced by three mechanisms – a local response, spinal reflex as well as hypothalamus influence. The impulses from the heat loss centre of the anterior hypothalamus increase the impulse discharge in the sympathetic cholinergic fibres to the sweat glands. As a result, sweating starts suddenly, and the rate of sweating progressively increases with the increase in environmental temperature.

Rate of sweating, which is practically zero in cold weather, may reach a maximum of 700 mL/h in bad weather. In very hot climate, sweat secretion may be greater than 10 L/day. Such a heavy sweating causes marked loss of body water and NaCl. This happens because body homeostasis mechanisms give priority to temperature regulation over water and electrolyte regulation. Therefore, in acute heat stress, death may occur due to severe dehydration and salt loss leading to circulatory failure.

Acclimatization of sweating mechanism is an adaptation which occurs following prolonged exposure to high environmental temperature. Acclimatization is very useful in conserving body NaCl as explained next.

The composition of sweat produced by glandular epithelial cells is modified by the ductal cells when sweat passes through the ducts. The NaCl concentration in primary secretion from the glandular cells is about 60 mEq/L. When the rate of sweat formation is low, the primary secretion passes slowly through the ducts, and during this time, most of the NaCl is reabsorbed by the ductal cells and the Na^+ concentration in the sweat may be as low as 5 mEq/L. On exposure to high-temperature environment, the sympathetic stimulation of the gland is very strong and so the rate of secretion becomes high. The primary secretion quickly passes through the ducts, and so the time available for Na^+ reabsorption is decreased. As a consequence, more NaCl is lost in the sweat, to the extent of 15–30 g/day. However, a prolonged exposure to high environmental temperature leads to acclimatization which leads to gradual decrease in NaCl concentration in the sweat, so that even at a high rate of sweat secretion, its Na^+ concentration remains low.

Mechanism of acclimatization: Acclimatization occurs due to increased secretion of aldosterone (stimulated due to slight decrease in NaCl levels of body fluids because of excessive sweating before acclimatization). Aldosterone increases absorption of Na^+ and Cl^- from the duct. This reduces excretion of salt to 3–5 g/day compared with 15–30 g/day before acclimatization.

3. Panting Panting refers to rapid shallow breathing which increases heat loss by increasing water vaporization in the mouth and respiratory passages. In some animals, like dogs, panting is an effective means of heat loss. Because the breathing is shallow, it produces little disturbance in the arterial pCO_2 or pH.

II. Mechanisms decreasing heat production and heat gain from environment

1. Anorexia and lethargy A rise in ambient temperature produces anorexia and lethargy. Anorexia results in decreased food intake which decreases heat production because of decrease in SDA of food. Lethargy decreases muscular activity which decreases heat of activity.

2. Behavioural responses Behavioural responses include shelter in shade or a cooler place and preference for cold food and drinks. These acts decrease heat gain from the environment.

B. Mechanisms Activated by Cold

I. Mechanisms conserving heat are:

1. Cutaneous vasoconstriction As mentioned earlier (see page 1201), the immediate reflex response to cold is cutaneous vasoconstriction, which reduces the heat loss from the body core to the surface and thus conserves heat.

Mechanism: Like vasodilatation, cutaneous vasoconstriction is produced through:

- Direct local effect of cold
- Local spinal reflex, evoked through peripheral thermoreceptors
- Hypothalamus-controlled cutaneous vasoconstriction
  Impulses from 'heat production and conservation centre' (which is located in the posterior hypothalamus) increase the sympathetic discharge to the cutaneous vessels causing extreme vasoconstriction. The effect of increased sympathetic

discharge is particularly prominent in the hands, feet and ear lobules where closure of A-V anastomoses (present in the skin) reduces the cutaneous blood flow to as low as 1 mL/100 g skin weight/min. As a result, the practically bloodless skin prevents heat loss by becoming an insulating barrier between the warm core of the body and the cold environment.

2. Piloerection Piloerection, i.e. cold-induced erection of the body hair, as mentioned earlier, entraps a layer of air in the hair, which acts as an insulator and thus reduces the cutaneous heat loss.

3. Behavioural responses Behavioural responses which help heat conservation are as follows:

Curling up while sleeping: It reduces the body surface area in contact with the environment.

Putting on warmer clothes also prevents heat loss.

II. Mechanisms increasing heat production Mechanisms increasing heat production include those given next.

1. Shivering thermogenesis When the heat loss prevented by cutaneous vasoconstriction is not sufficient to cope up with the environmental cold, heat production is increased by shivering (for details, see page 1200). Shivering is evoked in response to impulses from the 'heat production and conservation centre' located in the posterior or caudal hypothalamus.

2. Chemical (nonshivering) thermogenesis Chemical (nonshivering) thermogenesis refers to increased heat production due to increased cellular metabolism. It is associated with uncoupling of oxidative phosphorylation, i.e. the oxidation of foodstuffs is associated with release of heat rather than generation of ATPs. Chemical thermogenesis occurs because of the following effects:

i. Increased sympathetic stimulation and increased secretion of catecholamines (epinephrine and norepinephrine) occurs as a part of response to cold.

Role of brown fat: The amount of chemical thermogenesis occurring in response to increased catecholamine secretion is proportional to the amount of brown fat in the tissues, because the brown fat contains a large number of special mitochondria where the uncoupled oxidation occurs. Adults do not have brown fat; therefore, heat production by this mechanism is increased by only 10%–15%. However, in infants (who have brown fat in the interscapular region, around the neck, behind the sternum and around the kidneys), increased secretion of catecholamines may increase heat production by 100%.

ii. Increased secretion of thyroxine also promotes chemical thermogenesis. After several weeks of exposure to severe cold, hyperplasia of the thyroid gland and increased secretion of thyroxine can be demonstrated. This occurs because the cold temperature stimulates hypothalamic release of TRH, which in turn stimulates the secretion of TSH and thyroxine. Consequently, thyroxine secretion in winters is somewhat greater than in summers. In infants, even short exposure to cold increases thyroxine secretion.

3. Behavioural responses Behavioural responses associated with increased heat production are as follows:

i. ***Hyperphagia*** helps in increased heat production because of SDA of food.

ii. ***Hyperactivity***, e.g. in the form of rubbing of palms, also increases heat production.

iii. ***Seeking out sources of heat***, e.g. standing out in the sun, or heat fire and also consumption of hot food and hot drinks, helps in gaining heat.

Applied Aspects

Abnormalities of Body Temperature Regulation

Fever Fever, also known as *pyrexia*, refers to an increase in the body temperature above the normal range. It is the most common symptom/sign of the ill health.

Causes

Common causes of fever are as follows:

1. *Infections* caused by bacteria, viruses, protozoa (e.g. malaria) and other infecting agents are usually associated with fever.
2. *Tissue destruction*, as in myocardial infarction, uninfected neoplasms, serum sickness and rheumatism, etc., is also associated with fever.
3. *Pyrexia of unknown origin (PUO):* This term is used when the cause of fever cannot be ascertained.
4. *Hypersensitivity reactions* such as serum sickness are associated with fever.
5. *Neoplastic conditions* are also associated with fever.
6. *Stress* is also associated with fever.
7. *Genetic mutations in genes*; for pyrin (protein present in neutrophils), type 1 TNF receptors (involved in inflammation), mevalonate kinase (involved in synthesis of cholesterol) and the gene encoding for ryanodine receptors (RyR) lead to hyperthermia (see page 104).

Pathogenesis Fever develops when the hypothalamic set point is reset at a higher temperature by the pyrogens as explained next (Fig. 12.4.7).

Role of pyrogens: Toxins liberated from the infecting organism and tissue destruction act on the phagocytic cells (monocytes, macrophages and Kupffer cells) to produce cytokines that act as *endogenous pyrogens*. The pyrogens are polypeptides and include interleukin-1 (IL-1) and other cytokines, which act on the anterior hypothalamus to increase the production of prostaglandin E_2. Prostaglandin E_2 acts on the hypothalamus to increase the thermostat 'set point'. This explains how drugs like aspirin, which prevents the formation of prostaglandin E_2 from arachidonic acid, act as antipyretics (which lower the temperature).

Production of fever: Once the thermostat set point is raised by the pyrogens, the heat-producing mechanisms and heat-conserving mechanisms of the body are activated till the body temperature equals the elevated hypothalamic thermostat set point, i.e. till fever is produced. Because of these mechanisms, during production of fever, there occurs:

- Shivering (which produces heat) occurs.
- Skin vessels are constricted to minimize heat loss.
- Rate of metabolism is increased which increases further heat production.
- Chills are felt in fever when the heat-generating and heat-conserving mechanisms are active.

Termination of fever: When the causes producing pyrogens are removed, the set point of hypothalamic thermostat is reset back to normal. At this juncture, since the body temperature is

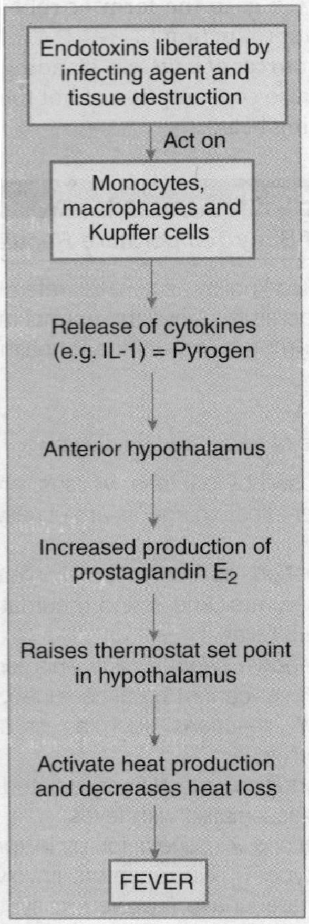

Fig. 12.4.7 Pathogenesis of fever.

higher than the set point of thermostat, the heat production is decreased and mechanisms of heat loss are activated. Because of these mechanisms, during termination of fever, there occurs:

- Cutaneous vasodilatation
- Profuse sweating

This sudden change in febrile condition associated with profuse sweating and red and hot skin is called *crisis* or *flush*.

Treatment of fever includes:

Nonsteroidal anti-inflammatory drugs (NSAIDs) such as aspirin are used. Aspirin acts by inhibiting the enzyme cyclooxygenase-2 (COX-2), thus inhibiting the production of prostaglandins from arachidonic acid.

Antibiotics can be given depending on infection by causative organisms.

Beneficial effects of fever include:

- *Inhibition of growth of bacteria, viruses* and other infecting organisms occurs at high body temperature. Because of this effect, artificial flu therapy was used to treat infections before the advent of antibiotics.
- *Antibody production* is increased when body temperature is raised.
- *Growth of some tumours* is slowed down by the increased body temperature.

Harmful effects of fever:

Fever is a catabolic state associated with:

- Dehydration, negative nitrogen balance, loss of NaCl and alkalosis (because of hyperventilation) may occur.
- Permanent damage to the brain, kidney and liver may occur when the core temperature is more than 41°C (hyperpyrexia) for a prolonged period.
- Death may occur due to heat stroke when temperature rises above 43°C.

Heat Exhaustion and Heat Stroke

Heat exhaustion refers to a condition of circulatory failure caused by excessive sweating following prolonged exposure to heat. It is characterized by dehydration, salt loss, decreased blood volume and decreased arterial pressure and syncope (fainting).

Heat stroke usually occurs when heavy physical work is performed in hot and humid environment. In this condition, normal response to increased ambient temperature (sweating) is impaired, and core temperature increases to the point of tissue damage. Convulsion, loss of consciousness and even death may occur when body temperature exceeds 41°C.

Hypothermia

Hypothermia results when the ambient temperature is so low that the body's heat-generating mechanisms (e.g. shivering and metabolism) cannot adequately maintain core temperature near the set point. Infants and old people develop hypothermia more easily than the adults.

It has been observed that:

- At a rectal temperature of 28°C, the body's ability to spontaneously return the temperature is lost.
- Humans can tolerate body temperature of 21–24°C without permanent ill effects, i.e. if rewarmed with external heat, they return to a normal state.

Effects of hypothermia on body include:

- Slowing of metabolic and physiological processes
- Retardation of glucose metabolism
- Slowing of respiration and heart rate
- Lowering of blood pressure
- Slowing of reflexes and occurrence of muscular rigidity
- Loss of consciousness
- Death, which may occur when temperature remains below 25°C for some time

Treatment includes:

- Depending on the cause of hypothermia, if the clothes are wet, then remove the wet clothes, dry the person and cover with warm blankets or give warm compressions.
- First, warm the trunk region and not the extremities (hands and feet) because it can result in a shock-like condition.
- Keep the room warm.
- Drugs like physostigmine can be used in severe cases.

Accidental hypothermia occurs due to prolonged exposure to cold air or cold water, e.g. after ship wreck or accidents in high mountains. It is a serious condition and requires careful monitoring and prompt rewarming.

Induced hypothermia: The fact that the human body can tolerate hypothermia (of 21–24°C) for quite some time without ill effects has been explained for use in heart and brain surgery. The induction of hypothermia during surgery is made easier with the use of anaesthesia and muscle relaxants, both of which abolish shivering.

Poikilothermia

Poikilothermia refers to a condition in which the individual is not able to maintain core body temperature during fluctuations in the environmental temperature. That is, with increase in the environmental temperature, the body temperature increases, and with the decrease in environmental temperature, the body temperature decreases. Such a condition of impaired thermoregulation occurs in hypothalamic lesions and brainstem lesions that interrupt descending hypothalamic fibres to the spinal cord.

Malignant Hyperthermia

Malignant hyperthermia is caused in susceptible individuals by inhalation anaesthesia. It is characterized by a massive increase in oxygen consumption and heat production by skeletal muscle, which causes a rapid rise in body temperature. In susceptive individuals, a defective ryanodine receptor leads to excess Ca^{2+} release during muscle contraction triggered by stress (see page 104).

Self-Assessment

1. Discuss about body heat balance and its maintenance.
2. Discuss the role of hypothalamus in regulation of body temperature.
3. Describe the following:
   - Mechanism of sweating
   - Pathophysiology of fever
4. Write notes on the following:
   - Thermoneutral zone
   - Hypothermia
   - Malignant hyperthermia

Clinical Cases

Case 1

A 15-year-old girl student staying in the hostel had high-grade fever and was shivering and feeling cold; she was brought to the emergency by the warden. The history revealed that there were a lot of mosquitoes in the hostel.

Examination showed oral temperature 39.60°C, pulse rate 138/min, respiratory rate 26/min, blood smear for malarial parasite negative and X-ray chest clear.

Q1. What is the pathogenesis of fever?
Q2. What is the reason for shivering?
Q3. What are the causes for fever?
Q4. What are the beneficial effects of fever?
Q5. What are the harmful effects of fever if not treated timely?

Case 2

A young labourer working at the construction site in extreme hot and humid conditions developed high-grade fever and jerky body movements; he was brought to the emergency in a confused state.

Examination showed body temperature 40.80°C, pulse rate 140/min regularly irregular and BP 100/54 mm Hg, and the patient was in a dehydrated state.

Q1. What is this condition called?
Q2. What is the cause for this condition?
Q3. What is the treatment?
Q4. What other investigations are required?
Q5. What are the ill effects if not treated?

Case 3

A 3-year-old male child went out of home and was exposed to extreme cold and windy weather for about 6–7 hours; he was brought by the police to the hospital emergency in a state of shivering; he could not speak properly, was confused and was not able to tell his parents' names.

Examination revealed rectal temperature 34.20°C, pulse weak and feeble, respiration slow, and fingers and toes cyanosed.

Q1. What is this condition?
Q2. What is the pathophysiology of this condition?
Q3. What is the reason for cyanosis?
Q4. What is the treatment?
Q5. What precaution should be followed while treating such cases?

12.5 Physiology of Growth and Behavioural Development

CHAPTER OUTLINE

GROWTH AND DEVELOPMENT

The terms growth and development are intimately interdependent and interacting with each other. Growth per se refers to the increase in the physical size, as the child grows to adulthood, whereas development refers to maturity, i.e. improvement in the capability of the tissue. They are, therefore, termed together to signify a process of maturation, in both quality and quantity.

GROWTH CURVES

Growth of different parts of the body does not follow a uniform pattern. The patterns of growth of different parts are described in the form of different growth curves (Fig. 12.5.1).

1. General growth curve General growth curve shows two growth spurts – one in infancy and another around puberty (Fig. 12.5.1A). General growth refers to increase in height, weight and growth of the skeletal muscle, blood volume, respiratory system, cardiovascular system, GIT and excretory system.

Infancy growth spurt Weight and height are generally considered a good index of the child's growth potential and a delicate measure of the individual's health.

The first spurt of growth occurring in infancy is characterized by increase in birth weight to two times by 6 months of age, three times at 1 year of age and four times at 2 years of age. After this, the weight increases by about 2 kg/year till about 12 years of age.

Height increases in increments of 2–2.5 cm/month in the first year of postnatal life. Thereafter, it slows down (Table 12.5.1).

Adolescent growth spurt Adolescent growth spurt is characterized by rapid increase in weight gain, about 3.5 kg/year, between 12 and 18 years of age (Table 12.5.1). During this period, rapid growth of bones is brought about by the various endocrinal influences. After this, the rate of growth again slows down. *Height* increase during adolescent growth of spurt varies between 4 and 7 cm/year depending on the genetic potential and endocrinal factors (Table 12.5.1).

2. Neural growth curve Neural growth curve shows that the brain, spinal cord and visual apparatus grow very rapidly after birth (Fig. 12.5.1B). At the end of the first year of postnatal life, the brain has already achieved two-thirds and by the end of the second year four-fifths of adult size. By 5 years of age, the brain is almost fully developed and the child is ready for education and training. The measurement of head circumference (which also increases with the growth of the brain) is thus very important up to 3–5 years of age to get information of the developing brain inside.

3. Lymphoid growth curve The growth of lymphoid organs such as tonsils, adenoids, thymus, spleen, lymph nodes and lymphoid tissue of the intestine is very rapid in infancy and childhood and is followed by a partial involution at puberty (Fig. 12.5.1C). Because of this reason, the size of tonsils and adenoids at the age of 8–10 years is larger than in the adults. It is important to recognize that more enlargement of tonsils is not an indication for removing them surgically.

4. Gonadal growth curve The gonads and accessory organs of reproduction remain in dormancy in childhood and grow at a remarkable rate around puberty. Thus, gonadal growth pattern is essentially opposite to the neural growth pattern (Fig. 12.5.1D).

FACTORS AFFECTING GROWTH

Marked differences existing between the growth and development patterns of various races and communities and different individuals in the same race and community are determined by various factors, which affect the growth.

1. Genetic factors The ultimate growth pattern of an individual is largely determined by the genetic inheritance, either maternal or paternal.

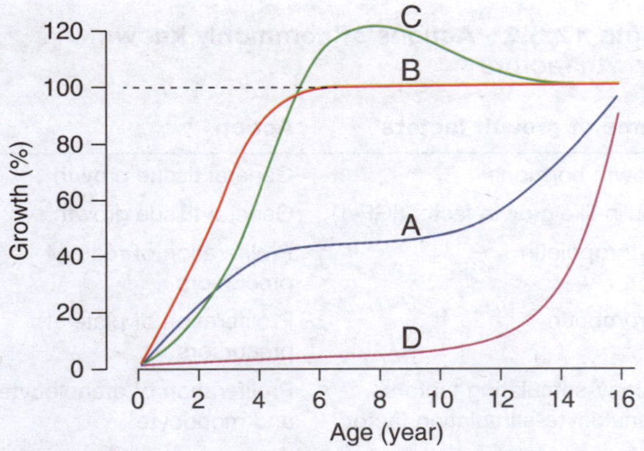

Fig. 12.5.1 Different growth curves: **A**, general growth curve; **B**, neural growth curve; **C**, lymphoid growth curve; and **D**, gonadal growth curve.

Table 12.5.1 Mean weight and height at different ages in Indian children

Age	Weight (kg) Male	Weight (kg) Female	Height (cm) Male	Height (cm) Female
Birth	2.8	2.7	48.5	47.7
3 months	4.5	4.5	60.2	58.5
6 months	6.2	6.0	65	63.6
9 months	7.9	7.5	68.7	67.6
1 year	8.9	8.4	73.9	72.8
3 years	12.6	12	88.8	87.2
6 years	16.3	16	108.5	107.4
9 years	21.5	21.3	123.7	122.9
12 years	28.5	29.8	138.3	139.2
15 years	39.6	36.8	155.5	149.6
18 years	47.4	42.4	163.1	151.7

Source: Indian Council of Medical Research (ICMR).

2. Hormonal factors The important hormones which affect the growth and development are as follows:

i. ***Growth hormone (GH)*** secreted by the anterior pituitary plays an important role in the growth and thus determines the height of an individual during childhood (see page 672). Therefore, deficiency of GH produces growth retardation known as *pituitary dwarfism*. For details, see page 676.

ii. ***Insulin-like growth factor-1 (IGF-1)***, as the name indicates, chemically resembles insulin. It is one of the polypeptides which are collectively known as somatomedins. IGF-1, like GH, promotes protein synthesis and epiphyseal growth. Some of its actions are opposite to those of GH. For details, see page 672.

iii ***Thyroxine*** plays an important role in the growth and development by its direct action, and also indirectly by potentiating the release of GH and somatomedins (see page 690). Congenital deficiency of thyroxine results in a clinical condition called 'cretinism', which is characterized by retardation of physical as well as mental growth. For details, see page 695.

iv. ***Sex hormones:*** The oestrogens and androgens cause maturation and are important in the adolescent age. The anabolic actions of sex hormones, adrenal androgens, GH and IGF-1 seem to potentiate each other, producing a marked growth spurt during puberty. For details, see page 797.

v. ***Insulin*** is an anabolic hormone and thus its role in growth and development cannot be overemphasized. Congenital deficiency of insulin results in juvenile diabetes mellitus. Retardation of growth is one of the characteristic features of juvenile diabetes mellitus. For details, see page 770.

Relative importance of different hormones at various stages of growth is as follows (Fig. 12.5.2):

- *Thyroxine* is essential for growth in late fetal life and first few years of postnatal life (Fig. 12.5.2A).
- *GH* in contrast to thyroxine does not seem to be of critical importance during fetal and early postnatal life. Infants with congenital deficiency of GH have normal height and weight up to about 2 years of age, after which a decrease in the velocity of growth becomes apparent (Fig. 12.5.2B).
- *Insulin*, being an anabolic hormone, remains important during fetal as well as postnatal growth (Fig. 12.5.2C).
- *Sex hormones* are most essential around puberty and play an important role in the development of gonads as well as general growth (Fig. 12.5.2D).

3. Nutritional factors The major ingredients of diet, i.e. proteins, fats, carbohydrates, minerals and vitamins, are important for optimal growth, both pre- and postnatally. Protein and its various amino acids are essential for laying down the new tissues, for wear and tear and for specific metabolic functions. Their requirements are increased during active periods of growth.

Lack of nutritional factors affects normal growth even when the genetic and hormonal factors are normal. Undernutrition and malnutrition in childhood is responsible for

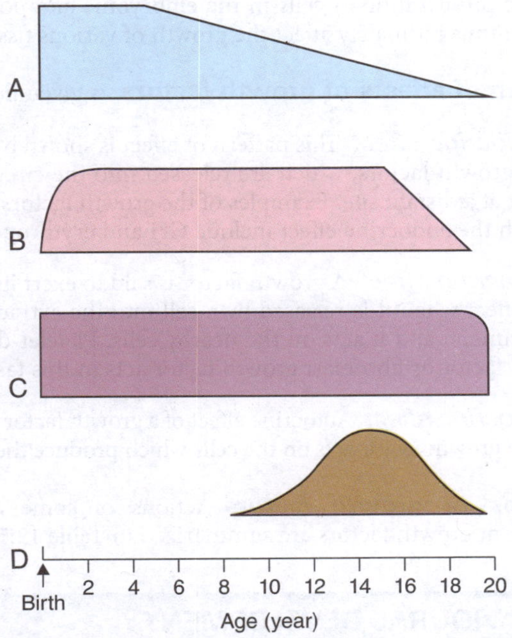

Fig. 12.5.2 Relative importance of different hormones at various stages of growth: **A**, thyroxine; **B**, growth hormone; **C**, insulin; and **D**, sex hormones.

smaller status, poor muscular development and generalized apathy in underdeveloped countries.

4. Illnesses Congenital anomalies compatible with life are likely to retard the growth of the child. Acute illnesses temporarily depress growth. Chronic long-standing illnesses, including long-standing infections, can markedly interfere with the normal pattern of physical and mental growth and can produce permanent growth retardation.

5. Emotional factors Lack of love and security and a disturbed child–parent relationship result in various psychological and behavioural problems during childhood and adolescence, which result in distortion of normal development and achievement of maturity.

6. Internal milieu Normal metabolism and coordinate functioning of all the organs result in optimum growth. Disturbed internal metabolism in various liver and kidney diseases precludes normal growth.

7. Environmental factors The environment influences the growth pattern right from the intrauterine life. Faulty position of the fetus, faulty implantation of the ovum, rubella syndrome, etc., are among the earliest environmental factors influencing growth. Birth injuries during a difficult labour and other factors during the natal period interfere with the normal development. Exposure to various seasonal variations has a similar effect. The countries in temperate zone have a small average height because of suboptimal environment. Lack of sunshine and poor personal hygiene also affect the normal growth.

8. Socioeconomic factors Socioeconomic factors also play an important role in growth and development of a child.

GROWTH FACTORS

Growth factors refer to a number of polypeptides which regulate the proliferation of cells in the embryonic and postnatal life and thus ultimately affect the growth of various tissues.

Pattern of effects of growth factors is given next.

1. Endocrine effect This pattern of effect is shown by some of the growth factors, which are released into the circulation and act at a distant site. Examples of the growth factors acting through the endocrine effect include GH and erythropoietin.

2. Paracrine effect A growth factor is said to exert its paracrine effect when it is released by a cell into the extracellular environment, and it acts on the nearby cells. Platelet-derived growth factor or fibroblast growth factor acts in this fashion.

3. Autocrine effect Autocrine effect of a growth factor means that the growth factor acts on the cells which produce them.

Actions of growth factors Actions of some of the important growth factors are summarized in Table 12.5.2.

Table 12.5.2 Actions of commonly known growth factors

Name of growth factors	Action
Growth hormone	General tissue growth
Insulin-like growth factor (IGF-1)	General tissue growth
Erythropoietin	Proliferation of red cell precursors
Thrombotin	Proliferation of platelet precursors
Colony-stimulating factors, granulocyte-stimulating factor	Proliferation of granulocyte and monocyte
Lymphokines	Proliferation of lymphocytes
Epidermal growth factor (EGF)	Proliferation of epithelial cells, fibroblasts and glial cells
Platelet-derived growth factor	Growth of vascular smooth muscle
Fibroblast growth factor	Proliferation of fibroblast, endothelial cells and vascular smooth muscle
Nerve growth factor	Growth and maintenance of neurons

BEHAVIOURAL DEVELOPMENT

Behavioural development of a child is studied through various responses which the child exhibits, following a natural or experimental stimulus. The developmental status depends not only on the age but also on the environment. The age determines the proper physical and biochemical growth of various constituent organs, and the environment determines the experiences during the process of learning. Hence, both the factors are essential to determine a particular behaviour which in other words could be called a milestone in the developmental process.

BEHAVIOUR PATTERN

Behaviour pattern can be divided into four groups, for the sake of convenience, to observe the development in different age groups (Gesell).

1. Motor behaviour Motor behaviour is of two types:

Gross motor behaviour is the behavioural response in ventral suspension, supine, prone, sitting, standing and walking postures.

Fine motor behaviour is seen in the form of grasp and manipulation of the objects, e.g. cube, pellet and string.

2. Adaptive behaviour This includes sensory and motor adjustments to objects and coordination of eyes and hands to adjust with the simple problem situations which are set before the infant.

3. Language behaviour This includes all visible and audible forms of communication whether by facial expression, gestures, postural movements, vocalization of words, phrases or sentences and mimicry. Articulate speech depends on social milieu and readiness of sensory, motor and cortical structures.

4. Personal–social behaviour A child's individual reaction depends primarily on the neuromotor maturity and the social culture in which the child lives. These include bladder and bowel control, feeding abilities, sense of priority, self-dependence in play, cooperativeness and emotional responsiveness to various stimuli.

DEVELOPMENTAL AND INTELLIGENT QUOTIENT

Developmental quotient (DQ) represents the proportion of normal development that is present at any given age. The measurement of the former depends on the achievement of the adaptive behaviour, e.g. prehension, locomotion and manipulation.

$$DQ = \frac{\text{Maturity age}}{\text{Chronological age}} \times 100$$

Intelligent quotient (IQ): The child can make use of his/her intellectual capabilities at the age of 5–6 years, because mental development is almost complete by this age. Therefore, IQ can be applied only at this age, unlike DQ which can be tested at any age after birth.

$$IQ = \frac{\text{Mental age}}{\text{Chronological age}} \times 100$$

MILESTONES

Some of the important developmental milestones at different ages are depicted in Table 12.5.3.

Table 12.5.3 Developmental milestones at different ages

Milestone (motor)	Age (weeks)
Holding of head with bobbing	12
Head control	16
Sitting with support	20
Sitting without support	26
Standing with support	32
Standing without support	36–40
Crawling on belly	30
Crawling on knees	32
Walking with support	45
Walking without support	52

Self-Assessment

1. Discuss the various growth curves and factors affecting growth.
2. Discuss about behavioural development.
3. Write notes on the following:
   - Developmental and intelligent quotient
   - Milestones
   - Growth factors

12.6 Physiology of Fetus, Neonate and Childhood

CHAPTER OUTLINE

INTRODUCTION

An infant or a child is not a miniature or small adult; rather, the difference between a child and an adult is more than that of the size. The physiological responses to environmental stresses, diseases and drugs are a lot different in a child and an adult. It is because of the fact that some of the organs develop during different stages of infancy or childhood, and in other organs, the function is not as well developed as in an adult. The difference is maximum between a newborn and an adult, and this gap gradually narrows down with the growth of a newborn into an adult. There exist both quantitative and qualitative differences between physiological responses of a child and adult in each organ system. Therefore, this section discusses some basic differences and specific details of systemic physiology of the fetus, neonate and childhood and how it changes during progress towards adulthood.

ROLE OF PLACENTA IN FETAL PHYSIOLOGY

UTERINE AND PLACENTAL CIRCULATION DURING PREGNANCY

Uterine Circulation

As described on page 819, the blood supply to the uterus comes through uterine arteries and fluctuates cyclically along with the menstrual cycle to fulfil the metabolic demands of myometrium and endometrium. During pregnancy, the uterine blood flow increases parallel to the increase in fetal weight and uterine size (Fig. 12.6.1A). During early pregnancy, a rise in the levels of oestrogen and progesterone leads to an increase in uterine blood flow which meets the increased O_2 demand. Eventually, the placenta develops and becomes the circulatory link between the mother and the fetus. Owing to increasing demand of O_2 with the progression of pregnancy, more and more O_2 is extracted from the uterine blood and consequently in later part of pregnancy, the O_2 saturation of uterine blood falls (Fig. 12.6.1B). As shown in Fig. 12.6.1A, the uterine blood flow increases tremendously (200–300 mL/min/kg of uterine mass including the fetus) during late pregnancy. To provide for it, the maternal cardiac output increases by 2–2.5 L/min near full term. Eighty per cent of the uterine blood flow enters the placenta. Just before parturition, there occurs a sharp decline in uterine blood flow, but the significance of this is not yet known.

Placental Circulation

Placenta, which forms the circulatory link between the mother and the fetus, also works as *fetal lung*, *fetal gut* and *fetal kidney*. It consists of two major portions (Fig. 12.6.2):

Maternal portion of the placenta is in fact a large blood sinus. The maternal blood flows through the uterine arteries into the maternal sinuses and back through the uterine veins of the mother.

Fetal portion of the placenta consists of placental villi. The fetal blood flows through umbilical arteries into the capillaries of placental villi and back through an umbilical vein into the fetus.

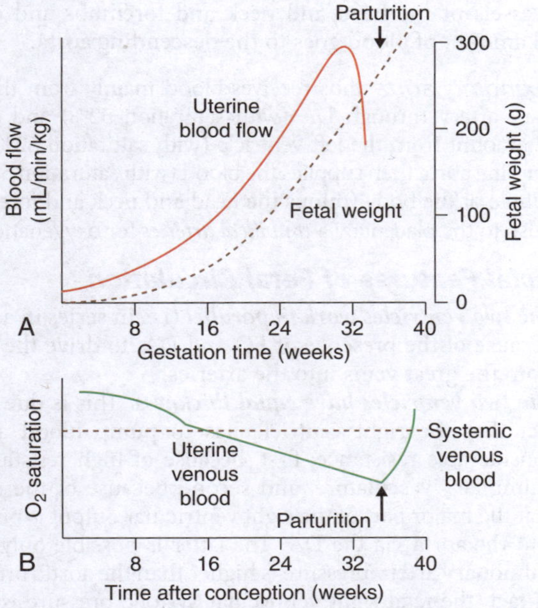

Fig. 12.6.1 Uterine circulation during pregnancy: **A**, changes in uterine blood flow; and **B**, changes in the amount of O_2 in the venous blood.

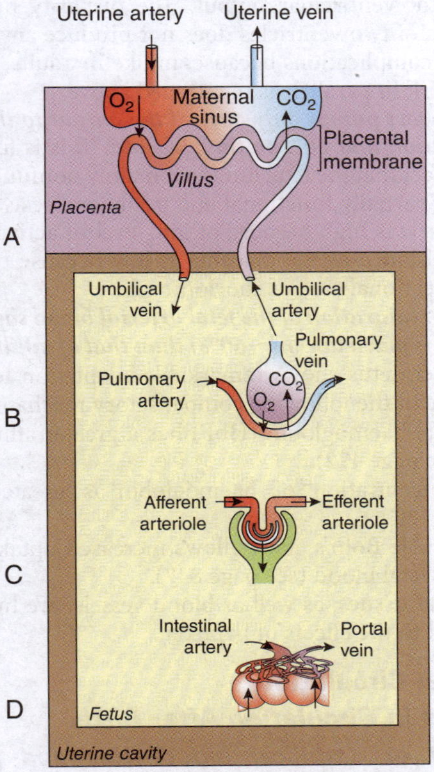

Fig. 12.6.2 Placental circulation: **A**, diagrammatic depiction of exchange across placental membrane between mother and fetal blood; **B**, diagrammatic depiction of gas exchange across pulmonary alveolus during extrauterine life. Observe the similarity with the process in placenta. For practical purposes, the umbilical artery can be compared with pulmonary artery and umbilical vein to pulmonary vein. **C**, diagrammatic depiction of nutrient absorption from the gut during extrauterine life. A similar process occurs in placenta where umbilical artery can be compared with intestinal artery and umbilical vein to portal vein. **D**, diagrammatic depiction of glomerular filtration during extrauterine life. In the fetus, a similar process takes place at placenta where the umbilical artery can be compared with afferent arteriole and umbilical vein to efferent arteriole.

EXCHANGE BETWEEN MATERNAL AND FETAL BLOOD ACROSS PLACENTAL MEMBRANE

As shown in Fig. 12.6.2, the placental villi containing fetal blood in capillaries project into and are then bathed by the blood in the maternal sinuses. Hence, in the placenta, the maternal and fetal blood do not mix with each other but are separated by the so-called placental membrane which consists (from fetal side) of the following layers (Fig. 9.4.6, page 842):

- Endothelium and basement membrane
- Surrounding mesenchymal tissue (connective tissue)
- Cytotrophoblast and its basement membrane
- Syncytiotrophoblast

All exchange of O_2, nutrients and waste products between the maternal and the fetal blood takes place through the placental membrane barrier.

1. Gaseous Exchange at Placenta: Placenta as Lung

As shown in Fig. 12.6.2A, O_2 is taken up by the fetal blood and CO_2 is discharged into the maternal circulation across the placental membrane in a fashion analogous to O_2 and CO_2 exchange in the lungs across the alveolocapillary membrane (Fig. 12.6.2B). However, it is important to note that the placental membrane (Fig. 9.4.6) is much thicker and less permeable than the alveolar membrane (Fig. 5.4.6), and, therefore, the exchange is much less efficient. Table 12.6.1 shows the values of gaseous interchange in the placenta.

2. Placental Transfer of Nutrients: Placenta as Gut

See page 846.

3. Excretion of Waste Products Through Placenta: Placenta as Kidney

See page 846.

SYSTEMIC PHYSIOLOGY OF FETUS, NEWBORN AND CHILDHOOD

CARDIOVASCULAR PHYSIOLOGY

Fetal Circulation

Pattern of Fetal Circulation

Pattern of fetal circulation shown in Fig. 12.6.3 and represented diagrammatically in Fig. 12.6.4 is as follows:

Umbilical vein brings oxygenated blood from the placenta, which acts as lungs for the fetus (see above). This blood is

Table 12.6.1 Values of pO_2 and pCO_2 in the maternal and umbilical cord blood

Blood vessel	pO_2 (mm Hg)	pCO_2 (mm Hg)
Uterine artery	95	36
Uterine vein	50	40
Umbilical artery	20	50
Umbilical vein	35	43

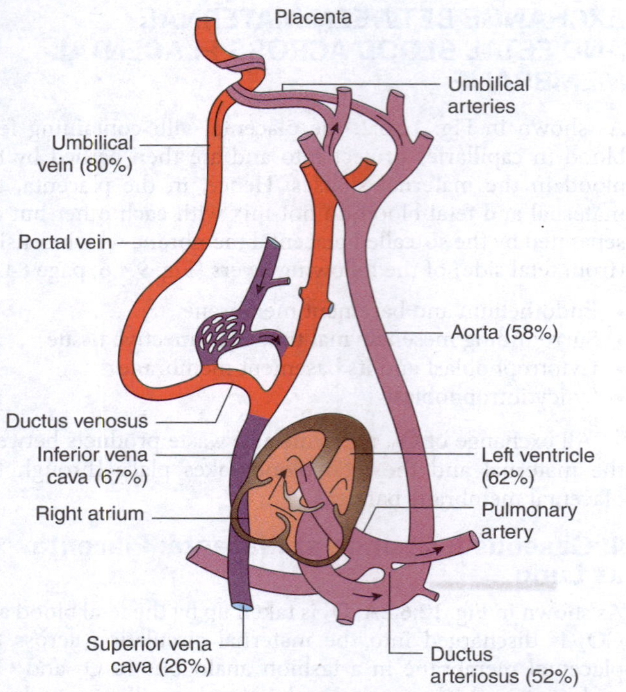

Fig. 12.6.3 Pattern of fetal circulation with pO_2 in different components.

80% saturated with O_2 (compared with 98% saturation in the arterial circulation in adults). The umbilical vein, before supplying the blood to the liver, bypasses some of the blood to the inferior vena cava through ***ductus venosus*** (Fig. 12.6.3).

Inferior vena cava thus receives some blood (80% saturated with O_2) from the umbilical vein through ductus venosus, and other blood from the hepatic veins and systemic veins draining from the trunk and inferior extremities (26% saturated with O_2). The mixed blood from the inferior vena cava (with approximate 67% saturation) then enters the right atrium.

Right atrium receives blood from the inferior vena cava (saturation 67%) as well as the superior vena cava (saturation 26%). The fate of blood entering the right atrium is very different from that in adults:

- From the right atrium, majority of the blood coming from the inferior vena cava (saturation 67%) passes to the left atrium directly through the *foramen ovale* (FO; an opening in the interatrial septum), and joins the blood coming from the pulmonary vein (saturation 42%). The mixed blood from the left atrium (saturation 62%) passes on to the left ventricle.
- From the right atrium, most of the blood coming from the superior vena cava (26% saturation) and a small amount of that coming from the inferior vena cava (saturation 67%) pass into the right ventricle. This mixed blood from the right ventricle (saturation 52%) is pumped into the pulmonary artery. But, since the fetal lungs are collapsed, their vascular resistance is very high. Hence, only a small fraction of blood passes through the lungs to reach the left atrium via the pulmonary veins. Bulk of the pulmonary artery blood enters the descending aorta directly by a vascular connection called the *ductus arteriosus* (DA).

Left ventricle pumps the blood (with saturation 62%) into the ascending aorta, from where most of the blood goes into the vessels of the head and neck and forelimbs and only a small amount of blood goes to the descending aorta.

Descending aorta thus receives blood mainly from the pulmonary artery through DA (with saturation 52%) and only a small amount from the left ventricle (with saturation 62%). The descending aorta then supplies the blood (with saturation 58%) to the whole of the body (minus the head and neck and forelimbs) and also to the placenta via *umbilical arteries* for oxygenation.

Special Features of Fetal Circulation

1. ***The two ventricles work in parallel*** (i.e. in series in adults), because of the presence of FO and DA, to drive the blood from the great veins into the arteries.
2. ***The two ventricles have equal thickness.*** This is due to the fact that the right ventricle has to pump blood against considerable resistance, first, because of high resistance of pulmonary vasculature, and second because of the reason that the major part of the right ventricular output is pumped into the aorta via the DA. The latter is possible only if the pulmonary artery pressure is higher than the aortic pressure. In fact, the fetal right ventricular systolic pressure is a few millimetres higher than the left ventricular pressure.
3. ***The two ventricles do not have similar cardiac output.*** The left ventricular output is approximately 20% greater than the right ventricular output. The disparity between the outputs of two ventricles does not produce any haemodynamic complications because, unlike in adults, the ventricles work in parallel, as mentioned above.
4. ***Fetal heart pumps only 40% of the output to the systemic circulation and 60% to the placenta.*** This is first because of the fact that the fetal lungs are mainly nonfunctional, the liver is partially functional and peripheral resistance of fetal vessels is high because of low level of activity. Second, the resistance of the placenta is low because of the large cross-sectional area of chorionic villi.
5. ***Oxygen saturation of the fetal arterial blood supplying the tissues is much lower (~60%) than that of adults (~98%).*** However, fetus shows remarkable adaptation to low pO_2, because of the following compensatory mechanisms:
   i. Fetal haemoglobin (HbF) has a greater affinity for O_2 (see page 422).
   ii. Concentration of haemoglobin is greater in fetus (18–20 g%).
   iii. Double Bohr's effect allows increased uptake of O_2 by the fetal blood (see page 847).
   iv. Fetal tissues, as well as blood vessels, are highly resistant to the effects of hypoxia.

Neonatal Circulation

Changes in Circulation After Birth

1. Arrest of umbilical blood flow and placental transfusion Factors responsible for arrest of umbilical blood flow and placental transfusion are given next.

i. Vasoconstriction of umbilical vessels Immediately after birth, there occurs sudden and marked reduction in blood flow through the umbilical vessels. It results from vasoconstriction of the umbilical vessels in response to:

- Mechanical stimulation
- Exposure to cold air
- Secretion of catecholamines from the infant's adrenal medulla due to stress

ii. Tying and cutting of the umbilical cord The process which is initiated by nature by producing vasoconstriction is completed by the doctor by tying and cutting the umbilical cord.

Precautions to be taken while tying the umbilical cord are as follows:

- Milking of the umbilical cord should not be done, because it can send so much blood to the infant that its circulation may get overloaded.
- Infant should be held at or slightly below the level of the vagina, as it leads to transfer of an additional 60–80 mL of blood to the infant, which is very useful.
- Optimum time to tie the umbilical cord is 40–60 seconds after birth. Tying earlier than this will prevent the transfer of additional blood from the placenta for the infant, and delay in tying may be associated with risk of blood flow from the infant to the placenta producing haemorrhagic anaemia.

2. Closure of foramen ovale Factors leading to closure to FO are given next.

i. Reduction in inferior vena cava–left atrial pressure gradient The valve of FO is held open before the birth by the pressure and momentum of blood flowing up to the inferior vena cava. After birth, closure of the umbilical circulation immediately decreases the volume of blood flowing up the inferior vena cava and causes contraction of ductus venosus within 1–3 hours after birth. Consequently, there occurs a reduction in the inferior vena cava–left atrial pressure gradient favouring functional closure of the valve of FO.

ii. Decrease in right atrial and right ventricular pressure Following arrest of umbilical flow, after birth, the infant develops asphyxia (i.e. pO_2 is lowered and pCO_2 is raised). Fetal asphyxia leads to an intense peripheral chemoreceptor discharge resulting in initiation of breathing. The infant gasps several times and the lungs expand. The inflation of lungs after birth causes a 10% decrease in pulmonary vascular resistance. The decreased resistance causes a large drop in the afterload of the right ventricle and lowers the right atrial and right ventricular pressure. The drop in the right-sided pressure causes pressure in the left atrium to exceed the pressure in the right atrium. This pressure reversal causes the flap-like valve to close over the FO.

The valve then normally fuses to the interatrial septum over the next few days.

Closure of the FO prevents the right-to-left flow of venous blood and thus improves the oxygenation of systemic arterial blood.

3. Changes in pulmonary circulation Rapid fall in pulmonary artery pressure, which occurs following inflation of previously collapsed lungs (as described above), is accompanied with a 6- to 10-fold increase in pulmonary blood flow. In the fetus, the pulmonary arterial pressure is slightly higher than that in the aorta and most of the output from the right heart passes through the DA to the aorta. After birth, the position is reversed, for the aortic pressure rises and pulmonary artery pressure falls so that blood flow through the DA, which remains partially open for many hours after birth, occurs from the aorta to the pulmonary trunk, i.e. in the reverse direction to that which takes place in the fetus (Fig. 12.6.4A and B).

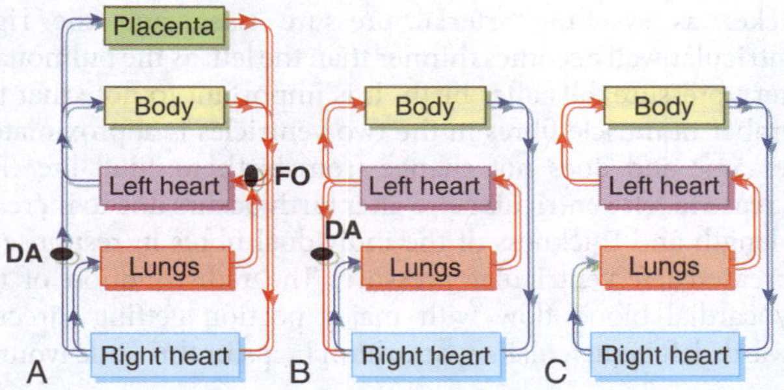

Fig. 12.6.4 Diagrammatic depiction of circulatory pattern: **A**, fetus; **B**, newborn; and **C**, adult. DA, ductus arteriosus; FO, foramen ovale.

4. Closure of ductus arteriosus The DA is almost as large as the ascending aorta of the mature fetus and has a thick, smooth muscle wall. The closure of ductus occurs in three steps:

- Vasoconstriction with partial patency
- Complete functional closure
- Permanent sealing with fibrous tissue

i. Vasoconstriction of DA occurs rapidly during the first few hours after birth but final functional closure takes place gradually over the next 1–3 days.

Factors responsible for constriction of ductus are as follows:

- Rise in pO_2 of neonatal blood which occurs following inflation of the lungs after birth causes constriction of ductus (this is consistent with the higher incidence of persistent patency of the ductus associated with fetal distress at birth and with delivery at high altitude)
- Vasoconstrictor effect of catecholamines released due to stress of birth
- Fall in levels of prostaglandins PGE and PGF_2, which help in keeping the DA patent during fetal life because of their vasodilator effect (therefore, inhibitors of prostaglandin synthesis like aspirin and indomethacin have been used clinically to promote closure of patent ductus arteriosus [PDA] in premature babies)

Blood flow through constricted ductus after birth: For the first hour after birth, flow continues through the ductus in the fetal direction (i.e. right-to-left shunt from the pulmonary artery to the aorta), but subsequently the flow reverses due to reduction in pulmonary pressure and rise in aortic pressure (as described above).

Flow of blood through this constricted but slightly patent ductus is responsible for the murmur which may be heard by careful auscultation in the immediate neonatal period. The murmur, though continuous, reaches a crescendo with each second heart sound.

ii. Functional closure of the ductus with complete muscular contraction occurs gradually over the next 1–8 days.

iii. Permanent sealing of the ductus lumen occurs 2–3 weeks after birth by replacement of musculature with fibrous tissue.

5. Changes in cardiac muscle During fetal life, the two ventricles have almost similar thickness, because the pressure in the pulmonary artery is slightly greater than the aortic pressure. However, after birth, the left ventricular wall rapidly grows thicker as systemic arterial pressure rises, and the right ventricular wall becomes thinner than the left, as the pulmonary artery pressure falls after birth. It is important to note that the number of muscle fibres in the two ventricles is approximately the same and does not change from birth to adult life. The increase in left ventricular size after birth occurs due to increase in length and thickness of the individual fibres in response to increased left ventricular pressure. The redistribution of the myocardial blood flow with major portion getting directed towards left ventricular myocardium helps in this endeavour.

Status of Cardiovascular System After Birth

1. ***Heart rate:*** Immediately after birth, the heart rate of an infant is approximately 140 beats/min. During infancy and childhood, heart rate decreases gradually and the adult values are reached only at puberty (Table 12.6.2).
   Sinus arrhythmia, i.e. variation in heart rate during two phases of respiration, can be observed in infants and children even during normal quiet breathing. In adults, it is observed only during deep breathing.
2. ***Blood pressure:*** At birth, the mean arterial blood pressure is approximately 80 mm Hg. During the next few hours, it declines to about 65 mm Hg. Thereafter, the blood pressure gradually increases throughout infancy and childhood to reach the adult values by the end of pubertal growth (Table 12.6.3).
3. ***Blood volume*** at birth is 300 mL (or 90 mL/kg).
4. ***Cardiac output*** at birth is about 550 mL/min (which is two times as much in relation to body weight as in the adult).
5. ***Electrocardiography (ECG):*** At birth, the ECG record shows all the normal waves; however, the right ventricular preponderance is indicated by mild right-axis deviation. After a few months of postnatal life, the right-axis deviation is no more evident. Left ventricular preponderance, indicated by mild left-axis deviation, is established between the ages of 6 and 8 years.

Table 12.6.2 Heart rate values in relation to age

Age	Heart rate (beats/min)
Birth	140–150
1 month	130–140
1 year	110–115
5 years	105–110
10 years	95–100
15 years	80–85
Adults	70–80
Old age	Up to 100

Table 12.6.3 Blood pressure values in relation to age

	Blood pressure (mm Hg)	
Age	**Systolic**	**Diastolic**
Birth	70–90	30–45
15 days	70	45
1 month	75	85
1 year	85	55
5 years	100	60
12 years	105	62
17 years	115	68
Adult	120	80
Old age	140	90

Applied Aspects

Congenital Heart Diseases

Congenital heart diseases occur either due to defective development of the embryonic heart or due to defect in the closure of three channels of communication (ductus venosus, DA and FO) after birth. A few common congenital heart diseases are described briefly.

1. Atrial Septal Defect

Atrial septal defect (ASD) results from failure of FO to close. A very small symptomless defect is not uncommon. A large defect causes problem due to shunting of a large volume of blood from the left atrium to the right atrium, and then to the right ventricle and pulmonary arteries. Thus, initially the right ventricle is overburdened, and later on pulmonary hypertension may develop. In ASD, oxygen-rich blood passes from the left atrium through opening in the septum and mixes with oxygen-poor blood in the right atrium.

Types: There are four major types of ASDs:

i. ***Ostium secundum ASD*** is the most common type. It is caused when a part of atrial septum fails to close completely.
ii. ***Ostium primum ASD:*** In this, there is a defect in the atrioventricular canal and is associated with cleft in one of the leaflets of the mitral valve.
iii. ***Sinus venosus ASD:*** This defect occurs at the junction of the superior vena cava and the right atrium, where pulmonary veins open into the heart. As a result, the pulmonary veins open into the right atrium instead of into the left atrium.
iv. ***Coronary sinus ASD:*** This defect lies within the walls of the coronary sinus where it passes behind the left atrium.

Signs and symptoms include:

- *Poor growth*
- *Tiredness on playing*
- *Fatigue*
- *Rapid and shallow breathing*
- *Frequent lung infection*

Diagnosis: *On examination, heart murmur occurs due to extra amount of blood flow through the pulmonary valve.*

Investigations *include:*

- *X-ray chest* shows heart enlargement due to handling of a large amount of blood by the right atrium and right ventricle.
- *Electrocardiogram (ECG)* shows arrhythmia.
- *Echocardiogram:* An echocardiogram can show pattern of blood flow through atrioseptal opening.
- *Cardiac catheterization* is an investigative procedure that gives detailed information about the structures inside the heart.

Treatment may include:
- *Medication* may be prescribed, for example, diuretics help the kidneys to remove excess fluid.
- *Surgical repair:* Usually, surgical repair is done if ASD is not closed on its own with time.
- *Device closure* is frequently done for ostium secundum ASD using septal occluders.

2. Ventricular Septal Defect

Ventricular septal defect (VSD) occurs due to defective development of interventricular septum. It is the most common congenital cardiac defect occurring in 1:500 live births. It is an acyanotic heart defect with left-to-right (L → R) shunt. The VSD may be small and isolated or may be a part of a complex congenital heart disease.

3. PDA

It is also an acyanotic congenital defect with left-to-right (L → R) shunt, as the blood flows from a high-pressure vessel (aorta) to a low-pressure vessel (pulmonary artery).

4. Tetralogy of Fallot

It occurs due to defective development of an embryonic heart, and, as the name indicates, consists of four components:
- VSD
- Overriding of the aorta at the level of VSD
- Pulmonary stenosis (subvalvular)
- Right ventricular hypertrophy

Due to pulmonary stenosis and large VSD, the right ventricular pressure is elevated and leads to right-to-left (R → L) shunt resulting in mixing of unoxygenated and oxygenated blood that is pushed through the overridden aorta. Thus, there occurs tissue hypoxia which produces cyanosis (bluish discolouration of the skin) and clubbing of the fingers in infancy or after the first year of life. Capacity for physical exercise is limited.

Signs and symptoms may include:
- *Cyanosis* along with poor feeding and poor weight gain
- *Rapid shallow breathing*
- *Presystolic murmur*

Diagnosis: VSD can be detected by cardiac auscultation and echocardiography.

Treatment depends on severity; most of these holes close on their own with time; however, the symptoms can be treated with:
Medication such as diuretics and ACE inhibitors
Supportive care
Surgical treatment that includes percutaneous VSD closure

RESPIRATORY PHYSIOLOGY

Fetal Respiration

Placenta as Lung

As described earlier (see page 847), the placenta acts as the site of gas exchange for the fetus before birth.

Oxygen and Carbon Dioxide Transport in the Fetus

See page 847.

Fetal Breathing Movements

Though gaseous exchange does not occur in the fetal lung, the breathing movements do occur during fetal life. Since the lungs are filled with fluid with a viscosity and density many times that of air, the breathing movements lead to only small alterations in pulmonary volume. Thus, there is little mixing of amniotic fluid and lung fluids. It has been suggested that the purpose of these breathing movements in utero is to exercise and train the respiratory muscles for their function after birth. Ultrasound scanning technique reveals fetal breathing movements as early as 11 weeks of gestation. Initially irregular, they gradually become more regular.

Fetal Pulmonary Blood Flow and Peripheral Chemoreceptors

Pulmonary blood flow, during fetal life, is just a fraction of the right ventricular outflow because, due to high pulmonary vascular resistance, most of the right ventricular output is diverted to the aorta through the DA.

Peripheral chemoreceptors are fully developed in a fetus before birth. However, due to some unexplained mechanisms, there is no chemoreceptor discharge in spite of very low pO_2 in the fetal blood.

Pulmonary Surfactant

See page 394.

Respiratory Adjustments at Birth

Birth is the most traumatic event that the respiratory system must withstand during the entire life span of an individual. It involves sudden transfer from a situation in which no breathing effort is necessary to one in which continual breathing effort is indispensable.

Initiation of breathing The essential changes which occur while shifting from perinatal respiration to postnatal respiration are summarized as follows:

Pulmonary fluid, which fills the airway in the fetus, keeps the respiratory system at approximately functional residual capacity (FRC). Hence, a major requirement after birth is speedy replacement of fluid by the air so that the respiratory movements can be easier and more useful in terms of gas exchange. From the lungs, fluid is removed by the following forces:
- Part of this vital task is accomplished when the thorax is squeezed while passing through birth passages during delivery.
- Part of the fluid is absorbed into the pulmonary capillaries and lymphatics after birth, and some fluid is removed by evaporation.

Alveolar epithelium, which has got a fluid secretory function in the prenatal period, changes its function to fluid reabsorption after birth.

Factors which stimulate first breath after the birth have been an interesting area of research and speculation, and probably are as follows:
- Squeezing of the thorax during birth
- Lower temperature outside as compared with that inside the uterus
- Sound, light, gravity and tactile and painful stimuli
- Fall in arterial pO_2 and rise in pCO_2 (asphyxia) due to suspension of fetal respiration for a small period during birth and mainly following arrest of umbilical flow (see page 1214), which is the main stimulant for initiation of breathing

All the above-stated factors are mediated through nerves, so these may be depressed if the mother receives general anaesthesia during labour, as the fetus is also anaesthetized.

Intrapleural pressure generated during the first few breaths is very high, about 60 mm Hg, since the lungs are partly fluid filled. The intense efforts required to expand the lungs slowly decrease and normalize in 2 weeks. During this period, *surfactant* is also produced lowering the surface tension which stabilizes the alveoli and allows the lung volume to increase steadily during the first few weeks of life.

Effects of initial breathing: After the first gasping breath, the normal breathing pattern is gradually established within hours of the breathing. The neonate recovers from hypoxia, hypercapnia and acidosis present throughout fetal life and aggravated markedly by the process of birth and subsequent ligation of the umbilical cord.

Neonatal resistance to hypoxia: It may be mentioned that even when the breathing is not initiated up to 10 minutes after birth, the neonate shows normal postnatal growth and development. Resistance to such a prolonged and severe hypoxia is a peculiar feature of neonatal physiology and does not occur in later life.

Neonatal respiration and haematological changes: Haematological changes also take place after birth, because the adaptations in the form of high haemoglobin level and fetal type of haemoglobin which are necessary to cope with the hypoxic environment in the uterus (pO_2 of the oxygenated fetal blood is 30 mm Hg and that of the mother's blood in the placenta is 50 mm Hg) are no more required after birth. The haemoglobin level falls by haemolysis outplacing erythropoiesis, and the haemoglobin type changes to the adult variety soon after birth (see page 140).

To conclude, it can be said that one set of mechanisms makes it possible for the fetus to respire and survive in the uterus, and another set of mechanisms makes the sudden transmission from the hypoxic but sheltered uterine environment to the normoxic but harsh extrauterine environment a smooth journey. One can only marvel at the gently coordinated events involved in the process.

Applied Aspects

Birth asphyxia/perinatal asphyxia or neonatal asphyxia is a respiratory problem that occurs due to oxygen deficit to a newborn during delivery process. It generally results from interruption of placental blood flow leading to hypoxia, hypercarbia and acidosis.

Apgar score is a scoring system that helps to assess the general condition of the newborn immediately after birth (1–5 minutes). The Apgar test is done after delivery and scoring points are recorded (Table 12.6.4). For Apgar scoring, there are five criteria, and for each criterion, the scoring points are 0, 1 and 2 (2 being the best). The total score is calculated by adding the five values. The general condition is interpreted as:

- Normal/excellent condition: 7–10 scoring points
- Moderately depressed: 4–6 scoring points
- Severely depressed: 0–3 scoring points

Table 12.6.4 Apgar score for assessment of status of newborn general condition

Criteria	Score 0	Score 1	Score 2
***A:* Appearance (skin colour)**	Pale or blue	Pink body and blue extremities	Pink body and pink extremities
***P:* Pulse** (heart rate)	Absent	<100 beats/min	>100 beats/min
***G:* Grimace** (reflex response)	Absent	Minimal response	Prompt response
***A:* Activity** (muscle tone)	Absent	Some flexion in extremities	Active and spontaneous
***R:* Respiration**	Absent	Slow and irregular	Good with cry

Table 12.6.5 Respiratory rate and tidal air in relation to age

Age	Respiratory rate (/min)	Tidal air volume (mL)
Premature	40–80	10–12
Full term/newborn	30–60	16–18
1 year	20–40	48
2 years	20–30	90
5 years	20–25	175
10 years	15–20	400
15 years	15–20	400

Status of Respiratory System After Birth

1. ***Number of alveoli in the lungs:*** About 20 million alveoli are present in the lungs at birth, and their number increases to the adult value of 300 million alveoli by the age of 8–10 years. After this age till the end of pubertal growth, the lungs increase in size because of increase in the size of alveoli rather than increase in their number.
2. ***Respiratory rate*** of a newborn is very high (30–60/min) and gradually decreases during infancy and childhood. The adult values of respiratory rate are reached at about 10 years of age (Table 12.6.5).
3. ***Tidal air volume*** at birth in a premature infant is 10–12 mL, whereas in a full-term newborn, it is 16–18 mL and keeps on increasing throughout childhood, till the pubertal growth is completed (Table 12.6.5).
4. ***Vital capacity*** also continues to increase throughout childhood. It reaches about 3.3 L at the age of 15 years.
5. ***Minute ventilation*** at birth is about 140 mL/min. This is two times as great as that of an adult in relation to body weight.
6. ***FRC*** in a newborn is only half that of an adult in relation to body weight.

Applied Aspects

Respiratory distress syndrome (RDS) or neonatal breathing disorder, also used to be called hyaline membrane disease, commonly occurs in premature infants due to lack of surfactant in the lungs. For details, see page 395.

BLOOD AND IMMUNE MECHANISMS

Erythropoiesis, Leucopoiesis and Thrombopoiesis

- *At 2 weeks of gestation*, erythropoiesis begins in the mesenchymal tissue of yolk sac. Large RBCs with low haemoglobin concentration are produced at this stage.

- *At second and third months of gestation*, the chief sites of erythropoiesis, leucopoiesis and thrombopoiesis are the liver and spleen.
- *After 4 months of gestation*, the chief site for erythropoiesis is the bone marrow.
- *In postnatal life*, the bone marrow remains the only site of erythropoiesis. However, the extramedullary regions (liver and spleen) remain the potential sites of erythropoiesis when the entire bone marrow has been damaged (myelosclerosis). For details, see page 132.

Fetal Haemoglobin and Adult Haemoglobin

Characteristic features of HbF and adult haemoglobin (HbA) are described on page 140. The salient point to be noted is that HbF has a higher affinity than the HbA. Up to 32 weeks of gestation, fetus RBCs contain only HbF, after which HbA begins to be synthesized in low concentration. Consequently, by 36 weeks of gestation, the fetal RBCs contain 90% HbF and 10% HbA. After birth, synthesis of HbF practically ceases; consequently, its concentration in the newborn's blood declines linearly. At about 3–4 months of age, almost all the RBCs contain HbA, and HbF is completely absent from the blood.

Characteristics of Blood in Newborn

1. ***Haemoglobin*** concentration is high (16–18 g%). It is related to low pO_2 of the fetal blood. Changes in Hb seen with age are depicted in Table 12.6.6.
2. ***RBC count*** at birth is about 5.5–6.6 million/mm^3, which gradually decreases to 3–4 million/mm^3 by approximately 10–12 weeks of age due to absence of hypoxic stimulus of fetal life, and returns to normal within another 2–3 months (Table 12.6.5).
3. ***WBC count at birth*** is nearly 20,000/mm^3 with preponderance of neutrophils (70%). It decreases to about 12,000/mm^3 with marked decrease in neutrophils (30%) by the end of 1 month. From the first month to 1 year of life, lymphocytes predominate. Normal adult values of WBC count are reached at 5–10 years of age (Table 12.6.6).
4. ***Coagulation factors:*** *At birth*, though all the clotting factors and fibrinolysins are present in plasma, the levels of prothrombin and factors V, VII and X are subnormal.
   In the first week of postnatal life, the levels of these clotting factors may decrease to a level to produce the so-called *haemorrhagic diseases of newborn*, which is characterized by bleeding from the umbilicus, GIT and other internal organs. Premature infants are more prone to it. This occurs primarily because of deficiency of vitamin K and consequently decreased synthesis of vitamin K–dependent clotting factors by immature hepatocytes. That is why to prevent this disease, injection of vitamin K is given immediately after birth as prophylaxis.
   At about 2–12 months of age, the adult values of all the clotting factors are reached.
5. ***Immunological functions:*** The newborn is competent to produce both T lymphocyte– and B lymphocyte–mediated response.
   IgG levels: During intrauterine life, IgG levels are actively transferred from the maternal blood to the fetus. Consequently, at birth, the newborn's plasma level of IgG is even higher than the maternal plasma level (Table 12.6.7). However, soon the IgG levels decline rapidly to reach a level of 400–500 mg% within 1 week compared with greater than 1200 mg% at birth. At about 4 months of age, the infant's immunological apparatus starts manufacturing IgG and adult levels are reached by the age of 8 months.
   IgA and IgM are not transferred to the fetus; consequently, their levels are much lower at birth as compared with the mother's levels (Table 12.6.7). After birth, IgM begins to rise rapidly, reaching 30 mg/dL by the end of 1 week and 45 mg/dL at 6 months of age. IgA levels also begin to rise in infancy, but adult levels are reached by the age of 12–16 years.

Applied Aspects

Physiological Anaemia

At birth, the cord blood shows a high concentration of erythropoietins, high Hb concentration (18 g/dL) and high RBC count (5.5–6.5 million/mm^3). It is related to low pO_2.

After birth, the hypoxic stimulus present throughout intrauterine life disappears and the pO_2 is raised. Consequently, after 1 week of life, there occurs complete cessation of RBC production in the bone marrow. As a result, by 10–12 weeks of life, the Hb concentration may fall to as low as 9–10 g/dL and RBC count may be as low as 3–4 million/mm^3. This produces the so-called *physiological anaemia* of the newborn, which cannot be prevented even by administration of haematinics. The disappearance of erythropoietin and reticulocytes from the infant's blood supports the explanation that physiological anaemia of newborn is related to disappearance of hypoxic stimulus after birth.

Table 12.6.6 Hb concentration, RBC count and WBC count in relation to age

Age	Hb concentration (g%)	RBC count (million/mm^3)	TLC per mm^3	DLC	
				Poly (%)	Lymphocyte (%)
1 day	18	6.0	20,000	70	20
1 month	16	4.7	12,000	30	60
3 months	10	4.0	11,000	35	55
1 year	12.5	4.5	10,000	45	50
5 years	13.0	4.7	8000	55	40
10 years	13.0	4.7	8000	60	35

Table 12.6.7 Levels of IgG, IgA and IgM (mg%) in maternal and fetal blood (at birth)

Immunoglobulin	Maternal blood (mg/dL)	Fetal blood (mg/dL)
IgG	1000	1230
IgA	350	7
IgM	125	15

NERVOUS SYSTEM

Neural growth is completed by 4–5 years of age (see page 1208):

- At the end of 1 year, 50% of postnatal growth is completed.
- At the end of 3 years, 75% of postnatal growth is completed.
- At the end of 5 years, 90% of postnatal growth is completed.

CNS weight:body weight ratio is as follows:

- At birth, 1:10
- At 5 years, 1:20
- In an adult, 1:50

Myelination begins during fetal life, but continues for several years postnatally.

Blood–brain barrier is not well developed at birth. This accounts for higher levels of protein, sugar and white cell count in CSF of newborn compared with those in later childhood. This also explains the occurrence of kernicterus in an infant at that level of serum bilirubin which is harmless in an adult.

Visual apparatus becomes fully developed by 5 years of age. Salient points to be noted are as follows:

- *Macula and fovea* of the retina are structurally and functionally differentiated by 4–6 months of age.
- *Colour perception* is fully developed by the age of 4–6 months.
- *Size of the eyeball* at birth is small, so the infant is hypermetropic. Adult size is obtained by 5 years, when the child becomes emmetropic.
- *Visual acuity* becomes 6/6 by the age of 5–6 years.

Auditory apparatus is almost fully developed at term. Therefore, response to loud noise can be elicited just after birth.

Taste sensation is present at birth, but becomes sharp by the age of 2–3 months.

Visceral reflexes involved in swallowing, micturition, defaecation, sneezing and coughing are fully developed at birth.

Deep reflexes: Most of the tendon jerks can be elicited at birth except the ankle jerk. The Babinski's sign appears only a few weeks after birth and can be elicited during the next 1–2 years.

GASTROINTESTINAL PHYSIOLOGY

GIT: During Fetal Life

Placental Transfer of Nutrients: Placenta as Gut

As mentioned earlier, the transfer of nutrients to the fetus occurs from the maternal blood through the placenta (see Fig. 12.6.2D and page 1213).

During fetal life, constant and plentiful supply of glucose reaches from the mother. Due to deficiency of enzymes like glucokinase and those for glycogenolysis and gluconeogenesis, the fetus is incapable of regulating blood sugar on its own. Thus, fetal glucose is regulated by maternal blood glucose level. Furthermore, large amounts of free fatty acids and amino acids are transported to the fetus across the placenta, but they are used for tissue formation rather than for energy production.

Fetal Gastrointestinal Tract

After 20 weeks, fetus ingests and absorbs large quantities of amniotic fluid.

At 24 weeks, fetal GIT functions approach those of a normal newborn infant. Small quantities of *meconium* are continuously formed in the GIT and excreted from the bowels into the amniotic fluid. The meconium consists of unabsorbed residue of amniotic fluid and secretions from GIT mucosa and glands.

GIT: After Birth

The fetus gets the nutrient supply from the maternal blood through the placenta, which is suddenly cut off after ligation of the cord. Since the newborn has to produce its own nutrient supply, the gastrointestinal function is fairly well developed at birth. Some of the salient features of GIT physiology of newborn are given next.

Digestive and Absorptive Functions

Salivary secretion, though present since birth, increases over the next 6 months, due to maturation of the salivary glands.

Gastric HCl concentration is very high on the first postnatal day but within the next 10–15 days, the gastric acid secretion almost ceases. After a gap of 3–4 months, gastric acid secretion starts once again. The initial fall in gastric acidity may be due to some gastrogenic hormone, which is supplied to the infant in utero either from the mother or from the placenta. The influence of this secretagogue is most marked during the first 2 days of the birth, and then it rapidly decreases.

Pancreatic juice contains adequate concentration of lipase and proteolytic enzymes at birth. But the concentration of α-amylase is very low at birth and begins to increase a few months later. Therefore, a newborn is not able to utilize starch in the early postnatal life, rather may get severe diarrhoea.

Intestinal absorption of fats is less; thus, milk with high fat content is inadequately utilized. However, due to presence of disaccharidases, the absorption of disaccharides is very efficient. Similarly, monosaccharides are also well absorbed right from birth.

Liver Functions

The newborn has to fulfil the caloric requirements from carbohydrate-poor, fat-rich milk diet and a number of adaptive changes in the hepatic enzymes help in this transition.

Liver functions Liver functions are quite deficient during the first few days as the liver of newborn:

- Poorly conjugates bilirubin causing its less excretion
- Poorly performs gluconeogenic function, decreasing blood glucose level to 30–40 mg%
- Inadequately synthesizes plasma proteins producing hypoproteinaemia
- Inadequately synthesizes clotting factors producing even haemorrhagic disease of newborn, sometimes, especially in premature babies

Fetal liver glycogen and blood glucose During late fetal life, the activity of glycogen synthetase in the fetal liver increases. As a result, the fetal liver is very rich in glycogen at birth. After ligation of the cord, the blood sugar level of the infant begins to fall and may reach 60 mg/dL within 1 hour. Hypoglycaemia induces the secretion of glucagon, catecholamines and glucocorticoids. Presence of hepatic glucose-6-phosphatase in high concentration in the full-term infant helps to convert glycogen into glucose and, therefore, blood glucose recovers soon. However, the enzyme involved in gluconeogenesis takes a few days to develop fully and thus accounts for occurrence of hypoglycaemia during the first few days of life (as mentioned above). The problem of neonatal hypoglycaemia is more pronounced in premature babies.

Hepatic bilirubin excretion *During fetal life*, the RBCs have a life span of approximately 70 days, and thus about 1.4% of circulating red cell mass is destroyed every day producing a large amount of bilirubin. However, the plasma bilirubin level usually remains below 1 mg/dL. Furthermore, even during pathological state like Rh incompatibility when the production of bilirubin is markedly increased, the plasma bilirubin level does not exceed 5 mg/dL. This happens because of the fact that the lipid-soluble unconjugated bilirubin can cross the placental barrier.

After birth, in the early postnatal life, the hepatic conjugation enzyme UDP-glucuronyltransferase is not fully active, so conjugation with glucuronic acid is poor and so is the bilirubin excretion (as also mentioned earlier).

This explains the occurrence of physiological jaundice in the first week of postnatal life. However, soon the enzyme activity begins to rise rapidly, and by the age of 15 days, it even exceeds the adult level (Fig. 12.6.5). There seems to be some variation in the rate of increase of the hepatic conjugation enzyme activity. That is why some babies develop more severe physiological jaundice (with plasma bilirubin as high as 18 mg/dL) than others. Furthermore, the risk of neonatal jaundice is more in premature neonates and those suffering from Rh incompatibility. Such infants are under the risk of developing kernicterus, since the blood–brain barrier is not well developed at birth (see 'Nervous System').

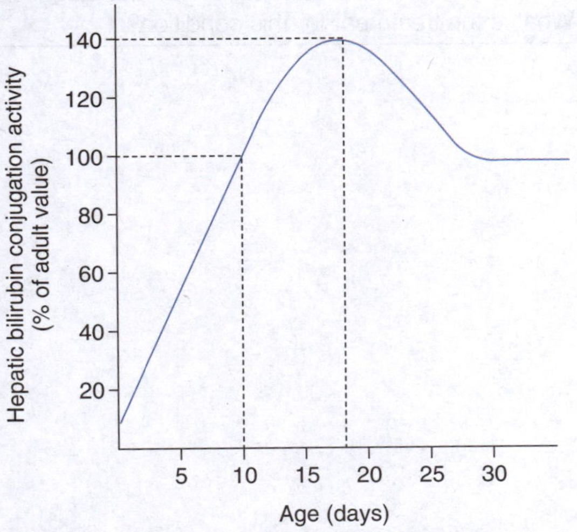

Fig. 12.6.5 Changes in rate of hepatic conjugation of bilirubin during neonatal period.

RENAL PHYSIOLOGY, AND FLUID AND ACID–BASE BALANCE

Anatomically, the development of nephrons is fairly complete at birth, and no new nephrons are formed in the postnatal life. However, functionally, the kidneys in infancy are immature and can manage to maintain normal blood chemistry as long as there is no homeostatic disturbance. In other words, there is very little margin of safety; hence, important problems of infancy are dehydration, overhydration and acidosis, explained as follows:

1. ***The fluid intake and fluid excretion*** in an infant is about 500 mL/day representing nearly 50% of the ECF volume. In contrast, an average adult takes and excretes about 2000 mL of fluid per day, which represents only 15% of ECF volume (the daily average urinary volume at different age groups is shown in Table 12.6.8). Furthermore, the ECF volume of the newborn infant per kilogram body weight is nearly double than the adult. Therefore, even a slight alteration of fluid balance due to diarrhoea, infection or solute overload may lead to rapidly developing fluid balance abnormalities.
2. ***Power of urinary concentration in an infant is poor.*** This is because of two main reasons:
   - At birth, 20% of the loop of Henle fails to reach the medulla in contrast to 1%–2% in adults.
   - Rate of urea secretion is low and so the osmolar gradient in medullary pyramids is slight. In turn, the low urea secretion of the neonate is because of the fact that the rate of deamination is low as more amino acids are utilized for tissue formation.

   Because of poor power of urinary concentration, the infant up to 1 year of age continues to pass iso-osmolar urine or even dilute urine in the face of severe dehydration. During infancy, the maximum urinary specific gravity may be only 1.008. Normal adult values of urinary concentration are reached by the age of 5–6 years.
3. ***Power of H^+ excretion is also poor in infancy.*** This is because of the fact that there is lesser glomerular filtration of phosphates, as well as inadequate synthesis of ammonia by the tubular cells. Furthermore, the rate of metabolism in infants is two times more in relation to body mass as in adults, i.e. two times as much acid is normally formed which produces tendency towards acidosis in infants.

Important Note

It is once again repeated that all the above-mentioned facts underline the risk of dehydration, overhydration and acidosis during infancy and the need for urgent treatment.

Table 12.6.8 Average daily urinary volume in relation to age

Age	Urine volume (mL)
1 day	15–50
10 days	50–300
1 month	250–400
1 year	400–500
5 years	600–750
10 years	700–1500
15 years	1500–2000

TEMPERATURE REGULATION IN NEWBORN AND INFANTS

The temperature regulation mechanisms, as described in Chapter 12.4 (see page 1198), are operative in newborns and even in premature babies. The salient points which need special mention for temperature regulation in newborns and infants are as follows:

1. ***Maintenance of body temperature presents greater problems in newborns and infants*** because of the following reasons:
   - *Surface area* in relation to the body weight is greater than adults.
   - *Basal metabolic rate (BMR)*, throughout the childhood, is relatively higher than the adult values.
   - *Sweating mechanism* is not fully developed during infancy.
2. ***Thermoneutral zone*** (see page 1202) for naked newborn infants (32–34°C in term infants and 35°C in premature infants) is higher than for the naked adult (26–28°C) (see Fig. 12.4.6). The fact underlines two important implications:
   - Infants have poor tolerance to cold.
   - While adjusting the temperature of the incubator for premature babies and of the labour room in general, the thermoneutral zone of the infant should be kept in mind.
3. ***Nonshivering or chemical thermogenesis*** is the most effective mechanism against cold in infants. Presence of brown adipose tissue in infants accounts for this fact (for details, see page 1205).

SEXUAL GROWTH AND DEVELOPMENT

See page 987.

Self-Assessment

1. Discuss the cardiovascular changes after birth.
2. Discuss about characteristic features of respiratory physiology in the fetus.
3. Discuss the characteristics of blood and immune system during fetal life.
4. Describe the following:
   - Changes in the central nervous system after birth
   - Liver functioning during fetal life
5. Write notes on the following:
   - Atrial septal defect
   - Fetal circulation
   - Apgar score
   - Physiological anaemia after birth

Clinical Cases

Case 1

A 9-year-old girl presented with very slow physical growth, getting tired early while playing with friends and having breathlessness.

Examination showed pulse rate 120/min and irregular, BP 100/60 mm Hg and respiration rate 22/min. Auscultation of the chest revealed cardiac murmur and whooshing sound. X-ray chest depicted an enlarged heart and ECG showed arrhythmia.

Q1. What is the probable diagnosis?
Q2. What further tests should be done to confirm the diagnosis?
Q3. What is pathophysiology of the disease?
Q4. What is the treatment plan?

Case 2

A 1-month-old male baby was brought to the paediatric OPD with complaints of feeding difficulties, shortness of breath, becoming blue when crying and not gaining weight, and his skin colour was not like that of normal babies.

Examination showed low weight, greyish colour of the skin and cyanosis; auscultation of the chest revealed loud murmur, and the probable diagnosis was a case of tetralogy of Fallot.

Q1. What are the components of this condition?
Q2. What is the reason for cyanosis in this condition?
Q3. What further tests should be carried out to confirm the diagnosis?
Q4. What should be the treatment plan?

Case 3

A 3-day-old male baby born premature at 32 weeks of gestation had difficulty in breathing, the respiratory rate was very high, and crackling sounds were heard during breathing.

Depending on signs and symptoms and premature birth, the probable diagnosis was neonatal respiratory distress syndrome.

Q1. What is the pathophysiology of this condition?
Q2. What is the reason for cyanosis?
Q3. What tests should be done to confirm the diagnosis?
Q4. What is the treatment for this condition?

Geriatric Physiology

12.7

CHAPTER OUTLINE

INTRODUCTION

AGEING

Ageing is a natural process. No one knows when old age begins. The biological age of the person is not identical with his/her chronological age. Ageing merely stands for growing old, whereas senescence is an expression used for the deterioration in the vitality or the lowering of the biological efficiency that accompanies ageing. From a physiological standpoint, human ageing is characterized by a progressive constriction of the homeostatic reserve of every organ system. This decline, often referred to as homeostenosis, is gradual and progressive, although the rate and extent of decline vary.

The decline of each organ system appears to occur independently of changes in other organ systems and is influenced by diet, environment and personal habits as well as by genetic factors.

In other words, ageing can be defined as the time-related deterioration of the physiological functions necessary for survival and fertility. The science of ageing is often referred to as *gerontology*. The scientists studying the science of ageing are known as *gerontologists*, and the branch of medicine dealing with the problems of ageing is called *geriatric medicine*.

AGE-RELATED CHANGES IN DIFFERENT ORGAN SYSTEMS

I. CARDIOVASCULAR CHANGES

Changes in Heart

1. ***Myocardium*** may show the following changes:
   - Deposition of yellow–brown lipofuscin pigment occurs.
   - Degenerative changes in the myofibrils and mitochondria occur.
   - Fibrotic lesions and sometimes amyloid deposits occur.
   - Capillary density may be decreased.
2. ***Valves*** show thickening and structural changes making the:
   - Aortic valve somewhat stenotic
   - Mitral valve slightly incompetent
3. Functional changes in the heart of elderly include:
   - *Heart rate* in resting conditions is unchanged, but the maximum heart rate during exercise declines.
   - *Maximum cardiac output* in response to exercise is decreased at the rate of 1% per year after the age of 40 years.
4. ***SA node automaticity*** and baroreceptor sensitivity is decreased with age. This leads to impaired blood pressure response to standing and volume depletion.
5. ***Electrocardiogram*** does not show any significant change with age. Therefore, any significant change in ECG of an elderly individual should be considered pathological.

Changes in Blood Vessels and Blood Pressure

Blood vessels show a gradual decrease in the number of elastic fibres and a progressive change in the characteristics of elastic tissue. There occurs deposition of calcium salts in the elastic and muscular type of arteries, as well as deposition of more collagen fibres resulting in decrease in the distensibility of the blood vessels.

Blood pressure: Systolic blood pressure is raised because of loss of elasticity in the aorta and its major branches, but there is little change in the diastolic blood pressure, resulting in widening of pulse pressure.

Blood flow to the various organs such as the heart, brain and especially kidney is decreased.

II. CHANGES IN RESPIRATORY SYSTEM

Structural changes in lungs: Alveoli become flatter and shallow, whereas alveolar ducts enlarge. The number of alveoli declines gradually due to progressive loss of interalveolar septa.

Pulmonary compliance is increased due to decrease in elasticity of the lungs.

Compliance of the thoracic cage and mobility of the ribs are decreased due to calcification of costal cartilages.

Pulmonary blood vessels show age-related increase in wall thickness.

Functional changes occurring as a result of aforementioned changes in the lungs and thoracic cage are as follows:

- *Functional residual capacity* of the lungs is increased by 50%.
- *Residual volume* is increased by 100%.
- *Vital capacity*, FEV_1, MBC and diffusion capacity for oxygen are significantly decreased.
- Respiratory response to hypoxia and hypercapnia is sluggish in the elderly.
- *Airways become more susceptible to collapse*, especially during expiration, because of reduced elastic recoil of thoracic cage. The collapse is more likely during exercise because of the high expiratory flow rate.
- *Arterial pCO_2 and pO_2*: The arterial pCO_2 is not changed, but arterial pO_2 is decreased by 10%–15% due to an increase in physiological dead space. But it has no serious detrimental effect on the body.
- *Impairment of bronchiolar escalator function*, which occurs in old age, causes a more serious problem, especially in smokers.

To summarize, the respiratory functions of the elderly show an overall impairment of ventilation, diffusion, ventilation/perfusion mismatch as well as regulation.

III. GASTROINTESTINAL TRACT CHANGES

Age-related changes noted in relation to GIT include:

1. ***Diminution of masticatory efficiency*** occurs due to teeth problems. With advancing age, teeth show *attrition* due to loss of first enamel and then even dentine and cement. In addition, several teeth are lost as a result of caries or periodontal diseases.
2. ***Difficulty in swallowing (dysphagia)*** may occur in extreme old age, because of frequent weakness of pharyngeal musculature and abnormal relaxation of the cricopharyngeal muscle. Disordered oesophageal motility, especially at the lower end of the oesophagus, may further compound this problem.
3. ***Reduction in gastric secretion*** leading to *achlorhydria* is seen in 25% of the individuals older than 60 years. It results from age-related mucosal atrophy. Decreased gastric acidity causes decreased Ca^{2+} absorption from an empty stomach. Achlorhydria also results in deficiency of iron and vitamin B_{12}.
   The secretion of pancreatic amylase is not affected in old age. Thus, as a whole, digestion and absorption of foodstuffs do not seem to be affected in old age, except for the deficiency of iron and vitamin B_{12}.
4. ***Age-related changes in the small intestine*** include reduction in villus height and reduction in lactase activity in the brush border. These changes decrease absorptive capacity in the elderly. However, there is no marked decrease in the digestive or absorptive processes. Therefore, nutritional deficiency in an elderly individual cannot be attributed to malabsorption and actually reflects deficient intake of the nutrients.
5. ***Changes in the liver*** include decrease in the number but increase in the size of hepatocytes, and an increase in fibrous tissue. But, because of large reserves, the hepatic function is maintained at the normal level even after 70 years of age. However, synthetic functions of the liver such as protein synthesis, microsomal mixed function and oxidase activity required for hepatic metabolism of drugs and steroids are reduced in old age. Consequently, all the liver function tests show normal results except for a decrease in albumin/globulin ratio. Pigment excretion also remains normal.
6. ***Colon motility*** may be decreased in extreme old age resulting in constipation.

IV. RENAL AND GENITOURINARY CHANGES

1. ***Kidneys*** show progressive reduction in weight. Functional renal changes include:
   - *Decreased GFR* occurs in the elderly because of 30%–40% decrease in the number of renal glomeruli by the age of 80 years. It leads to impaired excretion of certain drugs, which may produce toxicity at doses well tolerated in younger individuals.
   - *Decrease in tubular function*, both secretory and absorptive activity, leads to decreased urinary concentration and dilution abilities. This leads to delayed response to salt or fluid restriction/overload. There occurs nocturia. Maximum urinary osmolality is about 750 mOsm/kg (specific gravity 1.0) at the age of 80 years.
   - *Renal function* becomes borderline. Because of the large renal reserves, plasma concentration of creatinine and other nitrogenous waste products is not elevated. However, any type of circulatory stress may precipitate renal failure.
2. ***Prostate enlargement*** in elderly males is a frequent cause of increased residual urine volume. It may take the form of a disease (urinary incontinence or urinary retention).
3. ***Vaginal/urethral mucosal atrophy*** occurring in elderly females leads to dyspareunia and bacteriuria.

V. CHANGES IN ENDOCRINAL SYSTEM

Endocrinal changes have even been implicated as the underlying mechanism of ageing. Age-related decrease in endocrinal function may occur due to any of the following changes:

- Decrease in plasma concentration of hormone due to decreased production or due to decrease in the concentration of binding proteins involved in the transport of hormone
- Decreased responsiveness of the target cells
- Alteration in the number or sensitivity of the hormone receptors
- Diminished response to physiological stimuli for secretion of the hormone

Age-Related Changes Occurring in the Endocrinal System

Age-related changes occurring in the endocrinal system are as follows:

1. ***Thyroid hormone*** secretion is definitely decreased. Up to a 50% decrease in the production is noted by the age of 80 years.

2. ***Impaired glucose homeostasis*** is frequently seen in old age. This seems to be due to diminished sensitivity of tissues to insulin, as the plasma levels of insulin are unaffected. It has been observed that 2 hours after the administration of glucose load, plasma glucose is about 30 mg% higher at the age of 70 years than in young adults.
3. ***Reproductive hormones*** show most consistent age-related changes. In females, plasma levels of oestrogen and progesterone are decreased after menopause. In males, testosterone levels are decreased around the age of 70 years.
4. ***Anterior pituitary hormone*** secretion is not decreased.
   - *FSH and LH* levels in females are rather increased due to negative feedback effect exerted by the decreased plasma levels of oestrogen and progesterone.
   - *Gonadotropin* levels in males are raised because of negative feedback effect of lowered testosterone levels. The raised gonadotropin level induces an increase in testicular Leydig cell volume. But, because of the age-related changes, even the higher Leydig cell volume is not able to achieve the normal testosterone output.
5. ***ADH, renin and aldosterone*** levels are decreased in the old age. Changes in these hormones affect the renal functions, especially urinary concentration and dilution mechanism.
6. ***Vitamin D*** absorption and activation are decreased with age, and contributes to *osteoporosis* occurring in old age.

VI. CHANGES IN BLOOD AND IMMUNE MECHANISMS

1. ***Blood volume and blood cells:*** The blood cells (red blood cells, white blood cells and platelets) of elderly individuals are not significantly different from those of young individuals.
2. ***Haemopoietic marrow reserve*** is gradually decreased because of its replacement with fatty marrow as age advances. Long bones are first affected, followed by flat bones and, lastly, the vertebrae.
3. ***Anaemia*** in elderly usually occurs due to deficiency of iron and vitamin B_{12}.
4. ***Senile purpura*** occurs due to defect in the capillary endothelium. Platelet count and function of blood coagulation usually remain normal in old age.
5. ***Raised ESR*** (up to 40 mm in the first hour), seen in elderly, is related to increased plasma fibrinogen levels.
6. ***Immunological function*** is markedly depressed in old age. Both cell-mediated immunity and humoral immunity decline.
   - *Reduced immune surveillance* by T lymphocytes, at least in part, explains the greater incidence of malignancy in old age.
   - *Involution of the thymus* is a well-known age-related change.
   - *T-cell autoreactivity and autoantibody titre* are, however, increased, probably due to diminished tolerance to antigens normally recognized as self.

VII. CHANGES IN MUSCULOSKELETAL SYSTEM

1. ***Muscular power***, characteristically, reduces progressively with ageing due to loss of muscle fibres (decreased lean body mass). The loss of muscle fibres is much greater than the number explained by loss of motor neurons in the CNS. Muscle fibres show deposition of lipofuscin and many other degenerative changes with age.
2. ***Muscle twitch*** reveals a prolongation of latency, contraction period and relaxation period. The maximum tension developed in a muscle in elderly is much less than in young adults.
3. ***Osteoarthritis***, i.e. age-related degenerative changes in the joints, starts at the age of 40 years and becomes well marked by the age of 60–70 years.
4. ***Osteoporosis***, i.e. age-related decrease in bone density, is a characteristic feature of ageing. It is more marked in postmenopausal women than in men of the same age group. Osteoporosis predisposes the elderly to fractures.
5. ***Changes in stature and posture*** occur mainly due to changes in the vertebral column, as long bones of the limbs do not show any significant change. Initially, there occurs thinning of the intervertebral disc only; osteoporotic changes cause a decrease in the height of individual vertebra after the age of 50–60 years. As a result of these changes, the height decreases progressively from 50 years onwards, with a prominent change at 70–80 years. Furthermore, kyphosis and slight flexion at the hip and knee make an aged person look still smaller. A decrease of about 5 cm in height is reported to occur from 20 to 80 years of age, which increases to 10 cm by the age of 90 years.

VIII. CHANGES IN SKIN AND HAIR

1. ***Wrinkling of the skin*** due to decreased elasticity, increased thinning of the epidermis and dermis, and decreased subcutaneous fat are the hallmark of ageing.
2. ***Greying of hair***, due to loss of melanin pigment, is universal in ageing.
3. ***Baldness*** in males is quite common, though growth of beard is not affected.
4. ***Loss of axillary and pubic hair*** in females occurs due to decreased levels of adrenal androgens.
5. ***Increase in facial hair growth*** may occur in females due to unopposed action of the residual adrenal androgens in the absence of oestrogens.
6. ***Sweat glands*** decrease in size and number; therefore, secretion of sweat as well as sebaceous glands is decreased.

IX. CHANGES IN CENTRAL NERVOUS SYSTEM

Both structural and functional changes in CNS are quite common with ageing.

1. ***Brain atrophy and neuronal loss*** is the most obvious change. By the age of 70 years, there may be 45% cell loss in the cerebral cortex, and 25% loss in the cerebellum. Atrophy of frontal lobes leading to shrinkage of gyri and enlargement of sulci is quite common.
2. ***Degenerative changes*** may occur in the substantia nigra and lentiform nucleus. Degeneration in the spinal cord occurs to a lesser extent than in the brain.
3. ***Other histological changes*** include accumulation of lipofuscin granules in almost all the neurons and glial cells, loss of synapses and gradual loss of dendrites.
4. ***Cerebral blood flow*** is decreased by 40% at the age of 70 years, and oxygen utilization is reduced by 25%.
5. ***Functions of neurotransmitters are impaired.*** Specifically, cholinergic deficit has been demonstrated in *Alzheimer disease* (see also page 1091) and dopaminergic deficit in

Parkinson disease (see also page 918). Milder forms of cholinergic deficit may be responsible for *senile dementia*, and some degree of dopaminergic deficit may be responsible for *hypokinesia* of old age. Decrease in catecholamine synthesis may be responsible for depression in old age.

6. ***Reflexes*** tend to be sluggish or even absent. The ankle jerk is lost in most of the elderly individuals. Decreased righting reflexes result in increased body sway in old age.
7. ***Sleep changes*** occur in the form of decrease in stages 3 and 4 of non-REM sleep, whereas the total duration of sleep may not be decreased much. Very old people may not go into stage 4 of sleep at all and have early awakening. Numerous brief arousals occur and account for a feeling of no sleep or insomnia.

X. CHANGES IN AUTONOMIC NERVOUS SYSTEM

There is also an age-related impairment of ANS function associated with the increased sensitivity to humoral factors. Common manifestations of decreased ANS function are as follows:

1. ***Impaired temperature regulation*** in elderly individuals occurs because of the fact that exposure to moderate cold or hot environment does not produce expected vasoconstriction and shivering, or vasodilatation and sweating, respectively. Consequently, elderly are more prone to get hypothermia on exposure to cold and hyperthermia on exposure to heat.
2. ***Postural hypotension*** is of frequent occurrence in elderly. It is known to occur because of partial failure of baroreceptor mechanism.

XI. CHANGES IN SPECIAL SENSES

i. Age-Related Ocular Changes

Age-related ocular changes are as follows:

1. ***Presbyopia*** refers to age-related physiological insufficiency of accommodation, leading to failing vision for near or progressive increase in near point. It is as consistent an ageing effect as menopause in females. It usually starts at the age of 40 years, and by the age of 50 years, most of the normal individuals need glasses for near work. Decrease in the accommodating power of the crystalline lens with increasing age leads to presbyopia. It occurs due to:
   - Decrease in the elasticity and plasticity of the crystalline lens
   - Age-related decrease in the power of ciliary muscles
2. ***Age-related cataract*** or the senile cataract refers to opacification of the crystalline lens, leading to progressively decreasing vision. Its age of onset and maturation is influenced by the hereditary and environmental factors.
3. ***Age-related corneal degeneration*** manifests as a ring-shaped, whitish opacity near the limbus, which is called *arcus senilis*.
4. ***Age-related macular degeneration (ARMD)*** is a cause of irreversible blindness in many elderly individuals after the age of 70 years.
5. ***Dry eye*** may occur in elderly individuals, more so in postmenopausal females because of age-related decrease in tear secretion.

ii. Age-Related Changes in Ears

Age-related changes in ears are as follows:

1. ***Presbyacusia***, i.e. age-related impairment of hearing, especially for higher frequencies occurring due to degenerative changes in the organ of Corti (hair cells), ganglion cells as well as of temporal cortex, is not uncommon. Other factors contributing to presbyacusia are loss of elasticity of the tympanic membrane and basilar membrane, loss of neurons in the cochlea and atrophy of stria vascularis. The impaired sensitivity often leads to difficulty in understanding speech and the disturbances of localization of sounds.
2. ***Otosclerosis***, characterized by age-related decrease in motility of middle ear ossicles, is another cause of deafness in old age.
3. ***Impairment of postural reflexes*** may occur due to age-related degenerative changes in hair cells of the crista ampullaris, and decreased endolymph production because of atrophy of the stria vascularis.

iii. Age-Related Changes in Taste and Smell

Age-related changes in taste and smell are as follows:

1. ***Impairment in taste sensation*** in elderly is attributed to a decrease in the number of taste buds, from an average of 250 buds per papilla in childhood to about 90 buds per papilla by the age of 80 years.
2. ***Impairment in sensation of smell*** in the elderly is attributed to the decrease in smell receptors and partly to the loss of neurons in cerebral cortical centres.

THEORIES OF AGEING

Many theories have been put forward to explain the process of ageing, but none is able to explain all the queries. Most of the theories fall in one of the two main groups:

- Genetic theories of ageing
- Random damage theories

I. GENETIC THEORIES OF AGEING

These theories consider ageing to be the inevitable result of the genetic programme. The enthusiasm for genetic theories is fuelled by the following observations:

- Dramatic species-specific differences are present in maximal life span. For example, every dog grows old in about 10 years, whereas a human being takes about 60 years to reach the same level of senescence. Obviously, the difference lies in the genetic programme of two species.
- There is a strong correlation with the survival among the monozygotic compared with that among the dizygotic twins.
- Ageing cannot be prevented altogether, suggesting thereby that the gradual impairment of function is genetically programmed.
- The fact that a single mutation can prolong life span by more than 50% in some nematodes and mice is a very strong pointer to the role of genetics in ageing.

However, all genetic theories must account for the fact that evolutionary selection pressure is minimal following completion of reproduction.

Of the many genetic theories, some important ones are given next.

1. Programmed senescence theory Programmed senescence theory of ageing holds that ageing follows a biological timetable, perhaps a continuation of one that regulates childhood growth and development. According to *programmed senescence theory*, ageing is the result of the segmental switching on and off of certain genes, with senescence being defined as the time when age-associated deficits are manifested.

2. Mutation theory This theory suggests that, since animals usually succumb to natural forces long before reaching their maximal life span, ageing might reflect mutations that impair long-term survival. These mutations would accumulate in the genome because there is no selection pressure to delete them.

3. Theory of pleiotropic antagonism This theory proposes that ageing may be caused by the late and deleterious effects of the genes that are conserved because of the survival advantages they confer prior to reproduction.

4. Theory of ecological niches This theory applies to ecological niches, where extrinsic hazards are relatively low. In such an environment, evolution might select the mutations that retard the ageing process, since these might allow an animal to produce and protect many more litters. In support of this theory, the rate of ageing in an isolated class of *Virginia opossum* was calculated to be roughly half of that seen in their less-fortunate cousins.

Many genetic theories previously postulated to mediate ageing which have not been borne out include:

Isomatic mutation theory: This theory postulated that ageing would result from cumulative spontaneous mutations.
The error catastrophe theory: This theory postulated that ageing would result from errors in the synthesis of proteins critical to the synthesis of genetic material or protein-synthesizing machinery.
Intrinsic mutagenesis theory: According to this theory, ageing is the result of ongoing intrinsic DNA rearrangements.

II. THE 'RANDOM DAMAGE' THEORIES OF AGEING

All the 'random damage' theories are based on the possibility that the balance between ongoing damage and repair is disrupted. These theories differ in the emphasis placed on the increased damage (e.g. by free radicals, oxidation or glycation) versus deficient repair, as well as in the mechanisms that might mediate each. However, all share the observation that cell and organ repair capacity declines with age.

The 'random damage' theories include those given next.

1. Free radical theory Oxidation reactions in the cells are associated with the formation of free radicals, such as superoxide and hydroxyl radicals. For free radical scavenging, *antioxidant mechanisms* exist in the body in the form of glutathione, vitamin E, vitamin A and vitamin C. When these antioxidant mechanisms are overwhelmed, there occurs damage by the free radicals. The free radicals can possibly damage vital macromolecules such as DNA and proteins, and cause peroxidation of lipids in the membranes around cells and organelles. Although free radical theory is very popular, and antioxidants are being prescribed overenthusiastically by the physicians, neither has lipid peroxidation been demonstrated at the cellular level, nor has the beneficial effect of antioxidants been proven.

2. Cell replication theory Depending on the replicating capabilities, the cells in the body can be divided into three categories:

- *Cells which continuously replicate* include blood cells, epidermis cells and gastrointestinal cells.
- *Cells which replicate only under stress* (e.g. injury) include endothelial cells, hepatocytes and fibroblasts.
- *Cells which do not replicate at all* include neurons, myocardial and skeletal muscle cells.

It has been stated that replicating cells have a definite replicating limit. The cell replication theory suggests that ageing may represent a stage of life when replication of cell ceases, i.e. when repair is not capable to cope up with the damage.

Subsequent researches revealed that this replicative senescence was due to arrest of the cell cycles at the G_1/S phase, the point at which DNA synthesis begins. Recently, cell replication has also been linked to the length of *telomeric DNA*. With each cell division, roughly 50 of the total 2000 base pairs of the telomere are lost. Telomeric shortening might thus result in loss of gene accessibility, which is caused by metabolism. Together with cytoplasmic factors mediating arrest of DNA synthesis, telomeric shortening could also limit the cell's ability to divide and thereby replace cells loss to apoptosis.

3. Cross-linking theory This theory highlights that an accumulation of cross-linked proteins damages cells and tissues, slowing down bodily processes, and results in ageing. In a process called *nonenzymatic glycosylation or glycation*, glucose molecules attach themselves to proteins, setting in motion a chain of chemical reactions that ends in the proteins binding together or cross-linking, thus altering their biological and structural roles. The process is slow but increases with time.

Cross-links, which have been termed *advanced glycosylation end products* (AGEs), seem to toughen tissues and may cause some of the deterioration associated with ageing. AGEs have been linked to stiffening of the connective tissue (collagen), hardened arteries, clouded eyes, loss of nerve function and less efficient kidneys. These are deficiencies that often accompany ageing. They also appear at younger ages in people with diabetes, who have high glucose levels. Diabetes, in fact, is sometimes considered an accelerated model of ageing. Its complications mimic not only the physiological changes but also the expectances that can accompany old age. As a result, much research on cross-linking has focused on its relationship with diabetes, as well as ageing.

MODULATING THE PROCESS OF AGEING

The quest for staying youthful and preventing ageing has led to many trials on modulating the process of ageing. However, ageing has proved to be an almost inevitable process. The only measures that have shown some progress in this regard are caloric restriction and exercise.

Caloric restriction To date, the only intervention known to delay ageing and prolong the life span is caloric restriction, which has been proved in experimental animals. Although the underlying mechanism is still not determined, it is specific to caloric restriction rather than to the reduction of any dietary compound (e.g. fat intake) or supplementation with vitamins or antioxidants. Furthermore, the effects of caloric restriction in humans are still unknown.

Exercise There is still no conclusive evidence to document that exercise prevents ageing or not. However, definitely, exercise improves work capacity as assessed from maximum oxygen uptake. Physical exercise also improves cardiac performance and reduces musculoskeletal disability. It is also reported to prevent age-related decline in resting metabolic rate.

Self-Assessment

1. Discuss about theories of ageing.
2. Discuss the age-related cardiovascular changes and their effects.
3. Describe the following:
   - Effects of ageing on the central nervous system
   - Functional changes in the respiratory system with ageing
4. Write notes on the following:
   - Presbyacusia
   - Role of caloric restriction in ageing
   - Cross-linking theory of ageing

12.8 Physiology of Yoga

CHAPTER OUTLINE

INTRODUCTION

Yoga is a holistic practice originating from the ancient India. Yoga is basically a Sanskrit word 'Yuga' meaning union that integrates physical postures (asanas), breath control (pranayama), meditation and ethical principles to promote overall health and well-being. It encompasses a wide range of techniques aimed at harmonizing the body, mind and spirit, and creates a balance between the body and the mind to attain holistic health and self-enlightenment. Since 2015, every year on 21 June, 'International Yoga Day' is celebrated worldwide to increase the public awareness regarding various advantages of yoga practice.

TYPES OF YOGA

The common types of yoga are as follows:

1. ***Hatha yoga:*** Hatha yoga is a gentle form of yoga that focuses on physical postures and breathing exercises to channel the vital energy. In Sanskrit, hatha means force. It is often a good starting point for beginners.
2. ***Vinyasa yoga:*** Also known as flow yoga, vinyasa yoga involves linking breath with movement in a dynamic sequence of poses and it is like dancing movements.
3. ***Ashtanga yoga:*** Ashtanga yoga is a rigorous and structured style that follows a specific sequence of postures, typically practiced in a fast-paced manner to build strength, flexibility and stamina. During ashtanga yoga practice, internal heat is produced and a lot of sweating occurs that detoxify the body.
4. ***Iyengar yoga:*** Developed by B.K.S. Iyengar, this style emphasizes precise alignment and the use of props (such as blocks, straps and blankets) to help practitioners perform poses with greater ease and effectiveness.
5. ***Bikram yoga:*** Also known as hot yoga, Bikram yoga involves a series of 26 poses practiced in a heated room at about 101°F temperature. The heat is believed to enhance flexibility and detoxification.
6. ***Kundalini yoga:*** Kundalini yoga incorporates dynamic movements, breathing techniques, chanting and meditation to awaken and channel the energy believed to reside at the base of the spine (kundalini energy).
7. ***Yin yoga:*** Yin yoga focuses on passive, long-held poses that target the connective tissues, such as ligaments, tendons and fascia. It aims to improve flexibility and promote relaxation.
8. ***Restorative yoga:*** Restorative yoga utilizes props extensively to support the body in gentle poses held for extended periods. It is deeply relaxing and rejuvenating, making it suitable for stress relief and recovery.
9. ***Yoga nidra:*** Also known as yogic sleep, yoga nidra is a guided meditation practice that induces deep relaxation and a state of conscious sleep, allowing practitioners to access deeper layers of the mind.
10. ***Jivamukti yoga:*** Jivamukti yoga incorporates vigorous vinyasa sequences with spiritual teachings, chanting, music and meditation, aiming to promote physical, mental and spiritual well-being.

These are few examples, and there are many other styles and variations of yoga practiced worldwide, each with its own unique emphasis and approach.

PHYSIOLOGICAL ASPECTS OF YOGA

Yogic exercises, also known as yoga asanas or postures, have been studied extensively for their effects on human physiological parameters. Some of the well-documented effects on various body system are described next.

A. EFFECTS ON CARDIORESPIRATORY SYSTEM

Yoga has been shown to improve cardiovascular health by the following effects:

1. ***Reduced resting heart rate:*** Regular practice of yoga postures has been associated with a decrease in resting heart rate. This is believed to be due to the relaxation response induced by yoga, which helps to calm the sympathetic nervous system and increase vagal tone, leading to a slower resting heart rate.

2. ***Lower blood pressure:*** Yoga asanas have been found to help in lowering blood pressure (both systolic and diastolic) in individuals with hypertension. The combination of physical postures, breathing techniques and meditation reduces the stress and promotes relaxation, which in turn can lead to a decrease in blood pressure.
3. ***Improved cardiac function:*** Certain yoga postures involve movements that gently stretch and strengthen the muscles of the chest and improve circulation. Practices like pranayama (breathing exercises) can enhance lung function and oxygen uptake, which benefits overall cardiac functions by increasing venous return, cardiac contractility and cardiac output.
4. ***Enhanced circulation:*** Yoga asanas promote blood flow throughout the body, including to the extremities. Poses that involve inversions, such as headstands and shoulder stands, can help improve venous return to the heart which leads to increase in cardiac output and overall cardiovascular health
5. ***Improved respiratory function:*** Pranayama, or yogic breathing exercises, can improve respiratory function by increasing tidal volume, vital capacity and total lung capacity, enhancing oxygenation of tissues and promoting respiratory functions.

B. EFFECTS ON MUSCULOSKELETAL SYSTEM

Yoga asanas, or postures, have profound effects on the musculoskeletal system, offering various benefits for muscles, joints and overall structural health. The main effects include:

1. ***Improved flexibility:*** Yoga involves a wide range of stretching and lengthening movements that target muscles and connective tissues throughout the body. Regular practice leads to increased flexibility and range of motion in joints, promoting better overall mobility and reducing the risk of injuries. Many yoga asanas support the body weight in different positions, which helps to build strength, particularly in the core muscles, arms, legs and back. Poses such as plank and warrior poses and balances like tree pose can enhance muscular strength and endurance.
2. ***Enhanced muscle tone:*** Yoga postures engage muscles in a balanced and harmonious way, leading to improved muscle tone, not only of the superficial muscles but also of deeper stabilizing muscles.
3. ***Joint health:*** Yoga movements promote gentle traction and compression of joints, which can help improve joint health and function. Regular practice can alleviate stiffness, reduce inflammation and enhance synovial fluid production, which lubricates the joints and reduces friction.
4. ***Posture correction:*** Many yoga asanas focus on aligning the body properly, improving posture and correcting postural imbalances. By strengthening the muscles that support the spine and promoting awareness of body alignment, yoga helps individuals to maintain a more upright and balanced posture in daily activities.
5. ***Pain relief:*** Certain yoga asanas are used as complementary therapy for managing musculoskeletal disorders such as arthritis, back pain, neck pain and joint discomfort.
6. ***Prevention of osteoporosis:*** Regular weight-bearing yoga poses, such as standing poses and arm balances, stimulate bone growth and density, thus helping in preventing osteoporosis and maintaining bone health in ageing process.
7. ***Injury rehabilitation:*** Gentle, controlled movements can help in restoring mobility, strength and function for individuals recovering from musculoskeletal injuries or surgeries and also reducing the risk of reinjury.

C. EFFECTS ON NEUROENDOCRINE SYSTEM

Yoga asanas, or postures, have significant effects on the neuroendocrine system, which is a complex network involving the nervous system and various endocrine glands. The important effects of yoga asanas on the neuroendocrine system include:

1. ***Stress reduction:*** One of the most well-documented effects of yoga on the neuroendocrine system is to reduce stress. Stress activates the hypothalamic–pituitary–adrenal (HPA) axis, leading to the release of stress hormones such as cortisol and adrenaline. Yoga practices, including asanas, pranayama (breathing exercises) and meditation, promote relaxation and activate the parasympathetic nervous system, which counteracts the stress response.
2. ***Hormonal balance:*** Regular practice of yoga asanas regulates hormone levels in the body. Studies have shown that yoga may influence the secretion of hormones such as cortisol, insulin, thyroid hormones and reproductive hormones like oestrogen and testosterone. The hormonal balance is the most important for maintaining overall health and well-being.
3. ***Improved mood:*** Yoga practices have been shown to enhance mood and emotional well-being by modulating neurotransmitter levels in the brain. Yoga poses that involve an increased blood flow to the brain stimulate the release of neurotransmitters like serotonin and dopamine, which are associated with feelings of happiness and contentment.
4. ***Enhanced cognitive function:*** Yoga asanas that involve concentration, balance and coordination can stimulate neural pathways in the brain, leading to improved cognitive function. Regular practice of yoga has been linked to better attention, memory and executive function, which are essential for learning and problem solving.
5. ***Better sleep quality:*** Asanas that promote relaxation and stress reduction, combined with breathing exercises and meditation, calm the mind, induce a state of relaxation and help to improve sleep quality and duration.
6. ***Regulation of autonomic nervous system:*** The autonomic nervous system controls involuntary bodily functions such as heart rate, digestion and respiratory rate. Asanas and breathing techniques promote balance between the sympathetic and the parasympathetic divisions of the autonomic nervous system, leading to overall physiological equilibrium.
7. ***Pain management:*** Chronic pain can affect the neuroendocrine system, leading to dysregulation of stress hormones and neurotransmitters. Yoga asanas can help to alleviate pain by promoting relaxation, reducing muscle tension and modulating pain perception through the release of endorphins, the body's natural pain suppressing pathways.

D. EFFECTS ON METABOLIC ACTIVITY

Yoga asanas, or postures, can have several beneficial effects on metabolic activity. The documented effects are as follows:.

1. ***Improvement in insulin sensitivity:*** Yoga practices, including asanas, pranayama (breathing exercises) and meditation, have been shown to improve insulin sensitivity

in individuals with or at risk of type 2 diabetes. Enhanced insulin sensitivity allows cells to utilize glucose more efficiently, helping to regulate blood sugar levels.

2. ***Reduction in blood glucose levels:*** Regular practice of yoga has been associated with lower fasting blood glucose levels and improved glucose tolerance. This can be beneficial for individuals with diabetes or prediabetes in managing their condition and reducing the risk of complications.
3. ***Weight management:*** Certain yoga asanas can help with weight management by increasing calorie expenditure, improving metabolism and promoting mindful eating behaviours. Additionally, yoga practices can reduce stress, which is often associated with emotional eating and weight gain.
4. ***Lipid profile improvement:*** Yoga has been shown to positively influence lipid profiles, including reducing levels of total cholesterol, LDL cholesterol (often referred to as 'bad' cholesterol) and triglycerides, while increasing HDL cholesterol (often referred to as 'good' cholesterol). These improvements can help lower the risk of atherosclerosis and cardiovascular disease.
5. ***Reduction in inflammation:*** Chronic inflammation is a risk factor for metabolic syndrome and other metabolic disorders. Yoga practices have been found to reduce markers of inflammation in the body, such as C-reactive protein (CRP) and proinflammatory cytokines. By decreasing inflammation, yoga can help improve the overall metabolic health.
6. ***Regulation of appetite:*** Yoga asanas and mindfulness practices can influence appetite-regulating hormones such as leptin and ghrelin. Balancing of these hormones can help to regulate hunger and satiety signals, leading to better appetite control and weight management.
7. ***Enhanced digestive function:*** Certain yoga poses can stimulate digestion and improve gastrointestinal function by enhancing blood flow to the gastrointestinal tract, and promoting improvement of digestion, that contributes to better nutrient absorption and metabolic efficiency.
8. ***Stress reduction:*** Chronic stress is closely linked to metabolic dysregulation and the development of metabolic syndrome. Yoga practices, including relaxation techniques such as meditation and deep breathing, help in reducing stress hormone levels (such as cortisol) and promote a state of relaxation, which can have positive effects on metabolic health.

Overall, incorporating yoga asanas into a healthy lifestyle can contribute to improved metabolic health by enhancing insulin sensitivity, regulating blood glucose levels, managing weight, improving lipid profiles, reducing inflammation, optimizing digestive function and reducing stress. However, it is essential to combine yoga practice with other lifestyle modifications, such as a balanced diet and regular physical activity, for comprehensive metabolic health benefits.

E. EFFECTS ON IMMUNE SYSTEM

Yoga asanas, or postures, can have several beneficial effects on the immune system, the body's defence mechanisms against pathogens and infections. These occur due to:

1. ***Decreased inflammation:*** Chronic inflammation is a risk factor for various cardiovascular diseases. Some studies suggest that yoga practices may help to reduce inflammation markers in the body, contributing to a better cardiovascular health. Some studies suggest that regular yoga practice may enhance immune function by reducing inflammation and promoting the activity of immune cells. This could potentially lead to fewer instances of infections and improved overall health effects of yoga asanas on the immune system.
2. ***Stimulation of lymphatic system:*** Yoga poses can stimulate the lymphatic system. The lymphatic system helps in removal of toxins, waste products and pathogens from the body, supporting immune function and overall health.
3. ***Stress reduction:*** Chronic stress can weaken the immune system by elevating levels of stress hormones such as cortisol, which suppress immune function. Yoga practices, including asanas, pranayama (breathing exercises) and meditation, promote relaxation and activate the parasympathetic nervous system, reducing stress levels and supporting immune mechanism.

F. EFFECTS ON COGNITIVE FUNCTIONS

Yoga asanas, or postures, can have several beneficial effects on cognitive functions, which include various mental processes such as attention, memory, executive function and overall cognitive performance. Here are some ways in which yoga asanas influence cognitive functions:

1. ***Increased mindfulness:*** Yoga encourages mindfulness, which involves paying attention to the present moment without judgement. Practicing yoga asanas requires focus on breath, body sensations and alignment, promoting mindful awareness. Enhanced mindfulness has been associated with improved attention, cognitive flexibility and emotional regulation.
2. ***Enhanced attention and concentration:*** Yoga asanas require concentration and focus to maintain proper form, balance and coordination. Regular practice of yoga improves attentional control and concentration, which are essential for sustaining focus on tasks and activities in daily life.
3. ***Improved memory:*** Yoga asanas and pranayama (breathing exercises) practices that involve concentration and mindfulness exercises have been shown to enhance memory function. Mindful awareness promotes encoding and retrieval processes in the brain and leads to better memory consolidation and recall.
4. ***Stress reduction:*** Chronic stress can impair cognitive functions such as memory, attention and executive function. Yoga practices help to reduce stress levels by activating the parasympathetic nervous system and lowering cortisol levels. Therefore, reduced stress contributes to improved cognitive performance and mental clarity.
5. ***Enhanced executive function:*** Executive functions refer to higher-order cognitive processes involved in goal-oriented behaviour, problem solving, planning and self-regulation. Yoga practices that promote mindfulness, such as asanas and meditation, have been associated with improvements in executive function, including cognitive flexibility, inhibitory control and working memory.
6. ***Brain plasticity:*** Yoga asanas that involve challenging physical movements and balance require the activation of various brain regions involved in motor control, coordination and execution.

ROLE OF YOGA IN PREVENTING AGEING

Ageing is a natural process. Yoga asanas, or postures, can play a role in promoting healthy ageing by addressing various physical, mental and emotional aspects of well-being. Incorporating yoga into one's lifestyle can help mitigate some of the effects associated with ageing. The following are the ways of yoga asanas which help in preventing the ageing process:

1. ***Maintaining flexibility and mobility:*** Regular practice of yoga postures helps to maintain and improve flexibility and joint mobility, which naturally decline with age. Yoga stretches and strengthens muscles, ligaments and tendons, promoting better range of motion and reducing the risk of stiffness and immobility associated with ageing.
2. ***Promoting strength and balance:*** Many yoga asanas require strength and balance, which are essential for maintaining functional independence during ageing. Yoga asanas that challenge balance and build strength reduce the risk of falls and injuries, thereby supporting healthy ageing.
3. ***Improving posture:*** Yoga emphasizes proper alignment and posture, which can deteriorate over time due to factors such as sedentary behaviour and muscle imbalances. By practicing yoga asanas that promote spinal health and core strength, individuals can maintain good posture and reduce the risk of age-related postural issues.
4. ***Enhancing respiratory function:*** Pranayama, or yogic breathing exercises, improve respiratory function and lung capacity, which tend to decline with age. By practicing deep breathing techniques and breath awareness, individuals can enhance oxygenation of tissues, improve respiratory efficiency and support overall vitality.
5. ***Reducing stress and promoting relaxation:*** Chronic stress accelerates the ageing process by contributing to cellular damage and inflammation. Yoga practices, including relaxation techniques such as meditation and deep breathing, help to reduce stress levels, activate the parasympathetic nervous system and promote relaxation, thereby supporting healthy ageing at the cellular level.
6. ***Boosting circulation and heart health:*** Yoga poses that involve gentle rhythmic movements promote circulation and cardiovascular health, which are essential for maintaining vitality and preventing age-related cardiovascular issues. Improved blood flow supports the delivery of oxygen and nutrients to cells and tissues, promoting overall health and longevity.
7. ***Cognitive benefits:*** Yoga practices have been shown to enhance cognitive function, including memory, attention and executive function. By stimulating neural pathways and promoting neuroplasticity, yoga can help maintain cognitive vitality and reduce the risk of age-related cognitive decline.
8. ***Promoting emotional well-being:*** Yoga fosters emotional resilience and mental well-being by cultivating mindfulness, self-awareness and acceptance. By managing stress, anxiety and depression, individuals can maintain a positive outlook on life and navigate the challenges of ageing with greater ease.
9. ***Fostering social connections:*** Participating in yoga classes and community events provides opportunities for social interaction and connection, which are important aspects of healthy ageing. Building and maintaining social relationships can contribute to emotional well-being, cognitive function and overall quality of life in later years.

Overall, incorporating yoga asanas into a regular wellness routine can support healthy ageing by promoting physical vitality, mental clarity, emotional resilience and social engagement. Although yoga cannot stop the ageing process entirely, it can help individuals age gracefully and maintain a high quality of life as they grow older.

Self-Assessment

1. Describe the types of yoga.
2. Discuss the physiological aspects of yoga on the cardiorespiratory system.
3. Discuss the effects of yoga on cognitive functions.
4. Describe role of yoga in ageing.

Index

B

C

D

G

H

N

U

V

W

X

Y

Z